The Complete Directory for People with Disabilities

2008

Sixteenth Edition

The Complete Directory for People with Disabilities

A Comprehensive Source Book for Individuals and Professionals

A Sedgwick Press Book

Grey House Publishing

PUBLISHER: Leslie Mackenzie
EDITORIAL DIRECTOR: Laura Mars-Proietti

PRODUCTION MANAGER: Karen Stevens
PRODUCTION ASSISTANT: Anthony Del Vecchio, Alysia Giglio, Erica Irish, Karynn Kettinq, Gerald Simpson

MARKETING DIRECTOR: Jessica Moody

A Sedgwick Press Book
Grey House Publishing, Inc.
185 Millerton Road
Millerton, NY 12546
518.789.8700
FAX 518.789.0545
www.greyhouse.com
e-mail: books @greyhouse.com

First edition published 1991
Sixteenth edition published 2007

The complete directory for people with disabilities : products, resources, books, services.—1992-2005
1022p.; 29cm

Other title: Directory for people with disabilities
Title varies.
Annual

1. People with disabilities—Services for—United States—Directories. 2. People with disabilities—Services for—United States—Periodicals. 3. Disabled Persons—United States—Bibliography. 4. Disabled Persons—United States—Directory. 5. Information Services—United States—Bibliography. 6. Information Services—United States—Directory. 7. Mental Retardation—Rehabilitation—United States—Bibliography. 8. Mental Retardation—Rehabilitation—United States—Directory. 9. Rehabilitation—United States—Bibliography. 10. Rehabilitation—United States—Directory. I. Title: Directory for people with disabilities.
HV1553.C58
362.4/048/02573 92-658843
Printed in the USA
ISBN 13: 1-59237-194-5 softcover

Table of Contents

Introduction

Article: *Therapeutic Riding Programs for People with Disabilities*
Glossary of Disability-Related Terms

SECTION 1: Resources for People with Disabilities, by General Categories

Arts & Entertainment 1

Assistive Devices
Automobile 6
Bath 11
Bed 14
Communication 15
Chairs 20
Cushions & Wedges 22
Dressing Aids 24
Health Aids 25
Hearing Aids 27
Kitchen & Eating Aids 29
Lifts, Ramps & Elevators 31
Major Catalogs 36
Miscellaneous 41
Office Devices & Workstations 44
Scooters 46
Stationery 50
Visual Aids 51
Walking Aids: Canes, Crutches & Walkers 52
Wheelchairs
  Accessories 54
  General 56
  Pediatric 59
  Powered 59
  Racing 60

Associations 61

Camps by State 80

Clothing
Dresses & Skirts 97
Footwear 97
Jackets 98
Miscellaneous & Catalogs 99
Robes & Sleepwear 101

Shirts & Tops 102
Slacks & Pants 103
Undergarments 103

Computers
Assistive Devices 105
Braille Products 110
Information Centers & Databases 111
Keyboards, Mouses & Joysticks 117
Scanners 118
Screen Enhancement 119
Speech Synthesizers 119
Software: Math 121
Software: Miscellaneous 123
Software: Professional 132
Software: Reading & Language Arts 133
Software: Vocational 137
Word Processors 138

Conferences & Shows 140

Construction & Architecture
Associations, Publications & Videos 144

Education
Aids for the Classroom 147
Associations 160
Directories 163
Educational Publishers 164
State Agencies 166
Magazines & Journals 172
Newsletters 176
Professional Texts 178
Testing Resources 208
Treatment & Training 215

Exchange Programs 217

Foundations & Funding Resources
Listings by State 221
Funding Directories 264

Government Agencies
Federal 270
Listings by State 272

Independent Living Centers by State 317

Law
Associations & Referral Agencies 382
Resources for the Disabled 384

Libraries & Research Centers by State 393

Media, Print
Children & Young Adults 423
Community 428
Employment 430
General Disabilities 431
Parenting: General 451
Parenting: Specific Disabilities 457
Parenting: School 458
Parenting: Spiritual 458
Professional 460
Vocations 463
Pamphlets 464

Media, Electronic
Audio/Visual 468
Web Sites 472

Toys & Games 477

Travel & Transportation
Newsletters & Books 480
Programs 481
Tours 483
Vehicle Rentals 485

Veteran Services
National and Listings by State 487

Vocational & Employment Programs by State 506

Rehabilitation, Facilities, Acute by State 540

Rehabilitation, Facilities, Post-Acute by State 568

Rehabilitation Facilities, Sub-Acute by State 632

SECTION 2: Resources for People with Disabilities, by Specific Disability Categories

Blind & Deaf
Associations 652
Camps 652
Print & Non-Print Resources 652
Support Groups 663

Cognitive
Associations 654
Camps 656
Print & Non-Print Resources 660
Support Groups 677

Dexterity
Associations 678
Print & Non-Print Resources 678

Aging
Associations 680
Print & Non-Print Resources 684

Hearing
Associations 691
Camps 697
Print & Non-Print Resources 699
Sports 716
Support Groups 716

Mobility
Associations 717
Camps 720
Print & Non-Print Resources 721
Sports 729
Support Groups 733

Specific Disorders, including Cancer, Cerebral Palsy, Diabetes, Epilepsy, Respiratory Ailments, Spina Bifida, etc.
Associations 734
Camps 739
Print & Non-Print Resources 751
Sports 779
Support Groups 780

Speech & Language
Associations 784
Camps 785
Print & Non-Print Resources 785

Visual
Associations 791

Camps 800
Print & Non-Print Resources 802
Sports 824
Support Groups 824

Entry & Publisher Index 825
Geographic Index 894
Disability & Subject Index 913

Introduction

Welcome to the 16th edition of *The Complete Directory for People with Disabilities,* designed to assist the millions of Americans who, according to the American with Disabilities Act (ADA), have a mental or physical impairment that substantially limits one or more major life activity, and the network of individuals who support the disabled community.

A recent survey by the *International Center for Disability Information* estimates that 58 million Americans are living with a disability, up from an estimated 43 million in 1987 when the ADA was being drafted. Further research issued by the *ICD* and the *National Institute on Disability and Rehabilitation Research* indicates that 20% of the population has one or more disability and about 10% of that number live with severe disabilities.

Experts tell us that the number of disabled Americans continues to rise due to increased longevity, medical advances, and growing awareness of emerging syndromes, among other factors. With this rise in the number of disabled individuals, comes a strengthened commitment of physicians, healthcare workers, parents, and disabled individuals themselves to enable this growing population to participate in society as fully as possible, regardless of age or income.

This 16th edition of *The Complete Directory for People with Disabilities* provides unequaled coverage of the resources, products and services for disabled individuals and their families, all designed to help disabled individuals successfully attend school, live and work side-by-side with the non-disabled population.

New features of this edition include:

- New article outlining **Therapeutic Horseback Riding Programs** for people with disabilities, written by the president of the *New York Therapeutic Riding Center*
- **Glossary of Terms** often used in the disability community
- A new section of resources that are arranged by 8 disability categories:
  *** Blind & Deaf * Cognitive * Dexterity * Aging ***
  *** Hearing * Mobility * Speech & Language * Visual ***
- Canadian resources

The widely-acclaimed *Complete Directory for People with Disabilities* is an invaluable resource for all those committed to empowering individuals with disabilities. It contains thousands of resources, products and services for people with disabilities. All those with a disability, from vision problems to physical disabilities to asthma, will find ways in this Directory to succeed at work, in school, and in their community. Coverage extends from Associations that provide important support for families, individuals and professionals, to Products that enable and enhance the lifestyle of people with disabilities. Listings include Camps, Living Facilities, Print and Electronic Resources and much more. The comprehensive Table of Contents is a guide through the 33 chapters and 115 subchapters contained in this rich resource.

We utilized many resources to update this edition, including phone, fax, and Internet research. This 16th edition includes 9,099 entries with descriptions and key contacts, 8,061 fax numbers, 5,830 e-mail addresses and 7,347 web sites.

The careful research and compilation of the best data available is a year–long effort. As the reputation of *The Complete Directory for People with Disabilities* among educators, librarians and the disability community continues to grow, professionals and organizations send us new information and editorial feedback. Their cooperation and support are largely responsible for the strength of this directory.

We are confident that this resource will save hours of research time. Information on this subject is scattered, and searching the Internet is time consuming with results that are often overwhelming and unedited. *The Complete Directory for People with Disabilities* provides comprehensive, critical and immediate information in just one source that can be accessed quickly and easily.

In addition to the detailed listings, this edition includes three indexes to provide quick, easy access to the data:

> **Disability & Subject Index**: Organized alphabetically by hundreds of topics relevant to people with disabilities, this index groups together all listings on a particular subject (i.e., autism or language disorders), regardless of type.
>
> **Entry Index**: This alphabetical list of all entries saves time searching for an organization or group that may be repeated in several chapters.
>
> **Geographic Index:** Organizes listings alphabetically by state.

The Complete Directory for People with Disabilities is also available as an Online Database, as well as in a customized, downloadable database. Other health resource titles by Grey House include *The Complete Learning Disabilities Directory, The Complete Directory for People with Chronic Illness* and *The Complete Mental Health Directory*. As always, we welcome your comments, and look forward to another year of serving the disability community.

Therapeutic Riding Programs for People with Disabilities

By Richard Brodie

Therapeutic horseback riding programs have been developed to enable people with disabilities to ride horses for therapeutic and recreational purposes. The concept of therapeutic horseback riding dates back to ancient Greece, where it was employed to rehabilitate injured warriors. Therapeutic riding programs began in Europe and England in the 1950's, and were started in the United States in the 1970's. Over the years, these programs have spread rapidly, to the point where there are now over 600 therapeutic riding programs in this country. Most of these programs are in suburban and rural areas, although there are therapeutic riding programs in major urban centers such as New York City, Boston, Chicago and Los Angeles.

Therapeutic horseback riding is being utilized for children and adults with a wide range of disabilities. These disabilities include cerebral palsy, muscular dystrophy, multiple sclerosis, spinal cord injury, traumatic brain injury, mental retardation, developmental disabilities, autism and blindness.

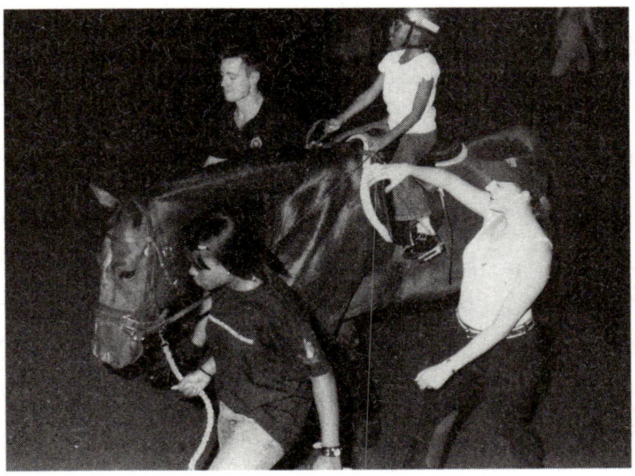

The growing popularity of therapeutic horseback riding in the United States is due to several factors:

1) the great pleasure that people with disabilities derive from engaging in horseback riding as a recreational activity, and

2) the specific rehabilitation benefits of therapeutic riding which include:

- improving balance, posture, coordination and mobility
- strengthening muscles and mobilizing trunk and pelvis
- increasing attention span and promoting communication skills
- improving confidence and self-esteem

The medical profession strongly supports the field of therapeutic riding. Howard A. Rusk, M.D., a pioneer in the rehabilitation of the physically disabled, and founder of the world-renowned Rusk Institute of Rehabilitation Medicine of NYU Medical Center stated: "The riding programs, I have always felt, are extremely helpful in severely disabled persons and truly therapeutic. They are a great asset in helping the disabled."

David Feldman, M.D., Chief of Pediatric Orthopedic Surgery at the Hospital for Joint Diseases in Manhattan, also feels that therapeutic riding is valuable in many ways for children with disabilities. "It encourages confidence, a feeling of freedom and mobility and is beneficial for their musculature, as well as for posture and hip positioning. Therapeutic riding is a wonderful adjunctive therapy in these children's lives," he said.

One of the most exciting areas within the field of therapeutic riding is hippotherapy. Hippo is the Greek word for horse, and hippotherapy is a medical treatment that uses the movement of the horse to produce specific therapeutic goals for the patient. Hippotherapy is utilized for children and adults with mild to severe movement disorders. Hippotherapy is performed by a licensed physical therapist or occupational therapist who directs the horse's 'movement to aid the client.

The North American Riding for the Handicapped Association, Inc. (NARHA) is the main accrediting body for therapeutic riding. To see a list of accredited programs in your area, visit www.narha.org.

The American Hippotherapy Association (AHA) is the main accrediting body for hippotherapy clinicians. To contact hippotherapy clinicians in your area, visit www.americanhippotherapyassociation.org.

Richard Brodie is President of the New York Therapeutic Riding Center, which has been conducting therapeutic horseback riding programs for children and adults with disabilities living in the 5 boroughs of New York City for the past 10 years. The New York Therapeutic Riding Center is based at the Chateau Stables in Manhattan. For more information, visit www.volunteersolutions.org/uwnyc/org/3307916.html

Glossary of Disability-Related Terms

DO·IT

Accessible: In the case of a facility, readily usable by a particular individual; in the case of a program or activity, presented or provided in such a way that a particular individual can participate, with or without auxiliary aid(s); in the case of electronic resources, accessible with or without adaptive computer technology.

Access barriers: Any obstruction that prevents people with disabilities from using standard facilities, equipment and resources.

Accessible Web design: Creating World Wide Web pages according to universal design principles to eliminate or reduce barriers, including those that affect people with disabilities.

Accommodation: An adjustment to make a program, facility, or resource accessible to a person with a disability.

Adaptive technology: Hardware or software products that provide access to a computer that is otherwise inaccessible to an individual with a disability.

ALT attribute: HTML code that works in combination with graphical tags to provide alternative text for graphical elements.

Alternative keyboard: A keyboard that is different from a standard computer keyboard in its size or layout of keys.

Americans with Disabilities Act of 1990 (ADA): A comprehensive federal law that prohibits discrimination on the basis of disability in employment, public services, public accommodations and services operated by private entities, and telecommunications .

American Standard Code for Information Interchange (ASCII): Standard for unformatted plain text which enables transfer of data between platforms and computer systems.

Applet: Computer program that runs from within another application.

Assistive technology: Technology used to assist a person with a disability, e.g., wheelchair, handsplints, computer-based equipment.

Binary files: Electronic files with formatting information that is software dependent.

Braille: System of embossed characters formed by using a Braille cell, a combination of six dots consisting of two vertical columns of three dots each. Each simple Braille character is formed by one or more of these dots and occupies a full cell or space. Some Braille may use eight dots.

Browser: Software designed to access and display information available on the World Wide Web. Browsers may be graphical or text-based. Text-only browsers cannot display images, sound clips, video and plug-in features that graphical browsers can. Talking browsers are also available for use by people who have difficulty reading text due to a learning disability or visual impairment.

Captioned film or videos: Transcription of the verbal portion of films or videos displayed to make them accessible to people who are deaf.

Captioning: Text that is included with video presentations or broadcasts that enables people with hearing impairments to have access to the audio portion of the material.

Closed Circuit TV Magnifier (CCTV): Camera used to magnify books or other materials to a monitor or television.

Communication device: Hardware that allows a person who has difficulty using their voice clearly to use words or symbols for communication. May range in complexity from a simple picture board to complex electronic devices that allow personalized, unique construction of ideas.

Compensatory tools: Adaptive computing systems that allow people with disabilities to use computers to complete tasks that they would have difficulty doing without a computer, e.g., reading, writing, communicating, accessing information.

Digital: Computer formatted data or information.

Disability: Physical or mental impairment that substantially limits one or more major life activities; a record of such an impairment; or being regarded as having such an impairment (Americans with Disabilities Act of 1990).

Discrimination: Act of making a difference in treatment or favor on a basis other than individual merit.

Electronic information: Any digital data for use with computers or computer networks including disks, CD-ROMs, World Wide Web resources.

Facility: All or any portion of a physical complex, including buildings, structures, equipment, grounds, roads, and parking lots.

FM Sound Amplification System: Electronic amplification system consisting of three components: a microphone / transmitter, monaural FM receiver and a combination charger / carrying case. It provides wireless FM broadcast from a speaker to a listener who has a hearing impairment.

Graphical User Interface (GUI): Program interface that presents digital information and software programs in an image-based format as compared to a character-based format.

Hardware: Physical equipment related to computers.

Hearing impairments: Complete or partial loss of ability to hear caused by a variety of injuries or diseases including congenital defects.

Helper: An external program that can be called up by a Web browser to display specially formatted material, such as word processed documents, spreadsheet documents or video / sound pieces. The Helper program is launched by the Web browser as a separate application to view or play the file.

Host: Any computer which holds Internet resources for access by others, or the computer that maintains your Internet access and electronic mail account.

HTML validation: Process that analyzes HTML documents identifies HTML errors and non-standard codes.

HyperText Transfer Protocol (HTTP): Communication protocol used by the World Wide Web to transfer text, graphics, audio, and video.

Hyperlink, hypertext: Highlighted word or graphic on a Web page that when selected allows the user to jump to another part of the document or another Web page.

Hypertext Markup Language (HTML): Programming language or code used to create World Wide Web pages.

Image map: Picture or graphic on a Web page in which hyperlinks are embedded.

Input: Any method by which information is entered into a computer.

Internet: Computer network connecting government, education, commercial, other organization and individual computer systems.

Interpreter: Professional person who assists a deaf person in communicating with hearing people.

Java: Programming language used to create programs or applets that work with some World Wide Web browsers to include features with animation or other characteristics not available through standard HTML.

Joystick: A device consisting of a lever that allows a pointer to move up, right, left, or down and serves as an alternative to a mouse. It usually includes buttons to enable mouse clicks.

Keyboard emulation: A method of having an alternative device and/or software, such as a switch-based system, serve the role of a keyboard.

Keyguard: A plastic or metal shield that covers a keyboard with holes over the keys. It allows use of a keyboard without undesired activation of surrounding keys.

Large print books: Most ordinary print is six to ten points in height (about 1/16 to 1/8 of an inch). Large type is 14 to 18 points (about 1/8 to 1/4 of an inch) and sometimes larger. The format of large print books is also proportionately larger (usually 8 1/2 x 11 inches).

Lynx: Text-based World Wide Web browser.

Mainstreaming, inclusion: The inclusion of people with disabilities, with or without special accommodations, in programs, activities, and facilities with their non-disabled peers.

Major life activities: Functions such as caring for oneself, performing manual tasks, walking, seeing, hearing, speaking, breathing, learning, working, and participating in community activities (Americans with Disabilities Act of 1990).

Mobility impairment: Disability that affects movement ranging from gross motor skills such as walking to fine motor movement involving manipulation of objects by hand.

Mouse emulation: A method of having an alternative device and/or software, such a switch based system, serve the role of a mouse.

Multimedia: In terms of electronic information, any data which is presented through several formats including text, graphics, moving pictures and sound.

Onscreen keyboard: See *Virtual Keyboard*.

Optical character recognition (OCR): Technology system that scans and converts printed materials into electronic text.

Output: Any method of displaying or presenting electronic information to the user through a computer monitor or other device.

Peripheral Neuropathy: A condition caused by damage to the nerves in the peripheral nervous system which includes nerves that run from the brain and spinal cord to the rest of the body.

Physical or mental impairment: Any physiological disorder or condition, cosmetic disfigurement, or anatomical loss affecting one or more of the following body systems: neurological; musculoskeletal; special sense organs; respiratory, including speech organs; cardiovascular; reproductive; digestive; genitourinary; hemic and lymphatic; skin; and endocrine; or any mental or psychological disorder, such as mental retardation, organic brain syndrome, emotional or mental illness, and specific learning disabilities (Americans with Disabilities Act of 1990).

Plug-in: Separate program written to be launched by a specific Web browser to display or run special elements in Web pages, such as animation, video, or audio.

Qualified individual with a disability: An individual with a disability who, with or without reasonable modification to rules, policies, or practices, the removal of architectural, communication, or transportation barriers, or the provision of auxiliary aids and services, meets the essential eligibility requirements for the receipt of services or the participation in programs or activities provided by a public entity (Americans with Disabilities Act of 1990).

Reader: Volunteer or employee of an individual with a disability (e.g., visual impairment, learning disability) who reads printed material in person or records to audio-tape.

Reading system: Hardware and software designed to provide access to printed text for people with visual impairments, mobility impairments, or learning disabilities. Character recognition software controls a scanner that takes an image of a printed page, converts it to computer text using recognition software and then reads the text using a synthesized voice.

Refreshable Braille Display: Hardware connected to a computer that echoes screen text on a box that has cells consisting of pins that move up and down to create Braille characters.

Repetitive Stress Injury (RSI): This disability may be chronic or acute and usually is described as pain caused by overuse of extremities, usually hands and wrists.

Scanning input: A switch-based method of controlling a computer. Activations of a switch will, in order, bring up a control panel that upon subsequent switch activations, allow a user to focus in on a desired control or keystroke. Custom scanning layouts can be created for a variety of purposes and programs and may also be used in a communication device.

Screen enlargement: Hardware and/or software that increases the size of characters and text on a computer screen.

Screen reader: Software used to echo text on a computer screen to audio output, often used by people who are blind, with visual impairments, or with learning disabilities.

Screen resolution: Refers to the clarity or sharpness of an image. For computer monitors, this term indicates the number of dots on the screen used to create text and graphics. Higher resolution means more dots, indicating increased sharpness and potentially smaller text.

Section 508 of the Rehabilitation Act: Legislation that requires Federal Agencies to develop, procure, and use accessible electronic and information technology.

Sensory impairment: A disability that affects touch, sight and/or hearing.

Server: Any computer that stores information that is available to other users, often over the Internet.

Sign language: Manual communication commonly used by deaf. The gestures or symbols in sign language are organized in a linguistic way. Each individual gesture is called a sign. Each sign has three distinct parts; the handshape, the position of the hands, and the movement of the hands. American Sign Language (ASL) is the most commonly used sign language in the United States. Deaf people from different countries speak different sign languages.

Specific Learning Disability: Disorder in one or more of the basic psychological processes involved in understanding or in using language, spoken or written, which may manifest itself in difficulties listening, thinking, speaking, reading, writing, spelling, or doing mathematical calculations. Frequent limitations include hyperactivity, distractibility, emotional instability, visual and/or auditory perception difficulties and/or motor limitations, depending on the type(s) of learning disability.

Speech impairment: Problems in communication and related areas such as oral motor function, ranging from simple sound substitutions to the inability to understand or use language or use the oral-motor mechanism for functional speech.

Speech input or speech recognition: A method of controlling a computer and creating text by dictation. Speech input software is combined with a microphone.

Standard HTML: Version of HTML accessible by all browsers.

Streaming multimedia: A method of transferring audio and/or video via a network from a server to an end user's computer. During the transmission, the material is displayed or played on the target computer.

Switch input: A method of controlling a computer or communication device. It is most often used with Morse code or scanning methods, but may also be used for controlling household appliances and related controls. Switches are available in a nearly endless array of sizes, shapes, and activation methods.

Tag: HTML code that prescribes the structure and formatting of Web pages.

Telecommunications Device for the Deaf (TDD) or Teletypewriter (TTY): A device which enables someone who has a speech or hearing impairment to use a telephone when communicating with someone else who has a TDD/TTY. TDD/TTYs can be used with any telephone, and one needs only a basic typing ability to use them.

Trackball: A mouse alternative that is basically an upside-down mouse. Useful for some people with mobility impairments because it isolates pointer movement from button clicking.

Traumatic Brain Injury (TBI): Open and closed head injuries resulting in impairments in one or more areas, including cognition; language; memory; attention; reasoning; abstract thinking; judgment; problem-solving; sensory, perceptual, and motor abilities; psychosocial behavior; physical functions; information processing; and speech. The term does not apply to brain injuries that are congenital, degenerative, or induced by birth trauma.

Universal design: Designing programs, services, tools, and facilities so that they are useable, without modification, by the widest range of users possible, taking into account a variety of abilities and disabilities.

Universal design of instruction: The design of instructional materials and activities that make learning achievable by students with a wide variety of abilities and disabilities.

Universal Resource Locator (URL): Address used to locate a specific resource on the Internet. DO-IT's URL is *http://www.washington.edu/doit/*.

Vocational Rehabilitation Act of 1973: Act prohibiting discrimination on the basis of disability which applies to any program that receives federal financial support. Section 504 of the Act is aimed at making educational programs and facilities accessible to all students. Section 508 of the Act requires that electronic office equipment purchased through federal procurement meets disability access guidelines.

Virtual keyboard: Software used to emulate a keyboard. A picture of a keyboard is displayed on a computer screen and the user points and clicks on the pictures of keys to enter text.

Vision impairments: Complete or partial loss of ability to see, caused by a variety of injuries or diseases including congenital defects. Legal blindness is defined as visual acuity of 20/200 or less in the better eye with correcting lenses, or widest diameter of visual field subtending an angular distance no greater than 20 degrees.

Word prediction: Software that reduces the number of keystrokes needed to type words and sentences. As characters are entered on either a standard, alternative or virtual keyboard, suggested completions of the word that has been started are provided to the user.

World Wide Web (WWW, W3, or Web): Hypertext and multimedia gateway to the Internet.

Grants and gifts funds DO-IT publications, videotapes, and programs to support the academic and career success of people with disabilities. Contribute today by sending a check to DO-IT, Box 355670, University of Washington, Seattle, WA 98195-5670.

Your gift is tax deductible as specified in IRS regulations. Pursuant to RCW 19.09, the University of Washington is registered as a charitable organization with the Secretary of State, State of Washington. For more information, call the Office of the Secretary of State, 800-322-4483.

About DO-IT

DO-IT (Disabilities, Opportunities, Internetworking, and Technology) helps individuals with disabilities transition to college and careers. Primary funding for DO-IT is provided by the National Science Foundation, the U.S. Department of Education, and the State of Washington. For more information, to be placed on the mailing list, or to request materials in an alternate format, contact:

DO-IT
University of Washington
Box 355670
Seattle, WA 98195-5670
doit@u.washington.edu
http://www.washington.edu/doit/
206-221-4171 (FAX)
206-685-DOIT (voice/TTY)
888-972-DOIT (voice/TTY) WA, outside Seattle
509-328-9331 (voice/TTY) Spokane
Director: Sheryl Burgstahler, Ph.D.

DO·IT

University of Washington
College of Engineering
Computing & Communications
College of Education

User Guide

Descriptive listings in *The Complete Directory for People with Disabilities* are organized into 24 chapters, by either resource type or disability category type. You will find the following types of listings throughout the book:

- National Agencies & Associations
- State Agencies & Associations
- Camps & Exchanges Programs
- Manufacturers of Assistive Devices, Clothing, Computer Equipment & Supplies
- Print & Electronic Media
- Living Centers & Facilities
- Libraries & Research Centers
- Conferences & Trade Shows

Below is a sample listing illustrating the kind of information that is or might be included in an Association entry. Each numbered item of information is described in the paragraphs on the following page.

---

1 → 1234

2 → **Advocacy Center for Seniors with Disabilities**

3 → 1762 South Major Drive
New Orleans, LA 98087

4 → **800-000-0000**

5 → **058-884-0709**

6 → **Fax: 058-884-0568**

7 → **TDD: 800-000-0001**

8 → **email: info@sadvoc.com**

9 → **www.sadvoc.com**

10 → Barbara Pierce, Executive Director
Diane Watkins, Marketing Director
Robert Goldfarb, Administrative Assistant

11 → The mission of the Center is to advance the dignity, equality, self-determination and choices of senior citizens with disabilities. It provides referrals, publishes information, including a monthly newsletter, offers workshops and consultation on legal, social, travel, and medical issues. The Center works with various local organizations to help seniors with disabilities stay active in their community.

12 → Founded 1964

13 → 18 pages

14 → Monthly

User Key

1 → **Record Number**: Entries are listed alphabetically within each category and numbered sequentially. The entry numbers, rather than page numbers, are used in the indexes to refer to listings.

2 → **Organization Name**: Formal name of company or organization. Where organization names are completely capitalized, the listing will appear at the beginning of the alphabetized section. In the case of publications, the title of the publication will appear first, followed by the publisher.

3 → **Address**: Location or permanent address of the organization.

4 → **Toll Free Number**: This is listed when provided by the organization.

5 → **Phone Number**: The listed phone number is usually for the main office of the organization, but may also be for the sales, marketing, or public relations office as provided by the organization.

6 → **Fax Number**: This is listed when provided by the organization.

7 → **TDD Number**: This is listed when provided. It refers to Telephone Device for the Deaf.

8 → **E-Mail**: This is listed when provided by the organization and is generally the main office e-mail.

9 → **Web Site**: This is also referred to as an URL address. These web sites are accessed through the Internet by typing *http://* before the URL address.

10 → **Key Personnel**: Name and titles of department heads of the organization.

11 → **Organization Description**: This paragraph contains a brief description of the organization and their services.

12 → **Year Founded:** The year in which the organization was established or founded. If the organization has changed its name, the founding date is usually for the earliest name under which it was known.

13 → **Number of Pages**: Number of pages if the listing is a publication.

14 → **Frequency:** The frequency of the listing if it is a publication.

Resources for the Disabled

1 **American Art Therapy Association (AATA)**
5999 Stevenson Avenue
Alexandria, VA 22304
703-212-2238
888-290-0878
e-mail: info@arttherapy.org
www.arttherapy.org

Edward J Stygar Jr, Executive Director
Organization of professionals who believe the art process is a beneficial and healing process.

2 **American Association of Music Therapy**
8455 Colesville Road
Suite 1000
Silver Spring, MD 20910
301-589-3300
FAX: 301-589-5175
e-mail: info@musictherapy.org
www.musictherapy.org

Andrea Farbman Ed D, Executive Director
Music Therapy is an established healthcare profession that uses music to address physical, emotional, cognitive, and social needs of individuals of all ages. Music therapy improves the quality of life for persons who are well and meets the needs of children and adults with disabilities or illnesses.

3 **American Dance Therapy Association (ADTA)**
2000 Century Plaza
Suite 108
Columbia, MD 21044
410-997-4040
FAX: 410-997-4048
e-mail: info@adta.org
www.adta.org

Patricia Gardner, Office Manager
Elissa Q White, President of the Board
Dance-movement therapy is a psychotherapeutic use of movement as a process which furthers the emotional, cognitive and physical integration of the individual.

4 **American Journal of Art Therapy**
Vermont College of Norwich University
Montpelier, VT 05602
802-828-8540
FAX: 802-828-8585
e-mail: mzimmerm@norwich.edu

Gladys Agell PhD ATR-BC HLM, Editor
Discusses the graphic and plastic arts as they contribute to human understanding, psycotherapy, rahabilitation and education. *$ 32.00*
35-40 pages Quarterly
ISSN 0007-47 4

5 **American Music Therapy Association (AMTA)**
8455 Colesville Road
Suite 1000
Silver Spring, MD 20910
301-589-3300
FAX: 301-589-5175
e-mail: info@musictherapy.org
www.musictherapy.org

Andrea H Farbman, Executive Director
Judy Simpson, Director Government Relations
AMTA's purpose is the progressive development of the therapeutic use of music in rehabilitation, special education and community settings. Predecessors to the American Music Therapy Association included the National Association for Music Therapy founded in 1950 and the American Association for Music Therapy founded in 1971. AMTA is committed to the advancement of education, training, professional standards, credentials and research in support of the music therapy profession.

6 **Arena Stage**
11101 Sixth Street
Washington, DC 20024
202-554-9066
FAX: 202-484-6279
e-mail: info@arenastage.org
www.arenastage.org

Thomas C Fichandler, Founding Executive Director
Stephen Richard, Chief Executive Officer
A pioneer in providing access to theater for people with disabilities and the birthplace of Audio Description. Offers infrared assistive listening devices (both loop and headset), program books in Braille, large print and wheelchair accessible seating with adjacent companion seating. Audio cassette format available upon request. Sign Interpretation and Audio Description are offered at selected performances. Cafe menus and shop lists in Braille. Wheelchair-accessible with lifts and ramps.

7 **Art Therapy SourceBook**
McGraw-Hill Company
2460 Kerper Boulevard
Dubuque, IA 52001
563-588-1451
800-338-3987
FAX: 614-755-5654
www.mhhe.com/hper/physed

Kurt Strand, Vice President
An overview of the uses of art as a mentally therapeutic tool. *$18.00*
272 pages 1998
ISBN 1-565658-84-1

8 **Art and Disabilities**
Brookline Books
39 University Road
Brookline, MA 02445
617-734-6772
800-666-2665
FAX: 617-734-3952
e-mail: brooklinebooks@brooklinebooks.com
www.brooklinebooks.com

William H Walters, Author
Esther Isabe Wilder, Author
A step-by-step guide to establishing creative arts centers for people with disabilities. Includes philosophy and making creative arts centers happen.

9 **Art and Healing: Using Expressive Art to Heal Your Body, Mind, and Soul**
Three Rivers Press

The author believes creating a visual image through any medium can produce physical and emotional benefits for both the creator as well as those who view it. *$17.00*
256 pages 1999
ISBN 0-609803-16-6

10 **Art for All the Children: Approaches to Art Therapy for Children with Disabilities**
2600 South 1st Street
Springfield, IL 62704
217-789-8980
800-258-8980
FAX: 217-789-9130
e-mail: books@ccthomas.com
www.ccthomas.com

Frances E Anderson, author
Michael Thomas, President
This second edition is for art therapists in training and for in-service professionals in art therapy, art education and special education who have children with disabilities as a part of their case/class load. *$56.95*
398 pages Paperback
ISBN 0-398060-07-X

11 **Clinical Applications of Music Therapy in Developmental Disability, Pediatrics and Neurology**
Taylor & Francis
47 Runway Drive
Suite G
Levittown, PA 19057
215-269-0400
FAX: 215-625-2940

Harold Stecker, President
Music therapists from Brooklyn to Belgium reflect on how music one plays or listens to has the ability to penetrate the anguish of grief, pain, and even the cognitive distortions of schizophrenia and Alzheimer's disease. *$34.95*

312 pages 1999
ISBN 1-853027-34-0

12 **Contemporary Art Therapy with Adolescents**
Taylor & Francis
47 Runway Drive
Suite G
Levittown, PA 19057
215-269-0400
FAX: 215-625-2940

Harold Stecker, President
Reviews contemporary theories on adolescent development and therapy and offers solutions to the treatment of young people. *$ 26.95*
285 pages 1999
ISBN 1-853026-37-9

13 **Creative Arts Resources Catalog**
MMB Music
3526 Washington Avenue
Saint Louis, MO 63103
314-531-9635
800-343-3771
FAX: 314-531-8384
e-mail: mlg@mmbmusic.com
www.mmbmusic.com

Marcie Lee Goldberg, VP Sales/Marketing
Publisher and distributor of creative arts therapy materials in the areas of music, dance, art, drama, and poetry. Free catalog contains hundreds of books, recordings, and videos.

14 **Dancing from the Inside Out**
Fanlight Productions
4196 Washington Street
Suite 2
Boston, MA 02131
617-469-4999
800-937-4113
FAX: 617-469-3379
e-mail: fanlight@fanlight.com
www.fanlight.com

Anthony Sweeney, Marketing Director
Nicole Johnson, Publicity Coordinator
Ben Achtenberg, Owner
This eloquent new video looks at the lives and work of three talented dancers who dance professionally with the acclaimed AXIS Dance Troupe, which includes both disabled and non-disabled dancers. They discuss the process they went through in adapting to their disability and how they came to re-discover physical expression through dance. *$ 195.00*

15 **Disability and Social Performance: Using Drama to Achieve Successful Acts**
Brookline Books
39 University Road
Brookline, MA 02445
617-734-6772
800-666-2665
FAX: 617-734-3952
e-mail: thestore@brooklinebooksmith.com
www.brooklinebooks.com

William H Walters, Author
Esther Wilder, Author
This book makes a major contribution to the understanding of disability, people with disabilities and the creative power they possess which can be unleashed through performance. *$17.95*

16 **Facts: Music for Blind and Physically Handicapped Individuals**
National Library Service for the Blind
1291 Taylor Street NW
Washington, DC 20542
202-707-5100

e-mail: nls@loc.gov
www.loc.gov/nls

Frank Cylke, Executive Director
Annual

17 **Freedom to Create**
National Institute of Art and Disabilities
551 23rd Street
Richmond, CA 94804
510-620-0290
FAX: 510-620-0326
e-mail: admin@niadart.org

Elias Katz, Author
Patricia Coleman, President
Presents philosophy and practical experiences enabling teachers to stimulate creativity in the visual arts for students with and without disabilities.

18 **Friends-In-Art**
American Council of the Blind
1155 15th Street NW
Suite 1004
Washington, DC 20005
202-467-5081
800-424-8666
FAX: 202-467-5085
e-mail: info@acb.org
www.acb.org

Melanie Brunson, Executive Director
Chris Grey, President
Aims to enlarge the art experience of blind people, encourages blind people to visit museums, galleries, concerts, the theater and other enjoyable public places, offers consultation to program planners in establishing accessible art and museum exhibits and presents Performing Arts Showcases at the American Council of the Blinds' national convention.

19 **Guide to the Selection of Musical Instruments**
MMB Music
3526 Washington Avenue
Saint Louis, MO 63103
314-531-9635
800-543-3771
FAX: 314-531-8384
e-mail: info@mmbmusic.com

Marcia Goldberg, President
A marvelous resource book to aid therapists teaching disabled to play musical instruments. *$7.75*

20 **In-Definite Arts Society**
7140C Fairmount Drive SE
Calgary, AB, ZZ T2H
403-253-3174
FAX: 403-255-2234
e-mail: ida@indefintearts.com
www.indefinitearts.com

Jarrett Hladly, Contact
Promotes opportunities for people with developmental disabilities to express themselves and to grow and develop through their involvement in art.

21 **Institute for Therapy Throughout the Arts**
Division 3 of Oakton College
7701 Lincoln Avenue
Skokie, IL 60077
847-635-1600

www.oakton.edu
In its twentieth year of service, ITA provides creative arts therapies for adults and children with special needs through the use of music, art, drama and or dance. Services include: assessment, treatment planning, one-to-one services and group therapy. ITA also offers adaptive lessons to students with special needs and workshops on topics related to the expressive arts therapies.

22 **Instrumental Music for Dyslexics: A Teach ing Handbook**
Whurr Publishers

Describes dyslexia in layman's terms and explains how the various problems that a dyslexic may have can affect all aspects of learning to play a musical instrument. It alerts the music teacher with a problem pupil to the possibilities of that pupil having some form of dyslexia. It offers suggestions as to how to teach dyslexics, with particular reference to piano teaching, and it suggests ways in which the music teacher may contribute to the welfare of a dyslexic pupil. *$ 34.95*

200 pages 2002
ISBN 1-861562-91-8

23 **Kaleidoscope: Exploring the Experience of Disability Through Literature & the Fine Arts**
United Disability Services
701 S Main Street
Akron, OH 44311
330-762-9755
FAX: 330-762-0912
TTY:330-379-3349
e-mail: mshiplett@udsakron.org
www.udsakron.org

Mildred Shiplett, Editorial Coordinator
Gail Willmott, Senior Editor
Phyllis Boerner, Publication Director
This magazine explores the experiences of disability through the lens of creative arts. Unlike rehabilitation, advocacy or independent living journals, this journal challenges and transcends stereotypical, patronizing and sentimental attitudes about disability. Offers a variety of articles, fiction, art and poetry relating to issues of disability, literature and the fine arts. *$10.00*
64 pages BiAnnually

24 **Manual of Sequential Art Activities for Classified Children and Adolescents**
Charles C Thomas
2600 S 1st Street
Springfield, IL 62704
217-789-8980
800-258-8980
FAX: 217-789-9130
e-mail: books@ccthomas.com
www.ccthomas.com

Charles C Thomas, Publisher
Michael Thomas, President
Offers information to the special education professional on art therapy and management. *$41.95*
246 pages Softcover
ISBN 0-39805 -85-6

25 **Mozart Effect: Tapping the Power of Music to Heal the Body, Strengthen the Mind**
Perennial Currents

Offers dramatic accounts of how doctors, shamans, musicians, and others use music to deal with everything from anxiety to cancer and chronic pain, from dyslexia to mental illness. *$14.00*
352 pages 2001
ISBN 0-060937-20-3

26 **Music Therapy**
Future Horizons

Provides an overview of music therapy as it applies to cognitive, communication, and social goals for children with autism. *$19.95*
123 pages 2000
ISBN 1-885477-53-8

27 **Music Therapy and Leisure for Persons with Disabilities**
Sagamore Publishing

Explores the use of musical therapy in order to enhance the development of independent leisure skills with a variety of special populations. Suggestions are provided for alternative avenues through musical experiences enabling individuals to achieve their greatest potential for independence and a high quality of life. *$19.95*
2002
ISBN 1-571675-11-6

28 **Music Therapy for the Developmentally Disabled**
Pro-Ed Publications
8700 Shoal Creek Boulevard
Austin, TX 78757
512-451-3246
800-897-3202
FAX: 512-451-8542
e-mail: info@proedinc.com
www.proedinc.com

Donald Hammill, Owner
Included are practical guidelines, case samples and step-by-step instructions that enable a music therapist to bring about dramatic improvements in developmentally disabled adults and children. *$40.00*
269 pages Hardcover
ISBN 0-890791-90-2

29 **Music Therapy in Dementia Care**
Jessica Kingsley Publishers

A comprehensive look at music therapy as a means of improving memory, health, and identity in those suffering from dementia, particularly Alzheimer's. For music therapists and those involved in psychogeriatry. *$29.95*
256 pages 2000
ISBN 1-853027-76-6

30 **Music Therapy, Sensory Integration and the Autistic Child**
Jessica Kingsley Publishers

Examines the human physiologic function, the brain, information processing, functional adaption, and how that might be affected by music interventions in persons with sensory integration difficulties. *$23.95*
256 pages 2001
ISBN 1-843107-00-7

31 **Music and Dyslexia: Opening New Doors**
Whurr Publishers

Dyslexic musicians can succeed provided only that they are given sufficient encouragement and understanding *$34.95*
200 pages 2001
ISBN 1-861562-05-5

32 **Music for the Hearing Impaired**
MMB Music
3526 Washington Avenue
Saint Louis, MO 63103
314-531-9635
800-543-3771
FAX: 314-531-8384
e-mail: info@mmbmusic.com

Marcia Goldberg, President
A resource manual and curriculum guide. It is the product of a four-year developmental music program, placing emphasis on the needs of those with severe and profound losses. *$29.95*

33 **Music: Physician for Times to Come**
Quest Books
306 West Geneva Road
Wheaton, IL 60187
630-665-0130
800-669-9425
FAX: 630-665-8791
e-mail: orders@questbooks.net
www.questbooks.net

Elisabeth Trumpler, Manager
A resource guide for various types of music and their theraputic oputcome.
365 pages 2000
ISBN 0-835607-88-7

34 **National Arts and Disability Center (NADC)**
Tarjan Center at UCLA
300 UCLA Medical Plaza
Suite 3310
Los Angeles, CA 90095
310-794-1141
FAX: 310-794-1143
e-mail: oraynor@mednet.ucla.edu
nadc.ucla.edu

Olivia Raynor Ph.D., Director
Beth Stoffmacher, Technical Assistance Coordinator
NADC has a database and website which deals with access to and participation in the arts by people with disabilities.

35 **National Association for Drama Therapy**
15 Post Side Lane
Pittsford, NY 14534
585-381-5618
FAX: 585-383-1474
e-mail: nadt@mgmtsol.com
www.nadt.org

Sherry Diamond, President
Kate Hurd, Vice President

36 **National Endowment for the Arts: Office for AccessAbility**
1100 Pennsylvania Avenue NW
Washington, DC 20506
202-682-5400
FAX: 202-682-5496
e-mail: webmgr@arts.endow.gov
www.nea.gov/resources/accessibility/index.htm

Dana Gioia, Chairman
Joy Kiser, Manager
The National Endowment for the Arts Office for AccessAbility is the advocacy-technical assistance arm of the Arts Endowment to make the arts accessible for people with disabilities, older adults, veterans, and people living in institutions.

37 **National Federation of the Blind: Music Division**
National Association of Blind Musicians
1740 Tamarack Lane
Janesville, WI 53545
608-752-8749
e-mail: lmentink@tds.net
www.nfb.org

Linda Mentink, President
Mary Brunoli, First Vice President
Karen McDonald, Second Vice President
Blind persons dedicated to advancing employment and entertainment opportunities in various music fields. Offers support and information regarding copyright, publishing, promotion and other career details.

38 **National Theatre Workshop of the Handicapped (NTWH)**
535 Greenwich Street
New York, NY 10013
212-206-7789
FAX: 212-206-0200
e-mail: stully@ntwh.org
www.ntwh.org

Jason Matthews, Director Admissions
Rick Curry, Executive Director
Steve Tully, Director of Development

39 **National Theatre of the Deaf**
139 North Main Street
West Hartford, CT 06107
860-236-4193
FAX: 860-236-4163
TTY:860-236-4193
e-mail: ntd-info@ntd.org
www.ntd.org

Paul Winters, Executive Director
Professional development of deaf actors, national theatrical touring company of deaf and hearing actors.

40 **New Music Therapist's Handbook**
Berklee Press Publications

New developments in the field of music therapy. Includes an introduction to the profession, guidelines for setting up a practice, new clinical applications, and helpful case studies. *$29.95*
256 pages 2000
ISBN 0-634006-45-2

41 **Non-Traditional Casting Project**
1560 Broadway
Suite 1600
New York, NY 10036
212-730-4750
FAX: 212-730-4820
e-mail: info@ntcp.org
www.ntcp.org

Sharon Jensen, Executive Director
Nancy Kim, Program Manager

42 **Open Road**
102 Brook Lane
Boulder Creek, CA 95006
510-222-6662
FAX: 831-338-3210

Staff, author
Teresa Tucker, Manager
Arts, Music, Sports, and Field Trips for disabled individuals.
2 pages Monthly

43 **Pied Piper: Musical Activities to Develop Basic Skills**
Jessica Kingsley Publishers

Describes 78 enjoyable music activities for groups of children or adults who may have learning difficulties. The emphasis is on using music, rather than learning songs or rhythms, so group members do not need any special skills to be able to participate. Full details are given about any equipment required for the games, as well as suggestions for variations or modifications. *$21.95*
96 pages 2001
ISBN 1-853029-94-

44 **Something Magical**
Educational Productions
9000 SW Gemini Drive
Beaverton, OR 97008
503-644-7000
800-950-4949
FAX: 503-350-7000
e-mail: custserve@edpro.com
www.edpro.com

Linda Freedman, President/Co-Owner
Molly Krumm, Marketing Director
In 1984 two teachers and one music therapist decided that a collaboration between their two schools would be mutually beneficial. The result is recorded in this heart-warming documentary.

45 **Start with the Arts**
1300 Connecticut Avenue NW
Suite 700
Washington, DC 20036
202-628-2800
800-933-8721
FAX: 202-737-0725
e-mail: info@vsarts.org
www.vsarts.org

Soula Antoniou, Executive Director
Tanya L Travers, Marketing Manager
$59.00

46 **Teaching Basic Guitar Skills to Special Learners**
MMB Music
3526 Washington Avenue
Saint Louis, MO 63103
314-531-9635
800-543-3771
FAX: 314-531-8384
e-mail: info@mmbmusic.com

Marcia Goldberg, President
The first-of-its-kind guitar book for use with persons who have difficulty learning to play via traditional methods. *$16.00*

47 **Theatre Without Limits**
VSA Arts of Maine
PO Box 4002
Portland, ME 04101
207-761-3861
FAX: 207-761-4740
e-mail: me@vsarts.org
vsartsmaine.org

Kippy Rudy, Executive Director
Video demonstrates how to make theatrical performances accessible to people who are blind, deaf, or who have other disabilities.

48 **VSA Arts**
JFK Center for the Performing Arts
818 Connecticut Avenue NW
Suite 600
Washington, DC 20006
202-628-2800
800-933-8721
FAX: 202-737-0725
TTY: 202-737-0645
e-mail: info@vsarts.org
www.vsarts.org

Soula Antoniou, Executive Director
Tanya L Travers, Marketing Manager
VSA Arts is an international nonprofit agency that promotes education and lifelong learning opportunities in the arts for people with disabilities. We promote the arts for children and adults with disabilities, strengthening the human spirit and improving quality of life for everyone.

49 **We Are PHAMALY**
4196 Washington Street
Suite 2
Boston, MA 02131
617-469-4999
800-937-4113
FAX: 617-469-3379
e-mail: info@fanlight.com
www.fanlight.com

Sandy St Louis, Distribution Director
Kelli English, Publicity Coordinator
Ben Achtenberg, Owner
Stands for Physically Handicapped Musical Actors League. This dynamic troupe doesn't cut any corners or make any comprmises. The musicals they perform are chosen for their appeal to the audience, not because they are easy for the performers, who have a variety of sensory and mobility handicaps.
$199.00

ISBN 1-572954-08-6

Automobile

50 Ability Center
Contact Technologies
11600 Western Avenue
Stanton, CA 90680
714-890-8262
877-938-8267
FAX: 714-901-1492
e-mail: info@abilitycenter.com
www.abilitycenter.com

Terry Barton, Manager
Offers rear or side entry designed with painstaking craftsmanship using steel.

51 Acc-u-trol
Ahnafield Corporation
2444 Production Drive
Indianapolis, IN 46241
317-241-2444
800-636-8060
www.ahnafield.com

Bruce Ahnafield, President
Jeff Ahnafield, Sales Manager
Computer-controlled device that operates all secondary accessory functions. These functions may include ignition, lift and door operation, windows, wipers, lights and flashers.

52 Arcola Mobility
51 Kero Road
Carlstadt, NJ 07072
201-507-8500
800-ARC-OLA1
FAX: 201-507-5372
e-mail: brianp@arcolasales.com
www.arcolasales.com

Tony Perez, Sales Represen/Mobility Vehicle
Brian Pruiksma, Lifts/Ramps/Etc Sales Rep
Arcola sells new and used accessible vehicles and adaptive driving equipment including hand controls, wheelchair lifts and securement systems. Daily, weekly and monthly vehicle rentals available. Stairway lift, porch elevators and ramps for the home sold and rented.

53 Automobile Lifts for Scooters, Wheelchairs and Powerchairs
Bruno Independent Living Aids
PO Box 84
Oconomowoc, WI 53066
262-567-4990
800-882-8183
FAX: 262-953-5501
e-mail: service@bruno.com
www.bruno.com

Patrick Foy, National Sales Manager
Karla Branham Shaw, Marketing
Michael Bruno, Owner
Over 18 different styles of automobile lifts for scooters, wheelchairs and powerchairs for nearly any car, van, truck or sport utility vehicle that can raise most scooters or wheelchiars under 200 pounds and powerchairs up to 300 pounds. All Bruno lifts are eligible for reimbursement of up to $1000.00 from GM, Saturn, Ford, and Chrysler under the terms of their Mobility Programs.

54 Ball Bearing Spinner
Kroepke Kontrols
PO Box 288
Ellicottville, NY 14731
718-885-1100
FAX: 718-885-1110
e-mail: kroepke@mail.idt.net
www.kroepkekontrols.com
One-lever-fingertip control which is custom designed for each car but does not interfere with normal operation of your car and ball joints for perfect alignment. Can be installed by any car dealer or mechanic in 2 hours. *$44.00*

55 Blinker Buddy II Electronic Turn Signal
HARC Mercantile
1111 W Centre Avenue
Portage, MI 49024
269-324-1615
800-445-9968
FAX: 269-324-2387
e-mail: info@harc.com
www.harcmercantile.com

Ronald Slager, President
Sounds a loud tone and flashes a light when the turn signal is on.
$79.95

56 Braun Corporation
PO Box 310
Winamac, IN 46996
574-946-6153
800-843-5438
FAX: 574-946-4670
www.braunlift.com

Jeff Ruff, Executive VP Sales
William Roth, President
Manufactures wheelchair lifts and lowered floor minivans as well as many other mobility products.

57 Chevy Lowered Floor
Ahnafield Corporation
2444 Production Drive
Indianapolis, IN 46241
317-241-2444
800-636-8060
FAX: 317-636-8098
www.ahnafield.com

Jeff Ahnafield, Sales Manager
Bruce Ahanfield, President
Full size Chevy van lowered floor from 4 to 12 depths.

58 Classic
Ricon
7900 Nelson Road
Panorama City, CA 91402
818-267-3000
800-322-2884
FAX: 818-267-3001
e-mail: sales@riconcorp.com
www.riconcorp.com

William Baldwin, Chief Executive Officer
Deluxe van conversion with equipment and accessories to offer freedom to the physically challenged.

59 DW Auto & Home Mobility
1208 N Garth Avenue
Columbia, MO 65203
573-449-3859
800-568-2271
FAX: 573-449-4187
e-mail: info@dwauto.com
www.dwauto.com

Sheila Lynch, Business Manager
Shawn Bright, Owner
Paratransit conversions and personalized conversions for the physically challenged. Home elevators and lifts. Scooter, wheelchairs and DME.

60 Dodge Lowered Floor
Ahnafield Corporation
2444 Production Drive
Indianapolis, IN 46241
317-241-2444
800-636-8060
FAX: 317-636-8098
www.ahnafield.com

Jeff Ahnafield, Sales Manager
Bruce Ahanfield, President
Full size Dodge van lowered floor from 4 to 12 depths.

61 Drive Master Company
37 Daniel Road W
Fairfield, NJ 07004
973-808-9709
FAX: 973-808-9713
e-mail: sales@drivemaster.net
www.drivemaster.net

Peter B Ruprecht, President
Tina Knapik, VP Operations Manager
Full service mobility center, raised tops/doors, drop floors, custom driving equipment, distributor of name brand devices and systems for full sized and mini vans. Sister company Van Master rents mobility equipped vans.

62 **Dual Brake Control**
Kroepke Kontrols
PO Box 288
Ellicottville, NY 14731
718-885-1100
FAX: 718-885-1110
e-mail: kroepke@mail.idt.net
www.kroepkekontrols.com
One lever fingertip brake controls, precision machines of the finest quality steel, are inconspicuous and do not take up lots of leg room. *$105.00*

63 **Entervan**
Braun Corporation
PO Box 310
Winamac, IN 46996
574-946-6153
800-THE-LIFT
www.entervan.com

William Roth, President
The Entervan accessible features are designed to blend seamlessly into the original design of the Chrysler minivan. In fact, you'll find the Entervan to be virtually indistinguishable from other minivans on the road, with the only differences being the easily accessible qualities of the van.

64 **Escort II XL**
Worldwide Mobility Products
720 N Golden Street
Suite B6
Gilbert, AZ 85233
480-497-4692
800-848-3433
FAX: 480-497-3834
e-mail: www.mobliftl@msn.com
www.worldwide-mobility.com

Greg Maloy, Owner
Automatically lifts and secures for transportation a fully assembled, three-wheel, electric scooter. *$1625.00*

65 **Foot Steering**
Drive Master Company
37 Daniel Road W
Fairfield, NJ 07004
973-808-9709
FAX: 973-808-9713
e-mail: sales@drivemaster.net
www.drivemaster.net

Peter Ruprecht, President
Custom installed system to steer a vehicle with your foot.

66 **Foot Steering System**
Ahnafield Corporation
2444 Production Drive
Indianapolis, IN 46241
317-241-2444
800-636-8060
FAX: 317-636-8098
www.ahnafield.com

Jeff Ahnafield, Sales Manager
Bruce Ahnafield, President

67 **Ford Lowered Floor**
Ahnafield Corporation
2444 Production Drive
Indianapolis, IN 46241
317-241-2444
800-636-8060
FAX: 317-636-8098
www.ahnafield.com

Jeff Ahnafield, Sales Manager
Bruce Ahanfield, President
Full size Ford van lowered floor from 4 to 12 depths.

68 **Gresham Driving Aids**
30800 S Wixom Road
Wixom, MI 48393
248-624-1533
800-521-8930
FAX: 248-624-6358
www.greshamdrivingaids.com

Larry Pratt, Sales Manager
Bill Dillon, Owner
Offers a full-service package to physically challenged individuals including lowered floors, raised roofs and doors and high-quad driver control systems. Dealer for Braun, Ricon, Crow River and Bruno wheelchair lifts.

69 **Hand Brake Control Only**
Kroepke Kontrols
PO Box 288
Ellicottville, NY 14731
718-885-1100
FAX: 718-885-1110
e-mail: kroepke@mail.idt.net
www.kroepkekontrols.com
One lever, fingertip brake controls that are custom designed to fit each car, completely adjustable and offer positioning operation at your fingertips. *$130.00*

70 **Hand Control Systems**
Wright-Way
175 E Interstate 30
Garland, TX 75043
972-240-8839
800-241-8839
FAX: 972-240-0412
e-mail: mobility@wrightwayinc.com
www.wrightwayinc.com

Sales Dept
Various automobile control systems that use hand, foot and steering aids for the disabled, including complete vehicle modifications.

71 **Hand Dimmer Switch**
Gresham Driving Aids
30800 S Wixom Road
Wixom, MI 48393
248-624-1533
800-521-8930
FAX: 248-624-6358
www.greshamdrivingaids.com

Bill Dillon, Owner
This switch is recommended for left leg handicaps or when a right leg handicap uses a left foot throttle. *$36.25*

72 **Hand Dimmer Switch with Horn Button**
Gresham Driving Aids
30800 S Wixom Road
Wixom, MI 48393
248-624-1533
800-521-8930
FAX: 248-624-6358
www.greshamdrivingaids.com

Bill Dillon, Owner
Attaches to the handle of control with a chrome plated steel insulated switch box, giving an instant warning without removing your hand from the steering wheel. *$28.75*

73 **Hand Gas & Brake Control**
Kroepke Kontrols
PO Box 288
Ellicottville, NY 14731
718-885-1100
FAX: 718-885-1110
e-mail: kroepke@mail.idt.net
www.kroepkekontrols.com
Driving controls that are attached by a control level right on to the gas and brake pedals for easy maneuvering and convenience. *$220.00*

74 **Hand Operated Parking Brake**
Gresham Driving Aids
30800 S Wixom Road
Wixom, MI 48393
248-624-1533
800-521-8930
FAX: 248-624-6358
www.greshamdrivingaids.com

Bill Dillon, Owner

Converts foot parking brake to a hand operation for easy access and maneuverability. *$30.20*

75 **Hand Parking Brake**
Kroepke Kontrols
PO Box 288
Ellicottville, NY 14731
718-885-1100
FAX: 718-885-1110
e-mail: kroepke@mail.itd.net
www.kroepkekontrols.com

One lever fingertip brake controls for your car that offer easy installment, complete adjustability, complete independence and more. *$25.00*

76 **Handicapped Driving Aids**
Handicapped Driving Aids of Michigan
4020 2nd Street
Suite 30
Wayne, MI 48184
734-595-4400
FAX: 734-595-4520

Jeff Stys, Manager

Automobiles and vans customized, modified and equipped with industry approved handicapped equipment for ease of operation.

77 **Headlight Dimmer Switch**
Kroepke Kontrols
PO Box 288
Ellicottville, NY 14731
718-885-1100
FAX: 718-885-1110
e-mail: kroepke@mail.idt.net
www.kroepkekontrols.com

One lever, fingertip controls for the disabled driver. *$23.00*

78 **Horizontal Steering**
Drive Master Company
37 Daniel Road W
Fairfield, NJ 07004
973-808-9709
FAX: 973-808-9713
e-mail: sales@drivemaster.net
www.drivemaster.net

Peter Ruprecht, President
Christina Ruprecht, VP
Shelby Wells, Sales Manager

Horizontal steering system is customized to meet the needs of the high-level, spinally injured and all others who experience limited arm strength and range of motion.

79 **Horn Control Switch**
Kroepke Kontrols
PO Box 288
Ellicottville, NY 14731
718-885-1100
FAX: 212-885-1110
e-mail: kroepke@mail.idt.net
www.kroepkekontrols.com

One lever, fingertip controls that do not interfere with the normal operation of your car. *$23.00*

80 **Institute for Driver Rehabilitation**
156 E Commodore Boulevard
Jackson, NJ 08527
609-734-8000
800-866-1529
FAX: 732-928-2449

Debra Jackrel, President
Ted Jackrel, Program Director
Peter Goddard, Executive Director

Driver evaluation training for the physically/mentally challenged offering state certified driving instructors. Door-to-door pickup at home, work or rehab centers.

81 **Joystick Driving Control**
Ahnafield Corporation
2444 Production Drive
Indianapolis, IN 46241
317-241-2444
800-636-8060
FAX: 317-636-8098
www.ahnafield.com

Jeff Ahnafield, Sales Manager
Bruce Ahnafield, President

Single lever, two axis, remote control system for steering, brakes, and accelerator.

82 **Key Holders, Ignition & Door Keys**
Gresham Driving Aids
30800 S Wixom Road
Wixom, MI 48393
248-624-1533
800-521-8930
FAX: 248-624-6358
www.greshamdrivingaids.com

Bill Dillon, Owner

Easy for arthritic hands to handle. Easily installed. *$18.70*

83 **Kneelkar**
Mednet
555 Industrial Park Drive
Battle Creek, MI 49015
269-964-7920
FAX: 269-962-8841

Anthony Vandillin, Owner

Offers the ultimate van conversions with equipment that is easily installed and accessible for the physically challenged.

84 **Latchloc Automatic Wheelchair Tiedown**
Ahnafield Corporation
2444 Production Drive
Indianapolis, IN 46241
317-241-2444
800-636-8060
FAX: 317-636-8098
www.ahnafield.com

Jeff Ahnafield, Sales Manager
Bruce Ahanfield, President

An independent wheelchair tiedown system utilized primarily by individuals who drive from their wheelchairs.

85 **Left Foot Accelerator**
Gresham Driving Aids
30800 S Wixom Road
Wixom, MI 48393
248-624-1533
800-521-8930
FAX: 248-624-6358
www.greshamdrivingaids.com

Bill Dillon, Owner

A custom pedal designed for left-foot usage. Stainless steel cross bar attaches above the throttle pedal and leaves right pedal free for right foot use. *$80.50*

86 **Left Foot Gas Pedal**
Kroepke Kontrols
PO Box 288
Ellicottville, NY 14731
718-885-1100
FAX: 212-885-1110
e-mail: kroepke@mail.itd.net
www.kroepkekontrols.com

One lever, fingertip controls that offer custom design, easy installment and complete freedom for the disabled driver. *$90.00*

87 **Left Hand Shift Lever**
Gresham Driving Aids
PO Box 930334
Wixom, MI 48393
248-624-1533
800-521-8930
FAX: 248-624-6358
www.greshamdrivingaids.com

Bill Dillon, Owner

Converts steering wheel lever or automatic transmission selector lever to left hand usage for right arm handicaps. *$34.50*

88 **Low Effort and No Effort Steering**
Drive Master Company
37 Daniel Road
Fairfield, NJ 07004
973-808-9709
FAX: 973-808-9713
e-mail: sales@drivemaster.net
www.drivemaster.net

Peter B Ruprecht, President
Christina M Ruprecht, General Manager
J Shelby Wells, Sales Manager

Reduced effort steering modifications available for nearly all vehicles. Additional products are pedal extensions which are 1 inch to 4 inch clamp-on aluminum blocks and 6 inch to 12 inch adjustable fold-down pedals.

89 **Mini-Bus and Mini-Vans**
Arcola Bus Sales
51 Kero Road
Carlstadt, NJ 07072
201-507-8500
800-ARC-OLA1
FAX: 201-507-5372
e-mail: info@arcolasales.com
www.arcolamobility.com

Tony Perez, Mobility Sales Representative
Brian Pruiksma, Sales Representative
Andrew Rolfe, Owner
Offers a virtually unlimited choice of chassis size, body style, floor plan and optional features. We provide transporters for almost every use, including school buses, vans, mini-coaches, medium-duty buses and personalized vans for the disabled.

90 **Mini-Rider**
Ricon
7900 Nelson Road
Panorama City, CA 91402
818-267-3000
800-322-2884
FAX: 818-267-3001
e-mail: sales@riconcorp.com
www.riconcorp.com

William Baldwin, Chief Executive Officer
Deluxe van conversions.

91 **Mobility Vehicle Stairlifts and Ramps**
Arcola Bus Sales
51 Kero Road
Carlstadt, NJ 07072
201-507-8500
800-ARC-OLA1
FAX: 201-507-5372
e-mail: info@arcolasales.com
www.arcolamobility.com

Tony Perez, Mobility Sales Representative
Brian Pruiksma, Accessibility Products
Andrew Rolfe, Owner
Arcola Mobility is a leading dealer of personal, accessible mini and full-size vans with custom conversions and modifications available. We offer a complete line of adaptive driving equipment, including wheelchair lifts, ramps, hand controls, steering devices, scooter lifters, car top wheelchair carriers and power transfer seats. In addition to new custom vehicles, we also have an extensive selection of used vehicles for the physically challenged.

92 **Monarch Mark 1-A**
Access Mobility Systems
21104 70th Avenue W
Edmonds, WA 98026
425-771-4659
800-854-4176
FAX: 425-771-3946
e-mail: info@accessams.com
www.accessams.com

Jennifer Richardson, Owner
System of hand controls which incorporates a popular method of operation by pushing the control handles directly toward the brakes.

93 **Monmouth Vans, Access and Mobility**
5105 Route 33
34
Wall Township, NJ 07727
732-919-1444
800-221-0034
FAX: 732-919-0256
e-mail: gmorton@avmvans.comom
www.monmouthvans.com

Eugene Morton, President
Raymond Morton, VP
Arthur Smith, Sales Manager
Full vehicle modifications for driving and for transport of people with disabilities. Access equipment for buildings, e.g. ramps, stair lifts, pool lifts, automatic door openers and patient transfer lifts, pride jazzy portable and modular wheelchairs and scooters. Large selection of modified vans in stock.

94 **New Quad Grip**
Gresham Driving Aids
30800 S Wixom Road
Wixom, MI 48393
248-624-1533
800-521-8930
FAX: 248-624-6358
www.greshamdrivingaids.com

Bill Dillon, Owner
Automobile aids for the disabled. *$40.25*

95 **PAC Unit**
Ahnafield Corporation
2444 Production Drive
Indianapolis, IN 46241
317-241-2444
800-636-8060
FAX: 317-636-8098
www.ahnafield.com

Jeff Ahnafield, Sales Manager
Bruce Ahnafield, President
Low effort accelerator and brake remote serves hand control.

96 **Pedal Ease**
Ahnafield Corporation
2444 Production Drive
Indianapolis, IN 46241
317-241-2444
800-636-8060
FAX: 317-636-8098
www.ahnafield.com

Jeff Ahnafield, Sales Manager
Bruce Ahnafield, President
Low effort accelerator and brake remote serves foot control.

97 **Portable Hand Controls**
Ahnafield Corporation
2444 Production Drive
Indianapolis, IN 46241
317-241-2444
800-636-8060
FAX: 317-636-8098
www.ahnafield.com

Jeff Ahnafield, Sales Manager
Bruce Ahanfield, President

98 **Portable Vehicle Controls**
Contact Technologies
1033 Business Center Circle
Newbury Park, CA 91320
805-498-8157
FAX: 805-498-2747
Fully portable, integrated, automotive hand control unit.

99 **Power Seat Base (6-Way)**
Ricon
7900 Nelson Road
Panorama City, CA 91402
818-267-3000
800-322-2884
FAX: 818-267-3001
www.riconcorp.com

William Baldwin, Chief Executive Officer
Facilitates a driver's self-transfer from a wheelchair to the driving seat and allows optimal driving positioning.

100 **Quad Grip with Pin**
Gresham Driving Aids
30800 S Wixom Road
Wixom, MI 48393
248-624-1533
800-521-8930
FAX: 248-624-6358
www.greshamdrivingaids.com

Bill Dillon, Owner
Automobile aids for the disabled. *$40.25*

101 **Rampvan**
Independent Mobility Systems
4100 W Piedras Street
Farmington, NM 87401
505-326-4538
800-467-8267
FAX: 505-326-4846
e-mail: info@ibraunmobility.com
www.ims-vans.com

Greg Anesi, President
Fully accessible minivan conversions with automatic doors and ramps, manufactured by Toyota, Chrysler, Dodge and Ford minivans.

102 **Recreation Vehicles**
Lazy Days RV Center
6130 Lazy Days Boulevard
Seffner, FL 33584
813-246-4777
800-626-7800
FAX: 813-246-4408
www.lazydays.com

Jack Graham
Don Wallace, President
Customized recreational vehicles for people with disabilities. Specializing in wheelchair accessible bathrooms.

103 **Reduced Effort Steering**
Ahnafield Corporation
2444 Production Drive
Indianapolis, IN 46241
317-241-2444
800-636-8060
FAX: 317-636-8098
www.ahnafield.com

Jeff Ahnafield, Sales Manager
Bruce Ahanfield, President

104 **Right Hand Turn Signal Switch Lever**
Gresham Driving Aids
30800 S Wixom Road
Wixom, MI 48393
248-624-1533
800-521-8930
FAX: 248-624-6358
www.greshamdrivingaids.com

Bill Dillon, Owner
Converts signal switch to right hand usage for left arm handicaps. *$34.50*

105 **Slim Line Brake Only**
Gresham Driving Aids
30800 S Wixom Road
Wixom, MI 48393
248-624-1533
800-521-8930
FAX: 248-624-6358
www.greshamdrivingaids.com

Bill Dillon, Owner
A chrome plated steel handle, contour shaped, with a left hand or right hand unit available. *$155.25*

106 **Slim Line Control**
Gresham Driving Aids
30800 S Wixom Road
Wixom, MI 48393
248-624-1533
800-521-8930
FAX: 248-624-6358
www.greshamdrivingaids.com

Bill Dillon, Owner
A plated, strong, compact unit designed to be easily transferred from car to car. Built of heavy steel tubing, welded and chrome plated and contour-shaped for maximum driving room. *$201.25*

107 **Slim Line Control: Brake and Throttle**
Gresham Driving Aids
30800 S Wixom Road
Wixom, MI 48393
248-624-1533
800-521-8930
FAX: 248-624-6358
www.greshamdrivingaids.com

Bill Dillon, Owner
Brake is actuated by pushing the control lever directly towards the brake. Throttle is actuated by moving the lever at right angles to the brake movement, toward the seat. The weight of the operator's hand is sufficient to hold the throttle at any designed speed. *$300.00*

108 **Steering Backup System**
Ahnafield Corporation
2444 Production Drive
Indianapolis, IN 46241
317-241-2444
800-636-8060
FAX: 317-636-8098
www.ahnafield.com

Jeff Ahnafield, Sales Manager
Bruce Ahanfield, President

109 **Superarm Lift**
Handicaps
4335 S Santa Fe Drive
Englewood, CO 80110
303-781-2062
800-782-4335
FAX: 303-761-6811
e-mail: Forest77@earthlink.com
www.handicapsinc.com

Geraldine O'Dell, Owner
Wheelchair lifts made for vans and motor homes. No platform is necessary and no doorways are blocked by lift that is simple and safe to use. We also make hand driving controls & other driving equipment.

110 **The HANDYBAR**
Maxi Aids
42 Executive Boulevard
Farmingdale, NY 11735
631-752-0521
800-522-6294
FAX: 631-752-0689
e-mail: sales@maxiaids.com
www.maxiaids.com
For those who have trouble getting in and out of a car. Sturdy bar slides into door striker and allows you better support to lift yourself out of the car. Stores easily under car seat.

111 **Tim's Trim**
25 Bermar Park
Rochester, NY 14624
585-429-6270
888-468-6784
FAX: 585-429-6355
e-mail: timstriminc@yahoo.com
www.theoptionstore.com

Timothy A Miller, President
Offers vehicle modifications, drop floors, raised tops/doors, driving equipment, touch pads and lifts. Also is a member of NEMDA and QAP certified

112 **Transportation Equipment for People with Disabilities**
Drive Master Company
37 Daniel Road W
Fairfield, NJ 07004
973-808-9709
877-282-8267
FAX: 973-808-9713
e-mail: sales@drivemaster.net
www.drivemaster.net

Peter Ruprecht, President
Wheelchair lifts and ramps, hand and foot controls, steering and braking modifications, complete van conversions, home modifications, wheelchairs and scooters and wheelchair accessible van rentals.

113 **Tri-Post Steering Wheel Spinner**
Gresham Driving Aids
30800 S Wixom Road
Wixom, MI 48393
248-624-1533
800-521-8930
FAX: 248-624-6358
www.greshamdrivingaids.com

Bill Dillon, Owner
Three nylon posts, adjustable for proper fit to drivers hand, to control the wheel, for use by persons with weak or limp wrists. *$40.25*

114 **Ultra-Lite XL Hand Control**
Drive Master Company
37 Daniel Road W
Fairfield, NJ 07004
973-808-9709
FAX: 973-808-9713
e-mail: sales@drivemaster.net
www.drivemaster.net

Peter Ruprecht, President
Allows the driver to operate gas and brake by hand— push for brake— pull for gas. Can be installed in nearly every vehicle.

115 **Vantage Mini-Vans**
Vantage Mini-Vans
5202 S 28th Place
Phoenix, AZ 85040
602-243-2700
FAX: 602-304-2804
e-mail: info@vantagemobility.com
www.vantagemobility.com

Doug Eaton, Sales Executive
Personalized vehicles with lowered floors and swing-away ramps.

116 **Voice Choice**
Ahnafield Corporation
2444 Production Drive
Indianapolis, IN 46241
317-241-2444
800-636-8060
FAX: 317-636-8098
www.ahnafield.com

Jeff Ahnafield, Sales Manager
Bruce Ahnafield, President
Voice recognition system for accessories.

117 **Voice Scan**
Ahnafield Corporation
2444 Production Drive
Indianapolis, IN 46241
317-241-2444
800-636-8060
FAX: 317-636-8098
www.ahnafield.com

Jeff Ahnafield, Sales Manager
Bruce Ahnafield, President
Voice feedback control for accessories.

118 **Warp Drive**
Ahnafield Corporation
2444 Production Drive
Indianapolis, IN 46241
317-241-2444
800-636-8060
FAX: 317-636-8098
www.ahnafield.com

Jeff Ahnafield, Sales Manager
Bruce Ahnafield, President
Low effort steering wheel attachment accelerator and brake hand control serves system.

119 **Wheelers Accessible Van Rentals**
6614 W Sweetwater Avenue
Glendale, AZ 85304
623-776-8830
800-456-1371
FAX: 623-412-9920
e-mail: info@WheelersVanRentals.com
www.WheelersVanRentals.com

Tammy Smith, Manager
Daily, weekly and monthly rentals. Locations throughout the US.

120 **XL Steering**
Ahnafield Corporation
2444 Production Drive
Indianapolis, IN 46241
317-241-2444
800-636-8060
FAX: 317-636-8098

Jeff Ahnafield, Sales Manager
Bruce Ahnafield, President
Extra light, small diameter, remote steering system.

Bath

121 **ARJO Inc.**
50 North Gary Avenue
Roselle, IL 60172
630-307-2756
800-323-1245
FAX: 888-594-2756
e-mail: info@arjousa.com
www.arjo.com

Lorena Chevrie, Marketing Communications
Ross Scavuzzo, President
Alexis LaSalvia, Marketing Comm. Specialist
ARJO offers a complete line of patient bathing, showering and lift/transport systems, bariatric solutions, and accompanying skin care products for long-term and acute care facilities.

122 **Adaptive Design Shop**
12847 Point Pleasant Drive
Fairfax, VA 22033
703-631-1585
800-351-2327
FAX: 775-256-2556
e-mail: info@email.com
www.adaptivedesignshop.com

Joe Rickerson, Marketing Director
Offers various adjustable models of bath and shower chairs, as well as adjustable toilet and commode supports for toddlers through adults. Call for a free brochure. Prices range from $200 to $800.

123 **Adjustable Bath Seat**
Arista Surgical Supply Company/AliMed
297 High Street
Dedham, MA 02026
781-329-2900
800-223-1984
FAX: 781-329-8392
e-mail: arista@alimed.com
www.aristasurgical.com

Julian Cherubini, President
Bath seat that fits easily in any size tub. Easily adjustable to any height for easier maneuverability. *$44.00*

124 **Adjustable Raised Toilet Seat & Guard**
Frohock-Stewart
39400 Taylor Parkway
N Ridgeville, OH 44035
440-329-6000
800-343-6059
FAX: 800-329-6270

A Mixon Iii, Chief Executive Officer
The seat features an exclusive pivot locking system so it won't slip or tip and the adjustable guard rail fits all toilets.

125 **BIT Talking Scale Bathroom Scale**
Sense-Sations
919 Walnut Street
Philadelphia, PA 19107
215-627-0600
800-876-5456
FAX: 215-922-0692

Patricia Johnson, Chief Executive Officer
Push the on button and the scale will invite you to jump on and discover how much weight you have lost or gained. *$91.50*

126 **Bath Fixtures**
Crane Plumbing/Fiat Products
1000 Industrial Drive
Suite 2a
Bensenville, IL 60106
630-350-7575
FAX: 630-350-7775
www.craneplumbing.com

Dave Pardue, Owner
Manufacturers plumbing fixtures for the disabled. Products include toilets, lavatories, showers and tub/shower units.

127 **Bath Products**
Snug Seat
PO Box 1739
Matthews, NC 28106
704-882-0666
800-336-7684
FAX: 704-882-0751
e-mail: information@snugseat.com
www.snugseat.com

Steve Scribner, VP
Kirk MacKenzie, President
Offers a wide range of products to meet the transportation, mobility, seating and bath aid needs for people of all ages. From car seats and standers for children with special needs to versatile wheelchairs that offer adults customized options and the freedom to go anywhere with confidence.

128 **Bath Shower & Commode Chair**
Clarke Health Care Products
1003 International Drive
Oakdale, PA 15071
724-695-2122
888-347-4537
FAX: 724-695-2922
e-mail: info@clarkehealthcare.com
www.clarkehealthcare.com

Susan Grabel, Marketing
Gerard Clarke, Owner
Aquatic Stainless steel shower/commode chairs and powered bathlifts. Mobeli portable grab bars, Dolomite rollators, Arco bed rails, Care bags for hygiene collection, DecPac portable ramps, Ableware eating, hygiene and dressing aids.

129 **Bath Supports**
Columbia Medical Manufacturing
13577 Larwin Circle
Santa Fe Springs, CA 90670
562-282-0264
800-454-6612
FAX: 310-305-1718
e-mail: info@columbiamedical.com
www.columbiamedical.com

Gary Werschmidt, President
Annie Chen, Marketing Communications Manager
Offers a full line of toilet supports, positioning commodes, wrap-around bath supports, reclining bath chairs and vehincle restraint systems for children from 20 to 102 pounds.

130 **Bath and Shower Bench 3301B**
Mada Medical Products
625 Washington Avenue
Carlstadt, NJ 07072
201-460-0454
800-526-6370
FAX: 201-460-3509
e-mail: dianelind@mail.madamedical.com
www.madainternational.com

Diane Lind, Operations Manager
Jeffrey Adam, Vice President
The bath and shower bench is corrosion resistent, has a cross brace design and angled legs to prevent tipping, and seat height adjustments.

131 **BathEase**
3815 Darston Street
Palm Harbor, FL 34685
727-786-2604
888-747-7845
FAX: 727-786-2604
e-mail: bathease@aol.com
www.bathease.com

Thomas Fitz Gerald, President/CEO
Terry Stickler, Director R&D
Gerry Grondin, Production Manager
BathEase is the original, standard size, residential style, acrylic bathtub with a door. Ideal for use in private homes by all who are ambulatory, the award winning design was specially created as an aid to daily living for the elderly and physically challenged. *$ 1897.00*

132 **Bathtub Safety Rail**
Arista Surgical Supply Company/AliMed
297 High Street
Dedham, MA 02026
212-679-3694
800-223-1984
FAX: 212-696-9046
e-mail: arista@alimed.com
www.aristasurgical.com
Made of stainless steel, this safety rail fits in any size bathtub and offers safety and independence at bathing time. *$55.00*

133 **Braun Corporation**
Braun Corporation
PO Box 310
Winamac, IN 46996
574-946-6153
800-843-5438
FAX: 574-946-4670
www.braunlift.com

Carolyn Watts, Public Affairs Contact
William Roth, President
Offers a variety of assistive devices for the bath and surrounding environment.

134 **Can-Do Products Catalog**
Independent Living Aids
PO Box 9022
Hicksville, NY 11802
516-937-1848
800-537-2118
FAX: 516-937-3906

Marvin Sandler, President
Fran Hennelly, Sales Director
84 pages Quarterly

135 **Commode**
Maxi Aids
42 Executive Boulevard
Farmingdale, NY 11735
631-752-0521
800-522-6294
FAX: 631-752-0689
e-mail: sales@maxiaids.com
www.maxiaids.com
Adjustable seat height for patient comfort. *$65.95*

136 **DSI**
16141 Runnymede Street
Van Nuys, CA 91406
818-782-6793
FAX: 818-782-6485
e-mail: sales@drivingsystems.com
www.drivingsystems.com

Greg Paquin, Marketing Manager
Bill Butt, Vice President
Designer grab bars with ergonomic grip. Available in colors and custom shapes. New fold down shower seat. Support grips extend out from the wall 24 or 30. Concealed fastener and modular components for many design possibilities. Price ranges from $30.00 to $280.00.

137 **Deluxe Bath Bench with Adjustable Legs**
Maxi Aids
42 Executive Boulevard
Farmingdale, NY 11735
631-752-0521
800-522-6294
FAX: 631-752-0689
e-mail: sales@maxiaids.com
www.maxiaids.com
Bath bench with back support and adjustable legs. *$ 49.95*

138 **Electric Leg Bag Emptier and Tub Slide Shower Chair**
RD Equipment
230 Percival Drive
West Barnstable, MA 02668
508-362-7498
FAX: 508-362-7498
e-mail: info@rdequipment.com
www.rdequipment.com

Richard J Dagostino, Inventor/President
Diana M Pontieri, Sales Manager

Designed for independence, this small, lightweight, battery-operated valve attaches to the bottom of the leg bag. A simple flip of the switch empties the leg bag, allowing the user to take in unlimited amounts of fluids. Tub Slide Shower Chair is a complete bathroom care system, with no need of costly renovations. Eliminates all transfers in the bathroom. *$200.00*

139 Freedom Bath
Arjo Inc.
50 North Gary Avenue
Roselle, IL 60172
630-307-2756
800-323-1245
FAX: 888-594-2756
e-mail: info@arjousa.com
www.arjo.com

Lorena Chevrie, Marketing Communications
Ross Scavuzzo, President
Residents can relax on a semi-reclining seat and enjoy the soothing deluxe whirlpool system. Freedom Bath offers a revolutionary solution with its unique Roll-Door.

140 Great Big Safety Tub Mat
Maxi Aids
42 Executive Boulevard
Farmingdale, NY 11735
631-752-0521
800-522-6294
FAX: 631-752-0689
e-mail: sales@maxiaids.com
www.maxiaids.com
Tub mat provides security against falls in the bath and shower. *$16.95*

141 Long Handled Bath Sponges
Therapro
225 Arlington Street
Framingham, MA 01702
508-872-9494
800-257-5376
FAX: 508-875-2062
e-mail: info@theraproducts.com
www.theraproducts.com

Karen Conrad, Owner
Plastic-handled, 18-inch bath sponge. Handle may be heated and bent for easy reach. *$2.50*

142 Modular Wall Grab Bars
Frohock-Stewart
39400 Taylor Parkway
N Ridgeville, OH 44035
440-329-6000
FAX: 440-365-7483

A Mixon Iii, Chief Executive Officer
Engineered for strength and beauty, these bars can be assembled in various combinations to fit any bath or shower.

143 Portable Shampoo Bowl
Ambulatory Cosmetology Technicians
12762 Brookhurst Street
Suite 532
Garden Grove, CA 92840
949-833-1432

Shirley D Smith
A bowl designed to allow a person who is in a wheelchair or sitting on a regular chair to shampoo hair.

144 Prelude
Arjo Inc.
50 North Gary Avenue
Roselle, IL 60172
630-307-2756
800-323-1245
FAX: 888-594-2756
e-mail: info@arjousa.com
www.arjo.com

Lorena Chevrie, Marketing Communications
Ross Scavuzzo, President
Prelude shower cabinet allows patients to be showered in comfort and privacy, at the same time as protecting staff from excessive splashing.

145 SLIDER Bathing System
Assistive Technology
21279 Protecta Drive
Elkhart, IN 46516
574-522-7201
800-478-2363
FAX: 574-293-0202
e-mail: info@pvcdme.com
www.pvcdme.com
The SLIDER bathing system eliminates costly roll-in shower renovations, bathroom transfers and other family members don't lose access to a bathtub. The SLIDER works with any standard built-in tub and rolls directly over any commode. The SLIDER utilizes 5 inch lock casters and has two swing-away arm rests for lateral transfers. Sliding gear functions in either direction. The SLIDER bathing system...a cost effective alternative to bathroom renovation.

146 Suregrip Bathtub Rail
Frohock-Stewart
39400 Taylor Parkway
N Ridgeville, OH 44035
440-329-6000
FAX: 440-365-7483

A Mixon Iii, Chief Executive Officer
Compact and versatile, the bars have a soft-touch, contoured, white vinyl gripping area for added safety.

147 Talking Bathroom Scale
Independent Living Aids
PO Box 9022
Hicksville, NY 11802
516-937-1848
800-537-2118
FAX: 516-937-3906
e-mail: can-do@independentliving.com
www.independentliving.com

Marvin Sandler, President
Talking scale. *$59.95*

148 Terry-Wash Mitt: Medium Size
Therapro
225 Arlington Street
Framingham, MA 01702
508-872-9494
800-257-5376
FAX: 508-875-2062
e-mail: info@theraproducts.com
www.theraproducts.com

Karen Conrad, Owner
Includes a thumb socket and a palm pocket to hold a bar of soap. *$8.00*

149 Toilet Guard Rail
Maxi Aids
42 Executive Boulevard
Farmingdale, NY 11735
631-752-0521
800-522-6294
FAX: 631-752-0689
e-mail: sales@maxiaids.com
www.maxiaids.com
Made of chrome-plated, heavy gauge steel. Fits securely to the toilet for maximum sturdiness. *$43.95*

150 Transfer Tub Bench
Arista Surgical Supply Company/AliMed
297 High Street
Dedham, MA 02026
781-329-2900
800-223-1984
FAX: 781-329-8392
e-mail: aristasurgical@juno.com
www.aristasurgical.com

Julian Cherubini, President
Curved padded backrest for comfortable support. Backrest also assists patient during lateral transfer. *$64.00*

151 Tri-Grip Bathtub Rail
Maxi Aids
42 Executive Boulevard
Farmingdale, NY 11735
631-752-0521
800-522-6294
FAX: 631-752-0689
e-mail: sales@maxiaids.com
www.maxiaids.com
Two gripping heights for easy bathtub entrance or exit. *$36.95*

152 **Tub Slide Shower Chair**
RD Equipment
230 Percival Drive
West Barnstable, MA 02668
508-362-7498
FAX: 508-362-7498
e-mail: info@rdequipment.com
www.rdequipment.com

Richard J Dagostino, Proprietor/Inventor
Diana M Pontieri, Sales Manager
The tub slide shower chair was designed for the elderly and disabled to make any bathroom (at home or when travelling) accessible with little or no renovations. Go from the bed, to the commode and over to the bathtub for a shower using one product. No transfers in the bathroom whatsoever. *$2000.00*

Bed

153 **ASSISTECH**
2738 N Campbell Avenue
Tucson, AZ 85719
520-883-8600
866-674-3549
FAX: 520-883-3172
e-mail: info@azhearing.com
www.azhearing.com

Oliver Simoes, Owner
Sells hearing, visual and mobility aid devices. *$39.00*

154 **Adjustable Bed**
Golden Technologies
401 Bridge Street
Old Forge, PA 18518
570-451-7477
800-624-6374
FAX: 570-451-7494
e-mail: info@goldentech.com
www.goldentech.com

Rich Golden, CEO
Fred Kiwax, VP
Bob Golden, President
Trouble-free gear motor, safety features, dual massage, variable speed timer and more, for the ultimate sleep experience.

155 **Bye-Bye Decubiti Air Mattress Overlay**
Ken McRight Supplies
7456 S Oswego Avenue
Tulsa, OK 74136
918-492-9657
FAX: 918-492-9694

Ken McRight, President
Originally designed for hospital beds, converts any bed into an exceptionally therapeutic, flotation unit when used between the conventional mattress and pad. The complete overlay is comprised of five individually inflatable, 100 percent natural rubber, ventilated sections enclosed within separate pockets of a soft fleece cover. Conforms to any configuration of electric or manual beds. *$731.50*

156 **Cervical Support Pillow**
Wise Enterprises
5017 El Don Drive
Rocklin, CA 95677
916-624-3848
888-947-3368
FAX: 916-624-3848
e-mail: wisent@pacbell.net
www.wisent.com/pillows.htm

Tom Wise, Owner
These hypoallergenic, antimicrobial fiber pillows support the neck in a natural position. Standard, midsize and petite pillows support the neck while sleeping on the back or side. The compact travel pillow offers support while sitting or lying down. The cervical roll has a gentle center and firm ends to ensure maximum comfort and proper support. Position the roll under the neck, back or knees. Standard and midsize fits adults, petite fits children and small adults.

157 **Dual Security Bed Rail**
Maxi Aids
42 Executive Boulevard
Farmingdale, NY 11735
631-752-0521
800-522-6294
FAX: 631-752-0689
e-mail: sales@maxiaids.com
www.maxiaids.com

Sleep without worry! Dual rails for double the safety. Steel with Powder Coat. Rails adjust up and down.

158 **Foam Decubitus Bed Pads**
Profex Medical Products
PO Box 140188
Memphis, TN 38114
800-325-0196
FAX: 901-454-9850
e-mail: wallaceswain@profexmed.com
www.profexmed.com

Convoluted foam provides extra back support and comfort for wheelchair users.

159 **Hard Manufacturing Company**
230 Grider Street
Buffalo, NY 14215
716-893-1800
800-873-4273
FAX: 716-896-2579
e-mail: currier@hardmfg.com
www.hardmfg.com

Kevin Currier, Corporate Sales
William Godin, President
Manufacturer of pediatric cribs and age appropriate youth beds. Free catalog.

160 **Jackson Cervipillo**
Wise Enterprises
5017 El Don Drive
Rocklin, CA 95677
916-624-3848
888-947-3368
FAX: 916-624-3848
e-mail: wisent@pacbell.net
www.wisent.com/pillows.htm

Tom Wise, Owner
The Jackson Cervipillo confortably supports the neck vertebrae when sleeping on the side or on the back. Pillow measures 7 in diameter and is 17 long. A machine-washable cover is available separately.

161 **NeckEase**
Wise Enterprises
5017 El Don Drive
Rocklin, CA 95677
916-624-3848
888-947-3368
FAX: 916-624-3848
e-mail: wisent@pacbell.net
www.wisent.com/pillows.htm

Tom Wise, Owner
Microwave NeckEase for penetrating heat that sooths stiff necks and shoulders, easing tension. NeckEase features a unique filling of organic, long grain rice and aromatic herbs and spices. When heated, this filling provides soothing, moist aromatherapy. Heat lasts about 30-45 minutes. Available in two sizes: small fits snugly around the neck, applying gentle pressure at the base of the skull; Large may be worn for a snug fit, or loosely for application on the shoulder and upper back.

162 **Permaflex Home Care Mattress**
BG Industries
8550 Balboa Boulevard
Suite 214
Northridge, CA 91325
818-894-0744
800-822-8288
www.bgind.com

Larry Lankard, President
Mattress with flame retardant upholstery material, water-repellant, anti-microbial and tear-resistant cover, for extra comfort.

163 **SleepSafe Beds**
3135 Dillons Mill Road
Callaway, VA 24067
540-334-1600
866-852-2337
FAX: 540-334-2100
www.sleepsafebed.com
Perfect for adult home or home care use. Offering twin or full size bed frames in classic style, these beds offer an attractive alternative to a hospital bed. Keeps the user safe during rest and electrically adjusts smoothly for user comfort and caregiver ease of use.

164 **Sonic Alert Bed Shaker**
ASSISTECH
2738 N Campbell Avenue
Tucson, AZ 85719
520-883-8600
866-674-3549
FAX: 520-883-3172
www.azhearing.com

Oliver Simoes, Owner
$49.00

165 **Vibes Bed Shaker**
ASSISTECH
2738 N Campbell Avenue
Tucson, AZ 85719
520-883-8600
866-674-3549
FAX: 520-883-3172
www.azhearing.com

Oliver Simoes, Owner

166 **Vibration Watch/Countdown Timer**
Global Assistive Devices
4950 N Dixie Highway
Oakland Park, FL 33334
954-776-1373
FAX: 954-776-8136
TTY:954-776-1373
e-mail: info@globalassistive.com
www.globalassistive.com

Peggy Hewitt, Marketing Manager
This useful innovation reminds you and alerts you. Use for medical conditions. It can even be used as a travel alarm. Unique Auto Repeat Countdown Timer resets itself each time it reaches zero.

167 **Waterproof Sheet-Topper Mattress and Chair Pad**
Pillow Talk
348 Pond Road
Freehold, NJ 07728
732-780-9483
FAX: 732-780-0279
e-mail: info@pillowtalkusa.com
www.pillowtalkusa.com

Jack Fajerman, President
Dorothy Faferman, Owner
This soft pad lies on the top sheet, absorbing accidents from incontinence, pregnancy or medical problems. Waterproof barrier locks out moisture, soiling and stains and eliminates midnight linen changes and the resulting laundry. Available in bed sizes W/4 Anchor, twin, full, queen, king, and crib.

Communication

168 **ADA Hotel Built-In Alerting System**
HARC Mercantile
1111 W Centre Avenue
Portage, MI 49024
269-324-1615
800-445-9968
FAX: 269-324-2387
e-mail: info@harc.com
www.harcmercantile.com

Ronald Slager, President
Ronald Damstra, Technical Sales Manager
Visual alerting system for ADA compliance for multihousing/rooms facilities, like hospitals, dorms, senior housing for persons who are hard of hearing or deaf. Alerts to five conditions: smoke, door bell, telephone ring, wake up and House central alarm.

169 **Access Control Systems: NHX Nurse Call System**
Aiphone Corporation
1700 130th Avenue NE
Bellevue, WA 98005
425-455-0510
800-692-0200
FAX: 425-455-0071
e-mail: info@aiphone.com
www.aiphone.com

Tak Kanie, President
AIPHONE manufactures audio and video intercom systems for home or business to help the physically disabled answer doors and communicate through physical barriers; also ADA-compliant emergency call intercom stations for use in public facilities and an Environmental Control System for persons with limited mobility.

170 **Adaptek Systems**
2320 Brighton Henrietta Town Line R
Rochester, NY 14623
800-685-4566
FAX: 585-475-9889
Developers of a voice output module designed to work with the Kurzweil voice-recognition system. The device provides voice output of what the computer hears for persons with visual impairments.

171 **Akron Resources**
20 La Porte Street
Arcadia, CA 91006
626-254-9005
FAX: 626-254-9266
www.akron.com

Lisa Avalos, Operations Manager
Paul Brassard, Owner
Manufacturers of infrared amplification systems for televisions or stereos. $29-$69.00.

172 **Amplified Handsets**
HARC Mercantile
1111 W Centre Avenue
Portage, MI 49024
269-324-1615
800-445-9968
FAX: 269-324-2387
e-mail: info@harc.com
www.harcmercantile.com

Ronald Slager, President
Choices of touch activated, electronic control, rotary (thumb wheel) volume control, that can directly replace old handset, stocked in round and square styles. This also includes an electric transmitter with variable settings. *$39.95*

173 **Amplified Phones**
HARC Mercantile
1111 W Centre Avenue
Portage, MI 49024
269-324-1615
800-445-9968
FAX: 269-324-2387
e-mail: info@harc.com
www.harcmercantile.com

Ronald Slager, President
Low frequency ringer, indicator light, enhances or amplifies sound, some that automatically return to normal dial tone when phone receiver is hung up, lighted easy to read dial pad and volume control boosts incoming sound. *$95.00*

174 **Amplified Portable Phone**
HARC Mercantile
1111 W Centre Avenue
Portage, MI 49024
269-324-1615
800-445-9968
FAX: 269-324-2387
e-mail: info@harc.com
www.harcmercantile.com

Ronald Slager, President
Portable amplified phones. *$199.00*

175 **Artificial Larynx**
HARC Mercantile
1111 W Centre Avenue
Portage, MI 49024
269-324-1615
800-445-9968
FAX: 269-324-2387
e-mail: info@harc.com
www.harcmercantile.com

Ronald Slager, President
For people unable to use their larynx, a hand-held speaking aid that simulates the natural vibrations of voice. *$220.00*

176 **Assistive Technology**
333 Elm Street
Dedham, MA 02026
781-461-8200
800-793-9227
FAX: 781-461-8213
e-mail: customercare@assistivetech.com
www.assistivetech.com

Jane Oles, Customer Service Manager
Roxanne Varteressian, Marketing Specialist
James Lewis, President
A premiere developer of innovative technology solutions for people with physical and learning disabilities. Breakthrough products enable people of all ages and abilities to live and learn independently. Supportive material for teachers, clinicians and those with disabilities.

177 **BESTspeech**
Berkeley Speech Technologies
2246 6th Street
Berkeley, CA 94710
510-841-5083
FAX: 510-841-5093
e-mail: webmaster@bst.com
www.bestspeech.com
This text-to-speech facility is useful to persons who are blind or vision impaired and may be used by those with speech, hearing and learning difficulties.

178 **Big Red Switch**
AbleNet
2808 Fairview Avenue N
Saint Paul, MN 55113
800-322-0956
FAX: 651-294-2259
e-mail: customerservice@ablenetinc.com
www.ablenetinc.com

Mary Kay Walch
Five inches across the top and activates no matter where on its surface it is touched. It is made of shatterproof plastic and contains a cord storage compartment. Also available in green, yellow and blue. *$42.00*

179 **Cornell Communications**
7915 N 81st Street
Milwaukee, WI 53223
414-351-4660
800-558-8957
FAX: 414-351-4657
e-mail: sales@cornell.com
www.cornell.com

David D Thompson, Account Executive
Pauline Haack, Customer Service
Janet Marien, Account Executive
Cornell's Rescue Assistance Systems allow personnel to request emergency assistance. Applications include handicapped evacuations, parking garages and elevators. Voice, intercom and visual only signaling systems are available.

180 **Davis Center**
200 Valley Road
Suite 205
Mt. Arington, NJ 07856
973-398-2710
FAX: 973-398-2721
e-mail: info@thedaviscenter.net
www.thedaviscenter.com

Dorinne S Davis, President
Sound-based therapies that help hearing, learning, speech and well-being. Complete hearing, speech and CAP testing.

181 **Flashing Lamp Telephone Ring Alerter**
Independent Living Aids
PO Box 9022
Hicksville, NY 11802
516-937-1848
800-537-2118
FAX: 516-937-3906
e-mail: can-do@independentliving.com
www.independentliving.com

Marvin Sandler, President
Once your phone is plugged into the Telephone Ring Alerter, the lamp light will flash with each ring, alerting you that there is a phone call. *$62.00*

182 **Gabbi Talk Phone**
Sense-Sations
919 Walnut Street
Philadelphia, PA 19107
215-627-0600
FAX: 215-922-0692

Patricia Johnson, Chief Executive Officer
The talking telephone for mistake-free dialing lets the individual know what numbers they have dialed. *$28.50*

183 **Headmaster Plus**
Prentke Romich Company
1022 Heyl Road
Wooster, OH 44691
330-262-1984
800-262-1984
FAX: 330-263-4829
e-mail: info@prentrom.com
www.prentrom.com

Dave Moffatt, President
A headpointing system that takes the place of a mouse and allows individuals who cannot use their hands but have good head control access to the computer. A transmitting unit sits atop the monitor and sends signals to the user's headset. The user puffs into a tube connected to the headset to make selections. Typing can be done with optional on-screen keyboards. *$1195.00*

184 **Ideal-Phone**
IDEAMATICS
1364 Beverly Road
Suite 101
McLean, VA 22101
703-903-4972
800-247-IDEA
FAX: 703-903-8949
e-mail: ideamatics@ideamatics.net
www.ideamatics.org

David L Danner, President
Pamela Danner, Owner
Integrates the personal computer and the telephone into a single, efficient workstation. It is ideal for mobility-impaired persons and others who need a hands-free operation of the phone. The Ideal-Phone includes one PC Board, a Plantronics headset, software for access and logging and complete documentation. It can be integrated into programs or pops-up over any application. MS-DOS based, version 3.0 or higher are available. *$195.00*

185 **IntelliKeys**
IntelliTools
1720 Corporate Circle
Petaluma, CA 94954
707-773-2000
800-889-6687
FAX: 707-773-2001
e-mail: tech@intellitools.com
www.intellitools.com

Arjan Khalsa, Chief Executive Officer
Card and cable to create keyboard port on Apple IIe computer to allow use of IntelliKeys alternative keyboard.

186 **LPB Communications**
960 Brook Road
Norristown, PA 19401
856-365-8080
FAX: 856-365-8999
e-mail: lpbsales@lpbinc.com
www.lpbinc.com

John Devecka, VP Sales

Limited area AM and FM broadcast systems for hearing assistance and language translation manufacturing since 1960. Systems for small conference halls, churches and Olympic stadiums. Components or complete system. *$400.00*

187 Language, Learning & Living
Prentke Romich Company
1022 Heyl Road
Wooster, OH 44691
330-262-1984
800-262-1984
FAX: 330-263-4829
e-mail: info@prentrom.com
www.prentrom.com

Dave Moffatt, President
A Minspeak application program designed for adolescent and adult individuals with developmental disabilities and associated learning difficulties. The software is used with Prentke Romich Company augmentative communication devices. *$355.00*

188 Large Button Speaker Phone
HARC Mercantile
1111 W Centre Avenue
Portage, MI 49024
269-324-1615
800-445-9968
FAX: 269-324-2387
e-mail: info@harc.com
www.harcmercantile.com

Ronald Slager, President
Speakerphone with or without remote control. *$395.00*

189 Large Print Telephone Dial
Maxi Aids
42 Executive Boulevard
Farmingdale, NY 11735
631-752-0521
800-522-6294
FAX: 631-752-0689
e-mail: sales@maxiaids.com
www.maxiaids.com
Pressure sensitive dial with numbers that are easy to see for the disabled. *$69.00*

190 Large Print Touch-Telephone Overlays
Maxi Aids
42 Executive Boulevard
Farmingdale, NY 11735
631-752-0521
800-522-6294
FAX: 631-752-0689
e-mail: sales@maxiaids.com
www.maxiaids.com
Pressure-sensitive and easy to apply overlays that make everyday phones accessible. *$49.00*

191 Liberator
Prentke Romich Company
1022 Heyl Road
Wooster, OH 44691
330-262-1984
800-262-1984
FAX: 330-263-4829
e-mail: info@prentrom.com
www.prentrom.com

Dave Moffatt, President
A portable electronic communication device that uses Minspeak so that symbols are used to represent words, sentences or phrases. Liberator can be accessed by pressing keys, optical headpointing and a wide variety of switch activated scans. It can be configured with 8, 32 or 128 locations. It offers a variety of unique features to permit the most effective communication possible. $7,345-$8,575.

192 Metropolitan Washington Ear
35 University Boulevard E
Silver Spring, MD 20901
301-681-6636
FAX: 301-681-5227
e-mail: info@washear.org
www.washear.org

Nancy Knauss, Executive Director
Multi-media reading service for blind and visually impaired. Offering 24 hour audio radio reading, dial-in newspapers and web casting, as well as audio description at theaters, museums and films.

193 Mini Teleloop
HARC Mercantile
1111 W Centre Avenue
Portage, MI 49024
269-324-1615
800-445-9968
FAX: 269-324-2387
e-mail: info@harc.com
www.harcmercantile.com

Ronald Slager, President
Home induction loop amplifier for use with hearing aids equipped with T-Coil. *$159.95*

194 Multiple Phone/Device Switch
HARC Mercantile
1111 W Centre Avenue
Portage, MI 49024
269-324-1615
800-445-9968
FAX: 269-324-2387
e-mail: info@harc.com
www.harcmercantile.com

Ronald Slager, President
Used to switch phone lines between two devices. *$34.95*

195 Personal FM Systems
HARC Mercantile
1111 W Centre Avenue
Portage, MI 49024
269-324-1615
800-445-9968
FAX: 269-324-2387
e-mail: info@harc.com
www.harcmercantile.com

Ronald Slager, President
Wireless FM systems transmit sound via a radio carrier wave. *$599.95*

196 Personal Infrared Listening System
HARC Mercantile
1111 W Centre Avenue
Portage, MI 49024
269-324-1615
800-445-9968
FAX: 269-324-2387
e-mail: info@harc.com
www.harcmercantile.com

Ronald Slager, President
Wireless method of listening to TV and radio with individually controlled amplification. *$199.00*

197 Phone-TTY
1246 Route 46 W
Parsippany, NJ 07054
973-299-6627
888-332-3889
FAX: 973-299-7768
e-mail: phonetty@aol.com
www.phone-tty.com

Anna M Terrazzino, Executive Director
Develops and promotes better communications for the deaf using ordinary telephone equipment and current technology. Installs computerized phone-television equipment in the homes of individuals who are deaf, enabling these individuals to communicate with local police, hospitals, answering services and news services.

198 Prentke Romich Company
1022 Heyl Road
Wooster, OH 44691
330-262-1984
800-262-1984
FAX: 330-263-4829
e-mail: info@prentrom.com
www.prentrom.com

Barry Romich, Chairman
Joe Durbin, President
Cherie Weaver, Marketing Coordinator
The Prentke Romich Company is a full service company offering easy, yet powerful communication aids. The company believes in supporting customers before and after the sale by offering funding assistance, distance learning training, extended warranty, service assistance and much more. Visit our website to view our full line catalog, read about our success stories and to sign up for our online newsletter.

199 **Push to Talk Amplified Handset**
HARC Mercantile
1111 W Centre Avenue
Portage, MI 49024
269-324-1615
800-445-9968
FAX: 269-324-2387
e-mail: info@harc.com
www.harcmercantile.com

Ronald Slager, President
Replacement receiver which is hearing aid compatible and is designed for high noise conditions. *$79.95*

200 **Ring-a-Lite**
Tellus Business Services
1120 SW Sampson Road
Lees Summit, MO 64081
816-554-3777
FAX: 816-765-3301
e-mail: telus@birch.net
www.birch.net/~telus/ring.htm

Ralph Taylor, Partner
Ron Toles, Owner
Allows persons to see a telephone ringing, eliminating missing calls. This easy to use unit connects directly to existing telephone connections and also works to signal incoming TDD messages. *$39.95*

201 **Room Valet Visual-Tactile Alerting System**
HARC Mercantile
1111 W Centre Avenue
Portage, MI 49024
269-324-1615
800-445-9968
FAX: 269-324-2387
e-mail: info@harc.com
www.harcmercantile.com

Ronald Slager, President
ADA compliant built-in visual-tactile alerting system. The Room Valet is fully supervised and has power failure back up. Alerts to in-room smoke, building alarm, door, phone and alarm clock. Designed for permanent installation.

202 **Silent Call Communications**
5095 Williams Lake Road
Waterford, MI 48329
248-673-7353
800-572-5227
FAX: 248-673-7360
e-mail: silentcall@ameritech.net
www.silentcall.com

George Elwell, President
Suzie Wright, Office Manager
Alerting devices such as paging systems and smoke detectors for deaf and deaf-blind people.

203 **Sonic Alert**
Harris Communications
15155 Technology Drive
Eden Prairie, MN 55344
952-906-1180
800-825-6758
FAX: 952-906-1099
e-mail: info@harriscomm.com
www.harriscomm.com

Bill Williams, National Sales Manager
Lori Foss, Marketing Director
Robert Harris, Owner
Offers visual alerting devices that provide safety and convenience by turning vital sound into flashing light: telephone ring signalers, doorbell signalers, baby cry signalers and wake up alarms. Free catalog available.

204 **Sound Induction Receiver**
HARC Mercantile
1111 W Centre Avenue
Portage, MI 49024
269-324-1615
800-445-9968
FAX: 269-324-2387
e-mail: info@harc.com
www.harcmercantile.com

Ronald Slager, President
Sound induction receiver to be used with any loop system. *$67.00*

205 **SpeakEasy Communication Aid**
AbleNet
2808 Fairview Avenue N
Saint Paul, MN 55113
800-322-0956
FAX: 612-379-9143
e-mail: customerservice@ablenetinc.com
www.ablenetinc.com
SpeakEasy is a digitalized voice output communication Aid that is ideal for anyone who is beginning to develop communication skills such as making choices and identifying symbols. It holds 12 messages totaling four minutes and 20 seconds of recording time. It measures 7 1/2 inch by 1 3/4 inch and weighs only one pound. Activate messages using the built-in keyboard or via external switch. *$399.00*

206 **Speakwriter 2000**
HumanWare
6140 Horseshoe Bar Road
Suite P
Loomis, CA 95650
916-652-7253

Talking typewriter.

207 **Speech Discrimination Unit**
HARC Mercantile
1111 W Centre Avenue
Portage, MI 49024
269-324-1615
800-445-9968
FAX: 269-324-2387
e-mail: info@harc.com
www.harcmercantile.com

Ronald Slager, President
Speech Adjust-A-Tone improves speech discrimination for use with telephone and/or TV and radio. *$189.95*

208 **Speechmaker-Personal Speech Amplifier**
HARC Mercantile
1111 W Centre Avenue
Portage, MI 49024
269-324-1615
800-445-9968
FAX: 269-324-2387
e-mail: info@harc.com
www.harcmercantile.com

Ronald Slager, President
Portable, body worn, personal speech amplifier for people with a weak voice. *$316.00*

209 **Standard Touch Turner Sip & Puff Switch**
Access to Recreation
8 Sandra Court
Newbury Park, CA 91320
805-498-7535
800-634-4351
FAX: 805-498-8186
e-mail: customerservice@accesstr.com
www.accesstr.com

Don Krebs, President
A page turning device.

210 **Step-by-Step Communicator**
AbleNet
2808 Fairview Avenue N
Saint Paul, MN 55113
800-322-0956
FAX: 612-379-9143
e-mail: customerservice@ablenetinc.com
www.ablenetinc.com
Allows you to record a series of messages (as many as you want up to the 75 second limit). It has a 2 1/2 inches diameter switch surface and is 3 inches at its tallest point. Angled switch surface makes it easy to see and access. *$129.00*

211 **Strobe Light Signalers**
HARC Mercantile
1111 W Centre Avenue
Portage, MI 49024
269-324-1615
800-445-9968
FAX: 269-324-2387
e-mail: info@harc.com
www.harcmercantile.com

Ronald Slager, President

Strobe alerts. Plugs into receivers for signaling systems. *$39.95*

212 **TTY's: Telephone Device for the Deaf**
HARC Mercantile
1111 W Centre Avenue
Portage, MI 49024
269-324-1615
800-445-9968
FAX: 269-324-2387
e-mail: info@harc.com
www.harcmercantile.com

Ronald Slager, President
With or without printer. *$239.00*

213 **TalkTrac Wearable Communicator**
Ablenet
2808 Fairview Avenue N
Saint Paul, MN 55113
800-322-0956
FAX: 612-379-9143
e-mail: customerservice@ablenetinc.com
www.ablenetinc.com
The TalkTrac Wearable Communicator is a personal, portable communication aid that is wearable on the wrist. TalkTrac features: simple to use, 75 seconds of recording time, four 3/4 x 1/2 message locations, rechargeable, water resistant, adjustable 9" band, Boardmaker compatible.

214 **Talking Calculators**
ASSISTECH
2738 N Campbell Avenue
Tucson, AZ 85719
520-883-8600
866-674-3549
FAX: 520-883-3172
e-mail: info@assistivedevices.net
www.azhearing.com

Oliver Simoes, Owner

215 **Talking Clocks**
HARC Mercantile
1111 W Centre Avenue
Portage, MI 49024
269-324-1615
800-445-9968
FAX: 269-324-2387
e-mail: info@harc.com
www.harcmercantile.com

Ronald Slager, President
Talking clocks with loud alarms, high and low volume control, choices of sound effects, hourly report options. Other languages are available. *$20.50*

216 **Talking Watches**
HARC Mercantile
1111 W Centre Avenue
Portage, MI 49024
269-324-1615
800-445-9968
FAX: 269-324-2387
e-mail: info@harc.com
www.harcmercantile.com

Ronald Slager, President
Digital display, hourly reports, alarm with rooster crow, in English or Spanish. *$20.25*

217 **Telecaption Adapter**
HARC Mercantile
1111 W Centre Avenue
Portage, MI 49024
269-324-1615
800-445-9968
FAX: 269-324-2387
e-mail: info@harc.com
www.harcmercantile.com

Ronald Slager, President
Caption opens up the world of television to hearing impaired people. Viewers can read on the screen what they may not be able to hear. Closed captions are the dialogue and sound effects of a TV program or home video printed on the screen, similar to subtitles. *$ 159.95*

218 **Touch Turner-Page Turning Devices**
Touch Turner Company
13621 103rd Avenue NE
Arlington, WA 98223
360-651-1962
888-811-1962
FAX: 360-658-9380
e-mail: touchturner@worldnet.att.net
www.touchturner.com

Karen Rieger, President
Turns pages in either direction powered by flashlight batteries or AC Adapter. Works with soft or hard bound books and magazines.

219 **Unity**
Prentke Romich Company
1022 Heyl Road
Wooster, OH 44691
330-262-1984
800-262-1984
FAX: 330-263-4829
e-mail: info@prentrom.com
www.prentrom.com

Dave Moffatt, President
A Minspeak application program available for the Liberator and Delta Talker communication devices. Provides single word vocabulary to people of all ages at varying stages of language development, who may be either cognitively intact or challenged. *$355.00*

220 **Vantage**
Prentke Romich Company
1022 Heyl Road
Wooster, OH 44691
330-262-1984
800-262-1984
FAX: 330-263-4829
e-mail: info@prentrom.com
www.prentrom.com

Dave Moffatt, President
Vantage is a portable communication aid that features the Unity Enhanced vocabulary software and a large high quality dynamic display. Vantage also employs the recently upgraded 4.0 operating system that makes system settings quick and easy. Vantage has synthesized speech powered by DECtalk Software, Spelling and Word Protection software, built-in visor (flip-up protective cover), digitized speech capability and built-in computer access and ECU controls. 15 and 45 location keyguards available. *$6295.00*

221 **Vibrotactile Personal Alerting System**
HARC Mercantile
1111 W Centre Avenue
Portage, MI 49024
269-324-1615
800-445-9968
FAX: 269-324-2387
e-mail: info@harc.com
www.harcmercantile.com

Ronald Slager, President
Composed of a small wireless personal device that receives coded signals and a group of transmitters that send them. *$195.95*

222 **Viewstar**
Viewstar
15303 Ventura Boulevard
Sherman Oaks, CA 91403
818-382-4104

Leonard Weinstein, Technical Director
A stand-alone CCTV system for single view reading, writing and examining small objects. *$1545.00*

223 **Voice Amplified Handsets**
HARC Mercantile
1111 W Centre Avenue
Portage, MI 49024
269-324-1615
800-445-9968
FAX: 269-324-2387
e-mail: info@harc.com
www.harcmercantile.com

Ronald Slager, President

Designed for the person who has a weak speaking voice. Control increases the level of the user's voice and can increase as much as 30%. *$65.00*

224 WalkerTalker
Prentke Romich Company
1022 Heyl Road
Wooster, OH 44691
330-262-1984
800-262-1984
FAX: 330-263-4829
e-mail: info@prentrom.com
www.prentrom.com

Dave Moffatt, President
A portable direct selection communication device for active persons. The 16 location keyboard and speakers are carried in a belt that straps comfortably around the waist. The keyboard can be removed from its pouch to use by activating keys. Two versions are available, standard memory and expanded memory. *$1195.00*

Chairs

225 Adjustable Chair
Bailey Manufacturing Company
PO Box 130
Lodi, OH 44254
330-948-2655
800-321-8372
FAX: 800-224-5390
e-mail: baileymfg@baileymfg.com
www.baileymfg.com

Adelle McClendon, Customer Service
Sandy Mooney, Customer Service
Judie Butler, Dealer Contact
The seat and footboard of this versatile chair can be adjusted to accommodate children of various sizes. A classroom-suitable variation of this model is also available.

226 Adjustable Clear Acrylic Tray
Bailey Manufacturing Company
118 Lee Street
Suite 130
Lodi, OH 44254
330-948-1080
800-321-8372
FAX: 800-224-5390
e-mail: baileymfg@attmail.com
www.baileymfg.com

Larry Strimple, President
Adjusts for height and depth and is equipped with a spill rim for easy to clean edges.

227 Adjustable Rigid Chair
Kuschall North America
1811 Lefthand Circle
Suite B
Longmont, CO 80501
303-682-2571
888-682-2571
FAX: 866-651-6973
www.kuschallna.com

Terry Mulkey, Owner
The Champion 3000 is a fully adjustable rigid frame chair weighing only 21 pounds with a new clamping system that adjusts seat height and angle without tools.

228 Adjustable Tee Stool
Bailey Manufacturing Company
118 Lee Street
Suite 130
Lodi, OH 44254
330-948-1080
800-321-8372
FAX: 800-224-5390
e-mail: baileymfg@attmail.com
www.baileymfg.com

Larry Strimple, President
May be used to encourage balance as well as develop integrative and perceptual motor skills.

229 AirLift Toileting System
Mobility
5726 La Jolla Boulevard
Suite 104
La Jolla, CA 92037
858-456-8121
866-456-8121
FAX: 858-456-8139
e-mail: info@mobilityinc.net
www.mobilityinc.net

Steve Winston, VP Sales
Eric Proffitt, VP Marketing
The Mobility AirLift toileting system makes it easy and painless to get on and off the toilet. With or without an assistant, the AirLift absorbs the user's weight, providing gentle lowering to a sitting position and smooth lifting to a standing position.

230 BackSaver
BackSaver Products Company
53 Jeffrey Avenue
Holliston, MA 01746
508-429-5940
800-251-2225
FAX: 508-429-8698
e-mail: stevek@backsaver.com
www.backsavercorp.com

Steven Kusmin, Sales Director
Eliminates slouching and extra pressure on your back and thighs which impairs circulation.

231 Better Back
Orthopedic Products Corporation
4100 1/2 Glencoe Avenue
Marina Del Rey, CA 90292
323-584-6977
FAX: 310-306-0177

An orthopedic multi-purpose seat.

232 Carendo
Arjo Inc.
50 North Gary Avenue
Roselle, IL 60172
630-307-2756
800-323-1245
FAX: 888-594-2756
e-mail: info@arjousa.com
www.arjo.com

Lorena Cherie, Marketing Communications
Ross Scavuzzo, President
The Carendo hygiene chair has been designed for caregivers.

233 Century 50/60XR Sit
Arjo Inc.
50 North Gary Avenue
Roselle, IL 60172
630-307-2756
800-323-1245
FAX: 888-594-2756
e-mail: info@arjousa.com
www.arjo.com

Lorena Cherie, Marketing Communications
Ross Scavuzzo, President
This bathing system has a built-in cleaning/disinfectant injection system with adjustable flowmeter. The incorporation of an automatic hot water alarm/shut-off system, and digital temperature monitors, helps to assure resident safety and comfort.

234 Convert-Able Table
Rehab and Educational Aids for Living
187 S Main Street
Dolgeville, NY 13329
800-696-7041
FAX: 315-429-3071
e-mail: rdesign@tweny.rr.com
www.realdesigninc.com

Kris Wohnsen, Sales
This table has push button height adjustment and interchangeable tops so it can become a desk, art easel or a sensory stimulation bowl.

235 **Evac + Chair Emergency Wheelchair**
Evac + Chair Corporation
PO Box 2396
New York, NY 10021
212-369-4094
FAX: 212-369-3710
e-mail: sales@evac-chair.com
www.evac-chair.com

Robert McLean, Sales Manager
Gravity driven evaluation chair allows one nondisabled person to smoothly glide a seated passenger down fire stairs and across landings to exit on a combination of wheels and track belts. Pivots in own width for tight landing turns. Aluminum; weight 19 pounds. Compactly stores on wall mount, 38 by 20 by 9 inches. Maximum capacity 330 pounds. Self braking features. No installation, works on all fire exit stairs. *$950.00*

236 **Folding Shower Chair By INVOCARE**
Maxi Aids
42 Executive Boulevard
Farmingdale, NY 11735
631-752-0521
800-522-6294
FAX: 631-752-0689
e-mail: sales@maxiaids.com
www.maxiaids.com
Folds quickly and easily for storage and travel and provides comfort and support when bathing and showering. Contoured, durable plastic seat and backrest and built in holder for an optional hand held shower.

237 **Golden Technologies**
401 Bridge Street
Old Forge, PA 18518
570-451-7477
800-624-6374
FAX: 800-628-5165

Bob Golden, President

238 **High-Low Chair**
Rehab and Educational Aids for Living
187 S Main Street
Dolgeville, NY 13329
800-696-7041
FAX: 315-429-3071

Kris Wohnsen, Sales
A high chair and mobile floor sitter in one. The high-low chair comes with colorful upholstered wipe clean seat and height adjustable tray. The chair has a single lever adjustment to change the seat height. Lateral and head supports are available as options. *$ 1199.00*

239 **Ladybug Corner Chair**
Rehab and Educational Aids for Living
187 S Main Street
Dolgeville, NY 13329
800-696-7041
FAX: 315-429-3071
For children 0-3 years. This chair is adjustable for long legs for conventional sitting.

240 **Lumex Recliner**
Graham-Field Health Products
2935 Northeast Parkway
Atlanta, GA 30360
770-447-1609
800-347-5678
FAX: 800-726-0601
e-mail: cs@grahamfield.com
www.grahamfield.com

Irwin Selinger, Chief Executive Officer
Combines therapeutic benefits of position change with attractive appearance.

241 **Modular QuadDesk**
Gpk
535 Floyd Smith Drive
El Cajon, CA 92020
619-593-7381
800-468-8679
FAX: 619-593-7514
e-mail: info@gpk.com
www.gpk.com

Rajesh Kanwar, President

Worktable specially dsigned for people in wheelchairs who lack grip strength, or cannot learn or reach. Small or medium.

242 **Mulholland Positioning Systems**
839 Albion Ave
PO Box 70
Burley, ID 83318
208-878-3840
800-543-4769
FAX: 208-878-3841
e-mail: info@mulhollandinc.com
www.mulhollandinc.com

John Oderkirk, Marketing
Larry Mulholland, Owner
Provides a full line of standing aids, seating systems, adaptive components and bath aids.

243 **Prime Engineering**
Prime Engineering
4202 W Sierra Madre Avenue
Fresno, CA 93722
559-276-0991
800-827-8263
FAX: 800-800-3355
e-mail: info@primeengineering.com
www.primeengineering.com

Peggy Woodward, Sales
Bruce Boegel, Manager
Prime Engineering is a leading manufacturer of adult and pediatric standing devices and patient transfer equipment. Products include the all-new Support Standing System, Granstand III MSS Standing System Kidstand III MSS Standing System Superstand Multi-Position Pediatric Stander, the Lift, the CindyLift and the Original Lift Walker.

244 **Roll Chair**
Bailey Manufacturing Company
118 Lee Street
Suite 130
Lodi, OH 44254
330-948-1080
800-321-8372
FAX: 800-224-5390
e-mail: baileymfg@attmail.com
www.baileymfg.com

Larry Strimple, President
The padded roll helps maintain proper hip abduction and prevents scissoring of the legs.

245 **Safari Tilt**
Convaid Products
PO Box 4209
Palos Verdes Peninsula, CA 90274
310-618-0111
888-266-8243
FAX: 310-618-8811
e-mail: custservice@convaid.com
www.convaid.com

Mervyn Watkins, President
A semi-contour seat provides positioning with 5-45 degree tilt adjustment. One step design folds compactly into a lightweight chair.

246 **Spatial Tilt Custom Chair**
Redman Powerchair
1660 S Research Loop
Suite 126
Tucson, AZ 85710
520-546-6002
800-727-6684
FAX: 520-546-5530

Don Redman, Owner
Custom chair designed for comfort with a solid seat and back with modifications available for seat depth, height or width.

247 **Special Needs 5**
Baby Jogger Company
8575 Magellan Parkway
Suite 1000
Richmond, VA 23227
804-726-1327
800-241-1848
FAX: 804-262-6277
e-mail: bfetzer@babyjogger.com
www.babyjogger.com/p6.asp

Billy Fetzer, Sales Representative
David Boardman, President
Special need mobility devices give passengers smooth rides indoors and outdoors. The light weight, aluminum frame supports up to 200 pounds. Modifications available.

248 Transfer Bench with Back
Frohock-Stewart
39400 Taylor Parkway
North Ridgeville, OH 44035
440-329-6000
FAX: 440-365-7483

A Mixon Iii, Chief Executive Officer
This bench with air-cushioned seat sections has a full, reversible backrest for safety and comfort.

Cushions & Wedges

249 Action Products
22 N Mulberry Street
Hagerstown, MD 21740
301-797-1414
800-228-7763
FAX: 301-733-2073
e-mail: service@actionproducts.com
www.actionproducts.com

Dee Price, Customer Service Manager
Troy McKnight, President
Michael Bredal, VP Sales North America
Wheelchair pads, mattress pads, positioning cushions and insoles that aid in the prevention and cure of pressure sores by reducing pressure. All products are made of Akton viscoelastic polymer that does not leak, flow or bottom out. Manufacturer of the Xact line of positioning cushions for patients with high risk of skin breakdown.

250 Adjustable Wedge
Bailey Manufacturing Company
118 Lee Street
Suite 130
Lodi, OH 44254
330-948-1080
800-321-8372
FAX: 800-224-5390
e-mail: baileymfg@attmail.com
www.baileymfg.com

Larry Strimple, President
Orthopedically and neurologically disabled children can freely move arms and hands while lying on this adjustable wedge.

251 Back Machine
Kingstar International America
PO Box 10157
Chicago, IL 60610
312-951-1115
FAX: 312-943-1727
www.kingstar.com

Robin Morgenstern, President
Musa Hammad, Manager
A nine position adjustable lumbar support that is compact and lightweight, portable and able to fit most chairs, adaptable for different body sizes and will not lose its shape. The inner spring design will give the spinal column over-all support to compensate for stress, fatigue and improper posture.

252 Back-Huggar Pillow
Bodyline Comfort Systems
3730 Kori Road
Jacksonville, FL 32257
904-262-4068
800-874-7715
FAX: 904-262-2225
e-mail: info@bodyline.com
www.bodyline.com

John Fiore, Owner
Exclusive design makes almost any seat more comfortable by exerting soothing pressure against back muscles and discs.

253 BetaBed Pressure Pad
Huntleigh Healthcare
40 Christopher Way
Eatontown, NJ 07724
732-935-0975
800-223-1218
FAX: 732-578-9889
www.huntleigh-healthcare.com

Robert Angel, President/CEO
Alternating pressure pad system automatically relieves tissue damaging pressure every 2 minutes.

254 Bye-Bye Decubiti (BBD)
Ken McRight Supplies
7456 S Oswego Avenue
Tulsa, OK 74136
918-492-9657
FAX: 918-492-9694

Ken McRight, President
The BBD therapeutic wheelchair cushions have been market-proven since 1951 — in the prevention and cure of pressure sores (decubiti). These natural rubber inflatable products have recently been expanded to include pediatric, sports and double-valve models. Moderately priced, they offer a viable and cost-effective alternative in the market. $84.00-$112.00

255 Dynamic Systems
235 Sunlight Drive
Leicester, NC 28748
828-683-3523
FAX: 828-683-3511
e-mail: dsi@sunmatecushions.com
www.sunmatecushions.com

Cathy Caldwell, Customer Service
Ellie Brown, Executive Officer Manufacturing
Lewis McCrain, General Manager
SunMate orthopedic foam sheets and cushions, pudgee pads for pressure relief and skin breakdown prevention, laminar wheelchair cushions and Foam-in-Place Seating for custom molding seat inserts. Sample packs and literature available upon request.

256 Econo-Float Water Flotation Cushion
Jefferson Industries
1985 Rutgers University Boulevard
Lakewood, NJ 08701
732-905-9001
800-257-5145
FAX: 732-905-9899

Charles Landa, General Manager
An inexpensive, yet effective approach to the problem of pressure ulcers for patients confined to wheelchairs, geriatric chairs, etc. *$15.00*

257 Econo-Float Water Flotation Mattress
Jefferson Industries
1985 Rutgers University Boulevard
Lakewood, NJ 08701
732-905-9001
800-257-5145
FAX: 732-905-9899

Charles Landa, General Manager
Helps prevent and treat pressure ulcers by reducing and distributing pressure over the patient's bony prominences while supporting the body evenly over a greater surface area. *$39.00*

258 Enhancer Cushion
ROHO Group
100 N Florida Avenue
Belleville, IL 62221
618-277-9150
800-851-3449
FAX: 618-277-9561
e-mail: mail@therohogroup.com
www.therohogroup.com

Jackie Wiegert, Corporate Marketing
Tom Olesky, Chief Executive Officer
Uses AIR IN PLACE progressive positioning for enhanced midline channeling of the femurs, lateral stability and tissue protection.

259 **Flex-Air Pressure Relief System**
Relax-A-Flex
211 River Street
Bennington, VT 05201
802-447-1166
800-782-8889
FAX: 802-442-6875

Jeff Wilkinson, Owner
Solves mattress problems.

260 **Functional Forms**
Consumer Care Products
1446 Pilgrim Road
Plymouth, WI 53073
920-893-4614
FAX: 800-977-2256
e-mail: ccpi@consumercareinc.com
www.consumercareinc.com

Terry Grall, Owner
These blocks, wedges, rolls, cervical pillows, head and leg supports and barrel rolls in resilient high density foam covered with durable antibacterial, antistatic, flame resistant, nonabsorbent vinyl are used to attain individualized support for the most difficult positioning needs for children and adults. Unique sizes allow fitting for almost any person. Use during exercise, feeding, therapy, recreation and rest at home, school and health care facilities. Packages available.

261 **GT Wheelchair Cushion**
Relax-A-Flex
211 River Street
Bennington, VT 05201
802-447-1166
800-782-8889
FAX: 802-442-6875

Jeff Wilkinson, Owner
The specially designed gel pads in this cushion help relieve pressure on the back.

262 **Gaymar Industries**
Gaymar Industries
10 Centre Drive
Orchard Park, NY 14127
716-662-2551
800-828-7341
FAX: 800-993-7890
e-mail: pmatteliano@gaymar.com
www.gaymar.com

Steve Snyder, VP Marketing
Peggy Matteliano, Communications Specialist
Thomas Stewart, Chief Executive Officer
Gaymar offers a complete line of support surfaces, including low-air-loss mattresses, specialty foam mattresses, turning mattresses, air overlays and fluid therapy beds. These products economically prevent and treat bedsores. Clinical and reimbursement professionals are available to answer any question related to bedsores (decubitus ulcers). Also offers a complete line of temperature control devices. The T-Pump delivers warm therapy to effectively dilate vessels and increase blood flow.

263 **Geo-Matt for High Risk Patients**
Span-America Medical Systems
70 Commerce Center
Greenville, SC 29615
864-288-8877
800-888-6752
FAX: 864-288-8692
www.spanamerica.com

James Ferguson, Chief Executive Officer
Helps prevent pressure sores in high risk patients.

264 **High Profile Single Compartment Cushion**
ROHO Group
100 N Florida Avenue
Belleville, IL 62221
618-277-9150
800-851-3449
FAX: 618-277-9561
e-mail: mail@therohogroup.com
www.therohogroup.com

Jackie Wiegert, Corporate Marketing
Tom Olesky, Chief Executive Officer
With 4 inch cells, the HIGH PROFILE is the cushion of choice for individuals who suffer from ischemic ulcers (pressure sores) or who have a history of tissue breakdown.

265 **Inflatable Back Pillow**
Corflex
669 East Industrial Park Drive
Manchester, NH 03109
603-623-3344
800-426-7353
FAX: 603-623-4111
e-mail: sales@corflex.com
www.corflex.com

Paul Lorenzetti, Owner
Folds flat to fit into its own carrying case, this inflatable back pillow ensures comfort while at home or traveling.

266 **Jobri**
520 N Division Street
Konawa, OK 74849
580-925-4100
800-432-2225
FAX: 800-769-0520
e-mail: support@jobri.com
www.jobri.com

Mike Deaton, Customer Service Manager
Brian Gourley, Chief Executive Officer

267 **Lumex Cushions and Mattresses**
Graham-Field Health Products
2935 Northeast Parkway
Atlanta, GA 30360
770-447-1609
800-347-5678
FAX: 800-726-0601
www.grahamfield.com

Irwin Selinger, Chief Executive Officer
Line of cushions and pillows give comfort and independence to the physically challenged.

268 **Medpro Static Air Chair Cushion**
Medpro
1950 Rutgers University Boulevard
Lakewood, NJ 08701
800-257-5145
FAX: 732-905-9899

Jody Gorran, President
Provides a protective layer of air beneath the patient helping prevent and treat pressure ulcers. *$94.95*

269 **Medpro Static Air Mattress Overlay**
Medpro
1950 Rutgers University Boulevard
Lakewood, NJ 08701
800-257-5145
FAX: 732-905-9899

Jody Gorran, President
Supports the patient on a cushioned network of air designed to redistribute the patient's weight reducing tissue interface pressure. Medpro's design incorporates a series of 65 air-breather vents that maintain air circulation. Medpro effectively reduces pressure and helps prevent and treat pressure ulcers. *$164.95*

270 **Mini-Max Cushion**
ROHO
100 N Florida Avenue
Belleville, IL 62221
618-277-9150
800-850-7646
FAX: 618-277-6518
e-mail: mail@rohogroup.com
www.therohogroup.com

Julie Petry, Corporate Marketing
Tom Olesky, Chief Executive Officer
Designed for the active individual with low risk of skin breakdown. The unique air cells of the MINI-MAX provide significant shock and impact absorption, skin protection and stability.

271 **NEXUS Wheelchair Cushioning System**
ROHO
100 N Florida Avenue
Belleville, IL 62221
618-277-9150
800-850-7646
FAX: 618-277-6518
e-mail: mail@rohogroup.com
www.therohogroup.com

Julie Petry, Corporate Marketing
Tom Olesky, Chief Executive Officer
A unique modular cushion that mates a contoured polyurethane foam base with a dry flotation support pad. It is designed to give the user positioning and stability, while offering maximum protection to the ischia, sacrum and coccyx.

272 **Nek-Lo, Nek-Lo Hot and Cold Pillow-Perfect, Body Buddy, Hugg-L-O Pillow**
Rinz-L-O Pillow Company
340 W Maplehurst Street
Ferndale, MI 48220
248-548-3993
800-594-9093
FAX: 248-548-0447
e-mail: rinzlo@netzero.net

G Rick Rinz, President
Ken Mack, Office Manager
Phill McAllister, Sales Manager
Nek-Lo a U-shaped cervical pillow; Nek-Lo Hot and Cold - U-shaped pillow with hot/cold pack; Pillow-Perfect - uses your conventional pillow to insert cover that has cervical support form piece; Magne-Aid and Magne-Systems - magnetic therapy braces, Hugg-L-O pillow V shaped body positioning, Hugg-L-O Extra pillow is 4 inches longer than original Hugg-L-O pillow. *$12.98*

273 **Pediatric Seating System**
ROHO
100 N Florida Avenue
Belleville, IL 62221
618-277-9150
800-850-7646
FAX: 618-277-6518
e-mail: rohoinc@rohoinc.com
www.rohoinc.com

Julie Petry, Corporate Marketing
Tom Olesky, Chief Executive Officer
ROHO Cushions for kids use individual air cells, creating the most versatile and dynamic cushioning products available. These cushions are designed to specifically fit pediatric wheelchairs.

274 **Quadtro Cushion**
ROHO
100 N Florida Avenue
Belleville, IL 62221
618-277-9150
800-851-3499
FAX: 618-277-9561
e-mail: mail@therohogroup.com
www.therohogroup.com

Julie Petry, Corporate Marketing
Tom Olesky, Chief Executive Officer
For individuals who require special positioning of the pelvis or thighs and are at risk of skin breakdown, the Quadtro, with 4 inch cell height and air in place, progressive positioning is the cushion of choice.

275 **Silicone Padding**
Spenco Medical Group
PO Box 2501
Waco, TX 76702
254-772-6000
800-433-3334

Steven Smith, Chief Executive Officer
For the management of pressure sores, this padding provides a special support system which allows even distribution of pressure and cool, comfortable, well-ventilated support.

276 **Soft-Touch Convertible Flotation Mattress**
Medpro
1950 Rutgers University Boulevard
Lakewood, NJ 08701
800-257-5145
FAX: 732-905-9899

Jody Gorran, President
Gives the patient the option to choose between water and gel flotation depending on the needs of the patient. The mattress helps prevent and treat pressure ulcers by spreading the patient's weight over a greater surface area. $164.95-$239.95.

277 **Soft-Touch Gel Flotation Cushion**
Medpro
1940 Rutgers University Boulevard
Lakewood, NJ 08701
732-905-9001
800-257-5145
FAX: 732-905-9899

Jody Gorran, President
Acts like an additional layer of fatty tissue beneath the patient to help prevent and treat pressure sores. *$99.95*

278 **Spenco Medical Group**
PO Box 2501
Waco, TX 76702
254-772-6000
800-433-3334
e-mail: spenco@spenco.com
www.spenco.com

Mark B Connors, VP Sales/Marketing
Patty Smith, Controller
Steven B Smith, CEO
Wheel chair cushions, silicore mattress pads, wound dressings, second skin blister and burn pads, polysorb insoles, elbow, knee and wrist supports and walking shoes.

279 **Stop-Leak Gel Flotation Mattress**
Jefferson Industries
1989 Rutgers University Boulevard
Lakewood, NJ 08701
732-905-9001
800-257-5145
FAX: 732-905-9899

Charles Landa, General Manager
Protects persons from messy leaks while it protects from pressure ulcers. *$54.00*

280 **Sun-Mate Seat Cushions**
Dynamic Systems
235 Sunlight Drive
Leicester, NC 28748
828-683-3523
FAX: 828-683-3511
e-mail: dsi@sunmatecushions.com
www.sunmatecushions.com

Pamela Price, Customer Service
Ellie Brown, Executive Officer Manufacturing
Charles Yost, Chief Executive Officer
Line of cushions, pads and accessory items for personal comfort of the disabled. SunMate Orthopedic foam cushions and sheets that contours slowly to give uniform pressure distribution and soft spring back. Liquid SunMate for Foam-in-Place Seating (FIPS) to make custom molded seat inserts.

281 **Twin-Rest Seat Cushion & Glamour Pillow**
Better Sleep
57 Industrial Road
Berkeley Heights, NJ 07922
908-464-2200
FAX: 908-464-0058

William Emery Jr, President
Makes any seat more comfortable because it is ingeniously designed to soothe sensitive areas while at work, in the car or at home.

Dressing Aids

282 **Button Aid**
Maxi Aids
42 Executive Boulevard
Farmingdale, NY 11735
631-752-0521
800-522-6294
FAX: 631-752-0689
e-mail: sales@maxiaids.com
www.maxiaids.com
Makes buttoning possible with the use of only one hand. *$9.95*

283 **Clothing Identification Kit**
Sense-Sations
919 Walnut Street
Philadelphia, PA 19107
215-627-0600
FAX: 215-922-0692

Patricia Johnson, Chief Executive Officer
This kit contains labels and tells you what is on the hanger. *$7.75*

284 Deluxe Sock and Stocking Aid
Therapro
225 Arlington Street
Framingham, MA 01702
508-872-9494
800-257-5376
FAX: 508-875-2062
e-mail: info@theraproducts.com
www.theraproducts.com

Karen Conrad, Owner
Flexible plastic, lined with blue nylon to reduce friction and outside with beige terry cloth to hold sock firmly until it is on the foot. *$12.95*

285 Dressing Stick
Maxi Aids
42 Executive Boulevard
Farmingdale, NY 11735
631-752-0521
800-522-6294
FAX: 631-752-0689
e-mail: sales@maxiaids.com
www.maxiaids.com
Helps put on coats, sweaters and garments even when arm and shoulder movement is limited. *$7.95*

286 Elastic Shoelaces
Therapro
225 Arlington Street
Framingham, MA 01702
508-872-9494
800-257-5376
FAX: 508-875-2062
e-mail: info@theraproducts.com
www.theraproducts.com

Karen Conrad, Owner
The elastic laces allow the wearer to slip tied shoes on and off. *$4.25*

287 Featherweight Reachers
Therapro
225 Arlington Street
Framingham, MA 01702
508-872-9494
800-257-5376
FAX: 508-875-2062
e-mail: info@theraproducts.com
www.theraproducts.com

Karen Conrad, Owner
Useful in dressing or retrieving objects. *$17.95*

288 Heavy Duty Sock Tuckers
Sense-Sations
919 Walnut Street
Philadelphia, PA 19107
215-627-0600
FAX: 215-922-0692

Patricia Johnson, Chief Executive Officer
This device keeps socks and hosiery paired throughout the laundering cycles. *$1.50*

289 Mirror Go Lightly
AbleNet
2808 Fairview Avenue N
Saint Paul, MN 55113
800-322-0956
FAX: 612-379-9143
e-mail: customerservice@ablenetinc.com
www.ablenetinc.com
Framed in plastic, the mirror can be tilted to provide either a normal or magnified image or to direct its lights at, or away from, the user. *$22.00*

290 Molded Sock and Stocking Aid
Therapro
225 Arlington Street
Framingham, MA 01702
508-872-9494
800-257-5376
FAX: 508-875-2062
e-mail: info@theraproducts.com
www.theraproducts.com

Karen Conrad, Owner
Sock or stocking is pulled over the molded plastic and then can be put on more easily. *$13.25*

291 Say What
Maxi Aids
42 Executive Boulevard
Farmingdale, NY 11735
631-752-0521
800-522-6294
FAX: 631-752-0689
e-mail: sales@maxiaids.com
www.maxiaids.com
Braille the tag with information that the wearer wants on the tag and place the tag on a hanger. The custom-identification program makes it easier for the user to remember and identify just the right clothes. *$4.95*

Health Aids

292 AMI
PO Box 808
Groton, CT 06340
860-536-3735
800-248-4031
FAX: 860-536-4362
e-mail: sales@aquamassage.com
www.amiaqua.com

David Cote, President
Dow Cote, Domestic Sales Manager
The Aqua PT provides the major benefits of Hydrotherapy, Massage Therapy and Dry Heat Therapy. 36 water jets provide continuous full body or localized massage while the client remains CLOTHED AND DRY! Adjustable water pressure, temperature and pulsation frequency can massage in either a two direction travel mode for musculoskeletal pain management or a one direction mode, flowing water from head to foot for a contrast massage-relax therapy. $25,000 to $30,000.

293 Absorbent Dressing Powder
Baxter Healthcare Corporation
1 Baxter Parkway
Deerfield, IL 60015
847-948-2000
FAX: 847-948-3948
www.baxter.com

Robert Parkinson Jr, Chief Executive Officer
Powder dressing for the treatment of pressure sores and other skin ulcers.

294 American Medical Industries
330 E 3rd Street
Suite 2
Dell Rapids, SD 57022
605-428-5501
FAX: 605-428-5502
e-mail: sales@americanmedicalindustries.com
www.ezhealthcare.com

Dan Anderson, CEO
EZ-Swallow, EZ-Health, EZ-Home Care, Kleen-Handz, Kleen-Scent, EZ-Irrigator, EZ-VU, Pureshark, Gobot and AMI are all trademarks of American Medical Industries. Healthcare products made easy.

295 BIPAP S/T Ventilatory Support System
Respironics
1010 Murry Ridge Lane
Murrysville, PA 15668
724-387-5200
FAX: 724-387-5012
e-mail: customerservice@respironics.com
www.respironics.com

John Miclot, Chief Executive Officer
Gerald McGinnis, Chairman
Daniel Bevevino, VP/CFO
Respironics, a recognized resource in the medical device market, provides innovative products and unique designs to the health care provider while helping them to grow and manage their business efficiently.

296 Bed Rails
Mada Medical Products
625 Washington Avenue
Carlstadt, NJ 07072
201-460-0454
800-526-6370
FAX: 201-460-3509
e-mail: dianelind@mail.madamedical.com
www.madainternational.com

Jeffrey Adam, Vice President
Chrome plated steel rails and crossbars, all welded construction, telescopic side rail length adjustable, and a standard rail height of 16 inches.

297 Coast to Coast Home Medical
3381 Fairlane Farms Road
Suite 4d
Wellington, FL 33414
561-792-4009
800-330-6316

Keri Suess, Owner
Home-delivered medical supplies for diabetes, respiratory, arthritis and impotence supplies.

298 Drew Karol Industries
PO Box 1066
Greenville, MS 38702
662-378-2188
FAX: 601-378-3188
e-mail: dki@techinfo.com

Andrew Hoszowski, President
Orally operated toothbrush and dental care system for persons with limited or complete loss of hand or arm use - wheelchair accessible. *$600.00*

299 Duraline Medical Products
PO Box 67
Leipsic, OH 45856
419-943-2044
800-654-3376
FAX: 419-943-3637
e-mail: duraline@q1.net
www.dmponline.com

Kathy Peck, General Manager
An assortment of quality incontinence products for adults and children.

300 Duro-Med Industries
1778 W Cherry Street
Jesup, GA 31545
912-427-7358
800-526-4753
FAX: 800-479-7968

Mike Mazza, President
Manufacturers of a complete line of home health care products. Featured products are patient gowns, back and seat cushions, pillows and a complete line of aids for daily living.

301 Easy Ply
BioMedical Life Systems
PO Box 1360
Vista, CA 92085
800-726-8367
FAX: 760-727-4220
e-mail: information@bmls.com
www.bmls.com
This disposable electrode has a cloth backing of a super-breathable medical tape that allows for comfort and a longer life.

302 Electronic Stethoscopes
HARC Mercantile
1111 W Centre Avenue
Portage, MI 49024
269-324-1615
800-445-9968
FAX: 269-324-2387
e-mail: info@harc.com
www.harcmercantile.com

Ronald Slager, President
High production fidelity with a number volume control wheels. *$454.95*

303 Fold-Down 3-in-1 Commode
Mada Medical Products
625 Washington Avenue
Carlstadt, NJ 07072
201-460-0454
800-526-6370
FAX: 201-460-3509
e-mail: dianelind@mail.madamedical.com
www.madainternational.com

Jeffrey Adam, Vice President
The Fold-Down commode is constructed of heavy duty, 1 inch diameter, steel tubing with X frame, has folding features convenient for storage and transport, easily removable back rest, and full length armrests.

304 Grab Bars and Tub Rails
Mada Medical Products
625 Washington Avenue
Carlstadt, NJ 07072
201-460-0454
800-526-6370
FAX: 201-460-3509
e-mail: dianelind@mail.madamedical.com
www.madainternational.com

Jeffrey Adam, Vice President
Several models made of heavy walled steel, available in knurled steel or white epoxy paint, various lengths and round flanges for either vertical or horizontal mounting.

305 Healing Dressing for Pressure Sores
Baxter Healthcare Corporation
1 Baxter Parkway
Deerfield, IL 60015
847-948-2000
FAX: 847-948-3948
www.baxter.com

Robert Parkinson Jr, Chief Executive Officer
A dressing specifically designed to promote healing of pressure sores and other dermal ulcers.

306 Invacare Corporation
1 Invacare Way
Elyria, OH 44035
440-329-6000
800-333-6900
FAX: 440-329-6568
e-mail: info@invacare.com
www.invacare.com

Lara Mahoney, Manager, Public Relations
The world's leading manufacturer and distributor of innovative home and long-term care medical products which promote recovery and active lifestyles.

307 MADAMIST 50/50 PSI Air Compressor
Mada Medical Products
625 Washington Avenue
Carlstadt, NJ 07072
201-460-0454
800-526-6370
FAX: 201-460-3509
e-mail: dianelind@mail.madamedical.com
www.madainternational.com

Jeffrey Adam, Vice President
The new compressor rated at 50 PSI is designed to drive humidifiers, nebulizers, mist tents and is ideal to administer pentamidine aerosol therapy.

308 MedDev Corporation
730 N Pastoria Avenue
Sunnyvale, CA 94085
408-730-9702
800-543-2789
FAX: 408-730-9732
e-mail: info@meddev-corp.com
www.meddev-corp.com

Suzanne Gray, Owner
Aids to rehabilitate hands following injury or illness, including patented complementary FingerHelper, ThumbHelper and Iso HandHelper models. Med Dev also manufactures Soft Touch foam exercisers and the FiddlLink exerciser for digital dexterity. The Ultimate Hand Helper, an ergonomically designed hand excerciser, is curved to conform to the shape of the hand.

309 **Medi-Grip**
Therapro
225 Arlington Street
Framingham, MA 01702
508-872-9494
800-257-5376
FAX: 508-875-2062
e-mail: info@theraproducts.com
www.theraproducts.com

Karen Conrad, Owner
Reasonably priced, nonskid material. This nonslip material is available in marine blue, desert sand and burgundy rolls 12 inches x 144 inches. *$11.95*

310 **Pocket Otoscope**
HARC Mercantile
1111 W Centre Avenue
Portage, MI 49024
269-324-1615
800-445-9968
FAX: 269-324-2387
e-mail: info@harc.com
www.harcmercantile.com

Ronald Slager, President
Simple, durable and dependable pocket otoscope uses standard replaceable parts. *$24.00*

311 **Standard 3-in-1 Commode**
Mada Medical Products
625 Washington Avenue
Carlstadt, NJ 07072
201-460-0454
800-526-6370
FAX: 201-460-3509
e-mail: dianelind@mail.madamedical.com
www.madainternational.com

Jeffrey Adam, Vice President
The standard commode is constructed of a heavy duty anodized aluminum frame, seat adjustment and an easily removable back rest.

312 **Strider**
Osborn Medical Corporation
PO Box 324
Utica, MN 55979
507-287-6554
800-535-5865
FAX: 507-932-5044
www.osbornmedical.com

Bill Davis, President
Strider allows you to exercise in most chairs found in your home. No more small, uncomfortable bicycle seats to sit on while exercising. With Strider, your hands are free to read the paper or your favorite book while you exercise.

313 **Talking Clinical Thermometer**
Maxi Aids
42 Executive Boulevard
Farmingdale, NY 11735
631-752-0521
800-522-6294
FAX: 631-752-0689
e-mail: sales@maxiaids.com
www.maxiaids.com

Audible clinical thermometer. *$199.95*

314 **Talking Thermometers**
Maxi Aids
42 Executive Boulevard
Farmingdale, NY 11735
631-752-0521
800-522-6294
FAX: 631-752-0689
e-mail: sales@maxiaids.com
www.maxiaids.com

Clearly announces temperature in Fahrenheit or Celcius. *$17.95*

315 **Transfer Bench**
Mada Medical Products
625 Washington Avenue
Carlstadt, NJ 07072
201-460-0454
800-526-6370
FAX: 201-460-3509
e-mail: dianelind@mail.madamedical.com
www.madainternational.com

Jeffrey Adam, Vice President
The transfer bench is a one piece bench with a wide base for stability, 1" diameter aluminum framework, corrosion resistant, and an adjustable seat.

Hearing Aids

316 **Auditech: DirectEar Transmitter and Headset**
PO Box 821105
Vicksburg, MS 39182
800-229-8293
FAX: 800-221-8639
e-mail: info@auditechusa.com
www.auditechusa.com

Turn up the volume when watching TV. The headset can also be used separately in public theaters and cinemas, that have infrared transmission. Additional headset receivers can be purchased. A neckloop can also be added to the headset. *$219.00*

317 **Auditech: Personal PA Value Pack System**
PO Box 821105
Vicksburg, MS 39182
800-229-8293
FAX: 800-221-8639
e-mail: info@auditechusa.com
www.auditechusa.com

Reliable hearing assistance. This wireless FM system broadcasts to listeners with a hearing assistance system, helping them overcome background noise at a distance from the sound source. *$899.00*

318 **Auditech: Pocketalker Pro**
PO Box 821105
Vicksburg, MS 39182
800-229-8293
FAX: 800-221-8639
e-mail: info@auditechusa.com
www.auditechusa.com

Pocketalker Pro can help you hear virtually anywhere whether in a car, crowded restaurant or at a noisy gathering. It can work to reduce background noise and easily converts to the Telelink. *$ 140.00*

319 **Battery Device Adapter**
AbleNet
2808 Fairview Avenue N
Roseville, MN 55113
651-294-2200
800-322-0956
FAX: 651-294-2259
e-mail: customerservice@ablenetinc.com
www.ablenetinc.com

Mary Kay Walch
A cable which connects to and adapts battery-operated devices for external switch control. Two sizes are available to adapt devices with either AA or C and D size batteries. *$8.00*

320 **Custom Earmolds**
Lloyd Hearing Aid Corporation
PO Box 1645
Rockford, IL 61110
815-964-4191
800-323-4212
FAX: 815-964-8378
e-mail: info@lloydshearingaid.com
www.lloydhearingaid.com

Andrew Palmquist, President
Hearing aid molds, custom built to the exact fit of the customer. *$29.95*

321 **Digital Hearing Aids**
Lloyd Hearing Aid Corporation
4435 Manchester Drive
Rockford, IL 61109
815-964-4191
800-323-4212
FAX: 815-964-8378
e-mail: info@lloydshearingaid.com

Andrew Palmquist, President
Latest hearing technology. Huge discounts on most makes. *$7.50*

322 Doorbell Signalers
HARC Mercantile
1111 W Centre Avenue
Portage, MI 49024
269-324-1615
800-445-9968
FAX: 269-324-2387
e-mail: info@harc.com
www.harcmercantile.com

Ronald Slager, President
Doorbell signalers to alert with either louder chime or flashing light. *$29.99*

323 Double Gong Indoor/Outdoor Ringer
HARC Mercantile
1111 W Centre Avenue
Portage, MI 49024
269-324-1615
800-445-9968
FAX: 269-324-2387
e-mail: info@harc.com
www.harcmercantile.com

Ronald Slager, President
Loud outdoor ringer that attaches to the wall for outside applications. *$50.00*

324 Duracell & Rayovac Hearing Aid Batteries
Lloyd Hearing Aid Corporation
4435 Manchester Drive
Rockford, IL 61109
815-964-4191
800-323-4212
FAX: 815-964-8378
e-mail: info@lloydhearingaid.com

Andrew Palmquist, President
Batteries for hearing aids at discounted prices. As low as 45 cents each.

325 Harris Communications
Harris Communications
15155 Technology Drive
Eden Prairie, MN 55344
952-906-1180
800-825-6758
FAX: 952-906-1099
e-mail: info@harriscomm.com
www.harriscomm.com

Bill Williams, National Sales Manager
Robert Harris, Owner
A national distributor of assistive devices for the deaf and hard-of-hearing with many manufacturers represented. Catalog includes a wide range of assistive devices as well as a variety of books and video tapes related to deaf and hard-of-hearing issues. Products available for children, teachers, hearing professionals, interpreters and anyone interested in deaf culture, hearing loss and sign language.
180 pages Yearly

326 Hearing Aid Batteries
HARC Mercantile
1111 W Centre Avenue
Portage, MI 49024
269-324-1615
800-445-9968
FAX: 269-324-2387
e-mail: info@harc.com
www.harcmercantile.com

Ronald Slager, President
Hearing aid batteries in all popular sizes in mercury, zinc air, silver as well as Nicad and Varta and batteries for electrolarynx and infrared systems. $3.95-$25.00.

327 Hearing Aid Battery Testers
HARC Mercantile
1111 W Centre Avenue
Portage, MI 49024
269-324-1615
800-445-9968
FAX: 269-324-2387
e-mail: info@harc.com
www.harcmercantile.com

Ronald Slager, President
From pocket size to professional type battery testers which test mercury, zinc air, silver, specialty and general usage batteries. *$11.95*

328 Hearing Aid Dehumidifier
HARC Mercantile
1111 W Centre Avenue
Portage, MI 49024
269-324-1615
800-445-9968
FAX: 269-324-2387
e-mail: info@harc.com
www.harcmercantile.com

Ronald Slager, President
Removes moisture from hearing aids and valuables. Contains desiccant pack and humidity guide, all in a rugged, vinyl case which provides protection and is water resistant. *$6.00*

329 In the Ear Hearing Aid Battery Extractor
HARC Mercantile
1111 W Centre Avenue
Portage, MI 49024
269-324-1615
800-445-9968
FAX: 269-324-2387
e-mail: info@harc.com
www.harcmercantile.com

Ronald Slager, President
Ideal tool to use when battery is stuck in battery compartment in ITE and canal hearing aids. *$3.00*

330 Micro Audiometrics Corporation
655 Keller Road
Murphy, NC 28906
828-644-0771
800-729-9509
866-327-7226
FAX: 828-644-0772
e-mail: sales@microaud.com
www.microaud.com

Jason Keller, VP
Lance Ralph, Marketing
James Keller, Owner
Manufacturer and distributor of hearing testing instruments, including the complete line of Earscan.

331 Model E-90W Hearing Aid
Rhodes Hearing
PO Box 358
Brookport, IL 62910
618-564-2026

Mary Rhodes, President
This hearing aid slips directly into the ear. *$327.00*

332 Model F-188T Hearing Aid
Rhodes Hearing
PO Box 358
Brookport, IL 62910
618-564-2026

Mary Rhodes, President
Designed to fit behind your ear at the most natural hearing level for detecting both distance and sound direction. *$329.00*

333 Mushroom Inserts
Lloyd Hearing Aid Corporation
PO Box 1645
Rockford, IL 61110
815-964-4191
800-323-4212
FAX: 815-964-8378
e-mail: info@lloydhearingaid.com

Andrew Palmquist, President
A universal earplug useful in wearing behind the ear type hearing instruments. *$2.50*

334 Oval Window Audio
33 Wildflower Court
Nederland, CO 80466
303-447-3607
FAX: 303-447-3607
e-mail: info@ovalwindowaudio.com
www.ovalwindowaudio.com

Norman Lederman, Director R&D/Owner
Paula Hendricks, Educational Director

Manufacturer of induction loop hearing assistance technologies compatible with hearing aids already used by many hard of hearing people. Also multisensory sound systems for use in speech and music therapy and science classes.

Kitchen & Eating Aids

335 **Bagel Holder**
Maxi Aids
42 Executive Boulevard
Farmingdale, NY 11735
631-752-0521
800-522-6294
FAX: 631-752-0689
e-mail: sales@maxiaids.com
www.maxiaids.com
Holds bagels in place for easy slicing. *$3.95*

336 **Big Bold Timer Low Vision**
Maxi Aids
42 Executive Boulevard
Farmingdale, NY 11735
631-752-0521
800-522-6294
FAX: 631-752-0689
e-mail: sales@maxiaids.com
www.maxiaids.com
Sixty-minute mechanical timer with large, easy-to-read numbers for the vision impaired. *$9.95*

337 **Box Top Opener**
Sammons Preston Rolyan
W68n158 Evergreen Boulevard
Cedarburg, WI 53012
800-323-5547
FAX: 262-387-8748
e-mail: customersupport@sammonspreston.com
www.sammonspreston.com
This handy device exerts the pressure on those hard-to-open boxes of laundry/dishwasher soap, rice and prepared dinners. *$2.95*

338 **Capscrew**
Access with Ease
PO Box 1150
Chino Valley, AZ 86323
928-636-9469
800-531-9479
FAX: 928-636-0292
e-mail: KMJC@northlink.com
Remove lids and caps easily. Can be mounted on walls or cupboards. Non-slip surface grips small and large jars. *$7.95*

339 **Cool Handle**
Maxi Aids
42 Executive Boulevard
Farmingdale, NY 11735
631-752-0521
800-522-6294
FAX: 631-752-0689
e-mail: sales@maxiaids.com
www.maxiaids.com
A specially designed, heat-resistant handle, available in three sizes which can be affixed to the handles of most fry, sauce and saute pans. *$7.95*

340 **Cordless Receiver**
AbleNet
2808 Fairview Avenue N
Saint Paul, MN 55113
800-322-0956
FAX: 651-294-2259
e-mail: customerservice@ablenetinc.com
www.ablenetinc.com
The Cordless Receiver in conjunction with the Cordless Big Red Switch, can be used anywhere a switch is currently used to control battery or electrically-operated toys, games or appliances; augmentative communication systems; and computers (through a computer switch interface). *$79.00*

341 **Deluxe Long Ring Low Vision Timer**
Maxi Aids
42 Executive Boulevard
Farmingdale, NY 11735
631-752-0521
FAX: 631-752-0689
e-mail: sales@maxiaids.com
www.maxiaids.com
Bold black numerals on white background allows for easy reading at any distance. *$17.95*

342 **Deluxe Roller Knife**
Sammons Preston Rolyan
1000 Remington Blvd.
Suite 210
Bolingbrook, IL 60440
630-378-6000
FAX: 630-378-6010
e-mail: customerservice@sammonspreston.com
www.sammonspreston.com
Stainless steel blade rolls smoothly, cutting food cleanly. *$10.95*

343 **Dual Brush with Suction Base**
Sammons Preston Rolyan
4 Sammons Court
Bolingbrook, IL 60440
630-226-1300
800-228-3693
FAX: 262-387-8748
e-mail: customerservice@sammonspreston.com
www.sammonspreston.com
Two brushes clean the inside and outside of bottles and glasses at the same time using just one hand. *$14.50*

344 **Easy Pour Locking Lid Pot**
Maxi Aids
42 Executive Boulevard
Farmingdale, NY 11735
631-752-0521
800-522-6294
FAX: 631-752-0689
e-mail: sales@maxiaids.com
www.maxiaids.com
Baked enamel and dishwasher safe, the pot comes with an easy lid that locks in place for extra safety. *$24.95*

345 **Electric Can Opener & Knife Sharpener**
Maxi Aids
42 Executive Boulevard
Farmingdale, NY 11735
631-752-0521
800-522-6294
FAX: 631-752-0689
e-mail: sales@maxiaids.com
www.maxiaids.com
Features include a powerful magnetic lid holder, the ability to open odd-shaped cans, and easy operation for the physically challenged. *$19.95*

346 **Evio Plastics**
PO Box 2295
Sandusky, OH 44871
419-621-1105
FAX: 419-626-2183

Doug Didion, Admininstrator Director
Danny Thomas, Owner
Handi Holder is a plastic holder for 1/2 gallon paper cartons of milk or juice. It is used to pour milk or juice without spills by using the handle.

347 **Food Markers/Rubberbands**
Maxi Aids
42 Executive Boulevard
Farmingdale, NY 11735
631-752-0521
800-522-6294
FAX: 631-752-0689
e-mail: sales@maxiaids.com
www.maxiaids.com
These are durable plastic markers, easily identified by touch, texture, shape and form which help the visually impaired orient themselves to food location on the plate. *$11.95*

348 **Funnel**
Sense-Sations
919 Walnut Street
Philadelphia, PA 19107
215-627-0600
FAX: 215-922-0692

Patricia Johnson, Chief Executive Officer
Wide mouth funnel aids in pouring liquids or dry goods from container to container. *$1.25*

349 **Good Grips Cutlery**
Therapro
225 Arlington Street
Framingham, MA 01702
508-872-9494
800-257-5376
FAX: 508-875-2062
e-mail: info@theraproducts.com
www.theraproducts.com

Karen Conrad, Owner
Stainless steel utensils have a special twist built into the metal to facilitate bending of a spoon or fork at any angle for right or left handed people. *$7.50*

350 **H.E.L.P. Knife**
Maxi Aids
42 Executive Boulevard
Farmingdale, NY 11735
631-752-0521
800-522-6294
FAX: 631-752-0689
e-mail: sales@maxiaids.com
www.maxiaids.com
Adjustable food slicing system guides the knife for even, uniform slices while protecting the user. *$11.95*

351 **Handy-Helper Cutting Board**
Maxi Aids
42 Executive Boulevard
Farmingdale, NY 11735
631-752-0521
800-522-6294
FAX: 631-752-0689
e-mail: sales@maxiaids.com
www.maxiaids.com
Laminated cutting board with unique features to hold food in place with corner ledge for cutting and spreading. *$19.95*

352 **Innerlip Plates**
Therapro
225 Arlington Street
Framingham, MA 01702
508-872-9494
800-257-5376
FAX: 508-875-2062
e-mail: info@theraproducts.com
www.theraproducts.com

Karen Conrad, Owner
Food may be pushed to the side of the plate, then scooped up with a fork and spoon. Available in beige or blue. *$5.00*

353 **Jordan's Motility Solutions: Adapt-Able Utensils**
PO Box 132772
Tyler, TX 75713
903-526-2100
FAX: 903-526-2103
e-mail: info@disabilityaccessories.com
www.disabilityaccessories.com

Gene Howland, President
Adapt-Able eating utensils encourage independent eating for individuals with limited mobility. Angle and reach of utensils can be adjusted to address specific needs.

354 **Long Oven Mitts**
Sammons Preston Rolyan
4 Sammons Court
Bolingbrook, IL 60440
630-226-1300
800-228-3693
FAX: 262-387-8748
e-mail: customerservice@sammonspreston.com
www.sammonspreston.com
Protect hands and forearms from heat, flames and oven grates with these practical mitts that allow a longer reach and less bending. *$8.95*

355 **Magnetic Card Reader**
Maxi Aids
42 Executive Boulevard
Farmingdale, NY 11735
631-752-0521
800-522-6294
FAX: 631-752-0689
e-mail: sales@maxiaids.com
www.maxiaids.com
Produces audible labels so a recorded card can be taped on cans of food or a box of cake mix; even adding instructions for baking. *$159.95*

356 **Maxi-Aids Braille Timer**
Maxi Aids
42 Executive Boulevard
Farmingdale, NY 11735
631-752-0521
800-522-6294
FAX: 631-752-0689
e-mail: sales@maxiaids.com
www.maxiaids.com
Three raised dots at 15, 30 and 45, two raised dots at remaining five minute intervals and one raised dot at remaining two and a half minute intervals, offers ease of operation to make this a helpful aid for the visually impaired. *$12.95*

357 **Nosey Cup**
Therapro
225 Arlington Street
Framingham, MA 01702
508-872-9494
800-257-5376
FAX: 508-875-2062
e-mail: info@theraproducts.com
www.theraproducts.com

Karen Conrad, Owner
For those with a stiff neck or persons who can't tip their head back while drinking. *$6.00*

358 **Paring Boards**
Therapro
225 Arlington Street
Framingham, MA 01702
508-872-9494
800-257-5376
FAX: 508-875-2062
e-mail: info@theraproducts.com
www.theraproducts.com

Karen Conrad, Owner
Suction feet stabilize board and stainless steel prongs hold food in place for easy, one-handed cutting. *$32.50*

359 **PowerLink 2 Control Unit**
AbleNet
2808 Fairview Avenue N
Saint Paul, MN 55113
800-322-0956
FAX: 651-294-2259
e-mail: customerservice@ablenetinc.com
www.ablenetinc.com
The PowerLink 2 Control Unit allows switch operation of electrical appliances. It can be used to activate 1 or 2 appliances (up to 1700 watts combined). If 2 appliances are used, they will activate simultaneously. There are four modes of control on the PowerLink 2; direct mode, timed (seconds) mode, timed (minutes) mode and latch mode. Meets safety standards from Underwriters Laboratory (UL) and Canadian Standards Association (CSA) for electrical appliances. *$159.00*

360 **Sammons Preston Rolyan**
4 Sammons Court
Bolingbrook, IL 60440
630-226-1300
800-228-3693
FAX: 262-387-8748
e-mail: customerservice@sammonspreston.com
www.sammonspreston.com
Sammons Preston Rolyan is a leading provider of rehabilitation and assistive devices to help those with disabilities meet daily physical challenges and achieve their greatest level of independence. With one of the industry's largest catalogs, Sammons Preston Rolyan offers a wide range of products available.

Annually

361 **Slicing Aid**
Snug Seat
PO Box 1739
Matthews, NC 28106
704-882-0666
800-336-7684
FAX: 704-882-0751
e-mail: sales@snugseat.com
www.snugseat.com

Earlene Hucks, Marketing Coordinator
Kirk Mackenzie, Owner
The design of these knives allows a better working posture and makes optimal use of strength in the arms and hands.

362 **Small Appliance Receiver**
AbleNet
2808 Fairview Avenue N
Saint Paul, MN 55113
800-322-0956
FAX: 651-294-2259
e-mail: customerservice@ablenetinc.com
www.ablenetinc.com
The Small Appliance Receiver, in conjunction with the Cordless Big Red Switch, allows you to control small electrical appliances in the environment without a cord. It should only be used with low-wattage appliances (under 500 watts) which have two prong plugs (ie, radios, fans, lamps, blenders, etc.). It should not be used with heat generating appliances. *$32.00*

363 **Steel Food Guard**
Maxi Aids
42 Executive Boulevard
Farmingdale, NY 11735
631-752-0521
800-522-6294
FAX: 631-752-0689
e-mail: sales@maxiaids.com
www.maxiaids.com
Provides stable area to push against while eating. *$ 10.95*

364 **Thick-n-Easy**
Therapro
225 Arlington Street
Framingham, MA 01702
508-872-9494
800-257-5376
FAX: 508-875-2062
e-mail: info@theraproducts.com
www.theraproducts.com

Karen Conrad, Owner
Instant food thickener that sets in 30 seconds and will not become thicker even after refrigeration. *$6.50*

365 **Thumbs Up Cup**
Therapro
225 Arlington Street
Framingham, MA 01702
508-872-9494
800-257-5376
FAX: 508-875-2062
e-mail: info@theraproducts.com
www.theraproducts.com

Karen Conrad, Owner
This cup is designed for those with limited strength or coordination or arthritis. The two backward-tilt handles and thumb rests allow finger joints to be used to their greatest mechanical advantage. *$9.50*

366 **Un-Skru**
Multi-Marketing & Manufacturers
PO Box 1070
Littleton, CO 80160
303-794-5955
800-506-0248
e-mail: penlane@xpert.net
www.seniorshops.com/unskru.html

Janet Lane, President
This jar and bottle opener mounts permanently to the underside of a cabinet, shelf, table or counter so it is out of sight yet always ready to use. Opens all sizes of jar lids — easily and with little strength. *$7.95*

367 **Undercounter Lid Opener**
Sammons Preston Rolyan
4 Sammons Court
Bolingbrook, IL 60440
630-226-1300
800-228-3693
FAX: 262-387-8748
e-mail: customerservice@sammonspreston.com
www.sammonspreston.com
The gripper of this unit which installs under the counter can help unscrew any cap. *$5.75*

368 **Uni-Turner**
Sammons Preston Rolyan
4 Sammons Court
Bolingbrook, IL 60440
630-226-1300
800-228-3693
FAX: 262-387-8748
e-mail: customerservice@sammonspreston.com
www.sammonspreston.com
Odd shaped handles can be turned easily with one-handed, L-shaped Uni-Turner. *$16.50*

369 **Universal Hand Cuff**
Therapro
225 Arlington Street
Framingham, MA 01702
508-872-9494
800-257-5376
FAX: 508-875-2062
e-mail: info@theraproducts.com
www.theraproducts.com

Karen Conrad, Owner
Comfortable cuff with Velcro strap holds utensils, toothbrushes, etc. *$9.95*

Lifts, Ramps & Elevators

370 **Accessibility Lift**
Inclinator Company of America
601 Gibson Boulevard
Harrisburg, PA 17104
717-939-8420
800-343-9007
FAX: 717-234-0941
e-mail: isaks@inclinator.com
www.inclinator.com

Dotty Keith, Sales Manager
Stephen Nock, President
An economical lift for restricted usage that provides barrier-free access that can be used by churches, schools, lodging halls and meeting halls to meet compliance requirements, with the dignified convenience and freedom they deserve.

371 **Adjustable Incline Board**
Bailey Manufacturing Company
118 Lee Street
Suite 130
Lodi, OH 44254
330-948-1080
800-321-8372
FAX: 330-948-4439
e-mail: baileymfg@attmail.com
www.baileymfg.com

Larry Strimple, President
Incline board for the physically challenged with a foot board with non-slip tread.

372 **AlumiRamp**
855 E Chicago Road
Quincy, MI 49082
517-639-8777
800-800-3864
FAX: 517-639-4314
e-mail: ramps@alumiramp.com
www.alumiramp.com

Linda Burke, President
Doug Cannon, Customer Service
Pam Lippert, Customer Service
Complete line of modular and portable ramps for both home and vehicle use. Welded construction and non-skid extruded surfaces are featured on all our ramps.

373 **Area Access**
8117 Ransell Road
Falls Church, VA 22042
703-573-2111
800-333-2732
FAX: 703-207-0446
e-mail: c_wenn@hotmail.com
www.areaaccess.com

Cliff Wenn, Sales Manager
Barbara Spellman, Mobility Consultant
Scott Hobson, Owner
Serving the entire Mid-Atlantic with scooters, stairway lifts and elevators. Large inventory and fully stocked showrooms.

374 **Bruno Independent Living Aids**
Bruno Independent Living Aids
PO Box 84
Oconomowoc, WI 53066
262-567-4990
800-882-8183
FAX: 262-567-4341
e-mail: webmaster@bruno.com
www.bruno.com

Patrick Foy, National Sales Manager
Karla Branham Shaw, Marketing
Michael Bruno, Owner
An ISO 9001 Certified Manufacturer of automotive lifts for scooter, wheelchairs, and powerchairs, three and four wheel scooters, and straight and custom curve stairlifts.

375 **Butlers Wheelchair Lifts**
Flinchbaugh Company
390 Eberts Lane
York, PA 17403
717-848-2418
800-326-2418
FAX: 717-843-7385

Gregg Kenkins, President
Brian McMaster, President Sales
Greg E Ness, Sales Manager
This wheelchair lift can be equipped with an end ramp and guard. Automatically retractable, it locks firmly into place when the lift is in operation.

376 **Cheney's Liberty II**
Handi-Lift
730 Garden Street
Carlstadt, NJ 07072
201-933-0111
800-503-2003
FAX: 845-947-4522
www.handilift.com

Douglas Boydston, Owner
Economical lift for straight stairways.

377 **Classique**
Handi-Lift
730 Garden Street
Carlstadt, NJ 07072
201-933-0111
800-503-2003
FAX: 845-947-4522
www.handilift.com

Douglas Boydston, Owner
The Classique elevator answers access problems in churches, schools and small offices.

378 **Columbus McKinnon Corporation**
140 John James Audubon Parkway
Amherst, NY 14228
716-689-5400
800-888-0985
FAX: 716-696-3220

Larry Smith, Manager
Timothy Tevens, Chief Executive Officer
Supplies various lift and transfer systems for independent or attended applications including ceiling mounted or freestanding overhead track lifts and mobile floorbase units for homes, schools and healthcare facilities. Lift Systems for transferring between bed, chair, commode or bath are available with a variety of slings, scales and accessories.

379 **Curb-Sider Super XL**
Bruno Independent Living Aids
PO Box 84
Oconomowoc, WI 53066
262-567-4990
800-882-8183
FAX: 262-953-5501
www.bruno.com

Michael R Bruno, Chairman/CEO/Owner
The lift of choice for storing your fully or partially assembled scooter or power chair weighing up to 400 pounds in the rear of your van or minivan, SUV, pickup truck or some station wagon applications.

380 **Custom Lift Residential Elevators**
Waupaca Elevator Company
1726 N Ballard Road
Appleton, WI 54911
920-991-9082
800-238-8739
FAX: 920-991-9087
e-mail: csr@waupacaelevator.com
www.waupacaelevator.com

Bill Michael, Owner
Waupaca Elevator residential elevators and dumbwaiters add value, convenience and reliability to today's homes.

381 **Deluxe Convertible Exercise Staircase**
Sammons Preston Rolyan
4 Sammons Court
Bolingbrook, IL 60440
630-226-1300
800-228-3693
FAX: 262-387-8748
e-mail: customerservice@sammonspreston.com
www.sammonspreston.com
Here's an exercise staircase to fit any department configuration. Just reposition a few nuts and bolts to change from a straight to a corner type staircase.

382 **EZ Access Roll-Up Ramp for Scooters, Wheel chairs**
Maxi Aids
42 Executive Boulevard
Farmingdale, NY 11735
631-752-0521
800-522-6294
FAX: 631-752-0689
e-mail: sales@maxiaids.com
www.maxiaids.com
Easy to use heavy-duty ramp for temporary or permanent installation. Grooved, non-skid surface for improved traction. Perfect for scooters, manual and electric wheelchairs.

383 **Easy Pivot Transfer Machine**
Rand-Scot
401 Linden Center Drive
Fort Collins, CO 80524
970-484-7967
800-467-7967
FAX: 970-484-3800
e-mail: randscot@webaccess.net
www.easypivot.com

Joel Lerich, President
The Easy Pivot Patient Lifting System allows for strain-free, one-caregiver transfers of the disabled individual.

384 **Easy Stand**
Altimate Medical
PO Box 180
Morton, MN 56270
507-697-6393
800-342-8969
FAX: 507-637-3024

Alan Tholkes, Chief Executive Officer
Designed to make standing fast and simple. The easy to operate, hydraulic lift system provides a controlled lifting and lowering. With the convenience of simply transferring to the chair and reaching a standing position in seconds with no straps to struggle with.

385 **Economical Liberty**
Handi-Lift
730 Garden Street
Carlstadt, NJ 07072
201-933-0111
800-503-2003
FAX: 845-947-4522

Douglas Boydston, Owner
Installs quickly and easily on most straight stairways. It uses regular household current and mounts over the carpet or directly to the stairs without marring.

386 **Electra-Ride Elite**
Bruno Independent Living Aids
PO Box 84
Oconomowoc, WI 53066
262-567-4990
800-882-8183
FAX: 262-953-5501
www.bruno.com

Michael R Bruno, Chairman/CEO/Owner
The new Electra-Ride Elite installs to within 5 inches of the wall and has a 350 pound weight capacity. Bruno stairlifts can fit almost any custom curve or straight rail application and require no structural modification to the stairway. Plus, battery power allows for uninterupted operation even during a power outage.

387 **Electra-Ride III**
Bruno Independent Living Aids
PO Box 84
Oconomowoc, WI 53066
262-567-4990
800-882-8183
FAX: 262-953-5501
www.bruno.com

Michael R Bruno, Chairman/CEO/Owner
Bruno stairlifts can fit almost any custom curve or straight rail application and require no structural modification to the stairway. Plus, battery power allows for uninterrupted operation even during a power outage.

388 **Freedom Wheelchair Lifts**
580 Tc Jester Boulevard
Houston, TX 77007
713-864-1460

Carlos Saez, Owner

389 **Freedom Wheels**
580 TC Jester Boulevard
Houston, TX 77007
713-864-1460
FAX: 713-864-1469
e-mail: info@freedomwheels.com
www.freedomwheels.com/index.html

N Donnelly
Freedom Wheels, Inc. is committed to people with disabilities and personal transportation options for an independent lifestyle.

390 **Handi Home Lift**
Handi-Lift
730 Garden Street
Carlstadt, NJ 07072
201-933-0111
800-503-2003
FAX: 845-947-4522

Douglas Boydston, Owner
An outdoor lift designed to provide access over porch stairs or other steps that impede movement.

391 **Handi Prolift**
Handi-Lift
730 Garden Street
Carlstadt, NJ 07072
201-933-0111
800-503-2003
FAX: 845-947-4522

Douglas Boydston, Owner
Provides dependable vertical transportation for multi-level buildings.

392 **Handi-Ramp**
Handi-Ramp
510 North Avenue
Libertyville, IL 60048
847-680-7700
800-876-7267
FAX: 847-816-8866
e-mail: info@handiramp.com
www.handiramp.com

Thomas Disch, President/CEO
Mike Smith, Production Manager
Scott Longueil, Sales Manager
Provides a complete line of economical, ADA Compliant access ramping products. Line includes van attachable and wheelchair tie downs; aluminum or expanded metal folding portables; aluminum channels; portable, sectional ramp systems; semi-permanent ramps, platforms and systems. All ramp series are available in varied lengths and widths in combination with platforms and optional hand railing, single or double bar construction with return ends. Special Order ramps and ramp systems.

393 **Homecare Products EZ-Access Portable Ramps**
15824 SE 296th Street
Kent, WA 98042
800-451-1903
FAX: 800-630-2350
e-mail: ezaccess@homecareproducts.com
www.homecareproducts.com

Don Everard, VP Marketing
Deanne Sandvold, VP Sales
EZ-ACCESS Ramps bridge gaps over curbs and steps, allowing scooters and wheelchairs to continue on a smooth, safe course. Available in several different styles and sizes, ranging from a two-foot curb ramp to a 10-foot multi-purpose ramp. All ramps are made of anodized aluminum.

394 **Homewaiter**
Inclinator Company of America
601 Gibson Boulevard
Harrisburg, PA 17104
717-939-8420
800-343-9007
FAX: 717-234-0941
e-mail: isaks@inclinator.com
www.inclinator.com

Dotty Keith, Sales Manager
Stephen Nock, President
With its roller truck riding in a specially formed monorail, it is easy to install and highly adaptable to existing conditions. It can travel up to 35 feet, opening on any or all three sides at different stations, whether at counter level or floor level.

395 **Horcher Lifting Systems**
324 Cypress Road
Ocala, FL 34472
352-687-8020
800-582-8732
FAX: 866-378-3318
e-mail: us-office@horcher.com
www.horcher.com

David Schultz, General Manager
Sharon Harbert, Administrative Assistant
Barrier Free Lifts by Horcher leads the industry for excellence in patient transfers and technology for over 18 years. They offer state of the art ceiling track systems, floor base lifts and bathing systems such as the Unilift, PC-2, Diana, Lexa, and Raisa to achieve greater mobility.

396 **Inclinette**
Inclinator Company of America
601 Gibson Boulevard
Harrisburg, PA 17104
717-939-8420
800-343-9007
FAX: 717-234-0941
e-mail: isaks@inclinator.com
www.inclinator.com

Stephen Nock, President
Inclinette provides comfort and convenience in providing multi-floor access to persons who have difficulty climbing stairs.

397 **Lectra-Lift**
La-Z-Boy
1284 N Telegraph Road
Monroe, MI 48162
734-242-1444
FAX: 734-457-2005
www.lazboy.com

Gerald L Kiser, President
David M Risley, SVP/CFO
Patrick H Norton, Chairman

This power recliner has a single motor drive that operates three distinct cycles: lifting, leg elevation and full power recline.

398 **Liberty LT**
Handi-Lift
730 Garden Street
Carlstadt, NJ 07072
201-933-0111
800-503-2003
FAX: 845-947-4522

Douglas Boydston, Owner
Stair lift with dual armrests that lock into position. The comfortable, contoured seat is designed to swivel and move forward at the bottom or top landings to facilitate transfer.

399 **Lifts for Swimming Pools and Spas**
Aquatic Access
417 Dorsey Way
Louisville, KY 40223
502-425-5817
800-325-5438
FAX: 502-425-9607
e-mail: info@AquaticAccess.com
www.AquaticAccess.com

Linda Nolan, President
Liz Waters, Advertising
Ann Bryant, Customer Service/Sales
Aquatic Access manufacturers and sells water-powered lifts providing access to in-ground and above-ground swimming pools, spas, boats and docks. *$2310.00*

400 **Mecalift Sling Lifter**
Arjo Inc.
50 North Gary Avenue
Roselle, IL 60172
630-307-2756
e-mail: info@arjousa.com
www.arjo.com

Ross Scavuzzo, President
Alexis LaSalvia, Marketing Comm. Specialist

401 **One for All Lift All**
Amigo Mobility International
6693 Dixie Highway
Bridgeport, MI 48722
989-777-0910
800-692-6446
FAX: 989-777-8184
www.myamigo.com

Mike Galen, Controller
Shirley Beebe, Order/Sales Operations
Mike LeBrake, Product Manager
The Lift-All transports your wheelchair easily into the trunk of an automobile and neatly stores it for easy access.

402 **Out-Sider III**
Bruno Independent Living Aids
PO Box 84
Oconomowoc, WI 53066
262-567-4990
800-882-8183
FAX: 262-953-5501
www.bruno.com

Michael R Bruno, Chairman/CEO/Owner
Lets you carry your scooter fully assembled and keeps your trunk space available for other things.

403 **Parker Bath**
Arjo Inc.
50 North Gary Avenue
Roselle, IL 60172
630-307-2756
800-323-1245
FAX: 888-594-2756
e-mail: info@arjousa.com
www.arjo.com

Lorena Chevrie, Marketing Communications
Ross Scavuzzo, President
This involves no manual lifting, strain or stress for the caregiver.

404 **Patient Lifting & Injury Prevention**
ARJO Inc.
50 North Gary Avenue
Roselle, IL 60172
630-307-2756
800-323-1245
FAX: 888-594-2756
e-mail: info@arjousa.com
www.arjo.com

Alexis LaSalvia, Marketing Communications
Aids in patient lifting while protecting the caregiver from the risk of backstrain.

405 **Ramplette Telescoping Ramp**
Graham-Field Health Products
2935 Northeast Parkway
Atlanta, GA 30360
770-447-1609
800-347-5678
FAX: 800-726-0601
www.grahamfield.com

Irwin Selinger, Chief Executive Officer
A multi-functional, easily moved, economical ramp weighing 25 pounds.

406 **Rickshaw Exerciser**
Access To Recreation
8 Sandra Court
Newbury Park, CA 91320
805-498-7535
800-634-4351
FAX: 805-498-8186
e-mail: customerservice@accesstr.com
www.accesstr.com

Don Krebs, President
Marie Krebs, Office Manager
This Exerciser develops the muscle used most by those in wheelchairs. It develops the strength you need to lift yourself for pressure relief, doing transfers and pushing your wheelchair.

407 **Ricon Corporation**
7900 Nelson Road
Panorama City, CA 91402
818-899-7588
800-322-2884
FAX: 818-267-3001
www.riconcorp.com
Ricon corporation is a world leader in the manufacture of lifts and other mobility products for people with disabilities. The Ricon product line features the Activan(R) a lowered floor minivan conversion, wheelchair lifts power seat base and automatic door openers.

408 **Smart Leg**
Invacare Corporation
899 Cleveland Street
Elyria, OH 44035
440-329-6000
e-mail: info@invacare.com
www.invacare.com

A Malachi Mixon III, CEO
Gerald B Blouch, President/COO
Thomas R Miklich, CFO
An ingenious elevating leg rest that automatically extends to correctly fit every outstretched leg.

409 **Smooth Mover**
Dixie EMS
385 Union Avenue
Brooklyn, NY 11211
718-387-9305
800-347-3494
FAX: 718-387-9310
e-mail: customerSVC@dixieems.com
www.dixieems.com

Eva Silverstein, President
Patient mover is a board designed to transfer patients from bed to stretcher or table with one or two people. *$199.95*

410 SpectraLift
Inclinator Company of America
601 Gibson Boulevard
Harrisburg, PA 17104
717-939-8420
800-343-9007
FAX: 717-234-0941
e-mail: isaks@inclinator.com
www.inclinator.com

Dotty Keith, Sales Manager
Stephen Nock, President
A newly designed hydraulic wheelchair lift made of fiberglass construction suitable for commercial and residential use.

411 Spectrum Aquatics
7100 Spectrum Lane
Missoula, MT 59808
406-543-5309

Dave Murray, President

412 Spectrum Products Catalog
Spectrum Products
7100 Spectrum Lane
Missoula, MT 59808
406-542-9781
800-791-8056
FAX: 406-542-1158
e-mail: info@spectrumproducts.com
www.spectrumproducts.com

Gerri McConnell, President
Kelly Youbles, Inside Sales Market/Comm. Man.
Manufacturers of swimming pool disabled access products such as lifts, ramps, railings, ladders, and stainless steel hydrotherapy tanks for the swimming pool and medical therapy markets.

413 StairLIFT SC & SL
Inclinator Company of America
601 Gibson Boulevard
Harrisburg, PA 17104
717-939-8420
800-343-9007
FAX: 717-234-0941
e-mail: isaks@inclinator.com
www.inclinator.com

Stephen Nock, President
Simple, self-contained and efficient stair units.

414 Stairway Elevators
Bruno Independent Living Aids
1780 Executive Drive
Suite 84
Oconomowoc, WI 53066
262-567-4990
800-882-8183
FAX: 262-567-4341
e-mail: webmaster@bruno.com

Michael Bruno, Owner
Bruno offers a full line of stairway elevators, including the Electra-Ride II featuring access during power interruptions, convenient installation, comfort and a powerful drive system. The Electra-Ride which features battery-powered technology, a rail width of 25 inches and seat rotation for easy transfers. The Comfort-Ride AC stair lift which is battery operated, has a rail width of 7.25 inches and folded width of less than 14.5 inches.

415 Straight and Custom Curved Stairlifts
Bruno Independent Living Aids
PO Box 84
Oconomowoc, WI 53066
262-567-4990
800-882-8183
FAX: 262-953-5501
e-mail: webmaster@bruno.com
www.bruno.com

Patrick Foy, National Sales Manager
Karla Branham Shaw, Marketing
Michael Bruno, Owner
Bruno stairlifts can fit almost any curve or straight rail application and requires little or no structural modification to the stairway. Normal rail position for a Bruno inside turn is 7 to 8 inches from the wall or obstruction which is the tightest radius of any stairlift manufacturing company in the world. The Bruno inside turn is ideal for bi-level homes or staircases with mid-level doors. Bruno's unique battery power allows for uninterrupted operation even during a power outage.

416 SureHands Lift & Care Systems
982 County Route 1
Pine Island, NY 10969
845-258-6500
800-724-5305
FAX: 845-258-6634
e-mail: info@surehands.com
www.surehands.com

Thomas Herceg, President
Joyce Moraczewski, Marketing Coordinator
Carol Colegrove, Sales Coordinator
SureHands Lift & Care Systems offer a unique, patented and exlusive range of lift and transfer systems to meet private and institutional needs of individuals with motor disabilties. Includes permanent and portable models for homes, workplaces and recreation. The SureHands Body Support offers safe, easy and secure transfers for user and the opportunity for independent transfers for some. They are a back-saver for caregivers. All lifts are easily maintained and operated with mininum assistance.

417 Swing-A-Way
Braun Corporation
PO Box 310
Winamac, IN 46996
574-946-6153
800-THE-LIFT
FAX: 574-946-4670

William Roth, President
A swing lift for transporting patients from bed to bath and more. It features a gravity-down operation made possible by a newly designed pump module package. The new, quieter module features a built-in hand pump and a plastic reservoir for easy fluid checking. This is a vehicle lift not bath lift.

418 Thyssen Krupp Access
4001 E 138th Street
Grandview, MO 64030
816-763-3100
800-829-9760
FAX: 816-763-4467
e-mail: marketing@tkaccess.com
www.tkaccess.com

Michael Bolton, Marketing Supervisor
Bill Koch, VP Sales
Pat Schmidt, Business Development Specialist
Whether you want to open your facility or stay in the home you love, Thyssen Krupp Access has the perfect wheelchair lift, stair lift or elevator to suit your budget and needs. Our lifts have the best warranties. Our nationwide network of dealers are close by and ready to help.

419 Turning Automotive Seating (TAS)
Bruno Independent Living Aids
PO Box 84
Oconomowoc, WI 53066
262-567-4990
800-882-8183
FAX: 262-953-5501
www.bruno.com

Michael R Bruno, Chairman/CEO/Owner
Transfer in and out of a car, minivan, pickup truck and full size van without any lifting!

420 Vangater, Vangater II, Mini-Vangater
PO Box 310
Winamac, IN 46996
800-THE-LIFT
FAX: 574-946-7935
www.braunlift.com
Tri-fold and fold-in-half lifts represent a major innovation in the field of adapted van transportation.

421 **Versatrainer**
Pro- Max/ Division Of Bow- Flex Of America
2200 NE 65th Avenue
Vancouver, WA 98661
800-BOW-FLEX
FAX: 360-993-3610
www.bowflex.com

One exercise system for the disabled person that does everything. Incorporates full body strength, muscle development, cardiovascular conditioning, gives full muscle movement and balanced muscle development.

422 **Vertical Home Lift Sales**
2715 Seaboard Lane
Long Beach, CA 90805
562-634-5962
800-795-6227
FAX: 562-634-4120

Rick Pierce, Vertical Home Lift Sales
Betty Haskings, Office Manager
Jerry MacDonald, President
Sales and service of van and truck lifts. Sales and service of wheel chair lifts for vans and automobiles. Sales, installation and service of vertical home lifts, scooter lifts and pool lifts. Sales of scooters.

423 **Vestibular Board**
Bailey Manufacturing Company
118 Lee Street
Suite 130
Lodi, OH 44254
330-948-1080
800-321-8372
FAX: 330-948-4439
e-mail: baileymfg@attmail.com
www.baileymfg.com

Larry Strimple, President
Creates tilting in a rolling motion for reclining patients who need help developing balance.

424 **Wheelchair Carrier**
203 Matzinger Road
Toledo, OH 43612
419-478-4423
800-541-3213
FAX: 419-478-4425
e-mail: davidm@wheelchaircarrier.com
www.wheelchaircarrier.com

David Makulinsky, President
Mike Siler, Engineer
Wheelchair, scooter and powerchair carriers for hitch mount on vehicles, priced from $199 to $999.

Major Catalogs

425 **Access Store Products for Barrier Free Environments**
Access Store.Com
820 W 7th Street
Chico, CA 95928
530-879-5600
800-497-2003
FAX: 530-893-1560
e-mail: sales@accessstore.com
www.accessstore.com

Timothy Vander Heiden, President
Lisa Bantum, Sales Administrator
One of the largest online ADA Compliance Catalogs available. Offers everything from innovative barrier removal products to survey equipment, to unique specialty products.

426 **Access to Recreation**
8 Sandra Court
Newbury Park, CA 91320
805-498-7535
800-634-4351
FAX: 805-498-8186
e-mail: customerservice@accesstr.com
www.accesstr.com

Don Krebs, President
The Access to Recreation catalog is full of recreation and exercise equipment. One can find items such as electric fishing reels and other fishing and hunting equipment for the disabled sportsman. There are also adapted golf clubs, swimming pool lifts, wheelchair gloves and cuffs and bowling equipment. There are devices to help with embroidery, knitting and card playing, videos, books and practical aides such as wheelchair ramps and book.

64 pages Bi-Annually

427 **Achievement Products**
PO Box 9033
Canton, OH 44711
800-373-4699
FAX: 800-766-4303
e-mail: info@specialkidszone.com
www.specialkidszone.com

Teresa Cardon, VP
Offer a wide range of pediatric rehabilitation equipment and special education products including handwriting aids, weighted vests, positioning equipment, sensory integration products and adaptive furniture. Call for your free catalog.

428 **Adaptive Clothing: Adults**
Special Clothes
PO Box 333
E Harwich, MA 02645
508-430-2410
FAX: 508-430-2410
TTY:508-430-2410
e-mail: SPECIALCLO@aol.com
www.special-clothes.com

Judith Sweeney, President
Special Clothes produces a catalogue of garments for adults with disabilities and/or incontinence. Offerings include: undergarments, snap-crotch tee shirts, sleepwear, jumpsuits, bibs and some footwear. The catalogue is available without charge. Comparable to department store prices. Special Clothes produces a catalog of adaptive clothing for children in sizes from toddler through young adults. A full line of clothing is included from undergarments through wheelchair jackets and ponchos.

429 **Adaptive Technology Catalog**
Synapse Adaptive
14 Lynn Court
Suite S
San Rafael, CA 94901
415-455-9700
800-317-9611
FAX: 415-455-9801
e-mail: info@synapseadaptive.com
www.synapseadaptive.com

Martin Tibor, Owner
Rebecca Jones, Sales
Aaptive technology for individuals with disabilities, ADA compliant workstations, and ergonomic furniture.

430 **Adult Long Jumpsuit with Feet**
Special Clothes
PO Box 333
E Harwich, MA 02645
508-896-7939
FAX: 508-896-7939
e-mail: specialclo@aol.com
www.special-clothes.com

Judith Sweeney, President
Line of clothing for people with disabilities. Child and adult catalog available.

431 **Adult Short Jumpsuit**
Special Clothes
PO Box 333
E Harwich, MA 02645
508-896-7939
FAX: 508-896-7939
e-mail: specialclo@aol.com
www.special-clothes.com

Judith Sweeney, President
This pull-on jumpsuit provides comfort and full coverage without bulk. Wide leg ribbing ends at mid-thigh, with snaps at the crotch. We use fine quality, comfortable cotton knit. 100% cotton knit. Made in USA. Option: long sleeves - add $3.00. Colors: white, navy, teal, light blue, light pink, red, burgundy, royal blue and black. Sm & Med: $36.50/3 for $104.00; L & XL: $39.00/3 for $111.25; and XXL: $42.00/3 for $119.25.

432 **American Discount Medical**
459 Main St.
Suite 101-417
Trussville, AL 35173
205-467-6995
800-877-9100
FAX: 205-467-7095
e-mail: adm@information44.com
www.americandiscountmed.com

Tom Ruf, General Manager
Deeply discounts every major brand medical product available.

433 **Apria Healthcare**
26220 Enterprise Court
Lake Forest, CA 92630
949-639-2000
800-277-4288
e-mail: contact_us@apria.com
www.apria.com

Lawrence Higby, Chief Executive Officer
Lifts, chairs, bathroom aids, bedroom aids, eating utensils and independent living aids for the physically challenged.

434 **Armstrong Medical**
575 Knightsbridge Parkway
Lincolnshire, IL 60069
847-913-0101
800-323-4220
FAX: 847-913-0138
www.armstrongmedical.com

Warren Armstrong, President
Training aids, anatomical models, medical equipment, pediatrics equipment and rehabilitation equipment.

435 **Assistive Technology Journal**
1700 N Moore Street
Suite 1540
Arlington, VA 22209
703-524-6686
FAX: 703-524-6630

$32.50
Bi-Annually

436 **Assistive Technology Sourcebook**
Special Needs Project
324 State Street
Suite H
Santa Barbara, CA 93101
805-962-8087
800-333-6867
FAX: 805-962-5087
e-mail: books@specialneeds.com
www.specialneeds.com

Alexandra Enders, Editor
Marian Hall, Editor
Provides you with 18 chapters of practical information on all aspects of assistive technology for individuals with functional limitations. *$60.00*
576 pages

437 **Bailey**
Bailey Manufacturing
PO Box 130
Lodi, OH 44254
330-948-2655
800-321-8372
FAX: 330-948-4439
e-mail: baileymfg@attmail.com
www.baileymfg.com

Dave Bailey, Owner
Ambulation aids, balance aids, benches, chairs, exercise devices, tables, stools, rehabilitation and physical therapy equipment for the physically challenged.
70 pages

438 **Best 25 Catalog Resources for Making Life Easier**
Meeting Life's Challenges
9042 Aspen Grove Lane
Madison, WI 53717
608-824-0402
FAX: 608-824-0403
e-mail: help@MeetingLifesChallenges.com
www.MeetingLifesChallenges.com

Unique reference guide to locate thousands of useful and hard-to-find adaptive devices to make dressing, eating, cooking, grooming, communicating, playing, exercising, etc. easier, safer and less frustrating for people of all ages and disabilities. A comprehensive, up-do-date reference for people with disabilities, caregivers and healthcare professionals. *$8.95*
36 pages
ISBN 1-891854-03-8

439 **Body Suits**
Special Clothes
PO Box 333
E Harwich, MA 02645
508-430-2410
FAX: 508-430-2410
e-mail: specialclo@aol.com
www.special-clothes.com

Judith Bari, President
Bodysuits, Jumpsuits, back opening garments, incontinence wear, bibs. Features include snap crotches and g-tube pockets.

440 **Cambridge Career Products Catalog**
Cambridge Educational
PO Box 931
Monmouth Junction, NJ 08852
304-744-9323
800-468-4227
FAX: 800-329-6687
e-mail: lisa.schmuclei@films.com
www.cambridgeeducational.com

Lisa Schmuclei, Marketing Director
A full color catalog featuring hundreds of products designed to aid people in career exploration, selecting specific occupations and obtaining these jobs through resume and interview preparation.
64 pages BiAnnual

441 **Carolyn's Low Vision Products**
3938 S Tamiami Trl
Sarasota, FL 34231
941-373-9100
800-648-2266
e-mail: sales@carolynscatalog.com
www.carolynscatalog.com

Carolyn Tojek, President
Free mail-order catalog of items for visually impaired people. We also have a retail store.

442 **Communication Aids for Children and Adults**
Crestwood Communication Aids
6625 N Sidney Place
Milwaukee, WI 53209
414-352-5678
FAX: 414-352-5679
e-mail: crestcomm@aol.com
www.communicationaids.com

Ruth B Leff MS CCC, President/Language Pathologist
A free catalog of communication aids for children and adults with disabilities. Over 300 light and high tech switches and aids, and a large selection of adapted and voice-activated toys. Talking Pictures and Passports communication boards, easy to use and moderately priced talking aids.
32 pages Yearly

443 **Danmar Products**
221 Jackson Industrial Drive
Ann Arbor, MI 48103
734-761-1990
800-783-1998
FAX: 734-761-8977
e-mail: sales@danmarproducts.com
www.danmarproducts.com

Dan Russo, President
Suzanne Gubachy, Sales Manager
Amy Belleau, Sales Marketing
Manufactures adaptive equipment for persons with physical and mental disabilities, from seating and positioning equipment, flotation devices, toileting aids to hard and soft shell helmets.

444 **Dayspring Associates**
2111 Foley Road
Havre De Grace, MD 21078
410-939-5900
FAX: 410-939-6252

Benedict Schwartz, Manager

This publisher provides a directory of 1,000 rehabilitation aids.

445 **Disabilities Sourcebook**
Omnigraphics
615 Griswold Street
Detroit, MI 48226
313-961-1340
800-234-1340
FAX: 800-875-1340
www.omnigraphics.com

Paul Rogers, Publicity Associate
Georgiann Lauginger, Customer Service Manager
Peter Ruffner, President
$78.00
616 pages 2000
ISBN 0-780803-89-2

446 **Disability Bookshop Catalog**
PO Box 129
Vancouver, WA 98666
360-694-2462
800-637-2256
FAX: 360-696-3210
e-mail: twinpeak@pacifier.com
disabilitybookshop.virtualave.net/
Offers more than 400 hard-to-find titles covering a wide range of health topics for the general public, and matters of interest to people with disabilities. Catalog. *$4.00*
40 pages

447 **Dressing Tips and Clothing Resources for Making Life Easier**
Attainment Company
PO Box 930160
Verona, WI 53593
608-848-2640
800-327-4269
FAX: 608-845-8040
e-mail: info@attainmentcompany.com
www.attainmentcompany.com

Don Bastian, President
Brent Denu, Marketing Manager
Learn hundreds of simple tips and techniques to make dressing easier. Learn how to adapt/modify ready-to-wear garments to accommodate your special dressing needs. Find out how to locate more than 100 resources offering specially designed or easy-on/easy-off clothing for men, women, children and/or wheelchair users. You'll find everything you need to look your best. An invaluable resource for people with special dressing needs, people with disabilities, caregivers and healthcare professionals. *$19.00*
144 pages 2000
ISBN 1-578611-19-9

448 **Enrichments Catalog**
Sammons Preston Rolyan
4 Sammons Court
Bolingbrook, IL 60440
630-226-1300
800-323-5547
FAX: 630-226-1389
e-mail: spr@abilityone.com
www.sammonsprestonrolyan.com
Provides people with physical challenges with the products they need to help live their lives to the fullest. Includes items for everyday tasks and personal care; assistive products for home use; toileting and bathing aids; grooming and dressing devices; kitchen and dining aids. Also items for range of motion, mobility and exercise such as weights, therapy putty and exercise equipment; ergonomic gloves and supports; canes, crutches, walkers and wheelchair accessories. 36-page catalog.

449 **Equipment Shop**
PO Box 33
Bedford, MA 01730
781-275-7681
800-525-7681
FAX: 781-275-4094
e-mail: info@equipmentshop.com
www.equipmentshop.com

Kenneth D Larson, Owner
Pediatric therapy equipment including pezzi Gymnastik balls, Tripp Trapp chair, airex mats, tricycle accessories, sensory integration equipment and adaptive devices.

450 **Everest & Jennings**
Division of Graham-Field
2935 Northeast Parkway
Atlanta, GA 30360
770-368-4724
800-347-5678
FAX: 800-726-0601
e-mail: cs@everestjennings.com
www.everestjennings.com
Manufactures more than 200 items for persons with physical disabilities, including wheelchairs, seat cushions, shower chairs, grab bars and more.

451 **Express Medical Supply**
28 Seebold Spur
Fenton, MO 63026
636-349-8448
800-633-2139
FAX: 800-633-9188
e-mail: sales@exmed.net
www.exmed.net

Chris Winston, Manager
Bill Nahm, Manager
Offers a full line of medical and ostomy supplies. at discounted prices. Order by phone or online.

452 **FlagHouse Rehab Resources**
601 Flaghouse Drive
Hasbrouck Heights, NJ 07604
201-288-7600

George Carmel, President

453 **FlagHouse Special Populations**
601 FlagHouse Drive
Hasbrouck Heights, NJ 07604
201-288-7600
800-793-7900
FAX: 800-793-7922
e-mail: sales@flaghouse.com
www.flaghouse.com

Brigid de Lime, Sr Brand Manager
Diana Hohman, Brand Manager
Contains over 2,000 products of interest to therapy professionals.
Bi-Annually

454 **Freedom Rider**
Freedom Rider
PO Box 4187
Manchester, NH 03108
603-645-1811
888-253-8811
FAX: 603-645-1811
e-mail: info@freedomrider.com
www.freedomrider.com

Victoria Surr, President
A catalog of equipment for people with disabilities who ride and drive horses which includes instructional aids, vaulting equipment, and lots of hard to find items.

455 **HAC Hearing Aid Centers of America: HARC Mercantile**
Hearing Center
1111 W Centre Avenue
Portage, MI 49024
269-324-0301
800-445-9968
FAX: 800-413-5248
TTY: 800-445-9968
e-mail: info@harc.com
www.harcmercantile.com

Ronald Slager, President
Specializes in products for the hard of hearing and deaf as required under ADA including visual alerting products for fire, phone, door, wake up, phone amplification, TTY, FM and infrared listening systems.

456 **Harris Communications**
Harris Communications
15155 Technology Drive
Eden Prairie, MN 55344
952-906-1180
800-825-6758
FAX: 952-906-1099
e-mail: mail@harriscomm.com
www.harriscomm.com

Bill Williams, National Sales Manager
Robert Harris, Owner
A national distributor of assistive devices for the deaf and hard of hearing with many manufacturers represented. Catalog includes a wide range of assistive devices as well as a variety of books and videotapes related to deaf and hard-of-hearing issues. Products available for children, teachers, hearing professionals, interpreters and anyone interested in deaf culture, hearing loss and sign language.
180 pages Yearly

457 **Health and Rehabilitation Products**
Luminaud
8688 Tyler Boulevard
Mentor, OH 44060
440-255-9082
800-255-3408
FAX: 440-255-2250
e-mail: info@luminaud.com
www.luminaud.com

Thomas Lennox, President
Dorothy Lennox, VP
Switches for limited capability, stoma and trach covers, shower protectors and thermo-stim oral motor stimulator. Personal voice amplifiers for people with weak voices. Artificial larynges for people with no voices. Small electronic communication boards. Books for laryngectomies and speech pathologists.

458 **HealthCare Solutions**
Blue Chip II
3478 Hauck Road
Cincinnati, OH 45241
513-271-5115
800-417-5115
FAX: 513-527-3686

LK Barker, Director
Quality rehabilitation equipment sales and rental. Available equipment includes manual and powered mobility, positioning/seating equipment, vehicle modification, environmental controls, augmentative and alternative communication devices, adaptive computer access, ambulance aids and aids for daily living. Equipment provision is carried out through a total team approach.

459 **Hear You Are**
98 Us Highway 46
Budd Lake, NJ 07828
973-347-7662
FAX: 973-691-0611

Dorinne S Davis, President
A large catalog of various assistive and communication devices for people who are hearing impaired. *$3.00*
42 pages

460 **Hig's Manufacturing**
2917 Anthony Lane
Minneapolis, MN 55418
612-788-1183
FAX: 612-638-1341

James Murphy, Owner
Factory direct, lightweight aluminum, portable, 2 & 4-way folding, telescoping tracks, threshold, van, scooter and approach ramps.

461 **Huntleigh Healthcare**
40 Christopher Way
Eatontown, NJ 07724
732-935-0975
800-223-1218
FAX: 732-578-9889
www.huntleigh-healthcare.com

Robert Angel, President/CEO
Offers quality products including support surfaces, seating surfaces and intermittent pneumatic compression devices.

462 **Kleinert's**
3968 194th Trail
Golden Beach, FL 33160
305-937-0824
800-463-7337
FAX: 305-937-0825
e-mail: mbrier1930@aol.com
www.hygienics.com

Michael Brier, President/CEO
Offers a complete line of incontinence products and skin care products consisting of disposable and reuseable panties for women and pants for men. Also disposable liners.
16 pages Bi-Annual

463 **LS&S**
PO Box 673
Northbrook, IL 60065
847-498-9777
800-468-4789
FAX: 847-498-1482
TTY: 800-317-8533
e-mail: info@LSSproducts.com
www.LSSproducts.com

Melissa Balbach, Owner
Specializes in products for the blind, visually impaired, hearing impaired, and deaf. Free catalog upon request.

464 **Lighthouse Low Vision Products**
Lighthouse International
111 E 59th Street
New York, NY 10022
212-821-9200
800-829-0500
FAX: 212-821-9707
e-mail: info@lighthouse.org
www.lighthouse.org

Tara Cortes, President & CEO
This organization provides health care services related to vision loss; Career and academic services for people with vision loss; Music instruction and pre K curriculum for visually impaired students.

465 **Luminaud**
8688 Tyler Boulevard
Mentor, OH 44060
440-255-9082
800-255-3408
FAX: 440-255-2250
e-mail: info@luminaud.com
www.luminaud.com

Thomas Lennox, President
Dorothy Lennox, VP
Offers a line of artificial larynx, personal voice amplifiers, special switches, stoma covers and other communication, health and safety items.

466 **MOMS Catalog**
24700 Avenue Rockefeller
Valencia, CA 91355
800-232-7443
FAX: 888-874-4347
e-mail: moms@hdis.com
www.momscatalog.com
MOMS catalog features high quality, incontinence supplies, mobility products, bath safety products urological products, aids for daily living products, ostomy supplies and many other adpative items. MOMS offers low prices, excellent customer service and convenient home delivery to your doorstep.
52 pages

467 **Maxi Aids**
PO Box 3209
Farmingdale, NY 11735
631-752-0521
800-522-6294
FAX: 631-752-0689
e-mail: sales@maxiaids.com
www.maxiaids.com
Products specially designed for the blind, low vision, visually impaired, deaf, deaf-blind, hard of hearing, arthritic, diabetic and individuals with special needs.

468 New Vision Store
919 Walnut Street
Philadelphia, PA 19107
215-627-0600
e-mail: webmaster@thenewvisionstore.com
www.thenewvisionstore.com

Patricia Johnson, Chief Executive Officer
Catalog for individuals with visual impairments, listing visual aids, magnifiers, large print books and more.
30 pages

469 Pearson Performance Solutions
1 North Deerborne Street
16th Floor
Chicago, IL 60602
312-938-9200
800-922-7343
FAX: 312-242-4400
e-mail: pearsonreidlondonhouse@pearson.com
www.pearsonreidlondonhouse.com

Publishes human resource assessment instruments for employment settings. The instruments include job analysis procedures to identify important characteristics for job success and objective assessment procedures to evaluate applicants and employees on these characteristics.

470 Pearson Reid London House
1 N Dearborn Street
Floor 16
Chicago, IL 60602
312-938-9200

Adrea Allen, Manager

471 Potomac Technology
1 Church Street
Suite 101
Rockville, MD 20850
301-762-4005
800-433-2838
FAX: 301-762-1892
e-mail: info@potomactech.com
www.potomactech.com

Patricia Relihan, VP/Manager
This catalog offers a variety of products for the deaf and hard of hearing, such as: wake-up devices, alarm clocks, alerting systems, assistive listening devices, signalers, smoke detectors, TTY, telephones and telephone amplifiers. We also carry novelties, and educational books and videos.
24 pages

472 Prentke Romich Company Product Catalog
1022 Heyl Road
Wooster, OH 44691
330-262-1984
800-262-1984
FAX: 330-263-4829
e-mail: info@prentrom.com
www.prentrom.com

Cherie Weaver, Marketing Coordinator
Dave Moffatt, President
A full line, product catalog containing information on speech-output communication devices, environmental controls and computer access products.

473 Products for People with Disabilities
LS&S
PO Box 673
Northbrook, IL 60065
847-498-9777
800-468-4789
FAX: 847-498-1482
TTY: 800-317-8533
e-mail: info@LSSproducts.com
www.LSSproducts.com

Melissa Balbach, Owner
LS&S, LLC has a free catalog of products for the blind, deaf, visually and hearing impaired including: TTYs, computer adaptive devices, CCTVs, talking blood pressure, blood glucose and talking scales.

474 Rehabilitation Engineering and Assistive Technology Society of North America (RESNA)
1700 N Moore Street
Suite 1540
Arlington, VA 22209
703-524-6686
FAX: 703-524-6630
TTY:703-524-6639
e-mail: info@resna.org
www.resna.org

Thomas A Gorski, Executive Director
RESNA improves the potential of people with disabilities to achieve their goals through the use of technology. RESNA promotes research, development, education, advocacy and provision of technology; and by supporting the people engaged in these activities.

475 Sammons Preston Enrichments Catalog
Sammons Preston Rolyan
4 Sammons Court
Bolingbrook, IL 60440
630-226-1300
800-228-3693
FAX: 262-387-8748
e-mail: customerservice@sammonspreston.com
www.sammonspreston.com

Tony Napolitano, Director Marketing Services
Our Enrichnments Catalog offers products that make the tasks and challenges of living at home— bathing, getting dressed, getting around— a little easier. Choose from personal care items to kitchen and dining aids, household helpers to mobility devices, plus a complete selection of pain-reducing products, exercise items, health monitoring equipment and more.
40 pages Yearly

476 Sportaid
78 Bay Creek Road
Loganville, GA 30052
770-554-5033
800-743-7203
FAX: 770-554-5944
e-mail: info@sportaid.com
www.sportaid.com

Jimmy Green
Stacy Green, Owner
Offers an assortment of wheelchairs (everyday and racing), wheelchair sports equipment, replacement tires, hubs, spokes, pushrims, cushions and more. Call for free catalog.
68 pages Yearly

477 Store @ HDSC Product Catalog
Hearing, Speech & Deafness Center (HDSC)
1625 19th Avenue
Seattle, WA 98122
206-323-5770
FAX: 206-328-6871
e-mail: hsdc@hsdc.org
www.hsdc.org

Susie Burdick, Executive Director
32 pages Yearly

478 Ultratec
450 Science Drive
Madison, WI 53711
608-238-5400
800-482-2424
FAX: 608-238-3008
e-mail: service@ultratec.com
www.ultratec.com

Jackie Morgan, Director Marketing
Robert Engel, President
The world's largest manufacturer of text telephones and amplified telephones. Products include desktop TTYs with built-in printer, memory capabilities, as well as compact portable units for cellular and cordless use. Ultratec also manufactures public TTYs for pay phone accessibility.

Yearly

479 **WCI/Weitbrecht Communications**
2716 Ocean Park Boulevard
Suite 1007
Santa Monica, CA 90405
310-452-8613
800-233-9130
FAX: 310-450-9918
e-mail: sales@weitbrecht.com
www.weitbrecht.com

Donna Barwald, Sales Manager
Catalog featuring a wide range of assistive devices for the deaf, hard of hearing, mobility and speech impaired.
24 pages

480 **Walgreens Home Medical Center**
7173 Cermak Road
Berwyn, IL 60402
708-795-1295
800-323-2828
FAX: 708-795-1308

Paul Pankros RPh, Director
Stan Kozlowski, Manager
Hospital supplies and home medical equipment with nationwide direct mail delivery.

481 **Walton Way Medical**
1225 Walton Way
Augusta, GA 30901
706-722-0276
FAX: 706-722-0279

Michael Bower, President
Offers medical, therapeutic, urological, hygiene and skin care products for disabled persons.

Miscellaneous

482 **BeOK Key Lever**
Sammons Preston Rolyan
4 Sammons Court
Bolingbrook, IL 60440
630-226-1300
800-228-3693
FAX: 262-387-8748
e-mail: customerservice@sammonspreston.com
www.sammonspreston.com
Handy accessory helps position key to provide maximum leverage enabling the user to work the most stubborn lock. *$11.50*

483 **Big Lamp Switch**
Maxi Aids
42 Executive Boulevard
Farmingdale, NY 11735
631-752-0521
800-522-6294
FAX: 631-752-0689
e-mail: sales@maxiaids.com
www.maxiaids.com
This big, three-spoked knob replaces small rotating knobs which are a problem for those with arthritis or other limitations of the fingers. *$6.75*

484 **Bookholder: Roberts**
Therapro
225 Arlington Street
Framingham, MA 01702
508-872-9494
800-257-5376
FAX: 508-875-2062
e-mail: info@theraproducts.com
www.theraproducts.com

Karen Conrad, Owner
Gray plastic, ideal for hand free reading, adjusts to all sizes of books and prevents pages from flipping for the physically challenged. *$27.50*

485 **Brandt Industries**
4461 Bronx Boulevard
Bronx, NY 10470
718-994-0800
800-221-8031
FAX: 718-325-7995
e-mail: info@brandtind.com
www.brandtind.com

Neil Brandt, President
Kathy Rice, Order Expediter

486 **Bus and Taxi Sign**
Maxi Aids
42 Executive Boulevard
Farmingdale, NY 11735
631-752-0521
800-522-6294
FAX: 631-752-0689
e-mail: sales@maxiaids.com
www.maxiaids.com
Signs that the individual with a disability can use to attract the attention of bus or taxi drivers. *$3.75*

487 **Care Electronics**
4700 Sterling Drive
Suite D
Boulder, CO 80301
303-444-2273
888-444-8284
FAX: 303-447-3502
www.medicalshoponline.com

Tom Moody, President
Care Electronics manufactures safety monitoring systems for caregivers, home-health care, and nursing homes. WanderCARE monitors loved ones who tend to wander away from home. Care Deluxe Occupancy systems monitor patients in bed and in wheelchairs to help prevent falls. WetSENSE provides incontinence monitors.

488 **Child Convertible Balance Beam Set**
Bailey Manufacturing Company
118 Lee Street
Suite 130
Lodi, OH 44254
330-948-1080
800-321-8372
FAX: 330-948-4439
e-mail: baileymfg@attmail.com
www.baileymfg.com

Larry Strimple, President
This convertible set is used to develop balance in two stages.

489 **Child Variable Balance Beam**
Bailey Manufacturing Company
135 S Mount Zion Road
Lebanon, IN 46052
765-482-7775
800-321-8372
FAX: 800-224-5390
e-mail: baileymfg@attmail.com
www.baileymfg.com

Jaqueline Bailey, Owner
The four walking beams can be arranged in several different ways for variable balance training.

490 **Child's Mobility Crawler**
Bailey Manufacturing Company
118 Lee Street
Suite 130
Lodi, OH 44254
330-948-1080
800-321-8372
FAX: 330-948-4439
e-mail: baileymfg@attmail.com
www.baileymfg.com

Larry Strimple, President
Neurologically delayed or orthopedically impaired small children can perform crawling and coordination exercises while being comfortably supported by the crawler.

491 **Choice Switch Latch and Timer**
AbleNet
2808 Fairview Avenue N
Saint Paul, MN 55113
800-322-0956
FAX: 651-294-2259
e-mail: customerservice@ablenetinc.com
www.ablenetinc.com
A Choice Switch Latch and Timer allows one user to learn to make choices. It has two switch inputs and can control two devices. Once one device has been activated, the other will not function until the first one is turned off or completes its timed cycle. *$83.00*

492 **Cordless Big Red Switch**
AbleNet
2808 Fairview Avenue N
Saint Paul, MN 55113
800-322-0956
FAX: 651-294-2259
e-mail: customerservice@ablenetinc.com
www.ablenetinc.com
The Cordless Big Red Switch, when used in conjunction with either the Cordless Receiver or the Small Appliance Receiver, gives you cordless control of toys, games, and appliances in your environment. *$89.00*

493 **DEUCE Environmental Control Unit**
APT Technology
236a N Main Street
Shreve, OH 44676
330-567-2001
888-549-2001
FAX: 330-567-3073
e-mail: sales@apt-technology.com
www.apt-technology.com

Grace Miller, Office Manager
Allows a severely disabled person to control a variety of useful devices via a dual switch. DEUCE controls phone, 4 AC powered devices such as a radio, 4 switch controlled devices such as a page turner and up to 16 lights and or appliances distributed around the environment. Starts at $1,500.

494 **Dazor Manufacturing Corporation**
4483 Duncan Avenue
Saint Louis, MO 63110
314-652-2400
800-345-9103
FAX: 314-652-2069
e-mail: info@dazor.com
www.dazor.com

Kirk Cressey, Marketing Director
Bob Smith, National Sales Manager
Mark Hogrebe, President
Dazor is a US manufacturer of quality task lighting. Products include fluorescent, incandescent and halogen lighting fixtures. Illuminated magnifiers combine light and magnification to greatly enhance activities such as reading and make hobbies more enjoyable. All lamps come in a variety of mounting options to include desk bases, clamp on, floor stands and wall tracks. $95 - $450.

495 **Digi-Flex**
Therapro
225 Arlington Street
Framingham, MA 01702
508-872-9494
800-257-5376
FAX: 508-875-2062
e-mail: info@theraproducts.com
www.theraproducts.com

Karen Conrad, Owner
This is a unique hand and finger exercise unit. Recommended for use of individuation of fingers, web space and general strengthening of work hands. Available in a variety of resistances. *$ 17.50*

496 **Dorma Architectural Hardware**
PO Box Ac
Reamstown, PA 17567
800-523-8483
FAX: 717-336-2106
e-mail: archdw@dorma-usa.com
www.dorma-usa.com

Paul Kosakowski, President/CEO
Gary Phillips AHC, VP Regional Sales, East
Ken Theaker, VP Regional Sales, West
DORMA provides a complete line of door controls, including barrier-free units that comply with the Americans with Disabilities Act. A wide variety of surface applied and concealed closers, low energy operators, exit devices and electronic access control systems are available to address these equipments.

497 **Dual Switch Latch and Timer**
AbleNet
2808 Fairview Avenue N
Saint Paul, MN 55113
800-322-0956
FAX: 651-294-2259
e-mail: customerservice@ablenetinc.com
www.ablenetinc.com
A Dual Switch Latch and Timer allows two users to activate two devices at a time in the latch. Timed seconds or timed minutes mode of control. *$88.00*

498 **Foot Inversion Tread**
Bailey Manufacturing Company
118 Lee Street
Suite 130
Lodi, OH 44254
330-948-1080
800-321-8372
FAX: 330-948-4439
e-mail: baileymfg@attmail.com
www.baileymfg.com

Larry Strimple, President
Effective for correcting flat feet. These angled boards require the patient to walk on the outside of the foot instead of the arch.

499 **Foot Placement Ladder**
Bailey Manufacturing Company
118 Lee Street
Suite 130
Lodi, OH 44254
330-948-1080
800-321-8372
FAX: 330-948-4439
e-mail: baileymfg@attmail.com
www.baileymfg.com

Larry Strimple, President
Adjustable cross bars for different length steps. Reinforced metal crosses for easier climbing for the physically-disabled.

500 **Hospital Environmental Control System**
Prentke Romich Company
1022 Heyl Road
Wooster, OH 44691
330-262-1984
800-262-1984
FAX: 330-263-4829
e-mail: info@prentrom.com
www.prentrom.com

Dave Moffatt, President
Permits the non-ambulatory patient to operate a variety of electrical items in a single room. A large liquid crystal display is mounted in front of the user and they scan through the menu of operations and make a selection using a sip-puff switch. Options include nurse call, standard telephone functions, electric bed control, hospital television operation and electrical appliance on and off. *$3860.00*

501 **Knock Light**
HARC Mercantile
1111 W Centre Avenue
Portage, MI 49024
269-324-1615
800-445-9968
FAX: 269-324-2387
e-mail: info@harc.com
www.harcmercantile.com

Ronald Slager, President
Easily attaches to a door with velcro, portable. *$ 29.95*

502 Leg Elevation Board
Bailey Manufacturing Company
118 Lee Street
Suite 130
Lodi, OH 44254
330-948-1080
800-321-8372
FAX: 330-948-4439
e-mail: baileymfg@attmail.com
www.baileymfg.com

Larry Strimple, President
Includes seven positions to a 30 degree incline, three pillows with Velcro, easy carry hand slot and a natural finish.

503 Leveron
Lindustries
21 Shady Hill Road
Weston, MA 02493
781-237-8177

Willard H Lind, President/Owner
Louise T Lind, VP
Leveron is a doorknob lever handle for ease of operation. Leveron converts standard doorknobs to lever action without removing existing hardware. No gripping, twisting or pinching when hands are wet, arthritic or arms are full. Leveron provides convenience. Available in five colors: almond, satin brass, silver metallic, dark bronze and Hi-Glow (glows in the dark) at low cost to comply with ADA access requirements in public and private places. *$16.95*

504 Longreach Reacher
Therapro
225 Arlington Street
Framingham, MA 01702
508-872-9494
800-257-5376
FAX: 508-875-2062
e-mail: info@theraproducts.com
www.theraproducts.com

Karen Conrad, Owner
Reacher is useful when reaching, sitting or when standing. *$18.95*

505 Loop Scissors
Therapro
225 Arlington Street
Framingham, MA 01702
508-872-9494
800-257-5376
FAX: 508-875-2062
e-mail: info@theraproducts.com
www.theraproducts.com

Karen Conrad, Owner
Pliable, plastic handles that allow for easy and controlled cutting. *$14.25*

506 Pedal-in-Place Exerciser
Thoele Manufacturing
475 Country Road 100 North
Montrose, IL 62445
217-924-4553
FAX: 217-924-4553
www.axistive.com/thoele-manufacturing.html
A great in-home exerciser that can benefit quadraplegics, paraplegics, stroke patients or anyone with limited use of their arms and legs.

507 Plastic Card Holder
Therapro
225 Arlington Street
Framingham, MA 01702
508-872-9494
800-257-5376
FAX: 508-875-2062
e-mail: info@theraproducts.com
www.theraproducts.com

Karen Conrad, Owner
For those with reduced finger control. *$4.00*

508 Power Door
11240 Gemini Lane
Dallas, TX 75229
800-688-1758
FAX: 972-620-9875
e-mail: info@powerdoor.com
www.powerdoor.com

Jim Goldthwaite, National Sales Manager
Power door, low energy door operators.

509 ProtectaCap, ProtectaCap+PLUS, ProtectaChin Guard and ProtectaHip
Plum Enterprises
PO Box 85
Valley Forge, PA 19481
610-783-7377
800-321-PLUM
FAX: 610-783-7577
www.plument.com

Janice Carrington, President
Plum Enterprises award winning, exquiste, ergonomic protective wear keeps you safe from the dangers of falls. ProtectCap+Plus and ProtectHips are engineered for superior shock-absorption and designed for exquiste simplicity and amazing lightweight comfort. The perfect blend of style and function.

510 Quad Commander
Gpk
535 Floyd Smith Drive
El Cajon, CA 92020
619-593-7381
800-468-8679
FAX: 619-593-7514
e-mail: info@gpk.com
www.gpk.com-or-www.quadriplegia.com

Rajesh Kanwar, President
Joystick for people with quadriplegia.

511 Rocker Balance Square
Bailey Manufacturing Company
118 Lee Street
Suite 130
Lodi, OH 44254
330-948-1080
800-321-8372
FAX: 330-948-4439
e-mail: baileymfg@attmail.com
www.baileymfg.com

Larry Strimple, President
The rocker is used in developing activity, balance control and coordination.

512 Scott Sign Systems
PO Box 1047
Tallevast, FL 34270
941-355-5171
800-237-9447
FAX: 941-351-1787
e-mail: mail@scottsigns.com
www.scottsigns.com

Kathy Hannon, vice President
Call for a brochure.

513 Series Adapter
AbleNet
2808 Fairview Avenue N
Saint Paul, MN 55113
800-322-0956
FAX: 651-294-2259
e-mail: customerservice@ablenetinc.com
www.ablenetinc.com
Allows two-switch operation of any battery-operated device or electrical devices. *$13.00*

514 Signaling Wake-Up Devices
HARC Mercantile
1111 W Centre Avenue
Portage, MI 49024
269-324-1615
800-445-9968
FAX: 269-324-2387
e-mail: info@harc.com
www.harcmercantile.com

Ronald Slager, President
Wake up devices. Vibrating alarm clocks, available with flashing lights, louder alarm noises and more. *$29.50*

515 **Smoke Detector with Strobe**
HARC Mercantile
1111 W Centre Avenue
Portage, MI 49024
269-324-1615
800-445-9968
FAX: 269-324-2387
e-mail: info@harc.com
www.harcmercantile.com

Ronald Slager, President
Most of the smoke alarms are twice as loud, and have a 120+ candela strobe that will wake a person from a sound sleep. Mounting hardware for ceiling or wall. *$165.95*

516 **Spinal Network: The Total Wheelchair Reso urce Book**
Nine Lives Press

Nearly 600 pages of profiles, articles and resources on every topic of interest to wheelchair users. Subjects include health, coping, relationships, sexuality, parenthood, computers, sports, recreation, travel, personal assistance services, legal rights, financial strategies, employment, and media images. *$39.95*
586 pages 2002
ISBN 0-971522-30-8

517 **SteeleVest**
Steele
PO Box 7304
Kingston, WA 98346
360-297-4555
888-783-3538
FAX: 360-297-2816
e-mail: info@steelevest.com
www.steelevest.com

Sandra Steele, Manager
Vest developed by NASA provides an external cooling system.

518 **TV & VCR Remote**
AbleNet
2808 Fairview Avenue N
Saint Paul, MN 55113
800-322-0956
FAX: 651-294-2259
e-mail: customerservice@ablenetinc.com
www.ablenetinc.com
Controls a TV, a VCR or a TV that is connected through a VCR tuner. It may be programmed to control functions such as on and off, channel up, preprogrammed TV channels and, if desired, other TV functions such as mute and pause. *$82.00*

519 **Tactile Thermostat**
Sense-Sations
919 Walnut Street
Philadelphia, PA 19107
215-627-0600
FAX: 215-922-0692

Patricia Johnson, Chief Executive Officer
Large embossed numbers on cover ring and raised temperature setting knob. *$31.50*

520 **Therapy Putty**
Therapro
225 Arlington Street
Framingham, MA 01702
508-872-9494
800-257-5376
FAX: 508-875-2062
e-mail: info@theraproducts.com
www.theraproducts.com

Karen Conrad, Owner
Designed to exercise and strengthen hands, ranging from soft to firm for developing a stronger grasp. Available in two, four and six ounce sizes. Three ounce putty in unique clear fist shaped container.

521 **Transcription Services**
Access-USA
PO Box 160
Clayton, NY 13624
800-263-2750
FAX: 800-563-1687
e-mail: info@access-usa.com
www.access-usa.com

Deborah Haight, PICOE
Access-USA provides one-stop alternate format transcription services for almost any type of document-reports, schedules, menus, monthly statements, brochures, reports, etc. Items may be submitted on computer disk, hard copy or email. Alternate formats include Braille, large print, Braille and print, audio recordings, adapted disks as well as video services-open/closed captioning and video descriptions. Accessible products Braille Business Cards and ADA signage. Braille and print stickers.

522 **Uppertone**
535 Floyd Smith Drive
El Cajon, CA 92020
619-593-7381
800-468-8679
FAX: 619-593-7514
e-mail: sales@gpk.com
www.gpk.com

Rajesh Kanwar, President
Unassisted muscle strengthening and conditioning system for quads. *$2495.00*

523 **Visual Alerting Guest Room Kit**
HARC Mercantile
1111 W Centre Avenue
Portage, MI 49024
269-324-1615
800-445-9968
FAX: 269-324-2387
e-mail: info@harc.com
www.harcmercantile.com

Ronald Slager, President
ADA compliant visual alerting guest room kit for the hard of hearing and deaf. Includes visual smoke detector, phone alert, door knock sensor, tactile alarm clock and telephone amplifier. Variations include TTY.

524 **Window-Ease**
A-Solution
1332 Cobo Place NE
Albuquerque, NM 87106
505-256-0115
FAX: 505-256-3756
www.windowease.com

Robert Gorrell, President
Jeff Dodd, Sales
Device adapts horizontally and vertically sliding windows to ANSI A117.1 standards. 10:1 mechanical advantage at the crank arm opens a 50lb window with 5lbs force. Price ranges from $350.00-$450.00.

Office Devices & Workstations

525 **Combination File/Reference Carousel**
Center for Rehabilitation Technology
490 10th Street NW
Suite 118
Atlanta, GA 30318
404-712-5667
800-457-9555
FAX: 404-875-9409
e-mail: rerc-br@scsn.net

TW Gannaway, Executive VP
Anthony Stringer PhD
Offers two reading platforms and file holders joined on one easily rotated carousel. The carousel is easily rotated by head, mouth or handstick. Page retainer adjusts to hold open a variety of books and magazines. *$299.00*

526 **Don Johnston**
26799 W Commerce Drive
Volo, IL 60073
847-740-0749
800-999-4660
FAX: 847-740-7326
e-mail: info@donjohnston.com
www.donjohnston.com

Ruth Ziolkowski, President
A provider of quality products and services that enable people with special needs to discover their potential and experience success. Products are developed for the areas of Physical Access, Augmentative Communication and for those who struggle with reading and writing.

527 **Extensions for Independence**
555 Saturn Boulevard
Suite B-368
San Diego, CA 92154
866-632-7149
FAX: 866-632-7149
e-mail: info@mouthstick.net
www.mouthstick.net

Arthur Heyer, President
Develops, manufactures and markets special vocational equipment for the physically handicapped. Products: mouthsticks, computer mechanical aids: key locks and diskette loaders. Also, turntable desks, wheelchair portable desks, filing trays with slanted sides, telephone adapters, and motorized artist easel. All these products have been designed to solve the functional limitations of people with little or no use of hands and/or arms.

528 **Fairway Spirit Adaptive Golf Car: Model 4852**
Fairway Golf Cars
3225 Gateway Road
Suite 300
Brookfield, WI 53045
262-790-9363
888-320-4850
888-320-4850
FAX: 262-790-9396
www.fairwaygolfcars.com

John Perez, Sales and Marketing Director
Ed Gaffney, Owner
Fairway Spirit is designed to allow access to all aspects of the game of golf- even greens and tee. Spirit 4850 features a 48 volt electronic system to provide unsurpassed power, range and speed. Couple the drive system performance with ergonomic features like an adjustable seat with flip up arm rests, 360 degree swivel and an adjustable tilter position.

529 **Freedom Ryder Handcycles**
Brike International
20589 SW Elk Horn Court
Tualatin, OR 97062
503-692-1029
800-800-5828

Mike Lofgren, President
Brian Stewart, VP
The finest handcycle in the world. The cycles incorporate body, lean steering and the finest bicycle components to make this a three-wheeled vehicle without equal. Suitable for both recreation and competition. *$1995.00*

530 **Golf Xpress**
Emotorsports
4275 County Line Road 214
Chalfont, PA 18914
215-997-9555
877-494-6532
FAX: 215-997-9560
e-mail: mitch@golfxpress.com
www.golfxpress.com

Don Labowsky, President
Patented single-rider adaptive golf cart allows you to play golf seated or supported. Hit woods, irons, and putt from the car. Drives onto tees and greens and into traps without damaging the course.

531 **Infogrip: AdjustaCart**
1794 E Main Street
Ventura, CA 93001
805-652-0770
800-397-0921
e-mail: sales@infogrip.com

Liza Jacobs, President
Sit or stand while working with this easily adjustable desk. With a simple squeeze of a paddle the front surface travel range of 12 3/4. The front surface tilts 9 degrees toward and 15 degrees away from you. Anthro carts are made of 1" thick industrial grade particleboard shelves with high-pressure laminated 16 gauge steel tube legs that safely hold 150 pounds. Spring assisted mechanism. There are holes in 1: increment in the legs so that you can put the shelves and accessories where needed. *$629.00*

532 **Infogrip: BAT Personal Keyboard**
1794 E Main Street
Ventura, CA 93001
805-652-0770
800-397-0921
FAX: 805-652-0880
e-mail: sales@infogrip.com

Liza Jacobs, President
Infogrip has creative computer access solutions for people with all types of disabilities. Alternative keyboards and mice, switches, screen readers, magnifiers and educational software. We also have a retail store, Your Low Vision Store. We have three locations in Southern California offering the best selection of video magnifiers in the industry. *$200.00*

533 **Maxi Marks**
Maxi Aids
42 Executive Boulevard
Farmingdale, NY 11735
631-752-0521
800-522-6294
FAX: 631-752-0689
e-mail: sales@maxiaids.com
www.maxiaids.com
Braille writing and identification products. *$2.50*

534 **Pencil/Pen Weighted Holders**
Therapro
225 Arlington Street
Framingham, MA 01702
508-872-9494
800-257-5376
FAX: 508-875-2062
e-mail: info@theraproducts.com
www.theraproducts.com

Karen Conrad, Owner
Securely hold any pencil or pen. These weighted holders allow for more control along with proprioceptive feedback to encourage better writing skills.

535 **Perkins Brailler**
Maxi Aids
42 Executive Boulevard
Farmingdale, NY 11735
631-752-0521
800-522-6294
FAX: 631-752-0689
e-mail: sales@maxiaids.com
www.maxiaids.com
Can emboss 25 lines with 42 cells on an 11 x 11 1/2 sheet. *$495.00*

536 **PhoneMax Amplified Telephone**
Assistech
2738 N. Campbell Ave.
Tucson, AZ 85719
866-674-3549
866-674-3549
FAX: 520-883-3172
www.assistech.com

Oliver Simoes, President

537 **Raised Line Drawing Kit**
Maxi Aids
42 Executive Boulevard
Farmingdale, NY 11735
631-752-0521
800-522-6294
FAX: 631-752-0689
e-mail: sales@maxiaids.com
www.maxiaids.com
For writing script or drawing graphs by the use of special plastic paper. *$24.45*

538 **Reizen Braille Labeler**
Maxi Aids
42 Executive Boulevard
Farmingdale, NY 11735
631-752-0521
800-522-6294
FAX: 631-752-0689
e-mail: sales@maxiaids.com
www.maxiaids.com

Label everything in Braille with 3/8 or 1/2 wide labeling tape. *$47.95*

539 **Sharp Calculator with Illuminated Numbers**
Independent Living Aids
PO Box 9022
Hicksville, NY 11802
516-937-1848
800-537-2118
FAX: 516-937-3906
e-mail: can-do@independentliving.com
www.independentliving.com

Marvin Sandler, President
A trim desktop calculator with large illuminated numbers that can be carried anywhere. *$34.95*

540 **Signature and Address Self-Inking Stamps**
Independent Living Aids
PO Box 9022
Hicksville, NY 11802
516-937-1848
800-537-2118
FAX: 516-937-3906
e-mail: can-do@independentliving.com
www.independentliving.com

Marvin Sandler, President
Gives thousands of impressions before requiring re-inking. *$11.95*

541 **Steady Write**
Maxi Aids
42 Executive Boulevard
Farmingdale, NY 11735
631-752-0521
800-522-6294
FAX: 631-752-0689
e-mail: sales@maxiaids.com
www.maxiaids.com

Furnishes the writer with increased holding capacity and stabilizes the hand. *$6.95*

542 **Talking Desktop Calculators**
Maxi Aids
42 Executive Boulevard
Farmingdale, NY 11735
631-752-0521
800-522-6294
FAX: 631-752-0689
e-mail: sales@maxiaids.com
www.maxiaids.com

Unique voice synthesizers call out numerals and functions as they are keyed in or read out data stored in memory. *$467.95*

543 **Talking Electronic Organizers**
Independent Living Aids
PO Box 9022
Hicksville, NY 11802
516-937-1848
800-537-2118
FAX: 516-937-3906
e-mail: can-do@independentliving.com
www.independentliving.com

Marvin Sandler, President
Electronic, portable, personal organizers that talk the user through all the functions and are totally voice interactive. $199.95 and up.

544 **Television Remote Controls with Large Numbers**
Independent Living Aids
PO Box 9022
Hicksville, NY 11802
516-937-1848
800-537-2118
FAX: 516-937-3906
e-mail: can-do@independentliving.com
www.independentliving.com

Marvin Sandler, President
Large 5 1/2 inch x 8 1/2 inch unit that has easy to see and use buttons. Can be used on nearly every TV, VCR and cable boxes. *$39.95*

545 **Wheelchair Activity/Computer Table**
Maxi Aids
42 Executive Boulevard
Farmingdale, NY 11735
631-752-0521
800-522-6294
FAX: 631-752-0689
e-mail: sales@maxiaids.com
www.maxiaids.com

This powered height-adjustable table is a wheelchair accessible activity table or computer workstation that's as stylish as it is functional. Adjusts with the push of a button from 27-39 inches, powered by an extremely quiet motor. ADA compliant computer workstation for assistive technology and school computer labs.

Scooters

546 **Aerospace Compadre**
Aerospace America
900 Truman Parkway
Suite 189
Bay City, MI 48706
989-684-2121
800-237-6414
FAX: 989-684-4486

Murray Sutherland, President
Fully customized golf cart type vehicle for the physically impaired person. Fully equipped with hand controls, wheelchair rack, storage racks, head and tail lights and full safety belts. *$2500.00*

547 **Alante**
Golden Technologies
401 Bridge Street
Old Forge, PA 18518
570-451-7477
800-624-6374
FAX: 570-451-7494
e-mail: info@goldentech.com
www.goldentech.com

Rich Golden, CEO
Bob Golden, President
Bob Smith, VP Sales
Rear-wheel-drive vehicle that represents the best in powered mobility.

548 **Amigo Mobility International**
Amigo Mobility International
6693 Dixie Highway
Bridgeport, MI 48722
989-777-0910
800-692-6446
FAX: 800-334-7274
e-mail: info@myamigo.com
www.myamigo.com

Alison Newkirk, Sales Rep
Sandy Roth, Sales Rep
Allan Thieme, Chief Executive Officer
An industry leader in the power operated scooters, Amigo provides innovative, durable, and customized mobility solutions for the disabled, injured, and seniors worldwide. *$2495.00*

549 **Amphibious ATV Distributors**
Amphibious ATV Distributors
2760 Greendale Drive
Sarasota, FL 34232
941-379-6186
800-843-2811
FAX: 941-377-8979
e-mail: CBeach1419@aol.com
www.maxsixwheel.com

Clay Beach, Owner
A two and four passenger, all-terrain vehicle that can provide you with year round activities the whole family can enjoy. Accessible and drivable for the physically disabled. Used in hunting, fishing and outdoor activities on land and in the water. Many options and accessories available. Delivery anwyhere in the US and worldwide. $5,000-$9,000.

550 **Bravo! + Three-Wheel Scooter**
EZ-International
3275 Intertech Drive
Suite 500
Brookfield, WI 53045
262-790-5200
800-824-1068
FAX: 262-542-3990

Anne Tyler, Marketing Director
Richard Lang, Owner
Designed to increase your mobility indoors. The Bravo! plus has extendible rear wheels for outdoor use and comes with easy to use finger tip controls and a maintenance free gel-cell battery. Available in red, blue, green or light sand gray with an optional power seat lift. Call for complete line of 3 and 4-wheel electronic vehicles.

551 **Cruiser Bus Buggy 4MB**
Convaid Products
PO Box 2458
Palos Verdes Peninsula, CA 90274
310-618-0111
FAX: 310-618-8811
www.convaid.com

Mervyn Watkins, President
In sizes from infant through young adult, this positioning buggy is crash-tested.

552 **Cub, SuperCub and Special Edition Scooters**
Bruno Independent Living Aids
PO Box 84
Oconomowoc, WI 53066
262-567-4990
800-882-8183
FAX: 262-953-5501
e-mail: webmaster@bruno.com
www.bruno.com

Patrick Foy, National Sales Manager
Karla Branham Shaw, Marketing
Michael Bruno, Owner
Bruno Independent Living Aids, Inc. has over 12 different scooter models. Bruno Cub and SuperCub scooters, has front or rear-wheel drive, in both 3 and 4-wheel versions and comes in four different colors plus a pediatric version. Each scooter can handle up to 300 pounds. Bruno Special Edition scooters resemble a fire engine, police car, Humvee and motorcycle. $2,000-$5,000

553 **Electric Mobility Corporation**
PO Box 156
Sewell, NJ 08080
856-468-1000
800-257-7955
FAX: 856-468-3426
www.emobility.com

Scott Patrick, Manager
Manufactures Rascal Scooters.

554 **Explorer+ 4-Wheel Scooter**
EZ-International
3275 Intertech Drive
Brookfield, WI 53045
262-790-5200
800-824-1068
FAX: 262-790-5204
www.orthokinetics.com

Anne Tyler, Director Marketing
Richard Lang, Owner
A tough and rugged 4-wheel, rear-wheel drive, transaxle scooter designed to take you just about anywhere you want to go. Easy to use finger-tip controls and maintenance free gel-cell batteries and an extendible, take-apart frame, make the Explorer+ a perfect fit for people seeking greater mobility. Available in red, blue, green and gray, with an optional power seat lift. $3,499-$3,999.

555 **Featherlite**
No Boundaries
12882 Valley View Street
Suite 5
Garden Grove, CA 92845
714-891-5899
800-926-8637
FAX: 714-891-0658
www.noboundaries.tv

Norman Stein, Owner
Lightweight scooter folds in seconds without tools or bending down for hassle free travel on airplanes, cruise ships, trains, RVs, buses and more! Heaviest component weighs 27 pounds. Fits easily in almost any vehicle trunk.

556 **Invacare Fulfillment Center**
Invacare Corporation
1 Invacare Way
Elyria, OH 44035
440-329-6000
800-333-6900
FAX: 440-329-6568
e-mail: info@invacare.com
www.invacare.com

Susan Elder, Dir Marketing/Communications
A Mixon Iii, Chief Executive Officer
Invacare Corporation is the world's leading manufacturer and distributor of non-acute medical products which promote recovery and active lifestyles for people requiring home and other non-acute health care.

557 **Leisure Lift**
Leisure Lift
1800 Merriam Lane
Kansas City, KS 66106
800-255-0285
FAX: 913-722-2614
e-mail: leisure-lift@kc.rr.com
www.pacesaver.com

DuWayne E Kramer Jr, President
Leisure Lift offers light three wheel scooter models and seven power wheelchair models. *$2695.00*

558 **MVP+ 3-Wheel Scooter**
EZ-International
3275 Intertech Drive
Suite 500
Brookfield, WI 53045
262-790-5200
800-824-1068
FAX: 262-790-5204

Richard Land, Owner
The MVP+ is the rugged 3-wheel rear-wheel drive, transaxle scooter with finger tip controls, and featuring an extendible, take-apart frame for a perfect fit. The MVP+ comes with maintenance free gel-cell batteries and is available in red, blue, green or light sand gray, with an optional power seat lift. $2,599-$3,099.

559 **Motorized Stander**
Advanced Technology Corporation
1601 Charlotte Street
Kansas City, MO 64108
816-421-6688
800-785-9108
FAX: 816-221-8371
e-mail: advancedtech@prodigy.net

Joel Poindexter, Marketing Executive
Occupant-operated motorized vehicle that offers independence, increased mobility and ease of movement to disabled people.

560 **Moxie**
No Boundaries
12882 Valley View Street
Suite 5
Garden Grove, CA 92845
714-891-5899
800-926-8637
FAX: 714-891-0658
www.noboundaries.tv

Norman Stein, Owner
Disassembles into three parts in less than a minute. Heaviest component weighs 41 pounds. Portable, affordable and downright snazzy!

561 **Outdoor Independence**
Palmer Industries
PO Box 5707
Endicott, NY 13763
607-754-2957
800-847-1304
FAX: 607-754-1954
e-mail: palmer@palmerind.com
www.palmerind.com

Joanne Martone, Information Specialist
Lisa Carter, Sales Manager
Jack Palmer, President
The futuristic, electric three-wheeler designed to take you almost anywhere.

562 **Pace Saver Plus II**
Leisure-Lift
1800 Merriam Lane
Kansas City, KS 66106
800-255-0285

e-mail: leisure-lift@kc.rr.com
www.pacesaver.com
The scooter combines outdoor ruggedness with indoor maneuverability at a low price.

563 **Palmer Independence**
Palmer Industries
PO Box 5707
Endicott, NY 13763
607-754-2957
800-847-1304
FAX: 607-754-1954
www.palmerind.com

Lisa Carter, Manager
Jack Palmer, President
Futuristic electric outdoor three wheeler designed to take the rider almost anywhere.

564 **Palmer Twosome**
Palmer Industries
PO Box 5707
Endicott, NY 13763
607-754-2957
800-847-1304
FAX: 607-754-1954
e-mail: palmer@palmerind.com
www.palmerind.com

Joanne Martone, Information Specialist
Lisa Carter, Sales Manager
Jack Palmer, President
All electric two seat vehicle for those who can't pedal.

565 **Phantom Compact Size Scooter**
Maxi Aids
42 Executive Boulevard
Farmingdale, NY 11735
631-752-0521
800-522-6294
FAX: 631-752-0689
e-mail: sales@maxiaids.com
www.maxiaids.com
Travel in style-ideal/affordable compact scooter. Great for both indoor and outdoor use. Three wheel design allows for small 32.3 turning radius. Top speed 4 miles per hour and a cruising range of 15 miles. Large carry basket.

566 **Polaris Trail Blazer**
Polaris Industries
2100 Highway 55
Medina, MN 55340
763-542-0500
800-765-2747
www.polarisindustries.com

Bennett J Morgan, President/COO
Thomas Tiller, CEO
Michael Malone, VP
A four-wheeler that has many engineered innovations, features such as: full floorboards for full comfort, single lever breaking with auxiliary foot brake, electronic throttle control, parking brake and adjustable handlebars.

567 **Quickie 2**
Sunrise Medical/Quickie Designs
2382 Faraday Avenue
Suite 200
Carlsbad, CA 92008
760-930-1500
FAX: 760-930-1585
www.sunrisemedical.com

Michael Hammes, Chief Executive Officer
This custom, ultralight, folding, everyday scooter offers portability and performance plus modular flexibility.

568 **Rascal 3-Wheeler**
Electric Mobility Corporation
PO Box 156
Sewell, NJ 08080
856-468-1000
800-257-7955
FAX: 856-468-3426
www.emobility.com

Scott Patrick, Manager
For primarily outdoor use, this three wheeler provides extra strength, durability and reliability.

569 **Rascal ConvertAble**
Electric Mobility Corporation
PO Box 156
Sewell, NJ 08080
856-468-1000
800-257-7955
FAX: 856-468-3426
www.emobility.com

Scott Patrick, Manager
An electric vehicle that's a compact mobile chair one minute and a rugged outdoor scooter the next. Use both indoors and outdoors. Also available with joystick controls.

570 **Regal Scooters**
Bruno Independent Living Aids
1780 Executive Drive
Suite 84
Oconomowoc, WI 53066
262-567-4990
800-882-8183
FAX: 262-567-4341
e-mail: webmaster@bruno.com
www.bruno.com

Michael Bruno, Owner
This line includes the Regal Standard, the Regal Large Adult, the Regal Small Adult, the Regal Pediatric, The Regal Ten models 65 and 75, and The Regal Four. These scooters offer adjustable flip-up armrests, pneumatic tires front and rear, and more.

571 **Regent**
Golden Technologies
401 Bridge Street
Old Forge, PA 18518
570-451-7477
800-624-6374
FAX: 800-628-5165
e-mail: info@goldentech.com
www.goldentech.com

Bob Golden, President
Top-rated performance scooter, with extra features and economically priced.

572 **Roadster 20**
ATV Solutions
4700 W 60th Avenue
Unit 4
Arvada, CO 80003
303-450-2881
866-777-9727
888-867-1159
FAX: 303-450-2880
e-mail: sales@atvsolutions.com
www.atvsolutions.com

Andrew Miro, Owner
Great for indoor or outdoor use. The powerful, quiet drive system, independent front suspension and fully reclining high-back seat make for a smooth, quiet ride. The Roadster is loaded with great features at a bargain price.

573 **Safari Scooter**
Ranger All Seasons Corporation
PO Box 132
George, IA 51237
712-475-2811
800-225-3811
FAX: 712-475-3320
e-mail: sales@rangerallseason.com
www.rangerallseason.com

Randy Riecks, Sales Manager
Larry Kruse, Owner
Ranger all season Corporation is proud to introduce the "new" auto plug design. Incorporated with our patented take-apart design, it will revolutionize the scooter industry. Ranger is the first company to have this feature on scooters rated with a rider capacity up to 450 lbs. For more information, call toll free 800-225-3811.

574 **Scoota Bug**
Golden Technologies
401 Bridge Street
Old Forge, PA 18518
570-451-7477
800-624-6324
FAX: 570-451-7974
e-mail: info@goldentech.com
www.goldentech.com

Bob Golden, President
A lightweight, completely modular scooter, that disassembles and fits into most auto trunks.

575 **Sierra 3000/4000**
EZ-International
3275 Intertech Drive
Suite 500
Brookfield, WI 53045
262-790-5200
800-824-1068
FAX: 262-790-5204
e-mail: info@ez-international.com
www.ez-international.com

Richard Lang, Owner
Look to the Sierra 3000/4000 series vehicles for comfort, convenience and performance. Increased leg and foot room, adjustable seat height and arm width, as well as adjustable tiller angle provide maximum comfort. For convenience, the Sierra is equipped with integrated cargo and cup holders and thumb/finger controls with built in wrist rest. Advanced safety features such as stall and free-wheeling situation identification and correction, anti roll-back sensory device and audio/visual feedback.

576 **Solo Scooter**
Ranger All Seasons Corporation
PO Box 132
George, IA 51237
712-475-2811
800-225-3811
FAX: 712-475-3320
e-mail: sales@rangerallseason.com
www.rangerallseason.com

Randy Riecks, Sales Manager
Larry Kruse, Owner
The SOLO is Ranger's flagship model. Introduction of the SOLO 1991 set the standard for easy disassembly of a scooter. The SOLO has a long list of user friendly features including patented take-apart and tiller adjustment mechanisms, non-rusting aluminum frame, comfortable contoured seats as standard, color impregnated-not painted-ABS plastic bodies, charger plug conveniently located on the Accelerator box and many more. Available in ultra-quiet drive and four wheel models.

577 **SoloRider Industries**
7315 S Revere Parkway
Suite 604
Centennial, CO 80112
303-858-0505
800-898-3353
FAX: 303-858-0707
e-mail: info@solorider.com
www.solorider.com

Roger Pretekin, President
Don Conty, Sr VP/Marketing
Tom Durbin, VP Sales
Manufactures and distributes the AteeA- the revolutionary single rider specifically designed to meet the needs of individuals with disabilities.

578 **Sportster 10**
ATV Solutions
4700 W 60th Avenue
Unit 4
Arvada, CO 80003
303-450-2881
866-777-9727
888-867-1159
FAX: 303-450-2880
e-mail: sales@atvsolutions.com
www.atvsolutions.com

Andrew Miro, Owner
Sportster 10 is our most maneuverable scooter, ideal for riders who must operate in tight spaces. Equipped with all of the great features of the Roadster 20, this three-wheeler is an exceptional buy.

579 **Systems 2000**
BioMedical Life Systems
PO Box 1360
Vista, CA 92085
760-727-5600
800-726-8367
FAX: 760-727-4220
e-mail: information@bmls.com
www.bmls.com

Richard Saxon, Chief Executive Officer
This five-mode TENS device has four adjustable modulations, plus conventional settings and comes with a five-year warranty.

580 **Terra-Jet: Utility Vehicle**
TERRA-JET USA
PO Box 918
Innis, LA 70747
225-492-2249
800-864-5000
FAX: 225-492-2249
e-mail: terra.jet@terra.jet.com
terra.jet.com

Larry Rabalaus, President
Michelle Radalais, Secretary/Treasurer
TERRA-JET utility vehicles are unique in their ability to traverse many different types of terrain in remote areas otherwise inaccessible. It has a multitude of uses for industry, sportsmen or the whole family. Uniquely designed, industrial duty construction of low maintenance and low fuel consumption. $8,675-$21,995.

581 **Terrier Tricycle**
TRIAID
PO Box 1364
Cumberland, MD 21501
301-759-3525
800-306-6777
FAX: 301-759-3525
e-mail: sales@triaid.com
www.triaid.com

Iain A MacDonald, Sales Director
Ann M Hutter, Sales Executive/Manager
Provides fun therapy and actively encourages participation, awareness and the building of self confidence. Designed for children from about five years it features ATB styling, 16 inch wheels, adjustable steering stop and a supportive saddle. Handlebar and seat adjustments combine with a broad wheelbase to ensure the rider is in the optimum position to pedal and the tricycle gives good stability and confident handling. Support accessories are available.

582 **Trekker 40**
ATV Solutions
4700 W 60th Avenue
Unit 4
Arvada, CO 80003
303-450-2881
866-777-9727
888-867-1159
FAX: 303-450-2880
e-mail: sales@atvsolutions.com
www.atvsolutions.com

Andrew Miro, Owner
Our biggest, toughest scooter. With a huge 450 pound capacity and five inches of ground clearance, this machine is ideal for the daily outdoor user. The high top speed means you get there fast and the four-wheel suspension makes the ride smooth and comfortable.

583 **Tri-Lo's**
TRIAID
PO Box 1364
Cumberland, MD 21501
301-759-3525
800-306-6777
FAX: 301-759-3525
e-mail: sales@triaid.com
www.triaid.com

Iain A MacDonald, Sales Director
Ann M Hutter, Sales Executive/Manager
Available in three sizes, these tricycles provide fun therapy for children from 2-15 years. Propelled by hand cranks, the Tri-Lo's are highly recommended by therapists for spina bifida children and any other child where the use of the lower limbs is restricted. The Tri-Lo's feature a robust frame with allowance for growth, low foot platform for ease of transfer, padded seat and back cushion, padded armrests, two forms of braking and an anti-tipping device. *$740.00*

584 **Tri-Wheelers**
Braun Corporation
PO Box 310
Winamac, IN 46996
574-946-6153
800-843-5438
FAX: 574-946-4670

William Roth, President
Provides convenience features, producing a high efficiency performance with ultra-smooth operation.

585 **Triumph 3000/4000**
EZ-International
3275 Intertech Drive
Suite 500
Brookfield, WI 53045
262-790-5200
800-824-1068
FAX: 262-790-5204

Richard Lang, Owner
The Triumph 3000/4000 series vehicles provide unique comfort and convenience features found nowhere else. Digital Dash with soft touch keypad, deluxe seat with suspension and integral cargo and cup holders are just a few of these features. Equipped with TOPS 24 (Total Ortho Power System) ensuring maximum power, performance and reliability. Luxurious options such as velour or allante seat fabrics, stylized wheels, metallic or pearl color options and digital controls are all standard. $2,899-$3,39

586 **Triumph Scooter**
EZ-International
3275 Intertech Drive
Suite 500
Brookfield, WI 53045
262-790-5200
800-824-1068
FAX: 262-790-5204
e-mail: info@ez-international.com
www.ez-international.com

Richard Lang, Owner
The sleek, rugged, three-wheel, rear-wheel drive, transaxle scooter with up-top controls, designed to help increase mobility and become more active. The Triumph is designed for both indoor and outdoor use. Available in red, blue, green or gray, with an optional power seat lift. $2,899-$3,399.

Stationery

587 **Address Book**
Sense-Sations
919 Walnut Street
Philadelphia, PA 19107
215-627-0600
FAX: 215-922-0692

Patricia Johnson, Chief Executive Officer
The big print address book is the first personal book to provide enlarged writing spaces, making it easier to write down and retrieve information. *$12.50*

588 **Big Print Address Book**
Access with Ease
PO Box 1150
Chino Valley, AZ 86323
928-636-9469
800-531-9479
FAX: 928-636-0292
e-mail: KMJC@northlink.com

Karen Clymer, President
Oversized organizer makes locating information easier for those with limited vision. The 7 1/2 inch by 9 1/2 inch plastic coil bound book has more than 500 listings with laminated alphabet tabs. *$16.95*

589 **Bold Line Paper**
Sense-Sations
919 Walnut Street
Philadelphia, PA 19107
215-627-0600
FAX: 215-922-0692

Patricia Johnson, Chief Executive Officer
This pad consists of 100 sheets of paper with bold lines to help guide the writing of an individual with limited vision. *$2.50*

590 **Braille Notebook**
Maxi Aids
42 Executive Boulevard
Farmingdale, NY 11735
631-752-0521
800-522-6294
FAX: 631-752-0689
e-mail: sales@maxiaids.com
www.maxiaids.com
Made of heavy-duty board, covered with waterproof imitation leather and three rings for binding, including braille paper and titles. *$12.95*

591 **Braille: Desk Calendar**
Maxi Aids
42 Executive Boulevard
Farmingdale, NY 11735
631-752-0521
800-522-6294
FAX: 631-752-0689
e-mail: sales@maxiaids.com
www.maxiaids.com
Schedule appointments, remember birthdays or write messages for a particular day. *$39.95*

592 **Braille: Greeting Cards**
Sense-Sations
919 Walnut Street
Philadelphia, PA 19107
215-627-0600
FAX: 215-922-0692

Patricia Johnson, Chief Executive Officer
Birthday, anniversary, get well, sympathy and Christmas cards offering braille print for the blind. *$.95*

593 **Clip Board Notebook**
Sense-Sations
919 Walnut Street
Philadelphia, PA 19107
215-627-0600
FAX: 215-922-0692

Patricia Johnson, Chief Executive Officer
Kit includes a pack of Bold Line paper and black ink pen. *$5.95*

594 **Deluxe Signature Guide**
Maxi Aids
42 Executive Boulevard
Farmingdale, NY 11735
631-752-0521
800-522-6294
FAX: 631-752-0689
e-mail: sales@maxiaids.com
www.maxiaids.com
Rods supported by two rubber blocks facilitate writing. *$1.25*

595 **Highlighter and Note Tape**
Therapro
225 Arlington Street
Framingham, MA 01702
508-872-9494
800-257-5376
FAX: 508-875-2062
e-mail: info@theraproducts.com
www.theraproducts.com

Karen Conrad, Owner
A great way to highlight and draw attention to words without damaging original. Price ranges from $4.00-$7.00.

596 **Letter Writing Guide**
Independent Living Aids
PO Box 9022
Hicksville, NY 11802
516-937-1848
800-537-2118
FAX: 516-937-3906
e-mail: can-do@independentliving.com
www.independentliving.com

Marvin Sandler, President
Sturdy plastic sheet with 13 apertures corresponding to standard line spacing. *$3.49*

597 **Lettering Guide Value Pack**
Independent Living Aids
PO Box 9022
Hicksville, NY 11802
516-937-1848
800-537-2118
FAX: 516-937-3906
e-mail: can-do@independentliving.com
www.independentliving.com

Marvin Sandler, President
Included in this useful pack are four durable plastic lettering and number guides for tracing letters when the individual is unable to write letters unassisted. *$6.29*

Visual Aids

598 **Aluminum Adjustable Support Canes for the Blind**
Maxi Aids
42 Executive Boulevard
Farmingdale, NY 11735
631-752-0521
800-522-6294
FAX: 631-752-0689
e-mail: sales@maxiaids.com
www.maxiaids.com
Adjustable canes for the visually impaired. *$17.95*

599 **Audio Book Contractors**
PO Box 40115
Washington, DC 20016
202-363-3429
FAX: 202-363-3429
e-mail: flogibsonABC@aol.com
www.audiobookcontractors.com

Flo Gibson, President
Over 950 titles of unabridged classic books on audio cassettes in sturdy vinyl covers with picture and spine windows. Discounted prices for disabled patrons.

600 **Beyond Sight, Inc.**
5650 S Windermere Street
Littleton, CO 80120
303-795-6455
FAX: 303-795-6425
e-mail: jim@beyondsight.com
www.beyondsight.com

Jim Misener, President
Products for the blind and visually impaired including talking clocks, watches and calculators. They also carry a large selection of braille products, magnifiers, reading machines and computer equipment. New products include: Accucheck Voicemate and PureFocus vision spray and GPS Talk, the first talking GPS system for the blind.

601 **Big Number Pocket Sized Calculator**
Independent Living Aids
PO Box 9022
Hicksville, NY 11802
516-937-1848
800-537-2118
FAX: 516-937-3906
e-mail: can-do@independentliving.com
www.independentliving.com

Marvin Sandler, President
A handy pocket size calculator with big numbers that fits easily into purse or pocket. *$14.95*

602 **Braille Compass**
Maxi Aids
42 Executive Boulevard
Farmingdale, NY 11735
631-752-0521
800-522-6294
FAX: 631-752-0689
e-mail: sales@maxiaids.com
www.maxiaids.com
The visually impaired can tell the direction by using this compass. *$42.95*

603 **Braille Plates for Elevator**
Maxi Aids
42 Executive Boulevard
Farmingdale, NY 11735
631-752-0521
800-522-6294
FAX: 631-752-0689
e-mail: sales@maxiaids.com
www.maxiaids.com
The plates have curing type pressure sensitive material applied for metal to metal bonding. *$79.95*

604 **Braille Touch-Time Watches**
Independent Living Aids
PO Box 9022
Hicksville, NY 11802
516-937-1848
800-537-2118
FAX: 516-937-3906
e-mail: can-do@independentliving.com
www.independentliving.com

Marvin Sandler, President
White dial with black numerals and hands makes telling time possible quickly and easily for the visually impaired. *$44.95*

605 **Circline Illuminated Magnifer**
Dazor Manufacturing Corporation
11721 Dunlap Industrial Drive
Maryland Heights, MO 63043
314-652-2400
800-345-9103
FAX: 314-652-2069
e-mail: info@dazor.com
www.dazor.com

Kirk Cressey, Marketing Director
Bob Smith, National Sales Manager
Provides even, shadow free light under the magnifying lens with a 22-watt circline fluorescent. The magnifier is mounted on a floating arm that allows you to position the light source and lens with the touch of a finger.

606 **Extra Loud Alarm with Lighter Plug**
HARC Mercantile
1111 W Centre Avenue
Portage, MI 49024
269-324-1615
800-445-9968
FAX: 269-324-2387
e-mail: info@harc.com
www.harcmercantile.com

Ronald Slager, President
Battery operated, easy to read, digital clock with extra loud alarm. *$45.00*

607 **Low Vision Telephones**
2738 N. Campbell Ave.e
Tucson, AZ 85719
520-883-8600
866-674-3549
FAX: 520-883-3172
e-mail: info@assistivedevices.net
assistivedevices.net/about.htm

Oliver Simeos, President

608 **Magni-Cam & Primer**
Innoventions
9593 Corsair Drive
Conifer, CO 80433
303-797-6554
800-854-6554
FAX: 303-727-4940
e-mail: magnicam@magnicam.com
www.magnicam.com/

Charleen Freeman, Sales Manager
Mark Freeman, President
Magni-Cam and Primer are hand-held, light weight, inexpensive auto-focus electronic magnification systems designed to meet the reading and writing needs of those with low vision. The systems present the image in black and white or in color with three different view modes. Connects to any TV monitor in minutes. Systems read any surface with no distortion. A battery powered system is available, providing total portability and flexibility.

609 **Magnifier Bookweight**
Levenger
420 South Congress Avenuenue
Delray Beach, FL 33445
561-276-4141
800-667-8034
FAX: 800-544-6910
e-mail: cservice@levenger.com
www.levenger.com
The Magnifier Bookweight features an optical quality magnifier and is long enough to enlarge the full width of most book pages while holing the pages open. This magnifier is encased in embossed leather and enlarges approximately four lines of text at a time to twice the original size.

610 **Man's Low-Vision Quartz Watches**
Independent Living Aids
PO Box 9022
Hicksville, NY 11802
516-937-1848
800-537-2118
FAX: 516-937-3906
e-mail: can-do@independentliving.com
www.independentliving.com

Marvin Sandler, President
An inexpensive, easy-to-read watch with chrome case. *$27.95*

611 **Men's/Women's Low Vision Watches & Clocks**
Maxi Aids
42 Executive Boulevard
Farmingdale, NY 11735
631-752-0521
800-522-6294
FAX: 631-752-0689
e-mail: sales@maxiaids.com
www.maxiaids.com
Choose from a wide range of watches from braille automatic to quartz pocket watches.

612 **MonoMouse Electronic Magnifiers**
Maxi Aids
42 Executive Boulevard
Farmingdale, NY 11735
631-752-0521
800-522-6294
FAX: 631-752-0689
e-mail: sales@maxiaids.com
www.maxiaids.com
Simple and affordable magnifier for people with Low Vision. Just about the size of a standard computer mouse. Allows you to read books, newspapers, product labels, etc. on either a computer or TV screen.

613 **Rigid Aluminum Cane with Golf Grip**
Maxi Aids
42 Executive Boulevard
Farmingdale, NY 11735
631-752-0521
800-522-6294
FAX: 631-752-0689
e-mail: sales@maxiaids.com
www.maxiaids.com
A straight, tubular, heavy gauge aluminum rigid cane for blind and visually impaired persons. *$12.95*

614 **Stretch-View Wide-View Rectangular Illuminated Magnifier**
Dazor Manufacturing Corporation
11721 Dunlap Industrial Drive
Maryland Heights, MO 63043
314-652-2400
800-345-9103
FAX: 314-652-2069
e-mail: info@dazor.com
www.dazor.com

Kirk Cressey, Marketing Director
Bob Smith, National Sales Manager
Provides shadow-free illumination or a highlighting effect under the magnifying lens with an 18-watt compact fluorescent light source. The magnifier is mounted on a floating arm that allows you to position the light source and lens with the touch of a finger.

615 **Timex Easy Reader**
Independent Living Aids
PO Box 9022
Hicksville, NY 11802
516-937-1848
800-537-2118
FAX: 516-937-3906
e-mail: can-do@independentliving.com
www.independentliving.com

Marvin Sandler, President
An easy-to-read large face watch that's water resistant. *$29.95*

616 **Unisex Low Vision Watch**
Independent Living Aids
PO Box 9022
Hicksville, NY 11802
516-937-1848
800-537-2118
FAX: 516-937-3906
e-mail: can-do@independentliving.com
www.independentliving.com

Marvin Sandler, President
Unisex watch with large numbers and wide hands. Gold-toned case with either expansion or leather band. *$31.95*

Walking Aids: Canes, Crutches & Walkers

617 **Air Lift Oxygen Carriers**
Air Lift Unlimited
1212 Kerr Gulch Road
Evergreen, CO 80439
303-526-4700
800-776-6771
FAX: 303-526-4774
e-mail: info@airlift.com
www.airlift.com

Lori Fortier, Office Manager
Michael Moore, President
Air Lift offers a full line of carriers for portable liquid and cylinder oxygen systems. These versatile carriers meet the needs of oxygen-dependent individuals and parents with oxygen-dependent children seeking more comfortable and convenient ways to transport oxygen. Carriers include backpacks, fanny packs, shoulder/hand bags and carriers for wheelchairs, scooters and walkers. All carriers feature non-flammable, washable fabric and adjustable straps; liquid carriers feature mesh pouches.

618 **Aluminum Crutches**
Arista Surgical Supply Company
297 High Street
Dedham, MA 02026
781-329-2900
800-223-1984
FAX: 781-329-8392
e-mail: arista@alimed.com
www.aristasurgical.com

Julian Cherubini, President
Lightweight aluminum crutches with wood underarms and handgrips. *$25.00*

619 **Aluminum Walking Canes**
Maxi Aids
42 Executive Boulevard
Farmingdale, NY 11735
631-752-0521
800-522-6294
FAX: 631-752-0689
e-mail: sales@maxiaids.com
www.maxiaids.com
Lightweight but strong, these walking canes are made of a heavy gauge aluminum tube with safety locknuts and heavy-duty rubber tips. *$10.75*

620 **Crutches**
Mada Medical Products
625 Washington Avenue
Carlstadt, NJ 07072
201-460-0454
800-526-6370
FAX: 201-460-3509
e-mail: dianelind@mail.madamedical.com
www.madainternational.com

Jeffrey Adam, Vice President
All aluminum construction, underarm crutch with double pushbutton height adjustment.

621 **Deluxe Nova Wheeled Walker & Avant Wheeled Walker**
Sammons Preston Rolyan
W68n158 Evergreen Boulevard
Cedarburg, WI 53012
800-323-5547
FAX: 262-387-8748
e-mail: customersupport@sammonspreston.com
www.sammonspreston.com
Lightweight and simple to handle with an easy-to-operate braking system. *$425.40*

622 **Deluxe Standard Wood Cane**
Arista Surgical Supply Company/AliMed
297 High Street
Dedham, MA 02026
781-329-2900
800-223-1984
FAX: 781-329-8392
e-mail: arista@alimed.com
www.aristasurgical.com

Julian Cherubini, President
A standard old-fashioned wooden cane for the physically challenged. *$10.00*

623 **EasyStand 6000 Glider**
Access To Recreation
8 Sandra Court
Newbury Park, CA 91320
805-498-7535
800-634-4351
FAX: 805-498-8186
e-mail: customerservice@accesstr.com
www.accesstr.com

Don Krebs, President
Provides dynamic leg motion for individuals who are unable to stand upright or walk on their own.

624 **Freedom Three Wheel Walker**
Mada Medical Products
625 Washington Avenue
Carlstadt, NJ 07072
201-460-0454
800-526-6370
FAX: 201-460-3509
e-mail: dianelind@mail.madamedical.com
www.madainternational.com

Jeffrey Adam, Vice President
The freedom walker has ultra light touch, locking loop brakes and sure grip hand grips.

625 **Liberty Lightweight Aluminum Stroll Walker**
Mada Medical Products
625 Washington Avenue
Carlstadt, NJ 07072
201-460-0454
800-526-6370
FAX: 201-460-3509
e-mail: dianelind@mail.madamedical.com
www.madainternational.com

Jeffrey Adam, Vice President
The Liberty walker has a spring loaded push down braking system, adjustable handle height with locking system, a 12" wide fully padded seat, and a removable shopping basket.

626 **Maxi Superior Cane**
Maxi Aids
42 Executive Boulevard
Farmingdale, NY 11735
631-752-0521
800-522-6294
FAX: 631-752-0689
e-mail: sales@maxiaids.com
www.maxiaids.com
Convenient folding cane designed for optimum balance. Tapered joints provide rigidity when open, and are made of heavy gauge aluminum. *$17.50*

627 **Out-N-About American Walker**
742 Market Street
Oregon, WI 53575
608-835-9255
FAX: 608-835-5234

Luann Smith, President
The lightweight Out-N-About is easy to handle. The four wheel design provides greater support and stability than any other walking aids. Its large rubber tires move effortlessly over most surfaces, indoors and out. The small turning radius makes it ideal for getting through confined spaces and narrow doorways. The attractive, burgundy colored, tubular steel frame is extremely durable. The Out-N-About folds flat and stands alone for easy storage. Made in USA.

628 **Patriot Extra Wide Folding Walkers**
Mada Medical Products
625 Washington Avenue
Carlstadt, NJ 07072
201-460-0454
800-526-6370
FAX: 201-460-3509
e-mail: dianelind@mail.madamedical.com
www.madainternational.com

Jeffrey Adam, Vice President
The extra wide walkers have padded foam hand grips, two-stage push button folding mechanism, dual width adjustment, height adjustment, and nonskid tips.

629 **Patriot Folding Walker Series**
Mada Medical Products
625 Washington Avenue
Carlstadt, NJ 07072
201-460-0454
800-526-6370
FAX: 201-460-3509
e-mail: dianelind@mail.madamedical.com
www.madainternational.com

Jeffrey Adam, Vice President
The patriot walker has high density, padded foam hand grips, high strength 1" lightweight, anodized, dull silver aluminum tube construction, adjustable height with push-button lock security, nonskid tips, and a single button folding mechanism.

630 **Patriot Reciprocal Folding Walkers**
Mada Medical Products
625 Washington Avenue
Carlstadt, NJ 07072
201-460-0454
800-526-6370
FAX: 201-460-3509
e-mail: dianelind@mail.madamedical.com
www.madainternational.com

Jeffrey Adam, Vice President
The reciprocal folding walkers have padded foam hand grips, adjustable height with snap-in security, double front cross brace, and nonskid tips.

631 **Prone Support Walker**
Consumer Care Products
PO Box 684
Sheboygan, WI 53082
920-893-4614
FAX: 920-459-9070

Terry Grall, President
Alice Maffongelli, Customer Service

This walker, in five sizes for children to adults, facilitates semi-prone to full upright mobility and dynamic weight bearing. The walker requires the user to push off the floor teaching the user to work with the floor and achieving a more efficient gait. Options such as tray, back support, and hip pads allow adaptation to most needs. $750-$1,300.

632 Push-Button Quad Cane
Arista Surgical Supply Company/AliMed
297 High Street
Dedham, MA 02026
781-329-2900
800-223-1984
FAX: 781-329-8392
e-mail: arista@alimed.com
www.aristasurgical.com

Julian Cherubini, President
A reliable walking cane offering independence to the physically challenged user. *$25.00*

633 Quad Canes
Mada Medical Products
625 Washington Avenue
Carlstadt, NJ 07072
201-460-0454
800-526-6370
FAX: 201-460-3509
e-mail: dianelind@mail.madamedical.com
www.madainternational.com

Jeffrey Adam, Vice President
There are large and small base quad canes with high density foam grips.

634 Rand-Scot
401 Linden Center Drive
Fort Collins, CO 80524
970-484-7967
800-467-7967
FAX: 970-484-3800
TTY: 800-467-7967
e-mail: info@randscot.com
www.randscot.com

Joel Lerich, President
Ed Kalin, Sales Marketing Director
Erin Thames, Materials Manager
Manufactures the Easy Pivot patient lift, the BBD wheelchair cushion line and Saratoga Exercise products for the disabled. Offers a line of patient lifts and standers for the disabled. Rand-scot products are designed to help the disabled acheive independence, comfort, and stamina. A video or dvd is available at no charge for potential users, $800-$3,000.

635 Secret Agent Walking Stick
Gold Violin
1717-2B Allied Streetreet
Suite I
Charlottesville, VA 22903
434-923-3277
877-648-8400
www.goldviolin
The Secret Agent Walking Stick features a built-in flashlight, a red reflector and a built-in secret pill compartment. this folding aluminum cane is height adjustable and has a derby-style handle and a non-skid rubber tip. A nylon carrying case is included. The walking stick comes in a choich of gold, bronze, or black shaft with a faux burled walnut handle.

636 StairClimber
Martin Technology
29 N Main Street
Gloversville, NY 12078
518-725-1837
800-800-1410
FAX: 518-725-9522

Michael Lewy, Owner
A walker-capable person can climb and descend stairs with this walker-designed StairClimber.

637 Standing Aid Frame with Rear Entry
Consumer Care Products
PO Box 684
Sheboygan, WI 53082
920-893-4614
FAX: 920-459-9070

Terry Grall, President
Alice Maffongelli, Customer Service

This rugged stander, made of natural hardwood in sizes for one to twelve year olds, allows weight bearing in an upright position. Table, upper trunk and/or head support, hip pads and casters allow individualized fitting. The new hinged rear entry option makes entry into this stander easy and quick for parents, teachers and therapists. $572-$1,800.

638 Stick Canes
Mada Medical Products
625 Washington Avenue
Carlstadt, NJ 07072
201-460-0454
800-526-6370
FAX: 201-460-3509
e-mail: dianelind@mail.madamedical.com
www.madainternational.com

Jeffrey Adam, Vice President
Mada's stick canes are adjustable with a locking security system.

639 Torso Support
Grandmar
5675-C Landregan Street
Emeryville, CA 94608
510-428-0441

John Cains, President
An aid for people who are unable to maintain an upright position in an automobile or a wheelchair.

640 Ventura Enterprises
35 Lawton Avenue
Danville, IN 46122
317-745-2989
FAX: 317-745-3179
www.venturaenterprises.com

Linda Plunkett, President
Manufacturer of everyday living mobility aids. Products include carrying aids for walkers and wheelchairs and also wheelchair cushions.

641 WCIB Heavy-Duty Folding Cane
Maxi Aids
42 Executive Boulevard
Farmingdale, NY 11735
631-752-0521
800-522-6294
FAX: 631-752-0689
e-mail: sales@maxiaids.com
www.maxiaids.com
A four section aluminum folding cane with a golf-type grip handle and flexible wrist loop. Available in 34-60 lengths. *$17.95*

642 Walker Leg Support
Sammons Preston Rolyan
W68n158 Evergreen Boulevard
Cedarburg, WI 53012
800-228-3693
FAX: 262-387-8748
e-mail: customerservice@sammonspreston.com
www.sammonspreston.com
For lower extremity trauma. An alternative to crutches that allows safe, stable ambulation and frees hands and arms for daily tasks. *$11.50*

Wheelchairs: Accessories

643 Advantage Wheelchair & Walker Bags
Laurel Designs
1805 Mar West Street
Apt A
Belvedere Tiburon, CA 94920
FAX: 415-435-1451
e-mail: laureld@ncal.verio.com

Janet Sawyer, Co-Owner
Lynn Montoya, Co-Owner
Wheelchair sport packs include: long, short, neon, multi-color and blowin' in the wind socks. Prices range from $20.00 to $60.00.

644 **Automatic Wheelchair Anti-Rollback Device**
Alzheimer's Store
Ageless Design
3197 Trout Place Road
Cumming, GA 30041
678-947-4001
800-752-3238
FAX: 678-947-8411
e-mail: cs@alzstore.com
www.alzstore.com

As a wheelchair user transfers to and from the chair, a pair of brake arms grabs the tires to prevent the chair from rolling backwards. Once the individual is seated, the device switches to stand-by modeand the wheelchair returns to standard funcion.

645 **Battery Operated Cushion**
DA Schulman
7701 Newton Avenue N
Brooklyn Park, MN 55444
763-561-2908

Battery-operated, dynamic cushion for wheelchairs.

646 **Dual-Mode Charger**
Lester Electrical
625 W a Street
Lincoln, NE 68522
402-477-8988
FAX: 402-474-1769
e-mail: sales@lesterelectrical.com
www.lesterelectrical.com

Ken Jeffcoat, Director Sales/Marketing
Bob Haahr, Cust Service Manager
James Carrier, President
Fully automatic battery charger.

647 **Equalizer 1000 Series**
Helm Distributing
1516 Nicholas Road
Dayton, OH 45418
937-268-7415
FAX: 937-268-9525
e-mail: info@helmdistributing.com
www.helmdistributing.com

Pruett B Helm, President and Owner
Weight training equipment designed with the wheelchair user in mind. *$7050.00*

648 **Equalizer 5000 Home Gym**
Helm Distributing
1516 Nicholas Road
Dayton, OH 45418
937-268-7415
FAX: 937-268-9525
e-mail: info@helmdistributing.com
www.helmdistributing.com

Bob Helm, President
Exercise machine for the able-bodied and the disabled, but specifically designed with a wheelchair user in mind. *$4250.00*

649 **Featherspring**
712 N 34th Street
Seattle, WA 98103
206-545-8585
FAX: 206-547-8589
www.featherspring.com

Peter Rothschild, President
Foot supports for wheelchair users to prevent and treat cold feet, sore heels, swollen feet and weak ankles. *$199.95*

650 **Lifestand**
Frank Mobility Systems
1003 International Drive
Oakdale, PA 15071
724-695-7822
888-426-8581
FAX: 724-695-3710
e-mail: Dallery@msn.com
www.lifestandusa.com

Jacques A Dallery, President
Werner Frank, Owner
Lifestand offers a full line of standing wheelchairs for manual operation. Power assisted are fully motorized. *$7000.00*

651 **Mat Factory**
760 W 16th Street
Bldg E
Costa Mesa, CA 92627
949-645-3122
800-628-7626
FAX: 949-645-0966
e-mail: info@matfactoryinc.com
www.matfactoryinc.com

Roger Maloney, President
Peggy Maloney, Owner
The Safety Deck II is an interlocking grid system made from recycled rubber tires and recycled PVC. The tiles are set directly on top of the ground and permit grass to grow through the holes and cover the surface. The system provides safe, non-barrier access for wheelchairs over grass. Once the grass has covered the tiles the only maintenance required is watering and mowing. Safety Deck II also allows for beach and sand access.

652 **One Thousand FS**
Fortress
PO Box 489
Clovis, CA 93613
559-322-5437
FAX: 559-323-0299

Add-on power system installs in minutes, enabling the driver to relax and drive anywhere with smooth, silent electric power.

653 **Pac-All Wheelchair Carrier**
Pac-All Carriers
2321 Carolton Road
Maitland, FL 32751
407-830-6604
800-628-6672
FAX: 407-339-2847

LE Angel
No more lifting and no more pain wheelchair carrier. VA approved. Made in USA.
$158 - $226.40

654 **Scooter & Wheelchair Battery Fuel Gauges and Motor Speed Controllers**
Curtis Instruments
200 Kisco Avenue
Mount Kisco, NY 10549
914-666-2971
FAX: 914-666-2188
e-mail: mikolaya@curtisinst.com
www.curtisinstruments.com

Stuart Marwell, Chief Executive Officer
Provides a readable, accurate indication of battery in easy to read type of display. Innovative, efficient motor speed controllers for single or dual PM motor vehicles.

655 **Tilt-N-Table**
Osterguard Enterprises c/o Jim's Shop
3228 W Olive Avenue
Fresno, CA 93722
559-275-4695

Jim Ii, Owner
These are lightweight tables for wheelchairs that are angle and height adjustable to your changing needs.

656 **Wheel Life News**
University of Virginia, Rehab Engineering Centers
3363 University Station
Charlottesville, VA 22903
434-924-0311

John Casteen Iii, President
Features tie downs and other adaptive technology for persons with disabilities.

657 **Wheelchair Accessories**
Diestco Manufacturing Company
PO Box 6504
Chico, CA 95927
530-893-3136
800-795-2392
FAX: 530-893-2635
e-mail: info@diestco.com
www.diestco.com

Chris Cawthon, VP Sales/Marketing
Dan Diestel, Owner

Diestco makes innovative accessories for wheelchairs, scooters and walkers. Products include canopies, backpacks, cupholders, pouches, threshhold ramps, laptrays and others.

658 Wheelchair Aide
Graham-Field
400 Rabro Drive
Hauppauge, NY 11788 631-348-1364

This is a heavy-duty wheelchair comfort tray which surrounds the wheelchair user and provides a large, smooth surface for dining, writing, hobbies or work. The heavy gauge plastic tray is easy to clean and attaches with two Velcro straps.

659 Wheelchair Back Pack and Tote Bag
Med Covers
1639 Green Street
Suite D
Raleigh, NC 27603 919-829-5777

Accessories are specifically designed with the wheelchair user in mind. The Back Pack has a main roomy pouch for larger items and has a full length zipper with four sliders for convenient access.

660 Wheelchair Roller
Access To Recreation
8 Sandra Court
Newbury Park, CA 91320 805-498-7535
800-634-4351
FAX: 805-498-8186
e-mail: customerservice@accesstr.com
www.accesstr.com

Don Krebs, President
The McClain Wheelchair Roller allows you to build strength and stamina in the comfort of your own home.

661 Wheelchair Work Table
Bailey Manufacturing Company
118 Lee Street
Lodi, OH 44254 330-948-1080
800-321-8372
FAX: 330-948-4439
e-mail: baileymfg@attmail.com
www.baileymfg.com

Larry Strimple, President
An adjustable height, functional, individual cut-out work table featuring a wood-grain laminate, scratch resistant top with chrome plated steel legs.

Wheelchairs: General

662 Bariatric Wheelchairs Regency FL
Gendron
Lugbill Road
Archbold, OH 43502 419-445-6060
800-537-2521
www.gendroninc.com

Steven Cotter, VP Sales/President
Bariatric wheelchairs, for users weighing up to seven hundred pounds. Manual and power styles built to order for specific needs.

663 Big Bounder Power Wheelchair
21st Century Scientific, Inc
4915 Industrial Way
Coeur D Alene, ID 83815 208-667-8800
800-448-3680
FAX: 208-667-6600
e-mail: 21st@wheelchairs.com
www.wheelchairs.com

RD Davidson, Sales/Marketing Director
Ron Prior, Owner
Manufactured for the bariatric in virtually any dimension. Its powerful motors and rugged frame can accommodate users up to 1000 lb. 21st Century Scientific, Inc's unique construction can reduce the overall width of the chair. This may make the difference between using normal doorways or remodeling a home. $10,695.

664 Breezy
Sunrise Medical/Quickie Designs
2382 Faraday Avenue
Carlsbad, CA 92008 760-930-1500
FAX: 760-930-1585
www.sunrisemedical.com

Michael Hammes, Chief Executive Officer
This lightweight chair is durable, comfortable and flexible enough to meet the needs of a wide range of wheelchair users.

665 Champion 1000
Kuschall of America
3601 Rider Trail S
Earth City, MO 63045 314-512-7000
800-654-4768
FAX: 800-542-3567
Ultralight wheelchair designed to improve mobility. $1,689

666 Champion 2000
Kuschall of America
3601 Rider Trail S
Earth City, MO 63045 314-512-7000
800-654-4768
FAX: 800-542-3567
Rigid chair that folds side-to-side. $1,765

667 Champion 3000
Kuschall of America
3601 Rider Trail S
Earth City, MO 63045 314-512-7000
800-654-4768
FAX: 800-542-3567
The high-performance chair built for perfectionists. $1,695

668 Choosing a Wheelchair: A Guide for Optimal Independence
Patient-Centered Guides
101 Morris Street
Sebastopol, CA 95472 707-829-0515
800-294-4747
FAX: 800-997-9901
e-mail: order@oreilly.com
www.patientcenters.com

Linda Lamb, Editor
Shawnde Paull, Marketing
Tim O'Reilly, Chief Executive Officer
With the right wheelchair, quality of life increases dramatically and even people with severe disabilities can have a considerable degree of independence and activity. Choosing the wrong chair can indeed the tantamount to confinement. This book describes technology, options, and the selection process to help you identify the chair than can provide you with optimal independence.
$9.95
186 pages Paperback
ISBN 1-565924-11-8

669 Convaid
PO Box 4209
Palos Verdes Peninsula, CA 90274 310-618-0111
888-266-8243
FAX: 310-618-2166
e-mail: convaid@convaid.com
www.convaid.com

Merv Watkins, Owner
Five different styles of wheelchairs.

670 Custom
Fortress
PO Box 489
Clovis, CA 93613 559-322-5437
FAX: 559-323-0299

Ultralight aluminum wheelchair that can be customized to customer's requests. Fifteen frame colors, eight seat widths and depths, along with thirteen rear wheel combinations are just a few of the features offered at the standard package price.

671 **Custom Durable**
21279 Protecta Drive
Elkhart, IN 46516
574-522-7199
800-933-0256
FAX: 574-293-0202

Dawn Slabach, President
Wheelchairs; accessories.

672 **Edge**
Fortress
PO Box 489
Clovis, CA 93613
559-322-5437
FAX: 559-323-0299
An ultra lightweight aircraft aluminum wheelchair that is suitable for sports, school or the workplace.

673 **Etac USA: F3 Wheelchair**
2325 Parklawn Drive
Suite J
Waukesha, WI 53186
800-678-3822
FAX: 262-796-4605
e-mail: etac1usa@execpc.com
www.execpc.com/~etac1usa
A swedish wheelchair designed to provide function, comfort and flexibility. Seat frame and upholstery are adjustable to fit each individual. Swing away, detachable footrests are standard. Available in frame widths from 14, 18 and 20 inch. Numerous accessories are available in order to individualize each chair. Lifetime warranty on frame for original user.

674 **Evacu-Trac**
Garaventa Canada
PO Box L-1
Blaine, WA 98230
360-332-2231
800-663-6556
This emergency evacuation chair is designed for safety and fast operation.

675 **Folding Chair with a Rigid Feel**
Kuschall of America
3601 Rider Trail S
Earth City, MO 63045
314-512-7000
800-654-4768
FAX: 800-542-3567
The Champion 1000 is a new concept in folding chairs. Even though it's ultra light, it has the feel and performance of a rigid chair.

676 **Formula Series Active Mobility Wheelchairs**
Everest & Jennings
3233 Mission Oaks Boulevard
Camarillo, CA 93012
805-389-7450

This is a new series of lightweight wheelchairs designed for the active user.

677 **Freestyle II**
Fortress
PO Box 489
Clovis, CA 93613
559-322-5437
FAX: 559-323-0299
Effort-sparing, ultra-lightweight aircraft aluminum construction and design allow for easy propelling over various rolling surfaces.

678 **Gadabout Wheelchairs**
Gadabout Wheelchairs
1165 Portland Avenue
Rochester, NY 14621
585-338-1000
800-828-4242

Michael Fonte, Owner
Enjoy independence with the wheelchair that is lightweight, portable, convenient, comfortable and sturdy.

679 **Gem Wheelchair & Scooter Service: Mobility & Homecare**
17639 Union Tpke
Flushing, NY 11366
718-463-3800
800-943-3578
FAX: 718-969-8300
e-mail: mywheelsturning@aol.com
www.wheelchairsusa.com

Jeff Bochner, President
GEM sells and services all makes and models of manual and motorized wheelchairs, power scooters, ramps, stairway lifts, and homecare products including diapers, chux, and bathroom safety equipment. Clients are in all five New York City Boroughs and Nassau County. Medicare and Medicaid accepted, pick-up and delivery, loaner equipment, and while-u-wait repair services available. Gem also buys and sells used equipment.

680 **Gendron**
Lugbill Road
Archbold, OH 43502
419-445-6060
800-537-2521
FAX: 419-446-2631

Steven Cotter, VP Sales/President
Manufacturer of wheelchairs for a variety of other applications, specializing in bariatric mobility products.

681 **HiRider**
Gaymar Industries
10 Centre Drive
Orchard Park, NY 14127
716-662-2551
800-828-7341

Thomas Stewart, Chief Executive Officer
A wheelchair that provides mobility in both sitting and standing positions.

682 **INVACARE IVC Tracer EX2 Wheelchair**
Maxi Aids
42 Executive Boulevard
Farmingdale, NY 11735
631-752-0521
800-522-6294
FAX: 631-752-0689
e-mail: sales@maxiaids.com
www.maxiaids.com
Durable low maintenace wheelchair with 24 rear wheels and 8 casters.

683 **Innovative Products**
4351 W College Avenue
Appleton, WI 54914
920-738-9090
800-424-3369
FAX: 920-738-9050

Art Fochs, Vice President
Wheelchairs; accessories.

684 **Liberty**
Fortress
PO Box 489
Clovis, CA 93613
559-322-5437
FAX: 559-323-0299
Ultra lightweight wheelchair provides a comfortable fit and leaves people able to function as normally as possible in daily activities.

685 **Lightweight Breezy**
Motion Design
2382 Faraday Avenue
Suite 200
Carlsbad, CA 92008
760-930-1500
FAX: 760-930-1585
www.sunrisemedical.com

Michael Hammes, Chief Executive Officer
A lightweight wheelchair. *$750.00*

686 Majors Medical Equipment
14601 Old Lima Road
Suite 100
Fort Wayne, IN 46818
260-637-8586
800-611-5552
e-mail: majorsmedical@majorsmedical.com

Larry Bobay, Owner
America's largest selection of wheelchairs and homecare equipment.

687 Natural Access
PO Box 5729
Santa Monica, CA 90409
310-392-9864
800-411-7789
FAX: 310-392-3874
e-mail: national@superlink.net
www.landeez.com

John Egan, Owner
Provides the Landeez all-terrain wheelchair, that can roll easily on sand, gravel and snow for outdoor fun. The entire chair can fit inside a travel bag!

688 Patient Transport Chair
Mada Medical Products
625 Washington Avenue
Carlstadt, NJ 07072
201-460-0454
800-526-6370
FAX: 201-460-3509
e-mail: dianelind@mail.madamedical.com
www.madainternational.com

Jeffrey Adam, Vice President
Mada's lightweight design transport chair is constructed of heavy gauge chrome-plated, steel tubing with reinforced cross braces.

689 Posture-Glide Lounger
Graham-Field Health Products
2935 Northeast Parkway
Atlanta, GA 30360
770-447-1609
800-347-5678
FAX: 800-726-0601
www.grahamfield.com

Irwin Selinger, Chief Executive Officer
Provides all day comfort and safe, independent mobilization with feet or hands. The ergonomically engineered seat back provides correct support.

690 Prairie Cruiser
Wheelchairs of Kansas
PO Box 32
Ellis, KS 67637
785-726-4950
800-537-6454
FAX: 800-337-2447
e-mail: workinfo@go2wok.com
www.wheelchairsofkansas.com
A large-frame powerchair constructed of high quality, stress tested stainless steel to insure durability and peak performance.

691 Redman Apache
Redman Powerchair
3840 S Palo Verde Road
Tucson, AZ 85714
520-546-6002
800-727-6684
FAX: 520-546-5530

Don Redman, Owner
These ultralight, active use wheelchairs offer quick release rear wheels, adjustable arm height and detachable arm swing-away.

692 Redman Crow Line
Redman Powerchair
3840 S Palo Verde Road
Tucson, AZ 85714
520-546-6002
800-727-6684
FAX: 520-546-5530

Don Redman, Owner
Reclining wheelchair that reclines a full 90 degrees to flat and can be stopped anywhere on the axis.

693 Rolls 2000 Series
Invacare Corporation
899 Cleveland Street
Elyria, OH 44035
440-329-6000
800-333-6900
e-mail: info@invacare.com
These wheelchairs are the first light-weight wheelchairs designed for rental use.

694 Skyway
Skyway Machine
4451 Caterpillar Road
Redding, CA 96003
530-243-5151
800-332-3357
FAX: 530-243-5104
e-mail: sales@skywaywheels.com
www.skywaytuffwheels.com

Parrey Cremeans, Sales Manager
Bart Weems, Sales/Customer Service
Ken Coster, President
For over 20 years Skyway has been the world leader in composite wheels. Supplying over 650 different wheel combinations for wheelchairs, lawn and garden products, bicycles and a large assortment of wheeled devices. Wheel sizes range from 4 inch to 24 inch diameter.

695 Stand-Up Wheelchairs
Lifestand
PO Box 232171
Encinitas, CA 92023
800-782-6324
FAX: 610-586-0847
e-mail: dallery@msn.com

Jacques A Dallery, President
Offers a complete line of manual, electric and stand-up wheelchairs for the disabled.

696 Standard Wheelchair
Mada Medical Products
625 Washington Avenue
Carlstadt, NJ 07072
201-460-0454
800-526-6370
FAX: 201-460-3509
e-mail: dianelind@mail.madamedical.com
www.madainternational.com

Jeffrey Adam, Vice President
Mada's standard wheelchairs are designed and built for long-lasting, reliable operation. Each wheelchair is constructed of heavy gauge, chrome plated, steel framework and tube in tube construction at stress points. Mada's state-of-the art engineering uses the most modern components to provide the strength needed while keeping the chair's weight down.

697 Surf Chair
2052 S Peninsula Drive
Daytona Beach, FL 32118
386-253-0986
800-841-6610
FAX: 386-253-7600

Wheelchairs; accessories.

698 Vista Wheelchair
Arista Surgical Supply Company/AliMed
297 High Street
Dedham, MA 02026
781-329-2900
800-223-1984
FAX: 800-437-2966
e-mail: aristasurgical@juno.com
www.aristasurgical.com

Julian Cherubini, President
Vista has a rugged cold-rolled steel frame, durable vinyl upholstery and steel bearings to assure a smooth ride. *$220.00*

699 Wheelchair with Shock Absorbers
Iron Horse Productions
3114 Strawberry Lane
Port Huron, MI 48060
810-987-6700
800-426-0354
The Iron Horse is a revolutionary concept in wheelchair design that offers comfort, indoors and outdoors. *$2375.00*

Wheelchairs: Pediatric

700 **Commuter & Kid's Commuter**
Fortress
PO Box 489
Clovis, CA 93613
559-322-5437
FAX: 559-323-0299
The first of a new generation of power wheelchairs. These chairs feature direct drive power yet are foldable, transportable and affordable.

701 **Convaid**
2830 California Street
Torrance, CA 90503
310-618-0111
888-266-8243
FAX: 310-618-2166
e-mail: convaid@earthlink.net
www.convaid.com

Merv Watkins, President
Rodolfo Restelli, Controller
Nathan Watkins, Executive VP
Convaid manufactures Mobile Positioning Systems for children. The Expedition, Safari Tilt, Cruiser, EZ Rider and Metro offer a noninstitutional styling and are lightweight and compact-folding. The steel/aluminum structure is engineered for maximum comfort and durability. The mobile positioning lines come with more than 20 positioning features and a full range of positioning adaptations. All chairs have been successfully crash-tested and offer a limited lifetime warranty (except the Metro).

702 **Imp Tricycle**
TRIAID
PO Box 1364
Cumberland, MD 21501
301-759-3525
800-306-6777
FAX: 301-759-3525
e-mail: sales@triaid.com
www.triaid.com

Iain A MacDonald, Sales Director
Ann M Hutter, Sales Executive/Manager
Provides fun therapy and actively encourages participation, awareness and the building of self confidence. Designed for children from about 3 years, it features ATB styling, 12 inch wheels, adjustable steering stop and a supportive saddle. Handlebar and seat adjustments combine with a broad wheelbase to ensure the rider is in the optimum position to pedal and the tricycle gives good stability and confident handling. Support accessories are available. *$590.00*

703 **Kid's Custom**
Fortress
PO Box 489
Clovis, CA 93613
559-322-5437
FAX: 559-323-0299
Custom pediatric mobility needs. This ultra light-weight chair is tailored fit to each child, to make wheeling fun and encourages kids to be active because they feel free, safe and secure.

704 **Kid's Edge**
Fortress
PO Box 489
Clovis, CA 93613
559-322-5437
FAX: 559-323-0299
This wheelchair offers multiple options, features and modifications at no upcharge.

705 **Kid's Liberty**
Fortress
PO Box 489
Clovis, CA 93613
559-322-5437
FAX: 559-323-0299
Offers a broad range of seat heights, widths and depths, back heights and numerous other modifications to accommodate the specific and unique requirements of children.

706 **Kid-Friendly Chairs**
Vector Mobility
5030 E Jensen Avenue
Fresno, CA 93725
800-441-0358
FAX: 559-441-0359
Manual base offers the lowest available floor to seat height, growth capability, one-third the parts of a conventional chair and no welds to break. The power unit features standard shapes and personality designs from elephants to inch worms and autos to rainbows, lowest seat height, and smallest turning radius on the market.

707 **Seven Fifty-Five FS**
Fortress
PO Box 489
Clovis, CA 93613
559-322-5437
FAX: 559-323-0299
Unharness the curiosity of childhood with the modular power/base seating system that sets kids free. This device is engineered and built especially for children.

708 **TMX Tricycle**
TRIAID
PO Box 1364
Cumberland, MD 21501
301-759-3525
800-306-6777
FAX: 301-759-3525
e-mail: sales@triaid.com
www.triaid.com

Iain A MacDonald, Sales Director
Ann M Hutter, Sales Executive/Manager
Provides fun therapy and actively encourages participation, awareness and the building of self confidence. Designed for children from about eight years, it features ATB styling, 20 inch wheels, adjustable steering stop and a supportive saddle. Handlebar and seat adjustments combine with a broad wheelbase to ensure the rider is in the optimum position to pedal and the tricycle gives good stability and confident handling. Support accessories are available. *$795.00*

Wheelchairs: Powered

709 **Bounder Plus Power Wheelchair**
21st Century Scientific
4915 Industrial Way
Coeur D Alene, ID 83815
208-667-8800
800-448-3680
FAX: 208-667-6600
e-mail: 21st@wheelchairs.com
www.wheelchairs.com

RD Davidson, Sales/Marketing Director
Jeanie L Saville, Sales Associate
Ron Prior, Owner
Available in widths of 16 to 20 inches for users up to 500 pounds with a 2 year warranty on the entire chair. It offers all the standard features of a BOUNDER, plus reinforced rear wheel mounts, reinforced caster barrels, and super duty upholstery (with double liner and web straps under every screw). The BOUNDER Plus also features tandem cross struts, middle vertical support strut, seat rails supported at five points and back upholstery attached with machine screws.

710 **Bounder Power Wheelchair**
21st Century Scientific
4915 Industrial Way
Coeur D Alene, ID 83815
208-667-8800
800-448-3680
FAX: 208-667-6600
e-mail: 21st@wheelchairs.com
www.wheelchairs.com

RD Davidson, Sales/Marketing Director
Jeanie L Saville, Sales Associate
Ron Prior, Owner
Available in a variety of widths from 16 to 18 inches for users up to 250 pounds. The rugged frame is constructed with steel tubing. The standard 12 position Adjustable Front Forks, made of 1/4 inch thick steel, provides impact dampening and seat tilt adjustment. A Dual Group 27 Sliding Battery Box provides extended range and easy battery maintenance. *$8695.00*

711 **Damaco D90**
Damaco
20542 Plummer Street
Chatsworth, CA 91311
800-432-2434
FAX: 818-709-5282

Portable power unit that fits manual wheelchairs with large rear wheels. Weighing just 22 pounds, the power system can be removed and stored in a matter of seconds. *$2495.00*

712 **Geronimo**
Redman Powerchair
3840 S Palo Verde Road
Suite 202
Tucson, AZ 85714
520-546-6002
800-727-6684
FAX: 520-546-5530

Don Redman, Owner
Wheelchair offering direct drive, two year electronic guarantee and micro controls.

713 **Jet 3 Ultra Power Wheelchair**
Maxi Aids
42 Executive Boulevard
Farmingdale, NY 11735
631-752-0521
800-522-6294
FAX: 631-752-0689
e-mail: sales@maxiaids.com
www.maxiaids.com

Delivers a broad range of standard performance features like Active-Trac Suspension and a powerful 50 amp PG VSI controller on a very compact and maneuverable frame.

714 **One Thousand FS**
Fortress
PO Box 489
Clovis, CA 93613
559-322-5437
FAX: 559-323-0299

Add-on power system installs in minutes, enabling the driver to relax and drive anywhere with smooth, silent electric power.

715 **Permobil Max 90**
Permobil
30 Ray Avenue
Burlington, MA 01803
781-272-7410
FAX: 781-229-9841

The power wheelchair for those needing an easily maneuverable and quiet indoor chair but who also need to use their chair outdoors.

716 **Permobil Super 90**
Permobil
30 Ray Avenue
Burlington, MA 01803
781-272-7410
FAX: 781-229-9841

The power wheelchair is designed for travel over uneven and hilly terrain outdoors and indoors.

717 **Power for Off-Pavement**
Redman Powerchair
3840 S Palo Verde Road
Suite 202
Tucson, AZ 85714
520-546-6002
800-727-6684
FAX: 520-546-5530

Don Redman, Owner
Power-drive wheelchair has a solid seat and can handle safely and securely knolls and off-pavement terrain.

718 **Reclining Power Wheelchairs**
LaBac Systems
4965 Kingston Street
Denver, CO 80239
303-914-9914
800-445-4402

Josh Barnum, President
Power recline seating systems for wheelchairs, offering more comfort and dependability for the physically challenged.

Wheelchairs: Racing

719 **Eagle Sportschairs**
2351 Parkwood Road
Snellville, GA 30039
770-972-0763
800-932-9380
FAX: 770-985-4885
e-mail: bewing@bellsouth.net
www.eaglesportschairs.com

Barry Ewing, Owner
Marty Frierson, Sales
The Eagle line of custom lightweight performance chairs includes a range of options to fit all racing and sport needs including; track, baseball, quad-rugby, tennis, field events and waterskiing. Also popular for daily use. We are able to customize any chair to accommodate size and disability and all frames have a full five year warranty.

720 **East Penn Manufacturing Company**
East Penn Manufacturing Company
PO Box 147
Lyon Station, PA 19536
610-682-6361
FAX: 610-682-4781
e-mail: eastpenn@eastpenn-delu.com

Harold Eberly, VP Sales
Daniel Langdon, President
Specially engineered for demanding deep-cycle applications Gelled electrolyte Deka Dominator Batteries provides maintenance-free operation, longer battery life and hours of reliable performance. Their excellent recharge characteristics provide quick turn around time.

721 **Invacare Top End**
4501 63rd Circle
Pinellas Park, FL 33781
727-522-8677
800-532-8677
FAX: 727-522-1007
www.invacare.com

Mary Carol Peterson, Marketing
Al Crisp, Manager
Manufacturers of light weight, rigid, sport-specific wheelchairs such as the Eliminator line of racing chairs,T-3 tennis and softball chairs, and the Terminator for quad rugby and basketball. The Excelerator, XLT three-wheel hand cycle for adults and juniors. Check out our full line of wheelchairs to fit every need. $1,895-$2,495

General Disabilities

722 **ACS Federal Healthcare**
5270 Shawnee Road
Alexandria, VA 22312
703-310-0158
FAX: 703-310-0126
goliath.ecnext.com/coms2/product-compint
Project RSVP supports the SSA's initiative to expand operations vocational rehabilitation services through a national network of private providers. Rehabilitation companies interested in gaining access to a new client base, acquiring a new funding stream, and developing creative service delivery and entrepreneurial partnerships, may benefit from such a program.

723 **AHEAD Association**
107 Commerce Center Drive
Suite 204
Huntersville, NC 28078
704-947-7779
FAX: 704-948-7779
e-mail: ahead@ahead.org
www.ahead.org

Carol Funckes, President
Mike Shuttic, President-Elect
Jim Marks, Treasurer
The premiere professional association committed to full participation of persons with disabilities in postsecondary education. AHEAD values diversity, personal growth and development and creativity. Promotes leadership and exemplary practices. Provides professional development and disseminates information. Orchestrates resources through partnership and collaboration. AHEAD dynamically addresses current and emerging issues with respect to disability, and education to achieve universal access.

724 **Abilities!**
201 I U Willets Road
Albertson, NY 11507
516-465-1400
FAX: 516-747-5400
www.ncds.org

Kevin McGilloway, CEO
Stephen V Murphy, President
Ralph F Palleschi, President and COO
Helps the business community develop effective, low-cost corporate policies and practices for integrating people with disabilities in the workplace.

725 **Acupressure Institute**
1533 Shattuck Avenue
Berkeley, CA 94709
510-845-1059
800-442-2232
FAX: 510-845-1496
e-mail: info@acupressure.com
www.acupressure.com

Michael Reed Gach, Executive Director
Since 1976 the Acupressure institute has offered comprehensive acupressure trainings in the traditional Asian Bodywork Therapy (ABT)such as Thai massage and Shiatsu massage to students from around the world. In comparing other Acupressure schools, our trainings provide high quality education to support each student'sprofessional and personal goals, in a setting that encourages communication, respect, and confidentiality and safety for everyone.

726 **Advocacy Center**
590 South Avenue
Rochester, NY 14620
585-546-1700
800-650-4967
FAX: 585-546-7069
TTY: 585-546-1700
e-mail: info@advocacycenter.com
www.advocacycenter.com

Steven Voellinger, President
Paul Shew, Executive Director
Joyce Steel, Program Coordinator
Is a non profit organization located in New York State that educates, supports, and advocates with people who have disabilities, their families and circles of support. A diverse consumer-driven organization leading New York State in shaping the future through the development of innovative, outcome-oriented, and quality initiatives for people with disabilities, their families, and circle of support.

727 **Advocacy Center for Persons with Disabilities**
2671 W Executive Center Circle
Suite 100
Tallahassee, FL 32301
850-488-9071
800-342-0823
FAX: 850-488-8640
TTY: 800-346-4127
e-mail: info@advocacycenter.org
www.advocacycenter.org

Gary Weston, Executive Director
Hubert Grisson, President
The Advocacy Center for Persons with Disabilites Inc., is a non-profit organization providing protection and advocacy services in the State of Florida. The Center's mission is to advance the dignity, equality, self-determination and expressed choices of individuals with disabilities.

728 **Advocates for Children of New York**
151 W 30th Street
5th Floor
New York, NY 10001
212-947-9779
FAX: 212-947-9790
e-mail: info@advocatesforchildren.org
www.advocatesforchildren.org

Jamie A. Levitt, President
Majorie M Glover, Secretary
Barry Ford, Treasurer
AFC works on behalf of children from infancy to age 21 who are at greatest risk for school-based discrimination and/or academic failure. These include children with disabilities, ethnic minorities, immigrants, homeless children, foster care children, limited English proficient children and those living in poverty.

729 **Alliance for Technology Access**
1304 Southpoint Boulevard
Suite 240
Petaluma, CA 94954
707-778-3011
FAX: 707-765-2080
TTY:707-778-3015
e-mail: atainfo@ataccess.org
www.ataccess.org

Mary Lester, Executive Director
Russ Holland, Program Director
Lois Symington, President
The ATA is a growing national network of technology resource centers, organizations, individuals and companies. ATA encourages and facilitates the empowerment of people with disabilities to participate fully in their communities. Through public education, information and referral, capacity building in community organizations, and advocacy/policy efforts, the ATA enables millions of people to live, learn, work, define their futures, and achieve their dreams.

730 **American Academy of Environmental Medicine**
7701 E Kellogg Drive
Suite 625
Wichita, KS 57207
316-684-5500
FAX: 316-684-5709
e-mail: centraloffice@aaem.com
www.aaem.com

Gerald D. Natzke D.O., President
Philip D. Ranheim MD FAAEM, President Elect
James W. Willoughby D.O., Secretary
Environmental Medicine is the comprehensive, proactive and preventive strategic approach to medical care dedicated to the evaluation, management, and prevention of the adverse consequences resulting from Environmentally Triggered Illnesses.

731 **American Academy of Pediatrics**

141 Northwest Point Boulevard
Elk Grove Village, IL 60007
847-434-4000
FAX: 847-434-8000
e-mail: csc@aap.org
www.aap.org

Jay Berkelhamer, MD, President
Renee R Jenkins, MD, President-Elect
Errol R. Alden, MD, Executive Director
Organization of 60,000 pediatricians committed to the attainment of optimal physical, mental, and social health and well-being for all infants, children, adolescents and young adults.

732 **American Association of Children's Residential Centers**

11700 W Lake Park Drive
Milwaukee, WI 53224
877-332-2272
FAX: 877-362-2272
e-mail: mskarich@alliance1.org
www.aacrc-dc.org

Brian Carroll MSW, LICSW, President
William Powers MHA, MPA, Secretary
Margaret Vimont LCSW, Treasurer
The American Association of Children's Residential Centers believes that children and adolescents, and their families, are entitled to treatment which offers the maximum opportunity for growth and change. AACRC believes that clinically crafted residential treatment options, ranging from community based homes through institutional environments, are essential components in a comprehensive system of behavioral health care.

733 **American Association of Oriental Medicine**

PO Box 162340
Sacramento, CA 95816
916-443-4770
866-455-7999
FAX: 916-443-4766
e-mail: editor@aaom.org
www.aaom.org

Leslie Mcgee, President
Martin Herbkersman, Vice President
P. Shane Burras, Treasurer
The AAOM represents and advocates on behalf of the professional Oriental Medicine provider in order to ensure that the well-being of the public is protected, and to ensure that Oriental Medicine providers are given their rightful place in the healthcare system.

734 **American Association of People with Disabilities**

1629 K Street NW
Suite 503
Washington, DC 20006
202-457-0046
800-840-8844
FAX: 202-457-0473
e-mail: aapd@aol.com
www.aapd-dc.org

Helena Berger, Chief Operating Officer
Jacqueline Brown, Executive Assistant
Diane DeAngelis, Director, Marketing
The largest national nonprofit cross-disability member organization in the United States, dedicated to ensuring economic self-sufficiency and political empowerment for the more than 56 million Americans with disabilities. AAPD works in coalition with other disability organizations for the full implimentation and enforcement of disability nondiscrimination laws, particularly the Americans With Disabilities Act (ADA) of 1990 and the Rehabilitation Act of 1973.

735 **American Board of Chelation Therapy**

70 West Huron Street
Chicago, IL 60610
312-266-7246
FAX: 312-266-3685

Jack Hank, Executive Director
Established protocol for chelation therapy and certifies physicians trained in chelation therapy. Will provide the names of board-certified physicians

736 **American Board of Professional Disability Consultants**

1350 Beverly Road
Suite 115-327
Mc Lean, VA 22101
703-952-0024
FAX: 703-952-0028

Taras Cerkevitch, Operations Director
Mark Long, Development Director
Bashar Islam, Owner
Certifies physicians, psychologists, attorneys, and counselors as specialists in disability and personal injury.

737 **American Botanical Council**

6200 Manor Road
Austin, TX 78723
512-926-4900
800-373-7105
FAX: 512-926-2345
e-mail: abc@herbalgram.org
www.herbalgram.org

Mark Blumenthal, Founder/Executive Director
Wayne Silverman, Phd, Chief Administrative Officer
The American Botanical Council (ABC) is the leading independent, nonprofit, international member-based organization providing education using science-based ad traditional information to promote the responsible use of herbal medicine.

738 **American Camping Association**

5000 State Road 67 N
Martinsville, IN 46151
765-342-8456
800-428-2267
FAX: 765-342-2065
www.acacamps.org

Ann Sheets, President
Dawn Ewing, VP
Peg Smith, CEO
The American Camp Association is a community of camp professionals who, for nearly 100 years, have joined together to share our knowledge and experience and to ensure the quality of camp programs. Because of our diverse 7,000 plus emmbership and exceptional programs, children and adults have the opportunity to learn powerful lessons in cmmunity, character-building, skill development, and healthy-living—-lessons that can be learned nowhere else.

739 **American Chiropractic Association**

1701 Clarendon Boulevard
Arlington, VA 22209
703-276-8800
FAX: 703-243-2593
e-mail: memberinfo@acatoday.org
www.acatoday.org

Kevin Corcoran, Executive VP
Janet Ridgely, VP Administration
Dean Millard, Director, Information Systems
The ACA is a professional organization representing Doctors of Chiropratic. Its mission is to preserve, protect, improve, and promote the chiropractic profession and the services of Doctors of Chiropratic for the benefit of the patients they serve. The purpose of the ACA is to provide leadership in health care and a positive vision for the chiropractic profession and its natural approach to health and wellness.

740 **American College of Advancement in Medicine**

24411 Ridge Route Drive
Suite 115
Laguna Hills, CA 92653
949-309-3520
800-439-6891
FAX: 949-309-3538
e-mail: info@acam.org
www.acam.org

Sharon Urch, Chief Executive Officer
Regina Wenger, Event Planning
Drew McGray, Interactive Services
The American College for Advancement in Medicine (ACAM)is a not-for-profit society dedicated to educating physicians and other health care professionals on the latest findings and emerging procedures in preventive/nutritional medicine. ACAM's goals are to improve skills, knowledge and diagnostic procedures as they relate to complimentary and alternative medicine; to support research; and to develop awareness of alternative methods of medical treatment.

741 **American College of Nurse Midwives**
8403 Colesville Road
Suite 1550
Silver Spring, MD 20910
240-485-1800
FAX: 240-485-1818
e-mail: info@acnm.org
www.acnm.org

Katherine Camacho Carr, President
Melissa Avery, Vice President
Claire M. Westdahl, Treasurer
The American College of Nurse-Midwives (ACNM) is the oldest women's health care organization in the U.S. ACNM provides research, accredits midwifery education programs, administers and promotes continuing education programs, establishes clinical practice standards, creates liasons with state and federal agencies and members of Congress.

742 **American Counseling Association**
5999 Stevenson Avenue
Alexandria, VA 22304
703-823-9800
800-347-6647
FAX: 703-823-0252
TTY: 703-823-6862
e-mail: webmaster@counseling.org
www.counseling.org

Marie Wakefield, President
Richard Yep, Executive Office
Theresa Holmes, Executive Office
The American Counseling Association is a not-for-profit, professional and educational organization that is dedicated to the growth and enhancement of the counseling profession.

743 **American Herbalists Guild**
141 Nob Hill Road
Cheshire, CT 06410
203-272-6731
FAX: 203-272-8550
e-mail: ahgoffice@earthlink.net
www.americanherbalistsguild.com

Aviva Jill Romm RH (AHG), CPM, President
Roy Upton RH(AHG), Vice President
Kp Khalsa, RH(AHG), Treasurer
Founded in 1989 as a non-profit, educational organization to represent the goals and voices of herbalists specializing in the medicinal use of plants. Our primary goal is to promote a high level of professionalism and education in the study and practice of theraputic herbalism.

744 **American Holistic Medical Association**
Po Box 2016
Edmonds, WA 98020
425-967-0737
FAX: 425-771-9588
e-mail: ahma@holisticmedicine.org
www.holisticmedicine.org

Lawrence B. Palevsky MD,FAAP,ABHM, President
Robert Wickiewicz MD, Secretary
Andrea Girman MD, Treasurer
The mission of the AMHA is to support practitioners in their evolving personal and professional development as healers and to educate physicians about holistic medicine.

745 **American Massage Therapy Association**
500 Davis Street
Suite 900
Evanston, IL 60201
847-864-0123
877-905-2700
FAX: 847-864-1178
e-mail: info@amtamassage.org
www.amtamassage.org

Mary Beth Braun, President
M K Brennan, VP
Liz Lucas, Executive Director
AMTA works to establish massage therapy as integral to the maintenance of good health and complementary to other therapeudic processes; to advance the profession through ethics and standards, certification, school accreditation, continuing education, professional publications, legislative efforts, public education, and fostering the development of members.

746 **American Occupational Therapy Association**
4720 Montgomery Lane
Po Box 31220
Bethesda, MD 20824
301-652-2682
800-789-2682
FAX: 301-652-7711
TTY: 800-377-8555
e-mail: praota@aota.org
www.aota.org

M Carolyn Baum, President
Charles Christiansen, VP
Mary Binderman, Manager
Settings include schools, hospitals, skilled nursing facilities, home health, outpatient rehabilitation clinicss, psychiatric facilities and community health programs.

747 **American Organization for Bodywork Therapies of Asia**
1010 Haddonfield Berlin Road
Suite 408
Voorhees, NJ 08043
856-782-1616
FAX: 856-782-1653
e-mail: office@aobta.org
www.aobta.org

Debra Howard, President
Beverly Sonen, Vice President
Stuart Watts, Treasurer
The American Organization for Bodywork Therapies of Asia (AOBTA) is a professional membership organizaton which promotes Asian Bodywork Therapy and its practitioners while honoring a diversity of disciplines. AOBTA serves its community of members by supporting appropriate credentialing; defining scope of practice and educational standards; and providing resources for training, professional development and networking. AOBTA advocates public policy to protect its members.

748 **American Public Health Association**
800 i Street NW
Washington, DC 20001
202-777-2742
FAX: 202-777-2533
e-mail: comments@apha.org
www.apha.org

Georges C Benjamin MD, FACP,, Executive Director
Olivia Pokras MHS PHD, Elected Member
Diana Conti, Ex-Officio Member
Founded in 1872, APHA is the oldest, largest and most diverse organization of public health professionals in the world. The association works to protect all Americans and their communities from preventable, seruious health threats. APHA represents a broad array of health officials, educators, environmentalists, policy-makers and health providers at all levels working both within and outside governmental organizations and educational institutions.

749 **American Red Cross: National Headquarters**
2025 E Street NW
Washington, DC 20006
202-303-4498
800-733-2767
FAX: 202-303-4498
e-mail: usa@redcross.org
www.redcross.org

Mark W. Everson, President/CEO
Carlos Gutierrez, Board of Governors
Michael Leavitt, Board of Governors
Today, in addition to domestic disaster relief, the American Red Cross offers compassionate services in five other areas: community services that help the needy; support and comfort for military members and their families; the collection, processing and distribution of lifesaving blood and blood products; educational programs that promote health and safety; and international relief and development programs.

750 **American Self-Help Clearinghouse**
Saint Clares Hospital
St Clares Health Services
Denville, NJ 07834
973-586-5000
800-367-6274
FAX: 973-326-9467
e-mail: info@selfhelpgroups.org
www.selfhelpgroups.org

Edward J Madara MS, Director
Provides information on national self-help groups and offers training and technical assistance to exisiting and new self-help groups and clearinghouses. It has compiled a national database of over 800 of these model groups. Provides information on resource groups such as Violence Anonymous, Batterers Anonymous, and Stalkers' Victims Support Groups.

751 **American Society for the Alexander Techniq ue**
PO Box 60008
Florence, MA 01062
413-584-2359
800-473-0620
FAX: 413-584-3097
e-mail: info@amsat.ws
www.amsat.ws

Ralph Zito, Chair
Clare Maxwell, Treasurer
Patricia Gallup, Member At Large
The Alexander Technique is a proven, effective self help method for improving balance and coordination and increasing movement awareness by eliminating habitual reactions of misuse in every day activities. AmSats mission is to define, maintain and promote the Alexander Technique at its highest standard of professional practice and conduct.

752 **American Society of Bariatric Physicians**
2821 S Parker Road
Suite 625
Aurora, CO 80014
303-770-2526
877-266-6834
FAX: 303-779-4834
e-mail: info@asbp.org
www.asbp.org

Judith Robinson PhD, CAE, Interim Executive Director
Harold C Seim MD, MPH, FASBP, Director of Medical Education
Karen Brenning, Membership Services Coordinator
The American Society of Bariatric Physicians is an international association and allied health care professionals with special interest and experience in the comprehensive treatment of overweight, obesity and related disorders.

753 **American Society of Clinical Hypnosis**
140 N Bloomingdale Road
Bloomingdale, IL 60108
630-980-4740
FAX: 630-351-8490
e-mail: info@asch.net
www.asch.net

Catherine Kasper, Executive Director
To provide and encourage education programs to further, in every ethical way, the knowledge, understanding, and application of hypnosis in health care; to encourage research and scientific publication in the field of hypnosis; to promote the further recognition and acceptance of hypnosis as an important tool in clinical health care and focus for scientific research; to cooperate with other professional societies that share mutual goals, ethics, and interests

754 **American Society of Teachers of the Alexander Technique**
PO Box 60008
Florence, MA 01062
413-584-2359
800-473-0620
FAX: 413-584-3097
e-mail: info@amsat.ws
www.amsat.ws

Ralph Zito, Chairman
Clare Maxwell, Treasurer
Patricia Gallup, Member At Large
A proven approach to self-care, the Alexander Technique is a method that people of all ages and abilities can learn to relieve the pain and stress caused by everyday misuse of the body. You learn how to strip away the movement habits and tensions patterns at the root of your discomfort. You learn how to balance your own body and take charge of your own health. You learn how to sit, stand and move-with safety, efficiency and ease.

755 **Association for Applied Psychophysiology and Biofeedback**
10200 West 44th Avenue
#304
Wheat Ridge, CO 80033
303-422-8436
800-477-8892
FAX: 303-422-8894
e-mail: aapb@resourcenter.com
www.aapb.org

Richard Gevirtz, PhD, President
Alan Glaros, PhD, President Elect
Jay Gunkelman, QEEGT, Treasurer
Provides names and phone numbers of local chapters. Mission is to advance the development, dissemination and utilization of knowledge about applied psychophysiology and biofeedback to improve health and the quality of life through research, education, and practice.

756 **Association for Persons in Supported Employment**
1627 Monument Avenue
Richmond, VA 23220
804-278-9187
FAX: 804-278-9377
e-mail: apse@apse.org
www.apse.org

Teresa Grossi, President
Ron Rucker, Vice President
Laura Owens, Secretary
Supported employment enables people with disabilities who have not been successfully employed to work and contribute to society. Focuses on a person's abiliities and provides the supports the individual needs to be successful on a long-term basis.

757 **Association for Persons with Severe Handicaps (TASH)**
1025 Vermont Avenue
Floor 7
Washington, DC 20005
202-263-5600
FAX: 202-637-0138
e-mail: info@tash.org
www.tash.org

Barbara Trader, Executive Director
Gerri A. Hanna, Program Director
Najai Gainous, Executive Assistant
International association of people with disabilities, their family members, other advocates and professionals, fighting for a society in which inclusion of all people in all aspects of society is the norm.

758 **Association of Educational Therapists**
100 Bush St.
Suite 1500
San Francisco, CA 94104
415-982-2389
800-286-4267
FAX: 415-982-9204
e-mail: aet@aetonline.org
www.aetonline.org

Stacy Turner, Administrator
Educational Therapy offers children and adults with learning disabilities and other learning challenges a wide range of intensive, individualized interventions designed to remediate learning problems.

759 **Association of University Centers on Disabilities**
AUCD
1010 Wayne Avenue
Suite 920
Silver Spring, MD 20910
301-588-8252
FAX: 301-588-2842
e-mail: kmusheno@aucd.org
www.aucd.org

Royal P. Walker Jr. JD, President
Michael McCormick, PhD, Director
M. Bryce Fifield, PhD, Treasurer
The central office for the 61 University Centers for Excellence programs and 21 Mental Retardation and Developmental Disabilities Research Centers and is their representative to the federal government. UCEDD's are located at major universities and teaching hospitals in all 50 states, the District of Columbia and many US territories. UCCED's target their activities to support the independence, productivity and integration into the community of individuals with developmental disabilities.

760 **Association on Higher Education and Disability (AHEAD)**
107 Commerce Center Drive
Suite 204
Huntersville, NC 08078
704-947-7779
FAX: 704-948-7779
e-mail: ahead@ahead.org
www.ahead.org

Richard Allegra, Director of Professional Dev.
Tri Do, Operations Manager
Michael Hamlin, Program Assistant
International, multicultural organization of proessionals committed to full participation in higher education for persons with disabilities. Plans and develops training programs, workshops, publications and conferences. Founded in 1977 to address the need and concern for upgrading the quality of services and support available to persons with disabilities in higher education.

761 **Bastyr University Natural Health Clinic**
3670 Stone Way N.
Seattle, WA 98103
206-834-4100
FAX: 206-834-4107
www.bastyrcenter.org
Bastyr Center is the teaching clinic of Bastyr University, which is a leading expert in natural medicine. We provide a team care approach that involves one licensed, experienced practicioner and two or three students, all invested in the outcome of your care. Working together with you to discover your own unique route to wellness. By offering the latest scientific information as well as the wisdom of ancient healing we can safeguard the health of the whole family.

762 **Beach Center on Families and Disability**
University of Kansas
1200 Sunnyside Avenue
Room 3136
Lawrence, KS 66045
785-864-7600
FAX: 785-864-7605
TTY:785-864-3434
e-mail: beachcenter@ku.edu
www.beachcenter.org

Ann Turnbull, Co-Founder, Co-Director
Rud Turnbull, Co-Founder, Co-Director
Robert Hemenway, Chief Executive Officer
A federally funded center that conducts research and training in the factors that contribute to the successful functioning of families with members who have disabilities.

763 **Birth Defect Research for Children**
930 Woodcock Road
Suite 225
Orlando, FL 32803
407-895-0802
800-313-2232
FAX: 407-245-7087
e-mail: staff@birthdefects.org
www.birthdefects.org

Betty Mekdeci, Manager
A nonprofit organization that provides information about birth defects of all kinds to parents and professionals. Offers a library of medical books and files of information on less common categories of birth defects and is involved in research to discover possible links between environmental exposures and birth defects.

764 **Bonnie Prudden Myotherapy**
PO Box 65240
Tucson, AZ 85728
520-529-3979
800-221-4634
FAX: 520-529-6679
e-mail: info@bonnieprudden.com
www.bonnieprudden.com

Enid Whittaker, Associate Director
Provides a list of Certified Myotherapists, clinics where Myotherapy is offered, as well as informational brochures on Myotherapy workshops and products.

765 **Brain Injury Association of America**
8201 Greensboro Drive
Suite 611
McLean, VA 22102
703-761-0750
800-444-6443
FAX: 703-761-0755
e-mail: shconnors@biausa.org
www.biausa.org

Susan H Connors, President/CEO
Mark J. Ashley ScD, CCC-SLP, Chairperson
Wayne Gordon PhdD, Vice Chairperson
Founded in 1980, the Brain Injury Association of America (BIAA) is the leading national organization serving and representing individuals, families and professionals who are touched by a life-altering, often devistating, traumatic brain injury (TBI) Together with its network of more then 40 charted state affiliates, as well as hundreds of local chapters and support groups across the country, the BIAA provides information, education and support to assist the 5.3 million living with brain injuries

766 **Brain Injury Association of New York State**
10 Colvin Avenue
Albany, NY 12206
518-459-7911
800-228-8201
FAX: 518-482-5285
e-mail: info@bianys.org
www.bianys.org

Michael Kaplen Esq., President
Judith Avner, Executive Director
Judith Sandman, Director Membership and Developm
(BIANYS) is a statewide non-profit membership organization that advocates on behalf of individuals with brain injury and their families, and promotes prevention. Established in 1982, BIANYS provides education, advocac, and community support services that lead to improved outcomes for children and adults with brain injuries and their families. BIANYS also offers chapters and support groups throughout the state, prevention programs, mentoring programs, speakers bureau and publications library.
1982

767 **Brain Injury Association of Texas**
316 W. 12th Street
Suite 405
Austin, TX 78701
512-326-1212
800-392-0040
512-326-8088
FAX: 512-478-3370
e-mail: info@biatx.org
www.biatx.org

Eric Makowski, President
Jonas Schwartz, Treasurer
Rose Pelzel, Secretary
The Brain Injury Association of Texas is an organization which arose from the mutual frustration and sense of helplessness experienced by families in their search for appropriate facilities and support to return loved ones who had sustained brain injuries to maximum functioning potential. It was organized in 1982 as the Texas Head Injury Association by a group of family members and health care professionals in an effort to meet the needs of the survivors of brain injury.
1982

768 **CAPP National Parent Resource Center Federation for Children with Special Needs**
59 Temple Place
Suite 664
Boston, MA 02111
617-542-7860
866-815-8122
FAX: 617-542-7832
e-mail: info@ppal.net
www.ppal.net

Donna Welles, Executive Director
Lisa Lambert, Assistant Director
Diane Haynes, Director Operations
A parent-run resource system designed to further the needs and goals of family-centered, community-based coordinated care for children with special health needs and their families. Offers written materials, training packages, workshops and presentations for parents and professionals on special education, health care financing and other topics.

769 **CARF Rehabilitation Accreditation Commission**

4891 E Grant Road
Tucson, AZ 85712

520-325-1044
888-281-6531
FAX: 520-318-1129
www.carf.org

Brian Boon PhD, President/CEO

CARF serves as the standards-setting and accrediting body for rehabilitation and life enhancement programs and services. The independent, not-for-profit commission promotes quality, value, and optimal outcomes of services through a consultative accreditation process that centers on enhancing the lives of the persons served. At present, CARD has accredited more than 19,000 programs and services in the US, Canada, and Sweden in the areas of adult day services, behavioral health, and medical rehab.

770 **California State Oriental Medical Association (CSOMA)**

703 Market Street
Suite 250
San Francisco, CA 94103

800-477-4564
FAX: 415-357-1940
e-mail: info@csomaonline.org
www.csomaonline.org

Greg Sperber DAOM BMMS LAc, President
Jim Bloomfield LAc, Treasurer
Laurie Terzo LAc, Secretary

A professional organization of licensed acupuncturists and supporters of Oriental medicine dedicated to the preservation and advancement of the art, science, and practice of Oriental medicine in a caring and ethical manner, thereby enhancing the health and well-being of the general public.

771 **Canine Companions for Independence**

National Offices
PO Box 446
Santa Rosa, CA 95402

707-577-1700
800-572-2275
FAX: 707-577-1711
TTY: 707-577-1756
e-mail: info@caninecompanions.org
www.caninecompanions.org

Ted Rogahn, President
Anne Gittinger, Vice President
William R. White III, Treasurer

A nonprofit organization that enhances the lives of people with disabilities by providing highly trained assistance dogs and ongoing support to ensure quality partnerships.

772 **Canine Helpers for the Handicapped**

5699 Ridge Road
Lockport, NY 14094

716-433-4035
FAX: 716-439-0822
e-mail: chhdogs@aol.com
www.caninehelpers.netfirms.com

Beverly Underwood, Executive Director/Founder

A nonprofit organization devoted to training dogs to assist people with disabilities to lead more independent, secure lives.

1983

773 **Case Management Society of America**

6301 Ranch Drive
Little Rock, AR 72223

501-225-2229
FAX: 501-221-9068
e-mail: cmsa@cmsa.org
www.cmsa.org

Connie Commander RN,BS,CCM,, President
Peter Moran RN,C,BSN,MS,CCM, President Elect
Deborah Gutteridge MS, Vice-President

The Case Management Society of America is an international, non-profit organization founded in 1990 dedicated to the support and development of the profession of case management through educational forums, networking opportunities and legislative involvement.

1990

774 **Center for Assistive Technology and Environmental Access**

490 Tenth Street NW
Atlanta, GA 30332

404-894-4960
800-726-9119
FAX: 404-894-9320
e-mail: catea@coa.gatech.edu
www.catea.org

Carrie Bruce, Research Scientist
Elizabeth Bryant, Project Director II
Charlie Drummond, Administrative Assistant

CATEA supports individuals with disabilities of any age within the State of Georgia and beyond through expert services, research, design and technological development, information dissemination, and educational programs.

775 **Center for Disability Resources**

University of South Carolina
8301 Farrow Road
Columbia, SC 29208

803-935-5231
FAX: 803-935-5059
www.uscm.med.sc.edu/cdrhome

Dr Richard Ferrante, Executive Director
Donald Wuori, MD

Information on early intervention and the elderly. Our mission is to enhance the well being and quality of life of persons with disabilities and their families. We collaborate with person's with disabilities and their families to develop new knowledge and best practices, trian leaders, and effect system change.

776 **Center for Mind/Body Studies**

5225 Connecticut Avenue NW
Suite 414
Washington, DC 20015

202-966-7338
FAX: 202-966-2589
e-mail: center@cmbm.org
www.cmbm.org

James S. Gordon, MD, Founder And Director
Donald de Laski, JD, CPA, Secretary/Treasurer
Lane Evans, Director

The Center for Mind-Body Medicine is a non-profit educational organization dedicated to reviving the spirit and transforming the practice of medicine. The Center is working to create a more effective, comprehensive and compassionate model of healthcare and education. The Center's model combines the precision of modern science with the best of the world's healing traditions.

777 **Center for Universal Design**

NC State University
Campus
Box 8613
Raleigh, NC 27695

919-515-3082
800-647-6777
FAX: 919-515-8951
e-mail: cud@ncsu.edu
www.design.ncsu.edu/cud

Nilda Cosco, Director
Richard C Duncan, MRP. Dir. of Universal Design
Nancy Hitchcock, BA, BS, MPH, Information Specialist

A federally funded resource center that works toward improving housing for people with disabilities. Provides technical assistance, training and publications on accessible housing and universal design.

778 **Change**

1413 Park Road NW
Washington, DC 20010

202-387-3725
FAX: 202-387-3729
e-mail: changeinc@hotmail.com
innercity.org/columbiaheights/agencies/change

Gracie Rolling, Executive Director
Therman Walker, President
Preston Hursey Jr., Vice President

Offers counseling/assessment, emergency food and clothing referrals, rental assistance and job assistance to disabled persons in the District of Columbia area.

779 Child and Parent Resource Institute

600 Sanatorium Road
London, Ontario, ZZ N6H
519-858-2774
FAX: 519-858-3913
www.cpri.thehealthline.ca

Anne Stark, Administrator
Provides services to children and youth from 0-18 years of age with complex mental health and/or developmental challenges on a short term residential and community basis.

780 Children's Alliance

420 Capitol Avenue
Frankfort, KY 40601
502-875-3399
FAX: 502-223-4200
e-mail: bart@childrensallianceky.org
www.childrensallianceky.org

Bart Baldwin, President
Melissa Lawson, Director of Member Services
Michelle Sanborn, Director of Public Policy
An association of individuals and human services organizations committed to being a voice for at-risk children and families. Interacts with the legislative and executive branches of government and assists members in developing services that most effectively meet the needs of at-risk children and families.

781 Children's National Medical Center

111 Michigan Avenue NW
Washington, DC 20010
202-884-5000
800-884-5433
FAX: 202-884-4492
e-mail: tbear@cnmc.org
www.cnmc.org

Edwin K. Zechman, Jr., President
Raymond S. Sczudlo, Esq, VP/Chief Legal Officer
John W. Thomas, Chief Operating Officer
Our mission is to be preeminent in providing health care services that enhance the health and well-being of children regionally, nationally and internationally. Through leadership and innovation, Children's will create solutions to pediatric health care problems. To meet the unique health care needs of children, adolescents and their families, Children's will excel in Care, Advocacy, Research and Education.

782 Clay Tree Society

838 Old Victoria Road
BC, ZZ V9R
250-753-5322
FAX: 250-753-2749
www.claytree.org

Kate Bocsky, Office Manager
Juli Stevenson, Executive Director
Non-profit society providing day programming for 75 adults with various developmental disabilities governed by an elected Board of Directors and funded by Community Living British Columbia and BC Gaming.

783 College of Maharishi Vedic Medicine Health Center

1000 N 4th Street
Fairfield, IA 52557
641-472-7000
800-369-6480
FAX: 641-472-1179
e-mail: admissions@mum.edu
www.mum.edu

Maharishi Mahesh Yogi, Founder
Provides referrals consultations to the Fairfield community and to visitors from around the world at its clinic on the Maharishi University of Management campus. Staff physicians are medical doctors with years of experience practicing Maharishi Vedic Medicine.

784 Community Enterprises

441 Pleasant Street
P.O. Box 598
Northampton, MA 01061
413-584-1460
FAX: 413-584-1460
www.communityenterprises.com

Richard Benne, President/CEO
Joseph E. April, Vice-Chair
Joanne Carlisle, Clerk
Provide supported education services in a community college setting; supported employment including job training, placement and follow-up; transitional services from group homes and other settings to supported living within the community.

785 DB-Link

Teaching Research
345 N. Monmouth Avenue
Monmouth, OR 97361
503-838-8391
800-438-9376
FAX: 503-838-8150
e-mail: dblink@tr.wou.edu
www.tr.wou.edu/dblink

John Reiman, Director
Gail Leslie, Project Coordinator
Peggy Malloy, Project Librarian
TRI has nearly 70 staff members in its main office in Monmouth and a branch office in Eugene, Oregon. Specific areas of work include studies examining the relationship between teaching and learning, model development and training in early childhood education, technical assistance in special education, research and development work in the area of traumatic brain injury and national technical assistance and information dissemination for deaf-blind individuals and their families.

786 Department of Physical Medicine & Rehabilitation at Sinai Hospital

2401 W Belvedere Avenue
Baltimore, MD 21215
410-601-5584
FAX: 410-601-9692
lifebridgehealth.org

Scott E Brown MD, Chief Physical Med/Rehab Dept
Gerald Felsenthal MD
As one of largest, most comprehensive and most highly respected providers of health-related services to the people of the Northwest Baltimore region, LifeBridge heath advocates preventive services, wellness and fitness services and programs to educate and support the communities it serves. LifeBridge is dedicated to advancing the health of the community through a variety of health and wellness programs and services.

787 Disability Community Small Business Development Center

2568 Packard Street
Ann Arbor, MI 48104
734-971-0277
FAX: 734-971-0826
TTY:734-971-0826
e-mail: cilstaff@aacil.org
www.aacil.org

James Magyar, President/CEO
Shirley Coombs, CFO
Dana Emerson, Director of Operations
The Ann Arbor Center for Independent Living utilizes the independent living model, a well-demonstrated and effective four-pronged advocacy and service delivery strategy. Fueled by a consumer-driven philosophy, we provide four core services required of all Centers for Independent Living along with several other servies. The four core services are: Information and Referral, Peer Support, Advocacy, and Independent Living Skill Development.

788 Disabled Children's Relief Fund

PO Box 89
Freeport, NY 11520
516-377-1605
FAX: 516-377-3978
e-mail: dc1605@aol.com
www.dcrf.com

Jerome H Blue PhD, President
National not-for-profit organization that provides modest grants for disabled children with preference given to those with no health insurance. Grants are provided for assistive devices, equipment and rehabilitative services.

789 Disabled and Alone/Life Services for the Handicapped

61 Broadway
Suite 510
New York, NY 10006
212-532-6740
800-995-0066
FAX: 212-532-3588
e-mail: info@disabledandalone.org
www.disabledandalone.org

Leslie Park, Chairman
Rex L. Davidson, Vice President
William G. Shannon, Treasurer
A national nonprofit humanitarian organization whose primary concern is the well-being of handicapped persons, particularly when their families can no longer care for them. Disabled and Alone 1) Helps families do sensible planning for and with their disabled children; 2) Provides advocacy and oversight when the parents cannot do so; 3) Advises families, attorneys and financial planners about life planning for a family member with a disability.

790 **ERIC Clearinghouse on Disabilities and Special Education**
Council for Exceptional Children
1110 N Glebe Road
Suite 300
Arlington, VA 22201
888-232-7733
FAX: 703-264-9494
TTY:866-915-5000
www.ericec.org

Drew Allbritten MD, Executive Director
ERIC Clearinghouse on Disabilities and Gifted Education gathers and disseminates educational information on all disabilities and on giftedness across all age levels. As part of the ERIC network, the clearinghouse acquires, selects, abstracts, and indexes the professional literature on disabilities and giftedness for the ERIC database. The Clearinghouse also develops publications, including digests, research syntheses, and bibliographies

791 **Educational Accessibility Services**
Wayne State University
5221 Gullen Mall
Detroit, MI 48202
313-577-1851
FAX: 313-577-4898
TTY:313 577-3365
e-mail: eas@teadmin.sa.wayne.edu
www.eas.wayne.edu

Jan Collins-Eaglin PhD, Director, ASC, CAPS and EAS
Jane Depriester-Morandini, Interim Assistant Director, EAS
Caprice Ellene Quinn MA, CRC, Learinig Specialist EAS
A powerful advocating force for students with disabilities at the university. Our purpose is to provide students with the resources they need to succeed and to support their participation in all University programs and activities with dignity and independence.

792 **Environmental Dental Association**
10160 Aviary Drive
San Diego, CA 92131
858-586-1208
800-388-8124
FAX: 858-586-1220
e-mail: info@enviromentaldental.com
Organization of alternative dentists concerned about the toxic effects of dental materials and procedures.

793 **Esalen Institute**
55000 Highway 1
Big Sur, CA 93920
831-667-3000
FAX: 831-667-2724
e-mail: info@esalen.org
www.esalen.org

Michael Murphy, Chairman
Gordon Wheeler, Manager
Founded in 1962 as an alternative education center devoted to the exploration of the world of unrealized human capacities that lies beyond the imagination. Blends East/West philosophies, experiential/didactic workshops, and a steady influx of philosophers, psychologists, artists, and religious thinkers.
1962

794 **Family Resource Center on Disabilities**
20 E Jackson Boulevard
Room 300
Chicago, IL 60604
312-939-3513
800-952-4199
FAX: 312-939-7297
TTY: 312-939-3519
e-mail: that-user-name@frcd.org
www.frcd.org

Gail Jones, President
Charlotte Jardins, Executive Director
Not-for-profit advocacy organization dedicated to improving services for all children with disabilities by providing support and services to affected families, informing parents of their rights, and helping parents become advocates for their children. Offers family support services, training, seminars and information and referral services. Publishes monthly newsletter.

795 **Family Voices**
2340 Alamo SE
Suite 102
Albuquerque, NM 87106
505-872-4774
888-835-5669
888-835-5669
FAX: 505-872-4780
e-mail: kidshealth@familyvoices.org
www.familyvoices.org

Sophie Arao- Nguyen Ph.D, Executive Director
Rachel Rodriguez, Assistant Executive Director
Nora Wells, Director of National Programs
Not-for-profit voluntary organization dedicated to ensuring that children's health issues are addressed as public and private healthcare systems undergo change in communities, states and the nation. National grassroots clearinghouse for information and education in ways to assure and improve health care for children with disabilities and chronic conditions. Provides materials including pamphlets, a newsletter and one-page papers on important topics.

796 **Favarh/Farmington Valley ARC**
225 Commerce Drive
Po Box 1099
Canton, CT 06019
860-693-6662
FAX: 860-693-8662
e-mail: favarh@favarh.org
www.favarh.org

Lyn Fierri, President
Stephen E. Morris MPA, Executive Director
Provides a variety of programs and services to adults with developmental, physical or mental disabilities and their families throughout the Farmington Valley communities of Avon, Burlington and more. Favarh's programs are designed to enhance the personal, social, emotional, vocational and living capabilities of persons with disabilities.

797 **Fedcap Rehabilitation Services**
211 W 14th Street
New York, NY 10011
212-727-4200
FAX: 212-727-4374
TTY:212-727-4384
e-mail: info@fedcap.org
www.fedcap.org

Susan Fonfa, Executive Director
Michael Brenner, President Executive Committee
Mark O'Donoghue, VP Executive Committee
Fedcap helps NYC work. Since 1935, we have helped people with all types of disabilities and barriers to employment join the workforce, while providing vital services to business and government.

798 **Federation for Children with Special Needs**
1135 Tremont Street
Suite 420
Boston, MA 02120
617-236-7210
800-331-0688
FAX: 617-572-2094
e-mail: fcsninfo@fcsn.org
www.fcsn.org

Daniel Heffernan Esq, President Board of Directors
Jane Wolfson, Director of Development
Rich Robison, President
Provides information, support and assistance to parents of children with disabilities, their professional partners and their communities. We are committed to listning to and learning from families and encouraging full participation in community life by all people, especially those with disabilities.

799 **Federation of Families for Children's Mental Health**
9605 Medical Center Drive
Suite 280
Rockville, MD 20850
240-403-1901
FAX: 240-403-1909
e-mail: ffcmh@ffcmh.org
www.ffcmh.org

Sandra Spencer, Executive Director
Ashawnda Flemming, Chief Operating Officer
Ralph Kiilu, Fiscal Officer
The FFCMH, a nationally family-run organization serves to provide advocacy at the national level for the rights of children and youth with emotional, behavioral and mental health challenges and their families. Provide leadership and technical assistance to a nation-wide network of family run organizations. Collaborate with family run and other child serving organizations to transform mental health care in America.

800 **Feingold Association of the US**
554 E Main Street
Suite 301
Riverhead, NY 11901
631-369-9340
800-321-3287
FAX: 631-369-2988
e-mail: help@feingold.org
www.feingold.org

Danielle Robinson, Office Manager
An organization of families and professionals, the Feingold Association of the United States is dedicated to helping children and adults apply proven dietary techniques for better behavior, learning and health.

801 **Feldenkrais Guild of North America (FGNA)**
5436 N. Albina Avenue
Portland, OR 97217
503-221-6612
800-775-2118
FAX: 503-221-6616
e-mail: guild@feldenkrais.com
www.feldenkrais.com

Barbara Greenfield, Executive Director
Maria Whisenand, Ethics Chair
This is the organization which sets the standards for and certifies all FELDENKRAIS practitioners in North America. In order to practice, a practitioner must be a graduate of an FGNA accredited program (a minimum of 800 instruction hours over a three to four year period), and agree to follow both the Code of Professional Conduct and the Standards of Practice. FGNA may be contacted for further information about the FELDENKRAIS METHOD or for a list of FELDENKRAIS practitioners sorted by region.

802 **Focus Alternative Learning Center**
126 Dowd Avenue
Po Box 452
Canton, CT 06019
860-693-8809
FAX: 860-693-0141
e-mail: info@focus-alternative.org
www.focus-alternative.org

Donna Swanson MSN, CS, APRN, Executive Director
Jen Haggerty MA, Clinical Coordinator
Sandy Kissel RN, BSN, MSN, Nurse Clinician
A private non profit, licensed clinical and learning center specialized in the treatment of creatively wired and socially challenged kids. We treat kids on the autism spectrum who suffer from high anxiety, experience processing difficulties and learning problems.

803 **George Washington University Health Resource Center**
2121 K Street NW
Suite 220
Washington, DC 20037
202-973-0904
800-544-3284
FAX: 202-973-0908
e-mail: askheath@gwu.edu
www.heath.gwu.edu

Dr Pamela Ekpone, Director
Zavolia Willis, Assistant Director
Dan Gardner, Publications Manager
National clearinghouse for information about education after high school for people with disabilities. Also serves as an information exchange about educational support services, policies, procedures, adaptations and opportunities on American campuses, vocational-technical schools, adult education programs, independent living centers and other training entities after high school.

804 **Goodwill Industries International**
15810 Indianola Drive
Rockville, MD 20855
301-530-6500
800-741-0186
FAX: 301-530-1516
e-mail: Contactus@goodwill.org
www.goodwill.org

George W Kessinger, President and CEO
Edward A Osborne, Chair, Board of Directors
Strives to achieve the full participation in society of disabled persons and other individuals with special needs by expanding their opportunities and occupational capabilities through a network of 179 autonomous, nonproft, community-based organizations providing services throughout the world in response to local needs.

805 **Haldimand-Norfolk Resource Education and C ounseling**
101 Nanticoke Creek Parkway
Box 5054
Townsend, ON, ZZ N0A
519-587-2441
800-265-8087
FAX: 519-587-4798
www.hnreach.on.ca

Promote and support community well-being by providing co-ordinated access, planning, programs and services for individuals and families.

806 **Health Action**
315 Meigs Rd.
Suite A-276
Santa Barbara, CA 93109
805-685-4670
FAX: 805-685-4710
www.healthaction.net

Dr. Roger Jahnke, Chief Executive Officer
Rebecca Mclean, Co Founder
Our mission is to foster innovation in health care that will increase health status, increase customer satisfaction, increase profitability, increase clinical efficacy and eliminate error, support provider efficiency and enhance clinical outcomes, and empower consumer self-managed care.

807 **Health Resource Center for Women with Disabilities**
Rehabilitation Institute of Chicago
345 E Superior Street
Chicago, IL 60611
312-238-1000
800-354-7342
FAX: 312-238-1205
e-mail: webmaster@ric.org
www.rehabchicago.org

Joanne C. Smith MD, MBA, President/CEO
Edward B. Case, Exec. Vice President/CFO
Nancy E. Paridy, JD, Senior Vice President
RIC has earned a worldwide reputation as being a leader in patient health care, advocacy, research and educating health professionals in physical medicine and rehabilitation. People from around the globe choose RIC because of our expertise in treating a range of conditions, from the most complex conditions including cerebral palsy, spinal cord injury, stroke and traumatic brain injury, to the more common, such as arthritis, chronic pain, and sports injuries.

808 **Homeopathic Educational Services**
2124B Kittredge Street
Berkeley, CA 94704
510-649-0294
800-359-9051
FAX: 510-649-1955
e-mail: mail@homeopathic.com
www.homeopathic.com

Dana Ullman, Director and Owner

Resource center for homeopathic products and services including books, tapes, research, medicines, medicine kits, software for the general public and the health professional and correspondence courses.

809 **Human Ecology Action League (HEAL)**

PO Box 509
Stockbridge, GA 30281
404-248-1898
FAX: 404-248-0162
e-mail: healnatnl@aol.com
members.aol.com/HEALNatnl/index.html

Katherine P Collier, Membership Coordinator/Manager
HEAL is a nonprofit education and information organization. It is primarily a member service organization. It is overseen by a volunteer Governing Board, and has its business office in Atlanta Georgia. HEAL is solely funded by memberships and by donations.

810 **IL Center: Cape Organization for Rights of the Disabled**

1019 Iyannough Road
Suite 4
Hyannis, MA 02601
508-775-8300
800-541-0282
FAX: 508-775-7022
TTY: 800-541-0282
e-mail: coreen@cape.com
www.cordonline.org

Pamela Burkley, Executive Director
The Cape Organization for the Rights of the Disabled (CORD) has been aggresively working since 1984 to advance the independence, productivity, and integration of people with disabilities including deaf and hard of hearing people, into mainstream society.
1984

811 **Institute for Scientific Research**

1000 Technology Drive
Suite 1000
Fairmont, WV 26554
304-366-2577
877-363-5482
FAX: 304-366-2699
e-mail: info@isr.us
www.wvhtf.org

James Estep, President
Raymond A Oliverio, Executive Vice President
Jonathan Elder, CPA, Chief Financial Officer
Institute for Scientific Research, Inc. performs cutting-edge research across a variety of scientific and engineering disciplines. Our people participate in world-class projects from concept through development, in some of today's most fascinating scientific fields.

812 **Institute of Transpersonal Psychology**

1069 E Meadow Circle
Palo Alto, CA 94303
650-493-4430
FAX: 650-493-6835
e-mail: itpinfo@itp.edu
www.itp.edu

Charles Randall, Interim President
Brigitte Lindsey, Exec. Assistant To President
Paul Roy, Academic Vice President
The Institute of Transpersonal Psychology is a private, non-sectarian graduate school accredited by the Western Association of Schools and Colleges. For over twenty-five years the Institute has remained a leader at the forefront of psychological research and education, probing the mind, body, spirit connection. The Institute's challenging and transformative educational paradigm has attracted students from all over the world.

813 **International Association of Machinists**

9000 Machinists Place
Upper Marlboro, MD 20772
301-967-4500
FAX: 316-522-7989
e-mail: websteward@goiam.org
www.goiam.org

Steve Rayni, President
R Buffenbarger, Chief Executive Officer
Placement programs for persons with disabilities.

814 **International Association of Yoga Therapists**

115 South McCormick Street
Suite 3
Prescott, AZ 86303
928-541-0004
FAX: 928-541-0182
e-mail: mail@iayt.org
www.iayt.org

Janice Gates, President
Eleanor Criswell Ed.D, Vice President
Matthew J. Taylor PT, PhD, Treasurer/Research Committee
IAYT supports research and education in Yoga and serves Yoga practitioners, Yoga teachers, Yoga therapists, health care professionals, and researchers worldwide. Our mission is to establish Yoga as a recognised and respected therapy in the Western world. IAYT also serves members, the media, and the general public as a comprehensive source of information about contemporary Yoga education, research, and statistics.

815 **International Chiropractors Association**

1110 N Glebe Road
Suite 650
Arlington, VA 22201
703-528-5000
800-423-4690
FAX: 703-528-5023
e-mail: chiro@chiropractic.org
www.chiropractic.org

Dr. John Maltby, President
Ronald Hendrickson, Executive Director
Established in 1926 to empower humanity in the expression of maximum health, wellness and human potential through the universal chiropractic expression and utilization. Strives to advance chiropractics throughout the world as a distinct health care profession predicated upon its unique philosophy, science and art.
1926

816 **International Clinic of Biological Regeneration**

PO Box 509
Florissant, MO 63032
314-921-3997
800-826-5366
FAX: 314-921-8485
e-mail: info@icbr.com
www.icbr.com

C Tom Smith, President
The International Clinic of Biological Regeneration (ICBR) is a leading international cell therapy center that has been in continuous operation since 1981. During this time, Dr. Smith has constantly improved theraputic results of the treatment by selecting newer, safer and more effective formulations as delveloped by leading European research centers.
1981

817 **International College of Applied Kinesiology**

6405 Metcalf Avenue
Suite 503
Shawnee Mission, KS 66202
913-384-5336
FAX: 913-384-5112
e-mail: info@icak.com
www.icak.com

Terry Underwood, Executive Director
Jennifer Palmer, Associate Executive Director
Allison Burwell, Conference Manager
Referral service for applied kinesiologists. AK is a system that evaluates structural, chemical and mental apsects of health using manual muscle testing combined with other standard methods of diagnosis. It is a non invasive stystem of evaluating body function that is unique in the healing arts, and has become a dynamic movement in health care in its relatively short existance.

818 **International Women's Health Coalition**

333 7th Avenue
6th Floor
New York, NY 10001
212-979-8500
FAX: 212-979-9009
e-mail: info@iwhc.org
www.iwhc.org

Kati Marton, Chiar
Thomas W. Merrick PhD, Vice Chair
Maria Plata, Vice Chair

Information and pamphlets on sexually transmitted diseases and other health concerns. IWHC works to generate health and population policies, programs, and funding that promote and protect the rights and health of girls and women worldwide.

819 **Job Accommodation Network**
PO Box 6080
Morgantown, WV 26506
304-293-7186
800-526-7234
FAX: 304-293-5407
e-mail: jan@jan.wvu.edu
www.jan.wvu.edu

DJ Hendricks, Director
JAN's mission is to facilitate the employment and retention of workers with disabilities by providing employers, employment providers, people with disabilities, their family members and other interested parties with information on job accomodations, self-employment and small business opportunities and related subjects. JAN's efforts are in support of the employment, including self-employment and small business ownership, of people with disabilities.

820 **Joni and Friends**
PO Box 3333
Agoura Hills, CA 91376
818-707-5664
800-523-5777
FAX: 818-707-2391
TTY: 818-707-9707
e-mail: jafmin@joniandfriends.org
www.joniandfriends.org

Joni Eareckson Tada, Founder
Doug Mazza, President & COO
Billy C. Burnett, VP/Chief Financial Officer
A nonprofit organization seeking to accelerate Christian ministry with people affected by disabilities. JAF educates churches and the community worldwide concerning the needs of the disabled and how those needs can be met. We sponsor family retreats for families with disabled members. Wheels for the World collects, restores and distributes used wheelchairs to disadvantaged populations around the world.
1979

821 **Juvenile Diabetes Foundation International**
120 Wall Street
19th Floor
New York, NY 10005
212-785-9500
800-533-2873
FAX: 212-785-9595
e-mail: info@jdrf.org
www.jdrf.org

Larry Soler, Vice President
Laura Whitton, Manager
Ronnie Tepp, National Manager
The world's leading nonprofit, nongovernmental funder of diabetes research. It was founded in 1970 by parents of children with diabetes. JDF's mission is to find a cure for diabetes and its complications through the support of research. JDF also sponsors international workshops and conferences for biomedical researchers, individual chapters offer support groups and other activities for families affected by diabetes. JDF has more than 110 chapters and affiliates worldwide. Quarterly newsletter.
1970

822 **Lambton County Developmental Services**
339 Centre Street
Box 1210
Petrolia, Ontario, ZZ N0N
519-882-0933
888-779-0061
FAX: 519-882-3386
e-mail: lcds@oasisonline.ca
www.lcds.on.ca
A network of caring people, working together to provide services for people with developmental disabilities to facilitate the achievement of their life dreams.

823 **LoSeCa Foundation**
215-1 Carnegie Drive
Albert, AB, ZZ T8N
780-460-1400
FAX: 780-459-1380
www.loseca.ca
A non-profit organization that provides support services to adults with developmental disabilities

824 **MCC Supportive Care Services**
103 2776 Bourquin Circle W
Abbotsford, BC, ZZ V2S
604-850-6608
800-622-5455
FAX: 604-850-2634
e-mail: office@mccscs.com
mccscs.com
A service provider, advocate and resource for persons living and dealing with mental, physical and/or emotional disabilities.

825 **Maharishi Ayur-Veda Medical Center**
1734 Jasmine Avenue
Fairfield, IA 52556
641-469-6706
800-864-8714
FAX: 641-472-2496
e-mail: theraj@theraj.com
www.theraj.com
The RAJ opened its doors in April 1993 and soon gained a reputation as America's premier Ayurveda Health Center. It is the only such facility outside of India specifically built to offer traditional Ayurveda rejuvenation treatments.
1993

826 **Mainstream**
300 S Rodney Parham Road
Suite 5
Little Rock, AR 72205
501-280-0012
FAX: 501-280-9267
TTY:501-280-9262
e-mail: mainstreamlr@earthlink.net
www.mainstreamilrc.com

Rita Byers, Executive Director
Non-profit organization that works with employers and service providers around the country to increase employment opportunities for persons with disabilities.

827 **March of Dimes Birth Defects Foundation**
1275 Mamaroneck Avenue
White Plains, NY 10605
914-997-4488
800-996-2724
FAX: 914-997-4763
www.modimes.org
The mission of the March of Dimes is to improve the health of babies by preventing birth defects and infant mortality. The MOD Resource Center provides information and referral services to the public from 9:00 am to 8:00 pm EST.

828 **Metametrix Clinical Laboratory**
4855 Peachtree Industrial Boulevard
Suite 201
Norcross, GA 30092
770-446-5483
800-221-4640
FAX: 770-441-2237
e-mail: inquiries@metametrix.com
www.metametrix.com/

J Alexander Bralley PhD, Chief Executive Officer
Robert M. David PhD, Laboratory Director
Richard S. Lord PhD, Director, Science And Education
Metametrix Clinical Laboratory has been a pioneer and leader in the development of nutritional, metabolic, and toxicant analyses since 1984. Metametrix is committed to helping health care professionals identify nutritional influences on health and disease, and is recognized internationally for its laboratory procedures in nutritional and biochemical testing.

829 **Mind-Body Clinic**
824 Boylston Street
Chestnut Hill, MA 02467
617-732-9130
FAX: 617-732-9111
e-mail: mindbody@partners. org
www.mbmi.org/home/default.asp

Gregory L. Fricchione MD, Director
Herbert Benson MD, Director Emeritus
Marylin Wilcher, Senior Vice President
The Benson-Henry Institue for Mind Body Medicine is a world leader in the study, advancement, and clinical practice of mind/body medicine. The BHI provides outpatient medical services, training for health professionals, corporate and school-based programs, women's health services, and affiliation for national and international health care systems.

830 Mind/Body Health Services

393 Dixon Road
Boulder, CO 80302
303-440-8460
FAX: 303-440-7580
e-mail: luzie@joanborysenko.com
www.joanborysenko.com

Joan Borysenko, President
Luzie Mason, Assistant
publish free annual newsletter/cataloge:Circle of Healing. Information about the works of Joan Borysenko.

831 Mississippi Society for Disabilities

500 G Woodrow Wilson Drive
Po Box 4948
Jackson, MS 39296
601-362-2585
800-962-2400
FAX: 601-982-1951
www.mississippicap.com

Presley Posey, Executive Director
Provides a broad spectrum of programs and services to meet the needs of Mississippi children and adults with disabilities, thus enabling them to achieve maximum independence and gain the greatest possible quality of life.

832 Muscular Dystrophy Association

3300 E Sunrise Drive
Tucson, AZ 85718
520-529-2000
800-572-1717
FAX: 520-529-5383
e-mail: mda@mdausa.org
www.mdausa.org

Robert Ross, Chief Executive Officer
Chris Rosa, PhD, Member of the Board
MDA provides comprehensive medical services to tens of thousands of people with neuromuscular diseases at some 230 hospital-affiliated clinics across the country. The Association's worldwide research program, which funds over 400 individual scientific investigations annually, represents the largest single effort to advance knowledge of neuromuscular diseases and to find cures and treatments for them. In addition, MDA conducts far-reaching educational programs for the public and professionals.

833 National Association for Holistic Aromatherapy

3327 W Indian Trail Road
Pmb 144
Spokane, WA 99208
509-325-3419
FAX: 509-325-3479
e-mail: info@naha.org
www.naha.org

Kelly Holland Azzaro, VP
Michele Miller, President
The NAHA is an educational, nonprofit organization dedicated to enhancing public awareness of the benefits of true aromatherapy. It offers aromatherapy courses and acts as a referral service.

834 National Association of Developmental Disabilities Councils

225 Reinekers Lane
Suite 650b
Alexandria, VA 22314
703-739-4400
FAX: 703-739-6030
e-mail: info@nacdd.org
www.nacdd.org

Karen Flippo, Executive Director
Phyllis Guinivan, Council Services Liason
Pat Brown, Office Manager
The National Association of Councils on Developmental Disabilities (NACDD) is a national, member-driven organization consisting of 55 State and Territorial Councils. NACDD places high value on meaningful participation and contribution by Council members and staff of all Member Councils, and we advocate and continually work towards positive system change on behalf of individuals with developmental disabilities and their families.

835 National Association of Protection and Advocacy Systems

900 2nd Street NE
Suite 211
Washington, DC 20002
202-408-9514
FAX: 202-408-9520
e-mail: info@ndrn.org
www.napas.org

Curtis L. Decker J.D., Executive Director
Joanna Solkoff, Executive/Public Policy Assis.
Voluntary national membership association of protection and advocacy systems and client assistance programs. Promoting and strengthening the role and performance of its members in providing quality legally based advocacy services.

836 National Association of State Directors of Developmental Disabilities Services (NASDDDS)

113 Oronoco Street
Alexandria, VA 22314
703-683-4202
FAX: 703-683-8773
e-mail: klebeau@nasddds.org
www.nasddds.org

Nancy Thaler, Executive Director
Robert M Gettings, Senior Advisor to Exec. Director
Charles R Moseley EdD, Director of Special Projects
A nonprofit organization devoted to improving and expanding services to persons with developmental disabilities. The primary aims of the association are to: facilitate an exchange of information regarding the most advanced and efficacious methods of providing care and training to this population and represent the interests of state programs for persons with mental retardation/developmental disabilities in the development and implementation of federal programs.

837 National Association of the Physically Handicapped

754 Staeger Street
Akron, OH 44306
330-724-1994
800-743-5008
e-mail: trumanjm@aol.com
www.naph.net

Jim Truman, National President
The NAPH advances the social, economic, and physical welfare of the physically handicapped in the United States. NAPH proposes and supports legislation to provide more educational and rehabilitation opportunities, tax relief, employment, and other benefits for the physically handicapped. Data and information relating to the physically handicapped are collected and studied and reported to members. NAPH supports efforts to make all public buildings accessible to the physically handicapped.
1958

838 National Business & Disability Council

201 I U Willets Road
Albertson, NY 11507
516-465-1516
FAX: 516-465-3730
e-mail: info@business-disability.com
www.nbdc.com

Michael J McGowan
Laura M Francis
Dedicated to increasing the employment of people with disabilities through a coordinated effort of N America's largest employers. Believing that people with disabilities bring value to the workplace. Provides the leadership necessary to infuse effective employment practices for workers with disabilities in our global economy.

839 National Center for Education in Maternal and Child Health

Georgetown University
PO Box 571272
Washington, DC 20057
202-784-9770
FAX: 202-784-9777
e-mail: mchlibrary@ncemch.org
www.ncemch.org

Rochelle Mayer, Research Professor and Director
Provides information on children with special health needs, child health and development, adolescent health, nutrition, violence and injury prevention and other issues of maternal and child health for health professionals and the public.

840 **National College of Naturopathic Medicine**
049 SW Porter Street
Portland, OR 97201
503-552-1555
FAX: 503-499-0022
e-mail: wkeppler@ncnm.edu
www.ncnm.edu

William Keppler, President
Pauline Baumannn, Chair of the Board
NCNM offers two graduate professional degrees in accredited and recognized programs that prepare you for licensed practice in many states and provinces: Doctor of Naturopathic Medicine, a four-year program of clinical sciences and holistic methods of healing and disease prevention, instilled with the ancient principle of the healing power of nature. Master of Science in Oriental Medicine, a four-year program that delves deeply into thousands of years of classical Chinese methods of diagnostics.

841 **National Council on Disability**
1331 F Street NW
Suite 850
Washington, DC 20004
202-272-2004
FAX: 202-272-2022
TTY:202-272-2074
e-mail: ncd@ncd.gov
www.ncd.gov

John R Vaughn, Chairperson
Patricia Pound, First Vice Chairperson
Glenn B. Anderson PhD, Second Vice Chairperson
Federal agency led by 15 members appointed by the President of the United States and confirmed by the United States Senate. The overall purpose of the National Council is to promote policies, programs, practices and procedures that guarantee equal opportunities to persons with disabilities.

842 **National Council on Independent Living**
1710 Rhode Island Avenue NW
5th Floor
Washington, DC 20036
202-207-0341
877-525-3400
FAX: 202-207-0341
e-mail: ncil@ncil.org
www.ncil.org

Kelly Buckland, President
Dan Kessler, Vice President
Frank Shible, Treasurer
Advances the independent living philosophy and advocates for the human rights of and services for people with disabilities to further their full integration and participation in society. The National Council on Independent Living (NCIL) is the oldest cross disability, grassroots organization run by and for people with disabilities.

843 **National Deaf Education Network and Clearinghouse**
Gallaudet University
800 Florida Avenue NE
Washington, DC 20002
202-651-5000
FAX: 202-651-5101
TTY:202-651-5101
e-mail: michael.wynne@gallaudet.edu
clerccenter.gallaudet.edu

Michael Wynne, Admissions Contact
Katherine Jankowski, Schools Programs Contact
Erving Jordan, President
Gallaudet University's Laurent Clerc National Deaf Education Center shares the concerns of parents and professionals about the achievement of deaf and hard of hearing students in different learning environments across the country. We all know that deaf and hard of hearing students can and do excel, but we also know that not all deaf and hard of hearing students are achieving their full potential.

844 **National Dissemination Center for Children and Youth with Disabilities (NICHCY)**
PO Box 1492
Washington, DC 20013
202-884-8200
800-695-0285
FAX: 202-884-8441
e-mail: nichcy@aed.org
www.nichcy.org

Suzanne Ripley, Director
Provides free information to assist parents, educators, caregivers, advocates and others in helping children and youth with disabilities become participating members of the community. In addition to a wealth of printed materials, the Center disseminates materials on cassette, computer disc and in Spanish. The Center can also provide personal responses to specific questions.

845 **National Early Childhood Technical Assistance Center**
8040 Unc-Ch
Chapel Hill, NC 27599
919-962-2001
FAX: 919-966-7463
TTY:919-843-3269
e-mail: nectac@unc.edu
www.nectac.org

Pascal Trohanis, Director
Lynne Kahn, Associate Director
Shelley deFosset, Associate Director
Assists states and other designated governing jurisdictions as they develop multidisciplinary, coordinated and comprehensive services for children with special needs.

846 **National Easter Seal Society**
230 W Monroe Street
Suite 1800
Chicago, IL 60606
312-726-6200
FAX: 312-726-1494
TTY:312 726 4258
www.easterseal.com

Janet D Jamieson, Communications Manager
James Williams Jr, Chief Executive Officer
The mission of the Society is to help people with disabilities achieve independence. Easter Seals provides quality rehabilitation services, technological assistance and disability prevention, advocacy and public education programs. A nationwide network of affiliate societies serving each of the 50 United States, the District of Columbia and Puerto Rico, all of which work together to serve more than 1 million people each year. There are 160 chapters offering more than 400 programs nationwide.

847 **National Federation of the Blind: Merchants Division**
National Federation of the Blind
1800 Johnson Street
Baltimore, MD 21230
410-659-9314
FAX: 410-685-5653
e-mail: nfb@nfb.org
www.nfb.org

Marc Maurer, President
Fred Schroeder, First Vice President
Peggy Elliott, Second Vice President
Membership organization of blind persons employed in either self-employment work or the Randolph-Sheppard vending program. Provides information regarding rehabilitation, social security, tax and other issues which directly affect blind merchants. Serves as advocacy and support group.

848 **National Federation of the Blind: Blind Industrial Workers Division**
National Federation of the Blind
1800 Johnson Street
Baltimore, MD 21230
410-659-9314
FAX: 410-685-5653
e-mail: nfb@nfb.org
www.nfb.org

Marc Maurer, President
Fredric Schroeder, First Vice President
Peggy Elliott, Second Vice President
Membership organization of blind persons employed in industrial and manufacturing work or in government job programs for the blind. Dedicated to protecting the rights of blind workers in salary, job stability, advancement, and labor issues.

849 **National Federation of the Blind: Computer Science Division**
National Federation of the Blind
1800 Johnson Street
Baltimore, MD 21230
410-659-9314
FAX: 410-685-5653
e-mail: nfb@nfb.org
www.nfb.org

Marc Maurer, President
Fredric Schroeder, First Vice President
Peggy Elliott, Second Vice President
National organization of blind persons knowledgeable in the computer science and technology fields. Works to develop new technologies, to secure access to current technology and to develop new ways of using current or new technologies by the blind.

850 **National Federation of the Blind: Public Employees Division**
1800 Johnson Street
Baltimore, MD 21230
410-659-9314
FAX: 410-685-5653
e-mail: nfb@nfb.org
www.nfb.org

Marc Mauer, President
Fredric Schroeder, First Vice President
Peggy Elliott, Second Vice President
Organization of blind persons holding local, state or federal jobs. Focuses on issues such as changes in governmental hiring and retention practices, new job skills needed for the future, government employment downsizing, new electronic means of finding public sector jobs, self-advocacy and career planning strategies.

851 **National Federation of the Blind: Science and Engineering Division**
National Federation of the Blind
1800 Johnson Street
Baltimore, MD 21230
410-659-9314
FAX: 410-685-5653
e-mail: nfb@nfb.org
www.nfb.org

Marc Maurer, President
Fredric Schroeder, First Vice President
Peggy Elliott, Second Vice President
Blind persons with expertise and experience in fields such as genetics, telecommunications, biology, chemistry, physics and nuclear physics or mechanical, electronic and chemical engineering. This is a strong support group to encourage blind persons in pursuit of these careers, many of which have been considered not possible for the blind in the past.

852 **National Federation of the Blind: Writers Division**
National Federation of the Blind
1800 Johnson Street
Baltimore, MD 21230
410-659-9314
FAX: 410-685-5653
e-mail: nfb@nfb.org
www.nfb.org

Marc Maurer, President
Fredric Schroeder, First Vice President
Peggy Elliott, Second Vice President
Blind writers in all styles, including poetry, short story, fiction, non-fiction, magazine writing and theatrical work offer encouragement and support to blind writers and authors. Issues cover various aspects of this business, including selling your work, publishing, technology, motivation and discovering writing and publishing resources.

853 **National Guild of Hypnotists**
PO Box 308
Merrimack, NH 03054
603-429-9438
FAX: 603-424-8066
e-mail: ngh@ngh.net
www.ngh.net

Dr. Dwight F Damon, President
The National Guild of Hypnotists, Inc. is a not-for-profit, educational corporation in the State of New Hampshire. Founded in Boston, Massachusetts in 1951, the Guild is a professional organization comprised of dedicated individuals committed to advancing the field of hypnotism. We provide an open forum for the free exchange of ideas concerning hypnotism. The Guild is a resource for members and a vehicle for legal and legislative action.

1951

854 **National Information Center for Children**
PO Box 1492
Washington, DC 20013
202-884-8200
800-695-0285
FAX: 202-884-8441
www.nichy.org

Susan Ripley, Manager
Information on disabilities and disibility-related issues for family, educators and professionals related to children and youth.

855 **National Institute on Disability and Rehabilitation Research**
400 Maryland Avenue SW
Washington, DC 20202
202-401-0689
800-872-5327
FAX: 202-401-0689
TTY: 800-437-0833
e-mail: customerservice@inet.ed.gov
www.ed.gov

Lacy B Ward Jr, VP
Daniel Holt, Director
Conducts comprehensive and coordinated programs of extramural research and related activities to maximize the full inclusion, social integration, employment and independent living of disabled individuals of all ages. Provides funding for programs to assist ADA compliance, including Regional Disability and Business Technical Assistance Centers, Materials Development Projects, and Peer Training Projects.

856 **National Maternal and Child Health Bureau**
Po Box 2910
Merrifield, VA 22116
301-443-2170
800-275-4772
FAX: 703-821-2098
e-mail: ctibbs@hrsa.gov
www.ask.hrsa.gov

Michael A Mucci, Director
Peter C Van Dyck MD, Associate Administrator
Offers information, books and pamphlets to professionals, parents and children facing health issues or disabilities.

857 **National Mental Health Association**
2000 N Beauregard Street
6th Floor
Alexandria, VA 22311
703-684-7722
800-969-6642
FAX: 703-684-5968
TTY: 800-433-5959
e-mail: infoctr@nmha.org
www.nmha.org

Michael Faenza, President and CEO
Nonprofit organization addressing all issues related to mental health and mental illness. With more than 340 affiliates nationwide, NMHA works to improve the mental health of all Americans, especially the 54 million individuals with mental disorders, through advocacy, education, research and service.
1909

858 **National Organization on Disability**
910 16th Street NW
Suite 600
Washington, DC 20006
202-293-5960
FAX: 202-293-7999
TTY:202-293-5968
e-mail: ability@nod.org
www.nod.org

Tom Ridge, Chairman
Michael R. Deland, President
Arlene E. Anns, Publisher
The National Organization on Disability promotes the full and equal participation of men, women and children with disabilities in all aspects of American life. Founded in 1982, NOD is the leading national disability organization concerned with all disabilites, all age groups and all disability issues.

1982

859 National Rehabilitation Association (NRA)

633 South Washington Street
Alexandria, VA 22314
703-836-0850
FAX: 703-836-0848
TTY:703-836-0849
e-mail: info@nationalrehab.org
www.nationalrehab.org

Linda Winslow, Executive Director
Dedicated to advocating, supporting, and enhancing the lives of individuals with disabilities and their families. disseminates up-to-date information, conducts educational seminars, and provides opportunities through knowledge and diversity for professionals in the field of rehabilitation. Produces educational materials and sponsors an annual training conference with exhibits displaying the latest in rehabilitation technologies, awards, and provides access to a nationwide employment network.

860 National Rehabilitation Information Center (NARIC)

8201corporate Drive
Suite 600
Landover, MD 20785
301-459-5900
800-346-2742
FAX: 301-459-4263
TTY:301 459 5984
e-mail: naricinfo@heitechservices.com
www.naric.com

Mark X Odum, Director
For 20 years, the staff of the NARIC has collected and disseminated the results of federally funded research projects. NARIC's literature collection, which also includes commercially published books, journal articles and audiovisuals, averages around 200 new documents per month. Funded by the National Institute on Disability and Rehabilitation Research to serve anyone, professional or lay person, who is interested in disability and rehabilitation.

861 National Respite Locator Service

800 Eastowne Drive
Suite 105
Chapel Hill, NC 27514
919-490-5577
FAX: 919-490-4905
TTY:919 490 5577
e-mail: awilcow@chtop.org
www.respitelocator.org

Angela Wilcox, Director
Michael Mathers, Executive Director
Linda Baker, Director
Dedicated to assisting parents, caregivers and professionals find temporary relief services in their state and local area. Provides appropriate referrals for further assistance and has a leaflet describing the organization.

862 National Vaccine Information Center

204 Mill Street
Suite B1
Vienna, VA 22180
703-938-3783
FAX: 703-938-5768
www.nvic.org

Barbara Loe Fisher, Co-Founder/President
Kathi Williams, Co-Founder/Vice President
Vicki Debold PhD, RN, Board Member
A national nonprofit educational organization dedicated to preventing, through public education, vaccine injuries and deaths. NVIC represents vaccine consumers and health care providers, including parents whose children suffered illness or died following vaccination. NVIC supports the right of vaccine consumers to have access to the safest and most effective vaccine as well as the right to make informed, independent vaccination decisions.

863 National Women's Health Network

514 10th Street NW
Suite 400
Washington, DC 20004
202-347-1140
FAX: 202-347-1168
e-mail: nwhn@nwhn.org
www.nwhn.org

Kimberly Lau, Chairperson
Judith Costlow, Action Vice Chair
Jyl Boline, Administrative Vice Chair
The National Women's Health Network improves the health of all women by developing and promoting a critical analysis of health issues in order to affect policy and support consumer decision-making. The Network aspires to a health care system that is guided by social justice and reflects the needs of diverse women.

864 Native American Protection and Advocacy

Po Box 306
Window Rock, AZ 86515
928-871-4151
800-862-7271
FAX: 928-871-5036
www.nativelegalnet.org

Therese Yanan, Executive Director
The Native American Protection & Advocacy which helps protect, promote, and expand the legal and human rights of Native Americans with disabilities. There are several goals for this organization, including quality legal representation for individuals with disabilities in various areas such as abuse and neglect, special education, civil rights and discrimination and employment.

865 New York Therapeutic Riding Center

306 East 71 Street
New York, NY 10021
212-535-3917
212-535-3917
www.nytrc.org

Richard Brodie, President
The Therapeutic Riding Center has been conducting therapeutic horseback riding progams for children and adults with disabilites living in New York City for 10 years. Its riding facility is located at the well-equipped Chateau Stables, and staffed by volunteers with experience in physical therapy, osteopathy, art therapy and other areas designed to deal with various aspects of disabled individuals.

866 North America Riding for the Handicapped Association

PO Box 33150
Denver, CO 80233
303-452-1212
800-369-7433
FAX: 303-252-4610
e-mail: narha@narha.org
www.narha.org

Sheila Kemper dietrich, Chief Executive Officer
Elizabeth Konstanty, Executive Assistant
Joyce Coniglio, Accountant
National nonprofit equestrian organization dedicated to serving individuals with disability by giving disabled individuals the opportunity to ride horses. Establishes safety standards, provides continuing education and offers networking opportunities for both its individuals and center members. Produces educational materials including fact sheets, brochures, booklets, audio-visual tapes, a directory and NARHA's magazine Strides.

867 North Hastings Community Integration Assoc iation

2 Alice Street
Bancroft, ON, ZZ K0L
613-332-2090
FAX: 613-332-4762
e-mail: nhcia@northcom.net

Jane Mayberry, Executive Director
Dave Buttineau, Community Support Coordinator
Supports people with an intellectual disability and their families.

868 Nurse Healers: Professional Associates International

Box 419
Craryville, NY 12521
518-325-1185
877-326-4774
FAX: 509-693-3537
e-mail: nh-pai@therapeutic-touch.org
www.therapeutic-touch.org

Dolores Krieger, Founder
Diane May RN, Coordinator
Sue Conlin, Treasurer

Cooperative among health professionals interested in healing. Sets the standards for the practice and teaching of Therapeutic Touch. Voluntary, not-for-profit organization.

869 Opportunity Plus of NC

PO Box 35481
Charlotte, NC 28235
704-376-4735
FAX: 704-376-4738
e-mail: info@opportunity-plus.org
www.opportunity-plus.org

Don Olin, President
Dallas Bolan, Executive Director
Opportunity Plus of North Carolina was founded 25 years ago to serve the needs of people with disabilities in the Charlotte metropolitan area and its contiguous counties. Our goal is to treat each person as an individual. Customized career paths are developed by discovering hidden potentials, addressing specific needs and removing hurdles.

870 PACER Center (Parent Advocacy Coalition for Educational Rights)

8161 Normandale Boulevard
Minneapolis, MN 55437
952-838-9000
800-537-2237
FAX: 952-838-0199
TTY: 952-838-0190
e-mail: pacer@pacer.org
www.pacer.org

Paula F Goldberg, Executive Director
Mission is to expand opportunities and enhance the quality of life of children and young adults with disabilities and their families based on the concept of parents helping parents. Offers workshops, individual assistance and written information. Provides programs and materials that assist multicultural families, programs for students, schools and professionals with disability awareness puppet and child abuse prevention programs. Computer Resource Center/Software Lending Library available.
1977

871 PEAK Parent Center

611 N Weber Street
Suite 200
Colorado Springs, CO 80903
719-531-9400
800-284-0251
FAX: 719-531-9452
e-mail: info@peakparent.org
www.peakparent.org

Barbara Buswell, Executive Director
PEAK Parent Center is a federally-designated Parent Training and Information Center (PTI). As a PTI, PEAK supports and empowers parents, providing them with information and strategies to use when advocating for their children with disabilities. PEAK works one-on-one with families and educators helping them realize new possibilities for children with disabilities by expanding knowledge of special education and offering new strategies for success.

872 Pacific Institute of Aromatherapy

PO Box 6723
San Rafael, CA 94903
415-479-9120
FAX: 415-479-0614
e-mail: osa_pia@yahoo.com
www.pacificinstituteofaromatherapy.com

Kurt Schnaubelt, Owner
To elevate the status of aromatherapy toward a classic discipline of learning and to present substance not currently availiable. Understanding the chemical composition and pharmacology of essential oils will lead to the most successfull aromatherapy treatments today. Insight into the biology of essential oils transcends the chemical worldview and will become the tool to design superior healing strategies.

873 Parent Professional Advocacy League

59 Temple Place
Suite 664
Boston, MA 02111
617-542-7860
866-815-8122
FAX: 617-542-7832
e-mail: info@ppal.net
www.ppal.net

Lisa Lambert, Interim Director
Carol Gramm, Education & Training Coordinator
Carol Mattina, PRN Line Coordinator
An organization that promotes a strong voice for families of children and adolescents with mental health needs. PAL advocates for supports, treatment and policies that enable families to live in their communities in an environment of stability and respect.

874 Parent to Parent

3805 Presidential Parkway
Suite 207
Atlanta, GA 30340
770-451-5484
800-229-2038
FAX: 770-458-4091
e-mail: info@parenttoparentofga.org
www.parenttoparentofga.org

Esther Sherberger, Director
Debra Tucker, Executive Director
Dedicated to strengthening, supporting, and empowering families by establishing one to one parent to parent contacts. Enhances the ability of parents to access services and resources for children with special needs by providing information, resources, and referrals to appropriate services; supports and empowers families to participate in parent programs and disability issues. Educational materials consist of a quarterly newsletter and a fact sheet containing managed care information.

875 Parents Helping Parents (PHP)

3041 Olcott Street
Santa Clara, CA 95054
408-727-5775
FAX: 408-727-0182
e-mail: info@php.com
www.php.com

Mary Ellen Peterson, CEO
Joanna Jaegar, Board Chair
Tom Downey, Board Treasurer
Dedicated to assisting children with any type of special need: mental, physical, emotional, or learning disability. Mission is to help children with special needs receive love, hope, respect, and services needed to achieve their full potential by strengthening their families and the professionals who serve them. Developed and implemented numerous programs; produce a variety of educational and support materials, including information packets, brochures, database and a quarterly newletter.

876 Parents for Residential Reform

Federation For Children With Special Needs
1135 Tremont Street
Suite 420
Boston, MA 02120
617-236-7210
800-672-7084
FAX: 617-572-2094
e-mail: pfrr@fcsn.org
www.pfrr.org

Andrea Watson, Founder and Project Coordinator
Rich Robison, President
Parents of children with special needs, whose children require intensive residential education settings, face a myriad of unique circumstances in their efforts to provide ongoing support to their children. PFRR provides information on placement, restraint medication, IEP, standardized testing, transition, parent/peer connections, workshops, trainings and the maze of state and federal agencies. We educate on the rights of parents, and their young people who are receiving services.

877 People First International

PO Box 12642
Salem, OR 97309
503-362-0336
FAX: 503-585-4718
e-mail: people1@people1.org
www.people1.org

Steven Kramer, President
Ruth Morris, VP
Rodney Carver, VP

Self-advocacy organization of developmentally disabled people who have joined together to learn how to speak for themselves. People first offers support, a united voice and advocacy to its members. Offers information and helps develop service projects in the communities they live in. Offers information and assistance to countries around the world in starting new chapters. Offers participation on DD boards, ARC boards, Transit Boards, and other boards in the community.

878 People First of Canada
120 Maryland Street
Suite 5
Winnipeg, Manitoba, ZZ R3G
204-784-7362
FAX: 204-784-7364
e-mail: info@peoplefirstofcanada.ca
www.peoplefirstofcanada.ca

Shelley Rattai, Executive Director
Catherine Allix, National Community Inclusion
An organization designed to support those disabled individuals in our communities who feel their disability is preventing them from opportunties available to non-disabled individuals.

879 People-to-People Committee for the Handicapped
1020 Ashton Road
Ashton, MD 20861
301-774-7446
FAX: 301-493-0510
e-mail: ngvb096@prodigy.com

David Brigham, Chairman
Individuals concerned about that circumstances of handicapped people throughout the world. Disseminates information, acts as a consultant in promoting exchange activities, coordinates special assistance in developing countries and more.

880 People-to-People Committee on Disability
501 E Armour Boulevard
Kansas City, MO 64109
816-531-4701
FAX: 816-561-7502
e-mail: ptpi@ptpi.org
www.ptpi.org/programs/disability.jsp

Mary Eisenhower, President/CEO
Marc L Bright, Exec VP/Program Director
Ernst Honegger, Vice Chairman
Individuals concerned about the circumstances of handicapped people throughout the world. Disseminates information, acts as a consultant in promoting exchange activities, coordinates special assistance projects in developing countries and more.

881 People-to-People International: Committee for the Handicapped
501 E Armour Boulevard
Kansas City, MO 64109
816-531-7231
800-676-7874
FAX: 816-561-7502
e-mail: ptpi@ptpi.org
www.ptpi.org

Marc L Bright, Deputy CEO/Executive VP
Mary Eisenhower, Chief Executive Officer
Rosanne Rosen, Senior VP of Operations
Goals of this committee include: betterment of the handicapped through international unity; educating those with and without handicaps through technical assistance; opening access doors through sensory aids, prosthetic devices and travel tips; and coordination of major international cultural exchanges.

882 Portland Naturopathic Clinic: NCNM National Health Centers Eastside Clinic
National College of Naturopathic Medicine
049 SW Porter Street
Portland, OR 97201
503-552-1555
FAX: 503-827-8460
www.ncnm.edu

William J Keppler, President
Established in 1956, NCNM is the oldest and one of the best known colleges of its type in the world. Because 90 percent of global health care involves methods other then conventional western medicine, NCNM's participation in international medical education and research is routinely solicited.

883 Quan Yin Healing Arts Center
455 Valencia Street
San Francisco, CA 94103
415-861-4964
FAX: 415-861-0579
e-mail: qyhacinfo@aol.com
www.quanyinhealingarts.com

Carla Wilson, Executive Director
Joanna Cullom, Office Manager
Alicia Diaz, Front Desk
The mission of Quan Yin Healing Arts Center is to provide accessable high quality, affordable acupuncture and Chinese medicine regardless of income. Collaborating with other healthcare providers, we support a holistic philosophy, empowering the individual to take responsibility for their health and well being.

884 Rehabilitation International
25 E 21st Street
4th Floor
New York, NY 10010
212-420-1500
FAX: 212-505-0871
e-mail: RI@riglobal.org
www.rehab-international.org

Michael Fox, President
Tomas Lagerwall, Manager
RI and its members develop and promote initiatives to protect the rights of people with disabilities and improve rehabilitation and other crucial services for disabled people and their families. RI also works toward increasing international collaboration and advocates for policies and legislation recognizing the rights of people with disabilities and their families, including the establishment of a UN Convention on the Rights and Dignity of Persons with Disabilities.

885 Rehabilitation Services
1490 E Beltline Avenue SE
Grand Rapids, MI 49506
616-940-0040
FAX: 616-940-8151
e-mail: jbaker@hopenetwork.org
www.hopenetworkrehab.org

Margaret Kroese, Executive Director
Mary Baily, Admissions Manager
Amanda Lake, Admissions Manager
An office of Hope Netowrk, one of the largest, private, nonprofit organization of its kind in Michigan. The purpose is to assist people with brain injuries and/or physical disabilities in achieving an optimal level of self determinations, dignity, and independence as they develop and attain goals to overcome environmental barriers and mobilize adaptive skills.

886 Rehabilitation Services Administration of the District of Columbia
810 1st Street NE
10th Floor
Washington, DC 20002
202-442-8663
FAX: 202-442-8742
e-mail: rsa.dhs@dc.gov
www.rsa.dhs.dc.gov/rsa/site/default.asp

Elizabeth B Parker, Administrator
Provides comprehensive vocational and independent living services to persons with disabilities to promote their opportunities for employment, economic self-sufficiency and independence. RSA works with communities, businesses and organizations in an effort to ensure that individuals attain integrated employment in the mainstream of society.

887 Rolf Institute
5055 Chaparral Court
Suite 103
Boulder, CO 80301
303-449-5903
800-530-8875
FAX: 303-449-5978
e-mail: seecof@aol.com
www.rolf.org

Ida P Rolf, Founder
G. Thomas Manzione PhD, Executive Director
Brigette Lause, Membership Services Coordinator

Established in 1971, The Rolf Institute is a nonprofit corporation, organized and existing under the laws of California and Colorado. It is recognized by the US Government as a tax-exempt educational and scientific research organization.
1971

888 **Ronald McDonald House**
1500 17th Street
Huntington, WV 25701
304-529-1122
FAX: 304-529-2970
e-mail: margaret@mchouse.org
www.mchouse.org

Margaret Wilson, Manager
A home-away-from-home, a temporary lodging facility for the families of seriously ill children being treated at nearby hospitals. Each house is run by a local nonprofit agency comprised of members of the medical community, McDonald's owners, businesses and civic organizations and parent volunteers.

889 **St. Paul Abilities Network**
4915 51 Avenue
PO Box 457
St. Paul, Alberta, ZZ T0A
780-645-3441
866-645-3900
FAX: 780-645-1885
e-mail: mail@spanet.ab.ca
www.stpaulabilitiesnetwork.ca

Tim Bear, Executive Director
Jack McIntyre, Director Residential Services
Provides support and opportunities to encourage the development of an individual's full potential through education, advocacy and community partnerships.

890 **Teacher Preparation and Special Education**
2134 G Street NW
Suite 416
Washington, DC 20052
202-994-6160
800-449-7343
FAX: 202-994-8613
e-mail: gsehdcom@gwu.edu
gsehd.gwu.edu

Jay Shotel, Professor of Special Education
Administers the Education of the Handicapped Act and related programs for the education of handicapped children, including grants to institutions of higher learning and fellowships to train educational personnel. Grants to states for the education of handicapped children, research and demonstration.

891 **Technology and Media Division**
Council For Exceptional Children
1110 N Glebe Road
Suite 300
Arlington, VA 22201
703-620-3660
888-232-7733
FAX: 703-264-9494
TTY: 866-915-5000
e-mail: service@cec.sped.org
www.cec.sped.org

Mary Ruth Coleman, President
Susan Fowler, President Elect
Stan Dublinske, Treasurer
The CEC is the largest international professional organization dedicated to improving educational outcomes for individuals with exceptionalities, students with disabilities, and/or the gifted. CEC advocates for appropriate governmental policies, sets professional standards, provides continual professional development, advocates for newly and historically underserved individuals with exceptionalities, and helps professionals obtain conditions and resources necessary for effective practice.

892 **Thresholds Psychiatric Rehabilitation Centers**
4101 N Ravenswood Avenue
Chicago, IL 60613
773-880-6260
888-997-3422
888-997-3422
FAX: 773-880-6279
TTY:773-880-6263
e-mail: thresholds@thresholds.org
www.thresholds.org

Margot Anderson, President
Ryan Cahill, Vice President
Chris Segal, Treasurer
A nationally-recognized psychosocial rehabilitation agency serving persons with severe and persistent mental illness. The agency offers its programming at 22 service locations and more than 40 residential facilities throughout Chicago and Northern Illinois. Also offers specialized programming for older adults, young adults, parents, the homeless and the hearing impaired and mentally ill.
Sliding scale

893 **Trager International**
13801 W Center Street Suite C
P.O. Box 1009
Burton, OH 44021
440-834-0308
FAX: 440-834-0365
e-mail: info@trager-us.org
www.trager-us.org

Anne Galbraith, President
Anna Marie Bowers, Administrative Director
Henry Bornstein, Vice President
The Trager approach is a pleasurable, gentle and effective approach to movement education and mind/body integration. The Trager approach helps release deep-seated physical and mental patterns and facilitates deep relaxation, increased physical mobility, and mental clarity. The benefits of a Trager session are long-lasting and cumulative, with subsequent sessions allowing for deeper and longer lasting changes.

894 **Universal Pediatric Services**
1115 N Warrior Lane
Waukee, IA 50263
515-987-3436
800-383-0303
FAX: 515-224-0630
e-mail: hrjay123@aol.com
www.upsi.net
Universal Pediatric Services, provides high tech care to medically fragile children and adults in the home setting. Emphasis is placed on the provision of services in the rural areas, the ability to service high tech needs and the promotion of primary nurse concept.

895 **Upledger Institute**
11211 Prosperity Farms Road
Suite D-325
Palm Beach Gardens, FL 33410
561-622-4334
800-233-5880
FAX: 561-622-4771
e-mail: edsrv@upledger.com
www.upledger.com

John Upledger DO, President/Founder
Lisa Upledger DC, CST-D,, Vice President
Roy Desjarlais LMT, CST-D, Vice President-Clinical Services
Health resource center dedicated to the advancement of complementary and innovative techniques.

896 **West Virginia Hospital Association**
100 Association Drive
Charleston, WV 25311
304-344-9744
FAX: 304-344-9745
www.wvha.com

Joseph Letnaunchun, President/CEO
John Eckhart, Account Rep., Shared Services
Janice Fink, Director of Accounting
For 80 years, the West Virginia Hospital Association, a not-for-profit statewide organization, has represented our member hospitals and health systems across the contiuum of care.

897 **Women to Women**
PO Box 306
Portland, ME 04112
800-798-7902
800-448-4919
FAX: 207-846-6167
e-mail: personalprogram@womentowomen.com
www.womentowomen.com

Marcelle Pick OB/GYN, NP, Co Founder/Director

Combination of alternative and conventional medicine in women's health, bring science and disipline to natural and preventative methods. Publishes the Creating Health Guide, a quarterly collection of articles written by the health care professionals at Women to Women.

898 World Institute on Disability

510 16th Street
Suite 100
Oakland, CA 94612
510-763-4100
FAX: 510-763-4109
TTY:510-208-9496
e-mail: wid@wid.org
www.wid.org

Kathy Martinez, Executive Director
A public policy center that is run by persons with disabilities. Research, training and public policy center promoting the civil rights and the full societal inclusion of people with disabilities.

899 Wyoming Institute for Disabilities (WIND)

1000 E University Avenue
Dept 4298
Laramie, WY 82071
307-766-2761
888-989-9463
FAX: 307-766-2763
TTY: 3077662720
e-mail: wind.uwyo.edu
wind.uwyo.edu

Keith Miller PhD, Executive Director
Ken B. Heinlein PhD, Associate Director
Terri Longhurst M.S., CFLE, Associate Director
WIND is committed to assisting individuals with developmental and other disabilities and thier families to achieve their desired quality of life by promoting and supporting full community inclusion, community membership, independence, productivity and social participation. The mission of WIND is to assist individuals with developmental and other disabilities and their families to achieve their desired quality of life.

900 YAI: National Institute for People with Disabilities

460 W 34th Street
New York, NY 10001
212-273-6100
FAX: 212-273-6200
www.yai.org

Joel M Levy, CEO
Philip H Levy, President/COO
Stephen E Freeman, Associate Executive Director
Mission is to build brighter futures for people with developmental and learning disabilities and thier families. Every person, at every age and level of disability, has the potential for growth. Each individual is entitled to the same dignity, respect, and opportunities as all other members of society. Firmly committed to helping the people we serve to achieve their potential for independence, individuality, productivity, and inclusion in their communities.
1957

Alabama

901 **Adventure Program**
Lakeshore Foundation
4000 Ridgeway Drive
Birmingham, AL 35209
205-313-7400
888-868-2303
FAX: 205-313-7475
e-mail: information@lakeshore.org
www.lakeshore.org

Jeffrey Underwood, President
Jill Collins, Director of Recreation/Athletics
Wynna Harris, Director of Aquatics/Fitness
The Lakeshore Foundation Advernture Program is a community resource, not only for individuals, but also for other organizations that serve people with disabilities. They organize adventures, assist with equipment, and make every effort to increase the accessibility of the outdoors. Certified Therapeutic recreation specialists coordinate the program.

902 **Camp Seale Harris Southeastern Diabetes Education Services**
500 Chase Park S
Suite 104
Hoover, AL 35244
205-402-0415
FAX: 205-402-0416
e-mail: info@southeasterndiabetes.org
www.southeasterndiabetes.org

Terry Ackley, Executive Director
A summer residential program that is located at Camp ASCCA (Alabama's Special Camp for Children and Adults), that encourages and motivates youth to reach their full potential despite diabetes, and teaches families how to serve as the primary educators and supporters for children and adolescents living with this illness.

Arizona

903 **Camp Civitan**
Civitan Foundation
3509 East Shea Blvd. #117
Phoenix, AZ 85028
602-953-2944
FAX: 602-953-2946
e-mail: info@campcivitan.org
www.campcivitan.org

Marianne Beram, Camp Director
Mike Beram, Assitant Director
Felicia Parker, Director Health Services
Camp for the physically and/or mentally challenged. Ages 12 and up. Week long summer sessions offered near Williams, Arizona. Activities include arts and crafts, hikes, sports, sing-a-longs, dances etc. $250 per week.

904 **Easter Seals Arizona**
2850 North 24th Street
Pheonix, AZ 85008
602-266-5976
800-626-6061
FAX: 480-222-4123
TTY: 480-222-4100
e-mail: info@azseals.org
www.az.easterseals.com

Michael Medoro, VP/COO
Michael Fitzgerald, President/CEO
Provides services to children and adults with disabilities and other special needs, and support to their families.

905 **Lions Camp Tatiyee**
PO Box 6910
Mesa, AZ 85216
480-380-4254
800-246-9771
FAX: 602-244-8667
e-mail: arizonalionscamp@cox.net
www.arizonalionscamp.com

Pamela Swanson, Executive Director
Camp is located in Lakeside, Arizona. Provides one-week sessions for campers with a wide variety of disabilities. May-August. Coed, ages 7-17 and seniors. Featured activities include arts and crafts, ceramics/pottery, climbing/rappelling, counselor training (CIT), drama, fishing, football, hiking, nature/environmental studies and team building.

California

906 **Camp Forrest**
Angel View Crippled Children's Foundation
12379 Miracle Hill Road
Desert Hot Springs, CA 92240
760-329-6471
FAX: 760-324-9024
e-mail: angelview44@aol.com
www.angelview.org

Mel Haber, President
David Thornton, Executive Director
Howard Gordon, Director
Camp is located in Joshua Tree, California. Offers to one-week sessions June-August to both able-bodied campers and those with a wide variety of disabilities. Coed, ages 10-25. Activities include archery, arts and crafts, cookouts, swimming, sports and games, hiking and star study.

907 **Camp Paivika**
Ability First
1300 E Green Street
Pasadena, CA 91106
626-396-1010
877-768-4600
FAX: 626-396-1021
e-mail: contactus@abilityfirst.org
www.abilityfirst.org

Kelly Kunsak, Camp Director
Stuart Wilkinson, President
Patricia Vick, Chairman
Camp is located in Crestline, California. A nonprofit camp owned and operated by Ability First to provide outdoor, recreational camping services for children and adults with physical and/or developmental disabilities. Located in the San Bernadino mountains, the camp has a dining lodge and rec room, four cabins, infirmary, program building and pool that are all fully accessible. Camp is available to rent during winter/spring for up to 80 people. Coed, ages 7-70.

908 **Camp Reach for the Sky**
American Cancer Society
2655 Camino Del Rio North
Suite 100
San Diego, CA 92108
619-299-4200
800-227-2345
FAX: 619-296-0928
e-mail: robby.medina@cancer.org
www.cancer.org

Stephen Sener, President
Richard Wender, Vice President
Robby Medina, Camp Administrator
One-week sessions for children who have had, or currently have, cancer. Coed, ages 8-18.

909 **Camp Ronald McDonald at Eagle Lake**
Eagle Lake Children's Charities
PO Box 172
Susanville, CA 96130
530-825-3158
916-734-4230
FAX: 530-825-3158
e-mail: vicky@campronald.org
www.campronald.org

Vicky Flaig MEd/RD, Camp Director
Is a fully accessible residential camp for kids with special needs. The goal of the camp is to provide confidence building experiences to children who are at risk, disadvantaged and/or living with physical or emotional disabilities.

910 **Camping Unlimited**
Camping Unlimited for Children
4610 Whitesands Ct.
El Sobrante, CA 94803
510-222-6662
FAX: 510-223-3046
e-mail: campkrem@campingunlimited.com
www.campingunlimited.com

Teresa Tucker, Executive Director
Camp is located in Boulder Creek, California. Offers one and two-week sessions June-August to campers with a variety of disabilities. Coed, ages 5-50. Camping unlimited also weekend programs and travel camps, year round progams and recreation.

911 **Costanoan**
Via Rehabilitation Services
2851 Park Avenue
Santa Clara, CA 95050
408-243-7861
FAX: 408-243-0452
e-mail: camp@viaservices.org
www.viaservices.org

Richard Frazier, Camp Director
Liya Murphy, Camp Registrar
Kay Walker, Chief Executive Officer
Camp Costanoan is a residential, respite and recreational camp for children and adults, ages 5 and older, with physical and/or developmental disabilities. Camp Costanoan enhances camper self-esteem, improves socialization skills and provides hands-on learning and therapeutic recreation opportunities. Additionally, Camp Costanoan provides respite for families of individuals with disabilities.

912 **Easter Seals Camp Harmon**
Easter Seals Central California
9010 Soquel Drive
Aptos, CA 95003
831-684-2166
800-400-0671
FAX: 831-684-1018
e-mail: jennifer@es-cc.org
www.centralcal.easterseals.com

Jennifer Johnson, Camping Services Coordinator
Camp is located in Boulder Creek, California. 6-10 day sessions for children and adults with physical and developmental disabilities. Coed, ages 8-65.

913 **Junior Wheelchair Sports Camp**
Santa Barbara Parks and Recreation Department
PO Box 1990
Santa Barbara, CA 93102
805-564-5418
FAX: 805-564-5480
www.sbparksandrecreation.org

Nancy Rapp, Executive Director
Sarah Clayton, Recreation Manager
Antonio Velasquez, Community Services Supervisor
This five-day camp is for children 5-19 years old that are physically disabled. Sports instruction in aquatics, tennis, track and field, basketball, archery and new sports activities introduced each year. The camp counselors and instructors are also physically disabled to provide the children with a role model. Fee based on fundraising efforts.

914 **Pilgrim Pines Camp**
United Church Of Christ
39570 Glen Road
Yucaipa, CA 92399
909-797-1821
800-616-6612
FAX: 909-797-2691
e-mail: info@pilgrimpinescamp.org
www.pilgrimpinescamp.org

Gail Benson, Executive Director
Renee Smith, Summer Camp Director
Shelley Wallace, Guest Services Manager
Christian camp offering one-week sessions for campers with developmental disabilities. Coed, ages 10-Adult. Also families.

Colorado

915 **Breckenridge Outdoor Education Center**
PO Box 697
Breckenridge, CO 80424
970-453-6422
FAX: 970-453-4676
e-mail: boec@boec.org
www.boec.org

Bruce Fitch, Executive Director
Bob Bond, Wilderness Program Director
Cindy Wetherald, Associate Program Director
Provides year-round adventure based wilderness and adaptive ski programs for people with disabilities. The Center excels in offering challenging, rewarding outdoor experiences individually designed to the abilities and needs of participants.

916 **Camp Paha**
City of Lakewood
480 South Allison Parkway
Lakewood, CO 80226
303-987-7000
FAX: 303-987-4863
TTY:303-987-7716
e-mail: joabur@lakewood.org
www.lakewood.org

Jo Burns, Executive Director
Zane Devan, Manager
Camp Paha is a day camp for children ages 6-17 and young adults ages 18-25 with disabilities. We provide programs for campers with all disability types: developmental, physical, emotional, behavioral, and learning. Camp Paha offers safe, quality, fun and challenging activities. Camp provides campers and opportunity to participate in aquatics, sports, games, nature, music, drama, hiking, arts and crafts, and field trips into the community.

917 **Challenge Aspen**
PO Box M
Aspen, CO 81612
970-923-0578
800-530-3907
FAX: 970-923-7338
e-mail: possibilities@challengeaspen.com
www.challengeaspen.com

Houston Cowan, Executive Director
Amanda Boxtel, Special Projects Mgr/Co-Founder
Sarah Williams, Program Director
Challenge Aspen provides recreational and cultural experiences for individuals who have mental or physical disabilities. Challenge Aspen offers a variety of recreational programs to fit a diversity of needs and interests. We offer both summer, winter and special events for both adults and children.

918 **Colorado Lions Camp**
PO Box 9043
Woodland Park, CO 80866
719-687-2087
FAX: 719-687-7435
e-mail: lionscampco@aol.com
www.coloradolionscamp.org

Bruce Wadman, President
Glen Scofield, Vice President
Jim Pierie, Executive Director
Outdoor recreational camping for the handicapped. All normal camp activities offered. 1 to 4 staff supervision with a nurse or doctor in attendance.

919 **Easter Seals Colorado Rocky Mountain Villa**
PO Box 115
Empire, CO 80043
303-569-2333
FAX: 303-569-3857
e-mail: info@eastersealscolorado.org
co.easterseals.com/

Lynn Robinson, President
Shirley Barenberg, Vice President
Nancy Hanson, VP
Camp is located in Empire, Colorado. One-week sessions June-August for children and adults with a wide variety of disabilities. Coed, ages 7-70. Single adults, families.

920 **Glacier View Ranch**
Rocky Mountain Conference of the
Seventh Day Adventist Church
2520 South Downing Street
Denver, CO 80210
303-733-3771
FAX: 303-733-1843
e-mail: webmaster@rmcsda.com
www.rmcsda.org

Dorothy Opp, President
James Brauer, Religious Leader
Marlene Perry, Youth Coordinator
Camp is located in Ward, Colorado. One-week sessions June and July. Programs for campers with asthma/respiratory aliments. Coed, ages 7-17.

921 **Rocky Mountain Village**
Easter Seals Colorado
PO Box 115
Empire, CO 80438
303-569-2333
FAX: 303-569-3857
e-mail: info@eastersealscolorado.org
www.eastersealsco.org

Roman Kratczyk, Director
Sessions are conducted for both developmentally and physically disabled children and adults. Activities include swimming, horseback riding, outdoor education, zigline challenge course elements.

922 **Sky Ranch Lutheran Camp**
805 S Shields Street
Fort Collins, CO 80521
970-493-5258
FAX: 970-493-7960
e-mail: info@doubler.org
www.fortnet.org/skyranch

Ralph Yernberg, Executive Director
Joel Abenth, Director Program Ministries
Stephanie Dugger, Development Assistant
Daily Bible study and worship for disabled campers.

Connecticut

923 **Easter Seal Camp Hemlocks**
85 Jones Street
PO Box 100
Hebron, CT 06248
860-228-9496
800-874-7687
FAX: 860-228-2091
TTY: 312-726-4258
e-mail: info@eastersealscamphemlocks.org
www.eastersealscamphemlocks.org/

Denise Hornbecker, Vice President
Sunny Ku, Camp Director
Camp is located in Hebron, Connecticut. One and two-week sessions June-August for campers with a variety of disabilities. Coed, ages 6-80. Families, seniors, single adults.

Florida

924 **Camp Thunderbird**
Florida Fund For Special Children
380 Semoran Commerce Place
Suite B-204 PO Box 1300
Apopka, FL 32704
407-889-4503
FAX: 407-889-5710
e-mail: contact@questinc.org
www.questinc.org

Katie Porta, President
Shirley O'Brien, Executive Director
Rob Hungate, Chairman
Residential summer camping program for children and adults with a developmental disability. Campers enjoy swimming, sports, nature hikes, canoeing, etc. One and two-week sessions June-August. Coed, ages 8-80.

925 **Florida Lions Camp**
Lions of Multiple District 35
2819 Tiger Lake Road
Lake Wales, FL 33898
863-696-1948
FAX: 863-696-2398
e-mail: flc@gte.net
www.lionscampfl.org

Rob Cage, Camp Program Director
Carissa Moen, Co-Summer Director
Hugo Paleaz, Aquatics Director
One-week sessions June-August for children with a variety of disabilities. Coed, ages 5-21. A variety of traditional summer camp activities which include: swimming, canoeing, fishing, hiking, camping out and cooking over a fire, games, arts & crafts, singing & dancing, hay-wagon rides, challenge course and much more. Activities are adapted to the age and ability of each camper to ensure maximum participation, safety and fun.

Georgia

926 **Camp Twin Lakes**
600 Means Street
Suite 110
Atlanta, GA 30318
404-231-9887
FAX: 404-577-8854
e-mail: info@camptwinlakes.org
www.camptwinlakes.org

Eric M Robbins, Executive Director
Daniel Matthews, Camp Director
Frank Beall, Special Projects Coordinator
One-week sessions June-August for children with a variety of medical problems. Coed, ages 8-18.

Hawaii

927 **Camp Erdman YMCA**
YMCA Camp H R Erdman
69-385 Farrington Highway
Waialua, HI 96791
808-637-4615
FAX: 808-637-8874
e-mail: jheimowitz@ymcahonolulu.org
www.camperdman.net

Josh Heimowitz, Executive Director
Elizabeth Staib-King, Senior Program Director
Mandy MacMahan, Resident/Family Program Director
Traditional Resident Camp program is five nights and six days of fun-filled activities that will create positive lifetime memories. Camp activitiesinclude: arts & crafts, swimming, kayaking, hiking, challenge course, snorkeling, athletics, nature, dance & drama, beach writing and archery . Traditional Resident Camp Experience (Ages 6-15) serving the needs of the disabled.

Illinois

928 **Camp Little Giant**
Southern Illinois University
206 Touch of Nature Road
Makanda, IL 62958
618-453-1121
FAX: 618-453-1188
e-mail: tonec@tonec.siu.edu
www.pso.siu.edu/tonec

Vicki Lang, Therapeutic Rec Specialist
David Gename, Manager
One and two week sessions for campers with a variety of disabilities. Coed, ages 8-80.

929 **Camp New Hope**
PO Box 764
Mattoon, IL 61938
217-895-2341
FAX: 217-895-3658
e-mail: cnhinc@rr1.net
www.myfavoritecamp.org

Kim Carmack, Executive Director
Terri Taylor, Program Coordinator
Advocacy services, social and recreational services and a summer camp for the disabled. The camp accommodates people of widely diverse needs and abilities including access for wheelchair users. Co-ed, for those 8 years and older, including adults. Facilities include a mini golf area; pontoon boat; fishing deck; playground; trails; swimmming pool; and sleeping cabins with air conditioning.

930 **Easter Seals of Bartholomew County**
Easter Seals
230 W Monroe Street
Suite 1800
Chicago, IL 60606
312-726-6200
800-221-6827
FAX: 312-726-1494
TTY: 312-726-4258
e-mail: info@easterseals.com
www.easterseals.com

James E Williams Jr, President/CEO
Joanne Cloonan, Project Manager Executive Office
Serves the needs of disabled persons and allows them to experience the joys and challenges unique to summer camp. Activities include: campfire sing-a-longs to boating, nature walks, swimming, and arts and crafts.

931 **Easter Seals: UCP Timber Pointe Outdor Center**
Easter Seals
230 W Monroe Street
Suite 1800
Chicago, IL 60606
312-726-6200
FAX: 312-726-1494
e-mail: info@easterseals-ucp.org
www.easterseals.com

Kurt Podeszwa, Director of Camping/VP
Wayne Baum, President
One and two-week sessions for campers with a wide variety of disabilities. Coed, ages 6-99. Campers experience different activities each day such as arts and crafts, music, horses, field sports, outdoor nature, swimming, canoeingand fishing. Every night there is a different activity: skit night, casino night, boat night (campers go out on the lake on pontoon boats), night swim, camp fires, and of course, everyone's favorite - a dance on the last night.

932 **Jewish Council for Youth Services**
JCYS Camp Red Leaf
26710 West Nippersink Road
Ingleside, IL 60041
847-740-5010
FAX: 847-740-5014
e-mail: info@jcys.org
www.jcys.org/redleaf

Anthony Warner, Director
Valerie Ravenna, Assistant Director
Joe Knudsen, Coach
Located on the grounds of JCYS Camp Henry Horner, JCYS Camp Red Leaf is designed to serve youth and adults with developmental disabilities, emotional and behavioral needs for ages 9 and upward. Various levels of care are availiable for specific ages and needs during the Camp's specialized sessions. The highly adaptable summer programs at JCYS Camp Red Leaf strive to increase self-esteem, promote interaction, improve social skills, and encourage independence in a natural environment.

933 **Touch of Nature Environmental Center**
1206 Touch Of Nature Road
Makanda, IL 62958
618-453-1121
FAX: 618-453-1188
e-mail: tonec@tonec.siu.edu
http://www.ton.siu.edu/

Vicki Lang, Camp Director
Chilang Lawless, Camp Registrant
David Gename, Manager
Providing a traditional camping experience for non-traditional campers, including recreational and outdoor programs for adults and children with various developmental, mental and physical disabilities as well as learning and behavioral disorders.

934 **YMCA Camp Duncan**
Tourette Syndrome Camp Organization
6933 North Kedzie
Suite 816
Chicago, IL 60645
773-465-7536
847-546-8086
FAX: 847-546-3550
e-mail: info@ymcacampduncan.org
www.tourettecamp.com/

Rona Roffey, Camp Director
Tammy Welninski, Day Camp Director
Addie Smits, Director Group Services
The Tourette Syndrome/TS Camp USA, founded in 1994, is a residential camping program designed for girls and boys ages 8 - 16+ whose primary diagnosis is TS, and to a lesser degree, OCD and ADD/ADHD. The TS Camp is held at YMCA Camp Duncan which is located 30 miles north of Chicago. The goal of the camp is to allow children with TS an opportunity to meet other children, share similar experiences and coping mechanisms in a fun, safe and positive environment.

Indiana

935 **Bradford Woods/Camp Riley**
Indiana University
5040 State Road 67 N
Martinsville, IN 46151
765-342-2915
FAX: 765-349-1086
TTY:765-349-5117
e-mail: bradwood@indiana.edu
www.bradwoods.org

John Koenig, Executive Director
One and two-week sessions for children with a variety of disabilities. Coed, ages 8-18.

936 **Camp Millhouse**
25600 Kelly Road
South Bend, IN 46614
574-233-2202
FAX: 574-233-2511
e-mail: leabee37@comcast.net
www.campmillhouse.org

Lea Anne Pitcher, Director
Nestled in a rustic clearing surrounded by 45 acres of woods, Camp Millhouse is a retreat for children and young adults with mental and physical disabilities. Hiking trails, nature studies, crafts, swimming, and stories around the bonfire make up activities campers long remember. One-week session. Co-ed, ages 4 to 30.

937 **Easter Seal Crossroads Rehabilitation Cent er**
4740 Kingsway Drive
Indianapolis, IN 46205
317-466-1000
FAX: 317-466-2000
TTY:317-479-3232
www.eastersealcrossroad.org

David Brandt, Chairman of the Board
James Vento, President
David Bussard, Director
A community resource working in partnership with children and adults with disabilities or special needs and their families to promote growth, independence and dignity.

938 **Easter Seals ARC of Northeast Indiana**
4919 Coldwater Road
Fort Wayne, IN 46825
260-456-4534
800-234-7811
FAX: 260-745-5200
e-mail: info@esarc.org
http://neindiana.easterseals.com/

Bill Martin, Chairperson
Nikki Holm, Senior Vice Chairperson
Stephen Hinkle, President

939 Easter Seals of Wayne & Union Counties
National Easter Seals
PO Box 86
Centerville, IN 47330
765-855-2482
FAX: 765-855-2482
e-mail: easterseals@juno.com
eastersealswu.tripod.com

Pat Bowers, Executive Director
Providing programs and services for youth and adults with disabilities in Wayne and Union Counties, Indiana. Limited to our service area.

940 Happiness Bag
3833 Union Road
Terre Haute, IN 47802
812-234-8867
FAX: 812-238-0728
e-mail: jmexdir@aol
www.happinessbag.org

Richard Shagley, President of the Board
Jodi Moan, Executive Director
Serves developmentally disabled age 5-adult; day and residential camp program; after school program; scouting; Special Olympic anticipation (basketball, athletics, bowling, softball and aquatics); and a bowling league.

941 Isanogel Center
7601 W Isanogel Road
Muncie, IN 47304
765-288-1073
FAX: 765-288-3103
TTY:765-288-1073
e-mail: isanogel@comcast.net
www.isanogelcenter.org

Tanner Underwood, President of the Board
Karen Kovac, Executive Director
One and two-week sessions June-August for special needs children through adults. Coed, ages 5-99.

Iowa

942 Camp Courageous of Iowa
PO Box 418
Monticello, IA 52310
319-465-5916
FAX: 319-465-5919
e-mail: info@campcourageous.org
www.campcourageous.org

Charlie Becker, Executive Director
Jeanne Muellerleile, Camp Director
A year round residential and respite care facility for individuals with special needs. Campers range in age from 1-99 years old. Activities include traditional activities like canoeing, hiking, swimming, nature and crafts plus adventure activities like caving, rock climbing, etc. Campers with disabilities have opportunities to succeed at challenging activities. This feeling of self-worth can transfer to home, work or school environments.

943 Camp Tanager
1614 West Mount Vernon Road
Mount Vernon, IA 52314
319-363-0681
FAX: 319-365-6411
e-mail: dpirrie@tanagerplace.org
www.camptanager.org

Donald Pirrie, Director
Offers camp experiences for children 7 to 12 whose special social, economic or medical needs might not otherwise allow them to enjoy a summer camp experience. This private, non-profit camp serves over 600 children each summer with the staff-camper ratio being 1:6.

944 Camp Wyoming
9106 42nd Avenue
Wyoming, IA 52362
563-488-3893
FAX: 563-488-3895
e-mail: campwyo@netins.net
www.campwyoming.net

Kevin Cullum, Executive Director
Robyn Meyers, Assistant Director
Paul Scott, Maintenance Director
Mainstreaming available June through August. Youth and adults with mild to moderate mental and physical disabilities can take part in a one week experience of fun and fellowship in early July.

945 Easter Seals Camp Sunnyside
Easter Seals Iowa
401 Northeast 66th Avenue
PO Box 4002
Des Moines, IA 50333
515-289-1933
FAX: 515-289-1281
TTY:515-289-4069
e-mail: mtope@eastersealsia.org
www.ia.easterseals.org

Marcia Tope, Camp Director
Donna Elbrecht, President
Each summer from June through August, campers with disabilities ages five and up, take part in one week camping sessions, gaining skills and independence by participating in activities like swimming, horseback riding, canoeing, fishing, camping and more. Coed, ages 4-95. Accepts seniors and single adults. Financial assistance available.

946 Riverside Lutheran Bible Camp
3001 Riverside Road
Story City, IA 50248
515-733-5271
800-372-7748
FAX: 515-733-4096
e-mail: rlbc@riversidelbc.org
www.riversidelbc.org

Dave McDermott, Director
Jan McDermott, Associate Director
Dan Scharnhorst, Program Coordinator
Helps disabled people to develop, renew and nurture their relationship with Jesus Christ in a unique Christian environment.

947 Wesley Woods Camp & Retired Center
Iowa United Methodist Conference Center
10896 Nixon Street
Des Moines, IA 50125
515-961-4523
866-684-7753
FAX: 515-974-8950
e-mail: wesleywoods.camp@iaumc.org
www.gbgm-umc.org/wesleywoods/

Dick Faris, Director Camp/Retreat Ministries
Kathy Potter, Camps Registrar
Deke Rider, Program Coordinator
Camp is located in Indianola, Iowa. Half-week and one-week sessions June-August for campers with developmental disabilities. Coed, ages 18-99.

Kentucky

948 Bethel Mennonite Camp
2773 Bethel Church Road
Clayhole, KY 41317
606-666-4911
FAX: 606-666-4216
e-mail: grow@bethelcamp.org
www.bethelcamp.org

Roger Voth, Director
Ruth Voth, Director
A non profit ministry thay meets a wide variety of needs.

949 **Easter Seal Camp KYSOC**
Kentucky Easter Sales Society
1902 Easter Day Road
Carrollton, KY 41008
502-732-5333
800-888-5377
FAX: 502-732-0783
e-mail: fun@kysoc.org
www.cardinalhill.org

Karry Gillihan, President
Beth Monarch, Vice President
Sallie Price, Director
Our services include: Adult day care services; audiology services; developmental intervention; medical day hospital; nursing; occupational therapy; physical therapy; psychological counseling; social services/case management and speech-language therapy.

950 **Life Adventure Camp**
Life Adventure Camp of the Bluegrass
570 Milner Road
Versailles, KY 40383
859-873-3271
FAX: 859-873-2410
e-mail: info@clevelandhome.org
www.lifeadventurecamp.org

Claudeca Clark, President
Essie Rogers, Equine Center Director
Wilderness camp for children, male and female, ages 9-18, with emotional and behavioral problems. Half week and one week sessions June-August.

Louisiana

951 **Camp Challenge**
PO Box 641253
Kenner, LA 70064
504-347-2267
e-mail: info@campc.org
www.campchallenge.org

Carl Klutz, Director
Cecil Klutz, Director
Camp Challenge is a grass roots non-profit organization dedicated to giving ill children and their siblings ages 6 through 18 a summer camp experience. Camp is open to all children who reside in Louisiana and have a form of cancer and chronic hematological disorders. These children do not have to pay for camp, it is free for all campers.

952 **LA Lions Camp for Disabled/Diabetic Youth**
LA Lions League Crippled Child
292 L. Beauford Dr.
Anacoco, LA 71403
337-239-6567
FAX: 337-239-9975
e-mail: lalions@lionscamp.org
lionscamp.org/index.html

Raymond E Cecil III, Director
Carol Laughlin, Executive Director
One-week sessions June-August for disabled children. Coed, ages 7-19.

Maine

953 **Camp Waban**
5 Dunaway Drive
Sanford, ME 04073
207-324-7955
FAX: 207-324-6050
e-mail: waban@gwi.netn.org
www.waban.org

Neal Meltzer, Executive Director
Gervaise Flynn, Assistant Executive Director
Paula Leavitt, Clinical Director
Camp is a non profit corporation organized to develop and operate programs which promote the general welfare and education of children and adults with developmental disabilities.

954 **Pine Tree Camp**
Pine Tree Society
149 Front Street
PO Box 518
Bath, ME 04530
207-443-3341
FAX: 207-397-5324
e-mail: info@pinetreesociety.org
www.pinetreesociety.org

Deborah Regan, President
Anne Marsh, Executive Director
Dawn Willard-Robinson, Program Management Director
Provides direct service programs statewide to people with disabilities.

Maryland

955 **Camp Greentop**
League Serving People With Disabilities
1111 East Cold Spring Lane
Baltimore, MD 21239
410-323-0500
FAX: 410-323-3298
TTY:410-435-4298
e-mail: leaguelink@leagueforpeople.org
www.campgreentop.org

Janice Frey-Angel, Chief Executive Officer
Toni Carter, Medical Day Program Director
Stephen Freeman, Wellness Director
Camp is located in Sabillasville, Maryland. Summer residential camp located in the Catoctin Mountain National Park. Since 1937, Greentop has been serving children and adults with physical and multiple disabilities in a completely accessible camp setting. Campers enjoy a traditional camping program. Medical facilities staffed 24 hours a day. Half-week/one/two-week sessions June-August. ACA/MD Youth Camp.

956 **Camp JCC**
Jewish Community Center of Greater Washington JCC
6125 Montrose Road
Rockville, MD 20852
301-881-0100
FAX: 301-881-6549
e-mail: campjcc@jccgw.org
www.jccgw.org

Diane Kendall, Camp Director
John Verstandig, President
Camp JCC serves children with disabilities alongside their neighbors and friends. The American Camping Association has presented a National award to Camp JCC for its extraordinary model inclusion program. We also offer a program designed especially for 13-21 year olds with severe to profound disabilities. In order for us to afford to do these things, we count on contributions to our Inclusion Fund. Four and eight-week sessions general day camp program offering June-August for children.

957 **Camp Superkids**
American Lung Association of Maryland
11350 McCormick Road
Executive Plaza 1, Suite 600
Hunt Valley, MD 21031
410-560-2120
800-642-1184
e-mail: hdougherty@marylandlung.org
www.marylandlung.org

Heather Dougherty, Camp Director
Marianne Hiteshew, Medical Director
Ceal Curry, Medical Director
Overnight asthma camp for children 7 1/2 to 12 years of age. During the week of camp the kids will participate in arts and crafts, nature hikes, karate, swimming, sport activities and much more. Along with these activities there are 2 sessions a day of asthma education.

958 **Easter Seals Camp Fairlee Manor**
Easter Seals DE/ MD Eastern Shore
22242 Bay Shore Road
Chestertown, MD 21620
410-778-0566
FAX: 410-778-0567
e-mail: fairlee@esdeo.org
www.de.easters.com

Dan Tabacheck, Director

One-week sessions June-August for campers with disabilities. Coed, ages 8-99, families, seniors, single adults.

959 **Maryland National Capital Park and Planning Commission**
Special Populations Division
6611 Kenilworth Avenue
Riverdale, MD 20737
301-454-1740
FAX: 301-454-1750
e-mail: webmanager@mncppc.org
www.mncppc.org

Samuel Parker, Chairman
William M Eley Jr, Vice Chairman
Laurie Verge, Program Director
Offers year round and seasonal activities and programs for individuals with disabilities and families including day camps, horseback riding, beep ball, aquatics, special events and much more.

960 **Milldale Camp**
J CC Of Baltimore
3506 Gwynnbrook Avenue
Owings Mills, MD 21117
410-429-4900
FAX: 410-578-0102
e-mail: milldale@jcc.org
www.campmilldale.org

Jodi Fishman, Camp Director
Jessica Witenstein-Weaver, Special Needs Coordinator
Camp is located in Reisterstown, MD. Four and eight week sessions, June - August. Inclusion program for children entering grades 5-13 with learning, developmental, social, emotional and physical disabilities. Self-contained program for teenagers with disabilities ages 14-21 focusing on recreational and vocational activities, including weekly field trips.

Massachusetts

961 **AU Kamp for Kids**
Abilities Unlimited
61 Union Street
PO Box 219
Westfield, MA 01086
413-562-5678
FAX: 413-562-1239
e-mail: info@abilitiesunlimited.org
www.abilitiesunlimited.org

C. David Scanlin PhD, Executive Director
Two-week sessions July-August for children and young adults with a variety of disabilities. Coed, ages 3-22.

962 **Camp Ramah in New England (Summer)**
39 Bennett Street
Palmer, MA 01069
413-283-9771
FAX: 413-283-6661
www.campramahNE.org

Howard Blas, Director
Rabbi Ed Gelb, Camp Director
8 week sleep-away camp for Jewish adolescents with developmental disabilities. Full camping program includes swimming, Hebrew singing and dancing, sports, arts and crafts, daily services, Kosher food and Jewish studies classes. Some mainstreaming and vocational opportunities.

963 **Camp Ramah in New England (Winter)**
35 Highland Circle
Needham, MA 02494
781-449-7090
FAX: 781-449-6331
e-mail: joels@campramahne.org
www.campramahne.org

Joel Stavsky, Director
8 week sleep-away camp for Jewish adolescents with developmental disabilities. Full camping program includes swimming, Hebrew singing and dancing, sports, arts and crafts, daily services, Kosher food and Jewish studies classes. Vocational program for select group of former campers.

964 **Easter Seals Massachusetts-Agassiz Village**
484 Main Street
6th Floor
Worcester, MA 01608
508-757-2756
800-922-8290
FAX: 508-831-9768
TTY: 800-564-9700
e-mail: camp@eastersealsma.org
www.eastersealsma.org

Kirk Joslin, Chief Executive Officer
Stefanie Morissette, Camp Manager
Mission is to help children and adults with disabilities expand their independence.

965 **Four-H Camp Howe**
PO Box 326
Goshen, MA 01032
413-549-3969
FAX: 413-577-0760
e-mail: office@camphowe.com
www.camphowe.com

Terrie Campbell, Camp Director
One and two-week sessions June-August for children with a variety of disabilities. Coed, ages 7-17.

966 **Handi-Kids**
470 Pine Street
Bridgewater, MA 02324
508-697-7557
FAX: 508-697-1529
e-mail: info@handikids.org
www.handikids.org

Ginny Pitts, Executive Director
Mary Gallant, Program Director
Jane Pariseau, Theraputic Riding Director
A therapeutic recreational facility in Bridgewater, Massachusetts offering after-school programs, special events, school vacation full-week and summer day camp programs. Every individual is welcome. Two-week sessions July-August.
Sliding Scale

Michigan

967 **Camp Roger**
The American Camping Association
8356 Belding Road
Rockford, MI 49341
616-874-7286
FAX: 616-874-5734
e-mail: office@camproger.org
www.camproger.org

Doug Vanderwell, Executive Director
Phil Warners, Director Outdoor Education
Kathy Collins, Executive Assistant
Camp Roger provides a fun top-notch summer program for disabled campers. Campers learn to love the woods, the water and the trails, getting to enjoy a wide variety of activities all designed to be fun, to build friendships, and develop self confidence.

968 **Echo Grove Camp**
The Salvation Army
1101 Camp Road
(248) 628-3108
Leonard, MI 48367
248-628-3108
FAX: 248-628-7055
e-mail: info@echogrove.org
www.echogrove.org/

Dale Johnson, Camp Director
Since 1921, the Army's Echo Grove Camp has offered a structured camping program for children, adults and seniors referred through Corps Community Centers. During the course of Echo Grove's 12 week season, the camp includes programs geared for every need and interest. In addition to outdoor recreation, camps may include religious, musical and skill-building instruction.

969 **Fowler Center**
2315 Harmon Lake Road
Mayfield, MI 48744
989-673-2050
FAX: 989-673-6355
e-mail: info@thefowlercenter.org
www.thefowlercenter.org/

John S Fowler, Chairman and Founder
Half-week, one-week and two-week sessions. June-August for campers with disabilities. Coed, ages 6-99, families, seniors.

970 **Indian Trails Camp**
0-1859 Lake Michigan Drive Northwes
Grand Rapids, MI 49534
616-677-5251
FAX: 616-677-2955
e-mail: lynnyntema@indiantrailscamp.org
www.indiantrailscamp.org

Lynn Gust, Executive Director
Patty Primozich, Camp Director
Lance Davis, Program Director
Year round residential camping program for children and adults with physical disabilities. One and two-week sessions. Coed, ages 6-70.

971 **YMCA Camp Copneconic**
Flint Michigan YMCA
10407 North Fenton Road
Fenton, MI 48430
810-629-9622
FAX: 810-629-2128
e-mail: fritzcheek@campcopneconic.org
www.campcopneconic.org

John Carlson, Executive Director
Matt Langdon, Associate Executive Director
Shelly Hilton, Director School Programs
Camp is located in Fenton, Michigan. Summer sessions for campers with diabetes. Coed, ages 3-16 and seniors.

Minnesota

972 **Camp Courage**
Courage Center Headquarters
3915 Golden Valley Road
Minneapolis, MN 55422
763-520-0520
FAX: 763-520-0577
www.courage.org

Jan Malcolm, Chief Executive Officer
Nancy Larkin, Chief Operating Officer
Alice Johnson, Chief Financial Officer
Camp is located in Maple Lake, Minnesota. Summer sessions for campers with a variety of disabilities. Coed, ages 6-99, families, seniors.

973 **Camp Friendship**
Friendship Ventures
10509 108th Street Northwest
Annandale, MN 55302
952-852-0101
800-450-8376
FAX: 952-852-0123
e-mail: fv@friendshipventures.org
www.friendshipventures.org

Laurie Tschetter, Program Director
Camp Friendship offers resident camp programs for children, teenagers and adults with developmental, physical or multiple disabilities, special medical conditions, Down Syndrome, Williams Syndrome, autism or other conditions. Summer camp offers archery, sailing, horseback riding, biking, fishing, creative arts, adventure challenge programs and other activities. Weekend camps and longer available. Other services available throughout the year. Coed, ages 5-90, families, seniors.

974 **Camp New Hope**
10509 108th Street Northwest
Annadale, MN 55302
952-852-0101
800-450-8376
FAX: 952-852-0123
e-mail: fv@friendshipventures.org
www.campnewhopemn.org

Lori Bittner, Director
CNH is a private, non-profit organization which provides quality educational, recreational and leisure opportunities to children and adults with mental, physical and other developmental disabilities. Stimulating programs and quality care. Half-week and one-week sessions June-September. Coed, ages 6-99, families, seniors, single adults.

975 **Camp Winnebago**
19708 Camp Winnebago Road
Caledonia, MN 55921
507-724-2351
FAX: 507-724-3786
e-mail: director@CampWinnebago.org
www.campwinnebago.org

Theresa Burroughs, Executive Director
Al Fravert, President
Rick Frank, Vice President
Offers one week summer sessions for children and adults with developmental disabilities. Also, integrated youth sessions to allow friends and siblings to attend with traditional campers. Respite week-ends are offered monthly throughout the year. Travel vacations are also offered as an option. Publishes a newsletter and makes a video available. Coed, ages 6-99, families, seniors, singles adults.

Missouri

976 **Camp Cub Creek Science Camp**
Bear River Ranch
16795 Highway East
Rolla, MO 65401
573-458-2125
FAX: 573-458-2126
e-mail: director@bearriverranch.com
www.bearriverranch.com

Lori Martin, Executive Director
Scott Martin, Owner
Rachel Martin, Assistant Program Director
Coed summer camp for children and adults with developmental disabilites.

977 **Camp Lakewood**
YMCA of the Ozarks
13528 State Highway AA
Potosi, MO 63664
573-438-2154
FAX: 573-438-5752
e-mail: camplakewood@ymcastlouis.org
www.ymcaoftheozarks.org/CampLakewood/

Shawn Moriarty, Camp Director
Libby Staley, Program Director
Nicholas Beheler, Assistant Program Director
The YMCA day camp for children ages 6-8. Children are under the direction and supervision of their counselors and engage in small group and camp-wide activities and work on developing their skills and self-confidence.

978 **Concerned Care Recreation Day Camp**
Clayton County Developmental Disabilities Board
920 South Kent Street
Suite B
Liberty, MO 64068
816-474-3026
FAX: 816-474-3029
e-mail: ccareinc@crn.org
www.macdds.org/Counties/clay.html

John Whalen, Director
Jim Humpman, Assistant Director
Karl Morris, Executive Director
Summer sessions for campers with developmental disabilities. Coed, ages 7-16.

979 **Wonderland Camp Foundation**
18591 Miller Circle
Rocky Mount, MO 65072
573-392-1000
FAX: 573-392-3605
e-mail: wondcamp@advertisnet.com
www.wonderlandcamp.org

Allen Moore, Chief Executive Officer
Marcela Trujillo, Program Director
One-week sessions May-January for mentally/physically challenged campers and respite care. Coed, ages 6-80, families, seniors, single adults.

Nebraska

980 **Camp Easter Seals**
Easter Seals Nebraska
638 North 109th Plaza
Omaha, NE 68154
402-345-2200
800-650-9880
FAX: 402-345-2500
e-mail: mtufte@ne.easterseals.com
www.ne.easterseals.com

Karen Ginder, President/CEO
Val Mcpherson, Development Director
Mike Tufte, Camp Respite/Recreation Director
Offers a variety of services to help people with disabilities address life's challenges and achieve personal goals.

981 **Eastern Nebraska 4-H Camps and Centers**
University of Nebraska
4-H Youth Development
Lincoln, NE 68583
402-472-2805

e-mail: 4hcampea@unl.edu
4h.unl.edu

Elizabeth Birnstihl, 4-H Program Administrator
Vickie Greve, 4-H Youth Development Specialist
Kathy Potthoff, 4-H Program Coordinator
Beautiful modern facilities overlooking Platte River for the disabled campers.

New Hampshire

982 **Camp Allen**
56 Camp Allen Road
Bedford, NH 03110
603-622-8471
FAX: 603-626-4295
e-mail: mary@campallennh.org
www.campallennh.org/

Mary Constance, Executive Director
Debra Schulte, Office Manager
A residential summer camp for individuals with disabilities. All of the activities are conducted by individual coordinators under the supervision of Program Director. Some of the activities include, aquatics, arts, crafts, games and nature programs. All camp events, special events, evening programs, and field trips are scheduled throughout the summer and are structured to meet the individual abilities and needs of each camper.

983 **Camp Dartmouth-Hitchcock**
Dartmouth-Hitchcock Medical Center Pediatrics
1 Medical Center Drive
Lebanon, NH 03756
603-650-5000

e-mail: pediatric.residency.program@hitchcock.org
http://www.dhmc.org/

John F Modlin, Chairman
Jody Stygles, Manager
To provide high quality health care and comfort to the ill, to prevent illness among the well, and to advance health care through education, research, community service and the improvement of clinical practice.

984 **Easter Seal Camp: New Hampshire**
555 Auburn Street
Manchester, NH 03103
603-623-8863
800-870-8728
FAX: 603-625-1148
e-mail: dgordon@eastersealsnh.org
nh.easterseals.com

Robert Kelly, Camp Director
Larry Gammon, President
Christine McMahon, Senior Vice President/CFO
Mission is to create solutions that change the lives of children and adults with disabilities or special needs or their families. From campfire sing-a-longs and late night ghost stories, to boating, nature walks, swimming, and arts and crafts, Easter Seals camps provide the same excitement and activity available at other summer camp programs. Easter Seals campers experience the joys and challenges of camp in a fully-accessible setting.

985 **Easter Seals NH Camp Sno-Mo**
Easter Seals NH Camping Programs
200 Zachary Road
Building 2
Manchester, NH 03103
603-623-8863

e-mail: dgordon@eastersealsnh.org
www.eastersealsnh.org/services/camping

Robert Kelly, Camp Director
Van Davis, President
Douglas Gordon, Director Recreation
Easteer Seals Camp Sno-Mo is an intergrated camp, bringing together disabled invidual ages (1-24) with able bodied boy scouts. Our emphasis is on positive social interaction while finding an individual level of sucess in all passes of the camping process.

New Jersey

986 **Aldersgate Center**
PO Box 122
Swartswood, NJ 07877
973-383-5978
FAX: 973-383-4428
e-mail: aldersgate@tellurian.net
www.aldersgatenj.com

Declan Thompson, Director
Richard Thompson, Grounds/Facilities Manager
Dale Card, Finance
Camp is located in Newton, New Jersey. Summer sessions for campers with developmental disabilities. Coed, ages 6-18 and families, single adults.

987 **Camp Jotoni**
ARC of Somerset County
141 South Main Street
Manville, NJ 08835
908-725-8544
FAX: 908-753-7868
e-mail: bonnies@thearcofsomerset.org
www.thearcofsomerset.org

Judy Miao, Executive Director
Bonnie C Sovinee, Development Director
Chris Gunning, Residential Director
Sponsored by the Arc of Somerset County, Camp Jotoni is a day and residential camp for children and adults with developmental disabilities. Campers are ages five to adult. Set on 15 acres in Somerset County, the camp features a junior Olympic size pool, cabins, dining hall, playgrounds, open air pavilions, unspoiled woods, and wildlife. Coed, ages 5-99.

988 **Camp Merry Heart**
Easter Seals New Jersey
1 Kimberly Road
East Brunswick, NJ 08816
732-257-6662
FAX: 732-257-7373
TTY:732-257-4442
e-mail: ahumanick@njeasterseals.com
www.njeasterseals.com

Brian J Fitzgerald, President
Alexander Humanick, Executive Director
Daniel Tabacheck, Camping Coordinator
An organized program of swimming, arts and crafts, boating, nature study and travel offered to campers with a variety of disabilities. Coed, ages 5-80, families, seniors. Fall and spring travel programs for adults.

989 **Camp Sun'N Fun**
The Arc of Gloucester
1555 Gateway Boulevard
Woodbury, NJ 08096
856-848-8648
FAX: 856-848-7753
e-mail: webmaster@thearcgloucester.org
www.thearcgloucester.org

Ana Rivera, Executive Director
Camp is located in Williamstown, New Jersey. Summer sessions for campers with developmental disabilities. Coed, ages 8-88. Activities include swimming, arts & crafts, nature, sports, games, music, dance and drama.

990 **Cerebral Palsy Center Summer Program**
Cerebral Palsy of New Jersey
1005 Whitehead Road Extension
Suite 1
Ewing, NJ 08638
888-322-1918
FAX: 609-882-4054
TTY:609-882-0620
e-mail: info@cpofnj.org
www.cpofnj.org/

Patrick Colligan, Executive Director
Raymond Freeman, Manager of Housing
Kristina Callender, Residential Services NJ/North
Cerebral Palsy of New Jersey offers a wide array of services and support to children and adults with disabilities and to their families. Whether they're offering assistance in school or the workplace or helping out at home, CP of New Jersey's staff is trained and knowledgeable. Together they form a network that allows people with disabilities to achieve their goals.

991 **Cross Roads Outdoor Ministries**
29 Pleasant Grove Road
Port Murray, NJ 07865
908-832-7264
FAX: 908-832-6593
e-mail: crossroadsom@yahoo.com
www.crossroadsretreat.com/

Andrew Molnar, Director
Marie Skweir, Religious Leader
Program for ages 6-15 offers Bible study, worship, swimming, crafts, hiking, canoeing and campfires. Special education program for those with developmental disabilities.

992 **New Jersey Camp Jaycee**
The Arc of New Jersey
985 Livingston Avenue
North Brunswick, NJ 08902
732-246-2525
FAX: 732-214-1834
e-mail: info@campjaycee.org
www.campjaycee.org

Thomas Baffuto, Executive Director
Victor M Mankoski, Coordinator of Camping Services
Camp Jaycee is located on 185 acres of forests, fields and streams located in the lovely Pocono Mountains, a short distance from the New Jersey border. Sessions for children and adults with autism and developmental disabilities. Goals of Camp Jaycee are centered around developing social skills, improving self esteem, increasing confidence, learning in a fun environment, developing physical fitness, and establishing meaningful relationships with new friends. Coed, ages 7-85.

New Mexico

993 **Santa Fe Mountain Center**
PO Box 449
Tesuque, NM 87574
505-983-6158
FAX: 505-983-0460
e-mail: info@santafemc.org
www.sf-mc.com

Sky Gray, Executive Director
Marge Kelley, Associate Director
Jenn Jevertson, Adventure Program Manager
Camp sessions offered to disabled campers from the ages of 1-20.

New York

994 **Camp Aldersgate**
Med Camps Coordinator
1375 Broadway
4th Floor
New York, NY 10018
212-391-5208
FAX: 212-391-5207
e-mail: info@aldersgateny.org
www.aldersgateny.org

Elizabeth Chiafair, Executive Assistant
Adam Weinstein, Executive Director
A private nonprofit social service agency allied with the United Methodist Church which co-sponsors a series of summer medical camps with Med Camps of Arkansas, Inc., and thirteen various health agencies. The camps allow children and youth, ages 6-16, who have various medical conditions and physical disabilities to enjoy traditional camping experiences adapted to their abilities. The Camp also offers respite care, senior citizens programs, West Side Clinic and the Children's Center. Coed.

995 **Camp Venture**
100 Convent Road
PO Box 402
Nanuet, NY 10954
845-624-3862
FAX: 845-624-7064
e-mail: jenkahn@campventure.org
www.campventure.org

Daniel Lukens, Executive Director
In more than a dozen Rockland neighborhoods, residential, employment, rehabilitation or recreation programs have arisen to help people with disabilities contribute to the life of the community. There are, for instance, more than a dozen Community Residential Facilities, Venture Industries, Venture Day Treatment, Day Habilitation, Venture Chorus, after school programs and more.

996 **Camp Whitman on Seneca Lake**
150 Whitman Road
PO Box 278
Dresden, NY 14441
315-536-7753
FAX: 315-536-2128
e-mail: camp@campwhitman.org
www.campwhitman.org

Thomas D Montgomery, Executive Director
Sam Edwards, Camp Operator
Chris Ruthven, Property Manager
Summer sessions for young people and adults with developmental disabilities. Coed, ages 10-adult.

997 **Clover Patch Camp**
Center for the Disabled
55 Helping Hand Lane
Glenville, NY 12302
518-384-3081
FAX: 518-384-3001
e-mail: cloverpatchcamp@cftd.org
www.cloverpatchcamp.org

Christopher Schelin, Program Administrator
Laura Taylor, Camp Director
Camp is located in Scotia, NY. Summer sessions for campers with a variety of disabilities. Coed, ages 5-85.

998 **Henry Kaufmann Campgrounds Staten Island**
1131 Manor Road
Staten Island, NY 10314
718-761-1423

Jeffrey Alan Coopersmith, Director
Morris W Offit, President
Susan K Stern, Chair
Disabled campers.

999 **Kamp Kiwanis**
New York District Kiwanis
9020 Kiwanis Road
Taberg, NY 13471
315-336-4568
FAX: 315-336-3845
e-mail: kamp@kiwanis-ny.org
www.kiwanis-ny.org/kamp

Orlando Marrazzo Jr, President
Rebecca Lopez, Executive Director/CEO
Donald Herring, Foundation Secretary
Kamp Kiwanis is a mainstream camp for underprivileged youth with and without special needs. 20 campers with disabilities are integrated into weekly sessions. Coed, ages 8-14, seniors and single adults.

1000 Ninety-Second Street Y Camps Nesher Program
1395 Lexington Avenue
New York, NY 10128 212-415-5500

e-mail: mmandel@92y.org
www.92y.org

Melanie S Mandel, Director of Program
Sol Adler, Executive Director
After-school recreation programs for children ages 4-20 with developmental disabilities.

1001 Programs for Children 3 to 5 with Disabili lities
New York State Education Department
1 Commerce Plaza
Suite 1624
Albany, NY 12234 518-473-2878
FAX: 518-486-7693
e-mail: schyer@mail.nysed.gov
www.vesid.nysed.gov/specialized

Micheal Plotvker, Manager
Richard Mills, Commissioner of Education
James DeLorenzo, State Coordinator Special Ed
The Mission of the Office of Vocational and Educational Services for Individuals with Disabilities (VESID) is to promote educational equity and excellence for students with disabilities and provide the highest quality vocational rehabilitation and independent living services to all eligible persons as quickly as those services are required to enable them to work and live independent, self-directed lives.

1002 Programs for Children Birth to 2 with Disa abilities
New York State Department of Health
Empire State Plaza
Corning Tower Bldg, Room 287
Albany, NY 12237 518-473-7016
FAX: 518-486-1090
e-mail: bjh08@health.state.ny.us
www.nichcy.org/stateshe/ny.htm

Bradley Hutton, Director
The Early Intervention Program offers a variety of therapeutic and support services to eligible infants and toddlers with disabilities and their families.

1003 Programs for Children with Special Health Care Needs
New York State Department of Health
ESP Corning Tower Building
Room 208
Albany, NY 12237 518-474-2001
FAX: 518-474-5445
e-mail: sjs11@health.state.ny.us
www.health.state.ny.us/nysdoh/child/

Susan Slade, Director
Patricia Hess, Manager
The Children with Special Health Care Needs Program (CSHCN) is a statewide public health program that provides information and referral services for health and related areas for families of CSHCN. This program is a referral linkage system to provide for those children ages birth to 21 who have, or are suspected of having, a serious or chronic physical, developmental, behavioral, or emotional condition who require a health or related service of a type or amount beyond what is generally required.

1004 Rochester Rotary Sunshine Camp
Rochester Rotary Club
100 Meridian Centre
Suite 304
Rochester, NY 14618 585-546-7435
FAX: 585-546-8675
e-mail: sknipper@rochester.com
www.rochester.com

Tracey Dreisbach, Executive Director
Stacy Morabito, Financial Director
Linda Garland, Executive Assistant
Camp is located in Rush, New York. Camping sessions for children and young adults with a variety of disabilities. Ages 7-21.

1005 Wagon Road Camp
Children's Aid Society Summer Camps
105 East 22nd Street
New York, NY 10010 212-949-4800
914-238-4761
FAX: 212-477-3705
e-mail: ellenl@childrensaidsociety.org
www.childrensaidsociety.org

Yahaira Jimenez, Camp Director
Ellen Lubel, Public Relations Director
C Warren Moses, Chief Executive Officer
Wagon Road Day Camp is a co-ed program for children ages 6-13 with a variety of disabilities held within Chappaqua, New York. Uniquely qualified specialists in Project Adventure activities, athletics, horsemanship, theater arts, nature/ecology studies and arts/crafts complement the day camp staff. Special events including Carnival, Olympics, Crazy Hat Day, Western Day, and optional sleepovers add to the summer excitement providing children with an enriching multicultural experience.

North Carolina

1006 Camp Sky Ranch
634 Sky Ranch Road
Blowing Rock, NC 28605 828-264-8600
FAX: 828-265-2339
e-mail: jsharp1@triad.rr.com
www.campskyranch.com

Jack Sharp, Director
Betty Sharp, Director
A private, residential camp for the developmentally delayed. This season is the camp's 56th year of providing a real camping experience for the handicapped. Camp Sky Ranch was the first private camp for the handicapped in the Southeast. Activities include: swimming, boating, horseback riding, and more. Campers must be able to walk, dress and feed themselves, and toilet trained.

1007 Mount Shepherd Retreat Center
1045 Mount Shepherd Road Ext
Asheboro, NC 27205 336-629-4085
FAX: 336-629-4880
e-mail: mtsheph@asheboro.com
www.mtshepherd.org/directions.php

Kent L Shrader, Executive Director
Vicky Matthew, Administrator
Camping for children with developmental disabilities. Coed, ages 14 to Adults. Mount Shepherd Retreat Center offers a year-round camping program. Our summer program attracts children and youth from around the region and across the state. We also offer facilities for you or your group to get away from it all and enjoy a weekend retreat on the grounds.

1008 Stone Mountain School
126 Camp Elliott Road
Black Mountain, NC 28711 828-669-8639
888-631-5994
FAX: 828-669-2521
e-mail: info@stonemountainschool.com
www.stonemountainschool.com

Sam Moore, Executive Director
Sue Miller, Public Relations
Eric Morlino, Program Supervisor
Year round therapeutic wilderness school for emotionally disturbed boys grades 6-12. Certified mental health program, licensed by the department of facility services and certified special education school.

Ohio

1009 Akron Rotary Camp
4460 Rex Lake Drive
Akron, OH 44319
330-644-4512
FAX: 330-644-1013
e-mail: rotarycamp@akronymca.org
www.akronymca.com/camp/rotary/

Dan Reynolds, Executive Director
Alexander Kuzmetsov, Camp Counselor
Amanda Grobler, Office Administrator
The Rotary Camp for Children with Special Needs, in cooperation with the Akron Area YMCA, offers camping experiences for children and adults with disabilities. Rotary Camp is American Camping Association (ACA) accredited and provides a nurturing and enriching atmosphere where campers develop friendships, skills and memories that will last a lifetime. Coed, ages 6-17.

1010 Beech Brook
3737 Lander Road
Pepper Pike, OH 44124
216-831-2255
877-546-1225
FAX: 216-831-0436
e-mail: debra_rex@beechbrook.org
www.beechbrook.org

Mario Tonti, President
Paula Atwood, Vice President
Debra Rex, Executive Director
Residential and day treatment center. Treatment center for emotionally disturbed children, including residential and day treatment; foster care; adoption; adn community based programs.

1011 Camp Allyn
Stepping Stones Center
5650 Given Road
Cincinnati, OH 45243
513-831-4660
FAX: 513-831-5918
e-mail: ssc@steppingstonescenter.org
www.steppingstonescenter.org

Susan Radabaugh, Executive Director
Dennis Carter, Associate Director
Fred Fischer, President
A camp in Batavia, Ohio for children and adults with disabilities. Coed, ages 7-60. Campers participate in crafts, swimming, hiking, nature, sports and motor activities. Camp sessions range from 3 to 10 days, are theme oriented, and geared to individual abilities and interests.

1012 Camp Courageous
12701 Waterville Swanton Road
Whitehouse, OH 43571
419-534-4980
B66-740-8117
FAX: 419-535-5809
e-mail: cherylt@campcourageous.com
www.campcourageous.com

Steve Kiessling, Camp Director
Emily Ohlrich, Assistant Camp Director
Jenny Nowak, Camp Coordinator
Camp Courageous provides residential camping services for people with developmental disabilities from ages 7-75 years old. Our six day, 5 night programs give campers a chance to experience activities such as: aquatics, arts and crafts, animal programs, sports skills, hiking, recreational and leisure education programs, nature studies, drama, cookouts and campfires.

1013 Camp Stepping Stone
Stepping Stones Center
5650 Given Road
Cincinnati, OH 45243
513-831-4660
FAX: 513-831-5918
e-mail: ssc@steppingstonescenter.org
www.steppingstonescenter.org

Susan Radabaugh, Executive Director
Clifford Dornette, President
Fred Fischer, Vice President
Nonprofit United Way affiliated camp serving all disabilities and charging on a sliding scale.

1014 Happiness Day at Parmadale
Catholic Charities Services
7911 Detroit Avenue
Cleveland, OH 44102
216-334-2963
800-869-6525
FAX: 216-334-2905
TTY: 440-845-7700
e-mail: mjscott@clevelandcatholiccharities.org
www.clevelandcatholiccharities.org/camping/

Marilyn Scott, Camp Program Administrator
Dennis McNulty, Disability Services Director
Camp is located in Parma, Ohio. Summer sessions for children and young adults with developmental disabilities. Coed, ages 6-21.

1015 Happiness Day at St. Augustine Academy
Cleveland Catholic Charities
7911 Detroit Road
Cleveland, OH 44102
216-334-2963
FAX: 216-334-2905
e-mail: gwanous@st-aug-academy.org
www.clevelandcatholiccharities.org/camping/

Georgianne Wanous, Executive Director
Fr. Joseph McNulty, Disability Ministry Director
Sr. Corita Ambro, Program Director
Serves mentally retarded campers with multiple handicaps.

1016 Happiness Day at the Center for Pastoral Leadership
Catholic Charities Services
7911 Detroit Avenue
Cleveland, OH 44102
216-334-2958
FAX: 216-334-2983
e-mail: lbtaylor@clevelandcatholiccharities.org
www.clevelandcatholiccharities.o rg/camping/

Tana Minneti, Camp Director
Eilean Klear, Camping Programs Director
Lynette Taylor, Camp Registrar
Camp is located in Wickliffe, Ohio. Summer sessions for children and young adults with developmental disabilities. Coed, ages 6-21.

1017 Leo Yassenoff JCC Day Camps
1125 College Avenue
Columbus, OH 43209
614-231-2731
FAX: 614-231-8222
e-mail: rfox@columbusjcc.org
www.columbusjcc.org

Carol Folkerth, Executive Director
Mike Klapper, Program Director
Summer camping sessions for children and young adults with developmental, physical, emotional, mental and learning disabilities. Coed, ages 3-25.

1018 Recreation Unlimited
7700 Piper Road
Ashley, OH 43003
740-548-7006
FAX: 740-747-2640
e-mail: info@recreationunlimited.org
www.recreationunlimited.org

Laura Smith, Program Director
Paul Huttlin, Executive Director/CEO
Camping sessions for children and adults with a variety of disabilities. Coed, ages 5-99, families, seniors and single adults.

Oregon

1019 Easter Seals Oregon Camping Program
5757 SW Macadam Avenue
Portland, OR 97239
503-228-5108
800-556-6020
FAX: 503-228-1352
e-mail: info@or.easterseals.com
or.easterseals.com

David Cheveallier, CEO and President
Camp is located in Corbett, Oregon. Summer sessions for children and adults with a variety of disabilities. Coed, ages 6-90.

1020 Gales Creek Diabetes Camp
Gales Creek Camp Foundation
6975 SW Sandburg Street
Suite 150
Portland, OR 97223
503-968-2267
FAX: 503-443-2313
e-mail: info@galescreekcamp.org
www.galescreekcamp.org

Cheryl Sheppard, Executive Director
Eric Hanson, Development Specialist
James Wolfe, Program Specialist
Camp is located in Forest Grove, Oregon. Summer sessions for children with diabetes. Coed, ages 6-16, family and pre-school family camps also available.

1021 Mt Hood Kiwanis Camp
Kiwanis Club of Montavilla
9320 SW Barbur Boulevard
Suite 165
Portland, OR 97219
503-452-7416
FAX: 503-452-0062
e-mail: information@mhkc.org
www.mhkc.org

Gene Nudelman, Executive Director
Charlene Dickinson, Administrator
Dianne Zellner, President
Camp is located in Government Camp, Oregon. Summer sessions for children and adults with a variety of disabilities. Coed, ages 9-35.

1022 Upward Bound Camp: Evans Creek
American Camping Association
PO Box C
Stayton, OR 97383
503-897-2447
FAX: 503-897-4116
e-mail: ubc@open.org
www.upwardboundcamp.org

Jerry Pierce, Executive Director
Laura Pierce, Director
Camping Christian for children and adults with a variety of disabilities. Ages 12-99, seniors and single adults.

Pennsylvania

1023 Achieva
711 Bingham Street
Pittsburgh, PA 15203
412-995-5000
888-272-7229
FAX: 412-995-5001
e-mail: contact@achieva.info
www.achieva.info

Marsha Blanco, CEO/President
Ray Rykaceski, Executive Vice President
Gary Horner, CFO
Life-long services for people with disabilities.

1024 Briarwood Day Camp
1380 Creek Road
Furlong, PA 18925
215-598-7143
FAX: 215-602-1060
e-mail: bruceatcamp@aol.com
www.briarwood-camp.com

Ted Levine, Owner
A comprehensive day camp providing lunch and transportation for children with disabilities.

1025 Camp AIM Lloyd Institute
2 Chatham Center
Suite 1500
Pittsburgh, PA 15219
412-454-0243
FAX: 412-281-6622
e-mail: mlloyd@lloydinstitute.com
www.lloydinstitute.com

Michael E Lloyd, Founder
Is a solid six week summer day program of adaptive aquatics, physical education, music expression, crafts, songs, special events, self-help, and socialization skills learning.

1026 Camp ARC Spencer
A RC of Beaver county
3582 Brodhead Road
Suite 202
Monaca, PA 15061
724-775-1602
800-272-0567
FAX: 724-775-2905
e-mail: arcbeaver@achieva.info
www.achieva.info

Jacqueline Finney, Executive Director
Camp is located in Fombell, Pennsylvania. Summer sessions for children and adults with developmental disabilities. Coed, ages 5-99.

1027 Camp Can Do
Easter Seals Southeastern PA
468 N Middletown Road
Media, PA 19063
610-565-2353
FAX: 610-565-5256
www.easterseals-sepa.org

Carl Webster, Chief Executive Officer
Lexy Chapel, Assistant Director
Donna Keiths, Executive Director
Camp is located in Kulpsville, Pennsylvania. Summer sessions for children and young adults with a variety of disabilities. Coed, ages 5-21

1028 Camp Dunmore
Easter Seals Southeastern PA
468 N Middletown Road
Media, PA 19063
610-565-2353
FAX: 610-565-5256
www.easterseals-sepa.org

Carl Webster, Chief Executive Officer
Lexy Chapel, Assistant Director
Donna Keiths, Executive Director
Summer sessions for children and young adults with a variety of disabilities. Coed, ages 5-21.

1029 Camp Keystone
Rr 1
Box 1515
Gouldsboro, PA 18424
570-842-4521
570-795-0029
FAX: 570-842-2158
e-mail: glance@keycommresp.com
www.campkey.com

Gloria J Lance, Director
Joy Smith, Executive Director
Keystone serves both children and adults with a variety of disabilities in various residential settings. Support services include 24 hour supervision, on site nursing services, special and therapeutic recreation programs and psychological and psychiatric services. Ages 6-66, seniors and single adults.

1030 Camp Lee Mar
805 Redgate Road
Dresher, PA 19025
215-658-1708
FAX: 215-658-1710
e-mail: gtour400@aol.com
www.leemar.com

Ariel J Segal, Executive Director
Lee Morone, Director
Seven week summer camp for children and young adults with mild to moderate developmental disabilities. 5-21 years of age

1031 Camp Surefoot
Easter Seals Southeastern PA
468 N Middletown Road
Media, PA 19063
610-565-2353
FAX: 215-945-4073
www.easterseals-sepa.org

Carl Webster, Director
Donna Keiths, Executive Director

Camp is located in Levittown, Pennsylvania. Sessions for children and young adults with a variety of disabilities. Coed, ages 5-21.

1032 Handi Camp

Handi Vangelism Ministries International
PO Box 122
Akron, PA 17501
717-859-4777
FAX: 717-859-4505
e-mail: info@hvmi.org
wwww.hvmi.org

Tim Sheetz, Executive Director
Deb Clark, Director of Counseling Ministrys
Kathy Sheetz, Executive Secretary
Christian, overnight camping program for people with disabilities, ages 7-50, in Eastern PA and Southern NJ. Sponsored by Handi Vangelism Ministries International.

1033 Helping Hands

415 Hoffmansville Road
Bechtelsville, PA 19505
610-754-6491
FAX: 610-754-7157
e-mail: hhandsinc@comcast.net
www.helpinghands.com

Bruce Waters, Executive Director
Provides vocational and recreational programs for individuals with developmental disabilities. Offers support and information to parents, caregivers, and individuals impacted by disabilities.

1034 Innabah

712 Pughtown Road
Spring City, PA 19475
610-469-6111
877-UMC-CAMP
FAX: 610-469-0330
e-mail: camp@innabah.org
www.innabah.org

Christy Heflin, Executive Director
Sessions for children and young adults with developmental disabilities. Ages 4-18, families and seniors.

1035 Ken-Crest Services

502 W Germantown Pike
Suite 200
Plymouth Meeting, PA 19462
610-825-9360
FAX: 610-825-4127
e-mail: kencrest@kencrest.org
www.kencrest.org

William Nolan, Chief Executive Officer
Mary Ellen Caffrey, Director Childrens Services
Ken-Crest provides services and supports for people who have developmental disability or who are at risk for disability across southeastern Pennsylvania and Delaware. Ken-Crest's community-based programs span the entire age continuum. Services for children include assessment, early intervention, therapies and parent education. For adults, Ken-Crest provides a full range of residential, employment, healthcare and therapy services.

1036 Living Waters

Penn West Conference Ucc
320 S Maple Avenue
Greensburg, PA 15601
724-834-0344
FAX: 724-834-0324
www.pennwest.org

Alan McLarty, Conference Minister/Manager
Linda Miller, Associate Conference Minister
Camp is located in Schellsburg, Pennsylvania. Sessions for children and adults with developmental disabilities, ages 6-96 and families.

1037 Make-a-Friend

3975 Conshohocken Avenue
Philadelphia, PA 19131
215-879-1000
FAX: 215-879-8424
sepa.easterseals.com

Mission is to create solutions that change lives of children and adults with disabilities or other special needs and their families.

1038 Souderton Special Needs Day Camp

149 E Cherry Lane
Souderton, PA 18964
215-723-6061

Donna Huff
Charles Amuso, Administrator
Field trips and special events for disabled campers.

1039 Variety Club Camp

PO Box 609
Worcester, PA 19490
610-584-4366
FAX: 610-584-5586
e-mail: varietyclubcamp@hotmail.com
http://www.montcopa.org/montcoworks

Andrew Pack, Executive Director
Stephanie Curran, Office Manager
Year-round camping and recreation facility for children with special needs and their families. Includes summer camping, aquatics, weekend retreats and other specialty programs. Coed, ages 5-21.

1040 Wesley Woods

Rr 1
Box 155
Grand Valley, PA 16420
814-436-7802
FAX: 814-436-7669
e-mail: wesleywoods@tbscc.com
www.wesleywoods.com

Fred Hunt, President
Alice Rentz, Vice President
Harold Burns, Director
Exceptional children's camp for children with emotional and intellectual handicaps.

1041 Woodlands

134 Shenot Road
Wexford, PA 15090
724-935-6533
FAX: 724-934-9610
e-mail: info@woodlandsfoundation.org
www.woodlandsfoundation.org

Peter Clakeley, Executive Director
Jessica Schlie, Program Director
Summer camping sessions and collaborative opportunities with charities serving individuals with disability and chronic illness. Year-round weekend retreats and aquatic programs for children and young adults with a variety of disabilities. Coed, ages 7-21.

Rhode Island

1042 Aldersgate Center

1043 Snake Hill Road
North Scituate, RI 02857
401-568-4350
FAX: 401-568-1840
e-mail: info@campaldersgate.com
www.campaldersgate.com

Jennifer Carpenter, Executive Director
Summer sessions for children and adults with asthma/respiratory ailments. Coed, ages 7-99 and families.

1043 Canonicus Camp

American Baptist Churches Rhode Island
PO Box 330
Exeter, RI 02822
401-294-6318
800-294-6318
FAX: 401-294-7780
e-mail: camp@canonicus.org
www.canonicus.org

Elizabeth Lussier, Director of Administration
Linda Martin, Conferencing Coordinator
Colleen Tolhurst, Registrar
Summer sessions for children with asthma/respiratory ailments. Coed, ages 4-18.

South Carolina

1044 **Burnt Gin Camp**
SC Department of Health and Environmental Control
2600 Bull Street
Columbia, SC 29201
803-737-0400
FAX: 803-898-0613
www.scdhec.net/hs/mch/burntgin/hsbgin1.hpm

Marie Aimone, Camp Director
Charles Way, Manager
A residential camp for children who have physical disabilities and/or chronic illnesses. Camper/staff ratio is 2:1. Five seven-day sessions for 7-15 year olds and one six-day sesssion for 16-19 year olds. Limited to residents of South Carolina.

1045 **Camp Gravatt**
1006 Camp Gravatt Road
Aiken, SC 29805
803-648-1817
FAX: 803-648-7453
e-mail: gravattguest@mindspring.com
www.bishopgravatt.org

Laurin Yeargin, Camp Gravatt Director
Linda Rybicki, Gravatt Administrator
Project adventure includes swimming, fishing, music and art and more in which disabled campers participate. Enjoy the fun and adventure of exploring a river in a canoe in the new canoe program.

Tennessee

1046 **Camp Discovery**
Tennessee Jaycee Fund
PO Box 10206
Knoxville, TN 37939
615-331-6345
FAX: 615-293-4497
e-mail: directorjayceecamp.org
www.jayceecap.org

Dawn Hickman, Director
Paula Petty, Camp Caretaker
Serves children with skin conditions including: Epidermolysis Bullosa, Psoriasis, Alopecia, Vitiligo, Eczema, Scleroderma, Congential Nevus, Ehlers-Danlos, Ichthyosis, Ectodermal Dysplasia and more. The Camp is located at 400 Camp Discovery Lane in Gainsboro, TN.

1047 **Easter Seals Camp**
6300 Benders Ferry Road
Mount Juliet, TN 37122
615-444-2829
FAX: 615-444-8576
e-mail: camp@eastersealstn.com
www.eastersealstn.com

Leslie Sohls, Executive Director
Penny Williams, Office Manager
Summer sessions for children and adults with various disabilities, ages 6-99.

Texas

1048 **Camp CAMP**
PO Box 27086
San Antonio, TX 78227
210-292-3566
FAX: 210-292-3576
e-mail: campmail@campcamp.org
www.campcamp.org

Susan Osborne, Family Services Director
Janice Bob, Development Director
Suzanne Reily, Training Director
Camping for children and young adults with a variety of disabilities. Coed, ages 5-21. Respite services throughout calendar year. Adult camp ages 22-45.

1049 **Camp John Marc**
Special Camps for Special Kids
2824 Swiss Avenue
Dallas, TX 75204
214-360-0056
FAX: 214-368-2003
e-mail: mail@campjohnmarc.org
www.campjohnmarc.org

Carol Touchstone, Chairman
Vance C Gilmore, Executive Director
Camp is located in Meridian, Texas. Year-round camping for children with a variety of disabilities. Coed, ages 6-16 and families.

1050 **Camp Summit**
2915 L B J Fwy
Suite 185
Dallas, TX 75234
972-484-8900
FAX: 972-620-1945
www.campsummittx.org

Lisa Braziel, Camp Director
Carla Weiland, Chief Executive Officer
Camp is located in Argyle, Texas. Camping for children and adults with a variety of disabilities. Coed, ages 6-99.

1051 **Camp for All**
Vicki La Rue
10500 Northwest Fwy
Suite 220
Houston, TX 77092
713-686-5666
FAX: 713-686-1242
e-mail: houstonoffice@campforall.org
www.campforall.org

Vicki Rue, President/CEO
Janet Johnson, Camp Director
Teri Todd, Operations Manager
Fully-accessible year round camp facility is located in Burton, Texas. Camping for children and adults with a variety of disabilities. Coed, ages 5-35 and up and families.

Utah

1052 **Camp Kostopulos**
Kostopulos Dream Foundation
2500 Emigration Cyn
Salt Lake City, UT 84108
801-582-0700
FAX: 801-583-5176
e-mail: kdf@campk.org
www.campk.org

Gary Ethington, Executive Director
Summer camping for children and adults ages 7-65 with a variety of disabilities. Year round recreation on site and community based activities.

Vermont

1053 **Bennington School Summer Program**
192 Fairview Street
Bennington, VT 05201
802-447-1557
FAX: 802-447-3234
e-mail: admissions@benningtonschoolinc.org
www.benningtonschoolinc.org

Patrick Ramsay, Director Admissions
Jeffrey LaBonte, Executive Director
A 115 bed residential treatment center serving emotionally and behaviorally disordered adolescent male and female students. Offers fully accredited on-grounds educational and summer programs in a beautiful rural setting with many recreational and cultural opportunities.

1054 **Camp Thorpe**
680 Capen Hill Road
Goshen, VT 05733 802-247-6611
e-mail: cthorpe@sover.net
www.campthorpe.org

Lyle Jepson, Director
Focuses on meeting the needs of each individual camper; showing each of them that they have the ability and potential. Also provides positive camping experience for children challenged with handicapping conditions.

Virginia

1055 **American Diabetes Summer Camp**
American Diabetes Association
1701 N Beauregard Street
Alexandria, VA 22311 703-549-1500
800-342-2383
e-mail: webmaster@diabetes.org
www.diabetes.org

Lynn B Nicholas, Chief Executive Officer
Alan Cherrington, President
Catherine Tibbetts, President
The American Diabetes Association is the nation's leading nonprofit health organization providing diabetes research, information, advocacy and year round programs for children with diabetes.

1056 **Camp Dickenson**
Holsten Conference Camping
801 Camp Dickson Lane
Fries, VA 24330 276-744-7241
FAX: 276-744-7241
e-mail: cdickenson@tcia.net

Chuck Jones, Director
Randy Pasqua, Executive Director
Charles Maynard, Director of Development
Camp is located in Fries, Virginia. Camping for children and adults with developmental disabilities. Coed, ages 5-18, families, seniors and single adults.

1057 **Camp Easter Seal: East/West**
Easter Seals Virginia
201 E Main Street
Salem, VA 24153 540-777-7325
800-365-1656
FAX: 540-777-2194
www.va.easter-seals.org

Kim Hutchinson, President
Tristan Robertson, Director
Summer camp sessions for children and adults ages 5-99 with physical disabilities, cognitive disabilities and sensory impairments. Therapeutic recreation activities including swimming, fishing, sports, horseback riding, rock climbing, and more. Twenty-six-day speech therapy camp children with disabilities ages 8-16. Twelve-day Spina Bifida Self Help Skills Camp.

1058 **Camp Holiday Trails**
400 Holiday Trails Lane
Charlottesville, VA 22903 434-977-3781
FAX: 434-977-8814
e-mail: holidaytrails@nexet.net
avenue.org/cht

Tina LaRoche, Director
Private, nonprofit camp for children with special health needs and various chronic illnesses. Residential, 2-week sessions are open June - August; camperships are available. Coed 7-17, nationwide and international. Canoeing, swimming, horseback riding, arts and crafts, drama, ropes course, etc. 24-hr. medical supervision by doctor and nursing staff. Air conditioned cabins.

1059 **Camp Virginia Jaycee**
2494 Camp Jaycee Road
Blue Ridge, VA 24064 540-947-2972
800-865-0092
FAX: 540-947-2043
e-mail: ewerness@campvirginiajaycee.com
www.campvirginiajaycee.com

Everett M Werness, President
Cathy Filicky, Camp Director
Peggy Ashe, Camp Registrar
Summer camping for children and adults with developmental disabilities. Coed, ages 7-70. Weekend respite camps for children and adults with mental retardation.

1060 **Civitan Acres**
Eggleston Services
1161 Ingleside Road
Norfolk, VA 23502 757-858-8011
757-722-5831
FAX: 757-627-4760
TTY: 757-852-9310
e-mail: info@egglestonservices.org
www.egglestonservices.org/programs_ca.html

Mr Jeffrey Parker, Chairman
Mr Edward Blair, Vice Chairman
Camping for children and adults with developmental disabilities. Coed, ages 5-99.

1061 **Loudoun County Special Recreation Programs**
Loudoun County Local Government
215 Depot Ct SE
Leesburg, VA 20175 703-777-0343
FAX: 703-771-5354
e-mail: prcs@loudoun.gov
www.loudoun.gov

Diane Ryburn, Director
Cynthia Welsh, Executive Director
Offers and promotes integration opportunities for individuals with disabilities. Coordinates ADA issues and Very Special Arts and Special Olympics for Loudoun County. Summer camps, sports, socials and community trips.

Washington

1062 **Camp Killoqua**
Camp Fire U SA
4312 Rucker Avenue
Everett, WA 98203 425-258-5437
FAX: 425-252-2267
e-mail: info@campfireusasnohoneish.org
www.campfireusasnohomish.org/killoqua

Carol Johnson, Director
Dave Surface, Executive Director
Camp is located in Stanwood, Washington. Camping for children with developmental disabilities. Coed, ages 6-17.

1063 **Volasuca Volunteers of America**
Volunteers of America
2802 Broadway Ave
Everett, WA 98201 425-259-3191
FAX: 425-258-2838
e-mail: info@voaww.org
www.voaww.org

Tom Robinson, President/CEO
Kelly Holderman, Director, Human Resource
Michael Frederick, Chief Financial Officer
Camp is located in Sultan, Washington. Summer sessions for children and adults with a variety of disabilities. Coed, ages 6-13, families and single adults.

West Virginia

1064 **Stepping Stones**
400 Mylan Park Lane
Morgantown, WV 26501
304-983-7837
800-982-8799
FAX: 304-983-8037
www.steppingstonescenter.net

Susan Fox, Executive Director
Jack Porter, President
Non-profit organization that serves individuals with disabilities. Programs include recreation, summer camps, technology and speech therapy.

Wisconsin

1065 **Easter Seal Camp Wawbeek**
Easter Seals Wisconsin
101 Nob Hill Road
Room 301
Madison, WI 53713
608-277-8288
800-422-2324
FAX: 608-277-8333
TTY: 608-277-8031
e-mail: wawbeek@wi-easterseals.org
www.eastersealswisconsin.com

Kelly Housman, Program Director
Nance Roepke, Executive Director
Christine Fessler, Chief Executive Officer
Disabled campers. Offers adventure programs, camp sessions for other health agencies, family camp opportunities and year round respite sessions. Coed, ages 8-99.

1066 **Lutherdale Bible Camp**
N7891 Us Highway 12
Elkhorn, WI 53121
262-742-2352
FAX: 262-742-3169
e-mail: lutherdale@lutherdale.org
www.lutherdale.org

Jeffrey Bluhm, Executive Director
Jenn Box, Program Assistant
Summer camping for people with developmental disabilities. Coed, ages 9-18 and families, seniors.

1067 **Wisconsin Badger Camp**
PO Box 723
Platteville, WI 53818
608-348-9689
FAX: 608-348-9737
e-mail: wiscbadgercamp@centurytel.net
www.badgercamp.org

Brent Bowers, Executive Director
Carissa Miller, Camp Director
Mission is to serve people with developmental disabilities by providing quality outdoor recreational experience. All developmentally disabled individuals, regardless of the severity of their disability or inability to pay are welcome.

Dresses & Skirts

1068 Budget Cotton/Poly Open Back Gown
Buck & Buck
3111 27th Avenue S
Seattle, WA 98144
206-722-4196
800-458-0600
FAX: 800-317-2182
e-mail: info@buckandbuck.com
www.buckandbuck.com

Julie Buck, Owner
Short raglan sleeves, lace at neck and bodice over lapping snapback closure. *$11.00*

1069 Budget Flannel Open Back Gown
Buck & Buck
3111 27th Avenue S
Seattle, WA 98144
206-722-4196
800-458-0600
FAX: 800-317-2182
e-mail: info@buckandbuck.com
www.buckandbuck.com

Julie Buck, Owner
3/4 raglan sleeve, lace at neck and bodice. *$13.00*

1070 Cotton/Poly Nancy Frocks
Buck & Buck
3111 27th Avenue S
Seattle, WA 98144
206-722-4196
800-458-0600
FAX: 800-317-2182
e-mail: info@buckandbuck.com
www.buckandbuck.com

Julie Buck, Owner
Comes in short and long sleeves, assorted florals and plaids. *$35.00*

1071 Dusters
Buck & Buck
3111 27th Avenue S
Seattle, WA 98144
206-722-4196
800-458-0600
FAX: 800-317-2182
e-mail: info@buckandbuck.com
www.buckandbuck.com

Julie Buck, Owner
Three types: Floral, Budget Better. Snap front styles and gathered yokes, flannel $16.00-$24.00.

1072 Flannel Gowns
Buck & Buck
3111 27th Avenue S
Seattle, WA 98144
206-722-4196
800-458-0600
FAX: 800-317-2182
e-mail: info@buckandbuck.com
www.buckandbuck.com

Julie Buck, Owner
Comes in long or short with a deep button-front opening for ease of slipping on. Shorter long length. *$16.50*

1073 Fleece Cape/Poncho
Laurel Designs
1805 Mar West Street
Apt A
Belvedere Tiburon, CA 94920
FAX: 415-435-1451
e-mail: laureld@ncal.verio.com
www.laureldesigns.co.uk

Janet Sawyer, Co-Owner
Lynn Montoya, Co-Owner
Warm and cozy high insulated cape with hood for wheelchair users, zip front, velcro side closure, self belt. All sizes and a variety of colors. *$53.00*

1074 Float Dress
Buck & Buck
3111 27th Avenue S
Seattle, WA 98144
206-722-4196
800-458-0600
FAX: 800-317-2182
e-mail: info@buckandbuck.com
www.buckandbuck.com

Julie Buck, Owner
A safe bet for everyone from a size medium to a 6X. Gathered yoke front and back and literally yards of fabric for fullness. Comes in cotton or polyester. *$34.00*

1075 Muu Muu
Buck & Buck
3111 27th Avenue S
Seattle, WA 98144
206-722-4196
800-458-0600
FAX: 800-317-2182
e-mail: info@buckandbuck.com
www.buckandbuck.com

Julie Buck, Owner
Comes in long and short styles, assorted bright floral prints. $20.00-$22.00.

1076 Polyester Nancy Frocks
Buck & Buck
3111 27th Avenue S
Seattle, WA 98144
206-722-4196
800-458-0600
FAX: 800-317-2182
e-mail: info@buckandbuck.com
www.buckandbuck.com

Julie Buck, Owner
Comes in short and long sleeves, assorted florals. *$ 35.00*

Footwear

1077 Acrylic Leg Warmers
Buck & Buck
3111 27th Avenue S
Seattle, WA 98144
206-722-4196
800-458-0600
FAX: 800-317-2182
e-mail: info@buckandbuck.com
www.buckandbuck.com

Julie Buck, Owner
Recommended for large or swollen legs where knee socks are too restrictive. *$7.00*

1078 Adult Acorn Polartec Socks
Special Clothes
PO Box 333
E Harwich, MA 02645
508-430-2410
FAX: 508-430-2410
e-mail: specialclo@aol.com
www.special-clothes.com

Judith Sweeney, President
These plush socks are made of Polartec fleece for unparalleled softness and comfort. The mid-calf length keeps feet and lower legs warmer than any conventional sock and the fabric has 2 way stretch to minimize binding. Polartec fleece is a remarkable light-weight fabric which breathes and insulates. Machine washable, of course. 100% Polartec fleece. Made in USA. Colors: solid black or charcoal print. *$18.00*
Per pair

1079 Adult Acorn Slippers
Special Clothes
PO Box 333
E Harwich, MA 02645
508-430-2410
FAX: 508-430-2410
e-mail: specialclo@aol.com
www.special-clothes.com

Judith Sweeney, President

These great looking, beautifully made slipper shoes keep chilly feet warm and comfortable. The sole is cut of fine suede leather, and the uppers and insoles are soft, plush polartec fleece. The knit cuff at the ankle opens wide to slip on easily, yet is snug enough to keep the slippers in place. Machine washable. Polartec fleece, suede sole, acrylic cuff. Made in USA. Colors: burgundy with navy cuff or dark green with navy cuff. *$30.00 Per pair*

1080 Booties with Non-Skid Soles
Buck & Buck
3111 27th Avenue S
Seattle, WA 98144
206-722-4196
800-458-0600
FAX: 800-317-2182
e-mail: info@buckandbuck.com
www.buckandbuck.com

Julie Buck, Owner
Acrylic knit or quilted cotton/poly and shearling inner. *$17.00*

1081 Foot Snugglers
Buck & Buck
3111 27th Avenue S
Seattle, WA 98144
206-722-4196
800-458-0600
FAX: 800-317-2182
e-mail: info@buckandbuck.com
www.buckandbuck.com

Julie Buck, Owner
Quilted poly/cotton outers lined with plush shearling pile, provide a thick, comfortable cushion which helps minimize the pressure points on tender areas. *$23.00*

1082 Lok-Tie Shoe Laces
Laurel Designs
1805 Mar West Street
Apt A
Belvedere Tiburon, CA 94920
FAX: 415-435-1451
e-mail: laureld@ncal.verio.com

Janet Sawyer, Co-Owner
Lynn Montoya, Co-Owner
Specially designed slide locks laces in place. Can be used with one hand. Stretch laces allow maximum comfort. *$4.00*

1083 TRU-Mold Shoes
42 Breckenridge Street
Buffalo, NY 14213
716-881-4484
800-843-6653
FAX: 716-881-0406
www.trumold.com

Husain Syed, Production Manager
Custom made, fully molded shoes, relieve pressure in sensitive areas by taking all of the weight off the painful areas.

1084 Terrycloth Slippers
Buck & Buck
3111 27th Avenue S
Seattle, WA 98144
206-722-4196
800-458-0600
FAX: 800-317-2182
e-mail: info@buckandbuck.com
www.buckandbuck.com

Julie Buck, Owner
Lined cotton/poly terrycloth upper with sewn-on, non-skid sole. *$18.00*

1085 Velcro Booties
Buck & Buck
3111 27th Avenue S
Seattle, WA 98144
206-722-4196
800-458-0600
FAX: 800-317-2182
e-mail: info@buckandbuck.com
www.buckandbuck.com

Julie Buck, Owner
The high-domed toe, and extra-wide, non-skid sole design accommodates virtually every foot related problem. *$18.00*

1086 Velcro Sneaker
Buck & Buck
3111 27th Avenue S
Seattle, WA 98144
206-722-4196
800-458-0600
FAX: 800-317-2182
e-mail: info@buckandbuck.com
www.buckandbuck.com

Julie Buck, Owner
Two velcro straps, nylon upper, rubber sole. *$22.00*

1087 Washable Shoes
Buck & Buck
3111 27th Avenue S
Seattle, WA 98144
206-722-4196
800-458-0600
FAX: 800-317-2182
e-mail: info@buckandbuck.com
www.buckandbuck.com

Julie Buck, Owner
Vinyl upper with velcro closure, nonskid sole. *$18.00*

Jackets

1088 Fleece Bed Jacket
Buck & Buck
3111 27th Avenue S
Seattle, WA 98144
206-722-4196
800-458-0600
FAX: 800-317-2182
e-mail: info@buckandbuck.com
www.buckandbuck.com

Julie Buck, Owner
Full snap front opening and collar. Assorted bright colors and pastel prints. *$22.00*

1089 Jackets
Special Clothes
PO Box 333
E Harwich, MA 02645
508-430-2410
FAX: 508-430-2410
e-mail: specialclo@aol.com
www.special-clothes.com

Judith Sweeney, President
Available styles include a unique, back opening jacket designed to fit easily over contractures and for wheelchair comfort. Prices range from $72.00-$89.00.

1090 Rain Poncho
Laurel Designs
1805 Mar West Street
Apt A
Belvedere Tiburon, CA 94920
FAX: 415-435-1451
e-mail: laureld@ncal.verio.com
www.laureldesigns.com

Janet Sawyer, Co-Owner
Lynn Montoya, Co-Owner
A favorite, this rain poncho slips on in a hurry to keep you dry. All sizes and a variety of colors. *$39.00*

1091 Wheelchair Ponchos
Special Clothes
PO Box 333
E Harwich, MA 02645
508-430-2410
FAX: 580-430-2410
e-mail: specialclo@aol.com
www.special-clothes.com

Judith Sweeney, President
These ponchos are cut shorter in the back for wheelchair comfort. Prices range from $76.00-$95.00.

Miscellaneous & Catalogs

1092 **Adaptive Clothing: Adults**
Special Clothes
PO Box 333
E Harwich, MA 02645
508-430-2410
FAX: 508-430-2410
e-mail: specialslo@aol.com
www.special-clothes.com

Judith Sweeney, President
Special Clothes produces a catalogue of garments for adults with disabilities and/or incontinence. Offerings include: undergarments, snap-crotch tee shirts, sleepwear, jumpsuits, bibs and some footwear. The catalogue is available without charge. Comparable to department store prices. Special Clothes produces a catalog of adaptive clothing for children in sizes from toddler through young adults. A full line of clothing is included from undergarments through wheelchair jackets and ponchos.

1093 **Adrian's Closet**
PO Box 9506
Rancho Santa Fe, CA 92067
800-831-2577
e-mail: adrians@electriciti.com
Fashions for the physically challenged child. Clothing offers Velcro closures, front pockets, concealed back openings and fashions for seated posture.

1094 **Adult Long Jumpsuit with Feet**
Special Clothes
PO Box 333
E Harwich, MA 02645
508-430-2410
FAX: 580-430-2410
e-mail: specialclo@aol.com
www.special-clothes.com

Judith Sweeney, President
A full, snap crotch for full access. For safety, feet have non-skid bottoms. 100% cotton knit. Made in USA. Also, identical in style, but are made of fleece for extra warmth. Fleece fabric is soft 100% cotton, and is available in medium blue only. Made in USA. Options on fleece jumpsuits available for additional charge. Long knit jumpsuit with feet: #A2051; long fleece jumpsuit: #A2032; long fleece jumpsuit with feet: #A2052.

1095 **Adult Short Jumpsuit**
Special Clothes
PO Box 333
E Harwich, MA 02645
508-430-2410
FAX: 508-430-2410
e-mail: specialclo@aol.com
www.special-clothes.com

Judith Sweeney, President
This pull-on jumpsuit provides comfort and full coverage without bulk. Wide leg ribbing ends at mid-thigh, with snaps at the crotch. We use fine quality, comfortable cotton knit. 100% cotton knit. Made in USA. Option: long sleeves - add $3.00. Colors: white, navy, teal, light blue, light pink, red, burgundy, royal blue and black. Sm & Med: $36.50/3 for $104.00; L & XL: $39.00/3 for $111.25; and XXL: $42.00/3 for $119.25.

1096 **Bibs**
Special Clothes
PO Box 333
E Harwich, MA 02645
508-430-2410
FAX: 580-430-2410
e-mail: specialclo@aol.com
www.special-clothes.com

Judith Sweeney, President
A variety of bib styles are available to protect clothing inconspicuously.

1097 **Body Suits**
Special Clothes
PO Box 333
E Harwich, MA 02645
508-430-2410
FAX: 508-430-2410
e-mail: specialclo@aol.com
www.special-clothes.com

Judith Sweeney, President
These are one piece garments that can be used to protect skin under braces, to add warmth and to shield incisions. Prices range from $18.25-22.50.

1098 **Buck and Buck Clothing**
3111 27th Avenue S
Seattle, WA 98144
206-722-4196
800-458-0600
FAX: 206-722-1144
e-mail: julie@buckandbuck.com
www.buckandbuck.com

Julie & Bill Buck, Co-Owners
Clothing for the disabled and elderly.
88 pages Yearly 1981

1099 **Carolyn's Catalog**
3938 S Tamiami Trail
Sarasota, FL 34207
941-373-9100
800-648-2266
e-mail: sales@carolynscatalog.com
www.carolynscatalog.com

Carolyn Tojek, President
Free, mail-order catalog of items for visually impaired people.

1100 **Clothing Solutions**
1525 W Alton Avenue
Santa Ana, CA 92704
714-427-0781
800-336-2660
FAX: 800-683-6510
e-mail: info@clothingsolutions.com
www.clothingsolutions.com

Jim Lechner, Owner
The nation's leading designer and manufacturer of assistive clothing for men and women. Free 56 page catalog available by calling 800-500-0260. 100% guarantee on all products.

1101 **Cotton Stockings**
Buck & Buck
3111 27th Avenue S
Seattle, WA 98144
206-722-4196
800-458-0600
FAX: 800-317-2182
e-mail: info@buckandbuck.com
www.buckandbuck.com

Julie Buck, Owner
Come in regular and snug-fit, cover leg to mid-thigh and work well for swollen legs.

1102 **Easy Dressing Fashions: JC Penney**
6501 Legacy Drive
Plano, TX 75024
972-431-8676
FAX: 972-431-9103

Natalie Torre, Marketing Manager
This is an entire collection of women's and men's fashions that are designed for easy wear, easy care and complete comfort. Plus, a selection of women's apparel with velcro brand wavelock fasteners.

1103 **Exquisite Egronomic Protective Wear**
Plum Enterprises
PO Box 85
Valley Forge, PA 19481
610-783-7377
FAX: 610-783-7577
e-mail: lynn@plument.com
www.plument.com

Janice Carrington, President
Egronomic Protective Wear; ProtectaCap custom-fitting headgear has earned an unparalleled reputation for quality, safety, and comfort. ProtectaCap+Plus technologically-advanced protective headgear closes the gap between hard and soft helmets. Comes with optional ProtectaChin Guard and new sporty design. Protecthip protective undergarment is the intelligent, innovative solution to the problem of hip injuries for both men and women. Ladies' styles are covered with attractive stretch lace.

1104 Fashion Ease
1541 60th Street
Brooklyn, NY 11219
718-853-6376
800-221-8929
FAX: 718-436-2067
e-mail: fashionease.com@aol
www.fashionease.com

Stacey Samuels, Customer Service Agent
Abraham Klein, Owner
Adaptive apparel and footwear for people who require ease in dressing. Free catalogue.
64 pages Yearly

1105 Forde's Functional Fashions
8020 East Drive
Suite #137
North Bay Village, FL 33141
305-754-4457
800-531-7705
FAX: 305-757-5447
e-mail: fashions@fordes.com
www.fordes.com

Patricia Forde MA RN CEAC, President
A fashion forward line of easy to wear clothing and accessories for men, women and children. Items include, sportswear, outerwear, ponchos, robes, sleepwear, dresses, wheelchair bags, walker bags and more. Hard to find specialty items for many special needs. Designs for people who use wheelchairs. Velcro closures if buttons are a problem. Fun clothing protectors too. Choose from our terrific assortment of fabrics and colors to suit all your fashion needs in simply functional style.

1106 Headliner
Designs for Comfort
4310 Highborne Drive NE
Marietta, GA 30066
770-565-8246
800-443-9226
FAX: 877-350-0501
e-mail: headliner@mindspring.com

Curt Maurer, President
A patented cap and hairpiece combination, the Headliner is both a quick, stylish coverup and an upbeat wig alternative for women experiencing hair care problems or hair loss. Ideal for social gatherings and outdoor activities as well as for sleeping and hospital stays. *$ 25.00*

1107 Knee Socks
Buck & Buck
3111 27th Avenue S
Seattle, WA 98144
206-722-4196
800-458-0600
FAX: 800-317-2182
e-mail: info@buckandbuck.com
www.buckandbuck.com

Julie Buck, Owner
Comes in regular and large size. *$3.50*

1108 Laurel Designs Catalog
Laurel Designs
1805 Mar W Street
Apt A
Belvedere Tiburon, CA 94920
415-435-1891
FAX: 415-435-1451
e-mail: laureld@ncal.verio.com
www.laureldesigns.com

Janet Sawyer, Owner
Lynn Montoya, Owner
Clothing for wheelchair users including rain wear, panchos and fleece capes. Other items include quality carrying bags for wheelchairs, walkers, crutches, accessories, and cookbooks of four ingredients only recipes. Home remodeling video 'Building & Remodeling for Accessibility', reacher and large print dictionary.
8 pages BiAnnual

1109 M&M Health Care Apparel Company
Fashion Collection
1541 60th Street
Brooklyn, NY 11219
718-871-8188
800-221-8929
FAX: 718-436-2067
e-mail: fashionease@aol.com

Stacey Samuels, Customer Service Agent
Abraham Klein, Owner
Specialized clothing for disabled people.

1110 No-Run Nylon Stockings
Buck & Buck
3111 27th Avenue S
Seattle, WA 98144
206-722-4196
800-458-0600
FAX: 800-317-2182
e-mail: info@buckandbuck.com
www.buckandbuck.com

Julie Buck, Owner
A full-length, heavy-weight stocking. *$2.25*

1111 Professional Fit Clothing
831 N Lake Street
Suite 1
Burbank, CA 91502
818-563-1975
800-422-2348
FAX: 818-563-1834
e-mail: kurt@professionalfit.com
www.professionalfit.com

Tom Pirruccello, President
Kurt Rieback, Owner
Professional fit clothing caters to homes that care for people with developmental disabilities and individuals who are physically challenged. Our clothing is fashionable, affordable and can be adapted to each person's special needs. There is a free catalog.
20 pages

1112 Quilted Waterproof Bib
Buck & Buck
3111 27th Avenue S
Seattle, WA 98144
206-722-4196
800-458-0600
FAX: 800-317-2182
e-mail: info@buckandbuck.com
www.buckandbuck.com

Julie Buck, Owner
Made with a nylon backing, these attractive bibs will not soak through like most others, protecting clothing from stains. *$15.00*

1113 Special Clothes Adult Catalogue
Special Clothes
PO Box 333
E Harwich, MA 02645
508-430-2410
FAX: 508-430-2410
e-mail: specialclo@aol.com
www.special-clothes.com

Judith Sweeney, President
Produces a catalogue of adaptive clothing for adults with disabilities. Offers include undergarments, casual bottoms, jumpsuits, sleepwear, swimwear, footwear and bibs. Prices are comparable to deparment store prices. The catalogue is free.
1-14 pages

1114 Special Clothes for Special Children
Special Clothes
PO Box 333
E Harwich, MA 02645
508-430-2410
FAX: 508-430-2410
e-mail: specialclo@aol.com
www.special-clothes.com

Judith Sweeney, President

Offers a variety of clothes for disabled children ranging from casual unisex clothes to undergarments. Clothing offers velcro closures, adjustable waistbands, drop-front briefs, wheelchair ponchos and more.

1115 **Specialty Care Shoppe**
16126 E 161st Street S
Bixby, OK 74008
918-366-1208
FAX: 918-366-9445
e-mail: deb@specialtycareshoppe.com
www.specialtycareshoppe.com

Deb Marshall, Owner
Catalog of attractive, affordable clothing and accessories for adults with special needs. Includes items for edema, incontinence, alzheimers, limited mobility, and hand impairment.

1116 **Super Stretch Socks**
Buck & Buck
3111 27th Avenue S
Seattle, WA 98144
206-722-4196
800-458-0600
FAX: 800-317-2182
e-mail: info@buckandbuck.com
www.buckandbuck.com

Julie Buck, Owner
This sock has been improved to stretch laterally throughout the foot area as well as at the top. *$3.75*

1117 **Swimwear**
Special Clothes
PO Box 333
E Harwich, MA 02645
508-430-2410
FAX: 508-430-2410
e-mail: specialclo@aol.com
www.special-clothes.com

Judith Sweeney, President
Cotton lycra swimsuits are available in boys and girls styles from size toddler-teen. One piece, designed to completely cover a diaper.

1118 **Trisha's of Acton**
PO Box 599
Acton, MA 01720
978-263-9318
877-955-5551
FAX: 978-263-4555
e-mail: trishas@tiac.net
www.trishasofacton.com

K Julie McCarthy, President
Clothing and accessories that provide dignity, freedom of movement and independence for the physically challenged.

1119 **Wishing Wells Clothing Collection**
11684 Ventura Boulevard
Suite 965
Studio City, CA 91604
818-840-6919
FAX: 818-760-3878
e-mail: FABC@dawnwells.com
www.dawnwells.com

Dawn Wells, Owner
Lorraine Parker, General Manager
Features designs full of back overlap construction and all velcro closures clothing.

Robes & Sleepwear

1120 **Adult Snap Front Sleeper**
Special Clothes
PO Box 333
E Harwich, MA 02645
508-430-2410
FAX: 508-430-2410
e-mail: specialclo@aol.com
www.special-clothes.com

Judith Sweeney, President
This soft, comfortable one piece garment is designed for easy dressing and full access. The top fastens down the front with snaps. The bottom section folds up from the back, and snaps to the waist. 100% cotton knit. Made in USA. Option, short sleeves - add $1.00. Colors: white, navy, teal, light blue, light pink, red, burgudy, royal blue and black. Sm & Med: $36.50/ 3 for $104.00; L & XL: $39.00/ 3 for $111.25; XXL: $42.00/3 for $119.75.

1121 **Chamois Shower Robe**
Buck & Buck
3111 27th Avenue S
Seattle, WA 98144
206-722-4196
800-458-0600
FAX: 800-317-2182
e-mail: info@buckandbuck.com
www.buckandbuck.com

Julie Buck, Owner
Totally covers a man or woman being wheeled to and from the shower or bath. Having test washed several fabrics, the chamois beat terry cloth for comfort, durability and faster drying time in the laundry. *$34.00*

1122 **Creative Designs**
Barbara Arnold
3704 Carlisle Court
Modesto, CA 95356
209-523-3166
800-335-4852
e-mail: robes4you@aol.com
www.robes4you.com

Barbara Arnold, Owner
Designer of the original Change-A-Robe and the new Handi-Robe, which allows the wearer to put it on without having to stand up. Robes are designed especially for physically challenged, disabled individuals, and wheelchair users.

1123 **Flannel Pajamas**
Buck & Buck
3111 27th Avenue S
Seattle, WA 98144
206-722-4196
800-458-0600
FAX: 800-317-2182
e-mail: info@buckandbuck.com
www.buckandbuck.com

Julie Buck, Owner
$18.00

1124 **Fleece Robe**
Buck & Buck
3111 27th Avenue S
Seattle, WA 98144
206-722-4196
800-458-0600
FAX: 800-317-2182
e-mail: info@buckandbuck.com
www.buckandbuck.com

Julie Buck, Owner
All with full-length, snap-front openings, patch pockets, short and long. Short: $39.00.

1125 **His & Hers**
Wishing Wells Collection
11684 Ventura Boulevard
Suite 965
Studio City, CA 91604
818-840-6919
FAX: 818-760-3878
e-mail: FABC@dawnwells.com
www.dawnwells.com

Dawn Wells, Owner
This sleep shirt is designed for him or her.

1126 **Nightshirts**
Buck & Buck
3111 27th Avenue S
Seattle, WA 98144
206-722-4196
800-458-0600
FAX: 800-317-2182
e-mail: info@buckandbuck.com
www.buckandbuck.com

Julie Buck, Owner

Come in flannel or cotton patterns and prints in sizes S-XL, for men. *$16.00*

1127 Open Back Nightshirts
Buck & Buck
3111 27th Avenue S
Seattle, WA 98144
206-722-4196
800-458-0600
FAX: 800-317-2182
e-mail: info@buckandbuck.com
www.buckandbuck.com

Julie Buck, Owner
Come in cotton or flannel (sizes S-XL). *$18.00*

1128 Terrycloth Robes
Buck & Buck
3111 27th Avenue S
Seattle, WA 98144
206-722-4196
800-458-0600
FAX: 800-317-2182
e-mail: info@buckandbuck.com
www.buckandbuck.com

Julie Buck, Owner
Two pockets, sash belts, assorted colors. *$36.00*

Shirts & Tops

1129 Adult Pull-On Feeding Bib
Special Clothes
PO Box 333
E Harwich, MA 02645
508-430-2410
FAX: 508-430-2410
e-mail: specialclo@aol.com
www.special-clothes.com

Judith Sweeney, President
This basic bib does a great job of protecting clothing from messy food and drink spills. It is constructed of sturdy, rib knit neckband which slips on comfortably. The front pocket catches food particles and is fastened at both sides with velcro for easy cleaning. 100% nylon with neckband of 100% cotton rib. Made in USA. Colors: white or light blue. One size: 17 inches wide, & 23 inches from shoulder to bottom. *$15.00*

1130 Avoid Eye Strain, Feel it T-Shirt
Sense-Sations
919 Walnut Street
Philadelphia, PA 19107
215-627-0600
FAX: 215-922-0692

Patricia Johnson, Chief Executive Officer
This slogan is printed in raised writing boldly across the front of our T-shirt. *$5.95*

1131 Basic Rear Closure Sweat Top
Buck & Buck
3111 27th Avenue S
Seattle, WA 98144
206-722-4196
800-458-0600
FAX: 800-317-2182
e-mail: info@buckandbuck.com
www.buckandbuck.com

Julie Buck, Owner
Top opens completely down the back for ease of dressing with velcro tab closures. *$20.50*

1132 Cotton Full-Back Vest
Buck & Buck
3111 27th Avenue S
Seattle, WA 98144
206-722-4196
800-458-0600
FAX: 800-317-2182
e-mail: info@buckandbuck.com
www.buckandbuck.com

Julie Buck, Owner
Wide shoulder straps that don't slide off shoulders. *$4.50*

1133 Dutch Neck T-Shirt
Buck & Buck
3111 27th Avenue S
Seattle, WA 98144
206-722-4196
800-458-0600
FAX: 800-317-2182
e-mail: info@buckandbuck.com
www.buckandbuck.com

Julie Buck, Owner
Stretchy neck makes it easy to get over the head. *$ 5.50*

1134 Open Back T-Shirts
Buck & Buck
3111 27th Avenue S
Seattle, WA 98144
206-722-4196
800-458-0600
FAX: 800-317-2182
e-mail: info@buckandbuck.com
www.buckandbuck.com

Julie Buck, Owner
Velcro tabs down the back. *$8.00*

1135 Printed Rear Closure Sweat Top
Buck & Buck
3111 27th Avenue S
Seattle, WA 98144
206-722-4196
800-458-0600
FAX: 800-317-2182
e-mail: info@buckandbuck.com
www.buckandbuck.com

Julie Buck, Owner
Comes in assorted colors, plain or with animal motifs. *$33.00*

1136 Rear Closure Shirts
Buck & Buck
3111 27th Avenue S
Seattle, WA 98144
206-722-4196
800-458-0600
FAX: 800-317-2182
e-mail: info@buckandbuck.com
www.buckandbuck.com

Julie Buck, Owner
Velcro tabs down the back on T-shirts and dress shirts. *$24.00*

1137 Rear Closure T-Shirt
Buck & Buck
3111 27th Avenue S
Seattle, WA 98144
206-722-4196
800-458-0600
FAX: 800-317-2182
e-mail: info@buckandbuck.com
www.buckandbuck.com

Julie Buck, Owner
Closes down the back with velcro tabs. *$8.50*

1138 Serape
Laurel Designs
1805 Mar West Street
Apt A
Belvedere Tiburon, CA 94920
FAX: 415-435-1451
e-mail: laureld@ncal.verio.com

Janet Sawyer, Co-Owner
Lynn Montoyo, Co-Owner
This unique sleeveless thermal vest is designed for active wheelchair persons. Multi-colored, one size fits all. *$30.00*

1139 T Shirt is Done in Braille: Read Gently
Sense-Sations
919 Walnut Street
Philadelphia, PA 19107
215-627-0600
FAX: 215-922-0692

Patricia Johnson, Chief Executive Officer
This slogan is printed in raised writing and braille dots. *$5.95*

Slacks & Pants

1140 **Comanche Pants**
Wheelies Manufacturing
33 NE Main Street
PO Box 97496
Winston, OR 97496
541-679-2318
FAX: 541-673-8719

Alice King, Store Manager
Leslie Bozovich, Customer Service
An innovative answer to dressing a person who cannot stand. These pants are sculptured to provide total coverage. A new freedom in dressing; easy for attendant or for self-dressing. They can be put on a seated person right in the chair with no lifting or standing. *$35.00*

1141 **Jumpsuits**
Special Clothes
PO Box 333
E Harwich, MA 02645
508-430-2410
FAX: 508-430-2410
e-mail: specialclo@aol.com
www.special-clothes.com

Judith Sweeney, President
Several styles of one-piece garments are available for dressing ease. Front opening styles are designed for easy access. Prices range from $32.20-$44.00.

1142 **Knit Pants**
Special Clothes
PO Box 333
E Harwich, MA 02645
508-430-2410
FAX: 508-430-2410
TTY:508-430-2410
e-mail: specialclo@aol.com
www.special-clothes.com

Judith Sweeney, President
Offers the best in comfort and convenience. Designed with a longer crotch and wider seat for a great fit. The elasticized waistband contains a hidden drawstring for size adjustments, and pockets are placed low for easy access while sitting. Order a full snap crotch (Option #1), for full access. Available in soft, 100% cotton knit. Made in USA. Colors: Light blue, teal, light pink, burgundy, navy and black. Sm & Med: $41.00; L & XL $45.00; XXL $48.00. Add full snap crotch.

1143 **Pants & Slacks**
Special Clothes
PO Box 333
E Harwich, MA 02645
508-430-2410
FAX: 508-430-2410
e-mail: specialclo@aol.com
www.special-clothes.com

Judith Sweeney, President
A variety of pant and skirt styles is available in sizes 2 toddler - 18 teen. These include straight leg and baggy jeans, drop front pleated dress pants, knit pants, shorts and skirted leggings. Prices range from $16.50-$44.00.

1144 **Side Velcro Slacks**
Buck & Buck
3111 27th Avenue S
Seattle, WA 98144
206-722-4196
800-458-0600
FAX: 800-317-2182
e-mail: info@buckandbuck.com
www.buckandbuck.com

Julie Buck, Owner
Slacks open down both sides from waist to hip with velcro tab closures at sides. *$25.00*

1145 **Side-Zip Sweat Pants**
Buck & Buck
3111 27th Avenue S
Seattle, WA 98144
206-722-4196
800-458-0600
FAX: 800-317-2182
e-mail: info@buckandbuck.com
www.buckandbuck.com

Julie Buck, Owner
Out-seam zippers un-zip 3/4 of the way down the sides to enable dressing a resident with severe leg contractures. *$32.00*

1146 **Trunks**
Buck & Buck
3111 27th Avenue S
Seattle, WA 98144
206-722-4196
800-458-0600
FAX: 800-317-2182
e-mail: info@buckandbuck.com
www.buckandbuck.com

Julie Buck, Owner
Come in cotton or nylon, flare leg, full cut. *$4.00*

Undergarments

1147 **Adult Absorbent Briefs**
Special Clothes
PO Box 333
E Harwich, MA 02645
508-430-2410
FAX: 508-430-2410
e-mail: specialclo@aol.com
www.special-clothes.com

Judith Sweeney, President
Soft, comfortable, 100% cotton knit brief is seven layers thick at the crotch. Sides of the brief are a non-bulky single layer. The waistband elastic is enclosed in a soft cotton knit casing and does not touch the skin. Comfortable cotton rib knit bands circle the leg. This brief will not replace a diaper, but provides absorbency for light incontinence.

1148 **Adult Lap Shoulder Bodysuit**
Special Clothes
PO Box 333
E Harwich, MA 02645
508-430-2410
FAX: 508-430-2410
TTY:508-430-2410
e-mail: specialclo@aol.com
www.special-clothes.com
Bodysuit styles fasten at the crotch with sturdy snaps to stay neatly tucked. All are made of soft, absorbent 100% cotton knit for maximum comfort. They are cut wide at the hip and seat for full coverage, and will accomodate a diaper if necessary. Soft knit rib circles the neck and leg. This cool tank style slips on easily. Deep armholes are banded with rib knit. all styles: Small/Medium $33.00/3 for $94.00; Large/X Large $38.00/3 for $108.00; XX Large $41.00/3 for $116.00. A choice of 9 colors.

1149 **Adult Sleeveless Bodysuit**
Special Clothes
PO Box 333
E Harwich, MA 02645
508-430-2410
FAX: 508-430-2410
e-mail: specialclo@aol.com
www.special-clothes.com

Judith Sweeney, President
Bodysuit styles fasten at the crotch with sturdy snaps to stay neatly tucked. All are made of soft, absorbent 100% cotton knit for maximum comfort. They are cut wide at the hip and seat for full coverage, and will accomodate a diaper if necessary. Soft knit rib circles the neck and leg. This cool tank style slips on easily. Deep armholes are banded with rib knit. All styles: Small/Medium $33.00/3 for $94.00; Large/X-Large $38.00/3 for $108.00; XX Large $41.00/3 for $116.00. A choice of 9 colors.

1150 **Adult Swim Diaper**
Special Clothes
PO Box 333
E Harwich, MA 02645
508-430-2410
FAX: 508-430-2410
e-mail: specialclo@aol.com
www.special-clothes.com

Judith Sweeney, President
This pant is made of soft, silent, light-weight, impermeable fabric- waterproof and secure. It is a containment brief, designed to be used in the pool in place of cloth or disposable diapers, which can become waterlogged or disintegrate in the water. Waist and legbands should be snug for proper fit, so please consult sizing chart before ordering. Darlex with lining of 100% cotton knit. Lycra waist and legbands. Made in USA.

1151 **Adult Tee Shoulder Bodysuit**
Special Clothes
PO Box 333
E Harwich, MA 02645
508-430-2410
FAX: 508-430-2410
TTY:508-430-2410
e-mail: specialclo@aol.com
www.special-clothes.com
Styles fasten at the crotch with sturdy snaps to stay neatly tucked. All are made of soft, absorbent 100% cotton knit for maximum comfot. They are cut wide at the hip and seat for full coverage, and will accommodate a diaper if necessary. Soft knit rib circles the neck and leg. This bodysuit looks like a regular tee shirt, but snaps at the crotch for a neat appearance. Small/Medium $33.00/3 for $94.00; Large/X Large $38.00/3 fpr $108.00; XX Large $41.00/3 for $116.00. Choice of 9 colors.

1152 **Adult Waterproof Overpant**
Special Clothes
PO Box 333
E Harwich, MA 02645
508-430-2410
FAX: 508-430-2410
e-mail: specialclo@aol.com
www.special-clothes.com

Judith Sweeney, President
Overpants are made of a soft, silent, lightweight fabric which is waterproof and very secure. It is designed to be used over our Adult Absorbent Brief, or cloth diapers. It is completely latex-free and is an excellent non-allergenic substitute for rubber or vinyl pants. Waist and legbands should be snug to minimize leakage, so please consult the sizing chart before ordering. Darlex with lining of 100% cotton. Lycra waist and legbands. Made in USA.

1153 **Adult Wet Wrap Swim Vest**
Special Clothes
PO Box 333
E Harwich, MA 02645
508-430-2410
FAX: 508-430-2410
e-mail: specialclo@aol.com
www.special-clothes.com

Judith Sweeney, President
This vest is made of neoprene - the same material used in wet suits - and it effectively insulates the torso to retain body heat. Muscles relax, enhancing the quality of recreational swimming or water therapy. The wrap design allows full freedom of movement. Made of Neoprene in the USA. Note: Vest provides warmth ony. It is not a flotation device. Wet wrap sizes: Adult small, adult medium and adult large.

1154 **Briefs**
Special Clothes
PO Box 333
E Harwich, MA 02645
508-430-2410
FAX: 508-430-2410
e-mail: specialclo@aol.com
www.special-clothes.com

Judith Sweeney, President
A variety of unique brief styles available for easy access and practicality.

1155 **Cloth Diapers**
Angel Fluff Diaper Company
PO Box 1131
Lewisburg, TN 37091
931-359-9604
800-996-2644
FAX: 931-359-8420
e-mail: custserv@angelfluff.com
www.angelfluff.com
Top quality cloth diapers.

1156 **Nylon Snip Slip**
Buck & Buck
3111 27th Avenue S
Seattle, WA 98144
206-722-4196
800-458-0600
FAX: 800-317-2182
e-mail: info@buckandbuck.com
www.buckandbuck.com

Julie Buck, Owner
Just snip with scissors at the appropriate hem length and it's ready to wear. *$12.00*

1157 **Nylon Stretch Bra**
Buck & Buck
3111 27th Avenue S
Seattle, WA 98144
206-722-4196
800-458-0600
FAX: 800-317-2182
e-mail: info@buckandbuck.com
www.buckandbuck.com

Julie Buck, Owner
Front hook closure with built-up shoulder straps. *$ 16.00*

1158 **Panties**
Buck & Buck
3111 27th Avenue S
Seattle, WA 98144
206-722-4196
800-458-0600
FAX: 800-317-2182
e-mail: info@buckandbuck.com
www.buckandbuck.com

Julie Buck, Owner
Come in nylon or cotton, band leg for comfort. *$4.00*

1159 **Safe and Dry-Feel and Sure-Toddler Dry**
Hygienics Direct Company
3968 194th Trail
Golden Beach, FL 33160
305-937-0824
888-463-7337
e-mail: mbrier1930@aol.com
www.hygenics.com

Michael Brier, President
A variety of stress incontinence disposable liners which absorb 8-10 oz. of fluid packaged in 20 and 40 counts. Also available are patented knit nylon panties in medium, large and extra large sizes. All products are priced for the mass market.

1160 **Support Plus**
99 West Street
Suite 500
Medfield, MA 02052
508-359-2910
800-229-2910
FAX: 508-359-0139
www.supportplus.com

Ed Janos, President
Offers a selection of support undergarments, braces and shoes for the physically challenged and medical professionals.

Assistive Devices

1161 **Ability Research**
PO Box 1721
Minnetonka, MN 55343
952-939-0121
FAX: 952-890-8393
e-mail: ability@skypoint.com
www.abilityresearch.com

John Severson, President
Manufacturers and marketers of assistive technology equipment.

1162 **Adaptivation**
2225 W 50th Street
Suite 100
Sioux Falls, SD 57105
605-335-4445
800-723-2783
FAX: 605-335-4446
e-mail: info@adaptivation.com
www.adaptivation.com

Amy Koch, Marketing Director
Manufacturers of switches, voice output devices and enviromental controls.

1163 **Adaptive Device Locator System**
Academic Software
3504 Tates Creek Road
Lexington, KY 40517
859-552-1020
FAX: 253-799-4012
e-mail: asistaff@acsw.com
www.acsw.com

Warren E Lacefield PhD, President
Penelope Ellis, Marketing Director
Sylvia P Lacefield, Graphic Artist
Employs a unique, goal-oriented approach to aid individuals in identifying adaptive devices with potential to support various physical limitations. Devices are categorized in seven databases: Existence, Travel, In-situ Motion, Environmental Adaptation, Communication, and Sports & recreation. ADLS provides its users with device descriptions, pictures and lists of sources for locating products and product information. *$200.00*

1164 **Analog Switch Pad**
Academic Software
331 W 2nd Street
Lexington, KY 40507
859-233-2332
800-842-2357
FAX: 859-231-0725

Warren E Lacefield PhD, President
Penelope Ellis, Marketing Director
A touch-activated, force-adjustable, low-voltage DC, electronic switch designed to control battery-operated toys, environmental controls, and computer access interfaces. This device features a large activation area that is soft and compliant to the touch. Force sensitivity is adjusted by a small dial from approximately 1 ounce to 32 ounces activation pressure, applied over an area ranging from the size of a fingertip to the size of the entire switch surface. *$149.00*

1165 **Arkenstone: The Benetech Initiative**
480 S California Avenue
Palo Alto, CA 94306
650-475-5440
FAX: 650-475-1067
e-mail: wynn@freedomscientific.com
www.freedomscentific.com

Lee Hamilton, President/CEO
Roberta G Brosnaha, General Manager/VP
Offers various models of ready-to-read personal computers for the disabled.

1166 **Augmentative Communication Systems (AAC)**
Z YG O Industries
PO Box 1008
Portland, OR 97207
503-684-6006
800-234-6006
FAX: 503-684-6011
e-mail: zygo@zygo-usa.com
www.zygo-usa.com

Lawrence Weiss, President
Full range of AAC systems and assistive technology including computer-based systems and computer access programs and devices.

1167 **Away We Ride IntelliKeys Overlay**
Soft Touch
4300 Stine Road
Suite 401
Bakersfield, CA 93313
661-396-8676
877-763-8868
FAX: 661-396-8760
e-mail: softtouch@funsoftware.com
www.funsoftware.com

Roxanne Butterfield
Joyce Meyer, President
Four full color preprinted overlays to use with Away We Ride. Just put them on an IntelliKeys keyboard and you are ready to go.

1168 **BIGmack Communication Aid**
AbleNet
2808 Fairview Avenue N
Roseville, MN 55113
651-294-2200
800-322-0956
FAX: 651-294-2222
e-mail: customerservice@ablenetinc.com
www.ablenetinc.com

Dave Binziazk, Director
A single message communication aid, BIGmack has 75 seconds of memory and has a 5 inches in diameter switch surface. *$86.00*

1169 **C2ILMAX**
Image Systems
12975 16th Avenue N
Suite 300
Minneapolis, MN 55441
952-935-1171
800-462-4370
FAX: 952-935-1386
e-mail: custserv@imagesystemscorp.com
www.imagesystemscorp.com

Dennis Stollenwerk, General Sales
LCD or CRT displays designed for applications requiring a larger viewing area and high to ultrahigh resolution.

1170 **Close-Up 6.5**
Norton- Lambert Corporation
PO Box 4085
Santa Barbara, CA 93140
805-964-6767
e-mail: sales@norton-lambert.com
www.norton-lambert.com

Jeannie Vesely, Marketing Coordinator
Remotely controls PC's via modem. Telecommute from your home or laptop PC to your office PC. Run applications, update spreadsheets, print documents remotely and access networks on remote PCs. Features: fast screen and file transfers, synchronize files, unattended transfers, multi-level security, transaction logs, automated installation. *$199.00*

1171 **Concepts on the Move Advanced Overlay CD**
Soft Touch
4300 Stine Road
Suite 401
Bakersfield, CA 93313
661-396-8676
877-763-8868
FAX: 661-396-8760
e-mail: softtouch@softtouch.com
www.softtouch.com

Jo Myer, President
Joyce Meyer, President

Use this overlay CD with Concepts on the Move Advanced Preacademics. Overlays match the concepts and graphics in the program. Includes standard overlays with all the choices and SoftTouch's changeable format overlays. Print and laminate the blank templates. Then print and laminate the picture keys in all three sizes - small, medium and large. Includes Overlay Printer by IntelliTools for easy printing.

1172 **Concepts on the Move Basic Overlay CD**
Soft Touch
4300 Stine Road
Suite 401
Bakersfield, CA 93313
661-396-8676
877-763-8868
FAX: 661-396-8760
e-mail: softtouch@softtouch.com.com
www.softtouch.com

Roxanne Butterfield, Marketing
Joyce Meyer, President
Use this Overlay CD with Concepts on the Move Basic Preacademics. Overlays match the conepts and graphics in the program. Includes standard overlays with all the choices and SoftTouch's changeable format overlays. Print and laminate the blank templates. Then print and laminate the picture keys in all three sizes - small, medium and large. It is easy and fast to place the images on the blank templates.

1173 **Darci Too**
WesTest Engineering Corporation
810 W Shepard Lane
Farmington, UT 84025
801-451-9191
FAX: 801-451-9393
e-mail: mary@westest.com
www.westest.com

Mary L Lynds, Manager
Robert Lessman, President
A universal device which allows people with physical disabilities to replace the keyboard and mouse on a personal computer with a device that matches their physical capabilities. DARCI TOO works with almost any personal computer and provides access to all computer functions. *$995.00*

1174 **EZ Touch Panel**
1120 W Avenue J
Lancaster, CA 93534
661-723-6523
800-869-8521
FAX: 661-723-2114
www.words-plus.com

Jess Dahlan, President
Momoko Deran, Chief Executive Director
Walt Wolosz, Manager
Touch screen input is the most direct and intuitive method for picture-based communication for those with the required motor skills. *$399.00*

1175 **Expanded Keyboard Emulator**
Words Plus
1220 W Avenue J
Lancaster, CA 93534
661-723-6523
800-869-8521
FAX: 661-723-2114
e-mail: info@words-plus.com
www.words-plus.com

Jeff Dalhen, President
Janet Aviles, Customer Service Supervisor
Walt Wolosz, Manager
Provides DUAl word prediction, abbreviation expansion (macrocapability), five different methods of voice output, keyboard control, RAM-resident and the ability to run in graphics mode and access to commercial software applications.

1176 **Eyegaze Computer System**
LC Technologies
1483 Chain Bridge Road
Suite 104
McClean, VA 22101
703-385-7133
800-393-4293
FAX: 703-288-3727
www.eyegaze.com

Nancy Cleveland, Medical Coordinator
Enables people with physical disabilities to do many things with their eyes that they would otherwise do with their hands.

1177 **Fall Fun IntelliKeys Overlay**
Soft Touch
4300 Stine Road
Suite 401
Bakersfield, CA 93313
661-396-8676
877-763-8868
FAX: 661-396-8760
e-mail: softtouch@funsoftware.com
www.funsoftware.com

Roxanne Butterfield, Marketing
Joyce Meyer, President
Seven full color preprinted overlays to use with Fall Fun. Just put them on an IntelliKeys keyboard and you are ready to go.

1178 **FingerFoniks**
Words- Plus
1220 W Avenue J
Lancaster, CA 93534
661-723-6523
800-869-8521
FAX: 661-723-2114
e-mail: info@words-plus.com
www.words-plus.com

Ginger Woltosz, Vice President
Tim Ross, Manager
Walt Wolosz, Manager
One-pound, hand-held, communicator incorporating synthesized and recorded speech. The user makes words and sentences by pressing sound (phoneme) keys on a membrane keyboard. *$995.00*

1179 **Five Green & Speckled Frogs IntelliKeys Overlay**
Soft Touch
4300 Stine Road
Suite 401
Bakersfield, CA 93313
661-396-8676
877-763-8868
FAX: 661-396-8760
e-mail: softtouch@funsoftware.com
www.funsoftware.com

Roxanne Butterfield, Marketing
Joyce Meyer, President
Seven full color preprinted overlays to use with Five Green and Speckled Frogs. Just put them on an IntelliKeys keyboard and you are ready to go.

1180 **GW Micro**
725 Airport North Office Park
Fort Wayne, IN 46825
260-489-3671
FAX: 260-489-2608
e-mail: sales@gwmicro.com
www.gwmicro.com

Dan Weirich, Owner
Chris Park, Sales Manager
Computer hardware and software products for people with disabilities.

1181 **Infogrip: ErgoPOD Model 500**
1794 E Main Street
Ventura, CA 93001
805-652-0770
800-397-0921
FAX: 805-652-0880
e-mail: sales@infogrip.com
www.infogrip.com

Liza Jacobs, President
Aaron Gaston, Vice President
ErgoPOD Model 500 provides a workstation solution to computer users who work from a reclining position. Model 500 straddles a bed or recliner and can hold up to 21" monitors anywhere on its surface, and will securely position the monitor at angles up to 60 degrees. The adjustable keyboard mechanism and motorized height adjustment make ergonomic configuration easy — even for the most demanding cases. *$ 1895.00*

1182 IntelliKeys IIe
Intelli Tools
1720 Corporate Circle
Petaluma, CA 94954
707-773-2000
800-899-6687
FAX: 707-773-2001
e-mail: info@intellitools.com
www.intellitools.com

Caroline Van Howe, Marketing Director
Ed Koenit, Chief Financial Officer
Arjan Khalsa, Chief Executive Officer
Card and cable to create keyboard port on Apple IIe computer to allow use of IntelliKeys alternative keyboard. *$129.95*

1183 Internal I/O Port Adapter
AbleNet
2808 Fairview Avenue N
Roseville, MN 55113
651-294-2200
800-322-0956
FAX: 651-294-2259
e-mail: customerservice@ablenetinc.com
www.ablenetinc.com

Mary Kay Walch, Executive Director
A converting cable designed to provide a 9-pin joystick port for Apple II+ and older model computers. *$18.00*

1184 Jelly Bean Switch
AbleNet
2808 Fairview Avenue N
Roseville, MN 55113
651-294-2200
800-322-0956
FAX: 612-379-9143
e-mail: customerservice@ablenetinc.com
www.ablenetinc.com

Cheryl Volkman, Chairman of the Board
A momentary touch switch made of shatterproof plastic, small and sensitive to 2-3 ounces of pressure, this switch is provided audible feedback when activated and is a compact version of the Big Red Switch. *$42.00*

1185 KeyWiz
Words+
42505 10th Street W
Suite 109
Lancaster, CA 93534
800-869-8521
FAX: 661-266-8969
www.words-plus.com

Phil Lawrence, Vice President
Rachel Nielsen, Customer Support
A software and hardware product designed to operate on an IBM compatible PC. The software provides word prediction, abbreviation expansion and access to commercial software applications. *$695.00*

1186 Keyguards for IntelliKeys
Intelli Tools
1720 Corporate Circle
Petaluma, CA 94954
707-773-2000
800-899-6687
FAX: 707-773-2001
e-mail: info@intellitools.com
www.intellitools.com

Beta Davis, Director Sales Operations
Lari Castle, Supervisor
Arjan Khalsa, Chief Executive Officer
Acrylic keyguards for each of IntelliKeys six standard overlays. *$250.00*

1187 Large Print Keyboard Labels
Hooleon Corp
PO Box 589
Melrose, NM 88124
505-253-4503
800-937-1337
FAX: 505-253-4299
e-mail: sales@hooleon.com
www.hooleon.com

Shannen Aikman, Admin. Manager/Sales
Joan Crozier, President/Sales
Frona Hollaway, Sales
Pressure sensitive labels for computer keyboards.

1188 LinkPower 50
Words+
1220 W Avenue J Lancaster
Palmdale, CA 93543
661-723-6523
800-869-8521
FAX: 661-723-2114
e-mail: ifo@words-plus.com
www.words-plus.com

Ginger Woltosz, Vice President
Tim Ross, Manager
Walt Wolosz, Manager
AC-to-DC switching power converter provides a continuous, independent multi-output, multi-voltage power supply to any augcom device, laptop computer, pointing device, voice synthesizer, cellular phone, or other battery-operated device directly from a wheelchair. *$449.00*

1189 MessageMate
Words+
42505 10th Street W
Suite 109
Lancaster, CA 93534
661-723-2114
800-869-8521
FAX: 661-266-8969
e-mail: info@words-plus.com
www.words-plus.com

Ginger Woltosz, Vice President
Tim Ross, Manager
Lightweight, hand-held communicator providing high-quality analog recording capability using either direct select keyboards or 1 to 2 switch access. Price ranges from $549.00 to $999.00.

1190 Monkeys Jumping on the Bed IntelliKeys Overlay
Soft Touch
4300 Stine Road
Suite 401
Bakersfield, CA 93313
661-396-8676
877-763-8868
FAX: 661-396-8760
e-mail: softtouch@funsoftware.com
www.funsoftware.com

Roxanne Butterfield, Marketing
Joyce Meyer, President
Seven full color preprinted overlays to use with Monkeys Jumping. Just put them on an IntelliKeys keyboard and you are ready to go.

1191 Morse Code Equalizer
Words+
42505 10th Street W
Suite 109
Lancaster, CA 93534
661-723-6523
800-869-8521
FAX: 661-723-2114
e-mail: info@words-plus.com
www.words-plus.com

Ginger Woltosz, Vice President
Tim Ross, Manager
Walt Wolosz, Manager
Provides complete word processing and voice output communications with single or dual switch Morse code inputs. Originally designed for a blind user with only eyelid movement. The system can be used by both sighted and visually impaired persons. *$1395.00*

1192 Mouthsticks
Sammons Preston Rolyan
4 Sammons Court
Bolingbrook, IL 60440
630-226-1300
800-323-5547
FAX: 630-226-1389
e-mail: spr@abilityone.com
www.sammonsprestonrolyan.com

Steve Brown, Director
Wide offering of mouthsticks featuring various functions (BK 5380, 5381, 5383, 5385, 6002, or BK 5370 series).

1193 **Old MacDonald's Farm IntelliKeys Overlay**
Soft Touch
4300 Stine Road
Suite 401
Bakersfield, CA 93313
661-396-8676
877-763-8868
FAX: 661-396-8760
e-mail: softtouch@funsoftware.com
www.funsoftware.com

Roxanne Butterfield, Marketing
Joyce Meyer, President
Extend your students' learning with more than 45 pre-made overlays that support all of the skills learned at the farm. Use with the IntelliKeys keyboard. Simply print and use. Print an extra set to make off computer activities, too. Note: Requires Overlay Maker or Overlay Printer by IntelliTools.

1194 **Perfect Solutions**
10513 Versailles Boulevard
Wellington, FL 33467
561-790-1070
800-726-7086
FAX: 561-790-0108
e-mail: perfect@gate.net
www.perfectsolutions.com

Andrew Kramer, President
Peter Flanagan, Owner
A computer for every student and it speaks! Wireless laptop computers starting at $290.00 are ideal for students to carry with them all day. Text-to-speech and web browsing are available. *$290.00*

1195 **Phillip Roy**
PO Box 130
Indian Rocks Beach, FL 33785
727-593-2700
800-255-9085
FAX: 727-595-2685
e-mail: info@philliproy.com
www.philliproy.com

Ruth Bragman PhD, President
Phil Padol, Vice President
Phillip Roy, Manager
Offers multimedia materials appropriate for use with individuals with disabilities. Programs range from preschool through the adult level. Many of the programs are high interest topics/low vocabulary, ideal for transition and employability skills. Materials are also available which focus on social and personal development. Call for a free catalog.

1196 **Rodeo IntelliKeys Overlay**
Soft Touch
4300 Stine Road
Suite 401
Bakersfield, CA 93313
661-396-8676
877-763-8868
FAX: 661-396-8760
e-mail: softtouch@funsoftware.com
www.funsoftware.com

Roxanne Butterfield, Marketing
Joyce Meyer, President
Four full color preprinted overlays to use with The Rodeo. Just put them on an IntelliKeys keyboard and you are ready to go.

1197 **SS-Access Single Switch Interface for PC's with MS-DOS**
Academic Software
331 W 2nd Street
Lexington, KY 40507
859-233-2332
800-842-2357
FAX: 859-231-0725

Warren E Lacefield PhD, President
Penelope Ellis, Marketing Director
A general purpose single switch hardware and software interface for DOS and the IBM and compatible PC family. It is designed to be easy to install, simple to use, and compatible with the widest possible range of computers and application software programs. SS-ACCESS! connects to one of the PC serial ports and provides a jack to connect an external switch. The DOS version of the software works by sending a user defined keystroke to the PC keyboard buffer whenever the switch is pressed. *$ 90.00*

1198 **Simplicity**
Words+
42505 10th Street W
Suite 109
Lancaster, CA 93534
661-266-8500
800-869-8521
FAX: 661-266-8969
www.words-plus.com

Phil Lawrence, VP
Rachel Nielsen, Customer Support
Swing-down mount for portable computers and other devices is made from high-quality aircraft aluminum. Simplicity contains very few moving parts and installs in minutes, providing a positive, secure support for computer/device in both the stored and overlap position. *$595.00*

1199 **Slim Armstrong Mounting System**
AbleNet
2808 Fairview Avenue N
Roseville, MN 55113
651-294-2200
800-322-0956
FAX: 651-294-2259
e-mail: customerservice@ablenetinc.com
www.ablenetinc.com
Slim Armstrong is a mounting system strong enough to hold up to five pounds in any position. Mix and match parts to create the system length you desire. *$188.00*

1200 **Smart Modem**
H AR C Mercantile
1111 West Center
Portage, MI 49024
269-324-1615
800-445-9968
FAX: 269-324-2387
e-mail: info@harc.com
www.harcmercantile.com

Ronald Slager, President
Smart modem makes your computer accessible to a TTY. *$349.00*

1201 **SoftTouch Favorites IntelliKeys Overlay**
Soft Touch
4300 Stine Road
Suite 401
Bakersfield, CA 93313
661-396-8676
877-763-8868
FAX: 661-396-8760
e-mail: softtouch@softtouch.com
www.softtouch.com

Roxanne Butterfield, Marketing
Joyce Meyer, President
Four full color preprinted overlays to use with SoftTouch Favorites. Just put them on an IntelliKeys keyboard and you are ready to go.

1202 **Songs I Sing at Preschool IntelliKeys Over lay**
Soft Touch
4300 Stine Road
Suite 401
Bakersfield, CA 93313
661-396-8676
877-763-8868
FAX: 661-396-8760
e-mail: support@softtouch.com
www.softtouch.com

Joyce Meyer, Director
Roxanne Butterfield, Marketing
Pre-made overlays for use with Songs I Sing at Preschool. Simply print and use with an IntelliKeys keyboard. Print an extra set to make off computer activities, too.

1203 **String Switch**
AbleNet
2808 Fairview Avenue N
Roseville, MN 55113
651-294-2200
800-322-0956
FAX: 651-294-2259
e-mail: customerservice@ablenetinc.com
www.ablenetinc.com
Ideal for students who have limited finger and hand mobility, as well as those with minimal strength. *$28.00*

1204 **Switch Basics IntelliKeys Overlay**
Soft Touch
4300 Stine Road
Suite 401
Bakersfield, CA 93313
661-396-8676
877-763-8868
FAX: 661-396-8760
e-mail: softtouch@softtouch.com
www.softtouch.com

Joyce Meyer, President
Roxanne Butterfield, Marketing
Four preprinted overlays to use with Switch Basics. Just put them on an IntelliKeys keyboard and you're ready to go.

1205 **Symbi-Key Computer Switch Interface**
AbleNet
1081 10th Avenue SE
Minneapolis, MN 55414
800-322-0956
FAX: 651-294-2254
e-mail: hresources@ablenetinc.com
www.ablenetinc.com

Cheryl Volkam, President/CEO
The Symbi-Key can be programmed to simulate any key stroke or a series of keystrokes (up to 5 per key) for single switch access to software programs whether or not it was designed for switch access. Works well in DOS and all versions of Windows providing access to any IBM program. *$299.00*

1206 **Teach Me Phonemics Blends Overlay CD**
Soft Touch
4300 Stine Road
Suite 401
Bakersfield, CA 93313
661-396-8676
877-763-8868
FAX: 661-396-8760
e-mail: softtouch@softtouch.com
www.softtouch.com

Roxanne Butterfield, Marketing
Joyce Meyer, President
Teach Me Phonemics Blends Overlay CD contains over 40 IntelliKeys overlays for use with Teach Me Phonemics - Blends program. Choose either 4-item or 9-item layout to match the presentation you use in the program. Print extra copies of the overlays for off computer activites, too.

1207 **Teach Me Phonemics Medial Overlay CD**
Soft Touch Incorporated
17117 Oak Street
Suite C
Omaha, NE 68130
402-334-8477
877-763-8868
FAX: 402-334-8478
e-mail: support@softtouch.com
www.softtouch.com

Joyce Meyer, President
Roxanne Butterfield, Marketing
Teach Me Phonemics Medial Overlay CD contains over 40 IntelliKeys overlays for use with Teach Me Phonemics - Medial program. Choose either 4-item or 9-item layout to match the presentation you use in the program. Print extra copies of the overlays for off computer activites, too.

1208 **Teach Me Phonemics Overlay Series Bundle**
Soft Touch
4300 Stine Road
Suite 401
Bakersfield, CA 93313
661-396-8676
877-763-8868
FAX: 661-396-8760
e-mail: softtouch@funsoftware.com
www.softtouch.com

Roxanne Butterfield, Marketing
Joyce Meyer, President
Teach Me Phonemics Overlay Series Bundle includes one copy of each Teach Me Phonemics Overlay CD - Initial, Medial, Final and - four CD's in all.

1209 **Teach Me to Talk Overlay CD**
Soft Touch
4300 Stine Road
Suite 401
Bakersfield, CA 93313
661-396-8676
877-763-8868
FAX: 661-396-8760
e-mail: softtouch@softtouch.com
www.softtouch.com

Roxanne Butterfield, Marketing
Joyce Meyer, President
For older version of Teach Me to Talk. Mac only version with red label and PC only version with yellow label. More than 48 pre-made overlays that match the activities on Teach Me to Talk. Simply print and use with an IntelliKeys keyboard. Print an extra set to make off computer activities, too.

1210 **Teach Me to Talk: USB-Overlay CD**
Soft Touch
4300 Stine Road
Suite 401
Bakersfield, CA 93313
661-396-8676
FAX: 661-396-8676
e-mail: softtouch@softtouch.com
www.softtouch.com

Joyce Meyer, President
Roxanne Butterfiled, Marketing
Revised version of Teach Me to Talk Overlays for the newest version that is USB IntelliKeys compatible. This CD contains more than 48 overlays that match the activities and updated graphics of Teach Me to Talk. Includes Overlay Printer by IntelliTools for easy printing.

1211 **Teen Tunes Plus IntelliKeys Overlay**
Soft Touch
4300 Stine Road
Suite 401
Bakersfield, CA 93313
661-396-8676
877-763-8868
FAX: 661-396-8760
e-mail: softtouch@softtouch.com
www.softtouch.com

Roxanne Butterfield, Marketing
Joyce Meyer, President
Seven full color, preprinted overlays to use with Teen Tunes Plus. Just put them on an IntelliKeys keyboard and you're ready to go.

1212 **TouchCorders Holder**
Soft Touch
4300 Stine Road
Suite 401
Bakersfield, CA 93313
661-396-8676
877-763-8868
FAX: 661-396-8760
e-mail: support@softtouch.com
www.softtouch.com

Roxanne Butterfield, Marketing
Joyce Meyer, President
The TouchCorders Holder enables you to position up to 4 TouchCorders for sequencing, spelling, communication, story telling and more. The TouchCorders Holder holds TouchCorders snugly and keeps them in place even when you are offering multiple choices to students in a group setting. The sturdy triangular shape presents TouchCorders at a 30-degree angle for better visual and physical access.

1213 **Turtle Teasers IntelliKeys Overlay**
Soft Touch
4300 Stine Road
Suite 401
Bakersfield, CA 93313
661-396-8676
877-763-8868
FAX: 661-396-8760
e-mail: softtouch@funsoftware.com
www.funsoftware.com

Roxanne Butterfield, Marketing
Joyce Meyer, President
Seven full color preprinted overlays to use with Turtle Teasers. Just put them on the IntelliKeys keyboard and you're ready to go.

1214 **U-Control II**
Words+
42505 10th Street W
Suite 109
Lancaster, CA 93534
800-869-8521
FAX: 661-266-8969
e-mail: info@word+.com
www.words-plus.com

Jeff Dhalan, President
Janet Aviles, Customer Support
Works with the Words+ system (EX Keys, Morse WSKE, Scanning WSKE, Talking Screen) to provide wireless, portable control of items which are already infrared-controlled such as a TV, VCR, CD player, etc. *$395.00*

1215 **Universal Switch Mounting System**
AbleNet
2808 Fairview Avenue N
Roseville, MN 55113
651-294-2200
800-322-0956
FAX: 651-294-2259
e-mail: customerservice@ablenetinc.com
www.ablenetinc.com

Mary Kate Walch, Director
Mounting system that allows switch placement in any position. A single lever locks all joints securely in place. Extends to 20 1/2 inches and holds up to five pounds. A mounting system for quick and easy positioning. *$210.00*

1216 **VISION**
Artic Technologies
1000 John R Roadrive
Suite 108
Troy, MI 48083
248-588-7370
FAX: 248-588-2650
e-mail: info@artictech.com
www.artictech.com
The premier access system for blind users of IBM personal computers.

1217 **WinSCAN: The Single Switch Interface for PC's with Windows**
Academic Software
3504 Tates Creek Road
Lexington, KY 40517
859-522-1020
FAX: 253-799-4012
e-mail: asistaff@acsw.com
www.acsw.com

Warren E Lacefield, President
Penelope Ellis, Marketing Director/COO
A general purpose single-switch control interface for Windows. It provides single-switch users independent control access to educational and productivity software, multimedia programs, and recreational activities that run under Windows 3.1 and higher versions on IBM and compatible PC's. The user can navigate through Windows; choose program icons and run programs, games, and CD's; even surf the Internet with WinSCAN and his or her adaptive switch. *$349.00*

1218 **Words+ Equalizer**
Words Plus
1220 W Avenue J
Lancaster, CA 93534
661-723-6523
800-869-8521
FAX: 661-723-2114
e-mail: info@words-plus.com
www.words-plus.com

Ginger Woltosz, Vice President
Walt Wolosz, Manager
A hardware/software product designed to operate on an IBM compatible PC. The software provides an intelligent word prediction scheme, a calculator, music, plus the ability to draw and play games. Equalizer is a dedicated augmentative communication system designed for use by individuals with severe motor disability. *$1395.00*

1219 **Words+ IST (Infrared, Sound, Touch)**
Words+
42505 10th Street W
Suite 109
Lancaster, CA 93534
661-723-6523
800-869-8521
FAX: 661-723-2114
e-mail: info@words-plus.com
www.words-plus.com

Phil Lawrence, VP
Rachel Nielsen, Customer Support
Walt Wolosz, Manager
A unique switch that is activated by slight movement or faint sound. The switch provides user control when connected to a device driven by a single switch. Individuals are currently accessing a wide variety of communication and computer systems with movement using the IST switch. Price ranges from $295.00 to $495.00.

Braille Products

1220 **Access Systems International**
415 English Avenue
Monterey, CA 93940
831-373-6291
FAX: 831-375-5313

Developers of Braille printers.

1221 **Braille Blazer**
Blazie Engineering
11800 31st Court N
St Petersburg, FL 33716
800-444-4443
FAX: 727-803-8001

Braille printer.

1222 **Braille Keyboard Labels**
Hooleon Corporation
PO Box 589
Melrose, NM 88124
928-634-7515
800-937-1337
FAX: 505-253-4299
e-mail: sales@hooleon.com
www.hooleon.com

Barry Green, Sales Manager
Joan Crozier, President/Sales
Also large print keyboard labels and large print with Braille.

1223 **Braille N' Speak**
Blazie Engineering
11800 31st Court N
St Petersburg, FL 33716
800-444-4443
FAX: 727-803-8001
A compact, portable talking device with a seven-key braille keyboard, may be used as a talking computer terminal, a braille to print transcriber and a word processor.

1224 **Brailon Thermoform Duplicator**
American Thermoform Corporation
1758 Brackett Street
La Verne, CA 91750
909-593-6711
FAX: 909-593-8001
e-mail: atc@atcbrleqp.com
www.atcbrleqp.com

Ruth Haggen, Vice President
Gary Nunnelly, Owner
This copy machine, for producing tactile images, copies any brailled or embossed original, by a vacuum forming process. This model is for the reproduction of teaching aids and mobility maps.

1225 **Computer Paper for Brailling**
Maxi Aids
42 Executive Boulevard
Farmingdale, NY 11735
631-752-0521
800-522-6294
FAX: 631-752-0689
e-mail: sales@maxiaids.com
www.maxiaids.com

Elliot Zaretsky, Contact
Specially made paper for braille printing. 1,000 sheets/case *$69.95*

1226 **Duxbury Braille Translator**
Duxbury Systems
270 Littleton Road
Suite 6
Westford, MA 01886
978-692-3000
FAX: 978-692-7912
e-mail: info@duxsys.com
www.duxburysystems.com

Dan Thibert, Operation Manager
Joe Sullivan, President
A complete line of easy to use word processing and Braille translation software available for Windows (including NT) and Macintosh. Applications for anyone wanting to produce or communicate with Braille; signs, note cards, textbooks, business communications and forms, telephone bills, etc. Simple to use, FREE technical support. Free one year upgrades. DBT is for producing Braille in English, Spanish, French, Portuguese, Italian, Latin, Greek, German and other languages. *$600.00*

1227 **Enabling Technologies Company**
1601 NE Braille Place
Jensen Beach, FL 34957
772-225-3687
800-777-3687
FAX: 772-225-3299
e-mail: enabling@brailler.com
www.brailler.com

Dede Haskins, Vice President
Greg Schenk, Marketing Executive
Manufactures the most complete line of American made Braille embossers, including desktop or portable models capable of producing high quality single sided or interpoint Braille. Also carries a complete line of adaptive technology aids for the blind community at affordable prices.

1228 **Freedom Scientific Blind/ Low Vision Group**
11800 31st Court N
Saint Petersburg, FL 33716
727-803-8000
800-444-4443
FAX: 727-803-8001
www.freedomscientific.com

Lee Hamilton, President
Developer and manufacturer of assistive technology products for blind and visually impaired individuals. Software: JANS for Windows, ScreenReader, Magic Screen Magnifier, Open Book Scanning and Reading Software. Hardware: Braille Wireless, personal note takers: Braille 'n Speak, BrailleLite, Type 'n Speak, Type Lite, Braille Embossers, Computer Braille Displays. Training and tutorials available. *$16.95*

1229 **Hooleon Corporation**
PO Box 589
Melrose, NM 88124
928-634-7515
800-937-1337
FAX: 928-634-4620
e-mail: sales@hooleon.com
www.hooleon.com

Barry Green, Sales Manager
Joan Crozier, President/Sales
Large print and combination Braille adhesive keytop labels for computer keyboards. Helps visually impaired computer users access correct key strokes either by sight or by touch. Raised Braille meets ADA specifications and large print fills key top surface.

1230 **Infogrip: Large Print/Braille Keyboard Labels**
1794 E Main Street
Ventura, CA 93001
805-652-0770
800-397-0921
FAX: 805-652-0880
e-mail: sales@infogrip.com
www.infogrip.com

Liza Jacobs, President
Makes a standard keyboard more accessible for visually impaired individuals with large print or Braille keyboard labels. Characters on the large print labels are .5" by .25", about 3 times larger than standard keyboard characters. Braille labels are available as clear labels with Braille dots or large print with Braille. Each set includes all the keys used on a standard Windows keyboard. *$29.00*

1231 **Raised Dot Computing**
Duxbury Systems Incorporated
270 Littleton Road
Suite 6
Westford, MA 01886
978-692-3000
FAX: 978-692-7912
e-mail: info@duxsys.com
www.duxburysystems.com

Joe Sullivan, President
Peter Sullivan, VP/Software Development
Software for the visually impaired.

1232 **Touchdown Keytop/Keyfront Kits**
Hooleon Corporation
PO Box 589
Melrose, NM 88124
505-253-4503
800-937-1337
FAX: 505-253-4299
www.hooleon.com

Barry Green, Sales Manager
Joan Crozier, President
These kits enlarge the key legends of a computer and include Braille for easy recognition.

Information Centers & Databases

1233 **ABLEDATA**
8630 Fenton Street
Suite 930
Silver Spring, MD 20910
301-608-8998
800-227-0216
FAX: 301-608-8958
TTY: 301-608-8912
e-mail: abledata@orcmacro.com
www.abledata.com

Katherine Belknap, Project Director
David Johnson, Publications Director
Tuanita Hardy, Information Specialist
ABLEDATA is an electronic database of assistive technology and rehabilitation equipment products for children and adults with physical, cognitive and sensory disabilities. ABLEDATA staff can perform database searches or the database can be searched on the ABLEDATA website database printouts, informer consumer guides and fact website sheets are available at cost from the office or free from the website.

1234 **ATTAIN**
Division of Disability Aging & Rehab Services
32 E Washington Street
Suite 1400
Indianapolis, IN 46204
317-232-1147
800-528-8246
FAX: 317-486-8809
e-mail: attain@attaininc.org
www.attaininc.org

Gary R Hand, Executive Director
Peter Bisbecos, Manager

Nonprofit organization that creates system change by expanding the availability of community-based technology-related activities, outreach services, empowerment and advocacy activities through the development of a comprehensive, consumer-responsive, statewide program to serve individuals with disabilities, of all ages and all disabilities, their families, caregivers, educators and service providers. Provides trainings, information and referrals, system change and assessments for equipment needs.

1235 Aloha Special Technology Access Center

710 Green Street
Honolulu, HI 96813
808-523-5547
FAX: 808-536-3765
e-mail: astachi@yahoo.com
www.geocities.com/astachi

Ali Sildert, President
Computer technology center.

1236 Audiogram/Clinical Records Manager

98 Us Highway 46
Budd Lake, NJ 07828
973-347-7662
FAX: 973-691-0611
www.daviscenter.com

Torine Davis, Director
Keeps track of client audiogram history and can print or view client with audiogram. The company no longer works with hearing aids. *$414.75*

1237 Birmingham Alliance for Technology Access Center

Birmingham Independent Living Center
206 13th Street S
Birmingham, AL 35233
205-251-2223
FAX: 205-251-0605
TTY:205-251-2223
e-mail: bilc@bellsouth.net
www.birminghamilc.org

Phil Klebine, President
Graham Sisson, Vice President
Daniel Kessler, Executive Director
Computer technology center.

1238 Bluegrass Technology Center

961 Beasley Street
Suite 103a
Lexington, KY 40509
859-294-4343
800-209-7767
TTY:606-491-8700
e-mail: office@bluegrass-tech.org
www.bluegrass-tech.org

Jennifer Bell, President
Angie Youngs Jayarante, Vice President
Jean Isaacs, Executive Director
Provides assistive technology information, consulting and training for education, health professionals, consumers and parents of consumers. Maintains extensive lending library of assistive devices and adapted toys. Statewide training such as; AAC, how to obtain funding for assistive technology, augmentative and alternate communication, equipment implementation strategies, specific to hardware and software, etc.

1239 CHID Combined Health Information Database

National Institute of Health
PO Box C
Rockville, MD
301-402-8714
FAX: 301-770-5164

Richard Pike
A computerized bibliographic database, developed and managed by health-related agencies of the Federal Government.

1240 CITE: Lighthouse for Central Florida

215 E New Hampshire Street
Orlando, FL 32804
407-898-9243
FAX: 407-898-0672
e-mail: info@cite-fl.com
www.centralflordilighthouse.org

Lee Masehi, Executive Director
CITE promotes the independence of adults and children with blindness, low vision and other disabilities through technology, education, support and advocacy.

1241 Carolina Computer Access Center

PO Box 247
Cramerton, NC 28032
704-342-3004
FAX: 704-342-1513
e-mail: bellsluth.net
ccac.ataccess.org

Linda Schilling, Executive Director
Nonprofit, community-based technology resource center for people with disabilities, providing information about and demonstration of the technology tools that enable individuals with disabilities to control and direct their own lives. Services and programs include: assessments, demonstrations, resource information, lending library, workshops and outreach.

1242 Center for Accessible Technology

2547 8th Street
Suite 12a
Berkeley, CA 94710
510-841-3224
FAX: 510-841-7956
e-mail: info@cforat.org
www.cforat.org

Dmitri Belser, Executive Director
Eric Smith, Administrative Director
The Center is a grassroots, consumer-based agency with programs that connect people with all types of disabilities, family members, educators, therapists and others with computer-based tools. Services include assessment, ongoing training, curriculum adaption, classes, demonstrations and a newsletter.

1243 Center for Applied Special Technology

40 Harvard Mill Square
Suite 3
Wakefield, MA 01880
781-245-2212
781-245-9320
FAX: 781-245-5212
e-mail: cast@cast.org
www.cast.org

Stephen P Crosby, Chairman
Sally Bowles, Director
David Rose, Executive Director
Expands opportunities for individuals with special needs through innovative use of computers and related technology. We pursue this mission through research and product development that further universal design for learning.

1244 Center for Assistive Technology & Inclusive Education Studies

PO Box 7718
Ewing, NJ 08628
609-771-3016
FAX: 609-637-5179
e-mail: caties@tcnj.edu
caties.tcnj.edu

Amy G Dell, Executive Director
Computer technology center offering resource time, workshops, technology, training and evaluations.

1245 Center on Evaluation of Assistive Technology

National Rehabilitation Hospital
102 Irving Street NW
Washington, DC 20010
202-877-1000
TTY:202-726-3996
e-mail: justin.m.carter@medstar.net
www.nrhrehab.org

Thomas J Collamore, Director
Edward B Healton, Senior Vice President
Edward Eckenhoff, Chief Executive Officer
The center develops ways of collecting, producing and distributing information to help users, prescribers and third-party payers make intelligent selections of devices.

1246 Compuserve: Handicapped Users' Database

5000 Arlington Centre Boulevard
Columbus, OH 43220
614-457-8600
FAX: 614-538-4023

Audrey Weil, General Manager
John Miller, Chief Executive Officer
This nationwide database with bulletin boards provides information for persons with disabilities and the issues and technologies that are of interest to them.

1247 **Computer & Web Resources for People With Disabilities**
Alliance for Technology Access
1304 Southpoint Boulevard
Suite 240
Petaluma, CA 94954
707-778-3011
FAX: 707-765-2080
TTY:707-778-3015
e-mail: atainfo@ataaccess.org
www.ataccess.org

Mary Lester, Executive Director
A guide to maneuvering the growing world of computers, both the mainstream and the assistive technology.

ISBN 0-897933-00-1

1248 **Computer Access Center**
6234 W 87th Street
Los Angeles, CA 90045
310-338-1597
FAX: 310-338-9318
e-mail: info@cac.org
www.cac.org

Mary Ann Glicksman, Executive Director
Joanne Orenski, Financial Administrator
Computer technology center.

1249 **Computer Center for Visually Impaired People: Division of Continuing Studies**
Baruch College
1 Bernard Baruch Way
New York, NY 10010
646-312-1000
FAX: 646-312-5101
e-mail: caps@baruch.cuny.edu
www.baruch.cuny.edu/ccvip

Karen Gourgey, Director
Judith Gerber, Manager
Offers courses, tutors, equipment and assistance.

1250 **Computer and Web Resources for People with Disabilities**
Hunter House Publishers
PO Box 2914
Alameda, CA 94501
510-865-5282
800-266-5592
FAX: 510-865-4295
e-mail: ordering@hunterhouse.com
www.hunterhouse.com

Kiran S Rana, Publisher
Part One describes conventional and assistive technologies and gives strategies for accessing the Internet. Part Two features easy-to-use charts organized by key access concerns, and provides detailed descriptions of software, hardware, and communication aids. Part Three is a gold mine of Web resources, publications, support organizations, government programs, and technology vendors. *$27.95*

ISBN 0-897933-01-X

1251 **Computer-Enabling Drafting for People with Physical Disabilities**
County College of Morris
214 Center Grove Road
Randolph, NJ 07869
973-328-5000
888-226-8001
FAX: 973-328-5286
www.ccm.edu

Edward Yaw, President
Brandi Robinson, Vice President
Computer service.

1252 **Computers to Help People**
913 Acewood Boulevard
Apt 109
Madison, WI 53714
608-257-5917
FAX: 608-257-3480
e-mail: techorlochpi.org
www.chpi.org

Carl Durocher, Assistive Technologies Manager
Johnny R Lee, Operations Manager
John J Boyer, Executive Director
A center for assistive technology, assessment, consulting and training, specializing in computer access products for persons with sensory or mobility impairments. Also provides a print-to-braille service with a specialty in technical writing.

1253 **DIRLINE**
National Library of Medicine
8600 Rockville Pike
Bethesda, MD 20894
301-496-6308
888-346-3656
FAX: 301-496-4450
e-mail: custserv@nml.nih.gov
www.nlm.nih.gov/

Robert Mehnert, Manager
18,000 listings of organizations that serve as information resources, including libraries, professional associations and government agencies.

1254 **Developmental Disabilities Council**
647 Main Street
70802
Baton Rouge, LA 70801
225-342-6804
800-922-3425
FAX: 225-342-1970
www.ladc.org

Sandee Winchell, Executive Director
Computer technology center.

1255 **Employment Resources Program**
330 South Grand Avenue W
Springfield, IL 62704
217-523-2587
800-447-4221
FAX: 217-523-0427

Ceceila Haasis, Employment Resource Program Mgr
An information and referral service that encourages inquiries from professionals, individuals with disabilities, family members, organizations or anyone requesting information pertaining to disabilities. The staff at DRN uses both computer listings and in-house library files to provide the programs services. The DRN program is funded by a grant from the Illinois Department of Rehabilitation Services.

1256 **Functional Skills Screening Inventory**
Functional Resources
3905 Huntington Drive
Amarillo, TX 79109
806-353-1114
FAX: 806-353-1114
e-mail: webmaster@winfssi.comnhsc.edu
www.winfssi.com

Ed Hammer PhD, Owner
Heather Becker PhD, Owner
Assesses the individual's level of functional skills and identifies supports needed by educational, rehabilitation and residential programs serving moderately and severely disabled persons. Includes enviromental assessments as well as profiles of jobs and training sites.

1257 **High Tech Center**
Sacremento State
6000 J Street
Sacramento, CA 95819
916-278-7915
FAX: 916-278-3660
e-mail: sswd@csus.edu
www.csus.edu/sswd/services
The Center offers assesment and training in adaptive hardware/software for eligible students with disabilities at Sacremento State upon referral from the Office of Services to Students with Disabilities.

1258 **Idaho Assistive Technology Project**
129 W 3rd Street
Moscow, ID 83843
208-885-3557
800-432-8324
FAX: 208-885-3628
e-mail: rseiler@uidaho.edu
www.idahoat.org

Ron Seiler, Director
Sue House, Information And Referral
The Idaho assistive technology project (IATP) is a federally funded program managed by the center on disabilities and human development at the university of Idaho. The goal of the IATP is to increase the availability of assistive technology devices and services for Idahoans with disabilities. The IATP offers free trainings and technical assistance, a low-interest loan program, assistive technology assessments for children and agriculture workers, and free informational materials.

1259 **Increasing Capabilities Access Network**
26 Corporate Hill Drive
Little Rock, AR 72205
501-666-8868
800-828-2799
FAX: 501-666-5319
www.arkansas-ican.org

Barry Valetich, Project Director
Barbara Gullett, Executive Director
A consumer responsive statewide systems change program promoting assistive technology for persons of all ages with disabilities. The program provides information on new and existing technology and maintains an equipment exchange free of charge. Training on assistive technology is also provided.

1260 **International Center for the Disabled**
340 E 24th Street
New York, NY 10010
212-585-6000
FAX: 212-585-6161
e-mail: info@icdrehab.org
www.icdrehab.org

Michael Burks, Chairman
Wen Lu, Secretary/Treasurer
Les Halpert, Chief Executive Officer
The ICD is a comprehensive outpatient rehabilitation facility, providing medical rehabilitation, behavioral health and vocational services to children and adults with a broad range of physical, communication, emotional and cognitive disabilities.

1261 **Kentucky Assistive Technology Service Network**
8412 Westport Road
Louisville, KY 40242
502-429-4484
800-327-5287
FAX: 502-429-7114
e-mail: katsnet@iglow.com
www.katsnet.org

Ronji Dearborn, Information/Referral Specialist
Statewide network of four regional assistive technology centers with a central coordinating office in Louisville and two regional centers in eastern Kentucky. Network services include but are not limited to assistive technology of services, loan of assistive devices, funding information and referral, assessment and evaluations, consultations on appropriate technologies, training, and technical assistance.

1262 **Learning Independence Through Computers**
1001 Eastern Avenue
Baltimore, MD 21202
410-659-5462
FAX: 410-659-5472
e-mail: lincmd@aol.com
www.linc.org

Susan Pompa, Associate Director
Mary Salkever, Executive Director
Computer technology center.

1263 **MEDLINE**
Dialog Corporation
11000 Regency Parkway
Suite 10
Cary, NC 27518
919-462-8600
800-334-2564
FAX: 919-468-9890
www.dialog.com

David Brown, General Manager
Mike Eastwood, Vice President
Bibliographic citations to biomedical literature.

1264 **Maine CITE**
University of Maine at Augusta
46 University Drive
Augusta, ME 04330
207-621-3000
877-862-1234
FAX: 207-621-3293
e-mail: umaweb@maine.edu
www.uma.maine.edu/cs/

Robert Stewart, Telecommunications Manager
Lauren Dubois, Director Computer Services
Pat Lynch, Manager
Computer technology center.

1265 **Maryland Technology Assistance Program**
Maryland Department of Disabilities
2301 Argonne Drive
Suite T-17
Baltimore, MD 21218
410-554-9230
800-832-4827
FAX: 410-554-9237
e-mail: mdtap@mdtap.org
www.mdtap.org

Jessica Voilmer, Office Manager
Assistive technology center. Information and referral, equipment display loans and demonstration, funding sources, alternative media, training, workshops and seminars. Rural outreach for individuals with disability in Maryland.

1266 **Minnesota STAR Program**
50 Sherburne Avenue
Room 309
Saint Paul, MN 55155
651-201-2640
888-234-1267
FAX: 651-282-6671
e-mail: star.program@state.mn.us
www.admin.state.mn.us/assistivetechnology

Chuck Rassbach, Executive Director
STAR's mission is to help all Minnesotans with disabilities gain access to and acquire the assistive technology they eed to live, learn, work and lay. The Minnesota STAR program is federally funded by the Rehabilitation Services Administration.

1267 **Mississippi Project START**
PO Box 1698
Jackson, MS 39215
601-987-4872
800-852-8328
FAX: 601-364-2349
e-mail: contactus@msprojectstart.org
www.msprojectstart.org

Steve Powers, Project Director
Project START is a Tech Act project established to bring about systems change in the field of assistive technology in the State of Mississippi. Activities include providing training opportunities for consumers and service providers on subjects such as state-of-the-art AT devices, their application and funding resources; referral information on AT evaluation centers; technical assistance to AT users; establishment of an AT equipment loan program and an Information and Referral Service.

1268 **National Technology Database**
American Foundation for the Blind/ AF B Press
11 Penn Plaza
Suite 300
New York, NY 10001
212-502-7600
800-232-5463
FAX: 412-741-0609
e-mail: afbinfo@afb.net
www.afb.org

Carl Augusto, President
This database includes resources for visually impaired persons.
$99.00

1269 New Jersey Department of Labor & Workforce Development
Office of the Commissioner
PO Box 110
Trenton, NJ 08625
609-292-2323
FAX: 609-633-9271
e-mail: cmycoff@dol.state.nj.us
www.state.nj.us/labor

David J Socolow, Commissioner-Designate
Marilyn D Davis, Deputy Commissioner
Kevin D Jarvis, Chief of Staff
Oversees various federal and state vocational rehabilitation services including sheltered workshops and independent living centers; adjudication of permanent disability claims filed with the Social Security Administration; oversees New Jesey's temporary disability program covering non-work related illnesses and injuries

1270 New Mexico Technology Assistance Program
New Mexico State Department of Education
435 Saint Michaels Drive
Suite D
Santa Fe, NM 87505
800-866-2253
FAX: 505-954-8608
TTY:800-659-4915
e-mail: aklaus@state.nm.us
www.nmtap.com

Andy Winnegar, Director
Examines and works to eliminate barriers to obtaining assistive technology in New Mexico. Has established a statewide program for coordinating assistive technology services; is designed to assist people with disabilities to locate, secure, and maintain assistive technology.

1271 Northern Illinois Center for Adaptive Technology
3615 Louisiana Road
Rockford, IL 61108
815-229-2163
e-mail: davegrass@eartlink.net
nicat.ataccess.org

Dave Grass, President
Computer technology center.

1272 OCCK
1710 W Schilling Road
Salina, KS 67401
785-827-9383
800-526-9731
FAX: 785-823-2015
e-mail: occk@occk.com
www.occk.com

Phyllis Anderson, Director Community Resource Dev.
Kathy Reed, Director Personal Supports
Carolee Miner, Chief Executive Officer
Computer technology center; training center for employment and independent living for people with disabilities; family support center. Kansas AgrAbility program coordinator, Kansas equipment exchange site.

1273 Parents, Let's Unite for Kids
516 N 32nd Street W
Billings, MT 59101
406-255-0540
800-222-7585
FAX: 406-255-0523
TTY: 406-657-2055
e-mail: pluk@info.org
www.pluk.org

Dennis Moore, Executive Director
Computer technology center. Parents, Let's Unite for Kids offers an assistive technology lab that is open to people of all ages. The lab is a computer and assistive technology demonstration site. There is no charge for services.

1274 Pathfinder Parent Training and Information Center
Pathfinder
1600 2nd Avenue NW
Minot, ND 58701
701-837-7500
800-245-5840
FAX: 701-837-7548
e-mail: ndpass1@minot.com
www.pathfinder.minot.com

Kathryn Erickson, Executive Director
A member of the National Parent Training and Information Program which helps parents to better understand their child's disability and to obtain information about the programs, services and resources available. The center provides referrals through their program, support for educational programs for children with disabilities and helps parents learn to communicate more effectively with those involved in their child's program.

1275 Pennsylvania's Initiative on Assistive Technology
Temple University
1601 N. Broad St.
Suite 610
Philadelphia, PA 19122
800-204-7428
FAX: 215-204-9371
TTY:866-268-0579
e-mail: ATinfo@temple.edu
www.disabilities.temple.edu

Amy S Goldman, Director
Pennsylvania's Initiative on Assistive Technology (PIAT) offers information and referral about assistive Technology (AT), device demonstrations, and awareness-level presentations. PIAT also operates Pennsylvania's AT Lending Library, a free, state-supported program that loans AT devices to Pennsylvanians of all ages. This program allows you to try a device for a limited time to be sure it meets your needs.

1276 Rehabilitation Engineering & Assistive Technology Society of North America (RESNA)
1700 N Moore Street
Suite 1540
Arlington, VA 22209
703-524-6686
FAX: 703-524-6630
TTY:703-524-6639
e-mail: info@resna.org
www.resna.org

Thomas A Gorski, Executive Director
Rosina Romano, Meetings/Membership Coordinator
Improves the potential of people with disabilities to achieve their goals through the use of technology and disability. Promotes research, development, education, advocacy and provision of technology, and by supporting the people engaged in theses activities.

1277 Resource Center for Independent Living
PO Box 210
Utica, NY 13503
315-797-4642
FAX: 315-797-4747
e-mail: burt.danovitz@rcil.com
www.rcil.com

Burton Danovitz, Executive Director
Services and advocacy for indiviuals with disabilities.

1278 SACC Assistive Technoloy Center
PO Box 1325
Simi Valley, CA 93062
805-582-1881
FAX: 805-582-2855
e-mail: dssaccca@aol.com

Debi Schultze, CEO
SACC connects children, adults and seniors with special needs to computers, technologies and resources. We provide information and referral, assessments, tutoring, presentations and outreach awareness.

1279 **South Dakota Department of Human Services: Computer Technology Services**
500 E Capitol Avenue
Pierre, SD 57501
605-000-1111
800-265-9684
FAX: 605-773-5483
TTY: 605-773-3195
e-mail: gary.goeden@state.sd.us

Gary Goeden
Jeff Pierce, Manager
Computer technology center.

1280 **Star Center**
1119 Old Humboldt Road
Jackson, TN 38305
731-668-3888
800-464-5619
FAX: 731-668-1666
e-mail: infostar@starcenter.tn.org
www.starcenter.tn.org

Judy Duke, Outreach Manager
Margaret Doumitt, Chief Executive Officer
Nation's largest assistive technology center dedicated to helping children and adults with disabilities achieve their goals for competitive employment, effective learning, returning to or starting school and independent living. Programs include: high-tech training, music therapy, art therapy, low vision evaluation, orientation and mobility evaluation and training, augmentative communication evaluation, vocational evaluations, assistive technology, job placement services and job skills training.

1281 **Students with Disabilities Office**
University of Texas at Austin
1 University Station
A5800
Austin, TX 78712
512-471-3434
FAX: 512-475-7730
www.utexas.edu/depts/dos/ssd

Jennifer Maedgen, Assistant Dean of Students
Sheldon Ekland-Olson, Chief Executive Officer

1282 **TASK Team of Advocates for Special Kids**
100 W Cerritos Avenue
Anaheim, CA 92805
714-533-8275
FAX: 714-533-2533
e-mail: taskca@aol.com

Marta Anchondo, Executive Director
Computer technology center.

1283 **Tech Connection**
35 Haddon Avenue
Shrewsbury, NJ 07702
732-747-5310
FAX: 732-747-1896
e-mail: tecconn@aol.com
www.techconnection.org

Joanne Castellano, Director
Offers a noncommercial center to examine and try computers, adapted equipment, alternative input devices, and a variety of software. Program of Family Resource Associates and a member of the Alliance for Technology Access (ATA), a growing national coalition of computer resource centers, professionals, technology developers and vendors, interacting with new technology to enrich the lives of people with disabilities. Tech Connection offers evaluations, for computer technology.

1284 **Tech-Able**
1114 Brett Drive SW
Suite 100
Conyers, GA 30094
770-922-6768
FAX: 770-922-6769
e-mail: techable@techable.org
www.techable.org

Carolyn Gonagill, Executive Director
Pat Hanus, Executive Assistant
Joe Tedesco, Assistive Tech Practitioner
Provide assistive technology to individuals with disabilities, toy-lending and software libraries, product demonstration, access to technology devices and fabrication of keyguards for keyboards. Low vision consultant on Thursdays; computer training for persons with disabilities.

1285 **Technical Aids & Assistance for the Disabled Center**
1950 W Roosevelt Road
Chicago, IL 60608
708-867-6060
800-346-2939
FAX: 312-421-3464
TTY: 312-421-3373

Andres Hernandez, Executive Director
Robert Kaige, Technologist
Provides consultation and technical advice on adaptive aids, software and hardware.

1286 **Technology Access Center of Tucson**
PO Box 13178
Tucson, AZ 85732
520-745-5588

e-mail: tactaz@aol.com
www.ed.arizona.edu/tact

Linda Bishop, Director Services
Sonia Rameriez, Service Coordinator
Linda Gonzalez, Manager
A resource center that provides assistive technology services for people with disabilities. Center personnel develop, provide and coordinate those services in communities throughout Middle Tennessee. Services are designed to assist people with disabilities to learn about, choose, acquire and use assistive technology devices. Services are offered to any child or adult with sensory, motor or cognitive disabilities, their family members, and professionals who serve them and employ them.

1287 **Technology Assistance for Special Consumers**
PO Box 443
Huntsville, AL 35804
256-532-5336
FAX: 256-532-2355
e-mail: tasc@hiwaay.net
www.ataccess.org

Linda Rags, Executive Director
T.A.S.C. is a computer resource center with 10 computers, which are equipped with special adaptations for those who are blind, visually impaired, or severely physically disabled. Our staff demonstrates and trains individuals on this equipment so that they can become more independent at home, school, and work. Over 2,500 pieces of educational software are available for individuals who are learning disabled, mentally retarded or who have developmental delays.

1288 **Tidewater Center for Technology Access Special Education Annex**
1415 Laskin Road
Virginia Beach, VA 23451
757-437-6542
FAX: 757-263-2801
e-mail: tcta@aol.com
tcta.access.org

Jane DeBord, Director
Myra Jessie Flint, Designee
Nonprofit organization providing persons with disabilities access, support, and knowledge—re: technology; organization contracts for consultations, workshops and training, or conventional and assistive technologies including computers, augmented communication devices and software; resources: extensive lending library of educational software; books and videotape library; yearly individual membership and corporate membership fees; working/presentation and evaluation fees available upon request.

1289 **Vermont Assistive Technology Project: Department of Aging & Disabilities**
Agency of Human Services
103 S Main Street
Weeks Building
Waterbury, VT 05671
802-241-2620
800-750-6355
FAX: 802-241-2174
TTY: 802-241-1464
e-mail: atinfo@dail.state.vt.us
www.dad.state.vt.us/atp

Julie L Tucker, Project Director
Betsy Ross, Administration
Dan Gilman, AT Access Specialist
Increase the awareness and change policies to insure assistive technology is available to all Vermonters with disabilities.

1290 Washington Technology Access Center
8705 232nd Place SW
Edmonds, WA 98026
425-883-4141
FAX: 425-776-3663

Grant Lord, Founder
The center was formed as a nonprofit organization to demonstrate how computer technology can transform limitations into opportunities for those with special needs. WTAC's mission is to increase the awareness, understanding and implementation of computer technology for persons with special needs, their friends, families, educators, rehabilitation and health professionals, public officials and employees.

1291 Xerox Imaging Systems/Adaptive Products Department
Personal Reader Department
9 Centennial Drive
Peabody, MA 01960
978-977-2000
800-248-6550
FAX: 978-977-2409
Offers information on new services, assistive devices and technology for blind, visually impaired, learning disabled and other print disabled individuals.

Keyboards, Mouses & Joysticks

1292 A4 Tech (USA) Corporation
5585 Brooks Street
Montclair, CA 91763
909-986-0966
FAX: 909-986-0626
e-mail: info@a4tech.com
www.a4tech.com
Manufacturers of a cordless mouse, trackballs and joysticks that emulate mouse controls, flatbed scanners, modified keyboards, and other specialty mouses.

1293 Abacus
3150 Patterson Avenue SE
Grand Rapids, MI 49512
616-698-0330
800-451-4319
FAX: 616-698-0325
e-mail: info@abacuspub.com
www.abacuspub.com

Arnie Lee, President
Designs a mouse software program that permits programs written for one computer to be run on another computer.

1294 Ability Center of Greater Toledo
5605 Monroe Street
Sylvania, OH 43560
419-885-5733
FAX: 419-882-4813
ww.abilitycenter.org

Tim Harrington, President
Manufactures keyboard wrist supports to help prevent repetitive motion disorders.

1295 Dreamer
TS Micro Tech
17109 Gale Avenue
City of Industry, CA 91745
626-839-8998
FAX: 626-839-8516
e-mail: sales@fancard.com
www.fancard.com

Steve Heung, Owner
An intelligent, add-on function keyboard providing single-keystroke access to multiple-keystroke functions.

1296 FlexShield Keyboard Protectors
Hooleon Corporation
PO Box 589
Melrose, NM 88124
928-634-7515
800-937-1337
FAX: 928-634-4620
e-mail: sales@hooleon.com
www.hooleon.com

Barry Green, Sales Manager
Joan Crozier, President
Transparent keyboard protectors allowing instant recognition of keytop legends. They have a matte finish to reduce glare.

1297 Infogrip: King Keyboard
1794 E Main Street
Ventura, CA 93001
805-652-0770
800-397-0921
FAX: 805-652-0880
e-mail: sales@infogrip.com
www.infogrip.com

Liza Jacobs, President
Aaron Gaston, Vice President
Giant alternative keyboard that plugs directly into a computer—no special interface is required. The keys are 1.25 inches in diameter, slightly recessed, and provide both tactile and auditory feedback. The King has a built-in keyboard so that you can rest on its surface without activating keys. This keyboard allows you to control both keyboard and mouse functions, so it's great for people who have difficulty maneuvering a standard mouse. *$130.00*

1298 Infogrip: Large Print Keyboard
1794 E Main Street
Ventura, CA 93001
805-652-0770
800-397-0921
FAX: 805-652-0880
e-mail: sales@infogrip.com
www.infogrip.com

Liza Jacobs, President
Aaron Gaston, Vice President
Standard Windows keyboard with large print keys. The keyboard and its keys are the same size as a standard keyboard; however, the print has been enhanced. The characters measure .5" by .25", about 3 times larger than standard keyboard characters. *$130.00*

1299 Infogrip: OnScreen
1794 E Main Street
Ventura, CA 93001
805-652-0770
800-397-0921
FAX: 805-652-0880
e-mail: sales@infogrip.com
www.infogrip.com

Liza Jacobs, President
OnScreen features word prediction/completion (with an editable dictionary), Key Dwell Timer (a timer that selects a key under the cursor), integrated Verbal Keys Feedback, Show and Hide Keys (turns on/off keys to prevent access and minimize confusion) a Smart Window (automatically re-positions the keyboard or panels off of the area in use). On Screen also offers edit, numeric, macro, calculator and Windows enhancement capabilities. *$200.00*

1300 IntelliKeys
Intelli Tools
1720 Corporate Circle
Petaluma, CA 94954
707-773-2000
800-899-6687
FAX: 707-773-2001
e-mail: info@intellitools.com
www.intellitools.com

Beth Davis, Director Sales Operation
Lari Castle, Supervisor
Arjan Khalsa, Chief Executive Officer
Alternative, touch-sensitive keyboards; plugs into any Macintosh or Windows computer. *$395.00*

1301 **IntelliKeys USB**
Intelli Tools
1720 Corporate Circle
Petaluma, CA 94954
707-773-2000
800-899-6687
FAX: 707-773-2001
e-mail: info@intellitools.com
www.intellitools.com

Paula Irons, Director Marketing/Communication
Arjan Khalsa, Chief Executive Officer
IntelliKeys alternative keyboard for USB computers and Windows 2000, Mac OSX. *$69.95*

1302 **Jouse**
Prentke Romich Company
1022 Heyl Road
Wooster, OH 44691
330-262-1984
800-262-1984
FAX: 330-263-4829
e-mail: info@prentrom.com
www.prentrom.com

Jennifer Monahan, Specialized Speech Technologist
Dave Moffatt, President
A joystick-operated mouse that is controlled with the mouth. Moving the joystick moves the cursor. Mouse button activations can be made with the sip and puff switch that is built into the joystick. Typing can be achieved through an on-screen keyboard. Nothing is attached to the operator. The adjustable Jouse arm mounts on a table or desktop and swings away when bumped. *$995.00*

1303 **Key Tronic KB 5153 Touch Pad Keyboard**
KeyTronic
PO Box 14687
Spokane Valley, WA 99214
800-262-6006
Integrates a regular full-function keyboard, a numeric keypad with a cursor key capability and a touch pad into one unit.

1304 **Liaison Computer Work Station**
Genesis One Technologies
343 W Milltown Road
Wooster, OH 44691
330-259-1304
888-221-5032
FAX: 775-252-4834
e-mail: sales@genesis.net
www.genesisone.net

Grace Miller, Office Manager
A full function computer work station for high level (C-2 to C-5) spinal cord injured users. It transparently emulates both keyboard and mouse, using rapid direct selection which commonly yields letter by letter typing rates of 15 to 20 words per minute. The user controls it via proportional IR remote control from the DU-IT controlled power wheelchair and chin or tongue/lip controller or via a desk-mounted proportional controller as a stand alone device. Full ECU features included. *$ 4685.00*

1305 **Magic Wand Keyboard**
In Touch Systems
11 Westview Road
Spring Valley, NY 10977
845-354-7431
800-332-6244
www.magicwandkeyboard.com

Jerry Crouch, President
Susan Crouch, Vice President
The magic wand keyboard allows your child to use a keyboard and mouse easily-no light beams, microphones, or sensors to wear of position. This miniature computer keyboard has zero-force keys that work with the slightest touch of a wand (hand-held of mouthstick). No strength required.

1306 **McKey Mouse**
In Touch Systems
11 Westview Road
Spring Valley, NY 10977
845-354-7431
www.prop.or.jp

Jerry Crouch, President
Microsoft compatible mouse for persons with little or no hand/arm movement; it's an option for the Magic Wand Keyboard and adds full mouse function without adding any extra devices.

1307 **PortaPower Plus**
Words+
42505 10th Street W
Suite 109
Lancaster, CA 93534
661-266-8500
800-869-8521
FAX: 661-266-8969
www.words-plus.com

Phil Lawrence, VP
Rachel Nielsen, Customer Support
Rechargeable battery pack designed to give longer life and remote usage time to laptop computers and other portable battery-operated devices and accessories. Requires a 12 volt auto adapter. *$149.00*

1308 **Step on It! Computer Control Pedals**
1290 Carmead Parkway
Suite 118
Sunnyvale, CA 94086
408-736-6086
FAX: 408-736-6083
www.bilbo.com

Sergei Burkov, President
Katie Sheinin, Manager
BILBO Innovations, Inc. manufactures and sells Step On It keyboard control pedals. Ergonomic foot switches to emulate keystrokes and mouse clicks. Designed for victims of Repetitive Strain Injury (RSI), Carpal Tunnel Syndrome (CTS), handicapped and disabled. *$99.00*

1309 **Unicorn Keyboards**
Intelli Tools
1720 Corporate Circle
Petaluma, CA 94954
707-773-2000
800-899-6687
FAX: 707-773-2001
e-mail: info@intellitools.com
www.intellitools.com

Paula Irons, Marketing Director
Arjan Khalsa, Chief Executive Officer
Alternative keyboards with membrane surface and large, user-defined keys. Large and small sizes are available. *$250.00*

Scanners

1310 **Scanmaster**
4 Townsend W
Suite 17
Nashua, NH 03063
603-882-5200
FAX: 603-880-3843

W Parr, Chief Executive Officer
A digital color scanner for desktop scanning. It allows the user to digitalize, modify, enhance and store images in color or black and white.

1311 **Scanning WSKE**
Words+
42505 10th Street W
Suite 109
Lancaster, CA 93534
661-723-6523
800-869-8521
FAX: 661-723-2114
www.words-plus.com

Ginger Woltosz, VP
Jeff Dahlen, Manager
Walt Wolosz, Manager
A software and a hardware product designed to operate on an IBM compatible PC. The software provides dual word prediction, abbreviation expansion, five different methods of voice output, and access to commercial software applications.

1312 **System 2000/Versa**
Words+
40015 Sierra Highway
Suite B145
Palmdale, CA 93550
800-869-8521
FAX: 661-266-8969
www.words-plus.com

Ginger Woltosz, VP
Tim Ross, Manager
Provides all of the strategies currently being used in AAC, from dynamic display color pictographic language, to dual-word prediction text language, in a single system.

1313 **Zygo Industries**
ZYGO Industries
PO Box 1008
Portland, OR 97207
503-598-7531
800-234-6006
FAX: 503-684-6011
e-mail: zygo@zygo-usa.com
www.zygo-usa.com

Lawrence Weiss, President/Owner

Screen Enhancement

1314 **Boxlight**
Boxlight Corporation
19472 Powder Hill Place NE
Suite 100
Poulsbo, WA 98370
360-779-7901
800-884-6464
e-mail: sales@boxlight.com
www.boxlight.com

Joanne Luttrell, Marketing
Herb Myers, President
BOXLIGHT is a global presentation solutions partner for trainers, educators and professional speakers. Solutions include projector sales, national rental service, technical support, repair, and presentation peripherals. For more information visit us online.

1315 **FDR Series of Low Vision Reading Aids**
Optelec U S
3030 Enterprise Court
Suite C
Vista, CA 92081
800-828-1056
FAX: 978-692-6073
e-mail: chrish@optelec.com
www.optelec.com

Annette Fasnacht, President
James Bailey, Vice President
The Low Vision Reading Aids features; high resolution, positive and negative display, a high-quality zoom lens, versatile swivel and a 12 inch or 19 inch high-resolution monitor, color or black and white, computer compatible, or portable.

1316 **InFocus**
AI Squared
PO Box 669
Manchester Center, VT 05255
802-362-3612
FAX: 802-362-1670
e-mail: zoomtext@alsquared.com

Benjermin Weiss, President
A memory-resident program that magnifies text and graphics - the entire screen, a single line or a portion of the screen.

1317 **Portable Large Print Computer**
Human Ware
175 Mason Circle
Concord, CA 94520
925-680-7100
800-722-3393
FAX: 925-681-4630
e-mail: us.info@humanware.com
www.humanware.com

Jim Halliday, President/Chief Executive Office
Sharon Spiker, Administrator
A portable large print computer which magnifies up to 64 times. It is linked to a PC and has a hand-held camera.

1318 **ZoomText**
A I Squared
PO Box 669
Manchester Center, VT 05255
802-362-3612
800-859-3612
FAX: 802-362-1670
e-mail: zoomtext@alsquared.com
www.aisquared.com

Benjermin Weiss, President
A RAM-resident program that enlarges screen characters up to eight times. It runs on IBM PC, XT, AT and PS/2.

Speech Synthesizers

1319 **Artic Business Vision (for DOS) and Artic WinVision (for Windows 95)**
Artic Technologies
55 Park Drive
Troy, MI 48083
248-588-7370
FAX: 248-588-2650
e-mail: info@artictech.com
www.artictech.com

Dale McDaniel, Vice President Marketing
Kathy Gargagliano, VP Operations
A speech processor for blind computer users featuring true interactive speech with spread sheets, word processors, database managers, etc. Now available with both Windows 3.1 and Windows 95 access. *$ 495.00*

1320 **Audapter Speech System**
Personal Data Systems
638 Sobrato Lane
Campbell, CA 95008
408-866-1126
FAX: 408-866-1128
e-mail: info@personaldatasystems.com
www.personaldatasystems.com

Robert Gallati, Director
Noel Runyan, President
A speech synthesizer. Its features include: intelligibility over 93 percent on the industry standard MRT test, fast response, 700-word-per-minute speech rate, speech halt control, compact unit with built-in speaker and serial interface.

1321 **Computerized Speech Lab**
Kay Elemetrics Corporation
2 Bridgewater Lane
Lincoln Park, NJ 07035
973-628-6200
800-289-5297
FAX: 973-628-6363
www.kayelemetrics.com

John Crump, President
Hardware/software for the acquisition, analysis/display, playback and storage of speech signals.

1322 **Digital Voice for Talking Database**
Hy-Tek Manufacturing Company
1980 W Us Highway 30
Sugar Grove, IL 60554
630-466-7664
FAX: 630-466-7678

William Bastian, Owner
This product adds speech to PC files. Uses include personnel identification and security, multilingual training, assembly instructions and reminders.

1323 **DynaVox Devices & Software**
Dyna Vox Systems
2100 Wharton Street
Suite 400
Pittsburgh, PA 15203
412-381-4883
800-344-1778
FAX: 412-381-5241
e-mail: sales@dynavoxsys.com
www.dynavoxsys.com

Joe Swenson, President
Allow non-speaking individuals to communicate their thoughts, ideas and feelings easily. The devices' built-in infrared technology also provides users with more independence, allowing them to access TVs, VCRs, and computers. DynaVox software helps turn Macintosh and Windows and computers into communication devices so clinicians can use their computers to conduct training and assessments.

1324 **Electronic Speech Assistance Devices**
Luminaud
8688 Tyler Boulevard
Mentor, OH 44060
440-255-9082
800-255-3408
FAX: 440-255-2250
e-mail: info@luminaud.com
www.luminaud.com

Thomas Lennox, President
Dorothy Lennox, Vice President
Offers a full line of speech aids, voice amplifiers, mini-vox amplifiers, laryngectomec products.

1325 **Hawk Communication Device**
Wayne County Regional Educational Service Agency
33500 Van Born Road
Wayne, MI 48184
734-334-1300
FAX: 734-334-1494
rvhs.net

Marlene Davis, Chief Executive Officer
The Hawk employs digital voice technology for high quality, natural voice output. The touch panel is divided into a three by three matrix for a total of nine selection areas. A bulletin microphone allows the recording of up to five seconds worth of digital speech into each of the nine selection areas. *$250.00*

1326 **In Cube Pro Voice Command**
Command Corporation
11080 Old Roswell Road
Suite 200
Alpharetta, GA 30004
770-360-1230

e-mail: webmaster@commandcorp.com
www.commandcorp.com
Continuous speech recognition system which can be used by people with disabilities. IN CUBE provides greatly increased capability, enhanced computer control and access. Blind and low-vision users gain voice access to the graphic user interface. Mobility-impaired people, including quadriplegics, benefit from voice window navigation and voice macro command input. Victims of various repetitive strain injuries RSI use IN CUBE to replace and eliminate repetitive keyboard and mouse operations. *$395.00*

1327 **Keywi**
Consultants for Communication Technology
35 Bell Avenue
Pittsburgh, PA 15205
412-761-6062
FAX: 412-761-7336
e-mail: cct@concommtech.com
www.concommtech.com

Kathleen H Miller, President/Owner
Keywi enables a laptop computer to become a complete communication device. Create entire conversations, call a friend on the telephone, manage your business or personal affairs. Requires minimal training. Multiple access methods-switch, mouse, joystick, keyboard. Custom vocabulary. Powerful word prediction abilities. *$495.00*

1328 **Laptalker**
Automated Functions
7700 Leesburg Pike
Suite 420
Falls Church, VA 22043
703-883-9797
FAX: 703-883-9798

R Morford, Owner
A portable talking computer that gives visually impaired people complete desk top PC compatibility.

1329 **Mega Wolf Communication Device**
Wayne County Regional Educational Service Agency
33500 Van Born Road
Wayne, MI 48184
734-334-1300

www.resa.net

Kimberly Kaminski, Assistant Operations
Marlene E Davis, Administrator
A low cost voice output communication device which is primarily intended to provide the power of speech to those individuals who are most severely challenged mentally and/or physically. The WOLF device is User programmable and uses the Texas Instruments' Touch and Tell case and touch panel; ADAMLAB electronics with synthesized (robotic) voice. For users able to point with approximately 6 ounces of pressure. *$400.00*

1330 **One-Step Communicator**
AbleNet
2808 Fairview Avenue N
Roseville, MN 55113
651-294-2200
800-322-0956
FAX: 651-294-2259
e-mail: customerservice@ablenetinc.com
www.ablenetinc.com

Dave Dinckik, Director
The One-Step Communicator has 20 seconds of memory and has an angled switch surface making it easy to see and access. The switch surface is 2 1/2 inches in diameter. Detachable mounting base makes it easy to position a single unit in a variety of locations. *$129.00*

1331 **Phone Manager**
Consultants for Communication Technology
508 Bellevue Ter
Pittsburgh, PA 15202
412-761-6062
FAX: 412-761-7336
e-mail: cct@concommtech.com
www.concommtech.com

Kathleen H Miller Phd, Partner
Jaime Oliva, Partner
Software that allows the user to dial an outgoing call directly from the computer, even with a single switch. Synthesized speech is sent through the phone line. The synthesizer then turns into a speaker phone enabling hands free, two way conversations. *$300.00*

1332 **Talking Screen**
Words+
42505 10th Street W
Suite 109
Lancaster, CA 93534
661-723-6523
800-869-8521
FAX: 661-723-2114
e-mail: info@words-plus.com
www.words-plus.com

Ginger Woltosz, Vice President
Tim Ross, Manager
Walt Wolosz, Manager
An augmentative communication program that allows the user to select graphic symbols on the display to produce speech output. Symbols can be used either singly or in sequence as picture abbreviations. *$ 1395.00*

1333 Turnkey Computer Systems for the Visually, Physically, and Hearing Impaired
E VA S
39 Canal Street
Westerly, RI 02891
401-596-3155
800-872-3827
FAX: 401-596-3979
e-mail: contact@evas.com
www.evas.com

Sara Swerdlick, Customer Service Manager
Gerald Swerdlick, Owner
Offers clear speech with pleasant inflection and tonal quality as well as variable pitch, intonation and voices.

1334 Voice-It
V XI Corporation Incorporated
1 Front Street
Rollinsford, NH 03869
603-742-2888
800-742-8588
FAX: 603-742-5065
e-mail: info@vxicorp.com
www.vxicorp.com

Richard Hale, President
Cheryl Keene, Senior Telecommunications Analys
Adds voice to popular spreadsheet and word processing applications on IBM PCs and compatibles, turning spreadsheets and word processing documents into talking documents.

1335 Window-Eyes
G W Micro
725 Airport North Office Park
Fort Wayne, IN 46825
260-489-3671
FAX: 260-489-2608
e-mail: sales@gwmicro.com
www.gwmicro.com

Daniel Weirich, Owner
Doug Geoffray, Owner
Provides access to available software automatically reading information important to the user while ignoring the rest. A screen reader for the windows operative system.

Software: Math

1336 AIMS Multimedia
Discovery Education
8145 Holton Drive
Florence, KY 41042
859-342-7200
FAX: 877-324-6830
e-mail: info@multimedia.com
www.aimsmultimedia.com

Mike Wright, Director
Lynn Fassett, Administrative Assistant
Cindy Vogt, Human Resources Executive
AIMS Multimedia is a leader in the production and distribution of trinaing and educational programs for the business and K-12 communities via YHS, interactive CD-ROM, DVD and Internet streaming video.

1337 Access to Math
Don Johnston
26799 W Commerce Drive
Volo, IL 60073
847-740-0749
800-999-4660
FAX: 847-740-7326
e-mail: info@donjohnston.com
www.donjohnston.com

Ruth Ziolkowski, President
This Macintosh Math Worksheet program is two products in one. For teachers, it makes customized worksheets in a snap. For students who struggle, it provides individualized on-screen lessons that contribute to success. *$79.00*

1338 Basic Math Competency Skill Building
Educational Activities Software
PO Box 754
Baldwin, NY 11510
516-867-7878
800-645-2796
FAX: 516-379-7429
e-mail: achieve@ea-software.com
www.ea-software.com

Alan Stern, Sales Director/Manager
Comprehensive MATH SKILLS software tutorials teach concepts ranging from rounding and tables to measuring area. MAC/WIN compatible. *$369.00*
Per Unit

1339 Basic Math: Detecting Special Needs
Allyn & Bacon
75 Arlington Street
Suite 300
Boston, MA 02116
617-848-6000
800-852-8024
FAX: 617-848-7490
www.adlongman.com

Thomas Longman, Founder
Describes special mathematics needs of special learners.
180 pages 1989
ISBN 0-205116-35-3

1340 Campaign Math
Mindplay
3130 N Dodge Boulevard
Tucson, AZ 85716
520-323-1303
800-221-7911
FAX: 520-322-0363
A complete program on the electoral process as well as a math package which teaches ratios, fractions and percentages.

1341 Fraction Factory
Queue
1450 Barnum Avenue
Suite 207
Bridgeport, CT 06610
203-335-0906
800-232-2224
FAX: 203-336-2481
e-mail: queueinc@aol.com
www.queueinc.com

1342 Information & Referral Services
Information + Referral Services
3130 N Dodge Boulevard
Tucson, AZ 85716
520-325-2111
800-632-3474
FAX: 520-323-2110
e-mail: inform@azinfo.org
www.azinfo.org

Leslie Ann Williams, Executive Director
Kim Millier, Vice President
Provides information about health and human services for people in Arizona over the telephone. Information specialists help callers clarify their needs, and provide referrals to the appropriate service agency.

1343 King's Rule
WINGS for Learning
1600 Green Hills Road
Scotts Valley, CA 95066
831-464-3600
FAX: 831-464-3600

Ani Stocks, Owner
A software mathematical problem solving game. Students discover mathematical rules as they work their way through a castle and generate and test a working hypothesis by asking questions.

1344 Learning About Numbers
C&C Software
5713 Kentford Circle
Wichita, KS 67220
316-683-6056
800-752-2086

Carol Clark, President
Three programs use the power of computer graphics to provide young children with a variety of experiences in working with numbers. *$50.00*

1345 **Math Rabbit**
Learning Company
100 Pine Street
Suite 1900
San Francisco, CA 94111
510-490-7311
800-825-4420
FAX: 408-263-3358
www.learningcompanyschool.com

Teaches early math concepts by matching objects to numbers, then adding and subtracting up to 18.

1346 **Math for Everyday Living**
Educational Activities Software
PO Box 754
Baldwin, NY 11510
516-867-7878
800-645-2796
FAX: 516-379-7429
e-mail: astearn@ea-software.com
www.ea-software.com

Alan Stern, Director of Sales
Real life math skills are taught with this tutorial and practice software program. Examples include Paying for a Meal (addition and subtraction), Working with Sales Slips (multiplication), Unit Pricing (division), Sales Tax (percent), Earning with Overtime (fractions) plus more. Software: CD-Rom, Windows, MAC, and DOS. *$159.00*

1347 **Math for Successful Living**
Siboney Learning Group
PO Box 220520
Saint Louis, MO 63122
314-909-1670
888-726-8100
FAX: 314-984-8063
e-mail: crichter@siboneylg.com
www.ea-software.com

Carrie Richter, Sales Coordinator
Bill Edwards, President
These programs include managing a checking account, budgeting, shopping strategies and buying on credit.

1348 **Optimum Resource Educational Software**
Optimum Resource
18 Hunter Road
Hilton Head Island, SC 29926
843-689-8000
FAX: 843-689-8008
e-mail: sticky@stickybear.com
www.stickybear.com

Chris Gintz, Chief Executive Officer
A complete topical curriculum of reading, math, keyboard skills and science programs that are age and skill specific. *$59.95*

1349 **Piece of Cake Math**
Queue Inc.
1 Control Drive
Shelton, CT 06484
203-446-8100
800-232-2224
FAX: 800-775-2729
e-mail: jdk@queueinc.com
www.queueinc.com

Jonathan Kantrowitz, Owner
Color, sound and animation combine forces in a program of five games focusing on basic mathematical operations.

1350 **Puzzle Tanks**
WINGS for Learning
1600 Green Hills Road
Scotts Valley, CA 95066
831-464-3600
FAX: 831-464-3600

Ani Stocks, Owner
A mathematical problem solving game that involves multi-step problems.

1351 **Right Turn**
WINGS for Learning
1600 Green Hills Road
Scotts Valley, CA 95066
831-464-3600
FAX: 831-464-3600

Ani Stocks, Owner
Requires students to predict, experiment and learn about the mathematical concepts of rotation and transformation.

1352 **RoboMath**
3130 N Dodge Boulevard
Tucson, AZ 85716
520-881-1794

Leslie Williams, Executive Director

1353 **Stickybear Math**
Optimum Resource
18 Hunter Road
Hilton Head Island, SC 29926
843-689-8000
FAX: 843-689-8008
e-mail: stickyb@stickybear.com
www.stickybear.com

Chris Gintz, Chief Executive Officer
Sharpen basic addition and subtraction skills with this captivating series of math exercises. *$59.95*

1354 **Stickybear Numbers**
Optimum Resource
18 Hunter Road
Hilton Head Island, SC 29926
843-689-8000
FAX: 843-689-8008
e-mail: sticky@stickybear.com
www.stickybear.com

Chris Gintz, Chief Executive Officer
Counting and number recognition are as easy as 1-2-3 with this award-winning program. *$59.95*

1355 **Stickybear Word Problems**
Optimum Resource
18 Hunter Road
Hilton Head Island, SC 29926
843-689-8000
FAX: 843-689-8008
e-mail: sticky@stickybear.com
www.stickybear.com

Chris Gintz, Chief Executive Officer
Hundreds of different word problems make it easy for students to practice basic math skills. *$59.95*

1356 **Stickybear's Math Splash**
Optimum Resource
18 Hunter Road
Hilton Head Island, SC 29926
843-689-8000
FAX: 843-689-8008
e-mail: sticky@stickybear.com
www.stickybear.com

Chris Gintz, Chief Executive Officer
Unique multiple activities keep the learning level high while children acquire skills in addition, subtraction, multiplication and division. *$59.95*

1357 **Stickybear's Math Town**
Optimum Resource
18 Hunter Road
Hilton Head Island, SC 29926
843-689-8000
FAX: 843-689-8008
e-mail: sticky@stickybear.com
www.stickybear.com

Chris Gintz, Chief Executive Officer
Children ages 5-10 gain proficiency in addition, subtraction, multiplication and division, as well as life skills and word problems. In English and Spanish, children sharpen skills both vertically and horizontally, clear crisp graphics and sound enable teachers to monitor and access skills and development. *$59.95*

1358 **Tomorrow's Promise: Mathematics**
Compass Learning
9920 Pacific Heights Boulevard
San Diego, CA 92121
858-587-0087
800-247-1380
FAX: 619-622-7873
www.compasslearning.com

Rajeev Turi, President

By integrating interdisciplinary content and real-world application of skills, this product emphasizes the practical value of fundamental math skills. It helps your students develop a problem-solving aptitude for ongoing mathematics achievement.

Software: Miscellaneous

1359 **Adventures in Musicland**
Electronic Courseware Systems
1713 S State Street
Champaign, IL 61820
217-359-7099
800-832-4965
FAX: 217-359-6578
e-mail: support@ecsmedia.com
www.ecsmedia.com

G Peters, President
Jodie Varner, Marketing Manager
This unique set of music games features characters from Lewis Carroll's, Alice in Wonderland. Players learn through pictures, sounds, and animation which help develop understanding of musical tones, composers, and musical symbols. Games include MusicMatch, Melody Mixup, Picture Perfect and Sound Concentration. *$49.95*

1360 **Ai Squared**
PO Box 669
Manchester Center, VT 05255
802-362-3612
800-859-0270
FAX: 802-362-1670
e-mail: zoomtext@aisquared.com
www.aisquared.com

Marilyn Petty, Director
Benjermin Weiss, President
Developers of software for the visually impaired.

1361 **All About You: Appropriate Special Interactions and Self-Esteem**
P CI Educational Publishing
PO Box 34270
San Antonio, TX 78265
210-377-1999
800-594-4263
FAX: 888-259-8284
www.pcicatalog.com

Jeff Clain, Chief Executive Officer
Janie McLane, Senior Vice President
This game offers parents and game players a new line of communication when discussing various issues such as learning to be thoughtful, respecting the rights and feelings of others, how to make and keep friends and more. *$49.95*

1362 **All Star Review**
Tom Snyder Productions
100 Talcott Avenue
6
Watertown, MA 02472
617-926-6000
800-342-0236
FAX: 800-304-1254
e-mail: ask@tomsnyder.com
www.tomsnyder.com

Rick Abrahams, Manager
This package turns group review into a baseball game for small and large groups.

1363 **Assistive Software Products**
Innovation Management Group
21350 Nordhuff Street
Suite 112
Chatsworth, CA 91311
818-701-1579
800-889-0987
FAX: 818-701-1581
e-mail: cs@imgpresents.com
www.imgpresents.com

Jerry Hussong, Vice President
IMG is the leading provider of programmable, infinitely sizeable, Onscreen Keyboards with Macro Panels, Text to Speech, Network Logon, and Word Prediction. CrossScanner adds switch scanning capabilities to Onscreen. Other products include: SmartClick for Hover and Dwell; Joystick-to-Mouse for Joystick/Game devices; and The Magnifier for screen magnification and cursor tracking.

1364 **At Home with Stickybear**
Optimum Resource
18 Hunter Road
Hilton Head Island, SC 29926
843-689-8000
FAX: 843-689-8008
e-mail: sticky@stickybear.com
www.stickybear.com

Chris Gintz, Chief Executive Officer
This dynamic new multifaceted program covers a wide range of preschool skills that go far beyond the strictly academic! At Stickybear's house, children discover the alphabet, numbers, shapes, colors; plus social skills, important safety messages and delightful off-screen activities that foster creativity. *$59.95*

1365 **Attainment Company**
I ET Resources
504 Commerce Parkway
PO Box 930160
Verona, WI 53593
608-845-7880
800-327-4269
FAX: 800-942-3865
e-mail: info@attainmentcompany.com
www.attainmentcompany.com

Brent Denu, Marketing Coordinator
Julie Denu, Technical Support
Theresa O'Connor, Office Manager
Augmentative/alternative communication, software, videos, print and hands-on materials for developmental and cognitive disabilities.

1366 **Attention Getter**
Soft Touch
4300 Stine Road
Suite 401
Bakersfield, CA 93313
661-396-8676
877-763-8868
FAX: 661-396-8760
e-mail: support @softtouch.com
www.funsoftware.com

Joyce Meyer, President
Roxanne Butterfield, Marketing
The whimsical photos morph to another photo and then to a third photo in categories. Paired with interesting sounds and music, the photo animations are so engaging that the student is motivated to activate the computer to see and hear the next one. This is a perfect vehicle to achieve goals aimed at attention getting, activating a switch or intentionality. Compatible with USB IntelliKeys keyboards.

1367 **Attention Teens**
Soft Touch
4300 Stine Road
Suite 401
Bakersfield, CA 93313
661-396-8676
877-763-8868
FAX: 661-396-8760
e-mail: support@softtouch.com
www.softtouch.com

Roxanne Butterfield, Marketing
Joyce Meyer, President
Attention Teens (formerly known as Loony Teens) is a program for teens with disabilities who need powerful input to get their attention. Attention Teens is a computer program to do just this. Paired with interesting sounds and music, the photo animations are so engaging that the student is motivated to activate the computer to see and hear the next one. Compatible with USB IntelliKeys keyboards.

1368 **Away We Ride**
Soft Touch
4300 Stine Road
Suite 401
Bakersfield, CA 93313
661-396-8676
877-763-8868
FAX: 661-396-8760
e-mail: support@softtouch.com
www.softtouch.com

Roxanne Butterfield, Marketing
Joyce Meyer, President
Software for children and teens. For Macintosh and PC.

1369 **Bailey's Book House**
Edmark Corporation
PO Box 97021
Redmond, WA 98073
425-556-8400
800-691-2986
www.edmark.com

Software for children.

1370 **Battenberg & Associates**
11135 Rolling Springs Drive
Carmel, IN 46033
317-843-2208

Offers various software programs that develop the user's visual memory, sequencing skills, word recognition, hand-eye coordination and more.

1371 **Behavior Skills: Learning How People Should Act**
Programming Concepts
PO Box 34270
San Antonio, TX 78265
210-377-1999
800-594-4263
FAX: 888-828-
www.pcieducation.com

Jeff Clain, Chief Executive Officer
Janie Haugen, Program Director
Helps players learn what behavior is acceptable and what behavior is not acceptable in the real world. *$49.95*

1372 **Blocks in Motion**
Don Johnston
26799 W Commerce Drive
Volo, IL 60073
847-740-0749
800-999-4660
FAX: 847-740-7326
e-mail: info@donjohnston.com
www.donjohnston.com

Ruth Ziolkowski, President
This unique art and motion program makes drawing, creating and animating fun and educational for all users. Based on the Piagetian Theory for motor-sensory development, this program promotes the concept that the process is as educational and as much fun as the end result. *$79.00*

1373 **CINTEX: Speak to Your Appliances**
NanoPac
4823 S Sheridan Road
Suite 302
Tulsa, OK 74145
918-665-0329
800-580-6086
FAX: 918-665-0361
e-mail: info@nanopac.com
www.nanopac.com

Silvio V Cianfrone CCSP, President
CINTEX, with a voice recognition program, will control up to 256 off/on appliances, dial and answer the phone, flash for call waiting, dial from a directory, control TV's, VCR's, stereos and more — all with your voice. CINTEX2 includes the necessary hardware and voice macros which you can use to immediately control your environment. You can tailor these macros to your personal needs and add new macros. Pops-up over current application allowing instant access. $695-$2,000.

1374 **Car Builder**
Optimum Resource
18 Hunter Road
Hilton Head Island, SC 29926
843-689-8000
FAX: 843-689-8008
e-mail: sticky@stickybear.com
www.stickybear.com

Chris Gintz, Chief Executive Officer
Richard Hefter, President
As design engineers, users build cars on screen, specifying chassis length, wheelbase, engine type, transmission, fuel tank size, suspension, steering, tires and brakes. All functional choices are interrelated and will affect the performance of the final design. *$ 59.99*

1375 **Center for Best Practices in Early Childhood**
32 Horrabin Hall
Macomb, IL 61455
309-298-1634
FAX: 309-298-2305
e-mail: l-robinson1@wiu.edu
www.wiu.edu/thecenter/

Linda Robinson, Assistant Director
A group of early childhood projects which focus on assistive technology for children ages birth to 8 with disabilities and their families. Services include technology training, curricula, books, software and online workshops.

1376 **Clock**
Compass Learning
203 Colorado Street
Austin, TX 78701
858-587-0087
800-247-1380
FAX: 619-622-7873
www.compasslearning.com

Rajeev Turi, President
An extremely simple, easy-to-use program for children who are learning how to read the time of day from clocks and digital displays. Apple and MS-DOS and Mac available. *$39.95*

1377 **Co:Writer**
Don Johnston
26799 W Commerce Drive
Volo, IL 60073
847-740-0749
800-999-4660
FAX: 847-740-7326
e-mail: info@donjohnston.com
www.donjohnston.com

Ketan Kothari, Chief Executive Officer
Ruth Ziolkowski, President
A writing description program that helps construct sentences. This is an easy-to-use, intelligent word prediction program that works in conjunction with any word processor or text application program to reduce the number of keystrokes necessary to complete an intended word or sentence. This invaluable program can help make the writing process easier, faster and even better for writers of all ages and ability levels. *$290.00*

1378 **Community Skills: Learning to Function in Your Neighborhood**
Programming Concepts
PO Box 34270
San Antonio, TX 78265
800-594-4263
FAX: 888-259-8284
e-mail: pciinfo@pcieducation.com
www.pcieducation.com

Janie Haugen, Program Director
Jeff McLean, President/CEO
Offers parents and educators a functional way to teach community life skills. *$49.95*

1379 **Companion Activities**
Soft Touch
4300 Stine Road
Suite 401
Bakersfield, CA 93313
661-396-8676
877-763-8868
FAX: 661-396-8760
e-mail: support@softtouch.com
www.softouch.com

Joyce Meyer, President
Roxanne Butterfield, Marketing
Print your own books, worksheets, flash cards, board games, matching games, bingo games, card games and many more. This CD offers numerous companion activities to different SoftTouch software titles. Activities range from very easy to difficult. Companion activities are great tools to reinforce learning. Use the work sheets - black and white and color - in the inclusion class for students with special needs.

1380 **Concepts on the Move Advanced Preacademics**
Soft Touch
4300 Stine Road
Suite 401
Bakersfield, CA 93313
661-396-8676
877-763-8868
FAX: 661-396-8760
e-mail: softtouch@funsoftware.com
www.funsoftware.com

Roxanne Butterfield, Marketing
Joyce Meyer, President
Choose from five concepts groups: categories, occupations, functions, goes with and prepositions. Use our Steps to Learning Design to choose how many concepts to present at one time and where to place each one in the scan array, on screen keyboard or IntelliKeys keyboard. Watch and listen as the concept morphs or changes and music plays. The words are also shown to reinforce emerging literacy skills. Compatible with USB IntelliKeys.

1381 **Cooking Class: Learning About Food Preparation**
Programming Concepts
PO Box B
San Antonio, TX 78265
800-594-4263
FAX: 218-480-5
e-mail: tciinfo@tcieducatio.com
www.tcieducation.com

Janie Haugen, Program Director
Jeff McLane, President/CEO
This game offers parents and educators a new way to teach basic preparation skills. Kitchen safety and sanitation are stressed throughout the game. *$49.95*

1382 **Dilemma**
Educational Activities Software
PO Box 754
Baldwin, NY 11510
516-867-7878
800-645-2796
FAX: 516-379-7429
e-mail: achieve@ea-software.com

Alan Stern, Sales Director/Manager
Realistic stories with a choice of different gripping endings, color graphics, a built-in dictionary and a user controlled reading rate make these computer programs compelling enough to interest all students. Comprehension and vocabulary questions follow each story. *$159.00*

1383 **Dino-Games**
Academic Software
331 W 2nd Street
Lexington, KY 40507
859-233-2332
800-842-2357
FAX: 859-231-0725

Warren E Lacefield PhD, President
Penelope Ellis, Marketing Director
Dino-Games are single switch software programs for early switch practice. Dinosaur games provide practice in pattern recognition, cause and effect demonstration, directionality training, number concepts and problem solving. They are compatible with most popular switch interfaces and alternate keyboards. For Macintosh, IBM and compatibles. DINO-LINK is a matching game; DINO-MAZE is a series of maze games; DINO-FIND is a game of concentration; and DINO-DOT is a collection of dot-to-dot games.

$39.95 per game

1384 **Directions: Technology in Special Education**
DREAMMS for Kids
273 Ringwood Road
Freeville, NY 13068
607-539-3027
FAX: 607-539-9930
www.dreamms.org
A CD containing all of 'Directions' past articles and information gathered from their newsletter which lists resources for assistive and adaptive computer tehnologies in the home, school and community. *$24.95*

1385 **ESI Master Resource Guide**
Educational Software Institute
4213 S 94th Street
Omaha, NE 68127
402-592-3300
800-955-5570
FAX: 402-592-2017
e-mail: info@edsoft.com
www.edsoft.com

Lee Myers, President
Kathy Cavanaugh, Catalog Manager
Educational Software Institute (ESI) provides a one-stop shop to purchase software titles by all of the best publishers. The ESI Master Gold Book catalog and CD-ROM represents more than 400 software publishers, with information on more than 8,000 software titles. Take the confusion out of software selection by calling ESI for all of your software needs - including competitive prices, software previews, knowledgeable assistance, and the largest selection available all in one place.
Yearly

1386 **EZ Keys**
Words+
42505 10th Street W
Suite 109
Lancaster, CA 93534
661-266-5800
800-869-8521
FAX: 661-266-8969
e-mail: info@words-plus.com
www.words-plus.com

Ginger Woltosz, Vice President
Tim Ross, Manager
A software and hardware product designed to operate on an IBM compatible PC. The software provides dual word prediction, abbreviation expansion, five different methods of voice output and access to commercial software applications. *$1395.00*

1387 **Early Games for Young Children**
Queue Incorporated
1 Control Drive
Shelton, CT 06484
203-446-8100
800-232-2224
FAX: 800-775-2729
e-mail: jdk@queueinc.com
www.queueinc.com

Jonathan Kantrowitz, Owner
Software that includes nine activities that entertain preschoolers in honing basic math and language skills.

1388 **Early Music Skills**
Electronic Courseware Systems
1713 S State Street
Champaign, IL 61820
217-359-7099
800-832-4965
FAX: 217-359-6578
e-mail: support@ecsmedia.com
www.ecsmedia.com

G Peters, President
Jodie Varner, Marketing Manager
A tutorial and drill program designed for the beginning music student. It covers four basic music reading skills: recognition of line and space notes; comprehension of the numbering system for the musical staff; visual and aural identification of notes moving up and down; and recognition of notes stepping and skipping up and down. *$ 39.95*

1389 Eating Skills: Learning Basic Table Manners
P CI Education Publishing
PO Box 34270
San Antonio, TX 78265
210-377-1999
800-594-4263
FAX: 210-377-1121
e-mail: pciinfo@pcieducation.com
www.pcieducation.com

Janie Haugen, Program Director
Jeff Clain, Chief Executive Officer
Offers parents and educators a functional way to teach and reinforce basic table manners. *$49.95*

1390 Electronic Courseware Systems
1713 S State Street
Champaign, IL 61820
217-359-7099
800-832-4965
FAX: 217-359-6578
e-mail: sales@ecsmedia.com
www.ecsmedia.com

Jodie Varner, Manager
G Peters, President
Offers a complete library of instructional software for music, math, science and social studies.

1391 Fall Fun
Soft Touch
4300 Stine Road
Suite 401
Bakersfield, CA 93313
661-396-8676
877-763-8868
FAX: 661-396-8760
e-mail: softtouch@fsofttouch.com
www.softtouch.com

Joyce Meyer, President
Roxanne Butterfield, Marketing
Your students can begin their day with the Pledge of Allegiance, Pumpkins, Owls, and Cats. Witches adorn Five Pumpkins Sitting on the Gate. Five Fat Turkeys out smart the pilgrims with song and antics. The owl and cat have songs of their own. A variety of activities reinforce concepts such as short, tall, first, second, third, same and different. Fall Fun includes cause and effect and easy to more difficult levels. Eight songs in all.

1392 Five Green & Speckled Frogs
Soft Touch
4300 Stine Road
Suite 401
Bakersfield, CA 93313
661-396-8676
877-763-8868
FAX: 661-396-8760
e-mail: softtouch@softtouch.com
www.softtouch.com

Roxanne Butterfield, Marketing
Joyce Meyer, President
Laugh, learn and sing with Five Humorous Frogs. Activities start with cause and effect and progress to teach directionality and simple subtraction. This classic song makes learning numbers and number worlds easy. Selections can be set to 2, 3, 4, 5, or 6 on-screen choices. Two games are included. One teaches direction on a number line. If the child moves the frog in the correct direction, the frog gets a point. The other game teaches beginning subtraction.

1393 Free and User Supported Software for the IBM PC: A Resource Guide
McFarland & Company
960 NC Highway 88 W
PO Box 677
Jefferson, NC 28640
336-246-4460
800-253-2187
FAX: 336-246-5018
e-mail: info@mcfarlandpub.com
www.mcfarlandpub.com
A selection of word processing, database management, spreadsheets, and graphics programs are described and evaluated. Describes how the program works and its strengths and weaknesses. Rating charts cover such aspects as ease of use, ease of learning, documentation, and general utility. *$27.50*
224 pages Paperback
ISBN 0-89950 -99-0

1394 GoalView: Special Education and RTI Studen t Management Information System.
Learning Tools International
2391 Circadian Way
Santa Rosa, CA 95407
707-521-3530
800-333-9954
FAX: 707-521-3531
e-mail: info@goalview.com
www.goalview.com

Cathy Zier, President/CEO
Katherine Del Carlo, National Sales Manager
An Web Based information system for students, educators and parents that enables accountability and achievement tracking; prepares IDEA compliant IEP's in minutes; provides over 250,000 education standards and special education goals and objectives in English and Spanish; generates Federal compliance reports; and creates IDEA GoalCard progress reports for students, schools and districts for every reporting period.

1395 HELP
V OR T Corporation
PO Box 60132
Palo Alto, CA 94306
650-322-8282
888-757-VORT
FAX: 650-327-0747
e-mail: sales@vort.com
www.vort.com

Tom Holt, Founder/Owner
A software version of HELP, covers over 650 skills in 6 developmental areas; cognitive, motor skills, language, gross motor, social and self-help.

1396 Handbook of Adaptive Switches and Augmentative Communication Devices
Academic Software
331 W 2nd Street
Lexington, KY 40507
859-233-2332
800-842-2357
FAX: 859-231-0725

Warren E Lacefield PhD, President/Author
Penelope Ellis, Marketing Director
Cindy L George, Author
This second edition contains physical descriptions and laboratory test data for a variety of commercially available pressure switches and augmentative communication devices and chapters on physical interaction, seating and positioning, and control access. It is an essential tool for assistive technology professionals and therapists who make decisions concerning physical access. *$60.00*
300 pages Hardcover

1397 HandiWARE
Microsystems Software
600 Worcester Road
Framingham, MA 01702
508-626-8511
800-828-2600
FAX: 508-879-1069
e-mail: infor@microsys.com
www.handiware.com

Terri McGrath, Sales/Marketing
Bill Kilroy, Product Manager
Adapted access software, assists persons with physical, hearing and visual impairments in accessing computers running DOS and Windows. HandiWARE is a suite of 8 software programs which provide users with screen magnification, alternate keyboard access, word prediction, augmentative communication, hands free telephone access, a visual beep. $20.00-$595.00.

1398 How to Write for Everyday Living
Educational Activities Software
PO Box 754
Baldwin, NY 11510
516-867-7878
800-645-2796
FAX: 516-379-7429
e-mail: achieve@ea-software.com

Alan Stern, Manager

An individualized Life Skills WRITING Software program emphasizing the reading, writing, communication and reference skills needed for real-life tasks: preparing a resume, an employment form, a business letter and envelope, a learner's permit, a social security application and banking forms. *$159.00*

1399 I KNOW American History
Soft Touch
4300 Stine Road
Suite 401
Bakersfield, CA 93313
661-396-8676
877-763-8868
FAX: 661-396-8760
e-mail: support@softtouch.com
www.softtouch.com

Joyce Meyer, President
Roxanne Butterfield, Marketing
The new I KNOW programs is the way students practice attending, choice making and turn-taking while uncovering learning puzzles. Each press reveals more of the image while the narrator reads the text on the screen. Offers three levels of language: short phrases, short sentences and longer sentences to match the student's learning level. Choose from the five topic areas: American Symbols, Westward Movement, Early Colonial Americans, Industrial Revolution and Biographies.

1400 I KNOW American History Overlay CD
Soft Touch
4300 Stine Road
Suite 401
Bakersfield, CA 93313
661-396-8676
877-763-8868
FAX: 661-396-8760
e-mail: softouch@softouch.com
www.softtouch.com

Roxanne Butterfield, Marketing
Joyce Meyer, President
Use this Overlay CD with I KNOW American History program. Includes standard overlays and SoftTouch's changeable overlays. Includes Overlay Printer by IntelliTools. Use Overlay Maker by IntelliTools (not included) to modify the overlays or to make additional learning materials.

1401 IntelliPics Studio 3
Intelli Tools
1720 Corporate Circle
Petaluma, CA 94954
707-773-2000
800-899-6687
FAX: 707-773-2001
e-mail: info@intellitools.com
www.intellitools.com

Beth Davis, Director Sales & Operations
Lori Castle, Supervisor
Arjan Khalsa, Chief Executive Officer
Multimedia authoring tool for both students and teachers to create activities, games, quizzes, slide shows, reports and presentations. *$395.00*

1402 KIDS (Keyboard Introductory Development Series)
Electronic Courseware Systems
1713 S State Street
Champaign, IL 61820
217-359-7099
800-832-4965
FAX: 217-359-6578
e-mail: sales@ecsmedia.com
www.ecsmedia.com

G Peters, President
Jodie Varner, Marketing Manager
A four disk series for the very young. Zoo Puppet Theater reinforces learning correct finger numbers for piano playing; Race Car Keys teaches keyboard geography by recognizing syllables or note names; Dinosaurs Lunch teaches placement of the notes on the treble staff; and Follow Me asks the student to play notes that have been presented aurally. *$49.95*

1403 Katie's Farm
Lawrence Productions
1800 S 53th Street
Galesburg, MI 49053
269-665-7075
800-421-4157
FAX: 269-665-7060
e-mail: sales@lpi.com
www.lpi.com

John W Lawrence, Chairman/Owner
Software for children ages four through eight.

1404 Keyboard Tutor, Music Software
Electronic Courseware Systems
1713 S State Street
Champaign, IL 61820
217-359-7099
800-832-4965
FAX: 217-359-6578
e-mail: sales@ecsmedia.com
www.ecsmedia.com

G Peters, President
Jodie Varner, Marketing Manager
Presents exercises for learning elementary keyboard skills including knowledge of names of the keys, piano keys matched to notes, notes matched to piano keys, whole steps and half steps. Each lesson allows unlimited practice of the skills. The program may be used with or without a midi keyboard attached to the computer. *$39.95*

1405 Keyboarding by Ability
Teachers Institute for Special Education
9933 NW 45th Street
Sunrise, FL 33351
954-235-7940
FAX: 866-843-0765
e-mail: tise@special-education-soft.com
www.special-education-soft.com

Gary Byowitz, Director
Allows the learning diabled or dyslexic student to acquire keyboarding skills through visually cued alphabetical approach designed and tested to meet the specific learning style needs of this unique population at every grade level. Package contains: IBM software, a set of lesson plans and instructional goals; supplamental graded data input exercises. *$148.95*

1406 Keyboarding for the Physically Handicapped
Teachers Institute for Special Education
4 Gabalin Court
Huntington Station, NY 11746
631-549-1715
FAX: 516-549-1715
e-mail: jackheller@aol.com
www.users.aol.com/jackheller

Jack Heller, Director/Owner
Customed designed touch typing programs for any student. A person needs order by the number of usable fingers on each hand (not counting the thumb), and whether or not a one finger or a head-pointer edition is wanted. Package includes IBM software; a complete set of lesson plans and instructional goals. *$149.95*

1407 Keyboarding with One Hand
Teachers Institute for Special Education
PO Box 2300
Wantagh, NY 11793
FAX: 516-781-4070
e-mail: jackheller@aol.com
www.users.aol.com/jackheller

Jack Heller, Director
This 22 lesson tutorial developed through 25 years of research, testing and teaching allows a student with one hand to aqure employable keyboarding skills using a touch system designed for the standard IBM PC keyboard. *$79.95*

1408 LPDOS Deluxe
Optelec U S
3030 Enterprise Court
Suite C
Vista, CA 92081
800-828-1056
FAX: 978-692-6073
e-mail: chrish@optelec.com
www.optelec.com

Annette Z Fasnacht, President
Robert Auger, General Manager
Large print software programs. *$595.00*

1409 Large Print DOS
Optelec U S
PO Box 796
Westford, MA 01886
978-692-9496
800-828-1056
FAX: 978-692-6073
www.optelec.com

Annette Fasnacht, President
James Bailey, Vice President

1410 Laureate Learning Systems
110 E Spring Street
Winooski, VT 05404
802-655-4755
800-562-6801
FAX: 802-655-4757
e-mail: info@llsys.com
www.laureatelearning.com

Michelle L Oakes, Administrative Assistant
Kathy Hollandsworth, Office Manager
Mary Wilson, Owner
Laureate publishes award-winning talking software for children and adults with disabilities. Programs cover cause and effect, language development, cognitive processing, and reading. High-quality speech, colorful graphics and amusing animation make learning fun. Accessible with touchscreen, single switch, keyboard and mouse. No reading required. Available on a hybrid CD-ROM for Windows and Macintosh. Visit our website for more information or call for a free catalog.

1411 Learning Company
222 3rd Avenue SE
Suite 400
Cedar Rapids, IA 52401
319-395-9626
888-242-6747
FAX: 319-395-0217
www.learningcompany.com

Barry O'Callaghan, Chief Executive Officer
Simon Calver, Chief Operating Officer
Software for children. For Macintosh or Windows (3.1 DOS or Windows 95, Windows 98 required).

1412 Little Red Hen
Compass Learning
9920 Pacific Heights Boulevard
San Diego, CA 92121
858-587-0087
800-247-1380
FAX: 619-622-7873
www.compasslearning.com

Rajeev Paulate, President
Eric Loeffel, Executive Vice President/COO
Children learn about the rewards of hard work when they discover who the Little Red Hen's friends miss out on freshly baked bread. Puzzles, rhymes, story writing and other interactive exercises enhance the creative learning process. *$34.95*

1413 Looking Good: Learning to Improve Your Appearance
Programming Concepts
PO Box 12428
San Antonio, TX 78212
800-594-4263
FAX: 218-480-5

Janie Haugen, Program Director
Jeff Mclane, President/CEO
This game offers a creative way to discuss all areas of grooming. *$49.95*

1414 Monkeys Jumping on the Bed
Soft Touch
4300 Stine Road
Suite 401
Bakersfield, CA 93313
661-396-8676
877-763-8868
FAX: 661-396-8760
e-mail: support@softtouch.com
www.softouch.com

Roxanne Butterfield, Marketing
Joyce Meyer, President
This program combines a favorite preschool song with number and color activities. Children and adults will enjoy engaging music and delightful animation. Students with cognitive delays respond to upbeat music and interesting sounds. Large graphics help learners focus on the action. Several important concepts are presented in enjoyable activity formats. Students learn cause and effect in Let's Play and Just for Fun.

1415 Morse Code WSKE
Words+
42505 10th Street W
Suite 109
Lancaster, CA 93534
661-723-6523
800-869-8521
FAX: 661-266-8969
e-mail: info@words-plus.com
www.words-plus.com

Ginger Woltosz, Vice President
Walt Wolosz, Manager
A software and hardware product designed to operate on an IBM compatible PC.

1416 Multi-Scan Single Switch Activity Center
Academic Software
331 W 2nd Street
Lexington, KY 40507
859-233-2332
800-842-2357
FAX: 859-231-0725

Warren E Lacefield PhD, President
Penelope Ellis, Marketing Director
A single switch activity center containing four educational games: Match, Maze, Dot-to-Dot, and Concentration, along with six graphics libraries; Dinosaurs, Sports, Animals, Independent Living, Vocations, and Cosmetology. MULTI-SCAN allows you to select a graphic library, choose games for each user, and adjust the difficulty level and other settings for each game. Other features allow you to save the game setups under each user's name and print out individual performance reports after sessions. *$154.00*

1417 Muppet Learning Keys
WINGS for Learning
1600 Green Hills Road
Scotts Valley, CA 95066
831-464-3600
FAX: 831-464-3600

Ani Stocks, Owner
Designed to introduce children to the world of the computer as they become familiar with letters, numbers and colors.

1418 My Own Pain
Soft Touch
4300 Stine Road
Suite 401
Bakersfield, CA 93313
661-396-8676
877-763-8868
FAX: 661-396-8760
www.softtouch.com

Roxanne Butterfield, Marketing Director
Joyce Meyer, President
Three activities - three levels. Press the switch and the paint brush chooses the color and paints the vehicle. Music reinforces the sounds when the picture is complete. A second activity allows the student to choose the color and paint the vehicle parts any color he or she wants. The third activity is a blueprint. Print the color that matches the one in the wire drawing. Color the drawing to complete the picture.

1419 Old MacDonald's Farm Deluxe
Soft Touch
4300 Stine Road
Suite 401
Bakersfield, CA 93313
661-396-8676
877-763-8868
FAX: 661-396-8760
e-mail: support@softtouch.com
www.softtouch.com

Roxanne Butterfield, Marketing
Joyce Meyer, President

Toddlers, preschoolers and early elementary students will be entertained and captivated by the six major activities and animations in the delightful program. Includes 18 real animation images or 9 cartoon like characters. The teacher or child can choose which animals they want to sing about. Some activities are designed for children within the normal population, others are designed for students with moderate and severe disabilities.

1420 **Please Understand Me: Software Program and Books**
Cambridge Educational
PO Box 931
Monmouth Junction, NJ 08852
609-671-1000
800-468-4227
FAX: 800-329-6687
e-mail: stesrv@films.com
www.cambridgeeducational.com

Promotes self-understanding while helping each student understand they are different from others. *$69.00*

209 pages BiAnnual
ISBN 0-927368-56-x

1421 **Pond**
WINGS for Learning
1600 Green Hills Road
Scotts Valley, CA 95066
831-464-3600
FAX: 831-464-3600

Ani Stocks, Owner
Software game that teaches pattern recognition and encourages observation, trial and error and the interpretation of data.

1422 **Print, Play & Learn #1 Old Mac's Farm**
Soft Touch Incorporated
4300 Stine Road
Suite 401
Bakersfield, CA 93313
661-396-8676
877-763-8868
FAX: 661-396-8760
e-mail: softtouch@software.com
www.softtouch.com

Roxanne Butterfield, Marketing Director
Joyce Meyer, President
Once your students have completed Old Mac's Farm, let them use the fun off-computer activities to continue learning. Over 25 activites with 250 sheets you print. Board games, dot-to-dot drawings, word puzzles, make a scene, flash cards. Concentration, sentence strips, worksheets and much more are availablefor techers to expand their teaching goals. This CD is full of activites to print and use.

1423 **Print, Play & Learn #7: Sampler**
Soft Touch
4300 Stine Road
Suite 401
Bakersfield, CA 93313
661-396-8676
877-763-8868
FAX: 661-396-8760
e-mail: support@softtouch.com
www.softtouch.com

Roxanne Butterfield, Marketing
Joyce Meyer, President
Print, Play and Learn Sampler gives you over 200 activites organized by training, easy, medium and hard levels so you can ready to help your student advance. Activites cover a wide range of basic knowledge, including colors, shapes, numbers, letters and much, much more. Note: Requires Overlay Maker or Overlay Printer by IntelliTools and a color printer.

1424 **Puzzle Power: Sampler**
Soft Touch
4300 Stine Road
Suite 401
Bakersfield, CA 93313
661-396-8676
877-763-8868
FAX: 661-396-8760
e-mail: support@softtouch.com
www.funsoftware.com

Joyce Meyer, President
Roxanne Butterfield, Marketing
Puzzle Power - Sampler offers a variety of puzzles in different themes. Each theme puzzle is followed by a puzzle of one item in this category. For example, first solve a puzzle for occupations. Then, solve a puzzle that is a baker. The pictures are large, clear and easily identifiable.

1425 **Puzzle Power: Zoo & School Days**
Soft Touch
4300 Stine Road
Suite 401
Bakersfield, CA 93313
661-396-8676
877-763-8868
FAX: 661-396-8760
e-mail: support@softtouch.com
www.softtouch.com

Roxanne Butterfield, Marketing Director
Joyce Meyer, President
Here is a program for all of our students who need puzzle skills, but cannot access commercial puzzles. Puzzle Power puzzles start with just two pieces and progress to 16 pieces. The pictures are large, clear and easily identifiable. Four different activites enable all students to be successful. Automatic Placement: the student just presses the switch or keyboard to place the pieces. Magnet Mouse: all the student needs to do is move the mouse and it drops into place.

1426 **Rodeo**
Soft Touch
4300 Stine Road
Suite 401
Bakersfield, CA 93313
661-396-8676
877-763-8868
FAX: 661-396-8760
e-mail: softtouch@funsoftware.com
www.funsoftware.com

Roxanne Butterfield, Marketing
Joyce Meyer, President
Rodeo action and familiar tunes for teens and preteens. Four activities invite students to learn, laugh, and sing as they go to the rodeo with up to six age-peer friends. Age-appropriate graphics with surprising animations reinforce the learning. The graphics are large and coorful, the melodies familiar, and the words descriptive of the action on the screen.

1427 **Shop Til You Drop**
Soft Touch
4300 Stine Road
Suite 401
Bakersfield, CA 93313
661-396-8676
877-763-8868
FAX: 661-396-8760
e-mail: softtouch@softtouch.com
www.softtouch.com

Roxanne Butterfield, Marketing
Joyce Meyer, President
Designed specifically for preteens and teens with moderate and severe disabilities, this program will become a staple for the classroom. The student goes shopping and can choose which outfits to put together. They may choose to purchase the outfit - of course, with mom's credit card. Another activity is a video arcade game about money. Shop 'Til You Drop can be adjusted from a single switch cause-and-effect program to row-and-column scanning to direct choice.

1428 **Songs I Sing at Preschool**
Soft Touch
4300 Stine Road
Suite 401
Bakersfield, CA 93313
661-396-8676
877-763-8868
FAX: 661-396-8760
e-mail: softtouch@funsoftware.com
www.funsoftware.com

Roxanne Butterfield, Marketing
Joyce Meyer, President
Songs I Sing at Preschool offers many options for the teacher and the student. Over the years, our software has used music because our students really respond to the sounds and rhythms of songs. Teachers select which songs to present, how many to present at one time and where to place each song on the overlay, keyboard or scan array.

1429 Stickybear Town Builder
Optimum Resource
18 Hunter Road
Hilton Head Island, SC 29926
843-689-8000
FAX: 843-689-8008
e-mail: stickyb@stickybear.com
www.stickybear.com

Chris Gintz, Chief Executive Officer
Children learn to read maps, build towns, take trips and use a compass in this simulation program. *$59.95*

1430 Stickybear Typing
Optimum Resource
18 Hunter Road
Hilton Head Island, SC 29926
843-689-8000
FAX: 843-689-8008
e-mail: stickyb@stickybear.com
www.stickybear.com

Chris Gintz, Chief Executive Officer
Sharpen typing skills with three challenging activities: Stickybear Keypress, Stickybear Thump and Stickybear Stories. *$59.95*

1431 Stickybear's Early Learning Activities
Optimum Resource
18 Hunter Road
Hilton Head Island, SC 29926
843-689-8000
FAX: 843-689-8008
e-mail: sticky@stickybear.com
www.stickybear.com

Chris Gintz, Chief Executive Officer
Two modes of play, structure and non-structured, allow youngsters to learn through prompted direction or by the discovery method. Lively animation and sound keep attention levels high and Stickybear's Early Learning Activities is bilingual, so youngsters can build skills in both English and Spanish. *$59.95*

1432 Stickybear's Kindergarden Activities
Optimum Resource
18 Hunter Road
Hilton Head Island, SC 29926
843-689-8000
FAX: 843-689-8008
e-mail: sticky@stickybear.com
www.stickybear.com

Chris Gintz, Chief Executive Officer
This dynamic new multifaceted program covers a wide range of preschool skills that go far beyond the stricktly academic! At Stickybear's house, children discover the alphabet, numbers, shapes, colors, plus - social skills, important safety messages and delightful off-screen activities that foster creativity. Over three hours of original music can be compose by a chid and saved for future use. *$59.95*

1433 Stickybear's Science Fair: Light
Optimum Resource
18 Hunter Road
Hilton Head Island, SC 29926
843-689-8000
FAX: 843-689-8008
e-mail: stickyb@stickybear.com
www.stickybear.com

Chris Gintz, Chief Executive Officer
The first in the new series of science-based programs Stickybear Science Fair: Light presents a content rich environment which allows students, ages 7-12 to explore, experiment with and understand light and it's properties. The program presents experiments, both structured and free-form, which allow users to work with prisms, lenses, color mixing, optical illusions and more. *$59.95*

1434 Storybook Maker Deluxe
Compass Learning
Evening Creek Drive N
Suite 200
San Diego, CA 92128
858-587-0087
800-247-1380
FAX: 619-622-7873
www.compasslearning.com

Rajeev Puri, President
Eric Loeffel, Chief Operating Officer
Martin Kenney Jr, Chief Executive Officer
Using Storybook Maker Deluxe and their imaginations, students can create and publish stories filled with exciting graphics. Students can write stories and watch as the text appears in the setting they've chosen. Engaging sounds and music, plus lively animations, provide positive learning reinforcement throughout the program. *$44.95*

1435 Super Challenger
Electronic Courseware Systems
1713 S State Street
Champaign, IL 61820
217-359-7099
800-832-4965
FAX: 217-359-6578
e-mail: support@ecsmedia.com
www.ecsmedia.com

Jodie Varner, Manager
G Peters, President
An aural-visual musical game that increases the player's ability to remember a series of pitches as they are played by the computer. The game is based on a 12-note chromatic scale, a major scale, and a minor scale. Each pitch is reinforced visually with a color representation of a keyboard on the display screen. Computer/software. *$39.95*

1436 Switch Basics
Soft Touch
4300 Stine Road
Suite 401
Bakersfield, CA 93313
661-396-8676
877-763-8868
FAX: 661-396-8760
e-mail: softtouch@funsoftware.com
www.funsoftware.com

Roxanne Butterfield, Marketing Director
Joyce Meyer, President
Discover whimsical animations and real life pictures while learning switch operations. Intriguing and humorous, nine different programs offer a multitude of learning experiences for all ages. Program options include: cause and effect, scanning, step scanning, row and column activites for one or two players. Watch the clouds roll away revealing African animals; visit the beauty salon or barber shop; work two to sixteen piece puzzles; or add swimming fish to a huge aquarium.

1437 Teach Me Phonemics Series Bundle
Soft Touch
4300 Stine Road
Suite 401
Bakersfield, CA 93313
661-396-8676
877-763-8868
FAX: 661-396-8760
e-mail: support@softtouch.com
www.funsoftware.com

Joyce Meyer, President
Roxanne Butterfield, Marketing
The Teach Me Phonemics Series Bundle includes one copy of each Teach Me Phonemics program - Initial, Medial, Final and Blends - four CD's in all.

1438 Teach Me Phonemics Super Bundle
Soft Touch
4300 Stine Road
Suite 401
Bakersfield, CA 93313
661-396-8676
877-763-8868
FAX: 661-396-8760
e-mail: softtouch@funsoftware.com
www.funsoftware.com

Roxanne Butterfield, Marketing
Joyce Meyer, President
Teach Me Phonemics Super Bundle includes all 4 Teach Me Phonemics programs and all 4 Teach Me Phonemics overlay CD's - eight CD's in all.

1439 Teach Me Phonemics: Blends
Soft Touch
4300 Stine Road
Suite 401
Bakersfield, CA 93313
661-396-8676
877-763-8868
FAX: 661-396-8760
e-mail: softtouch@funsoftware.com
www.funsoftware.com

Roxanne Butterfield, Marketing
Joyce Meyer, President
Teach Me Phonemics - Blends helps students explore words and hear the initial blend sounds. It features musical interludes and movement to engage the student. Teachers select the best combination options to motivate and engage the student. Options turn off and on the fly so you can quickly make changes to keep the student engaged.

1440 Teach Me Phonemics: Final
Soft Touch
4300 Stine Road
Suite 401
Bakersfield, CA 93313
661-396-8676
877-763-8868
FAX: 661-396-8760
e-mail: softtouch@funsoftware.com
www.funsoftware.com

Roxanne Butterfield
Joyce Meyer, President
Teach me Phonemics - Final helps students explore words and hear the final sounds. It features musical interludes and movement to engage the student. Options turn off and on the fly so you can quickly make changes to keep the student engaged.

1441 Teach Me Phonemics: Initial
Soft Touch
4300 Stine Road
Suite 401
Bakersfield, CA 93313
661-396-8676
877-763-8868
FAX: 661-396-8760
e-mail: softtouch@softtouch.com
www.softtouch.com

Roxanne Butterfield, Marketing
Joyce Meyer, President
Teach Me Phonemics - Initial helps students explore the words and hear the initial sounds. It features musical interludes and movement to engage the student. Teachers select the best combination options to motivate and engage the student. Options turn off and on the fly so you can quickly make changes to keep the student engaged.

1442 Teach Me Phonemics: Medial
Soft Touch
4300 Stine Road
Suite 401
Bakersfield, CA 93313
661-396-8676
877-763-8868
FAX: 661-396-8760
e-mail: softtouch@softtouch.com
www.softtouch.com

Roxanne Butterfield, Marketing
Joyce Meyer, President
Teach Me Phonemics - Medial helps students explore the words and hear the medial sounds. It features musical interludes and movement to engage the student. Teachers select the best combination options to motivate and engage the student. Options turn off and on the fly so you can quickly make changes to keep the student engaged.

1443 Teach Me to Talk
Soft Touch
4300 Stine Road
Suite 401
Bakersfield, CA 93313
661-396-8676
877-763-8868
FAX: 661-396-8760
e-mail: softtouch@softtouch.com
www.softtouch.com

Roxanne Butterfield, Marketing
Joyce Meyer, President
The first activity Teach Me to Talk is used as a springboard for the student to learn to speak the word. There are 150 real pictures. When a picture is chosen, it appears on a clear background with musical interludes, movement, written word and spoken word. It culminates by morphing to the corresponding black and white Mayer-Johnson symbol. The second activity Story Time, takes some of these nouns and puts them in four line poetry. This helps students hear the word in the midst of a sentence.

1444 Teen Tunes Plus
Soft Touch
4300 Stine Road
Suite 401
Bakersfield, CA 93313
661-396-8676
877-763-8868
FAX: 661-396-8760
e-mail: softtouch@softtouch.com
www.funsoftware.com

Joyce Meyer, President
Roxanne Butterfield, Marketing
Introduce switch use to older students with disabilities. Large intersting graphics, a variety of musical interludes, and surprising animations are combined with calm soothing music and beautiful pictures in the software specifically designed for preteens and teens with severe cognitive delays and/or physical disabilities, and older students learning to use a switch.

1445 There are Tyrannosaurs Trying on Pants in My Bedroom
Compass Learning
203 Colorado Street
Austin, TX 78701
858-587-0087
800-247-1380
FAX: 619-622-7873
www.compasslearning.com

Rajeev Puri, President
Eric Loeffel, Executive Vice President
In this popular story, Saturday chores turn into fun-filled frolicking when dinosaurs come for a visit. Sounds, music and animation make learning about phonics and vocabulary dyno-mite. *$34.95*

1446 Three Billy Goats Gruff
Compass Learning
203 Colorado Street
Austin, TX 78701
858-587-0087
800-247-1380
FAX: 619-622-7873
www.compasslearning.com

Rajeev Puri, President
Eric Loeffer, Executive Vice President/ OO
Motivating exercises and creative activities provide hours of learning fun while young students follow the adventure of The Three Billy Goats Gruff in this animated version of the timeless tale. *$ 34.95*

1447 Three Little Pigs
Compass Learning
203 Colorado Street
Austin, TX 78701
858-587-0087
800-247-1380
FAX: 619-622-7873
www.compasslearning.com

Rajeev Puri, President
Eric Loeffel, Executive Vice President
Help young students build reading comprehension and writing skills with this interactive version of the children's classic, The Three Little Pigs. Animated storytelling and creative activities inspire children to read, write and rhyme. *$34.95*

1448 TouchCorders
Soft Touch
4300 Stine Road
Suite 401
Bakersfield, CA 93313
661-396-8676
877-763-8868
FAX: 661-396-8760
e-mail: softtouch@funsoftware.com
www.funsoftware.com

Roxanne Butterfield, Marketing
Joyce Meyer, President

TouchCorders are the flexible and easty-to-use communicator designed by Jo Meyer and Linda Bidabe for reach classroom use. TouchCorders are sensitive to touch at every angle and give the student kinesthetic feedback. With the unique Add 'n Touch system, Jo connects the puzzles bases of 2 or more TouchCorders on the fly to present vocabulary, sequencing, story telling, social stories, concepts and other curriculum and communication opportunities.

1449 **TouchWindow Touch Screen**
Riverdeep Incorporated
100 Pine Street
Suite 1900
San Francisco, CA 94111
415-659-2000
800-542-4222
e-mail: edmarkteam@edmark.com
www.edmark.com

Barry Callaghan, Chairman/CEO
Simon Calver, Chief Executive Officer
Robert Kilgarriff, Sales Executive
Software for children. *$335.00*

1450 **Turtle Teasers**
Soft Touch
4300 Stine Road
Suite 401
Bakersfield, CA 93313
661-396-8676
877-763-8868
FAX: 661-396-8760
e-mail: softtouch@softtouch.com
www.softtouch.com

Joyce Meyer, President
Roxanne Butterfield, Marketing
Three Games, Three Levels from Easy, Medium to Hard. The Shell Game - easy: Watch one of the three turles get the tomato. Then watch carefully as they switch positions and pop shut. Choose incorrectly and the frog disappears until the correct one is displayed. The Pond - medium: Watch the tomato disappear somewhere in the pond scene. Tomato Dump - hard: Hit the shell and it turns into the tomato, giving a score. There are different difficulty levels to equalize all students.

1451 **Volcanoes**
Earthware Computer Services
2386 Spring Boulevard
Eugene, OR 97403
FAX: 541-342-3416
Simulation of volcano in which children play the role of the scientists. *$49.50*

1452 **What Was That!**
Compass Learning
203 Colorado Street
Austin, TX 78701
858-587-0087
800-247-1380
FAX: 619-622-7873
www.compasslearning.com

Rajeev Puri, President
Eric Loeffel, CEO
In this bedtime story, noises in the night send three brother bears scurrying out of bed. Thoughtful questions test young readers' comprehension, while games, voice recording, writing practice and other playful activities stimulate their creativity.

1453 **Wivik 3**
Prentke Romich Company
1022 Heyl Road
Wooster, OH 44691
330-262-1984
800-262-1984
FAX: 330-263-4829
e-mail: info@prentrom.com
www.prentrom.com

Dave Moffatt, President
On-screen keyboard provides access to any application in the latest Windows operating systems. Selections are made by clicking, dwelling or switch scanning. Enhancements include word prediction and abbreviation expansion.

1454 **You Tell Me: Learning Basic Information**
Programming Concepts
PO Box 34270
San Antonio, TX 78265
800-594-4263
FAX: 888-259-8284
e-mail: pciinfo@pcieducation.com
www.pcieducation.com

Janie Haugen, Program Director
Jeff McLane, President/CEO
This game teaches and reinforces basic information all individuals need to know. Questions asked in this game help prepare people to communicate personal identification information important to community survival. *$49.95*

Software: Professional

1455 **Acrontech International**
5500 Main Street
Williamsville, NY 14221
FAX: 716-854-4014
This company supplies software, audio mixers, and closed-caption televisions.

1456 **DPS with BCP**
V OR T Corporation
PO Box 60132
Palo Alto, CA 94306
650-322-8282
FAX: 650-327-0747
e-mail: sales@vort.com
www.vort.com

Tom Holt, Owner
This program uses unique DPS branching techniques to access goals and objectives.

1457 **Diagnostic Report Writer**
Parrot Software
190 Sandy Ridge Road
State College, PA 16803
800-727-7681
FAX: 814-237-7282

Fred Weiner, Owner
Creates a three page single-spaced diagnostic report for a child with a communication disorder from a list of questions; sections of the report include developmental and background history, oral peripheral exam, speech and language analysis, summary and recommendations.

1458 **Discriptive Language Arts Development**
Educational Activities Software
PO Box 754
Baldwin, NY 11510
516-867-7878
800-645-2796
FAX: 516-379-7429
e-mail: achieve@ea-software.com
www.ea-software.com

Alan Stern, Manager
This multimedia language arts development program provides instruction and application of fundamental English skills and concepts. *$395.00*

1459 **EZ Dot**
CAPCO Capability Corporation
1522 N Washington Street
Suite 200
Spokane, WA 99201
FAX: 509-535-1011
A critical software tool used in vocational counseling, job restructuring, recruitment and placement, better utilization of workers, and safety issues. This software offers occupational data by title, code, industry, GEO, DPT, or OGA. *$295.00*

1460 **EZ Keys for Windows**
Words+
42505 10th Street W
Suite 109
Lancaster, CA 93534
661-723-6523
800-869-8521
FAX: 661-266-8969
e-mail: info@words-plus.com
www.words-plus.com

Phil Lawrence, Vice President
Rachel Nielsen, Customer Support
Walt Wolosz, Manager
A software and hardware product designed to operate on an IBM compatible PC. The software provides dual word prediction, abbreviation expansion, five different methods of voice output and access to commercial software applications. *$1395.00*

1461 **Goals and Objectives**
JE Stewart Teaching Tools
PO Box 15308
Seattle, WA 98115
206-262-9538
FAX: 206-262-9538

J E Stewart, Owner
Goals and Objectives software helps teachers make student plans including IEP's, IPP's and IHP's. The system provides curricula for all students and programs to develop and evaluate plans, print reports and make data forms. Systems are available for Windows and Macintosh for $139.

1462 **Goals and Objectives IEP Program**
Curriculum Associates
PO Box 2001
N Billerica, MA 01862
978-667-8000
800-225-0248
FAX: 800-366-1158
e-mail: info@curriculumassociates.com
www.curriculumassociates.com

Frank Ferguson, President/Owner
Katherine Harvey, Vice President
BRIGANCE CIBS-R standardized scoring conversion software, is a teacher's tool that prints goal and objective pages of the IEP. In less than two minutes per student, a teacher types student data into the computer.

1463 **Nasometer**
Kay Elemetrics Corporation
2 Bridgewater Lane
Lincoln Park, NJ 07035
973-628-6200
800-289-5297
FAX: 973-628-6363
e-mail: sales@kaypentax.com
www.kaypentax.com

John Crump, President
Steve Crump, Direct Sales
Measures the ratio of acoustic energy for the nasal and real-time visual cueing during therapy. Used clinically in the areas of cleft palate, motor speach disorders, hearing impairment and palatal prosthetic fittings.

1464 **PSS CogRehab Software**
Psychological Software Services
6555 Carrollton Avenue
Indianapolis, IN 46220
317-257-9672
FAX: 317-257-9674
e-mail: nsc@netdirect.net
www.neuroscience.cnter.com

Nancy Bracy, Sales/Production
Odie Bracy, Executive Director
PSS CogRehab Software is a comprehensive and easy-to-use multimedia cognitive rehabilitation software available, for clinical and educational use with head injury, stroke LD/ADD and other brain compromises. The packages include 64 computerized therapy tasks which contain modifiable parameters that will accommodate most requirements. Exercises include attention and executive skills, multiple modalities of visuosatial and memory skills, simple, complex, proble-solving skills.
$260 - $2500

1465 **Parrot Easy Language Simple Anaylsis**
Parrot Software
PO Box 250755
W Bloomfield, MI 48325
248-788-8360
800-727-7681
www.parrotsoftware.com

Fred Weiner, Owner
Designed for grammatical analysis of language samples. The user types and translates language samples of up to 100 utterances.

1466 **TOVA**
Universal Attention Disorders
4281 Katella Avenue
Suite 215
Los Alamitos, CA 90720
714-821-9611
800-PAY-ATTN
FAX: 714-229-8782

Lawrence Greenberg, Developer
A computerized assessment which, in conjunction with classroom behavior ratings, is a highly effective screening tool for ADD. TOVA includes software, complete instructions, and supporting data including norms.

1467 **TTAP Outreach: Technology Team Assessment Process**

27 Horrabin Hall
Macomb, IL 61455
309-298-1634
FAX: 309-298-2305
e-mail: l_robinsonl@wiu.edu
www.mprojects.wiu.edu

Linda Robinson, Coordinator
Provides training to early childhood personnel and families on a team-based model for technology assessment. TTAP's procedures are designed to assess children's ability to use technology as a tool for achieving IEP/IFSP goals. Training and written materials are available.

1468 **Visi-Pitch III**
Kayelemetrics Corporation
2 Bridgewater Lane
Lincoln Park, NJ 07035
973-628-6200
FAX: 973-628-6363
e-mail: info@kayepentax.com
www.kayepentax.com

Robert McClurkin, Marketing Director
Steve Crump, Sales
John Crump, President
Assists the speech/voice clinician in assessment and treatment tasks across an expansive range of disorders.

Software: Reading & Language Arts

1469 **Choices, Choices 5.0**
Tom Snyder Productions
100 Talcott Avenue
6
Watertown, MA 02472
617-926-6000
800-342-0236
FAX: 800-304-1254
e-mail: ask@tomsnyder.com
www.tomsnyder.com

Rick Abrahams, Manager
Teaches students to take responsibility for their behavior. Helps students develop the skills and awareness they need to make wise choices and to think through the consequences of their actions.

1470 Circletime Tales Deluxe
Don Johnston
26799 W Commerce Drive
Volo, IL 60073
847-740-0749
800-999-4660
FAX: 847-740-7326
e-mail: info@donjohnston.com
www.donjohnston.com

Ruth Ziolkowski, President
This interactive CD-ROM introduces and reinforces pre-literacy concepts using nursery rhymes and songs familiar to many children. This English/Spanish program emphasizes listening to and learning basic concepts such as opposites, directionality, colors and counting. *$59.00*

1471 Community Exploration
Compass Learning
203 Colorado Street
Austin, TX 78701
858-587-0087
800-247-1380
FAX: 619-622-7873
www.compasslearning.com

Rajeev Puri, President
Eric Loeffel, Executive Vice President
An award-winning learning adventure takes students who are learning English as a second language on a field trip to the make-believe town of Cornerstone. More than 50 community locations come to life with sound and animation. While exploring places in this typical American community where people live, work and play, students also enhance important English language skills. Offers an exciting approach for any age student who needs to improve their English language proficiency. 4-12. *$19.95*

1472 Conversations
Educational Activities Software
PO Box 754
Baldwin, NY 11510
516-867-7878
800-645-2796
FAX: 516-379-7429
e-mail: achieve@ea-software.com
www.ea-software.com

Alan Stern, Manager
Using American digitalized voices, CONVERSATIONS provides 14 different dialogues in which the student can participate. The topics offer learners important information about American culture and the workplace. Available for DOS. *$195.00*

1473 Core-Reading and Vocabulary Development
Educational Activities
PO Box 87
Baldwin, NY 11510
516-223-4666
800-645-3739
FAX: 516-623-9282
e-mail: learn@edact.com
www.edact.com

Alfred Harris, President
Carol Stern, VP
Students begin with 36 basic words and progress to more than 200. Reading and writing activities are coordinated and integrated throughout the program for more substantial permanent learning. Five units covering readability levels from pre-primer to grade three.
Full Program

1474 Day at Play: A IKanDu Little Book
Don Johnston
26799 W Commerce Drive
Volo, IL 60073
847-740-0749
800-999-4660
FAX: 847-740-7326
e-mail: info@donjohnston.com
www.donjohnston.com

Ketan Kothari, Chief Executive Officer
Ruth Ziolkowski, President
One of the products in the UKanDu Little Book Series. This early literacy program consists of several four-page animated stories that help build language experience for emergent and early readers. Children fill-in-the-blank to complete a sentence on each page and then watch the page come alive with animation and sound. After completion, it can be printed to make a book. All children can be successful as there are no wrong answers. *$45.00*

1475 Friday Afternoon
13500 Evening Creek Drive N
Suite 200
San Diego, CA 92128
858-587-0087
800-247-1380
FAX: 619-622-7873
www.compasslearning.com

Rajeev Puri, President
Eric Loeffel, Chief Operating Officer
Martin Kenney Jr, Chief Executive Officer
Save hours of preparation time and dazzle your students with interesting new activities to supplement their classroom learning. With Friday afternoon, you'll produce flash cards, word puzzles, even customized bingo cards and more, all at the click of a mouse. MacIntosh diskette. *$99.95*

1476 How to Read for Everyday Living
Educational Activities Software
PO Box 754
Baldwin, NY 11510
516-867-7878
800-645-2796
FAX: 516-379-7429
e-mail: achieve@ea-software.com
www.ea-software.com

Alan Stern, Manager
Basic vocabulary and key words are taught and, when need, retaught using alternative teaching strategies. Passages that students read help put the vocabulary into context. Each lesson is followed by crossword and other puzzles check comprehension.

1477 Learning English: Primary
13500 Evening Creek Drive N
Suite 200
San Diego, CA 92128
858-587-0087
800-247-1380
FAX: 619-622-7873
www.compasslearning.com

Rajeev Puri, President
Eric Loeffel, Executive Vice President
Martin Kenney Jr, Chief Executive Officer
Four stories and rhymes help students familiarize themselves with essential English language concepts, recognize patterns in language and associate words with objects. *$49.95*

1478 Learning English: Rhyme Time
Compass Learning
13500 Evening Creek Drive N
San Diego, CA 92128
858-587-0087
800-247-1380
FAX: 619-622-7873
www.compasslearning.com

Rajeev Turi, President
Martin Kenney Jr, Chief Executive Officer
Using classic children's rhymes in an animated multimedia program, students work on language skills, vocabulary and comprehension.

1479 Lexia I, II and III Reading Series
Lexia Learning Systems
PO Box 466
Lincoln, MA 01773
781-259-8752
800-435-3942
FAX: 781-259-1349
e-mail: info@lexialearning.com
www.lexialearning.com

Henry Morgan, Director
Jonathan Bower, Chief Executive Officer

Lexia's software helps children and adults with learning disabilities master their core reading skills. Based on the Orton Gillingham method, Lexia Early Reading, Phonics Based Reading and SOS (Strategies for Older Students) apply phonics principles to help students learn essential sound-symbol correspondence and decoding skills. The Quick Reading Tests generate detailed skill reports in only 5-8 minutes per student to provide data for further instruction. Price: $40-400 per workstation.

1480 Memory Castle
WINGS for Learning
1600 Green Hills Road
Scotts Valley, CA 95066
831-464-3600
FAX: 831-464-3600

Ani Stocks, Owner
Introduces a strategy to increase memory skills via an adventure game. Set in a castle, the game requires memory, reading, spelling skills and more to win.

1481 On a Green Bus: A UKanDu Little Book
Don Johnston
26799 W Commerce Drive
Volo, IL 60073
847-740-0749
800-889-5242
FAX: 847-740-7326
e-mail: support@donjohnston.com
www.donjohnston.com

Ruth Ziolkowski, President
This early literacy program that consists of several create-your-own 4-page animated stories that help build language experience on each page and then watch the page come alive with animation and sound. After completing the story, students can print it out to make a book which can be read over and over again. Because there are no wrong answers, all children can have a successful literacy experience. *$ 45.00*

1482 Open Book
Freedom Scientific
11800 31st Court N
St Petersburg, FL 33716
727-803-8000
800-444-4443
FAX: 727-803-8001
e-mail: info@freedomscientific.com
www.freedomscientific.com

Lee Hamilton, Director
Software that reads scanned text allowed and includes other features that aid the vision-impaired. *$995.00*

1483 Optimum Resource Software
18 Hunter Road
Hilton Head, SC 29926
843-689-8000
FAX: 843-689-8008
e-mail: stickyb@stickybear.com
www.optimumlearning.com

Chris Gintz, Chief Executive Officer
Maureen Richards, Administration
Optimum Resource publishes over 100 K-12 education curriculum software titles under its varietal brands, StickyBear, MiddleWare, High School and Tools for Teachers.

1484 Out and About: A UKanDu Little Book
Don Johnston
26799 W Commerce Drive
Volo, IL 60073
847-740-0749
800-999-4660
FAX: 847-740-7326
e-mail: info@donjohnston.com
www.donjohnston.com

Ruth Ziolkowski, President
One of the products in the UKanDu Little Book Series. This early literacy program consists of several four-page animated stories that help build language experience for emergent and early readers. Children fill-in-the-blank to complete a sentence on each page and then watch the page come alive with animation and sound. After completion, it can be printed to make a book. *$45.00*

1485 Programs for Aphasia and Cognitive Disorders
Parrot Software
PO Box 250755
W Bloomfield, MI 48325
248-788-8360
800-727-7681
wwww.parrotsoftware.com

Fred Weiner, Owner
Over 50 different computer programs that facilitate language, memory and attention training. Programs are available for MS DOS, WINDOWS and Apple II.

1486 Punctuation Rules
Optimum Resource
18 Hunter Road
Hilton Head Island, SC 29926
843-689-8000
FAX: 843-689-8008
e-mail: sticky@stickybear.com
www.stickybear.com

Chris Gintz, Chief Executive Officer
Punctuation Rules is designed to help students improve their punctuation skills. Students work with appropriate level sentences which follow common rules of punctuation. The program covers material ranging from categories of sentences to forming possessives and allows students to gain strength in their ability to correctly use periods, commas, apostrophes, question marks, colons, hyphens, quotation marks, exclamation points and more. *$59.95*

1487 Quick Reading Test, Phonics Based Reading, Reading SOS (Strategies for Older Students)
Lexia Learning Systems
PO Box 466
Lincoln, MA 01773
781-259-8752
800-435-3942
FAX: 781-259-1349
e-mail: info@lexialearning.com
www.lexialearning.com

Jonathan Bower, Chief Executive Officer
Bob Baker, Sales Representative
Lexia's software helps children and adults with learning disabilities master their core reading skills. Based on the Orton Gillingham method, Phonics Based Reading and S.O.S. (Strategies for the Older Student) apply phonics principles to help students learn essential sound-symbol correspondence and decoding skills. The Quick Reading Tests generate detailed phonemic skills reports in only 5-8 minutes per student to provide teachers with accurate data to focus their instruction. Price: $67-$500.

1488 Quick Talk
Educational Activities Software
PO Box 754
Baldwin, NY 11510
516-867-7878
800-645-2796
FAX: 516-379-7429
e-mail: achieve@ea-software.com
www.ea-software.com

Alan Stern, Manager
Students will learn and use new vocabulary immediately: high-frequency, everyday vocabulary words are introduced and used contextually using human speech, graphics and text. Voice-interactive program (MS-DOS). *$65.00*

1489 Race the Clock
Mindplay
4440 S Williams Boulevard
Suite 206
Tucson, AZ 85716
520-888-0
800-888-7904
FAX: 520-322-0363
e-mail: mail@mindplay.com
www.mindplay.com
A matching game, uses the animation capabilities to teach verbs. The player chooses a matching game from a menu.

1490 **Reader Rabbit**
Learning Company
100 Pine Street
Suite 1900
San Francisco, CA 94111
800-825-4420
FAX: 877-278-7456
e-mail: SchoolCustomerService@riverdeep.net
www.learningcompanyschool.com
Supports young students in building fundamental reading readiness skills in a playful, multi-sensory environment.

1491 **Reading Comprehension Series**
Optimum Resource
18 Hunter Road
Hilton Head Island, SC 29926
843-689-8000
FAX: 843-689-8008
e-mail: sticky@stickybear.com
www.stickybear.com

Chris Gintz, Chief Executive Officer
The Reading Comprehension Series, includes six volumes for Windows, MacIntosh, DOS or Apple II computers. Packed with intriguing multi-level stories, each volume will capture the interest of children ages 8-14 while teaching them crucial reading comprehension skills. These open-ended programs are versatile and easy to use. *$59.95*

1492 **Simon Sounds it Out**
Don Johnston
26799 W Commerce Drive
Volo, IL 60073
847-740-0749
800-999-4660
FAX: 847-740-7326
e-mail: info@donjohnston.com
www.donjohnston.com

Don Johnston, Chief Executive Officer
Ruth Ziolkowski, President
This interactive phonics program enables students to learn and practice letter sounds with an instructional and nonthreatening on-screen tutor. This phonics program was designed by leading learning authorities and extensively tested in classrooms. Colorful graphics, digitalized sound and amusing animations reward students and motivate them to continue learning. *$59.00*
1998

1493 **Simon Spells**
Don Johnston
26799 W Commerce Drive
Volo, IL 60073
847-740-0749
800-999-4660
FAX: 847-740-7326
e-mail: info@donjohnston.com
www.donjohnston.com

Don Johnston, Founder
Ruth Ziolkowski, President
This innovative spelling program guides students through individualized instruction presented in a way that enables them to work at their own pace. Words are phonemically presented, as well as placed in the context of sentences so as to help increase vocabulary comprehension and spelling skills. Student progress is tracked and results are stored. *$59.00*

1494 **Sound Sentences**
Educational Activities Software
PO Box 754
Baldwin, NY 11510
516-867-7878
800-645-2796
FAX: 516-379-7429
e-mail: achieve@ea-software.com
www.ea-software.com

Alan Stern, Manager
This sound-interactive program breaks away from traditional language instruction. Instead of formal concentration on verb and basic vocabulary, students meet everyday English with colloquialisms they will hear in real life situations. They reinforce their knowledge of sentence structure while acquiring the ability to communicate in daily settings. (For MAC, MS-DOS and Windows). *$65.00*

1495 **Spelling Rules**
Optimum Resource
18 Hunter Road
Hilton Head Island, SC 29926
843-689-8000
FAX: 843-689-8008
e-mail: sticky@stickybear.com
www.stickybear.com

Chris Gintz, Chief Executive Officer
A curriculum based, easy-to-use program that provides students with the practice they need to build strong spelling skills. *$59.95*

1496 **Spelling Test Generator**
Optimum Resource
18 Hunter Road
Hilton Head Island, SC 29926
843-689-8000
FAX: 843-689-8008
e-mail: stickyb@stickybear.com
www.stickybear.com

Chris Gintz, Chief Executive Officer
Using more than 3000 of the most commonly encountered words in the English language, the Spelling Test Generator prepares spelling lists on the basis of difficulty, grade level, vowels, diphthongs, word origins and starting/ending letters or sounds. *$59.95*

1497 **Stickybear Parts of Speech**
Optimum Resource
18 Hunter Road
Hilton Head Island, SC 29926
843-689-8000
FAX: 843-689-8008
e-mail: stickyb@stickybear.com
www.stickybear.com

Chris Gintz, Chief Executive Officer
Children learn parts of speech with this exciting new program. *$59.95*

1498 **Stickybear Reading**
Optimum Resource
18 Hunter Road
Hilton Head Island, SC 29926
843-689-8000
FAX: 843-689-8008
e-mail: stickyb@stickybear.com
www.stickybear.com

Chris Gintz, Chief Executive Officer
Children build vocabulary and reading comprehension skills using hundreds of word/picture sets and thousands of put-together sentence parts. *$49.95*

1499 **Stickybear Reading Comprehension**
Optimum Resource
18 Hunter Road
Hilton Head Island, SC 29926
843-689-8000
FAX: 843-689-8008
e-mail: stickyb@stickybear.com
www.stickybear.com

Chris Gintz, Chief Executive Officer
This multi-level reading comprehension program helps children improve reading skills with 30 high-interest stories and question sets created by the Weekly Reader editors. *$59.95*

1500 **Stickybear Spellgrabber**
Optimum Resource
18 Hunter Road
Hilton Head Island, SC 29926
843-689-8000
FAX: 843-689-8008
e-mail: stickyb@stickybear.com
www.stickybear.com

Chris Gintz, Chief Executive Officer
Build spelling and vocabulary skills with three different activities: Picture Spell, Word Spell and Bear Dunk. *$59.95*

1501 **Stickybear Spelling**
Optimum Resource
18 Hunter Road
Hilton Head Island, SC 29926
843-689-8000
FAX: 843-689-8008
e-mail: sticky@stickybear.com
www.stickybear.com

Chris Gintz, Chief Executive Officer
Children ages 6 and up discover and practice critical spelling skills as they work with three unique action-packed activities, each with four graded levels of difficulty. The program is open-ended and teachers may add, change and modify the word lists for each individual. Stickybear Spelling contains more than 2000 recorded words. Levels may be set to allow students of different ages or abilities to compete effectively. *$59.95*

1502 Stickybear Spelling Rules
Optimum Resource
18 Hunter Road
Hilton Head Island, SC 29926
843-689-8000
FAX: 843-689-8008
e-mail: stickyb@stickybear.com
www.stickybear.com

Chris Gintz, Chief Executive Officer
Spelling Rules is designed to help students improve spelling accuracy and master the fundamentals - forming plurals (adding s, adding es, f, fe, to ves) and compound words, I before E rule, capitalization and many others. *$59.95*

1503 Stickybear's Reading Fun Park
Optimum Resource
18 Hunter Road
Hilton Head Island, SC 29926
843-689-8000
FAX: 843-689-8008
e-mail: stickyb@stickybear.com
www.stickybear.com

Chris Gintz, Chief Executive Officer
Children ages 4-8 discover and practice critical reading skills as the famous stickybear family guides users through unique, action-packed activities, each with multiple levels of difficulty and skills that address both the auditory and visual needs of budding readers. *$59.95*

1504 Stickybear's Reading Room
Optimum Resource
18 Hunter Road
Hilton Head Island, SC 29926
843-689-8000
FAX: 843-689-8008
e-mail: stickyb@stickybear.com
www.stickybear.com

Chris Gintz, Chief Executive Officer
The perfect combination of learning and fun, our award winning Stickybear's Reading Room provides colorful motivating thinking skills practice for children ages 4-8 with four unique bilingual learning activities. *$59.95*

1505 Tomorrow's Promise: Language Arts
Compass Learning
13500 Evening Creek Drive N
San Diego, CA 92128
858-587-0087
800-521-8538
FAX: 619-622-7873
www.compasslearning.com

Steve Allen, Alternate Channels Manager
Martin Kenney Jr, Chief Executive Officer
You'll strengthen students' grammar, usage and vocabulary skills and promote higher order thinking skills with this comprehensive Language Arts curriculum. It utilizes cross-curricular, thematic instruction engaging multimedia learning exercises that encourage writing, speaking and listening proficiency. Promotes higher order thinking skills. *$279.95*

1506 Tomorrow's Promise: Reading
Compass Learning
203 Colorado Street
Austin, TX 78701
512-478-9600
800-521-8538
www.compasslearning.com

Steve Allen, Alternate Channels Manager
This multimedia curriculum balances thematic, interactive exploration with core skills development, increasing your students' early reading proficiency, building a solid literacy foundation and fostering a lifelong love for reading. *$279.95*

1507 Tomorrow's Promise: Spelling
Compass Learning
203 Colorado Street
Austin, TX 78701
512-478-9600
800-678-1412
e-mail: support@compasslearning.com
www.compasslearning.com

Steve Allen, Alternate Channels Manager
Lovable characters and engaging multimedia effects put young students on a fast-track to early spelling proficiency with fourteen activities and three games. A full year's instruction on each CD includes 30 world lists per grade, in story context, or create word lists to suit your needs. This program addresses students' multiple learning styles and rewards students as they progress through each stage of spelling skill acquisition. *$99.95*

1508 Vocabulary Development
Optimum Resource
18 Hunter Road
Hilton Head Island, SC 29926
843-689-8000
FAX: 843-689-8008
e-mail: stickyb@stickybear.com
www.stickybear.com

Chris Gintz, Chief Executive Officer
A featured program in the middle school series. Vocabulary Development is designed to help students increase vocabulary as they strengthen reading skills. Students relate their current knowledge of vocabulary to the context in which they discover an unfamiliar word. Utilizing a variety of contextual aids, this program illustrates synonyms, antonyms, prefixes, suffixes, homophones, multiple meanings and context clues, allowing students to apply experience and context. *$59.95*

1509 Whoops
Cornucopia Software
PO Box 6111
Albany, CA 94706
510-528-7000
e-mail: supportstaff@practicemagic.com
www.practicemagic.com

Christina Morua, Manager
Checks spelling three ways. It checks words as they are typed, it checks an entire screen and highlights the errors and it reads ASCII text files from a disk and lists errors.

Software: Vocational

1510 Functional Literacy System
Conover Company
2926 Hidden Hollow Road
Oshkosh, WI 54904
920-231-4667
800-933-1933
FAX: 920-231-4809
e-mail: conover@execpc.com
www.conovercompany.com

Terry Schmitz, President
Assessment and skill building for basic functional literacy. This multimedia software program is adult in format and uses live action video taken in actual community settings to help learners become more capable of functioning independently. Twenty different programs are currently available. *$99.00*

1511 Learning Activity Packets
2926 Hidden Hollow Road
Oshkosh, WI 54904
920-231-4667
800-933-1933
FAX: 920-231-4809
e-mail: conover@execpc.com
www.conovercompany.com

Terry Schmitz, President
Bechky Schmitz, Vice President
Demonstrates how basic academic skills relate to 30 major career areas. LAPs provide valuable diagnostics in applied academic applications and demonstrates to users the importance of academics as they relate to the workplace. Software. *$99.00*

1512 **Microcomputer Evaluation of Careers & Academics (MECA)**
Conover Company
2926 Hidden Hollow Road
Oshkosh, WI 54904
920-231-4667
800-933-1933
FAX: 920-231-4809
e-mail: conover@execpc.com
www.conovercompany.com

Terry Schmitz, President
A cost-effective, technology-based, career development system which provides users with opportunities to get their hands dirty. The MECA system utilizes work simulations and is built around common occupational clusters. Each cluster, or career area, consists of hands-on WORK SAMPLES which provide a variety of career exploration and assessment experiences, linked to LEARNING ACTIVITY PACKETS, which integrate basic academic skills into the career planning and placement process. $580-$1,070.

1513 **OASYS**
Vertek
12835 Bel Red Road
Suite 112
Bellevue, WA 98005
425-455-9921
800-220-4409
FAX: 425-454-7264
e-mail: marketing@vertekinc.com
www.vertekinc.com

Gale Gibson, President
Jack Rosenoss, Vice President
A software system that matches a person's skills and abilities to occupations and employers.

1514 **Reading in the Workplace**
Educational Activities Software
PO Box 754
Baldwin, NY 11510
516-867-7878
800-645-2796
FAX: 516-379-7429
e-mail: achieve@ea-software.com
www.ea-software.com

Alan Stern, Manager
A job-based, reading software program using real-life problems and solutions to capture students' attention and improve their vocabulary and comprehension skills. Units include: automotive, clerical, health care and construction. *$295.00*

1515 **Stickybear Typing**
Optimum Resource
18 Hunter Road
Hilton Head Island, SC 29926
843-689-8000
FAX: 843-689-8008
e-mail: stickyb@stickybear.com
www.stickybear.com

Chris Gintz, Chief Executive Officer
The award winning Stickybear Typing program allows users to sharpen typing skills and achieve keyboard mastery with three engaging and amusing multi-level activities. *$59.95*

1516 **Vocational Interest Profile Report**
Cambridge Educational
90 Maccorkle Avenue SW
South Charleston, WV 25303
304-744-2055
800-468-4227
FAX: 800-329-6687
e-mail: melindab@citynet.net
www.cambridgeol.com

Melinda Ball, Marketing Director
Software that is designed to allow students to systematically define broad work categories that are of most interest. *$64.86*

ISBN 0-927368-59-5

1517 **Work-Related Vocational Assessment Systems**
Valpar International
12778 W North Avenue
Building A
Brookfield, WI 53005
262-797-0840
800-633-3321
FAX: 262-797-8488
e-mail: sales@valparint.com
www.valparint.com

Neal Gunderson, President
Patricia L Rastatter, VP Operations
Criterion-referenced to Department of Labor standards. Evaluate academic levels for reading, spelling, math and language, and various other aptitudes.

1518 **Workplace Skills: Learning How to Function on the Job**

Programming Concepts
PO Box 12428
San Antonio, TX 78212
800-594-4263
FAX: 218-480-5

Janie Haugen, Program Director
Jeff Mclane, President/CEO
Offers parents and educators a functional means by which to discuss all aspects of finding and keeping a job. *$49.95*

Word Processors

1519 **DARCI**
Wes Test Engineering Corporation
810 Shepard Lane
Farmington, UT 84025
801-451-9191
FAX: 801-451-9393
www.westest.com

Mary Lynds, Purchasing
Pam Burns, Office Manager
Robert Lessman, President
Provides transparent access to all computer functions by replacing the computer's keyboard with a smart joystick. *$975.00*

1520 **Eye Relief Word Processing Software**
SkiSoft Publishing Corporation
PO Box 364
Lexington, MA 02420
781-863-1876

e-mail: info@skisoft.com
www.skisoft.com

Ken Skier, President
Cynthia Skier, CFO
Large-type word processing program for visually-impaired PC users. *$295.00*

1521 **IntelliTalk**
Intelli Tools
1720 Corporate Circle
Petaluma, CA 94954
707-773-2000
800-899-6687
FAX: 707-773-2001
e-mail: tech@intellitools.com
www.intellitools.com

Beth Davis, Director Sales Operator
Lori Castle, Supervisor
Arjan Khalsa, Chief Executive Officer
Talking word-processing program available for MacIntosh, Apple IIe, IBM compatible and Windows computers. *$39.95*

1522 **Large Type**
PO Box 1088
Hewitt, NJ 07421
973-853-6585
800-736-2216
FAX: 928-832-2894

Donald Selwyn, Director

Display enlargement programs for visually impaired users. Consist of a variety of programs for different needs, ranging from basic to full-featured.

1523 Pegasus LITE

Words+
42505 10th Street W
Suite 109
Lancaster, CA 93534
661-723-6523
800-869-8521
FAX: 661-723-2114
e-mail: info@words-plus.com
www.words-plus.com

Phil Lawrence, Vice President
Rachel Nielsen, Customer Support
Walt Wolosz, Manager

Provides all of the strategies currently being used in AAC, from dynamic display color pictographic language, to dual-word prediction text language, in a single system. *$6995.00*

1524 Up and Running

Intelli Tools
5221 Central Avenue
Suite 205
Richmond, CA 94804
800-899-6687
e-mail: info@intellitools.com
www.intellitools.com

Beth Davis, Director Sales & Operations
Lori Castle, Supervisor

Instantly use hundreds of popular commercial software programs with this custom collection of setups and overlays. *$69.95*

1525 Write This Way

Compass Learning Incorporated
203 Colorado Street
Austin, TX 78701
512-447-8828
800-521-8538
FAX: 619-622-7873
www.compasslearning.com

Steve Allen, Alternate Channels Manager
Mike Campasso, Owner

An easy-to-use, versatile word processor designed with learning disabled or hearing-impaired individuals in mind. Apple or Mac available. *$99.95*

1526 Write: OutLoud

Don Johnston
26799 W Commerce Drive
Volo, IL 60073
847-740-0749
800-999-4660
FAX: 847-740-7326
e-mail: info@donjohnston.com
www.donjohnston.com

Don Johnston, Founder
Ruth Ziolkowski, President

The award-winning feasible and user friendly talking word processor with talking spell checker. Text-to-speech technology provides multi-sensory learning and positive reinforcements for writers of all ages and ability levels. *$99.00*

General

1527 **APSE Conference: Revitalizing Supported Employment, Climbing to the Future**
Association for Persons in Supported Employment
1627 Monument Avenue
Richmond, VA 23220
804-278-9187
FAX: 804-278-9377
e-mail: apse@apse.com
www.apse.org

Suzanne Hutcheson, President
Teresa Grossi, Vice President
Celane Whorter, Executive Director
A major conference on Supported Employment. The conference includes 130 sessions presented by nationally recognized leaders in the field. Conference attendees come from all 50 states, Canada and several foreign countries and include professionals in supported employment, occupational therapy, rehabilitation technology and other related fields.
July

1528 **Alexander Graham Bell Association for the Deaf and Hard of Hearing Annual Conference**
3417 Volta Place NW
Washington, DC 20007
202-337-5220
FAX: 202-337-8314
e-mail: info@agbell.org
www.agbell.org

K Todd Houston, Executive Director/CEO
Wendy Will, Executive Assistant
Garrett W Yates, Advertising/Exhibitor Sales
Over 60 booths offering information on resources and technology for the deaf and hard of hearing.
June

1529 **American Academy for Cerebral Palsy and Developmental Medicine Annual Conference**
555 E Wells Street
Suite 1100
Milwaukee, WI 53202
414-918-3014
FAX: 414-276-2146
e-mail: info@aacpdm.org
www.aacpdm.org

Tracy Burr, Executive Director
The Annual Meeting is a 3-day event, held in the Fall, designed to provide targeted opportunities for dissemination of information in the basic sciences, prevention, diagnosis, treatment, and technical advances as applied to persons with cerebral palsy and development disorders.
September

1530 **American Academy of Ophthalmology Annual Meeting**
655 Beach Street
San Francisco, CA 94109
415-561-8500
FAX: 415-561-8575
e-mail: meetings@aao.org
www.aao.org

Dunbar Hoskins, Executive Vice President
Offers the most comprehensive program with more than 2000 scientific presentations and six subspecialty day programs
October

1531 **American Association of the Deaf-Blind National Conference**
8630 Fenton Street
Suite 121
Silver Spring, MD 20910
301-495-4403
FAX: 301-495-4404
TTY:301-495-4402
e-mail: aadb-info@aadb.org
www.aadb.org

Elizabeth Spiers, Director of Information Services
A week of general meetings, workshops, tours and evening recreational activities.

1532 **American Association on Mental Retardation AAMR Annual Meeting**
444 N Capitol Street NW
Washington, DC 20001
202-387-1968
800-424-3688
FAX: 202-387-2193
e-mail: maria@aamr.org
www.aamr.org

M Doreen Croser, Executive Director
Maria A Alfaro, Meeting Planner/Web Associate
At The Crossroads: Ethics, Genetics, Leadership and Self-Determination, the annual meeting offers a full compliment of workshops, symposia, and multiperspective sessions that fill four days including social events.
May/June

1533 **American Board of Disability Analysts**
Disability Analyst
345 24th Avenue N
Suite 200
Nashville, TN 37203
615-327-2984
FAX: 615-327-9235
e-mail: americanbd@aol.com

Alexander E Horwitz MD, Executive Officer
Kenneth N Anchor PhD, President/Editor
Gabriel Sella MD, Continuing Education Coordinator

1534 **American Council of the Blind Annual Convention**
1155 15th Street NW
Suite 1004
Washington, DC 20005
202-467-5081
800-424-8666
FAX: 202-467-5085
e-mail: info@acb.org
www.acb.org

Melanie Brunson, Executive Director
Cynthia Towers, Convention Coordinator
Offers 50-75 booths of information for the blind.
June/July

1535 **American Diabetes Association Annual Conference**
National Call Center
1701 N Beauregard Street
Alexandria, VA 22311
703-379-7755
800-342-2383
www.diabetes.org/main/application/commercewf

Christina Pappas, Marketing Planner
Trade show featuring exhibits of equipment and supplies used by professionals involved in the treatment of diabetes.

1536 **American Physical Therapy Association**
1111 N Fairfax Street
Alexandria, VA 22314
703-684-2782
800-999-2782
FAX: 703-684-7343
TTY: 703-683-6748
e-mail: scottward@apta.org
www.apta.org

R. Scott Ward, President
John D. Barnes, Chief Executive Officer
The American Physical Therapy Association (APTA) is a national professional organization representing more than 66,000 members. Its goal is to foster advancements in physical therapy practice, research, and education.

1537 **American Rehabilitation Counseling Association**
American Counseling Association
5999 Stevenson Avenue
Alexandria, VA 22304
703-823-9800
800-347-6647
FAX: 703-823-0252
TTY: 703-823-6862
e-mail: webmaster@counseling.org
www.counseling.org

Richard Yep, Executive Director
Robin Hayes, Conventions/Meetings

March/April

1538 American Speech-Language-Hearing Association
10801 Rockville Pike
Rockville, MD 20852
301-897-5700
800-638-8255
FAX: 240-333-4705
TTY: 301-897-5700
e-mail: convention@asha.org
www.asha.org

Lawrence Higdon, President
Arlene A Pietranton, Executive Director
Joanne Jessen, Publications Director
Exhibits by companies specializing in alternative and augmentative communication products, publishers, software and hardware companies, and hearing aid testing equipment manufacturers. Speech-Language Pathologist Professionals who identify, asses, and treat speech and language problems. Audiologists are hearing health care professionals who specialize in preventing, identifying and assesing hearing disorders as well as providing audiologic treatment including hearing aids and more. *$.80*

1539 American Spinal Injury Association Annual Scientific Meeting
2020 Peachtree Road NW
Atlanta, GA 30309
404-355-9772
FAX: 404-355-1826
e-mail: asia-office@shepherd.org
www.asia-spinalinjury.org

Marca L Sipski-Alexander MD, President
Glenn Rechtine MD, Preseident Elect
Amie Jackson, Secretary-Treasurer
Professional association for physicans and other health professionals working in all aspects of spinal cord injury. Also holds an annual scientific that surveys the latest advancements in the field.
May

1540 Association for Education & Rehabilitation of the Blind & Visually Impaired Intl Conference
1703 N Beauregard Street
Suite 440
Alexandria, VA 22311
703-671-4500
877-492-2708
FAX: 703-671-6391
e-mail: aer@aerbvi.org
www.aerbvi.org

Gregory L Goodrich, President
Barbara Sherr, Acting Director
Mark Richert, Owner
Dedicated to rendering support and assistance to the professionals who work in all phases of education and rehabilitation of blind and visually impaired children and adults.
July

1541 Attention Deficit Disorders Association, Southern Region: Annual Conference
12345 Jones Road
Suite 287-7
Houston, TX 77070
281-897-0982
FAX: 281-894-6883
e-mail: addaoffice@pdq.net
www.adda-sr.org

Pam Esser, President
Mission is to: provide a resource network; to support individuals impacted by attention deficit disorders; to advocate for the development of community resources and services that meet the educational, social, and health care needs of all individuals with ADD/ADHD.
February

1542 Blazing Toward a Cure Annual Conference
National Parkinson Foundation
1501 NW 9th Avenue
Miami, FL 33136
305-547-6666
800-327-4545
FAX: 305-243-5595
e-mail: contact@parkinson.org
www.parkinson.org

Daniel Arty, President
Alan M Slewett, Secretary
Jose Garcia-Pedrosa, Executive Director
Purpose is to find the cause and cure for Parkinson's Disease and related neurodegenerative disorders through research, education and dissemination of current information to patients, caregivers and families.
July/August

1543 Blind Childrens Center Annual Meeting
4120 Marathon Street
Los Angeles, CA 90029
323-664-2153
800-222-3567
FAX: 323-665-3828
e-mail: info@blindchildrenscenter.org
www.blindchildrenscenter.org

Laurie Headley, Contact
Midge Horton, Executive Director
A family-centered agency which serves children with visual impairments from birth to school-age. The center-based and home-based services help the children to acquire skills and build their independence. The Center utilizes its expertise and experience to serve families and professionals worldwide through support services, education and research.
September

1544 Blinded Veterans Association National Convention
477 H St NW
Washington, DC 20001
202-371-8880
800-669-7079
FAX: 202-371-8258
e-mail: bva@bva.org
www.bva.org

Thomas H Miller, Executive Director
Annette Mongelli, Conventions Coordinator
Helps veterans and their families meet the challenges of blindness.Offers two main service programs without cost to blinded veterans. Field service program provides counseling to veterans and families and information on benefits and rehabilitation.
August

1545 Children and Adolescents with Emotional and Behavioral Disorders
Virginia Commonwealth University, Medical College
PO Box 980489
Richmond, VA 23298
804-828-1831
FAX: 804-828-2645

Cynthia R Eillis MD, Program Chair
Catherine Howard, Executive Director
October

1546 Closing the Gap's Annual Conference
PO Box 68
Henderson, MN 56044
507-248-3294
FAX: 507-248-3810
e-mail: info@closingthegap.com
www.closingthegap.com

Dolores Hagen, President
Topics will cover a broad spectrum of technology as it is being applied to all disabilities and age groups in education, rehabilitation, vocation and independent living. People with disabilities, special educators, rehabilitation professionals, administrators, service/care providers, personnel managers, government officials, and hardware/software developers will share their experiences and insights at what has become known as the most significant networking experience of the year.
October

1547 Contemporary Issues in Behavioral Health Care
American Assn. of Children's Residential Centers
11700 W Lake Park Drive
Milwaukee, WI 53224
877-332-2272
FAX: 877-362-2272
e-mail: mskarich@alliance1.org
www.aacrc-dc.org

William P Marton, President
Maggie Skarich, National Coordinator

One-day program that will address accrediation as it relates to current behavioral health care challenges held in Pasadena, CA.
October

1548 Council for Exceptional Children Annual Convention and Expo
1110 N Glebe Road
Suite 300
Arlington, VA 22201
703-245-0600
888-232-7733
FAX: 703-264-9494
TTY:866-915-5000
e-mail: service@cec.sped.org
www.cec.sped.org

Jim McCormick, President
Drew Allbritten, Executive Director
Bruce Ramirez, Manager
Works to improve the educational success of children with disabilities and/or gifts and talents.
April

1549 Eye Bank Association of America Annual Meeting
1015 18th Street NW
Suite 1010
Washington, DC 20036
202-775-4999
FAX: 202-429-6036
e-mail: malene@restoresight.org
www.restoresight.org

Patricia Acken-O'Neill Esq, President/CEO
Patricia Hardy, Meetingds Assistant
A four day program, which includes a series or presentations in administrative, hospital development, scientific and technical fields that are relative to eye banking.
June

1550 Handicapped Student Program Postsecondary Education Association
107 Commerce Center Drive.
Suite 204
Huntersville, NC 28078
704-947-7779
FAX: 704-948-7779
e-mail: ahead@ahead.org
www.ahead.org

Ed Suddeth, Executive Director
July

1551 Joint Conference with ABMPP Annual Conference
American Board of Disability Analysts
345 24th Avenue N
Suite 200
Nashville, TN 37203
615-327-2984
FAX: 615-327-9235
e-mail: americanbd@aol.com

Kenneth Anchor, President
Joint Conference with ABMPP Annual Conference Charleston, South Carolina.
May

1552 Lowe's Syndrome Association Conference
18919 Voss Road
Dallas, TX 75287
612-869-5693
FAX: 612-866-3222
e-mail: info@lowesyndrome.org
www.lowesyndrome.org

Jane Gallery, President
An international conference held approximately every two years where family, friends, medical and other professionals gather to exchange ideas and information. Next Conference held in 2008.
June

1553 National Council on the Aging Conference
Conference Department
409 3rd St SW
Washington, DC 20024
202-362-1464
800-424-9046
FAX: 202-479-0735
e-mail: info@ncoa.org
www.ncoa.com

James P Firman, President
Offers ideas and programs to increase your program and administrative skills through NCOA's professional development tracks and offering of continuing education units.
May

1554 National Managed Health Care Congress
71 2nd Avenue
3rd Floor
Waltham, MA 02451
781-663-6000
FAX: 781-663-6422
e-mail: SMeehan@iirusa.com
www.nmhcc.com

Megan Antonelli, Event Director
Shawn Meehan, Exhibit/Underwriter Sales
Attracts nearly 7,000 delegates, thereby reinforcing its status as the nation's largest conferences for all managed care constituencies.
April

1555 Prader-Willi Alliance of New York Annual Conference
PO Box 1114
Niagara Falls, NY 14304
585-442-1655
800-442-1655
FAX: 585-271-2782
e-mail: alliance@prader-willi.org
www.prader-willi.org

Daniel D Angiolillo, President
Elinor G Baller, Secretary
Through conferences, publications, electronic communication and networking (parent-to-parent, parent-to professional, and professional-to-professional), the Prader-Willi Alliance provides a valuable resource for individuals and families sharing the same concerns.
July

1556 RESNA Annual Conference
1700 N Moore Street
Suite 1540
Arlington, VA 22209
703-524-6686
FAX: 703-524-6630
TTY:703-524-6639
e-mail: conference@resna.org
www.resna.org

Thomas A Gorski, Executive Director
Rosina Romano, Meetings/Membership Coordinator
A multidisciplinary association for the advancement of rehabilitation and assistive technologies, holds an annual conference in June. The conference brings together a large number of rehabilitation professionals, products and services from around the world and has something to offer for both professionals and consumers. The conference provides an informative and thought provoking forum for anyone with interests in rehabilitation technology.
June

1557 Rehabilitation International
25 E 21st Street
4th Floor
New York, NY 10010
212-420-1500
FAX: 212-505-0871
e-mail: Rehabintl@rehab-international.org
www.rehab-international.org

Michael Fox, President
Tomas Lagerwall, Manager
Michele Morgan, Program Coordinator
Worldwide network of people with disabilities, service providers and government agencies working together to improve the quality of life for the disabled people and their families, has more than 200 member organizations in 90 nations.

1558 Rehabilitation Technology Association Conference
PO Box 1004
Institute, WV 25112
304-766-4602
800-624-8284
FAX: 304-766-2689

Betty Jo Tyler, RTA Coordinator
Dave Whipp, Information Manager

Holds annual conference in the spring. Publishes a quarterly newsletter and houses the Project Enable computerized bulletin board system.

1559 Santa Barbara Wheelchair Sports Conference

Santa Barbara Parks and Recreation Department
PO Box 1990
Santa Barbara, CA 93102
805-564-5421
FAX: 805-564-5480

Mariana de Sena RT CTRS, Recreation Supervisor
Richard Johns, Manager
Offers a yearly conference, offers programs and services for individuals with a physically disabling condition, head injured individuals that may be visually and hearing impaired. Offers excursions, outings, competition, recreation, etc.

1560 SubAcute Care: American SubAcute Care Association Annual Convention/Expo

PO Box 17413
Washington, DC 20041
FAX: 703-318-7568

Sherlyn Remley, Exhibit Sales
Jim Wasson, Exhibit Sales
Totally dedicated to servicing the subacute arena and its major entities. Features 100+ booths and over 75 exhibitors.
March

1561 Tourette Syndrome Association Conference

4240 Bell Boulevard
Bayside, NY 11361
718-224-2999
800-237-0717
FAX: 718-279-9596
e-mail: ts@tsa-usa.org
www.tsa-usa.org

Judit Ungar, President
Gary Frank, Executive Vice President
More than 400 attendees coming together for this biennial conference that brings together members of the TS community and their families, educators, TS advocates, physicians, researchers, allied professionals, and TSA staff member to interact, socialize, share ideas, discuss issues of concern, learn from experts, and in many instances meet face to face for the first time.
Spring

1562 United Cerebral Palsy Association Development Conference

1660 L St NW
Suite 700
Washington, DC 20036
202-776-0406
800-872-5827
FAX: 202-776-0414
TTY: 202-973-7197
e-mail: webmaster@ucp.org
www.ucpa.org

Stephen Bennett, President/CEO
National, not-for-profit self-help organization dedicated to providing information and support to individuals with cerebral palsy and other disabilities, and their families. Supports more than 160 local affiliates; these affiliates provide a variety of programs and services for affected families, including support groups. Offers several educational and support materials, including a quarterly magazine, regular newsletters, and research reports.

1563 Winter Conference

American Board of Disability Analysts
345 24th Avenue N
Suite 200
Nashville, TN 37203
615-327-2984
FAX: 615-327-9235
e-mail: americanbd@aol.com

Kenneth Anchor, President
Joint Conference: American Board of Disability.
February

1564 Young Onset Parkinson Conference

National Parkinson Foundation
1501 NW 9th Avenue
Miami, FL 33136
305-547-6666
800-327-4545
FAX: 305-243-4403
e-mail: contact@parkinson.org
www.parkinson.org

Daniel Arty, President
Alan M Slewett Esq, Secretary
Jose Garcia-Pedrosa, Executive Director
Purpose is to find the cause and cure for Parkinson's Disease and related neurodegenerative disorders through research, education and dissemination of current information to patients, care-givers and families.
Annual

Associations

1565 Adaptive Environments Center
180-200 Portland Street
Suite 1
Boston, MA 02114
617-695-1225
FAX: 617-482-8099
e-mail: info@adaptiveenvironments.org
www.adaptenv.org

Marie Trottier, Board President
Karen Murray, Information Specialist
Kathy Gips, Director Training
Develops educational programs and materials on universal design, Americans with Disabilities Act, home adaptation, and more. Central Adaptive Environments publication list also available.

1566 Building Owners and Managers Association International
1201 New York Avenue NW
Suite 300
Washington, DC 20005
202-408-2662
FAX: 202-408-2699
www.boma.org

Patricia Areno CAE, Senior Vice President
Conducts seminars nationwide and publishes resource guidebooks for building owners and managers on ADA requirements for commercial facilities and places of public accommodation.

1567 Mark Elmore Associates Architects
42 East Street
Suite 104
Crystal Lake, IL 60014
815-455-7260
800-801-7766
FAX: 815-455-2238
e-mail: mark@elmore-architects.com
www.elmore-architects.com

Mark Elmore, President
Architectural designs for accessible residential and commercial buildings. ADA compliance reviews.

1568 National Conference on Building Codes and Standards
505 Huntmar Park Drive
Suite 210
Herndon, VA 20170
703-437-0100
FAX: 703-481-3596
e-mail: membership@ncsbcs.org
www.ncsbcs.org

Debbie Becker, Administrative Assistant
Kevin Egilmez, Project Manager
Serves as a forum in the interchange of information and provides technical services, education and training to our members to enhance the public's social and economic well being through safe, durable, affordable, accessible and efficient buildings.

1569 National Council of Architectural Registration Boards (NCARB)
1801 K Street NW
Suite 1100-K
Washington, DC 20006
202-783-6500
FAX: 202-783-0290
e-mail: customerservice@ncarb.org
www.ncarb.org

Lenore M Lucey, Executive Vice President
Research service in print and online information. Large collection of books and periodicals on the building/architectural environments.

1570 Overcoming Mobility Barriers International
1022 S 4st Street
Omaha, NE 68105
402-342-5731
FAX: 402-342-5731

Kay Neil, Executive Director
Members are government officials, service consumers and providers, and other persons interested in removing mobility barriers for elderly, handicapped and disadvantaged persons. Advises and works in conjunction with other groups and government agencies to establish safety standards for special equipment used in retrofitting vehicles and works to retrain drivers in the use of nonconventional driving controls. Addresses such problems as possible allocation of fuel to social service agencies.

1571 Paradigm Design Group
Paralyzed Veterans of America
801 Eighteenth Street NW
Washington, DC 20006
202-872-1300
800-424-8200
FAX: 202-416-7647
e-mail: info@pva.org
www.pva.org

Carol Lopez, Director of Architecture
Del Mcneal, Executive Director
Randy Pleza, President
Specialized firm providing architectural consulting services related to accessible designs. Experience includes product design and building codes and standards.

1572 United States Access Board
1331 F Street NW
Suite 1000
Washington, DC 20004
202-272-0080
800-872-2253
FAX: 202-272-0081
TTY: 800-993-2822
e-mail: info@access-board.gov
www.access-board.gov

Dave Yanchulis, Public Affairs Specialist
Leland Schwartz, Owner
Offers information and referrals on architectural accessibility for architects, designers, government agencies, building owners and consumers. A list of free publications is available on request. The Access Board also enforces the Architectural Barriers Act, which covers buildings and facilities designed, built or altered since 1968 with certain federal funds or leased by federal agencies. Publications: Access Currents, bi-monthly newsletter.

Publications & Videos

1573 Access Currents
United States Access Board
1331 F Street NW
Suite 1000
Washington, DC 20004
202-272-0080
800-872-2253
FAX: 202-272-0081
TTY: 800-993-2822
e-mail: info@access-board.gov
www.access-board.gov

Jan Tuck, Chair
David L Bibb, Vice Chair
Leland Schwartz, Owner
Offers information and referrals on architectural accessibility for architects, designers, government agencies, building owners and consumers. A list of free publications is available on request.
bi-monthly

1574 Access Equals Opportunity
Council of B BB s Foundation
4200 Wilson Boulevard
Suite 800
Arlington, VA 22203
703-276-0100
FAX: 703-525-8277
e-mail: media@cbbb.bbb.org
www.bbb.org

Charlie Underhill, Chief Operating Officer
Steven J Cole, Chief Executive Officer

These six Title III compliance guides for existing small businesses offer creative cheap and easy suggestions for complying with the public accommodations section of the ADA. Each guide is industry specific for: retail stores, car sales/service, restaurants/bars, medical offices and fun/fitness centers. They include suggestions for readily achievable removal of architectural barriers; effective communication; and guidance for nondiscriminatory policies or procedures. *$2.50*

1575 Access House
Northside Mental Health Center
1109 E 139th Avenue
Tampa, FL 33613
813-972-2289

Cecil Woodside, Director
Barrier free regulations for design and construction.

1576 Access for All
Hospital Audiences
220 W 42nd Street
Frnt 3
New York, NY 10036
212-575-7660
FAX: 212-575-7669
e-mail: info@hostau.org
www.hospitalaudiences.org

Tricia Hennessey, Access Director
Max Daniels, Manager
Provides physical and program accessibility information for people with disabilities to New York City cultural institutions including theaters, museums, galleries, etc.

1577 Accessible Home of Your Own
Accent Books & Products
PO Box 700
Bloomington, IL 61702
309-378-2961
800-787-8444
FAX: 309-378-4420
e-mail: acmtlvng@aol.com
www.accentonliving.com

Raymond C Cheever, Publisher
Betty Garee, Editor
This guide includes 14 articles that have appeared in the magazine on the popular subject of how to make a disabled persons home more accessible. *$5.95*
52 pages Paperback
ISBN 0-91570 -29-9

1578 Adaptable Housing: A Technical Manual for Implementing Adaptable Dwelling
H UD U SE R
PO Box 23268
Washington, DC 20026
202-708-3178
800-245-2691
FAX: 202-708-9981
TTY: 800-927-7589
e-mail: helpdesk@huduser.org
www.huduser.org

Patrick J Tewey, Director
William Reeder, Director
An illustrated manual describing methods for implementing adaptability in housing. *$3.00*

1579 Adaptive Environments Center Home Assessment Form

374 Congress Street
Suite 301
Boston, MA 02210
617-695-1225
FAX: 617-482-8099
e-mail: info@adaptiveenvironment.org
www.adaptenv.org

Allen Crocker, President
Valerie Fletcher, Executive Director
A handy checklist for evaluating a disabled person's abilities and his/her home limitations to determine what accessibility modifications will be most effective. *$5.00*

1580 Consumer's Guide to Home Adaptation
Adaptive Environments Center
374 Congress Street
Suite 301
Boston, MA 02210
617-695-1225
FAX: 617-482-8099
e-mail: info@AdaptiveEnvironments.org
www.adaptiveEnvironments.org

Valerie Fletcher, Executive Director
Ana Gomez, Coordinator Design/Communication
Mike DiLorenzo, Publications Coordinator
A workbook that enables people with disabilities to plan the modifications necessary to adapt their homes. Describes how to widen doorways, lower countertops, etc. *$12.00*
52 pages Paperback

1581 Design for Acessibility
National Endowment for the Arts Office
1100 Pennsylvania Avenue NW
Washington, DC 20506
202-682-5485
FAX: 202-682-5715
e-mail: webmgr@arts.endow.gov
www.arts.gov

Paula Terry, Director
Joy Kiser, Manager
A handbook for compliance with Section 504 of the Rehabilitation Act of 1973 and the Americans with Disablities Act of 1990 including technical assistance on making arts programs accessible to staff, performers and audience.
101 pages 1987
ISBN 0-160042-83-6

1582 Directory of Accessible Building Products
N AH B Research Center
400 Prince Georges Boulevard
Upper Marlboro, MD 20774
301-249-4000
800-638-8556
FAX: 301-430-6180
www.nahbrc.org

Pamela Eggleston, Program Manager
Mike Luzier, President
Contains descriptions of more than 200 commercially available products designed for use by people with disabilities and age-related limitations. Paperback. *$5.00*
104 pages Yearly

1583 Do-Able Renewable Home
A AR P Fulfillment
601 East Street NW
Washington, DC 20049
202-434-2277
800-424-3410
FAX: 202-434-3443
e-mail: member@aarp.org
www.aarp.org

William Novelli, Chief Executive Officer
Marie Smith, President
Describes how individuals with disabilities can modify their homes for independent living. Room-by-room modifications are accompanied by illustrations.

1584 ECHO Housing: Recommended Construction and Installation Standards
601 East Street NW
Washington, DC 20049
888-687-2277
www.aarp.org

William Bill Novelli, Chief Executive Officer
Marie Smith, President
Illustrated design, construction, and installation standards for temporary dwelling units for elderly people on single family residential property.

1585 Electronic House: Enhanced Lifestyles with Electronics
Electronic House
111 Speen Street
Suite 989
Framingham, MA 01701
508-820-1515
800-375-8015
FAX: 508-663-1599
e-mail: kmoyes@ehpub.com
www.electronichouse.com

Kenneth Moyes, Owner/Chief Executive Officer
Julie Jacobson, Vice President
Dedicated to home automation. Featuring both extravagant and affordable smart homes that can be controlled with one touch. EH covers electronic systems that give homeowners more security, entertainment, convenience, and fun. Articles cover whole house control and subsystems like residential lighting, security, home theater, energy management and telecommunications. *$23.95*
84 pages BiMonthly
ISSN 0886-66 3

1586 Fair Housing Design Guide for Accessibility
National Council on Multifamily Housing Industry
1201 15th & M Street NW
Washington, DC 20005
202-266-8200
800-368-5242
FAX: 202-266-8400
www.nahb.com

David F Wilson, President
David L Pressly Jr, Vice President
Specifically tailored to address the needs of architects and builders. The book includes a detailed technical analysis of the legislation's impact on multifamily design, highlights potential construction problems, and identifies possible solutions. *$29.95*

1587 Ideas for Making Your Home Accessible
Accent Books & Products
PO Box 700
Bloomington, IL 61702
309-378-2961
800-787-8444
FAX: 309-378-4420
e-mail: acmtlvng@aol.com
www.accentonliving.com

Raymond C Cheever, Publisher
Betty Garee, Editor
Offers over 100 pages of tips and ideas to help build or remodel a home. Includes many special devices and where to get them. *$7.50*
94 pages Paperback
ISBN 0-91570 -08-6

1588 North Carolina Accessibility Code
North Carolina Department of Insurance
PO Box 26387
Raleigh, NC 27611
919-661-5880
e-mail: lwright@ncdoi.net

Laurel W Wright, Chief Acessiability Section
Making buildings and facilities accessible to and usable by the physically handicapped. *$20.00*
678 pages Triannually

1589 Removing the Barriers: Accessibility Guidelines and Specifications
A PP A
1643 Prince Street
Alexandria, VA 22314
703-684-1446
FAX: 703-549-2772
e-mail: webmaster@appa.org
www.appa.org

Wayne Leroy, Vice President
Steve Glazner, Communications Director
E Medlin, Executive Vice President
Offers site accessibility, building entrances, doors, interior circulation, restrooms and bathing facilities, drinking fountains and additional resources. *$45.00*
125 pages
ISBN 0-91335 -59-9

1590 Smart Kitchen/How to Design a Comfortable, Safe & Friendly Workplace
Ceres Press
PO Box 87
Woodstock, NY 12498
845-679-5573
888-804-8848
FAX: 845-679-5573
e-mail: cem620@aol.com
www.healthyhighways.com

David Goldbeck, Director/Owner
This book provides information about designing kitchens that may be helpful to people with disabilities as well as safe and energy efficient. *$16.95*
132 pages Paperback

1591 United Spinal Association
7520 Astoria Boulevard
East Elmhurst, NY 11370
718-803-3782
800-444-0120
FAX: 718-803-0414
e-mail: info@unitedspinal.org
www.unitedspinal.org

Peter F Addesso, President
Association news and articles on architecture and barrier-free design, legislation and other current events affecting veterans.
Monthly

Aids for the Classroom

1592 **AEPS Child Progress Record: For Children Ages Three to Six**
Brookes Publishing
PO Box 10624
Baltimore, MD 21285
410-337-9580
800-638-3775
FAX: 410-337-8539
e-mail: custserv@brookespublishing.com
www.brookespublishing.com

Anastasia Worchester, Publicity Manager
Tracy Gray, Educational Sales Manager
Paul Brooks, Owner
This chart helps monitor change by visually displaying current abilities, intervention targets, and child progress. In packages of 30. *$21.00*
8 pages Gate-fold
ISBN 1-557662-51-7

1593 **AEPS Curriculum for Three to Six Years**
Brookes Publishing
PO Box 10624
Baltimore, MD 21285
410-337-9580
800-638-3775
FAX: 410-337-8539
e-mail: custserv@brookespublishing.com
www.brookespublishing.com

Jeff Brookes, Exhibits Coordinator
Tracy Gray, Educational Sales Manager
Dante Washington, Account Sales Manager
$49.00
304 pages Spiral-bound
ISBN 1-557661-88-X

1594 **AEPS Data Recording Forms: For Children Ages Three to Six**
Brookes Publishing
PO Box 10624
Baltimore, MD 21285
410-337-9580
800-638-3775
FAX: 410-337-8539
e-mail: custserv@brookespublishing.com
www.brookespublishing.com

Paul Brooks, Owner
These forms can be used by child development professionals on four separate occasions to pinpoint and then monitor a child's strengths and needs in the six key areas of skill development measured by the AEPS Test. Packages of 10. *$24.00*
36 pages Saddle-stiched
ISBN 1-557662-49-5

1595 **AEPS Family Interest Survey**
Brookes Publishing
PO Box 10624
Baltimore, MD 21285
410-337-9580
800-638-3775
FAX: 410-337-8539
e-mail: custserv@brookespublishing.com
www.brookespublishing.com

Clary Creighton, Exhibits Coordinator
Tracy Gracy, Educational Sales Manager
Paul Brooks, Owner
This is a 30-item checklist that helps families to identify interests and concerns to address in a child's IEP/IFSP. Comes in packages of 30. *$15.00*
8 pages Saddle-stiched
ISBN 1-557660-98-0

1596 **Advanced Language Tool Kit**
Educators Publishing Service
625 Mount Auburn Street
Suite 3
Cambridge, MA 02138
617-547-6706
800-225-5750
FAX: 888-440-2665
e-mail: feedback@epsbooks.com
www.epsbooks.com

Charles Heinle, Vice President
Alexandra S Bigelow, Author
Gunnar Voltz, President
Provides an overview of the structure, organization, and sound units that are needed to develop skills for advanced reading and spelling. The kit contains a teacher's manual and threee packs of cards. *$60.00*
ISBN 0-838885-48-9

1597 **Affix & Root Cards**
Educators Publishing Service
625 Mount Auburn Street
Suite 3
Cambridge, MA 02138
617-547-6706
800-225-5750
FAX: 888-440-2665
e-mail: feedback@epsbooks.com
www.epsbooks.com

Charles H Heinle, Vice President
Alexandra S Bigelow, Author
Gunnar Voltz, President
These cards are specially designed to reinforce the adolescent's knowledge of reading, spelling and vocabulary and should be used in conjunction with language-training materials found in the Alphabetic Phonics and Gillingham curricula. Color-coded cards present word parts, definitions, and example words. *$29.70*
140 Cards
ISBN 0-838803-24-5

1598 **All Kinds of Minds**
Educators Publishing Service
PO Box 9031
Cambridge, MA 02139
617-547-6706
800-225-5750
FAX: 888-440-2665
e-mail: feedback@epsbooks.com
www.epsbooks.com

Charles H Heinle, Vice President
Alexandra S Bigelow, Author
Gunnar Voltz, President
A Young Student's Book about Learning Abilities and Learning Disorders is mainly a fictitious account of five appealing and realistic characters, each of whom has one or more learning disorders. Young readers will easily identify with the experiences of the characters as they appear in a variety of situations, and, at the level, there are suggestions for overcoming the effects of learning disorders. *$24.75*
296 pages
ISBN 0-838820-90-5

1599 **American Sign Language Handshape Cards**
T J Publishers, Distributor
817 Silver Spring Avenue
Suite 206
Silver Spring, MD 20910
301-585-4440
800-999-1168
FAX: 301-585-5930
e-mail: tjpubinc@aol.com

Angela K Thames, President
Jerald A Murphy, Vice President
Durable flashcards illustrate basic handshapes, classifiers and the American manual alphabet. An instructional booklet describes games for differing skill levels to improve vocabulary, increase hand and eye coordination, sign recognition and usage. *$16.95*

1600 **Assistive Technology in the Schools: A Guide for Idaho Educators**
Idaho Assistive Technology Project
129 West 3rd Street
Moscow, ID 83843
208-885-3559
800-432-8324
FAX: 208-885-3628
e-mail: rseiler@uidaho.edu
www.educ.uidaho.edu/idatech

Jill Iris, Training Coordinator
Ron Seiler, Project Coordinator
$15.00

1601 **Asthma Action Cards: Child Care Asthma/Allergy Action Card**
Asthma and Allergy Foundation of America
1125 20th Street NW
Suite 402
Washington, DC 20036
202-466-7643
FAX: 202-466-8940
e-mail: info@aafa.org
www.aafa.org

Bill Lin, Executive Director
Includes necessary information a provider needs to care for a young child who has asthma and allergies. The card includes a medication plan, a list of the child's specific signs and symptoms that indicate the child is having trouble breathing, and steps on how to handle an emergency situation.

1602 **Asthma Action Cards: Student Asthma Action Card**
Asthma and Allergy Foundation of America
1233 20th Street NW
Suite 402
Washington, DC 20036
202-466-7643
800-727-8462
e-mail: info@aafa.org
www.aafa.org

Chris Ward, President
Ben C Hadden, VP Finance & Treasurer
Bill Lin, Executive Director
Tool for communicating school aged children's and teen's asthma managment plan to school personnel. Includes sections for asthma triggers, daily medications, and emergency directions.

1603 **Auditech: Classroom Amplification System Focus CFM802**
PO Box 821105
Vicksburg, MS 39182
800-229-8293
FAX: 800-221-8639
e-mail: info@auditechusa.com
www.auditechusa.com
The SOUNDFOCUS FM System is designed to cover background noise and compensate for distance. Students find it easier to focus their attention and not strain to be heard. Two speaker system. *$1052.00*

1604 **Auditech: Personal FM Educational System**
PO Box 821105
Vicksburg, MS 39182
800-229-8293
FAX: 800-221-8639
e-mail: info@auditechusa.com
www.auditechusa.com
Personal FM Educational System is a portable system for classroom use. The teacher wears a microphone. Students use a portable receiver which works clearly and easily. For users who have a hearing problem, a switch, a necklooop telecoil coupler is available. *$679.00*

1605 **Auditory-Verbal Therapy for Parents and Professionals**
Alexander Graham Bell Association
3417 Volta Place NW
Washington, DC 20007
202-337-5220
FAX: 202-337-8314
e-mail: info@agbell.org
www.agbell.org

Jessica Ripper, Senior Director Marketing/Commun
Todd Houston, Executive Director
To teach children to listen, process spoken language and talk, auditory-verbal therapy develops language and speech through listening with effective use of hearing aids and partnership of parents, children and professionals. *$39.95*
313 pages Paperback

1606 **Barrier Free Education**
Center for Assistive Technology & Env Access
490 10th Street NW
Atlanta, GA 30332
404-894-4960
800-726-9119
FAX: 404-894-9320
www.catea.org

Elizabeth Bryant, Project Director
Math and science activities pose unique accommodation challenges for students with disabilities. The Barrier Free Education resource on accessible science experiments was developed for high school chemistry and physics students with physical or visual disabilities under the National Science Foundation's Program for Persons with Disabilities.

1607 **Beginning Reasoning and Reading**
Educators Publishing Service
625 Mount Auburn Street
Suite 3
Cambridge, MA 02138
617-547-6706
800-225-5750
FAX: 888-440-2665
e-mail: feedback@epsbooks.com
www.epsbooks.com

Charles H Heinle, Vice President
Alexandra S Bigelow, Author
Gunnar Volta, President
This workbook develops basic language and thinkink skills that build the foundation for reading comprehension. Workbook exercises reinforce reading as a critical activity. *$10.45*

ISBN 0-838830-01-3

1608 **Book of Possibilities: Elementary Edition**
AbleNet
2808 Fairview Avenue N
Roseville, MN 55113
651-294-2200
800-322-0956
FAX: 651-294-2259
e-mail: customerservice@ablenetinc.com
www.ablenetinc.com

Cheryl Volkan, President/CEO
Activity ideas for all elementary age switch users to be included in a variety of math, science, language arts, social studies, spelling and reading activities. A valuable how to resource for every educator that serves students with severe disabilities. *$27.00*

1609 **Book of Possibilities: Secondary Edition**
AbleNet
2808 Fairview Avenue N
Roseville, MN 55113
651-294-2200
800-322-0956
FAX: 651-294-2222
e-mail: customerservice@ablenetinc.com
www.ablenetinc.com

Cheryl Volkam, President/CEOr
Suggestions for including secondary age switch users in a variety of school experiences throughout the day. Includes sections on secondary academics, general classroom activities like giving tests or reports and noncurricular activities like school plays and sports events. A valuable how to resource for educators that serve students with severe disabilities. *$27.00*

1610 **Buy!**
JE Stewart Teaching Tools
PO Box 15308
Seattle, WA 98115
206-262-9538
FAX: 206-262-9538

J E Stewart, Owner
Teaches 50 words as they appear in commercial and community situations such as clinic, sale, receipt, price and cleaner. These words are functional at school, on the job and shopping. *$32.50*
116 pages
ISBN 1-877866-05-9

1611 **Catalog for Teaching Life Skills to Persons with Development Disability**
P CI Educational Publishing
PO Box 34270
San Antonio, TX 78265
210-377-1999
800-594-4263
www.pcicatalog.com

Jeff Clain, Chief Executive Officer
Janie Haugen Mclane, Senior Vice President/Founder
Leslie Boulet, Senior Marketing Manager

Over 200 educational products that help individuals learn and maintain the life skills they need to succeed in an inclusive society.

1612 Childs Spelling System: The Rules

Educators Publishing Service
PO Box 9031
Cambridge, MA 02139
617-547-6706
800-225-5750
FAX: 888-440-2665
e-mail: feedback@epsbooks.com
www.epsbooks.com

Charles H Heinle, Vice President
Alexandra S Bigelow, Author
Gunnar Voltz, President
This book presents reasonable explanations of spelling rules, makes suggestions for more effective teaching and provides lists of examples and exceptions. Basic spelling rules are listed on inside front cover. *$7.15*
32 pages
ISBN 0-838801-12-9

1613 Classroom GOAL: Guide for Optimizing Auditory Learning Skills

Alexander Graham Bell Association
3417 Volta Place NW
Washington, DC 20007
202-337-5220
FAX: 202-337-8314
e-mail: info@agbell.org
www.agbell.org

Todd Houston, Executive Director
This reader-friendly teacher's guide filled with tips, source materials and sample charts and plans is designed for educators who have yearned for a resource that explains how to incorporate auditory goals into academic learning for students with different degrees of hearing loss. *$34.95*
Paperback

1614 Classroom Notetaker: How to Organize a Program Serving Students with Hearing Impairments

Alexander Graham Bell Association
3417 Volta Place NW
Washington, DC 20007
202-337-5220
FAX: 202-337-8314
e-mail: info@agbell.org
www.agbell.org

Todd Houston, Executive Director
This detailed manual for instructors, administrators and staff notetakers promotes classroom notetaking within long-term educational programs as absolutely vital for students who are deaf and hard of hearing from elementary school to college. *$24.95*
127 pages Paperback

1615 Community Services for the Blind and Partially Sighted Store: Sight Connection

Community Service for the Blind
9709 3rd Avenue NE
Suite 100
Seattle, WA 98115
206-525-5556
800-458-4888
FAX: 206-525-0422
e-mail: csbstore@csbps.com
www.sightconnection.com

June Mansfield, Chief Executive Officer
Over 300 practical products for living with vision loss selected by certified vision rehabilitation specialists from Community Services for the Blind and Partially Sighted. Easy-to-use online store features large print, large photos, secure transactions, and links to other vision-related resources. Free store catalog available by mail in large print, Braille, audiotape or PC disk. Phone and mail orders welcome. Store open 9-5, M-F, Pacific Time.

1616 Community Signs

JE Stewart Teaching Tools
PO Box 15308
Seattle, WA 98115
206-262-9538
FAX: 206-262-9538

J E Stewart, Owner
Teaches 50 words like go, fire, rest room, men, women, danger and walk needed to successfully navigate our environment. *$ 32.50*

1617 Comprehensive Assessment of Spoken Language (CASL)

AGS
PO Box 99
Circle Pines, MN 55014
800-328-2560
FAX: 800-471-8457
e-mail: agsmail@agsnet.com
www.agsnet.com

Kevin Brueggeman, President
Robert Zaske, Market Manager
CASL is an individually and orally administered research-based, theory-drive oral language assessment battery for ages 3 through 21. Fifteen tests measure language processing skills - comprehension, expression, and retrieval - in four language structure categories: lexical/semantic, syntactic, supralinguistic and pragmatic. *$299.95*

1618 Creative Arts Therapy Catalogs

MMB Music
3526 Washington Avenue
Saint Louis, MO 63103
314-531-9635
800-543-3771
FAX: 314-531-8384
e-mail: info@mmbmusic.com
www.mmbmusic.com

Marcia Lee Goldberg, President
Catalogs of books, videos, recordings for the creative arts and wellness (music, art, dance, poetry, drama, therapies, photography).

1619 Cursive Writing Skills

Educators Publishing Service
625 Mount Auburn Street
Suite 3
Cambridge, MA 02138
617-547-6706
800-225-5750
FAX: 888-440-2665
e-mail: feedback@epsbooks.com
www.epsbooks.com

Charles H Heinle, Vice President
Alexandra S Bigelow, Author
Gunnar Volta, President
These two books, written by Diana King, for grades 7-adult for right and left-handed students. Books include exercises to establish good posture; pencil grip and paper position for both lower case and upper case letters, students also practice joining letters and copying. *$ 7.15*

ISBN 0-83881 -05-

1620 Don Johnston

26799 West Commerce Drive
Volo, IL 60073
847-740-0749
800-999-4660
FAX: 847-740-7326
e-mail: info@donjohnston.com
www.donjohnston.com

Don Johnston, Leader
Ruth Ziolkowski, President
A provider of quality products and services that enable people with special needs to discover their potential and experience success. Products are developed for the areas of Physical Access, Augmentative Communication and for those who struggle with reading and writing.

1621 Dyslexia Training Program

Educators Publishing Service
PO Box 9031
Cambridge, MA 02139
617-547-6706
800-225-5750
FAX: 888-440-2665
e-mail: feedback@epsbooks.com
www.epsbooks.com

Charles H Heinle, Vice President
Alexandra S Bigelow, Author
Gunnar Voltz, President

This program from the Texas Scottish Rite Hospital for grades 2-8 introduces reading and writing through a two-year, cumulative series of daily one-hour videotaped lessons and accompanying student's books and teacher's guides. It is presented in a structured multi-sensory sequence of alphabet, reading, spelling, cursive handwriting, listening, language history and review activities. Students are in a class of nor more than six who work with instructional tapes as teacher's guides are available.
$6.75 - $15

1622 Exceptional Teaching Inc.

5673 West Las Positas Boulevard
Suite 207
Pleasanton, CA 94588
925-598-0082
800-549-6999
FAX: 925-598-0086
e-mail: info@exceptionalteaching.com
www.exceptionalteaching.com

Helene Holman, Owner/manager
Susan Taylor, Order Information
Providing educational products for those with special needs via catalog and online store.

1623 Explode the Code Books 1-8

Educators Publishing Service
PO Box 9031
Cambridge, MA 02139
800-435-7728
800-225-5750
FAX: 888-440-2665
e-mail: feedback@epsbooks.com
www.epsbooks.com

Alexandra S Bigelow, Author
Gunnar Voltz, President
A program of workbooks helps children learn to read by teaching them to use the sounds of letters. This carefully sequenced program provides experience recognizing and combining sounds in order to read words, phrases, sentences and stories, as well as to build vocabulary. A set of fifty-four illustrated cards to practice the sounds taught in books 1-3 is now available. *$6.20*
Grades K-4, 1-3
ISBN 0-83881 -60-

1624 First Course in Phonic Reading

Educators Publishing Service
PO Box 9031
Cambridge, MA 02139
617-547-6706
800-225-5750
FAX: 888-440-2665
e-mail: feedback@epsbooks.com
www.epsbooks.com

Charles H Heinle, Vice President
Alexandra S Bigelow, Author
Gunnar Voltz, President
This book provides students with a basic foundation in phonics beginning with common consonants and short vowels, syllabication and spelling rules are also taught. There is a special emphasis on auditory and kinesthetic involvement. *$10.65*
Grades 2-3
ISBN 0-838801-24-2

1625 Food!

JE Stewart Teaching Tools
PO Box 15308
Seattle, WA 98115
206-262-9538
FAX: 206-262-9538

J E Stewart, Owner
Teaches 50 words like salt, pepper, hamburger, fruit, milk and soup, seen commonly on menus, packages and in directions used at home and at play. *$32.50*

1626 Fun for Everyone

AbleNet
2808 Fairview Avenue N
Roseville, MN 55113
800-322-0956
FAX: 651-294-2254
e-mail: hresources@ablenetinc.com
www.ablenetinc.com

Cheryl Volkam, President/CEO

Today, simple technology allows children and adults with disabilities to participate in leisure activities they were limited or excluded from in the past. *$20.00*

1627 Fundamentals of Autism

Slosson Educational Publications
PO Box 280
East Aurora, NY 14052
716-652-0930
888-756-7766
888-756-7760
FAX: 800-655-3840
e-mail: slosson@slosson.com
www.slosson.com

Steven Slosson, President
John Slosson, VP
David Slosson, VP
The Fundamentals of Autism handbook provides a quick, user friendly, effective and accurate approach to help in identifying and developing educationally related program objectives for children diagnosed as autistic. These materials have been designed to be easily and functionally used by teachers, therapists, special education/learning disability resource specialists, psychologists and others who work with children diagnosed as autistic. *$56.00*
72 pages

1628 GO-MO Articulation Cards- Second Edition

Pro-Ed Publications
8700 Shoal Creek Boulevard
Austin, TX 78757
512-451-3246
800-897-3202
FAX: 800-397-7633
e-mail: feedback@proedinc.com
www.proedinc.com

Donald Hammill, Owner
The most popular system used for remedying defective speech articulation in children and adults. This popular card set was the first and is still the best therapy tool of its kind, as it continues to produce results and maintains the interest of students of all ages.

1629 Get Ready/Get Set/Go for the Code

Educators Publishing Service
PO Box 9031
Cambridge, MA 02139
617-547-6706
800-225-5750
FAX: 888-440-2665
e-mail: feedback@epsbooks.com
www.epsbooks.com

Charles H Heinle, Vice President
Alexandra S Bigelow, Author
Gunnar Voltz, President
Primers for the Explode the Code series teaches consonants through engaging activities which includes: tracking, tracing, matching, copying, and following directions. The Activities progress is difficulty, and the three-book series for grades K-1 is cumulative. A set of picture letter cards are available.
80-96 pages $4.50 - $5.50
ISBN 0-83881 -80-

1630 Gillingham Manaual

Educators Publishing Service
PO Box 9031
Cambridge, MA 02139
617-547-6706
800-225-5750
FAX: 888-440-2665
e-mail: feedback@epsbooks.com
www.epsbooks.com

Charles H Heinle, Vice President
Alexandra S Bigelow, Author
Gunnar Voltz, President
Basic hardcover instructional manual for multisensory, phonetic technique of teaching reading to children with specific language disability. A classic. Many associated teaching materials, including drill cards, and stories.

352 pages $17.55 - $69
ISBN 0-83880 -00-

1631 Guide to Teaching Phonics
Educators Publishing Service
625 Mount Auburn Street
Suite 3
Cambridge, MA 02138
617-547-6706
800-225-5750
FAX: 888-440-2665
e-mail: feedback@epsbooks.com
www.epsbooks.com

Charles H Heinle, Vice President
Alexandra S Bigelow, Author
Gunnar Voltz, President
This flexible teacher's guide presents multisensory procedures developed in association with the late Dr. Samuel Orton. They consist of 100 phonograms for teaching phonetic elements and their sequences in words for reading, writing and spelling. Also contains coordinated Phonics Cards. *$13.50*
96 pages
ISBN 0-838802-41-9

1632 Homemade Battery-Powered Toys
Special Needs Project
324 State Street
Suite H
Santa Barbara, CA 93101
805-962-8087
800-333-6867
FAX: 805-962-5087
e-mail: books@specialneeds.com
www.specialneeds.com

Hod Gray, Administrator/Owner
Laraine Gray, Coordinator
Describes how to make simple switches and educational devices for severely handicapped children. *$7.50*

1633 How the Student with Hearing Loss Can Succeed in College, Second Edition
Alexander Graham Bell Association
3417 Volta Place NW
Washington, DC 20007
202-337-5220
FAX: 202-337-8314
e-mail: info@agbell.org
www.agbell.org

Jim Reisler, President
Todd Houston, Executive Director
This revised book informs student who are deaf and hard of hearing about the mutual and co-equal effort that students and professionals must exert together to achieve success for students to be successful. *$28.95*
278 pages Paperback

1634 If it is to Be, it is Up to Me
AVKO Dyslexia Research Foundation
3084 West Willard Road
Clio, MI 48420
810-686-9283
866-285-6612
FAX: 810-686-1101
e-mail: avkoemail@aol.com
www.avko.org

Don Cabe, Executive Research Director
This book is designed for parents to use. It will prove to the student that he isn't dumb. It builds self-confidence as the student learns he can learn without studying. *$9.95*
112 pages
ISBN 1-56400 -42-1

1635 Implementing Cognitive Strategy Instruction Across the School
Brookline Books
39 University Road
Brookline, MA 02445
617-734-6772
800-666-2665
FAX: 617-734-3952
e-mail: milt@brooklinebooks.com
www.brooklinebooks.com

William H Walters, Author
Esther Isabe Wilder, Author
Describes basic classroom based programs planned and executed by teachers to focus and guide students with serious reading problems to be goal oriented, strategic and self-assessing. *$24.95*

ISBN 0-914797-75-1

1636 Inclusive Play People
Educational Equity Concepts
100 Fifth Avenue
8th Floor
New York, NY 10011
212-243-1110
FAX: 212-627-0407
TTY:212-725-1803
e-mail: information@edequity.org
www.edequity.org
Six sturdy multiracial wooden figures that provide a unique variety of nonstereotyped work and family roles and are inclusive of disabled and nondisabled people of various ages. For block building and dramatic play. *$25.00*

1637 Instruction of Persons with Severe Handicaps
McGraw-Hill School Publishing
220 East Danieldale Road
Desoto, TX 75115
972-224-1111
800-442-9685
FAX: 972-228-1982
www.mhschool.com

Joseph Gavigan, President
A complete introduction to the status of education as it pertains to people with severe handicaps.

1638 Integrating Transition Planning Into the IEP Process
Council for Exceptional Children
1110 North Glebe Road
Suite 300
Arlington, VA 22201
703-245-0600
888-232-7733
FAX: 703-264-9494
e-mail: president@cec.sped.org
www.cec.sped.org

Janice Burdick, President
Suzanne Martin, Immediate Past President
Bruce Ramirez, Manager
Helps students with disabilities make a smooth transition from school to adult life. *$15.70*
78 pages

1639 Keeping Ahead in School
Educators Publishing Service
PO Box 9031
Cambridge, MA 02139
617-547-6706
800-225-5750
FAX: 888-440-2665
e-mail: feedback@epsbooks.com
www.epsbooks.com

Charles H Heinle, Vice President
Alexandra S Bigelow, Author
Gunnar Voltz, President
This book helps students not only understand their own strengths and weaknesses but also more fully appreciate their individuality. He suggests specific ways to approach work, bypass or overcome learning disorders, and manage other struggles that may beset students in school. *$24.75*
320 pages Paperback
ISBN 0-838820-69-7

1640 KeyMath Teach and Practice
AGS
PO Box 99
Circle Pines, MN 55014
800-328-2560
FAX: 800-471-8457
e-mail: agsmail@agsnet.com
www.agsnet.com

Kevin Brueggeman, President
Robert Zaske, Market Manager
This set of materials provides all the tools needed to assess students' math skills...and the strategies to deal with problem areas. Three sets are available: Basic Concepts Package; Operations Package; and Applications Package. $219.95 each or $599.95 for whole set.

1641 Kim Marshall Series in English
Educators Publishing Service
625 Mount Auburn Street
Suite 3
Cambridge, MA 02138
617-547-6706
800-225-5750
FAX: 888-440-2665
e-mail: feedback@epsbooks.com
www.epsbooks.com

Charles H Heinle, Vice President
Alexandra S Bigelow, Author
Gunnar Voltz, President
These two books for grades 4-8 contain a total of 36 cumulative units in grammar, writing skills and word analysis. English-Part A reviews writing skills and usage, while English-Part B reviews word analysis and parts of speech. There is a teacher's manual designed to accompany each book.
104 pages $8 - $8.95

1642 Kim Marshall Series in Math
Educators Publishing Service
625 Mount Auburn Street
Suite 3
Cambridge, MA 02138
617-547-6706
800-225-5750
FAX: 888-440-2665
e-mail: feedback@epsbooks.com
www.epsbooks.com

Charles H Heinle, Vice President
Alexandra S Bigelow, Author
Gunnar Voltz, President
These two books for grades 4-8 contain 35 units that cover basic computation skills, Roman numerals, English and metric measurements, graphing, fractions and basic geometry. There is a teacher's manual designed to accompany each book.
104 pages $10.45 - $11.60

1643 Kim Marshall Series in Reading
Educators Publishing Service
PO Box 9031
Cambridge, MA 02139
617-547-6706
800-225-5750
FAX: 888-440-2665
e-mail: feedback@epsbooks.com
www.epsbooks.com

Charles H Heinle, Vice President
Alexandra S Bigelow, Author
These two books for grades 4-6 contain 186 interesting stories with comprehension questions that encourage careful reading and stimulate thinking. Because of the wide appeal of the stories, these books can be used to meet the needs of a variety of students. *$8.00*
104 pages Grades 4-6

1644 Kim Marshall Series in Vocabulary
Educators Publishing Service
625 Mount Auburn Street
Suite 3
Cambridge, MA 02138
617-547-6706
800-225-5750
FAX: 888-440-2665
e-mail: feedback@epsbooks.com
www.epsbooks.com

Charles H Heinle, Vice President
Alexandra S Bigelow, Author
Gunnar Voltz, President
This approachable vocabulary program for grades 4-8 consists of 900 words chosen to be interesting and useful and to broaden vocabulary and improve spelling. The two books in the series each contain 18 units, and every one of these units introduces 25 words followed by 5 pages of exercises and a weekly test. A teacher's manual is available for each book. *$9.75*
128 pages

1645 Lakeshore Learning Materials
2695 East Dominguez Street
Carson, CA 90895
310-537-8600
800-421-5354
FAX: 800-537-5403
e-mail: lakeshore@lakeshorelearning.com
www.lakeshorelearning.com

Michael Kaplan, Chief Executive Officer
Offers books, resources, testing materials, assessment information and special education materials for the professional in the field of special education.
190 pages

1646 Language Parts Catalog
Educators Publishing Service
PO Box 9031
Cambridge, MA 02139
617-547-6706
800-225-5750
FAX: 888-440-2665
e-mail: feedback@epsbooks.com
www.epsbooks.com

Charles H Heinle, Vice President
Alexandra S Bigelow, Author
Gunnar Voltz, President
Informatively and humorously explains the various aspects of language and how they operate, asking students to imagine that they are reading a catalog featuring different parts to order that can help them improve their language abilities. *$9.00*

ISBN 0-838819-80-X

1647 Language Tool Kit
Educators Publishing Service
625 Mount Auburn Street
Suite 3
Cambridge, MA 02138
617-547-6706
800-225-5750
FAX: 888-440-2665
e-mail: feedback@epsbooks.com
www.epsbooks.com

Charles H Heinle, Vice President
Alexandra S Bigelow, Author
Gunnar Voltz, President
This kit teaches reading and spelling to students in grades 1-3 with specific language disability. It contains 163-426 cards and a comprehensive 32-page teacher's manual. Also available in Spanish. *$30.00*
32 pages English Edition
ISBN 0-838885-20-3

1648 Language, Speech and Hearing Services in School
American Speech-Language-Hearing Association
10801 Rockville Pike
Rockville, MD 20852
301-897-5700
800-638-8255
FAX: 301-571-0457
e-mail: actioncenter@asha.org
www.asha.org

John E Bernthal, President
Arlene Peitranton, Executive Director
Joanne Jessen, Publications Director
Professional journal for clinicians, audiologists and speech-language pathologists. *$30.00*

1649 Learning American Sign Language
Harris Communications
15155 Technology Drive
Eden Prairie, MN 55344
952-906-1180
800-825-6758
FAX: 952-906-1180
e-mail: info@harriscomm.com
www.harriscomm.com

Robert Harris, President/CEO/Owner
Offers over 700 titles on ASL including books, videotapes, CDs & DVDs. Free catalog available. *$78.95*
350 pages Video & Book

1650 Learning to Listen
Educators Publishing Service
PO Box 9031
Cambridge, MA 02139
617-547-6706
800-225-5750
FAX: 888-440-2665
e-mail: feedback@epsbooks.com
www.epsbooks.com

Charles H Heinle, Vice President
Alexandra S Bigelow, Author
Gunnar Voltz, President
A program to improve classroom listening skills in a variety of situations. Presents students in grades 7-9 with instruction and 33 exercises on eight basic listening skills. After reading about a particular skill, students practice it by listening to a selection and then answering questions about the selection in writing. A teachers manual is available to accompany the student book. *$6.20*
48 pages
ISBN 0-838820-61-1

1651 Learning to Sign in My Neighborhood
T J Publishers
2544 Tarpley Road
Suite 108
Carrollton, TX 75006
972-416-0800
800-999-1168
FAX: 301-585-5930
e-mail: tjpubinc@aol.com

Angela K Thames, President
Jerald A Murphy, Vice President
Beautifully illustrated coloring book lets children learn signs from kids just like themselves! Recommended for ages 4 and up, let children have fun while they learn signs for words typically used in day-to-day activities. *$3.50*
32 pages Softcover
ISBN 0-93266 -36-1

1652 Learning to Use Cursive Handwriting
Educators Publishing Service
625 Mount Auburn Street
Suite 3
Cambridge, MA 02138
617-547-6706
800-225-5750
FAX: 888-440-2665
e-mail: feedback@epsbooks.com
www.epsbooks.com

Charles H Heinle, Vice President
Alexandra S Bigelow, Author
Gunnar Voltz, President
This multisensory program with instructions for introducing, teaching, practicing and reviewing lower- and upper-case cursive letters; masters, with letter forms and lined and patterned writing paper; and wall cards, for lower- and upper-case letters. *$ 10.60*
96 pages Manual
ISBN 0-838802-53-2

1653 Learning to Use Manuscript Handwriting
Educators Publishing Service
625 Mount Auburn Street
Suite 3
Cambridge, MA 02138
617-547-6706
800-225-5750
FAX: 888-440-2665
e-mail: feedback@epsbooks.com
www.epsbooks.com

Charles H Heinle, Vice President
Alexandra S Bigelow, Author
Gunnar Voltz, President
This multisensory program contains a manual with instructions for introducing teaching, practicing and reviewing lower- and upper-case manuscript letters; masters with letter forms and lined and patterned writing paper; and wall cards for lower- and upper-case letters. *$10.30*
76 pages Paperback
ISBN 0-838802-50-8

1654 Let's Read: A Linguistic Reading Program
Educators Publishing Service
625 Mount Auburn Street
Suite 3
Cambridge, MA 02138
617-547-6706
800-225-5750
FAX: 888-440-2665
e-mail: feedback@epsbooks.com
www.epsbooks.com

Charles H Heinle, Vice President
Alexandra S Bigelow, Author
Gunnar Volta, President
This linguistic approach to teaching reading emphasizes the basic relationship of spelling to sound, presenting like concepts together, providing reading materials for practice, and building on previously mastered skills for grades 1-3. Word lists and teacher's manuals are available for Let's Read books 1-4, and Let's Look workbooks accompany the texts.
$10.35 - $19.15

1655 Literacy Program
Educators Publishing Service
PO Box 9031
Cambridge, MA 02139
617-547-6706
800-225-5750
FAX: 888-440-2665
e-mail: feedback@epsbooks.com
www.epsbooks.com

Charles H Heinle, Vice President
Alexandra S Bigelow, Author
Gunnar Voltz, President
This one year course, developed by the Scottish Rite Hospital, consists of 160 one hour videotaped lessons accompanied by student workbooks, designed for high schoolers and adults who read below a sixth grade level. This program uses multisensory applications to teach alphabet, reading, cursive writing, spelling, math and listening comprehension with frequent new activities. This is an ideal series for a community adult reading program. Grades 1-4.
$2.25 -$18

1656 Literature Based Reading
Oryx Press
4041 North Central Avenue
Suite 700
Phoenix, AZ 85012
602-265-2651
800-279-6799
FAX: 800-279-4663
Series offering children's books and activities to enrich the K-5 curriculum.

1657 Living an Idea: Empowerment and the Evolution of an Alternative School
Brookline Books
39 University Road
Brookline, MA 02445
617-734-6772
800-666-2665
FAX: 617-734-3952
e-mail: thestrore@brooklinebooksmith.com
www.brooklinebooks.com

William H Walters, Author
Esther Isabe Wilder, Author
This book is about the creation and 14 year evolution of a public alternative inner-city high school. The school lived an idea - empowerment. Students were encouraged to participate in shaping many aspects of their education, teachers were responsible for running the school, and parents invited to help govern. *$27.95*

ISBN 0-91479 -68-9

1658 Low Tech Assistive Devices: A Handbook for the School Setting
Therapro Inc.
225 Arlington Street
Framingham, MA 01702
508-872-9494
800-257-5376
FAX: 508-875-2062
e-mail: info@theraproducts.com
www.theraproducts.com

Karen Conrad, Founder/Owner
A how-to book with step by step directions and detailed illustrations for fabrication of frequently requested low-tech assistive devices. *$45.00*
320 pages Paperback

1659 MTA Readers
Educators Publishing Service
625 Mount Auburn Street
Suite 3
Cambridge, MA 02138
617-547-6706
800-225-5750
FAX: 888-440-2665
e-mail: feedback@epsbooks.com
www.epsbooks.com

Charles H Heinle, Vice President
Alexandra S Bigelow, Author
Gunnar Voltz, President
Illustrated readers for grades 1-3 that accompany the MTA Reading and Spelling Program (Multisensory Teaching Approach). Phonetic elements in a structured, but entertaining context.
48+ pages $4.65 - $11.65
ISBN 0-83882 -33-3

1660 Making School Inclusion Work: A Guide to Everyday Practice
Brookline Books
39 University Road
Brookline, MA 02445
617-734-6772
800-666-2665
FAX: 617-734-3952
www.brooklinebooks.com

William H Walters, Author
Esther Isabe Wilder, Author
This book tells the reader how to conduct a truly inclusive program, regardless of ethnic or racial background, economic level and physical or cognitive ability. *$24.95*
254 pages
ISBN 0-914791-96-4

1661 Making the Writing Process Work: Strategie s for Composition and Self-Regulation
Brookline Books
PO Box 1047
Cambridge, MA 02139
617-734-6772
800-666-2665
FAX: 617-734-3952
e-mail: thestore@brooklinebooksmith.com
www.brooklinebooks.com

William H Walters, Author
Esther Isabe Wilder, Author
This book is geared toward students who have difficulty organizing their thoughts and developing their writing. The specific stategies teach students how to approach, organize, and produce a final written product.. *$24.95*
240 pages Paperback
ISBN 1-571290-10-9

1662 Manual Alphabet Poster
TJ Publishers
2544 Tarpley Road
Suite 108
Carrollton, TX 75006
972-416-0800
800-999-1168
FAX: 972-416-0944
e-mail: TJPubinc@aol.com
www.TJpublishers.com

Pat O'Rourke, President
Poster presents the manual alphabet. *$4.50*

1663 Many Faces of Dyslexia
40 York Road
4th Floor
Baltimore, MD 21204
410-296-0232
FAX: 410-296-5069
www.interdys.org

Megan Cohen, Executive Director
Gives information on the teaching and rehabilitation techniques for people with dyslexia. *$16.50*
Paperback

1664 Match-Sort-Assemble Job Cards
Exceptional Education
PO Box 15308
Seattle, WA 98115
206-262-9538

Jeff Stewart, Owner
Teaches workers to use a series of symbolic cues to control their own production cycles. *$565.00*
Class Set

1665 Match-Sort-Assemble Pictures
Exceptional Education
PO Box 15308
Seattle, WA 98115
206-262-9538

Jeff Stewart, Owner
People with profound, severe and moderate mental retardation have immediate access with MSA Pictures. Students work with pictures (and if necessary a template) to match, sort, assemble and disassemble parts that vary in shape, length and diameter. *$426.00*
Class Set

1666 Match-Sort-Assemble SCHEMATICS
Exceptional Education
PO Box 15308
Seattle, WA 98115
206-262-9538

Jeff Stewart, Owner
Students with moderate and mild mental retardation and those who have completed MSA Pictures are ready for MSA Schematics. It increases abstraction and displacement of instruction from the work clearly and simply. *$495.00*
Class Set

1667 Match-Sort-Assemble TOOLS
Exceptional Education
PO Box 15308
Seattle, WA 98115
206-262-9538
FAX: 475-486-4510

JE Stewart, Owner
Students and clients learn to use the tools required for many jobs in light industry. Mastery of the production cycle with independence, endurance and the ability to learn new tasks through pictures and schematics and basic hand functions will help clients acquire and maintain employment in a competitive field. *$595.00*
Class Set

1668 Meeting-in-a-Box
Asthma and Allergy Foundation of America
1233 20th Street NW
Suite 402
Washington, DC 20036
202-466-7643
800-7AS-THMA
FAX: 202-466-8940
e-mail: info@aafa.org
www.aafa.org

Chris Ward, President
Bill Mclin, Executive Director
A series of self-contained, comprehensive kits that contain all the necessary components for a successful asthma presentation.

1669 More Food!
JE Stewart Teaching Tools
PO Box 15308
Seattle, WA 98115
206-262-9538
FAX: 206-262-9538

J E Stewart, Owner
Teaches 50 more words found in restaurants, grocery stores, cookbooks such as pizza, carrot, tacos, oysters and pineapple. These words are functional at home, going shopping and during leisure. *$32.50*

1670 More Work!
J E Stewart Teaching Tools
PO Box 15308
Seattle, WA 98115
206-262-9538
FAX: 206-262-9538

J E Stewart, Owner
Teaches 50 words as they appear on parts, tools, job instructions, signs and labels, such as fill, grasp, release, lock, search, position and select. These words are functional in school and on-the-job. *$32.50*

1671 Multisensory Teaching Approach
Educators Publishing Service
PO Box 9031
Cambridge, MA 02139
617-367-2700
800-225-5750
FAX: 617-547-0412
www.epsbooks.com

Comprehensive multisensory program in reading, writing, spelling, alphabet and dictionary skills for remedial and regular instruction. Based on Orton-Gillingham and Alphabetic Phonics. A complete program organized in kits, with additional classroom materials, supplementary materials, and handwriting programs.
$110 - $140
ISBN 0-83888 -10-9

1672 Peabody Articulation Decks
AGS
PO Box 99
Circle Pines, MN 55014
651-287-7220
800-328-2560
FAX: 763-786-9007
e-mail: agsmail@agsnet.com
www.agsnet.com

Keith Powel, Special Education Transition Coo
Robert Zaske, Marketing Manager
Complete kit of playing-card sized PAD decks let students focus on the 18 most commonly misarticulated English consonants and blends. *$115.95*

ISBN 0-88671 -75-4

1673 Phonemic Awareness in Young Children: A Classroom Curriculum
Brookes Publishing
PO Box 10624
Baltimore, MD 21285
410-337-9580
800-638-3775
FAX: 410-337-8539
e-mail: custserv@brookespublishing.com
www.brookespublishing.com

Clary Creighton, Exhibits Coordinator
Tracy Gray, Educational Sales Manager
Paul Brooks, Owner
This is a supplemental, whole-class curriculum for improving pre-literacy listening skills. It contains activities that are fun, easy to use, and proven to work in any kindergarten classroom - general, bilingual, inclusive, or special education. This program takes only 15-20 minutes a day. *$24.95*
208 pages Spiral-bound 1997
ISBN 1-557663-21-1

1674 Phonics for Thought
Educators Publishing Service
PO Box 9031
Cambridge, MA 02139
617-367-2700
800-225-5750
FAX: 617-547-0412
www.epsbooks.com

$8.00
Paperback

1675 Phonological Awareness Training for Reading
Pro-Ed Publications
8700 Shoal Creek Boulevard
Austin, TX 78757
512-451-3246
800-897-3202
FAX: 800-397-7633
e-mail: feedback@proedinc.com
www.proedinc.com

Joshua Jeffrey, Marketing Custodian
Courtney King, Marketing Coordinator
Donald Hammill, Owner
Designed to increase the level of phonological awareness in young children. Can be taught individually or in small groups and takes about 12 to 14 weeks to complete if children are taught in short sessions three or four times a week. *$129.00*

1676 Play!
JE Stewart Teaching Tools
PO Box 15308
Seattle, WA 98115
206-262-9538
FAX: 206-262-9538

J E Stewart, Owner
Teaches 50 more words as they appear at recreation sites, on signs and labels and in newspapers and magazines, such as movie, visitor, ticket, gallery and zoo. These words are functional in school and at leisure. *$32.50*

1677 Power Breathing Program
Asthma and Allergy Foundation of America
1125 15th Street NW
Suite 502
Washington, DC 20005
202-466-7643
FAX: 202-466-8940
e-mail: info@aafa.org
www.aafa.org

Bill McLin, Executive Director
Devoloped the only asthma education program specifically designed for and pre-tested with teens. Teens with asthma have special challenges. This interactive program covers everything from the basics of asthma to dealing with their asthma in social situations, in college, and on the job. Includes everything you need to present this three-four session program. *$295.00*

1678 Primary Phonics
Educators Publishing Service
625 Mount Auburn Street
Suite 3
Cambridge, MA 02138
617-547-6706
800-225-5750
FAX: 888-440-2665
e-mail: feedback@epsbooks.com
www.epsbooks.com

Charles H Heinie, Vice President
Alexandra S Bigelow, Author
Gunnar Voltz, President
A program of storybooks and coordinated workbooks that teaches reading for grades K-2. A structured phonetic approach. Contains 8 student workbooks, with 8 sets of 10 coordinated storybooks; consonant workbooks; initial consonant blend workbooks; picture dictionary, and coloring book. *$3.65*
$3.65 - $26.35
ISSN 0838-83 0

1679 Programmed Phonics Books 1-2 & Cassettes
Educators Publishing Service
625 Mount Auburn Street
Suite 3
Cambridge, MA 02138
617-547-6706
800-225-5750
FAX: 888-440-2665
e-mail: feedback@epsbooks.com
www.epsbooks.com

Charles H Heinle, Vice President
Gunnar Voltz, President
This self-instructing program is for children who are having difficulty with the word recognition phase of reading vocabulary that exceeds their reading vocabulary. The books review consonants and all consonant blends. A teacher's guide and script includes dictation, which is also available on cassettes. *$7.70*
88 pages $7.50 - $45
ISSN 0838-83 0

1680 Reading for Content
Educators Publishing Service
PO Box 9031
Cambridge, MA 02139
617-547-6706
800-225-5750
FAX: 888-440-2665
e-mail: feedback@epsbooks.com
www.epsbooks.com

Charles H Heinle, Vice President
Alexandra S Bigelow, Author
Gunnar Voltz, President

This four book series for grades 3-6 has been completely revised and updated so that the reading passages are more current and interesting. Each book contains 43 one-page reading questions. A detachable answer sheet and progress graph are involved in each book.
96 pages $7.75 each

1681 Reading from Scratch
Educators Publishing Service
PO Box 9031
Cambridge, MA 02139
617-367-2700
800-225-5750
FAX: 617-547-0412
www.epsbooks.com
Contains multisensory reading and spelling material and oral and written lessons and exercises in syntax, grammar, and precomposition topics. Complete set.
$6.25 - $49.30
ISBN 0-83888 -75-5

1682 Reasoning and Reading Levels I and II
Educators Publishing Service
625 Mount Auburn Street
Suite 3
Cambridge, MA 02138
617-547-6706
800-225-5750
FAX: 888-440-2665
e-mail: feedback@epsbooks.com
www.epsbooks.com

Charles H Heinle, Vice President
Alexandra S Bigelow, Author
Gunnar Voltz, President
Three four-unit workbooks are based on the belief that reasoning, language, and reading comprehension go hand in hand. The four units are word meaning, sentence menaing, paragraph meaning and reasoning skills. Completely revised.
$10.45 each

1683 Recipe for Reading
Educators Publishing Service
PO Box 9031
Cambridge, MA 02139
617-367-2700
800-435-7728
FAX: 888-440-2665
e-mail: feedback@epsbooks.com
www.epsbooks.com

Alexandra S Bigelow, Author
Charles Heinle, Vice President
A basic reading manual with 21 storybooks and 7 workbooks for grades K-3. For remedial work. Multisensory, phonetically structured. program also includes sequence chart, a record progress, and writing paper of assorted sizes.
$4.50 - $56.25
ISSN 0838-84 1

1684 Resourcing: Handbook for Special Education Resource Teachers
Council for Exceptional Children
1110 North Glebe Road
Suite 300
Arlington, VA 22201
703-245-0600
888-cec-sped
FAX: 703-264-9494
e-mail: service@cec.sped.org
www.cec.sped.org

Jim McCormick, President
Jamie Hopkins, Vice President
Bruce Ramirez, Manager
Everything you need to know to be a resource for other teachers and support personnel who work with special education students. *$12.00*
64 pages

1685 Rewarding Speech
Speech Bin
1965 25th Avenue
Vero Beach, FL 32960
772-770-0007
800-477-3324
FAX: 772-770-0006
e-mail: thespeechbin@aol.com
www.speechbin.com

Jan J Binney, Senior Editor
Reproducible reward certificates for children. *$12.95*
32 pages

1686 Rule-ette
Educators Publishing Service
31 Smith Place
Cambridge, MA 02138
617-547-6706
800-225-5750
FAX: 888-440-2665
e-mail: feedback@epsbooks.com
www.epsbooks.com

Charles H Heinle, Vice President
Alexandra S Bigelow, Author
Gunnar Voltz, President
A spelling card game that teaches basic spelling rules. The game was developed for grades 3-Adult. *$14.65*
Ages 3-Adult
ISBN 0-838806-72-

1687 SAYdee Posters
Speech Bin
1965 25th Avenue
Vero Beach, FL 32960
772-770-0007
800-477-3324
FAX: 772-770-0006
e-mail: info@speechbin.com
www.speechbin.com

Jan J Binney, Senior Editor
Colorful speech and language posters. *$20.00*
24 pages
ISBN 0-93785 -47-5

1688 Second Course in Phonic Reading
Educators Publishing Service
625 Mount Auburn Street
Suite 3
Cambridge, MA 02138
617-547-6706
800-225-5750
FAX: 888-440-2665
e-mail: feedback@epsbooks.com
www.epsbooks.com

Charles H Heinle, Vice President
Alexandra S Bigelow, Author
Gunnar Voltz, President
Two structured phonetic workbooks to teach reading for grades 2-3 and 4-5. Book 1 focuses on sounds of the letters, phonogram combinations, word families, and spelling rules. Book 2 develops comprehension and vocabulary skills. *$10.65*
Per Book
ISSN 0838-81 6

1689 Sequential Spelling I-VII
AVKO Educational Research Foundation
3084 West Willard Road
Clio, MI 48420
810-686-9283
FAX: 810-686-1101
www.avko.org

Don McCabe, Executive Research Director
Spelling books for individuals to classrooms. Builds from easier words of a word family to important power words that build self-confidence. Each of the seven levels contains 180 spelling lessons that teach phonics through the backdoor of spelling. Students learn the patterns without having to learn rules or studying. Teachers have no papers to correct.
72 pages $8.95 each
ISBN 1-56400 -11-6

1690 Signing Naturally Curriculum
Harris Communications
15155 Technology Drive
Eden Prairie, MN 55344
952-906-1180
800-825-6758
FAX: 952-906-1099
e-mail: info@harriscomm.com
www.harriscomm.com

Robert Harris, President/Owner
Bill Williams, National Sales
A series based on the functional approach that is the most popular and widely used sign language curriculum designed for teaching American Sign Language. Book and videotape set for level 1 & 2. Teacher's curriculum is also available.

1691 Small Wonder
AGS
PO Box 99
Circle Pines, MN 55014
800-328-2560
FAX: 800-471-8457
e-mail: agsmail@agsnet.com
www.agsnet.com

Robert Zaske, Marketing Manager
Kevin Brueggeman, President
This infant through toddler program offers a delightful array of activities to teach babies about themselves, others, their surroundings and the world outside. Level One - zero to 18 months; Level Two 18-36 months. Discount price of $389.95 when both levels ordered. *$229.95*

ISBN 0-91347 -62-5

1692 Solving Language Difficulties: Remedial Routines
Educators Publishing Service
625 Mount Auburn Street
Suite 3
Cambridge, MA 02138
617-547-6706
800-225-5750
FAX: 888-440-2665
e-mail: feedback@epsbooks.com
www.epsbooks.com

Charles H Heinle, Vice President
Alexandra S Bigelow, Author
Gunnar Voltz, President
A basic workbook for children in grades 4-6 who have a specific language disability. It can be used in any corrective reading program. It deals extensively with syllables, syllable division, prefixes, suffixes, accent and other important topics. *$9.75*
176 pages
ISBN 0-838803-26-1

1693 Sound Workbook
Educators Publishing Service
PO Box 9031
Cambridge, MA 02139
617-547-6706
800-225-5750
FAX: 888-440-2665
e-mail: feedback@epsbooks.com
www.epsbooks.com

Charles H Heinle, Vice President
Alexandra S Bigelow, Author
Gunnar Voltz, President
This workbook for grades 1-2 reinforces the teaching of specific vowel combinations. *$5.50*
44 pages
ISBN 0-838817-08-4

1694 Sound-Off 1-5
Educators Publishing Service
625 Mount Auburn Street
Suite 3
Cambridge, MA 02138
617-547-6706
800-225-5750
FAX: 888-440-2665
e-mail: feedback@epsbooks.com
www.epsbooks.com

Charles H Heinle, Vice President
Alexandra S Bigelow, Author
Gunnar Voltz, President
These five workbooks for grades K-2 cover the introduction of consonants and final consonant blends and consonant diagraphs, vowel-consonant-e combinations, and vowel + r combinations. There is a teacher's guide for each book. *$5.50*
32-48 pages Per Book
ISBN 0-83885 -34-

1695 Speech Bin
Abilitations
3155 Northwoods Parkway
Norcross, GA 30071
800-850-8602
FAX: 800-845-1535
e-mail: orders@sportime.com
www.speechbin.com

Cecilia Cruse MS OTR/L, Education Director
Debbie Kissel, New Product Development
Activities, worksheets and games to encourage practice of speech and language skills. *$25.00*
128 pages
ISBN 0-93785 -42-4

1696 Speech-Language Delights
1965 25th Avenue
Vero Beach, FL 32960
772-770-0007

1697 Spell of Words
Educators Publishing Service
625 Mount Auburn Street
Suite 3
Cambridge, MA 02138
617-547-6706
800-225-5750
FAX: 888-440-2665
e-mail: feedback@epsbooks.com
www.epsbooks.com

Charles H Heinle, Vice President
Gunnar Voltz, President
This book can be used with any student, from grade 7-adult, who needs help in spelling. It covers syllabication, word building with prefixes, word patterns, phonograms, suffixes, plurals and possessives. Chapters contain explanations of spelling rules, exercises and suggestions for short compositions. *$9.25*
128 pages Grades 7-Adult
ISBN 0-838801-55-2

1698 Spellbinding 2
Educators Publishing Service
625 Mount Auburn Street
Suite 3
Cambridge, MA 02138
617-547-6706
800-225-5750
FAX: 888-440-2665
e-mail: feedback@epsbooks.com
www.epsbooks.com

Charles H Heinle, Vice President
Alexandra S Bigelow, Author
Gunnar Voltz, President
Spellbinding 2 adds practice exercises with more complicated spelling problems and introduces new areas of study. The manuals give answers to exercises and include a large number of new dictations. *$11.55*
96+ pages Each
ISBN 0-838814-75-1

1699 Spellbound
Educators Publishing Service
PO Box 9031
Cambridge, MA 02139
617-547-6706
800-225-5750
FAX: 888-440-2665
e-mail: feedback@epsbooks.com
www.epsbooks.com

Charles H Heinle, Vice President
Alexandra S Bigelow, Author
Gunnar Voltz, President
This workbook begins with teaching simple, consistent rules and then moves on to those that are more difficult. By an inductive process, students use their own observations to confirm the spelling rules they learn. Each portion of the text is followed by exercises for drill and kinesthetic reinforcement. *$8.65*
144 pages Grades 7-Adult
ISBN 0-838801-65-X

1700 Spelling Dictionary
Educators Publishing Service
625 Mount Auburn Street
Suite 3
Cambridge, MA 02138
617-547-6706
800-225-5750
FAX: 888-440-2665
e-mail: feedback@epsbooks.com
www.epsbooks.com

Charles H Heinle, Vice President
Alexandra S Bigelow, Author
Gunnar Voltz, President

This handy reference is a dictionary/thesaurus of words most frequently used by student writers in the elementary grades. Words are listed without definitions, and synonyms are offered for commonly used words like said, big, good, etc. Children can add their own words at the bottom of each page. *$4.50*

52 pages
ISBN 0-838820-56-5

1701 Spelling Workbooks Emphasizing Rules and Generalization for Corrective Drill
Educators Publishing Service
625 Mount Auburn Street
Suite 3
Cambridge, MA 02138
617-547-6706
800-225-5750
FAX: 888-440-2665
e-mail: feedback@epsbooks.com
www.epsbooks.com

Charles H Heinle, Vice President
Alexandra S Bigelow, Author
Gunnar Voltz, President
Includes exercises for children in grades 7-12 who have reading difficulties and closely associated spelling weaknesses. The material is divided into phonetic drills, spelling rules and generalizations, syllable concepts, and punctuation symbols. There are frequent review exercises. Similar programs are available for grades 4-6 ($11.70). *$12.25*

144 pages Grades 7-12
ISBN 0-838800-90-4

1702 Starting Over
Educators Publishing Service
625 Auburn Street
3rd Floor
Cambridge, MA 02138
617-547-6706
800-225-5750
FAX: 888-440-2665
e-mail: feedback@epsbooks.com
www.epsbooks.com

Charles H Heinle, Vice President
Alexandra S Bigelow, Author
Gunnar Voltz, President
This comprehensive program is for a student who is ready to try to learn to read again, or for those who are learning English as a second language. Employs multisensory phonics, whole words, and language experience techniques to teach the building of words, vocabulary, and sentences. *$24.00*

ISBN 0-838881-65-5

1703 Structure of Words
Educators Publishing Service
PO Box 9031
Cambridge, MA 02139
617-547-6706
800-225-5750
FAX: 888-440-2665
e-mail: feedback@epsbooks.com
www.epsbooks.com

Charles H Heinle, Vice President
Alexandra S Bigelow, Author
Gunnar Voltz, President
Designed to help students in grades 7-12 learn to spell by using logic as well as memorization and drill, and to help them pronounce and arrive at the meanings of unfamiliar words. The consistent theme throughout is that of spelling, gradually shifting into the analysis of word structure and the development of a rich vocabulary. *$21.15*

96 pages Grades 7-12
ISBN 0-838801-35-8

1704 Studio 49 Catalog
MMB Music
3526 Washington Avenue
Saint Louis, MO 63103
314-531-9635
800-543-3771
FAX: 314-531-8384
e-mail: info@mmbmusic.com
www.mmbmusic.com

Marcia Lee Goldberg, President
Michelle Greenlaw, Vice President
Percussion instruments for school, therapy, church and family.

1705 Syracuse Community-Referenced Curriculum Guide for Students with Disabilties
Brookes Publishing
PO Box 10624
Baltimore, MD 21285
410-337-9580
800-638-3775
FAX: 410-337-8539
e-mail: custserv@brookespublishing.com
www.brookespublishing.com

Paul Brooks, Owner
Serving learners from kindergarten through age 21, this field-tested curriculum is a for professionals and parents devoted to directly preparing a student to function in the world. it examines the role of community living domains, functional academics, and embedded skills and includes practical implementation strategies and information for preparing students whose learning needs go beyond the scope of traditional academic programs. *$54.95*

416 pages Spiral-bound
ISBN 1-557660-27-1

1706 Teaching Individuals with Physical and Multiple Disabilities
McGraw-Hill, School Publishing
220 East Danieldale Road
Desoto, TX 75115
800-442-9685
FAX: 972-228-1982
www.mhschool.com

Joseph Gavigan, President
Focuses on the functional needs of the handicapped and the teaching skills of background teachers that they need to help them reach the highest possible level of self-sufficiency.

410 pages

1707 Teaching Students Ways to Remember
Brookline Books
39 University Road
Brookline, MA 02445
617-558-8010
800-666-2665
FAX: 617-558-8011
e-mail: milt@brooklinebooks.com
www.brooklinebooks.com
Teaches techniques for improving or strengthening memory. *$21.95*

ISBN 0-914797-67-0

1708 Teaching Test-Taking Skills: Helping Students Show What They Know
Brookline Books
39 University Road
Brookline, MA 02445
617-558-8010
800-666-2665
FAX: 617-558-8011
e-mail: milt@brooklinebooks.com
www.brooklinebooks.com
Test-taking skills that, when used effectively, contribute to test-wise performance and help students work productively with test materials. *$21.95*

ISBN 0-914797-76-X

1709 Tools for Transition
AGS
PO Box 99
Circle Pines, MN 55014
800-328-2560
FAX: 800-471-8457
e-mail: agsmail@agsnet.com
www.agsnet.com

Robert Zaske, Marketing Manager
This program prepares students with learning disabilities for postsecondary education. *$129.95*

1710 **VAK Tasks Workbook: Visual, Auditory and Kinesthetic**

Educational Tutorial Consortium
4400 South 44th Street
Lincoln, NE 68516
402-489-8133
FAX: 402-489-8160
e-mail: etc@altel.net
www.etc-ne.com

T Cross, Owner

A workbook emphasizing the multisensory approach to teaching vocabulary and spelling. It is intended for middle-grade and older students working with prefixes, roots, suffixes, homonyms, and the spelling of easily confused endings. Includes spelling posters. *$7.00*

96 pages Paperback

1711 **Volunteer Transcribing Services**

205 East 3rd Avenue
Suite 200
San Mateo, CA 94401
650-344-8664
FAX: 650-632-3510

Alanah Hoffman, Coordinator

VTS is a nonprofit California corporation that produces large print school books for visually impaired students in grades K-12.

1712 **Word Attack Manual**

Educators Publishing Service
625 Auburn Street
3rd Floor
Cambridge, MA 02138
617-547-6706
800-225-5750
FAX: 888-440-2665
e-mail: feedback@epsbooks.com
www.epsbooks.com

Charles H Heinle, Vice President
Alexandra S Bigelow, Author
Gunnar Voltz, President

This manual and test booklet are designed to develop word recognition and spelling skills for students in grades 6-10. Contents include lessons on syllables, syllabication and accent, consonants and consonant blends, diagraphs, diphthongs, prefixes, suffixes, and compound words, and using the dictionary. *$21.15*

176 pages Grades 6-10
ISBN 0-838881-00-5

1713 **Word Demons**

Educators Publishing Service
625 Mount Auburn Street
Suite 3
Cambridge, MA 02138
617-547-6706
800-225-5750
FAX: 888-440-2665
e-mail: feedback@epsbooks.com
www.epsbooks.com

Charles H Heinle, Vice President
Alexandra S Bigelow, Author
Gunnar Voltz, President

This spelling game helps students master the 86 non-phonetic words that are demons for the child in grades 2-4 with a language disability. *$14.40*

Grades 2-4
ISBN 0-838803-28-8

1714 **Word Elements: How They Work Together**

Educators Publishing Service
625 Mount Auburn Street
Suite 3
Cambridge, MA 02138
617-547-6706
800-225-5750
FAX: 888-440-2665
e-mail: feedback@epsbooks.com
www.epsbooks.com

Charles H Heinle, Vice President
Alexandra S Bigelow, Author
Gunnar Voltz, President

This vocabulary workbook teaches common word elements - prefixes, suffixes, and roots and their meanings for grades 6-8. *$ 10.65*

112 pages Grades 6-8
ISBN 0-838815-50-2

1715 **Word Mastery**

Educators Publishing Service
625 Mount Auburn Street
Suite 3
Cambridge, MA 02138
617-547-6706
800-225-5750
FAX: 888-440-2665
e-mail: feedback@epsbooks.com
www.epsbooks.com

Charles H Heinle, Vice President
Alexandra S Bigelow, Author
Gunnar Voltz, President

This phonics classic introduces over 3,500 words and supplements any reading program with its straightforward phonics instruction. It teaches students in grades 1-3 the letters of the alphabet with key words, and follows with vowels, consonants, vowel combinations, consonant diagraphs and blends, and phonetic rules. *$8.95*

124 pages Grades 1-3
ISBN 0-838820-00-X

1716 **Wordly Wise A,B,C**

Educators Publishing Service
PO Box 9031
Cambridge, MA 02139
617-547-6706
800-225-5750
FAX: 888-440-2665
e-mail: feedback@epsbooks.com
www.epsbooks.com

Charles H Heinle, Vice President
Alexandra S Bigelow, Author
Gunnar Voltz, President

This series of three vocabulary books for grades 2-4 presents 8-12 words in each lesson with brief definitions, illustrations and sentences using each word in context. Exercises reinforce learning by teaching students to use words precisely in a variety of situations. Keys and tests are available for each book.

64 pages $5.50 each
ISSN 0838-84 8

1717 **Work!**

JE Stewart Teaching Tools
PO Box 15308
Seattle, WA 98115
206-262-9538
FAX: 206-262-9538

J E Stewart, Owner

Teaches 50 words as they appear on parts, tools, job instructions, signs, labels such as: hard hat, assembly, clamp, cut, drill, package and schedule. These words are functional in school and on-the-job. *$32.50*

1718 **Working Together & Taking Part**

A GS
PO Box 99
Circle Pines, MN 55014
800-328-2560
FAX: 800-471-8457
e-mail: agsmail@agsnet.com
www.agsnet.com

Kevin Brueggeman, President
Robert Zaske, Market Manager

Two programs to build children's social skills in grades 3-6 through folk literature. Has 31 activity-rich lessons, teaching skills like: following rules, accepting differences, speaking assertively and helping others. Discount price of $279.00 when ordering both. *$149.95*

1719 **Writing Skills 1 and 2**

Educators Publishing Service
625 Mount Auburn Street
Suite 3
Cambridge, MA 02138
617-547-6706
800-225-5750
FAX: 888-440-2665
e-mail: feedback@epsbooks.com
www.epsbooks.com

Charles H Heinle, Vice President
Alexandra S Bigelow, Author
Gunnar Voltz, President
Students practice writing sentences and developing paragraphs through writing about their ideas and personal experiences. A logical sequence takes students from individual sentences to basic paragraphs of 5 sentences, expanded paragraphs, and essays. *$7.50*
64 pages Grades 4-6, 7-9
ISBN 0-83882 -50-

1720 **Writing Skills for the Adolescent**
Educators Publishing Service
PO Box 9031
Cambridge, MA 02139
617-547-6706
800-225-5750
FAX: 888-440-2665
e-mail: feedback@epsbooks.com
www.epsbooks.com

Charles H Heinle, Vice President
Alexandra S Bigelow, Author
Gunnar Voltz, President
Teaches the writing process in a series of logical steps as students learn to write and improve sentences, they work on grammar, which is taught in terms of writing. Meanwhile, they learn to generate ideas to compose topic sentences and to use transitional words. They gradually progress from paragraph writing to essay writing. *$10.65*
96 pages Paperback
ISBN 0-838817-04-1

Associations

1721 **AVKO Dyslexia Research Foundation**
3084 West Willard Road
Clio, MI 48420
810-686-9283
FAX: 810-686-1101
e-mail: avkoemail@aol.com
www.avko.org

Don McCabe, Executive Research Director
Devorah Wolf, Board President
Comprised of individuals interested in helping others learn to read and spell. Develops and sells materials for teaching dyslexics or others with learning disabilities using a method involving audio, visual, kinesthetic and oral (multi-sensory) techniques.

1722 **Alliance for Parental Involvement in Education**
PO Box 59
East Chatham, NY 12060
518-392-6900
FAX: 518-392-6900
e-mail: allpie@taconic.net
www.croton.com/allpie
A nonprofit organization to encourage and assist parental involvement in education, public, private and home. Offers a newsletter, a book catolog, retreats, workshops, and a lending library.

1723 **Alternative Work Concepts**
PO Box 11452
Eugene, OR 97440
541-345-3043
FAX: 541-345-9669
e-mail: awc@efn.com
www.alternativeworkconcepts.org

Liz Fox, Executive Director
To promote individualized, integrated, and meaningful employment opportunities in the community for adults with multiple disabilities; to improve the quality of life and provide continuous opportunities for personal growth for these individuals; and to assist businesses with workforce diversification.

1724 **American Council for Headache Education (ACHE)**
19 Mantua Road
Mount Royal, NJ 08061
856-423-0258
FAX: 856-423-0082
e-mail: achehq@talley.com
www.achenet.org

Linda McGillicuddy, Executive Director
Nonprofit, patient-health, professional partnership dedicated to advancing the treatment and management of headaches and to raising the public awareness of headache as valid, biologically based illness.

1725 **American School Counselor Association**
American Counselling Association
1101 King Street
Suite 625
Alexandria, VA 22314
703-683-2722
800-306-4722
FAX: 703-683-1619
e-mail: asca@schoolcounselor.org
www.schoolcounselor.org

Richard Wong, Executive Director
Kathleen Rakestraw, Director of Communications
Carolyn Stone, Board President
ASCA focuses on providing professional devleopment, enhancing school counseling programs, and research effective school counseling practices. Mission is to promote excellence in professional school counseling and the development of all students.

1726 **Association on Higher Education and Disability**
107 Commerce Center Drive
Suite 204
Huntersville, NC 28078
704-947-7779
FAX: 704-948-7779
TTY:617-287-3882
e-mail: ahead@ahead.org
www.ahead.org

Ethan Smith, President
Stephan Smith, Executive Director
Higher education for people with disabilities. A vital resource, promoting excellence through education, communication and training.

1727 **CARF Rehabilitation Accreditation Commission**
CARF International
4891 East Grant Road
Tucson, AZ 85712
520-325-1044
888-281-6531
FAX: 520-318-1129
e-mail: postmaster@carf.org
www.carf.org

Brian Boon PhD, President/CEO
Independent, nonprofit commission promotes quality services for people with disabilities and others in need of rehabilitation. CARF establishes customer-focused standards to help organizations measure and improve the quality of their rehabilitation programs and services. When reviewing a rehabilitation program or service, CARF applies standards that have been developed and accepted by peers in the field.

1728 **CEC-Division for Early Childhood**
Council for Exceptional Children
1110 North Glebe Road
Suite 300
Arlington, VA 22201
888-232-7733
FAX: 703-264-9494
e-mail: service@cec.sped.org
www.cec.sped.org

Jim McCormick, President
Drew Allbritten, Executive Director
Bruce Ramirez, Manager
A division of The Council for Exceptional Children. Promotes education for young children and infants with special needs, initiates programs that cooperatively involve parents in their children's education, stimulates communication and joint activity among early childhood organizations, sponsors professional development and disseminates research findings and information addressing issues of early childhood education and more.

1729 **Clearinghouse for Specialized Media and Technology**
California Department of Education
1430 North Street
Sacramento, CA 95814
916-324-4244
FAX: 916-323-9732
www.cde.ca.gov/re/pn/sm

David Supkofl, Manager

Assists schools and students in the identification and acquisition of textbooks, reference books and study materials in aural media, braille, large print and electronic media access technology.

1730 Council for Exceptional Children
1110 North Glebe Road
Suite 300
Arlington, VA 22201
703-245-0600
888-232-7733
FAX: 703-264-9494
e-mail: president@cec.sped.org
www.cec.sped.org

Janice Burdick, President
Suzanne Martin, Immediate Past President
Bruce Ramirez, Manager
The largest international organization dedicated to improving educational success for individuals with exceptionalities. CEC sets professional standards, advocates for appropriate government policies, provides continual professional development and advocates for newly and historically underserved individuals with exceptionalities. Helps professionals obtain conditions and resources necessary for effective practice.

1731 Educational Referral Service
Doctor Yvonne Jones and Associates
2222 Eastlake Avenue E
Seattle, WA 98102
206-325-2600
FAX: 206-328-9172

Yvonne Jones
Specializes in matching children with the learning environments that are best for them and works with families to help them identify concerns and establish priorities about their child's education.

1732 Institute on Disability/UCED
University of New Hampshire
10 West Edge Drive
Suite 101
Durham, NH 03824
603-862-4320
FAX: 603-862-0555
e-mail: contactiod@unh.edu
www.iod.unh.edu

Jan Nisbet, Director
Nancy Cicolini, Office Manager
Janice Mutschler, Manager
This mission of the Institute is to improve the knowledge, policy and practice related to the economic and social participation of persons with disabilities. The Institute provides a blend of programs that address the needs of local schools, community services and state and federal agencies. The Institute's goal is to increase the ability of the State of New Hampshire to foster inclusion of persons with disabilities into their communities.

1733 International Association of Parents and Professionals for Safe Alternatives in Childbirth
RR 4
Box 646
Marble Hill, MO 63764
573-238-2010
FAX: 573-238-2010
e-mail: napsac@clas.org
www.napsac.org

Lee Stewart, President
David Stewart, Executive Director
Dedicated to exploring, implementing, and establishing safe, family-centered childbirth programs that meet the social and emotional needs of families as well as provide the safe, appropriate aspects of medical science.

1734 International Childbirth Education Association
PO Box 20048
Minneapolis, MN 55420
952-854-8660
FAX: 952-854-8772
e-mail: info@icea.org
www.icea.org

Doris Olson, President
Sandra Anderson, Educator
Offer teaching certificates, seminars, continuing education workshops, and a mail order center.

1735 International Dyslexia Association
40 York Road
4th Floor
Baltimore, MD 21204
410-296-0232
FAX: 410-321-5069
e-mail: info@interdys.org
www.interdys.org

Anne Vickers, Executive Director
Thrace Mears, Admissions Director
John W Weaver, Advancement Director
Provides free information and referral services for diagnosis and tutoring for parents, educators, physicians, and individuals with dyslexia. 48 countries. Membership includes yearly journal and quarterly newsletter. Call for conference dates.

1736 International Organization for the Education of the Hearing Impaired
Alexander Graham Bell Association
3417 Volta Place NW
Washington, DC 20007
202-337-5220
FAX: 202-337-8314
TTY:202-337-5221
e-mail: info@agbell.org
www.agbell.org

Todd Houston, Executive Director
Professional educators of the hearing impaired make up the members of this organization which promotes the excellence in teaching the hearing impaired child.

1737 Jewish Guild for the Blind
JGB Audio Library
15 West 65th Street
New York, NY 10023
212-769-6200
800-284-4422
FAX: 212-769-6266
e-mail: info@jgb.org
www.JGB.org

Alan Morse, President
James M Dubin, President/CEO
Peter Williamson, Director of Communications
Full service vision care agency for children, adults and elderly people who are blind or visually impaired.

1738 Job Accommodation Network
Office of Disability and Employment Policy
PO Box 6080
Morgantown, WV 26506
800-232-9675
800-526-7234
FAX: 304-093-5407
TTY: 877-781-9403
e-mail: jan@jan.wvu.edu
www.jan.wvu.edu

DJ Hendricks, Director
International toll-free consulting service that provides information about job accommodations and the employability of people with disabilities. Also provides information regarding the Americans with Disabilities Act (ADA).

1739 Michigan Psychological Association
2105 University Park Drive
Suite C1
Okemos, MI 48864
517-347-1885
FAX: 517-347-1896
e-mail: mpa@acd.net
www.michpsych.org

Judith Kovach, Executive Director
Pamela Steffy, Managing Director
Tena Park, Administrative Assistant
Nonprofit organization of over 1000 psychologists, working to advance psychology as a science and a profession and to promote the public welfare by encouraging the highest professional standards, offering public education and providing a public service, and by participating in the public policy process on behalf of the profession and health care consumers.

1740 National Association of Colleges and Employers
62 Highland Avenue
Bethlehem, PA 18017
610-868-1421
800-544-5272
FAX: 610-868-0208
www.naceweb.org

Vanessa Strauss, President
Shawn Vanderziel, Director Human Resources
Sandra Dalious, Human Resources Manager
A national association with services for career planning, placement and recruitment professionals.

1741 National Association of Private Special Education Centers
1522 K St NW
Suite 1032
Washington, DC 20005
202-408-3338
FAX: 202-408-3340
e-mail: napsec@aol.com
www.napsec.org

Sherry L Kolbe, Executive Director
Jonathan Cartagena, Communications Coordinator
Rebecca Kantz, Membership Services Coordinator
Membership directory offering information on NAPSEC member schools nationwide available.

1742 National Center for Homeopathy
801 North Fairfax Street
Suite 306
Alexandria, VA 22314
703-548-7790
FAX: 703-548-7792
e-mail: info@homeopathic.org
http://nationalcenterforhomeopathy.org/

Jean Hoagland, President
Shirley Grassflower, Vice President
Sharon Stevenson, Executive Director
Provides information, referral lists, and courses to professionals.

1743 National Clearinghouse for Professions in Special Education
Council for Exceptional Children
1110 North Glebe Road
Suite 300
Arlington, VA 22201
703-245-0600
FAX: 703-264-9494
www.cec.sped.org

Janice Burdick, President
Bruce Ramirez, Manager
Designed to encourage individuals to seek careers in the various fields related to the education of children and youth with disabilities.

1744 National Council on Rehabilitation Education
2012 W. Norwood Drive
Carbondale, IL 62901
618-549-3267
FAX: 618-457-3632
www.rehabeducators.org

Charles Arokiasamy MD, Administrative Secretary
Brooke Beckege, Assistant Administrative Secreta
John Welty, Chief Executive Officer
Members include academic institutions and organizations, professional educators, researchers, and students. Assists in the documentation of the effect of education in improving services to persons with disabilities; determines the skills and training necessary for effective rehabilitation services; develops role models, standards and uniform licensure and certification requirements for rehabilitation personnel.

1745 National Education Association of the United States
1201 16th Street NW
Washington, DC 20036
202-833-4000
FAX: 202-822-7974
www.nea.org

John Wilson, Chief Executive Officer
Offers information to educational professionals.

1746 National Society for Experiential Education
19 Mantua Road
Mt. Royal, NJ 08061
856-423-3427
FAX: 856-423-3420
www.nsee.org

Karen Roloff, President
Clinton Stockwell, Executive Director
National nonprofit organization which advocates experiential learning and works with college administrators and high school and college internship programs.

1747 President's Committee for People with Intellectual Disabilities
Administration for Children & Families
370 L Enfant Promenade SW
Washington, DC 20447
202-619-0634
FAX: 202-205-9519
www.acf.hhs.gov/programs/pcpid

Sally Atwater, Executive Director
Dalls Rob Sweezy, Chairperson
MJ Karimi, Executive Director Assistant
Prepares an annual report to the president of the United States addressing issues concerning citizens with intellectual disabilities.

1748 Rifin Family/Daughters of Israel
JGB Audio Library for the Blind
15 West 65th Street
New York, NY 10023
212-769-6200
800-284-4422
FAX: 212-769-6266
e-mail: info@JGB.org
www.JGB.org

Peter Wiliamson, Director of Communication
Wanda Figueroa-Kilroy, Executive Vice President
Alan Morse, Manager

1749 SSD (Services for Students with Disabilities)
College Board
45 Columbus Avenue
New York, NY 10023
212-713-8000
FAX: 212-713-8277
www.collegeboard.com

Gaston Caperton, President
National, nonprofit membership association dedicated to preparing, inspiring and connecting students to college and opportunity. Founded in 1900, the association is composed of more than 3,800 schools, colleges, universities and other educational organizations. Services for Students with Disabilities (SSD) provides special arrangements to minimize the possible effects of disabilities on test performance through it's Admissions Testing Program (ATP).

1750 Target Teach
Evans Newton
15941 North 77th Street
Ste. 1
Scottsdale, AZ 85260
480-998-2777
800-443-0544
FAX: 480-951-2895
e-mail: info@evansnewton.com
www.evansnewton.com

Jocklyn Smith, Director
Gary Davis, Director of Curriculum and Instr
Jamie Piotti, Chief Executive Officer
Aligns and monitors Special Education Instructional Materials to tests that are used to measure the effectiveness of Special Education Instructional Programs.

1751 United Cerebral Palsy Research and Educational Foundation
UCP National
1660 L Street NW
Suite 700
Washington, DC 20036
202-776-0406
800-872-5827
FAX: 202-776-0414
e-mail: webmaster@ucp.org
www.ucpa.org

Stephen Bennett, President
Grants are awarded to institutions or organizations on behalf of a principal investigator in support of biomedical and bioengineering research in areas which have a significant relationship to cerebral palsy. While most research on central nervous system structure, function and disorder may be useful, the Foundation requires that research proposals address issues of relevance to cerebral palsy.

Directories

1752 **BOSC: Directory of Facilities for People with Learning Disabilities**
Books on Special Children
PO Box 3378
Amherst, MA 01004
413-256-8164
FAX: 413-256-8896
e-mail: irene@boscbooks.com
www.boscbooks.com

Michael Young, President
Directory of schools, independent living programs, clinics and centers, colleges and vocational programs, agencies and commercial products. Five sections in special post binder that can be updated annually. Hardcover. *$70.00*
300+ pages Yearly
ISSN 0961-3888

1753 **Complete Directory for Pediatric Disorders**
Sedgwick Press/Grey House Publishing
PO Box 860
Millerton, NY 12546
518-789-8700
800-562-2139
FAX: 518-789-0556
e-mail: books@greyhouse.com
www.greyhouse.com

Leslie Mackenzie, Publisher
Laura Mars, Editorial Director
Jessica Moody, Marketing Director
An annual directory for professionals, parents and caregivers. Provides valuable information on more than 200 pediatric conditions, disorders, diseases and disabilities, including informative descriptions and a wide variety of resources, from associations to publications. *$145.00*
702 pages Annual
ISBN 1-891482-41-6

1754 **Complete Directory for People with Chronic Illness**
Sedgwick Press/Grey House Publishing
PO Box 860
Millerton, NY 12546
518-789-8700
800-562-2139
FAX: 518-789-0556
e-mail: books@greyhouse.com
www.greyhouse.com

Leslie Mackenzie, Publisher
Laura Mars, Editorial Director
Jessica Moody, Marketing Director
This directory is structured around the ninety most prevalent chronic illnesses. Each chronic illness chapter includes an informative description, plus a comprehensive listing of resources and support services available for people diagnosed with chronic illness and their network of supportive individuals. *$165.00*
Annual

1755 **Complete Learning Disabilities Directory**
Sedgwick Press/Grey House Publishing
PO Box 860
Millerton, NY 12546
518-789-8700
800-562-2139
FAX: 518-789-0556
e-mail: books@greyhouse.com
www.greyhouse.com

Leslie Mackenzie, Publisher
Laura Mars, Editorial Director
Jessica Moody, Marketing Director
A comprehensive educational guide offering over 6,500 listings on associations and organizations, schools, government agencies, testing materials, camps, products, books, newsletters, legal information, classroom materials and more. Includes separate chapters on ADD and Literacy, as well as informative articles. *$145.00*
702 pages Annual
ISBN 1-891482-41-6

1756 **Complete Mental Health Directory**
Sedgwick Press/Grey House Publishing
PO Box 860
Millerton, NY 12546
518-789-8700
800-562-2139
FAX: 518-789-0556
e-mail: books@greyhouse.com
www.greyhouse.com

Leslie Mackenzie, Publisher
Laura Mars, Editorial Director
Jessica Moody, Marketing Director
This directory offers comprehensive information covering the field of behavioral health, with critical information for both the layman and the mental health professional. It covers, in depth, 25 specific mental disorders, and includes informative descriptions and a complete list of resources.
Annual

1757 **Diabetes: Caring for Your Emotions as Well as Your Health**
Harper Collins Publishers/ Basic Books
10 East 53rd Street
New York, NY 10022
212-207-7000
800-242-7737
FAX: 212-207-7203

Jane Friedman, Chief Executive Officer
This book offers suggestions for adaptation, relationships with medical personnel, family strategies, employment questions, technology and support groups. *$15.00*

ISBN 1-852300-47-7

1758 **Dictionary of Special Education and Rehabilitation**
Love Publishing Company
9101 East Kenyon Avenue
Suite 2200
Denver, CO 80237
303-221-7333
FAX: 303-221-7444
e-mail: lpc@lovepyblishing.com
www.lovepublishing.com

Ann Vernon, Author
Stan Love, Owner
A valuable basic resource in the field. It incorporates hundreds of additions and changes. *$39.95*
Paperback
ISBN 0-891082-43-3

1759 **Directory for Exceptional Children**
Porter Sargent Publishers
11 Beacon Street
Suite 1400
Boston, MA 02108
617-523-1670
800-342-7470
FAX: 617-523-1021
e-mail: orders@portersargent.com
www.portersargent.com

Porter Sergent Steft, author
John Yonce, General Manager
Daniel Mckeever, Senior Editor
Leslie A Weston, Production Manager
A comprehensive, objective survey of 3000 schools, facilities and organizations across the country serving children and young adults with developmental, emotional, physical and mental disabilities. *$75.00*

1120 pages Trienniel
ISBN 0-875581-50-1

1760 Educators Resource Directory
Sedgwick Press/Grey House Publishing
PO Box 860
Millerton, NY 12546
518-789-8700
800-562-2139
FAX: 518-789-0545
e-mail: books@greyhouse.com
www.greyhouse.com

Leslie Mackenzie, Publisher
Laura Mars, Editorial Director
Jessica Moody, Marketing Director
Gives education professionals immediate access to Associations and Organizations, Conferences and Trade Shows, Educational Research Centers, Employment Opportunities and Teaching Abroad, School Library Services, Scholarships, Financial Resources and much more. *$ 145.00*
591 pages Annual
ISBN 1-930956-48-7

1761 Enhancing Children's Communication: Research & Foundations
Enhancing Childrens Communication Research & Found
PO Box 10624
Baltimore, MD 21285
410-337-9580
800-638-3775
FAX: 410-337-8539
e-mail: custserv@brookespublishing.com
www.brookespublishing.com

Jeff Brookes, Director
Paul Brooks, Owner
This groundbreaking book provides helpful insights, unique perspectives, and innovative strategies that are needed to intervene successfully with children whose developmental disabilities affect their use of communication and language. *$43.00*
448 pages 1992
ISBN 1-557660-76-X

1762 Exceptional Children: An Introductory Survey of Special Education
McGraw-Hill School Publishing
220 East Danieldale Road
Desoto, TX 75115
972-224-1111
800-442-9685
FAX: 972-228-1982
www.mhschool.com

Joseph Gavigan, President
The focus of this survey is on observable characteristics of exceptional persons, and the instructional practices which foster their fullest development.
704 pages

1763 Increasing and Decreasing Behaviors of Persons with Severe Retardation and Autism
Research Press
PO Box 9177
Champaign, IL 61826
217-352-3273
800-519-2707
FAX: 217-352-1221
e-mail: rp@researchpress.com
www.researchpress.com

Russell Pence, President
These well-organized manuals are written for teachers, aides and persons responsible for designing or evaluating behavioral programs. Offers specific guidelines for arranging and managing the learning environment as well as standards for evaluating and maintaining success. In Volume Two of this series, chapters address more restrictive procedures including physical restraint, punishment, time-out and overcorrection. Set of two volumes. *$32.95*
428 pages Item 2650
ISBN 0-878222-65-0

1764 Teaching Special Students in Mainstream
Books on Special Children
PO Box 305
Congers, NY 10920
845-638-1236
FAX: 845-638-0847
e-mail: irene@boscbooks.com

Overview of mainstream, team of professionals managing classroom behavior, tips for teachers, social acceptance and handling of specific differences. *$33.00*
515 pages Softcover

1765 Young Children with Special Needs
McGraw-Hill School Publishing
220 East Danieldale Road
Desoto, TX 75115
972-224-1111
800-442-9685
FAX: 972-228-1982
www.mhschool.com

Glenn Evans, Chief Executive Officer
Phyllis Hsiao Hillwig, Chief Operating Officer
Joseph Gavigan, President
This text examines development in the critical areas of motor, self-help, cognitive, language, social, emotional and play skills.

526 pages

Educational Publishers

1766 AFB Press
American Foundation for the Blind / AFB Press
11 Penn Plaza
New York, NY 10001
212-502-7600
FAX: 212-502-7772
e-mail: afborders@abdintl.com
www.afb.org

Carl R Augusto, President/CEO
Maureen Matheson, Assistant Director
Develops, publishes, and sells a wide variety of informative books, pamphlets, periodicals, and videos for students, professionals, and researchers in the blindess and visual impairment fields, for people professionally involved in making the mainstream community accessible, and for blind and visually impaired people and their families; publication and video orders.

1767 American Association for Counseling & Development
American Counseling Association
5999 Stevenson Avenue
Alexandria, VA 22304
703-823-9800
800-347-6647
FAX: 800-473-2329
e-mail: webmaster@counseling.org
www.counseling.org

Marie Wakefield, President
Richard Yep, Executive Director
Offers tools and books for the professional.

1768 Brookes Publishing Company
PO Box 10624
Baltimore, MD 21285
410-337-9580
800-638-3775
FAX: 410-337-8539
www.brookespublishing.com

Paul H Brooks, President/Owner

1769 Brookline Books
39 University Road
Brookline, MA 02445
617-734-6772
800-666-2665
FAX: 617-734-3952
e-mail: thestore@brooklinebooksmith.com
www.brooklinebooks.com

William H Walters, Author
Esther Isabe Wilder, Author
Offers books for teachers and parents on law and legislation, education, integration and mainstreaming for the disabled, their families, caregivers and teachers.

1770 Brooks/Cole Publishing Company
511 Forest Lodge Road
Pacific Grove, CA 93950
831-373-0728
800-354-9706
FAX: 831-375-6414

Offers books in Special Education for those preparing to be special educators and for in-service professionals.

1771 **Charles C Thomas Publisher**

2600 South 1st Street
Springfield, IL 62704
217-789-8980
800-258-8980
FAX: 217-789-9130
e-mail: books@ccthomas.com
www.ccthomas.com

Michael Thomas, President
Publishes specialty titles and textbooks in medicine, dentistry, nursing, and veterinary medicine, as well as a complete line in the behavioral sciences, criminal justice, education, special education, and rehabilitation. Aims to accommodate the current needs for information.

1772 **Eric Clearinghouse on Disabilities and Gifted Education**

Council for Exceptional Children
1110 N Glebe Road
Suite 300
Arlington, VA 22201
703-245-0600
FAX: 703-264-9494
www.cec.sped.org

Janice Burdick, President
Bruce Ramirez, Manager
Provides information on special and gifted education. Provides referrals, offers patient networking services and provides information on current research programs. Focuses its efforts on prevention, identification, assessment, intervention and enrichment both in special settings and within mainstream communities. Offers a variety of materials including brochures and Spanish language matereials.

1773 **Gallaudet University Press**

Gallaudet University-Denison House
800 Florida Avenue NE
Washington, DC 20002
202-651-5000
800-621-2736
FAX: 202-651-5489
e-mail: bookstore.mailorder@gallaudet.edu
http://gupress.gallaudet.edu

Angelu Jorge-Quinones, Board of Trustees
Erving Jordan, President
Offers informational resources for the deaf, parents of the deaf, professionals, special educators and more. Produces a yearly catalog of materials on sign language and deafness.

1774 **Greenwood Publishing Group**

88 Post Road W
Westport, CT 06880
203-226-3571
FAX: 203-222-1502
e-mail: webmaster@greenwood.com
www.greenwood.com

David A Copeland, Author
Kirstin Olsen, Author
Wayne Smith, President

1775 **Grey House Publishing**

185 Millerton Road
Millerton, NY 12546
518-789-8700
800-562-2139
FAX: 518-789-0545
e-mail: books@greyhouse.com
www.greyhouse.com

Richard Gottlieb, President
Leslie Mackenzie, Publisher
Laura Mars, Editorial Director
Grey House Publishing publishes directories, handbooks and reference works for public, high school and academic libraries and the business and health communities. Most titles are available as online databases.

1776 **Information from HEATH Resource Center**

National Clearinghouse on Postsecondary Education
1 Dupont Circle NW
Suite 800
Washington, DC 20036
202-939-9320
800-544-3284
FAX: 202-833-5696
e-mail: heath@ace.nche.edu
www.HEATH-resource-center.org

The HEATH Resource Center operates the national clearinghouse on postsecondary education for individuals with disabilities. Support from the US Department of Education enables the Center, a program of the America Council on Education, to serve as an information exchange on educational support services; adaptations; and opportunities at American campuses, vocational-technical schools, adult education programs, independent living centers, and other postsecondary training entities.

1777 **McGraw-Hill Company**

2460 Kerper Boulevard
Dubuque, IA 52001
563-588-1451
800-553-4920
www.mcgraw-hill.com

Dana Kramer, Director
Kurt Strand, Vice President
Offers a catalog of testing resources and materials for the special educator.

1778 **National Association of School Psychologists**

4340 East West Highway
Suite 402
Bethesda, MD 20814
301-657-0270
FAX: 301-657-0275
e-mail: lnealis@naspweb.org
www.nasponline.org

Libby Kuffner Nealis, Director Public Policy
Susan Gorin, Executive Director
Represents over 22,500 school psychologists and related professionals. It serves its members and society by advancing the profession of school psychology and advocating for the rights, welfare, education and mental health of children, youth and their families.

1779 **Oryx Press**

4041 North Central Avenue
Suite 700
Phoenix, AZ 85012
602-265-2651
800-279-6799
FAX: 800-279-4663

1780 **PEAK Parent Center**

611 N Weber Street
Suite 200
Colorado Springs, CO 80903
719-531-9400
800-284-0251
FAX: 719-531-9452
e-mail: info@peakparent.org
www.peakparent.org

Barbara Buswell, Executive Director
PEAK Parent Center is a federally-designated Parent Training and Information Center (PTI). As a PTI, PEAK supports and empowers parents, providing them with information and strategies to use when advocating for their children with disabilities. PEAK works one-on-one with families and educators helping them realize new possibilities for children with disabilities by expanding knowledge of special education and offering new strategies for success.

1781 **Pro-Ed**

8700 Shoal Creek Boulevard
Austin, TX 78757
512-451-3246
800-897-3202
FAX: 800-397-7633
e-mail: feedback@proedinc.com
www.proedinc.com

Donald Hammill, Owner
Courtney King, Marketing Coordinator

Publishes, produces and sells books, curricular therapy materials and journals dedicated to psychology, special education and speech, language and hearing.

1782 Research Press
PO Box 9177
Champaign, IL 61826
217-352-3273
800-519-2707
FAX: 217-352-1221
e-mail: rp@researchpress.com
www.researchpress.com

Dennis Wiziecki, Marketing Department
Mark Amendola, Author
Russell Pence, President

1783 Special Needs Project
324 State Street
Suite H
Santa Barbara, CA 93101
805-962-8087
800-333-6867
FAX: 805-962-5087
www.specialneeds.com

Hod Gray, Founder

1784 Waterfront Books Publishing Company
85 Crescent Road
Burlington, VT 05401
800-639-6063
e-mail: helpkids@waterfrontbooks.com
www.waterfrontbooks.com

Sherrill N Musty, Owner

State Agencies: Alabama

1785 Alabama Department of Education: Division of Special Education Services
Alabama Department of Education
PO Box 302101
50 North Ripley Street
Montgomery, AL 36104
334-242-9700
www.alsde.edu

Bill East, Assistant Director

1786 Getting Ready for the Outside World (G.R.O.W.)
River View School
551 Route 6a
East Sandwich, MA 02537
508-888-0489
FAX: 508-833-7001
www.riverviewschool.org

Jeanne Pacheco, Director Admissions/Placement
Maureen Brenner, Principal
The G.R.O.W. Program is a unique ten month transitional prgoram (1-3 years) for high school graduates with diagnosed learning disabilities who share a common hisotry of lifelong difficulty with academic achievement and the development of friendships. This post secondary program is designed to further develop academic, vocational and life skills, to enable students to function as independently as possible.

State Agencies: Alaska

1787 Alaska Department of Education: Office of Special Education
801 West 10th Street, Suite 200
PO Box 110500
Juneau, AK 99811
907-465-2800
FAX: 907-465-4156
TTY:907-465-2815
www.eed.state.ak.us

Myrna Howe, State Director
Karen Rehfeld, Executive Director
Administers special educational programs through the Division of Education Program Support to the disabled residing in the Alaska area.

State Agencies: Arkansas

1788 Arkansas Department of Special Education
4 Capitol Mall
Suite 105-C
Little Rock, AR 72201
501-682-1121
800-NAT-URAL
FAX: 501-682-4313
www.arkansas.com

Diane Sydoriak MD, Associate Director Special Educa
Barbara Pardue, Executive Director
Provides oversight of all educational programs for children and youth with disabilities, ages 3 to 21. Provides technical assistance to all public agencies providing educational services to this population.

State Agencies: Arizona

1789 Arizona Department of Education
State of Arizona
1535 West Jefferson Street
Phoenix, AZ 85007
602-271-0945
800-352-4558
FAX: 602-542-5404
e-mail: essdesk@ade.az.gov
www.ade.az.gov

Joanne Phillips, State Director Special Education
Joe Sambo, Office Manager
Robert Plummer, Manager

State Agencies: California

1790 California Department of Education: Special Education Division
721 Capitol Mall
Sacramento, CA 95814
916-324-4244
FAX: 916-657-4770

Jack O'Connell, Superintendent
Leo Sandoval, Director Special Education
David Supkofl, Manager
Through consultants, coordinates the establishment and operations of special public school programs for blind and partially sighted pupils. The staff includes two regionally based consultant specialists in the education of visually impaired children, and the eligible age for help is 3-21.

State Agencies: Colorado

1791 Colorado Department of Education: Special Education Service Unit
Colorado Department of Education
201 East Colfax Avenue
Denver, CO 80203
303-698-2121
FAX: 303-866-6811
www.cde.state.co.us

William Maloney, Commissioner
Laura Reilly, Chief Executive Officer
Provides consultation on materials and educational services for visually handicapped children, supervises volunteer services, transcribes textbooks for visually handicapped students.

State Agencies: Connecticut

1792 **Connecticut Department of Education: Bureau of Special Education**
Connecticut Department of Education
25 Industrial Park Road
Middletown, CT 06457
860-632-1485
FAX: 860-632-8870
www.ctserc.org

Marianne Kirner, Executive Director
Carol Sullivan, Assistant Director
Commitment is to serve as a centralized resource for professionals, families, and community members regarding education and early intervention/prevention for all of Connecticut's children and youth and their families, particularly children with special needs, at-risk learners, and diverse learners. SERC strives for the highest possible level of excellence assistance initiatives, family education and support, and information and materials dissemination.

1793 **Connecticut State Board of Education and Services for the Blind**
State of Connecticut Agency
184 Windsor Avenue
Windsor, CT 06095
860-602-4000
800-842-4510
FAX: 860-602-4030
e-mail: brian.sigman@po.state.ct.us
www.besb.state.ct.us

Brian Sigman, Executive Director
Keith Maynard, Plant Manager
Provides consultation for the education of visually disabled children, provides Braille instruction, independent living skills training, vocational rehabilitation services and community outreach and advocacy.

State Agencies: Delaware

1794 **Department of Public Instruction: Exceptional Children & Special Programs Division**
Department of Education
401 Federal Street
Suite 2
Dover, DE 19903
302-735-4210
FAX: 302-739-2388

Martha Toomey, Director

State Agencies: DC

1795 **District of Columbia Public Schools: Special Education Division**
825 North Capitol Street NE
7th Floor
Washington, DC 20002
202-442-4800
202-442-5517

Paul L Vance MD, Superintendent
Committed to providing a continuum of services that offers students with disabilities the opportunity to actively participate in the learning environment of their neighborhood school.

1796 **National Clearinghouse on Family Support and Children's Mental Health**
1 Dupont Circle NW
Suite 800
Washington, DC 20036
202-939-9320
800-544-3284
FAX: 202-833-4760
e-mail: heatah@ace.nche.edu

State Agencies: Florida

1797 **Florida Department of Education: Bureau of Exceptional Education And Student Services**
325 West Gaines Street
Suite 614
Tallahassee, FL 32399
850-245-0475
FAX: 850-245-0953
www.fldoe.org

Jeanine Blomberg, Commissioner
Bambi Lockman, Bureau Chief
Myra Rogers, Administrative Assistant
The Department of Education strives to improve educational services for students with special needs.

State Agencies: Hawaii

1798 **Hawaii Department of Education: Special Needs**
Hawaii Department of Education
3430 Leahi Avenue
Honolulu, HI 96815
808-941-3894
FAX: 808-732-3701

Margaret Donovan MD, State Administrator
Provides consultation on educational services for local schools, offers psychological testing and evaluation, maintains resource rooms in district schools and more for the blind and handicapped throughout the state.

State Agencies: Illinois

1799 **Activities for Developing Pre-Skill Concepts In Children with Autism**
Autism Society of North Carolina Bookstore
505 Oberlin Road
Suite 230
Raleigh, NC 27605
919-743-0204
800-442-2762
FAX: 919-743-0208
e-mail: dcoffey@autismsociety-nc.org
www.autismsociety-nc.org

Darla Coffey, Bookstore Manager
Jill Keel, Executive Director
Chapters include auditory development, concept development, social development and visual-motor integration. *$36.00*

1800 **Illinois State Board of Education: Department of Special Education**
100 North 1st Street
Springfield, IL 62777
217-782-6601
FAX: 217-782-0372
e-mail: pstadeke@spr6.isbe.il.us
www.isbe.net

Gail Lieberman, Policy Advisor
Mission is to advance the human and civil rights of people with disabilities in Illinois. Statewide advocacy organization providing self-advocacy assistance, legal services, education and public policy initiatives. Designated to implement the federal protection and advocacy system; has broad statutory power to enforce the rights of people with physical and mental disabilities, including developmental disabilities and mental illnesses.

State Agencies: Indiana

1801 **Indiana Department of Education: Special Education Division**
Indiana Department of Education
229 State House
Indianapolis, IN 46204
317-232-6610
FAX: 317-232-8004
e-mail: webmaster@doe.state.in.us
www.ideanet.doe.state.in.us

Robert Marra, Assistant State Director
Provides consultation on educational services for local schools, offers psychological testing and evaluation, maintains resource rooms in district schools and more for the blind and handicapped throughout the state.

State Agencies: Iowa

1802 **Iowa Department of Public Instruction: Bureau of Special Education**
Grimes State Office Building
400 East 14th Street
Des Moines, IA 50319
515-281-3176
FAX: 515-242-6019
www.state.ia.us/educate/

Lana Michelson, Bureau Chief

State Agencies: Kansas

1803 **Kansas State Board of Education: Special Education Outcomes Team**
Kansas State Board of Education
120 SE 10th Avenue
Topeka, KS 66612
785-296-6054
785-296-3201
www.kansped.org

Colleen Riley, Director Team Leader
Carol Dermyer, Assitant Director
Provides consultation on educational services for local schools, offers psychological testing and evaluation, maintains resource rooms in district schools and more for the blind and handicapped throughout the state.

State Agencies: Kentucky

1804 **Kentucky Department of Education: Division of Exceptional Children's Services**
500 Mero Street
Room 805
Frankfort, KY 40601
502-564-4970
FAX: 502-564-6721
e-mail: marmstro@kde.state.ky.us
www.kde.state.ky.us

Johnny Grissom, Associate Commissioner
Judy Mallory, Executive Director
Provides consultation on educational services for local schools, offers psychological testing and evaluation, maintains resource rooms in district schools and more for the blind and handicapped throughout the state.

State Agencies: Louisiana

1805 **Louisiana Department of Education: Office of Special Education Services**
Louisiana Department of Education
PO Box 94064
Baton Rouge, LA 70804
225-383-4761
877-453-2721
FAX: 504-342-5880
www.doe.state.la.us

Cecil J Picard, State Superintendent
Kim Fitch, Director Human Resources
George Nelson, President

State Agencies: Massachusetts

1806 **Massachusetts Department of Education: Program Quality Assurance**
Massachusetts Department of Education
350 Main Street
Malden, MA 02148
781-388-3300
FAX: 617-388-3476

Pamela Kaufamann, Administrator

State Agencies: Maryland

1807 **Maryland State Department of Education: Division of Special Education**
200 West Baltimore Street
Baltimore, MD 21201
410-333-2490
FAX: 410-333-8165
www.msde.state.md.us

Richard Steinke, State Director
Provides consultation on educational services for local schools, offers psychological testing and evaluation, maintains resource rooms in district schools and more for the blind and handicapped throughout the state.

State Agencies: Michigan

1808 **Michigan Department of Education: Special Education Services**
Michigan Department of Education
PO Box 30008
608 West Allegan Street
Lansing, MI 48909
517-373-3654
FAX: 517-373-7504
e-mail: mdeweb@michigan.gov
www.michigan.gov/mde

Jeremy Hughes, Superintendent
Bobbie Butler, Manager
Provides consultation on educational services for local schools, offers psychological testing and evaluation, maintains resource rooms in district schools and more for the blind and handicapped throughout the state.

1809 **Services for Students with Disabilities**
University of Michigan
G664 Haven Hall
Ann Arbor, MI 48109
734-768-5000
FAX: 734-936-3947
e-mail: sgoodin@umich.edu
www.umich.edu/~sswd/

Sam Goodin, Director
Stuart Segal, Associate Director
Offers information to parents and students.

State Agencies: Minnesota

1810 Community Supports for People with Disabilities (CSP)
South Central Technical College (SCTC)
1920 Lee Boulevard
North Mankato, MN 56003
507-389-7200
800-722-9359
www.southcentral.edu

Christensen Tami, Executive Director
Keith Stover, President
Human services program available as a physical or online program, designed for those wanting to earn a certificate, diploma or associate degree as a Direct Support Professional for use in the health and human services industries. The program comprises eight courses relating to professional services and support for people with disabilities.

1811 Professional Development Programs
1675 Greeley Street South
Suite 101
Stillwater, MN 55082
651-439-8865
FAX: 651-439-0421
e-mail: programs@pdppro.com
www.pdppro.com

Eileen Richter, Director
Alexis Richter, Administrator
Sponsors cutting edge and popular continuing education workshops and symposia of interest to professionals who provide services to children and adults with special needs.

State Agencies: Missouri

1812 Missouri Department of Elementary and Secondary Education: Special Education Programs
Missouri Department of Elementary and Secondary Ed
PO Box 480
Jefferson City, MO 65102
573-751-5739
FAX: 573-526-4404
e-mail: doug.roach@dese.mo.gov
www.dese.mo.gov/divspeced

Pam Williams, Director
The Division of Special Education provides assistance to public school districts in the supervision, establishment, and improvement of programs of instruction for children with disabilities. The division operates the Missouri School for the Deaf, School for the Blind and State Schools for the Severely Handicapped. The division also supports a statewide system of sheltered workshops for adults with disabilities.

State Agencies: Mississippi

1813 Mississippi Department of Education: Office of Special Services
Mississippi Department of Education
PO Box 771
359 North West Street
Jackson, MS 39201
601-432-1200
FAX: 601-359-2198
e-mail: sthompson@mde.k12.ms.us
www.mde.k12.ms.us

Carolyn Black, Director
Key priorities are: reading, early literacy, student achievement, teachers/teaching, leadership/principals, safe and orderly schools, parent relations/community involvement, and technology.

State Agencies: Montana

1814 Department of Public Health Human Services
PO. Box 202501
Helena, MT 59620
406-444-4429
888-231-9393
FAX: 406-444-3921
www.opi.mt.gov.

Robert Runkel, Executive Director
Linda Mcculloch, Superintendent
Provides consultation on educational services for local schools, offers psychological testing and evaluation, maintains resource rooms in district schools and more for the blind and handicapped throughout the state.

State Agencies: North Carolina

1815 North Carolina Department of Public Instruction: Exceptional Children Division
301 North Wilmington Street
Raleigh, NC 27601
919-715-1565
FAX: 919-715-1569
e-mail: lharris@dpi.state.nc.us
www.publicschools.org

Lowell Harris, Director
Provides consultation on educational services for local schools, offers psychological testing and evaluation, maintains a continuum of educational sources in local schools for disabled children.

State Agencies: North Dakota

1816 North Dakota Department of Education: Special Education
600 East Boulevard Avenue
Bismarck, ND 58505
701-328-2455
FAX: 701-328-4149
www.dpi.state.nd.us

Robert Rutten, Director
Jeanette Kolberg, Assistant Director
Bryan Klipfel, Manager
Provides consultation on educational services for local schools, offers psychological testing and evaluation, maintains resource rooms in district schools and more for the blind and handicapped throughout the state.

State Agencies: Nebraska

1817 Nebraska Department of Education: Special Populations Office
Department of Education
PO Box 94987
Lincoln, NE 68509
402-471-2471
FAX: 402-471-5022
www.nde.state.ne.us/SPED/sped.html

Gary Sherman, Executive Director
Assists school districts in establishing and maintaining effective special education programs for children with disabilities (date of diagnosis through the school year when a child reaches 21). Major function: provide technical assistance to school districts and to parents of children with disabilities, assist programs in meeting state and federal special education regulations. Also responsible for assuring that the rights of children with disabilities and their parents are protected.

State Agencies: New Hampshire

1818 New Hampshire Department of Education: Bureau for Special Education Services
New Hampshire Department of Education
101 Pleasant Street
Concord, NH 03301
603-271-3494
FAX: 603-271-1953
www.ed.state.nh.us

Lyonel Tracy, Commissioner
Paul Ezen, Deputy Commissioner
Provides educational leadership and services which promote equal educational opportunites, quality practices and programs that enable NH residents to become fully productive members of society.

1819 New Hampshire Technology Partnership Project: Institute on Disability
Institute of Disability of the University of NH
Concord Center Ferry Street
Concord, NH 03301
603-228-2084
800-238-2048
FAX: 603-228-3270
TTY: 603-224-0630
e-mail: sd@cisunix.unh.edu
www.nhassistivetechnology.org

Jan Nisbet, Director
Mary Schuh, Executive Director
Eve Fralick, Associate Director
The goal of the New Hampshire Assistive Technology Partnership Project is to increase access to assistive technology through the creation and support of consumer driven systems for the provision of state-of-the-art assistive techology products and services for citizens in the state of New Hampshire.

State Agencies: New Jersey

1820 New Jersey Department of Education: Office of Special Education Program
New Jersey Department of Education
PO Box 500
Trenton, NJ 08625
609-292-8853
FAX: 609-984-8422
www.nj.gov/njded/specialed/

Barbara Gantwerk, Director
Alfred Murray, Executive Director

State Agencies: New Mexico

1821 New Mexico State Department of Education
300 Don Gaspar Avenue
Santa Fe, NM 87501
505-827-6508
FAX: 505-827-6696
www.sde.state.nm.us

Bill Trant, Assistant Director
Judy Parks, Assistant Director
Provides consultation on educational services for local schools, offers psychological testing and evaluation, maintains resource rooms in district schools and more for the blind and handicapped throughout the state.

State Agencies: Nevada

1822 Nevada Department of Education: Special Eduction Branch
700 East 5th Street
Suite 113
Carson City, NV 89701
775-884-6125
FAX: 775-687-9123
www.doe.nv.gov

Frankie McCabe, Director Office for Special Ed.
The Office of Special Ed and School Improvement Program of the Nevada State Department of Education is responsible for management of state and federal programs providing educational opportunities for students with diverse learning needs. Included are such programs as: special education/disabled (IDEA); disadvantaged/at-risk programs (Title I/IASA); early childhood programs (Title I/ESEA); early childhood programs; migrant education; English language learners; NRS 395 student placement program.

State Agencies: New York

1823 New York State Education Department
1606 One Commerce Plaza
Albany, NY 12234
518-474-5548
FAX: 518-473-5387
e-mail: nysed@mail.gov
www.nysed.gov

Tom Neveldine, Assistant Commissioner
Provides vocational rehabilitation and educational services for eligible individuals with disabilities throughout New York State. Services include evaluation, counseling, job placement, and referral to other agencies.

State Agencies: Ohio

1824 Ohio Department of Education: Division of Special Education
Ohio Department of Education
25 South Front Street
Columbus, OH 43215
614-466-2650
877-644-6338
FAX: 614-387-0964
www.ode.state.oh.us

Mike Armstrong, Director
Provides technical assistance to educational agencies for the development and implementation of educational services to meet the needs of students with disabilities and/or those who are gifted. Provides information to parents. Administers state and federal funds allocated to educational agencies for the provision of services to students with disabilities and/or those who are gifted.

State Agencies: Oklahoma

1825 Oklahoma State Department of Education
2500 North Lincoln Boulevard
Suite 411
Oklahoma City, OK 73105
405-521-3301
FAX: 405-522-3503
www.sde.state.ok.us

Misty Kimbrough, Executive Director
Sandy Garrett, Administrator
Provides consultation on educational services for local schools, offers psychological testing and evaluation, maintains resource rooms in district schools and more for the blind and handicapped throughout the state.

State Agencies: Oregon

1826 **Oregon Department of Education: Office of Special Education**
Oregon Department of Education:
255 Capitol St NE
Salem, OR 97310
503-986-4614
FAX: 503-378-5156
www.ode.state.or.us/sped/index/htm

Nancy Latini, Assistant Superintendent
Heidi Cockrell, Executive Assistant
Katy Coba, Executive Director
State agency ensuring provision of special education services to children with disabilities from birth to age 21.

State Agencies: Pennsylvania

1827 **Pennsylvania Department of Education: Bureau of Special Education**
333 Market Street
7th Floor
Harrisburg, PA 17126
717-783-6913
FAX: 717-783-6139
e-mail: 00specialed@psupen.psu.edu
www.pde.state.pa.us

Linda Rhen, Administrator
John Tommasini, Assistant Director
Provides effective and efficient administration of the Commonwealth of Pennsylvania's resources dedicated to enabling school districts to maintain high standards in the delivery of special education services and programs for all exceptional students.

State Agencies: Rhode Island

1828 **Rhode Island Department of Education: Office of Special Needs**
265 Westminster Street
Providence, RI 02903
401-784-9500
FAX: 401-222-6030
www.ride.ri.gov

Thomas Dipaola, Director
Alfred Moscola, Manager
Provides consultation on educational services for local schools, offers psychological testing and evaluation, maintains resource rooms in district schools and more for the blind and handicapped throughout the state.

State Agencies: South Carolina

1829 **South Carolina Assistive Technology Program (SCATP)**

Center for Disability Resources
Midlands Center
8301 Farrow Road
Columbia, SC 29203
803-935-5263
800-915-4522
FAX: 803-935-5342
e-mail: evelyne@cdd.sc.edu
www.sc.edu/scatp

Evelyn Evans, Project Director
Janet Jendron, Program Coordinator
Marie Queen, Executive Director
SCATP is a federally funded project concerned with getting technology into th hands of people with disabilities so that they might live, work, learn and be a more independent part of the community.

1830 **South Carolina Department of Education: Office of Exceptional Children**
1429 Senate Street
Columbia, SC 29201
803-734-8806
FAX: 803-734-4824
e-mail: sdurant@sde.state.sc.us
www.scschools.com

Susan Durant, State Director
Provides consultation on educational services for local schools, offers psychological testing and evaluation, maintains resource rooms in district schools and more for the blind and handicapped throughout the state.

State Agencies: South Dakota

1831 **South Dakota Department of Education & Cultural Affairs: Office of Special Education**
700 Governors Drive
Pierre, SD 57501
605-773-3131
FAX: 605-773-6139

Deboarh Barnett, State Director
Dorothy Liegl, Manager

State Agencies: Tennessee

1832 **Tennessee Department of Education**
710 James Robertson Parkway
Nashville, TN 37243
615-741-2851
888-212-3162
FAX: 615-532-9412
www.state.tn.us/education

Joseph Fisher, Executive Director
Provides consultation on educational services for local schools, offers psychological testing and evaluation, maintains resource rooms in district schools and more for the blind and handicapped throughout the state.

State Agencies: Texas

1833 **Texas Education Agency**
1701 North Congress Avenue
Austin, TX 78701
512-463-9734

www.tea.state.tx.us

Shirley J Neeley, Commissioner of Education
Provides consultation on educational services for local schools, offers psychological testing and evaluation, maintains resource rooms in district schools and more for the blind and handicapped throughout the state.

1834 **Texas Education Agency: Special Education Unit**
1701 Congress Avenue
Austin, TX 78701
512-463-8532
FAX: 512-463-9434
e-mail: wmccain@tmail.tea.state.tx.us
www.tea.state.tx.us/Cate

Gene Lenz, Deputy Associate Commissioner
Shirley Neeley, Administrator

1835 **Texas School of the Deaf**
1102 South Congress Avenue
Austin, TX 78704
512-462-5353
800-332-3873
www.tsd.state.tx.us

Claire Bugen, Administrator
Betty Bounds, Assistant Superintendent

Promote quality educational opportunities and achievement for the deaf students of Texas by providing a comprehensive educational and residential program and a complete array of consultative services for parents and professionals throughout the state.

State Agencies: Utah

1836 **Utah State Office of Education: At-Risk and Special Education Service Unit**
Utah State Office of Education
250 East 500 South
PO Box 144200
Salt Lake City, UT 84114
801-538-7500
www.usoe.k12.ut.us

Patti Harrington, Manager
Provides consultation on educational services for local schools, offers psychological testing and evaluation, maintains resource rooms in district schools and more for the blind and handicapped throughout the state.

State Agencies: Virginia

1837 **Virginia Department of Education: Division of Pre & Early Adolescent Education**
Virginia Department Of Education
James Monroe Bldg 101 N 14th Street
PO Box 2120
Richmond, VA 23219
804-340-0072
FAX: 804-371-2456
www.pen.k12.va.us

Austin Tuning, Lead Specialist Special Educatio
Provides consultation on educational services for local schools, offers psychological testing and evaluation, maintains resource rooms in district schools and more for the blind and handicapped throughout the state.

State Agencies: Washington

1838 **Superintendent of Public Instruction: Special Education Section**
PO Box 47200
Olympia, WA 98504
360-725-6000
FAX: 360-586-0247
www.k12.wa.us

Douglas Gill, Executive Director
Provides leadership, service and support for the development and implementation of research-based curriculum to assure that all learners achieve at all levels.

State Agencies: West Virginia

1839 **West Virginia Department of Education: Office of Special Education**
1900 Kanawha Boulevard East
Room 6
Charleston, WV 25305
304-558-0549
FAX: 304-558-3741
wvde.state.wv.us

Katherine Boyer, Director
Mary Nunn, Assistant Director
Sarah Hamrick, Executive Director
Provides consultation on educational services for local schools, offers psychological testing and evaluation, maintains resource rooms in district schools and more for the blind and handicapped throughout the state.

State Agencies: Wyoming

1840 **Wyoming Department of Education**
2300 Capitol Avenue
Cheyenne, WY 82002
307-777-7690
FAX: 307-777-6234
www.k12.wy.us

Sharon Davarno, State Director
Trent Blankenship, State Superintendent
Mission is to lead, model, and support continuous improvement of education for everyone in Wyoming.

Magazines & Journals

1841 **Adapted Physical Activity Programs**
Human Kinetics
PO Box 5076
Champaign, IL 61825
800-747-4457
FAX: 217-351-2674
e-mail: orders@hkusa.com
www.humankinetics.com

Patty Lehn, Publicity Manager
Alexis Koontz, Publicity Associate
Human Kinetics produces a variety of resources for adapted physical education practitioners, including books on activities, a research journal and higher education references. *$24.00*
Quarterly
ISSN 0736-58 9

1842 **Advance for Providers of Post-Acute Care**
Merion Publications
2900 Horizon Drive
PO Box 61556
King of Prussia, PA 19406
610-278-1400
800-355-5627
FAX: 610-278-1421
www.advanceweb.com
A free magazine for providers of post-acute care.

1843 **CEC Catalog**
Council for Exceptional Children
1110 North Glebe Road
Suite 300
Arlington, VA 22201
703-245-0600
888-232-7733
FAX: 703-264-9494
e-mail: president@cec.sped.org
www.cec.sped.org

Janice Burdick, President
Bruce Ramirez, Manager
Semi-annual catalog from the Council for Exceptional Children offering books, guides, materials, products and services for the special educator.
18 pages

1844 **Case Manager Magazine**
Elsevier Health
360 Park Avenue South
New York, NY 10010
212-989-5800
journals.elsevierhealth.com

Catherine M Mullahy, Editor in Chief
John Ragazzi, President
This national magazine is for medical case managers, social workers, counselors and home health professionals who work with people with serious injury or illness. It is a membership benefit of CMSA, the national association for case managers.
$55.00

84 pages BiMonthly

1845 Catalyst
The Catalyst
1259 El Camino Real
Suite 275
Menlo Park, CA 94025
800-647-0314
e-mail: info@thecatalyst.us
www.thecatalyst.us

Sue Swezey, Editor
Digest of news and information on the use of computers in special education. *$15.00*
20 pages Quarterly

1846 Clinical Connection
American Advertising Dist of Northern Virginia
708 Pendleton Street
Alexandria, VA 22314
703-549-5126
FAX: 703-548-5563

Georgina Ruley, Publisher
Roger Parks, Owner
Covers speech language pathology.

1847 College and University
AACRAO
1 Dupont Circle NW
Suite 520
Washington, DC 20036
202-293-9161
FAX: 202-872-8857
e-mail: info@aacrao.com
www.aacrao.org

Joseph Roof, President
Luz Barreras, Vice President
Scholarly research journal. American Association of Collegiate Registrars and Admissions Offers (AACRAO) is a nonprofit, voluntary, professional, educational association of degree-granting, postsecondary institutions, government agencies, private educational organizations and education-oriented businesses in the United States and abroad. $50 per year US; $60 per year international.
30 pages Quarterly
ISSN 0010-0889

1848 Continuing Care
Stevens Publishing Corporation
5151 Belt Line Road
10th Floor
Dallas, TX 75254
972-687-6700
FAX: 972-687-6769
e-mail: custserv@stevenspublishing.com
www.stevenspublishing.com

Craig Stevens, President/CEO
A national magazine for case management and discharge planning professionals published monthly except for December. *$119.00*
34 pages Monthly

1849 Counseling Psychologist
American Psychological Association
2455 Teller Road
Thousand Oaks, CA 91320
805-499-9734
800-818-7243
FAX: 805-499-0871
e-mail: info@sagepub.com
www.sagepub.com
Thematic issues in the theory, research and practice of counseling psychology. *$78.00*
Bi-Monthly

1850 Counseling and Values
American Counseling Association
5999 Stevenson Avenue
Alexandria, VA 22304
703-823-9800
800-347-6647
FAX: 800-473-2329
TTY: 703-823-6862
www.counseling.org

Dennis Engels, Editor
Richard Yep, Executive Director
Counseling and Values is the official journal of the Association for Spiritual, Ethical, and Religious Values in Counseling (ASERVIC), a member association of the American Counseling Association. Counseling and Values s a professional journal of theory, research, and informed opinion concerned with the relationships among psychology, philosophy, religion, social values, and counseling. *$12.00*
TriAnnual

1851 Directions: Technology in Special Education
DREAMMS for Kids
273 Ringwood Road
Freeville, NY 13068
607-539-3027
FAX: 607-539-9930
www.dreamms.org

Janet P Hosmer, Contact
Provides technology tips to ease home instruction and use; describes and reviews adaptive educational software and hardware; reviews pertinent literature and audio and videotapes; describes adaptive and assistive technology devices; provides on-line service information for the disabled; announces upcoming educational and technology conference; and reports on new Department of Education legislation. *$14.95*
Monthly

1852 Early Intervention
Early Childhood Intervention Clearinghouse
223 South Third St.et
Springfield, IL 62704
217-522-4655
800-852-4302
FAX: 217-522-4670
e-mail: clearinghouse@eosinc.com
www.eiclearinghouse.org

Chet Brandt, Executive Director
Patricia Taylor, Project Associate
Features articles, conference calendar, material reviews and news concerning early childhood intervention and disability.
4 pages Quarterly

1853 Exceptional Children
Council for Exceptional Children
1110 North Glebe Road
Suite 300
Arlington, VA 22201
703-245-0600
FAX: 703-264-9494
e-mail: service@cec.sped.org
www.cec.sped.org

Jim McCormick, President
Drew Allbritten, Executive Director
Bruce Ramirez, Manager
Articles include research, literature surveys and position papers concerning exceptional children, special education and mainstreaming. *$58.00*
96 pages BiMonthly

1854 Focus on Autism and Other Developmental Disabilities
Pro-Ed Publications
8700 Shoal Creek Boulevard
Austin, TX 78757
512-451-3246
800-897-3202
FAX: 800-397-7633
e-mail: feedback@proedinc.com
www.proedinc.com

Donald Hammill, Owner
Courtney King, Marketing Coordinator
Practical management, treatment and planning strategies; a must for persons working with individuals with autism and other developmental disabilities. *$43.00*
64 pages Quarterly

1855 Focus on Exceptional Children
Love Publishing Company
9101 East Kenyon Avenue
Suite 2200
Denver, CO 80237
303-221-7333
FAX: 303-221-7444
e-mail: lpc@lovepublishing.com
www.lovepublishing.com

Scott Thomas, Manager
Stan Love, Owner

Contains research and theory-based articles on special education topics, with an emphasis on application and intervention, of interest to teachers, professors and administrators. *$36.00*
Monthly 1969

1856 HomeCare Magazine
Trimedia Publications
Stuart Ranch Road
Malibu, CA 90265
866-212-1154
800-543-4116
FAX: 402-505-7173
e-mail: kcavallo@interec.com
www.homecaremag.com

Stacy Branning, Publisher
The business magazine of the home medical equipment industry offering information on legislation and regulations affecting the homecare industry, monthly profiles of suppliers, operational tips, newest products in the industry, advice on sales, government regulations. *$ 65.00*
120 pages Monthly

1857 I Wonder Who Else Can Help
AARP
601 East Street NW
Washington, DC 20049
202-434-2277
800-687-2277
FAX: 202-434-3443
e-mail: member@aarp.org
www.aarp.org

William Novelli, Chief Executive Officer
Contains information about crisis counseling, needs and resources, written in lay terms.

1858 International Rehabilitation Review
Rehabilitation International
25 East 21st Street
New York, NY 10010
212-420-1500
FAX: 212-505-0871
e-mail: rehabintal@aol.com

Barbara Duncan, Editor
Kathy Marchael, Editorial Assistant
Tomas Lagerwall, Manager
International overview of activities and programs in vocational and medical rehabilitation, prosthesis and orthotics and special education. *$30.00*
TriAnnual

1859 Intervention in School and Clinic
Pro-Ed Publications
8700 Shoal Creek Boulevard
Austin, TX 78757
512-451-3246
800-897-3202
FAX: 512-451-8542
e-mail: info@proedinc.com
www.proedinc.com

Donald Hammill, Owner
A hands-on, how-to resource for teachers and clinicians working with students for whom minor curriculum and environmental modifications are ineffective. *$35.00*
64 pages

1860 Journal for Vocational Special Needs Education
University of Wisconsin
1025 West Johnson Street
Madison, WI 53706
608-263-9250
FAX: 608-262-3050
e-mail: jgugerty@education.wisc.edu
www.cew.wisc.edu/jvsne/

John Gugerty, Co-Editor
Articles on vocational education for special needs population, including persons with physical and mental disabilities. *$16.00*

1861 Journal of Applied School Psychology
Haworth Press
10 Alice Street
Binghamton, NY 13904
607-722-5857
800-429-6784
FAX: 607-722-6362
e-mail: orders@haworthpress.com
www.haworthpress.com

Charles Maher, Editor
Roger Hall, Director
William Cohen, Owner
This journal disseminates the latest and the highest quality information to all professionals who provide special services in the schools and related educational settings. *$60.00*
BiAnnually

1862 Journal of Counseling & Development
American Counseling Association
5999 Stevenson Avenue
Alexandria, VA 22304
703-823-9800
800-347-6647
FAX: 800-473-2329
TTY: 703-823-6862
www.counseling.org

A Scott McGowan, Editor
Carolyn Baker, Publications Director
Richard Yep, Executive Director
Publishes archival material, also publishes articles that have broad interest for a readership composed mostly of counselors and other mental health professionals who work in private practice, schools, colleges, community agencies, hospitals, and government. An appropriate outlet for articles that: critcally intergrate published research; examine current professional and scientific issues; report research, new techniques, innovatetive programs and practices; and examine ACA as an organization. *$140.00*
128 pages Quarterly

1863 Journal of Emotional and Behavioral Disorders
Pro-Ed Publications
8700 Shoal Creek Boulevard
Austin, TX 78757
512-451-3246
800-897-3202
FAX: 800-397-7633
e-mail: feedback@proedinc.com
www.proedinc.com

Donald Hammill, Owner
Courtney King, Marketing Coordinator
An international, multidisciplinary journal featuring articles on research, practice and theory related to individuals with emotional and behavioral disorders and to the professionals who serve them. *$39.00*
64 pages Quarterly

1864 Journal of Learning Disabilities
Pro-Ed
8700 Shoal Creek Boulevard
Austin, TX 78757
512-451-3246
800-897-3202
FAX: 800-397-7633
e-mail: feedback@proedinc.com
www.proedinc.com

Joshua Jeffrey, Marketing Custodian
Courtney King, Marketing Coordinator
Donald Hammill, Owner
An international, multidisciplinary publication containing articles on practice, research and theory related to learning disabilities. Published bi-monthly. *$49.00*
Magazine

1865 Journal of Motor Behavior
Heldref Publications
1319 18th Street NW
Washington, DC 20036
202-296-6267
800-365-9753
FAX: 202-293-6130
e-mail: subscribe@heldref.org
www.heldref.org

Emilli Pawlowsky, Marketing Manager
Laura Rosse, Assistant Marketing Manager
Douglas Kirkpatrick, Publisher
A professional journal aimed at psychologists, therapists and educators who work in the areas of motor behavior, psychology, neurophysiology, kinesiology, and biomechanics. Offers up-to-date information on the latest techniques, theories and developments concerning motor control. *$77.00*

115 pages Quarterly 1969

1866 Journal of Musculoskeletal Pain
Haworth Press
10 Alice Street
Binghamton, NY 13904
607-722-5857
800-429-6784
FAX: 607-722-6362
e-mail: orders@haworthpress.com
www.haworthpress.com

Sandy Sickels, Vice President
Becky Minerbaum, Advertising Manager
S Harrington-Miller, Advertising
This journal serves as a central resource for the dissemination of information about musculoskeletal pain. *$75.00*
110 pages Quarterly

1867 Journal of Postsecondary Education & Disability
AHEAD
107 Commerce Center Drive
Suite 204
Huntersville, NC 28078
704-947-7779
FAX: 704-948-7779
TTY:617-287-3882
e-mail: ahead@ahead.org
www.ahead.org

Jim Kessler, President
Stephan J Smith, Executive Director
Provides in-depth examination of research, issues, policies and programs in postsecondary education.

1868 Journal of Prosthetics and Orthotics
330 John Carlyle Street
Suite 210
Alexandria, VA 22314
703-836-7116
FAX: 703-836-0838
e-mail: info@abcop.org
www.abcop.org

William Detoro, President
Stephen Fletcher, Secretary Treasurer
Tyler Wilson, Executive Director
Provides the latest research and clinical thinking in orthotics and prosthetics, including information on new devices, fitting techniques and patient management experiences. Each issue contains research-based information and articles reviewed and approved by a highly qualified editorial board. *$60.00*
64 pages Quarterly
ISSN 1040-88 0

1869 Journal of Reading, Writing and Learning Disabled International
Hemisphere Publishing Corporation
1900 Frost Road
Suite 101
Bristol, PA 19007
215-785-5800
FAX: 215-785-6616
Articles on reading, writing and learning disabilities, including mainstreaming issues. *$9.00*

1870 Journal of School Health Association
7263 State Route 43
PO Box 708
Kent, OH 44240
330-678-1601
FAX: 330-678-4526
e-mail: asha@ashaweb.org
www.ashaweb.org

Susan Wooley, Executive Director
Thomas Reed, Manager
This is a monthly journal which offers information to professionals and parents on school health. Membership dues, $95.00.

1871 Journal of Special Education
Pro-Ed
8700 Shoal Creek Boulevard
Austin, TX 78757
512-451-3246
800-897-3202
FAX: 800-397-7633
e-mail: feedback@proedinc.com
www.proedinc.com

Donald Hammill, Owner
Courtney King, Marketing Coordinator
Internationally known as the prime research journal in special education. JSE provides research articles of special education for individuals with disabilities, ranging from mild to severe. Published quarterly. *$39.00*
Magazine

1872 Journal of Vocational Behavior
Academic Press, Journals Division
525 B Street
Suite 1900
San Diego, CA 92101
619-231-0926
FAX: 619-231-0928
www.academicpress.com/jvb

Jasna Markovac, Vice President
The Journal of Vocational Behavior publishes empirical and theoretical articles that expand knowledge of vocational behavior and career development across the life span. Research presented in the journal encompasses the general categories of career choice, implementation, and vocational adjustment and adaptation. The articles are also valuable for applications in counseling and career development programs in colleges and universities, business and industry, government, and the military. *$7.00*

1873 MDA Newsmagazine
Muscular Dystrophy Association
3275 West Ina Road
Suite 155
Tucson, AZ 85741
520-795-3434
FAX: 520-795-3989
e-mail: tusconservices@mdausa.org

Kelly Larkin, Executive Director
Presents news related to muscular dystrophy and other neuromuscular diseases including research, personal profiles, fundraising activities and patient services.

1874 Measurement and Evaluation in Counseling and Development
American Association for Counseling & Development
5999 Stevenson Avenue
Alexandria, VA 22304
800-347-6647
FAX: 800-473-2329
TTY:703-823-6862
www.counseling.org

William D Schafer, Editor
Journal with professional articles on testing and evaluation. *$23.00*
Quarterly

1875 Our World
National Center for Learning Disabilities
381 Park Avenue S
Room 1401
New York, NY 10016
212-545-7510
800-575-7373
888-575-7373
FAX: 212-545-9665
e-mail: help@ncld.org
www.ld.org

James H Wendorf, Executive Director
Marica Griffith, Marketing Executive
Contains features, articles, human interest news and information and information, and other practical material to benefit the millions of children and adults with learning disabilities and their families, as well as educators and other helping professionals. Magazine.
Quarterly

1876 Psychiatric Staffing Crisis in Community Mental Health
Nat l Council for Community Behavioral Healthcare
12300 Twinbrook Parkway
Suite 320
Rockville, MD 20852
301-984-6200
FAX: 301-881-7159
www.nccbh.org

Dale Klatszaer, Board Chair
Linda Rosenberg, Chief Executive Officer

Find out some of the simple, low-cost ways you can increase workplace satisfaction among staff psychiatrists and compete successfully for their talents. *$20.00*

1877 Readings: A Journal of Reviews and Commentary in Mental Health
American Orthopsychiatric Association
Box 871104
Tempe, AZ 85287
480-727-7518
FAX: 480-965-8544
e-mail: americanortho@gmail.com
www.americanortho.com

Gary Melton, President
Nicole Bruno, Director
Reviews of recent books in mental health and allied disciplines. Includes essay reviews and brief reviews. *$25.00*
32 pages Quarterly

1878 Rehab Pro
3540 Soquel Avenue
Suite A
Santa Cruz, CA 95062
831-464-4892
800-240-9059
FAX: 831-576-1417
e-mail: glenn@btfenterprises.com
www.rehabpro.org

Glenn Zimmerman, Executive Director
Alan Gale, Executive Manager
The magazine is to promote the profession and to inform the public about the activities of the national organization, its state chapter affiliates, and the work of its special interest sections.
38 pages BiMonthly

1879 Remedial and Special Education
Pro-Ed Publications
8700 Shoal Creek Boulevard
Austin, TX 78757
512-451-3246
800-897-3202
FAX: 800-397-7633
e-mail: feedback@proedinc.com
www.proedinc.com

Donald Hammill, Owner
Courtney King, Marketing Coordinator
A professional journal that bridges the gap between theory and practice. Emphasis is on topical reviews, syntheses of research, field evaluation studies and recommendations for the practice of remedial and special education. Published six times a year. *$39.00*
64 pages

1880 Teaching Exceptional Children
Council for Exceptional Children
1110 North Glebe Road
Suite 300
Arlington, VA 22201
703-245-0600
FAX: 703-264-9494
www.cec.sped.org

Janice Burdick, President
Bruce Ramirez, Manager
Journal designed for teachers of gifted students and students with disabilities, featuring practical methods and materials for classroom use. *$58.00*
96 pages BiMonthly

Newsletters

1881 Alert
Association on Handicapped Student Service Program
PO Box 21192
Columbus, OH 43221
614-365-5216
FAX: 614-365-6718
Keeps members informed about Association activities, current legislative issues, innovative programs, and more. *$30.00*

1882 Camp Virginia Jaycee Newsletter
Dare Care Charity
2494 Camp Jaycee Road
Blue Ridge, VA 24064
540-947-2972
800-865-0092
FAX: 540-947-2043
e-mail: ewerness@campvirginiajaycee.com
www.campvirginiajaycee.com

Everett M Werness, President
Cindy Rinker, Camp Director
Summer camping for children and adults with developmental disabilities. Coed, ages 7-70. Weekend respite camps for children and adults with mental retardation.
8 pages quarterly

1883 Counseling Today
American Counseling Association
5999 Stevenson Avenue
Alexandria, VA 22304
703-823-9800
800-473-2329
FAX: 703-823-0252
www.counseling.org

Richard Yep, Executive Director
Jonathan Rollins, Editor
Aims to serve individuals active in porfessional counseling, in the school and university, in the workplace and the marketplace, as well as other citizens, community leaders and policy makers who appreciate the importance of the role of professional counselors in today's society.
Monthly

1884 Counselor Education and Supervision
American Counseling Association
5999 Stevenson Avenue
Alexandria, VA 22304
703-823-9800
FAX: 800-473-2329
e-mail: webmaster@counseling.org
www.counseling.org

Margaret L Fong, Editor
Richard Yep, Executive Director
Dedicated to the growth and development of the counseling profession and those who are served. *$18.00*
Quarterly

1885 Counterpoint
National Association of State Directors of Special
10860 Hampton Road
Fairfax Station, VA 22039
703-519-3800
FAX: 703-503-8627
Newspaper designed for teachers of disabled and gifted students, featuring practical methods and materials for classroom use. *$36.00*
Quarterly

1886 Disability Compliance for Higher Education
LRP Publications
PO Box 24668
West Palm Beach, FL 33416
561-622-6520
800-341-7874
FAX: 215-784-9639
e-mail: custserve@lrp.com
www.lrp.com

Kenneth Kahn, Chief Executive Officer
Jim Nartini, Vice President
The only newsletter that is dedicated to the exclusive coverage of disability issues that affect colleges and universities. *$195.00*
8 pages Monthly

1887 Disability Resources Monthly
Disability Resources
4 Glatter Lane
Centereach, NY 11720
631-585-0290
FAX: 631-585-0290
e-mail: pubs@disabilityresources.org
www.disabilityresources.org

Avery Klauber, Director

A newsletter that monitors, reviews and reports on resources for independent living. A monthly newsletter that features short topical articles, news items and reviews of books, pamphlets, periodicals, videotapes, on-line services, organizations and other resources for and about people with disabilities. It is intended primarily for librarians, social workers, educators, rehabilitation specialists, disability advocates, ADA coordinators and other health and social service professionals. *$33.00*

4 pages Monthly 1993
ISSN 1070-72 0

1888 **Early Childhood Reporter**
LRP Publications
747 Dresher Road
Horsham, PA 19044
215-784-0912
800-341-7874
FAX: 215-784-9014
e-mail: custserve@lrp.com
www.lrp.com

Kenneth Kahn, Founder/President
Monthly reports with information on federal, state, and local legislation affecting the implementation of early intervention and preschool programs for children with disabilities. *$145.00*
12-16 pages $10 shipping

1889 **Healthline**
CV Mosby Company
11830 Westline Industrial Drive
Saint Louis, MO 63146
314-872-8370
800-325-4177
FAX: 314-432-1380
e-mail: journal.service@mosby.com
www.mosby.com

Paul Insel, Editor
Health and fitness information for healthcare professionals and the general public alike.
Monthly

1890 **Help Newsletter**
Learning Disabilities Association of Arkansas
7509 Cantrell Road
Suite 103c
Little Rock, AR 72207
501-666-8777
FAX: 501-666-8777
e-mail: info@ldaarkansas.org
www.ldaarkansas.org

Dana Jackson, Executive Director
Kristen Joyner, Director Development
Information on how to overcome obstacles and to achieve in spite of learning disabilities. *$30.00*
8 pages Quarterly

1891 **International Rolf Institute**
5055 Chaparral Court
Suite 103
Boulder, CO 80301
303-449-5903
800-530-8875
FAX: 303-449-5978
www.rolf.org
Information, practitioner training and certification.

1892 **Learning Disabilities Consultants Newsletter**
Learning Disabilities Consultants
PO Box 716
Bryn Mawr, PA 19010
610-446-6126
800-869-8336
FAX: 610-446-6129
e-mail: rcooper-ldr@comcast.net

Richard Cooper, Director
Newsletter providing information about learning disabilities and differences. It contains both local and national news items and includes in each issue articles about various aspects of learning problems encountered in both children and adults. *$10.00*
6 pages 5x Year

1893 **MA Report**
National Allergy and Asthma Network
3554 Chain Bridge Road
Suite 200
Fairfax, VA 22030
703-385-4403
FAX: 703-352-4354

Offers information on medical breakthroughs, patient care, public awareness, activities and events focusing on the allergy and asthma patient. This newsletter is the only Monthly Asthma Report that a patient will need to keep fully informed with medical articles written by experts in the field.
Monthly

1894 **NYALD News**
New York Association for the Learning Disabled
90 South Swan Street
Albany, NY 12210
518-465-6115

Kelly Jarrard, Executive Director
Michael Vacek, Manager
Newsletter offering information on the learning disabled in the New York area.
Monthly

1895 **O&P Almanac**
American Orthotic & Prosthetic Association
1666 K Street NW
Suite 440
Washington, DC 20006
571-431-0876
FAX: 571-431-0899
e-mail: info@aopanet.org
www.aopanet.org

Lisa Gough, Editor-in-Chief
Carrie Parsons, Managing Editor
Offers in-depth coverage on orthotics and prosthetics to current professional, government, business and reimbursement activities affecting the orthotics and prosthetics industry. *$59.00*
80 pages Monthly

1896 **Occupational Therapy in Health Care**
Haworth Press
10 Alice Street
Binghamton, NY 13904
607-722-5857
800-429-6784
FAX: 800-895-0582
e-mail: getinfo@haworthpress.com
www.haworthpress.com

Bill Palmer, VP/Publications Director
Rebecca Browne, Administrative Manager
William Cohen, Owner
Each issue focuses on significant practices and concerns involving occupational therapy and therapists. *$75.00*

1897 **Ohio Coalition for the Education of Children with Disabilities**
165 West Center Street
Suite 302
Marion, OH 43302
740-382-5452
800-374-2806
FAX: 740-383-6421
e-mail: ocecd@gte.net
www.ocecd.org

Margret Burley, Executive Director
Lee Ann Derugen, Co-Director
Martha Lause, Librarian
Forum is a newsletter reporting on educational, legislative and other developments affecting persons with disabilities.
8 pages

1898 **SAMHSA News**
U S Department of Health and Human Services
200 Independence Avenue SW
Washington, DC 20201
202-690-7650
877-696-6775
www.samhsa.gov

Mark Weber, Associate Administrator
Deborah Goodmad, Public Affairs Specialist
This quarterly agency newsletter reports on information on substance abuse, mental health treatment and prevention programs of the Substance Abuse and Mental Health Services Administration.

Quarterly

1899 **Sibling Information Network Newsletter**
AJ Pappanikou Center
253 Farmington Avenue
Suite 262
Farmington, CT 06030
860-679-1500
866-623-1315
FAX: 860-679-1571
www.uconnucedd.org

Mary Beth Bruder, Director
Contains information aimed at the varying interested of our membership. Program descriptions, requests for assistance, conference announcements, literature summaries and research reports. *$8.50*

1900 **Sibpage**
AJ Pappanikou Center
263 Farmington Avenue
Suite 262
Farmington, CT 06030
860-679-1500
866-623-1315
FAX: 860-679-1571
www.uconnucedd.org

Mary Beth Bruder, Director
Jill Cotter, Instructor
Developed specifically for children containing games, recipes, pen pals, and articles written by siblings relating to developmental disabilities.
4 pages

1901 **Special Edge**
Resources in Special Education
1107 9th Street
4th Floor
Sacramento, CA 95814
916-492-9990
877-493-7833
FAX: 415-565-3012
e-mail: rise@wested.org
Provides education news, collaborative programs, amendments to the laws, tools for accommodations, resource information, a calendar of events, and more.
BiMonthly

1902 **Special Education Report**
LRP Publications
1901 North Moore Street
Suite 1106
Arlington, VA 22209
703-516-7002
FAX: 703-516-9313
www.lrp.com

Patrick Harden, Manager
Current, pertinent information about federal legislation, regulations, programs and funding for educating children with disabilities. Covers federal and state litigation on the Individuals with Disabilities Education Act and other relevant laws. Looks at innovations and research in the field. *$266.00*
8 pages BiWeekly
ISSN 0194-22 5

1903 **Topics in Early Childhood Special Education**
Pro-Ed Publication
8700 Shoal Creek Boulevard
Austin, TX 78757
512-451-3246
800-897-3202
FAX: 800-397-7633
e-mail: info@proedinc.com
www.proedinc.com

Donald Hammill, Owner
Courtney King, Marketing Coordinator
Designed for professionals helping young children with special needs in areas such as assessment, special programs, social policies and developmental aids. *$43.00*

Quarterly

1904 **Treatment Review**
AIDS Treatment Data Network
611 Broadway
Room 613
New York, NY 10012
212-253-7922
800-734-7104
FAX: 212-260-8869
e-mail: network@atdn.org
www.atdn.org

Mark Harrington, Executive Director
Max Setulveda, Financing Manager
Individual members recieve treatment education, counseling, referrals and case management support. Services are available in both English and Spanish. The Treatment Review newsletter includes descriptions of approved, alternative and experimental treatments, as well as announcements of seminars and forums on treatments and clinical trials.
Quarterly

1905 **VIP Newsletter**
201 S. University
Mt Pleasant, MI 48858
989-779-9966
FAX: 989-779-0015
e-mail: bcf@blindchildrensfund.org
www.blindchildrensfund.org
Blind Children's Fund, author
Karla Storrer, Executive Director
Didi Duncan, Outreach Director
Provides parents and professionals with information, materials and resources that help them succesfullly teach and nurture blind, visually and multi-impaired infants and preschoolers. *$10.00*
194

Professional Texts

1906 **A Teacher's Guide to HCU**
Arizona Department of Health Services
150 North 18th Avenue
Suite 310
Phoenix, AZ 85007
602-271-0945
FAX: 602-542-1235
e-mail: piowebmaster@azdhs.gov
www.azdhs.gov

Susan Gerard, Director
Robert Plummer, Manager
Resource book for preschool teachers and school staff on homocysteinuria basics and classroom activities. *$2.50*

1907 **A Teacher's Guide to Isovaleric Acidemia**
150 North 18th Avenue
Phoenix, AZ 85007
602-542-1000
FAX: 602-542-0883
www.azdhs.gov

Susan Gered, Director
Resource book for preschool teachers and school staff on isovaleric acidemia basics and classroom activities. *$2.50*

1908 **A Teacher's Guide to MSUD**
Arizona Department of Health Services
1740 West Adams Street
Phoenix, AZ 85007
602-271-0945
FAX: 602-542-1235
e-mail: piowebmaster@azdhs.gov
www.azdhs.gov

Susan Gerard, Director
Susan Gerard, Director
Resource book for preschool teachers and school staff on MSUD basics and classroom activities. *$2.50*

1909 **A Teacher's Guide to Methylmalonic Acidemia**
Arizona State Department of Health Services
1740 West Adams Street
Phoenix, AZ 85007
602-542-1073
FAX: 602-542-1235
e-mail: piowebmaster@azdhs.gov
www.azdhs.gov

Susan Gerard, Director
Resource book for preschool teachers and school staff on methylmalonic acidemia basics and classroom activities. *$2.50*

1910 **A Teacher's Guide to PKU**
Arizona Department of Health Services
1740 West Adams Street
Phoenix, AZ 85007
602-542-1886
FAX: 602-542-1890
e-mail: piowebmaster@azdhs.gov
www.azdhs.gov

Susan Gerard, Director
Margaret Tate, Manager
Resource book for preschool teachers and school staff on PKU basics, NutraSweet warning, and classroom activities. *$2.50*
13 pages

1911 **A Teacher's Guide to Propionic Acidemia**
Arizona Department of Health Services
1740 West Adams Street
Phoenix, AZ 85007
602-271-0945
FAX: 602-542-1235
e-mail: piowebmaster@azdhs.gov
www.azdhs.gov

Susan Gerard, Director
Robert Plummer, Manager
Resource book for preschool teachers and school staff on propionic acidemia basics and classroom activities. *$2.50*

1912 **ADD Challenge: A Practical Guide for Teachers**
Research Press
PO Box 9177
Champaign, IL 61826
217-352-3273
800-519-2707
FAX: 217-352-1221
e-mail: rp@researchpress.com
www.researchpress.com

Russell Tence, President
$15.95
196 pages
ISBN 0-878223-45-2

1913 **ADHD in the Classroom: Strategies for Teachers**
Guilford Publication
72 Spring Street
New York, NY 10012
212-431-9800
800-365-7006
FAX: 212-966-6708
e-mail: info@guilford.com

Bob Matloff, President
Designed specifically to help teachers with their ADHD students, thereby providing a better learning environment for the entire class. *$95.00*

ISBN 0-898629-85-3

1914 **ADHD in the Schools: Assessment and Intervention Strategies**
72 Spring Street
New York, NY 10012
212-431-9800
800-365-7006
FAX: 212-966-6708
e-mail: info@guilford.com
www.guilford.com

Seymour Weingarten, Editor-in-Chief
Judith Grauman, Managing Editor
Bob Matloff, President
The landmark volume emphasizes the need for a team effort among parents, community-based professionals, and educators. Provides practical information for educators that is based on empirical findings. Chapters Focus on how to identify and assess students who might have ADHD, the relationship between ADHD and learning disabilities; how to develop and supplement classroom-based programs. Communication strategies to assist physicians and the need for community-based treatments *$36.00*
269 pages Paperback
ISBN 0-898622-45-X

1915 **AEPS Curriculum for Birth to Three Years**
Brookes Publishing
PO Box 10624
Baltimore, MD 21285
410-337-9580
800-638-3775
FAX: 410-337-8539
e-mail: custserv@brookespublishing.com
www.brookespublishing.com

Paul Brooks, Owner
Directly linked to IEP/IFSP goals developed for a child from the AEPS test measure, the AEPS curriculum provides a complete set of learning activities to facilitate children's acquisition of functional skills. *$59.95*
496 pages
ISBN 1-557660-96-4

1916 **Access to Health Care: Number 1&2**
World Institute on Disability
510 16th Street
Suite 100
Oakland, CA 94612
510-763-4100
510-209-9493
FAX: 510-763-4109
e-mail: wid@wid.org
www.wid.org

Kathy Martinez, Executive Director
These health policy bulletins analyze health care needs. Volume 1 focuses on a wide range of information relevant to addressing the adequacy of the health care system for persons with disabilities or chronic illness. *$6.50*
63 pages Paperback

1917 **Access to Health Care: Number 3&4**
World Institute on Disability
510 16th Street
Suite 100
Oakland, CA 94612
510-763-4100
FAX: 510-763-4109
e-mail: wid@wid.org
www.wid.org

Stanley K Yarnell, Chairman
Martin B Schulter, Vice Chairman
These policy bulletins focus on the capacity of the private and public health insurance systems to respond to the health care needs of persons with disabilities or chronic illness. *$6.50*
91 pages Paperback

1918 **Activity-Based Approach to Early Intervention, 2nd Edition**
Brookes Publishing
PO Box 10624
Baltimore, MD 21285
410-337-9580
800-638-3775
FAX: 410-337-8539
e-mail: custserv@brookespublishing.com
www.brookespublishing.com

Clary Creighton, Exhibits Coordinator
Tracy Gray, Educational Sales Manager
Paul Brooks, Owner
Activity-based intervention shows how to use natural and relevant events to teach infants and young children, of all abilities, effectively and efficiently. *$24.00*

240 pages
ISBN 1-55766 -87-5

1919 **Adapted Physical Education for Students with Autism**
Charles C Thomas Publisher
2600 South 1st Street
Springfield, IL 62704
217-789-8980
800-258-8980
FAX: 217-789-9130
e-mail: books@ccthomas.com
www.ccthomas.com

Michael Thomas, President
Focuses on the physical education needs and curriculum for autistic children. Available in cloth, paperback and hardcover. *$23.95*
142 pages Paper
ISBN 0-398060-85-1

1920 **Adapting Early Childhood Curricula for Children with Special Needs**
McGraw-Hill School Publishing
220 East Danieldale Road
Desoto, TX 75115
972-224-1111
800-442-9685
FAX: 972-228-1982
www.mhschool.com

Joseph Gavigan, President
Offers information on educating the disabled.

1921 **Adapting Instruction for the Mainstream: A Sequential Approach to Teaching**
McGraw-Hill School Publishing
220 East Danieldale Road
Desoto, TX 75115
972-224-1111
800-442-9685
FAX: 972-228-1982
www.mcgrawhill.com

Joseph Gavigan, President.
Todd Painter, Assistant Director
This text gives both regular and special education teachers everything they need to help mildly handicapped students succeed in the mainstream.
226 pages

1922 **Adaptive Education Strategies Building on Diversity**
Brookes Publishing Company
PO Box 10624
Baltimore, MD 21285
410-337-9580
800-638-3775
FAX: 410-337-8539
e-mail: custserv@brookespublishing.com
www.brookespublishing.com

Tracy Gray, Educational Sales Manager
Paul Brooks, Owner
Based on more than two decades of systematic research, this comprehensive manual provides a road map to the effective implementation of adaptive education. *$35.00*
304 pages Paperback 1992
ISBN 1-557880-84-0

1923 **Advanced Sign Language Vocabulary: A Resource Text for Educators**
Charles C Thomas Publisher
2600 South 1st Street
Springfield, IL 62704
217-789-8980
800-258-8980
FAX: 217-789-9130
e-mail: books@ccthomas.com
www.ccthomas.com

Janice Ahmad, Author
Edward Allen, Author
Michael Thomas, President
This book is a collection of advanced sign language vocabulary for use by educators, interpreters, parents or anyone wishing to enlarge their sign vocabulary. *$48.95*
202 pages Paperback 1991
ISBN 0-398057-22-2

1924 **Advances in Cardiac and Pulmonary Rehabilitation**
Haworth Press
10 Alice Street
Binghamton, NY 13904
607-722-5857
800-429-6784
FAX: 607-722-6362
e-mail: orders@haworthpress.com
www.haworthpress.com

Sandy Sickels, Vice President
Becky Minerbaum, Advertising Manager
William Cohen, Owner
Enhance your rehabilitation program with this authoritative volume. *$34.95*
74 pages Hardcover
ISBN 0-866869-86-3

1925 **Aging Brain**
Taylor & Francis Group
325 Chestnut Street
Suite 800
Philadelphia, PA 19106
215-625-8900
800-354-1420
FAX: 215-625-8914
www.taylorandfrancisgroup.com

Kevin Bradley, Chief Executive Officer
Elderly treatment.
225 pages Paperback
ISBN 0-85066 -78-0

1926 **Aging and Rehabilitation II**
Springer Publishing Company
11 West 42nd Street
15th Floor
New York, NY 10036
212-431-4370
877-687-7476
FAX: 212-941-7842
e-mail: Contactus@springerpub.com
www.springerpub.com

Sheri Sussman, Vice President
Anette Imperati, Marketing/Sales Director
Ursula Springer, President
Current, multidisciplinary investigations of various practice issues. Leading experts in the field use a practical perspective to provide specific comments on interventions. The scope of this work encompasses the autonomy of elderly disabled, mobility, mental health and value issues, as well as basic aspects in rehabilitation of the elderly. *$41.95*
367 pages Hardcover
ISBN 0-82617 -80-3

1927 **Alphabetic Phonics Curriculum**
Educators Publishing Service
625 Mount Auburn Street
Suite 3
Cambridge, MA 02138
617-547-6706
800-225-5750
FAX: 888-440-2665
e-mail: feedback@epsbooks.com
www.epsbooks.com

Charles H Heinle, Vice President
Alexandra S Bigelow, Author
Gunnar Voltz, President
Ungraded multisensory curriculum for teaching phonics and the structure of language. Uses Orton-Gillingham approach to teach handwriting, spelling, reading, reading comprehension, and oral and written expression. program includes basic manual, workbooks, tests, teachers' guides, drill cards and all cards. *$28.15*

ISSN 8388-42

1928 **Alternative Educational Delivery Systems**
National Association of School Psychologists
4340 E West Highway
Suite 402
Bethesda, MD 20814
301-657-0270
FAX: 301-657-0275

Susan Gorin, Executive Director

A book offering information to the professional on how to enhance educational options for all students.

1929 Alternative Teaching Strategies

Special Needs Project
324 State Street
Suite H
Santa Barbara, CA 93101
805-962-8087
800-333-6867
FAX: 805-962-5087
www.specialneeds.com

Hod Gray, Founder

Offers help for teachers who teach behaviorally troubled students.

1930 Antecedent Control: Innovative Approaches to Behavioral Support

Brookes Publishing
PO Box 10624
Baltimore, MD 21285
410-337-9585
800-638-3775
FAX: 410-337-8539
e-mail: custserv@brookespublishing.com
www.brookespublishing.com

Melissa Behm, President

This book explains the theory and methodology of antecedent control. The treatment techniques in this book are effective for both children and adults.

416 pages Paperback 1998
ISBN 1-55766 -34-3

1931 Applied Rehabilitation Counseling

Springer Publishing Compn
11 West 42nd Street
15th Floor
New York, NY 10036
212-431-4370
877-687-7476
FAX: 212-941-7842
e-mail: contactus@springerpub.com
www.springerpub.com

Annette Imperati, Marketing/Sales Director
Sheri Sussman, Vice President
Ursula Springer, President

This comprehensive text describes current theories, techniques, and their applications to specific disabled populations. Perspectives on varying counseling approaches such as psychodynamic, existential, gestalt, behavioral and psychoeducational orientations are systematically outlined in an easy-to-follow format. Practical applications for counseling are emphasized with attention given to strategies, goal-setting and on-going evaluations. *$29.95*

400 pages Softcover
ISBN 0-82615 -70-4

1932 Art-Centered Education and Therapy for Children with Disabilities

Charles C Thomas
2600 South 1st Street
Springfield, IL 62704
217-789-8980
800-258-8980
FAX: 217-789-9130
e-mail: books@ccthomas.com
www.ccthomas.com

Michael Thomas, President

This book has been written to help both the regular education, and art and special education teachers, both pre- and in-service, better understand some of the issues and realities of providing education and remediation to children with disabilities. The book is also offered as model concept that has govern the author's personal and professional career of over thirty years. *$35.95*

284 pages Paperback
ISBN 0-398060-06-1

1933 Assessing the Handicaps/Needs of Children

Books on Special Children
PO Box 3378
Amherst, MA 01004
413-256-8164
FAX: 413-256-8896
e-mail: irene@boscbooks.com
www.boscbooks.com

Papers on treatment, rehab and social support in assessing the needs of mentally retarded children. *$66.00*

260 pages Hardcover
ISBN 0-12218 -02-0

1934 Assessment & Management of Mainstreamed Hearing-Impaired Children

Pro-Ed Publications
8700 Shoal Creek Boulevard
Austin, TX 78757
512-451-3246
800-897-3202
FAX: 800-397-7633
e-mail: feedback@proedinc.com
www.proedinc.com

Donald Hammill, Owner
Courtney King, Marketing Coordinator

The theoretical and practical considerations of developing appropriate programming for hearing-impaired children who are being educated in mainstream educational settings are presented in this book.

1935 Assessment Log & Developmental Progress Charts for the Carolina Curriculum

Brookes Publishing
PO Box 10624
Baltimore, MD 21285
410-337-9580
800-638-3775
FAX: 410-337-8539
e-mail: custserv@brookespublishing.com
www.brookespublishing.com

Clary Creighton, Exhibits Coordinator
Tracy Gray, Educational Sales Manager
Paul Brooks, Owner

This 28-page booklet allows the progress of children with skills in the 12-36 month development range to be easily recorded. Available in packages of 10. *$23.00*

28 pages Saddle-stiched
ISBN 1-557662-21-5

1936 Assessment and Remediation of Articulatory and Phonological Disorders

McGraw-Hill School Publishing
220 East Danieldale Road
Desoto, TX 75115
972-224-1111
800-442-9685
FAX: 972-228-1982
www.mhschool.com

Joseph Gavigan, President

Offers comprehensive coverage of articulation disorders.

1937 Assessment in Mental Handicap: A Guide to Assessment Practices & Tests

Brookline Books
39 University Road
Brookline, MA 02445
617-734-6772
800-666-BOOK
FAX: 617-734-3952
e-mail: thestore@brooklinebooksmith.com
www.brooklinebooks.com

William H Walters, Author
Esther Isabe Wilder, Author

Helps professionals understand the rationale and uses for assessment practices, and provides details of appropriate instruments within each type: adaptive behavior scales, assessment of behavioral disturbances, early development and Plagetian tests. *$20.00*

Hardcover
ISBN 0-91479 -31-X

1938 Assessment of Children and Youth

Longman Education/Addison Wesley
1185 Avenue of the Americas
New York, NY 10036
212-782-3300
800-322-1377
FAX: 800-333-3328
www.longman.awl.com

Ginny Blanford, Editor

Introductory text for preservice and in-service special educators on assessment, based on the principle that every child is unique. Comprehensive coverage of both formal and informal assessment instruments. *$50.00*

640 pages Paperback
ISBN 0-80131 -02-5

1939 Assessment of Individuals with Severe Disabilities
Brookes Publishing Company
PO Box 10624
Baltimore, MD 21285
410-337-9580
800-638-3775
FAX: 410-337-8539
e-mail: custserv@brookespublishing.com
www.brookespublishing.com

Clary Creighton, Exhibits Coordinator
Tracy Gray, Educational Sales Manager
Paul Brooks, Owner
This expanded text offers instructors guidelines to design a comprehensive educational assessment for individuals with severe disabilities. *$34.00*
432 pages Paperback 1991
ISBN 1-557660-67-0

1940 Assessment of the Technology Needs of Vending Facilitiy Managers In Tennessee
Mississippi State University
PO Box 6189
Mississippi State, MS 39762
662-325-8122
800-675-7782
FAX: 662-325-8989
www.blind.msstate.edu/
Moore, Maxson, Cavenugh, Johnson, Pearson, author
Kelly Schaefer, Publications Manager
Thomas Adkins, Executive Director
This report summarizes the results and recommendations of a survey conducted of vending facility managers throughout the state of Tennessee who participate in the Randolph-Sheppard program. *$15.00*
39 pages Paperback

1941 Assessment: The Special Educator's Role
Brooks Publishing Company
511 Forest Lodge Road
Pacific Grove, CA 93950
831-373-0728
FAX: 831-375-6414
e-mail: bc-info@brookscole.com
www.brookespublishing.com
Aimed at students with little or no classroom experience in assessment, the book focuses on the integration of dynamic, curriculum-based and norm-referenced data for diagnostic decisions and program planning.
580 pages Casebound
ISBN 0-53421 -32-1

1942 Asthma Management and Education
Asthma and Allergy Foundation of America
1233 20th Street NW
Suite 402
Washington, DC 20005
202-466-7643
FAX: 202-466-8940
e-mail: info@aafa.org
www.aafa.org

Todd Houston, Director
Bill McLin, Executive Director
One session, two hour program developed to educate allied health professionals about up-to-date asthma care and patient education, information and materials. Includes hands on experience with peak flow meters and demonstrations of medical devices.

1943 Aston-Patterning
PO Box 3568
Incline Village, NV 89450
775-831-8228
FAX: 775-831-8955
e-mail: info@astonenterprises.com
www.astonenterprises.com

Jane Davis, Administrative Assistant
J Aston, Owner
Integrated system of movement education, body assessment, environmental modification and fitness training.

1944 Attention Deficit Disorder in Children and Adolescents
Charles C Thomas
2600 South 1st Street
Springfield, IL 62704
217-789-8980
800-258-8980
FAX: 217-789-9130
e-mail: books@ccthomas.com
www.ccthomas.com

Mikal Aasved, Author
Howard Earle, Author
Michael Thomas, President
Presents an analysis of case studies of children and adolescents with attentional deficits and hyperactivity, demonstrating causal factors in these disorders and suggesting treatment strategies both in psychological and medical practice. Written as a review and summary of twenty years of private practice. *$35.95*
292 pages Paperback
ISBN 0-39806 -12-2

1945 Aural Habilitation
Alexander Graham Bell Association
3417 Volta Place NW
Washington, DC 20007
202-337-5220
FAX: 202-337-8314
e-mail: info@agbell.org
www.agbell.org

Gayla Hutsell, Chief Programs Officer
Todd Houston, Executive Director
This classic text for professionals, educators and parents discusses verbal learning and aural habilitation of young children with hearing losses to ensure that each child is educated in the best setting. It discusses communication, normal development of spoken language, speech audiologic assessment, hearing aids and use of residual hearing, and program designs for individualized needs, including the assessment and planning of IEPs. *$26.95*
324 pages

1946 Behavior Analysis in Education: Focus on Measurably Superior Instruction
Brooks Publishing Company
PO Box 10624
Baltimore, MD 21285
410-337-9580
800-638-3775
FAX: 410-337-8539
e-mail: custserv@brookespublishing.com
www.brookespublishing.com

Clary Creighton, Exhibits Coordinator
Tracy Gray, Educational Sales Manager
Paul Brooks, Owner
Designed to disseminate measurably superior instructional strategies to those interested in advancing sound, pedagogically effective, field-tested educational practices, this book is intended for graduate-level courses and seminars in special education and/or psychology focusing on behavior analysis and instruction.
512 pages Casebound
ISBN 0-53422 -60-9

1947 Behavior Modification
Sage Publications
2455 Teller Road
Thousand Oaks, CA 91320
805-499-0721
800-818-7243
FAX: 805-499-0871
www.sagepublications.com

Blaise R Simqu, Chief Executive Officer
Stephen Barr, Senior Vice President
Describes in detail for replication purposes assessment and modification techniques for problems in psychiatric, clinical, educational and rehabilitation settings. *$53.00*
640 pages Quarterly

1948 Behavioral Disorders
Council for Exceptional Children
1110 North Glebe Road
Suite 300
Arlington, VA 22201
703-245-0600
866-915-5000
FAX: 703-264-1637
e-mail: services@cec.sped.org
www.cec.sped.org

Jamie Hopkins, President
Drew Allbirtten, Executive Director
Bruce Ramirez, Manager
Provides professionals with a means to exchange information and share ideas related to research, empirically tested educational innovations and issues and concerns relevant to students with behavioral disorders. Individual, $20; Institution, $50.
Quarterly

1949 **Behind Special Education**
Love Publishing Company
9101 East Kenyon Avenue
Suite 2200
Denver, CO 80237
303-221-7333
FAX: 303-221-7444
e-mail: lpc@lovepub.com
www.lovepublishing.com

Ann Vernon, Author
Stan Love, Owner
This new work is a critical analysis of the nature of disability, special education, school organization and reform progress. *$24.95*
ISBN 0-89108 -17-4

1950 **Biomedical Concerns in Persons with Down's Syndrome**
Paul H Brookes Publishing Company
PO Box 10624
Baltimore, MD 21285
410-337-9580
800-638-3775
FAX: 410-337-8539
e-mail: custserv@brookespublishing.com
www.brookespublishing.com

Karen G Radke, Marketing Director
Clary Creighton, Exhibits Coordinator
Paul Brooks, Owner
Written by leading authorities and spanning many disciplines and specialties, this comprehensive resource provides vital information on biomedical issues concerning individuals with Down's Syndrome. *$45.00*
336 pages Hardcover 1992
ISBN 1-557660-89-1

1951 **Breaking Barriers**
AbleNet
2008 Fairview Avenue N
Roseville, MN 55113
800-322-0956
FAX: 651-294-2259
e-mail: customerservice@ablenetinc.com
www.ablenetinc.com

Cheryl Volkam, President/Chief Executive Office
A practical resource for parents, caregivers, teachers and therapists. *$15.00*

1952 **Building the Healing Partnership: Parents, Professionals and Children**
Brookline Books
39 University Road
Brookline, MA 02445
617-734-6772
800-666-BOOK
FAX: 617-734-3952
e-mail: thestore@brooklinebooksmith.com
www.brooklinebooks.com

William H Walters, Author
Esther Isabe Wilder, Author
Successful programs understand that the disabled child's needs must be considered in the context of a family. This book was specifically written for practitioner's who must work with families but who have insufficient training in family systems assessment and intervention. It is a valuable blend of theory and practice with pointers for applying the principles. *$24.95*
Paperback
ISBN 0-91479 -63-8

1953 **Career Assessment Inventories Learning Disabled**
C FK R Career Materials
PO Box 99
Meadow Vista, CA 95722
800-525-5626
FAX: 800-770-0433
e-mail: ffrerry@cfkr.com
www.cfkr.com

Francis Ferry, Operation Manager
Takes personality, ability and interest into account in pointing learning disabled students of all ages toward intelligent and realistic career choices. Contains binder with paperback teaching guide plus 50 interest inventories and 50 abilities inventories. *$50.00*

1954 **Caring for Children with Chronic Illness**
11 West 42nd Street
New York, NY 10036
212-431-4370
877-687-7476
FAX: 212-941-7842
e-mail: marketing@springerpub.com
www.springerpub.com

Annette Imperati, Marketing/Sales Director
Ursula Springer, President
A critical look at the current medical, social, and psychological framework for providing care to children with chronic illnesses. Emphasizing the need to create integrated, interdisciplinary approaches, it discusses issues such as the roles of families, professionals, and institutions in providing health care, the impact of a child's illness on various family structures, financing care, the special problems of chronically ill children as they become adolescents and more. *$36.95*
320 pages Hardcover
ISBN 0-82615 -00-1

1955 **Carolina Curriculum for Infants and Toddlers with Special Needs, 2nd Edition**
Brookes Publishing
PO Box 10624
Baltimore, MD 21285
410-337-9580
800-638-3775
FAX: 410-337-8539
e-mail: custserv@brookespublishing.com
www.brookespublishing.com

Clary Creighton, Exhibits Coordinator
Tracy Gray, Educational Sales Manager
Paul Brooks, Owner
This book includes detailed assessment and intervention sequences, daily routine integration strategies, sensorimotor adaptations, and a sample 24-page assessment log that shows readers how to chart a child's individual progress. *$40.00*
384 pages Spiral-bound
ISBN 1-55766 -74-3

1956 **Carolina Curriculum for Preschoolers with Special Needs**
Brookes Publishing
PO Box 10624
Baltimore, MD 21285
410-337-9580
800-638-3775
FAX: 410-337-8539
e-mail: custserv@brookespublishing.com
www.brookespublishing.com

Clary Creighton, Exhibits Coordinator
Tracy Gray, Educational Sales Manager
Paul Brooks, Owner
This curriculum provides detailed teaching and assessment techniques, plus a sample 28-page assessment log that shows readers how to chart a child's individual progress. This guide is for children between 2 and 5 in their developmental stages who are considered at risk for developmental delay or who exhibit special needs. *$34.00*

352 pages Spiral-bound
ISBN 1-55766 -32-8

1957 Challenge of Educating Together Deaf and Hearing Youth: Making Manistreaming Work
Charles C Thomas
2600 South 1st Street
Springfield, IL 62704
217-789-8980
800-258-8980
FAX: 217-789-9130
e-mail: books@ccthomas.com
www.ccthomas.com

Michael Thomas, President
Those who have this challenge of education: teachers, administrators, other professionals, parents, and concerned individuals will benefit from this book. Also available in cloth. *$28.95*
198 pages Softcover
ISBN 0-398063-91-5

1958 Challenged Scientists: Disabilities and the Triumph of Excellence
Greenwood Publishing Group
88 Post Road West
Suite 5007
Westport, CT 06880
203-226-3571
800-225-5800
FAX: 203-222-1502
www.greenwood.com

Wayne Smith, President
This volume points out how the increasing need for scientists in this country can be lessened by utilizing a long overlooked pool of scientific talent in those persons who are scientifically oriented but who happen to have physical or sensory disabilities. Hardcover. $49.95-$55.00.
208 pages
ISBN 0-275938-73-5

1959 Child Care and the ADA: A Handbook for Inclusive Programs
Brookes Publishing
PO Box 10624
Baltimore, MD 21285
410-337-9580
800-638-3775
FAX: 410-337-8539
e-mail: custserv@brookespublishing.com
www.brookespublishing.com

Clary Creighton, Exhibits Coordinator
Tracy Gray, Educational Sales Manager
Paul Brooks, Owner
This book is designed for educators and administrators in child care settings. It offers a straightforward discussion of the Americans with Disabilities Act including children with disabilities in community programs. *$25.95*
240 pages Paperback
ISBN 1-55766 -85-5

1960 Child with Disabling Illness
Lippincott, Williams & Wilkins
227 East Washington Square
Philadelphia, PA 19106
215-521-8300
800-777-2295
FAX: 301-824-7390
www.lpub.com

J Lippincott, Chief Executive Officer
$108.50
700 pages

1961 Childhood Behavior Disorders: Applied Research & Educational Practice
Pro-Ed Publications
8700 Shoal Creek Boulevard
Austin, TX 78757
512-451-3246
800-897-3202
FAX: 800-397-7633
e-mail: feedback@proedinc.com
www.proedinc.com

Donald Hammill, Owner
Courtney King, Marketing Coordinator
The only comprehensive overview of childhood behavior disorders. This book gives you the how and why for helping children with behavior disorders.

1962 Childhood Disablity and Family Systems
Haworth Press
10 Alice Street
Binghamton, NY 13904
607-722-5857
800-429-6784
FAX: 607-722-6362
e-mail: orders@haworthpress.com
www.haworthpress.com

William Cohen, President/Owner
Maevin B Sussman PhD, Co-Editor
S Harrington-Miller, Advertising
Focuses on what the presence of a disabled child means to a family. Those professionals involved in teaching, research, and direct care with families having disabled children will value the coverage of such topics as the contemporary context of disability, ethical issues, family effects, and care systems. *$74.95*
246 pages Hardcover
ISBN 0-866566-71-6

1963 Children and Youth Assisted by Medical Technology in Educational Settings, 2nd Edition
Brookes Publishing
PO Box 10624
Baltimore, MD 21285
410-337-9580
800-638-3775
FAX: 410-337-8539
e-mail: custserv@brookespublishing.com
www.brookespublishing.com

Clary Creighton, Exhibits Coordinator
Tracy Gray, Educational Sales Manager
Paul Brooks, Owner
Contains detailed daily care guidelines and emergency-response techniques, including information on working with a range of students who have the HIV infection, that rely on ventilators, that utilize tube feeding, or require catheterization. Also covers every aspect of planning for inclusive classrooms, including information on personnel training, entrance planning and transition, legal requirements, and transportation issues. *$52.00*
432 pages Spiral-bound 1997
ISBN 1-55766 -36-3

1964 Children's Needs Psychological Perspective
National Association of School Psychologists
8455 Colesville Road
Suite 1000
Silver Spring, MD 20910
301-681-3223
FAX: 301-608-2514
This very popular monograph was developed with the recognition that many factors beyond the classroom and the child's own personal characteristics influence school success.
637 pages

1965 Choices: A Guide to Sex Counseling for the Physically Disabled Adult
Krieger Publishing Company
PO Box 9542
Melbourne, FL 32902
321-724-9542
800-724-0025
FAX: 321-951-3671
e-mail: info@krieger-publishing.com
www.krieger-publishing.com

R Krieger, Owner
Provides rehabilitation professionals with the basic information necessary for limited sexuality counseling of physically disabled adults. *$14.50*
132 pages
ISBN 0-898749-03-4

1966 Choosing Options and Accommodations for Children
Brookes Publishing
PO Box 10624
Baltimore, MD 21285
410-337-9580
800-638-3775
FAX: 410-337-8539
e-mail: custserv@brookespublishing.com
www.brookespublishing.com

Clary Creighton, Exhibits Coordinator
Tracy Gray, Educational Sales Manager
Paul Brooks, Owner

Bridging the gap between the philosophy and practice of inclusive education, this important manual provides a practical assessment and planning process for the inclusion of students with disabilities in general education classrooms. *$29.00*

192 pages
ISBN 1-55766 -06-5

1967 **Classroom Success for the LD and ADHD Child**
John F Blair Publishing
1406 Plaza Drive
Winston Salem, NC 27103
336-768-1374
800-222-9796
FAX: 336-768-9194
e-mail: southern@blairpub.com
www.blairpub.com

Suzanne Stevens, author
Carolyn Sakowski, President
John F. Blair, Publisher
This book offers suggestions on teaching techniques, adapting texts, recognition of children with disabilities and testing, grading and mainstreaming the learning disabled and ADHD child. *$12.95*

314 pages Paperback
ISBN 0-895871-42-4

1968 **Clinical Management of Childhood Stuttering, 2nd Edition**
Pro-Ed Publications
8700 Shoal Creek Boulevard
Austin, TX 78757
512-451-3246
800-897-3202
FAX: 800-397-7633
e-mail: feedback@proedinc.com
www.proedinc.com

Donald Hammill, Owner
Courtney King, Marketing Coordinator
Updates and integrates recent findings in childhood stuttering into a broad range of therapeutic strategies for assessing and treating the young dysfluent child. *$38.00*

336 pages

1969 **Cognitive Approaches to Learning Disabilities**
Pro-Ed Publications
8700 Shoal Creek Boulevard
Austin, TX 78757
512-451-3246
800-897-3202
FAX: 800-397-7633
e-mail: feedback@proedinc.com
www.proedinc.com

Joshua Jeffrey, Marketing Custodian
Courtney King, Marketing Coordinator
Donald Hammill, Owner
The first to bridge the gap between cognitive psychology and information processing theory in understanding learning disabilities. *$39.00*

495 pages Hardcover

1970 **Cognitive Strategy Instruction That Really Improves Children's Academic Skills**
Brookline Books
34 University Road
Brookline, MA 02445
617-743-6772
800-666-BOOK
FAX: 617-734-3952
www.brooklinebooks.com

William H Walters, Author
Esther Isabe Wilder, Author
A concise and focused work that summarily presents the few procedures for teaching strategies that aid academic subject matter learning: decoding reading comprehension, vocabulary, math, spelling and writing. Learning unrelated facts and science. Completely revised in 1995. *$27.95*

Paperback
ISBN 1-571290-07-9

1971 **Collaborating for Comprehensive Services for Young Children and Families**
Brookes Publishing Company
PO Box 10624
Baltimore, MD 21285
410-337-9580
800-638-3775
FAX: 410-337-8539
e-mail: cutserv@brookespublishing.com
www.brookespublishing.com

Clary Creighton, Exhibits Coordinator
Tracy Gray, Educational Sales Manager
Paul Brooks, Owner
Taking collaboration a step beyond basic implementation, this useful book shows agency and school leaders how to coordinate their efforts to stretch human services dollars while still providing quality programs. Provides the building blocks needed to establish a local interagency coordinating council. *$37.00*

272 pages 1992
ISBN 1-557661-03-0

1972 **Collaborative Teams for Students with Severe Disabilities**
Brookes Publishing
PO Box 10624
Baltimore, MD 21285
410-337-9580
800-638-3775
FAX: 410-337-8539
e-mail: custserv@brookespublishing.com
www.brookespublishing.com

Clary Creighton, Exhibits Coordinator
Tracy Gray, Educational Sales Manager
Paul Brooks, Owner
How can educators, parents and therapists work together to ensure the best possible educational experience for students with severe disabilities? This resource describes how a collaborative team can successfully create exciting learning opportunities for students, while teaching them to participate fully at home, school, work and play. *$ 30.00*

304 pages
ISBN 1-55766 -88-3

1973 **Communicating with Parents of Exceptional Children**
Love Publishing Company
9101 East Kenyon Avenue
Suite 2200
Denver, CO 80237
303-221-7333
FAX: 303-221-7444
www.lovepublishing.com

Stan Love, Owner
This book shows how teachers can facilitate parent involvement with children's education. It presents the mirror model of parent involvement, family, dynamics, how to listen actively to parents, values and perceptions, problem-solving, parent conferences and training groups. *$19.95*

ISBN 0-89108 -67-4

1974 **Communication & Language Acquisition: Discoveries from Atypical Development**
Brookes Publishing
PO Box 10624
Baltimore, MD 21285
410-337-9580
800-638-3775
FAX: 410-337-8539
e-mail: custserv@brookespublishing.com
www.brookespublishing.com

Clary Creighton, Exhibits Coordinator
Tracy Gray, Educational Sales Manager
Paul Brooks, Owner
This text demonstrates how the study of language acquisition in children with atypical development promotes advances in basic theory. *$44.00*

352 pages Hardcover 1997
ISBN 1-557662-79-7

1975 Communication Skills for Working with Elders
Springer Publishing Company
11 West 42nd Street
New York, NY 10036
212-431-4370
877-687-7476
FAX: 212-941-7842
e-mail: marketing@springerpub.com
www.springerpub.com

Annette Imperati, Marketing/Sales Director
Ursula Springer, President
How aging and illness affects communication. *$17.95*
160 pages Softcover
ISBN 0-82615 -20-7

1976 Communication Unbound
Teachers College Press
14781 Memorial Drive
Suite 2115
Houston, TX 77079
415-738-4323
FAX: 415-738-4329
e-mail: tcc.orders@aidcvt.com
www.tcp.com

Michael Mcgann, Administrator
Complete title is 'Communication Unbound: How Facilitated Communication is Challenging the Traditional Views of Autism and Ability/Disablity'. Reveals the wonder of expression by people who have been trapped in silence and diminished by presumptions of their incompetence. *$18.95*
240 pages Paperback
ISBN 0-087737-21-4

1977 Complete Handbook of Children's Reading Disorders: You Can Prevent or Correct LDs
Gallery Bookshop
PO Box 270
Mendocino, CA 95460
707-937-2665
FAX: 707-937-3737
e-mail: info@gallerybooks.com
www.gallerybooks.com

Linda Pack, Manager
Tony Miksak, Owner
The complete handbook of children's reading disorders. *$34.95*
732 pages Paperback
ISBN 0-80772 -83-3

1978 Comprehensive Assessment in Special Education
Charles C Thomas
2600 South 1st Street
Springfield, IL 62704
217-789-8980
800-258-8980
FAX: 217-789-9130
e-mail: books@ccthomas.com
www.ccthomas.com

Michael Thomas, President
D Sexton, Author
The purpose of this book is to incorporate (1) detailed approaches to assessment, (2) assessment fundamentals, (3) traditional and emerging assessment, (4) today's special assessment concerns. *$104.95*
578 pages Hardcover
ISBN 0-398056-45-5

1979 Computer Access/Computer Learning
Special Needs Project
324 State Street
Suite H
Santa Barbara, CA 93101
805-962-8087
800-333-6867
FAX: 805-962-5087
www.specialneeds.com

Hod Gray, Founder
A resource manual in adaptive technology and computer training. *$22.50*

1980 Consulting Psychologists Press
1055 Joaquin Road
2nd Floor
Mountain View, CA 94043
650-969-8901
800-624-1765
FAX: 650-969-8608
www.cpp-db.com
Catalog offering job assessment software, career development reports, educational assessment information and books for the professional.

1981 Counseling Persons with Communication Disorders and Their Families
Pro-Ed Publications
8700 Shoal Creek Boulevard
Austin, TX 78757
512-451-3246
800-897-3202
FAX: 800-397-7633
e-mail: feedback@proedinc.com
www.proedinc.com

Donald Hammill, Owner
Courtney King, Marketing Coordinator
A learning manual for speech-language pathologists and audiologists on how to deal with the emotional issues facing them in their work with clients with communication disorders and their families. *$ 29.00*
187 pages

1982 Creating Positive Classroom Environments: Strategies for Behavior Management
Brooks / Cole Publishing Company
511 Forest Lodge Road
Pacific Grove, CA 93950
831-373-0728
800-354-9706
FAX: 831-375-6414
e-mail: bc-info@brookscole.com
www.brookescole.com
A hands-on text that offers an approach to classroom management that encourages situation-specific decision making. Presenting research-based information on how to establish an effective behavior management system in both regular and special education settings, the book centers on ways to help students manage their own behavior, rather than on ways their behavior can be managed by teachers, peers, parents or other adults.
448 pages Paperbound
ISBN 0-53422 -54-4

1983 Critical Voices on Special Education
State University of New York Press
194 Washington Avenue
Suite 305
Albany, NY 12210
518-472-5000
800-666-2211
FAX: 518-472-5038
e-mail: info@sunypress.edu
www.sunypress.edu

James Peltz, Interim Director
Janice Vunk, Assistant to the Director
Problems and progress concerning the mildly handicapped. *$21.95*
265 pages Paperback
ISBN 0-79140 -20-3

1984 Cultural Diversity, Families and the Special Education System
Teachers College Press
1234 Amsterdam Avenue
New York, NY 10027
212-678-3929
800-575-6566
FAX: 212-678-4149
e-mail: tcpress@tc.columbia.edu
www.teacherscollegepress.com

Mary Lynch, Manager
This timely and thought-provoking book explores the quadruple disadvantage faced by the parents of poor, minority, handicapped children whose first language is not that of the school they attend. *$22.95*

296 pages Paperback
ISBN 0-807731-19-6

1985 Curriculum Decision Making for Students with Severe Handicaps

Teachers College Press
Columbia University
New York, NY 10027
212-678-3929
800-575-6566
FAX: 212-678-4149
e-mail: tspress@ts.columbia.edu.
www.teacherscollegepress.com

Brian Ellerbeck, Executive Acquisitions Editor
Susan Liddicoat, Acquisitions Editor
Mary Lynch, Manager

The inclusion of severely handicapped students within the scope of public education has brought about many changes for teachers in special education, this book helps the professional to distinguish which avenues are the best to take. *$17.95*

192 pages Paperback
ISBN 0-807728-61-6

1986 Deciphering the System: A Guide for Families of Young Disabled Children

Brookline Books
34 University Road
Brookline, MA 02445
617-734-6772
800-666-BOOK
FAX: 617-734-3952
e-mail: brooklinebooks@brooklinebooks.com
www.brooklinebooks.com

William H Walters, Author
Esther Isabe Wilder, Author

This book informs parents of disabled children (0-5) of their rights and the service system, e.g., ways to manage the cumulating information, tips on IEP and IFSP meetings and the educational assessment process, and how parents can work with multiple service providers. It includes contributions from both parents and professionals who have experience with the service system. *$21.95*

ISBN 0-914797-87-5

1987 Defining Rehabilitation Agency Types

Mississippi State University
PO Box 6189
Mississippi State, MS 39762
662-325-2001
800-675-7782
FAX: 662-325-8989
www.blind.msstate.edu

Kelly Schaefer, Dissemination Specialist
Elton Moore, Executive Director

Relationships of participant selection and cost factors of service delivery across rehabilitation agency types. A national survey of state agencies for the blind was conducted to examine factors that define the characteristics of different agencies; similar programs were grouped together. Classification criteria were developed to distinguish agencies into logical groups based on line of authority, funding and operating procedures. *$10.00*

15 pages Paperback

1988 Designing and Using Assistive Technology: The Human Perspective

Brookes Publishing
PO Box 10624
Baltimore, MD 21285
410-337-9580
800-638-3775
FAX: 410-337-8539
e-mail: custserv@brookespublishing.com
www.brookespublishing.com

Clary Creighton, Exhibits Coordinator
Tracy Gray, Educational Sales Manager
Paul Brooks, Owner

Presented here is a holistic perspective on how and why people choose and use AT. Features personal insights and the latest research on design and development. *$31.00*

352 pages Paperback 1998
ISBN 1-55766 -14-9

1989 Developing Cross-Cultural Competence:Guide to Working with Young Children & Their Families

Brookes Publishing
PO Box 10624
Baltimore, MD 21285
410-337-9580
800-638-3775
FAX: 410-337-8539
e-mail: custserv@brookespublishing.com
www.brookespublishing.com

Clary Creighton, Exhibits Coordinator
Tracy Gray, Educational Sales Manager
Paul Brooks, Owner

This enlightening book perceptively and sensitively explores cultural, ethnic, and language diversity in human services. For those who work with families whose infants and young children may have or be at risk for a disability or chronic illness. (Second Edition) *$ 32.00*

448 pages Paperback
ISBN 1-55766 -31-9

1990 Developing Individualized Family Support Plans: A Training Manual

Brookline Books
34 University Road
Brookline, MA 02445
617-734-6772
800-666-2665
FAX: 617-734-3952
e-mail: milt@brooklinebooks.com
www.brooklinebooks.com

William H Walters, Author
Esther Isabe Wilder, Author

This manual provides in-service training coordinators, administrators, supervisors and university personnel with a compact package of functional and practical methods to train professionals about implementing family-centered individualized family support plans (IFSP'S). Also, case studies provide concrete examples to aid in learning to write IFSP's. *$24.95*

ISBN 0-914797-69-7

1991 Developing Staff Competencies for Supporting People with Disabilities

Brookes Publishing
PO Box 10624
Baltimore, MD 21285
410-337-9580
800-638-3775
FAX: 410-337-8539
e-mail: custserv@brookespublishing.com
www.brookespublishing.com

Clary Creighton, Exhibits Coordinator
Tracy Gray, Educational Sales Manager
Paul Brooks, Owner

This timely second edition, now in a new easier to read format, gives service providers helpful strategies for increasing effectiveness and maintaining well-being while working in the rewarding yet challenging field of human services. *$34.00*

480 pages Paperback
ISBN 1-55766 -07-3

1992 Development of Language

McGraw-Hill, School Publishing
220 East Danieldale Road
Desoto, TX 75115
972-224-1111
800-442-9685
FAX: 972-228-1982
e-mail: mcgrawhill.com
www.mhschool.com

Cheri Scott, Director
Joseph Gavigan, President

An organizational book based on the developmental stages of language.

464 pages

1993 Developmental Disabilities of Learning
Gallery Bookshop
PO Box 270
Mendocino, CA 95460
707-937-2665
FAX: 707-937-3737
e-mail: info@gallerybooks.com
www.gallerybooks.com

Linda Pack, Manager
Tony Miksak, Owner
Manual for professionals on developmental and learning disabilities in the growing child. *$25.00*
224 pages Illustrated

1994 Developmental Disabilities: A Handbook for Occupational Therapists
Haworth Press
10 Alice Street
Binghamton, NY 13904
607-722-5857
800-429-6784
FAX: 607-722-6362
e-mail: orders@haworthpress.com
www.haworthpress.com

Sandy Sickels, Vice President
Becky Millerbaum, Advertising Manager
William Cohen, Owner
Provides broad coverage of the spectrum of problems confronted by patients with developmental disabilities and the many kinds of occupational therapy services these individuals need. Experts identify exemplary institutional and community service programs for treating patients with autism, cerebral palsy, epilepsy, and mental retardation. *$74.95*
268 pages Hardcover
ISBN 0-866569-59-6

1995 Developmental Disabilities: A Handbook for Interdisciplinary Practice
Brookline Books
34 University Road
Brookline, MA 02445
617-734-6772
800-666-BOOK
FAX: 617-734-3952
e-mail: brooklinebooks@brooklinebooks.com
www.brooklinebooks.com

William H Walters, Author
Esther Isabe Wilder, Author
Successful interdisciplinary team practice for persons with developmental disabilities that require each team member to understand and respect the contributions of the others. This handbook explains the professions most often represented on interdisciplinary teams: their natures, concerns and roles in the interdisciplinary context. *$29.95*
256 pages
ISBN 1-571290-03-6

1996 Developmental Variation and Learning Disorders
Educators Publishing Service
PO Box 9031
Cambridge, MA 02139
800-435-7728
FAX: 888-440-2665
e-mail: feedback@epsbooks.com
www.epsbooks.com

Charles H Heinle, Vice President
Alexandra S Bigelow, Author
Gunnar Voltz, President
Discusses seven major areas of development and four major areas of academic proficiency and then ties this information together by examining factors that predispose a child to dysfunction and disability, offering guidelines to assessment and management, and analyzing long-range outcomes and factors that promote resiliency for parents, educators and clinicians. *$69.00*
640 pages Cloth
ISBN 0-838819-92-3

1997 Digest of Neurology and Psychiatry
Institute of Living: Hartford Hospital
200 Retreat Avenue
Hartford, CT 06106
860-545-7841
800-673-2411
FAX: 860-545-2351
e-mail: fishe@harthosp.org
www.instituteofliving.org

Harold I Schwartz MD, Vice President
John Meehan, President
Abstracts and reviews of selected current literature in psychiatry, neurology and related fields.

1998 Disability Funding News
C D Publications
8204 Fenton Street
Silver Spring, MD 20910
301-588-6380
800-666-6380
FAX: 301-588-6385
e-mail: subscription@cdpublications.com
www.cdpublications.com

Jim Rogers, Editor
Michael Gerecht, President
Grantseeking tips and strategies for nonprofit, government administrators, plus proved fundraising ideas. Includes grant application critiques, ho-to advice, and private and public funding updates. *$ 199.00*
8 pages Weekly

1999 Disability and Rehabilitation
Taylor & Francis
7625 Empire Drive
Florence, KY 41042
859-371-9571
800-634-7064
FAX: 800-248-4724
www.taylorandfrancis.com

Mike Hunninghake, Journals Representative
Jeff Taylor, Owner
An international, multidisciplinary journal seeking to encourage a better understanding of all aspects of disability, and to promote the rehabilitation process. *$395.00*
Monthly
ISSN 0963-82 8

2000 Divided Legacy: A History of the Schism in Medical Thought, The Bacteriological Era
North Atlantic Books
1435 4th Street
Berkeley, CA 94710
510-559-8277
800-337-2665
FAX: 510-559-8279
e-mail: orders@northatlanticbooks.com
www.northatlanticbooks.com

Richard Grossinger, Publisher
Lindy Hough, Publisher
Concluding volume of Coulter's history of medical philosophy, from ancient times to today. Covers the orgins of bacteriology and immunology in world medicine; describes the clash between orthodox and alternative medicine.
1993

2001 Dual Relationships in Counseling
American Counseling Association
5999 Stevenson Avenue
Alexandria, VA 22304
703-823-9800
800-347-6647
FAX: 703-823-0252
e-mail: webmaster@counseling.org
www.counseling.org

Sam Gladding, President
Debra Bass, Marketing Coordinator
Richard Yep, Executive Director
Covers topics such as whether to accept a client, whether to reveal information, whether to refer a case, whether to consider factors you might not otherwise consider, and how to deal with gifts, invitations and social situations. *$23.95*

244 pages paperback 1992
ISBN 1-556200-90-0

2002 Early Communication Skills For Children wi th Down Syndrome

Woodbine House
6510 Bells Mill Road
Bethesda, MD 20817
301-897-3570
800-843-7323
FAX: 301-897-5838
e-mail: info@woodbinehouse.com
www.woodbinehouse.com

Irv Shapell, Owner

An expert shares her knowledge of speech and language development in young children and adolescents with Down syndrome. Intelligibility, hearing loss, apraxia and other factors that affect communications are discussed. It also covers speech-language assessments and alternative communication options and literacy. *$19.95*

368 pages 2003
ISBN 1-890627-27-5

2003 Early Intervention, Implementing Child & Family Services for At-Risk Infants

Pro-Ed Publications
8700 Shoal Creek Boulevard
Austin, TX 78757
512-451-3246
800-897-3202
FAX: 800-397-7633
e-mail: feedback@proedinc.com
www.proedinc.com

Donald Hammill, Owner
Courtney King, Marketing Coordinator

New directions and recent legislation have produced a need for this guide which is designed for professionals facing the challenge of program development for disabled and at-risk infants, toddlers and their families. *$36.00*

394 pages
ISBN 0-890796-21-1

2004 Ecology of Troubled Children

Brookline Books Publications
34 University Road
Brookline, MA 02445
800-666-2665
800-666-2665
FAX: 617-734-3952
e-mail: milt@brooklinebooks.com
www.brooklinebooks.com

William H Walters, Author
Esther Isabe Wilder, Author

Designed for frontline mental health clinicians working with children with serious emotional disturbances; shows how to make childrens' worlds more supportive by changing the places, activities and people in their lives. *$15.95*

256 pages
ISBN 1-571290-57-5

2005 Educating Children with Disabilities: A Transdisciplinary Approach, 3rd Edition

Brookes Publishing
PO Box 10624
Baltimore, MD 21285
410-337-9580
800-638-3775
800-638-3775
FAX: 410-337-8539
e-mail: custserv@brookespublishing.com
www.brookespublishing.com

Clary Creighton, Exhibits Coordinator
Tracy Gray, Educational Sales Manager
Paul Brooks, Owner

Widely respected textbook presents you with the strategies you need for developing an inclusive curriculum, integrating health care and educational programs and addressing needs and concerns. *$38.00*

512 pages 1996
ISBN 1-557662-46-0

2006 Educating Children with Multiple Disabilities: A Transdisciplinary Approach

Brookes Publishing
PO Box 10624
Baltimore, MD 21285
410-337-9580
800-638-3775
FAX: 410-337-8539
e-mail: custserv@brookespublishing.com
www.brookespublishing.com

Clary Creighton, Exhibits Coordinator
Tracy Gray, Educational Sales Manager
Paul Brooks, Owner

Emphasizing transdisciplinary cooperation between teachers, therapists, nurses and parents, this book describes a general model and specific techniques for effectively educating children with multiple disabilities. *$29.00*

496 pages Paperback
ISBN 1-557662-46-0

2007 Educating Students Who Have Visual Impairments with Other Disabilities

Brookes Publishing
PO Box 10624
Baltimore, MD 21285
410-337-9580
800-638-3775
FAX: 410-337-8539
e-mail: custserv@brookespublishing.com
www.brookespublishing.com

Clary Creighton, Exhibits Coordinator
Tracy Gray, Educational Sales Manager
Paul Brooks, Owner

This introductory text provides techniques for facilitating functional learning in students with a wide range of visual impairments and multiple disabilities. With a concentration on educational needs and learning styles, the authors of this multidisciplinary volume demonstrate functional assessment and teaching adaptations that will improve students' inclusive learning experiences. *$49.95*

552 pages Paperback
ISBN 1-557662-80-0

2008 Educating all Students in the Mainstream

Brookes Publishing Company
PO Box 10624
Baltimore, MD 21285
410-337-9580
800-638-3775
FAX: 410-337-8539
e-mail: custserv@brookespublishing.com
www.brookespublishng.com

Clary Creighton, Exhibits Coordinator
Tracy Gray, Educational Sales Manager
Paul Brooks, Owner

Incorporating the research and viewpoints of both regular and special educators, this textbook provides an effective approach for modifying, expanding, and adjusting regular education to meet the needs of all students. *$34.00*

304 pages 1989
ISBN 1-557660-22-0

2009 Educational Audiology for the Limited Hearing Infant and Preschooler, 3rd Edition

Charles C Thomas
2600 South 1st Street
Springfield, IL 62704
217-789-8980
800-258-8980
FAX: 217-789-9130
e-mail: books@ccthomas.com
www.ccthomas.com

Micheal Thomas, President
Donald Goldberg, Author
Nancy Coleffe-Schenck, Author

Offers information on current concepts and practices in audio-logic screening and evaluation, development of the listening function, development of speech, development of language, the role of parents, parent education, mainstreaming of the limited-hearing child, and program modifications for the severely learning disabled child. Also includes information on auditory assessment, sensory aides, cochlear implants, acoupedics and auditory verbal programs. *$69.95*

430 pages paperback 1997
ISBN 0-39806 -28-1

2010 Educational Care
Educators Publishing Service
625 Mount Auburn Street
Suite 3
Cambridge, MA 02138
617-547-6706
800-225-5750
FAX: 888-440-2665
e-mail: feedback@epsbooks.com
www.epsbooks.com

Charles H Heinle, Vice President
Alexandra S Bigelow
Gunnar Voltz, President
This book, written for both parents and teachers, is based on the view that education should be a system of care that is able to look after the specific needs of individual students. Using case studies, it analyzes various types of learning disorders and then suggests ways to help students with these problems. *$31.50*
325 pages
ISBN 0-838819-87-7

2011 Educational Intervention for the Student with Multiple Disabilities
Charles C Thomas
2600 South 1st Street
Springfield, IL 62704
217-789-8980
800-258-8980
FAX: 217-789-9130
e-mail: books@ccthomas.com
www.ccthomas.com

Donna Irons-Reavis, Author
Michael Thomas, Presidentm
This text will assist those who want to teach severely, multiply disabled students by providing information on general principles of education and classroom organization and managing the behavior of students. Also available in cloth $34.95 (ISBN# 0-398-05793-1) *$24.95*
140 pages Softcover
ISBN 0-398061-73-4

2012 Educational Prescriptions
Educators Publishing Service
625 Mount Auburn Street
Suite 3
Cambridge, MA 02138
617-547-6706
800-225-5750
FAX: 888-440-2665
e-mail: feedback@epsbooks.com
www.epsbooks.com

Charles H Heinle, Vice President
Alexandra S Bigelow, Author
Gunnar Voltz, President
This book provides specific recommendations for the classroom management of students who are experiencing subtle developmental and/or learning difficulties. Intended for regular classroom teachers, specific examples of accommodations teachers can make are provided for grades 1-3 and 4-6. *$13.50*
64 pages
ISBN 0-838819-90-7

2013 Effective Instruction for Special Education, 2nd Edition
Pro-Ed Publications
8700 Shoal Creek Boulevard
Austin, TX 78757
512-451-3246
800-897-3202
FAX: 800-397-7633
e-mail: info@proedinc.com
www.proedinc.com

Joshua Jeffrey, Marketing Custodian
Courtney King, Marketing Coordinator
Donald Hammill, Owner
This exciting and wide-ranging book provides special educators with effective methods for teaching students with mild and moderate learning and behavioral problems, as well as for teaching remedial students in general. *$37.00*
419 pages Paperback

2014 Effective Teaching Methods for Autistic Children
Charles C Thomas
2600 South 1st Street
Springfield, IL 62704
217-789-8980
800-258-8980
FAX: 217-789-9130
e-mail: books@ccthomas.com
www.ccthomas.com

Michael Thomas, President
$20.95
124 pages Paper
ISBN 0-398063-09-5

2015 Effectively Educating Handicapped Students
Longman Publishing Group
10 Bank Street
9th Floor
White Plains, NY 10606
914-287-8000
FAX: 914-421-5598
www.pearsoned.com

Kathryn Costello, President
For educators and other professionals who work with deaf and hearing impaired students in preschool and elementary programs. A developmental approach provides the foundation for several intervention methods including preparation for instruction, language, speech, audition and speechreading.
468 pages Paperback 1991
ISBN 0-801303-17-6

2016 Emotional Problems of Childhood and Adolescence
McGraw-Hill School Publishing
220 East Danieldale Road
Desoto, TX 75115
972-224-1111
800-442-9685
FAX: 972-228-1982
mhschool.com

Joseph Gavigan, President
For future special educators, psychologists and others who work with emotionally disturbed children and adolescents.

2017 Enabling & Empowering Families: Principles & Guidelines for Practice
Brookline Books
34 University Road
Brookline, MA 02445
617-734-6772
800-666-2665
FAX: 617-734-3952
e-mail: brooklinebooks@brooklinebooks.com
www.brooklinebooks.com

William H Walters, Author
Esther I Wilder, Author
Angela Deal MSW, Author
This book was written for practioners who must work with families but who have insufficient training in family systems assessment and intervention. The authors' system enables professionals to help the family identify its needs, locate the formal and informal resources to meet these needs and develop the abilities to effectively access these resources. *$24.95*
220 pages
ISBN 0-914797-59-X

2018 Enhancing Self-Concepts and Achievement of Mildly Handicapped Students
Charles C Thomas
2600 South 1st Street
Springfield, IL 62704
217-789-8980
800-258-8980
FAX: 217-789-9130
e-mail: books@ccthomas.com
www.ccthomas.com

Micheal Thomas, President
Carroll J Jones, Author

This book is aimed towards students who are learning disabled, mildly mentally retarded, and who have behavior disorders. Individuals should be aware that unless they appreciate and understand themselves, it is difficult to relate to the world around them. This is no less true of exceptional than nonhandicapped learners. This book provides a wonderfully complete window of insight into the most tenuous of human aspects, the self-concept. Also available in cloth at $55.95 (ISBN# 0-398-05760-5) *$39.95*

294 pages Paperback
ISBN 0-398061-91-2

2019 Evaluation and Educational Programming of Deaf-Blind/Severly Multihandicapped Students
Charles C Thomas
2600 South 1st Street
Springfield, IL 62704
217-789-8980
800-258-8980
FAX: 217-789-9130
e-mail: books@ccthomas.com
www.ccthomas.com

Michael Thomas, President
Offers information on the special education of deaf-blind students. *$41.95*
314 pages Softcover
ISBN 0-398055-15-7

2020 Evaluation and Treatment of the Psychogeriatric Patient
Haworth Press
10 Alice Street
Binghamton, NY 13904
607-722-5857
800-429-6784
FAX: 607-722-6362
e-mail: orders@haworthpress.com
www.haworthpress.com

Sandy Sickels, Vice President
Becky Minerbaum, Advertising Manager
William Cohen, Owner
This pertinent book assists occupational therapists and other health care providers in developing up-to-date psychogeriatric programs and understands details of treating the cognitively impaired elderly. *$74.95*
111 pages Hardcover
ISBN 1-560240-52-0

2021 Exceptional Children in Focus
McGraw-Hill School Publishing
220 East Danieldale Road
Desoto, TX 75115
972-224-1111
800-442-9685
FAX: 972-228-1982
www.mhschool.com

Joseph Gavigan, President
Todd Painter, Assistant Director
Combines a light, personal look at the problems of special educators experiences with the basic facts of exceptionality.
288 pages

2022 Exceptional Lives: Special Education in T oday's Schools, 4th Edition
Pearson Education
1 Lake Street
Upper Saddle River, NJ 07458
201-236-7000
FAX: 201-236-3400
www.pearsoned.com

John Fallon, Chief Executive Officer
Rod Bristow, President of Higher Education
George Werner, Chief Financial Officer
Comprehensive coverage is built upon six guiding principles: 1) high expectations for individuals with disabilities and their educators, 2) inclusion for all students, 3) relationships and friendships as essential outcomes of collaboration, 4) positive contributions by students with disabilities, 5) the importance of choice and self-advocacy for students with disabilities, and 6) full citizenship for all students with disabilities. Emphasizes the daily lives of students and educators. *$90.00*

592 pages 2003
ISBN 0-131126-00-8

2023 Facilitating Self-Care Practices in the Elderly
Haworth Press
10 Alice Street
Binghamton, NY 13904
607-722-5857
800-429-6784
FAX: 607-722-6362
e-mail: orders@haworthpress.com
www.haworthpress.com

Sandy Sickels, Vice President
Becky Minerbaum, Advertising Manager
William Cohen, Owner
This up-to-date book is a synthesis of current knowledge from published sources and expert consultants relating to three commonly occurring problems in home health care practice: self-administration of medications, family caregiving issues, and teaching the elderly. *$ 74.95*
185 pages Hardcover
ISBN 1-560240-13-X

2024 Family-Centered Early Intervention with Infants and Toddlers
Brookes Publishing
PO Box 10624
Baltimore, MD 21285
410-337-9580
800-638-3775
FAX: 410-337-8539
e-mail: cutserv@brookespublishing.com
www.brookespublishing.com

Clary Creighton, Exhibits Coordinator
Tracy Gray, Educatrional Sales Manager
Paul Brooks, Owner
This informative text provides professionals with insight and practical guidelines to help fulfill the federal requirements for provision of early intervention services. *$37.00*
368 pages Hardcover 1993
ISBN 1-557661-24-3

2025 Feeding Children with Special Needs
Arizona Department of Health Services
1740 West Adams Street
Phoenix, AZ 85007
602-542-1886
FAX: 602-542-1890
www.hs.state.az.us/cfhs/ons/

Margaret Tate, Manager
Guide designed to help develop a greater awareness of the special challenges involved in the nutrition and feeding concerns for children with special health care needs, and ways to approach the issues. *$5.00*

2026 Focal Group Psychotherapy
New Harbinger Publications
5674 Shattuck Avenue
Oakland, CA 94609
510-652-0215
800-748-6273
FAX: 510-652-5472
e-mail: customerservice@newharbinger.com
www.newharbinger.com

Lorna Garano, Director
Matthew McKay, Owner
Guide to leading brief, theme-based groups. This book offers an extensive week-by-week description of the basic concepts and interventions for 14 theme or focal groups for: codependency, rape victims, shyness, survivors of incest, agoraphobia, survivors of toxic parents, depression, child molesters, anger control, domestic violence offenders, assertiveness, alcohol and drug abuse, eating disorders, and parent training. *$59.95*
544 pages Cloth
ISBN 1-879237-18-0

2027 Free Hand: Enfranchising the Education of Deaf Children
TJ Publishers
2544 Tarpley Road
Suite 108
Carrollton, TX 75006
972-416-0800
800-999-1168
FAX: 301-585-5930
e-mail: TJPubinc@aol.com

Angela K Thames, President
Jerald A Murphy, VP
A select group of nationally prominent educators, linguists and researchers met at Hofstra University to consider the most vital and controversial question in education of the deaf: what role should ASL play in the classroom? Become part of that discussion with A Free Hand. *$16.95*
204 pages Softcover 1990
ISBN 0-93266 -40-X

2028 Functional Assessment Inventory Manual
Stout Vocational Rehab Institute
University of Wisconsin-Stout
Menomonie, WI 54751 715-232-1411
FAX: 715-232-2356
e-mail: botterbuschd@uwstout.edu

Ronald R Fry, Manager
Darlene Botterbusch, Program Assistant
The Functional Assessment is a systematic enumeration of a client's vocactionally relevant strengths and limitations. *$12.00*
96 pages Paperback
ISBN 0-916671-53-4

2029 Global Perspectives on Disability: A Curriculum
Mobility International U SA
132 East Broadway
Suite 343
Eugene, OR 97401 541-343-1284
FAX: 541-343-6812
e-mail: info@miusa.org
www.miusa.org

Susan Sygall, Executive Director
Melissa Mitchell, Public Relations Coordinator
Tracy Scharn, Project Assistant
Designed for secondary and higher education instructors. Includes five lesson plans covering disability awareness, disability rights and international perspectives on disability. Available in alternative formats. *$40.00*

2030 Glossary of Terminology for Vocational Assessment/Evaluation/Work
Rehabilitation Resource University
University of Wisconsin-Stout
Menomonie, WI 54751 715-232-1478
FAX: 715-232-2356

Ronald R Fry, Manager
Darlene Botterbusch, Program Assistant
This glossary contains 254 terms and their definitions. Primary focus is on the terminology related to the practice and professionals of vocational assessment, vocational evaluation and work adjustment. *$9.50*
40 pages Softcover

2031 Graduate Technological Education and the Human Experience of Disability
Haworth Press
10 Alice Street
Binghamton, NY 13904 607-722-5857
800-429-6784
FAX: 607-722-6362
e-mail: orders@haworthpress.com
www.haworthpress.com

Sandy Sickels, Vice President
Becky Minerbaum, Advertising Manger
William Cohen, Owner
This book examines graduate schools of theology and their limited familiarity with the study of disability — and the presence of people with disabilities in particular — on their campuses. This text offers critical research and illuminates new pathways for theologia and practice in the community of faith. It offers suggestions for incorporating disability studies into theological education and religious life. *$34.95*
115 pages Hardcover
ISBN 0-789060-08-6

2032 HIV Infection and Developmental Disabilities
Brookes Publishing
PO Box 10624
Baltimore, MD 21285 410-337-9580
800-638-3775
FAX: 410-337-8539
e-mail: cstserv@brookespublishing.com
www.brookespublishing.com

Tracy Gray, Educational Sales Manager
Clary Creighton, Exhibits Coordinator
Paul Brooks, Owner
A resource for service providers pinpointing the most crucial medical, legal and educational issues to control HIV infection. *$47.00*
320 pages
ISBN 1-557660-83-2

2033 Handbook for Implementing Workshops for Siblings of Special Children
Special Needs Project
324 State Street
Suite H
Santa Barbara, CA 93101 805-962-8087
800-333-6867
FAX: 805-962-5087
www.specialneeds.com

Hod Gray, Founder
Based on three years of professional experience, this handbook provides guidelines and techniques for those who wish to start and conduct workshops for siblings. *$40.00*

2034 Handbook for Speech Therapy
Psychological & Educational Publications
PO Box 520
Hydesville, CA 95547 707-768-1807
800-523-5775
FAX: 800-447-0907
e-mail: psych-edpublications@cck.net
www.psych-edpublications.com

Morrison Gardner, President
Basic handbook for beginning speech teachers, shows how speech sounds are made, what their individual characteristics are, how they relate to each other, what the most common errors are, and how to correct those errors.
143 pages paperback

2035 Handbook for the Special Education Administrator
Edwin Mellen Press
415 Ridge Street
Lewiston, NY 14092 716-754-4421
800-753-2788
FAX: 716-754-4056
e-mail: mellen@wzrd.com
www.mellenpress.com
Organization and procedures for special education. *$ 49.95*
96 pages Hardcover
ISBN 0-88946 -22-9

2036 Handbook of Developmental Education
Greenwood Publishing Group
88 Post Road West
Suite 5007
Westport, CT 06880 203-226-3571
FAX: 203-222-1502
www.greenwood.com

Duane L Dobbert, Author
Wayne Smith, President
This comprehensive handbook has brought together the leading practitioners and researchers in the field of developmental education to focus on the developmental learning agenda. Hardcover.

400 pages $65 - $75
ISBN 0-275932-97-4

2037 Handbook on Supported Education for People with Mental Illness
Brookes Publishing
PO Box 10624
Baltimore, MD 21285
410-337-9580
800-638-3775
FAX: 410-337-8539
e-mail: custserv@brookespublishing.com
www.brookespublishing.com

Clary Creighton, Exhibits Coordinator
Tracy Gray, Educational Sales Manager
Paul Brooks, Owner
Here you will find all necessary information that mental health professionals need in order to provide supported education services. There are specific suggestions on how to help people with mental illness return to or remain in college, trade school, or GED programs. Also addressed are funding and legal issues, accommodations, and specific interventions.
208 pages Paperback 1998
ISBN 1-55766 -52-1

2038 Head Injury Rehabilitation: Children
Taylor & Francis
47 Runway Drive
Suite G
Levittown, PA 19057
FAX: 215-785-5515
Rehabilitation guide for the help of children or adolescents that have suffered brain injury.
460 pages Cloth
ISBN 0-85066 -67-1

2039 Health Care Management in Physical Therapy
Charles C Thomas
2600 South 1st Street
Springfield, IL 62704
217-789-8980
800-258-8980
FAX: 217-789-9130
e-mail: books@ccthomas.com
www.ccthomas.com

Laura I Moriarty, Author
Joseph Antho Travers, Author
Michael Thomas, President
The focus of this book is on physical therapists as supervisors in health care settings of hospitals, nursing homes, home health agencies and in private practice. *$62.95*
328 pages Hardcover
ISBN 0-398056-42-0

2040 Health Care for Students with Disabilities
Brookes Publishing Company
PO Box 10624
Baltimore, MD 21285
410-337-9580
800-638-3775
FAX: 410-337-8539
e-mail: custserv@brookespublishing.com
www.brookespublishing.com

Clary Creighton, Exhibits Coordinator
Tracy Gray, Educational Sales Manager
Paul Brooks, Owner
This practical guidebook provides detailed descriptions of the 16 health-related procedures most likely to be needed in the classroom by students with disabilities. *$25.00*
304 pages Paperback 1990
ISBN 1-557660-37-9

2041 Helping Learning Disabled Gifted Children Learn Through Compensatory Play
Charles C Thomas
2600 South 1st Street
Springfield, IL 62704
217-789-8980
800-258-8980
FAX: 217-789-9130
e-mail: books@ccthomas.com
www.ccthomas.com

Micheal Thomas, President
James H Humphrey, Author
About 3% of the school population is gifted and 5 to 8% of this number suffer from learning disabilities. These children experience a great deal more trauma than the normal child. *$24.95*
164 pages Softcover
ISBN 0-398061-62-9

2042 Helping Students Grow
American College Testing Program
500 ACT Drive
PO Box 168
Iowa City, IA 52243
319-337-1000

www.act.org

Richard Ferguson, Chief Executive Officer
Designed to assist counselors in using the wealth of information generated by the ACT Assessment.

2043 How to Teach Autistic & Severely Handicapped Children
Autism Society of North Carolina Bookstore
505 Oberlin Road
Suite 230
Raleigh, NC 27605
919-743-0204
800-442-2762
FAX: 919-743-0208
e-mail: info@autismsociety-nc.org
www.autismsociety-nc.org

Ann Palmer, President
Darla Coffey, Bookstore Manager
Jill Keel, Executive Director
Book provides procedures for effectively assessing and teaching autistic and other severely handicapped children. *$8.00*

2044 How to Teach Spelling/How to Spell
Educators Publishing Service
625 Mount Auburn Street
Suite 3
Cambridge, MA 02138
617-547-6706
800-225-5750
FAX: 888-440-2665
e-mail: feedback@epsbooks.com
www.epsbooks.com

Charles H Heinle, Vice President
Alexandra Bigelow, Author
Gunnar Voltz, President
This is a comprehensive resource manual based on the Orton-Gillingham approach to reading and spelling. It recommends what and how much to teach at each grade level at the beginning of each lesson or section. There are four student manuals that accompany this. *$22.50*
Teachers Manual
ISBN 0-838818-47-1

2045 Human Exceptionality: Society, School, and Family
Allyn & Bacon
75 Arlington Street
Suite 300
Boston, MA 02116
617-848-6000
800-852-8024
FAX: 617-848-7490
www.ablongman.com
Examination of the definitions, classification, prevalence and characteristics of each category of exceptionality in relation to the major topics and issues of the field of special education.
615 pages
ISBN 0-20528 -39-0

2046 I Heard That!
3417 Volta Place NW
Washington, DC 20007
202-337-5220
866-337-5220
FAX: 202-337-8314
e-mail: info@agbell.org
www.agbell.org

Todd Houston, Executive Director
Provides a framework for teachers, clinicians and parents when writing objectives and designing activities to develop listening skills in children with hearing loss from newborn to 3 years. *$7.95*

36 pages

2047 I Heard That!2
Alexander Graham Bell Association
3417 Volta Place NW
Washington, DC 20007
202-337-5220
FAX: 202-337-8314
e-mail: info@agbell.org
www.agbell.org

Jessica Ripper, Senior Director
Todd Houston, Executive Director
Provides a framework for teachers, clinicians and parents when writing objectives and designing activities to develop listening skills in children who are deaf or hard of hearing. *$7.95*
36 pages

2048 Images of the Disabled, Disabling Images
Greenwood Publishing Group
88 Post Road West
Suite 5007
Westport, CT 06880
203-226-3571
FAX: 203-222-1502
e-mail: hr@greenwood.com
www.greenwood.com

Robert K Mueller, Author
Richard B Higgins, Author
Wayne Smith, President
Combines an examination of the presentation of persons with disabilities in literature, film and the media with an analysis of the ways in which these images are expressed in public policy concerning the disabled. *$55.00*
227 pages Hardcover
ISBN 0-275921-78-6

2049 Implementing Family-Centered Services in Early Intervention
Brookline Books
PO Box 1047
Cambridge, MA 02139
617-868-0360
800-666-2665
FAX: 617-868-1772
e-mail: thestore@brooklinebooksmith.com
www.brooklinebooks.com
This book describes a team-based decision-making workshop for implementing family-centered services in early interventions. Unlike a training curriculum, it focuses on the decisions that teams must make as they seek to become family-centered. *$19.95*
180 pages Paperback
ISBN 0-91479 -62-

2050 Including All of Us: An Early Childhood Curriculum About Disability
Educational Equity Concepts
100 5th Avenue
8th Floor
New York, NY 10011
212-243-1110
FAX: 212-627-0407
TTY:212-725-1803
e-mail: information@equity.org
www.edequity.org

Barbara Sprung, Author
The first nonsexist, multicultural, mainstreamed curriculum. Step-by-step activities incorporate disability into three curriculum areas: Same/Different (hearing impairment), Body Parts (visual impairment), and Transportation (mobility impairment). *$14.95*
144 pages
ISBN 0-93162 -00-4

2051 Including Students with Severe and Multiple Disabilites in Typical Classrooms
Brookes Publishing
PO Box 10624
Baltimore, MD 21285
410-337-9580
800-638-3775
FAX: 410-337-8539
e-mail: custserv@brookespublishing.com
www.brookespublishing.com

Clary Creighton, Exhibits Coordinator
Tracy Gray, Educational Sales Manager
Paul Brooks, Owner
This straightforward and jargon free resource gives instructors the guidance needed to educate learners who have one or more sensory impairments in addition to cognitive and physical disabilities. *$32.95*
224 pages Paperback
ISBN 1-55766 -39-8

2052 Including Students with Special Needs: A Practical Guide for Classroom Teachers
Allyn & Bacon
75 Arlington Street
Suite 300
Boston, MA 02116
617-848-6000
800-852-8024
FAX: 617-848-7490
e-mail: ab_webmaster@abacon.com
www.ablongman.com
Focuses on educating students with special needs in inclusive settings based on substantive admisistrative backing, support for general education teachers, and an understanding that sometimes not all needs can be met in a single location.
544 pages
ISBN 0-20528 -85-4

2053 Inclusive & Heterogeneous Schooling: Assessment, Curriculum, and Instruction
Brookes Publishing
PO Box 10624
Baltimore, MD 21285
410-337-9580
800-638-3775
FAX: 410-337-8539
e-mail: custserv@brookespublishing.com
www.brookespublishing.com

Clary Creighton, Exhibits Coordinator
Tracy Gray, Educational Sales Manager
Paul Brooks, Owner
Presents methods for successfully restructuring classrooms to enable all students, particularly those with disabilities, to flourish. Provides specific strategies for assessment, collaboration, classroom management, and age-specific instruction. *$34.95*
448 pages Paperback
ISBN 1-55766 -02-9

2054 Independent Living Approach to Disability Policy Studies
World Institute on Disability
510 16th Street
Suite 100
Oakland, CA 94612
510-763-4100
FAX: 510-763-4109
e-mail: wid@wid.org
www.wid.org

Stanley Yarnell, Chairman
Martin Schulter, Vice Chairman
This collection of essays and bibliographies attempts to build a framework for understanding how the relationship between public policy, disability studies and disability policy studies will impact us in the future. *$17.50*
240 pages Paperback

2055 Information & Referral Center
Mississippi State University
PO Box 6189
Mississippi State, MS 39762
662-325-2001
800-675-7782
FAX: 662-325-8989
www.blind.msstate.edu

Kelly Schaefer, Publications Manager
Elton Moore, Executive Director
A comprehensive website that includes information about client assistance programs, vocational rehabilitation agencies, low vision clinics and information about blindness and low vision. *$25.00*
150 pages

2056 Instructional Methods for Students
Allyn & Bacon
75 Arlington Street
Suite 300
Boston, MA 02116
617-848-6000
800-852-8024
FAX: 617-848-7490
www.ablongman.com

Instructional methods for students with learning and behavior problems.
450 pages 1986
ISBN 0-205087-35-3

2057 Interactions: Collaboration Skills for School Professionals
Longman Education/Addison Wesley
95 Church Street
White Plains, NY 10601
914-328-2090
800-322-1377
FAX: 800-333-3328
www.longman.awl.com

Thomas Longman, Founder
Shows school professionals how to develop and use the skills necessary for effective collaboration among teachers, school support staff, and parents of children with special needs. *$35.00*
270 pages Paperback
ISBN 0-80131 -21-2

2058 International Journal of Arts Medicine
MMB Music
3526 Washington Avenue
Saint Louis, MO 63103
314-531-9635
800-543-3771
FAX: 314-531-8384
e-mail: info@mmbmusic.com
www.mmbmusic.com

Marcia Lee Goldberg, President
Exploration of the creative arts and healing. Presents peer-reviewed articles clearly written by educators in the creative arts, as well as internationally prominent physicians, therapists and health care professionals.

2059 Interpreting Disability: A Qualitative Reader
Teachers College Press
Columbia University
New York, NY 10027
212-678-3929
800-575-6566
FAX: 212-678-4149
e-mail: Carol
www.tcpress.com

Mary Lynch, Manager
This book offers a collection of exemplary qualitative research affecting people with disabilities and their families. Instead of focusing upon methodological details, the chapters illustrate the variety of styles and formats that interpretive research can adopt in reporting its results. *$24.95*
328 pages Paperback
ISBN 0-807731-21-8

2060 Intervention Research in Learning Disabilities
Gallery Bookshop
PO Box 270
Mendocino, CA 95460
707-937-2665
FAX: 707-937-3737
e-mail: info@gallerybooks.com
www.gallerybooks.com

Linda Pack, Manager
Tony Miksak, Owner
Based on the Symposium on Intervention Research, this volume presents 12 papers addressing issues in intervention research, academic interventions, social and behavioral interventions, and postsecondary interventions. *$30.00*
347 pages

2061 Introduction to Learning Disabilities, 2nd Edition
Allyn & Bacon
75 Arlington Street
Suite 300
Boston, MA 02116
617-848-6000
800-852-8024
FAX: 617-848-7490
e-mail: ab_webmaster@abacon.com
vig.abacon.com
Presents the current state of research in the area of learning disabilities, as well as intervention ideas and programs. Includes updated material on the 1997 re-authorization of IDEA (Individuals with Disabilities Education Act) and expanded coverage of ADHD and its relationship to learning disabilities. Presents the latest information on the characteristics of persons with learning disabilities, causes, and educational interventions.
608 pages
ISBN 0-20529 -43-4

2062 Introduction to Mental Retardation
Allyn & Bacon
75 Arlington Street
Suite 300
Boston, MA 02116
617-848-6000
800-852-8024
FAX: 617-848-7490
e-mail: ab_webmaster@abacon.com
vig.abacon.com
A thorough overview of mental retardation with a level of knowledge suitable for an undergraduate or beginning graduate student.
350 pages Casebound 1986
ISBN 0-134879-27-9

2063 Introduction to Special Education: Teaching in an Age of Challenge, 4th Edition
Allyn & Bacon
75 Arlington Street
Suite 300
Boston, MA 02116
617-848-6000
800-852-8024
FAX: 617-848-7490
e-mail: ab_webmaster@abacon.com
vig.abacon.com
Provides an applied approach to children with disabilities through the use of specific research and suggestions to focus on how the educational practices impact the lives of children, their families, and their teachers.
640 pages cloth
ISBN 0-20526 -94-4

2064 Introduction to the Nature and Needs of Students with Mild Disabilities
Charles C Thomas
2600 South 1st Street
Springfield, IL 62704
217-789-8980
800-258-8980
FAX: 217-789-9130
e-mail: books@ccthomas.com
www.ccthomas.com

Laura I Moriarty, Author
Joseph Antho Travers, Author
Michael Thomas, President
Source of information for the special educator on the needs of students with mild disabilities. It has been designed as an introductory text for an undergraduate degree program in special education. The first chapter includes an overview of students who are at risk for academic failure. The remaining chapters are divided into three categorical units: students with mild mental retardation, behavior disorders, and learning disabilities.
300 pages Paperback
ISBN 0-398067-12-0

2065 Introduction to the Profession of Counseling
McGraw-Hill School Publishing
220 East Danieldale Road
Desoto, TX 75115
972-224-1111
800-442-9685
FAX: 972-228-1982
www.mhschool.com

Joseph Gavigan, President
Offers information, theories and techniques for counseling numerous cases from drug addiction to special populations.
464 pages

2066 Issues and Research in Special Education
Teachers College Press
PO Box 20
Williston, VT 05495
800-575-6566
FAX: 802-664-7626
www.teacherscollegepress.com

Marilen McConell, Director
Provides up-to-date research and discourse on a wide range of topics affecting professionals in the field of special education. *$38.00*

264 pages Hardcover
ISBN 0-807731-95-1

2067 Kendall Demonstration Elementary School Curriculum Guides
Gallaudet University Bookstore
800 Florida Avenue NE
Washington, DC 20002
202-651-5220
FAX: 202-651-5724
e-mail: bookstore.mailorder@gallaudet.edu
www.bookstore.gallaudet.edu

Priscilla O'Donnell, Manager
These guides provide detailed information to help teachers organize curriculums and education programs. Pre-school: $15.95, Health: $8.95, Language Arts: $13.75, Social Studies: $14.95, Math: $11.95, Science: $17.95, Auditory & Speech: $10.95.

2068 Language Arts: Detecting Special Needs
Allyn & Bacon
75 Arlington Street
Suite 300
Boston, MA 02116
617-848-6000
800-852-8024
FAX: 617-848-7490
www.ablongman.com

Describes special language arts needs of special learners.
180 pages paperback 1989
ISBN 0-205116-36-1

2069 Language Learning Practices with Deaf Children
Pro-Ed Publications
8700 Shoal Creek Boulevard
Austin, TX 78757
512-451-3246
800-897-3202
FAX: 800-397-7633
e-mail: feedback@proedinc.com
www.proedinc.com

Donald Hammill, Owner
Courtney King, Marketing Coordinator
This new edition describes the variety of language-development theories and practices used with deaf children without advocating anyone. *$38.00*
321 pages Hardcover

2070 Language and Communication Disorders in Children
McGraw-Hill School Publishn
220 East Danieldale Road
Desoto, TX 75115
972-224-1111
800-442-9685
FAX: 972-228-1982
www.mhschool.com

Joseph Gavigan, President
Comprehensive coverage encompassing all aspects of children's language disorders.
512 pages

2071 Learning Disabilities, Literacy, and Adult Education
Brookes Publishing
PO Box 10624
Baltimore, MD 21285
410-337-9580
800-638-3775
FAX: 410-337-8539
e-mail: custserv@brookespublishing.com
www.brookespublishing.com

Clary Creighton, Exhibits Coordinator
Tracy Gray, Educational Sales Manager
Paul Brooks, Owner
This book focuses on adults with severe learning disabilities and the educators who work with them. Described are the characteristics, demographics, and educational and employment status of adults with LD and the laws that protect them in the workplace and in educational settings.

450 pages Paperback 1998
ISBN 1-55766 -47-5

2072 Learning Disabilities: Concepts and Characteristics
McGraw-Hill School Publishing
220 East Danieldale Road
Desoto, TX 75115
972-224-1111
800-442-9685
FAX: 972-228-1982
www.mhschool.com

Cheri Scott, Director
Joseph Gavigan, President
Covers the conceptual basis of learning disabilities, identification, etiology and diagnosis.
448 pages

2073 Learning Disability: Social Class and the Cons of Inequality In American Education
Greenwood Publishing Group
88 Post Road West
Suite 5007
Westport, CT 06880
203-226-3571
FAX: 203-222-1502
www.greenwood.com

Wayne Smith, President
Presents a detailed historical description of the social and educational assumptions integral to the idea of learning disability.
167 pages $43.95 - $47.95
ISBN 0-313253-96-X

2074 Learning and Individual Differences
National Association of School Psychologists
8455 Colesville Road
Suite 1000
Silver Spring, MD 20910
301-681-3223
FAX: 301-608-2514

A multidisciplinary journal in education.

2075 Learning to See: American Sign Language as a Second Language
Gallaudet University Press
11030 South Langley Avenue
Chicago, IL 60628
800-621-2736
FAX: 800-621-8476
TTY:800-621-9347
gupress.gallaudet.edu

Sherman Wilcox, Co-Author
Phyliss Wilcox, Co-Author
This important book has been updated to help teachers teach American Sign Language as a second language, including information on Deaf culture, the history and structure of ASL, teaching methods and issues facing educators. *$19.95*
160 pages Softcover

2076 Legal-Ethical Considerations, Restrictions and Obligations for Clinicians
Charles C Thomas
2600 South 1st Street
Springfield, IL 62704
217-789-8980
800-258-8980
FAX: 217-789-9130
e-mail: books@ccthomas.com
www.ccthomas.com

Micheal Thomas, President
Legal-Ethical Considerations, Restrictions and Obligations for Clinicians who Treat Communicative Disorders is a clinical functioning of speech-language pathologists and audiologists is determined not only by their clinical skills but by their awareness of the legal-ethical restrictions and obligations they are required by law to consider in their relationships with their clients and their families *$51.95*

258 pages Softcover
ISBN 0-39806 -29-6

2077 Library Manager's Guide to Hiring and Serving Disabled Persons

Mc Farland & Company
PO Box 611
Jefferson, NC 28640
336-246-4460
800-253-2187
FAX: 336-246-5018
e-mail: infoinso@mcfarlandpub.com
www.mcfarlandpub.com

Krall Heinz Roscman, Director
Information for library staff on hiring and serving disabled persons. *$35.00*
171 pages Illustrated
ISBN 0-89950 -16-3

2078 Life-Span Approach to Nursing Care for Individuals with Developmental Disabilities

Brookes Publishing
PO Box 10624
Baltimore, MD 21285
410-337-9580
800-638-3775
FAX: 410-337-8539
e-mail: custserv@brookespublishing.com
www.brookespublishing.com

Clary Creighton, Exhibits Coordinator
Tracy Gray, Educational Sales Manager
Paul Brooks, Owner
This reference book was written by and for nurses. This guide addresses fundamental nursing issues such as health promotion, infection control, seizure management, adaptive and assistive technology, and sexuality. Also offered are in-depth case studies, helpful charts and tables, and problem-solving strategies. *$49.95*
464 pages Hardcover
ISBN 1-557661-51-0

2079 Look, Now Hear This: Combined Auditory Training and Speech-Reading Instruction

Charles C Thomas
2600 South 1st Street
Springfield, IL 62704
217-789-8980
800-258-8980
FAX: 217-789-9130
e-mail: books@ccthomas.com
www.ccthomas.com

Micheal Thomas, President
A manual on combined auditory training and speech reading instruction. Also available in cloth: $42.95 (ISBN# 0-398-03830-9) *$ 30.95*
230 pages Softcover
ISBN 0-398061-81-5

2080 Mainstreaming Deaf and Hard of Hearing Students: Questions and Answers

Gallaudet University Bookstore
800 Florida Avenue NE
Washington, DC 20002
202-651-5000
800-451-1073
FAX: 202-651-5489
www.gallaudet.edu

Erving Jordan, President
This booklet presents mainstreaming as one educational option and suggests some considerations for parents, teachers and administrators. *$6.00*
40 pages

2081 Mainstreaming Exceptional Students: A Guide for Classroom Teachers, 4th Edition

Allyn & Bacon
75 Arlington Street
Suite 300
Boston, MA 02116
617-848-6000
FAX: 617-848-7490
e-mail: ab_webmaster@abacon.com
vig.abacon.com

Covers the various categories of exceptional students and discusses educational strategies and classroom management.

464 pages paperback
ISBN 0-20515 -24-6

2082 Mainstreaming: A Practical Approach for Teachers

McGraw-Hill School Publishing
220 East Danieldale Road
Desoto, TX 75115
972-224-1111
800-442-9685
FAX: 972-228-1982
e-mail: custserv@mcgraw-hill.com
www.mhschool.com

Joseph Gavigan, President
Provides teachers, administrators and school psychologists with the background, techniques and strategies they need to offer appropriate services for mildly handicapped students in the mainstream classroom.

2083 Managing Diagnostic Tool of Visual Perception

Gallery Bookshop
PO Box 270
Mendocino, CA 95460
707-937-2665
FAX: 707-937-3737
e-mail: info@gallerybooks.com
www.gallerybooks.com

Linda Pack, Manager
Tony Miksak, Owner
For diagnosing specific perceptual learning abilities and disabilities. *$14.00*

ISBN 0-80580 -83-4

2084 Medical Rehabilitation

Lippincott, Williams & Wilkins
227 East Washington Square
Philadelphia, PA 19106
215-521-8300
800-777-2295
FAX: 301-824-7390
www.lpub.com

J Lippincott, Chief Executive Officer
Information for the professional on new techniques and treatments in the medical rehabilitation fields. *$80.50*
368 pages Illustrated
ISBN 0-88167 -85-5

2085 Mental & Physical Disability Law Digest

A BA Commission on Mental and Physical Disability
740 15th Street NW
9th Floor
Washington, DC 20005
202-662-1570
800-285-2221
FAX: 202-662-1032
e-mail: cmpdl@abanet.org
www.abanet.org/disability

John Parry, Executive Director
Amy Allbright, Managing Editor
Provides comprehensive, summary and analysis of federal and state disability and state disability laws from mental disability law and disability discrimination law perspectives. *$60.00*
376 pages
ISBN 1-590310-05-5

2086 Mental Health Concepts and Techniques for the Occupational Therapy Assistant

Lippincott, Williams & Wilkins
227 East Washington Square
Philadelphia, PA 19106
215-521-8300
800-777-2295
FAX: 301-824-7390
www.lpub.com

J Lippincott, Chief Executive Officer
This text offers clear and easily understood explanations of the various theoretical and practiced health models. *$36.00*

344 pages
ISBN 0-88167 -53-X

2087 Mental Health and Mental Illness
Lippincott, Williams & Wilkins
227 East Washington Square
Philadelphia, PA 19106
215-521-8300
800-777-2295
FAX: 301-824-7390
www.lpub.com

J Lippincott, Chief Executive Officer
Concise, comprehensive and completely up to date, this book presents the most current theory in mental health nursing for the student and the new practitioner. *$28.95*
480 pages
ISBN 0-39755 -73-7

2088 Mentally Ill Individuals
Mainstream
3 Bethesda Metro Center
Suite 830
Bethesda, MD 20814
301-961-9299
800-247-1380
FAX: 301-654-6714
e-mail: info@mainstreaminc.org

Charles Moster
Mainstreaming mentally ill individuals into the workplace. *$2.50*
12 pages

2089 Midland Treatment Furniture
Sammons Preston Rolyan
W68 N158 Evergreen Boulevard
Cedarburg, WI 53012
800-228-3693
FAX: 262-387-8748
e-mail: customerservice@sammonspreston.com
www.sammonspreston.com
This catalog has the biggest selection of OT/PT products anywhere. Whether you deal with larger or smaller caseloads, you need treatment furniture you can count on. Midland Treatment Furniture from SPR is designed and built to stand up to the heaviest use. From tilt tables and traction packages to mat platforms and parallel bars, you'll find the complete line of Midland Treatment Furniture inside this brochure. All products are assembled from premium materials and carefully crafted.
Free

2090 Multidisciplinary Assessment of Children With Learning Disabilities and Mental Retardation
Gallery Bookshop
PO Box 270
Mendocino, CA 95460
707-937-2665
FAX: 707-937-3737
e-mail: info@gallerybooks.com
www.gallerybooks.com

Linda Pack, Manager
Tony Miksak, Owner
Assessment of children with learning disabilities and mental retardation. *$24.00*
346 pages Illustrated
ISBN 0-93371 -62-1

2091 Multisensory Teaching of Basic Language Skills: Theory and Practice
Brookes Publishing
PO Box 10624
Baltimore, MD 21285
410-337-9580
800-638-3775
FAX: 410-337-8539
e-mail: custserv@brookespublishing.com
www.brookespublishing.com

Clary Creighton, Exhibits Coordinator
Tracy Gray, Educational Sales Manager
Paul Brooks, Owner
This book presents specific multisensory methods for helping students who are having trouble learning to read due to dyslexia or other learning disabilities. Recommended techniques are offered for teaching alphabet skills, composition, comprehension, handwriting, math, organization and study skills, phonological awareness, reading and spelling. *$59.00*
608 pages Hardcover 1999
ISBN 1-557663-49-1

2092 No Longer Immune: A Counselor's Guide to AIDS
American Counceling Association
5999 Stevenson Avenue
Alexandria, VA 22304
703-823-9800
800-347-6647
FAX: 800-473-2329
TTY: 703-823-6862
www.counseling.org

Richard Yep, Executive Director
Covers a broad range of issues such as working with specific populations, handling pre and post testing situations, coping with fear, grief and survivor guilt, struggling with spiritual issues and dealing with counter transference. *$26.95*
295 pages
ISBN 1-55620 -64-1

2093 Occupational Therapy Across Cultural Boundaries
Haworth Press
10 Alice Street
Binghamton, NY 13904
607-722-5857
800-429-6784
FAX: 607-722-6362
e-mail: orders@haworthpress.com
www.haworthpress.com

Sandy Sickels, Vice President
Becky Minerbaum, Advertising Manager
William Cohen, Owner
Examines the concept of culture from a unique perspective, that of individual occupational therapists who have worked in environments very different from those in which they were educated or had worked previously. *$74.95*
107 pages Hardcover
ISBN 1-560242-23-X

2094 Occupational Therapy Approaches to Traumatic Brain Injury
Haworth Press
10 Alice Street
Binghamton, NY 13904
607-722-5857
800-429-6784
FAX: 607-722-6362
e-mail: orders@haworthpress.com
www.haworthpress.com

Sandy Sickels, Vice President
Becky Minerbaum, Advertising Manager
William Cohen, Owner
Focuses on the disabled individual, the family, and the societal responses to the injured, this comprehensive book covers the spectrum of available services from intensive care to transitional and community living. *$74.95*
137 pages Hardcover
ISBN 1-560240-64-4

2095 Overcoming Dyslexia in Children, Adolescents and Adults
Pro-Ed Publications
8700 Shoal Creek Boulevard
Austin, TX 78757
512-451-3246
800-897-3202
FAX: 512-451-8542
e-mail: feedback@proedinc.com
www.proedinc.com

Donald Hammill, Owner
Courtney King, Marketing Coordinator
This book describes some forms of dyslexia in detail and then relates those problems to the social, emotional and personal development of dyslexic individuals. *$34.00*
350 pages Paperback

2096 Oxford Textbook of Geriatric Medicine
Oxford University Press
198 Madison Avenue
New York, NY 10016
212-726-6000
800-334-4249
FAX: 212-726-6440
www.oup.com/us

Laura Brown, Chief Executive Officer
Ellen Taus, Senior Vice President

This comprehensive text brings together extensive experience in clinical geriatrics with a strong scientific base in research. *$125.00*

784 pages

2097 PKU for Children: Learning to Measure

University of Washington PKU Clinic
PO Box 357920
Seattle, WA 98195
206-598-1800
877-685-3015
FAX: 206-685-1286
e-mail: pku@u.washington.edu
www.depts.washington.edu/pku

Ronald Scott, Medical Director
Lesson format for parents and teachers.

2098 Pain Centers: A Revolution in Health Care

Lippincott Williams And Wilkins
227 East Washington Square
Philadelphia, PA 19106
215-521-8300
800-777-2295
FAX: 301-824-7390
www.lpub.com

J Lippincott, Chief Executive Officer
$103.00

280 pages

2099 Parental Concerns in College Student Mental Health

Haworth Press
10 Alice Street
Binghamton, NY 13904
607-722-5857
800-429-6784
FAX: 607-722-6362
e-mail: orders@haworthpress.com
www.haworthpress.com

Sandy Sickels, Vice President
Becky Minerbaum, Advertising Manager
William Cohen, Owner
An instructive guide for parents and mental health professionals regarding the most important issues about psychological development in college students. *$74.95*

204 pages Hardcover
ISBN 0-866567-20-8

2100 Parents and Teachers

Alexander Graham Bell Association
3417 Volta Place NW
Washington, DC 20007
202-337-5220
866-337-5220
FAX: 202-337-8314
e-mail: info@agbell.org
www.agbell.org

Todd Houston, Executive Officer
This excellent book offers in-depth guidance to parents and teachers whose partnership can foster language in school-aged children with hearing impairments. The first section examines roles of parents, teachers, professionals and children in language acquisition, residual hearing and audiological management, language development stages and readying children for preschool. The second portion of the book presents specific objectives and teaching strategies to use at school and at home. *$27.95*

386 pages

2101 Patient and Family Education

Springer Publishing Company
11 West 42nd Street
15th Floor
New York, NY 10036
212-431-4370
877-687-7476
FAX: 212-941-7842
e-mail: contactus@springerpub.com
www.springerpub.com

Sheri Sussman, Vice President
Ursula Springer, President
This guide outlines the actual clinical content needed to develop, implement and maintain patient education programs. Conveniently arranged in one-hour long lesson plans, each disease or condition is organized in an easy-to-follow format. *$26.95*

272 pages Softcover
ISBN 0-82615 -41-7

2102 Person to Person: Guide for Professionals Working with the Disabled, 2nd Edition

Paul H Brookes Publishing Company
PO Box 10624
Baltimore, MD 21285
410-337-9580
800-638-3775
FAX: 410-337-8539
e-mail: custserv@brookespublishing.com
www.brookespublishing.com

Clary Creighton, Exhibits Coordinator
Tracy Gray, Educational Sales Manager
Paul Brooks, Owner
This second edition of an already-popular book helps professionals approach interactions with a people-first, disability second attitude. *$29.00*

288 pages Paperback 1992
ISBN 1-557661-00-6

2103 Personality and Emotional Disturbance

Taylor & Francis
47 Runway Drive
Suite G
Levittown, PA 19057
FAX: 215-785-5515
The brain injured person has unique needs. Recent findings have highlighted that it is the personality, behavioral and emotional problems which most prohibit a return to work, create the greatest burden for the long-term care and rehabilitation of physical and cognitive functions. *$72.00*

260 pages Cloth
ISBN 0-85066 -71-3

2104 Peterson's Guide to Colleges with Programs for Learning Disabled Students

Special Needs Project
324 State Street
Suite H
Santa Barbara, CA 93101
805-962-8087
800-333-6867
FAX: 805-962-5087
e-mail: books@specialneeds.com
www.specialneeds.com

Hod Gray, Administrator/Owner
Laraine Gray, Coordinator
The most complete and accurate guide to the more than 900 colleges with programs for the learning disabled. *$19.95*

406 pages

2105 Phenomenology of Depressive Illness

Human Sciences Press
233 Spring Street
New York, NY 10013
212-229-2859
800-221-9369
FAX: 212-463-0742
Provides the reader with a detailed knowledge of the clinical characteristics of depressive disorders that will permit judgement of the general ability of the various theoretical models of depressive disorders. *$42.95*

263 pages Cloth
ISBN 0-89885 -69-9

2106 Physical Disabilities and Health Impairments: An Introduction

McGraw-Hill School Publishing
220 East Danieldale Road
Desoto, TX 75115
972-224-1111
800-442-9685
FAX: 972-228-1982
www.mhschool.com

Joseph Gavigan, President
A comprehensive text which presents a wealth of up-to-date medical information for teachers.

2107 **Physical Education and Sports for Exceptional Students**

McGraw-Hill Company
2460 Kerper Boulevard
Dubuque, IA 52001
563-588-1451
800-338-3987
FAX: 614-755-5654
www.mhhe.com/hper/physed

Kurt Strand, Vice President
Physical education for exceptional students and teaching students with learning and behavior exceptionalities.
Cloth

2108 **Physical Management of Multiple Handicaps: A Professional's Guide**
Brookes Publishing Company
PO Box 10624
Baltimore, MD 21285
410-337-9580
800-638-3775
FAX: 410-337-8539
e-mail: custserv@brookespublishing.com
www.brookespublishing.com

Clary Creighton, Exhibits Coordinator
Tracy Gray, Educational Sales Manager
Paul Brooks, Owner
Comprehensive guide, takes a transdisciplinary approach to therapeutic/technological management of persons with multiple handicaps. *$36.00*
352 pages Hardcover
ISBN 1-557660-47-6

2109 **Physically Handicapped in Society**
Ayer Company Publishers
400 Bedford Street
Suite 322
Manchester, NH 03101
603-669-9307
888-267-7323
FAX: 603-669-7945
e-mail: stg@ncia.net
www.ayerpub.com

Kathy Train, Office Manager
Ellie Phipps, Customer Service
A group of 39 books. Biographies that offer studies on attitudes, sociological and psychological. Please write or call for catalog. *$965.00*
Hardcover
ISBN 0-40513 -00-3

2110 **Practicing Rehabilitation with Geriatric Clients**
Springer Publishing Company
11 West 42nd Street
New York, NY 10036
212-431-4370
877-687-7476
FAX: 212-941-7842
e-mail: marketing@springerpub.com
www.springerpub.com

Annette Imperati, Marketing/Sales Director
Ursula Springer, President
Physical therapy in the geriatric client, psychological and psychiatric considerations in the rehabilitation of the elderly. *$32.95*
256 pages Hardcover
ISBN 0-82616 -80-5

2111 **Pragmatic Approach**
Educators Publishing Service
625 Mount Auburn Street
Suite 3
Cambridge, MA 02138
617-547-6706
800-225-5750
FAX: 888-440-2665
e-mail: feedback@epsbooks.com
www.epsbooks.com

Charles H Heinle, Vice President
Alexandra S Bigelow, Author
Gunnar Voltz, President
Monograph on evaluation of children's performances on Slingerland Pre-Reading Screening Procedures to Identify First Grade Academic Needs. *$6.00*
56 pages
ISBN 0-838816-85-1

2112 **Preschoolers with Special Needs: Children At-Risk, Children with Disabilities, 2nd Edition**
Allyn & Bacon
75 Arlington Street
Suite 300
Boston, MA 02116
617-848-6000
800-852-8024
FAX: 617-848-7490
www.ablongman.com
Explores ways of providing preschool children with special needs and their families with a learning environment that will help them develop and learn. Emphasizes the needs of preschoolers age three to six and provides information to teachers and others who work with young children in all settings. Current models of curricula, which incorporate new features from research and practical expreiences with children who have special needs, are described and discussed. *$59.00*
336 pages cloth
ISBN 0-205358-79-9

2113 **Preventing Academic Failure**
Educators Publishing Service
625 Mount Auburn Street
Suite 3
Cambridge, MA 02138
617-547-6706
800-225-5750
FAX: 888-440-2665
e-mail: feedback@epsbooks.com
www.epsbooks.com

Charles H Heinle, Vice President
Alexandra S Bigelow, Author
Gunnar Voltz, President
Ungraded multisensory curriculum coordinating Orton-Gillingham and Merrill Linguistic reading techniques for language disabled students. Teaches phonics, spelling and reading to reinforce the development of language skills. A separate handwriting program is available. *$42.00*
284 pages Paperback
ISBN 0-838852-71-8

2114 **Preventing School Dropouts**
Pro-Ed Publications
8700 Shoal Creek Boulevard
Austin, TX 78757
512-451-3246
800-897-3202
FAX: 800-397-7633
e-mail: feedback@proedinc.com
www.proedinc.com

Donald Hammill, Owner
Courtney King, Marketing Coordinator
For secondary teachers, special education and regular, who have difficulty teaching youth in their classes. Presented are 120 tactics, specific instructional techniques, for helping adolescents to stay in school. Each tactic is written in a format that includes five sections. *$38.00*
509 pages

2115 **Prevocational Assessment**
Exceptional Education
PO Box 15308
Seattle, WA 98115
206-262-9538
FAX: 475-486-4510

J E Stewart, Owner
Use the PACG to assess your students in nine areas (attendance and endurance, learning and behavior, communication skills, social skills, grooming and eating and toileting) covering 46 specific workshop experiences. *$12.00*
16 pages Complete Set
ISBN 1-87786 -23-7

2116 **Progress Without Punishment: Approaches for Learners with Behavior Problems**
Teachers College Press
1234 Amsterdam Avenue
New York, NY 10027
212-678-3929
800-575-6566
FAX: 212-678-4149
www.teacherscollegepress.com

Carol Saltz, Director
Brian Ellerbeck, Executive Acquisitions Editor
Lee Bollinger, President
In this volume, the authors argue against the use of punishment, and instead advocate the use of alternative intervention procedures. *$17.95*
184 pages Paperback
ISBN 0-807729-11-6

2117 Promoting Postsecondary Education for Students with Learning Disabilities
Pro-Ed Publications
8700 Shoal Creek Boulevard
Austin, TX 78757
512-451-3246
800-897-3202
FAX: 800-397-7633
e-mail: feedback@proedinc.com
www.proedinc.com

Donald Hammill, Owner
Courtney King, Marketing Coordinator
Primarily designed for postsecondary service providers who are responsible for serving college students with learning disabilities. *$41.00*
440 pages

2118 Psychiatric Mental Health Nursing
Lippincott, Williams & Wilkins
227 East Washington Square
Philadelphia, PA 19106
215-521-8300
800-777-2295
FAX: 301-824-7390
www.lpub.com

J Lippincott, Chief Executive Officer
This text emphasizes and contrasts the roles of the generalist nurse and the psychiatric nurse specialist. *$52.00*
1120 pages Illustrated

2119 Psychoeducational Assessment of Visually Impaired and Blind Students
Pro-Ed
8700 Shoal Creek Boulevard
Austin, TX 78757
512-451-3246
800-897-3202
FAX: 800-397-7633
e-mail: feedback@proedinc.com
www.proedinc.com

Joshua Jeffrey, Marketing Custodian
Courtney King, Marketing Coordinator
Donald Hammill, Owner
Professional reference book that addresses the problems specific to assessment of visually impaired and blind children. Of particular value to the practitioner are the extensive reviews of available tests, including ways to adapt those not designed for use with the visually handicapped. *$29.00*
140 pages Paperback
ISBN 0-890791-08-2

2120 Reading and Deafness
Pro-Ed Publications
8700 Shoal Creek Boulevard
Austin, TX 78757
512-451-3246
800-897-3202
FAX: 800-397-7633
e-mail: feedback@proedinc.com
www.proedinc.com

Donald Hammill, Owner
Courtney King, Marketing Coordinator
Three areas are looked at in this book: deaf children's prereading development of real-world knowledge, cognitive abilities and linguistic skills. *$39.00*
422 pages

2121 Readings on Research in Stuttering
Longman Publishing Group
10 Bank Street
9th Floor
White Plains, NY 10606
914-993-5000
FAX: 914-421-5598
www.ablongman.com

Roth Wilkofsky, Systems Contact
Joanne Dresner, President
Collection of the key journal articles published on stuttering over the past decade, addressing trends in recent research in the field.
231 pages Paperback 1991
ISBN 0-801304-10-5

2122 Recreation Activities for the Elderly
Springer Publishing Company
11 West 42nd Street
15th Floor
New York, NY 10036
212-431-4370
877-687-7476
FAX: 212-941-7842
e-mail: marketing@springerpub.com
www.springerpub.com

Annette Imperati, Marketing/Sales Director
Joanne Dresner, President
Included in this volume are simple crafts that utilize easily obtainable, inexpensive materials, hobbies focusing on collections, nature, and the arts' and games emphasizing both mental and physical activity. *$23.95*
240 pages Softcover
ISBN 0-82616 -30-1

2123 Reference Manual for Communicative Sciences and Disorders
Pro- Ed Publications
8700 Shoal Creek Boulevard
Austin, TX 78757
512-451-3246
800-897-3202
FAX: 800-397-7633
e-mail: feedback@proedinc.com
www.proedinc.com

Donald Hammill, Owner
Courtney King, Marketing Coordinator
An indispensable guide to standards and values essential in the assessment of communication disorders. *$54.00*
393 pages

2124 Rehabilitation Counseling and Services: Profession and Process
Charles C Thomas
2600 South 1st Street
Springfield, IL 62704
217-789-8980
800-258-8980
FAX: 217-789-9130
e-mail: books@ccthomas.com
www.ccthomas.com

Michael Thomas, President
Gives information on the rehabilitation and counseling process, work evaluation, work adjustment and more. *$52.95*
376 pages Cloth
ISBN 0-39052 -24-4

2125 Rehabilitation Interventions for the Institutionalized Elderly
Haworth Press
10 Alice Street
Binghamton, NY 13904
607-722-5857
800-429-6784
FAX: 607-771-0012
e-mail: orders@haworthpress.com
www.haworthpress.com

William Cohen, Owner/Publisher
Gerontology professionals offer suggestions to enrich the quality of rehabilitation services offered to the institutionalized elderly. This volume examines up to the minute ideas, some that would have been unlikely even a few years ago, that focus exclusively on rehabilitation services for the institutionalized elderly. *$44.95*

77 pages Hardcover
ISBN 0-866568-33-6

2126 **Rehabilitation Nursing for the Neurological Patient**
Springer Publishing Company
11 West 42nd Street
15th Floor
New York, NY 10036
212-431-4370
877-687-7476
FAX: 212-941-7842
e-mail: marketing@springerpub.com
www.springerpub.com

Annette Imperati, Marketing/sales Director
Ursula Springer, President
A practical new reference written especially for practicing nurses who work with neurologically disabled persons. *$ 32.95*
240 pages

2127 **Rehabilitation Resource Manual: VISION**
Resources for Rehabilitation
22 Bonad Road
Winchester, MA 01890
781-368-9094
FAX: 781-368-9096

Susan Greenblatt
A desk reference that enables service providers, librarians and others to make effective referrals. Includes guidelines on establishing self-help groups, information on research and service organizations, and chapters on assistive technology, for special population groups and by eye condition. *$44.95*
Biennial

2128 **Rehabilitation Technology**
Haworth Press
10 Alice Street
Binghamton, NY 13904
607-722-5857
800-429-6784
FAX: 607-722-6362
e-mail: orders@haworthpress.com
www.haworthpress.com

Sandy Sickels, Vice President
Becky Minerbaum, Advertising Manager
William Cohen, Owner
Learn how the use of technological devices can enhance the lives of disabled children. Informs physical therapists, occupational therapists, and rehabilitation technologists about the devices that are available today and provides important background information on these devices. *$74.95*
173 pages Hardcover
ISBN 1-560240-33-4

2129 **Report Writing in Assessment and Evaluation**
Stout Vocational Rehab Institute
University of Wisconsin-Stout
Menomonie, WI 54751
715-232-1478
FAX: 715-232-2356

Ronald R Fry, Manager
Darlene Botterbusch, Program Assistant
This examines questions of who are you writing for and what does the referral source want. Defines characteristics of good reports, common problems, writing in different settings, types of reports, getting ready to write, and writing prescriptive recommendations. *$ 17.75*
188 pages Softcover

2130 **Resources for Rehabilitation**
22 Bonad Road
Winchester, MA 01890
781-368-9094
FAX: 781-368-9096

R Frances Weisse, President
Provides training and information to professionals and the public about disabilities and resources available to help. Publishes resource guides, professional publications and patient/client educational materials. Conducts custom designed training programs and workshops.

2131 **Restructuring High Schools for All Students: Taking Inclusion to the Next Level**
Brookes Publishing
PO Box 10624
Baltimore, MD 21285
410-337-9580
800-638-3775
FAX: 410-337-8539
e-mail: custserv@brookespublishing.com
www.brookespublishing.com

Clary Creighton, Exhibits Coordinator
Tracy Gray, Educational Sales Manager
Paul Brooks, Owner
Details the process of creating an inclusive, collaborate community of learners and teachers at the secondary level. *$29.95*
304 pages Paperback 1998
ISBN 1-557663-13-0

2132 **Restructuring for Caring and Effective Education: Administrative Guide**
Brookes Publishing
PO Box 10624
Baltimore, MD 21285
410-337-9580
800-638-3775
FAX: 410-337-8539
e-mail: custserv@brookespublishing.com
www.brookespublishing.com

Clary Creighton, Exhibits Coordinator
Tracy Gray, Educational Sales Manager
Paul Brooks, Owner
In this empowering book, leading general and special education schools reform experts synthesize the major school restructuring initiatives and describe the processes and rationale for changing the organizational structure and instructional practices of schools. *$ 29.00*
384 pages Paperback
ISBN 1-55766 -91-3

2133 **Scoffolding Student Learning**
Brookline Books
PO Box 1047
Cambridge, MA 02139
617-495-3682
800-666-2665
FAX: 617-868-1772
e-mail: thestore@brooklinebooksmith.com
www.brooklinebooks.com

William Walters, Author
Esther Isabe Wilder, Author
Collection of papers on the theory and practice of scoffolding—an interactive style of instructions that helps students develop more powerful thinking tools.. *$21.95*
180 pages Paperback
ISBN 1-571290-36-2

2134 **Selective Nontreatment of Handicapped**
Oxford University Press
2001 Evans Road
Cary, NC 27513
919-677-0977
800-451-7556
FAX: 919-677-2673
e-mail: humanres@oup-usa.org
www.us.oup.com

Thomas Carty, Senior Vice President
Information on selective nontreatment of handicapped newborns, moral dilemmas in neonatal medicine. *$17.95*
304 pages Paperback

2135 **Service Coordination for Early Intervention: Parents and Friends**
Brookline Books
34 University Road
Brookline, MA 02445
800-666-2665
800-666-2665
FAX: 617-734-3952
e-mail: thestore@brooklinebooksmith.com
www.brooklinebooks.com

William H Walters, Author
Esther I Wilder, Author
This book helps administrators and professionals to structure early intervention and ongoing services so that professionals work collaboratively with parents to promote the health, well being and development of children with special needs. *$19.95*

110 pages Paperback
ISBN 0-91479-91-3

2136 Services for the Seriously Mentally Ill: A Survey of Mental Health Centers
Nat'l Council for Community Behavioral Healthcare
12300 Twinbrook Parkway
Suite 320
Rockville, MD 20852
301-984-6200
FAX: 301-881-7159
www.nccbh.org

Linda Rosenberg, President/CEO
Dale K Klatzker, Board Chair
This ground-breaking report documents what administrators and practitioners have maintained for many years: community mental health organizations devote a significant percentage of the human and financial resources to serving the seriously mentally ill. *$30.00*

2137 Shop Talk
Research Press
PO Box 9177
Champaign, IL 61826
217-352-3273
800-519-2707
FAX: 217-352-1221
e-mail: rp@researchpress.com
www.researchpress.com

Russell Pence, President
A well-structured group training program that covers five crucial communication areas: social communication routines, identification information, basic language skills, language-related concepts and cognitive components. The authors emphasize direct cooperation between educators and parents by providing over 100 interesting activities that focus on the student's affective impact on others, unique identify as a person, self-care, grooming, leisure and ability to work independently. *$25.95*
236 pages Paperback
ISBN 0-878222-29-4

2138 Signed English Schoolbook
Gallaudet University Press
800 Florida Avenue NE
Washington, DC 20002
202-651-5488
FAX: 202-651-5489
gupress.gallaudet.edu

Karen Hyzy, Customer Service Manager
The Signed English Schoolbook provides vocabulary for teachers and others who serve school-age children and adolescents and covers the full range of school activities. *$13.95*
184 pages Softcover

2139 Social Studies: Detecting and Correcting Special Needs
Allyn & Bacon
75 Arlington Street
Suite 300
Boston, MA 02116
617-848-6000
800-852-8024
FAX: 617-848-7490
www.ablongman.com
Describes social studies and special needs for special learners.
180 pages 1990
ISBN 0-205121-51-9

2140 Social and Emotional Development of Exceptional Students: Handicapped
Charles C Thomas
2600 South 1st Street
Springfield, IL 62704
217-789-8980
800-258-8980
FAX: 217-789-9130
e-mail: books@ccthomas.com
www.ccthomas.com

Michael Thomas, President
Sixteen years after the passage of P.L. 94-142, the dream of special educators to educate the handicapped and nonhandicapped children and youth together resulting in increased academic gains and age-appropriate school skills for handicapped children and youth has not yet materialized. This book helps eliminate an existing void by providing teachers with understandable information regarding the social and emotional development of exceptional students. Also in cloth at $41.95 (ISBN# 0-398-05781-8) *$29.95*
218 pages Softcover
ISBN 0-398061-94-7

2141 Special Education Today
LifeWay Christian Resources Southern Baptist Conv.
127 9th Avenue N
Nashville, TN 37234
615-251-2089
800-458-2772
FAX: 651-251-5764
e-mail: specialed@lifeway.com
www.lifeway.com

Ellen Beene, Editor
Wade Stapleton, Manager
This unique quarterly publications ministers to people with special education needs and to their families, the church, and other caregivers. It offers a variety of helps and encouragement, including: What's working in churches, Suggestions for adapting teaching techniques, inspirational stories about people who have disabilities, Parenting and family issues, Ideas for reaching, witnessing, worship, and recreation. *$4.25*
36 pages Quarterly

2142 Special Education for Today
Allyn & Bacon
75 Arlington Street
Suite 300
Boston, MA 02116
617-848-6000
800-852-8024
FAX: 617-848-7490
www.ablongman.com

Thomas Longman, Founder
Nancy Forfyth, President
An undergraduate introduction to special education covering all major areas of exceptionality. Contains pedagogical features designed to make the book accessible to the undergraduate.
576 pages hardcover 1984
ISBN 0-138264-53-8

2143 Speech and the Hearing-Impaired Child
Alexander Graham Bell Association
3417 Volta Place NW
Washington, DC 20007
202-337-5220
866-337-5220
FAX: 202-337-8314
e-mail: info@agbell.org
www.agbell.org

Todd Houston, Executive Director
This textbook for professionals deals with basic theoretical issues in the acquisition of speech and the form of language (phonetics and phonology) in children with hearing losses. It provides a systematic framework to develop and evaluate speech target behaviors and their underlying subskills. *$29.95*
402 pages Paperback

2144 Speech-Language Pathology and Audiology: An Introduction
McGraw-Hill School Publishing
220 East Danieldale Road
Desoto, TX 75115
972-224-1111
800-442-9685
FAX: 972-228-1982
www.mhschool.com

Joseph Gavigan, President
Offers classroom-tested coverage of clinical objectives and functioning.
301 pages

2145 Spinal Cord Dysfunction
Oxford University Press
2001 Evans Road
Cary, NC 27513
919-677-0977
800-451-7556
FAX: 919-677-1303
e-mail: humanres@oup-usa.org
www.oup-usa.org

Henry Reece, Chief Executive Director
Thomas Carty, Senior Vice President

Offers information on restoration of function after spinal cord damage as seen from the point of view of identification of impaired or absent function in the nerve cells and processes which survive after the initial insult, intact but with impaired functions. *$95.00*
368 pages

2146 Strategies for Teaching Learners with Special Needs
McGraw-Hill School Publishing
220 East Danieldale Road
Desoto, TX 75115
972-224-1111
800-442-9685
FAX: 972-228-1982
www.mhschool.com

Joseph Gavigan, President
This is a text that helps special educators develop the full range of teaching competencies needed to be effective.
560 pages

2147 Strategies for Teaching Students with Learning and Behavior Problems
Allyn & Bacon
75 Arlington Street
Suite 300
Boston, MA 02116
617-848-6000
800-852-8024
FAX: 617-848-7490
www.ablongman.com

Thomas Longman, Founder
Provides descriptions of methods and strategies for teaching students with learning and behavior problems, managing professional roles, and collaborating with families, professionals, and paraprofessionals.
544 pages
ISBN 0-205113-89-3

2148 Students with Acquired Brain Injury: The School's Response
Brookes Publishing
PO Box 10624
Baltimore, MD 21285
410-337-9580
800-638-3775
FAX: 410-337-8539
e-mail: custserv@brookespublishing.com
www.brookespublishing.com

Clary Creighton, Exhibits Coordinator
Tracy Gray, Educational Sales Manager
Paul Brooks, Owner
This book is designed for school professionals and describes a range of issues that this population faces and presents proven means of addressing them in ways that benefit all students. Included topics are hospital-to-school transitions, effective assessment strategies, model programs in public schools, interventions to assist classroom teachers, and ways to involve family members in the educational program. *$29.95*
424 pages Paperback 1997
ISBN 1-55766 -85-1

2149 Students with Mild Disabilities in the Secondary School
Longman Group
1185 Avenue of the Americas
New York, NY 10036
212-782-3300

www.ablongman.com

Roth Wilkofsky, Chief Executive Officer
Provides methods and strategies for curriculum delivery to students with mild disabilities at the secondary school level.
2313G pages Paperback 1991
ISBN 0-801301-66-1

2150 Supporting and Strengthening Families
Brookline Books
34 University Road
Brookline, MA 02445
617-734-6772
800-666-2665
FAX: 617-734-3952
e-mail: thestore@brooklinebooksmith.com
www.brooklinebooks.com

William Walters, Author
Esther Isabe Wilder, Author
A collection of papers addressing the theory, methods, strategies, and practices involved in adopting an empowerment and family-centered resources approach to supporting families and strengthening individual and family functioning. *$30.00*
252 pages Paperback
ISBN 0-91479 -94-8

2151 TESTS
Slosson Educational Publications
PO Box 544
East Aurora, NY 14052
716-652-0930
888-756-7766
FAX: 800-665-3840
e-mail: slosson@slosson.com
www.slosson.com

Leslie Foote, Office Personnel
Peggy Meyer, Office Personnel
Steven Slosson, President
Slosson Educational Publications, Inc. offers educators an extensive selection of testing products, along with books on autism. ADED and other special needs materials. Our catalog includes 30 pages of speech-language testing and language rehabilitation products. The behavioral conduct. Special needs section includes checklist and scales on aberrant/disruptive behavior, tapes on ADD, as well as products for dyslexia and remediation of reversals.

2152 Teacher's Guide to Including Students with Disabilities in Regular Physical Education
Brookes Publishing
PO Box 10624
Baltimore, MD 21285
410-337-9580
800-638-3775
FAX: 410-337-8539
e-mail: custserv@brookespublishing.com
www.brookespublishing.com

Clary Creighton, Exhibits Coordinator
Tracy Gray, Educational Sales Manager
Paul Brooks, Owner
Provides simple and creative strategies for meaningfully including children with disabilities in regular physical education programs. *$39.00*
288 pages Paperback
ISBN 1-557661-56-1

2153 Teachers Working Together
Brookline Books
34 University Road
Brookline, MA 02445
617-734-6772
800-666-2665
FAX: 617-734-3952
e-mail: thestore@brooklinebooksmith.com
www.brooklinebooks.com

Hon Deshier, Author
Jean Schumaker, Author
Karen Harris, Author
This collection of papers describes collaboraborative efforts for such classroom settings as preschools, elementary, middle and high schools, for content area teaching and into the transition to work. Each chapter describes actual practice and analyzes what is required to accomplish this collaboration. *$19.95*
Paperback 1998
ISBN 1-57139 -66-4

2154 Teaching Adults with Learning Disabilities
Krieger Publishing Company
PO Box 9542
Melbourne, FL 32902
321-724-9542
800-724-0025
FAX: 321-951-3671
e-mail: info@krieger-publishing.com
www.krieger-publishing.com

James Gardner, Editor
Peter Lapaglia, Editor
R Krieger, Owner
Designed to teach literacy providers and classroom instructors how to recognize specific learning disability (LD) patterns and block reading, spelling, writing and arithmetic skills in students of all ages. One of the major problems faced by literary providers is keeping low-skill adults involved in basic education programs long enough to increase their literacy skills to the level of success. Shows instructors in adult education how to modify teaching strategies. *$25.50*

160 pages
ISBN 0-894649-10-8

2155 Teaching Disturbed and Disturbing Students: An Integrative Approach

Pro-Ed Publications
8700 Shoal Creek Boulevard
Austin, TX 78757
512-451-3246
800-897-3202
FAX: 800-397-7633
e-mail: feedback@proedinc.com
www.proedinc.com

Donald Hammil, Owner
Courtney King, Author

Using an integrative approach, this text provides teachers with step-by-step details of how to implement and use the methods and theories discussed in each chapter. *$37.00*

465 pages

2156 Teaching Every Child Every Day: Integrated Learning in Diverse Classrooms

Brookline Books
34 University Road
Brookline, MA 02445
617-734-6772
800-666-2665
FAX: 617-734-3952
e-mail: thestore@brooklinebooksmith.com
www.brooklinebooks.com

William H Walters, Author
Esther Isabe Wilder, Author

Collection of articles addressing various issues in teaching to diverse classrooms—varied in need for special educational services, English proficiency, and socioeconomic and racial backgrounds. *$19.95*

224 pages Paperback
ISBN 0-57129 -40-0

2157 Teaching Infants and Preschoolers with Handicaps

Mc Graw- Hill, School Publishing
220 East Danieldale Road
Desoto, TX 75115
972-224-1111
800-442-9685
FAX: 972-228-1982
www.mhschool.com

Joseph Gavigan, President

Builds a solid background in early childhood special education.

380 pages

2158 Teaching Language-Disabled Children: A Communication/Games Intervention

Brookline Books
34 University Road
Brookline, MA 02445
617-734-6772
800-666-2665
FAX: 617-734-3954
e-mail: thestore@brooklinebooksmith.com
www.brooklinebooks.com

William Walters, Author
Esther Isabe Wilder, Author
Barbara Hecht, Author

Describes exactly how to play the communication games. It does not simply exhort practitioners to give topic-relevant responses and take advantage of opportunities. It provides specific teaching methods and not simply a new perspective on language remeditation. *$22.95*

Hardcover
ISBN 0-91479 -38-7

2159 Teaching Learners with Mild Disabilities: Integrating Research and Practice

Brooke Publishing
PO Box 10624
Baltimore, MD 21285
410-337-9580
800-638-3775
FAX: 410-337-8539
e-mail: bc-info@brookscole.com
www.brookespublishing.com

Clary Creigthon, Exhibits Coordinator
Paul Brooks, Owner

The authors illustrate interactions among regular teachers, special education teachers and students with mild disabilities through the use of hypothetical case studies of students and teachers.

496 pages Paperbound
ISBN 0-53421 -02-0

2160 Teaching Mathematics to Students with Learning Disabilities

Pro-Ed Publications
8700 Shoal Creek Boulevard
Austin, TX 78757
512-451-3246
800-897-3202
FAX: 800-397-7633
e-mail: feedback@proedinc.com
www.proedinc.com

Donald Hammill, Owner
Courtney King, Marketing Coordinator

New trends in school mathematics have surfaced in the teaching world. Problem-solving, estimation and the use of computers are receiving considerably greater emphasis than in the past and these areas are included in the new text. *$38.00*

486 pages Paperback

2161 Teaching Mildly and Moderately Handicapped Students

Allyn & Bacon
75 Arlington Street
Suite 300
Boston, MA 02116
617-848-6000
800-852-8024
FAX: 617-848-7490
www.ablongman.com

A cross-categorical text providing teaching ideas and techniques. Focuses on the theme of learning as a constructive process in which the learner interacts with the environment, constructing new systems of knowledge, Behavioral techniques and research are also presented.

hardcover 1986
ISBN 0-138939-00-4

2162 Teaching Reading to Children with Down Syndrome: A Guide for Parents and Teachers

Woodbine House
6510 Bells Mill Road
Bethesda, MD 20817
301-897-3570
800-843-7323
FAX: 301-897-5838
www.woodbinehouse.com

Alison Oelwein, Illustrator
Irv Shapell, Owner

Guide includes lessons customized to meet the unique interests and learning style of each child. *$16.95*

371 pages Paperback
ISBN 0-933149-55-7

2163 Teaching Reading to Disabled and Handicapped Learners

Charles C Thomas
2600 South 1st Street
Springfield, IL 62704
217-789-8980
800-258-8980
FAX: 217-789-9130
e-mail: books@ccthomas.com
www.ccthomas.com

Michael Thomas, President

Designed as a text for undergraduate and graduate students, it's aim is to help the many children, adolescents, and adults who encounter difficulty with reading. It guides prospective and present special education teachers in assisting and teaching handicapped learners to read. The text integrates traditional methods with newer perspectives to provide and effective reading program in special education. *$37.95*

260 pages Paperback
ISBN 0-398062-48-X

2164 Teaching Reading to Handicapped Children
Love Publishing Company
9101 East Kenyon Avenue
Suite 2200
Denver, CO 80237
303-221-7333
FAX: 303-221-7444
e-mail: lpc@lovepublishing.com
www.lovepublishing.com

Stan Love, Owner
The author covers skills teaching through letter sound association, word identification, synthetic and analytic methods and others, plus testing and assessment. *$24.95*

ISBN 0-89108 -13-5

2165 Teaching Self-Determination to Students with Disabilities
Brookes Publishing
PO Box 10624
Baltimore, MD 21285
410-337-9580
800-638-3775
FAX: 410-337-8539
e-mail: custserv@brookespublishing.com
www.brookespublishing.com

Clary Creighton, Exhibits Coordinator
Tracy Gray, Educational Sales Manager
Paul Brooks, Owner
Basic skills for successful transition. This teacher-friendly source will help educators prepare students with disabilities with the specific skills they need for a satisfactory, self-directed life once they leave school. *$34.95*
384 pages Paperback 1997
ISBN 1-55766 -02-5

2166 Teaching Students with Learning Problems
McGraw-Hill School Publishing
220 East Danieldale Road
Desoto, TX 75115
972-224-1111
800-442-9685
FAX: 972-228-1982
mhschool.com

Joseph Gavigan, President
Expanded coverage of learning strategies, generalization training, self-monitoring techniques, and techniques for increasing the time students spend on academic tasks.
608 pages

2167 Teaching Students with Learning and Behavior Problems
Pro-Ed Publications
8700 Shoal Creek Boulevard
Austin, TX 78757
512-451-3246
800-897-3202
FAX: 512-302-9128
e-mail: lindyn@proedinc.com
www.proedinc.com

Donald Hammill, Owner
Judith Voress Ph.D, Periodicals Director
Lindy Jordaan, Marketing Coordinator
Popular, classic text with a comprehensive overview of best practices in assessing and instructing students with mild-to-moderate learning and behavior problems. *$44.00*
520 pages Paperback

2168 Teaching Students with Mild and Moderate Learning Problems
Allyn & Bacon Longman College Faculty
75 Arlington Street
Suite 300
Boston, MA 02116
800-852-8024
FAX: 617-848-7490
e-mail: info@ablongman.com
www.ablongman.com

Tom Smith, Author
Ed Polloway, Author
Provides teachers with skills for assisting students with mild to moderate handicaps in making successful transitions in school and community environments.
496 pages 1990
ISBN 0-205123-62-7

2169 Teaching Students with Moderate/Severe Disabilities, Including Autism
Charles C Thomas Publications
2600 South 1st Street
Springfield, IL 62704
217-789-8980
800-258-8980
FAX: 217-789-9130
e-mail: books@ccthomas.com
www.ccthomas.com

Micheal Thomas, President
This resource and guide was written to help teachers, parents, and other caregivers provide the best educational opportunities for their students with moderate and severe disabilities. The author addresses functional language and other language intervention strategies, vocational training, community based instruction, transition and postsecondary programming, the adolescent student with autism, students with multiple disabilities, parent and family issues, and legal concerns. *$58.95*
416 pages Paperback
ISBN 0-398067-01-5

2170 Teaching Students with Special Needs in Inclusive Settings
Allyn & Bacon
75 Arlington Street
Suite 300
Boston, MA 02116
617-848-6000
800-852-8024
FAX: 617-848-7490
www.ablongman.com

Nancy Forfyth, President
Thomas Longman, Founder
James Patton, Author
This text is intended to be a survey text providing practical guidance to general education teachers. It will help them to meet the diverse needs of students with disabilities.
544 pages
ISBN 0-20527 -16-6

2171 Teaching Young Children to Read
Brookline Books
PO Box 1047
Brookline, MA 02446
617-868-0360
800-666-2665
FAX: 617-868-1772
e-mail: thestore@brooklinebooks.com
www.brooklinebooks.com

Milt Budoff, Publisher
Detailed instructions on teaching reading to preschoolers. Gradually develops full fluency. *$16.95*
192 pages Paperback
ISBN 0-57129 -48-6

2172 Teaching the Bilingual Special Education Student
Ablex Publishing Corporation
PO Box 811
Stamford, CT 06904
FAX: 201-767-6717
This book focuses on teaching those students who are bilingual, handicapped and in need of special instruction. It responds to the complex and practical issues of teaching these students in an effective way.

ISBN 0-89391 -23-4

2173 Teaching the Learning Disabled Adolescent
Love Publishing Company
9101 East Kenyon Avenue
Denver, CO 80237
303-221-7333
FAX: 303-221-7444
e-mail: lovepublishing@compuserve.com

Stan Lover, Owner
This book gives expert strategies and methods for teaching learning disabled adolescents how, rather than what, to learn. *$34.95*

ISBN 0-89108 -94-5

2174 Teaching the Mentally Retarded Student: Curriculum, Methods, and Strategies
Allyn & Bacon
75 Arlington Street
Suite 300
Boston, MA 02116
617-848-6000
800-852-8024
FAX: 617-848-7490
www.ablongman.com

Tom Smith, Author
Ed Polloway, Author
Represents a comprehensive approach to curriculum, methods and strategies for teaching the mildly mentally retarded student.
640 pages hardcover 1987
ISBN 0-205102-62-X

2175 Technology and Handicapped People
Springer Publishing Company
11 West 42nd Street
15th Floor
New York, NY 10036
212-431-4370
877-687-7476
FAX: 212-941-7842
e-mail: contactus@springerpub.com
www.springerpub.com

Sheri Sussman, Vice President
Ursula Springer, President
Important information for concerned professionals about new rehabilitation techniques and treatments for handicapped people. *$29.95*
224 pages Hardcover
ISBN 0-82614 -10-8

2176 Textbooks and the Student Who Can't Read Them: A Guide for Teaching Content
Brookline Books
PO Box 1046
Cambridge, MA 02139
617-868-0360
800-666-2665
FAX: 617-868-1772
e-mail: thestore@brooklinebooks.com
www.brooklinebooks.com
Based on a careful analysis of 10 textbook programs, the author concisely and sensibly indicates the procedures that facilitate teachers' use of regular grade level textbooks with low-reading students. *$21.95*
Paperback
ISBN 0-91479 -57-3

2177 There's a Hearing Impaired Child in My Class
Gallaudet University Bookstore
800 Florida Avenue NE
Washington, DC 20002
202-651-5000
800-451-1073
FAX: 202-651-5489
www.bookstore.gallaudette.edu

Joseph Cachie
Erving Jordan, President
This complete package provides basic facts about deafness, practical strategies for teaching hearing impaired children, and the question-and-answer information for all students. *$16.95*
44 pages

2178 To Teach a Dyslexic
AVKO Educational Research Foundation
43-955 Port Maria Road
Bermuda Dunes, CA 92203
760-238-3900

e-mail: info@abko.org
www.abko.org

Don McCabe, Executive Research Director
A dyslexic tells how luck enabled him to learn to read and how his blissful ignorance and stubbornness enabled him to discover how to teach other dyslexics to read and write. *$14.95*
288 pages Paperback

2179 Toward Effective Public School Program for Deaf Students
Teachers College Press
Columbia University
525 West 120th Street
New York, NY 10027
212-678-3000
800-575-6566
FAX: 212-678-4149
www.tc.columbia.edu

Mary Lynch, Manager
This book translates research and data into useable recommendations and possible courses of action for organizing effective public school programs for deaf students. *$22.95*
272 pages Paperback
ISBN 0-807731-59-5

2180 Treating Cerebral Palsy for Clinicians by Clinicians
Pro-Ed Publications
8700 Shoal Creek Boulevard
Austin, TX 78757
512-451-3246
800-897-3202
FAX: 800-397-7633
e-mail: feedback@proedinc.com
www.proedinc.com

Donald Hammill, Owner
Courtney King, Marketing Coordinator
A clinical manual for professionals beginning to work with persons who have cerebral palsy. *$31.00*
312 pages

2181 Treating Disordered Speech Motor Control
Pro-Ed Publications
8700 Shoal Creek Boulevard
Austin, TX 78757
512-451-3246
800-897-3202
FAX: 512-451-8542
e-mail: feedback@proedinc.com
www.proedinc.com

Donald Hammill, Owner
Courtney King, Marketing Coordinator
This book about neuromotor disturbances of speech production is aimed at practicing professionals and advanced graduate students interested in the neuropathologies of communication. *$36.00*
410 pages

2182 Treating Families of Brain Injury Survivors
Springer Publishing Company
11 West 42nd Street
15th Floor
New York, NY 10036
212-431-4370
877-687-7476
FAX: 212-941-7842
e-mail: contactus@springerpub.com
www.springerpub.com

Annette Imperati, Marketing/Sales Director
Sheri Sussman, Vice President
Ursula Springer, President
Provides the mental health practitioner with a comprehensive program for helping families of head injury survivors cope with the change in their lives. Includes background on medical aspects of head injury, family structure functioning and special needs of various family members.
220 pages
ISBN 0-82616 -20-1

2183 Understanding and Teaching Emotionally Disturbed Children & Adolescents
Pro-Ed Publications
8700 Shoal Creek Boulevard
Austin, TX 78757
512-451-3246
800-897-3202
FAX: 800-397-7633
e-mail: feedback@proedinc.com
www.proedinc.com

Donald Hammill, Owner
Courtney King, Marketing Coordinator

The teacher's handbook provides information that will change misconceptions about children who are frequently labeled as emotionally disturbed. It also gives information about a wide variety of intervention methods and approaches for use in educational settings. *$41.00*
620 pages Hardover

2184 Using the Dictionary of Occupational Titles in Career Decision Making
Stout Vocational Rehab Institute
University of Wisconsin Stout
Menomonie, WI 54751
715-232-2470
FAX: 715-232-5008
e-mail: luij@uwstout.edu
www.svri.uwstout.edu

John Lui, Contact Person
This is a self-study manual for learning how to use the 1991 U.S. Department of Labor's Dictionary of Occupational Titles. It gives the DOT user a tool to understand the DOT and then put its information to work. Shows how to quickly obtain information about the work performed in 12,741 occupations listed and described in the DOT and the worker requirements for those occupations. *$24.00*
142 pages Softcover

2185 VBS Special Education Teaching Guide
Life Way Christian Resources Southern Baptist Conv
1 Lifeway Plaza
Nashville, TN 37234
615-251-2000
e-mail: specialed@lifeway.com
www.lifeway.com

Mike Harland, Director
James Draper Jr, President
This book contains teaching plans for five bible study sessions with reproducible handouts for learners. The plans use multisensory, experiential-based learning activities designed for adults and older youth who have mental retardation. Suggestions for Bible learning, crafts, recreation, snacks and theme interpretation are included. Designed primarily for Vacation Bible School, but may be used in camp/retreat settings. *$9.95*
56 pages Yearly

2186 Vermont Interdependent Services Team Approach (VISTA)
Brookes Publishing
PO Box 10624
Baltimore, MD 21285
410-337-9580
800-638-3775
FAX: 410-337-8539
e-mail: custserv@brookespublishing.com
www.brookespublishing.com

Clary Creighton, Exhibits Coordinator
Tracy Gray, Educational Sales Manager
Paul Brooks, Owner
A guide to coordinating educational support services. This manual enables IEP team members to fulfill the related services provisions of IDEA as they make effective support services decisions using a collaborative team approach. *$27.95*
176 pages Spiral bound
ISBN 1-55766 -30-4

2187 When You Have a Visually Impaired Student in Your Classroom: A Guide for Teachers
American Foundation for the Blind
11 Penn Plaza
Suite 300
New York, NY 10001
212-502-7600
800-232-5463
FAX: 212-502-7777
e-mail: afbinfo@afb.net
www.afb.org/store

Carl R Augusto, President/CEO
This guide provides information on students' abilities and needs, resources and educational team members, federal special education requirements, and technology materials used by students. *$9.95*
84 pages 2001
ISBN 0-891283-93-5

2188 Working Bibliography on Behavioral and Emotional Disorders
Natl. Clearinghouse for Alcohol & Drug Information
PO Box 2345
Rockville, MD 20847
301-468-2600
800-729-6686
FAX: 301-468-6433
e-mail: info@health.org
www.health.org

Lizabeth J Foster, Librarian/Info. Resource Manager
NCADI is a service of the U.S. Substance Abuse and Mental Health Services Administration. As the national focal point for information on alcohol and other drugs, NCADI collects, prepares, classifies, and distributes information about alcohol, tobacco and other drugs, prevention strategies and materials, research, treatment, etc.
40 pages

2189 Working Together with Children and Families: Case Studies
Brookes Publishing Company
PO Box 10624
Baltimore, MD 21285
410-337-9580
800-638-3775
FAX: 410-337-8539
e-mail: custerv@brookespublishing.com
www.brookespublishing.com

Clary Creighton, Exhibits Coordinator
Tracy Gray, Educational Sales Manager
Paul Brooks, Owner
Early interventionists will be able to bridge the gap between theory and practice with this edited collection of case studies. *$23.00*
336 pages 1993
ISBN 1-557661-23-5

2190 Working with Visually Impaired Young Students: A Curriculum Guide
Charles C Thomas
2600 South 1st Street
Springfield, IL 62704
217-789-8980
800-258-8980
FAX: 217-789-9130
e-mail: books@ccthomas.com
www.ccthomas.com

Micheal Thomas, President
The first step in the education process of a visually impaired child is the early identification and treatment by an eye care specialist. This book is geared to the age of birth through 3-years. Available in cloth, paperback and hardcover. *$36.95*
208 pages Paperback
ISBN 0-398068-75-5

Testing Resources

2191 AEPS Child Progress Report: For Children Ages Birth to Three
Brookes Publishing
PO Box 10624
Baltimore, MD 21285
410-337-9580
800-638-3775
FAX: 410-337-8539
e-mail: custserv@brookespublishing.com
www.brookespublishing.com

Clary Creighton, Exhibits Coordinator
Tracy Gray, Educational Sales Manager
Paul Brooks, Owner
This chart helps monitor change by visually displaying current abilities, intervention targets, and child progress. In packages of 30. *$18.00*

6 pages Gate-fold
ISBN 1-55766 -65-0

2192 AEPS Data Recording Forms: For Children Ages Birth to Three
Brookes Publishing
PO Box 10624
Baltimore, MD 21285
410-337-9580
800-638-3775
FAX: 410-337-8539
e-mail: custserv@brookespublishing.com
www.brookespublishing.com

Paul Brooks, Owner
These forms can be used by child development professionals on four separate occasions to pinpoint and then monitor a child's strengths and needs in the six key areas of skill development measured by the AEPS Test. Packages of 10. *$23.00*
36 pages Saddle-stiched
ISBN 1-55766 -97-2

2193 AEPS Measurement for Birth to Three Years
Brookes Publishing
PO Box 10624
Baltimore, MD 21285
410-337-9580
800-638-3775
FAX: 410-337-8539
e-mail: custserv@brookespublishing.com
www.brookespublishing.com

Clary Creighton, Exhibits Coordinator
Tracy Gray, Educational Sales Manager
Paul Brooks, Owner
This dynamic volume explains the Assessment, Evaluation and Programming System, provides the complete AEPS Test and parallel assessment/evaluation tools for families and includes the forms and plans needed for implementation. *$39.00*
352 pages

2194 AEPS Measurement for Three to Six Years
Brookes Publishing
PO Box 10624
Baltimore, MD 21285
410-337-9580
800-638-3775
FAX: 410-337-8539
e-mail: custserv@brookespublishing.com
www.brookespublishing.com

Clary Creighton, Exhibits Coordinator
Tracy Gray, Educational Sales Manager
Paul Brooks, Owner
$57.00
400 pages Spiral-bound
ISBN 1-55766 -87-1

2195 AIR: Assessment of Interpersonal Relations
Pro-Ed Publications
8700 Shoal Creek Boulevard
Austin, TX 78757
512-451-3246
800-897-3202
FAX: 512-451-8542
e-mail: feedback@proedinc.com
www.proedinc.com

Donald Hammill, Owner
Courtney King, Marketing Coordinator
A thoroughly researched and standardized clinical instrument assessing the quality of adolescents' interpersonal relationships in a hierarchical fashion, including global relationship quality and relationship quality with three domains: Family, Social and Academic. *$89.00*

2196 ALST: Adolescent Language Screening Test
Pro-Ed Publications
8700 Shoal Creek Boulevard
Austin, TX 78757
512-451-3246
800-897-3202
FAX: 800-397-7633
e-mail: feedback@proedinc.com
www.proedinc.com

Joshua Jeffrey, Marketing Custodian
Courtney King, Marketing Coordinator
Donald Hammill, Owner
Provides speech/language pathologists and other interested professionals with a rapid thorough method for screening adolescents (ages 11-17). *$119.00*

2197 Adaptive Mainstreaming: A Primer for Teachers and Principals, 3rd Edition
Longman Publishing Group
1185 Avenue of the Americas
New York, NY 10036
212-782-3300
www.ablongman.com
An introduction to education for handicapped and gifted students. Presents research-based rationales for teaching exceptional students in the least restrictive environment. Provides historical perspectives, offers realistic descriptions of prevailing practices in the field, and reviews trends and new directions.
366 pages Paperback 1988
ISBN 0-582285-04-6

2198 Ages & Stages Questionnaires
Brookes Publishing
PO Box 10624
Baltimore, MD 21285
410-337-9580
800-638-3775
FAX: 410-337-8539
e-mail: custserv@brookespublishing.com
www.brookespublishing.com

Clary Creighton, Exhibits Coordinator
Tracy Gray, Educational Sales Manager
Paul Brooks, Owner
ASQ is an economical and field-tested system for identifying whether infants and young children may require further developmental evaluation and offers a screening and tracking program that helps early intervention professionals, service coordinators, and administrators maximize financial resources while promoting the health and growth of the children they serve. Set includes 11 color-coded, reproducible questionnaires, 11 reproducible, age appropriate scoring sheets. *$135.00*

2199 American College Testing Program
500 ACT Drive
PO Box 168
Iowa City, IA 52243
319-537-1028
FAX: 319-537-1014
www.act.org

Richard L Ferguson, Chief Executive Officer
Michael Eisenstein, President/COO
An independent, nonprofit organization that provides a variety of educational services to students and their parents, to high schools and colleges, and to professional associations and government agencies.

2200 Assessing Students with Special Needs
Longman Publishing Group
10 Bank Street
9th Floor
White Plains, NY 10606
914-993-5000
www.ablongman.com

Thomas Longman, Founder
Joanne Dresner, President
Step-by-step guide to informal, classroom assessment of students with special needs.
174 pages Paperback 1990
ISBN 0-801301-77-7

2201 Assessment Log & Developmental Progress Charts for the CCPSN
Brookes Publishing
PO Box 10624
Baltimore, MD 21285
410-337-9580
800-638-3775
FAX: 410-337-8539
e-mail: custserv@brookespublishing.com
www.brookespublishing.com

Clary Creighton, Exhibits Coordinator
Tracy Gray, Educational Sales Manager
Paul Brooks, Owner
This 28-page booklet allows readers to actually chart the ongoing progress of each preschool child. Available in packages of 10. *$22.00*

28 pages Saddle-stiched
ISBN 1-55766 -39-5

2202 Assessment of Learners with Special Needs
Allyn & Bacon
75 Arlington Street
Suite 300
Boston, MA 02116
617-848-6000
800-852-8024
FAX: 617-848-7490
www.ablongman.com

Nancy Forfyth, President
Thomas Longman, Founder
The central goal of this book is to help teachers become sophisticated, informed test consumers in terms of choosing, using and interpreting commercially prepared tests for their special needs students.
508 pages Casebound 1989
ISBN 0-205227-33-3

2203 Benchmark Measures
Educators Publishing Service
625 Mount Auburn Street
Suite 3
Cambridge, MA 02138
617-547-6706
800-225-5750
FAX: 888-440-2665
e-mail: feedback@epsbooks.com
www.epsbooks.com

Charles H Heinle, Vice President
Alexandra S Bigelow, Author
Gunnar Voltz, President
Ungraded test containing three sequential levels that assess alphabet and dictionary skills, reading, handwriting and spelling, and correspond to the first three schedules of the Alphabetic Phonics curriculum. The tests can be used at any level to measure a student's general knowledge of phonics. *$64.40*
Kit

2204 CREVT: Comprehensive Receptive and Expressive Vocabulary Test
Pro-Ed Publications
8700 Shoal Creek Boulevard
Austin, TX 78757
512-451-3246
800-897-3202
FAX: 800-397-7633
e-mail: feedback@proedinc.com
www.proedinc.com

Donald Hammill, Owner
Courtney King, Marketing Coordinator
A new, innovative, efficient measure of both receptive and expressive oral vocabulary. The CREVT has two subtests and is based on the most current theories of vocabulary development, suitable for ages 4 through 17. *$174.00*
Complete Kit

2205 Carolina Curriculum for Preschoolers with Special Needs
Brookes Publishing
PO Box 10624
Baltimore, MD 21285
410-337-9580
800-638-3775
FAX: 410-337-8539
e-mail: custserv@brookespublishing.com
www.brookespublishing.com

Clary Creighton, Exhibits Coordinator
Tracy Gray, Educational Sales Manager
Paul Brooks, Owner
This curriculum provides detailed teaching and assessment techniques, plus a sample 28-page Assessment Log that shows readers how to chart a child's individual progress. This guide is for children between 2 and 5 in their developmental stages who are considered at risk for developmental delay or who exhibit special needs. *$35.95*

352 pages Spiral-bound
ISBN 1-557660-32-8

2206 DAYS: Depression and Anxiety in Youth Scale
Pro-Ed Publications
8700 Shoal Creek Boulevard
Austin, TX 78757
512-451-3246
800-897-3202
FAX: 512-451-8542
e-mail: feedback@proedinc.com
www.proedinc.com

Donald Hammill, Owner
Courtney King, Marketing Coordinator
A unique battery of three norm-references scales useful in identifying major depressive disorder and overanxious disorders in children and adolescents. *$129.00*
Complete Kit

2207 DOCS: Developmental Observation Checklist System
Pro- Ed Publications
8700 Shoal Creek Boulevard
Austin, TX 78757
512-451-3246
800-897-3202
FAX: 800-397-7633
e-mail: feedback@proedinc.com
www.proedinc.com

Donald Hammill, Owner
Courtney King, Marketing Coordinator
A three-part system for the assessment of very young children with respect to general development, adjustment behavior and parent stress and support. *$124.00*

2208 Daytime Development Center
Joseph Willard Health Center
3750 Old Lee Highway
Fairfax, VA 22030
703-246-7100
FAX: 703-246-7307

Susan Delauter, Program Coordinator
Allan Phillips, Director Early Intervention
Cheryl Clatterbuck, Manager
Offers assessments, evaluations and educational/therapeutic infant programs for parents and their children.
Sliding Scale

2209 Developmental Services Center
Therapeutic Nursery Program
4525 Lee Street NE
Washington, DC 20019
202-388-3216
FAX: 202-576-8799

Alice Anderson
Offers assessment information and evaluation for developmentally delayed students.

2210 Frames of Reference for the Assessment of Learning Disabilities
Brookes Publishing
PO Box 10624
Baltimore, MD 21285
410-337-9580
800-638-3775
FAX: 410-337-8539
e-mail: custserv@brookespublishing.com
www.brookespublishing.com

Clary Creighton, Exhibits Coordinator
Tracy Gray, Educational Sales Manager
Paul Brooks, Owner
New views on measurement issues. Here you'll find an in=depth look at the fundamental concerns facing those who work with children with learning disabilities - assessment and identification. *$55.00*
672 pages Hardcover
ISBN 1-55766 -38-3

2211 How to Conduct an Assessment
FSSI
3905 Huntington Drive
Amarillo, TX 79109
806-853-1114
FAX: 806-353-1114
e-mail: webamster@winfssi.com
www.winfssi.com

Ed Hammer, Director

2212 Inclusive & Heterogeneous Schooling: Assessment, Curriculum, and Instruction
Brookes Publishing
PO Box 10624
Baltimore, MD 21285
410-337-9580
800-638-3775
FAX: 410-337-8539
e-mail: custserv@brookespublishing.com
www.brookespublishing.com

Clary Creighton, Exhibits Coordinator
Tracy Gray, Educational Sales Manager
Paul Brooks, Owner
Presents methods for successfully restructuring classrooms to enable all students, particularly those with disabilities, to flourish. Provides specific strategies for assessment, collaboration, classroom management, and age-specific instruction. *$34.95*
448 pages Paperback
ISBN 1-557662-02-9

2213 K-BIT: Kaufman Brief Intelligence Test
AGS
5910 Rice Creek Parkway
Suite 1000
Shoreview, MN 55126
651-287-7220
800-328-2560
FAX: 800-471-8457
e-mail: agsmail@agsnet.com
www.agsnet.com

Kevin Brueggeman, President
Robert Zaske, Market Manager
Quick and easy-to-use, KBIT assesses verbal and non-verbal abilities through two reliable subtests - vocabulary and matricies. *$ 124.95*
Ages 4-90

2214 K-FAST: Kaufman Functional Academic Skills Test
AGS
5910 Rice Creek Parkway
Suite 1000
Shoreview, MN 55126
651-287-7220
800-328-2560
FAX: 800-471-8457
e-mail: agsmail@agsnet.com
www.agsnet.com

Robert Zaske, Market Manager
Helps assess a person's capacity to function effectively in society regarding functional reading and math skills. *$99.95*
Ages 15-85+

2215 K-SEALS: Kaufman Survey of Early Academic and Language Skills
AGS
5910 Rice Creek Parkway
Suote 1000
Shoreview, MN 55126
651-287-7220
800-328-2560
FAX: 800-471-8457
e-mail: agsmail@agsnet.com
www.agsnet.com

Kevin Brueggeman, President
Robert Zaske, Market Manager
An individually administered test of children's of both expressive and receptive skills, pre-academic skills and articulation. K-SEALS offers reliable scores usually in less than 25 minutes. *$ 179.95*
Ages 3-0; 6-11

2216 KLST-2: Kindergarten Language Screening Test Edition, 2nd Edition
Pro-Ed
8700 Shoal Creek Boulevard
Austin, TX 78757
512-451-3246
800-897-3202
FAX: 800-397-7633
e-mail: feedback@proedinc.com
www.proedinc.com

Donald Hammill, Owner
Courtney King, Marketing Coordinator
Identifies children who need further diagnostic testing to determine whether or not they have language deficits that will accelerate academic failure. *$94.00*

2217 Kaufman Test of Educational Achievement (K-TEA)
AGS
PO Box 99
Circle Pines, MN 55014
800-328-2560
FAX: 800-471-8457
e-mail: agsmail@agsnet.com
www.agsnet.com

Robert Zaske, Marketing Manager
Kevin Brueggeman, President
K-TEA is an individually administered diagnostic battery that measures reading, mathematics, and spelling skills. Setting the standards in achievement testing today, K-TEA Comprehensive provides the complete diagnostic information you need for educational assessment and program planning. The Brief Forum is indispensable for school and clinical psychologists, special education teachers when a quick a measure of achievement is needed. *$249.95*

2218 Life Centered Career Education: A Contemporary Based Approach, 4th Edition
Council for Exceptional Children
1110 N Glebe Road
Suite 300
Arlington, VA 22201
703-245-0600
888-232-7733
FAX: 703-264-9494
e-mail: president@cec.sped.org
www.cec.sped.org

Janice Burdick, President
Bruce Ramirez, Manager
Provides a framework for building 97 functional skill competencies appropriate for preparing for adult life and special education students. *$28.00*
175 pages

2219 Measure of Cognitive-Linguistic Abilities (MCLA)
Speech Bin
1965 25th Avenue
Vero Beach, FL 32960
772-770-0007
800-477-3324
FAX: 772-770-0006
e-mail: info@speechbin.com
www.speechbin.com

Jan J Binney, Senior Editor
A diagnostic test of cognitive-linguistic abilities of adolescents and adults with traumatically induced brain injuries. High level. Normed. *$89.00*
100 pages
ISBN 0-93785 -72-

2220 ONLINE
West Virginia Research and Training Center
PO Box 1004
Institute, WV 25112
304-766-9495
800-624-8284
FAX: 304-766-2689
e-mail: info@icdi.wvu.edu
www.icdi.wvu.edu

Clifford Lantz, President
A quarterly newsletter offering information about hardware technology, software (commercial and home grown); applications that work and bonuses such as an exchange program for copyright-free software. *$25.00*
Quarterly

2221 OWLS: Oral and Written Language Scales LC/OE & WE
AGS
PO Box 99
Circle Pines, MN 55014
800-328-2560
FAX: 800-471-8457
e-mail: agsmail@agsnet.com
www.agsnet.com

Kevin Brueggeman, President
Robert Zaske, Market Manager

One kit provides an assessment of listening comprehension while the other assesses oral expression tasks: semantic, syntactic, pragmatic, and supralinguistic aspects of language. Written Expression may be administered individually or in small groups.
$249.95

2222 PAT-3: Photo Articulation Test
Pro-Ed Publications
8700 Shoal Creek Boulevard
Austin, TX 78757
512-451-3246
800-897-3202
FAX: 800-397-7633
e-mail: feedback@proedinc.com
www.proedinc.com

Joshua Jeffrey, Marketing Custodian
Courtney King, Marketing Coordinator
Barbara Lippke, Author
This test consists of 72 color photographs. The first 69 photos test consonants and all but one vowel and one diphthong. The remaining pictures test connected speech and the remaining vowel and diphthong. *$144.00*
Complete Kit

2223 Peabody Early Experiences Kit (PEEK)
AGS
PO Box 99
Circle Pines, MN 55014
800-328-2560
FAX: 800-471-8457
e-mail: agsmail@agsnet.com
www.agsnet.com

Kevin Brueggeman, President
Robert Zaske, Market Manager
1,000 activities and all the materials you need to build youngsters' cognitive, social and language skills. Manuals, puppets, manipulatives, picture card deck, picture mini decks and more to teach early development concepts. *$789.95*

2224 Peabody Individual Achievement Test-Revised Normative Update (PIAT-R-NU)
AGS
PO Box 99
Circle Pines, MN 55014
800-328-2560
FAX: 800-471-8457
e-mail: agsmail@agsnet.com
www.agsnet.com

Kevin Brueggeman, President
Robert Zaske, Market Manager
PIAT-R-NU is an efficient individual measure of academic achievement. Reading, mathematics, and spelling are assessed in a simple, non-threatening format that requires only a pointing response for most items. This multiple choice format makes the PIAT-R ideal for assessing individuals who hesitate to give a spoken response, or have limited expressive abilities. *$289.98*

2225 Peabody Language Development Kits (PLDK)
AGS
PO Box 99
Circle Pines, MN 55014
800-328-2560
FAX: 800-471-8457
e-mail: agsmail@agsnet.com
www.agsnet.com

Kevin Brueggeman, President
Robert Zaske, Market Manager
The main goals of the Peabody Kit language program are to stimulate overall language skills in Standard English and, for each level of the program, advance children's cognitive skills about a year. *$ 649.95*
Level P
ISBN 0-88671 -25-1

2226 Pediatric Early Elementary (PEEX II) Examination
Educators Publishing Service
625 Mount Auburn Street
Suite 3
Cambridge, MA 02138
617-547-6706
800-225-5750
FAX: 888-440-2665
e-mail: feedback@epsbooks.com
www.epsbooks.com

Charles H Heinle, Vice President
Alexandra S Bigelow, Author
Gunnar Voltz, President
Assesses the second-fourth grade child's performance on thirty-two tasks in six specific areas of development: fine-motor function, language, gross-motor function, memory, visual processing, and delayed recall. At three points during the exam, the child is rated on selective attention and behavior and effect.
$15.40 - $93
ISBN 0-83888 -80-6

2227 Pediatric Exam of Educational-PEERAMID Readiness at Middle Childhood
Educators Publishing Service
625 Mount Auburn Street
Suite 3
Cambridge, MA 02138
617-547-6706
800-225-5750
FAX: 888-440-2665
e-mail: feedback@epsbooks.com
www.epsbooks.com

Charles H Heinle, Vice President
Alexandra S Bigelow, Author
Gunnar Voltz, President
Assesses the 4th-10th grade child's performance on thirty-one tasks in six specific areas: minor neurological indicators, fine-motor function, language, gross-motor function, temporal-sequential organization, and visual processing. Complete set.
$15.40 - $109
ISBN 0-83888 -99-3

2228 Pediatric Examination of Educational Readiness
Educators Publishing Service
PO Box 9031
Cambridge, MA 02139
617-547-6706
800-225-5750
FAX: 888-440-2665
e-mail: feedback@epsbooks.com
www.epsbooks.com

Charles H Heinle, Vice President
Alexandra S Bigelow, Author
Gunnar Voltz, President
Assesses the Pre-1st grade child's performance on twenty-nine tasks in six specific areas of development: orientation, gross-motor, visual-fine motor, sequential, linguistic and preacademic learning. The child is rated on ten dimensions of selective attention/activity processing efficiency and adaptation. Complete set.
$12.85 - $86.40
ISBN 0-83888 -80-1

2229 Pediatric Extended Examination at-PEET Three
Educators Publishing Service
625 Mount Auburn Street
Suite 3
Cambridge, MA 02138
617-547-6706
800-225-5750
FAX: 888-440-2665
e-mail: feedback@epsbooks.com
www.epsbooks.com

Charles H Heinle, Vice President
Alexandra S Bigelow, Author
Gunnar Volta, President
Assesses the preschool-age child's performance on twenty-eight tasks in five basic areas of development: gross-motor, language, visual-fine motor, memory, and intersensory integration. Complete set.
$13.75 - $126
ISBN 0-83888 -79-4

2230 Pre-Reading Screening Procedures
Educators Publishing Service
625 Mount Auburn Street
Suite 3
Cambridge, MA 02138
617-547-6706
800-225-5750
FAX: 888-440-2665
e-mail: feedback@epsbooks.com
www.epsbooks.com

Charles H Heinle, Vice President
Alexandra S Bigelow, Author
Gunnar Voltz, President
This revised group test, for grades K-1, evaluates auditory, visual and kinesthetic strengths in order to identify children who may have some form of dyslexia or specific language disability.
$ 18.00
Grades K-1
ISBN 0-83885 -23-4

2231 Preparing for ACT Assessment
American College Testing Program
PO Box 168
Iowa City, IA 52243 319-337-1000
www.act.org

Richard L Ferguson, Chief Executive Officer
Designed to help high school students ready themselves for the ACT Assessment's subject area tests, explains the purposes of the four tests, describes their content and format, provides tips and exercises to improve student's test-taking skills and includes a complete sample text with scoring key.

2232 Psycho-Educational Assessment of Preschool Children
National Association of School Psychologists
4340 East West Highway
Suite 402
Bethesda, MD 20814 301-657-0270
866-331-NASP
FAX: 301-657-4155
This is a contributed text on assessing specific skills of preschool children.
592 pages

2233 RULES: Revised
Speech Bin
1965 25th Avenue
Vero Beach, FL 32960 772-770-0007
800-477-3324
FAX: 772-770-0006
e-mail: info@speechbin.com
www.speechbin.com

Jan J Binney, Senior Editor
Treatment program for young children who have phonological disorders. *$43.95*
280 pages
ISBN 0-93785 -51-3

2234 Receptive-Expressive Emergent-REEL-2 Language Test, 2nd Edition
Pro-Ed Publications
8700 Shoal Creek Boulevard
Austin, TX 78757 512-451-3246
800-897-3202
FAX: 800-397-7633
e-mail: feedback@proedinc.com
www.proedinc.com

Donald Hammill, Owner
Courtney King, Marketing Coordinator
A revision of the popular scale used for the multidimensional analysis of emergent language. The REEL-2 is specifically designed for use with a broad range of at risk infants and toddlers in the new multidisciplinary programs developing under P.L. 99-457. *$79.00*

2235 Slingerland Screening Tests
Educators Publishing Service
PO Box 9031
Cambridge, MA 02139 617-547-6706
800-435-7728
FAX: 888-440-2665
e-mail: feedback@epsbooks.com
www.epsbooks.com

Charles H Heinle, Vice President
Alexandra S Bigelow, Author
Gunnar Voltz, President
These tests, by Beth Slingerland, for individuals or groups of children, grades 1-6, identify children who show indications of having specific language disability in reading, handwriting, spelling or speaking. Form D evaluates personal orientation in time and space as well as the ability to express ideas in writing.
$14.80 - $27.45
ISBN 0-83882 -02-2

2236 Spatial Orientation and Sequencing Development Remedial Activities
Psychological & Educational Publications
PO Box 520
Hydesville, CA 95547
800-523-5775
FAX: 800-447-0907
e-mail: psych-edpublications@cox.net
www.psych-edpublications.com

Morrison Gardner, President
Designed to be used to remediate those children who perform poorly on any one or more activities of the Test of Pictures test.
$59.95

2237 Speech Bin
1965 25th Avenue
Vero Beach, FL 32960 772-770-0007
800-477-3324
FAX: 772-770-0006
e-mail: info@speechbin.com
www.speechbin.com

Jan J Binney, Senior Editor
Catalog offering test materials, assessment information, books and special education resources for speech-language pathologists, occupational and physical therapists, audiologists, and other rehabilitation professionals in schools, hospitals, clinics and private practices.

ISSN 4773-324

2238 Stuttering Severity Instrument for Children and Adults
Psychological & Educational Publications
PO Box 520
Hydesville, CA 95547 707-768-1807
800-523-5775
FAX: 800-447-0907
e-mail: psych-edpublications@cox.net
www.psych-edpublications.com

Morrison Gardner, President
With this tool teachers can determine whether to schedule a child for therapy or to evaluate the effects of treatment.

2239 Taking Part: Introducing Social Skills to Young Children
AGS
PO Box 99
Circle Pines, MN 55014
800-328-2560
FAX: 800-471-8457
e-mail: agsmail@agsnet.com
www.agsnet.com

Kevin Brueggeman, President
Robert Zaske, Market Manager
The first social skills curriculum to be linked directly to an assessment tool. More than 30 lessons correlate with the skills assessed by the Social Skills Rating System, a multirater approach to assessing prosocial and problem behaviors. *$149.95*

2240 Test Accommodations for Students with Disabilities
Charles C Thomas
2600 S 1st Street
Springfield, IL 62704 217-789-8980
800-258-8980
FAX: 217-789-9130
e-mail: books@ccthomas.com
www.ccthomas.com

Michael Thomas, President
Considers legal questions, theoretical issues, and practical methods for meeting the assessment needs of students with diabilities. The book is comprised of ten chapters and includes test accommodations topics relating to federal and state regulations (including the IDEA Amendments Act of 1997), problems concerning reliability and validity, and practical strategies for planning test accomodations and adapting and modifying tests.
$51.95

340 pages Paperback 1998
ISBN 0-398068-45-3

2241 **Test Critiques: Volumes I-X**
Pro-Ed Publications
8700 Shoal Creek Boulevard
Austin, TX 78757
512-451-3246
800-897-3202
FAX: 800-397-7633
e-mail: feedback@proedinc.com
www.proedinc.com

Donald Hammill, Owner
Courtney King, Marketing Coordinator
Provides the professional and nonprofessional with in-depth, evaluative studies of more than 800 of the most widely used of these assessment instruments. *$649.00*

2242 **Test of Early Reading Ability Deaf or Hard of Hearing**
Pro- Ed Publications
8700 Shoal Creek Boulevard
Austin, TX 78757
512-451-3246
800-897-3202
FAX: 800-397-7633
e-mail: feedback@proedinc.com
www.proedinc.com

Donald Hammill, Author/Owner
Courtney King, Marketing Coordinator
This adaptation of the TERA-2 for simultaneous communication of American Sign Language is the ONLY individually administered test of reading designed for children with moderate to profound sensory hearing loss. *$169.00*
Complete Kit

2243 **Test of Language Development: Primary**
Pro-Ed Publications
8700 Shoal Creek Boulevard
Austin, TX 78757
512-451-3246
800-897-3202
FAX: 800-397-7633
e-mail: feedback@proedinc.com
www.proedinc.com

Donald Hammill, Owner
Coutney King, Marketing Coordinator
TOLD P:2 and TOLD 1:2 are the most popular tests of spoken language used by clinicians today. They are used to identify children who have language disorders and to isolate the particular types of disorders they have. Primary Edition for ages 1-4 to 8-11: Intermediate Edition for ages 8-6 to 12-11.

2244 **Test of Mathematical Abilities, 2nd Editio n**
Pro-Ed Publications
8700 Shoal Creek Boulevard
Austin, TX 78757
512-451-3246
800-897-3202
FAX: 512-451-8542
e-mail: feedback@proedinc.com
www.proedinc.com

Donald Hammill, Owner
Courtney King, Marketing Coordinator
Elizabeth McEntire, Author
The latest version was developed for use in grades 3 through 12. It measures math performance on the two traditional major skill areas in math as well as attitude, vocabulary and general application of math concepts in real life. *$84.00*

2245 **Test of Nonverbal Intelligence, 3rd Editio n**
Pro-Ed Publications
8700 Shoal Creek Boulevard
Austin, TX 78757
512-451-3246
800-897-3202
FAX: 800-397-7633
e-mail: feedback@proedinc.com
www.proedinc.com

Donald Hammill, Owner
Courtney King, Marketing Coordinator
Susan K Johnson, Author
A language-free measure of intelligence, aptitude and reasoning. The administration of the test requires no reading, writing, speaking or listening on the part of the test subject. The items included in this test are problem-solving tasks that increase in difficulty. Each item presents a set of figures in which one or more components is missing. The test items include one or more of the characteristics of shape, position, direction, rotation, contiguity, shading, size, movement or pattern. *$229.00*
Complete Kit

2246 **Test of Phonological Awareness**
Pro-Ed Publications
8700 Shoal Creek Boulevard
Austin, TX 78757
512-451-3246
800-897-3202
FAX: 800-397-7633
e-mail: feedback@proedinc.com
www.proedinc.com

Donald Hammill, Owner
Courtney King, Marketing Coordinator
Measures young children's awareness of the individual sounds in words. Children who are sensitive to the phonological structure of words in oral language have a much easier time learning to read than children who are not. *$143.00*

2247 **Test of Written Spelling, 3rd Edition**
Pro- Ed Publications
8700 Shoal Creek Boulevard
Austin, TX 78757
512-451-3246
800-897-3202
FAX: 800-397-7633
e-mail: feedback@proedinc.com
www.proedinc.com

Donald Hammill, Owner
Courtney King, Marketing Coordinator
This revised edition assesses the student's ability to spell words whose spellings are readily predictable in sound-letter patterns, words whose spellings are less predictable and both types of words considered together. *$74.00*

2248 **Woodcock Reading Mastery Tests**
Pearson
5601 Green Valley Drive
Bloomington, MN 55437
800-627-7271
e-mail: pearsonassessments@pearson.com
www.pearsonassessments.com

Christine Carlson, Product Manager
The Woodcock Reading Mastery Tests - Revised provides an interpretive system and age range to help you assess reading skills of children and adults. Two forms, G and II, make it easy to test and retest, or you can combine the results of both forms for a more comprehensive assessment. Revised with recent updates. *$329.95*

2249 **Young Children with Special Needs: A Developmentally Appropriate Approach**
Allyn & Bacon
75 Arlington Street
Suite 300
Boston, MA 02116
617-848-6000
800-852-8024
FAX: 617-848-7490
www.ablongman.com

Nancy Forfyth, President
Thomas Longman, Founder
This book is designed to prepare students in making curriculum decisions in order to care for and foster the development of young children with special needs in normal early childhood settings.

270 pages
ISBN 0-20518 -94-X

Treatment & Training

2250 ABLE Program MCC-Longview
500 SW Longview Road
Lees Summit, MO 64081
816-672-2366
FAX: 816-672-2719
TTY:816-672-2144
e-mail: joan.bergstrom@mcckc.edu.edu
mcckc.edu

Joan Bergstrom, Director
Kay Owens, Administrative Assistant
Intensive support services program for post secondary students with neurological disabilities. The ABLE Program can be reached at http://mcclcc.edu/home.asp?qlinks=ABLE+Program+at+Longview+C=Z

2251 Academy for Guided Imagery
30765 Pacific Coast Highway
Suite 369
Malibu, CA 90265
800-726-2070
FAX: 800-727-2070
www.academyofguidedimagery.com

David E Bresler, President
Aims to teach people to access and use the power of the mind/body connection for healing and to further understanding of the imagery process in human life and development. Also to provide systematic training and guidance to health professionals who are interested in the use of Guided Imagery in their practice.

2252 Asthma & Allergy Education for Worksite Clinicians
Asthma and Allergy Foundation of America
1233 20th Street NW
Suite 402
Washington, DC 20036
202-466-7643
800-727-8462
FAX: 202-466-8940
e-mail: info@aafa.org
www.aafa.org

Bill McLin, Executive Director
Eileen Marcus, VP Marketing/Communications
Developed to teach health professionals in the worksite about asthma and allergies and ultimately improve the health of the employees who have theses de\iseases. The program gives worksite clinicians the knowledge and tools they need to give employees guidance on how to control environmental factors both in the home and in the workplace, self-manage thier asthma and/or allergies and to determaine if ti is necessary for employees to see an allergist if symptoms persist.

2253 Asthma & Allergy Essentials for Children's Care Provider
Asthma and Allergy Foundation of America
1233 20th Street NW
Suite 402
Washington, DC 20036
202-466-7643
800-727-8462
FAX: 202-466-8940
e-mail: info@aafa.org
www.aafa.org

Bill McLin, Executive Director
Course gives child care providers the tools and knowledge they need to care for children with asthma and allergies. During the interactive, three hour program, a trained health professional teaches providers how to recognize the signs and symptoms of an asthma or allergy episode, how to institute environmental control measures to prevent these episodes, and how to properly use medication and the tools for asthma management. In areas of the country serviced by AAFA's 14 chapters.

2254 Asthma Care Training for Kids (ACT)
Asthma and Allergy Foundation of America
1125 15th Street NW
Suite 502
Washington, DC 20005
202-466-7643
FAX: 202-466-8940
e-mail: info@aafa.org
www.aafa.org

Bill McLin, Executive Director
Interactive program for children ages seven to 12 and their families. Children and their families attend three group sessions seperately to learn their own unique styles and then come together at the end of each session to share their knowledge.

2255 Ayurvedic Institute
11311 Menaul Boulevard NE
Suite A
Albuquerque, NM 87112
505-291-9698
800-863-7721
FAX: 505-294-7572
e-mail: registrar@ayurveds.com
www.ayurveda.com

Vasant Lad, President/Chairman of the Board
Wynn Werner, Administrator
Directed by Dr. Vasant Lad, trains people in Ayurveda.

2256 East Brunswick Adult and Community Education Program
Adult Life Skills
380 Cranbury Road
E Brunswick, NJ 08816
732-613-6984
FAX: 732-390-6432
e-mail: bmethven@ebnet.org
www.ebnet.org

Bernadette Methven LSW, Project Coordinator
Wayne Dyer, Adult Education Administrator
Offers education, training, and social programs for adults with developmental disabilities in an integrated adult/evening school environment. Residents of Middlesex County, New Jersey, ages 18 and over are eligible to register. Limited transportation is also available. Annual enrollment fee $40.00.

2257 Harriet & Robert Heilbrunn Guild School
JGB Audio Library for the Blind
15 West 65th Street
New York, NY 10023
212-769-6331
FAX: 212-769-6266
e-mail: info@JGB.org
www.JGB.org

Peter Williamson, Executive Director
Ken Stanley, Manager

2258 Howard School
1192 Foster Street
Atlanta, GA 30318
404-377-7436
FAX: 404-377-0884
e-mail: kschuller@yahoo.com
www.howardschool.org

Keren Schuller, Director of Admissions
Marifred Cilella, Head of School
Sandra Kleinman, Executive Director
Enrolls students whose language-learning disabilities and differences hinder their learning to their fullest potential. Goal is to help students simultaneously build basic academi skills, maximize academic progress, develop higher level thinking skills, gain self-advocacy strategies and become independent life-long learners. Average class size is less than 12 students.

2259 Lake Michigan Academy
West Michigan Learning Disabilities Foundation
2428 Burton Street SE
Grand Rapids, MI 49546
616-464-3330
FAX: 616-285-1935
e-mail: info@wmldf.org
www.wmldf.org

Andrea Goetz, Executive Director
Is a private day school for children with learning disabilities.

2260 **Mad Hatters: Theatre That Makes a World of Difference**

PO Box 50002
Kalamazoo, MI 49005
FAX: 269-385-5868

Bobbe A Luce, Executive Director
A nationally-known theater which has presented effective and innovative programs to more than 175,000 people in over 1,150 performances in the past 15 years. Our presentations and training programs are a proven method of changing attitudes and behaviors. The Mad Hatters is a leader in the field of sensitivity training to build community and foster the inclusion of all people in society. Fees: $500-$4000 per program, depending on topic and audience.

2261 **Sandhills Academy**

1500 Hallbrook Drive
Columbia, SC 29209
803-695-1400
FAX: 803-695-1214
e-mail: info@sandhillsacademy.com
www.sandhillsacademy.com

Anne Vickers, Executive Director
Thrace Mears, Admissions Director
John W Weaver, Advancement Director
Exists to provide educational programs and intellectual development for average to above average students, six to 15, who learn differently and to promote the development of self-awareness, joy in learning and a vision of themselves as life-long learners.

2262 **Senior Program for Teens and Young Adults with Special Needs**

Camp J CC
6125 Montrose Road
Rockville, MD 20852
301-230-3759
FAX: 301-881-6549
e-mail: jcccamp@jccgw.org
www.jccgw.org

The senior Program is a transitional program for teens and young adults with mental retardation, severe learning disabilities and multiple disabilities. Socialization, recreation and independent living skills are enhanced ina fun enviroment. Activities include art, music, recreational swim and more.

2263 **Vanguard School**

Valley Forge Specialized Educational Services
1777 North Valley Road
PO Box 730
Paoli, PA 19301
610-296-6700
FAX: 610-640-0132
www.vanguardschool-pa.org

Ernest Brattstrom, Principal
James Kirkpatrick, Chief Financial Officer
Donna Annechino, Admissions Director
An Approved Private School (APS) for students aged 2.7-21 years with traumatic brain injury (TBI), social/emotional disturbance (SED) and/or autism/pervasive developmental disorder.

2264 **Worthmore Academy**

1301 North Riley Avenue
Indianapolis, IN 46201
317-253-5367
FAX: 317-253-5824
www.familyeducation.com/IN/worthmore_academy

Brenda Jackson, Director
Sandy Foster, Assistant Director
A center for learning disabilities providing educational assessments, alternative educational programs, academic guidance and public awareness services available as follows: full-time day school, K-8th, 1 to 1 teacher student ratio; six week summer school, K-12th, 1 to 1 teacher student ratio; after school tutoring; adult tutoring, educational assessments, counseling and educational seminars.
1988

General

2265 American Institute for Foreign Study
River Plaza
9 West Broad Street
Stamford, CT 06902
203-399-5000
866-906-2437
FAX: 203-399-5590
e-mail: info@aifs.com
www.aifs.org

Anthony Cook, Executive Director
Organizes cultural exchange programs throughout the world for more than 50,000 students each year and arranges insurance coverage for our own participants as well as participants of other organizations. Also provides summer travel programs overseas and in the US ranging from one week to a full academic year.

2266 American Universities International Programs
307 S College Avenue
Fort Collins, CO 80524
970-495-0869
888-730-2847
FAX: 970-484-6997
e-mail: info@auip.com
www.auip.com

Linda Detling, Program Coordinator AUIP
Study abroad organization sending students to universities in Australia and New Zealand.

2267 American-Scandinavian Foundation
58 Park Avenue
New York, NY 10016
212-879-9779
FAX: 212-879-2301
e-mail: info@amscan.org
www.amscan.org

Jean Prahl, Director Training
Promotes international understanding through educational and cultural exchange between the United States and Denmark, Finland, Iceland, Norway and Sweden.

2268 Antioch College
150 E. South College Street
Yellow Springs, OH 45387
937-769-1340
FAX: 937-769-1350
e-mail: aea@antioch-college.edu
www.antioch-college.edu

Nancy Wilburn, Executive Asst to the President
Richard Jurasek, President
Education abroad offers numerous programs which can be included in undergraduate and graduate study programs.

2269 Army and Air Force Exchange Services
PO Box 660202
Dallas, TX 75266
214-312-2011
FAX: 214-312-3429
www.aafes.com

Management Recruiter, Contact
Brings a tradition of value, service, and support to its 11.5 million authorized customers at military installations in the United States, Europe and in the Pacific.

2270 Association for International Practical Training
10400 Little Patuxent Parkway
Suite 250
Columbia, MD 21044
410-997-2200
FAX: 410-992-3924
e-mail: aipt@aipt.org
www.aipt.org

Elizabeth Chazottes, President
Elizabeth Chazottes, Chief Executive Officer
Nonprofit organization dedicated to encouraging and facilitating the exchange of qualified individuals between the US and other countries so they may gain practical work experience and improve international understanding.

2271 Basic Facts on Study Abroad
International Education
809 United Nations Plaza
New York, NY 10017
212-883-8200
FAX: 212-963-3489
e-mail: publications@un.org

Allen Goodman, Chief Executive Officer
Information book including foreign study planning, educational choices, finances and study abroad programs. *$35.00*
30 pages

2272 Beaver College
Arcadia University
450 S Easton Road
Glenside, PA 19038
215-572-2901
888-232-8379
FAX: 215-572-2174
e-mail: cea@beaver.edu
www.beaver.edu/cea

Lorna Stern, Deputy Director
One of the largest college-based study abroad programs in the country. Prices from $8000.00 semester to $22000.00 a year.

2273 Buffalo State (SUNY)
University College at Buffalo State
1300 Elmwood Avenue, SW 140
Buffalo, NY 14222
716-878-4620
FAX: 716-878-3054
e-mail: intleduc@buffalostate.edu
www.buffalostate.edu/studyabroad

Dennis Ponton, Vp Academic Affairs
Provides international educational exchange opportunities for students of university age and older through its Office of International Education.

2274 Building Bridges: Including People with Disabilities in International Programs
Mobility International USA
132 East Broadway,Suite 343
Eugene, OR 97401
541-343-1284
FAX: 541-343-6812
e-mail: info@miusa.org
www.miusa.org

Susan Sygall, CEO/Executive Director
Empowers people with disabilities around the world through international exhange and international development to achieve their human rights. The international exchange programs usually last two-four weeks and are held throughout the year in the US and abroad. Activities include living with homestay families, leadership seminars, disability rights workshops, cross cultural learning and teambuilding activities such as river rafting and challenging courses.

2275 Davidson College, Office of Study Abroad
Davidson College
PO Box 7171
Davidson, NC 28035
704-894-2240
FAX: 704-892-2120
e-mail: kocampbell@davidson.edu
www.davidson.edu/academic/sasian/application.

Thomas W Ross Sr., President
Recognizes the value of study abroad for both the devlopment of worl understanding and the development of the student as a broadminded, objective and mature individual.

2276 High School Students Guide to Study, Travel, and Adventure Abroad
7 Custom House Street 3rd Floor
Portland, ME 04101
207-553-7600
FAX: 207-553-7600
e-mail: studyinfo@ciee.org
www.ciee.org

Cheryl Jeffries, Administrative Assistant

This guide provides high school students with all the information they need for a successful trip abroad. Included are sections to help students find out if they're ready for a trip abroad, make the necessary preparations and get the most from their experience. Over 200 programs are described including language study, summer camps, homestays, study tours and work camps. The program descriptions include information for people with disabilities.

ISSN 0312-11

2277 Higher Education Consortium for Urban Affairs (HECUA)

2233 University Avenue W
Suite 210
Saint Paul, MN 55114
651-646-8831
FAX: 651-659-9421
e-mail: info@hecua.org
www.hecua.org

Haroun Er. Rashid, Professor

HECUA offers college-level off-campus study programs in Latin America, Asia, Europe and the U.S. Internships, field projects and other forms of experimental learning are combined with academic study. Programs focus on issues of inequality and ways to bring about positive social change. HECUA has thirty years of experience and a national reputation for the best in teaching and learning that engages students in meaningful study and action. Students with disabilities welcome to apply.

2278 International Christian Youth Exchange

134 W 26th Street
New York, NY 10001
212-206-7307
FAX: 212-633-9085

Ed Gragert

Offers participants a unique experience to learn about another culture and make friends from different countries.

2279 International Partnership for Service-Learning and Leadership

815 2nd Avenue
New York, NY 10017
212-986-0989
FAX: 212-986-5039
e-mail: info@ipsl.org
www.ipsl.org

Nevin Brown, President

A not for profit educational organization incorporated in New York State serving students, colleges, universities, service agenices and related organizations around the world by fostering programs that link volunteer service to the community and academic study.

1982

2280 International University Partnerships

University of Pennsylvania
1011 South Drive
Indiana, PA 15705
724-357-2295
FAX: 724-357-2514
www.iup.edu

Dr. Robert Morris

Offers a variety of international educational exchange programs to students who wish to study overseas.

2281 Lake Erie College

Academic Programs Abroad
Painesville, OH 44077
440-352-3361
FAX: 440-352-3533
www.lec.edu

Catherine Shaw
Harold Laydon, President

Sends students abroad for a term or longer to develop intellectual awareness and individual maturity.

2282 Lane Community College

4000 E 30th Avenue
Eugene, OR 97405
541-463-3000
www.lanecc.edu

Larry Tardie, Chair

To be a learning centered community college that provides affordable, quality, lifelong educational opportunities that include: professional technical and lower division college transfer programs, employess skill upgrading, business development and career enhancement, foundational academic, language and life skills development, lifelong personal development and enrichment, and cultural and community services.

2283 Lions Clubs International

300 W 22nd Street
Oak Brook, IL 60523
630-571-5466
FAX: 630-571-8890
e-mail: districtadministration@lionsclub.org
www.lionsclubs.org

Mahendra Amarasuriya, International President

Over 46,000 individual clubs in over 194 countries and geographical areas which provide community service and promote better international relations. Clubs work with local communities to provide needed and useful programs for sight, diabetes and hearing.

2284 Lisle

900 County Road 269
Leander, TX 78641
800-477-1538
e-mail: lisle2@io.com
www.lisle.utoledo.edu

Barbara Bratton, Executive Director

Educational organization which works toward world peace and better quality of human life through increased understanding between persons of similar and different cultures.

2285 National 4-H Council

7100 Connecticut Avenue
Chevy Chase, MD 20815
301-961-2800
FAX: 301-961-2894
www.fourhcouncil.edu

Jill Bramble, Director National Partnerships

National, private sector non profit partner of 4-H and the Cooperative Extenisive System. Also manages the National 4-H Conference Center, which is a full service conference facility, and the National 4-H Supply Service which is the authorized agent for items bearing the 4-H name and emblem. Partners with 4-H at all levels national,state and local and provides training and support, curriculum development, fostering innovative programming and facilitating meetings and connections.

2286 New Directions for People with Disabilities

5276 Hollister Avenue
Suite 207
Santa Barbara, CA 93111
805-967-2841
FAX: 805-964-7344
e-mail: info@newdirectiontravel.org
www.newdirectionstravel.org

Dee Duncan, Executive Director/Founder

Provides high quality local, national, and international travel vacations and holiday programs for people with mild to moderate developmental disabilities. Through these programs, people with disabilities are increasingly understood, appreciated and more accepted as important and contributing members of our world.

2287 People to People International

501 E Armour Boulevard
Kansas City, MO 64109
816-531-4701
FAX: 816-561-7502
e-mail: ptpi@ptpi.org
www.ptpi.org

Mary Eisenhowser, President/CEO
Marc L Bright, Deputy CEO/Executive VP
Tracy Geise, Executive Assistant

Exchanges international understanding and friendship through educational, cultural and humantarian activities involving the exchange of ideas and experiences directly among people of different countries and diverse cultures. Is also dedicated to enhancing cross cultural communication within each communityand across communities and nations.

2288 **Rotary Youth Exchange**
Rotary International
One Rotary Center
1560 Sherman Ave.
Evanston, IL 60201
847-866-3000
FAX: 847-328-8554
www.rotary.org

Carl Wilhelm Stenhammar, International President
Wilfrid J. Wilkinson, President
Rotary a worlwide organization of business and professional leaders that provides humanitarian service, encourages high ethical standards in all vocations, and helps build goodwill and peace in the world. Approximately 1.2 million Rotarians belong to more than 31,000 Rotary clubs located in 167 countries.

2289 **Scandinavian Seminar**
24 Dickinson Street
Amherst, MA 01002
413-253-9736
FAX: 413-253-5282
e-mail: study@scandinavianseminar.org
www.scandinavianseminar.org

Jacqueline D Waldman, Chief Executive Officer
Student exchange program founded in 1949.

2290 **Sister Cities International**
1301 Pennsylvania Avenue NW
Suite 850
Washington, DC 20004
202-347-8630
FAX: 202-393-6524
e-mail: info@sister-cities.org
www.sister-cities.org

Patrick Madden, Executive Director
A non profit citizen diplomacy netowrk creating and strengthening partnerships between US and international communities in an effort to increase global cooperation at the municipal level, to promote cultural understnading and to stimulate economic development. Also leads the movement for local community development and volunteer action by motivating and empowering private citizens, municipal officials and business leaders to conduct long term programs of mutual benefits.

2291 **Southern Illinois University at Carbondale**
Washington Square D-Mail Code 6716
707 S Washington Street
Carbondale, IL 62901
618-453-4551
FAX: 618-453-4832
e-mail: twoolf@siu.edu
www.siuc.du

Fernando M. Trevino, Chancellor
Main emphasis in international programs abroad is school-to-school direct exchanges and exchanges through organizations such as the International Student Exchange Program.

2292 **State University of New York**
1400 Washington Avenue
Albany, NY 12222
518-442-5435
FAX: 518-442-5383
e-mail: ugadmissions@albany.edu
www.albany.edu

Kermit L Hall, President
Robert Andrea, Director of Undergraduate Adm.
Offers over 150 international educational exchange programs in 37 different countries. Broad mission of excellence in undergraduate and graduate education, research and public service engages 17,000 diverse students in nine schools and colleges across three campuses.

2293 **University of Minnesota at Crookston**
170 Owen Hall
2900 University Ave.
Crookston, MN 56716
218-281-6510
800-862-6466
FAX: 218-281-8050
e-mail: umcinfo@umn.edu
www.crk.umn.edu

Amber Evans-Dailey, Director of Admissions
A four-year college with innovative educational programs for the acquisition of technical skills and a liberal arts education.

2294 **University of Oregon**
5000 N Willamette Boulevard
Portland, OR 97203
503-943-8000
e-mail: webmaster@up.edu
www.up.edu

Jason McDonald, Dean of Admissions
Study/cultural experience is available in Tokyo and other Japanese cities as part of the Japan Studies Program at the University.

2295 **University of Oregon International Service**
1217 University Of Oregon
Eugene, OR 97403
541-346-1323
FAX: 541-346-5815
e-mail: dsaluski@uoregon.edu
www.uoregon.edu

Dave Frohmayer, President
International programs offered through the University of Oregon offer participants the opportunity to gain academic, cultural, and personal experience.

2296 **Western Washington University**
516 High Street
Bellingham, WA 98225
360-650-3353
FAX: 360-650-6555
www.wwu.edu

Karen Morse, President
Nurtures the intellectual, ethical, social, physical and emotional development of each student. It aims to teach learning skills useful in a rapidly changing and highly technical world to develop a consciousness of the challenges and responsibilities of living in a diverse and pluralistic society.

2297 **World Experience**
2440 S Hacienda Boulevard
Suite 116
Hacienda Heights, CA 91745
626-330-5719
800-633-6653
FAX: 626-330-5719
e-mail: weworld@worldexperience.org
www.worldexperience.org

Bobby Fraker, President
Offers a quality and affordable program for over two decades and continues to provide students and host families a youth exchange program based on individual attention, with the help of an international network of overseas directors and USA coordinators

2298 **World of Options**
Mobility International USA
132 E Broadway
Suite 343
Eugene, OR 97401
541-343-1284
FAX: 541-343-6812
e-mail: info@miusa.org
www.miusa.org

Susan Sygall, Executive Director
Empowering people with disabilities around the world through international exchange and international development to achieve their human rights. *$16.00*
338 pages
ISBN 1-880034-01-8

2299 **World of Options: A Guide to International Educational Exchange**
Mobility International USA
132 E. Broadway
Suite 343
Eugene, OR 97401
541-343-1284
FAX: 541-343-6812
e-mail: info@miusa.org
www.miusa.org

Susan Sygall, Executive Director

A Guide to International Educational Exchange, Community Service and Travel for People with Disabilities includes information travel and international programs, as well as personal experience stories from people with disabilities who have had successful international experiences. *$45.00*

600 pages 1997

ISBN 1-880034-24-7

2300 Youth for Understanding International Exchange

6400 Goldsboro Road
Suite 100
Bethesda, MD 20817
240-235-2100
FAX: 240-352-2104
e-mail: admissions@yfu.org
www.youthforunderstanding.org

Rachel Andreson, Founder
Samantha Brizzolara, Chair

Youth for Understanding (YFU) International Exchange, an educational, nonprofit organization, prepares young people for the opportunities and responsabilities in a changing, independent world. With YFU, students can choose a year, semenster, or summer program in one or more than 35 countries worldwide. More than 200,000 young people from more than 50 nations in Asia, Europe, North and South America, Africa and the Pacific have participated in YFU exchanges.

Alabama

2301 **Alabama Power Foundation**
600 18th Street N
17th Floor
Birmingham, AL 35203
205-326-8002
800-245-2244
FAX: 205-226-1441

Charles McCrary, Chief Executive Officer
Giving is limited to Alabama. No support is given for religious or political organizations, individuals or for operating funds that duplicate the United Way support.

2302 **Andalusia Health Services**
1208 West Bypass
Po Box 667
Andalusia, AL 36420
334-222-2030
FAX: 334-222-7844
e-mail: patty.ashworth@lifepointhospitals.com
www.andalusiachamber.com

Patty Ashworth, President
Dr. Ed Meadows, Executive Vice President
Daniel McMullen, Treasurer
Only offers grants to the residents of Covington County in Alabama who are pursuing a degree in a medical field.

2303 **Arc of Alabama**
Arc of United Inc.
300 S Hull Street
Montgomery, AL 36104
334-262-7688
866-243-9557
FAX: 334-834-9737
e-mail: info@thearcofalabama.com
www.thearcofalabama.com

Mike Sullivan, President
Leland Conner, Director
Tom Holmes, Executive Director
The Arc of Alabama is committed to securing for all people with mental retardation the opportunity to choose and realize their goals in regard to where and how they learn, live, work and play.

2304 **Blount Foundation**
4520 Executive Park Drive
Montgomery, AL 36116
334-244-4348

http://www.arhaonline.org/

D Joseph McInnes
Established in 1970, the Foundation was created to serve as the voice with which the Blount Companies address the need to provide financial assistance to a variety of activities and programs concerned with the general welfare of our country and its citizens. The Foundation has a strong commitment to corporate citizenship and endorses the concept that companies, as well as individuals, must contribute to the well-being of society.

Alaska

2305 **Arc of Alaska**
The Arc Of Anchorage
2211 Arca Drive
Anchorage, AK 99508
907-277-6677
800-258-2232
FAX: 907-272-2161
www.arc-anchorage.org

Gwen Lee, Chief Executive Officer

2306 **Rasmuson Foundation**
301 W Northern Lights Boulevard
Suite 400
Anchorage, AK 99503
907-297-2700
877-366-2700
FAX: 907-297-2770
e-mail: rasmusonfdn@rasmuson.org
www.rasmuson.org

Diane Kaplan, President
Jeff Clarke, Vice Presaident
Grants for Alaska 501C3 nonprofits only.

Arizona

2307 **Arizona Community Foundation**
2201 E Camelback Road
Suite 202
Phoenix, AZ 85016
602-381-1400
800-222-8221
FAX: 602-381-1575
e-mail: rking@azfoundation.org/
www.azfoundation.org

Robert L. King, President And Ceo
Deborah Whitehurst, Chief Operating Officer
Patricia Gardner, Executive Assistant

2308 **Arizonia Autism Resources**
The Arc Of Arizonia
5610 S Central Avenue
Phoenix, AZ 85040
602-243-1787
800-252-9054
www.autism-pdd.net/

Richard Young, Executive Director
The Arc, a national organization on mental retardaion, is committed to securing for all people with developmental disabilities the opportunity to choose and realize their goals in regard to where they live, learn, work and play.

2309 **Margaret T Morris Foundation**
PO Box 592
Prescott, AZ 86302
928-445-4010

http://www.archive.naccho.org/

Eugene P Polk, Trustee

Arkansas

2310 **Arc of Arkansas**
2004south Main Street
Little Rock, AR 72204
501-375-7770
FAX: 501-372-4621
www.arcark.org

Steve Hitt, Executive Director

2311 **Roy and Christine Sturgis Charitable Trust**
PO Box 7599
Little Rock, AR 72217
501-337-5109

Physically disabled, hospitals, child welfare and visually impaired are priorities of giving for this foundation.

2312 **Winthrop Rockefeller Foundation**
308 E 8th Street
Little Rock, AR 72202
501-376-6854
FAX: 501-374-4797
e-mail: webfeedback@wrfoundation.org
http://www.wrfoundation.org/

Sherece West, President

Mission is to improve the quality of life in Arkansas. It focuses its grantmaking efforts in three areas: education, economic development and civic affairs. Education projects funded in the past have included grants to schools that are working to involve teachers and parents in making decisions about what happens at their schools, projects that work to remove prejudice from the educational process and more. Major grants are made to support the development of new programs.

California

2313

2314 **Ahmanson Foundation**
9215 Wilshire Boulevard
Beverly Hills, CA 90210 310-278-0770
e-mail: info@theahmansonfoundation.org
http://www.theahmansonfoundation.org/

Leonard Walcott, Managing Director
Robert Ahmanson, President
The Foundation primarily gives in Southern California with major emphasis in Los Angeles County. The Foundation focuses on the arts and humanities, education, mental health and support for a broad range of social welfare programs.

2315 **Alice Tweed Touhy Foundation**
205 E Carrillo Street
Suite 219
Santa Barbara, CA 93101 805-962-6430

Harris Seed, President
Eleanor Van Cott, Executive VP
Rehabilitation, recreation and building funds are given to organizations only within the Santa Barbara area.

2316 **Alternating Hemiplegia of Childhood Foundation**
239 Nevada Street
Redwood City, CA 94062 650-365-5798
888-225-3353
FAX: 650-365-5798
e-mail: laegan6@sbcglobal.net
www.ahckids.org

Lynn Egan, Vice President
Voluntary not-for-profit organizations dedicated to promoting professional and public awareness of Alternating Hemiplegia of Childhood (AHC) and providing current information to affected individuals and their families. Supports ongoing medical research into the cause, treatment and potential cure of AHC. Disseminates information about this disorder to promote proper diagnosis and maintains a registry of families, affected chidren and physicians who are familiar with AHC.

2317 **Amateur Athletic Foundation of Los Angeles**
La84 Foundation
2141 W Adams Boulevard
Los Angeles, CA 90018 323-730-4600
FAX: 323-730-9637
e-mail: info@la84foundation.org
www.la84foundation.org

Anita Defrantz, President
Enables AAF to serve as an educational and research center for sport— a leading forum for the advancement of coaching, the exchange of ideas and exploration of important issues in sport.

2318 **Annuziata Sanguinetti Foundation**
420 Montgomery Street
5th Floor
San Francisco, CA 94104 415-477-1000

Eugene Ranghiasci
Hard-of-hearing, speech impaired and recreation. Serves only the San Francisco Bay area.

2319 **Apple Computer**
Worldwide Disability Solutions Group
2851 Park Avenue
Santa Clara, CA 95050 408-996-1010
800-692-7753
TTY:800-755-0601

Steven Jobs, Chief Executive Officer
Offers grants in the areas of education, health and in areas of company operations.

2320 **Arc of California**
1225 8th Street
Suite 210
Sacramento, CA 95814 916-552-6619
800-698-6619
e-mail: arcca@arccalifornia.org
www.arccalifornia.org

Shirley Dove, President
Pat Heineke, VP

2321 **Atkinson Foundation**
1720 S Amphlett Boulevard
Suite 100
San Mateo, CA 94402 650-357-1101
FAX: 650-357-1101
e-mail: atkinfdn@aol.com
www.atkinsonfdn.org

Elizabeth Curtis, Administrator
The Foundation focuses and awards grants to community service and civic organizations serving the residents of San Mateo County, California through programs that benefit children, youth, seniors, the disadvantaged and those in need of rehabilitation. Grants are also made to local churches and schools, and overseas for sustainable development, health education and family planning. No grants to individuals or for research, travel, special events, annual campaigns, media and publications.

2322 **Baker Commodities Corporate Giving Program**
4020 Bandini Boulevard
Los Angeles, CA 90023 323-268-2801
FAX: 323-268-5160
www.bakercommodities.com

James Andreoli, President

2323 **Bank of America Foundation**
315 Montgomery Street
8th Floor
San Francisco, CA 94104 415-622-3456
888-488-9802
FAX: 704-386-6444
www.bankamerica.com/foundation

Caroline Boitano
The Foundation will consider grants in four categories including: Health & Human Services, which provides support to health & human service organizations primarily through grants to the United Way campaigns; Education, with the focus on preparing people to become productive employees and participating citizens; Conservation & Environment, the improvement of California communities for the benefit of their citizens; and Culture & The Arts, supporting the leading performing and visual arts groups.

2324 **Bergen Brunswig Corporation Contributions Program**
4000 W Metropolitan Drive
Orange, CA 92868 714-385-1077
800-442-3040
FAX: 714-385-6948
www.amerisourceburgen.com

Jeanne Fisher, Executive Vice President

2325 **Blind Babies Foundation**
1200 Gough Street
San Francisco, CA 94109 415-922-9185
FAX: 415-771-9026

Dennak Murphy, Executive Director
Ken Gardner, Owner

Founded in 1949, provides services and programs that enable and empower families, professionals and the broader community to meet the unique needs of infants and preschool children who are blind or visually impaired. *$5.00*

2326 Bothin Foundation

1660 Bush Street
300
San Francisco, CA 94109 415-561-6540
FAX: 415-771-4064

Lyman J Casey, Executive Director
Eric Sloan, Manager
The broad purpose of this foundation is to support public charities located in the five counties of San Francisco, Marin, Sonoma, San Mateo and Santa Barbara. Bothin elects to support charitable organizations that promote youth, elderly, disabled, health care, minorities, community social services and the environment. Grants for the arts are made mainly to those groups predominantly serving youth or with heavy emphasis on youth participation.

2327 Briggs Foundation

PO Box 1510
Rancho Santa Fe, CA 92067 858-756-4875

Blaine A Briggs

2328 Burns-Dunphy Foundation

5 3rd Street
Suite 1200
San Francisco, CA 94103 415-421-6995
FAX: 415-882-7774

Walter Gleason
Cressey Nakagawa
Grants are given to promote wellness for the visually impaired, physically and mentally disabled and to promote research in these areas.

2329 California Community Foundation

445 S Figueroa Street
Suite 3400
Los Angeles, CA 90071 213-413-4130
FAX: 213-383-2046
e-mail: info@ccf-la.org
www.calfund.org

Jane Eisner, President
Areas of funding priority include grants for the disabled, child welfare, rehabilitation, developmentally disabled, employment projects, research and computer projects. Giving is limited to the greater Los Angeles area.

2330 California Endowment

1000 N Alameda Street
Los Angeles, CA 90012
800-449-4149
FAX: 213-928-8801
e-mail: questions@calendow.org
www.calendow.org

Arthur Chen, Chair of Board
Daniel Boggan, Vice Chair
California Endowment's mission is to expand access to affordable, quality health care for underserved individuals and communities, and to promote fundamental improvements in the health status of all Californians.

2331 Carrie Estelle Doheny Foundation

707 Wilshire Boulevard
Suite 4960
Los Angeles, CA 90017 213-488-1122
FAX: 213-448-1544
e-mail: doheny@dohenyfoundation.org
dohenyfoundation.org

Robert A Smith III, President
Nina S Shepherd, Chief Administrstive Officer

2332 Clorox Company Foundation East Bay Community Foundation

Dedomenico Building
200 Frank Ogawa Plaza
Oakland, CA 94612 510-836-3223
e-mail: cloroxfndt@eastbaycf.org
www.thecloroxcompany.com

Donald R Knauss, Ceo
Lawrence Peiros, Executive Vice President
Community Support Programs are offered to make the communities in which we live and work stronger, while providing measurable benefits to the Company and its shareholders. The Foundation's primary concern continues to be youth and K-12 education. The Foundation is helping our young people to improve their educational and job skills and develop their leadership potential.

2333 Coeta and Donald Barker Foundation

PO Box 936
Rancho Mirage, CA 92270 760-324-2656
http://archieve.naccho.org

Coeta Barker, Owner
Nancy Harris, Executive Admin
It is an independent organization that gives its attention to organizations that are charitable or nonprofit under the laws of the state of Oregon or California.

2334 Community Foundation of Santa Clara County

111 W Saint John Street
Suite 230
San Jose, CA 95113 408-264-2437

Peter Hero
Visually impaired, mentally and physically disabled, hard-of-hearing, special education, mental health and employment projects are areas of priority. Giving is limited to Santa Clara and surrounding counties.

2335 Crescent Porter Hale Foundation

655 Redwood Highway
Suite 301
Mill Valley, CA 94941 415-388-2333
http://compasspoint.org

Ulla Davis, Grants Administrator
Serves organizations in the San Francisco Bay Area who are involved in the following areas of concern: education in the fields of art and music; private elementary, high school and university education; capital funding; and other worthwhile programs which can be demonstrated as serving broad community purposes, leading toward the improvement of the quality of life.

2336 Darrow Foundation

1000 4th Street
Suite 570
San Rafael, CA 94901 415-453-0534
http://www.grantsca.com

Dewitt K Macdonald, Director
Peter Mitchell, Partner
Grants are given in the areas of child welfare, visually impaired, projects involving independence, mentally and physically disabled.

2337 David and Lucile Packard Foundation

300 2nd Street
Suite 200
Los Altos Hills, CA 94022 650-948-7658
www.packard.org

Carol Larson, President And Ceo
Brad Colby, Executive Assistant To Ceo

This foundation provides grants to nonprofit organizations in the following areas: conservation; population; science; children, familes, and communities; arts and organizational effectiveness; and philanthropy. It provides national and international grants and also has a special focus on the Northern California Counties.

2338 Deutsch Foundation

5454 Beethoven Street
Los Angeles, CA 90066
310-862-3000
877-340-7700
FAX: 310-862-3100
www.deutschinc.com

Mike Sheldon, Manager
Learning disabled, visually impaired, mental health, eye research, child welfare, speech and hearing impaired, physically disabled and independence projects are funded through this Foundation. Giving is limited to California.

2339 East Bay Community Foundation

De Domenico Building
200 Frank Ogawa Plaza
Oakland, CA 94612
510-836-3223
FAX: 510-836-3287
e-mail: areese@eastbaycf.org
http://www.ebcf.org

Sara Dubois, Director of Developement
A collection of funds created by many people, organizations and businesses, the Foundation helps those people and groups to support effective nonprofit organizations to the East Bay and beyond.

2340 Evelyn and Walter Hans Jr

1 Lombard Street
Suite 305
San Francisco, CA 94111
415-398-4474
FAX: 415-986-4779

Ira Hirschfield, President
Pamela David, Executive Director
A private foundation interested in programs which assist people who are hungry, homeless, or at risk of homelessness; enable older adults to maintain independent lives in the community and support Hispanic community development in San Francisco's Mission District. The Foundation also encourages proposals for corporate social responsibility efforts within the business community.

2341 Financial Aid for Study and Training Abroad

Reference Service Press
5000 Windplay Drive
Suite 4
El Dorado Hills, CA 95762
916-939-9620
FAX: 916-939-9626
e-mail: info@rspfunding.com
www.rspfunding.com

Gail Ann Schlachter, President
R David Weber, Editor In Chief
Sandy Perez, Business Manager
This directory, which Children's Bookwatch calls invaluable describes more than 1,100 financial aid opportunities available to support study abroad. Updated every 2 years. *$39.50*
300 pages
ISBN 1-588410-31-5

2342 Fireman's Fund Foundation

Firemans Fund Insurance Companies
777 San Marin Drive
Novato, CA 94998
415-899-2000
800-227-1700
FAX: 415-899-3600
e-mail: smurdy1@ffic.com
www.firemansfund.com

Susan Murdy, Executive Director
Provides discretionary grants to the disabled only in Marin and Sonoma counties in the San Francisco Bay area.

2343 Fred Gellert Foundation

95 Harriet Way
Tiburon, CA 94920
415-381-7575
FAX: 415-381-8526
e-mail: foundation@fredgellert.com
http://www.foundationcenter.org

Fred Gellert Jr, Chairman
Focuses on organizations and programs serving residents of San Mateo and San Francisco and Marin counties in California, with the exception of environmentally concerned organizations.

2344 Gallo Foundation

PO Box 1130
Modesto, CA 95353
209-579-3204
FAX: 209-341-3307
http://www.fundsnetservices.com

John Gallo, Senior VP Operations
Physically and mentally disabled, child welfare, Special Olympics, United Cerebral Palsy and Easter Seal Society are among the grants provided by this foundation.

2345 Glaucoma Research Foundation

251 Post Street
Suite 600
San Francisco, CA 94108
415-986-3162
800-826-6693
FAX: 415-986-3763
e-mail: question@glaucoma.org
www.glaucoma.org

Deirdre Porter, Executive Vice President
A national organization dedicated to protecting the sight of people with glaucoma through research and education. The Foundation conducts and supports research that contributes to improved patient care and a better understanding of the disease process. Provides education, advocacy and emotional support to patients and their families.

2346 Harden Foundation

PO Box 779
Salinas, CA 93902
831-442-3005

e-mail: jgrainger@hardenfoundation.org
www.hardenfoundation.org

Joseph C Grainger, Executive Director

2347 Harry and Grace Steele Foundation

441 N Newport Boulevard
Suite 30
Newport Beach, CA 92663
949-631-0418
FAX: 949-631-1255

Marie Kowert, Manager
Gives grants to qualified tax-exempt charitable organizations which are not private foundations. Tax-supported organizations of any kind, and applications from individuals are not accepted. Grants are made for altruistic purposes, charitable, benevolent or educational, primarily local giving.

2348 Henry J Kaiser Family Foundation

2400 Sand Hill Road
Menlo Park, CA 94025
650-854-9400
FAX: 650-854-4800
www.kff.org

Drew Altman, President/CEO
Sheila Burke, Chief Operating Officer
Tom Campbell, Professor of Business

2349 Henry W Bull Foundation

Santa Barbara Bank & Trust
PO Box 2340
Santa Barbara, CA 93120
805-564-6211
FAX: 805-884-1404

Janice Gibbons, VP/Senior Trust Officer
Alexia Quinn, Sr Trust Admin Assistant

Grant given to a wide range of organizations that include those which provide services for the disabled; arts, education, services for elderly and youth grants awarded two times a year. Grant size ranges from $500 to $5,000. Proposal deadlines April 1, Sept 1.

2350 Irvine Health Foundation

18301 Von Karman Avenue
Irvine, CA 92612
949-253-2959
e-mail: info@ihf.org
www.ihf.org

Edward B Kacic, President
Partricia Meredith, Program Director

2351 Joseph Drown Foundation

1999 Avenue of the Stars
Suite 2330
Los Angeles, CA 90067
310-277-4488
FAX: 310-277-4573
e-mail: staff@jdrown.org
www.jdrown.org

Norman Obrow, President
Giving is focused primarily in California. No support for religious purposes or to individuals.

2352 Junior Blind of America

5300 Angeles Vista Boulevard
Los Angeles, CA 90043
323-295-4555
800-352-2290
FAX: 323-296-0424
e-mail: info@juniorblind.org
www.juniorblind.org

Miki Jordan, President
Junior Blind provides programs and services for children and adults who are blind or visually impaired and their families to achieve independence and self-esteem. Progrmas include; Camp Bloomfield, Visions: Adventures in Learning, Infant-Family Program, Special Education School, Children's Residential Program, Davidson Program for Independence, and Student Transition and Enrichment Program.

2353 Kenneth T and Eileen L Norris Foundation

11 Golden Shore
Suite 450
Long Beach, CA 90802
562-435-8444
FAX: 562-436-0584
www.norrisfoundation.org

Ronald Barnes, Executive Director
Walter Zanino, Controller Trustee
The Foundation is primarily focused on medicine and education. To a lesser extent the foundation contributes to community programs including visually impaired, autism, mentally and physically disabled, deaf and mental health in the Southern California area. Average grant size in this area is $5,000-$10,000. Grants are also given in the area of culture and youth.

2354 Koret Foundation

33 New Montgomery Street
Suite 1090
San Francisco, CA 94105
415-882-7740
FAX: 415-882-7775
e-mail: info@koretfoundation.org
www.koretfoundation.org

Jeff Farber, Chief Executive Officer

2355 LJ Skaggs and Mary C Skaggs Foundation

1221 Broadway
21st Floor
Oakland, CA 94612
510-451-3300
FAX: 510-451-1527
www.skaggs.org

Marry Skaggs, Cbe President
Jayne Davis, Vice President
Joseph Martin, Director And Treasurer
The Foundation presently makes grants under four program categories: performing arts, social concerns, projects of historic interest and special projects.

2356 LK Whittier Foundation

Whittier Trust Company Foundations Office
625 Fair Oaks Drive
Suite 360
S Pasadena, CA 91030
626-441-5188
e-mail: lblinkenberg@whittiertrust.com
http://www.whittiertrust.com

Linda Blinkenberg, Foundations Director
Giving is primarily offered to preselected organizations. No grants are given to individuals.

2357 Legler Benbough Foundation

2550 5th Avenue
Suite 132
San Diego, CA 92103
619-235-8099
FAX: 619-235-8077
e-mail: peter@benboughfoundation.org
www.benboughfoundation.org

Peter K Elsworth, President
Thomas E Cisco, Treasurer
Hugh C Carter, Director

2358 Levi Strauss Foundation

1155 Battery Street
San Francisco, CA 94111
800-872-5384
www.levistrauss.com/responsibility/foundation
Has a funding initiative to support organizations which provide services for people with AIDS, and/or educational programs which help prevent the further spread of the HIV virus. The Foundation will assist in the development and enhancement of such services only in those communities where Levi Strauss & Co. has plants and distribution centers.

2359 Louis R Lurie Foundation

Louis R Lurie Foundation
555 California Street
Suite 5100
San Francisco, CA 94104
415-392-2470
http://www.foundationcenter.org

Nancy Terri, Contact
Visually impaired, hard-of-hearing and physically disabled in the San Francisco Bay Area and Metropolitan Chicago areas only.

2360 Luke B Hancock Foundation

360 Bryant Street
Palo Alto, CA 94301
650-321-5536
FAX: 650-321-0697
http://www.activistcash.com

Kimberly Hancock, Trustee
Thomas Hancock, Trustee
Has concentrated its resources over the past year on programs which provide job training and employment for at-risk youth. Consortium funding with other foundations in areas where there is unmet need; emergency and transitional funding; and selected funding for music education.

2361 Marin Community Foundation

5 Hamilton Landing
Suite 200
Novato, CA 94949
415-464-2500
FAX: 415-464-2555
e-mail: info@marincf.org
www.marincf.org

Thomas Peters, President And Ceo
Linda Compton, Assistant To President

2362 Mary A Crocker Trust

233 Post Street
Suite 201
San Francisco, CA 94108
415-982-0138
FAX: 415-982-0141
e-mail: staff@mactrust.org
www.mactrust.org

Established in 1889, the Foundation is interested in Bay Area programs such as environment, education and community relations.

2363 National Foundation of Wheelchair Tennis
940 Calle Amanecer
Suite B
San Clemente, CA 92673
714-361-3663
FAX: 714-361-6603
e-mail: nfwt@aol.com
http://www.nfwt.org

Bill Butler
Founded in January of 1980, the intention of this foundation is to assist the newly physically disabled individual to realize his full potential in society by enhancing his esteem, independence productivity and physical capabilities regardless of age, sex, creed or disability extent.

2364 Optometric Extension Program Foundation
1921 Carnegie Avenue
Suite 31
Santa Ana, CA 92705
949-250-8070
FAX: 949-250-8157
e-mail: rwilliams@oep.org
www.oep.org

Robert Williams, Executive Director
Offers continuing education in behavioral optometry for consumers and optometrists.

2365 Parker Foundation
4365 Executive Drive
Suite 1100
San Diego, CA 92121
858-677-1431
FAX: 858-677-1401
http://www.theparkerfoundation.org

Judy McDonald, Vice President
William Beamer, President
The assets are directed to projects which will contribute to the betterment of any aspect of the people of San Diego County, California and solely to entities which, among other things, are organized exclusively for charitable purposes and are operating in San Diego County, California.

2366 Pasadena Foundation
260 S Los Robles Avenue
Suite 119
Pasadena, CA 91101
626-796-2097
FAX: 626-583-4738
e-mail: pcfstaff@pasadenacf.org
www.pasadenacf.org

Jennifer Devoll, Executive Director
Vgee Ramiah, Director of Finance
The mission of the Pasadena Foundation is to improve the quality of life for citizens of the Pasadena area through support of nonprofit organizations that provide services beneficial to the community.

2367 RC Baker Foundation
PO Box 6150
Orange, CA 92863
714-750-8987

F Scott, Manager
Established in 1952, for general philanthropic purposes. The bulk of assistance and support has been to religious, scientific, educational institutions and youth organizations.

2368 Ralph M Parsons Foundation
1055 Wilshire Boulevard
Suite 1701
Los Angeles, CA 90017
213-482-3185
www.rmpf.org

Joseph Hurley, President
Edgar Jackson, Vice President
Robert Erburu, Chairman of the Board
The Foundation is concerned with the encouragement and support of projects and programs deemed beneficial to mankind in several major areas of interest such as: education; social impact; civic and cultural; health and special products. Only funds in Los Angeles County.

2369 Robert Ellis Simon Foundation
152 S Lousky Drive
Beverly Hills, CA 90212
310-275-7335

Joan Willens
Mental health and visually impaired grants are the main concerns of this organization.

2370 San Francisco Foundation
225 Bush Street
Suite 500
San Francisco, CA 94104
415-733-8500
FAX: 415-477-2783
e-mail: rec@sff.org
www.sff.org

Chris Nicholson, Director of Business Development
Sandra Hernandez, Chief Executive Officer
The Foundation's purpose is to improve life, promote greater equality of opportunity and assist those in need or at risk in the San Francisco Bay Area. The Foundation strives to protect and enhance the unique resources of the Bay Area, committed to equality of opportunity for all and the elimination of any injustice, seeks to enhance human dignity and seeks to establish mutual trust, respect and communication among the Foundation.

2371 Santa Barbara Foundation
15 E Carrillo Street
Santa Barbara, CA 93101
805-963-1873
FAX: 805-966-2345
e-mail: jrivera@sbfoundation.org
http://www.sbfoundation.org

Charles Slosser, President/CEO
Susanne Farwell, Director of Communications
James Rivera, VP Administration
The Foundations mission is to enrich the lives of the people of Santa Barbara County through philanthropy. The Foundation awards grants to nonprofits within the County in the areas of education, health, human services, personal development, cluture, recreation, community enhancement and environment. No support is given to individuals except through student aid.

2372 Sidney Stern Memorial Trust
PO Box 893
Pacific Palisades, CA 90272
310-459-2117

Peter Hooffers, Chair
Marvin Hoffenberg, Advisor
A Southern California-based foundation providing grants to nonprofit organizations for various projects. The foundation gives priority to the following areas of interest: education, health and science, community service projects, youth, services to the mentally and emotionally disabled, the arts, organizations and activities serving California. The Board prefers to make contributions to organizations that use the funds directly in the furtherance of their charitable and public purposes.

2373 Sierra Health Foundation
1321 Garden Highway
Sacramento, CA 95833
916-922-4755
FAX: 916-922-4024
e-mail: info@sierrahealth.org
http://www.sierrahealth.org

Gil Alvarado, Chief Financial Officer
Amy Birtwhistle, Program Assistant
The Foundation strives to establish a collaborative relationship with its grantees, and with other funders and foundations, through an open dialogue. The Foundation approaches each grant as a partnership, with opportunities for the grantee and grantor to work cooperatively to enhance the effectiveness of the grant project.

2374 **Silicon Valley Community Foundation**
1700 S El Camino Real
Suite 300
San Mateo, CA 94402
650-358-9369
FAX: 650-358-9817
e-mail: edcarson@siliconvalleycf.org
http://www.siliconvalleycf.org

Emmett Carson, President And Ceo
Lianne Araki, Executive Assistant
For more than 36 years, Peninsula Community Foundation has built involvement and investment in the community. Develops resources and imaginative programs that make it easy for Peninsula and Silicon Valley residents— from Daly City to San Jose, from the Pacific Ocean to the San Francisco Bay— to support the common good and connect with causes they care about.

2375 **Sonora Area Foundation**
PO Box 577
20100 Cedar Road North Suite E
Sonora, CA 95370
209-533-2596
FAX: 209-533-2412
www.sonora-area.org

Celeste Boyd, President
Clark Segertrom, Vica President

2376 **Stella B Gross Charitable Trust**
Bank of the West
PO Box 1121
San Jose, CA 95108
408-947-5203
e-mail: gpadilla@bankofthewest.com
http://www.compasspoint.org

Gabe Padilla, Trust Admin
Organization must be federal and state tax-exempt and reside within the bounds of Santa Clara County, California to be eligible.

2377 **Teichert Foundation**
3500 American River Drive
Sacramento, CA 95864
916-484-3011
FAX: 916-484-6506
www.teichert.com

Frederick A Teichert, Executive Director

2378 **Times Mirror Foundation**
202 W 1st Street
Los Angeles, CA 90012
213-237-3700
FAX: 213-237-2116
www.timesmirrorfoundation.org

Michelle Williams, Executive Director
Vanessa Briseno, Contributions Coordinator

2379 **WM Keck Foundation**
550 S Hope Street
Suite 2500
Los Angeles, CA 90071
213-680-3833
e-mail: info@wmkeck.org
www.wmkeck.org

Josh Pekarsky, Contact
Created to support accredited colleges and universities with particular emphasis on the sciences, engineering and medical research. The Foundation also maintains a Southern California Grant Program that provides support for non-profit organizations in the field of civic and community services, health care, precollegiate education and the arts.

2380 **Willam G Gilmore Foundation**
Family Caregiver Alliance
180 Montgomery Street
Suite 1100
San Francisco, CA 94104
415-434-3388
800-445-8106
FAX: 415-434-3508
e-mail: info@caregiver.org
http://www.caregiver.org

Kathy Murphy, President
Kathryn Lee, Vice President
Janice Oringer, Secretary

Colorado

2381 **Adolph Coors Foundation**
4100 E Mississippi Avenue
Suite 1850
Denver, CO 80246
303-388-1636
FAX: 303-388-1684
e-mail: generalinfo@acoorsfdn.org
www.coorsfoundation.org

Sally Rippey, Executive Director
Jeanne Bistranin, Senior Program Officer
Christina Coors, Program Officer
Applicant organizations must be classified as 501 and must operate within the United States. The areas covered by the Foundation are health, education, youth, community services, civic and cultural and public affairs.

2382 **Anschutz Family Foundation**
555 17th Street
Suite 2400
Denver, CO 80202
303-293-2338
FAX: 303-299-1235
e-mail: info@anschutzfamilyfoundation.org
http://www.anschutzfamilyfoundation.or g

Sue Anschutz Rodgers, President
Jeff W. Pryor, Executive Director
Michelle Sturm, Program Officer
The Foundation's interests are to support efforts helping the elderly, the young and the economically disadvantaged. The Foundation has supported over 600 public and private charities sharing in the concern for neighborhood strengthening and community cooperation.

2383 **Arc of Colorado**
8000 E Prentice Avenue
Suite D1
Greenwood Village, CO 80111
303-864-9334
800-333-7690
FAX: 303-864-9330
www.thearcofco.org

Marian Neely - Carlson, Treasurer

2384 **Bonfils-Stanton Foundation**
Daniels And Fisher Tower
1601 Arapahoe Street
Suite 500
Denver, CO 80202
303-825-3774
FAX: 303-825-0802
e-mail: dorthy@bonfils-stanton.org
www.bonfils-stantonfoundation.org

Dorothy Horrell, President
Susan France, Vice President
Linda Niven, Controller
Grants limited to Colorado 501 (c) (3) organizations. Grants are for general, charitable philanthropic activities within the State. Major categories include education, scientific (including hospital and health services), civic and cultural, community and human services. Organizations should request foundation guidelines before submitting a proposal.

2385 **Comprecare Foundation**
PO Box 740610
Arvada, CO 80006
303-629-8661

JR Gilsdorf, Executive Director

2386 Denver Foundation
950 S Cherry Street
Suite 200
Denver, CO 80246
303-300-1790
FAX: 303-300-6547
e-mail: information@denverfoundation.org
www.denverfoundation.org

David Miller, President
Julie Wilson, Executive Assistant
Rebecca Arno, Vice President
Neighbors helping neighbors, that's what the foundation is for. As Denver's only community foundation we've been accepting charitable donations since 1925. Those funds have been given back to the community in ongoing grants to nonprofit organizations - organizations that touch nearly every meaningful artistic, cultural, civic, health and human services interest of metro Denver's citizens.

2387 El Pomar Foundation
10 Lake Circle
Colorado Springs, CO 80906
719-633-7733
800-554-7711
FAX: 719-577-5702
www.elpomar.org

William J Hybl, Chairman/President/CEO
William R Ward, Vice Chairman

2388 Gates Family Foundation
3575 Cherry Creek North Drive
Suite 100
Denver, CO 80209
303-722-1881
FAX: 303-316-3038
e-mail: info@gatesfamilyfoundation.org
http://www.gatesfamilyfoundation.org

Charles Cannon, Vice Chair
Thomas Kaesemeyer, Executive Director
Diane Wallach, Board Chair
Purpose is to aid, encourage, initiate or carry on activities that will promote the health, well-being, security and education of all people. Because of a deep concern for and confidence in the future of Colorado, the foundation will invest primarily in institutions, projects and programs that will enhance the quality of life of those who live and work in the state, especially the Denver metropolitan area. Also finds ways to encourage greater cooperation between public and private sectors.

2389 Helen K and Arthur E Johnson Foundation
1700 Broadway
Suite 1100
Denver, CO 80290
303-861-4127
FAX: 303-861-0607
e-mail: info@johnsonfoundation.org
www.johnsonfoundation.org

John Alexander Jr, President
Cindy Willard, Program Officer
Suzanne Bruce, Program Associate
A nonprofit, grantmaking private foundation incorporated under the laws of the State of Colorado in 1948. The Foundation is a general purpose foundation whose grant program consists of a wide variety of creative efforts to solve problems and to enrich the quality of life. The areas of interest are: education, youth, health, community services, civic and culture and senior citizens. Grants limited to the state of Colorado.

2390 Kitzmiller-Bales Trust
110 East 3rd Street
Laird, CO 80758
970-332-3484

http://www.listings.allpages.com/

Robert U Hansen

2391 V Hunter Trust
650 S Cherry Street
Suite 535
Glendale, CO 80246
303-399-5450
FAX: 303-399-5499
http://www.avhuntertrust.org

George C. Gibson, President
W. Robert Alexander, Vice President
Bruce K. Alexander, Treasurer

Connecticut

2392 Aetna Foundation
151 Farmington Avenue
Hartford, CT 06156
860-273-6382

www.aetna.com/foundation

Diana Kinosh, Consultant

2393 Arc of Connecticut
1030 New Britain Avenue
West Hartford, CT 06110
860-953-8335

e-mail: arcct@aol.com
www.arcct.com

Lynn Warner, Executive Director
Peg Dignoti, Consultant
Dorothy Amundsen, Administrative Assistant

2394 Community Foundation of Southeastern Connecticut
147 State Street
New London, CT 06320
860-442-3572
FAX: 860-442-0584
e-mail: alice@cfsect.org
www.cfsect.org

Alice F Fitzpatrick, President
Jennifer O'Brien, Program Director

2395 Connecticut Mutual Life Foundation
140 Garden Street
Hartford, CT 06154
860-727-3000

Astrida Olds, Executive Director
Distinguished throughout its long history by unusual commitment to high principles of corporate purpose and business ethics. That commitment has been reflected not only in the firm belief that normal business functions must be carried out with a sense of responsibility beyond that required by the marketplace. Maintains an ongoing program of corporate contributions, a nationwide matching gifts plan for all employees on behalf of private and public education, skills training programs, and more.

2396 Cornelia de Lange Syndrome Foundation
302 W Main Street
Suite 100
Avon, CT 06001
860-676-8166
800-753-2357
FAX: 860-676-8337
e-mail: info@cdlsusa.org
www.cdlsusa.org

Julie Mairano, Executive Director
Provides information about birth defects caused by Cornelia de Lange Syndrome.

2397 Fidelco Guide Dog Foundation
PO Box 142
Bloomfield, CT 06002
860-243-5200
FAX: 860-243-7215
e-mail: training@fidelco.org
www.fidelco.org

Roberta C Kaman, Chairman
George J Salpietro, Vice Chairman
Nancy Levin, Vice President

Purpose is to breed, train and place Fidelco German Shepherd guide dogs with persons who are visually impaired throughout the Northeast. Provides in community training services to persons receiving guide dogs, reviews performance of the guide dog teams to see that satisfactory level of achievement is maintained, utilizes genetic processes and clinical methods to improve and refine the breed and maintains an ongoing program for development and improvement of training methods.

2398 GE Foundation
General Electric Company
3135 Easton Tpke
Fairfield, CT 06828
203-373-2211
FAX: 203-373-3029
e-mail: gefoundation@ge.com
www.gefoundation.com

Robert Corcoran, President
Believes that our greatest national resource is the work force. If we are to successfully compete in the global arena, then we become involved in improving the education of all of our citizens. The Foundation sets examples for others to emulate helping people with their international grant program to higher education and to health care for children in developing countries.

2399 General Electric Foundation
3135 Easton Tpke
Fairfield, CT 06828
203-373-2211
FAX: 203-373-3029
e-mail: gefoundation@ge.com
www.ge.com/foundation

Robert Corcoran, President
Roger Nozaki, Executive Director
Jeffrey Immelt, Chief Executive Officer
Blind, physically and mentally disabled and rehabilitation grants are among the priorities of the company.

2400 Hartford Foundation for Public Giving
550 Main Street
Hartford, CT 06103
860-543-8885
FAX: 860-722-6014
e-mail: danwaralghani@hotmail.com
www.hartnet.org

D Anwar Al Ghani, Chairman
Developmentally disabled, housing, deaf, recreation and education grants.

2401 Hartford Insurance Group
690 Asylum Avenue
Hartford, CT 06105
860-547-5000
www.thehartford.com

Ramani Ayer, President/CEO
Thomas Marra, Executive Vice President
Giving is primarily in the Hartford, CT area and in communities where the company has a regional office. No support is available for political or religious purposes. Grants are given in the areas of education, health and United Way organizations.

2402 Henry Nias Foundation
20 Carmen Road
Milford, CT 06460
203-874-2787
http://www.conntact.com

Charles D Fleischman, Vice President

2403 Jane Coffin Childs Memorial Fund for Medical Research
Jane Coffin Childs Memorial Fund
333 Cedar Street
LW300-SHM
New Haven, CT 06510
203-785-4612
FAX: 203-785-3301
www.jccfund.org

Kim Roberts, Administrative Director
The Fund awards fellowships to suitably qualified individuals for full time postdoctoral studies in the medical and related sciences bearing on cancer.

2404 John H and Ethel G Nobel Charitable Trust
Bankers Trust Company
1 Fawcett Place
Greenwich, CT 06830
203-629-7120
FAX: 203-629-7170

Paul J Bisset, Vice President

2405 Scheuer Associates Foundation
Robert Scheuer
960 Lake Avenue
Greenwich, CT 06831
203-861-6525
FAX: 203-622-5002

Thomas Scheuer, President
Robert Scheuer, Treasurer
B Scharbach, Owner

2406 Swindells Charitable Foundation Trust
Shawmut Bank
777 Main Street
242
Hartford, CT 06115
860-728-4900
FAX: 860-240-1210

Maggie Willard, Vice President
Joseph Giangreco, Personal Trust Association
Paul Spinella, Manager
Grants made to charitable organizations or societies incorporated for the relief of sick and suffering poor children and/or the relief of sick suffering and indigent aged men and women and/or the support of public charitable hospitals. Geographic area includes Hartford, CT area primarily. Application is required, deadlines are Feb. 1 and Aug. 1.

Delaware

2407 Arc of Delaware
1016 Centre Road
Suite 1
Wilmington, DE 19805
302-996-9400
www.arcde.org

Timothy F Brooks, President
Wesley E Perkins, Executive Vice President

2408 Laffey-McHugh Foundation
PO Box 2207
Wilmington, DE 19899
302-658-9141
http://equinerescue.info/

Thomas Lodge, Secretary

2409 Longwood Foundation
100 W 10th Street
Wilmington, DE 19801
302-654-2477
FAX: 302-654-2323
http://www.activistcash.com/

David D Wakefield, Executive Secretary
Offers grants to the mentally and physically disabled - capital, program, education and housing grants in the state of Delaware.

District of Columbia

2410 Albert L and Elizabeth T Tucker Foundation
1120 20th Street NW
Suite 300
Washington, DC 20036
202-457-1600
FAX: 202-457-1678

Nicholas S McConnell
James Schaller, President

2411 Alexander and Margaret Stewart Trust
Brawner Building
888 17th Street NW
Suite 610
Washington, DC 20006 202-785-9892
e-mail: DLustine@stewart-trust.org
http://www.stewart-trust.org

Doris Lustine, Executive Secretary
Wiliam Bierbower, Trustee
Grants are given only to the Washington, DC area organizations providing care or treatment to cancer patients or those with childhood afflictions.

2412 Arc of the District of Columbia
817 Varnum Street NE
Suite 229
Washington, DC 20017 202-636-2950
FAX: 202-635-7086
e-mail: arcdc@arcdc.net
www.arcdc.net

Robert A Andersen, President
Vincent C. Gray, Vice President
Mitchell T. Miller, Treasurer
Advocating for and providing services to persons with mental retardation.

2413 Charles Delmar Foundation
1918 16th Street NW
Washington, DC 20009 202-293-2494
FAX: 202-293-1788

Mareen D Hughes, President

2414 Eugene and Agnes E Meyer Foundation
The Meyer Foundation
1400 16th Street NW
Suite 360
Washington, DC 20036 202-483-8294
FAX: 202-328-6850
e-mail: meyer@meyerfdn.org
www.meyerfoundation.org

Julie Rogers, President
Katie Shaw, Executive Assistant
Kristen Conte, Vice President
Awards grants to projects dealing with the learning disabled, blind, mental health and vocational training in the Washington metropolitan area.

2415 Federal Student Aid Information Center
U S Department of Education
400 Maryland Avenue SW
Washington, DC 20202 202-275-5446
800-433-3243
www.answers.com

Theresa Shaw
Answers questions about Federal student aid from students, parents and Members of Congress, as well as financial aid administrators.

2416 GEICO Philanthropic Foundation Geico Corp.
Geico Corp.
Chevy Chase, MD 20815 301-986-2185
www.geico.com

Charles Davies, President
Thomas Wells, Director
Hospitals, physically disabled and Special Olympics.
1980

2417 Giant Food Foundation
PO Box 1804
Washington, DC 20013 202-331-0200
888-4MY-GIAN
FAX: 301-618-4667
www.giantfood.com

Barry F Scher, VP Public Relations
Luis Guinot, Partner
Offers grants in the areas of mental health, recreation, community and cultural programs, art, and educational programs for the health and prosperity of the greater Washington area.

2418 Jacob and Charlotte Lehrman Foundation
1027 33rd Street NW
Washington, DC 20007 202-338-8400
FAX: 202-338-8405
e-mail: info@lehrmanfoundation.org
www.lehrmanfoundation.org

Elizabeth Berry

2419 John Edward Fowler Memorial Foundation
1725 K Street NW
Suite 1201
Washington, DC 20006 202-728-9080
http://www.foundationcenter.org/

Suzanne Martin, Grant Consultant
Although not a program priority, the foundation does offer grants to the physically disabled in the Washington, DC area only.

2420 Joseph P Kennedy Jr Foundation
1133 19th Street Nw
12th Floor
Washington, DC 20036 202-393-1250
FAX: 202-824-0351
e-mail: info@jpkf.org
www.jpkf.org

Eunice Shriver, Executive Vice President
Edward Kennedy, President
Erika Hagensen, Executive Director
Has two firm objectives: to seek the prevention of mental retardation, and to improve the way society deals with its citizens who are already mentally retarded. The Foundation uses its funds in areas where a multiplier effect can be achieved through development of innovative models for the prevention and amelioration of mental retardation, through provision of seed money that encourages new researchers, and thorough use of the Foundation's influence to promote public awareness.

2421 Kiplinger Foundation
1729 H Street NW
Washington, DC 20006 202-887-6559
e-mail: foundation@kiplinger.com
http://tgci.com

Andrea Wilkes, Secretary
Austin Kiplinger, President
Limited to the greater Washington, DC area, the grants focus primarily on education, social welfare, cultural activities and community programs. Matching grants to eligible secondary or higher education institutions are provided on behalf of employees and retirees of Kiplinger Washington Editors, Inc. The Foundation does not fund scholarships.

2422 Morris and Gwendolyn Cafritz Foundation
1825 K Street NW
Suite 1400
Washington, DC 20006 202-223-3100
FAX: 202-296-7567
e-mail: info@cafritzfoundation.org
www.cafritzfoundation.org

Calvin Cafritz, President
Daniel Callahan, Vice Chairman And Treasurer
Grants are awarded to only 501(c)(3) organizations that are in the DC area. Grants are not awarded for capitol purposes, special events, endowments, or to individuals.

2423 Paul and Annetta Himmelfarb Foundation
4545 42nd Street NW
Suite 203
Washington, DC 20016 202-966-3796
http://www.himmelfarbfoundation.org/

Paul Himmelfarb, President

2424 Public Welfare Foundation
1200 U Street NW
Washington, DC 20009 202-965-1800

e-mail: reviewcommittee@publicwelfare.org
www.publicwelfare.org

Juliet Villarreal Garcia, Chair
Robert H Haskell, Vice Chair
C. Elizabeth Warner, Secretary And Treasurer
The foundation's funding is specifically targeted to economically disadvantaged populations. Proposals must fall within one of the following categories: criminal justice, disadvantaged elderly, disadvantaged youth, environment, health and population and reproductive health, human rights and global security, and community economic developmental and participation. Proposals should be addressed to the Review Committee.

Florida

2425 Able Trust
106 E College Avenue
Suite 820
Tallahassee, FL 32301 850-224-4493
FAX: 850-224-4496
e-mail: info@abletrust.org
www.abletrust.org

Sharon Griffith, President
Kristen Knapp, Vice President of Publications
Guenevere Crum, Director Grants Program
Provides grant funds to further employment for people with disabilities and employment-related programs for non-profit agencies in Florida. Assists agencies through educational conferences, and youth training programs. Provides businesses free resources for hiring people with disabilities.

2426 Arc of Florida
2898 Mahan Drive
Suite 1
Tallahassee, FL 32308 850-921-0460
800-226-1155
e-mail: info@arcflorida.org
www.arcflorida.org

John C Hall, Executive Director
Deborah Linton, Assistant Director
Promotes, for all people with mental retardation and other developmental disabilities, through education, awareness, research, advocacy and the support of families, friends and community.

2427 BCR Foundation
PO Box 13307
Pensacola, FL 32591 850-438-2509

Betty Rainwater, Director

2428 Bank of America Client Foundation
1800 2nd Street
Suite 750
Sarasota, FL 34236 941-957-0442
FAX: 941-957-3135
e-mail: djacobs@selbyfdn.org
www.selbyfdn.org

Debra Jacobs, President/CEO
Janet Noah, Grants Manager
Joan McArdle, Office Manager

2429 Baron de Hirschmeyer Foundation
407 Lincoln Road
Suite 6j
Miami Beach, FL 33139 305-672-0934

Polly Lux de Hirshmeyer, President

2430 Barron Collier Jr Foundation
2600 Golden Gate Parkway
Suite 200
Naples, FL 34105 239-262-2600
FAX: 239-262-1840

Lamar Gable, Director
Paul Marinelli, President

2431 Camiccia-Arnautou Charitable Foundation
Bill T Smith Jr
980 N Federal Highway
Suite 402
Boca Raton, FL 33432 561-368-5757
FAX: 561-368-8505

Bill Smith Jr, Owner

2432 Chatlos Foundation
PO Box 915048
Longwood, FL 32791 407-862-5077

e-mail: info@chatlos.org
www.chatlos.org

William J Chatlos, President
Funds nonprofit organizations in the USA and around the globe. Funding is provided in the following areas of giving: Bible Colleges/Seminaries, Religious Causes, Medical Concerns, Liberal Arts Colleges and Social Concerns. Category of placement is determined by the organizations overall mission rather than the project under consideration. The Foundation does not make scholarship grants directly to individuals but rather to educational institutions which in turn select recipients.
1953

2433 Dade Community Foundation
200 S Biscayne Boulevard
Suite 2780
Miami, FL 33131 305-371-2711
FAX: 305-371-5342
e-mail: ruth.shack@dadecommunityfoundation.org

Ruth Shack, President

2434 Dr. Jack Widrich Foundation
400 W Rivo Alto Drive
Miami Beach, FL 33139 305-673-5050

Jack Widrich, Owner

2435 EIS Foundation
550 SE Mizner Boulevard
Apt 507
Boca Raton, FL 33432 561-852-6854
FAX: 561-852-6884

Maurice L Schwarz, President

2436 Edyth Bush Charitable Foundation
PO Box 1967
Winter Park, FL 32790 407-647-4322
888-647-4322
FAX: 407-647-7716
e-mail: dodahowski@edythbush.org
www.edythbush.org

David A Odahowski, President/CEO
Mary Gretche Belloff, Vice Chairman
Funding is resrticted to 501c3 nonprofit organizations located and operating in Orange, Osceola, Seminole and Lake Counties, Florida. Visit www.edythbush.org for a list of funding policies.

2437 FPL Group Foundation
700 Universe Boulevard
Juno Beach, FL 33408 561-694-4000
800-222-4511
FAX: 561-694-4620

John L Kitchens
James Robo, President

2438 Florida Rock Industries Foundation
155 E 21st Street
Jacksonville, FL 32206
904-355-1781
FAX: 904-791-1810

HB Horner, Secretary
John Baker II, Chief Executive Officer

2439 Frank Stanley Beveridge Foundation
1340 N US Highway 1
Suite 102
Jupiter, FL 33469
800-600-3723
FAX: 561-748-0644
e-mail: administrator@beveridge.org
www.beveridge.org

Philip Caswell, President
Carole S Lenhart, CPA, VP/Treasurer
The mission of The Frank Stanley Beveridge Foundation, Inc. is to preserve and enhance the quality of life by embracing and perpetuating Frank Stanley Beveridge's philanthropic vision through grantmaking initiatives in support of The Stanley Park of Westfield, Inc. and programs in youth development, health, education, religion, art and environment primarily in Hampden and Hampshire Counties, Massachusetts.

2440 Jack Eckerd Corporation Foundation
PO Box 4689
Clearwater, FL 33758
727-395-6000
FAX: 727-395-7934
e-mail: serve@eckerd.com
www.eckard.com

Tamz Alderman, MCR, PR
Robert Sloan, Plant Manager
The foundation limits its giving to nonprofit, tax-exempt organizations located in Eckerd Drug Company's 13-state marketing area. The majority of our funds are committed to national health organizations, the United Way campaigns, and scholarship funding at various colleges of pharmacy.

2441 Jefferson Lee Ford III Memorial Foundation
9600 Collins Avenue
546487
Bal Harbour, FL 33154
305-885-5447
FAX: 305-868-2646

Herbert Kurras, Trustee
Suzanne Kingsbury, Trustee
Disabled children, hearing and speech center. Grants are only given to tax exempt organizations, no individual grants are offered.

2442 Jessie Ball duPont Fund
1 Independent Drive
Suite 1400
Jacksonville, FL 32202
904-353-0890
800-252-3452
FAX: 904-353-3870
e-mail: contactus@dupontfund.org
www.dupontfund.org

Sherry P Magill PhD, President
Davena Sawyer, Executive Assistant
Established under the terms of the will of the late Jessie Ball duPont. The fund is a national foundation having a special though not exclusive interest in issues affecting the South. The Fund works with the approximately 325 individual institutions to which Mrs. duPont personally contributed during the five-year period, 1960 through 1964.

2443 Joe and Emily Lowe Foundation
249 Royal Palm Way
Palm Beach, FL 33480
561-659-1203
FAX: 561-655-7130

Bernard Sterm, President
Emphasis is on Jewish welfare funds, the arts, museums, higher education including medical education, hospitals, medical research, aid to the handicapped, underprivileged children's organizations and women's projects. The funding is limited to the New York Metropolitan Area including New Jersey and Palm Beach County, Florida. No grants are made to individuals.

2444 John E & Nellie J Bastien Memorial Foundation
440 E Sample Road
Suite 209
Pompano Beach, FL 33064
954-942-3203

Carol Kearns, Manager

2445 Lost Tree Village Charitable Foundation
11555 Lost Tree Way
North Palm Beach, FL 33408
561-622-3780
FAX: 561-622-7558
www.losttreefoundation.org

2446 Publix Super Markets Charities
Publix Super Market Corporation Office
PO Box 407
Lakeland, FL 33802
863-688-1188
800-242-1227
www.publix.com

2447 Richard W Higgins Charitable Foundation M And I Marshall And Ilsley Bank
Marshall & Ilsley Trust of Florida
800 Laurel Oak Drive
Suite 100
Naples, FL 34108
877-202-9234

www.micorp.com

Georgia

2448 Community Foundation for Greater Atlanta
50 Hurt Plaza
Suite 449
Atlanta, GA 30303
404-688-5525

e-mail: aphilipp@atlcf.org
www.atlcf.org

Alicia Philipp, President
Juanita Sheppard, Executive Assistant
Rob Smulian, Vice President

2449 Florence C and Harry L English Memorial Fund
Sun Trust Bank Atlanta
PO Box 4418-Mail
Atlanta, GA 30302
404-588-8250
FAX: 404-724-3082
e-mail: raymond.king@suntrust.com
www.suntrustatlantafoundation.org

Raymond B King, Senior VP
Kay Miller, Foundation Administrator
Grants only made to Metro Atlanta non-profit organizations; no grants to churches or individuals.

2450 Georgia Power
96 Annex
Atlanta, GA 30396
888-655-5888
http://www.georgiapower.com

Michael Garrett, President And Ceo

2451 Grayson Foundation
PO Box 515
Grayson, GA 30017
770-554-1000
FAX: 770-554-1003
e-mail: graysonfoundation@yahoo.com
www.graysonfoundation.org

Sam B Grayson, President
Dan Hicks, Principal
Grayson Foundation enhances the quality of public educationfor the students of the Grayson cluster of schools by providing funds which enrich and extend educational oppurtunities.

2452 **Harriet McDaniel Marshall Trust in Memory of Sanders McDaniel**
Sun Trust Bank Atlanta
PO Box 4418-Mail
Atlanta, GA 30302
404-588-8250
FAX: 404-724-3082
e-mail: raymond.king@suntrust.com
www.suntrustatlantafoundation.org

Raymond B King, Senior Vice President
Kay Miller, Foundation Administrator
Grants only made to Metro Atlanta non-profit organizations, no grants to churches or individuals.

2453 **IBM Corporation**
4111 Northside Parkway NW
Atlanta, GA 30327
404-238-3996
e-mail: wwall@us.ibm.com
http://www.iiug.org

Wanda Wall
Manages disability programs (which leverage IBM resources through partnerships) designed to train persons with disabilities and assist them in gaining employment. Also, disseminates information regarding products and resources for persons with disabilities with those of other companies and organizations.

2454 **John H and Wilhelmina D Harland Charitable Foundation**
Two Piedmont Center
Suite 106
Atlanta, GA 30305
404-264-9912
FAX: 404-266-8834
http://foundationcenter.org

Jane G Hardesty, Executive Director

2455 **Lettie Pate Whitehead Foundation**
50 Hurt Plaza
Suite 1200
Atlanta, GA 30303
404-522-6755
FAX: 404-522-7026
e-mail: fdns@woodruff.org
www.lpwhitehead.org

P. Russell Hardin, President
Non-profit organization dedicated to the support of needy women in nine southeastern states.

2456 **Patterson-Barclay Memorial Foundation**
6487 Peachtree Industrial Boulevard
Suite A
Atlanta, GA 30360
770-458-9888
FAX: 770-452-7704

Hugh R Powell Jr, Secretary

2457 **Perkins-Ponder Foundation**
PO Box 4007
Macon, GA 31213

2458 **Rich Foundation**
11 Piedmont Center NE
Suite 204
Atlanta, GA 30305
404-262-2266
FAX: 404-262-4123

Anne Poland-Berg, Grant Consultant

2459 **SunTrust Bank, Atlanta Foundation**
Sun Trust Bank Atlanta
PO Box 4418
Atlanta, GA 30302
404-588-8250
FAX: 404-724-3082
e-mail: raymond.king@suntrust.com
www.suntrustatlantafoundation.org

Raymond B King, Senior VP
Kay Miller, Foundation Administrator

2460 **The Arc Of Georgia**
Po Box 2987
Atlanta, GA 30301
404-657-8904
888-303-0024
e-mail: info@thearcofgeorgia.org
http://www.thearcofgeorgia.org/

Deirdre O'Brien, President
Anita Robinson, Vice President

Hawaii

2461 **Arc of Hawaii**
3989 Diamond Head Road
Honolulu, HI 96816
808-737-7995
FAX: 808-732-9531
e-mail: info@thearcinhawaii.org
www.thearcinhawaii.org/

2462 **Atherton Family Foundation**
1164 Bishop Street
Suite 800
Honolulu, HI 96813
808-566-5524
888-731-3863
FAX: 808-521-6286
e-mail: foundations@hcf-hawaii.org
www.atherton.hawaiicommunityfoundation.org

Paul F. Morgan, Vice President
Joan Rohlfing, Vice President And Secretary
Supports educational projects, programs and institutions as the highest priority, with the enterprises of a religious nature and those concerned with health and social services given careful attention. The Foundation is one of the largest private resources in the State devoted exclusively to the support of activities of a charitable nature.

2463 **Clarence TC Ching Foundation**
841 Bishop Street
Suite 1619
Honolulu, HI 96813
808-521-8841
http://www.tgci.com/

Lawrence SL Ching, Chairperson And Trustee

2464 **GN Wilcox Trust**
Pacific Century Trust
PO Box 3170
Honolulu, HI 96802
808-538-4580

Peter Ho, Executive Vice President

2465 **Hawaii Community Foundation**
1164 Bishop Street
Suite 800
Honolulu, HI 96813
808-537-6333
888-731-3863
FAX: 808-521-6286
e-mail: webmaster@hcf-hawaii.org
http://www.hawaiicommunityfoundation.org

Thomas Atou, Program Officer

2466 **McInerny Foundation Bank Of Hawaii,Corporate Trustee**
Po Box 3170
Department 758
Honolulu, HI 96802
808-538-4945
800-272-7262
FAX: 808-538-4006
e-mail: pboyce@boh.com
http://www.tgci.com

Paula Boyce, Avp And Grants Administrator

2467 Sophie Russell Testamentary Trust Bank Of Hawaii

Po Box 3170
Honolulu, HI 96802
808-538-4944
FAX: 808-538-4006
e-mail: pboyce@boh.com

Paula Boyce, Asst. Vice President
Supports qualified tax-exempt charitable organizations, in the State of Hawaii only. Offers grants to the Humane Society and institutions giving nursing care and serving the physically and mentally handicapped.

Illinois

2468 Alfred Bersted Foundation

231 S Lasalle Street
Chicago, IL 60604
312-251-8850

M Catherine Ryan
Gregory Rothman, Owner
Grants are given to programs serving the mentally and physically disabled, and organizations included in the broader focus of the foundation. Grants are restricted to organizations in four Illinois counties: DuPage, Kane, McHenry and DeKalb.

2469 Alzheimer's Association

225 N Michigan Avenue
Floor 17
Chicago, IL 60601
312-335-8700
FAX: 866-699-1246
TTY:312-335-5886
e-mail: info@alz.org
www.alz.org

Evan Thompson, Chairman
Paul Attea, Vice Chaiman

2470 American Foundation for the Blind-Midwest

11 Penn Plaza
Suite 300
New York, NY 10001
212-502-7600
e-mail: afbinfo@afb.net
www.afb.org

Carl Augusto, President And Ceo

2471 American National Bank and Trust Company

33 N La Salle Street
Chicago, IL 60602
312-661-6000
FAX: 815-961-7745

Joan M Klaus, Foundation Director
Supports the endeavors of organizations working to meet the critical needs of the city and its surrounding communities. Success is greatly affected by the well-being of the communities the company serves, thus the foundation seeks to fulfill the social obligations both through financial funding and human resources. The Foundation funding categories include organizations and programs involved in economic development, education, community and social services, healthcare and culture and the arts.

2472 Ameritech Corporation Contributions Program

30 S Wacker Drive
34th Floor
Chicago, IL 60606
312-263-2805
FAX: 312-727-1496
www.ameritech.com

Michael E Kuhlin, Senior Director

2473 Amerock Corporation

PO Box 7018
Rockford, IL 61125
815-963-9631
800-618-9559
FAX: 815-969-6029
www.amerock.com

Robert Bailey, President
Grants are given to organizations promoting wellness, health and rehabilitation of the visually impaired and physically disabled.

2474 Arc of Illinois The Illinois Life Span Project

18207 Dixie Highway
Suite A
Homewood, IL 60430
708-206-3993
800-588-7002
FAX: 708-206-1171
e-mail: mike@illinoislifespan.org
www.illinoislifespan.org

Mike Kaminsky, Director
The Arc of Illinois is committed to empowering persons with disabilities to achieve full participation in community life thru informed choices.

2475 Benjamin Benedict Green-Field Foundation

18313 Greenleaf Ct
Tinley Park, IL 60487
708-444-4241
FAX: 708-614-0496
e-mail: kathy@greenfieldfoundation.org
www.greenfieldfoundation.org

Colin Fisher, President
A privately endowed grantmaking organization trying to improve the qaulity of life for children and the elderly in the city of chicago.

2476 Blowitz-Ridgeway Foundation

1701 E Woodfield Road
Suite 201
Schaumburg, IL 60173
847-446-1010
FAX: 847-446-6318

Tina M Erickson, Administrator
Provides limited program, capital and research grants to organizations aiding the physically and mentally disabled, and agencies serving children and youth. Grants generally limited to Illinois.

2477 Burlington Northern Santa Fe Foundation

5601 W 26th Street
Cicero, IL 60804
630-222-4815
FAX: 630-222-4857

Dick Russack, President

2478 Chicago Community Trust and Affiliates

111 E Wacker Drive
Suite 1400
Chicago, IL 60601
312-616-8000
FAX: 312-616-7955
TTY:312-853-0394
e-mail: info@cct.org
www.cct.org

Sandy Chears, Grants Manager
Donald Stewart, Chief Executive Officerl

2479 Community Foundation of Champaign County

404 W Church Street
Champaign, IL 61820
217-359-0125
FAX: 217-352-6494

Joan Dixon, Executive Director

2480 Dr. Scholl Foundation

1033 Skokie Boulevard
Suite 230
Northbrook, IL 60062
847-559-7430
www.drschollfoundation.com

Pamela Scholl, President

2481 Duchossois Foundation The Chamberlain Group Inc.
845 N Larch Avenue
Elmhurst, IL 60126
800-528-5880
FAX: 877-528-7633
e-mail: info@chamberlain.com
www.chamberlain.com

Established in 1984, the foundation returns dollars to the communities supporting its facilities and employees. Within these following areas, organizations are carefully selected on the basis of community needs and the organization's value and performance. Areas aimed at include: medical research, children/youth programs and cultural institutions.

2482 Evenston Community Foundation
1007 Church Street
Suite 108
Evanston, IL 60201
847-492-0990
e-mail: schastok@evanstonforever.org
www.evcommfdn.org

Sara Schastok, Executive Director

2483 Field Foundation of Illinois
200 S Wacker Drive
Suite 3860
Chicago, IL 60606
312-831-0910
FAX: 312- -
TTY:1

Aurie Pennick, Executive Director
The Foundation awards grants to institutions and agencies in the fields of health, welfare, education, cultural and conservation activities, and urban and community affairs, primarily serving the people of the Chicago metropolitan area.

2484 Francis Beidler Charitable Trust
53 W Jackson Boulevard
Suite 530
Chicago, IL 60604
312-922-3792

Thomas B Dorris, Director

2485 Fred J Brunner Foundation
9300 King Street
Franklin Park, IL 60131
847-678-3232
FAX: 847-678-0642

Pam Sthwegal, Director
Fred Brunner, Chief Executive Officer
General disability grants.

2486 George M Eisenberg Foundation for Charities
2340 S Arlington Heights Road
Suite 480
Arlington Heights, IL 60005
847-981-0545
FAX: 847-941-0548

James Marousis, Treasurer

2487 George Zoltan Lefton Family Foundation
George Zoltan Lefton Company
3622 S Morgan Street
Chicago, IL 60609
773-254-4344

Magda Lefton, Secretary

2488 Green Bay Foundation
Goldman, Sachs & Company
71 S Wacker Drive
Suite 1
Chicago, IL 60606
312-655-4600

General disability grants.

2489 Grover Hermann Foundation
6600 Sears Tower
233 South Wacker Drive
Chicago, IL 60606
312-258-5500
FAX: 312-258-5600
e-mail: rsafer@schiffhardin.com
www.schiffhardin.com

Ronald Safer, Managing Partner,
Provides funds for educational, health, public policy, community and religious organizations throughout the United States. Its major interests are in higher education and health.

2490 Harry F and Elaine Chaddick Foundation
The Chaddick Institute for Metropolitan Developmen
243 S Wabash Avenue
Suite 9000
Chicago, IL 60604
312-362-5731
FAX: 312-362-5506
www.condor.depaul.edu

Joseph P Scwieterman, Director

2491 Helen Brach Foundation
55 W Wacker Drive
Suite 701
Chicago, IL 60601
312-372-4417
FAX: 312-372-0290

Toni Perille, Assoc. Director

2492 John D and Catherine T MacArthur Foundation
Office Of Grants Managment
140 S Dearborn Street
Chicago, IL 60603
312-726-8000
FAX: 312-920-6258
TTY:312-920-6285
e-mail: 4answers@macfound.org
www.macfound.org

Lloyd Axworthy, President/ Vice Chancellor
Robert Denham, Chair

2493 LaSalle Chicago Community Trust
222 N Lasalle Street
Suite 1400
Chicago, IL 60601
312-372-3356
FAX: 312-580-7411
www.cct.org

Sandy Chears, Grants Manager
A community foundation established in 1915, which receives gifts and bequests from individuals, families or organizations interested in providing through the community foundation, financial support for the charitable agencies or institutions which serve the residents of metropolitan Chicago.

2494 Les Turne Amyotrophic Laterial Sclerosis Foundation
5550 W Touhy Avenue
Suite 302
Skokie, IL 60077
847-679-3311
FAX: 847-679-9109
e-mail: info@lesturnerals.org
www.lesturnerals.org

Jamie Weissburg, Associate Executive Director
Wendy Abrams, Executive Director
Voluntary health organization dedicated to raising funds for ALS research, patient services and public awareness. Provides educational materials for affected individuals and family members, health care professionals, and the general public. Program services include referrals and counseling; audio-visual aids and periodic newsletters. Offers support groups and patient networking to affected individuals, family members, and caregivers.

2495 Little City Foundation
1760 W Algonquin Road
Palatine, IL 60067
847-358-5510
FAX: 847-358-3291
www.littlecity.org

Alex Alexandrou, President
Fred Lebed, Vice President
Robyn Cook, Director Adult Services
Provides progressive community-based services and service coordination for children and adults with mental retardation or other developmental, emotional and behavioral challenges. Services include direct care with up to 24-hour per day support for children and adults, Foster Care, Families One, adoption opportunities, respite care, supported employment, studio and multidisciplinary fine arts, public education, and advocacy.

2496 MAGIC Foundation for Children's Growth
6645 North Avenue
Oak Park, IL 60302
708-383-0808
800-362-4423
FAX: 708-383-0899
e-mail: dianne@magicfoundation.org
www.magicfoundation.org

Dianne Tamburrino, Executive Director
This is a national nonprofit organization providing support and education regarding growth disorders in children and related adult disorders, including adult GHD. Dedicated to helping children whose physical growth is affected by a medical problem by assisting families of afflicted children through local support groups, public education/awareness, newsletters, specialty divisions and programs for the children.

2497 McDonald's Corporation Contributions Program
Mc Donalds Plaza
Oak Brook, IL 60523
630-623-3000
FAX: 630-623-5004
www.mcdonalds.com/countries/usa/community/ind

Jackie Meara, Supervisor Contributions
James Skinner, Chief Executive Officer

2498 Michael Reese Health Trust
20 N Wacker Drive
Suite 760
Chicago, IL 60606
312-726-1008
FAX: 312-726-2797
e-mail: wpalmer@healthtrust.net
www.healthtrust.net

Gregory S. Gross, President
Herbert S. Wander, Chairman

2499 Moen Foundation
First National Bank of Chicago
1 S Northwest Highway
Park Ridge, IL 60068
815-729-1850
FAX: 815-729-5047

2500 National Eye Research Foundation (NERF)
910 Skokie Boulevard
Suite 207a
Northbrook, IL 60062
847-564-4652
800-621-2258
FAX: 847-564-0807
e-mail: nerf1955@aol.com
www.rarediseases.org

Carolyn Asbury, Chair
Frank Sasinowski, Vice Chair
Kimberly Symonds, Secretary
Dedicated to improving eye care for the public and meeting the professional needs of eye care practitioners; sponsors eye research projects on contact lens applications and eye care problems. Special study sections in such fields as orthokertology, primary eyecare, pediatrics, and through continuing education programs. Provides eye care information for the public and professionals. Educational materials including pamphlets. Program activities include education and referrals.

2501 National Headache Foundation
820 N Orleans Street
Suite 217
Chicago, IL 60610
888-643-5552
e-mail: info@headaches.org
www.headaches.org/

Seymore D. Diamond, Executive Director
Headache physicians.

2502 OMRON Foundation Omron Electronics Llc
1 Commerce Drive
Schaumburg, IL 60173
847-843-7900
FAX: 847-843-7787
e-mail: info@omron.com
http://www.omron247.com/

2503 Oris B Hastings Charitable Foundation
PO Box 186
Cairo, IL 62914
618-734-2800

John G Holland, Owner

2504 Parkinson's Disease Foundation
833 W Washington Boulevard
Chicago, IL 60607
312-733-1893
FAX: 312-733-1896
e-mail: info@pdf.org
www.pdf.org

Robin Anthony Elliot, Executive Director
International voluntary not-for-profit organization dedicated to patient services; education of affected individuals, family members, and healthcare professionals; and promotion and support of research for Parkinson's Disease and related disorders. Offers an extensive referral service to guide affected individuals to proper diagnosis and clinical care. Provides referrals to genetic counseling and support groups; promotes patient advocacy; and offers a variety of educational and support materials
Quarterly

2505 Peoria Area Community Foundation
331 Fulton Street
Suite 310
Peoria, IL 61602
309-674-8730
FAX: 309-674-8754
e-mail: jim@communityfoundationci.org
www.communityfoundationci.org

Jim Sullivan, Executive Director
Connie Jo Alexander, Executive Assistant

2506 Polk Brothers Foundation
20 W Kinzie Street
Suite 1110
Chicago, IL 60610
312-527-4684
FAX: 312-527-4681
e-mail: questions@polkbrosfdn.org
www.polkbros.org

2507 Retirement Research Foundation
8765 W Higgins Road
Suite 430
Chicago, IL 60631
773-714-8080
FAX: 773-714-8089
e-mail: info@rrf.org
www.rrf.org

Marilyn Hennessy, President
Edward J. Kelly, Chairman
A private philanthropy with primary interest in improving the quality of life of older persons in the United States.

2508 Rush Hayward Masonic Fund
14 Bel Air Court
Champaign, IL 61820
217-352-7528

Ruth Hayword

2509 Sears-Roebuck Foundation
3333 Beverly Road
Chicago, IL
847-286-2500
www.sears.com

Alan Lacy, Chief Executive Officer

2510 Siragusa Foundation
875 N Michigan Avenue
Chicago, IL 60611
312-280-0833
FAX: 312-943-4489
www.siragusa.org

Irene S Phelps, President
Sharmila Rao Thakkar, Program Officer

2511 Square D Foundation
1415 S Roselle Road
Palatine, IL 60067
847-397-2600
FAX: 847-397-8814

Chris Richardson, Chief Executive Officer
Makes donations for operating support, capital development needs, and special projects to nonprofit organizations that have been granted exemption from the Federal Income Tax. The Foundation has a strong commitment to the following areas: health and welfare, education, civic and community affairs, and culture and the arts. Support of higher education is also made for scholarships, endowments for facility and acquisition or expansion of equipment or facilities, through Matching Gift Program.

2512 WP and HB White Foundation
540 W Frontage Road
Suite 33240
Northfield, IL 60093
847-446-1441

Margaret Blandford, Executive Director
The Foundation's funds are allocated on a continuing basis within the metropolitan area of Chicago where our founder's business prospered. The Foundation helps organizations specializing in the visually impaired, mental health, youth and recreation.

2513 Washington Square Health Foundation
875 N Michigan Avenue
Suite 3516
Chicago, IL 60611
312-664-6488
FAX: 312-664-7787
e-mail: washington@wshf.org
www.wshf.org

James M. Snyder, Executive Director
John C. York, Treasurer

2514 Wheat Ridge Ministries
1 Pierce Place
Suite 250
Itasca, IL 60143
630-766-9066
800-762-6748
FAX: 630-766-9622
www.wheatridge.org

Richard Herman, President

Indiana

2515 Arc of Indiana
107 N Pennsylvania Street
Suite 300
Indianapolis, IN 46204
317-977-2375
800-382-9100
FAX: 317-977-2385
e-mail: thearc@arcind.org
ww.arcind.org

Jeff Bassett Howe, Vice President
Judy Abbott, President
Arc of Indiana is commited to people with mental retardation and othe developmental disabilities realizing their goals of learning, living, working, and playing in the community.

2516 Ball Brothers Foundation
222 S Mulberry Street
Muncie, IN 47308
765-741-5500
FAX: 765-741-5518
e-mail: info@ballfdn.org
http://www.ballfdn.org

Jud Fisher, Executive Director
Neil Schmottlach, Program Officer
Mentally and physically disabled, only serving Indiana area.

2517 Community Foundation of Boone County
Boone County Community Network
PO Box 451
Zionsville, IN 46077
317-873-8726

e-mail: tlmmjh@tds.net
www.bccn.boone.in.us

Terry Mccain, Vice President

2518 Crown Point Community Foundation
PO Box 522
Crown Point, IN 46308
219-662-7252
FAX: 219-662-9493
e-mail: cpcf@sbcglobal.net
http://www.lakenetnwi.org

Patricia Huber-Salach, Executive Director
Crown Point Community Foundation is a not for profit organization that serves as a facilitataor for the community good, builds endowments, allocates grants and awards scholarships to better serve Crown Point and South Lake county area of Indiana.

2519 Eli Lilly & Co Corporate Contributions Pro
Lilly Corporate Center
Indianapolis, IN 46285
317-276-2000

www.lilly.com/about/overview/access/foundatio

Sidney Taurel, Chairman And Ceo
Robert W. Armstrong, Vice President

2520 John W Anderson Foundation
402 Wall Street
Valparaiso, IN 46383
219-462-4611

Wilfred Wilkins, Chairman
Willam N Vinovich, Vice Chairman
Physically and mentally disabled, recreation and youth agencies in Northwest Indiana area.

2521 Trabant North Knox
Bank One, Trust Group
111 Monument Circle
Suite 1501
Indianapolis, IN 46277
317-321-8030

Iowa

2522 Arc of Iowa
Po Box 1096
Cedar Rapids, IA 52406
515-210-6686
800-362-2927
FAX: 319-365-9938
e-mail: info@thearcofiowa.org
http://www.thearcofiowa.com

2523 Hall-Perrine Foundation
115 3rd Street SE
Suite 803
Cedar Rapids, IA 52401
319-362-9079
FAX: 319-362-7220
http://www.hallperrine.org
This foundation is dedicated tio improving the quality of life for peole in Linn County, IA by responding to the changing social, economic, and cultural needs of the community.

2524 **Homer G Barr Trust**
PO Box 798
Fort Dodge, IA 50501
515-955-0679
FAX: 515-955-0631
www.bankfirstamerican.com

Susan Ahlers Leman, VP & Wealth Advisor

2525 **Kent A Hall**
PO Box 520
Mason City, IA 50401
515-896-3888

e-mail: jean-blair@uiowa.edu
http://www.iowagrantsguide.org

Pat Hall, Trustee
Offers grants only to the area of Iowa for projects to help; Special Olympics, physically disabled and art and cultural affairs.

2526 **Mid-Iowa Health Foundation**
3900 Ingersoll Avenue
Suite 104
Des Moines, IA 50312
515-277-6411

e-mail: info@midiowahealth.org
http://www.midiowahealth.org

Kathryn Bradley, President
Ivan Johnson, Chair
Denise Swartz, Program Officer

2527 **Principal Financial Group Foundation**
711 High Street
Des Moines, IA 50392
800-986-3343
FAX: 515-246-5475
www.principal.com/

2528 **Siouxland Community Foundation**
505 5th Street
Suite 412
Sioux City, IA 51101
712-293-3303
FAX: 712-293-3303
e-mail: office@siouxlandcommunityfoundation.org
www.siouxlandcommunityfoundation .org

Joseph E. Twindwell, President
Daniel D. Dykstra, Vice President
Carolyn J. Ohlfest, Secretary

Kansas

2529 **Arc of Kansas**
3601 SW 29th Street
Topeka, KS 66614
785-271-8783
FAX: 785-272-4645
e-mail: mkeating@tarcinc.org
www.thearcks.org

2530 **Hutchinson Community Foundation**
PO Box 298
1 N. Main Street, Suite 501
Hutchinson, KS 67504
620-663-5293
FAX: 620-663-9277
www.hutchcf.org

Aubrey Abbott Patterson, President

Kentucky

2531 **Arc of Kentucky**
706 E Main Street
Suite A
Frankfort, KY 40601
502-875-5225
800-281-1272
FAX: 502-875-5226
e-mail: arcofky@aol.com
www.arcofky.org

Patty Dempsey, Executive Director
Linda Weinscott, Assistant Executive Director
The Arc of Kentucky helps in securing a positive future for individuals with mental retardation. The Arc values services and supports that enhance the quality of life through independence, friendship, choice and respect for individuals with mental retardation.

2532 **Omnicare Foundation**
1717 Dixie Highway
Suite 800
Ft Wright, KY 41011
859-426-3000
FAX: 859-426-3118

Cheryl D Hodges, Secretary
D Laney, Vice President

Louisiana

2533 **Arc of Louisiana**
8336 Kelwood Avenue
Baton Rouge, LA 70806
225-303-0463
FAX: 225-924-3935
e-mail: thearcla@thearcla.org
www.thearcla.org

2534 **Baton Rouge Area Foundation**
402 N 4th Street
Baton Rouge, LA 70802
225-387-6126
877-387-6126
FAX: 225-387-6153
www.braf,org

2535 **Community Foundation of Shreveport-Bossier**
401 Edwards Street
Suite 105
Shreveport, LA 71101
318-221-0582
FAX: 318-221-7463
e-mail: hickman@comfoundsb.org
www.comfoundsb.org
Paula Hickman, Executive Director
Public Foundation that makes grants only to 501C3 organizations.

Maine

2536 **UNUM Charitable Foundation Maine Association Of Non Profits**
565 Congress Street
Suite 301
Portland, ME 04101
207-871-1885
FAX: 207-780-0346
e-mail: technicalassistance@nonprofitmaine.org
http://www.nonprofitmaine.org

Lydia Badger, Membership Manager
Scott Schnapp, Executive Director
Jessica Lantos, Administrative Assistant

The Foundation encourages projects that: stimulate others in the private or public sector to participate in problem solving; advance innovative and cost-effective approaches for addressing defined, recognized needs; and demonstrate ability to obtain future project funding, if needed. The foundation generally limits its consideration of capital campaign requests to the Greater Portland, Maine area.

Maryland

2537 American Health Assistance Foundation
22512 Gateway Center Drive
Clarksburg, MD 20871
301-948-3244
800-437-2423
FAX: 301-258-9454
e-mail: janthony@ahaf.org
www.ahaf.org

Jane Anthony, Donor Services Coordinater

2538 American Occupational Therapy Foundation
4720 Montgomery Lane
Po Box 31220
Bethesda, MD 20824
301-652-6611
FAX: 301-656-3620
e-mail: aotf@aotf.org
www.aotf.org

Mindy Hecker, Director of Information
Jane Huntington, Executive Assistant
Martha Kirkland, Consultant

2539 Arc of Maryland
49 Old Solomons Island Road
Suite 205
Annapolis, MD 21401
410-571-9320
FAX: 410-974-6021
e-mail: info@thearcmd.org
www.thearcmd.org

Christine Marchand, Executive Director
Sarah Basehart, Assistant Director
Susan McGarry, Director of Finance

2540 Baltimore Community Foundation
2 E Read Street
9th Floor
Baltimore, MD 21202
410-332-4171
FAX: 410-837-4701
e-mail: questions@bcf.org
www.bcf.org

Thomas Wilcox, President And Ceo
Shauna'h Martin, Executive Assistant
Laurie Baker Crosley, Director
Makes grants in Baltimore City and Baltimore County; see website for how to apply.

2541 Candlelighters Childhood Cancer Foundation
PO Box 498
Kensington, MD 20895
301-962-3520
800-366-2223
FAX: 301-962-3521
e-mail: staff@candlelighters.org
www.candlelighters.org

Ruth Hoffman, Executive Director/Owner
Janine Lynne, Co-President
Ken Philips, Treasurer
An international organization providing information and support, and advocacy to parents of children with cancer and survivors of childhood cancer.Health and Education professionals also welcome as members.Network of local support groups. Information on disabilities related to treatment of childhood cancer. Publications.

2542 Children's Fresh Air Society Fund
Baltimore Community Foundation
2 E Read Street
Baltimore, MD 21202
410-332-4171
FAX: 410-837-4701
www.bcf.org

Thomas Wilcox, President
Makes grants to nonprofit camps to provide tuition for disadvantaged and disabled Maryland children to attend summer camp. See website for how to apply.

2543 Clark-Winchcole Foundation
3 Bethesda Metro Center
Suite 550
Bethesda, MD 20814
301-654-3607

Vincent Burke Jr., President
Supported tax-exempt charitable organizations operating in the metropolitan area of Washington, DC in the following areas: deaf, higher education and physically disabled.

2544 Columbia Foundation
10227 Wincopin Circle
Suite G15
Columbia, MD 21044
410-730-7840
FAX: 410-997-6021
e-mail: info@columbiafoundation.org
http://www.columbiafoundation.org/

Meg Moon Esq., Chair
Mary Ann Scully, Vice Chair
Dorothy V. Harris, Secretary

2545 Cystic Fibrosis Foundation
6931 Arlington Road
Bethesda, MD 20814
301-951-4422
800-344-4823
FAX: 301-951-6378
e-mail: info@cff.org
www.cff.org/

2546 Foundation Fighting Blindness
11435 Cronhill Drive
Owings Mills, MD 21117
800-683-5555
TTY:800-683-5551
e-mail: info@blindness.org
www.fightblindness.org

Gordon Gund, Chairman
Edward H Gollob, President
David B. Brint, Vice President
The urgent mission of The Foundation Fighting Blindness is to fund the research with will discover the causes, treatments, preventive methods and cures for Retinitis Pigmentosa, Macular Degeneration, Usher Syndrome, Stargart disease, and the entire spectrum of retinal degenerative diseases.

2547 George Wasserman Family Foundation
Grossberg Company
6707 Democracy Boulevard
Suite 300
Bethesda, MD 20817
301-571-1900
FAX: 301-571-1932

Janice W Goldsten, President
Anthony Cpa, Partner

2548 Harry and Jeanette Weinberg Foundation
7 Park Center Court
Owings Mills, MD 21117
410-654-8500
FAX: 410-654-4900
hjweinbergfoundation.org

Shale Stiller, President/Trustee
Donn Weinberg, VP/Trustee
Barry I. Schloss, Treasurer/Trustee

2549 Miracle-Ear Children's Foundation
5000 Cheshire Lane
Minneapolis, MN 55446
877-268-4264
FAX: 763-268-4365
www.miracle-ear.com

Nonprofit organization that provides hearing aids to children whose families to not qualify for public assistance. Provides hearing aid fittings and follow-up care and services free of charge through Miracle-Ear Hearing Centers. Provides information on alternative communication. Offers educational materials and brochures.

2550 National Federation of the Blind
1800 Johnson Street
Baltimore, MD 21230
410-659-9314
FAX: 410-685-5653
e-mail: f.wurtzel@comcast.net
www.nfb.org

Michael Barber, President
Deb Smith, Vice President
Joy Harris, Secretary

The largest consumer membership organization of the blind, founded in 1940, it has 50,000 members nationwide in 52 affiliates and over 700 local chapters. Provides public education about blindness, support services to the newly blinded, scholarships, publications about blindness, adaptive equipment for the blind, advocacy services, Newsline for the Blind, assistive technology information and Job Opportunities for the Blind.

2551 Ryland Group Corporate Giving Program
11000 Broken Land Parkway
Columbia, MD 21044
800-267-0998
FAX: 443-367-3500

Maurice M Simpkins, Vice President

2552 Sjogren's Syndrome Foundation
6707 Democracy Boulevard
Suite 325
Bethesda, MD 20817
301-530-4420
800-475-6473
FAX: 301-530-4415
e-mail: tms@sjogrens.org
www.sjogrens.org

Steven Taylor, Ceo
Sheriese Defruscio, Vice President

Provides patients practical information and coping strategies that minimize the effects of Sjogren's syndrome. In addition, the Foundation is the clearinghouse for medical information and is the recognized national advocate for Sjogren's syndrome.
$25.00
Monthly

Massachusetts

2553 Abbot and Dorothy H Stevens Foundation
PO Box 111
North Andover, MA 01845
978-688-7211
FAX: 978-686-1620

Josh Miner, Executive Director

2554 Arc Massachusetts
217 South Street
Waltham, MA 02453
781-891-6270
FAX: 781-891-6271
e-mail: arcmass@arcmass.org
www.arcmass.org

Beth Rutledge, Administrative Assistant
John Thomas, Deputy Director
Brenda Asis, Director of Development

Advocacy and education for individuals with intellectual and developmental disabilties.

2555 Bank of Boston Corporation Charitable Foundation
100 Federal Street
Boston, MA 02110
617-434-2659

Giving primarily to New England.

2556 Boston Foundation
75 Arlington Street
10th Floor
Boston, MA 02116
617-338-1700
FAX: 617-338-1604
e-mail: info@tbf.org
www.tbf.org

Paul Grogan, President

2557 Boston Globe Foundation
135 Morrissey Boulevard
Po Box 55819
Boston, MA 02205
617-929-2000
e-mail: sainsley@globe.com
www.botonglobe.com/foundation

Ainsley P. Steven, Publisher

The mission of the Boston Globe Foundation is to empower community-based organizations to effect real change in the ares of greatest need, where the Globe is uniquely postioned to add the most value. Priority focus areas: strengthen the reading, writing and critical thinking of young people, while fostering their inherent love of learning. Strengthen the roads that link people to culture. Strengthen the civic fabric of the city. Be responsive to the needs of our immediate community.

2558 Bushrod H Campbell and Ada F Hall Charity Fund
Palmer & Dodge
111 Huntington Avenue
Boston, MA 02199
617-239-0540
FAX: 617-227-4420

Brenda Taylor, Foundation Administrator

The fund's areas of interest include organizations and/or their projects supporting aid to the elderly, healthcare and population control. Medical research grants are administered through the Medical Foundation. No grants are awarded to individuals and the geographical area of support is limited to organizations located in Massachusetts within the area of Boston and Route 128.

2559 Clipper Ship Foundation
55 Court Street
Suite 520
Boston, MA 02108
617-426-2606
FAX: 617-426-2849
e-mail: agm@agmconnect.org
www.agmconnect.org/

Ron Ancrum, President
Miki Akimoto, Vice President

2560 Community Foundation of Western Massachusetts
PO Box 15769
Springfield, MA 01115
413-732-2858
FAX: 413-733-8565
e-mail: wmass@communityfoundation.org
www.communityfoundation.org

Kent W Faerber, President/CEO
Kristen Leutz, Director of Development

Provides a simple way to achieve the charitable objectives of donors most effectively; supports nonprofit organizations that offer programs in the arts, education, human services, healthcare, housing, and the environment; and works to improve the quality of life in our region.

2561 Frank R and Elizabeth Simoni Foundation
434 Providence Highway
Norwood, MA 02062
781-762-3449
FAX: 781-769-6166

Victor F Coletti, Vice President
Robert Donald, Manager

2562 **Friendly Ice Cream Corp Contributions Prog ram**
1855 Boston Road
Wilbraham, MA 01095
800-966-9970
www.friendlys.com

Barbara Miller, Director

2563 **Greater Worcester Community Foundation**
370 Main Street
Suite 650
Worcester, MA 01608
508-755-0980
e-mail: atlisi@greaterworcester.org
www.greaterworcester.org

Ann T Lisi, Executive Director
Joe Wiinikka-Lydon, Prgram Officer

2564 **Hyams Foundation**
50 Federal Street
9th Floor
Boston, MA 02110
617-426-5600
FAX: 617-426-5696
e-mail: info@hyamsfoundation.org
www.hyamsfoundation.org

Elizabeth B Smith, Executive Director
Sylvia R Johnson, Associate Director

2565 **Nathaniel and Elizabeth P Stevens Foundation**
PO Box 111
North Andover, MA 01845
978-688-7211
FAX: 978-686-1620

Elizabeth A Beland, Administrator

2566 **Raytheon Company Contributions Program**
870 Winter Street
Waltham, MA 02451
781-522-3000
e-mail: jonathan_d_kasle@raytheon.com
raytheon.com/

William Swanson, Chairman And Ceo
Industry leader in defense and government electronics, space, information technology, technical services, and business aviation and special mission aircraft.

2567 **Spero Charitable Foundation**
Shirley Spero
79 Florence Street
Suite 200
Chestnut Hill, MA 02467
617-244-3174
FAX: 617-244-3174

2568 **The TJX Foundation**
The TJX Companies
770 Cochituate Road
Framingham, MA 01701
508-390-3199
FAX: 508-390-2091

Christine A Strickland, Foundation Manager
Carol Meyrowitz, President & CEO

2569 **Vision Foundation**
8901 Strafford Circle
Knoxville, TN 37923
865-357-4603
FAX: 865-690-9322
e-mail: gordon@visionfoundation.net
www.visionfoundation.net

Rev. Adams, Prsident
Offers counseling, support groups, seminars and transportation for the blind providing 600 members.

Michigan

2570 **Ann Arbor Area Community Foundation**
301 North Main St.
Suite 300
Ann Arbor, MI 48104
734-663-0401
FAX: 734-663-3514
e-mail: info@aaacf.org
www.aaacf.org

Cheryl Elliott, President/CEO
Martha L Bloom, Vice President
Phil D'Anieri, Program Director
Interested in funding projects which will improve the quality of life for citizens of the Ann Arbor area. Eligible projects generally fall within these categories: education, culture, social service, community development, environmental awareness and health and wellness. The Foundation aims to support creative approaches to community needs and problems by making grants which will benefit the widest possible range of people.

2571 **Arc of Michigan**
State of Michigan
1325 S Washington Avenue
Lansing, MI 48910
517-487-5426
800-292-7851
FAX: 517-487-0303
e-mail: tcler429@aol.com
www.arcmi.org

Dohn Hoyle, Executive Director
Tom Lerchen, President
Norm Delisle, Vice President

2572 **Berrien Community Foundation**
2900 S State Street
Suite 2e
Saint Joseph, MI 49085
269-983-3304
FAX: 269-983-4939
e-mail: bcf@BerrienCommunity.org

Nanette M. Keisetz Ed.D, President

2573 **Blind Children's Fund**
201 S University Street
Mt. Pleasant, MI 48858
989-779-9966
FAX: 989-779-0015
e-mail: bcf@blindchildrensfund.org
www.blindchildrensfund.org

Karla Storrer, Executive Director
Provides parents and profesionsals informaion materials and resources that help them scuccesfullly teach and nurture blind, visually and multi-impaired infants and preschoolers.

2574 **Clarence & Grace Chamberlin Foundation**
600 Woodbridge Street
Detroit, MI 48226
313-567-1000
FAX: 313-567-1001
e-mail: jking@berrymoorman.com

John L King, President

2575 **Community Foundation of Monroe County**
28 South Macomb Street
Po Box 627
Monroe, MI 48161
734-242-1976
FAX: 734-242-1234
e-mail: ktheisen@cfmonroe.org
www.cfmonroe.org

Kristyn Theisen, Executive Director

2576 **Cowan Slavin Foundation**
7881 Dell Road
Saline, MI 48176
734-944-0469
FAX: 734-944-3529

Marjorie Bovee, Executive Director

2577 **Daimler Chrysler**
Automobility Program
PO Box 5080
Troy, MI 48007
800-255-9877
FAX: 248-925-3062
TTY:800-922-3826
www.dc-automobility.com

Jennifer Rossbach, Account Supervisor
Provides a cash reimbursement to assist in reducing the cost of adaptive driving equipment and conversion aids installed on new model Daimler Chrysler LLC vehicles. Up to a maximum of $1000 on Dodge Caravan, Grand Caravan, and Chrysler Town and Country vans and up to $750 on all other vehicles.

2578 **Frank & Mollie S VanDervoort Memorial Foun dation**
4646 Okemos Road
Okemos, MI 48864
517-349-7232

Ann L Gessert, Secretary

2579 **Fremont Area Foundation**
PO Box B
Fremont, MI 49412
231-924-5350
FAX: 231-924-5391
e-mail: info@tfacf.org
www.tfaf.org

Elizabeth Cherin, President And Ceo
Kathryn Huschke, Chief Program Officer
Kathleen Bower, Program Officer
A local nonprofit organization serving the residence of Newaygo County. We connect the needs of the community with those who have the conviction to make a lasting impact. Our mission is to improve the quality of life for the people of Newaygo County.

2580 **Grand Rapids Foundation**
161 Ottawa Avenue NW
Suite 209c
Grand Rapids, MI 49503
616-454-1751

e-mail: dsieger@grfoundation.org
www.grfoundation.org

Diana Sieger, President

2581 **Granger Foundation**
PO Box 22187
Lansing, MI 48909
517-393-1670

e-mail: elee@grangerconstruction.com
www.grangerfoundation.org

Alton Granger, President
Janice Granger, Trustee

2582 **Harvey Randall Wickes Foundation**
4800 Fashion Square Boulevard
Saginaw, MI 48604
989-799-1850
FAX: 989-799-3327

James Finkbeiner
Grants for rehabilitation.

2583 **Havirmill Foundation**
3503 Greenleaf Boulevard
Suite 203
Kalamazoo, MI 49008
269-375-1800
FAX: 269-375-1346

Jerry L Miller, President
Kenneth Miller, Owner

2584 **Kelly Services Foundation**
999 W Big Beaver Road
Troy, MI 48084
248-362-4444
FAX: 248-244-5518

Kelly Sylvested, Corporate Manager
Carl Camden, Chief Executive Officer

2585 **Kresge Foundation**
3215 W Big Beaver Road
Troy, MI 48084
248-643-9630
FAX: 248-643-0588
e-mail: info@kresge.org
www.kresge.org

Ripn Rapson, President And Ceo
Sharon Zimmerman, Executive Assistant
This foundation offers challenge grants for capital projects, most often for construction or renovation of buildings, but also for the purchase of major equipment and real estate. As challenge grants, they are intended to stimulate new, private gifts in the midst of an organized fund raising effort. Offers special opportunities to build capacity, both in providing enhanced facilities in which to present programs and in generating private support. Only charitable organizations may apply.

2586 **Lanting Foundation**
1575 S Shore Drive
Holland, MI 49423
616-355-2740

Arlyn Lanting, Partner

2587 **Ransom Fidelity Company Foundation**
702 Michigan National Tower
Lansing, MI 48933
517-482-1538
FAX: 517-482-1539
Grants for the schools, Native Americans, minorities, environmnt, youth and physically disabled.

2588 **Rollin M Gerstacker Foundation**
PO Box 1945
Midland, MI 48641
989-631-6097

E N Brandt, Vice President

2589 **Steelcase Foundation**
PO Box 1967
Grand Rapids, MI 49501
616-246-4695
FAX: 616-475-2200
e-mail: sbroman@steelcase.com

Susan Broman, Executive Director

Minnesota

2590 **Arc of Minnesota**
The Arc of Minnesota
770 Transfer Road
Suite 26
Saint Paul, MN 55114
651-523-0823
800-582-5256
e-mail: mail@arcmn.org
www.thearcofminnesota.org

Steve Larson, Executive Director
Monica Saby, Secretary
Your membership in The Arc of Minnesotta benefits persons with developmental disabilities and their families as they live, learn, work and play. Please join today!

2591 **Deluxe Corporation Foundation**
Deluxe Corporation
PO Box 64235
Saint Paul, MN 55164

e-mail: jenny.anderson@deluxe.com
www.deluxe.com

Jennifer A Anderson, Director Foundations
Lee J. Schramm, President

2592 **General Mills Foundation**

PO Box 9452
Minneapolis, MN 55440
800-248-7310
FAX: 763-764-8330
e-mail: corporate.response@genmills.com
www.generalmills.com/

2593 **Hugh J Andersen Foundation**

White Pine Building
342 5th Avenue N.
Bayport, MN 55003
651-439-1557
888-439-9508
FAX: 651-439-9480
e-mail: hjafdn@srinc.biz
www.srinc.biz/

Brad Kruse, Program Director

Established in 1962, this fund is a nonprofit charitable corporation classified as a private foundation. The Foundation was established as a general charitable fund, but now identifies projects that build individual and community capacity to be a priority. Giving is focused primarily in the counties of Washington, Minnesota, & St, Croix, Polk and Pierce of Wl. Grants are given in the areas of human services, health, education, arts and culture, community services and the environment.

2594 **James R Thorpe Foundation**

Bremer Tower
445 Minnesota Street
Suite 500
St Paul, MN 55101
651-228-9061
800-774-2655
FAX: 651-228-0379
e-mail: colleges@mnprivatecolleges.org
www.mnprivatecolleges.com

John Manning, Director of Marketing

2595 **Jay and Rose Phillips Family Foundation**

East Bridge Building
10 2nd Street NE
Suite 200
Minneapolis, MN 55413
612-623-1654
FAX: 612-623-1653
e-mail: phillipsfnd@phillipsfnd.org
www.phillipsfund.org

Amy Crawford, Executive Director
Arlene M. Reed, Admin. Assistant
Patrick Troska, Senior Program Officer

2596 **Minneapolis Foundation**

800 Ids Center
80 South Eighth Street
Minneapolis, MN 55402
612-672-3878
FAX: 612-672-3846
e-mail: email@mplsfoundation.org
www.mplsfoundation.org

Sandra Vargas, President And Ceo
Jenifer Thompson, Executive Assistant

2597 **Ordean Foundation**

424 W Superior Street
Duluth, MN 55802
218-726-4785

Stephen A Mangan, Executive Director

Grants are given for a variety of purposes including: treatment and rehabilitation for persons who are chronically or temporarily mentally ill, persons whose physical capacity is impaired by injury or illness, promotes mental and physical health of the elderly, provides for youth guidance programs designed to avoid delinquency, and provides relief, aid and charity to people with no or low incomes. Grants are only offered to certain cities and townships near and around St. Louis County/Duluth.

2598 **Otto Bremer Foundation**

445 Minnesota Street
Suite 2250
Saint Paul, MN 55101
651-227-8036
FAX: 651-312-3665
e-mail: obf@bremer.org
www.ottobremer.org

John Kostishack, Executive Director
Christine Tholkess, Program Officer

2599 **Rochester Area Foundation**

2200 2nd Street SW
Suite 300
Rochester, MN 55902
507-282-1027
FAX: 507-282-4938
e-mail: info@rochesterarea.org
www.rochesterarea.org

Steve Thornton, Executive Director
Chris Mart, Admin. Assistant
Jane Campion, Grants Admin.

Mississippi

2600 **Arc of Mississippi**

7 Lakeland Circle
Suite 600
Jackson, MS 39216
601-982-1180
800-717-1180
FAX: 601-982-5792
e-mail: info@arcms.org
www.arcms.org

Matt Nalker, Executive Director

Missouri

2601 **Allen P & Josephine B Green Foundation**

222 South Jefferson Street
Po Box 523
Mexico, MO 65265
573-581-5568
FAX: 573-581-1714
e-mail: nrcox@greenfdn.org
www.greenfdn.org

While the Foundation makes grants in a variety of fields, in the past its major support was in the field of medical research. During a 20-year period, 1951-71, it contributed over $900,000 to research in Parkinson's and related diseases of the nervous system; $600,000 for research in pediatric neurology and lesser amounts in other areas of medical research, but the board is now trending in other directions. Grants are limited to Missouri and none are offered to individuals.

2602 **Anheuser-Busch Inc.**

One Busch Place
St. Louis, MO 63118
800-342-5283
http://www.anheuser-busch.com/

2603 **Greater Kansas City Community Foundation and Affiliated Trusts**

1055 Broadway Street
Suite 130
Kansas City, MO 64105
816-842-0944
FAX: 816-842-8079
e-mail: info@gkccf.org
www.gkccf.org

Jodi Adams, Investment Accountant
George Bittner, Executive Vice President

2604 **Greater St. Louis Community Foundation**
319 N 4th Street
Suite 300
Saint Louis, MO 63102 314-588-8200
FAX: 314-588-8088
e-mail: dluckes@gstlcf.org
www.stlcf.org

David R Luckes, President/CEO
Marilyn J. Trauner, Executive Assistant
To improve the quality of life across the region by helping individuals, families and businesses make a difference through charitable giving.

2605 **H&R Block Foundation**
One H&R Block Way
Kansas City, MO 64105 816-854-4361
FAX: 816-854-8025
e-mail: foundation@hrblock.com
http://www.hrblockfoundation.org/

David P Miles, President
Carey Wilkerson Looney, Vice President Secretary
Robert Bloch, Program Officer
A charitable organization under the not-for-profit corporation law of the state of Missouri. Grants are made only to organizations which are tax exempt from Federal Income taxation and which are not classified as private foundations. Major emphasis is placed in the metropolitan areas of Kansas City, Missouri: and Columbus, Ohio. The goal is to provide proportionately significant support of relatively few activities, as opposed to minor support for a great many.

2606 **James S McDonnell Foundation**
1034 S Brentwood Boulevard
Suite 1850
Saint Louis, MO 63117 314-721-1532
FAX: 314-721-7421
www.jsmf.org

John T Bruer Md, President
Susan M Fitzpatrick, Vice President

2607 **Lutheran Charities Foundation of St. Louis**
211 N Broadway
Suite 1290
Saint Louis, MO 63102 314-231-2244
FAX: 314-231-0799
e-mail: info@lutheranfoundation.org
www.lutheranfoundation.org

Ann Vazquez, President/CEO
Donna Lucker, Foundation Secretary

2608 **Mary's Call**
Po Box 162
504 W. U.S. Hwy.24
Salisbury, MO 65281 660-388-5308

e-mail: maryscall@maryscall.com
www.maryscall.com

2609 **Oppenstein Brothers Foundation**
PO Box 13095
Kansas City, MO 64199 816-234-8671

Sheila K Rice, Program Officer

2610 **RA Bloch Cancer Foundation**
One H&R Block Way
Kansas City, MO 64105 816-854-5050
800-433-0464
FAX: 816-854-8024
www.blochcancer.org
Provides a hotline that matches newly diagnosed cancer patients with someone who has survived the same kind of cancer. Offers free infomration, resources and support groups, and distributes lists of multidisciplinary second opnion centers. Also supplies three books at no charge: Fighting Cancer; Cancer... There's Hope; and A Guide for Cancer Supporters. All services and books are free of charge.

2611 **Victor E Speas Foundation**
10434 Indiana Ave.
Kansas City, MO 64137 816-868-9300

e-mail: vccmetro@crn.org
www.vcckcmetro.org

Latricia Scott Adams, President

Nebraska

2612 **Arc of Nebraska**
1672 Van Dorn Street
Lincoln, NE 68502 402-475-4407

e-mail: arcneb@inebraska.com
www.arc-nebraska.org

Jill Meile, Secretary
Arc of Nebraska is commited to helping children and adults with disabilities secure the oppurtunity to choose and realize their goals of where and how they learn, live, work, and play.

2613 **Cooper Foundation**
870 Wells Fargo Center
1248 O Street
Lincoln, NE 68508 402-476-7571
FAX: 402-476-2356
e-mail: info@cooperfoundation.org
www.cooperfoundation.org

Art Thompson, President
Serves only Nebraska with the primary interest in education, arts and humanities and the human services area.

2614 **Slosburg Family Charitable Trust**
10040 Regency Circle
Suite 200
Omaha, NE 68114 402-391-7900
FAX: 402-391-6615

D David Slosburg, Treasurer/Owner

2615 **Union Pacific Foundation**
1400 Douglas Street
Omaha, NE 68179 402-544-5000
888-870-8777
www.up.com

James R. Young, Chair President And Ceo

Nevada

2616 **Conrad N Hilton Foundation**
100 W Liberty Street
Suite 840
Reno, NV 89501 775-323-4221
FAX: 775-323-4150
e-mail: cnhf@hiltonfoundation.org
www.hiltonfoundation.org

Edmund Cain, Vice President
Steven Hilton, President And Ceo
Our grant-making style is to initiate and develop major long-term projects and then seek out the organizations to implement them. As a consequence of this proactive approach, the Foundation does not generally consider unsolicited proposals. Our major projects currently include: blindness prevention and treatment, support the work of the Catholic Sisters, drug abuse prevention among youth, support of the Conrad N. Hilton College of Hotel and Restaurant Management, and much more.

2617 **EL Wiegand Foundation**
165 W Liberty Street
Reno, NV 89501 775-333-0300
FAX: 775-333-0314

Kristen A Avansino, President
Raymond Avansino Jr, Manager

2618 **Mark B Wallner Foundation**
1105 Cambria Way
El Dorado Hills, CA 95762 775-856-1166

Kimberly England, President

2619 **Nell J Redfield Foundation**
PO Box 61
Reno, NV 89504 775-323-1373
FAX: 775-323-4476

Gerald C Smith, Director

2620 **William N and Pennington Foundation**
441 W Plumb Lane
Reno, NV 89509 775-333-9100
FAX: 775-333-9111

Kent Green, Manager
William Pennington, Owner

New Hampshire

2621 **Agnes M Lindsay Trust**
660 Chestnut Street
Manchester, NH 03104

e-mail: admin@lindsaytrust.org
www.lindsaytrust.org

Susan Bouchard, Administrative Director
Funding for health and wefare organizations, special needs, mental health, blind, deaf and cultural programs to organizations, specifically for capital needs, not operating funds, located in the New England states of Maine, Massachusetts, New Hampshire and Vermont. We highly recommend you visit our web site.

2622 **Foundation for Seacoast Health**
100 Campus Drive
Suite 1
Portsmouth, NH 03801 603-422-8200

e-mail: ffsh@communitycampus.org
www.ffsh.org

Daniel C. Hoefle, Chair
Timothy Connors, Vice Chair
Patricia Barbour, Treasurer
Giving limited to Portsmouth, Rye, New Castle, Greenland, Newington, North Hampton, NH; and Kittery, Eliot, and York, ME.

New Jersey

2623 **American Express Foundation**
200 Vesey Street
New York, NY 10285 212-640-2000
FAX: 201-209-4303

Kenneth Chenault, Chief Executive Officer
Giving primarily in Arizona, California, Colorado, Florida, Georgia, Illinois, Minnesota, North Carolina, Nebraska, New York, Texas, Utah, Massachusetts and Pennsylvania. Also include international committees.

2624 **Arc of New Jersey**
985 Livingston Avenue
N Brunswick, NJ 08902 732-246-2525
FAX: 732-214-1834
e-mail: info@arcnj.org
www.arcnj.org

Thomas Baffuto, Executive Director
Celine Fortin, Assistant Director

2625 **Arnold A Schwartz Foundation**
15 Mountain Boulevard
Warren, NJ 07059 908-757-7800
FAX: 908-757-8039
e-mail: skunzmannewjerseylaw.net

Steven A. Kunzman, President

2626 **Campbell Soup Foundation**
PO Box 60f
Camden, NJ 08101 856-342-4800
FAX: 856-342-3878

John M Coleman, Chairman
James J Baldwin, Vice Chairman
Douglas Conant, Chief Executive Officer
Goal of this foundation is to match the company's assets with community needs in order to help forge solutions to community challenges. The Foundation believes that involvement at the community level can play a catalytic role in improving the quality of life. Giving is located in the areas of education, nutrition and health, cultural and youth related programs. The major focus of the foundation is on nutrition and health related matters, and places a high priority on Camden, New Jersey areas.

2627 **Children's Hopes & Dreams Wish Fulfillment Foundation**
280 Us Highway 46
Dover, NJ 07801 973-361-7348
800-IDR-EAM2
FAX: 973-361-6627
e-mail: info@chddover.org
www.childrenswishes.org

Victor Franklin Jr, President
Mariann Oswald, Executive Director
Provides continual support for children and their families through the International Pen-Pal Program and the Kid's Kare Packages program. All services are free. Fulfills the last dreams of children with life threatening illnesses.

2628 **Community Foundation of New Jersey**
PO Box 338
Knox Hill Road
Morristown, NJ 07963 973-267-5533
800-659-5533
FAX: 973-257-2903
www.cfnj.org

Hans Dekker, President
Patty Heath, Financial Assistant
Giving limited to the state of New Jersey.

2629 **Cowles Charitable Trust**
PO Box 219
Rumson, NJ 07760 732-936-9826

Gardner Cowles III, President

2630 **F Mason Perkins Trust**
210 Main Street
Hackensack, NJ 07601 201-646-5225
FAX: 201-646-9881

2631 **FM Kirby Foundation**
PO Box 151
Morristown, NJ 07963 973-538-4800
FAX: 973-538-4801
fdncenter.org/grantmaker/kirby/

F Kirby, President

2632 Fannie E Rippel Foundation
180 Mount Airy Road
Suite 200
Basking Ridge, NJ 07920 908-766-0404

e-mail: info@rippelfoundation.org
www.mharc.com/fundpri-rz.htm

Edward W Probert, President/CEO

2633 Fund for New Jersey
94 Church Street
Suite 303
New Brunswick, NJ 08901 732-220-8656
FAX: 732-220-8654
e-mail: info@fundfornj.org
www.fundfornj.org

Candace McKee-Ashmun, Vice Chairman
Mark Murphy, Executive Director

2634 Merck Company Foundation
PO Box 100
Whitehouse Station, NJ 08889 908-423-1000
FAX: 908-423-1987
www.merck.com

David A Ruth, Executive Vice President
Richard Clark, Chief Executive Officer

2635 Merrill Lynch & Company Foundation
2 World Financial Center
New York, NY 10281 212-236-5065

Eddy Bayardelle, Vice President

2636 Milton Schamach Foundation
411 Hackensack Avenue
Hackensack, NJ 07601 973-423-9494
FAX: 973-423-2376

Andrew Er Frommel Jr, Secretary/Treasurer

2637 Nabisco Foundation
7 Campus Drive
Parsippany, NJ 07054 973-682-5000
FAX: 973-503-3018

2638 Ostberg Foundation
PO Box 1098
Alpine, NJ 07620 201-569-6800
FAX: 201-569-6606

Charles Borhan

2639 Prudential Foundation
Prudential Financial
751 Broad Street
15th Floor
Newark, NJ 07102 973-802-6000
FAX: 973-802-3345
e-mail: community.resources@prudential.com
www.prudential.com

Gabriella Morris, President
Arthur Ryan, Chief Executive Officer
Gives priority to national programs that further our objectives and programs serving areas where The Prudential has a substantial employee presence. Places special emphasis on the home state of New Jersey and the headquarters city, Newark.

2640 Robert Wood Johnson Foundation
PO Box 2316
Princeton, NJ 08543 609-452-8701
FAX: 888-727-1966
e-mail: mail@rwjf.org
www.rwjf.org

Richard J Toth, Director Office/Proposal
Risa Lavizzo-Mourey, Chief Executive Officer
Our mission is to assure that all Americans have access to basic health care at reasonable cost, improve care and support for people with chronic health conditions, promote healthy communities and lifestyles and also, reduce the personal, social and economic harm caused by substance abuse.

2641 Victoria Foundation
946 Bloomfield Avenue
Glen Ridge, NJ 07028 973-748-5300
FAX: 973-748-0016
e-mail: icb@victoriafoundation.org
www.victoriafoundation.org

Catherine M McFarland, Executive Officer
Desire is to help individuals in need reach their potential remains. Provides emergency coal for needy families and treated rheumatic fever in children.

New Mexico

2642 Arc of New Mexico
3655 Carlisle Boulevard NE
Albuquerque, NM 87110 505-883-4630
800-358-6493
FAX: 505-883-5564
e-mail: arcnm@arcnm.org
www.arcnm.org

Randy Costales, Associate Director
Rebecca Schuman, Executive Director
Our mission is to improve the quality of life for individuals with developmental disabilities of all ages by advocating for equal opportunities and choices in where and how they learn, live, work, play and socialize. The Arc of New Mexico promotes self-determination, healthy families, effective community support systems and partnerships.

2643 Frost Foundation
511 Armijo Street
Apt A
Santa Fe, NM 87501 505-986-0208
FAX: 505-986-0430
www.frostfound.org

Mary Whited-Howell, President

2644 McCune Charitable Foundation
345 E Alameda Street
Santa Fe, NM 87501 505-983-8300
FAX: 505-983-7887
e-mail: mccune@nmmccune.org
www.nmmccune.org

Frances R Sowers, Associate Director
Sarah M Losinger, Chairman
Owen Lopez, Executive Director

2645 Santa Fe Community Foundation
PO Box 1827
Santa Fe, NM 87504 505-988-9715
FAX: 505-988-1829
e-mail: foundation@santafecf.org
www.santafecf.org

Amy S Duggan, Program Officer
Billie Blair, President

New York

2646 AT&T Foundation
32 Avenue of the Americas
24th Floor
New York, NY 10013 212-387-5400
FAX: 212-387-5097
e-mail: info@att.com
www.att.com/foundation/

Ronald Dabney, Communications Manager
Edward Whitacre, Chief Executive Officer

2647 Alavi Foundation of New York
500 5th Avenue
New York, NY 10110
212-944-8333
FAX: 212-921-0325
www.alavifoundation.org/
Purposes are charitable and philanthropic with an emphasis on education and civic concerns.
1973

2648 Altman Foundation
521 5th Avenue
Floor 35
New York, NY 10175
212-682-0970
www.foundationcenter.org/grantmaker/altman

Jane B O'Connell, President
Karen L Rosa, VP/Executive Director
John W Townsend, VP
For the benefit of such charitable and educational institutions in the City of New York as said directors shall approve. Foundation grants support programs and institutions that enrich the quality of life in the city, with a particular focus on initiatives that help individuals, families and communities benefit from the services and opportunities that will enable them to achieve their full potential.
1913

2649 Ambrose Monell Foundation
1 Rockefeller Plaza
Room 301
New York, NY 10020
212-586-0700
FAX: 212-245-1863
e-mail: info@monellvetlesen.org
www.monellvetlesen.org/

George Rowe Jr, President
Voluntary aiding and contributing to religious, charitable, scientific, literary, and educational uses and purposes, in New York, elsewhere in the US and throughout the world.

2650 American Chai Trust
41 Madison Avenue
40th Floor
New York, NY 10010
212-889-0575
FAX: 212-743-8120
e-mail: info@perlmanandperlman.com
www.perlmanandperlman.com

Sammy Mantilla, Systems Administrator

2651 American Foundation for the Blind
11 Penn Plaza
Suite 300
New York, NY 10001
212-502-7600
200-232-5463
FAX: 212-502-7777
e-mail: afbinfo@afb.net
www.afb.org

Carl R Augusto, President/CEO
Richard J O'Brien, Chairman
Dedicated to addressing issues of literacy, independent living, employment, and access through technology for the ten million Americans who are blind or visually impaired.

2652 Arthur Ross Foundation
20 E 74th Street
Suite 4c
New York, NY 10021
212-737-7311
FAX: 212-650-0332

Arthur Ross, President

2653 Artists Fellowship
47 5th Avenue
New York, NY 10003
646-230-9833
e-mail: info@artistsfellowship.org
www.artistsfellowship.org/

2654 Bell Atlantic Foundation
1095 Avenue of the Americas
Room 3200
New York, NY 10036
800-360-7955
FAX: 212-398-0951
www.horizon.com/foundation

Suzanne A Du Bose, President

2655 Bodman Foundation
767 3rd Avenue
Floor 4
New York, NY 10017
212-644-0322
FAX: 212-759-6510
e-mail: main@achelis-bodman-fnds.org
www.fdncenter.org/grantmaker/bodman

Joseph Dolan, Executive Director

2656 Brooklyn Home for Aged Men
PO Box 280062
Brooklyn, NY 11228
718-745-1638

Nancy K Munson, President

2657 Cancer Care
1180 Avenue of the Americas
New York, NY 10036
212-221-3300
800-207-0992
e-mail: clf@airmail.net
celebratinglife.org/

Sylvia Dunnavant, Executive Director

2658 Clark Foundation
415 Madison Ave.
10th Floor
New York, NY 10017
212-551-9100
FAX: 212-421-9325
e-mail: info@emcf.org
http://www.emcf.org

Nancy Roob, President
Susan Pichardo, Office Manager
Giving in New York and New York City.

2659 Commonwealth Fund
1 E 75th Street
New York, NY 10021
212-606-3800
FAX: 212-606-3500
e-mail: info@cmwf.org
http://www.commonwealthfund.org

Karen Davis, President
John Craig, Executive Vice President
A private foundation with the broad charge to enhance the common good. Carries out this mandate by supporting efforts that help people live healthy and productive lives, and by assisting certain groups with serious and neglected problems. Supports independent research on health and social issues and makes grants to improve heathcare practice and policy.
1918

2660 Community Foundation for Greater Buffalo
712 Main Street
Buffalo, NY 14202
716-852-2857
FAX: 716-852-2861
e-mail: gailj@cfgb.org
www.cfgb.org

Gail Johnstone, President

2661 Community Foundation of Herkimer &
1222 State Street
Utica, NY 13502
315-735-8212
FAX: 315-735-9363
e-mail: jdewar@foundationhoc.org
http://www.foundationhoc.org

Margret O'Shea, President/CEO
Susan Korosec, Director of Finance
Jan Squadrito, Senior Program Officer

2662 Community Foundation of the Capitol Region
6 Tower Place
Albany, NY 12203
518-446-9638
FAX: 518-446-9708
e-mail: info@cfcr.org
www.cfcr.org

James E. Prout, Chairman
Sheridan Biggs, Treasurer
Roy M. Hershey, Secretary

2663 Comsearch: Broad Topics
Foundation Center
79 5th Avenue
New York, NY 10003
212-620-4230
800-424-9836
FAX: 212-807-3677
www.fdncenter.org

Sara Engelhardt, President
Maureen Mackey, Executive Vice President
Subset publications of The Foundation Grants Index, are printouts of actual foundation grants, covering 26 key areas of grantmaking. This tool is designed for fundraisers who wish to examine grantmaking activities in a broad field of interest.
$55.00

2664 DE French Foundation
120 Genesee Street
Suite 503
Auburn, NY 13021
315-253-9321

J Douglas Pedley, President

2665 David J Green Foundation
599 Lexington Avenue
Suite 12
New York, NY 10022
212-371-4200
FAX: 212-371-5099

Barbara A McBride, Secretary
Michael Greene, Manager

2666 Easter Seals New York
29 W. 36th Street
4th Floor
New York, NY 10018
212-244-6053
800-727-8785
FAX: 212-244-6059
http://ny.easterseals.com/

John McGrath, Vice President
Hayrim Byun, Director
Offers resources and expertise that allow children and adults with disabilities to live with dignity and independence. A long standing commitment to serve those for whom no other resources exist. Statewide, provides innovative solutions that enhance the lives of people with disabilities, while heightening community awareness and acceptance.

2667 Edward John Noble Foundation
32 E 57th Street
Floor 19
New York, NY 10022
212-759-4212

Noble Smith, Executive Director
June Larkin, Owner

2668 Epilepsy Foundation of Long Island
506 Stewart Avenue
Garden City, NY 11530
516-739-7733
888-672-7154
www.epilepsyfoundation.org/

Richard E Daly, Executive Director
Elaine Lubelsky, CFO
Provides education, counseling and residential care to Long Island residents with epilepsy and related conditions.
1953

2669 Epilepsy Society of New York
305 7th Avenue
12th Floor
New York, NY 10001
212-633-2930
FAX: 212-633-2991
www.epilepsynyc.org

George H Smith, Executive Director
Tara Powers, President

2670 Episcopal Charities
1047 Amsterdam Avenue
New York, NY 10025
212-932-7376
FAX: 212-316-7431
e-mail: episcopalcharities@dioceseny.org
http://www.episcopalcharities-newyork.o rg

Mary Beth Sasso, Executive Director
Mark W. Hummell, Associate Director
Juliet Lowe-Tannis, Development Associate

2671 Esther A & Joseph Klingenstein Fund
787 7th Avenue
Floor 6
New York, NY 10019
212-492-6181
e-mail: kathleen.pomerantz@klingenstein.com
www.klingfund.org

Kathleen Pomerantz, President

2672 Fay J Lindner Foundation
1161 Meadowbrook Road
Merrick, NY 11566
516-292-1331

Ruth Torito, Director
Robert Goldberg, President

2673 Florence V Burden Foundation
630 5th Avenue
Suite 2900
New York, NY 10111
212-332-1100

Edward P H Burden, President
Publishes an annual or periodic report.

2674 Ford Foundation
320 E 43rd Street
New York, NY 10017
212-573-5000
FAX: 212-351-3677
e-mail: office-of-communications@fordfound.org
www.fordfound.org

Susan Berresford, President
A resource for innovative people and institutions worldwide. Goals are to: strenghthen democratic values; reduce poverty and injustice; promote international cooperation; and advance human achievement.

2675 Fortis Foundation
1 Chase Manhattan Plaza
New York, NY 10005
212-859-7000
http://ir.assurant.com

John Palms, Chairman of Board
Robert J. Blendon, Director

Grants are offered in healthcare fields, especially in medical research ($500-$5,000). New York City social, educational organizations also receive funds ($250-$5,000).

2676 **Foundation Center**

79 5th Avenue
New York, NY 10003 212-620-4230
800-424-9836
FAX: 212-807-3677
e-mail: communications@fdncenter.org
www.fdncenter.org

Sara Engelhardt, President
Macy Morin, Executive Vice President
Laura Cascio, Fulfillment Manager
The center disseminates current information on foundation and corporate giving through our national collections in New York City and Washington D.C., our field offices in San Francisco and our network of over 180 cooperating libraries in all 50 states and abroad.

2677 **Foundation Center Library Services**

Foundation Center
79 5th Avenue
New York, NY 10003 212-620-4230
800-424-9836
FAX: 212-807-3677
www.fdncenter.org

Sara Engelhardt, President
Macy Morin, Executive Vice President
The Center disseminates current information on foundation and corporate giving through our national collections in New York City and Washington D.C., our field offices in San Francisco and our network of over 180 cooperating libraries in all 50 states and abroad.

2678 **Foundation for Advancement in Cancer Therapy**

PO Box 1242
Old Chelsea Station
New York, NY 10113 212-741-2790

www.fact-ltd.org

Ruth Sackman, President
Pat Judson, Vice President
A clearinghouse for information regarding alternative cancer therapies, emphasizing nutritional and metabolic approaches.

2679 **Foundation for the Advancement of Innovative Medicine**

2 Executive Boulevard
Suite 206
Suffern, NY 10901 212-501-8143

www.faim.org

Peter Agho
A voice for innovative medicine's professionals, patients, and suppliers. Defines innovative medicine as a treatment or therapy of empirical clinical benefit that is yet outside the mainstream of conventional medicine. Complementary to conventional medicine, offering alternatives as an individual situation may warrant.
1989

2680 **Gebbie Foundation**

111 W 2nd Street
Suite 1100
Jamestown, NY 14701 716-487-1062
FAX: 716-484-6401
e-mail: info@gebbie.org
www.gebbie.org

John Mernio, Executive Director
Thomas J Faber, Program Officer
Jennifer Lewis, Reaserch Associate
Giving in Chautauqua County, and secondly, in neighboring areas of western New York. Giving is offered in other areas only when the project is consonant with program objectives that cannot be developed locally.

2681 **Gladys Brooks Foundation**

126 3rd Street
2nd Floor
Mineola, NY 11501

www.gladysbrooksfoundation.org
Jessica Rutledge, Manager
The purpose of this Foundation is to provide for the intellectual, moral and physical welfare of the people of this country by establishing and supporting nonprofit libraries, educational institutions, hospitals and clinics. The Foundation will make grants only to private, publicly supported, nonprofit, tax-exempt organizations.

2682 **Glickenhaus Foundation**

6 E 43rd Street
New York, NY 10017 212-953-7855

2683 **Graphic Controls Corporate Giving Program**

PO Box 1271
Buffalo, NY 14240 716-853-7500

Phyllis Rudz
John Bellotti, Plant Manager

2684 **Guide Dog Foundation for the Blind**

371 E Jericho Tpke
Smithtown, NY 11787 613-930-9000
800-548-4337
FAX: 631-930-9009
e-mail: info@guidedog.org
www.guidedog.org

Wells B Jones, Chief Executive Officer
Pam Vitale, Executive Assistant
Established in 1946, the Foundation provides rehabilitation for the blind by breeding and training guide dogs. A fully trained guide dog is given to blind applicants from all over the United States and some foreign countries. They train together as a team for 25 days on campus. All of these programs, including the cost of transportation and after-care programs, are given without cost to the blind recipients. Quarterly newsletter, video cassette, audio cassette.

2685 **Henry and Lucy Moses Fund**

405 Lexington Avenue
New York, NY 10174 212-554-7800
FAX: 212-554-7700
e-mail: klinhardt@mosessinger.com
www.mosessinger.com

Jill E. Anderson, Counsel

2686 **Herman Goldman Foundation**

61 Broadway
Floor 18
New York, NY 10006 212-797-9090

e-mail: goldfound@aol.com

Richard K Baron, Executive Director

2687 **Horace W Goldsmith Foundation**

375 Park Avenue
Suite 1602
New York, NY 10152 212-319-8700

James C Slaughter, CEO/Executive Director

2688 **International Paper Company Foundation**

2 Manhattanville Road
Purchase, NY 10577 914-397-4057
FAX: 914-397-1500
www.internationalpaper.com

Robert Amen, President
Martha Brooks, Chief Operation Officer

2689 Jedra Charitable Foundation
11011 Queens Boulevard
Apt 208
Forest Hills, NY 11375 718-263-4956

David Shechet, President

2690 Joseph Alexander Foundation
400 Madison Avenue
Room 906
New York, NY 10017 212-355-3688

2691 Kenneth & Evelyn Lipper Foundation
101 Park Avenue
6th Floor
New York, NY 10178 212-883-6333

Kenneth Lipper, Treasurer

2692 Long Island Alzheimer's Foundation
5 Channel Drive
Port Washington, NY 11050 516-767-6856
FAX: 516-767-6864
e-mail: info@liaf.org
www.liaf.org

Partricia Gallatin, Executive Director
Jen Brajevich, Executive Assistant

2693 Louis and Anne Abrons Foundation
First Manhattan Company
437 Madison Avenue
New York, NY 10022 212-756-3300
FAX: 212-832-6698

David Manischewitz, Chief Executive Officer

2694 Margaret L Wendt Foundation
40 Fountain Plaza
Suite 277
Buffalo, NY 14202 716-855-2146
FAX: 716-855-2149

Robert J Kresse, Secretary/Treasurer/Manager

2695 Marquis George MacDonald Foundation
270 Park Avenue
New York, NY 10017 212-270-6000

Donna M Bowers, Administrator
William Harrison Jr, Chief Executive Officer

2696 Metzger-Price Fund
230 Park Avenue
Suite 2300
New York, NY 10169 212-867-9500
FAX: 212-599-1759

Isaac A Saufer, Secretary/Treasurer
Charles Palella

2697 Milbank Foundation For Rehabilitation
654 Madison Avenue
Suite 1605
New York, NY 10065 212-687-7735
FAX: 212-697-5495

Carl Helstrom, Executive Director
Awarding grants from trust funds based on a competitive selection process or the preferences of the foundation managers and granters. The foundations mission is to integrate people with disabilities into all aspects of american life. Current priorities include, but are not limited to: consumer-focused initiatives that enable people with disablities to lead fulfilling,independent lives; innovative policy research and education on market-based approaches to health care and rehabilitation...

2698 Morgan Stanley Foundation
1585 Broadway Street
New York, NY 10036 212-761-4000

e-mail: mediainquiries@morganstanley.com
www.morganstanleyindividual.com

Jill Bobigan, Senior Vice President

2699 Mount Sinai Medical Center
1 Gustve L Levy Place
New York, NY 10029 212-241-6500

e-mail: barry.stimmel@mssm.edu
www.mountsinaimedicalcenter.org

Barry Stimmel, President
Autism Research

2700 National Foundation for Facial Reconstruction
317 E 34th Street
Room 901
New York, NY 10016 212-263-6656
FAX: 212-263-7534
e-mail: info@nffr.org
www.nffr.org

Whitney Burnett, Executive Director
Michele Golombuski, Associate Executive Director
Melissa Raskin, Director of Special Events
A nonprofit organization whose major purposes are to provide facilities for the treatment and assistance of individuals who are unable to afford private reconstructive surgical care, to train and educate professionals in this surgery, to encourage research in the field and to carry on public education.

2701 National Hemophilia Foundation
116 W. 32nd Street
11th Floor
New York, NY 10001 212-328-3700
FAX: 212-328-3777
e-mail: webmaster@hemophilia.org
www.hemophilia.org

Ray Stanhope, Chair of the Board
Brain K. Andrew, Treasurer
Eileen F. Bostwick, Secretary

2702 National Neurofibromatosis Foundation The Childrens Tumor Foundation
95 Pine Street
16th Floor
New York, NY 10005 212-344-6633
800-323-7938
FAX: 212-747-0004
e-mail: info@ctf.org
www.ctf.org

George Orfanakos, Vice President Development
Wendy Levine, Marathon Program Coordinator
A nonprofit 501 (c)(3) medical foundation, dedicated to improving the health and well-being of individuals and families affected by neurofibromatosis. The Foundation sponsors medical research, clinical services, public education programs and patient support services. It is the central source for up-to-date and accurate information about NF. It also assists patients and families with referrals to NF clinics and healthcare professionals specializing in NF. The goal is to find a cure for NF.

2703 Neisloss Family Foundation
1737 Veterans Highway
Suite 7
Central Islip, NY 11749 631-234-1600
FAX: 631-234-1066

Stanley Neisloss, President/Owner

2704 New York Community Trust
909 3rd Avenue
22nd Floor
New York, NY 10022
212-686-0010
FAX: 212-532-8528
e-mail: info@nycommunitytrust.org
www.nycommunitytrust.org

Lorie A Slutsky, President
Joyce M. Bove, Vice President

2705 New York Foundation
350 5th Avenue
Room 2901
New York, NY 10118
212-594-8009

www.nyf.org

Adriana Rocha

2706 Northern New York Community Foundation
Hsbc Building
120 Washington Street
Suite 400
Watertown, NY 13601
315-782-7110
FAX: 315-782-0047
e-mail: info@nnycf.org
www.nnycf.org

Alex C Velto, Executive Director
Louise Scarlett, Program Associate
Raises, manages and administers an endowment and collection of funds for the benefit of the community

2707 Parkinson's Disease Foundation
1359 Broadway
Suite 1509
New York, NY 10018
212-923-4700
800-457-6676
FAX: 212-923-4778
e-mail: info@pdf.org
www.pdf.org

Robin Elliott, Executive Director
Jeanne Rosner, Director Of Information
Yasnahia Cortorreal, Manager Of Administration
National not-for-profit organization dedicated to funding scientific research to investigate the cause and cure of Parkinson's disease and related disorders. The Foundation has a post-doctoral training program, Interntional Research Grant Program, and makes referrals to physicians who treat PD. Other services include supporting advocacy efforts, making referrals to self-help groups, conducting educational symposiums for patients and professionals.

2708 Reader's Digest Foundation
Readers Digest Association
Readers Digest Road
Pleasantville, NY 10570
914-238-1000
FAX: 914-238-4559
www.readersdigest.com

Claudia L Edwards, Executive Director
Thomas Ryder, Chief Executive Officer

2709 Research to Prevent Blindness
645 Madison Avenue
Floor 21
New York, NY 10022
212-752-4333
800-621-0026
e-mail: inforequest@rpbusa.org
www.rpbusa.org
National voluntary health foundation supported by foundations, corporations and voluntary gifts and bequests from individuals. Established to stimulate basic and applied research into the causes, prevention and treatment of blinding eye diseases.

2710 Rita J and Stanley H Kaplan Foundation
866 United Nations Plaza
Room 306
New York, NY 10017
212-688-1047
FAX: 212-688-6907

Rita J Kaplan, Director
Stanley Kaplan, President

2711 Robert Sterling Clark Foundation
135 E 64th Street
New York, NY 10021
212-288-8900
FAX: 212-288-1033
www.rsclark.org

Margaret Ayers, Executive Director
Darcy Hector, Program Officer
Laura Wolff, Program Officer
Giving primarily in New York with emphasis on advocacy, research, and public education aimed at informing New York City of state policies.

2712 Skadden Fellowship Foundation
4 Times Square
New York, NY 10036
212-735-3000
FAX: 212-735-2000
e-mail: info@skadden.com
www.skadden.com

Jamie Boucher, Attorney

2713 St. George's Society of New York
216 E 45th Street
Suite 901
New York, NY 10017
212-682-6110
FAX: 212-682-7945
www.stgeorgesociety.org

2714 Stanley W Metcalf Foundation
120 Genesee Street
Suite 503
Auburn, NY 13021
315-253-9321

www.ruralhousing.org

J Douglas Pedley, President

2715 Stonewall Community Foundation
119 W 24th Street
7th Floor
New York, NY 10011
212-367-1155
FAX: 212-367-1157
e-mail: stonewall@stonewallfoundation.org
www.stonewallfoundation.org

Ken Green, President
Mission is to promote the well being of lesbian, gay, bisexual, and transgender (LGBT) individuals and strengthen the LGBT community. We do this by increasing resources; targeting those resources strategically to areas of greatest need; and by serving as a catalyst and clearinghouse for ideas and solutions. Through grant-making donor-advised funds, endowment funds and charitable education, Stonewall supports LGBT organizations and helps donors realize their philanthropic goals.

2716 Surdna Foundation
330 Madison Avenue
30th Floor
New York, NY 10017
212-557-0010

e-mail: questions@surdna.org
www.surdna.org

Phillip Henderson, President
Justine Koch, Assistant Controller
Aisha Musto, Program Assistant

2717 The Dana Foundation The Dana Alliance For Brain Initiatives
745 5th Avenue
Suite 900
New York, NY 10151
212-223-4040
FAX: 212-317-8721
e-mail: danainfo@dana.org
www.dana.org/

Barbara E. Gill, Executive Director
Barbara D. Best, Director Member Relations
Karen Graham, Special Projects

2718 The William Randolph Hearst Foundations
300 W. 57th Street
26th Floor
New York, NY 10019
212-586-5404
FAX: 212-586-1917
www.hearstfdn.org

Ilene Mack, Program Director
Alison N. Yu, Program Officer
Mayra Cedeno, Grants Manager

2719 Tisch Foundation
655 Madison Avenue
Floor 8
New York, NY 10021
212-521-2930
FAX: 212-521-2983

Mark J Krinsky, Vice President

2720 Van Ameringen Foundation
509 Madison Avenue
New York, NY 10022
212-758-6221
www.vanamfound.org

Henry P Van Ameringen, President
George Rowe Jr, Vice President
Eleanor Sypher, Executive Director

2721 Western New York Foundation
11 Summer Street
4th Floor
Buffalo, NY 14209
716-839-4225
FAX: 716-883-4954
e-mail: info@wnyfoundation.org
www.wnyfoundation.org

Richard Moot, President
John Walsh, Vice President
John Moot, Secretary

2722 William T Grant Foundation
570 Lexington Avenue
18th Floor
New York, NY 10022
212-752-0071
FAX: 212-752-1398
e-mail: info@wtgrantfdn.org
www.wtgrantfoundation.org

Robert Granger, President
Sharon Brewster, Director

North Carolina

2723 Arc of North Carolina
343 Six Forks Road
Suite 320
Raleigh, NC 27609
919-782-4632
800-662-8706
FAX: 919-782-4634
e-mail: info@arcnc.org
www.arcnc.org

Betty Stanberry, President
Chris Egan, Senior Vice President
Donna Thomas, Secretary

2724 Bob & Kay Timberlake Foundation
1660 E Center Street Ext
Lexington, NC 27292
336-243-7777

Daniel Timberlake, President

2725 Broyhill Family Foundation
PO Box 500
Lenoir, NC 28645
828-758-6100

Hunt Broyhill, President

2726 Duke Endowment
100 North Tryon Street
Suite 3500
Charlotte, NC 28202
704-376-0291
FAX: 704-376-9336
e-mail: info@tde.org
www.dukeendowment.org

Eugene Cochrane, President
Deborah Brinkley, Administrative Assistant
Susan McConnell, Program Officer

2727 First Union Foundation
301 S College Street
Charlotte, NC 28288
704-383-0525
FAX: 704-374-2484

Judy Allison, Director

2728 Foundation for the Carolinas
217 S Tyron Street
Charlotte, NC 28202
704-973-4500
800-973-7244
e-mail: mmarsicano@fftc.org
www.fftc.org

Michael Marsicano, President And Ceo
Laura Meyer, Vice President
Pat Costner, Executive Assistant
Giving primarily to organizations serving the citizens of North and South Carolina.

2729 John H Wellons Foundation
PO Box 1254
Dunn, NC 28335
910-892-0887
FAX: 910-892-4888

John H Wellons, Senior President/Owner

2730 Kate B Reynolds Charitable Trust
The Kate B Reynolds Charitable Trust
128 Reynolda Vlg
Winston Salem, NC 27106
336-723-1456
800-485-9080
FAX: 336-723-7765
e-mail: joyce@kbr.org
www.kbr.org

Joyce Adger, Director
Susie Gordon, Administrative Assistant
Karen McNeil-Miller, President
Grants resricted to the state of North Carolina only.

2731 Kathleen Price and Joseph M Bryan Family Foundation
220 S Eugene Street
Greensboro, NC 27401
336-273-0080
FAX: 336-288-5458

Nancy H Poteet, Interim Director
Joseph M Bryan Jr, President
Only organizations or projects demonstrating direct benefits to North Carolina are eligible for consideration with emphasis on Greensboro and Guilford County and rural communities in North Carolina with financial need. The Foundation does not consider support for annual campaigns, conferences, video production, individuals, research, travel for band and sports teams. There are no discretionary or emergency funds.

2732 Mary Reynolds Babcock Foundation
2920 Reynolda Road
Winston Salem, NC 27106
336-748-9222
FAX: 336-777-0095
e-mail: info@mrbf.org
www.mrbf.org

Glenn Lavastian
For 1994, this foundation is committed to an extensive educational and planning process to better understand the Southeast and to articulate the role the foundation seeks to play in the region into the twenty-first century.

2733 Triangle Community Foundation
324 Blackwell Street
Suite 1220
Durham, NC 27701
919-474-8370
FAX: 919-941-9208
e-mail: info@trianglecf.org
www.trianglecf.org

Fred Stang, Director of Development
Robyn Fehrman, Program Officer
Andrea Bazan-Mason, President

North Dakota

2734 Alex Stern Family Foundation
609 1/2 1st Avenue N
Fargo, ND 58102
701-237-0170
FAX: 701-234-9724

Don Scott, Executive Director

2735 Arc of North Dakota
2500 Demers Ave.
Po Box 12420
Grand Forks, ND 58208
701-772-6191
877-250-2022
FAX: 701-772-2195
e-mail: thearc@arcuv.com
www.thearcuppervalley.com

Dianne Sheppard, Executive Director
Liz Tyree, President
Peggy Johnson, First Vice President

2736 North Dakota Community Foundation
309 N Mandan Street
Suite 2
Po Box 387
Bismarck, ND 58502
701-222-8349
e-mail: kdvorak@ndcf.net
www.ndcf.net

Kevin J Dvorak, President
Valerie Bren, Administrator

Ohio

2737 Akron Community Foundation
345 W Cedar Street
Akron, OH 44307
330-376-8522
www.akroncommunityfdn.org/

Jody Bacon, President
Paul Kunce, Program Officer

2738 Albert G and Olive H Schlink Foundation
49 Benedict Avenue Suite C
Po Box 640
Norwalk, OH 44857
e-mail: atty4u@accnorwalk.com
www.schlinkfoundation.org

2739 American Foundation Corporation
720 National City Bank Building
Cleveland, OH 44114
216-241-6664

William Murphy, President
Barbara Lattner, Manager

2740 Arc of Ohio
1335 Dublin Road
Suite 205c
Columbus, OH 43215
614-487-4720
800-875-2723
FAX: 614-487-4725
e-mail: info@thearcofohio.org
www.thearcofohio.org

Gary Tonks, Executive Director

2741 Cleveland Foundation
1422 Euclid Avenue
Suite 1300
Cleveland, OH 44115
216-861-3810
FAX: 216-861-1729
www.clevelandfoundation.org

J.T. Mullen, Vice President
Lisa Botoms, Program Director
Ronald Richard, President

2742 Columbus Foundation and Affiliated Organizations
1234 E Broad Street
Columbus, OH 43205
614-251-4000
FAX: 614-251-4009
e-mail: info@columbusfoundation.org
www.columbusfoundation.org

Doug Krilder, President
Carol Harmon, Director Of Communications
Lisa Schweitzer, Vice President

2743 Eleanora CU Alms Trust
Fifth Third Bank
9990 Montgomery Road
Dept 00864
Cincinnati, OH 45263
513-793-2200

Bryan Webb, Manager
Giving limited to Cincinnati, OH.

2744 Eva L And Joseph M Bruening Foundation
Foundation Managment Services
1422 Euclid Avenue
Suite 627
Cleveland, OH 44115
216-621-2901
FAX: 216-621-8198
e-mail: cstarkey@fmscleaveland.com
www.fmscleveland.com/

Cristin N. Sleshn, President
Janet Narten, Owner
Susan Althans, Senior Associate
Charitable foundation providing grants to noprofit organizations located inCuyahoga county Ohio. No grant are awarded to invividuals.

2745 Fred & Lillian Deeks Memorial Foundation
PO Box 1118
Cincinnati, OH 45201
937-339-2329
FAX: 937-339-1861

2746 GAR Foundation
PO Box 1500
Akron, OH 44309
330-576-2926
FAX: 330-294-5315
e-mail: info@garfdn.org
www.garfdn.org

2747 George Gund Foundation
1845 Guildhall Building
45 Prospect Ave. West
Cleveland, OH 44115
216-241-3114
FAX: 216-241-6560
e-mail: info@gundfdn.org
www.gundfdn.org

David Abbott, Executive Director
Marcia Egbert, Senior Program Officer
Robert Jaquay, Associate Director

2748 Greater Cincinnati Foundation
200 W 4th Street
Cincinnati, OH 45202
513-241-2880
FAX: 513-852-6886
e-mail: merchantk@greatercincinnatifnd.org
www.greatercincinnatifdn.org

Kathryn Merchant, President
Amy Cheney, Vice President
Karen Bond, Grants Manager

2749 HCR Manor Care Foundation
PO Box 10086
Toledo, OH 43699
419-252-5989
FAX: 419-252-5221
e-mail: foundation@hcr-manorcare.com
www.hcr-manorcare.com

Susan J Harless, President
Jennifer Steiner, Executive Director

2750 Harry C Moores Foundation
100 S 3rd Street
Columbus, OH 43215
614-227-8884

Mary B Cummins, Administrator

2751 Helen Steiner Rice Foundation
221 E 4th Street
Cincinnati, OH 45202
513-451-9241
800-877-2665
e-mail: hsrice@fuse.net
www.helensteinerrice.com

Virginia Ruehlman, Executive Director
Andrea Cornett, Administrator/Grant Coordinator

2752 Herbert W Hoover Foundation
220 Market Avenue
Canton, OH 44702
330-454-1010

Harry Nealy, Owner

2753 John P Murphy Foundation
50 Public Square
Suite 924
Cleveland, OH 44113
216-623-4770
FAX: 216-623-4773
www.fdncenter.org/grantmaker/jpmurphy/

Nancy W McCann, President
Robert R Broadbent, Vice President

2754 Nationwide Foundation
1 Nationwide Plaza
Columbus, OH 43215
877-422-6569
www.nationwide.com

Jerry Jurgensen, Ceo
Michael Miller, President

2755 Nordson Corporate Giving Program
28601 Clemens Road
Westlake, OH 44145
440-892-1580
e-mail: kladiner@nordson.com
www.nordson.com

Constance T Haqq, Executive Director
Cecilia Render, Manager

2756 Parker-Hannifin Foundation
6035 Parkland Boulevard
Cleveland, OH 44124
216-896-3000
FAX: 216-896-4057
www.parker.com

Tom Mackie, President

2757 Reinberger Foundation
27600 Chagrin Boulevard
Cleveland, OH 44122
216-292-2790
FAX: 216-292-4466

Robert N Reinberger, Executive Director

2758 Robert Campeau Family Foundation
7 W 7th Street
Cincinnati, OH 45202
513-579-7000
FAX: 513-579-7555

Terry Lundgren, Chief Executive Officer

2759 Sisler McFawn Foundation
PO Box 149
Akron, OH 44309
330-849-8887
FAX: 330-996-6215

Charlotte M Stanley, Grants Manager
Our trust restricts giving to certain programs and types of organizations. You can see recent giving has been by referring to the list of grants approved and paid during the past year. Call foundation office to request a guidelines brochure and list.

2760 Stark Community Foundation
Unizan Plaza 220 Market Avenu
Suite 920
Canton, OH 44702
330-454-5800
FAX: 330-454-5855
www.starkcommunityfoundation.org

Vicki Conley, Executive Director

2761 The Bahmann Foundation
8041 Hosbrook Road
Suite 210
Cincinnati, OH 45236
513-891-3799
FAX: 513-891-3722
e-mail: info@bahmann.org
www.bahmann.org

2762 The Stocker Foundation
401 Broadway
Suite C
Lorain, OH 44052
440-246-5719
FAX: 440-246-5720
e-mail: pobrien@stockerfoundation.org
www.stockerfoundation.org

Patricia O'Brien, Executive Director

2763 Toledo Community Foundation
608 Madison Avenue
Suite 1540
Toledo, OH 43604
419-241-5049
FAX: 419-242-5549
e-mail: toledocf@toledocf.org
www.toledocf.org

Dennis Johnson, President And Chair
Charles Stocking, Vice Chair
William Rose, Treasurer

2764 William J and Dorothy K O'Neill Foundation
30195 Chagrin Boulevard
Suite 310
Cleveland, OH 44124
216-831-9667
FAX: 216-831-3779
e-mail: oneillfdn@aol.com
www.oneillfdn.org

Catherine T Abbott, Director
William O'Neill, Owner

2765 Youngstown Foundation
Dollar Savings & Trust Company
PO Box 450
Youngstown, OH 44501
330-744-0320
FAX: 330-744-0344

Jerry Walsh, Executive Director

Oklahoma

2766 Anne and Henry Zarrow Foundation
401 S Boston Avenue
Suite 900
Tulsa, OK 74103
918-295-8004
FAX: 918-295-8049
e-mail: jgillert@zarrow.com
www.zarrow.com

Jeanne Gillert, Grants Manager
A broad-based funding foundation. However, ares of emphasis include Jewish causes, the indignant, the disenfranchised and the homeless. The Foundation meets on a quartely basis, in the months of February, April, September and November. Proposals are due on the first day of the following months:January, April, August and October. Any proposals recieved after the due date will be held until the next quarter's meeting.

2767 International Bio-Oxidative Medicine Foundation (IBOM)
1015 Waterwood Parkway
Suite G
Edmond, OK 73034
405-478-4266

Offers educational programs, referrals and a newsletter.

2768 Sarkeys Foundation
530 E Main Street
Norman, OK 73071
405-364-3703
FAX: 405-364-8191
e-mail: cheri@sarkeys.org
www.sarkeys.org

Cheri D Cartwright, Executive Director
Improves the quality of life in Oklahoma. Offers contributions in the areas of social services, arts and cultural programs, educational funding and health care and medical research. Funding only in agencies in the state of Oklahoma.

Oregon

2769 Arc of Oregon
1745 State Street
Salem, OR 97301
503-581-2726
877-581-2726
877-581-2726
FAX: 503-363-7168
e-mail: info@arcoregon.org
www.arcoregon.org

Marcie Ingledue, Executive Director
Brady Romtvedt, Ececutive Assistant
Guardianship, Advocacy and Planning Services. Oregon special needs trust; information and referral.

2770 Chiles Foundation
111 SW 5th Avenue
Suite 4050
Portland, OR 97204
503-222-2143

Giving in Oregon, with emphasis on Portland, and the Pacific Northwest.

2771 Jackson Foundation
PO Box 3168
Portland, OR 97208
503-275-6564

Robert H Depew, Vice President

2772 Leslie G Ehmann Trust
PO Box 3168
Portland, OR 97208
503-275-5929
800-522-9100
FAX: 503-275-4117
e-mail: william.dollan@usbank.com

William Dolan, Trustee

2773 Samuel S Johnson Foundation
PO Box 356
Redmond, OR 97756
541-548-8104
FAX: 541-548-2014
e-mail: info@tgci.com

Becky Johnson, President

Pennsylvania

2774 Acorn Alcinda Foundation
Rr 4
Box 710
Mifflintown, PA 17059
717-436-6597

Robert J Kennedy, President/Treasurer

2775 Air Products Foundation
7201 Hamilton Boulevard
Allentown, PA 18195
610-481-4911
FAX: 610-481-5900
www.airproducts.com

John Jones III, Chief Executive Officer
Giving primarily in areas of company operations throughout the US.

2776 Arc of Pennsylvania
Arc of United States
101 S 2nd Street
Suite 8
Harrisburg, PA 17101
717-234-2621
800-692-7258
FAX: 717-234-7615
www.thearcpa.org

Stephen Suroviec, Executive Director
Wendy Kramer, Administrative Assistant/Finance

2777 Arcadia Foundation
105 E Logan Street
Norristown, PA 19401
610-275-8460

Marilyn L Steinbright, President

2778 Brachial Plexus Palsy Foundation
210 Springhaven Circle
Royersford, PA 19468
610-792-0974
FAX: 610-792-0974
e-mail: contact@brachialplexuspalsyfoundation.org
www.brachialplexuspalsyfoundat ion.org

Thomas J Cirino, President
Michael F Cirino, Executive Director
Nonprofit organization dedicated to raising funds for support of families who hae children with brachial plexus injuries. Supports medical facilities that research and treat such injuries, holds fund-raising events to support further research, has support groups, and produces educational materials including a newsletter, Outreach, and brochures.

2779 **Claude Washington Benedum Foundation**
1400 Benedum
Pittsburgh, PA 15222 412-288-0360
FAX: 412-288-0366
e-mail: info@benedum.org
www.fdncenter.org/grantmaker/benedum

William Getty, President
Dwight Keating, Vice President
Giving limited to West Virginia and southwestern Pennsylvania.

2780 **Columbia Gas of Pennsylvania Corporate Giv ing**
650 Washington Road
Pittsburgh, PA 15228 412-572-7104
FAX: 412-572-7140
e-mail: info@columbiaenergygroup.com
www.columbiagaspamd.com/html/

Rosemary Martinelli, Manager Corporation

2781 **Connelly Foundation**
1 Tower Brg
Suite 1450
West Conshohocken, PA 19428 610-834-3222
FAX: 610-834-0866
e-mail: info@connellyfdn.org
www.connellyfdn.org

Josephine C Mandeville, Chief Executive Officer
Emily C Riley, Executive Vice President

2782 **Dolfinger-McMahon Foundation**
1 Liberty Place
Philadelphia, PA 19103 215-979-1768

Sharon Renz, Contact Person

2783 **Harry C Trexler Trust**
33 S 7th Street
Suite 205
Allentown, PA 18101 484-664-3500

Thomas Christman, Secretary Trustees
Thomas Gaughan, Executive Director
Giving limited to Lehigh County, Pennsylvania.

2784 **Henry L Hillman Foundation**
2000 Grant Building
Pittsburgh, PA 15219 412-338-3466
FAX: 412-338-3463
e-mail: foundation@hillmanfo.com

Ronald W Wertz, President

2785 **Howard Heinz Endowment**
625 Liberty Avenue
Pittsburgh, PA 15222 412-281-5777

Maxwell King, President

2786 **Hoxie Harrison Smith Foundation**
350 Pond View Road
Devon, PA 19333 610-688-0143
FAX: 610-688-0143

Bruce M Brown, Secretary/Treasurer

2787 **Jewish Healthcare Foundation of Pittsburgh**
Centre City Tower
Suite 2400
Pittsburgh, PA 15222 412-594-2550
FAX: 412-232-6240
e-mail: info@jhf.org
www.jhf.org

Karen W Feinstein, President

2788 **Juliet L Hillman Simonds Foundation**
330 Grant Street
Suite 2000
Pittsburgh, PA 15219 412-338-3466
FAX: 412-338-3463
e-mail: foundation@hillmanfo.com

Ronald W Wertz, President
David Rager, Program Manager

2789 **Oberkotter Foundation**
1600 Market Street
Suite 3600
Philadelphia, PA 19103 215-751-2601
FAX: 215-751-2678
e-mail: orders@oraldeaf.org
oraldeafed.org

George H Nofer, Executive Director

2790 **PECO Energy Company Contributions Program**
2301 Market Street
7toorh Floor
Philadelphia, PA 19103 215-841-4000
FAX: 215-841-4040

Anne Baker, Manager
Denis O'Brien, President

2791 **PNC Bank Foundation**
249 5th Avenue
Pittsburgh, PA 15222 412-762-2000
FAX: 412-768-3779
www.pncbank.com

Bill Kosis, Chief Executive Officer

2792 **Philadelphia Foundation**
1234 Market Street
Suite 1800
Philadelphia, PA 19107 215-563-6417
FAX: 215-563-6882
e-mail: parkow@philafound.org
www.philafound.org

R Andrew Swinney, President
Jeffery W Perkins, VP Finance/Administrator

2793 **Pittsburgh Foundation**
5 Ppg Place
Suite 250
Pittsburgh, PA 15222 412-391-5122
FAX: 421-391-7259
e-mail: trueheartw@pghfdn.org
www.pittsburghfoundation.org

William E Trueheart, President/CEO

2794 **Shenango Valley Foundation**
33 Chestnut Avenue
Sharon, PA 16146 724-347-3767
FAX: 724-983-9044
www.sv-foundation.org

Larry Haynes, Executive Director
Tony Bianco, Owner
Pooled Income Trust

2795 **Staunton Farm Foundation**
Centre City Tower
650 Smithfield Street
Suite 210
Pittsburgh, PA 15222 412-281-8020
FAX: 412-232-3115
e-mail: jschwager@stauntonfarm.org
www.stauntonfarm.org

Joani Schwager, Executive Director

2796 **Stewart Huston Charitable Trust**
Will of Stewart Huston
50 S 1st Avenue
Coatesville, PA 19320
610-384-2666
FAX: 610-384-3396
e-mail: admin@stewarthuston.org
www.stewarthuston.org

Scott G Huston, Executive Director

2797 **Teleflex Foundation**
630 W Germantown Pike
Suite 461
Plymouth Meeting, PA 19462
610-834-6378
FAX: 610-834-0248

Thelma A Fretz, Executive Director

2798 **USX Foundation**
600 Grant Street
Suite 685
Pittsburgh, PA 15219
412-433-5238
FAX: 412-433-6847

CD Mallick, General Manager
Patricia Funaro, Program Manager
Giving primarily in areas of company operations located within the United States.

2799 **WW Smith Charitable Trust**
3515 W Chester Pike
Suite E
Newtown Square, PA 19073
610-359-1811
FAX: 610-359-9717

Frances R Pemberton, Trust Administrator

2800 **William B Dietrich Foundation**
Duane Morrs Llt
30 S W 17th Street
Philadelphia, PA 19103
215-979-1919
FAX: 215-979-1020
www.duanemorrs.com

William B Dietrich, President

2801 **William Talbott Hillman Foundation**
2000 Grant Building
Pittsburgh, PA 15219
412-338-3466
FAX: 412-338-3463
e-mail: foundation@hillmanfo.com

Ronald W Wertz, President

2802 **William V and Catherine A McKinney Charitable Foundation**
20 Stanwix Street
Pittsburgh, PA 15222
412-644-8332
FAX: 412-644-6058

William M Schmidt, Senior Vice President

Rhode Island

2803 **Arc South County Chapter**
24 Salt Pond Road
Suite G3
Wakefield, RI 02879
401-789-4386
FAX: 401-789-4394

2804 **Arc of Northern Rhode Island**
The Homestead Group Administrative Offices
68 Cumberland Street
Woonsocket, RI 02895
401-597-6700
FAX: 401-597-6706
e-mail: info@thgri.org
www.arcofnri.org

George Beaubien, Public Relations Specialist

2805 **Arc-Down Syndrome Society of Rhode Island**
99 Bald Hill Road
Cranston, RI 02920
401-463-5751

2806 **Blackstone Valley Chapter RI Arc**
115 Manton Street
Pawtucket, RI 02861
401-727-0150
FAX: 401-727-0153
e-mail: contact@bvcriarc.org
www.bvcriarc.org

John Padien, Ceo
A private nonprofit organization providing residential, developmental, employment and recreational programs and services to more then 400 individuals with intellectual and related disabilities

2807 **Bristol County Chapter Arc**
PO Box 711
Bristol, RI 02809
401-846-0340
FAX: 401-253-7880

John Maher, Executive Director

2808 **Champlin Foundations**
300 Centerville Road
Suite 300s
Warwick, RI 02886
401-736-0370
FAX: 401-736-7248

David King, Director
Keith Lang, Executive Director
Giving in the Rhode Island area.

2809 **Cranston Arc**
111 Comstock Parkway
Cranston, RI 02921
401-941-1112
FAX: 401-941-2516
e-mail: webmaster@cranstocarc.org
www.cranstonarc.org

2810 **Horace A Kimball and S Ella Kimball Foundation**
23 Broad Street
Westerly, RI 02891
401-364-7799
www.hkimballfoundation.org

Thomas F Black III, President
Makes grants almost exclusively to Rhode Island operatives (charities) or those benefitting Rhode Island residents ans causes.

2811 **Kent County Arc**
3445 Post Road
Warwick, RI 02886
e-mail: mmadden@kentcountyarc.org
www.kentcountyarc.org

Mary Madden, Executive Director
Providing individuals with disabilties meaningful opportunities throughout their communities.

2812 **Newport County Arc**
PO Box 4390
Middletown, RI 02842
401-846-4600
FAX: 401-849-4267

Jack Maher, Executive Director

2813 **Rhode Island Arc**
99 Bald Hill Road
Cranston, RI 02920
401-463-9191
FAX: 401-463-9244
e-mail: riarc@compuserve.com
riarc@compuserve.com

James Healey, Executive Director

2814 Rhode Island Foundation
1 Union Station
Providence, RI 02903
401-274-4564
FAX: 401-331-8085
www.rifoundation.org

Ronald Gallo, President

2815 Westerly Chariho Arc
93 Airport Road
Westerly, RI 02891
401-596-2091
FAX: 401-596-3945
e-mail: info@oleancenter.org
www.oleancenter.org/

Brian Thorp, President Director
A non-profit organization representing and providing services and supports to persons with developmental disabilities and their families throughout Southern Rhode Island and Southeastern Connecticut.

South Carolina

2816 Arc of South Carolina
Arc of United States
1823 Gadsden Street
Columbia, SC 29201
803-748-5020
FAX: 803-779-0017
e-mail: info@arcsc.org
www.arcsc.org

Ron Kuebler, President
Jackie Robey, Vice President

2817 Center for Developmental Disabilities
University of South Carolina
8301 Farrow Road
Columbia, SC 29208
803-935-5231
FAX: 803-935-5059
e-mail: ddsnweb@ddsn.sc.gov
www.scsis.org

Denise Rivers, Project Coordinator
Donald Wuori, MD
A University Affiliated Program which develops model programs designed to serve persons with disabilities and to train students in fields related to disabilities.

2818 Colonial Life and Accident Insurance Company Contributions Program
1200 Colonial Life Boulevard W
Columbia, SC 29210
803-798-7000
FAX: 803-213-7245

Edwina Carns, Public/Community Relations
Donna Northam, Plant Manager

2819 Pickens County Arc
PO Box 1308
Easley, SC 29641
864-859-5416
FAX: 864-859-1157

Elaine Thena, Executive Director
Kaye Golden, Assistant Executive Director

Tennessee

2820 Arc Putnam County
453 Gould Drive
Cookeville, TN 38506
931-432-5981
FAX: 931-432-5987

2821 Arc of Anderson County
PO Box 4823
Oak Ridge, TN 37831
865-481-0550

Melanie Davis, Executive Director

2822 Arc of Davidson County
Arc of Tennessee
151 Athens Way
Suite 100
Nashville, TN 37228
615-248-5878
800-835-7077
FAX: 615-248-5879
e-mail: wrogers@thearctn.org
www.thearctn.org

Walter Rogers, Executive Director

2823 Arc of Hamilton County
4613 Brainerd Road
Chattanooga, TN 37411
423-624-6887
800-624-6887
FAX: 423-624-3974
e-mail: arcofhamilton@aol.com

Shawn Ellis, Executive Director
Constance Tiller, Deputy Director
Richard Burke, Board President
Provides assistance to individuals and families with mental retardation and related disabilities, in the form of advocacy, information, and support coordination

2824 Arc of Washington County
2700 S Roan Street
Suite 300b
Johnson City, TN 37601
423-928-9362
FAX: 423-928-7431
e-mail: bill@arcwc.org
www.arcec.org

Bill Schiers, Executive Director
Is a non-profit organization that serves individuals with disabilities and their families. They have an independent support coordination service, as well as, early intervention, family support and respite services.

2825 Arc of Williamson County
129 W Fowlkes Street
Franklin, TN 37064
615-790-5815
www.thearcofwilliamsoncounty.org

Sharon Bottorff, Executive Director

2826 Benwood Foundation
736 Market Street
Suite 1600
Chattanooga, TN 37402
423-267-4311
FAX: 423-267-9049

Corinne A Allen, Executive Director
Giving primarily in the Chattanooga area.

2827 Community Foundation of Greater Chattanooga
1270 Market Street
Chattanooga, TN 37402
423-265-0586
FAX: 423-265-0587
e-mail: info2@cfgc.org
www.cfgc.org

Peter T Cooper, President

2828 Education and Auditory Research Foundation
PO Box 330867
Nashville, TN 37203
615-627-2724
800-545-4327
FAX: 615-627-2728
e-mail: info@earfoundation.org
www.earfoundation.org

Michael Glasscock, President

Provides the general public support services promoting the integration of the hearing and balance impaired into mainstream society; to provide practicing ear specialists continuing medical education courses and related programs specifically regarding rehabilitation and hearing preservation; to educate young people and adults about hearing preservation and early detection of hearing loss, enabling them to prevent at an early age hearing and balance disorders.

2829 Montgomery County Arc
PO Box 2145rive
Clarksville, TN 37042
931-905-0900
FAX: 931-905-0900

Joann Wilson, President

2830 The Arc of Tennessee
151 Athens Way
Suite 100
Nashville, TN 37228
615-248-5878
800-835-7077
FAX: 615-248-5879
e-mail: pcooper@thearctn.org
www.thearctn.org

Walter Rogers, Executive Director
Peggy Cooper, Operations Manager
Advocacy, information, referral and support for people with intellectual and developmental disabilities and their families.

Texas

2831 Abell-Hangar Foundation
PO Box 430
Midland, TX 79702
432-684-6655
FAX: 423-684-4474
e-mail: ahf@abell-hanger.org

David L Smith, Chief Executive Officer
Giving limited to Texas, preferably within the Permian Basin.

2832 Albert & Bessie Mae Kronkosky Charitable Foundation
112 E Pecan Street
Suite 830
San Antonio, TX 78205
210-475-9000
888-309-9001
FAX: 210-354-2204
e-mail: kronfndn@kronkosky.org
www.kronkosky.org

Palmer Moe, Executive Director

2833 American Foundation for the Blind: Southwest
260 Treadway Plaza
Dallas, TX 75235
214-352-7222
FAX: 903-352-3214
e-mail: dallas@afb.net
www.afb.org

Mary Ann Siller, National Education Consultant
Judy Scott, Executive Director

2834 Arch and Stella Rowan Foundation
307 W 7th Street
Fort Worth, TX 76102
817-336-2679
FAX: 817-336-2679

Alice B Myatt, Secretary

2835 BA and Elinor Steinhagen Benevolent Trust
Chase Bank of Texas
PO Box 3928
Beaumont, TX 77704
FAX: 409-880-1437

Jean Monica, Vice President

2836 Brown Foundation
PO Box 130646
Houston, TX 77219
713-523-6867
FAX: 713-523-2917
e-mail: bfi@brownfoundation.org
www.brownfoundation.org
Giving primarily in Texas, with emphasis on Houston.

2837 Burlington Northern Foundation
777 Main Street
Fort Worth, TX 76102
817-878-2000
FAX: 800-677-4816

Beverly Edwards, President
Becky Blankenship, Administrator
Giving primarily in the areas of company operations, included, but not limited to the areas of civic service, culture and the arts, education, federated, human service and youth.

2838 Burnett Foundation
801 Cherry Street
Suite 1585
Fort Worth, TX 76102
817-877-3344

Thomas F Beech, Executive VP
V Agather, Executive Director

2839 CH Foundation
PO Box 94038
Lubbock, TX 79493
806-792-0448
FAX: 806-792-7824

Nelda Thompson, Secretary

2840 Cockrell Foundation
1000 Main Street
Suite 3250
Houston, TX 77002
713-209-7300
e-mail: foundation@cockrell.com
www.cockrell.com

Jennifer Delaney, Assistant to the Board
M Nancy Williams, Executive VP
Purpose is for giving for higher education at the University of Texas at Austin; support also for cultural programs, social services, youth services and health care. Limitations are giving in Houston, Texas and no grants are awarded to individuals.

2841 Communities Foundation of Texas
5500 Caruth Haven Lane
Dallas, TX 75225
214-750-4222
FAX: 214-750-4210
e-mail: jsmith@cftexas.org
www.cftexas.org

Michael J Redfearn, VP Finance
Marcia Williams-Godwin, VP Administration
Brent Christopher, Manager
Giving in the Dallas area.

2842 Community Foundation of the Metropolitan Tarrant County
306 W 7th Street
Suite 306
Fort Worth, TX 76102
817-877-0702
FAX: 817-877-1215
www.cfmtx.org

Homer M Dowd, President
Melissa Saniuk, Director of Finance

2843 Cullen Foundation
601 Jefferson Street
40th Floor
Houston, TX 77002
713-651-8837
FAX: 713-651-2374

Alan M Stewart, Executive Director
Grants are restricted to Texas-based organizations for programs in Texas, primarily in the Houston area.

2844 Curtis & Doris K Hankamer Foundation
9039 Katy Fwy
Suite 530
Houston, TX 77024 713-461-8140

Gregory A Herbst, Manager

2845 Dallas Foundation
900 Jackson Street
Dallas, TX 75202 214-741-9898
FAX: 214-741-9848
e-mail: info@dallasfoundation.org
www.dallasfoundation.org

Mary M Jalonick, Executive Director
Cathy McNally, Program Manager

2846 David D & Nona S Payne Foundation
436 Hughes Street
Pampa, TX 79065 806-665-7281

Adelaide S Colwell, Secretary
Mark Buzzard, Partner

2847 El Paso Natural Gas Foundation
PO Box 2511
Houston, TX 77252 713-420-3630
FAX: 713-420-5312
www.elpaso.com

Douglas Foshee, President/CEO
Bill Baerg, Manager And Investor Relations

2848 Epilepsy Foundation of Greater North Texas
2906 Swiss Avenue
Dallas, TX 75204 214-823-8809
800-447-7778
www.efgnt.org

Robert Miller, President
Kathlyn Hampton, Vice President

2849 Epilepsy Foundation of Southeast Texas
2630 Fountain View Drive
Suite 3210
Houston, TX 77057 713-789-6295
888-548-9716
FAX: 713-789-5628
e-mail: dstahlhut@efset.org
www.efset.org

Donna Stahlhut, Executive Director

2850 Epilepsy Foundation: Central and South Texas
10615 Perrin Beitel Road
Suite 602
San Antonio, TX 78217 210-653-5353
888-606-5353
www.efcst.org

Judy Allen, President
Neal Shaver, Vice President
Sindi Rosales, Executive Director

2851 Gil and Dody Weaver Foundation
500 W 7th Street
Suite 1714
Fort Worth, TX 76102 817-877-1712

William R Weaver

2852 Harris and Eliza Kempner Fund
2201 Market Street
Suite 601
Galveston, TX 77550 409-762-1603
FAX: 409-762-5435
www.kempnerfund.org

Barbara K Crews, Executive Director

2853 Henry & Tommy Lehmann Charitable Foundation
PO Box 223
Giddings, TX 78942 979-542-3636

Jake Jacobson, Chairperson

2854 Hesta Stuart Christian Charitable Trust
Bank One Texas N A
PO Box 2050
Fort Worth, TX 76113 817-884-4151

www.bankone.com

Robert Lansford, Trust Officer

2855 Hillcrest Foundation
Bank of America
PO Box 830241
Dallas, TX 75283 214-740-1728

Daniel Kelly, Vice President
Shannon James, Manager

2856 Hoblitzelle Foundation
5956 Sherry Lane
Suite 901
Dallas, TX 75225 214-373-0462

www.hoblitzelle.org

Paul W Harris, Executive Vice President

2857 Houston Endowment
600 Travis Street
Suite 6400
Houston, TX 77002 713-238-8100
FAX: 713-238-8101
www.houstonendowment.org

H Nelson III, President

2858 John G & Marie S Kennedy Memorial Foundati on
1700 First City Tower i I
Corpus Christi, TX 78478

2859 John S Dunn Research Foundation
3355 W Alabama Street
Suite 702
Houston, TX 77098 713-626-0368

Lloyd J Gregory Jr MD, Executive VP
John Dunn, President

2860 Kent Waldrep National Paralysis Foundation
16415 Addison Road
Suite 550
Addison, TX 75001 972-248-7100
877-724-2873
FAX: 972-248-7313
e-mail: info@spinalvictory.org
www.spinalvictory.org

Lisa Koen, Office Manager/Media Coordinator
Not-for-profit organization dedicated to raising funds for research to find a cure for paralysis caused by brain injury, spinal cord injury, or stroke. Educational materials include brochures and a quarterly newsletter.

2861 Lola Wright Foundation
PO Box 1138
Georgetown, TX 78627 512-869-2574

Wilford Flowers, President
Paul Hilgers, Vice President
Sandra Donnell, Manager

2862 **Marcia & Otto Koehler Foundation**
Bank of America
PO Box 121
San Antonio, TX 78291 210-637-8800

Gregg Muenster, Senior Vice President
Jesse Ramos, Manager

2863 **Meadows Foundation**
3003 Swiss Avenue
Dallas, TX 75204 214-826-9431
800-826-9431
e-mail: grants@mfi.org
www.mfi.org

Robert A Meadows, Chairman
John W Broadfoot, Director
Linda Evans, Chief Executive Officer

2864 **Moody Foundation**
2302 Post Office Street
Suite 704
Galveston, TX 77550 409-763-5333
FAX: 409-763-5564
www.moody.org

Peter M Moore, Grants Director
Francis Moody Dahlberg, Executive Director
Harold MacDonald, Chief Executive Officer

2865 **Pearle Vision Foundation**
2534 Royal Lane
Dallas, TX 75229 214-821-7770

Trina Parasiliti, Secretary
Leo Priolo, Owner

2866 **Rockwell Foundation**
1360 S Post Oak Road
Suite 780
Houston, TX 77056 713-629-9022
FAX: 713-629-7702

R Terry Bell, President

2867 **San Antonio Area Foundation**
110 Broadway Street
Suite 230
San Antonio, TX 78205 210-225-2243
FAX: 210-225-1980
e-mail: info@saafdn.org
www.saafdn.org

Raymond Carvajal, President
Pat Wilson, Vice President
Clarence Williams, Chief Executive Officer

2868 **Shell Oil Company Foundation**
PO Box 2099
Houston, TX 77252 281-544-7171
FAX: 713-241-3329
e-mail: info@shellfoundation.org
www.shellfoundation.org

Ah Myresty, Vice President
BL McHam, Executive Director
A not-for-profit foundation funded by donations from Shell Oil Company and other participating Shell companies and subsidiaries.

2869 **South Texas Charitable Foundation**
PO Box 2459
Victoria, TX 77902 512-573-4383

Rayford L Keller, Secretary

2870 **Sterling-Turner Foundation**
815 Walker Street
Suite 1543
Houston, TX 77002 713-237-1117
FAX: 713-223-4638
e-mail: jeannie.arnold@stfdn.org
www.sterlingturnerfoundation.org

Eyvonne Moser, Executive Director
Patricia Turner, Assistant Director

2871 **Swalm Foundation**
PO Box 1248
New Ulm, TX 78950 281-497-5280
FAX: 281-497-7340

Miriam Minkoff, Secretary

2872 **TLL Temple Foundation**
109 Temple Boulevard
Lufkin, TX 75901 936-639-5197
e-mail: wcorley@tlltf.com

A Wayne Corley, Executive Director
Buddy Zeagler, Assistant Executive Director

2873 **The Arc of Texas**
Arc of United States
8001 Centre Park Drive
Austin, TX 78754 512-454-6694
800-252-9729
FAX: 512-454-4956
e-mail: secretary@thearcoftexas.org
www.thearcoftexas.org

Therese Palombi

2874 **Vale-Asche Foundation**
2001 Kirby Drive
Suite 1010
Houston, TX 77019 713-520-7334
FAX: 713-520-6208

Vale-asche Russell, President

2875 **William Stamps Farish Fund**
1100 Louisiana Street
Suite 1250
Houston, TX 77002 713-757-7300

Terry Ward, Manager
Primary giving in Texas.

Utah

2876 **Arc of Utah**
155 S 300 W
Suite 201
Salt Lake City, UT 84101 801-364-5060
800-371-3060
FAX: 801-364-6030
e-mail: debowman@arcutah.org
www.arcutah.com

Douglas Hathaway, Executive Director
Melba Gibson, Donor Services Manager

2877 **Ben B and Iris M Margolis Foundation**
First Security Bank of Utah
PO Box 628
Salt Lake City, UT 84110 801-350-5583

Julie Webster

2878 Marriner S Eccles Foundation
79 S Main Street
Salt Lake City, UT 84111 801-532-0934

Shannon K Toronto

2879 Questar Corporation Contributions Program
PO Box 45433
Salt Lake City, UT 84145 801-324-5000
FAX: 801-324-5483
www.questar.com

Janice Bates, Director Community Affairs
Keith Rattie, Chief Executive Officer

Vermont

2880 Vermont Community Foundation
PO Box 30
Middlebury, VT 05753 802-388-3355
FAX: 802-388-3398
e-mail: info@vermontcf.org
www.vermontcf.org

Vicky Young, Chairman
Kathy Hoyt, Vice President
David Rahr, President

Virginia

2881 Arc of Virginia
2025 E Main Street
Suite 120
Richmond, VA 23223 804-649-8481
FAX: 804-649-3585
e-mail: thearc@arcofva.org
www.arcofva.org

Nita Grignol, President
Jeannie Cummins, Vice President
Clarissa Riely, Executive Director

2882 Bell Atlantic Foundation
1310 N Court House Road
Arlington, VA 22201 703-524-9761
FAX: 703-974-0131
www.foundation.verizon.com/04014.shtml
Concentrates efforts on programs that support its vision to produce more scientifically and technically literate population effecting measurable improvements in the way pre-collegiate science, math and technology education is delivered to and understood by students.

2883 Camp Foundation
PO Box 813
Franklin, VA 23851 757-562-3439

Bobby B Worrell, Chief Executive Officer

2884 Community Foundation of Richmond & Central Virginia
7325 Beaufont Springs Drive
Suite 210
Richmond, VA 23225 804-330-7400
FAX: 804-330-5992
www.tcfrichmond.org

Darcy S Oman, President

2885 Gannett Foundation
1100 Wilson Boulevard
30th Floor
Arlington, VA 22234 703-271-8330
FAX: 703-558-3819
e-mail: foundation@gannett.org
www.gannettfoundation.org

Irma Simpson, Manager

2886 John Randolph Foundation
PO Box 1606
Hopewell, VA 23860 804-458-2239
FAX: 804-458-3754
e-mail: jrfoundation@covad.net
www.johnrandolphfoundation.org

Lisa Sharpe, Executive Director
Diane Lowder, Assistant Director

2887 Norfolk Foundation
1 Commercial Place
Suite 1410
Norfolk, VA 23510 757-622-7951
FAX: 757-622-1751
e-mail: mmorris@norfolkfoundation.org
www.norfolkfoundation.org

Angelica Light, Executive Director
Man Edgerton, VP Development

2888 Robey W Estes Family Foundation
Robey W Estes Jr
PO Box 25612
Richmond, VA 23260 804-353-1900

Robey Estes Jr, Chief Executive Officer

2889 Virginia Beach Foundation
PO Box 4329
Virginia Beach, VA 23454 757-422-5249
FAX: 757-422-1849
fdncenter.org/grantmaker/vbf

Ted Clarkson, Executive Director

2890 W Alton Jones Foundation
232 E High Street
Charlottesville, VA 22902 434-245-5838
FAX: 434-295-1648
www.whn.org

Washington

2891 Arc of Washington State
2600 Martin Way E
Suite B
Olympia, WA 98506 360-357-5596
888-754-8798
FAX: 360-357-3279
e-mail: info@arcwa.org
www.arcwa.org

Sue Elliott, Executive Director
Jackie Thomason, Assistant Director

2892 Ben B Cheney Foundation
3110 Ruston Way
Suite A
Tacoma, WA 98402 253-572-2442
FAX: 253-572-2902
e-mail: Info@benbcheneyfoundation.org
www.bebncheneyfoundation.org

Brad Cheney, President

2893 **Glaser Foundation**
2601 Elliott Avenue
Seattle, WA 98121
206-728-1050
FAX: 206-728-1123

Martin Collier, Executive Director
Leslie Donald, Manager

2894 **Greater Tacoma Community Foundation**
PO Box 1995
Tacoma, WA 98401
253-383-5622
FAX: 253-272-8099
e-mail: info@gtcf.org
www.tacomafoundation.org

Margy McGroarty
Rose Lincoln, President

2895 **Greater Wenatchee Community Foundation**
PO Box 3332
Wenatchee, WA 98807
509-662-8580
FAX: 509-664-9569

Raymond Taylor, President/CEO

2896 **Inland Northwest Community Foundation**
221 N Wall Street
Suite 624
Spokane, WA 99201
509-624-2606
888-267-5606
FAX: 509-624-2608
e-mail: kwatkins@inwcomfound.org
www.inwcomfound.org

Kandace Watkins, Front Office/Operations Coordin.

2897 **Medina Foundation**
801 2nd Avenue
Suite 1300
Seattle, WA 98104
206-652-8783

e-mail: info@medinafoundation.org
www.medinafoundation.org

Tricia Mckay, Executive Director
Katie Heinrich, Programs/Operations Officer
Nick MacPhee, Programs Officer
A family foundation that works to foster positive change in the Greater Puget Sound area. The Foundation strives to improve the human condition by supporting organizations that provide critical services to those in need.

2898 **Norcliffe Foundation**
999 3rd Avenue
Suite 1006
Seattle, WA 98104
206-682-4820
FAX: 206-682-4821
e-mail: arline@thenorcliffefoundation.com
www.thenorcliffefoundation.com

Arline Hefferline, Foundation Manager
Geographic area of funding limited to the Puget Sound Region in and around Seattle, Washington.

2899 **Stewardship Foundation**
PO Box 1278
Tacoma, WA 98401
253-620-1340
FAX: 253-572-2721
e-mail: info@stewardshipfdn.org
www.stewardshipfdn.org

Cary A Paine, Executive Director
William T Weyerhaeuser, Chairman
Christian, evangelical organizations - national or international impact.

2900 **Weyerhaeuser Company Foundation**
PO Box Ch1132
Tacoma, WA 98477
253-474-8888
FAX: 253-924-3658

Karen Veitenhans, Finance Manager
Scott Gardner, Manager
Although the foundation does fund programs for disabled persons from time to time, it is not a specific priority for the foundation. Since it was formed in 1948, the foundation has given more than $81.1 million to nonprofit organizations and is one of the oldest funds for corporate philanthropy in the country. Nearly all of its contributions have been made within the communities where Weyerhaeuser employees live and work and awards approximately 600 grants annually.

West Virginia

2901 **Bernard McDonough Foundation**
311 4th Street
Parkersburg, WV 26101
304-424-6280
FAX: 304-424-6281

James Wakley, President
Bob Stephen, Executive Vice President

Wisconsin

2902 **Arc of Dane County**
1320 Mendota Street
Suite 111a
Madison, WI 53714
608-257-9738

e-mail: arcdane@chorus.net

Ken Hobbes, Executive Director

2903 **Arc of Dunn County**
Arc Of United States
538 Woodridge Court
Menomonie, WI 54751
715-235-7373
FAX: 715-233-3565
e-mail: thearc@wwt.net

Kathy Lausted, Executive Director
Joann Knutson, Residential Director
Advocating for the rights of citizens with disabilities.

2904 **Arc of Eau Claire**
515 S Barstow Street
Eau Claire, WI 54701
715-834-7204
FAX: 715-834-7416
e-mail: thearcec@execpc.com

Babara Shafer, Executive Director

2905 **Arc of Outagamie County**
633 W Wisconsin Avenue
Appleton, WI 54911
920-731-9831
FAX: 920-731-9850

Barb Vanharen, Executive Director

2906 **Arc of Racine County**
1220 Mound Avenue
Suite 319
Racine, WI 53404
262-634-6303
FAX: 262-635-2640

Sandra Engel, Executive Director

2907 **Arc of Wisconsin Disability Association**
600 Williamson Street
Suite J
Madison, WI 53703
608-251-9272
877-272-8400
FAX: 608-251-1403
e-mail: arcw@chorus.net
www.arc-wisconsin.org

Jim Hoegmeier, Executive Director
Ginny Lukken, Administrative Coordinator
The Arc-Wisconsin strives to be a major force in advocating and promoting self-determined quality of life opportunities for poeple with developmental and related disabilities and their families.

2908 Faye McBeath Foundation
1020 N Broadway
Milwaukee, WI 53202
414-272-2626
FAX: 414-272-6235
e-mail: info@fayemcbeath.org
www.fayemcbeath.org

Sarah M Dean, Executive Director

2909 Helen Bader Foundation
233 N Water Street
Milwaukee, WI 53202
414-224-6464
FAX: 414-244-1441
e-mail: info@hbf.org
www.hbf.org

Daniel J Bader, President

2910 Johnson Controls Foundation
PO Box 591
Milwaukee, WI 53201
414-476-2341
800-333-2222
FAX: 414-228-3200
e-mail: webmaster@jci.com
www.johnsoncontrols.com

John Barth, Chairman/Chief Executive Officer
John Fiori, Executive Vice President
John Jensen, President
Organized and directed to be operated for charitable purposes which include the distribution and application of financial support to soundly managed and operated organizations or causes which are fundamentally philanthropic.

2911 Lynde and Harry Bradley Foundation
1241 N Franklin Place
Milwaukee, WI 53202
414-291-9915
FAX: 414-291-9991
www.bradleyfdn.org

Michael W Grebe, President/CEO
Daniel Schmidt, Executive Vice President
The Foundation's programs support limited, competent government; a dynamic marketplace for economic, intellectual and cultural activity; a vigorus defense at home and abroad, of American ideas and institutions; and scholarly studies and academic achievement.

2912 Milwaukee Foundation
1020 N Broadway
Milwaukee, WI 53202
414-272-5805
FAX: 414-272-6235
e-mail: info@greatermkefdn.org
www.greatermilwaukeefoundation.org

Douglas M Jansson, Executive Director

2913 Northwestern Mutual Life Foundation
720 E Wisconsin Avenue
Milwaukee, WI 53202
414-665-1800
800-388-8123
FAX: 414-665-2199
www.northwesternmutual.com

Edward Zore, Chief Executive Officer
Fredric H Sweet, Executive Vice President

2914 Patrick and Anna M Cudahy Fund
PO Box 11978
Milwaukee, WI 53211
414-271-6020
FAX: 847-475-0679
e-mail: secretary@cudahyfund.org
www.cudahyfund.org

Judith L Borchers, Executive Director

2915 SB Waterman & E Blade Charitable Foundation
Marshall & Ilsley Trust Company
PO Box 2980
Milwaukee, WI 53201
414-287-8700
FAX: 414-298-8097

Thomas C Boettcher
Kenneth Krei, Chief Executive Officer

Wyoming

2916 Arc of Wyoming
PO Box 393
Casper, WY 82602
307-577-4913
FAX: 307-577-4014

Festi Moon, President
Toni Hutchison, Executive Director

Funding Directories

2917 AIDS Funding
Foundation Center
79 5th Avenue
New York, NY 10003
212-620-4230
800-424-9836
FAX: 212-807-3677
e-mail: ajt@fdncenter.org
www.fdncenter.org

Sara Engelhardt, President
Cheryl Loe, Director of Communications
Gives vital information on over 450 foundations, corporate giving programs, and public charities; more than twice the number of grantmakers appeared in the last edition. All the grantmakers listed have proven their commitment by funding projects such as direct relief, medical research, legal aid and other programs to empower AIDS victims and combat the disease. *$60.00*

ISBN 0-87954 -82-5

2918 Chronicle Guide to Grants
Chronicle Guide to Grants
1255 23rd Street NW
Washington, DC 20037
202-331-4267
800-287-6072
FAX: 202-659-2236

Edward R Weidlein, Publisher
A computerized research tool, on floppy disks or a CD-ROM, for immediate use on any IBM compatible personal computer. Offers electronic listings of 10,000 grants from hundreds of foundations, with a subscription that offers 1,000 plus new listings every two months. Each listing offers grant information as well as names, addresses and phone numbers of the grant-making organizations. *$295.00*

2919 College Student's Guide to Merit and Other No-Need Funding
Reference Service Press
5000 Windplay Drive
Suite 4
El Dorado Hills, CA 95762
916-939-9620
FAX: 916-939-9626
e-mail: findaid@aol.com
www.rspfunding.com

Gail Schlachter, Director/Owner
More than 1,200 funding opportunities for currently-enrolled or returning college students are described in this directory. *$32.00*

450 pages
ISBN 1-588410-41-2

2920 Community Health Funding Report
C D Publications
8204 Fenton Street
Silver Spring, MD 20910
301-588-6380
800-666-6380
FAX: 301-588-0591
e-mail: chf@cdpublications.com
www.cdpublications.com

Michael Gerecht, Publisher/President
Gives the widest range of funding information available anywhere, including public and private grant announcements, reports on successful health programs nationwide, interviews with grant officials, plus national news on health policy topics affecting various organizations. *$339.00*
18 pages BiWeekly

2921 Corporate Foundation Files
Foundation Center
79 5th Avenue
Department Ze
New York, NY 10003
212-620-4230
800-424-9836
FAX: 212-807-3677
www.fdncenter.org

Sara Engelhardt, President
Provides an even more updated in-depth examination of over 250 of America's top corporate foundations, grantmakers with assets of $1 million plus or annual giving of $100,000 or more. This book supplements information presented on leading corporate foundations and provides 4-6 page reports with full background data on each Corporation and foundation structure plus a complete grants analysis and listing of sample grants awarded to nonprofit organizations. *$125.00*

ISBN 0-87954 -36-1

2922 Corporate Foundation Profiles
Foundation Center
79 5th Avenue
Department Ze
New York, NY 10003
212-620-4230
800-424-9836
FAX: 212-807-3677
www.fdncenter.org

Sara Engelhardt, President
Offers foundation portraits, grants analysis and grants list. *$135.00*

2923 Crime and Justice
Foundation Center
79 5th Avenue
New York, NY 10003
212-620-4230
800-424-9836
FAX: 212-807-3677
e-mail: ajt@fdncenter.org
www.fdncenter.org

Sara Engelhardt, President
Cheryl Loe, Director of Communications
This comprehensive work examines foundation funding for programs involved with crime prevention, juvenile justice, law enforcement, correction facilities, rehabilitation and victim assistance. This book looks at significant developments in the criminal justice field, changing public perceptions of crime and cuts in governmental expenditures. *$35.00*

ISBN 0-87954 -90-6

2924 Directory of Financial Aids for Women
Reference Service Press
5000 Windplay Drive
Suite 4
El Dorado Hills, CA 95762
916-939-9620
FAX: 916-939-9626
e-mail: findaid@aol.com
www.rspfunding.com

Gail Ann Schlachter, Author/Owner
David R Weber, Author
Funding programs listed support study, research, travel, training, career development, or innovative effort at any level; descriptions of more than 1,700 funding programs - representing billions of dollars in financial aid set aside for women; also an annotated bibliography of 60 key directories that identify even more financial aid opportunities and a set of indexes that let you search the directory by title, sponser, researching, tenability, subject, and deadline. *$45.00*
578 pages Biennial 1999
ISBN 1-588410-00-5

2925 Directory of Japanese Giving
79 Fifth Avenue 16th Street
New York, NY 10003
212-620-4230
800-424-9836
FAX: 212-807-3677
e-mail: orders@fdncenter.org
www.fdncenter.org

Laura Cascio, Fulfillment Manager
Cheryl Lee, Director of Communications
Sara Engelhardt, President
Offers crucial information on the fastest growing sector of corporate philanthropy. *$190.00*

2926 Directory of New and Emerging Foundations
Foundation Center
79 5th Avenue
Department Ze
New York, NY 10003
212-620-4230
800-424-9836
FAX: 212-807-3677
e-mail: aj@fdncenter.org
www.fdncenter.org

Sara Engelhardt, President
Provides information on over 3,000 foundations that have incorporated as grantmaking institutions in the United States. *$95.00*

2927 Directory of Venture Capital Firms
Grey House Publishing
PO Box 860
Millerton, NY 12546
518-789-8700
800-562-2139
FAX: 518-789-0556
e-mail: books@greyhouse.com
www.greyhouse.com

Leslie Mackenzie, Publisher
Richard Gottlieb, President
This annual directory includes more than 2,000 active venture capital and private equity firms in both the US and overseas. Each detailed profile includes fund size, portfolio companies, investment criteria and key executives.
Annual

2928 Disability Funding News
C D Publications
8204 Fenton Street
Silver Spring, MD 20910
301-588-6380
800-666-6380
FAX: 301-588-6385
e-mail: info@cdpublications.com
www.cdpublications.com

Jim Rogers, Editor
Michael Gerecht, President
Offers comprehensive listings on federal grants, detailed listings of foundations, legal news, grant-seeking techniques and more. *$249.00*
18 pages SemiWeekly
ISSN 1069-13 9

2929 Federal Funding to Fight AIDS
Government Information Services
4301 Fairfax Drive
Suite 875
Arlington, VA 22203
703-465-9100
800-876-0226
FAX: 800-926-2012
Describes all the federal government grants and financial aid programs to fight the AIDS epidemic. Includes agency-by-agency description of $1.9 billion in available grants, including the name, address and telephone number of the federal official responsible for each program. *$57.00*

74 pages Special Report

2930 Federal Grants & Contracts Weekly
Capitol Publications
1333 H Street NW
Suite 100e
Washington, DC 20005
202-223-3000
800-655-5597
FAX: 703-736-6501

Pam Moore, Editor
Claudia Moran, Marketing Manager
Merle Morgan, President
The latest funding announcements of federal grants for project opportunities in research, training and services. Provides profiles of key programs, tips on seeking grants, updates on legislation and regulations, budget developments and early alerts to upcoming funding opportunities. *$369.00*
Weekly

2931 Financial Aid for Asian Americans
Reference Service Press
5000 Windplay Drive
Suite 4
El Dorado Hills, CA 95762
916-939-9620
FAX: 916-939-9626
e-mail: findaid@aol.com
www.rspfunding.com

Gail Ann Schlachter, President/Owner
R David Weber, Editor-in-Chief
This is the source to use if you are looking for financial aid for Asian Americans; nearly 1,000 funding opportunities are described. *$35.00*
336 pages 1999
ISBN 1-588410-02-1

2932 Financial Aid for Hispanic Americans
Reference Service Press
5000 Windplay Drive
Suite 4
El Dorado Hills, CA 95762
916-939-9620
FAX: 916-939-9626
e-mail: findaid@aol.com
www.rspfunding.com

Gail Ann Schlachter, Author/Owner
R David Weber, Author
Nearly 1,300 funding programs open to Americans of Mexican, Puerto Rican, Central American, or other Latin American heritage are described here. *$37.50*
472 pages 1999
ISBN 1-588410-03-X

2933 Financial Aid for Native Americans
Reference Service Press
5000 Windplay Drive
Suite 4
El Dorado Hills, CA 95762
916-939-9620
FAX: 916-939-9626
e-mail: findaid@aol.com
www.rspfunding.com

Gail Ann Schlachter, Author/Owner
R David Weber, Author
Detailed information is provided on 1,500 funding opportunities open to American Indians, Native Alaskans, and Native Pacific Islanders. *$37.50*
546 pages
ISBN 1-588410-04-8

2934 Financial Aid for Research and Creative Ac tivities Abroad
Reference Service Press
5000 Windplay Drive
Suite 4
El Dorado Hills, CA 95762
916-939-9620
FAX: 916-939-9626
e-mail: findaid@aol.com
www.rspfunding.com

Gail Ann Schlachter, Author/Owner
Described here are 1,200 funding programs (scholarships, fellowships, grants, etc.) available to support research, professional, or creative activities abroad. *$45.00*
378 pages
ISBN 1-588410-82-5

2935 Financial Aid for Veterans, Military Personnel and their Dependents
Reference Service Press
5000 Windplay Drive
Suite 4
El Dorado Hills, CA 95762
916-939-9620
FAX: 916-939-9626
e-mail: findaid@aol.com
www.rspfunding.com

Gail Ann Schlachter, Author/Owner
David R Weber, Author
According to Reference Book Review, this directory (with its 1,100 entries) is the most comprehensive guide available on the subject. *$40.00*
392 pages
ISBN 1-588410-43-9

2936 Financial Aid for the Disabled and their Families
Reference Service Press
5000 Windplay Drive
Suite 4
El Dorado Hills, CA 95762
916-939-9620
FAX: 916-939-9626
e-mail: info@rspfunding.com
www.rspfunding.com

Gail Ann Schlachter, Author/Owner
R David Weber, Author
Organized to easily identify funding opportunities not only by type, but by specific subject coverage, sponsoring organization, program title, residency requirements, where the money can be spent, and even deadline date; includes detailed program descriptions. Program profiles indicate purpose, eligibility, financial data, duration, special features, limitations, number awarded, and application. Complete contact information is also provided including fax numbers, toll-free, and email/website. *$37.50*
508 pages Every other yr. 1999
ISBN 1-588410-01-3

2937 Foundation & Corporate Grants Alert
Capitol Publications
1333 H Street NW
Suite 100e
Washington, DC 20005
202-223-3000
800-655-5597
FAX: 703-736-6501

Patricia Hagmann, Editor
Claudia Moran, Marketing Manager
Merle Morgan, President
A complete guide to foundation and corporate grant opportunities for nonprofit organizations. Tracks developments and trends in funding and provides notification of changes in foundations' funding priorities. *$245.00*
Monthly
ISSN 1062-46 6

2938 Foundation 1000
Foundation Center
79 5th Avenue
Department Ze
New York, NY 10003
212-620-4230
800-424-9836
FAX: 212-691-1828
www.fdncenter.org

Jeffrey Fulkenstein, Editor
Sara Engelhardt, President
Full profiles of all 1,000 grantmakers across the United States. *$195.00*

2939 Foundation Center's User-Friendly Guide
Foundation Center
79 5th Avenue
Department Ze
New York, NY 10003
212-620-4230
800-424-9836
FAX: 212-807-3677
www.fdncenter.org

Sara Engelhardt, President

This helpful book answers the most commonly asked questions about fundraising in an upbeat, easy-to-read style. Specifically designed for novice grantseekers, this publication will lead you through the maze of unfamiliar jargon and the wide range of research guides used successfully by professional grantseekers everyday. *$9.95*

ISBN 0-87954 -42-6

2940 Foundation Directory
Foundation Center
79 5th Avenue
Department Ze
New York, NY 10003
212-620-4230
800-424-9836
FAX: 212-807-3677
www.fdncenter.org

Sara Engelhardt, President
An expanded, updated version of the fundraising research classic, offers a chance to bolster your prospect files with newly gathered data on these influential funders: over 7,500 foundation entries and over 1,100 foundations covered for the very first time in a Foundation Directory. *$140.00*

ISBN 0-87954 -45-0

2941 Foundation Grants to Individuals
Foundation Center
79 5th Avenue
Department Ze
New York, NY 10003
212-620-4230
800-424-9836
FAX: 212-807-3677
www.fdncenter.org

Sara Engelhardt, President
The only publication that provides extensive coverage of foundation funding prospects for individual grantseekers. *$40.00*
Biennially

2942 From the State Capitals: Public Health
Wakeman/ Walworth
PO Box 7376
Alexandria, VA 22307
703-768-9600
FAX: 703-768-9690
e-mail: newsletters@statecapitals.com
www.statecapitals.com

Keyes Walworth, Publisher
Christine Ryan, Marketing Manager
Digest of state and municipal health care financing and cost containment measures, includes medical legislation, disease control, etc. *$245.00*
6 pages

2943 Guide to Federal Funding for Child Care and Early Childhood Development
Government Information Services
4301 Fairfax Drive
Suite 875
Arlington, VA 22203
703-465-9100
800-225-5750
FAX: 703-528-6060

James J Marshall, Publisher
Joel M Drucker, Associate Publisher
Describes more than 60 federal grant, loan and tax credit programs to assist child care and early childhood development programs. The guide describes more than $25 billion in federal aid for traditional day care, developmental programs such as Head Start and school-based early childhood education programs such as Even Start. *$169.00*
372 pages 3-Ring Binder

2944 Guide to Federal Funding for Hospitals and Health Centers
The Foundation Center
79 5th Avenue 16th Street
New York, NY 10003
212-620-4230
800-424-9836
FAX: 212-807-3677
www.fdncenter.org

Laura Cascio, Fulfillment Manager
Maggie Morth, Director of Communications
Describes approximately 150 federal grant and loan programs for hospitals, health centers, and other agencies involved in administering health services. *$297.00*
958 pages 3-Ring Binder

2945 Guide to Federal Funding for Volunteer Programs & Community Service
Government Information Services
4301 Fairfax Drive
Suite 875
Arlington, VA 22203
703-465-9100
800-225-5750
FAX: 703-528-6060

James J Marshall, Publisher
Joel M Drucker, Associate Publisher
Guide describes in detail roughly 60 federal programs that provide aid to establish and operate volunteer programs. *$85.00*
3-Ring Binder

2946 High School Senior's Guide to Merit and Ot her No-Need Funding
Reference Service Press
5000 Windplay Drive
Suite 4
El Dorado Hills, CA 95762
916-939-9620
FAX: 916-939-9626
e-mail: findaid@aol.com
www.rspfunding.com

Gail Schlachter, Director/Owner
Here's your guide to 1,100 funding programs that never look at income level when making awards to college bound high school seniors. *$29.95*
400 pages
ISBN 1-588410-44-X

2947 How to Pay for Your Degree in Business & Related Fields
Reference Service Press
5000 Windplay Drive
Suite 4
El Dorado Hills, CA 95762
916-939-9620
FAX: 916-939-9626
e-mail: findaid@aol.com
www.rspfunding.com

Gail Schlachter, Director/Owner
If you need funding for an undergraduate or graduate degree in business or related fields, this is the directory to use (500+ funding programs described). *$30.00*
290 pages
ISBN 1-588410-49-8

2948 How to Pay for Your Degree in Education & Related Fields
Reference Service Press
5000 Windplay Drive
Suite 4
El Dorado Hills, CA 95762
916-939-9620
FAX: 916-939-9626
e-mail: findaid@aol.com
www.rspfunding.com

Gail Schlachter, Director/Owner
Here's hundreds of funding opportunities available to support undergraduate and graduate students preparing for a career in education, guidance etc. *$30.00*
250 pages
ISBN 1-588410-63-3

2949 International Encyclopedia of Foundations
Foundation Center
79 5th Avenue
New York, NY 10003
212-620-4230
800-424-9836
FAX: 212-807-3677
e-mail: ajt@fdncenter.org
www.fdncenter.org

Sara Engelhardt, President
Cheryl Loe, Director of Communications

Compiled volume of useful and often hard-to-find information on the history and operation of major foundations located outside the U.S. One of the very few book-length accounts of international foundations in English, the book is made up of 146 historical sketches of the most significant foundations in 31 countries. *$75.00*

ISBN 0-31325 -83-6

2950 Japanese Corporate Connection: A Guide for Fundraisers

Foundation Center
79 5th Avenue
New York, NY 10003
212-620-4230
800-424-9836
FAX: 212-807-3677
e-mail: ajt@fdncenter.org
www.fdncenter.org

Sara Engelhardt, President
Cheryl Loe, Director of Communications
Shows how certain U.S. nonprofits have successfully approached major Japanese philanthropics. *$90.00*

2951 National Data Book of Foundations

Foundation Center
79 5th Avenue
Department Ze
New York, NY 10003
212-620-4230
800-424-9836
FAX: 212-807-3677
e-mail: fdnonline@fdncenter.org
www.fdncenter.org

Sara Engelhardt, President
Allyson Tuffs, Vice President
Gives fast access to vital information on 32,000 U.S. foundations, the most complete listing of grantmakers ever published. It reflects the broad scope of this important foundation locator. It can help you quickly develop a list of initial funding prospects from the largest national to the smallest local foundations. *$125.00*

ISBN 0-87954 -85-0

2952 National Directory of Corporate Giving

Foundation Center
79 5th Avenue
New York, NY 10003
212-620-4230
800-424-9836
FAX: 212-807-3677
e-mail: ajt@fdncenter.org
www.fdncenter.org

Sara Engelhardt, President
Cheryl Loe, Director of Communications
Offers over 2,000 corporate funders, current giving reviews and profiles of sponsoring companies. *$195.00*

2953 National Guide to Funding Religion

Foundation Center
79 5th Avenue
New York, NY 10003
212-620-4230
800-424-9836
FAX: 212-807-3677
www.fdncenter.org

Sara Engelhardt, President
Macy Morin, Executive Vice President
This book gives access to a fundraising guide designed specifically for them. This new subject directory brings together a group of 2,800 foundations and corporate direct giving programs, all of which have a history of funding churches, religious welfare and religious education programs. *$125.00*

ISBN 0-87954 -80-9

2954 National Guide to Funding for Children, Youth & Families

Foundation Center
79 Fifth Avenue 16th Street
New York, NY 10003
212-620-4230
800-424-9836
FAX: 212-807-3677
e-mail: orders@fdncenter.org
www.fdncenter.org

Sara Engelhardt, President
Cheryl Lee, Director of Communications
Caters specifically to development professionals for organizations serving the needs of children, youth and families. With over 2,400 listings of funding sources, both foundations and direct giving programs and over 8,000 sample grants. *$125.00*

ISBN 0-87954 -91-5

2955 National Guide to Funding for Elementary & Secondary Education

Foundation Center
79 5th Avenue
Department Ze
New York, NY 10003
212-620-4230
800-424-9836
FAX: 212-807-3677
www.fdncenter.org

Sara Engelhardt, President
This guide gathers together, in one convenient source, a list of grantmakers committed to improving pre-college education. This book provides full profiles for over 1,400 foundations and corporate direct giving programs. *$125.00*

ISBN 0-87954 -94-9

2956 National Guide to Funding for Libraries and Information Services

Foundation Center
79 5th Avenue
New York, NY 10003
212-620-4230
800-424-9836
FAX: 212-807-3677
e-mail: ajt@fdncenter.org
www.fdncenter.org

Sara Engelhardt, President
Cheryl Loe, Director of Communications
This guide features a long list of grantmakers that support facilities. This directory provides essential data on over 400 foundations and corporate direct giving programs. In addition, many of these grantmaker entries include grant lists. *$75.00*

ISBN 0-87954 -95-7

2957 National Guide to Funding for Women and Girls

Foundation Center
79 5th Avenue
New York, NY 10003
212-620-4230
800-424-9836
FAX: 212-807-3677
e-mail: ajt@fdncenter.org
www.fdncenter.org

Sara Engelhardt, President
Cheryl Loe, Director of Communications
Fundraisers who seek support for nonprofits that provide services and advocate women and girls can now turn to this new subject directory. This book offers grantseekers the benefit of over 700 foundations and corporate direct giving program entries. *$95.00*

ISBN 0-87954 -93-0

2958 National Guide to Funding in Aging

Foundation Center
79 5th Avenue
Department Ze
New York, NY 10003
212-620-4230
800-424-9836
FAX: 212-807-3677
www.fdncenter.org

Sara Engelhardt, President
Professional fundraisers recognize this book as the premier source of information on the agencies and foundations that support aging projects. This volume covers federal and state programs as well as foundations and other voluntary organizations. *$75.00*

ISBN 0-87954 -33-7

2959 National Guide to Funding in Arts and Culture

Foundation Center
79 5th Avenue
New York, NY 10003
212-620-4230
800-424-9836
FAX: 212-807-3677
e-mail: ajt@fdncenter.org
www.fdncenter.org

Sara Engelhardt, President
Cheryl Loe, Director of Communications

Designed specifically to meet the needs of development professionals in the field of arts and culture, this guide thoroughly prepares you for an informed grant search. With over 3,300 listings of foundations and corporate direct giving programs, the volume offers fundraisers in the field an excellent opportunity to increase their funding base. *$125.00*

ISBN 0-87954 -48-9

2960 National Guide to Funding in Health

Foundation Center
79 5th Avenue
New York, NY 10003
212-620-4230
800-424-9836
FAX: 212-807-3677
www.fdncenter.org

Sara Engelhardt, President
Macy Morin, Executive Vice President

Contains essential facts on more than 2,500 foundations and corporate direct giving programs, each with a history of awarding grant dollars to hospitals, universities, research centers, community-based facilities, rural health-care projects and a range of other health-related programs and projects. *$125.00*

ISBN 0-87954 -79-5

2961 National Guide to Funding in Higher Education

Foundation Center
79 5th Avenue
New York, NY 10003
212-620-4230
800-424-9836
FAX: 212-807-3677
e-mail: ajt@fdncenter.org
www.fdncenter.org

Sara Engelhardt, President
Cheryl Loe, Director of Communications

Designed for those seeking foundation support for higher education, this National Guide allows researchers to immediately find information on top funders in the field. This directory covers nearly 3,000 foundations, all with a history of awarding grants to colleges, universities, graduate programs and research institutes. *$125.00*

ISBN 0-87954 -90-1

2962 New York State Foundations

Foundation Center
79 5th Avenue
New York, NY 10003
212-620-4230
800-424-9836
FAX: 212-807-3677
www.fdncenter.org

Sara Engelhardt, President
Macy Morin, Executive Vice President

Provides a complete list of every grantmaking foundation in the state. *$150.00*

2963 Report on Disability Programs

Business Publishers
2601 University Boulevard W
Suite 200
Silver Spring, MD 20902
301-587-6300
800-274-6737
FAX: 301-589-8493
e-mail: custserv@bpinews.com
www.bpinews.com

Leonard Eiser, Publisher
Adam Goldstein, President
Melissa Reid, Marketing Manager

Follows all programs and funding sources in education, housing, job training, therapy, Social Security Supplemental Security Income, Medicare, Medicaid and more of importance to persons with disabilities. Also covers the latest on the Americans with Disabilities Act. Publishes a newsletter. *$327.00*

25x Year

2964 Source Book Profiles

Foundation Center
79 5th Avenue
New York, NY 10003
212-620-4230
800-424-9836
FAX: 212-807-3677
www.fdncenter.org

Sara Engelhardt, President
Macy Morin, Executive Vice President

Now the fundraising resource that publishes comprehensive portraits of the country's most influential foundations over a two-year cycle offers even more for your research dollars. A database publication which means that it is now more flexible and efficient than ever before, an even more essential part of your philanthropic library. *$350.00*

ISBN 0-87954 -83-3

2965 Student Guide

US Department of Education
400 Maryland Avenue SW
Washington, DC 20202
202-401-2000
800-872-5376
FAX: 202-401-0689
TTY: 800-437-0833
e-mail: customerservice@inet.ed.gov
www.ed.gov/prog_info/SFA/studentguide

William J Ryan, Acting Director
Margaret Spellings, Chief Executive Officer

Describes the major student aid programs the US Department of Education administers and gives detailed information about program procedures.

74 pages Annual

2966 Substance Abuse Funding News

C D Publications
8204 Fenton Street
Silver Spring, MD 20910
301-588-6380
800-666-6380
FAX: 301-588-6385
e-mail: info@cdpublications.com
www.cdpublications.com

Jim Rogers, Editor
Michael Gerecht, Publisher/President

Newsletter covers private and federal funding opportunities for alcohol, tobacco and drug abuse programs. Plus advice on grantseeking and proposal writing, tips from funding officials and reports on the latest federal and state initives to address substance abuse and related concerns.

18 pages 2x Month

Federal

2967 Administration on Children, Youth and Families
U S Department of Health and Human Services
370 L Enfant Promenade
Washington, DC 20201 202-690-7650
www.acf.dhhs.gov

Responsible for federal programs that promote the economic and social well-being of families, children, individuals and communities.

2968 Administration on Developmental Disabilities
U S Department of Health and Human Services
370 L Enfant Promenade SW
Mail Stop: HHH 405-D
Washington, DC 20447 202-690-6590
FAX: 202-205-8037
www.acf.hhs.gov/programs/add

Patricia Morrissey PhD, Commissioner
Faith McCormick, Director

Ensures that individuals with developmental disabilities and their families participate in the design of and have access to culturally competent services, supports, and other assistance and opportunities that promote independence, productivity, and integration and inclusion into the community.

2969 Administration on the Aging
U S Department of Health and Human Services
3330 Independence Avenue SW
Washington, DC 20201 202-690-7650
FAX: 202-357-3556
e-mail: AoAInfo@aoa.gov
www.aoa.gov

Josefina Carbonell, Commissioner

Administers the Older Americans Act of 1965 to assist states and local communities to develop programs for older persons.

2970 Americans with Disabilities Act Informatio n
US Department of Justice
950 Pennsylvania Avenue NW
Washington, DC 20530 202-646-5095
800-574-0301
FAX: 202-307-1197
www.ada.gov

In cooperation with many federal agencies, the ADA assures that Americans with disabilities have the same opportunities as all Americans. To this end, the Justice Department produces publications, sponsors programs and continually reviews the needs of individuals with disabilities.

2971 Committee for Purchase from People Who Are Blind or Severely Disabled
1421 Jefferson Davis Highway
Suite 10800
Arlington, VA 22202 703-603-7740
FAX: 703-603-0655
e-mail: info@jwod.gov
www.jwod.gov

Leon A Wilson Jr, Executive Director
Patrick Rowe, Deputy Executive Director
Robert M Hartt, Manager Legislative Affairs

A federal agency that administers the Javits-Wagner-O'Day Program, directing federal agencies to purchase products and services from nonprofit agencies that employ people who are blind or have other severe disabilities. Provides a wide range of vocational options to individuals with severe disabilities.

2972 Equal Opportunity Employment Commission
1801 L Street NW
Washington, DC 20036 202-663-4900
800-669-4000
e-mail: info@ask.eeoc.gov
www.eeoc.gov

Carim Dominguez, Chairman
Naomi C Earp, Vice Chairman
Ida Castro, Manager

This agency is responsible for drafting and implementing the regulations of Title I of the ADA.

2973 Federal Communications Commission
445 12th Street SW
Washington, DC 20554 202-418-0450
888-835-5322
888-225-5322
FAX: 866-418-0232
e-mail: fccinfo@fcc.gov
www.fcc.gov

Jennifer Simpson, Specialist
Gloria Thomas, Manager

Enforces ADA telecommunications provisions which require that companies offering telephone service to the general public must offer telephone relay services to individuals who use text telephones or similar devices. Also enforces closed captioning rules, hearing compatibility and access to equipment and services for people with disabilities.

2974 Health Care Financing Administration
200 Independence Avenue SW
Washington, DC 20201 202-690-6726
FAX: 202-690-6262

William Roper, Administrator
Thomas Scully, President

Through the Social Security administration, it administers the Medicare program under Title XVIII of the Social Security Act. Administers grants to the states for Medicaid under Title XIX of the Social Security Act for individuals who are medically indigent.

2975 National Coalition of Federal Aviation Employees with Disabilities
Federal Aviation Administration
6500 S Mac Authur Street
Oklahoma City, OK 73169 405-954-4709
FAX: 405-954-4490
TTY:405-954-4587
www.faa.gov/acr/ncfaed.htm

Becky Pritchett, Treasurer
Alan Jones, President of Aeronautical Center

NCFAED is working on: 1) improvement of work conditions for employees; 2) expansion on National Coalition to serve all FAA employees; 3) promote equal opportunity for people with disabilities in the FAA workplace; 4) assist the FAA in its commitment to remove physical and attudinal barriers which inhibit opportunities for people with disabilities; 5) align with internal and external organizations to attract future generations of people with disabilities to the FAA as employees.

2976 National Council on Disability
1331 F Street NW
Suite 850
Washington, DC 20004 202-272-2004
FAX: 202-272-2022
e-mail: info@ncd.gov
www.ncd.gov

Mark Quigley, Communications Director
Ethel Briggs, Executive Director

Federal agency led by 15 members appointed by the President of the United States and confirmed by the United States Senate. The overall purpose of the National Council is to promote policies, programs, practices and procedures that guarantee equal opportunity for all people with disabilities, regardless of the nature of severity of the disability; and to empower people with disabilities to achieve economic self-sufficiency, independent living and integration into all aspects of society.

2977 National Division of the Blind and Visually Impaired
330 C Street NW
Washington, DC 20001 202-205-8520

Chester Avery, Director

Develops methods, standards and procedures to assist state agencies in the rehabilitation of blind persons. Administers the Randolph-Sheppard Act, which assures priority for blind persons in the operation of vending facilities on federal property and serves as a program manager for the Helen Keller National Center for Youth who are deaf-blind.

2978 National Institutes of Health: National Eye Institute

31 Center Drive
Bethesda, MD 20892
301-496-5751
FAX: 301-496-9970
e-mail: kcl@nei.nih.gov
www.nei.nih.gov

Paul A Sieving, Director
Audrey Penn, Executive Director
Finances intramural and extramural research on eye diseases and vision disorders. Supports training of eye researchers.

2979 Office of Policy

Social Security Administration
2100 M Street NW
Washington, DC 20037
202-523-0412
800-772-1213
TTY:800-325-0778
e-mail: concepcion.mcneace@ssa.gov
www.ssa.gov/policy

Laurence Love, Acting Deputy Commissioner
Edward Demarco, Assitant Deputy Commissioner
Serge Harrison, Executive Officer
Administers grants to the states for social services under Title XX of the Social Security Act to welfare recipients and others likely to become them.

2980 Office of Special Education Programs: Department of Education

400 Maryland Avenue, SW
Washington, DC 20202
202-245-7468

e-mail: gblumenthal@acs.dhhs.gov
www.ed.gov/osers/osep

Alexa Posny, Director
Patty Guard, Deputy Director
The Office of Special Education Programs (OSEP) is dedicated to improving results for infants, toddlers, children and youth with disabilities ages birth through 21 by providing leadership and financial support to assist states and local districts.

2981 President's Committee on People with Intellecutual Disabilities

U S Department of Health and Human Services
370 L Enfant Promenade SW
Washington, DC 20447
202-619-0364
FAX: 202-205-9519
e-mail: gblumenthal@acf.dhhs.gov
www.acf.dhhs.gov/programs/pcmr

Dalls Rob Sweezy, Chairperson
Sally Atwater, Executive Director
Formerly the President's Committee on Mental Retardation, a federal advisory committee, estalished by the presidential executive order to adivse the President of the United States and the Secretary of the Department of Health and Human Services on issues concerning citizens with intellectual disabilities, coordinate activities between different federal agencies and assess the impact of their policies upon the lives of citizens with intellectual disabilities and their families.

2982 Rehabilitative Services Administration

U S Department of Education
400 Maryland Avenue, SW
Washington, DC 20202
202-245-7468
FAX: 202-205-9874
www.ed.gov

The Rehabilitation Services Administration (RSA) oversees formula and discretionary grant programs that help individuals with physical or mental disabilities to obtain employment and live more independently through the provision of such supports as counseling, medical and psychological services, job training and other individualized services.

2983 Social Security Administration

6401 Security Boulevard
Baltimore, MD 21235
410-965-6114
800-772-1213
www.socialsecurity.gov

Martha Mcsteen, Acting Commissioner
Bill Vitek, Manager
Administers old age, survivors, and disability insurance programs under Title II of the Social Security Act. Also administers the federal income maintenance program under Title XVI of the Social Security Act. Maintains network of local/regional offices nationwide.

2984 US Department of Education: Office of Civil Rights

300 C Street NW
Room 5414
Washington, DC 20202
202-208-5815
800-421-3481

John Sherrod, Executive Director
Prohibits discrimination on the basis of disability in programs and activities funded by the Department of Education. Investigates complaints and provides technical assistance to individuals and entities with rights and responsibilities under Section 504.

2985 US Department of Education: Office of Civil Rights

U S Department of Education
400 Maryland Avenue SW
Washington, DC 20202
202-401-2000
FAX: 202-401-0689
www.ed.gov

Margaret Spellings, Chief Executive Officer
Prohibits discrimination on the basis of disability in programs and activities funded by the Department of Education. Investigates complaints and provides technical assistance to individuals and entities with rights and responsibilities under Section 504.

2986 US Department of Justice

Civil Rights Division/ Disability Rights Section
950 Pennsylvania Avenue NW
Washington, DC 20530
202-514-3301
800-514-0301
FAX: 202-307-1197
www.ada.gov

John Wodatch, Chief
The US Department of Justice answers questions about the American Disabilities Act (ADA) and provides free publications by mail and fax through its ADA Information Line.

2987 US Department of Labor: Office of Federal Contract Programs

200 Constitution Avenue NW
Washington, DC 20210
202-693-5000
888-376-3227
FAX: 202-693-1304

Elaine Chao, Chief Executive Officer
Prohibits discrimination on the basis of disability and requires federal contractors and sub-contractors with contracts of $2,500 or more to take affirmative action to employ and advance individuals with disabilities.

2988 US Department of Transportation

400 7th Street SW
Washington, DC 20590
202-366-4000
FAX: 202-366-7149
www.dot.gov

Norman Mineta, Chief Executive Officer
Enforces ADA provisions that require nondiscrimination in public and private mass transportation systems and services.

2989 US Office of Personnel Management

1900 E Street NW
Washington, DC 20415
202-606-1381
FAX: 202-606-2532
e-mail: GENERAL@opm.gov
www.opm.gov

Linda M Springer, Director
Claudio Benedi, Manager
Establishes policies for employment of the handicapped within the federal service. Administers a merit system for the federal employment that includes recruiting, examining, training, and promoting people on the basis of knowledge and skills, regardless of sex, race, religion or other factors.

Alabama

2990 Alabama Council For Developmental Disabilities
RSA Union Building
100 N Union Street
PO Box 301410
Montgomery, AL 36130
334-242-3973
800-232-2158
FAX: 334-242-0797
e-mail: mjones@mh.state.al.us
www.acdd.org

Elmyra Jones, Executive Director
Joyce Carvana, Administrative Assistant
Serves as an advocate for Alabama's citizens with developmental disabilities and their families; to empower them with the knowledge and opportunity to make informed choices and exercise control over their own lives; and to create a climate for positive socialchange to enable them to be respected, independent and productive integrated members of society.

2991 Alabama Department of Public Health
20 Monroe Street
Suite 1552
Montgomery, AL 36104
334-206-5200
FAX: 334-206-5520
www.adph.org

William Son, State Health Officer
Donald Williamson, Administrator
Provides professional services for the improvement and protection of the public's health through disease prevention and the assurance of public health services to resident and transient populations of the state regardless of social circumstances or the ability to pay.

2992 Alabama Department of Rehabilitation Services
2129 E S Boulevrad
Montgomery, AL 36116
334-281-8780
800-441-7607
FAX: 334-281-1973
e-mail: sshiver@rehab.state.al.us
www.rehab.state.al.us

Steve Shivers, Commissioner/President
Jim Harris III, Assistant Commissioner

2993 Alabama Department of Senior Services
770 Washington Avenue
Montgomery, AL 36130
334-242-4363
877-425-2243
FAX: 334-242-5594
e-mail: ageline@adss.state.al.us
www.adss.state.al.us

Irene B Collins, Executive Director

2994 Alabama Disabilities Advocacy Program
University of Alabama
PO Box 870395
Tuscaloosa, AL 35487
205-348-4928
800-826-1675
FAX: 205-348-3909
e-mail: adap@adap.ua.edu
www.adap.net

Ellen Gillespie, Executive Director
Robin Lunceford, Marketing Coordinator
The federally mandate statewide protection and advocacy system serving eligible individuals with disabilities in Alabama. ADAP has five program components: Protection and Advocacy for persons with developmental disabilities (PADD), Protection and Advocacy for Individuals with Mental Illness (PAIMT), Protection and Advocacy of Individual Rights (PAIR), Protection and Advocacy for Assistive Technology (PAAT) and Protection & Advocacy For Beneficiaries of Social Security (PABSS).

2995 Alabama Division of Rehabilitation and Crippled Children
2129 E South Boulevard
Montgomery, AL 36116
334-281-8780
800-441-7607
FAX: 334-281-1973
e-mail: sshiver@rehab.state.al.us
www.rehab.state.al.us

Steve Shivers, President
Jim Harris III, Assistant Commissioner

2996 Alabama State Department of Human Resources
PO Box 250380
Montgomery, AL 36125
334-293-3100
FAX: 334-293-3453
e-mail: ogapi@dhr.state.al.us
www.dhr.state.al.us/fsd/Child_Care.asp

Terry Benton, Executive Director
Partners with communities to promtoe family stability and provide for the safety and self-sufficiency of vulnerable Alabamians.

2997 Client Assistance Program: Alabama
2129 E South Boulevard
Montgomery, AL 36116
334-281-8780
FAX: 334-281-1973
www.rehab.state.al.us

Lamona Lucas, Director
Steve Shivers, President

2998 Disability Determination Service: Birmingham
PO Box 830300
Birmingham, AL 35283
205-870-1205
FAX: 256-773-2296

Tammy Warren, Director
Janet Cox, Owner

2999 Governor's Committee on Employment of Persons with Disabilities
Division of Rehabilitation Service
PO Box 11586
Montgomery, AL 36111
334-281-8780
FAX: 334-613-3893

Lamona Lucas, Director
Steve Shivers, Manager

3000 Social Security: Mobile Disability Determination Services
Disability Determination Services
PO Box 2371
Mobile, AL 36652
251-433-2820
800-292-6743
FAX: 251-436-0599
www.ssa.gov

Tommy Warren, Executive Director
Jack Miller, Office Manager

3001 Workers Compensation Board Alabama
Alabama Dept of Industrial Relation
649 Monroe Street
Montgomery, AL 36131
205-362-9040
FAX: 334-261-3143
e-mail: director@dir.alabama.gov
dir.alabama.gov/contacts

Phyllis Kennedy, Director, DIR
Scottie Spates, Worker's Compensation Director

Alaska

3002 ATLA
2217 E Tudor Road
Suite 4
Anchorage, AK 99507
907-563-2599
800-723-2852
FAX: 907-563-0699
e-mail: atla@atla.biz
www.atla.biz

Kathy Privratsky, Executive Director
Rich Sanders, Program Manager
Mystie Rail, PR/Marketing
Assistive Technology sales and services. ATLA is Alaska's only assistive technology resource center.

3003 Alaska Commission on Aging
PO Box C
Juneau, AK 99811
907-465-3250
FAX: 970-465-1398
TTY:970-465-2205
www.alaskaaging.org

Linda Gohl, Director

3004 Alaska Department of Handicapped Children
1231 Gambell Street
Room 314
Anchorage, AK 99501
907-269-3400

Rita Schmidt, Chief

3005 Alaska Division of Mental Health and Developmental Disabilities
350 Main Street
110620
Juneau, AK 99801
907-465-3562
FAX: 907-465-2668
www.state.ak.us

Julie Neyhart, Director
The division plans for and provides appropriate prevention, treatment and support for families impacted by mental disorders or developmental disabilities while maximizing self-determination. Community based services are provided by grantees. Inpatient services are provided in two division operated facilities.

3006 Alaska Division of Vocational Rehabilitation
801 W 10th Street
Suite A
Juneau, AK 99801
907-465-2814
800-478-2815
FAX: 907-465-2856
www.labor.state.ak.us/ddr/home

Gale Finnott, Executive Director
Russ Cusack, Chief Rehabilitation Therapist
Provides comprehensive services to people with disabilities to assist in achieving an employment outcome.

3007 Client Assistance Program: Alaska
2900 Boniface Parkway
Suite 100
Anchorage, AK 99504
907-333-2211
800-478-0047
FAX: 907-333-1186
e-mail: akcap@alaska.com
www.home.gci.net/~alaskacap

Pam Stratton, Director
We provide informatory referral to other programs in Alaska that are funded under the Rehabilitation Act of 1973 as amended; Individual assistance or advocacy, if an individual with disability has applied for or received services from an agency funded under the Rehabilitation Act and has concerns or questions we will work with them to help resolve their concerns with the agency.

3008 Governor's Committee on Employment and Rehabilitation of People with Disabilities: Alaska
801 W 10th Street
Suite A
Juneau, AK 99801
907-465-2814
800-478-2815
FAX: 907-465-2856
e-mail: Velja_Elstad@labor.state.ak.us
www.labor.state.ak.us/dvr

Velja Elstad, Staff Liaison
Gale Finnott, Executive Director
Carries on a continuing program to promote the employment and rehabilitation of citizens with disabilities in the State of Alaska. Advocates for a comprehensive statewide system for access to assistive technology. Obtains and maintains cooperation with public and private groups and individuals in this field.

3009 Governor's Council on Disabilities and Special Education
3601 C Street, Suite 740
PO Box 240249
Anchorage, AK 99524
907-269-8990
888-269-8990
FAX: 907-269-8995
e-mail: millie_ryan@health.state.ak.us
www.hss.state.ak.us/gcdse/

Millie Ryan, Executive Director
Kathy Allely, Planner III

3010 Protection & Advocacy System: Alaska
Disability Law Center of Alaska
3330 Arctic Boulevard
Suite 103
Anchorage, AK 99503
907-565-1002
800-478-1234
FAX: 907-565-1000
e-mail: akpa@dlcak.org
www.dlcak.org

David Fleurant, Executive Director
Cynthia Hite, Business Manager
Deals with rights of the disabled. Works in conjunction with agencies, law offices and family members.

3011 Protection & Advocacy for Persons with Developmental Disabilities: Alaska
Advocacy Services of Alaska
615 E 82nd Avenue
Suite 101
Anchorage, AK 99518
FAX: 907-349-1002
e-mail: rtessardore@dlcakelcak.org

Rick Tessardore, Director

3012 Workers Compensation
Department of Labor + Workforce Developments
PO Box 115512
Juneau, AK 99811
907-465-2790
FAX: 907-465-2797
www.labor.state.ak.us

Clark Bishop, Commissioner
Paul Lisankie, Division Director

Arizona

3013 Arizona Department of Children's Rehabilitative Services
1740 W Adams Street
Suite 205
Phoenix, AZ 85007
602-271-0945

W Sundin Applegate
Robert Plummer, Manager

3014 Arizona Department of Economic Security
1717 W Jefferson Street
Phoenix, AZ 85007 602-542-5678

Linda J Blessing, Director
Lynne Smith, Chief Executive Officer
The Department of Economic Security is a human service agency providing services in six areas: Aging and Community Services, Benefits and Medical Eligibility, Child Support Enforcement, Children and Family Services, Developmental Disabilities and Employment and Rehabilitation Services.

3015 Arizona Department of Family Health Services
1740 W Adams Street
Phoenix, AZ 85007 602-271-0945
FAX: 602-542-1235
e-mail: piowebmaster@azdhs.gov
www.azdhs.gov

Susan Gerard, Director
Robert Plummer, Manager

3016 Arizona Department of Handicapped Children
1740 W Adams Street
Room 205
Phoenix, AZ 85007 602-271-0945
FAX: 602-542-2589

W Sundin Applegate, Chief
Robert Plummer, Manager

3017 Arizona Division of Aging and Adult Services
1789 W Jefferson Street
Phoenix, AZ 85007 602-542-4446
FAX: 602-542-6575
www.azdcs.gov/aaa

Rex Critchfield, Program Administrator

3018 Arizona Rehabilitation State Services for the Blind and Visually Impaired
4620 N 16th Street
Suite 100
Phoenix, AZ 85016 602-938-2422

Kenneth House, State Manager
Erik Markoff, Manager
Offers clients a conservation program, eye examinations, treatments, counseling, social work, psychological testing and evaluation, professional training, computer training and more for the visually impaired. The staff includes 56 full time employees.

3019 Developmental Disability Council: Arizona
1717 W Jefferson Street
Phoenix, AZ 85007 602-542-4049
800-352-8168
FAX: 602-547-5320

David Berns, Director
Nebal Chavez, Executive Director
Susan Madison, Manager

3020 Governor's Council on Developmental Disabilities
3839 N 3rd Street
Phoenix, AZ 85012 602-863-0484
866-771-9378
FAX: 602-277-4454
e-mail: jsnyder@azdes.gov
www.azgcdd.org

Crystal Snyder, Executive Director
The purpose of the council is to advocate for and assure that individuals with developmental disabilities and their families participate in the design of and have access to culturally competent services, supports and provides opportunities to become integrated and included in the community.

3021 International Dyslexia Association: Arizona Branch
PO Box 6284
Scottsdale, AZ 85261 480-941-0308
800-222-3123
e-mail: info@interdys.org
www.dyslexia-az.org

Kay Byrd, President
Provides free information and referral services for diagnosis and tutoring for parents, educators, physicians, and individuals with dyslexia. The voice of our membership is heard in 48 countries. Membership includes yearly journal and quarterly newsletter. Call for conference dates.

3022 Protection & Advocacy for Persons with with Disabilities: Arizona
Arizona Center for Disability Law
3839 N 3rd Street
Suite 209
Phoenix, AZ 85012 602-274-6287
800-927-2260
FAX: 602-274-6779
e-mail: center@azdisabilitylaw.or
www.azdisabilitylaw.org

Peri Jude Radecic, Director of Public Advocacy
Henry G Watkins, Executive Director
Judy Fox, Manager

3023 Social Security: Phoenix Disability Determination Services
Social Security Admission
1122 N 7th Street
Suite 100
Phoenix, AZ 85006
800-772-1213
TTY:800-325-0778
www.ssa.gov

3024 Social Security: Tucson Disability Determination Services
3500 N Campbell Avenue
Tucson, AZ 85719
800-772-1213
TTY:800-325-0778
www.socialsecurity.gov

Arkansas

3025 Arkansas Assistive Technology Projects
Increasing Capabilities Access
2201 Brookwood Drive
Suite 117
Little Rock, AR 72202 501-666-8868
800-828-2799
FAX: 501-666-5319
e-mail: aehurst@ars.state.ar.us
www.arkansas-ican.org

Barbara Gullett, Executive Director
Barry Vuletich, Supervisor
Linda Morgan, Occupational Therapist
A consumer responsive ,statewide program promoting assistive technology devices and sources for persons of all ages with all disabilities. Referral and information services provide information about devices, where to obtain them and their cost.

3026 Arkansas Division of Aging & Adult Services
Department of Human Services
PO Box 1437
Little Rock, AR 72203 501-682-2441
FAX: 501-682-8155
e-mail: ron.tatus@mail.state.ar.us
www.state.ar.us/dhs/aging

Herb Sanderson, Director
Coney Parker, Assistant Director
Sandra Barrett, Assistant Director

The division provides services geared for adults and the elderly including supervised living, home delivered meals, adult day care, senior centers, personal care, household chores, and adult protective services.

3027 Arkansas Division of Developmental Disabilities Services
PO Box 1437
Little Rock, AR 72203
501-682-8665
FAX: 501-682-8380

Mike McCreight, Director
Charlie Green, Manager
State agency to assist persons with developmental disabilities and their family in obtaining appropriate assistance and services.

3028 Arkansas Division of Services for the Blind
Department Of Health and Human Services
700 Main Street
Little Rock, AR 72201
501-682-5463
800-960-9270
FAX: 501-682-0366
e-mail: donnabirdwell@arkansas.gov
www.state.ar.us/dhs/dsd/newdsb/index.html

James Hudson, Executive Director
Katy Morris, Assistant Director
State program which offers services in the areas of health, counseling, social work, self help and education for the visually and multihandicapped. The staff includes 4 full time and 13 part time members including mobility specialists and rehabilitation teachers.

3029 Baptist Health Rehabilitation Institute
Baptist Heath
9601 Interstate 630 Exit 7
Little Rock, AR 72205
501-202-7011
FAX: 501-202-7259
www.baptist-health.com

Doug Weeks, Senior Vice President/Administra
Greg Craine, Vice President
Russell Harrington, President
Acute rehab facility serving patients with ortho, spinal cord injury, brain injury, CVA, arthritis, cardiac and generalized weakness; JCAHO and CARF accredited; 17 outpatient therapy centers throughout central Arkansas.

3030 Children's Medical Services
PO Box 1437, Slot S-380
Little Rock, AR 72203
501-682-2277
800-482-5850
FAX: 501-682-8247

Nancy Holder, Program Director
Iris Fehr, Nursing Director

3031 Developmental Disability Council: Arkansas
5800 West 10th Street
Suite 805
Little Rock, AR 72204
501-661-2519
FAX: 501-661-2399

Wilma Stewart, Director
David Taylor, Manager

3032 President's Committee on People with Disabilities: Arkansas
7th & Main Street
Little Rock, AR 72203

3033 Social Security: Arkansas Disability Determination Services
701 S Pulaski Street
Little Rock, AR 72201
501-682-3030
800-772-1213
FAX: 501-682-7553
www.socialsecurity.gov

Arthur Boutiette, Executive Director

California

3034 California Department of Aging
1300 National Drive
Suite 200
Sacramento, CA 95834
916-324-4244
FAX: 916-327-3902
www.aging.ca.gov

Lora Connoly, Chief Deputy Director
David Supkofl, Manager

3035 California Department of Handicapped Children
714 P Street
Room 323
Sacramento, CA 95814
916-445-4171

Maridee Gregory
Diana Bonta, Chief Executive Officer

3036 California Department of Rehabilitation
830 K Street
Sacramento, CA 95814
916-324-4244
TTY:916-445-3971
e-mail: doroa.bpremo@hwl.cahwnet.gov

Brenda Premo, Director
David Supkofl, Manager
Assists people with disabilities, particularly those with severe disabilities, in obtaining and retaining meaningful employment and living independently in their communities. The department develops, purchases, provides and advocates for programs and services in vocational rehabilitation, habilitation and independent living with a priority on serving persons with all disabilities, especially those with the most severe disabilities.

3037 California Governor's Committee on Employment of People with Disabilities
800 Capitol Mall
MIC 41
Sacramento, CA 95814
916-654-8055
800-695-0350
FAX: 916-654-9821
TTY: 916-654-9820
www.disabilityemployment.org
GCEPD works to eliminate the barriers that preclude equal consideration for employment opportunities for people with disabilities. The Governor's Committee is responsible for providing leadership to increase the numbers of people with disabilities in the California workforce.

3038 California Protection & Advocacy: (PAI) A Nonprofit Organization
Protection and Advocacy (PA I)
100 Howe Avenue
Suite 235n
Sacramento, CA 95825
916-488-9950
800-776-5746
FAX: 916-488-9960
e-mail: legalmail@pai-ca.org
www.pai-ca.org

Catherine Blakemore, Executive Director
Barbara Silda, Deputy Director
Eric Gelber, Manager
Advancing the human and legal rights of people with disabilities.

3039 California State Council on Developmental Disabilities
1507 21st Street
Suite 210
Sacramento, CA 95814
916-322-8481
FAX: 916-443-4957
e-mail: council@scdd.ca.gov
www.scdd.ca.gov

Alan Kerzin, Executive Director

3040 Client Assistance Program: California
CA Health and Human Services Agency, Dept of Rehab
2000 Evergreen Street
Sacramento, CA 95815
916-263-7367
800-952-5544
TTY:866-712-1085
e-mail: capinfo@dor.ca.gov
www.dor.ca.gov

Catherine Campisi, PhD, Director

3041 International Dyslexia Association: Central California Branch
4594 E Michigan Avenue
Fresno, CA 93703
559-251-9385
800-222-3123
FAX: 599-252-1216
e-mail: dyslexias@attbi.com
www.interdys.org

Joy Moody, President
Provides free information and referral services for diagnosis and tutoring for parents, educators, physicians, and individuals with dyslexia. The voice of our membership is heard in 48 countries. Membership includes yearly journal and quarterly newsletter. Call for conference dates. Other locations also available in California.

3042 Long Beach Department of Health and Human Services
2525 Grand Avenue
Long Beach, CA 90815
562-570-4000
FAX: 562-570-4049
e-mail: info@ci.long-beach.ca.us/health
www.ci.long-beach.ca.us/health

Ronald Aries, Director
Michael Johnson, Manager

3043 Los Angeles County Department of Health Services
313 N Figueroa Street
Los Angeles, CA 90012
800-427-8700
e-mail: webmaster@adhs.org
www.ladhs.org

Bridget A Ward, Director
Jennifer Cayanan, Staff Development Specialist

3044 Social Security: California Disability Determination Services
3164 Garrity Way
Richmond, CA 94806
800-772-1213
TTY:800-325-0778
www.ssa.gov

Sally Keen, San Francisco Regional PDF Coord

3045 Social Security: Fresno Disability Determination Services
Social Security
1052 C Street
Fresno, CA 93706
559-487-5391
800-772-1213
FAX: 510-970-2947
e-mail: sally.keen@ssa.gov
www.ssa.gov

Sally Keen, Regional PDF Coordinator

3046 Social Security: Oakland Disability Determination Services
238 11th Street
Oakland, CA 94607
800-772-1213
TTY:800-325-0778
www.ssa.gov

3047 Social Security: Sacramento Disability Determination Services
8351 Folsom Boulevard
Sacramento, CA 95826
916-381-9410
800-772-1213
FAX: 916-263-5310
TTY: 916-381-9445
www.ssa.gov

3048 Social Security: San Diego Disability Determination Services
1333 Front Street
San Diego, CA 92101
800-772-1213
FAX: 619-278-4303
TTY:800-325-0778
e-mail: josesanbria@ssa.gov
www.ssa.gov

Colorado

3049 Colorado Department of Aging & Adult Servi ces
1575 Sherman Street
10th Floor
Denver, CO 80203
303-866-3851
FAX: 303-620-2696
www.cdhs.state.co.us/ADRS/AAS

Jeanette Hensley, Director
A department providing services to the elderly.

3050 Colorado Developmental Disabilities Council
3401 Quebec Street
Suite 6009
Denver, CO 80207
720-941-0176
FAX: 720-941-8490
e-mail: cdppc.email@state.co.us
www.coddc.org

Marcia Tewell, Manager
The mission is to advocate in collaboration with and on behalf of people with developmental disabilities for the establishment and implementation of public policy which will further their independence, productivity and integration.

3051 Colorado Division of Mental Health
3520 W Oxford Avenue
Denver, CO 80236
303-866-7066
FAX: 303-762-4373

George Kawamura, Director
Keith Lagrenade, Chief Executive Officer

3052 Colorado Health Care Program for Children with Special Needs
4300 Cherry Creek South Drive
Denver, CO 80246
303-861-8228
800-886-7689
FAX: 303-753-9249
www.state.cdphe.co.us

Kathy Watters, Director
Arlene Miles, President
Provides information and state aid to children with disabilities.

3053 Eastern Colorado Services for the Disabled
211 W Main Street
Sterling, CO 80751
970-842-2413
FAX: 970-522-7121

Charles W Hayes, Executive Director
Marylu Walton, Administrative Assistant
Case coordination, infant stimulation, family support, residential and vocational programs.

3054 **International Dyslexia Association: Rocky Mountain Branch**
PO Box 461010
Glendale, CO 80246
303-721-9425
800-222-3123
e-mail: info@interdys.org
www.interdys.org

Lynn Kuhn, President
Provides free information and referral services for diagnosis and tutoring for parents, educators, physicians, and individuals with dyslexia in Utah, Colorado and Wyoming. The voice of our membership is heard in 48 countries. Membership includes yearly journal and quarterly newsletter. Call for conference dates.

3055 **Legal Center for People with Disabilities & Older People**
455 Sherman Street
Suite 130
Denver, CO 80203
303-722-0300
800-288-1376
FAX: 303-722-0720
e-mail: tlcmail@thelegalcenter.org
www.thelegalcenter.org

Mary Anne Harvey, Executive Director
Mark Ivandick, Manager
Uses the legal system to protect and promote the rights of people with disabilities and older people in Colorado through direct legal representation, advocacy, education and legislative analysis. The Legal Center is Colorado's Protection and Advocacy System. We are also the State Ombudsman for nursing homes and assisted living facilities. Call for a free publications and products list.

3056 **Workers Compensation Board Colorado**
Division of Labor
1515 Arapahoe Street
14th Floor
Denver, CO 80202
303-318-8441
888-390-7936
FAX: 303-318-8710
www.coworkforce.com/dwc/

Connecticut

3057 **Connecticut Board of Education and Service for the Blind**
184 Windsor Avenue
Windsor, CT 06095
860-602-4000
FAX: 860-602-4020
TTY:860-602-4002
e-mail: besb@po.state.ct.us
www.besb.state.ct.us

Patricia Wilson, Commissioner
Alan Sylvestre, Chairman
Keith Maynard, Plant Manager
Offers rehabilitative services and information for persons with legal blindness and childrenwhonare visually impaired that are residents of Connecticut.

3058 **Connecticut Commission on Aging**
210 Capitol Avenue
509
Hartford, CT 06106
860-240-5200
FAX: 860-240-5204
e-mail: coa@cga.ct.gov
www.cga.ct.gov/coa

Julie Evans Starr, Executive Director
Robert J Norton, Communications Director
Advocates on beha;f of elderly persons in Connecticut by regularly monitoring their status, assessing the impact of current and propsed initiatives, and conducting activities which promote the interests of these individuals and report to the Governor and the Legislature.

3059 **Connecticut Department of Children and Youth Services**
505 Hudson Street
Hartford, CT 06106
860-247-2732
FAX: 860-566-7947

Linda D Amario Rossi, Commissioner
Bruce Douglas, Executive Director

3060 **Connecticut Developmental Disabilities Council**
460 Capitol Avenue
Hartford, CT 06106
860-418-6160
800-653-1134
FAX: 860-418-6003
TTY: 860-418-6172
www.state.ct.us/ctcdd/

Edward T Preneta, Executive Director

3061 **Connecticut Office of Protection and Advocacy for Persons with Disabilities**
60 Weston Street
Suite B
Hartford, CT 06120
860-297-4300
800-842-7303
FAX: 860-566-8714
TTY: 860-566-2102
e-mail: OPA-Information@po.state.ct.us
www.ct.gov/opapd

James McGaughey, Executive Director
Gretchen Knaff, Assistant Director
Linda Mizzi, CI Director
Seeks to protect the rights of and to advocate for people with disabilities. The Consumer Information Section provides information, referral services and short-term advocacy assistance. The Case Services unit staff advocates for individuals who have been discriminated against based on disability or who have been denied needed services to which they are entitled to under state or federal law. Offers training & technical assistance to individuals and groups to promote self-advocacy.

3062 **Social Security: Hartford Area Office**
960 Main Street
2nd Floor
Hartford, CT 06103
860-493-1857
800-772-1213
FAX: 860-566-1795
TTY: 860-525-4967
www.ssa.gov

Jan Gilbert, Professional Relations Coord.

Delaware

3063 **Delaware Assistive Technology Initiative Center for Applied Science & Engineering**
Univ. of DE/Alfred I duPont Hospital for Children
1600 Rockland Road
PO Box 269
Wilmington, DE 19899
302-651-6790
800-870-3284
FAX: 302-651-6793
TTY: 302-651-6794
e-mail: dati@asel.udel.edu
www.dati.org

Beth Mineo-Mollica, Project Director
The Delaware Assistive Technology Initiative (DATI) connects Delawareans who have disabilities with the tools they need in order to learn, work, play and participate in community life safely and independently. The Delaware Assistive Technology Initiative's (DATI) endeavors to improve access to assistive technology for all Delawareans with disabilities.

3064 **Delaware Client Assistance Program**
United Cerebral Palsy Association
254 E Camden Wyoming Avenue
Camden, DE 19934
302-698-9336
800-640-9336
FAX: 302-698-9338
e-mail: capdir@magpage.com

Melissa Shahan, Executive Director
Provides advocacy services for persons involved with programs covered under the Rehabilitation Act of 1973 as amended, information and referrals on ADA, Title I.

3065 **Delaware Department of Health and Social Services**
Administration Building D HS S Campus
1901 N Dupont Highway
New Castle, DE 19720
302-577-4500
800-464-HELP
FAX: 302-577-4510
e-mail: dhssinfo@state.de.us
www.dhss.delaware.gov/dhss

Vincent Meconi, Secretary

3066 **Delaware Department of Public Instructing**
PO Box 1402
Dover, DE 19903
302-739-4686
800-433-5292
FAX: 302-739-3092

Dr. Pascal D Forgione Jr, Superintendent
A publicly funded, state agency that gives information about local facilities and administers supplemental funds for visually handicapped students in local schools. It also maintains special teachers of sight conservation and braille programs for both children and adults.

3067 **Delaware Developmental Disability Council**
410 Federal Street
Suite 2
Dover, DE 19901
302-739-3613
FAX: 302-739-2015
e-mail: arose@state.de.us

Christine O'Connor, Executive Director
Alexander Rose, Director of Social Services
Patricia Maichle, Manager

3068 **Delaware Division for the Visually Impaired**
1901 N Du Pont Highway
New Castle, DE 19720
302-577-4730
FAX: 302-255-4441
e-mail: dhssinfo@state.de.us
www.state.de.us

Debra Wallace, Executive Director
Ken Sutton, Program Spec/Staff Dev Officer
State agency serving the visually impaired persons from birth, with or without other handicaps. Services offered include educational, computer training, employment and pre-vocational training.

3069 **Delaware Industries for the Blind**
1901 N Dupont Highway
New Castle, DE 19720
302-255-9855
FAX: 302-255-4442
e-mail: awingrove@state.de.us
www.promoplace.com/dib

Alan B Wingrove, General Manager
Provides jobs for blind and visually impaired via sales of products and services.

3070 **Delaware Protection & Advocacy for Persons with Disabilities**
Arc of Delaware
144 E Market Street
Georgetown, DE 19947
302-856-6019
FAX: 302-856-6133
e-mail: challdover@aol.com

Becky Allen, Executive Director

3071 **Delaware Workers Compensation Board**
Industrial Accident Board de dept
4425 N Market Street
Wilmington, DE 19802
302-761-8200
www.delawareworks.com

James Cagle, Manager

3072 **Social Security: Wilmington Disability Determination**
U S Department of Health and Human Services
321 N Front Street
Wilmington, NC 28401
910-254-3456
800-453-9851
FAX: 910-254-3444
www.socialsecurity.gov

Allen J Murphy, Founder
Vickie O'Brien, Manager

District of Columbia

3073 **District of Columbia Department of Handicapped Children**
D C General Hospital
1900 Massachusetts Avenue SE
Building 10
Washington, DC 20003
202-675-5000
FAX: 202-675-7694

Jacqueline Mcmorris, Acting Chief
Nayab Ali, MD

3074 **District of Columbia Office on Aging**
441 4th Street NW
9th Floor
Washington, DC 20001
202-504-3400
FAX: 202-724-4979

Francis Smith, Executive Director
Serves the District of Columbia residents 60 years of age and older. Contact the Information and Assistance Unit for more information about innovative programs and services offered by the Office.

3075 **Information, Protection & Advocacy for Persons with Disabilities**
IPACHI
4455 Connecticut Avenue NW
Suite B
Washington, DC 20008
FAX: 202-966-6313

Vivianne Hardy-Townes, Executive Director
Ronald Tyson, Information/Referral
Offers services and support for persons with disabilities in the Washington, DC area.

3076 **Information, Protection and Advocacy Center for Handicapped Individuals**
4455 Connecticut Avenue NW
Suite B100
Washington, DC 20008
202-659-0215
FAX: 202-966-6313

Vivianne Hardy-Townes, Executive Director
Darell Hammond, Owner
Serves all persons with disabilities in the DC, Maryland and Virginia areas offering them legal representation and advocacy, information and referrals and several publications.

3077 **International Dyslexia Association of DC**
5914 Reservoir Heights Avenue
Alexandria, VA 22311
703-827-9019
800-222-3123
e-mail: info@interdys.org
www.interdys.org

Ruth R Tifford LCSW, President

The DC Capital Area Branch, provides support for individuals with dyslexia and their families in the Washington, DC metropolitan area, including parts of Maryland, Virginia and West Virginia. Our conferences, book sales and online information resources are designed to further the understanding of dyslexia and encourage the use of systematic, multisensory teaching methods enabling children and adults to reach their educational potential.

3078 Wage and Hour Division of the Employment Standards Administration
US Department of Labor
200 Constitution Avenue NW
Washington, DC 20210
202-693-5000
FAX: 202-693-1406
www.dol.gov

Elaine Chao, Chief Executive Officer
Administers regulations governing the employment of individuals with disabilities in sheltered workshops and the disabled workers industries.

3079 Washington Hearing and Speech Society
1934 Calvert Street NW
Washington, DC 20009
202-537-4010
e-mail: support@dcsha.org

Judyth Tinsley
Dianne Carthy, Manager
Offers individuals with hearing or speech impairments, in the DC area, speech, reading classes, audiological services and new aids.

3080 Well Mind Association of Greater Washington
18606 New Hampshire Avenue
Ashton, MD 20861
301-774-6617
FAX: 301-946-1402
Holistic mental health information and publications, public lectures in the Washington D.C. area, and nationwide referrals.

3081 Workers Compensation Board: District of Columbia
1200 Upshur Street NW
Washington, DC 20011

Florida

3082 ARC Gateway
3932 N 10th Avenue
Pensacola, FL 32503
850-434-2638
FAX: 850-438-2180
e-mail: aresc@aol.com
www.arc-gateway.org

Donna Fassett, Executive Director
To secure for all people with developmental disabilities the opportunity to choose and realize their goals of where and how they learn, live, work and play. ARC Gateway is committed to increasing the opportunities for all persons with, or at risk of, development disabilities the opportunity to choose where, how and with whom they live, learn, work and play.

3083 Advocacy Center for Persons with Disabilities
2671 W Executive Center Circle
Suite 100
Tallahassee, FL 32301
850-488-9071
800-342-0823
FAX: 850-488-8640
e-mail: info@advocacy.org
www.advocacycenter.org

Gary Weston, Executive Director
Hubert Grisson, President

3084 Assistive Technology Educational Network of Florida
1207 S Mellonville Avenue
Sanford, FL 32771
800-328-3678
FAX: 407-688-4593
e-mail: diane_penn@scps.k12.fl.us
www.aten.scps.k12.fl.us

Dee Wright, Executive Secretary
Diane Penn, MA, Technology Specialist
Provides state-wide information, awareness and training for students, family members, teachers and other professionals in the area of assisted technology; a quarterly newsletter and a network of specialists (Local Assistive Technology Specialists) trained by ATEN to provide support at the district level.

3085 Bureau of Education for Exceptional Children
Turlington Building
Tallahassee, FL 32399
850-245-0477
FAX: 850-245-0987

Shan Goff, Bureau Chief
Provides consultative services for the establishment and operation of school programs for visually impaired students. Provides assistance for in-service teacher training through state or regional workshops or technical assistance to individual programs.

3086 Department of Health & Rehabilitative Services
1317 Winewood Boulevard
Tallahassee, FL 32399
850-488-8304
FAX: 850-921-5830

Roderick Hall, Director
Beth Carter, Administrative Assistant
John Bryant, Manager
Offers counseling and referrals on rehabilitation facilities.

3087 Division of Workers Compensation
2012 Capital Circle SE
Tallahassee, FL 32399
850-413-1600
800-342-1741
FAX: 850-922-6779
www.fldfs.com

Tanner Hollaman, Manager

3088 Florida Adult Services
1317 Winewood Boulevard
Tallahassee, FL 32399
850-488-8922
FAX: 850-922-4193
www.myglorida.com/adultservices

Chris Schummacher, Director
Nancy Fulton, Executive Director

3089 Florida Department of Handicapped Children
4030 Esplanade Way
Suite 380
Tallahassee, FL 32399
850-488-8304
FAX: 850-488-3813
www.apd.myflorida.com

Shelly Branetley, Director
John Bryant, Manager

3090 Florida Department of Mental Health and Rehabilitative Services
1317 Winewood Boulevard
Tallahassee, FL 32399
850-488-8304
FAX: 850-487-2239

Rod Hall, Executive Director
John Bryant, Manager

3091 Florida Developmental Disabilities Council
124 Marriott Drive
Suite 203
Tallahassee, FL 32301
850-488-4180
800-580-7801
FAX: 850-922-6702
e-mail: admin@fddc.org
www.fddc.org

Debra Dowds, Executive Director

3092 Florida Division of Vocational Rehabilitation
2002 Old Saint Augustine Road
Building A
Tallahassee, FL 32301
850-488-6210
800-451-4327
FAX: 850-921-7215
TTY: 850-488-2867
e-mail: costin@vr.doe.state.fl.us

Bill Palmer, Director
Linda Parnell, Manager
State agency serving individuals with physical or mental disabilities that interfere with them keeping or maintaining employment.

3093 Florida's Protection and Advocacy Programs for Persons with Disabilities
2671 Executive Center Circle W
Suite 100
Tallahassee, FL 32301
850-488-9071
800-342-0823
FAX: 850-488-8640
TTY: 800-346-4127
www.advocacycenter.org
The Center is a non-profit organization providing protection and advocacy services in the State of Florida. The Center's mission is to advance the dignity, equality, self-determination and expressed choices of individuals with disabilities.

3094 International Dyslexia Association: Florida Branch
5005 W Laurel Street
Suite 100
Tampa, FL 33607
305-252-3474
800-222-3123
e-mail: jewasc@aol.com
www.interdys.org

Jean Schmidt, President
The Florida Branch is a non-p;rofit, scientific, educational organization committed to the study, prevention and treatment of language-based learning disabilities (dyslexia) for those in Florida and Puerto Rico. It is specifically concerned with the many children and adults with average or superior intelligence who experience difficulty in learning skills such as speaking, reading, writing, spelling and math.

3095 Social Security Administration
2002 Old Saint Augustine Road
Suite B12
Tallahassee, FL 32301
850-224-9337
800-772-1213
FAX: 850-942-8980
www.socialsecurity.gov

Carrie Tucker, Operations Supervisor
Sheila Lee, Management Support Specialist
Administers the Title II and Title XVII disability programs. To be insured for Title II benefits, applicants must have worked in covered employment for at least five of the last ten years prior to becoming disabled. To be eligible for Title XVII disability benefits, applicants must meet an income and resource test.

3096 Social Security: Miami Disability Determination
Social Security
11401 W Flagler Street
Miami, FL 33174
800-772-1213
FAX: 800-325-0778
www.ssa.gov

Robert L Meekins, Deputy General for Executive Ope

3097 Social Security: Orlando Disability Determination
Social Security
80 N Hughey Avenue
Federal Building, Room 159
Orlando, FL 32801
407-648-6673
800-342-2065
TTY:407-245-7057
www.ssa.gov

John C Massolio Jr, Founder
Neil Bush, President

3098 Social Security: Tampa Disability Determination
Social Security Administration
PO Box 340572
Tampa, FL 33694
813-878-2906
800-772-1213
e-mail: info@dbstampabay.org
www.dbsatampabay.org

Neil Bush, President
John C Massolio Jr, Founder

Georgia

3099 ADA Technical Assistance Program
Southeast Disability & Business Technical Assist.
490 10th Street NW
Atlanta, GA 30318
404-385-0636
800-949-4232
FAX: 404-385-0641
e-mail: sedbtacproject@law.sgr.edu
www.sedbtac.org

Amy Oliveras, Administrative Assistant
Shelley Kaplan, Director
Pam Williamson, Assistant Director
One of ten regional centers funded by NIDRR, to provide information and technical assistance to assist in voluntary compliance with the Americans with Disabilities Act, and accessible education-based information technology.

3100 Division of Birth Defects and Developmental Disabilities

12 Executive Park Drive NE
Atlanta, GA 30329
404-498-3800

3101 Georgia Advocacy Office
150 E Ponce De Leon Avenue
Suite 430
Decatur, GA 30030
404-885-1234
800-537-2329
FAX: 770-414-2948
e-mail: info@thegao.org
www.thegao.org

Ruby Moore, Executive Director
Protection and advocacy services for Georgians with disabilities.

3102 Georgia Client Assistance Program
Division of Rehabilitation Services
2 Peachtree Street NW
Room 23-307
Atlanta, GA 30303
404-605-1986
800-822-9727

Gail Greene, Executive Director
Helps eligible persons with complaints, appeals and understanding available benefits under the 1992 Rehabilitation Act Amendments and Title I of the Americans with Disabilities Act. CAP investigates complaints, mediates conflict, represents complainants in appeals, provides legal services if warranted, advocates for due process, identifies and recommends solutions to system problems, advises of benefits available under the 1992 Rehab Act Amendments and Americans with Disabilities Act.

3103 **Georgia Department of Aging**
878 Peachtree Street NE
Apt 318
Atlanta, GA 30309
404-656-4374
FAX: 404-730-7950

Fred McGinnis, Director
Andrea Fuller-Ruffin, Administrator

3104 **Georgia Department of Handicapped Children**
2600 Skyland Drive NE
Atlanta, GA 30319
770-980-5100

Linnette Jackson-Hunt, Manager
Frank Koues, Auditor

3105 **Georgia Division of Mental Health, Developmental Disabilities & Addictive Diseases**
2 Peachtree Street NW
22nd Floor
Atlanta, GA 30303
404-463-8037
FAX: 404-657-2310
e-mail: srhall1@dhr.ga.gov
mhddad.dhr.georgia.gov

Stephen Hall, Director, Office of DD
MHDDAD provides treatment and support services to people with mental illnesses and addictive diseases, and support to people with mental retardation and related developmental disabilities. MHDDAD serves people of all ages with the most severe and likely to be long-term conditions.

3106 **Georgia State Board of Workers' Compensation**
270 Peachtree Street NW
Atlanta, GA 30303
404-656-3875
800-533-0682
FAX: 404-657-1767
www.ganet.org/sbwc

Ron Simpson, Executive Director

3107 **Governor's Council on Developmental Disabilities**
Govenors Coucil on Development Disabilities
2 Peachtree Street NW
Atlanta, GA 30303
404-657-2126
888-275-4233
888-275-4233
FAX: 404-657-2132
TTY:404-657-3000
e-mail: eejacobson@dhr.state.ga.us
www.gcdd.org

Eric E Jacobson, Executive Director
Daniel Doughman, Program Director
Yao Seidu, Public Information Officer
Advocacy and support organization focusd on improving the lives of people with disabilities and their families.
Quartlery

3108 **International Dyslexia Association: Georgia Branch**
1951 Greystone Road NW
Atlanta, GA 30318
404-256-1232
800-222-3123
e-mail: jennifer@syllablesreadingcenter.com
www.interdys.org

Jennifer Hasser, President
The Georgi Branch was formed to increase public awareness about dyslexia in the State of Georgia. In addition, the Branch encourages teachers to train in multisensory language instruction. The Branch also provides a network for individuals with dyslexia, their families and professionals in the educational and medical fields.

3109 **Social Security: Atlanta Disability Determination**
401 W Peachtree Street
Suite 2860
Atlanta, GA 30308
800-772-1213
TTY:800-325-0778
www.socialsecurity.gov

3110 **Social Security: Decatur Disability Determination**
2853 Candler Road
Suite 8
Decatur, GA 30034
800-772-1213
TTY:800-325-0778
www.socialsecurity.gov

Hawaii

3111 **Assistive Technology Resource Centers of Hawaii**
414 Kuwili Street
Suite 104
Honolulu, HI 96817
800-532-7110
800-645-3007
FAX: 808-532-7120
e-mail: atrc-info@atrc.org
www.atrc.org

Barbara Fischlowitz-Leong, Executive Director
Provides information and referral to anyone interested in assistive technology devices and services. Operates equipment loan. Provides training to consumer and professional groups including self-advocacy skills for consumers and family members. Works to ensure that schools, vocational rehabilitation agencies and health insurers provide assessments, funding and training in the use of assistive technology devices and services for their clients. Low-interest loan programs available.

3112 **Diabetes Network of East Hawaii**
1221 Kilauea Avenue
Suite 70
Hilo, HI 96720
808-935-8658

Martha Ahyee, Executive Director

3113 **Disability and Communication Access Board**
919 Ala Moana Boulevard
Suite 101
Honolulu, HI 96814
808-586-8121
FAX: 808-586-8129
e-mail: dcab@doh.hawaii.gov
www.hawaii.gov/health/dcab

Francine Wai, Executive Director
Charlotte Townsend, Coordinator,Programs/Policy Dev.
Judy Paik, Program Specialist
Clearinghouse of information related to disability issues, lead agency in the community for dissemination of ADA information, systems advocacy provided through the introduction and lobbying of bills at the state legislation, review of blueprints for state and county renovation and new construction to make recommendations for physical accessibility; establishment of guidelines for communication access, including sign language interpreters and conducts state test to credential interpreters.

3114 **Hawaii Assistive Technology Training and**
414 Kuwili Street
Suite 104
Honolulu, HI 96817
808-532-7110

Barbara Fischlowitz'le, Executive Director

3115 **Hawaii Department for Children With Special Needs**
Department of Health
741a Sunset Avenue
Honolulu, HI 96816
808-733-9030
FAX: 808-733-8355
www.state.hi.us/doh/resource/family

Dr Patricia Hue, Chief Medical Officer
Karen Mak, Manager

3116 Hawaii Department of Health, Adult Mental Health Division
PO Box 3378
Honolulu, HI 96801
808-941-3894
FAX: 808-586-4745
www.amhd.org

Thomas W Hester MD, Chief

3117 Hawaii Department of Human Services
Hawaii Department of Human Serv
1901 Bachelot Street
Honolulu, HI 96817
808-941-3894
FAX: 808-586-4143
www.hoopono.com

Linda Lingel, Governor
Lillian Koller, Director
Provides services to blind and visually impaired persons in adjustment to blindness, vocational rehabilitation, low vision evaluation and assistance. Work Evaluation, operates Work Activities Center, Vending training and the Ho'opono Workshop, a sheltered workshop program for the blind and visually impaired persons.

3118 Hawaii Disability Compensation Division Department Labor and Industrial Relations
830 Punchbowl Street
Room 211
Honolulu, HI 96813
808-586-9161
FAX: 808-586-9219
hawaii.gov/labor

Gary Hamada, Administrator
Clyde Imada, Workers Comp Chief
Administers Hawaii's Workers' Compensation Program.

3119 Hawaii Disability Rights Center
900 Fort Street Mall
Suite 1040
Honolulu, HI 96813
808-949-2922
800-882-1052
FAX: 808-949-2928
e-mail: info@hawaiidisabilityrights.org
www.hawaiidisabilityrights.org

Henry Smith, President
Ann Collins, Vice President

3120 Hawaii Executive Office on Aging
250 S Hotel Street
Suite 406
Honolulu, HI 96813
808-586-0100
800-468-4644
FAX: 808-586-0185
e-mail: eoa@mail.health.state.hi.us
www2.hawaii.gov/eoa

Pat Sasaki, Executive Director
State unit on aging responsible for policy formulation, program development, planning, information dissemination, advocacy and other activities, for persons age 60 and over.

3121 Hawaii State Council on Developmental Disabilities
919 Ala Moana Boulevard
Honolulu, HI 96814
808-586-8100
FAX: 808-586-7543
e-mail: council@hiddc.org
www.hiddc.org

Waynette K Y Cabral, Executive Administrator
The mission of the council is to support people with developmental disabilities to control their own destiny and determine the quality of life they desire.

3122 International Dyslexia Association: Hawaii Branch
PO Box 61610
Honolulu, HI 96839
808-538-7007
FAX: 808-566-6837
e-mail: hida@dyslexia-hawaii.org
www.dyslexia-hawaii.org

Sue Voit, Co-president
Margaret Higa, Manager
Provides free information and referral services for diagnosis and tutoring for parents, educators, physicians, and individuals with dyslexia. The voice of our membership is heard in 48 countries. Membership includes yearly journal and quarterly newsletter. Call for conference dates.

3123 Social Security: Honolulu Disability Determination
Social Security
300 Ala Moana Boulevard
Honolulu, HI 96850
808-541-3600
800-772-1213
FAX: 800-825-0778
e-mail: hivrsbd@kestrok.com
www.ssa.gov

Neil Shim, Administrator

3124 State Planning Council on Developmental Disabilities
919 Ala Moana Boulevard
Suite 113
Honolulu, HI 96814
808-586-8121
FAX: 808-586-8129
e-mail: tiza100w@wonder.cm.cdc.gov

Francine Wai, Executive Director
Consists of 25 Hawaii residents appointed by the governor. The council addresses the needs of the people with developmental disabilities: specifically, develops a state plan that sets the priorities for persons with developmental disabilities.

Idaho

3125 Idaho Commission on Aging
3380 Americana Ter
Suite 120
Boise, ID 83720
208-334-3833
877-471-2777
FAX: 208-334-3033
www.idahoaging.com

Lois S Bauer, Administrator
Gioia M Frahm, Planner/Statistician
Cathy Hart, State Ombudsman

3126 Idaho Council on Developmental Disabilities
Health and Wellfare
802 W Bannock Street
Suite 308
Boise, ID 83702
208-334-6800
800-544-2433
FAX: 208-334-3417
e-mail: icdd@icdd.state.id.us
www.state.id.us/icdd

Marilyn B Sword, Executive Director

3127 Idaho Department of Handicapped Children
Statehouse
Boise, ID 83720
208-334-8000

Thomas Bruck, Chief
Sandy Frazier, Manager

3128 Idaho Disability Determinations Service
PO Box 21
Boise, ID 83707
208-327-7333
800-626-2681
FAX: 208-373-7287
www.accessidaho.org

Barbara Bauer, Director
Rogelio Valdez, Executive Director
Under contract with the Social Security Administration, makes determinations of medical eligibility for disability benefits.

3129 **Idaho Industrial Commission**
PO Box 83720
Boise, ID 83720
208-334-6000
800-950-2110
FAX: 208-334-2321
www.state.id.us

Mindy Montgomery, Director
Nancy Bedson, Administrative Assistant
Free rehabilitation services to workers' who have suffered on the job injuries in Idaho. Field offices throughout the state.

3130 **Idaho Mental Health Center**
1720 Westgate Drive
Boise, ID 83704
208-334-0800
FAX: 208-334-0828

Dr. Gary Payne, Director
Pat Fitzpatrick, Manager

Illinois

3131 **Attorney General's Office: Disability Rights Bureau & Health Care Bureau**
100 W Randolph Street
Chicago, IL 60601
312-814-3000
FAX: 312-814-3212
www.illinoisattorneygeneral.gov

Lisa Madigan, Manager
Raymond Throlkeld, Chief Health Care Bureau
Information on Illinois' Comprehensive Health Insurance Plan and architectural accessibility. Enforcement of Illinois' access law and standards and other disability rights laws. Information on initiatives such as: Opening the Courthouse Doors to People with Disabilities; the abuse, neglect or financial exploitation of people with disabilities and voter accessibility. Other information and referrals.

3132 **Client Assistance Program (CAP)**
Illinois State Board of Education
100 N 1st Street
1st Floor
Springfield, IL 62777
866-262-6663
800-641-3929
FAX: 217-524-1790
TTY: 217-782-1900
www.isbe.state.il.us/

Brenda J Holmes, Interim State Superintendent

3133 **Equip for Equality**
20 N Michigan Avenue
Suite 300
Chicago, IL 60602
312-341-0022
800-537-2632
FAX: 312-341-0295
TTY: 800-610-2779
e-mail: contactus@equipforequality.org
www.equipforequality.org

Zena Naiditch, President/CEO
Barry C Taylor, Legal Advocacy Director
The mission of Equip for Equality is to advance the human and civil rights of children and adults with physical and mental disabilities in Illinois. It is the only statewide, cross-disability, comprehensive advocacy organization providing self-advocacy assistance, legal services, and disability rights education while also engaging in public policy and legislative advocacy and conducting abuse investigations and other oversight activities.

3134 **Illinois Assistive Technology Project**
1 W Old State Capitol Plaza
Springfield, IL 62701
217-522-7985
800-852-5110
FAX: 217-522-8067
TTY: 217-522-9966
e-mail: iatp@iltech.org
www.iltech.org

Wilhelmina Gunther, Executive Director
Sue Castles, Info/Assistance Funding Advoc.
Directed by and for people with disabilities and their family members. As a federally mandated program, IATP strives to break down barriers and change policies that make getting and using technology difficult. IATP offers solutions to help people find what is available in products and services that will best meet their needs, where to find it, and how to get it.

3135 **Illinois Council on Developmental Disability**
State of Illinois Center
100 W Randolph Street
Chicago, IL 60601
312-814-2700
800-843-6154
FAX: 312-814-7441
e-mail: drs@dhs.state.il.us
www.dhs.state.il.us/ors

Robert Kilbury, Executive Director
Dennis Sienko, Manager

3136 **Illinois Department of Mental Health and Developmental Disabilities**
314 E Madison
Suite 3b
Springfield, IL 62701
217-782-2000
FAX: 217-785-3066

Carol Adams Phd, Secretary
Lori Stone, Director

3137 **Illinois Department of Rehabilitation**
622 E Washington Street
Springfield, IL 62701
217-782-7820
FAX: 217-557-0142

Susan Suter, Director
Timothy Martin, Manager

3138 **Illinois Department on Aging**
421 E Capitol Avenue
Suite 100
Springfield, IL 62701
217-785-2870
800-252-8966
FAX: 217-785-4477
e-mail: ilsenior@age084r1.state.il.us
www.state.il.us/aging

Charles D Johnson, Executive Director
Nikki Smith, Communications Director

3139 **International Dyslexia Association: Illinois Branch**
751 Roosevelt Road
Building 7
Glen Ellyn, IL 60137
630-469-6900
800-222-3123
FAX: 808-538-7007
e-mail: slonghall@aol.com
www.interdys.org

Susan Hall, President
Maria Leibold, Executive Director
Gail Oliphant, Manager
Provides free information and referral services for diagnosis and tutoring for parents, educators, physicians, and individuals with dyslexia in Illinois and Missouri. The voice of our membership is heard in 48 countries. Membership includes yearly journal and quarterly newsletter. Call for conference dates.

3140 **Social Security: Springfield Disability Determination**
2715 W Monroe Street
Springfield, IL 62704
217-862-6651
800-772-1213
TTY:217-862-6681
www.ssa.gov

3141 **Workers Compensation Board Illinois**
100 W Randolph Street
Suite 8-200
Chicago, IL 60601
FAX: 312-814-6523

John Hallock Jr, Director

Indiana

3142 Indiana Client Assistance Program
850 N Meridian Street
Suite 2c
Indianapolis, IN 46204 317-888-8366
800-622-4845

Richard Gordon, Owner

3143 Indiana Developmental Disability Council
143 W Market Street
Suite 404
Indianapolis, IN 46204 317-231-7100

Dan Parker, Executive Director

3144 Indiana Protection & Advocacy Services
4701 N Keystone Avenue
Suite 222
Indianapolis, IN 46205 317-722-5555
800-622-4845
FAX: 317-722-5564
e-mail: info@ipas.in.gov
www.in.gov/ipas

Thomas Gallagher, Executive Director
Milo Gray, Client & Legal Services Director
Gary Richter, Support Services Director
An independent state agency established to protect and promote the rights of individuals with disabilities through empowerment and advocacy.

3145 Indiana State Commission for the Handicapped
PO Box 1964
Indianapolis, IN 46206 317-233-1292

3146 International Dyslexia Association: Indiana Branch
2511 E 46th Street
Suite O2
Indianapolis, IN 46205 317-926-1450
800-222-3123
FAX: 317-705-2067
e-mail: inbofida@hotmail.com
www.inbofida.org

Mary Ian McAtter, President
The Indiana Branch was formed to help the members of the learning disabilities community in Indiana. Promotes understanding and facilitate treatment of the Specific Language Disability (Dyslexia) in children and adults, promotes teacher training and educational intervention strategies for dyslexic students and to foster effective teaching, supports research in the field and early identification of dyslexia, serves as a clearinghouse for information and to actively disseminate knowledge.

Iowa

3147 Governor's Developmental Disability Council
617 E 2nd Street
Des Moines, IA 50309 515-281-9082
800-452-1936
FAX: 515-281-9087
e-mail: jshoema@dhs.state.ia.us
www.state.ia.us/ddcouncil

Becky Maddy Harker, Executive Director
Rik Shannon, Public Policy Manager
Janet Shoeman, Program Planner/Contract Manager
The Council identifies, develops and promotes public policy and support practices through capacity building, advocacy, and systems change activities. The purpose is to ensure that people with developmental disabilities and their families are included in planning, decision making, and development of policy related to services and supports that affect their quality of life and full participation in communities of their choice.

3148 International Dyslexia Association: Iowa Branch
PO Box 11188
Cedar Rapids, IA 52410 319-551-2851
800-222-3123
e-mail: info@interdys.org
www.interdys.org

Terri Peterson, President
The purpose of the Iowa Branch of IDA (IDA-IA) is to increase awareness of dyslexia and promote services that address the importance of diagnosis and remediation for those not meeting their reading potential. Our goal is to provide services and assistance in a way that promotes unity, support, and cooperation among those who work with these individuals so that all communities in Iowa benefit from the skills and talents of its citizens.

3149 Iowa Child Health Specialty Clinics
100 Hawkins Drive
Room 247
Iowa City, IA 52242 319-356-1469
866-219-9119
FAX: 319-356-3715
www.uihealthcare.com/chsc

Jeffrey Lobas, Director
Brian Wilkes, Director Of Operations
Child Health Specialty Clinics has a mission to improve the health, development, and well-being of Iowa's children and youth with special health care needs in partnership with families, service providers, and communities.

3150 Iowa Commission of Persons with Disabilities
Department of Human Rights
321 E 12th Street
Des Moines, IA 50319 515-242-6171
888-219-0471
FAX: 515-242-6119
e-mail: dhr.disabilities@dhr.state.ia.us
www.state.ia.us/dhr/pd

Jill Abery, Administrator

3151 Iowa Compass
Center for Disabilities and Development
100 Hawkins Drive
Iowa City, IA 52242 319-353-6900
877-686-0032
FAX: 319-356-1343
TTY: 877-686-0032
e-mail: iowacompass@uiowa.edu
www.medicine.uiowa.edu/cdd

Jane Gay, Project Director
David Sorton, President
Mark Moser, Administrator
A statewide program provides free information and referral about disability related services and resources: advocacy, assistive technology, community services, early intervention, education, financial support, healthcare, legal aid, residential services and transportation.
BiMonthly

3152 Iowa Department for the Blind
524 4th Street
Des Moines, IA 50309 515-281-1333
800-362-2587
FAX: 515-281-1263
TTY: 515-281-1355
e-mail: harrisallen@blind.state.ia.us
www.blind.state.ia.us

Allen C Harris, Executive Director
Mission is to be the means for persons who are blind to obtain univeral access and full participation as citizens in whatever roles they may choose.

3153 **Iowa Department of Elder Affairs**
510 E 12th Street
Room 2
Des Moines, IA 50319
515-725-3333
800-532-3213
FAX: 515-725-3300
www.state.ia.us/elderaffairs

Mark Haverland, Executive Director
Sherry James, Executive Secretary

3154 **Iowa Department of Human Services**
1305 E Walnut Street
Des Moines, IA 50319
515-281-3974
800-972-2017
FAX: 515-242-6036
e-mail: joverla@dhs.state.ia.us
www.dhs.state.ia.us

Jim Overland, Bureau Chief

3155 **Iowa Protection & Advocacy for the Disabled**
950 Office Park Road
Suite 221w
W Des Moines, IA 50265
515-278-2502
800-779-2502
FAX: 515-278-0539
e-mail: info@ipna.org
www.ipna.org

Sylvia Piper, Executive Director

3156 **Social Security: Des Moines Disability Determination**
Social Security Administration
210 Walnut Street
Federal Building, Room 293
Des Moines, IA 50309
800-532-1223
TTY:515-281-1333
www.ssa.gov

Karen Brown, President

3157 **Workers Compensation Board Iowa**
1000 E Grand Avenue
Des Moines, IA 50319
515-281-5387

Kansas

3158 **Beach Center on Families and Disability**
University of Kansas
1200 Sunnyside Avenue
Lawrence, KS 66045
785-864-2700
FAX: 785-864-7605
e-mail: beachcenter@ku.edu
www.beachcenter.org

HR Turnbull, Director
Ann Turnbull, Co-Director
Robert Hemenway, Chief Executive Officer
A federally funded center that conducts research and training in the factors that contribute to the successful functioning of families with members who have disabilities.

3159 **International Dyslexia Association: Kansas/West Missouri Branch**
430 E Blue Ridge Boulevard
Kansas City, MO 64145
816-838-7323
www.interdys.org

Billie Calvery, President
Arden Murilo, VP
IDA members in Kansas and Missouri work to establish and maintain a presence for IDA with parents, schools, and teachers in order to help individuals with dyslexia. We maintain a list of individuals in Kansas and Missouri who have specialized training and who are available for diagnosis and remediation of reading, writing, and spelling problems, information for parents, information for teachers, an annual spring conference, newsletter dealing with state and local issues.

3160 **Kansas Advocacy and Protective Services**
3745 SW Wanamaker Road
Topeka, KS 66610
785-273-9661
877-776-1541
FAX: 785-776-5783
e-mail: michelle@ksadv.org
www.ksadv.org

Rocky Nichols, Executive Director
Tim Voth, Attorney
Michelle Rola, Director Operations
Protection and advocacy for persons with disabilities.

3161 **Kansas Client Assistance Program**
300 SW Oakley Avenue
Topeka, KS 66606
785-296-4454

3162 **Kansas Commission on Disability Concerns**
1430 SW Topeka Boulevard
Topeka, KS 66612
785-296-1722
800-295-5232
FAX: 785-296-0466
www.kcdcinfo.com

Martha Gabehart, Executive Director
Randy Fisher, Employment/Training Liaison
Kerrie Bacon, Legislative Liasion
KCDC believes that all people with disabilities are entitled to be equal citizens and partners in Kansas society. The purpose is to involve all segments of the Kansas Community through legislative advocacy, education and resource networking to ensure full and equal citizenship for all Kansans with disabilities.

3163 **Kansas Department on Aging**
503 S Kansas Avenue
Topeka, KS 66603
785-296-4986
800-432-3535
FAX: 785-296-0256
e-mail: wwwmail@aging.state.ks.us
www.agingKansas.org

Wilda Davison, Information And Referral
Barbara Conant, Public Information Officer
Services and information for Kansas seniors.

3164 **Kansas Developmental Disability Council**
Disability Rights Center of Kansas
635 SW Harrison Street
Suite 100
Topeka, KS 66603
785-273-9661
877-776-1541
TTY:877-335-3725
e-mail: info@drckansas.org
srskansas.org/rehab/text/CAP.html
To protect children and promote adult self-sufficiency.

Kentucky

3165 **Kentucky Council on Developmental Disability**
100 Fair Oakes Lane
Suite 4E-F
Frankfort, KY 40601
877-367-5332
FAX: 502-564-9826
e-mail: shelley.runkle@ky.gov
www.kcdd.ky.gov

Pat Seybold, Executive Director
Implementation of Developmental Disabilities Planning Council responsible under P.L. 101-496.

3166 **Kentucky Department for Mental Health and Mental Retardation Services**
100 Fair Oaks Lane
Suite 4E-B
Frankfort, KY 40621
502-564-4527
FAX: 502-564-5478
www.dmhmrs.chr.state.ky.us

John M Burt, Commissioner
Deborah Anderson, Staff Assistant
The Department for Mental Health and Mental Retardation Services contracts with fourteen regional community mental health and mental broads to provide an array of community based mental health services; operates three psychiatric hospitals and contracts with two additional hospitals; operates or contracts for 10 ICFs/MR; also operates two nursing facilities.

3167 **Kentucky Department for Mental Health:**
100 Fair Oaks Lane
Suite 4e-B
Frankfort, KY 40621
502-564-4527

3168 **Kentucky Department for the Blind**
PO Box 757
Frankfort, KY 40602
502-564-4754
800-321-6668
TTY:502-564-2929
e-mail: Wayne.Thompson@ky.gov
www.state.ky.us/agencies/wforce

Stephen Johnson, Executive Director
Provides career services and assistance to adults with severe visual handicaps who want to become productive in the home or work force. Also provides the Client Assistance Program established to provide advice, assistance and information available from rehabilitation programs to persons with handicaps.

3169 **Kentucky Office of Aging Services**
Cabinet for Health Services
275 E Main Street
5w-A
Frankfort, KY 40621
502-564-6930
FAX: 502-564-4595
www.chfs.ky.gov

Jerry Whitley, Manager
The Kentucky Office of Aging Services is the state agency directly responsible for programs and services for people with disabilities. Efforts are made to fully integrate the service response information that considers broad farmiliar implications.

3170 **Kentucky Protection & Advocacy Division**
100 Fair Oaks Lane
3rd Floor
Frankfort, KY 40601
502-564-2967
800-372-2988
FAX: 502-564-0848
e-mail: info@mail.pa.state.ky.us
www.kypa.net

Maureen Fitzgerald, Executive Director
Protecting the rights of persons with disabilities in Kentucky with a disability-related rights violation, providing information and referral, training and technical assistance.

3171 **Social Security: Frankfort Disability Determination**
Social Security
PO Box 1000
Frankfort, KY 40602
502-875-2232
800-928-8050
FAX: 502-226-4519
TTY: 502-226-4519
www.ssa.gov

Stephen Jones, Director
Burton Sisk, Manager

3172 **Social Security: Louisville Disability Determination**
Social Security
601 W Broadway
Suite 101
Louisville, KY 40202
502-582-6690
800-772-1213
www.socialsecurity.gov

Louisiana

3173 **Louisiana Assistive Technology Access Network**
PO Box 3455
Baton Rouge, LA 70821
225-342-6804
800-922-3452
FAX: 225-342-8823

Jill Revers, Project Director
Sandee Winchell, Executive Director
An information and training resource on Assistive Technology for the State of Louisiana. LATAN operates three regional centers to provide better access for consumers.

3174 **Louisiana Center for Dyslexia and Related Learning Disorders**
PO Box 2050
Thibodaux, LA 70310
985-448-4214
FAX: 985-448-4423
e-mail: karen.chauvin@nicholls.edu
www.nicholls.edu/dyslexia

Karen Chauvin, Director
Provides free information and referral services for diagnosis and tutoring for parents, educators, physicians and individuals with dyslexia. The voice of our membership is heard in 48 countries. Membership includes yearly journal and quarterly newsletter. Call for conference dates.

3175 **Louisiana Client Assistance Program**
225 Baronne Street
Suite 2112
New Orleans, LA 70112
800-960-7705
FAX: 504-522-5507
e-mail: advocacycenter@advocacyla.org
www.advocacyla.org

Diane Mirvis, CAP Director
Assistance to persons seeking, receiving or who have been denied rehabilitation services from Louisiana Rehabilitaton Services (LRS) or other projects, programs or facilities funded under the Rehabilitation Act (such as Vocational Rehabilitation, Independent Living or Supported Living). Must be a Louisiana resident and have a physical or mental disability.

3176 **Louisiana Department of Aging**
Office of Elderly Affairs
412 N 4th Street, 3rd Floor
PO Box 61
Baton Rouge, LA 70802
225-342-7100
FAX: 225-342-7133

Godfrey White, Executive Director
Serves as a focal point for Louisiana's senior citizens and administers a broad range of home and community based services through a network of 37 Area Agencies on Aging. Serve as the focal point for the development, implementation, and administration of the public policy for the state of Louisiana, and address the needs of the state's elderly citizens.

3177 **Louisiana Developmental Disability Council**
PO Box 3455
Baton Rouge, LA 70821
225-342-6804
800-922-DIAL
FAX: 225-342-1970
www.laddc.org

Sandee Winchell, Executive Officer

3178 **Louisiana Division of Mental Health**
PO Box 4049
Baton Rouge, LA 70821 225-342-2540
FAX: 225-342-5066

Cheryll Bowers-Scephens, Director
William Payne, Manager

3179 **Louisiana Learning Resources System**
2525 Wyandotte Street
Baton Rouge, LA 70805 225-355-6197
FAX: 225-357-3508

Dr. Charlene Bishop, Director
Bobbie Robertson, Administrator
Provides consultation on educational services for local schools, offers psychological testing and evaluation, maintains resource rooms in district schools and more for the blind and handicapped throughout the state.

3180 **Louisiana Protection & Advocacy for Persons with Developmental Disabilities**
225 Baronne Street
Suite 2112
New Orleans, LA 70112 504-566-1600
800-960-7705
FAX: 504-522-5507
e-mail: adce@advocacyla.org

Lois Simpson, Executive Director
Loretta Topey, Manager
Legal and advocacy services and training to persons whose legal issue is directly related to their disablity and has been designated an AC priority issue. Provides legal representation, counseling, information and referral, outreach, technical assistance, special subject speakers, and staff/professional training.

3181 **Protection & Advocacy of Individual Rights**
Advocate for Developmentally Disabled
225 Baronne Street
Suite 2112
New Orleans, LA 70112 504-522-2337
800-960-7705
FAX: 504-522-5507
e-mail: webmaster@advocacyla.org
www.advocacyla.org

Freddie Pincus, Vice President
Legal services and training to people whose legal issue is directly related to their disability and has been designated an AC priority issue. Provides legal representation, counseling, information and referral, outreach, technical assistance, special subject speakers, and staff/professional training.

3182 **Social Security: Baton Rouge Disability Determination**
Department of Social Services
755 N 3rd Street
Room 328
Baton Rouge, LA 70802 225-342-0286
800-772-1213
FAX: 225-219-9399
e-mail: adren.wilson@dss.state.la.us
www.ssa.gov

Shirley Williams, Director
Ann Williamson, Manager

3183 **Workers Compensation Board Louisiana**
PO Box 94040
Baton Rouge, LA 70804 225-342-7561
800-201-2494
FAX: 504-342-6555
www.laworks.net

Karen Winfrey, Executive Director

Maine

3184 **Maine Assistive Technology Projects**
University of Maine at Augusta
University Hts
Augusta, ME 04330 207-621-3000
FAX: 207-772-1302

Kathleen Powers, Project Director
Pat Lynch, Manager
A statewide program promoting assistive technology devices and services for persons of all ages with all disabilities.

3185 **Maine Bureau of Elder and Adult Services**
State of Maine
11 State House Station
Augusta, ME 04333 207-287-9200
FAX: 207-287-9229
www.maine.gov

Catherine Cobb, Director
Christine Gianopoulos, Executive Director

3186 **Maine Department of Health and Human Services**
221 State Street
Augusta, ME 04333 207-287-3707
FAX: 207-287-3005
e-mail: brenda.harvey@maine.gov
www.maine.gov

Brenda Harvey, Commissioner
Katherine Veilleux, Administrative Assistant
Provision of services to people with nental illness, mental retardation, substance abuse issues, children with special needs and people with developmental disabilities.

3187 **Maine Developmental Disability Council**
45 Memorial Circle
Suite 302
Augusta, ME 04330 207-622-6345
FAX: 207-622-6346
e-mail: mdf@mdf.org
www.mdf.org

Laurie Lachance, President/CEO

3188 **Maine Division for the Blind and Visually Impaired**
2 Anthony Avenue
Augusta, ME 04333 207-624-5120
800-760-1573
FAX: 207-624-5133
TTY: 800-698-4440
e-mail: harold.j.lewis@state.me.us
www.state.me.us/rehab

Harold Lewis, Director
Sandra Cavanaugh, Manager
Works to bring about full access to employment, independence and community integration for people with disabilities in Maine.

3189 **Maine Workers' Compensation Board**
27 State House Station
Augusta, ME 04333 207-287-3751
888-801-9087
FAX: 207-287-7198
www.state.me.us/wcb

Paul Dionne, Executive Director

3190 **Social Security: Maine Disability Determination**
40 Western Avenue
Augusta, ME 04330 207-622-1451
800-772-1213
TTY:207-623-4190
www.ssa.gov

Louis Tepin, Manager

Maryland

3191 **Health Resources & Services Administration : State Bureau of Health**
Federal Government
5600 Fishers Lane
Rockville, MD 20857
301-443-2216
888-275-4772
FAX: 301-443-1246
www.hrsa.gov

Elizabeth M Duke, Administrator
Through appropriated funds, supports education programs, credentialing analysis, and development of human resources needed to staff the U.S. health care system.

3192 **International Dyslexia Association: Maryland Branch**
International Dyslexia Association
8600 La Salle Road
Suite 382
Baltimore, MD 21286
410-296-0232
800-222-3123
FAX: 410-321-5069
e-mail: info@interdys.org
www.interdys.org

Nancy Hennessy, President
Guinevere Eden, Vice President
Megan Cohen, Executive Director
Nonprofit organization providing free information and referral services for diagnosis and tutoring for parents, educators, physicians, and individuals with dyslexia. The voice of our membership is heard in 48 countries. Membership includes yearly journal and quarterly newsletter. Call for conference dates.

3193 **Maryland Client Assistance Program Division of Rehabilitation Services**
2301 Argonne Drive
Baltimore, MD 21218
410-554-9361
800-638-6243
FAX: 410-554-9362
TTY: 800-735-2258
e-mail: cap@dors.state.md.us
www.dors.state.md.us/dors/programservices/cap

Beth Lash, CAP Director
Helps individuals with disabilities understand the rehabilitation process and receives appropriate and quality services from the Division of Rehabilitation Services and other programs and facilities providing services under the Rehabilitation Act of 1973.

3194 **Maryland Department of Aging**
State Office Building
301 W Preston Street
Suite 1007
Baltimore, MD 21201
410-767-1100
800-243-3425
FAX: 410-333-7943
e-mail: drb@mail.ooa.state.md.us
www.mdoa.state.md.us/

Dakota Burgess, Senior Information Program Manag
Jean Roesser, Manager

3195 **Maryland Department of Handicapped Children**
201 W Preston Street
Unit 50
Baltimore, MD 21201
410-396-4476

Judson Force, Director
Children's Medical Services is a joint federal/state/local program which assists in obtaining specialized medical, surgical and related habilitative/rehabilitative evaluation and treatment services for children with special health care needs and their families. To be eligible for the program's services, an individual must be a resident of Maryland, younger than 22 years, have or be suspected of having an eligible medical condition and meet both medical and financial criteria.

3196 **Maryland Developmental Disabilities Council**
217 E Redwood Street
Suite 1300
Baltimore, MD 21202
410-767-3670
800-305-6441
FAX: 410-333-3686
e-mail: brianc@md-council.org
www.md-council.org

Brian Cox, Executive Director
Catherine Lyle, Deputy Director
A public policy organization comprised of people with disabilities and family members who are joined by state officials, service providers and other designated partners. The Council is an independent, self-governing organization that represents the interests of people with developmental disabilities and their families.

3197 **Maryland Division of Mental Health**
2301 Argonne Drive
Baltimore, MD 21218
410-243-7495
FAX: 410-333-7482

Norma Pinette, Executive Director

3198 **Social Security: Baltimore Disability Determination**
711 W 40th Street
Rotunda Mall, Suite 415
Baltimore, MD 21211
800-772-1213
TTY:800-325-0778
www.socialsecurity.gov

3199 **Workers Compensation Board Maryland**
10 E Baltimore Street
Baltimore, MD 21202
410-864-5100
800-492-0479
e-mail: wcc@state.md.us
www.wcc.state.md.us

Sheldon Press, Vice Chairman
Mary Ahearn, Director

Massachusetts

3200 **Center for Public Representation**
22 Green Street
Northampton, MA 01060
413-587-6265
FAX: 413-586-5711
e-mail: info@cpr-ma.org
www.centerforpublicrep.org

Steven Schwartz, Executive Director
Robert Fleischner, Assistant Director

3201 **International Dyslexia Association of New England**
8600 La Salle Road
Suite 382
Baltimore, MD 21286
410-296-0232
800-222-3123
FAX: 410-321-5069
e-mail: info@interdys.org
www.interdys.org

Nancy Hennessy, President
Guinevere Eden, Vice President
Provides free information and referral services for diagnosis and tutoring for parents, educators, physicians, and individuals with dyslexia in Connecticut, Maine, New Hampshire, Rhode Island, and Vermont. The voice of our membership is heard in 48 countries. Membership includes yearly journal and quarterly newsletter. Call for conference dates.

3202 **Massachusetts Assistive Technology Partnership**
Children s Hospital Boston
1295 Boylston Street
Suite 310
Boston, MA 02215
617-267-9397
800-848-8867
FAX: 617-355-6345
e-mail: info@matp.org
www.matp.org

Marylyn Howe, Project Director
Pat Hill, Training Coordinator
A statewide program promoting assistive technology devices and services for persons with all disabilities.

3203 **Massachusetts Client Assistance Program**
Massachusetts Office on Disability
1 Ashburton Place
Room 1305
Boston, MA 02108
617-727-7440
800-322-2020
FAX: 617-727-0965
e-mail: barbara.lybarger@state.ma.us
www.state.ma.us

Barbara Lybarger, Assistant Director
Myra Berloff, Executive Director
Provides advocacy and information services.

3204 **Massachusetts Department of Mental Health**
25 Staniford Street
Boston, MA 02114
617-626-8000
FAX: 617-727-4350

Eileen Elias, Commissioner
Michele Anzaldi, Manager

3205 **Massachusetts Developmental Disabilities Council**
1150 Hancock Street
Quincy, MA 02169
617-770-7676
FAX: 617-770-1987
e-mail: adelia.deltrecco@state.ma.us
www.state.ma.us/mddc/

Adelia Deltrecco, Executive Assistant
Harold Lieberman, Administrative Assistant
Dan Shannon, Executive Director
Group of citizens which analyzes needs of people with severe, lifelong disabilities and works to improve public policy. MDDC produces several publications and has committees and a grants program to study and advocate for changes in the service system.

3206 **Social Security: Boston Disability Determination**
10 Causeway Street
Room 148, 1st Floor
Boston, MA 02222
800-772-1213
TTY:800-325-0778
www.socialsecurity.gov

Manuel J Vaz, Commissioner

3207 **Workers Compensation Board Massachusetts**
1 Ashburton Place
Room 211
Boston, MA 02108
617-727-2720
FAX: 617-727-3285
www.state.ma.us/dia

James J Campbell, Director
Russell Gilfus, Manager

Michigan

3208 **Department of Blind Rehabilitation**
Western Michigan University
1903 W Michigan Avenue
Kalamazoo, MI 49008
269-387-3248
e-mail: bldrehab@wmich.edu

Dr. William Wiener, Chairperson
Daniel Litynski, President

3209 **Michigan Association for Deaf and Hard of Hearing**
2929 Covington Court
Unit 200
Lansing, MI 48912
517-487-0066
800-968-7327
FAX: 517-487-0202
TTY: 517-487-2586
e-mail: yourear@madhh.org
www.madhh.org

Nancy Asher, Executive Director
L'Tonya Felder, Program Coordinator
SaDonna White, Interpreter/Project Coordinator
Substance abuse and anti violence prevention videos for deaf and hard of hearing students (alcohol, marijuana, inhalants) acted in sign language, voicing and captioning. HIV/AIDS prevention and information for the deaf and hard of hearing. Lending library books, videos and audio tapes. Accessibility to courts video and information. TTY distribution program.

3210 **Michigan Association for Deaf, and Hard of Hearing**
2929 Covington Court
Unit 200
Lansing, MI 48912
517-487-0066
800-968-7327
FAX: 517-487-2586
e-mail: yourear@madhs.org
www.madhs.org

Nancy Asher, Executive Director
Substance abuse prevention for deaf and hard of hearing students (alcohol, marijuana, inhalants) acted in sign language, voicing and captioning. HIV/AIDS prevention and information for the deaf and hard of hearing. Lending library books, videos and audio tapes. Accessibility in Courts video and information. TTY distribution Program.

3211 **Michigan Client Assistance Program**
PO Box 30008
Lansing, MI 48909
517-487-1755

Elmer Cerano, Executive Director

3212 **Michigan Coalition for Staff Development and School Improvement**
530 W Ionia Street
Suite C
Lansing, MI 48933
734-513-9080
800-444-2014
FAX: 517-371-1170

3213 **Michigan Commission for the Blind**
201 N. Washington Square
PO Box 30652
Lansing, MI 48909
800-292-4200
FAX: 517-335-5140
e-mail: turneys@michigan.gov
www.michigan.gov/mcb

Patrick Cannon, Director
The Michigan Commision for the blind is a state government agency that provides state-and federally funded training and other services to individuals who are legally blind (blind and visually impaired). Services are provided to people of all ages throughout the state of Michigan toward the goal of employment and/or independence.

3214 Michigan Commission for the Blind - Gaylord
209 W 1st Street
Suite 102
Gaylord, MI 49735
989-732-2448
800-292-4200
FAX: 989-731-3587
www.michigan.gov

Judy Terwilliger, Manager

3215 Michigan Commission for the Blind
Michigan Department of Labor and Economic Growth
PO Box 30652
Lansing, MI 48909
517-373-2062
800-292-4200
FAX: 517-335-5140
TTY: 517-373-4025
e-mail: cannonp@mi.gov
www.michigan.gov/mcb

Patrick Cannon, Executive Director
Bob Robertson, Administrative Services Director
The Commission for the Blind serves as the vocational rehabilitation agency for the blind. The Commission also operates a residential training center in kalamazoo, provides independent living services for Michigan's older blind population, low-vision services for the state's youth, a deaf/blind program, and entrepreneurial opportunities for blind persons through its Business Enterprise Program.

3216 Michigan Commission for the Blind Training Center
1541 Oakland Drive
Kalamazoo, MI 49008
269-337-3875
800-292-4200
FAX: 269-337-3872
e-mail: mossc@michigan.gov
www.michigan.gov/mcb

Melody Lindsey, Director
Roger Yake, Councilor
Residential facility that provides instruction to legally blind adults in braille, computers, handwriting, keyboarding, cane travel, adaptive kitchen skills, daily living, industrial arts and also crafts. Clients may also learn to use a variety of adaptive devices such as raised dot timers and watches, hand tools, talking calculators, tape recorders, reading machines and computers. Special training is also offered in vending stand operation, college preparation and job seeking skills.

3217 Michigan Commission for the Blind: Escanaba
305 Ludington Street
Escanaba, MI 49829
906-786-8602
800-323-2535
FAX: 906-786-4638
michigan.gov/mcb

Ed Haines, Rehabilitation Teacher/Counselor

3218 Michigan Commission for the Blind: Flint
125 E Union Street
Floor 7
Flint, MI 48502
810-760-2030
FAX: 810-760-2032
www.mfia.state.mi.us

Elizabeth White, Manager

3219 Michigan Commission for the Blind: Grand Rapids
350 Ottawa Avenue NW
Grand Rapids, MI 49503
616-356-0180
800-292-4200
FAX: 616-356-0199
www.mcp1.org

Patrick Cannon, Director
Bernie Kramer, Manager

3220 Michigan Council of the Blind and Visually Impaired (MCBVI)
Neal Freeling
1037 Winchester Avenue
Lincoln Park, MI 48146
313-381-7844
888-956-2284
e-mail: freeling@concentric.net

Neal Freeling, Information/Referral Specialist
Advocate for blind and visually impaired people throughout the state of Michigan.

3221 Michigan Department of Community Health
320 S Walnut
Lansing, MI 48913
517-373-3654
FAX: 517-335-3090
e-mail: mccullochs@michigan.gov
www.michigan.gov/mdch

Janet Olszewski, Director
A Edwin Dore, Chief Deputy Director
Bobbie Butler, Manager

3222 Michigan Department of Handicapped Children
3423 N Logan Street
Lansing, MI 48906
517-373-3654
FAX: 517-335-9222

Karen Schrock
Bobbie Butler, Manager

3223 Michigan Developmental Disability Council
1033 S Washington Avenue
Lansing, MI 48910
517-334-6123
FAX: 517-334-7353
TTY:517-334-7354
www.michigan.gov/ddcouncil

Vendella Collins, Executive Director
Todd Koopmans, Council Chairmain
Mitzi Allen, Administrative
The Michigan DD Council is a group of citizens from across the state. Its membership is made up of: people with developmental disabilities; people from families who have, among their members, people with developmental disabilities; and professionals from state and local agencies charged with assisting people with developmental disabilities.

3224 Michigan Office of Services to the Aging
PO Box 30026
Lansing, MI 48909
517-373-0219
FAX: 517-373-4092

Diane K Braunstein, Director
Tom Fogle, Executive Director
State unit on aging; allocates and monitors state and federal funds for the Older American Act services: nutrition, community services, administers home and community based waiver, develops programs through Area Agencies on Aging, advocates on behalf of seniors with legislature, governor, state departments, federal government, responsible for state planning of aging services, develops formula for distribution of state and federal funds.

3225 Michigan Protection & Advocacy Service
4005 Legacy Parkway
Suite 500
Lansing, MI 48911
517-487-1755
800-288-5923
FAX: 517-487-0827
e-mail: molsen@mpas.org
www.mpas.org

3226 Michigan Rehabilitation Services
PO Box 30010
Lansing, MI 48909
517-373-3390
800-605-6722
FAX: 517-373-0565
TTY: 517-373-4035
www.michigan.org

Jaye Balthazar, Manager

A state and federally funded program that helps persons with disabilities prepare for and fund a job that matches their interests and abilities. Assistance is also available to workers with disabilities who are having difficulty keeping a job. A person is eligible for MRS services if he or she has a disability, is unemployed and needs vocational rehabilitation services to prepare for and find a job or independent living services.

3227 **Social Security Administration**
5210 Perry Robinson Circle
Lansing, MI 48911
517-393-3876
800-772-1213
FAX: 517-393-4686
TTY: 800-366-3404
e-mail: mi.fo.lansing@ssa.gov
www.ssa.gov

Julie McCarthy, District Manager

3228 **State of Michigan/Bureau of Workers' Disability Compensation**
PO Box 30016
Lansing, MI 48909
888-396-5014
FAX: 517-322-1808
www.cis.state.mi.us/wkrcomp

3229 **Workers Compensation Agency**
PO Box 30016
Lansing, MI 48909
888-396-5041
FAX: 517-322-1808
e-mail: wcinfo@michigan.gov
www.michigan.gov/wca

Jack Nolish, Director
Bruno Czyrka, Deputy Director

Minnesota

3230 **International Dyslexia Association: Minnesota Branch**
International Dyslexia Association
5021 Vernon Avenue
PMB 159
Minneapolis, MN 55436
651-450-7589
800-222-3123
e-mail: info@interdys.org
www.interdys.org

Claire Eckley, President
UMBIDA-the Upper Midwest Branch of the International Dyslexia Association (IDA-serves the residents of Minnesota, North Dakota, South Dakota, and Winnipeg, Canada and offers: local educational conferences about dyslexia and related subjects, Orton-Gillingham training for teachers, tutors, and parents, Quarterly speaker series, member discounts on conferences, information line, and tutor referral.

3231 **Minnesota Assistive Technology Project**
STAR
50 Sherburne Avenue
Suite 309
Saint Paul, MN 55155
651-296-7138
800-657-3862
FAX: 651-282-6671
e-mail: star.program@state.mn.us
www.admin.state.mn.us/assistivetechnology

Chuck Rassbach, Executive Director
Nancy Stark, Manager
A statewide program promoting assistive technology devices and services for persons of all ages with all disabilities.

3232 **Minnesota Board on Aging**
444 Lafayette Road N
Saint Paul, MN 55155
651-296-2770
800-627-3529
FAX: 651-297-7855
e-mail: mba@sate.mn.us
www.mnaging.org

Jim Varpness, Director
Maria Gomez, Board Member
A state unit on aging for the state of Minnesota. Funds 14 area agencies on aging throughout the state that provide services at the local level. The mission is to keep older people in the homes or places of residence for as long as possible.

3233 **Minnesota Children with Special Needs, Minnesota Department of Health**
85 E 7th Place
PO Box 64882
Saint Paul, MN 55164
651-201-3650
800-728-5420
FAX: 651-201-3655
e-mail: mcshnweb@health.state.mn.us
www.health.state.mn.us/mcshn
Minnesota Children with Special Health Needs (MCSHN) provides leadership through partnerships with families and other key stakeholders to improve the access and quality of all systems impacting children and youth with special health care needs and their families.

3234 **Minnesota Department of Labor & Industry Workers Compensation Division**
443 Lafayette Road N
Saint Paul, MN 55155
651-284-5005
800-342-5354
FAX: 651-284-5727
e-mail: dli.workcomp@state.mn.us
www.doli.state.mn.us

Scott Brener, Manager
To reduce the impact of work related injuries for employees and employers. Advice is given and questions answered on the toll-free number.

3235 **Minnesota Disability Law Center**
430 1st Avenue N
Suite 300
Minneapolis, MN 55401
612-332-1441
800-292-4150
FAX: 612-334-5755
www.mndlc.org

Pamela Hoopes, Manager
Provides free, civil, legal assistance to Minnesotans with disabilities on issues related to their disability.

3236 **Minnesota Governor's Council on Developmental Disabilities GCDD**
370 Centennial Office Building
658 Cedar Street
Saint Paul, MN 55155
651-296-4018
877-348-0505
FAX: 651-297-7200
e-mail: admin.dd@state.mn.us
www.mncdd.org

Colleen Wieck PhD, Executive Director
The mission of the Minnesota Governor's Council on Developmental Disabilities is to provide information, education, and training to build knowledge, develop skills, and change attitudes that will lead to increased independence, productivity, self determination, integration and inclusion (IPSII) for people with developmental disabilities and their families.

3237 **Minnesota Mental Health Division**
Human Services Building
444 Lafayette Road N
Saint Paul, MN 55155
651-296-6117
e-mail: dhs.info@state.mn.us
www.dhs.state.mn.us/Provider/faqs/mental_heal

Edwin Swenson, Director
Kevin Goodno, Manager
Oversees the provision of services to people with mental illness in the state of Minnesota. Services are provided on the local level through a network of 87 county social service departments.

3238 **Minnesota Protection & Advocacy for Persons with Disabilities**
Minnesota Disability Law Center
430 1st Avenue N
Suite 300
Minneapolis, MN 55401
612-334-5784
800-292-4150
FAX: 612-334-5755
www.mnlegalservices.org/mdlc

Lisa Cohen, Administrator
Pamela Hoopes, Manager

3239 **Minnesota State Council on Disability (MSCOD)**
121 7th Place E
Suite 107
Saint Paul, MN 55101
651-361-7800
800-945-8913
FAX: 651-296-5935
e-mail: joan.willshire@state.mn.us
www.disability.state.mn.us

Joan Willshire, Executive Director
The MSCOD collaborates, advocates, advises and provide technical information to expand opportunities, increase the quality of life and empower all persons with disabilities. This mission is accomplished by: providing information, referral and technical assistance to thousands of individuals every year via email, letter or telephone; through trainings on a variety of disability related topics; through publications and its web site; and through its advocacy and advisory work.

3240 **Minnesota State Services for the Blind**
2200 University Avenue W
Suite 240
Saint Paul, MN 55114
651-642-0500
800-652-9000
FAX: 651-649-5927
www.mnssb.org

Lyle Lundquist, Senior Services Supervisor
Chuck Hamilton, Executive Director
Pam Brown, Workforce Development Director
State agency serving blind and visually impaired persons with rehabilitation, information access, assistive technology, training and job placement services. Extensive older blind program.

3241 **Social Security: St. Paul Disability Determination**
190 5th Street E
Sibley Building, Suite 800
Saint Paul, MN 55101
800-772-1213
TTY:800-325-0778
www.ssa.gov

Noreen Hale, Director

Mississippi

3242 **International Dyslexia Association: Mississippi Branch**
1604 Bistineau
Ruston, LA 71270
985-414-2575
800-222-3123
e-mail: info@interdys.org
www.interdys.org

Alice Higginbotham, President
It is the mission of the Louisiana Branch to provide information and resources to parents, educators, students and the community in a way that creates a clear and positive understanding of dyslexia and related language learning needs so that every individual has the opportunity to lead a productive and fulfilling life for the benefit of society.

3243 **Mississippi Assistive Technology Division**
PO Box 1698
Jackson, MS 39215
601-853-5100
FAX: 601-853-5158
www.mdrs.state.ms.us

Chris Geroux, Coordinator
Marie Gaddis, Administrative Assistant
Bob Richards, Manager
A statewide program promoting assistive technology devices and services for persons of all ages with all disabilities.

3244 **Mississippi Bureau of Mental Retardation**
1101 Robert E Lee Bldg
Jackson, MS 39201
601-359-1288
FAX: 601-359-6295

Ed LeGrand, Chief
Herb Loving, Executive Director

3245 **Mississippi Client Assistance Program**
Mississippi Department of Rehabilitation Services
PO Box 39110
Jackson, MS 39215
601-362-2585
FAX: 601-982-1951

Presley Posey, Executive Director
Advocacy program for clients/client applicants for state of MS vocational services.

3246 **Mississippi Department of Mental Health**
1101 Robert E Lee Bldg
Jackson, MS 39201
601-359-1288
FAX: 601-359-6295
www.dmh.state.ms.us

Herb Loving, Executive Director
Edwin Legrand, Assistant Director
Administers Mississippi's public programs of serving persons with mental illness, mental retardation, alcohol and substance abuse problems, and alzheimer's disease and related dementia.

3247 **Mississippi Division of Aging and Adult Services**
Mississippi Department Of Human Services
750 N State Street
Jackson, MS 39202
601-359-4500
800-345-6347
FAX: 601-359-3664
e-mail: webspinner@mdhs.state.ms.us
www.mdhs.state.ms.us/

Donald Taylor, Director
Protects the rights of older citizens while expanding their opportunities and access to quality services.

3248 **Mississippi State Department of Health**
Children s Medical Program
PO Box 1700
Jackson, MS 39215
601-987-3965
800-844-0898
FAX: 601-987-5560

Larry Clark, Director
Denise Faith, State Nursing Coordinator
Virginia Green MD, Medical Director
Financial assistance to families of children with physical handicaps. Rehabilitative in nature and has as its goal the correction or reduction of physical handicaps. Eligibility determined by diagnosis and provided to children from birth to age twenty-one. Financial eligibility is determined by factors of family income, family size, estimated cost of treatment and family liabilities. Categories include, but are not limited to: orthopedic, congenital heart defects, cerebral palsy, etc.

3249 **Mississippi: Workers Compensation Commission**
1428 Lakeland Drive
Jackson, MS 39216
601-987-4200
FAX: 601-987-4233
www.mwcc.state.ms.us

Ray Minor, Executive Director
Carla Clark, Division Director

Missouri

3250 Institute for Human Development
University of Missouri-Kansas City
2220 Holmes Street
Kansas City, MO 64108
816-235-1700
800-444-0821
FAX: 816-235-1762
e-mail: ellerbuschk@umkc.edu
www.ihd.umkc.edu

Carl Calkins, Director
Lora Lacey-Haun, Administrator
A statewide program promoting person-centered planning and services for persons of all ages with all disabilities.

3251 Missouri Division of Mental Retardation & Developmental Disabilities
Department of Mental Health
PO Box 687
Jefferson City, MO 65102
573-751-4054
FAX: 573-751-9207
e-mail: dmhmail@dmh.mo.gov
www.dmh.mo.gov

Bernard Simons, Division Director
Keith Schafer, Department Director

3252 Missouri Protection & Advocacy Services
925 S Country Club Drive
Jefferson City, MO 65109
573-893-3333
800-392-8667
FAX: 573-893-4231
e-mail: mopasjc@earthlink.net
www.moadvocacy.org

Shawn T Loyola, Executive Director
Linda Snider, Information Specialist
Connie Wright, Information Specialist
MO P&A provides protection of the rights of persons with disabilities in Missouri and assistance to clients who have disabilities through information, referral, advocacy or legal counsel. Informational brochures, Alliance newsletter, Client Assistance Program (CAP) Manual available upon request.

3253 Missouri Rehabilitation Services for the Blind
PO Box 88
Jefferson City, MO 65103
573-751-4249
800-592-6004
FAX: 573-751-4984
e-mail: mmerrick@mail.state.mo.us
www.dss.state.mo.us/dfs/rehab/rehab.htm

Mike Fester, Executive Director
Mike Merrick, Policy Development Coordinator
Offers services for the totally blind, legally blind, visually impaired, including counseling, educational, recreational, rehabilitation, computer training and professional training services.

3254 Social Security: Jefferson City Disability Determination
2401 E McCarty Street
Jefferson City, MO 65101
800-772-1213
www.ssa.gov

Dr. Don Gann, Director

3255 Workers Compensation Board Missouri
Department of Labor and Industrial Realtions
3315 W Truman Boulevard
Jefferson City, MO 65109
573-751-4231
FAX: 573-751-2012
e-mail: workerscomp@dolir.mo.gov
www.dolir.state.mo.us

Patricia Secrest, Director

Montana

3256 Addictive & Mental Disorders Division
555 Fuller Avenue
Helena, MT 59601
406-444-3964
FAX: 406-444-4435
www.dphhs.state.mt.us

Joyce Decunzo, Administrator
Joan Cassidy, Bureau Chief
Lou Thompson, MH Bureau Chief

3257 MonTECH
634 Eddy Avenue
Missoula, MT 59812
406-243-5511
877-243-5511
FAX: 406-243-4730
e-mail: montech@ruralinstitute.umt.edu
www.montech.ruralinstitute.umt.edu

Kathleen Laurin, Program Director
Chris Clasby, Program Coordinator
Specialzing in Assistive Technology and oversee a variety of AT related grants and contracts. The overall goal is to develop a comprehensive, statewide system of assistive technology related assistance. Striving to ensure that all people in Montana with disabilities have equitable access to assistive technology devices and services in order to enhance their independence, productivity and quality of life.

3258 Montana Advocacy Program
PO Box 1680
Helena, MT 59624
406-449-3266
800-245-4743
FAX: 406-449-2418
TTY: 800-245-4743
e-mail: advocate@mtadv.org
www.mtadv.org

Bernadette Franks-ongoy, Executive Director
Protects and advocates the human and legal rights of Montanans with mental and physical disabilities while advancing dignity, equality, and self-determination. Designated federal P&A, with AT, CAP, PADD, PAIMI and PAIR programs. Advocacy and legal services for abuse, neglect, rights violations, access, discrimination in employment, accommodations and housing, and assistance with vocational rehabilitation/visual services.

3259 Montana Blind & Low Vision Services
PO Box 4210
Helena, MT 59604
406-444-2590
FAX: 406-444-0230
www.dphhs.state.mt.us/dsd

Joe Mathews, Manager
Mission: promoting work and independence for Montanans with disabilities.

3260 Montana Council on Developmental Disabilit ies
PO Box 526
Helena, MT 59624
406-443-4332
FAX: 406-443-4192
e-mail: deborah@mtcdd.org
www.mtcdd.org

Deborah Swingley, Executive Director

3261 Montana Department of Aging
Capitol Station
Room 219
Helena, MT 59620
406-225-4411
FAX: 406-444-5529

Hank Hudson, Aging Coordinator
Jeff Sturm, President

3262 Montana Department of Handicapped Children
Cogswell Building
Helena, MT 59620
406-225-4411

Jeff Sturm, President

3263 **Montana Protection & Advocacy for Persons with Disabilities**
400 N Park Avenue
Helena, MT 59601
406-449-2344
800-245-4743
FAX: 406-449-2418
e-mail: advocate@mtav.org
www.mtadv.org

Bernadette Franks-Ongoy, Executive Director

3264 **Montana State Fund**
5 S Last Chance Gulch
PO Box 4759
Helena, MT 59601
406-444-6500
800-332-6102
FAX: 406-444-5963
e-mail: msfwebmaster@montanastatefund.com
www.montanastatefund.com

Ed Henrich, Chairman
Montana State Fund is committed to the health and economic prosperity of Montana through superior service, leadership and caring individuals, working in an environment of teamwork, creativity and trust.

3265 **Social Security: Helena Disability Determination**
10 W 15th Street
Suite 1600
Helena, MT 59601
406-411-1270
800-772-1213
TTY:406-441-1278
www.socialsecurity.gov

Nebraska

3266 **International Dyslexia Association: Nebraska Branch**
5921 Sunrise Road
Lincoln, NE 68510
402-488-7920
800-222-3123
e-mail: carolyn.brandle@ne-ida.com
www.interdys.org

Carolyn Brandle, President
The Nebraska Branch of the International Dyslexia Association is a 501(c)(3), non-profit organization dedicated to the study and treatment of dyslexia and related learning differences. This Branch was formed in 1981 to increase public awareness of dyslexia throughout Nebraska, and to serve individuals with dyslexia and their families. The organization includes professionals in the area of learning disabilities education, counseling and medicine as well as dylexics and their families and friends.

3267 **Nebraska Advocacy Services**
134 S 13th Street
Suite 600
Lincoln, NE 68508
402-474-3183
800-422-6691
FAX: 402-474-3274
e-mail: nas@nas-pa.org
www.nebraskaadvocacyservices.org

Timothy Shaw, Executive Director
Eric Evans, Deputy Director
Offers protection and advocacy services to people with developmental disabilities or mental illness. Direct assistance provided if issue within broad case priorities. Sliding scale fee. Information and referral at no cost.

3268 **Nebraska Client Assistance Program**
PO Box 94987
Lincoln, NE 68509
402-471-3656
800-742-7594
FAX: 402-471-0117
e-mail: victoria@cap.state.ne.us
www.cap.state.ne.us/

Victoria Rasmussen, Director
Frank Lloyd, Executive Director

3269 **Nebraska Commission for the Blind & Visually Impaired**
4600 Valley Road
Suite 100
Lincoln, NE 68510
402-471-2891
877-809-2419
FAX: 402-471-3009
e-mail: pearl.vanzandt@ncbvi.ne.gov
www.ncbvi.ne.gov

Pearl Van Zandt PhD, Executive Director
Carlos Servan, Deputy Director
Bob Deaton, Deputy Director
Offers services for the totally blind, legally blind, visually impaired, mentally retarded blind and more with health, counseling, educational, recreational, rehabilitation, computer training and professional training services.

3270 **Nebraska Department of Health & Human Services of Medically Handicapped Children's Prgm**
301 Centennial Mall S
5th Floor
Lincoln, NE 68508
402-471-5185
FAX: 402-471-6352
e-mail: roger.hillman@hhss.state.ne.us

Jeanne Garvin MD, Medical Director
Harlow Hyde, Program Specialist
Roland Snuttjer, Program Manager
Maternal and child health, Title V, children with special health care needs; community based, statewide programs to facilitate diagnoses and care of children with disabilities and chronic medical conditions.

3271 **Nebraska Department of Health and Human Services, Division of Aging Services**
PO Box 95044
Lincoln, NE 68509
402-471-5185
800-942-7830
FAX: 402-471-4619
www.hhss.ne.gov

Joan Weis, Director
Arti Cover, Manager

3272 **Nebraska Department of Mental Health**
301 Centennial Mall S
Lincoln, NE 68508
402-471-5185
FAX: 402-423-7045
www.nmhc-clinics.com

Arti Cover, Manager

3273 **Nebraska Planning Council on Developmental Disabilities**
Department of Health and Human Services
301 Centennial Mall S
PO Box 95026
Lincoln, NE 68509
402-471-2330
FAX: 402-471-0183
TTY:402-471-9570
e-mail: mary.gordon@hhss.ne.gov
www.hhs.state.ne.us/ddplanning

Mary Gordon, Director
The Council focuses on persons who experience a severe disability that occurs before the individual attains the age of 22, which includes persons with physical disabilities, mental/behavioral health conditions and persons that are served by the current state developmental disabilities system.

3274 **Nebraska Workers' Compensation Court**
State of Nebraska
PO Box 98908
Lincoln, NE 68509
402-471-6468
800-599-5155
FAX: 402-471-2700
e-mail: newcc@wcc.ne.gov
www.wcc.ne.gov/

Glenn Morton, Administrator
Su Davis, Public Information Manager

3275 Social Security: Lincoln Disability Determination
Department of Education
PO Box 94987
Lincoln, NE 68509
402-471-2295
800-772-1213
FAX: 471-362-
TTY: 402-471-3659
e-mail: flloyd@nde4.nde.state.ne.us
www.socialsecurity.gov

Frank Lloyd, Assistant Commissioner
Doug Christensen, Manager

Nevada

3276 Assistive Technology Center at NCEP: Nevada Community Enrichment Program
2820 W Charleston Boulevard
Las Vegas, NV 89102
702-259-1903
FAX: 702-259-1907

Terry Sjoberg Otr/l, Manager
Robert Hogan, Executive Director
Reggie Bennett, Independent Living Coordinator
Provides information, demonstration and training to adults and children with disabilities in the use of microcomputers and other assistive technology product systems and devices. ATC offers peer screening, pre-service financial and resource planning, low interest loan program, technology matching, rehabilitation engineering, outreach training, and maintains a product information database.

3277 Nevada Assistive Technology Project
3656 Research Way
Suite 32
Carson City, NV 89706
775-687-4452
888-337-3839
FAX: 775-687-3292
www.hr.state.nv.us

Kelleen Preston, Project Manager
Todd Butterworth, Chief
Serves all ages and all disabilities through partnerships with community organizations. The NATP provides training, advocacy, funding, information and referral services, a newsletter and weekly television show.

3278 Nevada Bureau of Services to the Blind and Visually Impaired
505 E King Street
Suite 501
Carson City, NV 89701
775-684-4244
FAX: 775-684-4186

Gayle Sherman, Chief
Offers services for the totally blind, legally blind, visually impaired, mentally retarded blind and more with health, counseling, educational, recreational, rehabilitation, computer training and professional training services.

3279 Nevada Developmental Disability Council
3656 Research Way
Suite 32
Carson City, NV 89706
775-687-4452
e-mail: rweathermon@dhr.state.nv.us
www.nevadaddcouncil.org

Richard Weathermon, Executive Director
Mary Bryant, Acting Council Chair
The mission of the Nevada Developmental Disabilities Council is to provide resources at the community level which promote equal opportunity and life choices for people with disabilities through which they may positively contribute to Nevada society.

3280 Nevada Disability Advocacy and Law Center -Sparks/Reno Office
1311 N McCarran Boulevard
Suite 106
Sparks, NV 89431
775-333-7878
800-992-5715
FAX: 775-788-7825
TTY: 702-788-7824
e-mail: reno@ndalc.org
www.ndalc.org

Anna Maria Carini, Office Coordinator
Jack Mayes, Executive Director
Nevada's protection and advocacy system for the human legal and service rights of individuals with disabilities. NDALC has offices in Reno/Sparks and Las Vegas, with services provided statewide.

3281 Nevada Division for Aging: Carson City
3416 Goni Road
Building D
Carson City, NV 89706
775-687-4210
800-992-0900
FAX: 775-687-4264
e-mail: dascc@aging.state.nv.us
www.aging.nv.state.us

Carol Fala, Administrator
Provides services for seniors in Nevada including community based care. advocacy and volunteer programs. Call write or e-mail for more information.

3282 Nevada Division for Aging: Las Vegas
3100 W Sahara Avenue
Suite 103
Las Vegas, NV 89102
702-486-3545
FAX: 702-486-3572
e-mail: dasvegas@aging.nv.gov
www.nvaging.net

Carol Sala, Administrator
Marilyn Wills, Deputy Administrator
Develops, coordinates and delivers a comprehensive support service system in order for Nevada' senior citizens to lead independent, meaningful and dignified lives.

3283 Nevada Division of Mental Health and Devel opmental Services
4126 Technology Way
Suite 201
Carson City, NV 89706
775-684-5943
FAX: 775-684-5966
e-mail: mhds@govmail.state.nv.us
www.mdhs.state.nv.us
Brandenburg , Director
Carlos Brandenberg, Administrator
Offers treatment, prevention, education, habitation and rehabilitation for mental disorders. Works with advocacy groups, families, agencies and the community.

3284 Social Security: Carson City Disability Determination
1170 Harvard Way
Reno, NV 89502
800-352-1605
800-772-1213
TTY:800-325-0778
www.socialsecurity.gov

Dan Mooney, Director

3285 State of Nevada Client Assistance Program
2450 Wrondel Way
Suite E
Reno, NV 89502
775-688-1440
800-633-9879
FAX: 775-688-1627

3286 Workers Compensation Board Nevada
6515 E Musser Street
Carson City, NV 89714
775-687-6492
FAX: 775-687-5786

New Hampshire

3287 **New Hampshire Workers Compensation Board**
46 Donovan Street
Concord, NH 03301
603-224-9222
FAX: 603-226-6903
www.nhprimex.org

Paul Genevose, Chief Executive Officer
Kathy Fortin, Manager

3288 **New Hampshire Assistive Technology Partnership Project**
Department of Education
State of New Hampshire
Concord, NH 03824
603-862-2260
FAX: 603-228-2468

Jan Nisbet, Director
Mary Schuh, Associate Director
Eve Fralick, Associate Director
The goal of the New Hampshire Assistive Technology Partnership Project is to increase access to assistive technology through the creation and support of consumer driven systems for the provision of state-of-the-art assistive technology products and services for citizens with disabilities in the state of New Hampshire.

3289 **New Hampshire Client Assistance Program**
57 Regional Drive
Concord, NH 03301
603-271-4175
FAX: 603-271-2837
www.state.nh.us/disability/caphomepage.html

Bill Hagy, Director

3290 **New Hampshire Commission for Human Rights**
2 Chenell Drive
Concord, NH 03301
603-271-2767
800-735-2964
FAX: 603-271-6339
e-mail: humanrights@nhsa.state.nh.us
www.state.nh.us

Katharine A Daly, Executive Director
Enforces New Hampshire law against discrimination in housing, employment or public accomodations. Disability discrimination is prohibited under New Hampshire law. Takes formal charges and investigates them.

3291 **New Hampshire Department of Mental Health**
State Office Park S
Concord, NH 03301
603-226-0111
FAX: 603-271-5058

Donald Shumway, Director
Paul Garmon
Tim Rourke, Religious Leader

3292 **New Hampshire Developmental Disabilities Council**
21 S Sruit Street
Suite 22
Concord, NH 03301
603-271-3236
800-852-3345
FAX: 271-115-
e-mail: NHDDCNCL@aol.com
www.nhddc.org

Gordon Allen, Executive Director
Leslie Nelson, Director of Policy/Planning
Jennifer Daniels, Administrative Assistant
Offers information, referral and support services to disabled persons. A federally funded state agency.

3293 **New Hampshire Division of Developmental Services**
Department of Health and Human Services
105 Pleasant Street
Concord, NH 03301
603-271-5034
FAX: 603-271-5166
e-mail: dpowers@dhhs.state.nh.us
www.dhas.srare.nh.us.

Matthew Ertas, Director
Michelle Rosado, Administrative Assistant
Developmental Services promotes opportunities for normal life experiences for persons with developmental disabilities and aquired brain disorders in all areas of community life: employment, housing, recreation, social relationships and community association. Services and supports are organized throught a central state office and twelve private nonprofit community area agencies. Family support is provided to families of children with chronic health conditions or are developmentally disabled.

3294 **New Hampshire Division of Elderly and Adult Services**
Bureau of Elderly & Adult Services
129 Pleasant Street
Concord, NH 03301
603-271-4680
800-351-1888
FAX: 603-271-4643
www.dhhs.state.nh.us

Douglas McNutt, Acting Bureau Chief
Mary Maggioncaida, Manager Program Development
The Bureau of Elderly and Adult Services provides a variety of social and long-term supports to adults age 60 and older and to adults between the ages of 18 and 60 who have a chronic illness or disability. These services range from home care, meals on wheels, care management, transportation assistance and assisted living to nursing home care.

3295 **New Hampshire Governor's Commission on Disability**
57 Regional Drive
Suite 5
Concord, NH 03301
603-271-2773
800-852-3405
FAX: 603-271-2837
www.nh.gov/disability

Carol Nadeau, Executive Director

3296 **New Hampshire Protection & Advocacy for Persons with Disabilities**
18 Low Avenue
Concord, NH 03301
603-224-4394
800-834-1721
FAX: 603-225-2077
e-mail: advocacy@drcnh.org
www.drcnh.org

Richard Cohen, Executive Director
Ron Lospennato, Legal Director
Legal services for individuals with disabilities; I & R.

3297 **Social Security: Concord Disability Determination**
70 Commercial Street
Suite 100
Concord, NH 03301
603-224-1939
800-772-1213
TTY:603-225-8475
www.ssa.gov

3298 **Workers Compensation Board New Hampshire**
95 Pleasant Street
Concord, NH 03301
603-271-3176
800-272-4353
FAX: 603-271-6149
e-mail: workerscomp@labor.state.nh.us
www.labor.state.nh.us

Kathryn Barger, Executive Director

New Jersey

3299 **Division of Developmental Disabilities**
PO Box 726
Trenton, NJ 08625
609-292-3742
800-932-9173
FAX: 609-292-6610
e-mail: advoca@njpanda.org
www.njpanda.org

James W Smith Jr, Extecutive Director

New Jersey's designated protection and advocacy system for poeple with disabilities and provides legal, nonlegal individual and systems advocacy.

3300 **International Dyslexia Association: New Jersey Branch**
NJIDA
PO Box 32
Long Valley, NJ 07853 908-879-1179
e-mail: riegpainting@msn.com
www.interdys.org

Francie M Matthews PhD, President
The New Jersey Branch of The International Dyslexia Association is a 501(c)(3) non-profit, scientific and educational organization which was formed to increase public awareness of dyslexia in New Jersey. We have been serving individuals with dyslexia, their families, and professionals in the field in this community for more than 25 years.

3301 **New Jersey Commission for the Blind and Visually Impaired**
153 Halsey Street
6th Floor, PO Box 47017
Newark, NJ 07101 973-648-2324
877-685-8878
FAX: 973-648-7364
e-mail: Vito.DeSantis@dhs.state.nj.us
www.state.nj.us/humanservices/cbvi

Vito J DeSantis, Executive Director
James W Smith, Jr, Acting Commissioner
Jose Morales, Manager
The mission of the New Jersey Commission for the Blind and Visually Impaired is to promote and provide services in the areas of education, employment, independence and eye health through informed choice and partnership with persons who are blind or visually impaired, their families and the community. Serves Bergen, Essex, Hudson, Morris, Passaic, Sussex and Warren Counties.

3302 **New Jersey Department of Aging**
S Broad and Front Street
Trenton, NJ 08608 609-292-3766

Ruth Leader, Director

3303 **New Jersey Department of Health/Special Child Health Services**
New Jersey Department of Health and Senior Service
PO Box 364
Trenton, NJ 08625 609-777-7778
FAX: 609-292-3580
e-mail: plisciotto@doh.state.nj.us

Gloria Rodriguez, Director
Pauline Lisciotto, Program Manager
Provides services for New Jersey children that will prevent or reduce the effects of a developmental delay, chronic illness or behavioral disorder.

3304 **New Jersey Division of Mental Health Services**
Department Human Services
50 E State Street
Trenton, NJ 08608 609-292-3717
800-382-6717
FAX: 609-341-3333
www.state.nj.us/humanservices

Lyn Gates, Bureau Chief
James Davy, Commissioner
Oversees the public mental health system for the state of New Jersey. Operates six regional and specialty psychiatric hospitals, and contracts with over 125 not-for-profit agencies to provide a comprehensive system of community mental health services throughout all counties in the state.

3305 **New Jersey Governor's Liaison to the Office of Disability Employment Policy**
PO Box 52
Trenton, NJ 08625 609-292-2323
FAX: 609-633-9271
e-mail: cmycoff@dol.state.nj.us
www.state.nj.us/labor

Mark B Boyd, Commissioner
Al Kirk, Assistant Director
Rick Shanberg, Program Assistant
The Division of Vocational Rehabilitation Services provides vocational rehabilitation services to prepare and place in employment eligilbe individuals with disabilities who, because of their disabling conditions, would otherwise be unable to secure and/or mantain employment

3306 **New Jersey Protection & Advocacy for Persons with Disabilities**
Trenton, NJ 08625 609-530-5200
FAX: 609-292-6610

Robert Nickolas, Director
Ida Castro, President

3307 **Regional ADA Technical Assistance Center**
United Cerebral Palsy Associations of New Jersey
354 S Broad Street
Trenton, NJ 08608 609-392-4004
800-949-4232
FAX: 609-392-7044
TTY: 609-392-7044
e-mail: BTACUPNJ@aol.com
home.earthlink.net/~dawwn/dbtac.htm

Richard Dodds, Contact Person
Jack Mudge, Executive Director

3308 **Social Security Administration**
635 S Clinton Avenue
Trenton, NJ 08611
800-772-1213
TTY:800-325-0778
www.ssa.gov
Social Security disability is a social insurance program that workers and employers pay for with their Social Security taxes. Eligibility is based on your work history, and the amount of your benefit is based on your earnings. Social Security also has a disability program for people with limited income and resources-the Supplemental Security Income (SSI) program. For more information on these federal programs, please call our nationwide toll-free number.

New Mexico

3309 **New Mexico Aging and Long-Term Services Department**
2550 Cerrillos Road
Santa Fe, NM 87505 505-827-7640
866-451-2901
FAX: 505-476-4836
www.nmaging.state.nm.us

Debbie Armstrong, Executive Director
Patsy Trujillo-Knaver, Deputy Secretary
Michael Spanier, Deputy Secretary
Information and services for seniors, people with disabilities and their families.

3310 **New Mexico Client Assistance Program**
1720 Louisiana Boulevard NE
Suite 204
Albuquerque, NM 87110 505-256-3100
800-432-4682
FAX: 505-256-3184
e-mail: info@nmpanda.org
www.nmpanda.org

James Jackson, Exeuctive Director

3311 **New Mexico Commission for the Blind**
2905 Rodeo Park Drive E
Building 4
Santa Fe, NM 87505
505-820-6860
FAX: 505-476-4475
e-mail: greg.trapp@state.nm.us
www.state.nm.us/cftb

Robert Stark, Executive Director
Offers services for the totally blind, legally blind, visually impaired, mentally retarded blind and more with health, counseling, educational, recreational, rehabilitation, computer training and professional training services.

3312 **New Mexico Department of Health: Children's Medical Services**
1190 S Saint Francis Drive
Santa Fe, NM 87505
505-827-2548
FAX: 505-827-1697
e-mail: lchristiansen@doh.state.nm

Lynn Christiansen, Program Manager
Title V MCH Program for children with special health care needs from birth to age 21 years. Services provided include: diagnosis, medical intervention, clinics and service coordination.

3313 **New Mexico Governor's Committee on Concerns of the Handicapped**
491 Old Santa Fe Trail
Santa Fe, NM 87501
505-986-4589
FAX: 505-827-6328

Paula Tackett, Executive Director

3314 **New Mexico Protection & Advocacy for Persons with Disabilities**
1720 Louisiana Boulevard NE
Suite 204
Albuquerque, NM 87110
505-256-3100
800-432-4682
FAX: 505-256-3184
e-mail: info@nmpanda.org
www.nmpanda.org

James Jackson, Executive Director

3315 **New Mexico Technology Assistance Program**
NMDVR/NMTAP
435 Saint Michaels Drive
Building D
Santa Fe, NM 87505
800-866-2253
FAX: 505-954-8608
TTY:800-659-4915
e-mail: andy.winnegar@state.mn.us
www.nmtap.com

Andy Winnegar, Director
Yvonne Hart, Planner Director
The New Mexico Technology Assistance Program (NMTAP) offers free services to New Mexicans with disabilities to help them get the assistive technology (AT)services they need. Our mission is to help persons with disabilities enhance their quality of life through the use of assistive technology.

3316 **New Mexico Workers Compensation Administration**
PO Box 27198
Albuquerque, NM 87125
505-841-6000
866-WOR-KOMP
FAX: 505-841-6866
www.state.nm.us/wca

Alan Varela, Director
Regulates workers' compensation in New Mexico.

3317 **Social Security: Santa Fe Disability Determination**
604 W San Mateo Road
Santa Fe, NM 87505
505-473-3707
800-772-1213
FAX: 505-827-3512
e-mail: terryb@oscar.state.nm.us
www.socialsecurity.gov

Terry Brigance, Director

3318 **Southwest Branch of the International Dyslexia Association**
International Dyslexia Association
PO Box 25891
Albuquerque, NM 87125
505-255-8234
800-222-3123
FAX: 505-262-8547
e-mail: swida@southwestida.com
southwestida.com

Linda Curry, President
Provides free information and referral services for diagnosis and tutoring for parents, educators, physicians, and individuals with dyslexia. The voice of our membership is heard in 48 countries. Membership includes yearly journal and quarterly newsletter. Call for conference dates.

3319 **Workers Compensation Board New Mexico**
PO Box 27198
Albuquerque, NM 87125
505-841-6000
FAX: 841-606-0

Steven Kennedy, Director
Alan Varela, Manager

New York

3320 **Albany County Department for Aging**
162 Washington Avenue
Albany, NY 12210
518-447-7198
FAX: 518-447-7188
e-mail: aging@albanycounty.com
www.albanycounty.com

Vincent Colonno, Director

3321 **International Dyslexia Association of NY: Buffalo Branch**
c/o Gow School
2491 Emery Road
South Wales, NY 14139
716-687-2030
800-222-3123
e-mail: bufida@gow.org
www.interdys.org

Timothy Madigan PhD, President

3322 **Jawonio Vocational Center**
Jawonio Vocational Center
260 N Little Tor Road
New City, NY 10956
845-634-4648
FAX: 845-634-7731
www.jawonio.org

Esther White, Associate Director Employment
Paul Tendler, Administrator
Offers vocational evaluation, training, counseling and job placement services.

3323 **NYS Commission on Quality of Care & Advocacy for Persons with Disabilities**
1 Empire State Plaza
Suite 1001
Albany, NY 12223
518-449-2825
800-522-4369
FAX: 518-473-6005
e-mail: webmaster@cqcapd.state.ny.us
www.cqcapd.state.ny.us

Gary O'Brien, Commissioner
RoseMary Lamb, Associate Advocate
Mark Keegan, Director QA/Investigations

3324 **NYSARC**
393 Delaware Avenue
Delmar, NY 12054
518-439-8311
800-724-2094
FAX: 518-439-1893
e-mail: info@nysarc.org
www.nysarc.org

Marc Brandt, Executive Director

3325 **National Alliance for the Mentally Ill of NY State**
260 Washington Avenue
Albany, NY 12210
518-462-2000
800-950-3228
FAX: 518-462-3811
e-mail: info@naminys.org
www.naminys.org

Ione Christian, President
J David Seay, Executive Director

3326 **New State Office of Mental Health Agency**
Office of Mental Health
44 Holland Avenue
Albany, NY 12229
518-473-6579
800-597-8481
FAX: 518-474-2149
www.omh.state.ny.us

Sharon Carpinello, Commissioner
Promoting the mental health of all New Yorkers with a particular focus on providing hope and recovery for adults with serious mental illness and children with serious emotional disturbances.

3327 **New York Client Assistance Program**
99 Washington Avenue
Suite 1002
Albany, NY 12210
518-869-1543
FAX: 518-474-2652
www.nls.org/caplist.htm

3328 **New York Department of Handicapped Children**
Department of Heath Education
PO Box 678
Albany, NY 12201
518-447-4691
FAX: 518-447-4573
e-mail: jcrucetti@albanycounty.com
www.health.state.ny.us

Thomas Blake, Acting Bureau Chief
James Crucetti, Commisioner

3329 **New York State Commission for the Blind**
52 Washington Street
Rensselaer, NY 12144
518-473-8072
FAX: 518-486-5819

Thomas Robertson, Associate Commissioner
Madeline Raciti, Manager
Offers services for the totally blind, legally blind, visually impaired, mentally retarded blind and more with health, counseling, educational, recreational, rehabilitation, computer training and professional training services.

3330 **New York State Commission on Quality of Care**
401 State Street
Schenectady, NY 12305
518-388-2892
FAX: 518-388-2890
e-mail: marcelc@cqc.state.ny.us
www.cqc.state.ny.us

Marcel Chaine, Director Advocacy Services
Gary O'Brien, Manager

3331 **New York State Congress of Parents and Teachers**
1 Wembley Court
Albany, NY 12205
518-452-8808
FAX: 518-452-8105
e-mail: office@nypta.com
www.nyspta.org

Penny Leask, President
Maria Dewald, First Vice President

3332 **New York State Office of Advocates for Persons with Disabilities**
1 Empire State Plaza
Suite 1001
Albany, NY 12223
518-449-7860
800-522-4369
FAX: 518-473-6005
e-mail: oapwdinfo@oapwd.org
www.oapwd.org

Gary O'Brien, Chair Commissioner
Provides information and referral services; administers NYS Tech Art Project; promotes implementation of disability-related laws.

3333 **New York State Office of Mental Health**
44 Holland Avenue
Albany, NY 12229
518-474-2568
800-597-8481
FAX: 518-474-1846
www.omh.state.ny.us

Sharon E Carpinello RN PhD, Commissioner
Promoting the mental health of all New Yorkers with a particular focus on providing hope and recovery for adults with serious mental illness and children with serious emotional disturbances.

3334 **New York State TRAID Project**
New York State Commisionon Qualityof Careand Advoc
1 Empire State Plaza
Suite 1001
Albany, NY 12223
518-449-7860
800-522-4369
FAX: 518-473-6005
www.oatwd.org

Lisa Rosano, Project Director

3335 **Parent to Parent of New York State**
500 Balltown Road
Schenectady, NY 12304
518-381-4350
800-305-8817
FAX: 518-393-9607
e-mail: p2pnys@adelphia.net
www.parenttoparentnys.org

Janice Fitzgerald, Executive Director
Mary Hebert, Manager
Tina Beauparlant, Education Specialist

3336 **Protection and Advocacy Agency of NY**
401 State Street
Schenectady, NY 12305
518-388-2892
800-624-4143
FAX: 518-388-2890
e-mail: marcelc@cqc.state.ny.us
www.cqc.state.ny.us

Marcel Chaine, Director Advocacy Services
Gary O'Brien, Manager

3337 **Regional Early Childhood Director Center**
875 E Main Street
Suite 240
Rochester, NY 14605
585-399-4617
800-462-4344
FAX: 585-271-4228
e-mail: amy_campbell@boces.monroe.edu
www.vesid.nysed.gov

Amy Campbell, Director
Michael Reif, Executive Director
Jill Jensen, Family Information Specialist
Provides information, support and referral assistance to parents and professionals who are concerned with chilren with special needs or handicapping condition between the ages of birth to five.

3338 **Schools And Services For Children With Autism Spectrum Disorders.**
116 E 16th Street
Floor 5
New York, NY 10003
212-677-4650
FAX: 212-254-4070
e-mail: info@resourcesnyc.org
www.resourcesnyc.org

Karen Schlesinger, Executive Director
Dianne Littwin, Publishing Director
This publication fun resource for children provides extreme coverage of services for children with autism, asbergez syndrome, and/or PDD.

3339 **Singeria/Metropolitan Parent Center**
15 W 65th Street
6th Floor
New York, NY 10023
212-496-1300
FAX: 212-496-5608
e-mail: intake@sinergiany.org
www.sinergiany.org

Harminia Mendez, Human Resources Executive

3340 **Social Security: Albany Disability Determination**
1 Clinton Avenue
Room 430, Federal Building
Albany, NY 12207
518-431-4051
800-772-1213
TTY:518-431-4050
www.ssa.gov

Thomas A Robertson, Assistant Commissioner

3341 **State Agency for the Blind and Visually Impaired**
52 Washington Street
Rensselaer, NY 12144
518-474-6812
866-871-3000
FAX: 518-486-5819
e-mail: info@ocfs.state.ny.us
www.ocfs.state.ny.us

Thomas Robertson, Associate Commissioner
Brian Daniels, Manager

3342 **State Education Agency Rural Representative**
Education Building Anx
Room 876
Albany, NY 12234
518-474-3936
FAX: 518-473-2860
e-mail: sspear@mail.nysed.gov
www.nysed.gov

Suzanne Spear, Supervisor

3343 **State Mental Health Representative for Children and Youth**
44 Holland Avenue
Albany, NY 12229
518-473-6328
e-mail: cocompz@omh.state.ny.us

David Woodlock, Deputy Commissioner

3344 **State Mental Retardation Program**
44 Holland Avenue
Albany, NY 12229
518-473-1997
FAX: 518-473-1271
www.omr.state.ny.us

Thomas Maul, Commissioner

3345 **United We Stand of New York**
594 Bushwick Avenue
Brooklyn, NY 11206
718-302-4313
FAX: 718-302-4315
e-mail: uwsofny@aol.com
www.uwsony.org

Lourdes Rivera-Putz, Executive Director
Lourdes Figueroa, Intake/Receptionist
Carmen Soltero, Outreach/Trainer
Assists families with improving the quality of life for all individuals with disabilities.

3346 **University Afiliated Program/Rose F Kennedy Center**
1971
Parkway South
Suite 10
Bronx, NY 10461
430-850-
www.aecom.yu.edu/cerc

Hebert J Cohen, Director

3347 **University of Rochester Medical Center**
601 Elmwood Avenue
Rochester, NY 14642
585-275-6772
FAX: 585-275-3366
e-mail: phil_davidson@urmc.rochester.edu
www.urmc.rochester.edu/strong/scdd

Philp W Davidson, Director
Susan Edwards, Manager

3348 **VESID**
New York State Education Department
1606 One Commerce Plaza
Room 1606
Albany, NY 12234
518-474-2714
FAX: 518-474-8802
www.vesid.nysed.gov

Dr Rebecca Cort, Deputy Commissioner
Vocational and educational services for individuals with disabilities.

3349 **VSA Arts of New York City**
18-05 215 Street
Suite 15N
Bayside, NY 11360
718-225-6305
FAX: 717-225-6305
e-mail: bbvsanyc@msn.com
www.vsarts.org

Dr Bebe Berenstein, Executive Director
Provides art, educational and creative expression experiences to thousands of children, youth, and adults with disabilities who reside in the five boroughs of New York City. It provides opportunities for people with disabilities to demonstrate their accomplishments in the arts and foster increased understanding and acceptance.

3350 **Westchester Institute for Human Development**
Cedarwood Hall
Valhalla, NY 10595
914-493-8150
e-mail: wihd@wihd.org
www.wihd.org

Ansley Bacon PhD, President/CEO
Alison Bailey MSEd, Administrative Operations
Maritza Molina MD, Medical Director
WIHD advances policies and practices that foster the healthy development and ensure the safety of all children, strengthen families and communities, and promote health and well-being among people of all ages with disabilities and special health care needs.

3351 **Workers Compensation Board New York**
20 Park Street
Albany, NY 12207
800-877-1373
877-632-4996
FAX: 718-802-6642
www.wcb.state.ny.us

Linda Spano, District Administrator
Pat Wright, District Manager

North Carolina

3352 Developmental Disability Services Section
Albemarle
Building 325n
Raleigh, NC 27699
919-733-7011
FAX: 919-733-9455
www.dhhs.state.nc.us/mhddsas/

Michael Moseley, Director
Sylvia Prumpler, Human Resource Manager
Makes policies and monitors public services and supports to people with mental illness, developmental disabilities and substance abuse throughout North Carolina.

3353 International Dyslexia Association: North Carolina Branch
1829 E Franklin Street
Franklin Square, Suite 1200 K
Chapel Hill, NC 27514
919-933-8880
800-222-3123
FAX: 828-963-1883
e-mail: edutherapy@earthlink.net
www.interdys.org

Susan Lowell MA BCET, President
The North Carolina Branch of The International Dyslexia Association (NCIDA) is a 501 (c)(3) non-profit, scientific and organization dedicated to educating the public about the learning disability, dyslexia. The North Carolina Branch has four objectives: to increase awareness in the dyslexic and general community; to network with other learning disability groups and legislators in education;to increase membership and provide services that will strengthen members presence in their communities

3354 North Carolina Workers Compensation Board
430 N Salisbury Street
Raleigh, NC 27603
919-676-2288
FAX: 919-715-0282
www.comp.state.nc.us/

J Bunn Jr, Director

3355 North Carolina Assistive Technology Project
1110 Navaho Drive
Suite 101
Raleigh, NC 27609
919-872-2298
FAX: 919-850-2792
e-mail: ncatp@minespring.com
www.ncatp.org

Ricki Cook, Project Director
Annette Lauber, Funding Specialist
Jacquelyne Gordon, Consumer Resource Specialist
The North Carolina Assistive Technology Project exists to create a statewide, consumer-responsive system of assistive technology services for all North Carolinians with disabilities. The project's activities impact children and adults with disabilities across all aspects of their lives.

3356 North Carolina Children & Youth Branch
North Carolina Publc of Health
1928 Mail Service Center
Raleigh, NC 27699
919-832-2839
FAX: 919-715-3187
e-mail: cathy.kluttz@nemail.net
www.nchealthychilderen.com

Carol Tant, Head Children/Youth Branch
Cathy Kluttz, Unit Manager Special Service
Dianne Tyson, Help Line Manager

3357 North Carolina Client Assistance Program
2806 Mail Service Center
Raleigh, NC 27699
919-855-3600
800-215-7227
FAX: 919-715-2456
e-mail: nccap@ncmail.net
cap.state.nc.us

Kathy Brack, Director
Frank Ashfield, Client Advocate
A federally funded program designed to assist individuals with disabilities in understanding and using rehabilitation services.

3358 North Carolina Developmental Disabilities
1001 Navaho Drive
Suite Gl103
Raleigh, NC 27609
919-850-2833
800-357-6916
FAX: 919-850-2895
e-mail: Holly.Riddle@ncmail.net
www.nc-ddc.org

Holly Riddle
A planning council established to assure that individuals with developmental disabilities and their families participate in the planning of and have access to culturally competent services, supports, and other assistance and opportunities that promote independence, productivity, and integration and inclusion into the community; and to promote, through systemic change, capacity building and advocacy activities, a consumer and family-centered comprehensive system.

3359 North Carolina Division of Aging
2101 Mail Service Center
Raleigh, NC 27699
919-733-3983
FAX: 919-733-0443
www.dhhs.state.nc.us/aging/home.htm

Karen Gottivi, Director

3360 North Carolina Industrial Commission
430 N Salisbury Street
Raleigh, NC 27603
919-733-3484
FAX: 919-715-0282
www.comp.state.nc.us

J Howard Bunn Jr, Chairman
Peg Dorer, Executive Director

3361 Social Security: Raleigh Disability Determination
4701 Old Wake Forest Road
Raleigh, NC 27609
919-790-2782
800-772-1213
FAX: 919-790-2773
TTY: 919-790-2773
e-mail: www.socialsecurity.gov
www.ssa.gov
Provides information on how to obtain social security through a disability.

North Dakota

3362 Division of Mental Health and Substance Abuse
1237 W Divide Avenue
Suite 1C
Bismarck, ND 58501
701-328-8920
800-755-2719
FAX: 701-328-8969
e-mail: dhsmhsas@nd.gov
www.nd.gov/humanservices

Jo Anne Hoesel, Director
Don Wright, Ass't. Director Substance Abuse
The Department of Human Services' Mental Health and Substance Abuse Services Division provides leadership for the planning, development, and oversight of a system of care for children, adults, and families with severe emotional disorders, mental illness, and/or substance abuse issues.

3363 North Dakota Workers Compensation Board
50 E Front Avenue
Bismarck, ND 58504
701-328-3800
800-777-5033
FAX: 701-329-9911
TTY: 701-328-3786
www.ndworkerscomp.com

Brent Edison, Director

3364 **North Dakota Client Assistance Program**
1237 W Divide Avenue
Suite 3
Bismarck, ND 58501
701-328-8947
800-207-6122
TTY:701-328-8968
e-mail: cap@state.nd.us
www.nd.gov/cap

Dennis Lyon, Chief Executive Officer
CAP assists clients and client applicants of North Dakota Vocational Rehabilitation services, Tribal Vocational Rehabilitation, or Independent Living services.

3365 **North Dakota Department of Aging**
600 E Boulevard Avenue
Dept 325
Bismarck, ND 58505
701-328-2455
800-451-8693
FAX: 701-328-4061
e-mail: dhsaging@state.nd.us
www.state.nd.us/humanservices/

Linda Wright, Director
Bryan Klipfel, Manager

3366 **North Dakota Department of Human Services**
600 E Boulevard Avenue
Dept 325
Bismarck, ND 58505
701-328-2310
800-472-2622
FAX: 701-328-3480
e-mail: dhseo@nd.gov
www.nd.gov/humanservices

Tamara Gallud-millner, Deputy Director
Provides services that help vulnerable North Dakotans of all ages to maintain or enhance their quality of life, which may be threatened by lack of financial resources, emotional crises, disabling conditions, or an inability to protect themselves. Also supports the provision of services and care as close to home as possible to maximize each person's independence while preserving the dignity of all individuals and respecting their constitutional and civil rights.

3367 **Protection & Advocacy Project**
1984
400 E Broadway Avenue
Suite 409
Bismarck, ND 58501
701-328-2950
800-472-2670
FAX: 701-328-3934
e-mail: panda@state.nd.us
www.ndpanda.org

Teresa Larsen, Executive Director
The Protection and Advocacy is a state agency whose purpose is to advocate for and protect the rights of people with disabilities. The Protection and Advocacy Project has programs to serve people with developmental disabilities, mental illnesses and other types of disabilities. The projects programs and services are free to eligible individuals.

3368 **Social Security: Bismarck Disability Determination**
1680 E Capitol Avenue
Bismarck, ND 58501
701-250-4200
800-772-1213
TTY:701-250-4620
www.ssa.gov

3369 **Workers Compensation Board North Dakota**
4007 State Street
Bismarck, ND 58503
701-328-3800

Ohio

3370 **Epilepsy Council of Greater Cincinnati**
895 Central Avenue
Suite 550
Cincinnati, OH 45202
513-721-2905
877-804-2241
FAX: 531-721-0799
e-mail: ecgc@fuse.net
www.epilespsyfoundation.org/cincinatti

Margie Frommeyer, Executive Director

3371 **International Dyslexia Association: Central Ohio Branch**
PO Box 16216
Columbus, OH 43216
614-899-5711
800-222-3123
e-mail: cybdischultz@columbus.rr.com
www.interdys.org

Cyndi Schultz, President
Provides free information and referral services for diagnosis and tutoring for parents, educators, physicians, and individuals with dyslexia. The voice of our membership is heard in 48 countries. Membership includes yearly journal and quarterly newsletter. Call for conference dates. Other locations available in Ohio state.

3372 **Ohio Bureau for Children with Medical Hand icaps**
Ohio Department of Health
PO Box 1603
Columbus, OH 43216
614-466-2115
800-755-4769
FAX: 614-728-3616
e-mail: bcmb@.odh.ohio.gov
www.odh.ohio.gov

James Bryant Md, Bureau Chief
Nick Baird, Director
Steven Kelley, Manager
Provides funding for the diagnosis, treatment and coordination of services for eligible Ohio children, under age 21, with medical handicaps; conducts quality assurance activities to establish standards of care and determine unmet needs of children with handicaps and their families; collaborates with public health nurses to increase access to care; and assists families to access and use third party resources. Conducts a separate program for adults with cystic fibrosis.

3373 **Ohio Bureau of Worker's Compensation**
30 W Spring Street
Columbus, OH 43215
800-644-6292
FAX: 877-520-6446
TTY:800-292-4833
e-mail: ombudsperson@bwc.state.oh.us
www.ohiobwc.com

William E Mabe, Administrator/CEO
To provide a quality, customer-focused workers' compensation insurance system for Ohio's employers and employees.

3374 **Ohio Client Assistance Program**
30 E Broad Street
Room 120
Columbus, OH 43215
614-466-6920
FAX: 614-752-4197

Donald Bishop, Executive Director

3375 **Ohio Department of Aging**
1982
50 W Broad Street
Floor 9
Columbus, OH 43215
614-466-5500
866-243-5678
888-243-5678
FAX: 614-466-5741
www.goldenbuckeye.com

Barbara E Riley, Director
John Ratliff, Public Information Officer
The department serves and represents about 2 million Ohioans age 60 & older. They advocate for the needs of all older citizens with emphasis on improving the quality of life, helping senior citizens live active, healthy, & independent lives, & promoting positive attitudes toward aging & older people. Committed to helping the frail elderly who choose to remain at home by providing home & community based services, their goal is to promote the level of choice, independence & self-care.

3376 Ohio Department of Mental Health
30 E Broad Street
Floor 8
Columbus, OH 43215
614-466-4775
877-275-6364
FAX: 614-466-1571
e-mail: uhricks@mh.state.oh.us
www.mh.state.oh.us

Michael Hogan, Director
Christine Vincenty, Manager

3377 Ohio Developmental Disability Council
8 E Long Street
12th Floor
Columbus, OH 43215
614-466-5205
800-766-7426
FAX: 614-466-0298
e-mail: david.zwyer@dmr.state.oh.us
www.ddc.ohio.gov

David Zwyer, Director
The Ohio Developmental Disabilities Council is one of 55 councils found in all states and territories which provides funding for systems change grant projects. The DD Council is a planning and advocacy agency that seeks to improve the lives of Ohioans with disabilities.

3378 Ohio Governor's Council on People with Disabilities
400 E Campus View Boulevard
Columbus, OH 43235
614-438-1393
800-282-4536
FAX: 614-438-1274
gcpd.ohio.gov

Robin Moore Cooper, Executive Committee Chair
Marcella Eblin, Secretary
The Governor's Council on People with Disabilities exists to: Advise the Governor and General Assembly on statewide disability issues, promote the value of diversity, dignity and the quality of life for people with disabilities, be a catalyst to create systemic change promoting awareness of disability-related issues that will ultimately benefit all citizens of Ohio, Educate and advocate for: partnerships at the local, state and national level, promotion of equality, access and independence.

3379 Ohio Legal Rights Service
8 E Long Street
5th Floor
Columbus, OH 43215
614-466-9956
800-282-9181
FAX: 614-448-8
www.state.oh.us/OLRS/

Carolyn Knight, Administrator

3380 Ohio Rehabilitation Services Commission
400 E Campus View Boulevard
Columbus, OH 43235
614-438-1200
800-282-4536
FAX: 614-438-1257
www.state.oh.us/rsc

John M Connelly, Executive Director
RSC is Ohio's state agency that provides vocational rehabilitation (VR) services to help people with disabilities become employed and independent. We also offer a variety of services to Ohio businesses, resulting in quality jobs for individuals who have disabilities.

3381 Social Security: Columbus Disability Determination
90 E Washington Bridge Road
Suite 160
Worthington, OH 43085
614-888-5339
800-772-1213
TTY:614-288-0226
www.socialsecurity.gov

Jo Anne B Barnhart, Commissioner
Mary B Chatel, Executive Director of Disability

3382 Workers Compensation Board Ohio
246 N High Street
Columbus, OH 43215
614-466-4110

Michele Frizzell, Manager

Oklahoma

3383 Oklahoma Workers Compensation Board
Department of Labor
400 N Lincon Boulevard
Oklahoma City, OK 73105
405-528-1500
888-269-5353
FAX: 405-528-5751
www.okdol.state.ok.us

Trey Davis, Chief of Staff
Brenda Reneau, Commissioner

3384 Oklahoma Client Assistance Program
2401 NW 23rd Street
Suite 90
Oklahoma City, OK 73107
405-521-3756
FAX: 405-522-6695
www.ohc.state.ok.us

James Sirmans, Director
Steve Stokes, Executive Director

3385 Oklahoma Department of Children with Disabilities
4001 N Lincoln Boulevard
4th Floor
Oklahoma City, OK 73105
405-521-2255
888-269-5353
FAX: 405-528-5751
www.okdol.state.ok.us

Trey Davis, Chief of Staff
Patrick McGuigun, Deputy Commissioner

3386 Oklahoma Department of Human Services Aging Services Division
PO Box 25352
Oklahoma City, OK 73125
405-521-2255
FAX: 405-521-2086
www.okdhs.org

Karey Garland, Director

3387 Oklahoma Department of Mental Health & Substance Abuse Services
PO Box 53277
Oklahoma City, OK 73152
405-522-3908
800-522-9054
FAX: 405-522-3650
www.odmhsas.org

Terry Cline PhD, Executive Director/Commissioner
State agency providing mental helath , substance abuse and domestic violence services.

3388 Oklahoma Department of Rehabilitation Services
3535 NW 58th Street
Suite 500
Oklahoma City, OK 73112
405-951-3400
800-845-8476
FAX: 405-951-3529
e-mail: jharlan@drs.state.ok.us
www.okrehab.org

Linda Parker, Executive Director
Jody Harlan, Public Information Administrator
Provides vocational rehabilitation, employment, education, independent living assistance and special services, and determines eligibility for disability benefits.

3389 Workers Compensation Board Oklahoma
1915 N Stiles Avenue
Oklahoma City, OK 73105
405-522-8600

Marcia Davis, Administrator

Oregon

3390 International Dyslexia Association: Oregon Branch
International Dyslexia Association
PO Box 3677
Portland, OR 97208
503-228-4455
800-530-2234
FAX: 503-228-3152
e-mail: info@orbida.org
www.orbida.org

Karen Brown, President
Charles Weswig, Vice President
Provides free information and referral services for diagnosis and tutoring for parents, educators, physicians, and individuals with dyslexia. The voice of our membership is heard in 48 countries. Membership includes yearly journal and quarterly newsletter. Call for conference dates.

3391 Office of Vocational Rehabilitation Servic es (OVRS)
500 Summer Street NE
E-87
Salem, OR 97301
503-945-5880
877-277-0513
FAX: 503-947-5025
TTY: 503-378-3933
www.oregon.gov/dhs/index.shtml

Stephaine Taylor, Administrator
Travis Wall, Planning and Program Manager
The mission of OVRS to assist Oregonians with disabilities to achieve and maintain employment and independence.

3392 Oregon Advocacy Center
620 SW 5th Avenue
5th Floor
Portland, OR 97204
503-243-2081
800-452-6094
FAX: 503-243-1738
e-mail: welcome@oradvocacy.org
www.oradvocacy.org

Robert Joondeph, Executive Director
Barbara Herget, Operations Director
The protection and advocacy system for Oregon.

3393 Oregon Client Assistance Program
620 SW 5th Avenue
Suite 500
Portland, OR 97204
503-243-2081
FAX: 503-243-1738
www.oradvocacy.org

Robert Joondeph, Executive Director

3394 Oregon Commission for the Blind
535 SE 12th Avenue
Portland, OR 97214
503-731-3221
888-202-5463
FAX: 503-731-3230
e-mail: linda.mock@state.or.us
www.cfb.state.or.us

Linda Mock, Administrator
Frank Armstrong, Representative of Blind Oregonia
Pat Donell, Executive Director

3395 Oregon Department of Mental Health
500 Summer Street NE
E86
Salem, OR 97301
503-945-5944
FAX: 503-945-5895
www.oregon.gov/DHS

Bob Nikkel, Assistant Director
Bruce Goldberg, Executive Director
Sets out the purpose and guides the activities of our large, complex organization. Vision is for better outcomes for clients and communities through collaboration, integration and shared responsibility.

3396 Oregon Technology Access for Life
3070 Lancaster Drive NE
Salem, OR 97305
503-361-1201
FAX: 503-370-4530
e-mail: info@accesstechnologiesinnc.com
www.accesstechnologiesinc.org

Laurie Brooks, Project Director
A statewide program promoting assistive technology devices and services for persons of all ages with all disabilities.

3397 Social Security: Salem Disability Determination
530 Center Street NE
Suite 30
Salem, OR 97301
800-722-1213
TTY:800-325-0778
www.socialsecurity.gov

Patrick P O'Caroll Jr, Inspector General

3398 Washington County Disability, Aging and Veteran Services
133 S East Second Avenue
Hillsboro, OR 97123
503-640-3489
FAX: 503-693-6124
www.co.washington.or.us/aging

Mary Lou Ritter, Director

Pennsylvania

3399 International Dyslexia Association: Pennsylvania Branch
PO Box 251
Bryn Mawr, PA 19010
610-527-1548
800-ABC-D123
FAX: 610-527-5011
e-mail: dyslexia@pbida.org
www.pbida.org

Jack Rogers, President
Mary Ellen Trent, Office Manager
Amy Ress, Manager
Provides free information and referral services for diagnosis and tutoring for parents, educators, physicians, and individuals with dyslexia. The voice of membership is heard in 48 countries. Membership includes yearly journal and quarterly newsletter, and Pennsylvania newsletter; discounts to conferences and events.

3400 Mental Health Association in Pennysylvania
1414 N Cameron Street
Harrisburg, PA 17103
717-236-8110
800-692-7443
FAX: 717-236-0192
e-mail: swalther@paonline.com
www.ttpinc.org

Ilene Shane, Executive Director

3401 Pennsylvania Workers Compensation Board
1171 S Cameron Street
Room 103
Harrisburg, PA 17104
717-939-9551
FAX: 717-772-0342

Joseph Brimmeier, Chief Executive Officer

3402 Pennsylvania Bureau of Blindness
Department of Pennsylvania
1621 N 6th Street
Harrisburg, PA 17102
717-236-3610
800-622-2842
FAX: 717-787-3210
www.dli.state.pa.us

Pamela Shaw, Director
Alfred Baker, President
Offers services for the totally blind, legally blind, visually impaired, mentally retarded blind and more with health, counseling, educational, recreational, rehabilitation, computer training and professional training services.

3403 Pennsylvania Client Assistance Program
1617 JFK Boulevard
Suite 800
Philadelphia, PA 19103
215-557-7112
888-745-2357
FAX: 215-557-7602
e-mail: info@equalemployment.org
www.equalemployment.org

Stephen S Pennington, Executive Director
Jamie C Ray, Assistant Director
The Pennsylvania Client Assistance Program is dedicated to ensuring that the rehabilitation system in Pennsylvania is open and responsive to your needs. CAP help is provided to you at no charge, regardless of income. CAP helps people who are seeking services from the Office of Vocational Rehabilitation, Blindness and Visual Services, Centers for Independent Living and other programs funded under federal law.

3404 Pennsylvania Department of Aging
555 Walnut Street
5th Floor
Harrisburg, PA 17101
717-783-1550
FAX: 717-783-6842
e-mail: aging@state.pa.us
www.aging.state.pa.us

Nora Dowd Eisenhower, Secretary

3405 Pennsylvania Department of Children with Disabilities
PO Box 90
Harrisburg, PA 17108
717-783-1289
FAX: 717-772-0323

Donna Wenger, Acting Director
Frank Maisano, Manager

3406 Pennsylvania Developmental Disabilities Council
569 Forum Building
Harrisburg, PA 17120
717-939-9551
FAX: 717-772-0738
e-mail: paddpc@aol.com

Graham Mulholland, Executive Director
Joseph Brimmeier, Chief Executive Officer

3407 Pennsylvania Protection & Advocacy for Persons with Disabilities
1414 N Cameron Street
Harrisburg, PA 17103
717-236-8110
800-692-7443
FAX: 717-236-0192
e-mail: ppa@ppaninc.org
www.ppainc.org

Ilene Shane, Executive Director
Provide advocacy, information and referral for persons with disabilities and mental illness issues.

3408 Public Interest Law Center of Philadelphia
125 S 9th Street
Suite 700
Philadelphia, PA 19107
215-627-7100
FAX: 215-627-3183
e-mail: pobint@aol.com

Michael Churchill, Chief Counsel
Judith Gramd, Director
A non-profit, public interest law firm with a Disabilities Project specializing in class action suits brought by individuals and organizations.

3409 Social Security: Harrisburg Disability Determination
555 Walnut Street
Harrisburg, PA 17101
717-782-3400
800-722-1213
TTY:717-783-8917
e-mail: ovr@dli.state.pa.us
www.ssa.gov

Susan Aldrete, Executive Director

3410 Workers Compensation Board Pennsylvania
1171 S Cameron Street
Room 103
Harrisburg, PA 17104
717-783-5421
800-482-2383
FAX: 717-772-0342
e-mail: ra-li-bwc-helpline@state.pa.us
www.dli.state.pa.us

John J Kupchinsky, Director

Rhode Island

3411 Department of Mental Health, Retardation and Hospitals of Rhode Island
Goverment of Rhode Isalnd
14 Harrington Road
Cranston, RI 02920
401-462-3201
FAX: 401-462-3204
www.mhrh.state.ri.us www.nhirh.ri.gov

Cathleen M Stanglei, Acting Director
Kathleen Spangler, Manager
State department responsible for creating and administering systems of care for individuals with disabilities, specifically focused on mental health and mental illness; developmental disabilities, substance abuse and long term hospital care.

3412 Rhode Island Department Health
3 Capitol Hl
Providence, RI 02908
401-222-2231
FAX: 401-222-6548
e-mail: library@doh.state.ri.us
www.health.state.ri.us

David R Gifford, Director
Patricia Nolan, Executive Director
Pamela Corcoran, Disability Health Program

3413 **Rhode Island Department of Elderly Affairs**
35 Howard Avenue
Cranston, RI 02920
401-462-3000
FAX: 401-222-3389
e-mail: larry@dea.state.ri.us
www.dea.state.ri.us

Corinne Cali Russo, Director

3414 **Rhode Island Department of Mental Health**
Cottage 405 Court B
Cranston, RI 02920
401-467-9200
FAX: 401-464-2005

Reed Cosper, Director
Robert Emerson, President

3415 **Rhode Island Developmental Disabilities Council**
400 Bald Hill Road
Suite 515
Warwick, RI 02886
401-732-3240
FAX: 401-737-3395
e-mail: riddc@riddc.org
www.riddc.org

Marie Citrone, Executive Director
Don Ouelette, Manager
The Rhode Island Developmental Disabilities Council works to make Rhode Island a better place for people with developmental disabilities to live, work, go to school, and be part of their community.

3416 **Rhode Island Governor's Commission on Disabilities**
John O Pastore Center
41 Cherrydale Court
Cranston, RI 02920
401-462-0100
FAX: 401-462-0106
e-mail: disabilities@gcd.state.ri.gov
www.disabilities.ri.gov

Bob Cooper, Executive Secretary
The Commision is responsible for: coordinating compliance by state agencies with federal and state disablity right laws; approving or modifying state and local goverment agency's open meeting accessibility for persons with disabilities transition plans; assisting local boards of canvassers to ensure accessible polling places locations; aproving or rejecting requests to waive the state building code's standards for accessibility at facilities to be leased by state agencies...

3417 **Rhode Island Parent Information Network**
175 Main Street
Unit 1
Pawtucket, RI 02860
401-727-4040
800-464-3399
FAX: 401-727-4040
e-mail: ripin@ripin.org
www.ripin.org

Vivian Weisman, Executive Director
Matthew Cox, Associate Exeutive Director
A nonprofit organization established by parents and concerned professionals providing culturally appropriate information, training and support for families and professionals designed to improve educational and life outcomes for all children. Serving the State of Rhode Island.

3418 **Rhode Island Protection & Advocacy for Persons with Disabilities**
Rhode Island Disability Law Center
349 Eddy Street
Providence, RI 02903
401-831-3150
FAX: 401-274-5568
e-mail: info@ridlc.org
www.ridlc.org

Raymond Bandusky, Executive Director

3419 **Rhode Island Services for the Blind and Visually Impaired**
40 Fountain Street
Providence, RI 02903
401-222-2300
800-752-8088
FAX: 401-222-1328
TTY: 401-277-3010
e-mail: thompson@ors.state.ri.us
www.ors.ri.gov

Raymond Carroll, Administrator
Stephen Brunero, Deputy Administrator
Offers services for the totally blind, legally blind, visually impaired, mentally retarded blind and more with health, counseling, educational, recreational, rehabilitation, computer training and professional training services.

3420 **Services for the Blind and Visually Impaired**
40 Fountain Street
Providence, RI 02903
401-222-2300
FAX: 401-222-1328
www.ors.ri.gov

Gary Wier, Deputy Administrator
Raymond Carroll, Administrator
Offers services for the blind and visually impaired.

3421 **Social Security: Providence Disability Determination**
Social Security
380 Westminster Street
3rd Floor
Providence, RI 02903
401-528-4501
800-772-1213
FAX: 401-273-6648
TTY: 401-273-6648
www.ssa.gov

John J Corson, Director

3422 **Workers Compensation Board Rhode Island**
1 Dorrance Plaza
Providence, RI 02903
401-458-5000
FAX: 401-421-3123

John Sabatini, Administrator
George Healy Jr, Manager

South Carolina

3423 **Protection & Advocacy for People with Disabilities**
3710 Landmark Drive
Suite 208
Columbia, SC 29204
803-782-0639
866-275-7273
FAX: 803-790-1946
e-mail: info@protectionandadvocacy-sc.org

Anne Trice, Director Administration
Gloria Prevost, Executive Director
An independent, nonprofit organization responsible for safe guarding rights of South Carolinians with disabilities and other handicapped individuals without regard to age, income, severity of disability, sex, race, or religion.

3424 **Social Security: West Columbia Disability Determination**
1835 Assembly Street
Columbia, SC 29201
803-929-7635
800-772-1213
TTY:800-325-0078
www.socialsecurity.gov

3425 **South Carolina Assistive Technology Project**
University of South Carolina
Columbia, SC 29208
803-779-0343
FAX: 803-935-5342
TTY:803-935-5263
e-mail: jjendron@usit.net
www.sc.edu/scatp/

Evelyn Evans, Project Director
Marie Queen, Executive Director
Mary Alice Bechtler, Program Coordinator
A statewide program promoting assistive technology devices and services for persons of all ages with all disabilities. Recently a statewide AT resource, demonstrations and equipment loan center and lab annual expo and training and workshops on a variety of disabilities and technology topics.

3426 **South Carolina Client Assistance Program**
Governor's Office oe Executive Policy & Programs
1205 Pendleton Street
Columbia, SC 29201
803-734-0285
FAX: 803-734-0546
TTY:803-734-1147
e-mail: lbarker@govpoepp.state.ce.us
www.govoepp.state.sc.us/cap

Larry Barker PhD, Director
The Client Assistance Program (CAP) helps citizens of the State by acting as advocates regarding services provided by the Vocational Rehabilitation Department (VR), Commission for the Blind, and all Independent Living programs and projects funded under the Rehabilitation Act of 1973. As advocates, CAP staff can investigate, negotiate, mediate, and pursue administrative, and other remedies to ensure that clients' rights are protected.

3427 **South Carolina Commission for the Blind**
PO Box 79
Columbia, SC 29202
803-733-8100
800-922-2222
FAX: 803-898-8852
www.sccb.state.sc.us

Nell Carney Md, Commissioner
Linda Johnston, Secretary
Clente Flemming, President
Offers services for the totally blind, legally blind, visually impaired, mentally retarded blind and more with health, counseling, educational, recreational, rehabilitation, computer training and professional training services.

3428 **South Carolina Department of Children with Disabilities**
2600 Bull Street
Columbia, SC 29201
803-898-2038

Ann Lee, Director
Peter Getz, Administrator

3429 **South Carolina Department of Mental Health and Mental Retardation**
PO Box 485
Columbia, SC 29202
803-898-8581
FAX: 803-898-8316
www.state.sc.us/dmh

Maureen Donnelly, Director
John J Connery, State Director

3430 **South Carolina Developmental Disabilities Council**
Office of the Governor
1205 Pendleton Street
Suite 450
Columbia, SC 29201
803-734-0465
FAX: 803-734-0465
TTY:803-734-1147
e-mail: jjennings@oepp.sc.gov
www.scddc.state.sc.us

Charles Lang, Executive Director
Jennifer Jennings, Program Information Coordinator
The mission of the South Carolina Developmental Disabilities Council is to provide leadership in advocating, funding and implementing initiatives which recognize the inherent dignity of each individual, and promote independence, productivity, respect and inclusion for all persons with disabilities and their families.

3431 **South Carolina Services Information System**
University of South Carolina
Columbia, SC 29208
803-935-5300
800-922-1107
FAX: 803-935-5342
e-mail: ddsnweb@ddsn.sc.gov
www.state.sc.us/ddsn/pubs/scsis/scsis.htm

Denise Rivers, Program Director
SCSIS provides information on aging and disability services in the State of South Carolina. Also, has a used equipment referral exchange where buyers and sellers are matched.

3432 **Workers Compensation Board: South Carolina**
PO Box 1715
Columbia, SC 29202
803-737-5700
FAX: 803-737-5764
e-mail: Gary
www.state.sc.us/wcc

Gary Thibault, Executive Director

South Dakota

3433 **South Dakota Advocacy Services**
221 S Central Avenue
Pierre, SD 57501
605-224-8294
800-658-4782
FAX: 605-224-5125
e-mail: sdas@sdadvocacy.com
www.sdadvocacy.com

Robert J Kean, Executive Director
Designated protection and advocacy progam for South Dakota providing legal, administrative, mediation and other services to elgible persons with disabilities in the state.

3434 **South Dakota Department of Aging**
700 Governors Drive
Pierre, SD 57501
605-773-3656
866-854-5465
FAX: 605-773-6834
www.state.sd.us/social/asa

Gail Ferris, Executive Director

3435 **South Dakota Department of Children's Special Health Services**
South Dakota State Department of Health
615 E 4th Street
Pierre, SD 57501
605-773-3011
800-305-3064
FAX: 605-773-5683
e-mail: barb.hemmelman@state.sd.us
www.state.sd.us/boh

Kayla Tinker, Office Director
Barb Hemmelman, Director
Gail Gray, Manager

3436 **South Dakota Department of Human Services Division of Mental Health**
South Dakota of Human Services
500 E Capitol Avenue
Pierre, SD 57501
605-000-1111
800-265-9684
FAX: 605-773-7076
e-mail: infomh@dhs.state.sd.us
www.state.sd.us/dhs/dmh

Jeff Peirce, Manager
Amy Iversen-Pollreisz, Director
Jennifer Fahey-Seale, Adult Svcs Program Specialist

3437 **South Dakota Developmental Disability Council**
Hillsview Plaza E Highway 34
Pierre, SD 57501
605-000-1111
FAX: 605-773-5483
e-mail: info@ddc
www.state.sd.us/dhs/ddc

Arlene Poncelet, Director
Jeff Pierce, Manager
To assist individuals with developmental disabilities to control their own destiny and to achieve the quality of life they desire.

3438 South Dakota Division of Rehabilitation
700 Governors Drive
Pierre, SD 57501
605-773-3423
FAX: 605-773-5483

David Miller, Director
Patrick Keating, Manager
Offers diagnosis, evaluation and physical restoration services, counseling, social work, educational and professional training, employment and rehabilitation services for the disabled.

3439 Workers Compensation Board: South Dakota
700 Governors Drive
Pierre, SD 57501
605-773-3681
FAX: 605-773-4211
e-mail: jamesmarsh@state.sd.us
www.sdjobs.org

James Marsh, Executive Director

Tennessee

3440 International Dyslexia Association: Tennessee Branch
3508 Hackworth Road
Knoxville, TN 37931
877-836-6432
800-222-3123
FAX: 865-693-3653
e-mail: tennessee_IDA@hotmail.com
www.tn-interdys.org

Martie Wood, President
The Tennessee Branch of the International Dyslexia Association (TN-IDA) was formed to increase awareness about Dyslexia in the state of Tennessee. TN-IDA supports efforts to provide information regarding appropriate language arts instruction to those involved with language-based learning differences and to encourage the identity of these individuals at-risk for such disorders as soon as possible.

3441 Social Security: Nashville Disability Determination
Social Security
4527 Nolensville Pike
Nashville, TN 37211
615-781-5800
800-772-1213
FAX: 615-781-5836
www.ssa.gov

3442 Tennessee Assistive Technology Projects
Doctor S Building
300
Nashville, TN 37243
615-322-1210

Eh Buddy White
Julie Oden, Manager
A statewide program promoting assistive technology devices and services for persons of all ages with all disabilities.

3443 Tennessee Client Assistance Program
Tennessee Protection and Advocacy
PO Box 121257
Nashville, TN 37212
615-298-1080
800-342-1660
FAX: 615-298-2046
e-mail: gethelp@tpainc.org
www.tpainc.org

Shirley Shea, Executive Director
Doris Lopez, Assistant Executive Director

3444 Tennessee Commission on Aging and Disability
500 Deaderick Street
8th Floor
Nashville, TN 37243
615-741-2056
FAX: 615-741-3309
e-mail: tnaging.tnaging@state.tn.us
www.state.tn.us/comaging

Kathy Zamata, Assistant Director
LaVerdia McCulloagh, Information/Assistant Coord.

3445 Tennessee Council on Developmental Disabilities
Parkway Towers Suite 130
404 James Robertson Pkwy
Nashville, TN 37243
615-532-6615
FAX: 615-532-6964
e-mail: tnddc@state.tn.us
www.state.tn.us/odd

Wanda Willis, Executive Director
Provides leadership to ensure independence, productivity, integration and inclusion of individuals with disabilities in the community through promotion of systems change. The council works with members of the community, including public and private aencies, business, legislators and policymakers, to create a future in which; people with disabilities are full included in the community and experience no barriers related to attitudes about their disabilities as they persue their goals.

3446 Tennessee Department of Children with Disabilities
436 6th Avenue N
Room 525
Nashville, TN 37243
615-741-0466

Judy Womack, Director
Haticile Buchanan, Manager

3447 Tennessee Department of Mental Health and Developmental Disabilities
425 5th Avenue N
Nashville, TN 37243
615-741-7213
FAX: 615-532-6514
e-mail: kay.horner@state.tn.us
www.state.tn.us/mental

Virginia Trotter Betts, Commissioner
Jill Hudson, Press Officer
Suzanne Hubbard, Executive Director

3448 Tennessee Division of Rehabilitation
400 Deaderick Street
Nashville, TN 37243
615-248-4996

Patsy Matthews, Commissioner
Randall Beasley, Manager
Offers rehabilitation, medical and therapeutic information and referrals to the disabled.

3449 Workers Compensation Board Tennessee
710 James Robertson Parkway
Nashville, TN 37243
615-741-2395
FAX: 615-532-5929
www.state.tn.us/labor-wfd/wcomp.html

Sueanne Head, Administrator

Texas

3450 Disability Policy Consortium
7800 Shoal Creek Boulevard
Suite 171e
Austin, TX 78757
512-454-4816
FAX: 512-458-9202
e-mail: dpctexas@advocacyinc.org
www.dpctexas.org

Mary Faithfull, Executive Director
Jonas Schwartz, Manager
An independent group of statewide advocacy organizations that strives to achieve the development and full implementation of public policy that promotes and supports the rights, inclusion, integration and independence of Texans with disabilities.

3451 Division of Special Education
1701 Congress Avenue
Austin, TX 78701
512-463-9414
FAX: 512-463-9560
e-mail: spedfrontdesk@tea.state.tx.us
www.tea.state.tx.us

Gene Lenz, Deputy Associate Commissioner
Kathy Clayton, Senior Director

3452 Easter Seal of Greater Dallas, TX
4443 N Josey Lane
Carrollton, TX 75010
972-394-8900
800-580-4718
www.easterseals.com

Elizabeth Hart, President/CEO
Bob Painter, Vice President
Nancy Hitzfelder, MD

3453 Easter Seals Greater NW Texas
2100 Circle Drive
Fort Worth, TX 76119
817-536-8693
888-288-8324
e-mail: info@easterseals.fw.org

Monica Crather, Chief Executive Officer

3454 El Valle Community Parent Resource Center
530 S Texas Boulevard
Suite J
Weslaco, TX 78596
956-969-3611
800-680-0255
e-mail: texasfiestaedu.org
www.tfepodder.org

Laura Reagan, Project Coordinator

3455 Grassroots Consortium
Greenroots Consortium
6202 Belmark Street
Houston, TX 77087
713-643-9576
FAX: 713-643-6291
Speckids@aol.com

Agnes A Johnson, Director

3456 International Dyslexia Association: Austin Branch
PO Box 92604
Austin, TX 78709
512-452-7658
800-222-3123
e-mail: info@interdys.org
www.interdys.org

Sharon McMichael, President
The Austin Area Branch of the International Dyslexia Association is a 501(c)(3) non profit organization dedicated to promoting reading excellence for all children through early identification of dyslexia, effective literacy education for adults and children with dyslexia, and teacher training.

3457 NAMI Texas
2800 S i H 35
Suite 140
Austin, TX 78704
512-693-2000
800-633-3760
FAX: 512-693-8000
e-mail: namitexas@texami.org
www.tx.nami.org

Joe Lovelace, Executive Director
NAMI Texas has a variety of programs directed to mental health consumers, family members, friends, professionals, other stake holders and the community at large to address the mental health needs of Texans. NAMI Texas works to inform the public about mental illness by distributing information about mental illness through every means of communication. Interviews are produced on television, stories are featured in newspapers, brochures are distributed, referrals are provided and more.

3458 Parent Connection
1020 Riverwood Court
Conroe, TX 77304
936-756-8321
800-839-8876
ParentCNCT@aol.com

3459 Parents Supporting Parents Network
601 N Texas Boulevard
Suite C
Weslaco, TX 78596
956-447-8408
888-857-8668
FAX: 956-973-9503
e-mail: cbtjr1@aol.com
www.thearcoftexas.org

Mike Bright, Executive Director
Rona Statman, Assistant Director
Leticia Padilla, Manager

3460 Partners Resource Network
1090 Longfellow Drive
Suite B
Beaumont, TX 77706
409-898-4684
800-866-4726
e-mail: path@partnerstx.org
www.PartnersTx.org

Leslie Vasquez, Program Director
Mary Ellen Peterson, Chief Executive Director
Janice Meyer, Executive Director

3461 Social Security: Austin Disability Determination
903 San Jacinto Boulevard
Austin, TX 78701
512-916-5404
800-772-1213
TTY:512-916-5958
www.ssa.gov

3462 Statewide Information at Texas School for the Deaf
1102 S Congress Avenue
Austin, TX 78704
512-462-5329
800-DEA-FTSD
FAX: 512-462-5663
e-mail: ercod@tsd.state.tx.us
www.tsd.state.tx.us

Betty Bounds, Director of Instructions
Claire Bugen, Superintendent

3463 Texas Advocates Supporting Kids with Disabilities
PO Box 162685
Austin, TX 78716
512-310-2102
FAX: 512-310-2102
e-mail: ASKTASK@aol.com
www.main.org/task/

3464 Texas Commission for the Blind
PO Box 12866
Austin, TX 78711
512-459-2500
800-252-5204
FAX: 512-459-2685

Terrell I Murphy, Executive Director
Offers services for the totally blind, legally blind, and visually impaired, with counseling, educational, recreational, rehabilitation, computer training and professional training services.

3465 Texas Commission for the Deaf and Hard of Hearing
D AR S
PO Box 12904
Austin, TX 78711
512-407-3250
FAX: 512-407-3299
TTY:512-407-3251
e-mail: david.meyers@tcdhh.state.tx.us
www.dars.state.tx.us

David Meyers, Assistant Director

3466 Texas Council for Developmental Disabilities
6201 E Oltorf Street
Suite 600
Austin, TX 78741
512-437-5432
800-262-0334
FAX: 512-437-5434
TTY: 512-437-5431
e-mail: tcdd@tcdd.state.tx.us
www.txddc.state.tx.us

Roger Webb, Executive Director
Carl Risinger, Operations Director
The Texas Council for Developmental Disabilities is a 27-member board dedicated to ensuring that all Texans with developmental disabilities, about 411,479 individuals, have the opportunity to be independent, productive and valued members of their communities. The mission of the Texas Council for Developmental Disabilities is to create change so that all people with disabilities are fully included in their communities and exercise control over their own lives.

3467 Texas Department of Human Services
701 W 51st Street
Austin, TX 78751
512-438-3011
888-834-7406
TTY:888-425-6889
e-mail: mail@dads.state.tx.us
www.dads.state.tx.us

Jim Hine, Division Director
Carlela Vogel, Vice Chair

3468 Texas Department of Mental Health & Mental Retardation
PO Box 12668
Austin, TX 78711
512-438-3011
FAX: 512-206-4560
www.mhmr.state.tx.us

Eduardo J Sanchez, Commissioner
Randy Fritz, Chief Operating Officer
Offers information and referrals.

3469 Texas Department on Aging
701 W 51st Street
Austin, TX 78751
512-438-3200
800-252-9240
e-mail: mail@tdoa.state.tx.us
www.dadds.state.tx.us

James Hine, Executive Director
John Willis, Director Ombudsman
Karl Urban, Deputy Director
The state's visible advocate and steward for a full range of services and opportunities that allow older Texans to live healthy, dignified and independent lives.

3470 Texas Federation of Families for Children's Mental Health
7701 N Lamar Boulevard
Suite 505
Austin, TX 78752
512-407-8844
866-893-3264
FAX: 512-407-8266
e-mail: info@txffcmh.org
www.txffcmh.org

Patti Derr, Executive Director
Pat Calley, Chairperson
S Barron, Director Operations
Texas Federation of Families for Children's Mental Health is an organization comprised of family members of with emotional, behavioral and mental health needs; supporting families and youth through advocacy, links to resources and training.

3471 Texas Governor's Committee on People with Disabilities
1100 San Jacinto Boulevard
Austin, TX 78701
512-463-5739
FAX: 513-463-5745
e-mail: ppound@governor.state.tx.us
www.governor.state.tx.us/disabilities

Pat Pound, Executive Director

3472 Texas Protection & Advocacy Services for Disabled Persons
Advocacy
7800 Shoal Creek Boulevard
Suite 171e
Austin, TX 78757
512-454-4816
800-252-9108
FAX: 512-323-0902
e-mail: infoai@advocacyinc.org
www.advocacyinc.org

Mary Faithfull, Executive Director
Shirley R DeBerry, Executive Assistant
Jonas Schwartz, Manager
A federally funded, independent, nonprofit agency that advocates for the legal, human and service rights of persons with disabilities. Publishes "Special Edition" newsletter, at a small fee and "It's a Good Idea!" a parent manual for $10, plus many other handouts free of charge.

3473 Texas Respite Resource Network
Station A
PO Box 7330
San Antonio, TX 78207
512-228-2794

e-mail: elizabethnewhouse@srhcc.org

Jennifer Cernoch, Director
Liz Newhouse, Assistant Director
A state clearinghouse and technical assistance network for respite in Texas. TRRN identifies, initiates and improves respite options for families caring for individuals with disabilities on the local, state and national levels. TRRN provides training/technical assistance to programs/groups wanting to establish respite services.

3474 Texas Technology Access Project
Center for Disabilities Studies
4030 W Braker Lane
Building 2
Austin, TX 78759
512-482-8682
800-828-7839
FAX: 512-232-0761
TTY: 512-232-0762
e-mail: john.moore@mail.utexas.edu
tatp.edb.utexas.edu/

John Moore, Project Director
Provides information, conducts training and technical assistance and works with policy makers to support children and adults with disabilities.

3475 Texas UAP for Developmental Disabilities
University of Texas
430 W Braker Lane
Building 2
Austin, TX 78753
512-471-4822
800-828-7839
FAX: 512-232-0761
e-mail: pseay@mail.utexas.edu
www.utexas.edu

Penny Seay, Executive Director
Bob Harkins, Manager

3476 Texas Workers Compensation Commission
4000 S Ih 35
Austin, TX 78704
512-804-4000
FAX: 512-440-3547

Robert Shipe, Executive Director

3477 **United Cerebral Palsy of Texas**
National Cerebral Palsy of American
5555 N Lamar Boulevard
Suite L139
Austin, TX 78751
512-472-8696
800-798-1492
FAX: 512-472-8026
e-mail: info@ucpa.org
www.ucpa.org

Jean Langendorf, Executive Director

Utah

3478 **Access Utah Network**
155 S 300 W
Suite 100
Salt Lake City, UT 84101
801-533-4636
800-333-8824
FAX: 801-533-3968
e-mail: access@utah.gov
www.accessut.org

Cecilia Giron, Information Specialist
Mark Smtih, Information Specialist I/Manager

3479 **Social Security: Salt Lake City Disability Determination**
Social Security
202 W 400 S
Salt Lake City, UT 84101
801-524-4115
800-772-1213
TTY:801-524-5047
www.ssa.gov

Wilkes R Barre, Program Director

3480 **Utah Assistive Technology Projects**
Utah State University
6855 Old Main Hl
Logan, UT 84322
435-797-0037
e-mail: garthe@coe.usu.edu

Marvin Fifield, Director
Dan Peterson, Manager
A statewide program promoting assistive technology devices and services for persons of all ages with all disabilities.

3481 **Utah Client Assistance Program**
205205 N 400 W
Salt Lake City, UT 84103
801-363-1347
800-662-9080
FAX: 801-363-1437
e-mail: info@disabilitieslawcenter
www.disabilitylawcenter.org

Nancy Friel, Chief of Client Assistance Progr
Fraser Nelson, Executive Director

3482 **Utah Department of Aging**
120 N 200 W
Salt Lake City, UT 84103
801-538-3910
877-424-4640
FAX: 801-538-4395
e-mail: dirdhs@utah.gov
www.hsdaas.utah.gov

Alan Ormsby, Director
Terri Ruesch, Assistant Director

3483 **Utah Department of Human Services: Division of Services for People with Disabilities**
Utah Department of Human Services
120 N 200 W
Room 411
Salt Lake City, UT 84103
801-538-4200
800-837-6811
FAX: 801-538-4279
e-mail: dirdhs@utah.gov
www.hsdspd.utah.gov

George Kelner, Executive Director
Paul Day, Associate Director
Information and referral services for people with disabilities, including DD/MR, brain injury and physical disabilities throughout the state of Utah.

3484 **Utah Department of Mental Health**
Utah Department of Human Services
120 N 200 W
Room 209
Salt Lake City, UT 84103
801-538-3939
FAX: 801-538-9892
www.hsmh.state.ut.us

James Ashworth, Chairman
Michael Crookston, Vice Chairman
Mark Payne, Manager

3485 **Utah Division of Services for the Disabled**
660 S 200 E
Suite 400
Salt Lake City, UT 84111
801-238-4560
800-284-1823
FAX: 801-359-5627

Wayne Peterson, Director
Don Uchida, Assistant Director
Bonnie Williams, Executive Director
Offers services for the totally blind, legally blind, visually impaired, mentally retarded blind and more with health, counseling, educational, recreational, rehabilitation, computer training and professional training services.

3486 **Utah Governor's Council for People with Disabilities**
155 S 300 W
Suite 100
Salt Lake City, UT 84101
801-533-4636
FAX: 801-533-3968
e-mail: alozano@utah.gov
www.gcpd.org/

Allison Lozano, Executive Director
Angela Allen, Administrative Secretary
Mark Smith, Manager

3487 **Utah Labor Commission**
160 East 300 South, Third Floor
PO Box 146630
Salt Lake City, UT 84114
801-530-6801
800-222-1238
FAX: 801-530-7609
e-mail: hmorrison@utah.gov
www.laborcommission.utah.gov

Shernie Hayashi, Labor Commissioner
Alan Hennebold, Deputy Commisioner
Heather Morrison, Director, Anti-Discrimination

3488 **Utah Protection & Advocacy Services for Persons with Disabilities**
Disability Law Center
205 N 400 W
Salt Lake City, UT 84103
801-363-1347
800-662-9080
FAX: 801-363-1437
e-mail: info@disabilitylawcenter.org
www.disabilitylawcenter.org

Fraser Nelson, Executive Director
Rob Denton Esq, Senior Attorney
Eric Dmitchell, Advocacy Director

Vermont

3489 **Disability Law Project**
57 N Main Street
Rutland, VT 05701
802-775-0021
800-769-7459
FAX: 802-775-0022
e-mail: nbreiden@vtlegalaid.org
www.vtlegalaid.org

Tom Garrett, Executive Director
Rachel Corey, Office Manager
Robert Clark, Manager
Legal services (protection and advocacy) for people with disabilities on legal issues arising from disability. Statewide. Adults and children. Employment, education, discrimination, housing, public benefits, health care.

3490 **Social Security: Vermont Disability Determination Services**
93 Pilgrim Park Road
Suite 6
Waterbury, VT 05676
802-241-2463
800-734-2463
FAX: 802-241-2492
www.ssa.gov

Trudy Lyon-Hart, Executive Director

3491 **Vermont Assistive Technology Projects**
103 S Main Street
Weeks Building
Waterbury, VT 05671
802-241-2620
800-750-6355
FAX: 802-241-2174
TTY: 802-241-1464
e-mail: atinfo@dail.state.vt.us
www.dad.state.vt.us/atp

Julie L Tucker, Project Director
Betsy Ross, Administrative Assistant
Increase awareness and change policies to insure assistive technology (AT) is available to all Vermonters with disabilities. Our Commitment is to enable Vermonters with disabilities to have greater independence, productivity, and confidence. To provide them with a clear and direct avenue toward integration and inclusion within the work force and community.

3492 **Vermont Client Assistance Program**
57 N Main Street
Rutland, VT 05701
802-775-0021
800-769-7459
www.vocrehabvermont.org/html/clientassistance

Patrick Flood, Commissioner
The Client Assistance Program (CAP) is an independent advocacy program to help if you are applying for or receiving services from one of the following sources: Division of Vocational Rehabilitation (VR); Vermont Center for Independent Living (VCIL); Division for the Blind and Visually Impaired (DBVI); Vermont Association of Business, Industry & Rehabilitation (VABIR); Vermont Association for the Blind and Visually Impaired (VABVI); Supported Employment Programs; Transition Programs.

3493 **Vermont Department of Aging**
103 S Main Street
Waterbury, VT 05671
802-241-2400

Patrick Flood, Manager

3494 **Vermont Department of Developmental and**
103 S Main Street
Waterbury, VT 05671
802-241-2614

Theresa Wood, Manager

3495 **Vermont Department of Disabilities, Aging and Independent Living**
Aging and Disabilities
103 S Main Street
Waterbury, VT 05671
802-241-2401
FAX: 802-241-2325
www.dad.state.vt.us

Patrick Flood, Commissioner

3496 **Vermont Department of Health: Children with Special Health Needs**
Vermont Department Of Health
PO Box 70
Burlington, VT 05402
802-863-7338
FAX: 802-863-7635
www.healthy.vermonters.org

Carol Hassler MD, Director
Steve Brooks, Administrator
Multidisciplinary clinics and family support for children with chronic conditions, birth to age 21 years.

3497 **Vermont Developmental Disabilities Council**
103 S Main Street
Waterbury, VT 05671
082-241-2220

e-mail: vtddc@upgate1.ahs.state.vt.us
www.ahs.state.vt.us/vtddc

Cynthia D LaWare, Secretary
The mission of VTDDC is to facilitate connections and to promote supports that bring people with developmental disabilities into the heart of Vermont Communities.

3498 **Vermont Division for the Blind and Visually Impaired**
103 S Main Street
Weeks IC, Room 109
Waterbury, VT 05671
802-241-2210
888-405-5005
FAX: 802-241-2128
e-mail: vtblind_request@lists.dad.state.vt.us
www.dad.state.vt.us/dbvi

Fred Jones, Director
Scott Langley, Program Service Chief
Offers services for the totally blind, legally blind, visually impaired, mentally retarded blind and more with health, counseling, educational, recreational, rehabilitation, computer training and professional training services.

3499 **Vermont Division of Disability & Aging Services**
103 S Main Street
Waterbury, VT 05671
802-241-2614
FAX: 802-241-4224
www.dail.state.vt.us

Theresa Wood, Deputy Commissioner

3500 **Vermont Protection and Advocacy**
141 Main Street
Suite 7
Montpelier, VT 05602
802-229-1355
800-834-7890
FAX: 802-229-1359
TTY: 800-889-2047
e-mail: info@vtpa.org
www.vtpa.org

Ed Paquin, Executive Director
AJ Ruben, Supervising Attorney
Advocacy and legal services for people with mental illness on legal issues arising, out of disabilities. Children and adults.

3501 **Workers Compensation Board Vermont**
Department of Labor
PO Box 20
Montpelier, VT 05620
802-828-2286
FAX: 802-828-2195
www.state.vt.us/ladind

Laura Collins, Commissioner

Virginia

3502 International Dyslexia Association: Virginia Branch
PO Box 17605
Richmond, VA 23226
804-285-1946
800-988-8336
FAX: 804-285-1946
e-mail: vbida@hotmail.com
www.interdys.org

Debra Farr, President
Carolyn Russ, Executive Assistant
The Virginia Branch of The International Dyslexia Association (VBIDA) is a 501(c)(3) non-profit, scientific and educational organization dedicated to the study and treatment of the learning disability, dyslexia. This Branch was formed to increase public awareness of dyslexia in the State of Virginia. We serve the entire state, with the exception of Northern Virginia, which is part of the DC-Capital Branch in Washington, DC. We have been serving individuals with dyslexia, their families.

3503 Virginia Department for the Blind and Vision Impaired
397 Azalea Avenue
Richmond, VA 23227
804-371-3140
FAX: 804-371-3351
e-mail: bowmanja@dbvi.virginia.gov
www.vdbvi.org

Joseph A Bowman, Commissioner
James Taylor, Chief Deputy Commissioner
Offers services for the totally blind, legally blind, visually impaired, mentally retarded blind and more with health, counseling, educational, recreational, rehabilitation, computer training and professional training services.

3504 Virginia Department of Mental Health
PO Box 1797
Richmond, VA 23218
804-340-0072
FAX: 804-786-3827

Joe Damico, Director Administrative Services

3505 Virginia Developmental Disability Council
101 N 14th Street
Floor 17
Richmond, VA 23219
804-225-3144
FAX: 804-225-3221

Sandra Reen, Director

3506 Virginia Office Protection and Advocacy for People with Disabilities
1910 Byrd Avenue
Suite 5
Richmond, VA 23230
804-225-2042
800-552-3962
FAX: 804-662-7057
e-mail: general.vopa@vopa.virginia.gov
www.vopa.state.va.us
Through zealous and effective advocacy and legal representation to: protect and advance legal, human, and civil rights of persons with disabilities; combat and prevent abuse, neglect, and discrimination; and promote independence, choice, and self-determination by persons with disabilities.

3507 Virginia Office for Protection & Advocacy
1910 Byrd Avenue
Suite 5
Richmond, VA 23230
804-225-2042
800-552-3962
FAX: 804-662-7077
www.vopa.state.va.us

V Collen Miller, Executive Director
An independent state agency that helps ensure that the rights of persons with disabiltiies in the Commonwealth are protected. The mission of DRVD is to provide zealous and effective advocacy and legal representation to protect and advance legal, human and civil rights of persons with disabilities, combat and prevent abuse, neglect and discrimination, and promote independence, choice and self-determination by persons with disabilities.

3508 Virginia Office for Protection and Advocacy
1910 Byrd Avenue
Suite 5
Richmond, VA 23230
804-225-2042
800-552-3962
FAX: 804-662-7057
e-mail: general.vopa@vopa.virginia.gov
www.vopa.state.va.us

V Colleen Miller, Executive Director
Annette Sannuti, Business Manager

3509 Virginia's Developmental Disabilities Plan ning Council

Stae Agency
202 N 9th Street
9th Floor
Richmond, VA 23219
804-786-0016
800-846-4464
FAX: 804-786-1118
e-mail: lindlekv@vbpd.state.va.us
www.vaboard.org

Barbara Ettner, Director Policy & Program
Heidi Lawyer, Director
Nan Pembeston, Administrator

Washington

3510 DSHS/Aging & Adult Disability Services Administration
PO Box 45600
Olympia, WA 98504
800-422-3263
TTY:800-737-7931
www.adsa.dshs.wa.gov

Kathy Leitch, Assistant Director
The Aging and Disability Services Administration assists children and adults with developmental delays or disabilities, cognitive impairment, chronic illness and related functional disabilities to gain access to needed services and supports by managing a system of long-term care and supportive services that are high quality, cost effective, and responsive to individual needs and preferences.

3511 International Dyslexia Association: Washington State Branch
PO Box 1247
Mercer Island, WA 98040
206-382-1020
800-222-3123
e-mail: wabida@drizzlw.com
www.wabita.org

Stacy Turner, President
Provides free information and referral services for diagnosis and tutoring for parents, educators, physicians, and individuals with dyslexia in Arkansas, Idaho, Montana and Washington state. The voice of our membership is heard in 48 countries. Membership includes yearly journal and quarterly newsletter. Call for conference dates.

3512 Social Security: Olympia Disability Determination
Social Security
402 Yauger Way SW
Olympia, WA 98502
800-772-1213
TTY:800-325-0778
www.ssa.gov

Laurie Watkins, Commissioner

3513 WA Department of Services for the Blind
402 Legion Way
Suite 100
Olympia, WA 98504
360-586-1224
800-552-7103
FAX: 360-586-7627
www.dsb.wa.gov

Luoana Durand, Executive Director
Erin Larson, Assistant Director
Vocational rehabilitation for the blind.

3514 **Washington Client Assistance Program**
2531 Rainier Avenue S
Seattle, WA 98144
206-721-5999
888-721-6072
FAX: 206-721-5980
www.capseattle.org

Jerry Johnson, Executive Director
Advocacy and information assistance for persons of disability seeking services through vocational rehabilitation or other program under the 1973 Rehabilitation Act as commented. We provide counseling.

3515 **Washington Department of Mental Health**
Department of Social and Health Services
1115 Washington Street
PO Box 45320
Olympia, WA 98504
360-902-8070
FAX: 360-902-7691
www.dshs.wa.gov

Richard E Kellogg, MHD Director

3516 **Washington Developmental Disability**
2600 Martin Way E
Suite F
Olympia, WA 98504
360-586-3560

3517 **Washington Governor's Committee on Disability Issues & Employment**
605 Woodland Square Loop SE
Lacey, WA 98503
360-438-3168
FAX: 360-438-3208
www.gcde.org

Toby Olson, Director

3518 **Washington Office of Superintendent of Public Instruction**
Old Capitol Building
PO Box 47200
Olympia, WA 98504
360-725-6000
TTY:360-644-3631
e-mail: webmaster@ospi.wednet.edu
www.k12.wa.us

Dr Terry Bergeson, State Superintendent
The Office of Superintendent of Public Instruction (OSPI) is the primary agency charged with overseeing K-12 education in Washington state. OSPI works with the state's 296 school districts to administer basic education programs and implement education reform on behalf of more than one million public school students.

3519 **Washington Protection & Advocacy System**
315 5th Avenue S
Suite 850
Seattle, WA 98104
206-324-1521
800-562-2702
FAX: 425-776-0601
e-mail: wpas@wpas-rights.org

Mark Stroh, Executive Director
WPAS is a private, non-profit right protection agency for persons with disabilities residin in Washington state. Our advocacy services include information referral, technical assistance, training, publications and systemic advocacy.

3520 **Washington State Developmental Disabilities Council**
2600 Martin Way East Suite F
PO Box 48314
Olympia, WA 98504
360-586-3560
800-634-4473
FAX: 360-586-2424
e-mail: edh@cted.wa.gov
www.ddc.wa.gov

Ed Holen, Executive Director

3521 **Workers Compensation Board Washington**
State of Washington
7273 Linderson Way SW
Tumwater, WA 98501
360-236-4018
800-547-8367
www.lni.wa.gov

Gary K Weeks, Director
Maxine Hayes, MD

West Virginia

3522 **Bureau of Employment Programs Division of Workers' Compensation**
State of West Virginia
409 Virginia Street E
Charleston, WV 25301
304-357-0130
800-628-4265
FAX: 304-357-0585
e-mail: pgrinste@wvbep.org
www.state.wv.us

Kent W Carper, Commissioner
Vern Cormick, Manager

3523 **Disability Determination Section**
500 Quarrier Street
Suite 500
Charleston, WV 25301
304-343-5055
800-344-5033
FAX: 304-353-4212

Jane Johnstone, Executive Director

3524 **Social Security: Charleston Disability Determination**
Social Security
500 Quarrier Street
Suite 300
Charleston, WV 25301
304-347-5217
800-772-1213
FAX: 304-353-4212
www.socialsecurity.gov

3525 **West Virginia Advocates**
1207 Quarrier Street
4th Floor
Charleston, WV 25301
304-346-0847
800-950-5250
FAX: 304-346-0867
www.wvadvocates.org

Clarice Hausth, Executive Director

3526 **West Virginia Client Assistance Program**
West Virginia Advocates
1900 Kanawha Boulevard E
Room 6
Charleston, WV 25305
304-346-0847
FAX: 304-346-0867
e-mail: vhuffman@access.k12.wv.us
wvde.state.wv.us/

Clarice Hausch, Executive Director

3527 **West Virginia Department of Aging**
PO Box 1100
Charleston, WV 25324
304-345-7303
888-825-7303
e-mail: hollygrove@juno.com

Patricia Bedford, Director

3528 **West Virginia Department of Children with Disabilities**
Children with Special Health Care Needs
350 Capital Street
Room 427
Charleston, WV 25301
304-558-5388
FAX: 304-558-2866

Cathy Capps, Director

3529 **West Virginia Department of Health**
1900 Capital Complex
Building 3
Charleston, WV 25305
304-558-0549
FAX: 304-558-1008

Taunja Willis-Miller, Secretary
Sarah Hamrick, Executive Director

3530 **West Virginia Developmental Disabilities Council**
110 Stockton Street
Charleston, WV 25312
304-558-0416
FAX: 304-558-0941
e-mail: jchankins@wvdhhr.org
www.wvddc.org

Steven Wiseman, Executive Director
Jonathan Hankins, Office Manager
6-8 pages Quarterly Newsl

3531 **West Virginia Division of Rehabilitation Services**
PO Box 547
Institute, WV 25112
304-766-2634

www.wvdrs.org

Deborah Lovely, Acting Director
DRS' mission is to enable and empower individuals with disabilities to work and to live independently.

Wisconsin

3532 **Disability Rights Wisconsin: Milwaukee Office**
6737 W Washington Street
Suite 3230
Milwaukee, WI 53214
414-733-4646
800-708-3034
888-758-6049
FAX: 414-773-4647
TTY:414-342-8700
www.disabilityrightswi.org
The protection and advocacy agency for people with disabilities in Wisconsin. DRW provides guidance, advice, investigation, negotiation and in some cases legal representation to people with disabilities and their families. Local and state level systems advocacy and training are also provided.

3533 **International Dyslexia Association: Wisconsin Branch**
WIBIDA
PO Box 284
Baraboo, WI 53913
608-355-0911
800-222-3123
FAX: 608-355-0911
e-mail: loral@centurytel.net
www.wis-dys.org

Lorinda L Clary, President
The International Dyslexia Association actively promotes effective teaching approaches and related clinical educational intervention strategies for dyslexics. We support and encourage interdisciplinary study and research. We facilitate the exploration of the causes and early identification of dyslexia and are committed to the responsible and wide dissemination of research-based knowledge.

3534 **Social Security: Madison Disability Determination**
6011 Odana Road
Madison, WI 53719
608-270-1141
800-772-1213
TTY:800-325-0778
www.ssa.gov

3535 **West Virginia Department of Health**
Building 3
Room 206
Charleston, WV 25305
304-558-0684
800-441-4576
FAX: 304-558-1130
e-mail: helmqp@dhfs.state.wi.us
wvdhhrsecretary@wvdhhr.org

Martha Yeager Walker, Cabinet Secretary
The Department of Health and Family Services operates the federal Title V Maternal and Child Health Block Grant Program for Children with Special Health Care Needs. The program provides program monitoring, consultation and technical assistance to five regional CSHCN centers throughout Wisconsin; a Birth Defects Monitoring and Surveillance Program and a Universal Newborn Hearing Screening Program.

3536 **Wisconsin Bureau of Aging**
State Office of Wisconsin
PO Box 7851
Madison, WI 53707
608-266-2536
FAX: 608-267-3203
e-mail: mcdowdb@dhfs.state.wi.us
www.dhfs.state.wi.us/aging

Donna Mcdowell, Executive Director
Gail Schwersenska, Section Chief
Keeps and updates information and printed materials on senior housing directories, nursing home listings, and home care agencies.

3537 **Wisconsin Coalition for Advocacy: Madison Office**
16 N Carroll Street
Suite 400
Madison, WI 53703
608-267-0214
800-928-8778
FAX: 608-267-0368

Kim Hogan, Intake Specialist
Mr Lynn Breedlove, Executive Director
The protection and advocacy agency for people with disabilities in Wisconsin. WCA provides guidance, advice, investigation, negotiation and in some cases legal representation to people with disabilities and their families. Local and state level systems advocacy and training are also provided.

3538 **Wisconsin Council on Developmental Disabilities (WCDD)**
201 W Washington Avenue
Suite 110
Madison, WI 53703
608-266-7826
FAX: 608-267-3906
TTY:608-266-6660
e-mail: hfswiscwcdd@dhfs.state.wi.us
www.wcdd.org

Jennifer Ondrejka, Executive Director
Helen Hartman, Office Manager
Statewide systems advocacy group for people with developmental disabilities in Wisconsin.

3539 **Wisconsin Governor's Committee for People with Disabilities**
1 W Wilson Street, Room 951
Madison, WI 53702
608-266-7974
866-278-6440
FAX: 608-266-3386
TTY: 608-267-9880
www.dhfs.state.wi.us

Sarah Lincoln, GCPD Staff Support
To advise the Governor and state agencies on problems faced by people with disabilities; to review legislation affecting people with disabilities; to promote effective operation of publicly-administered or supported programs serving people with disabilities; to promote the collection, dissemination and incorporation of adequate information about persons with disabilities for purposes of public planning at all levels of government.

3540 **Workers Compensation Board Wisconsin**
PO Box 7901
Madison, WI 53707
608-266-1340
FAX: 608-267-0394

Frances Huntley-Cooper, Administrator

Wyoming

3541 Social Security: Cheyenne Disability Determination
Social Security
821 W Pershing Boulevard
Cheyenne, WY 82002
307-777-7341
800-438-5788
FAX: 800-972-2372
www.ssa.gov/disability/professional/procontac

Vicky Johnson, Director
Jeff Graham, Manager

3542 WY Department of Health: Mental Health and Substance Abuse Service Division
6101 Yellowstone Road
Suite 220
Cheyenne, WY 82002
307-777-7094
FAX: 307-777-5580
TTY:307-777-5581
e-mail: wdh@state.wy.us
www.mentalhealth.state.wy.us

Mary Flanderka, Administrator
Korin Schmidt, Administrator For Policy
Rodger McDaniel, Deputy Director
State office responsible for purchase of service and program development policy.

3543 Workers Compensation Board Wyoming
122 W 25th Street
2nd Floor
Cheyenne, WY 82001
307-777-7159
FAX: 307-777-5946

3544 Wyoming Client Assistance Program
Protection and Advocacy System
320 W 25th Street
2nd Floor
Cheyenne, WY 82001
307-632-3496
877-854-5041
FAX: 307-638-0815
e-mail: wypanda@vcn.com
wypanda.vcn.com

Lee Beidlemam, Client Assistant
Jeanne A Thobro, Executive Director

3545 Wyoming Department of Aging
State Department of Wyoming
6101 Yellowstone Road
Room 259b
Cheyenne, WY 82002
307-777-7986
800-442-2766
FAX: 307-777-5340
www.httt://wdhss.state.wi.us/aging/index.htm

Beverly Morrow, Administrator
Ruth Davis, Excutive Secretary

3546 Wyoming Developmental Disability Council
122 W 25th Street
Cheyenne, WY 82001
307-777-7230
FAX: 307-777-5690

Lynn Achter, Director
Brenda Oswald, Manager

3547 Wyoming Protection & Advocacy for Persons with Disabilities
320 W 25th Street
2nd Floor
Cheyenne, WY 82001
307-632-3497
FAX: 307-638-0815

Jeanne Thobro, Manager

Alabama

3548 **Birdie Thornton Center**
The Arc Of Alabama
P O Box 1444 Street
Athens, AL 35612
256-236-0336
FAX: 256-230-9398
www.thearcofalabama.com/chapters/athens

Jodie Loftin, Program Director
The Arc of Alabama, Inc. provides the following services for members, local chapters, people with cognitive, intellectual and developmenta disabilites and their families, other disability organizations, and the general public: annual state convention, advocacy, information and referral, respite programs, local chapter support, newsletter and new chapter development.

3549 **Birmingham Independent Living Center**
206 13th Street South
Birmingham, AL 35233
205-251-2223
FAX: 205-251-0605
TTY:205-254-7333
e-mail: bilc@bellsouth.net
www.birminghamilc.org

Daniel Kessler, Executive Director
Carolyn Agee, Programs Coordinator
Bobbie Austin, Fiscal Manager
The mission of this Independent Living Center is to empower people with disabilities to fully participate in the community.

3550 **Independent Living Center of Alabaster**
120 Plaza Circle
Suite C
Alabaster, AL 35007
205-685-0570
FAX: 205-251-0605
TTY:205-685-0605
e-mail: alabasterilc@bellsouth.net
www.ilrgb.org/docs/locations

Dan Kessler, Director
The mission of this Independent Living Center is to empower people with disabilities to fully participate in the community.

3551 **Independent Living Center of Jasper**
300 Birmingham Avenue
Jasper, AL 35002
205-387-0159
FAX: 205-387-1594
TTY:205-387-1594
e-mail: ilcwalker@bellsouth.net
www.ilrgb.org/docs/locations

Dan Kessler, Director
The purpose of this Independent Living Center is to empower people with disabilities to fully participate in the community.

3552 **Independent Living Center of Mobile**
5304 B Overlook Road
- B
Mobile, AL 36618
251-460-0301
FAX: 251-341-1267
e-mail: ilc@ilcmobile.org
www.ilcmobile.org

Michael Davis, Executive Director
Ann Robertson, Assistant Director/Interpreter
Barbara Hattier, ILS/Transportation Coordinator
The mission of the Independent Living Center of Mobile is to foster and promote programs which empower persons with disabilities to attain their maximum degree of independence.

3553 **Montgomery Independent Living Center**
600 S Court Street
Montgomery, AL 36104
334-240-2520
FAX: 334-240-6869
e-mail: mcil@bellsouth.net

Scott Renner, Director
To empower people with disabilities to fully participate in the community.

Alaska

3554 **Access Alaska: ADA Partners Project**
121 W Fireweed Lane
Suite 105
Anchorage, AK 99503
907-222-6166
888-462-1444
888-462-1444
FAX: 907-222-6166
e-mail: monam@adapartners.org
www.adapartners.org

Jim Beck, Executive Director
Mona McAleese, Coordinator
The Partner's Project provides expert in-depth advise for implementing the Americans witht he Disabilities Act. The Project also maintains a statewide network of community based experts, most of whom experience disabilities, to provide interpretive guidance and training for business and local government.

3555 **Access Alaska: Fairbanks**
526 Gaffney Road
Suite 100
Fairbanks, AK 99709
907-479-7940
800-770-7940
FAX: 907-474-4052
TTY: 907-474-8619
e-mail: info@accessalaska.org
www.fairnet.org/agencies/accessak

David Jacobson, Executive Director
A local non profit agency using its resources to actively promote a society where persons with disabilities can live and work independently in the community of their choice.
1983

3556 **Access Alaska: Mat-Su**
897 Commercial Drive
Wasilla, AK 99687
907-357-2588
800-770-0228
FAX: 907-357-5585
e-mail: info@accessalaska.org
www.accessalaska.org

Jim Beck, Care Services Supervisor
Maxie Smith, Administration/Owner
Cheryl Unthicum, Service Coordinator
Provides independent living services to persons with significant disabilities. Mission is to encourage and promote the total integration of persons with disabilities into the community of their choice. Services include independent living skills training, information and referral, advocacy, peer support, case management services, care coordination, interim accessible transportation and at home modifications.

3557 **Alaska SILC**
1057 W Fireweed Lane
Suite 206
Anchorage, AK 99503
907-263-2004
888-294-7452
888-294-7452
FAX: 907-263-2012
e-mail: preinhart.silc@gci.net
www.alaskasilc.org

Patrick Reinhart, Executive Director
Runika Rollins, Office Manager
The Alaska Statewide Independent Living is committed to promoting a philosophy of consumer control, peer support, self help, self determination, equal access, and individual and systems advocacy, in order to maximize leadership, empowerment, independence, productivity, and to support full inclusion and integration of individuals with disabilities into the mainstream of American society.

3558 Arctic Access
Independent Living Center
PO Box 930
Kotzebue, AK 99752
907-442-2393
877-442-2393
FAX: 907-442-2393
TTY: 907-442-2393
e-mail: arcticac@otz.net
www.arcticaccess.org

Roger Wright Jr, Executive Director
Audrey Aanes, Member of the Board
The Arctic Access Independent Living Center provides services and opportunities for elders and others with disabilities so they may remain in their village and be as active as possible with their families and commuities in the North West Arctic and Bering Straits Regions of Alaska.
1993

3559 Hope Community Resources
540 W International Airport Road
Anchorage, AK 99518
907-561-5335
800-478-0078
FAX: 907-564-7429
e-mail: kjez@hopealaska.org
www.hopealaska.org

Stephen Lesko, Executive Director
Kris Jez, Deputy Director Public Relations
Tonja Rambow, Deputy Director Programs
providing a multitude of community services including independent living, assisted living, foster care, respite and employment services for people who experience developmental disabilities.

3560 Kenai Peninsula IL Center
3953 Bartlett Street
P.O. Box 2474
Homer, AK 99603
907-235-7911
800-770-7911
FAX: 907-235-6236
e-mail: ilc@xyz.net
www.peninsulailc.org

Joyanna Geisler, Executive Director
Offers peer counseling, disability education and awareness, attendant care registry and information on accessible housing.

3561 Kenai Peninsula IL Center: Seward
201 Third Avenue Suite 1
P.O. Box 3523
Seward, AK 99664
907-224-8711
FAX: 907-224-7793
e-mail: sewardilc@qci.net
www.peninsulailc.org

Joyanna Geisler, Executive Director
Lynn Hohl, Manager
Offers peer counseling, disability, education and awareness, attendant care registry and information on accessible housing.

3562 Keni Peninsula-Central Peninsula
47255 Princeton Avenue Suite 1
P.O. Box 1907
Soldotna, AK 99669
907-262-6333
FAX: 907-260-4495
e-mail: nadine@peninsulailc.org
www.peninsulailc.org

Joyanna Geisler, Executive Director
Offers peer counseling, disability education and awareness, attendant care registry and information on accessible housing.

3563 SE Alaska ILC: Ketchikan
602 Dock Street
Suite 107
Ketchikan, AK 99901
907-225-4735
888-452-7245
FAX: 907-225-4753
e-mail: ketchikan@sailinc.org
www.sailinc.org

Joan Keese, Director
Kara Lunde, Manager
Independent living is a philosophy and a movement of people with disabilities who work for self-determination, equal opportunities and self-respect.

3564 SE Alaska Independent Living Center (SAIL)
3225 Hospital Drive
Unit 300
Juneau, AK 99801
907-586-4920
800-478-7245
FAX: 907-586-4980
e-mail: info@sailinc.org
www.sailinc.org

Joan O Keefe, Executive Director
Robert Purvisainen, Vice President
Clark Gruening, President
SAIL's purpose is to empower consumers with disabilities by providing services and information to support them in making choices that will positively affect their independence and productivity. SAIL also serves all people with physical and mental disabilities regardless of race, ancestry, color, religion, age, marital status, sexual preference, gender and/or income.

3565 SE Alaska Independent Living: Sitka
514 Lake Street
Suite C
Sitka, AK 99835
907-747-6859
800-478-7245
FAX: 907-747-6783
e-mail: sitka@sailinc.org
www.sailinc.org

Joan O'Keese, Executive Director
Independent living is a philosophy and a movement of people with disabilities who work for self determination, equal opportunities and self-respect.

Arizona

3566 ASSIST! to Independence
PO Box 4133
Tuba City, AZ 86045
928-283-6261
888-848-1449
FAX: 928-283-6284
e-mail: assist01@frontiernet.net
www.ASSISTtoIndependence.org

Michael Blatchford, Executive Director
Elizabeth Pifer, Director Rehab Technology Svcs.
Priscilla Lane, Independent Livincg Svcs Coord
Native American owned and operated non-profit located on the Navagjo Nation. Programs: Center for Independent Living, Regional Resource Center for Assistive Technology, Functional Assessment Clinic, Sensory Integration Program, Special Needs Toy Lending Library.

3567 Arizona Bridge to Independent Living
1229 E Washington Street
Phoenix, AZ 85034
602-256-2245
800-280-2245
FAX: 602-254-6407
e-mail: boardofdirectors@abil.org
www.abil.org

Phil Pangrazio, Executive Director
Ann Pasco, Operations Director
Feng Chiou, Financial Director
ABIL offers and promotes programs designed to empower people with disabilities to take personal responsibility so they may achieve or continue independent lifestyles within the community.
1977

3568 Arizona Bridge to Independent Living: Phoenix
10000 N 31st Avenue
Suite D-405
Phoenix, AZ 85051
602-424-4100
800-280-2245
FAX: 602-424-4118
TTY: 602-296-0591
e-mail: boardofdirectors@abil.org
www.abil.org

Phil Pangrazio, Director
Darlene Clayton, Receptionist/Program Aide
Donna Lorti, Work Incentives Specialist
ABIL offers and promotes programs designed to empower people with disabilities to take personal responsibility so they may achieve or continue independent lifestyles within the community.

3569 Arizona Bridge to Independent Living: Mesa
2150 S County Club Drive
Suite 10
Mesa, AZ 85210
480-655-9750
800-280-2245
FAX: 480-655-9751
TTY: 480-655-9750
e-mail: azbridge@abil.org
www.abil.org

Phil Pangrazio, Director
Marie Adams, Receptionist/Program Aide
Diane Patton, Program Manager/Trainer
ABIL offers and promotes programs designed to empower people with disabilities to take personal responsibility so they may achieve or continue independent lifestyles within the community.

3570 Casa Del Rey
PO Box W
Parker, AZ 85344
928-669-9695
FAX: 928-669-5280

Shane Hall, President
Center for Independent Living

3571 Community Outreach Program for the Deaf
268 W Adams Street
Tucson, AZ 85705
520-792-1906
800-234-0344
FAX: 520-770-8544
TTY: 520-792-1906
e-mail: annel@ccs-ddp.org
www.copdaz.org

Anne Levy, Executive Director
Sue Henning-Mitchell, Deputy Director
Independent living centers offering peer counseling, disability education and awareness, advocacy and other services to the community.
1973

3572 Direct Center for Independence
1023 N Tyndall Avenue
Tucson, AZ 85719
520-624-6452
800-342-1853
FAX: 520-792-1438
TTY: 520-624-6452
e-mail: direct@directilc.org
www.directilc.org

Ann Meyer, Executive Director
Bennie Wik, Administrative Assistant
A consumer directed, community based advocacy organization that promotes independent living and offers a variety of programs for all people with disabilities. Through DIRECT's programs, people are encouraged to achieve their full potential and to participate in the community.
1980

3573 New Horizons: Prescott Valley
8085 E Manley Drive
Suite 1
Prescott Valley, AZ 86314
928-772-1266

Ken Edwards, Executive Director

3574 Services Maximizing Independent Living and Empowerment (SMILE)
1929 S Arizona Avenue
Suite 12
Yuma, AZ 85364
928-329-6681
FAX: 928-329-6715
e-mail: smile1929@adelphia.net
www.neiaw.com/smile/smileindex.htm

Cathryn Robins, Executive Director
Suzanne Canole, Chairman
Independent Living Center.
1998

3575 Sterling Ranch: Residence for Special Women
Sterling Ranch
PO Box 36
Skull Valley, AZ 86338
928-442-3289
FAX: 928-442-9272
e-mail: director@sterlingranch.info
www.sterlingranch.info

Russell Dryer, Executive Director
Trent Nichel, Manager
A nonprofit residence for women with developmental disabilities which has been in operation since 1947. As a small facility (19 residents) the orientation is personal and family-like. Offers activities that range from gardening, quilting, academics, sign-language, crafts and a myriad of field trips and excursions. Private rooms and spacious living on 4 1/2 acres.

Arkansas

3576 Arkansas Independent Living Council
523 South Louisiana Street
Suite 305
Little Rock, AR 72201
501-372-0607
800-772-0607
FAX: 501-372-0598
TTY: 501-372-0607
e-mail: 105344.1767@kcompuserve.com
www.ailc-ar.org

Rebecca Riggs, Executive Director
Elizabeth Virden-Simmons, Assistant Director
Richard Royal, Chair
The mission of the Arkansas Independent Living Council is to promote independence, including freedom of choice and full inclusion into the mainstream of society, for all Arkansans with disabilities.
Quarterly

3577 Delta Resource Center for Independent Living
1514 S Poplar
Pine Bluff, AR 71601
870-535-2222
800-824-0009
FAX: 870-534-8191
TTY: 870-535-2222
e-mail: drcil@sbcglobal.net

Billy Altom, Executive Director
Independent living center providing information and referrals, advocacy, peer counseling and independent living skills training to the Southeast region of Arkansas.

3578 Mainstream
300 S Rodney Parham Road
Suite 5
Little Rock, AR 72205
501-280-0012
FAX: 501-280-9267
TTY:501-280-9262
e-mail: mainstreamlrc@earthlink.net
www.mainstreamilrc.com

Rita Byers, Director
A non residential, consumer driven independent living resource center for persons with disabilities. Mainstream operates with conviction that people with disabilities have the right and responsibility to make choices, to control their lives and to participate fully and equally in the community.

3579 **Our Way**
10434 W 36th Street
Little Rock, AR 72204
501-225-5030
FAX: 501-225-5190

Wendy Harris, Project Manager
Carla Mithchell, Manager
Advocacy and information services. One bedroom apartments for mobility impaired and elderly 62 years or older persons.
Based on income

3580 **Sources for Community IL Services**
1918 N Birch Avenue
Fayetteville, AR 72703
479-442-5600
888-284-7521
888-284-7521
FAX: 479-442-5192
e-mail: sources@arsources.org
www.arsources.org

Richard Royal, Executive Director
Sources provides services, supports, and advocacy for persons with disabilities, their families, and the communities at large. We serve persons with all types of disabilities.

3581 **Spa Area Independent Living Services**
600 Main Street
Hot Springs, AR 71913
501-624-7710
FAX: 501-624-7003
www.arsales.org

Brenda Stinebuck, Executive Director
Provides services and advocacy by and for persons with all types of disabilities. The goal is to assist individuals with disabilities to achieve thier maximum potential within their families and communities.

California

3582 **Access Center of San Diego**
1295 University Avenue
Suite 10
San Diego, CA 92103
619-293-3500
800-300-4326
FAX: 619-293-3508
TTY: 619-293-7757
e-mail: louisf@accesscentersd.org
www.a2isd.org

Louis Frick, Executive Director
Sharon McCabe, Operations Manager
Roberto Frias, Program Director
The Access Center, through advocacy, education, and opportunity, promotes full inclusion by empowering and challenging people with disabilities to achieve their greatest potential.

3583 **Access To Independence Of Imperial Valley**
584 Main Street
Suite C
El Centro, CA 92243
760-353-4191
FAX: 760-353-4474
TTY:760-353-2802
e-mail: louisf@accesscentersd.org
www.accesscentersd.org

Louis Frick, Program Director
Denise Donaho-Smith, Manager
Access to Independence, through advocacy, education, and opportunity, promotes full inclusion by empowering and challenging people with disabilities to achieve their greatest potential.

3584 **Access To Independence Of North County**
209 E Broadway
Suite A
Vista, CA 92084
760-643-0447
FAX: 760-643-0453
TTY:760-435-9213
e-mail: info@accesscentersd.org
www.accesscentersd.org

Christina Mill, Program Manager
The Access Center, through advocacy, education and opportunity, promotes full inclusion by empowering and challenging people with disabilities to achieve their greatest potential.

3585 **Beaumont Senior Center: Community Access Center**
550 E 6th Street
Beaumont, CA 92223
951-769-8539
FAX: 909-769-2794
TTY:909-769-2794
e-mail: pmgr1@ilcac.org

Laurie Hoirup, Director
A non profit organization; one of 29 similar programs throughout the state of California CAC is a community resource, advocate, and educator for Riverside County residents with disabilities.

3586 **CAPH Independent Living Center**
3475 W Shaw Avenue
Suite 101
Fresno, CA 93711
209-927-6777
800-204-2274
FAX: 209-927-6778
TTY: 559-276-6779
e-mail: program_dir@earthlink.net
www.cil-fresno.org

Karen Pendleton, Director
Robert Hand, Executive Director
Independent living center.

3587 **California Foundation For Independent Living Centers**
4716 E Cesar E Chavez Avenue
Building A
Los Angeles, CA 90022
323-266-0453
FAX: 323-266-7992
TTY:323-266-3016
e-mail: cfilc@cfilc.org
www.cfilc.org

Eric Vasquez, Director
Frances Fontenelle, Manager
Community Rehabilitation Services, Inc. (CRS) is a private, non-profit agency established in 1974 to assist persons with disabilities within the East/North East areas of Los Angeles County to enhance their options for living independently. Any person who is 18 yrs of age or more with physical, sensory, mental/emotional or developmental disabilities can work with us to become more self-sufficient. Our intake procedures provide an orientation to the staff, facilities and services at CRS.

3588 **California Foundation for Independent Living Centers**
1029 J Street
Suite 120
Sacramento, CA 95814
916-325-1690
FAX: 916-325-1699
TTY:916-325-1695
e-mail: cfilc@cfilc.org
www.cfilc.org

Patricia Yeager, Executive Director
CFILC's mission is to support independent living centers in their local communities through advocating for systems change and promoting access and integration for people with disabilities.

3589 **California State Independent Living Council (SILC)**
1600 K Street
Suite 100
Sacramento, CA 95814
916-445-0142
866-866-7452
FAX: 916-445-5973
TTY: 916-445-5627
e-mail: neal@calsilc.org
www.calsilc.org

Michael C Collins, Director
To maximize options for independence for persons with disabilities

3590 Center for Independence Of The Disabled- Daly City

355 Gellert Boulevard
Suite 256
Daly City, CA 94015
650-991-5124
FAX: 650-757-2075
TTY:650-991-5182
e-mail: dalycity5@aol.com
www.cidbelmont.org

Kent Mickelson, Director
The Daly City Branch office fulfills its mission by serving disabled consumers in Brisbane, Colma, Daly City, El Granada, Half Moon Bay, Montara, Moss Beach, Pacifica, Pescadero, Princeton and South San Francisco. Our mission is to increase the social, educational, economic, social and political participants of persons with disabilities in San Mateo county, California.

3591 Center for Independence of the Disabled

875 Oneill Street
Belmont, CA 94002
650-595-0783
FAX: 650-595-0261
TTY:650-595-0743
e-mail: info@cidbelmont.org
www.cidbelmont.org

Kent Mickelson, Executive Director
Ray Pittsinger, Program Manager
Arsie Tuquero-Zacarias, Administrative Assistant
Increase the social, educational, and economic participation of persons with disabilities in San Mateo County, and to encourage, support, and provide options for self determination, equal access and freedom of choice.

3592 Center for Independent Living

2539 Telegraph Avenue
Berkeley, CA 94704
510-841-4776
FAX: 510-841-6168
TTY:510-848-3101
e-mail: jgarrett@cilberkeley.org
www.cilberkeley.org

Jan Garrett, Executive Director
Gerald Baptiste, Deputy Director
The Center for Independent Living, Inc (CIL) is a national leader in helping people with disabilities live independently and become productive members of society. Founded in 1972, CIL is a pioneer advocating for greater accessibility in communities, designing techniques in independent living and providing direct services to people with disabilities. A partial list of services includes Information and Referral, Personal Assistance Services, Independent Living Skills Training and Peer Counseling.

3593 Center for Independent Living: Oakland

610 16th Street
Suite 419
Oakland, CA 94612
510-763-9999
FAX: 510-763-4910
TTY:510-444-1837
e-mail: ddaviscil@yahoo.com
www.cilberkeley.org

Jan Garrett, Director
A national leader in supporting disabled people in their efforts to lead independent lives.

3594 Center for Independent Living: Tri-County

955 Myrtle Avenue
Eureka, CA 95501
707-445-8404
877-576-5000
FAX: 707-445-9751
TTY: 707-445-8405
www.tilnet.org

Chris Jones, Manager

3595 Center for Independent Living:Fresno

3475 Wesy Shaw Avenue
Suite 101
Fresno, CA 93711
559-276-6777
FAX: 559-276-6778
TTY:559-276-6779
e-mail: execdirector@cil-fresno.org
www.cil-fresno.org

Robert Hand, Executive Director

3596 Center for Independent Living; East Oakland

7200 Bancroft Avenue
Suite 9A
Oakland, CA 94612
510-635-4920
FAX: 510-635-4261
e-mail: cwood@cilberkeley.org

Jan Garrett, Director
A national leader in helping people with disabilities live independently and become productive, fully participating members of society.

3597 Center for Independent Living; Oakland

1470 Fruitvale Avenue
Oakland, CA 94601
510-536-2271
FAX: 510-261-2968
e-mail: ediazalvarezcil@yahoo.org

Jan Garrett, Director
Independent living center to maximise the options for independence for persons with disabilities.

3598 Center of Independent Living: Visalia

208 W Main Street
Suite 7
Visalia, CA 93291
559-622-9276
FAX: 559-622-9638
e-mail: f_phillips@cil-fresno.org
www.cil-fresno.org

Fran Phillips, Executive Directorram Manager
Renee Ezelle, Manager

3599 Central Coast Center for IL: San Benito

1029 J Street
Suite 120
Sacramento, CA 95814
916-325-1690
FAX: 916-325-1699
e-mail: cfile@cfilc.org
www.cfilc.org

Cheryl Bergan, Director
Kim Cantrell, Director
Patricia Yeager, Executive Director
To advocate for barrier-free access and equal opportunity for people with disabilities to participate in the community life by increasing the capacity of Independent Living Centers to achieve their missions.

3600 Central Coast Center for Independent Living

234 Capitol Street
Suites A & B
Salinas, CA 93901
831-757-2968
FAX: 831-757-5549
TTY:831-757-3949
e-mail: cccil@cccil.org
www.cccil.org

Elsa Quezada, Executive Director
CCCIL promotes the independence of people with disabilities by supporting their equal and full participation in community life. CCCIL provides advocacy, education and support to all people with disabilities, their families and the community.

3601 Central Coast Center: Independent Living - Santa Cruz Office

1395 41st Avenue
Suite B
Capitola, CA 95010
831-462-8720
FAX: 831-462-8727
TTY:831-462-8729
e-mail: cccilcap@cccil.org
www.cccil.org

Elsa Quezada, Director
CCCIL promotes the independence of eople with disabilities by supporting their equal and full participation in community life. CCCIL provides advocacy, education and support to all people with disabilities, their families and the community.

3602 Central Coast for Independent Living
1111 San Felipe Road
Suite 107
Hollister, CA 95023
831-636-5196
FAX: 831-637-0478
TTY:831-638-0826
e-mail: cccilQ@cccil.org
www.cccil.org

Elsa Quezada, Director
CCCIL promotes the independence of people with disabilities by supporting their equal and full particpation in community life. CCCIL provides advocacy, education and support to all people with disabilities, their families and the community.

3603 Central Coast for Independent Living: Watsonville
521 Main Street
Suite Y
Watsonville, CA 95076
831-786-0915
TTY:831-786-0915

Elsa Quezada, Director
An advocacy and information center organized by and for people with disabilities that strives to make our communities more accessible and to empower people with disabilities with information and skills to live fulfilling lives in our communities.

3604 Communities Actively Living Independent and Free
634 S Spring Street
2nd Floor
Los Angeles, CA 90014
213-627-0477
FAX: 213-627-0535
e-mail: info@calif-ilc.org
www.calif-ilc.org

Lilibeth Navarro, Founder/Executive Director
CALIF looks to achieve greater input, participation and control of over policies and services especially those for people with disabilities, including those that exclude them; addresses discrimination wherever it exists; encourages the meaningful participation of persons with disabilities in mainstream activities that enhance the positive image and experience disability; empowers people with disabilities by encouraging ongoing education and a broad knowledge of the history and heritage.

3605 Community Access Center
6848 Magnolia Avenue
Suite 150
Riverside, CA 92506
951-274-0358
FAX: 951-274-0833
TTY:951-274-0834
e-mail: execdir@ilcac.org
www.communityaccesscenter.org

Laurie Hoirup, Executive Director
A non-profit organization; one of 29 similar programs throughout the state of California. CAC is a community resource, advocate, and educator for Riverside County residents with disabilities.

3606 Community Access Center: Indio Branch
81-730 Hwy 111
Suite 2
Indio, CA 92201
760-347-4888
FAX: 760-347-0722
TTY:760-347-6802
e-mail: pmgr2@ilcac.org
www.ilcac.org

Raymond Martin, Program Manager
Velma Pacrem, Manager
Mission of the Center is to empower persons with disabilities to control their own lives, create an accessible community and advocate to achieve complete social, economic, and political integration. We implement this vision by providing information, supportive services and independent living skills training.

3607 Community Access Center: Perris
371 Wilderson Avenue
Perris, CA 92570
951-443-1158
FAX: 951-443-2608
TTY:951-443-1158
e-mail: spmgr@ilcac.org
www.ilcac.org

Community Access Center empowers persons with disabilities to control their own lives, create an accessible community and advocate to achieve complete social, economic, and political integration. CAC also implements this vision by providing information, suportive services and independent living skills training.

3608 Community Rehabilitation Services
844 E Mission Road
Suite B
San Gabriel, CA 91776
626-614-1570
FAX: 626-614-1590

Geneva Soloman, Manager
Services that includes physical therapy, occupational therapy, and speech therapy. Treating a wide variety of patients including those that have neurologic or orthopedic diagnosis.

3609 Community Resources for Independence
980 Hopper Avenue
Santa Rosa, CA 95403
707-528-2745
800-528-7703
FAX: 707-528-9477
TTY: 707-528-2151
e-mail: shobart@sonic.net
www.cri-dove.org

Sandy Hobart, Executive Director
Inga Lizdenyte-Phillips, Program Assistant
Non profit organization that offers a wide variety of ways that enable individuals or corporations to contribute to our efforts to advocate for people and serve people with disabilities in Sonoma, Napa, Mendocino and Lake counties.

3610 Community Resources for Independence: Mendocino/Lake Branch
415B Talmage Ave
Suite B
Ukiah, CA 95482
707-463-8875
FAX: 707-463-8878
TTY:707-463-4498
e-mail: cfilc@cfilc.org
www.cfilc.org

Joyce Larson, Certified Benefits Advocate
Tammy Rogers, Independent Living Advocate
Tanner Silva, Rural Outreach Director/Manager
Non profit organization that offers a wide variety of ways that enable individuals or corporarions to contribute to our efforts to advocate for people and serve people with disibilities in Sonoma, Napa, Mendocino, and Lake counties.
1995

3611 Community Resources for Independence: Napa Office
1040 Main Street
Suite 208
Napa, CA 94558
707-258-0270
FAX: 707-258-0275
TTY:707-257-0274
e-mail: cfilc@cfilc.org
www.cfilc.org

Vaughn Heldlas, Assistive Technology
Tyler Stanley, Independent Living Advocate
Sheila Oreilly, Manager
Non profit organization that offers a wide variety of ways that enable individuals or corporations to contribute to our efforts to advocate for people and serve people with disabilities in Sonoma, Napa, Mendocino and Lake counties.

3612 Community Resources for Independent Living Hayward
439 A Street
Hayward, CA 94541
510-881-5743
FAX: 510-881-1593
TTY:510-881-0218
e-mail: info@cril-online.org
www.cril-online.org

Elizabeth Pazdral, Executive Director
John Quinn, Interim Program Director
Wayland Wong, Independent Living Coordinator

CRIL offers independent living services at no charge to persons with disabilities living in southern and eastern Alameda county. CRIL is also a resource for disability awareness education and training, advocacy and technical advice.

3613 Community Resources for Independent Living
39155 Liberty Street
Suite A100
Fremont, CA 94538
510-794-5735
FAX: 510-794-5562
TTY:510-794-5562
e-mail: info@cril-online.org

3614 DRAIL (Disability Resource Agency for Independent Living)
4555 Precissi Lane
Stockton, CA 95207
209-477-8143
FAX: 209-477-7730
TTY:209-477-7734
e-mail: jeff@drail.org
www.drail.org

Jeff Vierra, Center Coordinator
George Lewis, Executive Director
Provides services to meet the diverse needs of people who have a variety of disabilities in all age groups.

3615 Dayle McIntosh Center: Laguna Niguel
24012 Calle De La Plata
Suite 210
Laguna Hills, CA 92653
949-460-7784
FAX: 949-855-8742
TTY:949-855-6749
www.daylemc.org

Tu Lynn Smylie, Director
Myvan Mguyen, Office Manager
Kyle Minnis, Field Coordinator
DMC advances empowerment and inclusion of all persons with disabilities. DMC is the largest Independent Living Center in California, and was named in memory of a young woman with a severe physical disability who worked to found the center.
1977

3616 Disability Resource Agency for Independent Living: Modesto
221 McHenry Avenue
Modesto, CA 95354
209-521-7260
FAX: 209-521-4763
TTY:209-521-1425
e-mail: dwight@drail.org
www.drail.org

Dwight Bateman, Executive Director
Fred Dickinson, Director of Services
DRAIL provides services to persons with disabilities that lead to increased self-sufficiency and independent living. DRAIL's mission is to empower persons with disabilities to achieve their goals and dreams, increase their independence and increase their advocacy skills to become self-advocates.

3617 Disabled Resources Center
2750 E Spring Street
Suite 100
Long Beach, CA 90806
562-427-1000
FAX: 562-427-2027
TTY:562-427-1366
e-mail: info@drcinc.org
www.drcinc.org

Jeanette Nishikawa, Executive Director
Dolores Nathan, Assistant Director
DRC provides services to all people with disabilities, regardless of their age, gender, ethnicity, sexual preference or disability type. DRC looks to empower people with disabilities to live independtly in the community, to make their own decisions about their lives and to advocate on their own behalf.
1976

3618 FREED
508 J Street
Marysville, CA 95901
530-742-4474
FAX: 530-742-4476
TTY:530-742-4474
e-mail: webmaster@freed.org
www.freed.org

Ann Guerra, Executive Director
Claudia Hidek, Program Manager
A non profit Independent Living Resource Center, the goal is to empower people with disabilities to exercise their civil rights in becoming active, productive members of the community. FREED's Mission is to eliminate barriers to full equality for people with disabilities through programs which promote independent living and effect systems change, while honoring dignity and self determination.

3619 FREED Center for Independent Living
900 E Main Street
Suite 201
Grass Valley, CA 95945
530-272-1732
FAX: 530-272-7793
TTY:530-272-1732
e-mail: contact-04@Freed.org
www.freed.org

Ann Guerra, Executive Director
A non profit Independent Living Resource Center, the goal is to empower people with disabilities to exercise their civil rights in becoming active, productive members of the community. FREED's Mission is to eliminate barriers to full equality for people with disabilities through programs which promote independent living and effect systems change, while honoring dignity and self determination.

3620 First Step Independent Living
1174 Nevada Street
Redlands, CA 92374
800-362-0312
e-mail: cvsfs@deltanet.com
Independent living center, empowers people with disabilities to become active, productive, members of the community.

3621 IL Resource Center: Ventura
1802 Eastman Avenue
Suite 112
Venutra, CA 93003
805-650-5993
FAX: 805-650-9278
TTY:805-650-5993
e-mail: jblack@ilrc-trico.org

Josephine Black, Director
An organization of, by and for persons with disabilities who reside or work in our service area. Our purpose is to assist and encourage individuals to achieve their optimal level of self-sufficiency while eliminating the architectural, communication and attitudinal barriers which prevent them from pull participation in the community.

3622 Independent Living Center Of Southern California
14407 Gilmore Street
101
Van Nuys, CA 91401
818-785-6934
FAX: 818-785-0330
TTY:818-785-6934
e-mail: ilcsc@ilcsc.org
www.ilcsc.org

Norma Jean Vescovo, Executive Director
A non-profit consumer based, non-residentail agency providing a wide range of services to a growing population of people with disabilities.

3623 Independent Living Center of Kern County
1631 30th Street
Bakersfield, CA 93301
661-325-1063
800-529-9541
FAX: 661-325-6702
TTY: 661-325-6702
e-mail: bonita@ilcofkerncounty.org
www.ilcofkerncounty.org

Bonita Coyle, Executive Director
A consumer-based consumer-directed non-profit agency assisting persons with disabilities to live independently in their community. The ILCKC presently offers a wide range of services to a growing population of persons with disabilities.

3624 Independent Living Center of Lancaster
1505 West Avenue J, #102
Lancaster, CA 93534
661-945-6602
FAX: 661-945-5690
TTY:661-945-6604
e-mail: ilcsc@ilcsc.org
www.ilcsc.org

Norma J Vescovo, Executive Director
ILCSC is a non-profit, consumer based, non-residential agency providing a wide range of services to a growing population of people with disabilities. ILCSC is dedicated to empowering persons with disabilities to exercise indpendence-pofessionally, personally and creatively-while striving to educate the community on their needs.

3625 Independent Living Center: San Gabriel Valley
Po Box 549
Claremont, CA 91711
909-445-0726
800-491-6722
FAX: 909-445-0727
TTY: 949-445-0729
e-mail: carol@ilc-car.org
www.ilc-clar.org

Carol Lane, CEO
Dedicated to expanding access to information and resources to help increase independence and enhance the quality of life for the East San Gabriel Valley residents with disabilities.

3626 Independent Living Resource Center, Inc.
1150 Laurel Lane
Suite 184
San Luis Obispo, CA 93401
805-593-0667
FAX: 805-549-7423
TTY:805-593-0667
e-mail: jblack@ilrc-trico.org
www.ilrc-trico.org

Josephine Black, Director
Juanita Lopez, Bilingual Info & Referral
Lisa Rubio, Community Living Advocate
Assists persons with disabilities through a comprehensive program of peer support, life skills trainging, advocacy and information and referral services while reducing barriers to access in the community. Other services provided include: Sign Language Interpreter Registry, Personal Assistant Registry & Referral, Communications Advocacy, Assistive Technology Services, Outreach, Benefits Assistance and Advocacy and many others.

3627 Independent Living Resource Center, Inc.
423 W Victoria Street
Santa Barbara, CA 93101
805-963-0595
FAX: 805-963-1350
TTY:8059630595
e-mail: jblack@ilrc-trico.org
www.ilrc-trico.org

Josephine Black, Executive Director
Kathleen Riel, Program Manager
Jennifer Griffin, Business/Grants Manager
A private, nonprofit organization founded by and for persons with disabilities to assist individuals to achieve optimal levels of self-sufficiency. Services include personal assistant referrals, peer and benefits counseling, advocacy, sign language interpreter/communication services, independent living skills training, information and referrals, community education and systems advocacy, housing and employment assistance.

3628 Independent Living Resource Center: San Francisco
649 Mission Street
3rd Floor
San Francisco, CA 94105
415-543-6222
FAX: 415-543-6318
TTY:415-543-6698
e-mail: info@ilrcsf.org
www.ilrcsf.org

Herb Levine, Executive Director
The ILRC Enables persons with persons with diabilites to take resposiblity for and control of their own lives to make decisions to reduce their dependence on people around them the ILRC Provides persons with disabilities the oppurtunties to develop the skills necessary to live their own lives. The ILRC Facilities independent living by making available on going support services thereby empowering persons with physical visual and or hearing disabilities to acheive self sufficiency.

3629 Independent Living Resource Center: Santa Maria Office
327 E Plaza Drive
Suite 3A
Santa Maria, CA 93454
805-925-0015
FAX: 805-349-2416
TTY:805-925-5892
e-mail: cridenour@ilrc-trico.org
www.ilrc-trico.org

Josephine Black, Executive Director
Laurie Colson Young, Assistance/Outreach Specialist
Jennie Morales, Interpreter Registry Coordinator
Peern and Benefit counseling, Independent living skills, Attendentr Recruitment/referral, American Sign language interpreting, Advocacy, housing and employment assistance information and referrals, Social Security benefit planning.

3630 Independent Living Resource of Contra Coast
3200 Clayton Road
Concord, CA 94519
925-363-7293
FAX: 925-363-7296

Bryan Balch, Manager
Offers workshops, services are accessible to individuals with cognitive disabilities, physical disabilities, deaf and hard of hearing, emotional disabilities, visual impairments, learing disabilities and seniors.

3631 Independent Living Resource of Fairfield
1545 Webster Street
Suite C
Fairfield, CA 94533
707-435-8174
FAX: 707-435-8177
e-mail: susanr@ilrcoco-sol.org
www.ilrcoco-sol.org

Susan Rotchyaus, Program Manager
To empower people with disabilities to: control their own lives, provide advocacy and support for individuals with disabilities to live independently, create an accessible community free of physical and attitudinal barriers.

3632 Independent Living Resource: Antioch
310 West 10th Street
Antioch, CA 94509
925-754-0539
www.ilrccc.org

Bryan M Balch, Executive Director
Paul Demange, Program Director
Non-profit organizations run and controlled by persons with disabilities. They are non-residential, community-based centers where people with disabilities can receive assistance with a variety of daily living issues and learn the skills they need to take controll of their lives from people who have had similar experiences living with a disability.

3633 Independent Living Resource: Concord
3200 Clayton Road
Concord, CA 94519
925-363-7293
FAX: 925-363-7296
e-mail: bryanb@ilrccc.org

Bryan Balch, Executive Director
To empower people with disabilities to: control their own lives, provide advocacy and support for individuals with disabilities to live independently, create an accessible community free of physical and attitudinized barriers.

3634 Independent Living Resources (ILR)
101 Broadway
Building #2A
Richmond, CA 94806
510-232-4942
e-mail: info@ilrccc.org

Bryan Balch
Provides services to meet the diverse needs of people who have a variety of disabilities in all age groups.

3635 Independent Living Service Northern California: Redding Office
1411 Yuba Street
Redding, CA 96001
530-242-8550
FAX: 530-241-1454
e-mail: info@ilsnc.org
www.ilsnc.org

Evan Le Vang, Executive Director
Jerry Towne, Manager
Independent Living Services of Northern California is a private non profit organization that provides support services to help empower community members with disabilities.

3636 Independent Living Services of Northern California
Jennifer Roberts Building
1161 East Avenue
Chico, CA 95926
530-893-8527
800-464-8527
FAX: 530-893-8574
e-mail: info@ilsnc.org
www.ilsnc.org

Evan LeVang, Executive Director
Independent Living Services of Northern California is a private, non profit organization that provides support services to help empower community members with disabilities.
1980

3637 Marin Center for Independent Living
710 4th Street
San Rafael, CA 94901
415-459-6245
FAX: 415-459-7047
e-mail: mcilbob@earthlink.net
www.marincil.org

Amy Reisch, Executive Director
A one stop resource center for seniors and people with disabilities, whose mission is to assist people with all types of disabilities to achieve their maximum level of sustainable independence as contributing, responsible and equal participants in society.

3638 Mother Lode Independent Living Center
67 Linoberg Street
Suite A
Sonora, CA 95370
209-532-0963
FAX: 209-532-1591
TTY:209-532-1591

Dwight Bateman, Director
Housing, advocay, benefits counseling and independent living skills.

3639 Placer Independent Resource Services
11768 Atwood Road
Suite 29
Auburn, CA 95603
530-885-6100
800-833-3453
FAX: 530-885-3032
e-mail: administrator@pirs.org
www.pirs.org

Susan Miller, Executive Director
A non profit independent living center whose mission is to advocate, empower, educate and provide services for people with disabilities enabling them to control their alternatives for independent living.

3640 Resources for Independent Living
420 I Street
Suite 3
Sacramento, CA 95814
916-446-3074
FAX: 916-446-2443
e-mail: monicag@ril-sacramento.org
www.ril-sacramento.org

Frances Gracechild, Executive Director
The only organization in Sacramento providing services to people with all forms of disability. RIL is dedicated to providing services and support to disabled people, so they can live happy and productive lives.

3641 Rolling Start
570 W 4th Street
Suite 107
San Bernardino, CA 92401
909-884-2129
FAX: 909-386-7446
TTY:909-884-7396
e-mail: rs.inc@verizon.net
www.rollingstart.com

Frances Bates, Executive Director
Rolling Start looks to empower and educate people with disabilities to achieve the independent life of their choice.

3642 Rolling Start: Victorville
15647 Village Drive
Suite A
Victorville, CA 92392
760-843-8435
FAX: 760-241-8787
TTY:760-843-7959
e-mail: calimom394@aol.com

Frances Bates, Director
Rolling Start looks to empower and educate people with disabilities to achieve the independent life of their choice.

3643 Service Center for Independent Living: Covina Office
Claremont
109 Spring Street
Box 1296
Claremont, CA 91711
909-621-6722
800-491-6722
FAX: 909-445-0727
TTY: 626-967-4401
e-mail: scilcovn@tstonramp.com
www.ilc-clar.org

Carol Lane, Executive Director/CEO
Private, non-profit, consumer-controlled, community based organizations providing services and advocacy by and for persons with all types of disabilities.

3644 Silicon Valley Independent Living Center: Gilroy Office

7415 Eigleberry Street
Suite C
Gilroy, CA 95020
408-847-1805
FAX: 408-842-2321
TTY:408-842-2591
e-mail: info@svilc.org
www.svilc.org

Cheryl L Cairns, Executive Director
Sheri Burns, Deputy Executive Director
Shobha Srinivasan, Development Services Director
SVILC strives to eliminate attitudinal, physical, and communication barriers faced by people with disabilities as they work towards independence and full integration in their communities. The programs and services available at SVILC meet a variety of independent living needs. In addition, SVILC offers classes, workshops, support groups, and recreational activities.

3645 Silicon Valley Independent Living Center
2306 Zanker Road
San Jose, CA 95131
408-894-9041
FAX: 408-894-9050
TTY:408-894-9012
e-mail: info@svilc.org
www.svilc.org

Cheryl Cairnes, Executive Director
Martha Bell, Director Of Community Services
Shobha Srinivasan, Development Services Director
SVILC strives to eliminate attitudinal, physical, and communication barriers faced by people with disabilities as they work towards independence and full integration in their communities. The programs and services available at SVILC meet a variety of independent living needs. In addition, SVILC offers classes, workshops, support groups, and recreational activities.

3646 **Southern California Rehabilitation Services**
7830 Quill Drive
Suite D
Downey, CA 90242
562-862-6531
FAX: 562-923-5274
TTY:562-869-0931
e-mail: scrs@scrs-ilc.org
www.scrs-ilc.org

Tim Whittier, Executive Director
Steve Brandt, Program Director
Southern California Rehabilitation Services empowers persons with disabilities to achieve their personalized goals through community education and individualized services that provide the knowledge, skills, and confidence building to maximize their quality of life. SCRS develops comprehensive programs, responding to the needs of the disability community, enabling them to lead healthy, independent, and productive lives. Most services are provided free of charge to all persons with disabilities.
1979

3647 **Through the Looking Glass**
2198 6th Street
Suite 100
Berkeley, CA 94710
510-848-1112
800-804-1616
FAX: 510-848-4445
e-mail: tlg@lookingglass.org
www.lookingglass.org

Megan Kirshbaum, Executive Director
Tina Evoyne Washington, Office Manager/Publications Dept
A disability community based nonprofit organization, which emerged from the independent living movement, and was founded in 1982 in Berkeley, California.

3648 **Tri-County Independent Living Center**
955 Myrtle Avenue
Eureka, CA 95501
707-445-8404
877-576-5000
FAX: 707-445-9751
TTY: 707-445-8405
e-mail: chrisjones@tilinet.org
www.tilinet.org

Chris Jones, Executive Director
Mari Dorenstreich, Independent Living Specialist
Promotes the philosophy of independent living, to connect individuals to services, and to create and accessible community, so that people with disabilities can have control over their lives and full access to the communities in which they live.

3649 **Westside Center for Independent Living**
12901 Venice Boulevard
Los Angeles, CA 90066
310-568-0107
888-851-9245
FAX: 310-390-4906
e-mail: wcil@wcil.org
www.wcil.org

Mary Ann Jones, Executive Director
A non-residential, public-benefit corporation to enable people with disabilities and seniors in the Los Angeles community to live more independent, self supporting and satisfying lives.
1976

Colorado

3650 **Atlantis Community**
201 S Cherokee Street
Denver, CO 80223
303-733-9324
FAX: 303-733-9324
TTY:303-733-0047
e-mail: adaptbabs@earthlink.net
www.atlantiscommunity.net

Tim Thornton, Co-Director
Terrance Turner, Co-Director
Babs Johnsona, Co-Administrator
Provide direct services, and to empower people with disabilities integrating, with full and equal rights, into all parts of society including employment, affordable, accessible, housing, transportation, recreation, communication, education, and public places while exercising and exerting choice and self determination.
1975

3651 **Center for Independence**
740 Gunnison Ave
Grand Junction, CO 81501
970-241-0315
800-613-2271
FAX: 970-245-3341
TTY: 970-245-3341
e-mail: info@cfigj.org
www.cfigj.org

Linda Taylor, Director
Gail Gutierrez, Executive Asst/Admin Coordinator
Serving people with disabilities since 1982.

3652 **Center for Independent Living**
740 Gunnison Ave.
Grand Junction, CO 81501
970-241-0315
800-613-2271
FAX: 970-245-3341
e-mail: info@cfigj.org
www.cfigj.org

Lindalle Taylor, Executive Director
The only state certified Independent Living Center on the Western Slope of Colorado, serving 11 counties.

3653 **Center for People with Disabilities**
615 Main Streetreet
Longmont, CO 80501
303-772-3250
FAX: 303-772-5125
TTY:303-772-3250
e-mail: davuid@cpwd-ilc.org
www.cpwd-ilc.org

David Bolin, Director
CPWD provides resources, information, and advocacy to assist people with disabilities in overcoming barriers to independent living.

3654 **Center for People with Disabilities (CPWD)**
1675 Range Street
Boulder, CO 80301
303-442-8662
FAX: 303-442-0502
e-mail: info@cpwd-ilc.org
www.cpwd-ilc.org

Andrew J Imparato, CEO and President
Lowel Aird, Executive Director
Provides resources, information, and advocacy to assist people with disabilities in overcoming barriers to independent living. CPWD's goal is an integrated community that equally welcomes all members.

3655 **Center for People with Disabilities: Pueblo**
1304 Berkley Avenue
Pueblo, CO 81003
719-546-1271
800-659-3656
FAX: 719-546-1374
e-mail: ivaleneamidei@yahoo.com
www.du.edu/~bfox2/ilcpueblo

Larry Williams, Executive Director
One of the 10 centers for independent living in Colorado founded under Title VII of the Rehabilitation Act of 1973 as amended in 1978. All new centers under this Independent Living (CIL) Title of the Act received initial and ongoing grants through this new Federal Program created by the Act.

3656 Colorado Springs Independence Center
21 E Las Animas Street
Colorado Springs, CO 80903
719-471-8181
FAX: 719-471-7829
TTY:719-471-2076
e-mail: info@csicindliving.org
www.csicindliving.org

Vicki Skoog, Executive Director
To empower persons with disabilities to maximize their independence within the community and to remove barriers which impact their quality of life, while encouraging them to live independently in their community.

3657 Connections for Independent Living
1024 9th Avenue
Suite E
Greeley, CO 80631
970-352-8682
800-887-5828
FAX: 970-353-8058
TTY: 970-352-8682
e-mail: pattid4z@yahoo.com

Beth Danielson, Executive Director
Certified IL Center, I and R advocacy, peer support, skills training, sign language interpretations, reader services, housing. Cross-disability, all ages.

3658 Denver CIL
777 Grant Street
Suite 100
Denver, CO 80203
303-837-1020
FAX: 303-837-0859

Greg Beran, Owner
Provides resources, information, and advocacy to assist people with disabilities in overcoming barriers to independent living.

3659 Disability Center for Independent Living
5900 E 39th Avenue
Suite 4
Denver, CO 80207
303-320-1345
FAX: 303-320-1355
TTY:303-320-1345
e-mail: crlrynlds@aol.com

Carol Reynolds, Executive Director
Independent living center providing quality services for people with disabilities.

3660 Disabled Resource Services
424 Pine Street
Suite 101
Fort Collins, CO 80524
970-482-2700
FAX: 970-407-7072
TTY:970-407-7060
e-mail: drs@fortnet.org
www.fortnet.org/drs

Nancy Jackson, Executive Director
Marge Grell, Assistant Director
To empower individuals with disabilities to achieve their maximum level of independence and to gain personal dignity within society. Disabled Resource Services, as a private non-profit state certified center for independent living, is dedicated to working with individuals with all types of disabilities in Larimer County to promote their independence and equality through services which support advocacy, awareness and access to their community.

3661 Disbled Resource Services
620 E Eisenhower Boulevard
Loveland, CO 80537
970-667-0816
FAX: 970-663-9526
e-mail: drs@jymis.com

Don Maroney, Director
To empower individuals with disabilities to achieve their maximum level of independence and to gain personal dignity within society.

3662 Greeley Center for Independence
2780 28th Avenue
Greeley, CO 80634
970-339-2444
800-748-1012
FAX: 970-339-0033
e-mail: gciinc@gci.org
www.gci.org

Hope Cassidy, Executive Director
Rob Rabe, Outpatient Services Director
Leslie Vail, Human Resources Director
Provides places of growth, transition and encouragement, where people with temporary and permanent disabilities can reach toward their maximum potential of personal independence and wellness.

3663 Independent Life Center
PO Box 612
356 Ranny Street
Craig, CO 81626
970-826-0833
888-526-0833
FAX: 970-826-0832
TTY: 970-826-0833
e-mail: info@indlife.org

Evelyn Tileston, Director
Provides resources, information, and advocacy to assist people with disabilities in overcoming barriers to independent living.

3664 Martin Luther Home Of Colorado
109 Cameron Drive
Building A
Fort Collins, CO 80525
970-206-1645
FAX: 970-223-1781

Molly Kennif, Executive Director
Providing a wide array of services to assist individuals and families in achieving positive life goals. Services to persons with disabilities and other special needs include community living options, training and employment options, spiritual growth and development options, training and counseling support.

3665 Pueblo Goodwill Industries
1020 Constitution Road
Pueblo, CO 81001
719-543-4483
FAX: 719-545-5134
TTY:719-543-4483
e-mail: customerservice@pueblogoodwill.com
www.pueblogoodwill.com

Debbie Mill, Director
Pueblo Goodwill Industries, Inc. is a community resource dedicated to assisting individuals with disabling and/or disadvantaging conditions in achieving their fullest potential by offering them, through networking and collaboration, enriching opportunities and choices geared toward wage earning and productive living. These opportunities and choices are provided through rehabilitative services, counseling, educational training, and employement.

3666 Southwest Center for Independence
835 E 2nd Avenue
Suite 200
Durango, CO 81301
970-259-1672
FAX: 970-259-0947
TTY:970-259-1672
e-mail: isabel@swcidur.org
swcidurango.org

Isabel Viana, Executive Director
Larry Wales, Housing Coordinator
Gail Swinderman, OIB Coordinator
Empowering individuals with disabilities and their families to achieve their maximum level of independence in work, play and other areas of life.

3667 Southwest Center for Independence: Cortez
6900 Cr Road 24.2
Cortez, CO 81321
970-565-7169
FAX: 970-565-9182
e-mail: swcidur@frontier.net

Isabel Viana, Executive Director
Maxine Carton, Independent Living Coordinator
Empowers individiuals with disabilities and their families to achieve their maximum level of independence in work, play and other areas of life.

Connecticut

3668 Center for Disability Rights
764 Campbell Avenue
Suite A
W Haven, CT 06516
203-934-7077
FAX: 203-934-7078
TTY:203-934-7079
e-mail: cdr7077@aol.com

Marc A Gallucci, Executive Director
Resources, information, and advocacy to assist people with disabilities in overcoming barriers to independent living.

3669 Center for Independent Living SC
26 Palmer's Hill Road
Stamford, CT 06902
203-353-8550
FAX: 203-353-1423
TTY:203-353-8550

Dana Canevari, Director
Provides resources, information, and advocacy to assist people with disabilities in overcoming barriers to independent living.

3670 Chapel Haven
1040 Whalley Avenue
New Haven, CT 06515
203-397-1714
FAX: 203-392-3698
www.chapelhaven.org

Betsey Parlato, President/CEO
Thayer Quoos, VP Residential Programs
Frank Hughes, VP Finance/Operations
Chapel Haven is committed to providing a lifelong program of individualized support services for adults with cognitive disabilities, enabling them to live independent and productive lives.

3671 Disabilities Network of Eastern Connecticut
238 W Town Street
Norwich, CT 06360
860-823-1898
FAX: 860-886-2316
e-mail: dnec@snet.net
www.disability-dnec.org

Carolyn Newcombe, Executive Director
The mission of the Disabilities Network is to empower persons with disabilities in Eastern Connecticut to live as independently as they choose, and to improve the quality of their lives, as well as to effect positive change that promotes the inclusion of all persons with disabilities within society.

3672 Disability Resource Center of Fairfield County: Stratford Office
80 Ferry Boulevard
Suite 210
Stratford, CT 06615
203-378-6977
FAX: 203-375-2748
TTY:203-378-3248
e-mail: info@drcfc.org
www.drcfc.org

Anthony Lacava, Executive Director
Stephanie Mastrolillo, Executive Assistant
The Disability Resource Center of Fairfield County DRCFC provides a comprehensive array of services both to the individuals and the communities of Fairfield County, Connecticut. These services embody the Independent Living philosophy...a philosophy that challenges the social attitudes and the physical barriers that stigmatize and exclude persons with disabilities from the community.
1981

3673 Independence Northwest Center for Independent Living
1183 New Haven Road
Suite 200
Naugatuck, CT 06770
203-729-0153
FAX: 203-729-2839
TTY:203-729-1281

Eileen Healy, Executive Director
Offers peer counseling, disability education and awareness.

3674 Independence Unlimited
151 New Park Avenue
Suite D
Hartford, CT 06106
860-523-5021
FAX: 860-523-5603
e-mail: contactus@independenceunlimited.org

Candace Low, Executive Director
Center for independent living that provides skills training, peer counseling, advocacy, transition from institutions to the community and a variety of other services.

3675 New Horizons Village
37 Bliss Road
Unionville, CT
203-675-4711
FAX: 203-675-4369
www.newhorizonsvillage.com

Michael Shaw, Director
Services offered Housing and other support systems for the physically disabled

Delaware

3676 Easter Seal Independent Living Center
24 Reads Way
New Castle, DE 19720
302-324-4488
FAX: 302-324-4481
e-mail: rbrouill@inet.net

Ray Brouillette, Contact
Private non-profit consumer-controlled, community-based organization providing services and advocacy by and for the persons with all types of disabilities. Their goal is to assist individuals with disabilities to achieve their maximum potential within their families and communities.

3677 Freedom Center for Independent Living
400 North Broad Street
Middletown, DE 19709
302-376-4399
FAX: 302-376-4395
TTY:302-376-4397
e-mail: info@fcilde.org
www.fcilde.org

Hector Gomez, Executive Director
Lillian Evans, Independent Living Specialist
FCILDE protects the Civil rights and promotes the empowerment of persons with disabilities and their families through the independent living philosophy.

3678 Independent Living
1800 N Broom Street
Apt 210
Wilmington, DE 19802
302-429-6693
FAX: 302-429-8031
TTY:302-429-8034

Susan Cycyk, Executive Director

Providing skilled support and caring guidance to adults with disabilities. Our case management services include: daily living skills training, medical coordination, transportation assistance, financial management, housing assistance, and vocational/educational planning.

3679 **Independent Resource Georgetown**
410 S Bedford Street
Suite 37
Georgetown, DE 19947
302-854-9330
FAX: 302-854-9408
TTY:302-854-9340
e-mail: pboyd@independentresource.org

Larry Henderson, Director
Pat Boyd, Manager
Provides independent living services to persons who experience a significant disability. Offers skills training, individually and in small groups, peer support/peer counseling and information and referral services. Strives to remove the architectural and attitudnal barriers through individual and systems advocacy.

3680 **Independent Resources**
52 Reads Way
New Castle, DE 19720
302-328-6704
FAX: 302-328-6705
Private, non-profit, consumer-controlled, community based organization providng services and advocacy by and for persons with all types of disabilities. The goal is to assist individuals with disabilities to achieve their maximum potential within their families and communities.

3681 **Independent Resources: Dover**
32 W Loockerman Street
Suite 104
Dover, DE 19904
302-735-4599
FAX: 302-735-5623
TTY:302-735-5629
e-mail: lhenderson@independentresources.org

Larry Henderson, Director
Private, non-profit, consumer-controlled, community based organization providing services and advocacy by and for persons with all types of disabilities. Their goal is to assist individuals with disabilities to achieve their maximum potential within their families and communities.

3682 **Independent Resources: Wilmington**
6 Denny Road
Suite 205
Wilmington, DE 19809
302-765-0191
FAX: 302-765-0195
e-mail: fox205007@aol.com

Larry Henderson, Executive Director
Private, non-profit, consumer-controlled, community based organization providing services and advocacy by and for persons with all types of disabilities. Their goal is to assist individuals with disabilities to achieve their maximum potential within their families and communities.

3683 **Martin Luther Homes of Delaware**
260 Chapman Road
Suite 104a
Newark, DE 19702
302-456-5995
877-366-7242
FAX: 302-456-5998
e-mail: info@mosaic.org

Terry Olson, Program Director
Provides services to adults with developmental disabilities who reside in homes and apartments. Services are designed to provide them with opportunities for choices and participation in the life of their communities. Supports are geared to assist each individual in becoming more independent in activities of daily living, vocational skills, community mobility and transportation, and recreation and leisure activities.

District of Columbia

3684 **Disability Rights Center**
2500 G Street NW
Washington, DC 20007
202-986-0375
FAX: 202-337-4939
e-mail: crippower@aol.com

Susan Ferris, Contact

3685 **District of Columbia Center for Independent Living**
1400 Florida Ave NE
Washington, DC 20002
202-388-0033
FAX: 202-398-3018
TTY:202-388-0277
e-mail: info@dccil.org
www.dccil.org

Richard A Simms, Executive Director
A consumer controlled, cross disability, community based, private non-profit organization that promotes independent life styles for persons with significant disabilities in the District Of Columbia.

3686 **National Council on Independent Living**
1710 Rhode Island Avenue NW
5th Floor
Washington, DC 20036
202-207-0334
877-525-3400
FAX: 202-207-0341
TTY: 703-525-4153
e-mail: ncil@ncil.org
www.ncil.org

John Lancaster, Executive Director
Oldest cross disability, grassroots organization run by and for people with disabilities.

Florida

3687 **Ability 1st**
1823 Buford Court
Tallahassee, FL 32308
850-575-9621
FAX: 850-575-5740
TTY:850-576-5245
e-mail: ability1st@ability1st.info
www.ability1st.info

Judith Barrett, Executive Director
Formerly the Center for Independent Living of North Florida, empowers persons with disabilities to live indepdently and participate actively in their community.

3688 **Adult Day Training**
Goodwill Industries- Suncoast
10596 Gandy Boulevard N
St Petersburg, FL 33702
727-523-1512
888-279-1988
FAX: 727-563-9300
TTY:727-579-1068
e-mail: gw.marketing@goodwill-suncoast.com
www.goodwill-suncoast.org

Cathy Roegiers, Program Manager
Lee Waits, President
An innovative program which uses job skills to teach self-help, daily living, communication, mobility, travel, decision-making, behavioral and social skills. This focus provides concrete, transferable experiences to help prepare individuals for greater community inclusion by achieving the highest possible degree of independence in their daily life, increasing their confidence and supporting their successful transitions to less structured, self-sufficient environments.

3689 **CIL Options-One Stop Career Center: Royal Palm Beach**
1030 Royal Plam Beach Boulevard
Royal Palm Beach, FL 33411
561-798-7997

Promotes independence for people with disabilities.

3690 CIL of Central Florida

720 N Denning Drive
Winter Park, FL 32789
407-623-1070
FAX: 407-623-1390
e-mail: info@cilorlando.org
www.cilorlando.org

Elizabeth Howe, Executive Director
A private non-profit organization that was founded in 1976 by Central Floridians dedicated to helping people with disabilities achieve their self-determined goals for independent living. CIL of Central Florida serves individuals with any type of disability of any age residing in Orange, Seminole, Osceola and Polk counties.

3691 CIL of Florida Keys

88005 Overseas Highway
Suite 17
Islamorada, FL 33036
305-852-0177
877-335-0187
FAX: 305-453-3488
e-mail: bpierce@cilkeys.org
www.cilkeys.org

Brenda Pierce, Executive Director
Aleisa McGuirl, Consumer Advocate
Offers assistance to persons with disabilities in acquiring independent living and self advocacy skills in order to obtain and maintain independence and self-sufficiency.

3692 CIL of Florida Keys-Key West

300 Southard Street
Suite 105
Key West, FL 33040
305-295-7945
FAX: 305-295-7945
e-mail: cilkeys@cilkeys.org
www.cilkeys.org

Brenda Pierce, Director
Offers assistance to persons with disabilities in acquiring independent living and self-advocacy skills in order to obtain and maintain independence and self-sufficiency.

3693 CIL of North Central Florida

222 SW 36th Terrace
Gainesville, FL 32607
352-378-7474
800-265-5724
FAX: 352-378-5582
TTY: 352-375-8448
e-mail: admin@cilncf.org
www.cilncf.org

William Kennedy, Director
Empowering people with disabilities to exert their individual rights to live as independently as possible, make personal life choices and achieve full community inclusion.

3694 Caring and Sharing Center for Independent Living

12552 Belcher Road S
Largo, FL 33773
727-577-0065
866-539-7550
FAX: 727-539-7588
TTY: 727-577-0065
e-mail: cascil@cascil.org
www.cascil.org

Michael Cook, Executive Director
Mary Jensen, Office Manager
Assist persons with all type of disabilities and their families, to achieve the greatest degree of self-determination in accessibility, advocacy, education, employment, and place of residence in keeping with the consumer's freedom of choice

3695 Caring and Sharing Center: Pasco County

24356 US Highway 19 N
Suite 300
Holiday, FL 34691
727-945-8933
877-422-7245
FAX: 727-945-8944
TTY: 727-945-8933
e-mail: cascil@cascil.org
www.cascil.org

Michael Cook, Executive Director
CASCIL assists persons with all types of disabilities and their families, to achieve the greatest degree of self-determination in accessibility, advocacy, education, employment and place of residence in keeping with the consumer's freedom of choice.

3696 Caring and Sharing: Gulf Port

5730 Shore Boulevard
Gulfport, FL 33707
727-384-6346
e-mail: cascil@cascil.org
www.cascil.org

Michael Cook, Executive Director
CASCIL assists persons with all types of disabilities and their families, to achieve the greatest degree of self-determination in accessibility, advocacy, education, employment and place of residence in keeping with the consumer's freedom of choice.

3697 Cathedral Center for Independent Living

3599 University Boulevard S
Jacksonville, FL 32216
904-789-9473

Susan Hughes, Administrator
Reza Taba, MD
Offers comprehensive rehabilitation.

3698 Center for Independent Living in Central Florida - Advocacy Living Skills Peer Support

720 N Denning Drive
Winter Park, FL 32789
407-623-1070
877-891-6448
FAX: 407-623-1390
TTY: 407-623-1885
e-mail: info@cilorlando.org
www.cilorlando.org

Gassie Jeanneatte, Program Director
Elizabeth Howe, Executive Director
Information and referral services, advocacy, living skills, peer support, employment.

3699 Center for Independent Living of Broward

4800 N State Road 7
Suite 102
Ft. Lauderdale, FL 33319
954-722-6400
888-722-6400
FAX: 954-735-1958
e-mail: cilb@cilbroward.org
www.cilbroward.org

Karen Dickerhoof, Executive Director
William Knight, Deputy Director
A non-profit organization whose mission is to offer assistance to people with disabilities in fulfilling the goals of independence and self sufficiency.

3700 Center for Independent Living of Florida Keys

103400 Overseas Highway
Suite 243
Key Largo, FL 33037
305-453-3491
877-335-0187
FAX: 305-453-3488
TTY: 305-453-3491
e-mail: cilkeys@cilkeys.org
www.cilkeys.org

Brenda Pierce, Director
Offers assistance to persons with disabilities in acquiring independent living and self-advocacy skills in order to obtain and maintain independence and self-sufficiency.

3701 Center for Independent Living of N Central Florida

3445 NE 24th Street
Ocala, FL 34470
352-368-3788
800-265-5724
FAX: 352-629-0098
e-mail: cilncf@cilncf.org
www.cilncf.org

Carol Terrillion, Site Coordinator

CILNCF empowers people with disabilities to exert our individuals rights to live as independently as possible, make personal life choices and achieve full community inclusion.

3702 Center for Independent Living of N Florida

1823 Buford Court
Tallahassee, FL 32308 850-575-9621
e-mail: cilnf@nettally.com

Janet Kahn, Executive Director
Offers assistance to persons with disabilities in acquiring independent living and self-advocacy skills in order to obtain and maintain independence and self-sufficiency

3703 Center for Independent Living of NW Florida

3600 N Pace Boulevard
Pensacola, FL 32505 850-595-5566
877-245-2457
FAX: 850-595-5560
e-mail: cilnwf@cilnwf.org
www.cilnwf.org

Susan Patterson, President
Frank Cherry, Executive Director
We provide resources and services for people with disabilities in Escarnbia, Santa Rosa, Okaloosa and Walton Counties. Equipment loan, home modifications, ramps, art class and many other services. We are the Gulf Coast demonstration & resource center for the Florida alliance for assistive services and technology.

3704 Center for Independent Living of North Central Florida

3774 W Gulf to Lake Highway
Lecanto, FL 34461 352-527-8399
877-232-8261
FAX: 352-527-9511
TTY: 352-527-8399
e-mail: jackson@cilncf.org
www.cilncf.org

Cathy Jackson, Site Coordinator
Empowers people with disabilities to exert their individual rights to live as independently as possible, make personal life choices and achieve full community inclusion.

3705 Center for Independent Living of S Florida

6660 Biscayne Boulevard
Miami, FL 33138 305-751-8025
800-854-7551
FAX: 305-751-8944
TTY: 305-751-8025
e-mail: info@soflacil.org
www.soflacil.org

Kelly Greene, Executive Director
Ubaldo Alvarez, Program Manager
Jackie , Information and Referral Special
A community based non for profit, independent living center serving people of all ages with any type of disability. Services: Basic education, GED preperation, American sign language advocacy, peer support, information and referral, independent living skills training, housing assistance, transportation assistance, home modiifications, transition from nursing facility to the community assisatnace filing ADA complaints, accessibility surveys, diability awareness traing.

3706 Center for Independent Living of SW Florida

2830 Winkler Avenue
Unit 201
Fort Myers, FL 33916 239-277-1447
888-343-6991
888-343-6991
FAX: 239-277-1647
TTY:239-277-3964
e-mail: cilfl@neosmart.com
www.cilfl.org

Linda Hendricks, Director
Ronald Muschonge, President
PRovides information and referral services, advocacy, independent living skills training, peer counseling and support for persons with significant disabilities.

3707 Coalition For Independent Living Options Inc.

6800 Forest Hill Boulevard
West Palm Beach, FL 33413 561-966-4288
800-683-7337
FAX: 561-641-6619
www.cilo.org
Promotes independence for people with disabilities.

3708 Coalition for Independent Living Option

6800 Forest Hill Boulevard
Greenacres, FL 33413 561-966-4288
800-683-7337
FAX: 561-641-6619
TTY: 561-641-6538
e-mail: cilo2000@bellsouth.net
www.cilo.org

Shelley Gottsagen, Executive Director
Independent living centers offer peer counseling, advocacy, information and referral and independent living skills development. CILO offers teen programs, an adaptive equipment loan closet, disability sensitivity training and accessibility studies and services for people who are crime victims, transition services for high school students and meal delivery programs.

3709 Coalition for Independent Living Options- One Stop Career Center

6800 Forest Hill Boulevard
West Palm Beach, FL 33413 863-462-5350
FAX: 863-462-5355
www.cilo.org
Promotes independence for people with disabilities.

3710 Disability Resource Center

625 Highway 231
Panama City, FL 32405 850-769-6890
FAX: 850-769-6891
TTY:850-769-1513
e-mail: drcpanamacity@knology.net
www.drcpc.org

Robert Cox, Director
We create new resources, ideas, and programs to assist people with disabilities.

3711 Disability Solutions for Independent Livin g

475 South Nova Road
Ormond Beach, FL 32174 386-671-1960
FAX: 386-671-1961
TTY:386-671-1960
e-mail: allysounQ@victorylanecil.org
www.victorylanecil.org

Allysoun Gallup, Director
Victory Lane CIL assists in providing educational opportunities for individuals with disabilities and our community regardng disability rights and personal responsibilities via: networking, collaboration, and grassroots advocacty efforts to enhance self-empowered individual living.

3712 Lighthouse Central Florida Inc.

215 E New Hampshire Street
Orlando, FL 32804 407-898-2483
FAX: 407-895-5255
e-mail: lvaneepoel@lcf-fl.org
www.lighthousecentralflorida.org

Lee Nasehi, Executive Director
Joyce Hildreth, CVRT, Associate Executive Director
Lee Van Eepoel, Case Management Supervisor
Lighthouse Central Florida promotes the independence of children and adults with blindness, low vision and other disabilities through technology, education, support and advocacy.

3713 Miami-Dade County Disability Services and Independent Living (DSAIL)

1335 NW 14th Street
Miami, FL 33125 305-547-5445
FAX: 305-547-7355

Edeline B Clermont, Director

Offers information and referral services serving all types of disabilities with the goal of assisting the disabled acquiring independence and control over their lives. Teaches independent living skills, job readiness and placement, home health care, sensitivity training, training in ASL and Braille, counsel people with disabilities or wide range of problems.

3714 North Central Florida Citrus County

1675 S Suncoast Boulevard
Homosassa, FL 34448
352-795-3144
800-476-5373
FAX: 352-628-3600
e-mail: sellfaster@eraamericanrealty.com
www.eraamericanrealty.com

Alma Warren, Executive Director
Dennis Pilon, Manager

3715 SCCIL at Titusville

725 Deleon Avenue
Titusville, FL 32780
407-268-2244
FAX: 706-724-6729
TTY:706-724-6324
e-mail: kswoil@csranet.com
www.virtualcil.net

Gerri Martin, Executive Director
Directory of Independent Living Centers throughout the United States.

3716 Self Reliance

8901 North Armenia Avenue
Tampa, FL 33604
813-375-3965
FAX: 813-375-3972
TTY:813-375-3972
e-mail: lfields@self-reliance.org
www.self-reliance.org

Joseph DiDomenico, Director
A cross disability agency providing services to both children and adults with disabilities to identify and overcome barriers to independence in their lives. Self Reliance also promotes independence through empowering persons with disabilities and improving the communities in which they live.

3717 Space Coast Center for Independent Living

803 N. Fiske Blvd.,
Cocoa Beach, FL 32922
321-784-9008
FAX: 321-784-3702
e-mail: sccil@bellsouth.net

Donna Taylor, Executive Director
Provides overall services for individuals with al types of disabilities. Offers peer support, advocacy, skills training, accessibility surveys, support groups, transportation, specialized equipment and sign language interpreter coordination services.

3718 Suncoast Center for Independent Living

2989 Fruitville Road
Suite 101
Sarasota, FL 34237
941-351-9545
FAX: 941-351-9875
e-mail: keith@scil4u.org
www.scil4u.org

Keith Kitchens, Executive Director
Evan Farrar, Consumer Advocate
A non-profit organizatio that assists persons with significant disabilities to live successfully in their communities. Also helps the disabled achieve their full potential with independent living services & advocating for the elimination of social and physical barriers that hinder integration in the community.

Georgia

3719 Arms Wide Open

871 Forest Path
Stone Mountain, GA 30088
770-413-2241
FAX: 770-498-2778
e-mail: hmkennet@aol.com
www.armswideopen.org

Ken Morris, Director
Mission is to provide the most economically needy members of the in-home chronic ill, aged, and disabled communities with supportive services.

3720 Bain, Inc. Center For Independent Living

316 W Shotwell Street
Bainbridge, GA 39819
229-246-0150
888-830-1530
FAX: 229-246-1715
TTY: 800-255-0135
e-mail: vharris@baincil.org
www.baincil.org

Neil Griffin, Board President
Virginia Harris, Executive Director
Established in 1995, a grass roots non profit advocacy organization founded by two disabled persons.

3721 DisABILITY LINK NW

411 Broad Street
Rome, GA 30161
706-314-0008
FAX: 706-314-0011
TTY:770-534-6656
e-mail: rrtuttle@disabilitylink.org

Donna Baxley, Director
disABILITY LINK NW is committed to promoting the rights of all people with disabilites.

3722 Disability Action Center for Georgia

755 Commerce Drive
Suite 105
Decatur, GA 30030
404-687-8890
800-239-2507
FAX: 404-687-8298
TTY: 404-687-9175
e-mail: info@disabilitylink.org
www.disabilitylink.org

Rebecca Ramag-Tuttle, President/CEO
Hilary Elliott, Assistant Director
Diana Allen, Program Manager
Offers the following services: self advocacy, systems advocacy, peer support, information & referral, independent living skills training and nursing facility transition services,

3723 Disability Connections

170 College Street
Macon, GA 31201
478-741-1425
800-743-2117
FAX: 478-755-1571
e-mail: dcinfo@disabilityconnections.com
www.disabilityconnections.com

Jerilyn Leverett, Director
A private non-profit organization that looks to enable all people with disabilities to attain and have access to all opportunities in life.

3724 Division of Rehabilitation Services

Georgia Department of Labor
410 Mall Boulevard
Suite B
Savannah, GA 31406
912-356-2537
FAX: 912-691-6816
TTY:912-356-2940
e-mail: www.dol.state.ga.us

Allen Beall, Regional Director
George Foley, Manager
Vocational rehabilitation services.

3725 Georgia's SILC

755 Commerce Drive
Suite 415
Decatur, GA 30033
770-270-6860
888-288-9780
FAX: 770-270-5957
TTY: 770-270-5671
e-mail: ppuckett@silcga.org
www.silcga.org

Patricia Puckett, Executive Director
Colleen Caffrey, Executive Assistant
The mission of the Statewide Independent Living Council of Georgia, Inc. is equal participation of people with disabilities within their communities.

3726 Living Independence for Everyone (LIFE)
17 Travis Street
Savannah, GA 31406
912-920-2414
800-948-4824
FAX: 912-920-0007
TTY: 912-920-2419
e-mail: info@lifecil.com
www.lifecil.com

Frances Todd, Director
Offers a wide range of resources, education, and advocacy to the community to help level the playing field for people with disabilities to create a world in which everyone can participate.

3727 Multiple Choices Center for Independent Living
999 Gaines School Road
Athens, GA 30605
706-549-1020
877-549-1020
FAX: 706-549-1060
e-mail: info@multiplechoices.us
www.multiplechoices.us

Peggy Chavis, Director
Mutliple Choices is dedicated to the empowerment of people of all ages and with all types of disabilities to live independently and to control their lives as much as possible. Serves people in Barrow, Clark, Elbert, Green, Jackson, Madison, Morgan, Oconee, Oglethorpe and Walton counties.

3728 North District Independent Living Program
311 Green St NW
Suite 209
Gainesville, GA 30501
770-535-5930

Sharon McCurry, Coordinator
Cindy Hanna, Executive Director
Information and referral, advocacy, peer counseling, service coordination and ADA consultation.

3729 Southeastern Paralyzed Veterans Of America (PVA)
4010 Deans Bridge Road
Hephzibah, GA 30815
706-796-6301
800-292-9335
FAX: 706-796-0363
e-mail: paravet@comcast.net
www.pva.org

David Vaughn, President
Works to maximize the quality of life for its members and all people with SCI/D as a leading adovocate for healthcare, SCI/D research and education, veteran's benefits, and rights, accessibility and the removal of architectural barriers, sports programs, and disability rights.

3730 Southwest District Independent Living Program
PO Box 1606
Albany, GA 31702
229-430-4170
FAX: 229-430-4466

Bill Layton, Director
Diane Davis, Executive Director
Offers peer counseling, disability education and awareness, attendant care registry, and information on accessible home for the disabled.

3731 Walton Option for Independent Living
948 Walton Way
PO Box 519
Augusta, GA 30903
706-724-6262
FAX: 706-724-6729
TTY:706-724-6262
e-mail: tjohnston@walteroptions.org
www.waltonoptions.org

Tiffany Johnston, Executive Director
Services include advocacy, assistive technology services, braille instruction, community education, home modifications, orientation and mobility services, peer support, and return to work services

3732 Walton Options For Independent Living (Warrington)
928 E 1 Warrenton Highway
PO Box 162
Warrenton, GA 30828
706-465-1148
FAX: 706-465-1168
TTY:706-465-1148
e-mail: tjohnston@waltonoptions.org
www.waltonoptions.org

Tiffany Johnston, Director
Empowers persons of all ages with all types of disabilities to reach their highest level of independence, including community inclusion and employment. Walton OPtions covers 30 counties in north eastern Georgia, and 10 counties in western South Carolina.

Hawaii

3733 Center For Independent Living- Kauai
PO Box 3529
Lihue, HI 96766
808-245-4034
FAX: 808-245-7218
e-mail: kcil@aloha.net
www.hiddc.org/kauai

Humberto Blanco, Administrator
Teri Yamashiro, IL Specialist
Offers peer counseling, disability education, attendant care registry, outreach services and advocacy.

3734 Center for Independent Living: E Hawaii
400 Hualani Street
Suite 16d
Hilo, HI 96720
808-935-3777
FAX: 808-961-6737
e-mail: cilwh@ilhawaii.net

Laura Tobosa, Contact
Provides an array of support services for people with all types of disabilities of any age.

3735 Hawaii Center for Independent Living-Maui
220 Imi Kala Street
Suite 103
Wailuku, HI 96793
808-242-4966
FAX: 808-244-6978
TTY:808-242-4968
e-mail: mcilogg@gte.net

Pat Lockwood, Contact
T Lay , Administrative Assistant
Offers disability education and awareness, advocacy and counseling.

3736 Hawaii Centers for Independent Living
414 Kuwili Street
Suite 102
Honolulu, HI 96817
808-522-5400
FAX: 808-522-5427
TTY:808-522-5415
e-mail: patl@pacificil.org
www.hawaii.cil.org

Patricia Lockwood, Executive Director
Our staff and Board of directors are excellent advocates with the disabled community. We will connect you with resources to make your own choices for housing, employment, and personal care and to find assistive devices and technology to improve quality of life. On both the islands of Oahu and Hawaii, we have a independent living specialist who is fluent in american sign language and is well known in the deaf community.

3737 Kailua Kona Center for Independent Living: West Hawaii

81-6627 Mamalahoa Highway
Suite B-5
Kealakekua, HI 96750
808-323-2221
FAX: 808-323-2383
TTY:808-323-2262
e-mail: cilwh@ilhawaii.net

Merle Martin, Contact
A nonprofit organization run by and for persons with disabilities. Information on housing referrals, financial benefits, advocacy, personal care attendants, services for elderly blind, and independent living skills counseling. Services are free to all disabled persons.

3738 Kauai Center for Independent Living

PO Box 3529
Lihue, HI 96766
808-245-4034
FAX: 808-245-7218
e-mail: kcil@mail.aloha.net

Laurao Tobosa, Program Coordinator
Provides a variety of support services for people with all types of disabilities.

Idaho

3739 American Falls Office: Living Independently for Everyone (LIFE)

2110 South Rollandet Avenue
Idaho Falls, ID 83402
208-529-8610
FAX: 208-529-6804
e-mail: deann@idlife.org
www.idlife.org

Dean Nielson, Executive Director
Tina Noreen, Programs Coordinator
Enables people with disabilities to manage their own lives, make their own choices, and give information and knowledge to assist in living with dignity and bravado.

3740 Dawn Enterprises

280 Cedar Street
PO Box 388
Blackfoot, ID 83221
208-785-5890
FAX: 208-785-3095
e-mail: dawnent2@if.rmci.net
www.orgsites.com/id/dawnent

Teresa Oakes, Director
Donna Butler, Assistant Director
A private non-profit organization that offers Employment, housing and Community Support Services to assist individuals with mental, physical, or social disabilities to achieve independence up to each person's maximum capability.

3741 Disability Action Center NW

East 124 Third Street
Suite 7
Moscow, ID 83843
208-883-0523
800-475-0070
FAX: 208-883-0524
e-mail: moscow@dacnw.org
www.dacnw.org

Mark Leeper, Organization Director
Gina Morris, Independent Living Advocate
Information and referrals, accessibility consultant, advocacy, personal care attendant registry, peer support groups, counseling and recreation opportunities and skills training. Also provides assistive technology services and information. *$45.00*

3742 Disability Action Center, NW

307 19th Street
Suite A-1
Lewiston, ID 83501
208-746-9033
FAX: 208-746-1004
TTY:208-746-9033
e-mail: lewiston@dacnw.org
www.dacnw.org

Mark Leeper, Director
Melissa Painter, Independent Living Advocate
Information and referrals, accessibility consultant, advocacy, personal care attendent registry, peer support groups, counseling and recreation opportunities and skills training. Also provides assistive technology services and information.

3743 Disability Action Center-N.W.

1323 E Sherman Avenue
Suite 7
Coeur D Alene, ID 83814
208-664-9896
800-854-9500
FAX: 208-666-1362
e-mail: cda@dacnw.org
www.dacnw.org

Amy Dreps, Site Coordinator
Cindy Nelson, Independent Living Advocate
Mark Leeper, Executive Director
Provides advocacy, peer counseling, information and referral, independent living skills and personal assistant services.

3744 Idaho Commission for the Blind and Visually Impaired

341 Washington Street
Po Box 83720
Boise, ID 83720
208-334-3220
800-542-8688
FAX: 208-334-2963
e-mail: mblackal@icbvi.state.id.us
www.icbvi.state.id.us

Mike Blackaller, Vocational Rehabilitation
Brian Jain, Independent Living
Nancy Wise, Sight Restoration
Empowers persons who are blind or visually impaired by providing vocational rehabilitation training, skills training and educational opportunities to achieve self fulfillment through quality employment and independent living; to serve as a resource to families and employers and to expand public awareness regarding the potential of all persons who are blind or visually impaired.

3745 Idaho Falls Office: Living Independently for Everyone (LIFE)

640 Pershing Avenue
Suite A
Pocatello, ID 83204
208-232-2747
800-631-2747
FAX: 208-232-2753
e-mail: deann@idlife.org
www.idlife.org

Dean Nielson, Executive Director
Tina Noreen, Programs Coordinator
Enables people with disabilities to manage their own lives, make their own choices, and give information and knowledge to assist in living with dignity and bravado.

3746 LIFE: Fort Hall

PO Box 4185
Fort Hall, ID 83203
208-478-3952

e-mail: wparker@if.rmci.net
www.ilru.org

Wnedy Parker, Director
Enables people with disabilities to manage their own lives, make thier own choices, and give information and knowledge to assist in living with dignity and bravado.

3747 **Living Independence Network Corporation**
2500 Kootenai Street
Boise, ID 83705
208-336-3335
FAX: 208-384-5037
e-mail: info@lincidaho.org
www.lincidaho.org

Roger Howard, Executive Director
A non-profit organization empowering people with disabilities to achieve their desired level of independence. LINC promotes personal growth and freedom of choice through advocacy, networking, public awareness and modification of environments.

3748 **Living Independence Network Corporation: Canyon County Satelite**
2922 Cleveland Boulevard
Suite 800
Caldwell, ID 83605
208-454-5511
FAX: 208-454-5515
TTY:208-454-5511
e-mail: info@lincidaho.org
www.lincidaho.org

Lonora Barney, Executive Director
A non-profit organizaition, empowers people with disabilities to achieve their desired level of independence.

3749 **Living Independent for Everyone (LIFE): Pocatello Office**
640 Pershing Avenue
Pocatello, ID 83201
208-232-2747
FAX: 208-232-2753
TTY:208-232-2747
e-mail: dean@if.rmci.net
www.idaholifecenter.org

Dean Nielson, Executive Director
Enables people with disabilities to manage thier own lives, make their own choices, and give information and knowledge to assist in living with dignity and bravado.

3750 **Living Independently Now Center Inc., Twin Falls**
132 Main Avenue S
Twin Falls, ID 83301
208-733-1712
FAX: 208-733-7711
e-mail: mheinrich@lincidaho.org
www.lincinc.org

Melva Heinrich, Executive Director
A non-profit organization empowering people with disabilities to achieve their desired level of independence. LINC promotes personal growth and freedom of choice through advocacy, networking, public awareness and modification of environments.

3751 **Living Independently Now Center, Inc.**
317 Happy Day Boulevard
Suite 130
Caldwell, ID 83607
208-454-5511
FAX: 208-454-5515
e-mail: linccc3info@aol.com
www2.state.id.us/silc/cils.htm

Lonora Barney, Executive Director
A non-profit organization, empowers people with disabilities to achieve their desired level of independence. LINC promotes personal growth and freedom of choice through advocacy, networking, public awareness and modification of environments.

3752 **Living Independently for Everyone (LIFE): Blackfoot Office**
Living Independently for Everyone (LIFE): Pocate
67 North Maple
PO Box 86
Blackfoot, ID 83221
208-785-9648
FAX: 208-785-2398
e-mail: bfoot@ida.net
www.idaholifecenter.org

Dean Nielson, Executive Director
Lucy Navo, Manager
Lori Galvan, Independent Living Advisor
Enable people with disabilities to manage their own lives, make their own choices, and give information and knowledge to assist in living with dignity and bravado.

3753 **Living Independently for Everyone: Burley**
2311 Park Avenue
Suite 7
Burley, ID 83318
208-678-7705
FAX: 208-678-7771
e-mail: lifetoni@pmt.org
www2.state.id.us/silc/Life.htm

Ruth Gneiting, President
Dean Nielson, Executive Director
Sandra Dressel, Program Coordinator/Manager
Enables people with disabilities to manage their own lives, make their own choices, and give information and knowledge to assist in living with dignity and bravado.

3754 **Southwestern Idaho Housing Authority**
1108 W Finch Drive
Nampa, ID 83651
208-467-7461
FAX: 208-463-1772

David W Patten, Executive Director
Offers housing for rent and section/8

Illinois

3755 **Access Living of Metropolitan Chicago**
115 West Chicago Avenue
Chicago, IL 60610
312-640-2100
800-613-8549
FAX: 312-640-2101
TTY: 312-253-7002
e-mail: generalinfo@accessliving.org
www.accessliving.org

Henry Chandler, Chairman
Marca Bristo, President/CEO
Joanne Crown, Life Director
Access Living is a cross disability organization governed and staffed by a majority of people with disabilities. Access Living fosters the dignity, pride, and self esteem of people with disabilities and enhances the options available to them so they may choose and maintain individualized and satisfying lifestyles.

3756 **Center on Deafness**
3444 Dundee Road
Northbrook, IL 60062
847-559-0110
FAX: 847-559-8199
TTY:847-559-9493
e-mail: cod@centerondeafness.org
www.centerondeafness.org

Patrick Palbicke, Technical Coordinator
Donna Gomez, Residential Services
Bonita Simon, Executive Director
COD is dedicated to providing quality services for persons who are deaf or hard of hearing and their families, through educational, vocational, and residential services in a therapuetic, community-based environment

3757 **Community Residential Alternative**
Coleman Tri- County Services
835 W Lincoln Street
Harrisburg, IL 62946
618-252-3204
FAX: 618-252-0884
TTY:618-269-4211
e-mail: ctscila6@hotmail.com
www.colemantricounty.com

Samantha Austin, Director
Six bed group home that provides a residential alternative for the developmentally disabled adult. This program is designed to promote independence in daily living skills, economic self-sufficiency, and integration into the community.

3758 **Division of Rehabilitation Services**
Department of Human Services
400 W Lawrence Avenue
Springfield, IL 62704
217-557-1601
800-843-6154
e-mail: ors@dhs.state.il.us
www.dhs.state.il.us

Rob Kilbury, Director
Carol Adams, Manager
Provides medical, therapeutic and counseling services for the disabled, as well as employment services.

3759 DuPage Center for Independent Living
739 Roosevelt Road Building 8
Suite 109
Glen Ellyn, IL 60137
630-469-2300
FAX: 630-469-2606
TTY:630-469-2300
e-mail: dcil@mcs.com
www.glen-ellyn.com/dcil

Leigh Ann Heenan, Executive Director
A non residential, community based, not for profit agency wich provides advocacy and services to persons with disabilities in DuPage County.

3760 Fox River Valley Center for Independent Living
730 W Chicago Street
Elgin, IL 60123
847-695-5818
FAX: 847-695-5892
e-mail: frvcil@frvcil.net

Marcia Savage, Executive Director
Provides services to people with disabilities in Kane, Kendall and McHenry counties. Our non-residential agency provides independent living skills training, advocacy, systemic + individual peer counseling, information and referral and housing services. Also provides technical assistance to businesses and agencies to work with people with disabilities. Locations in Elgin and Aurora. Please call for further details.

3761 Gaining Access to IL
205 N. Fourth Street
PO Box 486
Effingham, IL 62401
217-342-7110
FAX: 217-347-2562
TTY:217-342-7110
e-mail: gailcil@consolidated.net
www.silcofillinois.org

Debbie Beard, Executive Director
Dedicated to assisting persons with disabilities to achieve their own independent lifestyle.

3762 Illinois Department of Rehab Services
Department of Human Services
400 W Laurence 100
2nd Floor
Springfield, IL 62762
217-557-1601
800-843-6154
FAX: 217-558-4207
www.dhs.state.il.us/ors/

Rob Kilbury, Executive Director
Carol Adams, Manager
The state's lead agency serving individuals with disabilities. DRS works in partnership with people with disabilities and their families to assist them in making informed choices to achieve full community participation through employment, education, and independent living opportunities.

3763 Illinois Valley Center for Independent Living
18 Gunia Drive
La Salle, IL 61301
815-224-3126
800-822-3246
FAX: 815-224-3576
TTY: 815-224-8271
e-mail: ivcil@ivcil.com
www.ivcil.com

Donna Joerger, Executive Director
Brian M Szuda, Associate Director
A community-based, non-residential center for independent living dedicated to enhancing options available to persons with disabilities so they may choose and maintain individualized and satisfying lifestyles.

3764 Illinois and Iowa Center for Independent Living
PO Box 6156
Rock Island, IL 61204
309-793-0090
877-541-2505
FAX: 309-283-0097
e-mail: execdirector@iicil.com
www.iicil.com

Liz Sherwin, Executive Director
IICIl creates and maintains independence options for people with disabilities by advocating for civil rights, providing services, and promoting full participation of disabled individuals in all aspects of the community.

3765 Impact Center for Independent Living
2735 E Broadway
Alton, IL 62002
618-474-5333
FAX: 618-474-5309
e-mail: staff@impactcil.org
www.impactcil.org

Cathy Contarino, Executive Director
IMPACT promotes pride and respect for people with disabilities by sharing the tools that are necessary to take control of one's own life. IMPACT advocates full community participation, with supports, of all citizens.

3766 Jacksonville Area CIL: Havana
220 W Main
Havana, IL 62644
309-543-6680
FAX: 309-543-6711
TTY:309-543-6680

Becky McGinnis, Director
A non-profit organization, empowers people with disabilities to achieve their desired level of independence.

3767 Jacksonville Area Center for Independent Living
60 E Central Park Plaza
Jacksonville, IL 62650
217-245-8371
888-317-3287
888-317-3287
FAX: 217-245-1872
TTY:217-245-8371
e-mail: info@jacil.org
www.jacil.org

Becky McGinnis, Executive Director
Roger Deem, Administrative Assistant
JACIL is organized to serve people with disabilities in Morgan, Scott, Cass and Mason counties. JACIl is committed to enabling persons with disabilities to gain effective control and direction of their lives in the home, in the workplace and in the comunity.

3768 LIFE Center for Independent Living
2201 Eastland Drive
Suite 1
Bloomington, IL 61704
309-663-5433
888-543-3245
888-543-3245
FAX: 309-663-7024
TTY:309-663-0054
e-mail: gail@lifcil.org
www.lifecil.org

Gail Kear, Executive Director
Marianne Cavanaugh-Wozniak, Admin Services Coordinator
Disability advocacy, information & referral, independent living skills training, peer counseling, sign language interpreter referrals, braille & alternate formats, equipment loan. Services people with disabilities and their families and friends in DeWitt, Ford, Livingston, and McLean Counties in Illinois.

3769 LINC-Monroe Randolph Center
1514 S Main Street
Suite 4
Red Bud, IL 62278
618-282-3700
FAX: 618-282-2740
TTY:618-282-3700

Violette Nast, Director

3770 **Lake County Center for Independent Living**
377 N Seymour Avenue
Mundelein, IL 60060
847-949-4440
FAX: 847-949-4445
TTY:847-949-0641
e-mail: lccil@dls.org
www.lccil.org

Anita Gorski, Executive Director
Lake County Center for Indepdendent Living is a disability rights organization governed and staffed by a majority of people with disabilities. LCCIL offers services and advocacy that promote a fully accessible society, which expects participation by persons with disabilities.

3771 **Life Center for Independent Living**
741 West Washington Street
Suite 3
Pontiac, IL 61764
815-844-1132
FAX: 815-844-1148
www.lifecil.org

Dana Craig, Director
Community-based, not-for-profit, non-residential organization that was founded in 1985. LIFE Center promotes disability rights, equal access, and full community participation for persons with disaibilities.

3772 **Living Independently Now Center (LINC)**
120 East A Street
Belleville, IL 62220
618-235-9988
FAX: 618-233-3729
TTY:618-235-9988
e-mail: info@lincinc.org
www.lincinc.org

John Laker, Executive Director
Carolyn Durham, Assistant Director
Empowering persons with disabilities to live independently in the St. Clair, Monroe and Randolph counties.

3773 **Mosaic-Pontiac**
725 W Madison Street
Pontiac, IL 61764
815-842-4166
FAX: 815-842-4053
www.mosaicinfo.org

Rod Patterson, Executive Director
Providing a wide array of services to assist individuals and families in achieving positive life goals. Services to persons with disabilities and other special needs include community living options, training and employment options, spiritual growth and development options, training and counseling support.

3774 **Opportunities for Access: A Center for Independent Living**
4206 Williamson Place
Suite 3
Mount Vernon, IL 62864
618-244-9212
FAX: 618-244-9310
TTY:618-244-9575
e-mail: info@ofacil.org
www.ofacil.org

Michael Egbert, Executive Director
Serves, trains and provides information to persons with disabilities, family members and significant others and service providers. Services include: advocacy, information and referral, peer support, skills training, volunteer programs and other related services. Services are free. A cross disability community based, nonresidential, nonprofit organization serving Clay, Clinton, Edwards, Effingham, Fayette, Hamilton, Jasper, Jefferson, Marion, Wabash, Washington, Wayne and White Counties.

3775 **Options Center For Independent Living: Bourbonnais**
22 Heritage Drive
Suite 107
Bourbonnais, IL 60914
815-936-0100
FAX: 815-936-0117
TTY:815-936-0132
e-mail: optionscil@optionscil.com
www.optionscil.com

Kathy Jackson, Director
Options CIL believes that persons with disabilities have the right to make choices about their own lives and to experience life as active participants in society.

3776 **Options Center for Independent Living: Watseka**
130 Laird Littelfuse Road
Suite 103
Watseka, IL 60970
815-432-1332
FAX: 815-432-1360
TTY:815-432-4361
e-mail: options@daily-journal.com
www.optionscil.com

Kathy Petersen, Executive Director
Dorei Schoolman, Operations Manager
Promotes independent living for people with disabilities in Kankakee and Iroquis counties in Illinois. Offered free of charge are: advocacy information and referral, peer support, independent living skills training, personal assistant training and referral, community reintergration, elderly blind program, youth advocacy, free equipment/assistive technology loan, TTY training and distribution, and sign language interpreter referral.

3777 **PACE Center for Independent Living**
1317 E Florida Avenue
Urbana, IL 61801
217-344-5433
FAX: 217-344-2414
TTY:217-344-5024
e-mail: paceurbana@aol.com
www.incil.org

Nancy Hickey, Executive Director
Robin Arbiter, Program Director
PACE is a Center for Independent Living serving people with disabilities, their families, ad service providers. PACE also offers disability awareness and information to the community at large. PACE covers Champaign, Douglas, Vermilion, Edgar and Piatt counties.

3778 **Progress Center South**
400 Forest Boulevard
Park Forest, IL 60466
708-748-5156
FAX: 708-748-1630
TTY:708-748-5156
e-mail: info@progresscil.org
www.progresscil.org

Diane Coleman, Executive Director
John Jansa, Program Director
Progress Center is a community-based, non-profit, non rsidential, service and advocacy organization, operated for people with disabilities, by people with disabilities.

3779 **Progress Center for Independent Living**
7521 Madison Street
Forest Park, IL 60130
708-209-1500
FAX: 708-209-1735
TTY:708-209-1826
e-mail: info@progresscil.org
www.progresscil.org

Diane Coleman, Executive Director
John Jansa, Program Director
Offers peer counseling, attendant registry, information and referral services, advocacy, independent living skills, paid internships, housing assistance, national headquarters of Not Dead Yet.

3780 **RAMP Regional Access and Mobility Project**
202 Market Street
Rockford, IL 61107
815-968-7467
FAX: 815-968-7612
TTY:815-968-2401
e-mail: jrouse@rampcil.org
www.rampcil.org

Willie Wierman, President
Arles Hendershott Love, Vice President
Julie Bosma, Executive Director

Provides services and advocacy for people with disabilities. Services include information and referral, personal assistant services, sign language interpreters, 24 hour emergency sign language service, bus training, peer counseling, independent living skills training, accessibility assessments and information on the Americans with Disabilities Act (ADA) serving Boone, DeKalb, Stephenson and Winnebago counties in north central Illinois.

3781 Regional Access and Mobilization Project (RAMP)
530 S State Street
Suite 103
Belviderer, IL 61008
815-544-8404
FAX: 815-544-1896
TTY:815-544-8404
e-mail: myerk@rampcil.org
www.rampcil.org

Julie Bosma, Director
RAMP promotes an accessible society that allows and expects full participation by people with disabilities.

3782 Regional Access and Mobilization Project: DeKalb
1022 W Lincoln Highway
DeKalb, IL 60115
815-756-3202
FAX: 815-756-3556
TTY:815-756-2058
e-mail: myerk@rampcil.org
www.rampcil.org
RAMP promotes an accessible society that allows and expects full participation by people with disabilities.

3783 Soyland Access To Independent Living
1810 W South 3rd
Shelbyville, IL 62565
217-774-4322
866-415-0058
FAX: 217-774-4368
TTY: 217-774-4322
e-mail: sailsullQ@one-eleven.net
www.decatursail.org

William Kienzle, Director
A community-baes, non residential Center for Independent Living, is to promote and practice independent living for all persons with disabilities.

3784 Soyland Access to IL
1102 West Jackson
Sullivan, IL 61951
217-728-3186
800-358-8080
FAX: 217-728-2299
TTY: 217-523-6304
e-mail: jwooters@decatursail.com
decatursail.com

Jen Wooters, Executive Director
A community based non residential Center for Independent Living, it is to promote and practice independent living for all persons with disabilities.

3785 Soyland Access to Independent Living (SAIL)
2449 E Federal Drive
Decatur, IL 62526
217-876-8888
800-358-8080
FAX: 217-876-7245
e-mail: jwooters@decatursail.com
www.decatursail.com

Jeri Wooters, Executive Director
A community-based, non-residential Center for Independent Living, is to promote and practice independent living for all persons with disabilities. SAIL also strives to encourage and assist persons with disabilities to gain effective control of their lives by participation in all aspects of society to their fullest extent possible, especially in performing routine daily activities.

3786 Soyland Access to Independent Living: Charleston
757 Windsor Road
Charleston, IL 61920
217-345-7245
FAX: 217-345-7226
TTY:217-345-7245
e-mail: triplec@consolidated.net

Brendt Ramsey, Director
A community based non residential Center for Independent Living, is to promote and practice independent living for all persons with disabilities.

3787 Springfield Center for Independent Living
330 South Grand Avenue West
Springfield, IL 62704
217-535-2587
800-841-6167
FAX: 217-523-0427
TTY: 217-523-6304
e-mail: scil@scil.org
www.scil.org

Pete Roberts, Director
SCIL provides 4 core services: information and referral, independent living skills training, peer counseling and advocacy.

3788 Stone-Hayes Center for Independent Living
39 N Prairie Street
Galesburg, IL 61401
309-344-1306
888-347-4245
FAX: 309-344-1305
TTY: 309-344-1306
e-mail: stonehayes@misslink.net
www.incil.org

Catherine Holland, Executive Director
The purpose of INCIL is to facilitate the collaboration of all Centers for Independent Living in Illinois for promoting, through the Independent Living Movement, equal opportunities and civil rights for all persons with disaibilities.

3789 West Central Illinois Center for Independent Living
Illinois Network of Centers for Independent Living
131 North 4th Street
Quincy, IL 62301
217-223-0400
800-225-0407
FAX: 217-223-0479
TTY: 217-223-0475
e-mail: wcicil@adams.net

Julie Irvine, Director
Terry Solter, Contact
A not for profit organization providing services to people with disabilities to promote, increase and improve opportunities within the community. WCICIL's four core services are advocacy, Independent Living Skills Training, Information and Referral, and Peer Counseling. The counties served are: Adams, Brown, Hancock, Pike, McDonough and Schuyler.

3790 Will Grundy Center for Independent Living
2415-A West Jefferson Street
Joliet, IL 60435
815-729-0162
FAX: 815-729-3697
TTY:815-729-2085
e-mail: wgcil@sbcglobal.net
www.will-grundycil.org

Pam Heavens, Executive Director
Festus Fabilola, Program Manager
The Will Grundy Center for Indpendent Living strives for equality and empowerment of persons with disabilities in the Will and Grundy County areas. The Center is a cross disability, community based organization.

Indiana

3791 Assistive Technology Training and Information Center (ATTIC)
PO Box 2441
Vincennes, IN 47591
812-886-0575
877-962-8842
FAX: 812-886-1128
e-mail: attic1@aol.com

Ruth Kimberley, Executive Director
Patricia Stewart, Assistant Director
ATTIC provides support, information and education for individuals with disabilities and for families of children with special needs, and the professionals who assist these families.

3792 **Damar Homes Incorporated**
6234 Kentucky Avenue
Po Box 41
Indianapolis, IN 46113
317-856-5201
FAX: 317-856-2333
e-mail: info@damar.org
www.damar.org

Greg Johnson, CEO
Jim Dalton, COO
Carla Bill, Admissions Director
Provides Residential, Educational, Therapeutic and community living and support services.

3793 **Everybody Counts Center for Independent Living**
9111 Broadway
Suite A
Merrillville, IN 46410
219-769-5055
FAX: 219-769-5325
TTY:219-756-3323
e-mail: ecount@netnitco.net
www.lakenetnwi.org

Teresa Torres, Executive Director
A nonprofit corporation dedicated to the achievement of maximum independence and enhanced quality of life for persons with disabilities.

3794 **Four Rivers Resource Services**
PO Box 249
Linton, IN 47441
812-847-2231
FAX: 812-847-8836
e-mail: fourrivers@frrs.org
www.frrs.org

Stephen Sacksteder, Executive Director
FRRS is established to enable individuals with disabilities and other challenges to attain self independence and natural interdependence, inclusion in normal life experiences and opportunities, and general life enrichment, by working in partnership with them, their families and the communities in and around Greene, Sullivan, Daviess, and Martin Counties.

3795 **Future Choices Independent Living Center**
309 N High Street
Muncie, IN 47305
765-741-8332
866-741-3444
FAX: 765-741-8333
e-mail: futurechoicesinc@aol.com
www.futurechoices.org

Beth Quarles, Director
Provides unlimited options for minorities, youth, and hoosiers with disabilities.

3796 **Independent Living Center of Eastern Indiana (ILCEIN)**
201 S 5th Street
Richmond, IN 47374
765-939-9226
877-939-9226
FAX: 765-935-2215
TTY: 765-939-1309
e-mail: info@ilcein.org
www.ilcein.org

Tom Cooney, Executive Director
Christi Gigliotti, Administrative Director
Thomas B Glen, Jr, Program Director
Serving Fayette, Franklin, Henry, Decatur, Rush, Union and Wayne Counties.

3797 **Indianapolis Resource Center For Independent Living**
1426 W 29th Street
Suite 207
Indianapolis, IN 46208
317-926-1660
800-860-7181
FAX: 317-936-1687
TTY: 317-926-1660
e-mail: ircil@ircil.org
www.ircil.org

Melissa Madill, Director
ICIL provides services, support and information to people with disabilities to help insure equal access to all aspects of community life. IRCIL also provides educatiom amd advocacy to all members of the community to help increase awareness and break down barriers that impede inclusion.

3798 **League for the Blind and Disabled**
5821 S Anthony Boulevard
Fort Wayne, IN 46816
260-441-0551
800-889-3443
FAX: 260-441-7760
TTY: 800-889-3443
e-mail: the.league@verizon.net
www.the-league.org

David Nelson, President
Nancy Gasparini, Assistant Director
David Callister, Chief Executive Officer
Peer counseling, education, advocacy services training and support, independent living skills training, assistive equipment loaner program, youth services, orientation and mobility training, information and referral, disability awareness, Braille transcription, Center for Independent living, and public education.

3799 **Martin Luther Homes of Indiana**
Mosaic
26 N Brown Avenue
Terre Haute, IN 47803
812-235-3399
FAX: 812-235-1590
e-mail: abean@mlhs.com

Sally Montgomery, Chief Executive Officer
Anita Bean, Program Director
Providing a wide array of services to assist individuals and families in achieving positive life goals. Services to persons with disabilities and other special needs include community living options, training and employment options, spiritual growth and development options, training and counseling support.

3800 **Ruben Center for Independent Living**
4522 Indianapolis Boulevard
Suite 3
East Chicago, IN 46312
219-397-6494
FAX: 219-397-6496
TTY:219-397-6496
An independent living center providing support, information and education.

3801 **SILC, Indiana Council on Independent Living (ICOIL)**
PO Box 7083
Indianapolis, IN 46207
317-232-1303
800-545-7763
FAX: 317-232-6478
TTY: 317-232-1427
e-mail: nancy.young@fssa.in.gov

Nancy Young, Program Director
Jodi James, Silc Chairperson

3802 **Southern Indiana Center for Independent Living**
651 X Street
Bedford, IN 47421
812-277-9626
800-845-6914
FAX: 812-277-9628
e-mail: bsrimst@kiva.net

Albert Tolbert, Executive Director
Darlene Webster, Director
SICIL is a consumer controlled, community based, cross-disability, non-residential and not for profit organization that promotes and practices the philosophy of independent living: consumer control, peer support, self-help, self-determination, equal access, and individual and community advocacy. SICIL also promotes accesible and affordable housing, recreation and transportation.

3803 **Wabash Independent Living Center & Learning Center (WILL)**
4312 S 7th Street
Terre Haute, IN 47802
812-298-9455
877-915-9455
FAX: 812-299-9061
e-mail: info@thewillcenter.org
www.thewillcenter.org

Teresa A Mager, Executive Director
Darlena Gentry, Program Director/Business Mgr
Danny Wayne Beemer, Services Program Manager
The WILL Center is a nonprofit community based, nonresidential organization that is run by and for people with disabilities The WILL Center provides Systems Advocacy Information and Referral Independent Living Skills Training, Assistance in fionding anf obtaining affordable housing, Infromation on the Americans with Disabilities Act, and Assistive Technology Infromation

Iowa

3804 Black Hawk Center for Independent Living
312 Jefferson Street
Waterloo, IA 50701
319-291-7755
888-291-7754
888-291-7754
FAX: 319-291-7781
e-mail: bhcil@blackhawkcenter.org
www.blackhawkcenter.org

Dave Schumaker, Executive Director
BHCIL is a consumer controlled, private, non-residential, non-profit corporation. Provides services in the community when people with disabilities are unable to locate those services through existing agencies.

3805 Central Iowa Center for Independent Living
655 Walnut Street
Suite 131
Des Moines, IA 50309
515-243-1742
888-503-2287
FAX: 515-243-5385
e-mail: cicil@racoon.com
www.centraliowacil.com

Robert Jepson, Manager
CICIL is a community based, non-profit, non-residential program serving persons with disabilities. CICIL is dedicated to assisting all persons, regardless of disability in making choices about their own lives and in experiencing success as active participants in society.

3806 Evert Conner Rights & Resources CIL
730 S Dubuque Street
Iowa City, IA 52240
319-338-3870
800-982-0272
FAX: 319-338-8385
TTY: 319-338-3870
e-mail: info@ownersvoices.com

Chris O'Hanlon, Director
The power in our philosophy can be captured in 3 fundamental ideas: Choice, Community, and Expertise. We join with those who support human dignity in any form and we believe that those who offer financial and in other forms of support are, in no uncertain terms, making a valuable, prudent, and important social investment.

3807 Hope Haven
1800 19th Street
Rock Valley, IA 51247
712-476-2737
FAX: 712-476-3110
e-mail: vbrummel@hopehaven.org
www.hopehaven.org

David Vanningen, Executive Director/CEO
Calvin Helmus, Associate Director
Purpose is to assist persons with mental/physical/emotional disabilities to reach their potential based on Biblical convictions. Services group homes, supervised apartments, and vocational employment services.

3808 Independent Living: Iowa Everett Conner Center
730 S Dubuque Street
Iowa City, IA 52240
319-338-3870
FAX: 319-338-8385
e-mail: connerctr@aol.com

Chris O' Hanlon, Executive Director
An independent living center, non-profit, nonresidential, consumer run, community based. The center assists individuals with disabilities to maintain control over day to day activities and to advocate for themselves in order to achieve greater independence and full participation in an integrated society.

3809 League of Human Dignity
1520 Avenue M
Council Bluffs, IA 51501
712-323-6863
FAX: 712-323-6811
e-mail: cinfo@leagueofhumandignity.com
www.leagueofhumandignity.com

Michael Schafer, Contact
Christine Solomon, Manager
League of Human Dignity actively promotes the full integration of individuals with disabilities into society. To this end, the League will advocate their needs and rights, and provide quality services to involve these persons in becoming and remaining independent citizens.

3810 Martin Luther Homes of Iowa
22 Second Street NW
PO Box 15
Waukon, IA 52172
563-568-3992
FAX: 563-568-3992

Mary Lynn ReVoir, Administrator
Fred Naumann III, Communications
Richard Wicks, Executive Director
Providing a wide array of services to assist individuals and families in achieving positive life goals. Services to persons with disabilities and other special needs include community living options, training and employment options, spiritual growth and development options, training and counseling support.

3811 South Central Iowa Center for Independent Living
1907 7th Avenue SE
Suite 301
Oskaloosa, IA 52577
641-672-1867
800-651-7911
FAX: 641-672-1867
e-mail: nika.naylor@mahaska.org

Nika Naylor, Executive Director
Provides services, support and information to people with disabilities to help insure equal access to all aspects of community life.

3812 Three Rivers Center for Independent Living
505 6th Street
Sioux City, IA 51101
712-255-1065
866-253-3043
FAX: 712-255-1065
e-mail: bjdenny@aol.com

Brenda Denney, Director
Jeannie Theis, Program Coordinator
Jimmy Weber, Manager
Providing a wide array of services to assist individuals and families in achieving positive life goals.

Kansas

3813 Center for Independent Living Southwest Kansas
1802 E Spruce St
Garden City, KS 67846
620-276-1900
800-736-9443
FAX: 620-271-0200
e-mail: thorton@cilswks.org
www.cilswks.org

Troy Horton, Executive Director
The Center for Independent Living in Southwest Kansas is dedicated to helping people achieve full participation in society.

3814 **Center for Independent Living for SW Kansas**

2601 Central Avenue
Dodge City, KS 67801
620-227-6660
FAX: 620-227-8185
TTY:620-227-6660
e-mail: cilswks@gcnet.com
www.cilswks.org

Bonnie Ray, Independent Living Coordinator
Mary Jane Sandoval, Independent Living Advocate
Dedicated to helping people achieve full participation in society. Advocates for the choices, independence, and civil rights of people with disabilities

3815 **Coalition For Independence**

4911 State Avenue
Kansas City, KS 66102
913-321-5140
FAX: 913-321-5182
TTY:913-321-5216
e-mail: mail@cfi-kc.org
www.cfi-kc.org

Clark Byron, Executive Director
Dan German, Executive Assistant
Coalition for Independence looks to facilitate positive and responsible independence for all people with disabilities by acting as an advocate for individuals with disabilities, providing services, and promoting accessibility and acceptance.

3816 **Cowley County Developmental Services**

824 W Madison
PO Box 618
Arkansas City, KS 67005
620-442-5270
FAX: 620-442-5623

Martha Crane, Director
William P. Brooks, Executive Director
Offers peer counseling, attendant care registry and other services to the community.

3817 **Independence**

2001 Haskell Avenue
Lawrence, KS 66046
785-841-0333
888-824-7277
FAX: 785-841-1094
TTY: 785-841-1046
e-mail: webmaster@independenceinc.org
www.independenceinc.org

Tanya Dorf, Executive Director
Carol Hartmsn, Administrative Assistant
Services include individual and systems advocacy, assistance obtaining benefits, technical assistance, housing, assistance with modifications for accessibility, counseling, peer support, microcomputer training, transportation, community outreach and education, business management services for persons using attendants, a resource library, independent living skills training, assistive technology, information and referral, human diversity workshops and volunteer involvement.

3818 **Independence First**

2001 Haskell Avenue
Lawrence, KS 66046
785-841-0333
888-824-7277
FAX: 414-291-7525
TTY: 785-841-1046
e-mail: bobm@independenceinc.org
www.independenceinc.org

Tanya Dorf, Executive Director

3819 **Independent Connection**

1710 W Schilling Road
PO Box 1160
Salina, KS 67402
785-827-9383
800-526-9731
FAX: 785-823-2015
TTY: 785-827-7051
e-mail: occk@occk.com
www.occk.com

Shiela Nelson-Stout, Contact
Carolee Miner, Chief Executive Officer
Independent Connection believes that all people have the right to make their own decisions and exercise control over their own lives. People have the right to pursue success and take risks.

3820 **Independent Connection: Beloit**

501 W 7th
Beloit, KS 67420
785-738-5423
FAX: 785-738-3320
TTY:785-827-4081
e-mail: occk@occk.com
www.occk.com

Independent Connection believes that all people have the right to make their own decisions and exercise controll over their own lives. People have the right to persue success and take risks.

3821 **Independent Living Center of Northeast Kan sas**

521 Commercial Street
Suite C
Atchison, KS 66002
913-367-1830
888-845-2879
FAX: 913-367-1430
e-mail: ilcnek@sbcglobal.net
www.ilcnek.org

Ken Gifford, Executive Director
A not for profit agency providing services within the State of Kansas. ILCNEK looks to assist people with disabilities to live an integrated, quality life with dignity, respect, and independence.

3822 **Independent Living Resource Center**

3033 W 2nd Street N
Wichita, KS 67203
316-942-6300
800-479-6861
FAX: 316-942-2078
e-mail: jweigel@ilrcks.org
www.ilrcks.org

Judy Weigel, Executive Director
La Rae Santiagao, IL Services Manager
Using a self-help peer approach model, ILRC staff provides services, such as, independent living skills training, peer counseling, individual and systems advocacy, information and referral and service coordination to more than 400 people with disabilities annually in the counties of Bernalillo, Valencia, Cibola, Sandoval, Torrance, Guadalupe and DeBaca. Also provides funding for home modifications, vehicle modifications, assistive technology, adaptive devices, and professional counseling.

3823 **Kansas Services for the Blind & Visually Impaired**

2601 SW East Circle Drive N
Topeka, KS 66606
785-296-3311
800-547-5789
FAX: 785-291-3138
e-mail: rehab@srskansas.org
www.srskansas.org

Dianne Hemphill, Administrator
Dale Barnum, Director
Helps persons who are blind or visually to improve their quality of life. KSBVI provides people with an array of services and experiences aimed at overcoming not only the physical difficulties brought on by the loss of vision, but also the fear of change associated with vision loss. KSBVI can also help with job search and retention activities; life skills training; access to medical services; and technical assistance.

3824 **LINK: Colby**

505G N Franklin Avenue
Colby, KS 67701
785-462-7600
800-736-9418
FAX: 785-462-7679
TTY: 785-462-7600
e-mail: scarver@st-tel.net
www.linkinc.org

Scot Carver, Director
Promotes and supports the civil rights of people with disabilities and empowers them to achieve a life of independence and equality.

3825 LINK: Hays

2401 E 13th Street
Hays, KS 67601
785-625-6942
FAX: 785-625-2334
www.linkinc.org

Brian Atwell, Manager
Promotes and supports the civil rights of people with disabilities and empowers them to achieve a life of independence and equality.

3826 Osage City Resource Center for Independent Living

1137 Laing
Osage City, KS 66523
785-528-3105
800-580-7245
FAX: 785-528-3665
TTY: 785-528-3106
e-mail: rcil@rcilinc.org
www.rcilinc.org

Chad Wilkins, Contact
Mary Holloway, Chief Executive Officer
RCIL is committed to working with individuals, families, and communities to promote independent living and individual choice to persons with disabilities.

3827 Prairie IL Resource Center

103 West Second Street
Pratt, KS 67124
620-672-9600
FAX: 620-672-9601
e-mail: info@pilr.org
www.pilr.org

Chris Owens, Executive Director
Glenda Lickteig, Independent Living Specialist
The Center is directed by and serves people with disabilities. The Center also provides servies designed to empower an individual to participate in community life to the greatest extent possible, and tp experience a productive, dignified life.

3828 Prairie Independent Living Resource Center

17th S Main Street
Hutchinson, KS 67501
620-663-9920
888-715-6818
FAX: 620-663-4711
TTY:620-663-9920
e-mail: info@pilr.org
www.pilr.org

Chris Owens, Executive Director
Christi Ireland, Administrative Assistant
The center is directed by and serves people with disabilities. The center provides services designed to empower an individual to participate in community life to the greatest extent possible, and to experience a productive, dignified life.

3829 Resource Center for Independent Living: Emporia

625 Merchant Street
Suite 238
Emporia, KS 66801
620-342-1648
888-261-4024
FAX: 316-342-1821
e-mail: chad@rcilinc.org
www.rcilinc.org

Chad Wikins, Director
RCIL is committed to working with individuals, families, and communities to promote independent living and individual choice to persons with disabilities.

3830 Resource Center for Independent Living: Bu rlington

410 Cumberland Street
Burlington, KS 66839
316-364-2263
FAX: 620-364-2700
e-mail: chad@rcilinc.org
www.rcilinc.org

Chad Wilkins, Director
RCIL is committed to working with individuals, families, and communities to promote independent living and individual choice to persons with disabilities.

3831 Resource Center for Independent Living: El Dorado

615 1/2 N. Main
El Dorado, KS 67042
316-322-7853
800-960-7853
FAX: 316-322-7888
e-mail: chad@rcilinc.org
www.rcilinc.org

Chad Wilkins, Director
Doris Hammon, Manager
Marcie Adair, Office Assistant
RCIL is committed to working with individuals, families, and communities to promote independent living and individual choice to persons with disabilities.

3832 Resource Center for Independent Living: Fo rt Scott

Resource Center for Independent Living of Osage
602 Southdale
Kiowa, KS 67070
620-365-8144
877-944-8144
FAX: 620-365-7726
e-mail: chad@rcilinc.org
www.rcilinc.org

Chad Wilkins, Director
RCIL is committed to working with individuals, families, and communities to promote independent living and individual choice to persons with disabilities.

3833 Resource Center for Independent Living: Ot tawa

1302 S Main Street
Suite 8
Ottawa, KS 66067
785-242-1805
800-995-1805
FAX: 785-242-1448
e-mail: chad@rcilinc.org
www.rcilinc.org

Chad Wilkins, Director
RCIL is committed to working with individuals, families and communities to promote independent living anf individual choice to persons with disabilities.

3834 Southeast Kansas Independent Living: Yates Center

119 W. Butler
PO Box 129
Yates Center, KS 66783
620-625-2818
866-927-2818
FAX: 620-625-2585
e-mail: skilyc@skilonline.com
www.skilonline.com

Shari Coatney, Director
Gary Bates, Manager
A private not for profit corporation devoted to meeting the needs of individuals with disabilities and to serving them, their families and communities.

3835 Southeast Kansas Independent Living

1801 Main
P.O. Box 957
Parsons, KS 67357
620-421-5502
800-688-5616
FAX: 620-421-3705
TTY: 620-421-0983
e-mail: sharic@skilonline.com
www.skilonline.com

Shari Coatney, Chief Executive Officer
A private not for profit coporation devoted to meeting the needs of individuals with disabilities and to serving them, their families and communities.

3836 Southeast Kansas Independent Living: Pittsburg

104 W 6th Street
P.O. Box 1706
Pittsburg, KS 66762
620-231-6780
866-927-6780
FAX: 620-231-5920
TTY: 620-231-6780
e-mail: skilpittsburg@skilonline.com
www.skilonline.com

Shari Coatney, Director

A private not for profit corporation devoted to meeting the needs of individuals with disabilities and to serving them, their families and communities.

3837 Southeast Kansas Independent Living: Colum bus

125 E Maple Street
PO Box 645
Columbus, KS 66725
620-429-3600
866-927-3600
FAX: 620-429-3695
e-mail: skilcolumbus@skilonline.com
www.skilonline.com

Shari Coatney, President
SKIL is a private, not-for-profit corporation devoted to meeting the needs of individuals with disabilities and to serving them, their families and communities.

3838 Southeast Kansas: Chanute

106 E. Main
P.O. Box 645
Chanute, KS 66720
620-431-0757
866-927-0757
FAX: 620-431-7174
e-mail: skilchanute@skilonline.com
www.skilonline.com

Shari Coatney, Director
A private not for profit corporation devoted to meeting the needs of individuals with disabilities and to serving them, their families and comunities.

3839 Southeast Kansas: Fredonia

623 Monroe
P.O. Box 448
Fredonia, KS 66736
620-378-4881
866-927-4881
FAX: 620-378-4851
TTY: 620-378-4881
e-mail: skilfredonia@skilonline.com
www.skilonline.com

Shari Coatney, Director
Kelly Denny, Coordinator
A private not-for-profit corporation devoted to meeting the needs of individuals with disabilities and to serving them, their families and communities.

3840 Three Rivers IL Center

408 Lincoln
PO Box 408
Wamego, KS 66547
785-456-9915
800-555-3994
FAX: 785-456-9923
TTY: 785-456-9915
e-mail: reception@threerivervsinc.org
www.threeriversinc.org

Audrey Schremmer-Philip, Director
Three Rivers is a nonprofit organization promoting the self reliance of individuals with disabilities through education, advocacy, training and support.

3841 Three Rivers Independent Living Center: Centralia

PO Box 236
Centralia, KS 66415
785-857-3521
FAX: 785-857-3521
e-mail: reception@threeriversinc.org
www.threeriversinc.org

Audrey Schremmer-Philip, Director
Three Rivers is a non-profit organization promoting the self reliance of individuals with disabilities through, education, advocacy, training and support.

3842 Three Rivers Independent Resource Center

200 Southwind PI.
Suite 103
Manhattan, KS 66502
785-537-8985
877-714-7272
FAX: 785-537-3435
TTY: 785-537-8985
e-mail: reception@threeriversinc.org
www.threeriversinc.org

Audrey Phillips, Executive Director
Three Rivers is a non profit organization promoting the self reliance of individuals with disabilities through education, advocacy, training and support.

3843 Topeka Independent Living Resource Center

501 SW Jackson Street
Suite 100
Topeka, KS 66603
785-233-4572
FAX: 785-233-1561
TTY:785-233-4572
e-mail: tilrc@tilrc.org
www.tilrc.org

Michael Oxford, President
A civil and human rights organization that advocates for justice, equality and essential services for a fully integrated and accessible society for all people with disabilities.

3844 Whole Person: Nortonville

PO Box 117
Nortonville, KS 66060
913-886-2609
FAX: 913-886-2615
e-mail: info@thewholeperson.org
www.thewholeperson.org

Lon Swearingen, President
Grady Banker, VP
A private, non-residential, non-profit corporation providing Independent Living Services to residents of the states of Kansas and Missouri.

3845 Whole Person: Olathe

114 W Gregory Boulevard
Floor 1
Kansas City, MO 64114
816-561-0304
800-878-3037
FAX: 816-753-8163
TTY: 816-627-2201
e-mail: info@thewholeperson.org
www.thewholeperson.org

Lon Swearingen, President
Joseph Marvil, Vice President
David Robinson, Executive Director
A private, nonresidential, non-profit corporation providing Independent Living Services to residents of the states of Kansas and Missouri.

3846 Whole Person: Prairie Village

7301 Mission Road
Suite 135
Prairie Village, KS 67124
913-262-1294
877-767-8896
FAX: 913-262-2392
TTY: 913-393-9805
e-mail: ksdirector@thewholeperson.org
www.thewholeperson.org

Evelyn Harden, Director
The Whole Person assists people with disabilities to live independently and encourages change within the community to expand opportunities for independent living.

3847 Whole Person: Tonganoxie

10200 W Schilling Road
Salina, KS 67402
785-827-9383
FAX: 785-823-2015
TTY:785-827-7051
e-mail: ksdirector@thewholeperson.org
www.thewholeperson.org

Evelyn Harden, Director
The Whole Person assists people with disabilities to live independently and encourages change within the community to expand opportunities for independent living.

Kentucky

3848 Best Center for Independent Living
624 Eastwood Avenue
Bowling Green, KY 42103
270-796-5992
866-286-3608
FAX: 270-796-6630
e-mail: bestcil@bestcil.org
www.bestcil.org

Sharli Rogers, Executive Director
BCIL provides needed services to persons with all disabilities in South Central Kentucky.

3849 Center for Accessible Living
305 W Broadway
Suite 200
Louisville, KY 40202
502-589-6620
888-813-8497
FAX: 502-589-3980
TTY: 502-589-6690
e-mail: info@calky.org
www.calky.org

Jan Day, Executive Director
The mission of the center is to assist in providing an environment that supports the individual with disabilities in attaining independent living and the right to choose his or her personal degree of independence.

3850 Center for Accessible Living: Murray
1051 N 16th Street
Suite C
Murray, KY 42071
270-753-7676
888-261-6194
FAX: 270-753-7729
TTY: 270-767-0549
e-mail: jgallimore@calky.org
www.calky.org

Jeanne Gallimore, Executive Director
The mission of the center is to assist in providing an environment that supports the individual with disabilities in attaining independent living and the right to choose his or her personal degree of independence.

3851 Center for Community Alternatives
115 E Jefferson Street
Suite 300
Syracuse, NY 13202
315-422-5638
FAX: 315-471-4924
www.communityalternatives.org

Marsha Weissman, Executive Director
A private, not for profit agency whose primary mission is to develop effective alternatives to incarceration and to foster a more responsive juvenile and criminal justice system in order to help youth and adults live more productive and safe lives.

3852 Center for Independent Living Options
3031 Dixie Highway
Suite 103
Edgewood, KY 41017
859-341-4346
FAX: 859-341-1252
e-mail: ciloky@cilo.net
www.cilo.net

Lin Laing, Director
Steve Bradford, Executive Director
Independent Living Center

3853 Center for Independent Living: Kentucky Department for the Blind
Independent Living Office
409 N Miles Street
Rear
Elizabethtown, KY 42701
270-766-5126

e-mail: buel.stalls@mail.state.ky.us

Buel E Stalls Jr, Office Manager and IL Specialist
Nancy Bachuss, Manager
Offers peer counseling, attendant care registry and other services to the community as they relate to the blind community. The Murray office is an independent living regional office which covers 20 far western counties of Kentucky.

3854 Disability Coalition of Northern Kentucky
525 W Est 5th Street
Suite 219
Covington, KY 41011
859-431-7668
FAX: 859-431-7668
TTY:800-648-6057
e-mail: grader@fuse.net

Sarah Todvine, Executive Director
Kit Heea, Administrative Assistant
Groups working together on legislation issues concerning the people in Kentucky.

3855 Independence Place
824 E Euclid Avenue
Suite 101
Lexington, KY 40502
859-266-2807
877-266-2807
FAX: 859-335-0627
e-mail: info@independenceplaceky.org
www.independenceplaceky.org

Barry Hamilton, Executive Director
Amber D Haag, Consumer Services Director
The mission of Independence Place, is to educate and inform all persons regarding the Independent Living Philosophy for those with disabilities and for those living with disabilities. Our services include information and referral to resources, peer counseling, independent living skills training and public advocacy.

3856 Pathfinders for Independent Living
105 E Mound Street
Harlan, KY 40831
606-573-5777
FAX: 606-573-5739
e-mail: pathfinderil@kin.net

Sandra Goodwyn, Executive Director
They publish a newsletter called LifeLine 6-10 times a year. Most articles are written by Sandra Goodwyn. Editor is F.E. Goodwyn.

3857 SILC Department of Vocational Rehabilitation
209 Saint Clair Street
Frankfort, KY 40601
502-564-4440
800-372-7172
FAX: 502-564-6745
e-mail: sarahf.richardson@ky.gov
www.ovr.ky.org

Sarah Richardson, SILC Liaison
We recognize and respect the contributions of all individuals as a necessary and vital part of a productive society.

Louisiana

3858 New Horizons: Alexandria
3400 Jackson Street
Suite A
Alexandria, LA 71301
318-484-3596
888-361-3596
888-361-3596
FAX: 318-484-3640
e-mail: nhilc@nhilc.org
www.nhilc.org

Gale M McLean, Executive Director
Dimple Hughes, Manager
An association of adults with disabilities working to improve the quality of life for all who have disabilities.

3859 **New Horizons: Monroe**
2406 Ferrand
Suite 18
Monroe, LA 71201
318-323-4374
800-428-5505
FAX: 318-484-3640
e-mail: dholloway@nhilc.org
www.nhilc.org

Gale Dean, Director
New Horizons is a non-residential independent living center that offers a variety of programs and services for persons with disabilities.

3860 **New Horizons: Shreveport**
6670 Saint Vincent Avenue
Shreveport, LA 71106
860-675-4711
877-219-7327
FAX: 318-688-7823
e-mail: nhilc@nhilc.org
www.nhilc.org

Gale M Dean, Executive Director
New Horizons is an association of adults with disabilities working to improve the quality of life for all who have disabilities.

3861 **Resources for Independent Living: Baton Rouge**
New Orleans Resources for Independent Living
11931 Industriplex Boulevard
Suite 200
Baton Rouge, LA 70809
225-753-4772
800-505-2260
FAX: 225-753-4831
TTY: 225-753-4831
e-mail: contact@noril.org
www.noril.org

Yazonka Archaga, Executive Director
RIL provides quality services to individuals with disabilities to assist with living independent. RIL also offers services to inculde information and referral, advocacy, peer support and independent living skills training.

3862 **Resources for Independent Living: Baton Ro ge**
5700 Florida Boulevard
Baton Rouge, LA 70806
225-216-3844
FAX: 225-753-4831
e-mail: contact@noril.org

Yavnoka Archaga, Executive Director
RIL provides quality services to individuals with disabilities to assist with living independently; also offer a wide array of services to include information and referral, advocacy, peer support and independent living skills training.

3863 **Resources for Independent Living: Metairie**
3616 S I-10 Service Road W
Suite 111
Metairie, LA 70001
504-522-1955
877-505-2260
FAX: 504-522-1954
TTY: 504-522-1956
e-mail: contact@noril.org
www.noril.org

Yavonka Archaga, Executive Director
RIL provides quality services to individuals with disabilities to assist with living independently. RIL also offers an array of services to include information and referral, advocacy, peer support and independent living skills training.

3864 **Southwest Louisiana Independence Center: L ake Charles**
1202 Kirkman Street
Lake Charles, LA 70601
337-477-7194
888-403-1062
FAX: 337-477-7198
TTY: 337-477-7196
www.slic-la.org

Mitch Granger, Executive Director
SILC provides Information and Referral, Advocacy, Peer Counseling and other Independent Living Services, to develop community options for persons with significant disabilities in Southwest and Central Louisiana, and to assist them in achieving and maintaining self-sufficient, productive lives.

3865 **Southwest Louisians Independence Center: Lafayette**
850 Kaliste Saloom Rd.
Suite 118
Layfayette, LA 70506
337-269-0027
888-516-5009
FAX: 337-233-7660
TTY: 337-233-7660
e-mail: lafslic@catel.net
www.slic-la.org

Mitch Granger, Executive Director
SILC provides Information and Referral, Advocacy, Peer Counseling and other Independent Living Services, to develop community options for persons with significant disabilities in Southwest and South Central Louisiana, and to assist them in achieving and maintaining self-sufficient, productive lives.

3866 **Volunteers of America Supported Living Program**
3939 N Causeway Boulevard
Suite 3200
Metairie, LA 70002
504-836-8702
FAX: 504-835-0409

Carrie Reinecke, Executive Director
Provides supported living services including pca, respite, skills traning, day, night, and behavior companion.

3867 **W Troy Cole Independent Living Specialist**
1900 Lamy Lane
Suite H
Monroe, LA 71201
318-323-4374

Katherine Carnell, Manager

Maine

3868 **Alpha One: Aroostook**
Alpha One: South Portland
127 Main Street
South Portland, ME 04106
207-767-2189
800-640-7200
FAX: 207-799-8346
e-mail: aroostook@alphaonenow.com
www.alphaonenow.com

Darlene Stewart, Independent Living Specialist
Ketra S Crosson, Aroostook County Coordinator
Kelley Teague, Manager
Committed to being a leading enterprise providing the community with information, services and products that create opportunities for people with disabilities to live independently. Offers adaptive equipment loan program, independent living skills instruction, adapted driver evaluation and training, information and referral services, peer support, advocacy, access design consultation, and more.

3869 **Alpha One: Augusta**
242 Western Avenue
Augusta, ME 04330
207-623-1115
800-499-2357
FAX: 207-623-1369
www.alphaonenow.com

Steven Tremblay, Director
Works throughout the state of Maine. The Board of Directors, staff and a network of personal and professional connections assist people with disabilities to gain access to and achieve their own independent living goals. Wherever persons are in Maine, this network creates improved and increased opportunities for people with disabilities.

3870 Alpha One: Bangar
1048 Union Street
Suite 2
Bangor, ME 04401
207-441-6553
800-300-6016
FAX: 207-941-6410
e-mail: dfitzgibbons@alphaonenow.com
www.alphaone.org

Dennis Fitzgibbons, Executive Director
Kelly McTague, Branch Manager
Committed to being a leading enterprise providing the community with information, services and products that create opportunities for people with disabilities to live independently. Provides many services including adaptive and mobility equipment selection, peer support, advocacy, information and referral services, adapted drive evaluation and training, and consumer directed personal assistance.

3871 Alpha One: Main Office
127 Main Street
South Portland, ME 04106
207-767-5690
800-640-7200
FAX: 207-799-8346
e-mail: dfitzgibbons@alphaonenow.com
www.alpha-one.org

Dennis Fitzgibbons, Director
Steven Tremblay, Owner
Alpha One, directed by people with disabilities, is committed to being a leading enterprise providing the community with information, services and products that create opportunities for people with disabilities to live independently. Offer a variety of services including access design consultation, information and referrals, attendant services, independent living skills instruction and more.

3872 Motivational Services
PO Box 229
14 Glenridge Drive
Augusta, ME 04332
207-626-3465
FAX: 207-626-3469
TTY:2076212542
e-mail: rweiss@mocomaine.com
www.mocomaine.com

Richard Weiss PhD, Executive Director
Motivational Services has assisted adults recovering from significant mental illness living in the cities and towns of Kennebec County in Central Maine.

3873 Shalom House, Inc
PO Box 560
Portland, ME 04112
207-874-1080
FAX: 207-874-1077
TTY:207-842-6888
e-mail: generalmail@shalomhouseinc.org
www.shalomhouseinc.org

Joe Brannigan, Executive Director
Ric Hanley, President
Shalom House offers hope for adults living with severe mental illness by providing a choice of quality housing and support services that help people lead stab;e and fulfilling lives in the community.

Maryland

3874 Broadmead
13801 York Road
Cockeysville, MD 21030
410-527-1900
800-201-7165
TTY:800-201-7165
e-mail: hr@broadmead.org
www.broadmead.org

James E B Felter, Chairman
Rich Compton, Executive Director
A accredited not for profit continuing care retirement commuity, provides continuing care services to a diverse group of seniors in a warm, congenial community founded and operated in the spirit of the Religious Society of Friends.

3875 Eastern Shore Center for Independent Living
9 Sunburst Center
Cambridge, MD 21613
410-221-7701
FAX: 410-221-7714
TTY:410-221-7701
e-mail: escil@comcast.net
www.escil.org

Shirley Tarbox, Executive Director
ESCIL provides services to people with all disabilities regardless of age, religion, gender, ethnicity, race or national origin. In addition to the core services of information and referral, skills training, peer support and advocacy, ESCIL also offers assistance with accessibility modifications, Americans with Disabilities Act education and training, housing referrals and counseling, transportation referral and information, Brailling capabilities, Personal Attendent Services referral, and more.

3876 Freedom Center
1560 Opossumtown Pike
Frederick, MD 21702
301-846-7811
FAX: 301-846-9070
TTY:301-846-7811
e-mail: advocate@thefreedomcenter-md.org
www.thefreedomcenter-md.org

Jamey George, Executive Director
A walk in center for independent living, provides services and supports to empower individuals with disabilities to lead self-directed, independent, and productive lives in a barrier-free community.

3877 Housing Unlimited
1398 Lamberton Drive
Suite G1
Silver Spring, MD 20902
301-592-9314
FAX: 301-592-9318
e-mail: information@housingunlimited.org
www.housingunlimited.org
To address the housing crisis for adults with psychiatric disabilities who reside in Montgomery County, Maryland.

3878 Independence Now: Riverdale
6811 Kenilworth Avenue
Suite 504
Riverdale, MD 20737
301-277-2839
FAX: 301-277-4587
TTY:301-277-2839
e-mail: info@innow.org
www.innow.org

Patricia Laird, President
Catherine Raggio, Executive Director
Center for Independent Living serving Montgomery and Prine George's Counties in Maryland.

3879 Independence Now: Silver Spring
1400 Spring Street
Suite 400
Silver Spring, MD 20910
301-587-4162
FAX: 301-588-3951
e-mail: info@InNow.org
www.InNow.org

Catherine Raggio, Director
A nonprofit organization created by people with disabilities. Provides services that promote independence and the inclusion of people with disabilities in their communities. Serves Montgomery and Prince George's counties.

3880 Making Choices for Independent Living
3011 Montebello Ter
Baltimore, MD 21214
410-444-1400
888-560-2221
FAX: 410-444-0825
TTY: 800-735-2258
e-mail: mcil@mcil-md.org
www.mcil-md.org

Andrea Buonincontro, Executive Director
A non-profit agency of, by and for people with disabilities offering services and advocacy throughout the Baltimore Metropolitan Area.

3881 Resources for Independence
708 Fayette Street
Cumberland, MD 21503
301-784-1774
800-371-1986
FAX: 301-784-1776
e-mail: phcil2hereintown.net
www.rficil.org

Lori Magruder, Director
Private, non-profit, consumer-controlled, community-based organization providing services and advocacy by and for persons with all type of disabilities. Their goal is to create opportunities for independence, and to assist individuals with disabilities to achieve their maximum level of independent functioning within their families and communities.

3882 Resources for Independent Living
420 i Street
Suite 3
Sacramento, CA 95814
916-446-3074
FAX: 916-446-2443
e-mail: monicag@ril-sacramento.org
www.ril-sacramento.org

Monica Gracechild, Office Manager
The only organization in Sacramento providing services to peopl with all forms of disabilities. RIL is dedicated to providing services and support to disabled people so they can live happy and productive lives.

3883 Southern Maryland Center for LIFE
PO Box 657
Charlotte Hall, MD 20622
301-884-4498
FAX: 301-884-6099
e-mail: cflife@eartlink.net
www.somd.com

Gene Potts, Executive Director
Carrie Lanthier, Administrative Assistant
A non-profit community based organization which provides services to disabled people who live or work in the tri-county area. Our mission is to empower people with disabilities to lead self-directed, independent, and productive lives in their community.

Massachusetts

3884 ARC Of Cape Cod
PO Box 428
Hyannis, MA 02601
508-790-3667
888-593-8062
FAX: 508-775-5233
e-mail: arcofcapecod@hotmail.com
www.arcofcapecod.org

Robert Spongberg, Executive Director
Provides adults with developmental disabilities a full range of individual supports to assist them in becoming valued members of their community.

3885 Adlib Inc.
215 North Street
Pittsfield, MA 01201
413-442-7047
800-232-7047
FAX: 413-443-4338
TTY: 413-442-7158
e-mail: adlib@adlibcil.org

Joseph Castellani, Executive Director
Offers information and referral services, independent living skills training, peer counseling, individual and group advocacy services available to all people with disabilities. Access consultation provided to businesses, agencies and institutions in accordance to the Americans with Disabilities Act.

3886 American Red Cross of Cape Cod and Islands
American Red Cross in Washington DC
286 South Street
Hyannis, MA 02601
508-775-1540
FAX: 508-771-2209
e-mail: arc@cape.com
www.capecodandislandsredcross.org

Glen Beasley, Executive Director
Provides emergency response service and health and safety training to the residents of Cape Cod, Nantucket and Martha's Vineyard for 90 years.

3887 Boston Center for Independent Living
60 Temple Place, 5th Floor
Boston, MA 02111
617-338-6666
866-338-8085
888-338-8085
FAX: 617-338-6661
TTY:617-338-6662
e-mail: info@bostoncil.org
www.bostoncil.org

Bill Henning, Executive Director
Offers skills training, peer mentoring, advocacy training and information services to help persons with disabilities of all ages assume full control over their own life choices. Works with youth in schools to promote effective transition into adult independence. Empowers people by providing information in all aspects of daily living, including the statewide housing registry, personal care assistant program and ongoing assistance. Works with others to address social concerns effecting disabled.

3888 Cape Organization for Rights of the Disabled (CORD)
1019 Iyannough Road
Suite 4
Hyannis, MA 02601
508-775-8300
800-541-0282
FAX: 508-775-7022
e-mail: coreen@cape.com
www.cordonline.org

Coreen Brinckerhoff, Acting Director
CORD works to advance the independence, productivity, and integration of people with disabilities, inluding deaf and hard of hearing people, into mainstream society.

3889 Center for Living & Working: Fitchburg
76 Summer Street
Fitchburg, MA 01420
978-345-1568
TTY:978-345-1568
e-mail: centerlwA@centerlw.org
www.centerlw.org
The Center for Living and Working is a non-profit Independent Living Center which takes its direction from persons with disabilities. The Center advocates to empower persons with disabilities to take active roles in their lives and in their community in which they live. Also provides comprehensive amd innovative programs and services in order to maximize individual independence and opportunities.

3890 Center for Living & Working: Milford
100 Medway Road
Milford, MA 01757
508-473-2271
TTY:508-473-2271
e-mail: centerlw@centerlw.org
www.centerlw.org

Mike Kennedy, President
Ann Ruder, VP
The Center advocates to empower persons with disabilities to take active roles in their lives and in the community in which they live. Provides comprehensive and innovavtive programs and services in order to maximize individual independence and opportunities.

3891 Center for Living & Working: Worcester
484 Main Street
Suite 345
Worcester, MA 01608
508-798-0350
FAX: 508-797-4015
TTY:508-363-1226
e-mail: centerlw@centerlw.org
www.centerlw.org

Mike Kennedy, President
Jamie Ross, Executive Director
The Center advocates to empower persons with disabilities to take active roles in their lives and in the community in which they live. We provide comprehensive and innovative programs and services in order to maximize individual independence and opportunities.

3892 DEAF
215 Brighton Avenue
Allston, MA 02134
617-254-4041
800-886-5195
FAX: 617-254-7091
TTY: 617-254-4041
e-mail: info@deafinconline.org
www.deafinconline.org

Sharon Applegate, Executive Director
DEAF encourages and empowers Deaf and Hard of Hearing individuals to lead independent and productive lives.

3893 Independence Associates
10 Oak Street
2nd Floor
Taunton, MA 02780
508-880-5325
FAX: 508-880-6311
e-mail: indasspc@iacil.org
www.iacil.org

Constance Gallant, Executive Director
Provides comprehensive services which wll enhance the range of acceptable options available to the consumer and improve the quality of life of persons with disabilities; to work on behalf of the objective of the disablility rights and independent living movement.

3894 Independent Living Center of the North Shore and Cape Ann
27 Congress Street
Suite 107
Salem, MA 01970
978-741-0077
888-751-0077
FAX: 978-741-1133
TTY: 978-745-1735
e-mail: smcduff@ilcnsca.org
www.ilcnsca.org

Mary Margaret Moore, Executive Director
Kathy O'Brien, Associate Director
ILNSCA is a service and advocacy center run by and for people with disabilities. Offered services include independent living skills training, peer counseling, information and referral, and advocacy; home modification, vehicle modifications and assistive equipment limited funding; ADA technical assistance.

3895 Independent Living Center of Starvos: Spri ngfield
210 Old Farm Road
Amherst, MA 01002
413-256-0473
800-804-1899
FAX: 413-733-5473
TTY: 413-781-5555
e-mail: ebrancewicz@stavros.org
www.stavros.org

James Kruidenier, Director
Promoting independence and access in the communities for persons with disabilities and Deaf people.

3896 Independent Living Center of Stavros: Gree nfield
55 Federal Street
Suite 210
Greenfield, MA 01301
413-774-3001
FAX: 413-772-2556
TTY:413-772-2556
e-mail: jkruidenier@starvos.org
www.starvos.org

James Kruidenier, Director
Promoting independence and access in the communities for persons with disabilities and Deaf people.

3897 Independent Living Center of the Southeast
66 Troy Street
Suite 3
Fall River, MA 02720
508-679-9210
FAX: 508-677-2377
TTY:508-679-9210
e-mail: scil@secil.org
www.secil.org

Lisa M Titta, Executive Director
Liz Harbison, Program Coordinator
SCIL provides training, information and support to help consumers achieve individual goals, experience personal growth and participate fully in community life.

3898 Independent Living Center: Massachusetts
48 Boylston Street
Boston, MA 02116
617-727-5550
FAX: 617-727-4716

Dave Govostes, Manager

3899 Independent Living Center: Multi-Culural Center of Boston
110 Claybourne Sreet
Dorchester, MA 02124
617-288-9431
FAX: 617-288-2597
TTY:617-288-2707
e-mail: dunn@milcb.org
www.milcb.org

Suzeth Dunn, Executive Director
MCILCB strives to empower the consumers by providing critical information that enhances their ability to live independently and function productively within their households and their communities.

3900 Massachusetts Commission for the Blind
48 Boylston Street
Boston, MA 02116
617-727-5550
800-392-6450
FAX: 617-626-7685
www.mass.gov/mcb

Joseph Weisse, Director of Outreach/Info Svcs
Provides social and rehabilitative services to all legally blind residents of the Commonwealth of Massachusetts.

3901 MetroWest Center for Independent Living
280 Irving Street
Framingham, MA 01702
508-875-7853
FAX: 508-875-8359
e-mail: pspooner@m2wcil.org
www.mwcil.org

Paul Spooner, Executive Director
A community-based, consumer-controlled, cross disability center for independent living, serving the MetroWest area of Massachusetts. MWCIL is dedicated to working on behalf of the objectives of the disability rights and independent living movements, through the provision of comprehensive services to enhance the range of options available to, and improve the quality of life of persons with disabilities.

3902 Northeast Independent Living Program
20 Ballard Road
Lawrence, MA 01843
978-687-4288
FAX: 978-689-4488
TTY:978-687-4288
e-mail: info@nilp.org
www.nilp.org

Charles Carr, Executive Director
A consumer controlled Independent Living Center providing Advocacy and Services to people with all disabilities in the greater Merrimack Valley who wish to live as independently as possible in the commuity.

3903 Renaissance Clubhouse
176 Walker Street
Lowell, MA 01854
978-454-7944
FAX: 978-937-7867
e-mail: renclub@channel1.com

Elaine Walker, Director
Pammy Sadoie, Assistant Director
Offers daily structure, assistance wtih jobs, retirement, and housing.

3904 Southeast Center for Independent Living
Merrill Street
66 Troy Street
Fall River, MA 02720
508-679-9210
FAX: 508-677-2377
TTY:508-679-9210
e-mail: scil@secil.org
www.secil.org

Lisa M Pitta, Executive Director
Bill Boffa, Director Of Programs
The Philosophy of Independent Living, maintains that individuals with disabilities have the right to choose services and make decisions for themselves. This belief is the foundation and guiding principle of all of SCIL's policies and operations. SCIL provides training, information and support to help consumers achieve individual goals, experience personal growth and participate fully in community life.

3905 Student Independent Living Experience Massachusetts Hospital School
3 Randolph Street
Canton, MA 02021
781-828-2440
FAX: 781-821-4060
www.massjury.org
Offers young adults with disabilities an opportunity to participate in a group learning situation, where they will develop independent and transitional living skills through a residential or non-residential model.

Michigan

3906 Ann Arbor Center for Independent Living
2568 Packard Road
Ann Arbor, MI 48104
734-971-0277
FAX: 734-971-0826
TTY:734-971-0310
e-mail: cilstaff@aacil.org
www.aacil.org

Jim Magyar, President/CEOector
Tom Hoatlin, Development Director
Phil Zepeda, Manager
AACIL assists people with disabilities and their families in living full and productive lives. AACIL assures the equality of opportunity, full participation, independent living and economic self-sufficiency of people with disabilities in the community.

3907 Arc Detroit
51 W Hancock Street
Detroit, MI 48201
313-831-0202
FAX: 313-831-7974
e-mail: thearcdetroit@aol.com
www.arcmi.org

Tom Lerchen, President
Norm DeLisle, Vice President
Henry Johnson, Administrator
Exists to empower local chapters of The Arc to asure that citizens with developmental disabilities are valued and that they and their families csn participate fully in and contribute to the life of their community

3908 Arc/Muskegon
1145 Wesley Avenue
Muskegon, MI 49442
231-777-2006
FAX: 231-777-3507
www.arcmuskegon.org

Margaret O'Toole, Executive Director
Michele Rosema, Administrative Assistant
Offers information and referral, advocacy services and peer counseling.

3909 Bad Axe Center for Independent Living
610 Woodworth
Bad Axe, MI 48413
989-269-5421
888-772-0442
888-772-0442
FAX: 989-269-5422
e-mail: huron@bwcil.org
www.bwcil.org

Angela Hoff, Director
BWCIL is a consumer based organization designed to serve persons with disabilities who have physical, psychiatric, sensory, cognitive, and multiple disabilities through the provision of advocacy, information and referral, service provision, and the promotion of needed services so to maximize the individual's optimal level of independence.

3910 Bay Area Coalition for Independent Living
701 South Elmwood
Suite 17
Traverse City, MI 49684
231-929-4865
FAX: 231-929-4896
e-mail: steve@bacil.org

Steve Wade, Director
Independent living center that provides information and referral services, advocacy, independent living skills training and peer support to anyone with a disability.

3911 Blue Water CIL: Lapeer
392 Nepessing Street
Lapeer, MI 48446
810-664-9098
810-401-4448
FAX: 810-664-9037
e-mail: lapeer@bwcil.org
www.bwcil.org

Angela Hoff, Director
A consumer based organization that is designed to serve persons with disabilities who have physical, psychiatric, sensory, cognitive and multiple disabilities through the provision of advocacy, information and referral, service provision and the promotion of needed services so to maximize the individual's optimal level of independence.

3912 Blue Water CIL: Port Huron
310 Watrer Street
Port Huron, MI 48060
810-987-9337
800-527-5167
FAX: 810-987-9548
TTY: 810-987-9337
e-mail: stclair@bwcil.org
www.bwcil.org

Angela Hoff, Executive Director
Offers disability education, peer counseling, advocacy, transpotation, employment, substance abuse counseling, support groups and information on accessible housing.

3913 CIL of Mid-Michigan
201 Mulholland
#302B
Bay City, MI 48708
989-895-2359

e-mail: davert@cilmm.org
www.cilmm.org

Melissa Davert, Director
CILMM exists to assist people with disabilities in learning skills and giving guidance in order for them to make choices and decisions for themselves. CILMM also promotes and encourages independence for all people with disabilities. Serves Bay, Midland, Saginaw, Arenac, Clare, Gladwin, Gratiot and Isabella counties.

3914 Capital Area Center for Independent Living
1048 Pierpont Drive
Suite 9 And 10
Lansing, MI 48911
517-241-0393
877-834-9683
FAX: 517-241-0438
e-mail: cacil@cacil.org
www.cacil.org

Ellen Weaver, Executive Director
CACIL empowers people with disabilities to take control of their lives.

3915 Caro Center for Independent Living
1184 Cleaver Road
Suite 1000
Caro, MI 48723
989-673-3678
888-673-8006
FAX: 989-673-3678
e-mail: tuscola@bwcil.org
www.bwcil.org

Ralph Moore, IL Specialist/Manager
Offers disability, education, peer counseling, advocacy, transportation, employment, substance abuse conseling, support groups and information on accessible housing.

3916 Center for Community Access
4750 Woodward Avenue
Suite 213
Detroit, MI 48201
313-832-4783
FAX: 313-832-4793
e-mail: infor@centerforcommunityaccess.org

Michael Paul, Director
The Center for Community Access assists individuals with disabilities in the metropolitan Detroit area in maintaining their independence and gaining acess to the greater community through education, advocacy and celebrating the differences.

3917 Center for Handicapped Affairs
3815 W Saint Joseph Street
Suite D
Lansing, MI 48917
517-733-7830
FAX: 517-733-7849
Organization that supports a diverse range of people with disabilities through empowerment, advocacy, information and referral, and peer support.

3918 Center for Independent Living of Mid-Michigan
2568 Packard Street
Ann Arbor, MI 48104
734-971-0277
FAX: 734-971-0826
www.aacil.org

James Magyar, Executive Director
Comprised of over 51 percent of people with disabilities, and advocates for the rights of people with disabilities in the Mid-Michigan area. Call for information on disability issues or for assistance in obtaining services, within your community..

3919 Community Connections of Southwest Michiga n
133 E Napier
Suite 2
Benton Harbor, MI 49022
269-925-6422
800-578-4245
FAX: 269-925-7141
e-mail: kellis@miconnect.org
www.miconnect.org

Kathy Ellis, Director
Teaching and empowering people with disabilities to make choices about living independently., controlling and directing their own lives and asserting their rights and responisibilites.

3920 Cristo Rey Handicappers Program
1717 N High Street
Lansing, MI 48906
517-372-4700
FAX: 517-372-8499
e-mail: info@cristo-rey.com
www.cristo-rey.com

John Roy Castillo, Executive Director
Cindi Benavides, Program Coordinator
Social/recreational program, outreach, support and self sufficiency services, drop in area.

3921 Detroit Center for Independent Living
5555 Conner
Suite 2075
Detroit, MI 48213
313-923-1655
FAX: 313-923-1404
TTY:313-923-1404
e-mail: wayne@bwcil.org
www.bwcil.org

Richard Sides, Director
BWCIL is a consumer-based organization designed to serve persons with disabilities who have physical, psychiatric, sendory, cognitive, and multiple disabilities through the provision of advocacy, information and referral, service provision, and the promotion of needed services so to maximize the individual's optimal level of independence.

3922 DisAbility Connections
409 Linden Avenue
Jackson, MI 49203
517-782-6054
FAX: 517-782-3118
e-mail: monicas@disabilityconnect.org
www.disabilityconnect.org

Monica Salgat, Director
Disability Connections is a non-profit agency serving nearly 1,100 individuals and families each year. Each person is a resident of Jackson County, Michigan. Our mission is supporting Jackson County residents in their efforts to lead independent, fulfilling, productive lives.

3923 Disability Advocates of Kent County
3600 Camelot Drive SE
Grand Rapids, MI 49546
616-949-1100
FAX: 616-949-7865
TTY:616-949-1100
e-mail: contact@dakc.us
www.dakc.us

David Bulkowski, Executive Director
DAKC exists to advocate, assist, educate and inform on independent living options for persons with disabilities and to create a barrier free society for all.

3924 Disability Connection
1871 Peck
Muskegon, MI 49441
231-722-0088
FAX: 231-722-0066
TTY:231-722-0088
e-mail: annal@dcimi.org
www.dcilmi.org

Susan Cloutier-Myers, Executive Director
An organization that supports a diverse range of people with disabilities through empowerment, advocacy, information and referral, and peer support.

3925 Disability Network, Oakland/Macomb
13213 E 14 Mile Road
Sterling Heights, MI 48312
586-268-4160
FAX: 586-268-4720
e-mail: info@omcil.org
www.omcil.org

Kelley Wilson, Executive Director
Disability Network provides information and referral services, advocacy, independent living skills training and peer support to anyone with a disability

3926 Disability Resource Center of SW Michigan
200 W. Michigan
Room B
Battle Creek, MI 49017
269-288-0047
FAX: 269-345-0229
e-mail: jcooper@drccil.org
www.drccil.org

Joel Cooper, President/CEO
Crystal Haigh, I and R Coordinator
DRCCIL educates and empowers people with disabilities to create change in their ow lives, and advocates for social change to create inclusive communities. Serving Barry, Branch, Calhoun, Kalamazoo, St. Joseph and Van buren Counties.

3927 Grand Traverse Area Community Living Management Corporation
935 Barlow
Traverse City, MI 49686
231-922-9030
FAX: 231-941-3421
e-mail: jimmoore@chartermi.net
www.gtaclmc.org

Jim Moore, Director
Mary Jean Brick, Administrative Director
We are a training home for individuals with developmental disabilities over the age of 18

3928 Great Lakes Center for Independent Living
3850 2nd Street
Wayne, MI 48184
734-727-0901
FAX: 313-832-3850
e-mail: jmeece@glcil.org

Jeannie Meece, Executive Director
Issac Hood, Owner
Independent living skills training, de-institutionalization and empowerment training for persons with disabilities.

3929 Great Lakes/Macomb Rehabilitation Group
4 E Alexandrine Street
Apt 104
Detroit, MI 48201
313-832-3371
FAX: 313-832-3850
e-mail: jlcil@home.msen.com

Jeannie Meece-Brooks, Contact
Independent living center.

3930 JARC
30301 Northwestern Highway
Suite 100
Farmington Hills, MI 48334
248-538-6611
FAX: 248-538-6615
e-mail: jarc@jarc.org
www.jarc.org

Joyce Keller, Executive Director
Non-profit organization providing residential care and support services to adults with developmental disabilities. Operates 13 licensed homes and 5 unlicensed transition homes, and supports over 60 people who live on their own. JARC also offers an array of services to families of children and adults with any disability still living at home, including respite care, life planning, educational and social programming.

3931 Jackson Center for Independent Living
2319 West Main Street
Jackson, MI 49203
517-784-1723
FAX: 517-784-9921
e-mail: jcil@modempool.com

Jim Cyphers, Director
Perry Stahl, PR/Independent Living Specialist
Jim Cyphers, I&R/Human Resources/IL Advocate
Independent Living is the principal that individuals with any disability, to the fullest extent possible, shall work, live in their own homes, raise families, and participate in the everyday activities of life.

3932 Kalamazoo Center for Independent Living
517 E. Crosstown Parkway
Kalamazoo, MI 49001
616-345-1516
800-394-7450
FAX: 616-345-0229
www.drccil.org
Provides services to people with a variety of disabilities, including physical, neurological, psychiatric, learning, cognitive, and sensory disabilites.

3933 Lakeshore Center for Independent Living
426 Century Lane
Holland, MI 49423
616-396-5326
800-656-5245
FAX: 616-396-3220
TTY: 616-396-5326
e-mail: ruth@lcil.org
www.lcil.org

Ruth Stegeman, Executive Director
Rick Diamond, Program Coordinator
A cross-disability, community-based organization providing advocacy, education, and information and referral to persons with disabilities in Ottawa and Allegan counties.

3934 Livingston Center for Independent Living
3075 E Grand River Street
Suite 108
Howell, MI 48843
517-548-1741
FAX: 517-548-1751
e-mail: dianaus1@yahoo.com

Dan Durci, Director
Independent living skills training and empowerment training for persons with disabilities.

3935 Michigan Commission for the Blind: Independent Living Rehabilitation Program
411 E Genesee Avenue
Saginaw, MI 48607
989-758-1765
800-292-4200
FAX: 989-758-1405
www.mfia.state.mi.us

Leaman Jones, Supervisor
Patrick Cannon, Manager
Rehabilitation teaching, independent living skills for persons over 55 with severe vision loss.

3936 Michigan Commission for the Blind: Detroit
Cadillac Place
3038 W Grand Boulevard, Suite 4-450
Detroit, MI 48202
313-456-1646
FAX: 313-456-1645

Gwen McNeal, Supervisor
Promotes the inclusion of people with disabilites into our communities on a full and equal basis through empowerment, education, participation, and choice.

3937 Midland Center for Independent Living
1160 James Savage Road
Suite C
Midland, MI 48640
989-835-4041
800-782-4160
FAX: 989-835-8121
e-mail: info@dnmm.org
www.cilmm.org

Sara Kristol-Brando, Executive Director
Independent Living Center.

3938 Monroe Center for Independent Living
40 N Roessler Street
Monroe, MI 48162
734-242-5919
FAX: 734-242-7129
e-mail: lmaier@aacil.org
monroecil.tripod.com

Linda Maier, Director
Assists people with disabilities and their families in living full and productive lives. Assures the equality and opportunity, full participation, independent living and economic self-sufficency of people with disabilities in the community.

3939 Southeastern Michigan Commission for the Blind
4450 Grandy Street
Detroit, MI 48207
313-456-0334
800-292-4200
FAX: 313-456-1645
www.michigan.gov

Patrick Cannon, Executive Director
Pat Bragg, Manager
Vocational rehabilitation agency. Personal adjustment vocational assessment and training, job placement and follow-up services.

3940 **Superior Alliance for Independent Living (SAIL)**
129 W Baraga Avenue
Suite H
Marquette, MI 49855
906-228-5744
800-379-7245
FAX: 906-228-5573
e-mail: moey@upsail.com
www.upsail.com

Stoney Polman, Executive Director
David Carl, Independent Living Coordinator
SAIL promotes the inclusion of people with disbilities into our communities on a full and equal basis through empowerment, education, participation and choice.

Minnesota

3941 **Accessible Space**
2550 University Avenue
Suite 330N
Saint Paul, MN 55114
651-645-7271
800-466-7722
FAX: 651-645-0541
e-mail: info@accessiblespace.org
www.accessiblespace.org

Stephen Schaaf, President/CEO
Steven F Wiggins, Founder
Provides accessible, affordable community-based housing with support services at residential and apartment sites in 20 states. Support services offered in Minnesota, Montana, Nevada and North Dakota.

3942 **Accessnorth CIL of Northeastern MN: Aitkin**
105 4th Street, NW
Aitkin, MN 56431
218-927-3748
800-390-3681
FAX: 218-927-3749
TTY: 218-927-3748
e-mail: parson@accessnorth.net
www.accessnorth.net

Kim Tyler, Director
Assists individuals to live independently, pursue meaningful goals, and have equal opportunities and choices.

3943 **Accessnorth CIL of Northeastern MN: Duluth**
118 E Superior Street
Duluth, MN 55802
218-625-1400
888-625-1401
FAX: 218-625-1401
TTY: 218-625-1400
e-mail: roberta@accessnorth.net
www.accessnorth.net

Kim Tyler, Director
Assisting individuals with disabilities to live independently, puruse meaningful goals, and have equal opportunities and choices.

3944 **Center for Independent Living of NE Minnesota**
2104 East 6th Ave. E
Hibbing, MN 55746
218-262-6675
800-390-3681
FAX: 218-262-6677
TTY: 218-262-6675
e-mail: kim@accessnorth.net
www.accessnorth.net

Kimberly Tyler, Executive Director
Assisting individuals with disabilities to live independently, pursue meaningful goals, and have an equal opportunities and choices

3945 **Courage Center**
3915 Golden Valley Road
Minneapolis, MN 55422
763-520-0312
888-846-8253
FAX: 763-520-0577
TTY: 763-520-0245
e-mail: courageinfo@courage.org
www.courage.org

Jan Malcolm, CEO
Pete Berridge, VP, Human Resources
Mary Jensen Manager
A not for profit rehabilitation organization, empowers people with physical disabilities to reach for their full potential in every aspect of life.

3946 **Freedom Resource Center for Independent Living: Fergus Falls**
125 W Lincoln Avenue
Suite 17
Fergus Falls, MN 56537
218-998-1799
FAX: 218-998-1798
e-mail: joycew@freedomrc.org
www.freedomrc.org

Nathan Aalgaard, Executive Director
Freedom Resource Center assists people in working towards goals they establish for themselves.

3947 **Metropolitan Center for Independent Living**
1600 University Avenue W
Suite 16
Saint Paul, MN 55104
651-646-8342
FAX: 651-603-2006
TTY:651-603-2001
e-mail: margotsk@mcil-mn.org
www.mcil-mn.org

David Hancox, Executive Director
MCIL is dedicated to the full promotion of independent living philosophy by supporting individuals with disabilities in their personal efforts to pursue self-directed lives.

3948 **Minnesota Association of Centers for Independent Living**
519 2nd Street N
Saint Cloud, MN 56303
320-529-9000
888-529-0743
FAX: 320-529-0747
TTY:320-529-9000
e-mail: ilicil@independentlifestyles.org
www.macil.org

Cara Ruff, President
A non profit organization whose purpose is to advocate for the independent living needs of people with disabilities who are citizens of the State of Minnesota, to develop new resources, identify and provide access to existing resources which provide the services needed by persons with disabilities so that they may live independently in the situation and community of their choice.

3949 **OPTIONS**
123 S Main Street
Suite B
Crookston, MN 56716
218-281-5722
FAX: 218-281-5722
TTY:218-281-5722
e-mail: options3@rrv.net

Gordie Haug, Director
Provides people with disabilities advocacy, information, skills training and peer mentoring relationships to help them achieve their personal goals of how and where they live their lives.

3950 **Options Interstate Resource Center for Independent Living**
318 3rd Street NW
E Grand Forks, MN 56721
218-773-6100
800-726-3692
FAX: 218-773-7119
TTY: 218-773-6100
e-mail: options@myoptions.info
www.macil.org/options

Randy Sorensen, Executive Director
Located in Minnesota, but also serves North Dakota.

3951 **Perry River Home Care**
330 High Way Pen S
Saint Cloud, MN 56304
320-255-1882
FAX: 320-255-5137

Berna Florentine, CEO
Ken Figge, President
Courtney Salzi, Administrator
Offers skilled nursing services RN, LPN, TV Therapy, Pediatrics, Rehabilitation Services, PT, OT, ST, Paraprofessional staff, Home Health Aides, Homemakers, Personal Care Attendents, Companions, Live-ins, Sleep overs, Respite care, Extended hours.

3952 **SMILES**
820 Winnebago Avenue
Suite 1
Fairmont, MN 56031
507-235-3488
FAX: 507-235-3488
e-mail: smiles@smilescil.org
www.smilescil.org

Alan Augustin, Director
A non profit organization committed to providing a wide array of services that assists indivduals with disabilities that live independently, pursue meaningful goals, and enjoy the same opportunities and choices as all persons.

3953 **Southeastern Minnesota Center for Independent Living: Red Wing**
201 E 7th Street
Red Wing, MN 55066
651-388-0466
FAX: 651-385-0643
e-mail: semcil@semcil.org.com
www.semcil.org

Sharon Taft, Contact
Non profit organization that assists people with disabilities to become independent and productive community members.

3954 **Southeastern Minnesota Center for Independent Living: Rochester**
2720 N Broadway
Rochester, MN 55906
507-285-1815
888-460-1815
FAX: 507-288-8070
e-mail: semcil@semcil.org
www.semcil.org

Vicki Molle, Executive Director
A non profit organization that assists people with disabilities to become independent and productive community members.

3955 **Southern Minnesota Independent Living Enterprises and Services**
709 S Front Street
Mankato, MN 56001
507-345-7139
888-676-6498
888-676-6498
FAX: 507-345-8429
e-mail: smiles@smilescil.org
www.smilescil.org

Alan Augustin, Executive Director
Julie Birkemeyer, IL Skills Specialist
A nonprofit organization committed to providing a wide array of services that assist individuals with disabilities that live independently, puruse meaningful goals, and enjoy the same oportunities and choices as all persons.

3956 **Southwestern Center for Independent Living**
109 S 5th Street
Suite 700
Marshall, MN 56258
507-532-2221
800-422-1485
FAX: 507-532-2222
TTY: 507-532-2221
e-mail: swcil@swcil.com
www.swcil.com

Steve Thovson, Executive Director
SWCIL is dedicated to the ever changing needs of persons wih disabilities in southwestern Minnesota. SWCIL strives to provide services, supports, and resources, as defined necessary by consumers, that will lead to the creation or enhancement of independent living options. SWCIL is also committed to providing education and awareness to promote society acceptance, inculsion, and equal access for all persons with disabilities.

3957 **Vinland Center Lake Independence**
PO Box 308
Loretto, MN 55357
763-479-3555
FAX: 763-479-2605
e-mail: vinland@vinlandcenter.org
www.vinlandcenter.org

Carol Jackson, Executive Director
Duane Reynolds, Associate Director
Mary Roehl, Operations Director
A Minnesota based rehabilitation center which offers services in three distinct service areas: vocational rehabilitation; inclusive community programs; and for people with cognitive disabilities, specially adapted chemical dependency treatment.

Mississippi

3958 **Alpha Home Royal Maid Association for the Blind**
PO Box 30
Hazlehurst, MS 39083
FAX: 601-894-2993
e-mail: sigworks@teclink.net

Howard Becker, Director
Offers attendant care registry, information on accessible housing and referrals.

3959 **Gulf Coast Independent Living Center**
18 J M Tatum Industrial Drive
Hattiesburg, MS 39401
601-544-4860
FAX: 601-582-2544

Albert Holifield, Executive Director
Independent living center.

3960 **Jackson Independent Living Center**
300 Capers Avenue
Building 4
Jackson, MS 39203
601-961-4140
FAX: 601-354-6678
TTY:601-351-1585
e-mail: odhh@odhh.org
www.odhh.org

Denea Smith, Director
Timothy Jackson
Provides services to consumers with severe disabilities.

3961 **LIFE of Central Mississippi**
1304 Vine Street
Jackson, MS 39202
601-969-4009
800-748-9398
FAX: 601-969-1662
TTY: 800-748-9398
e-mail: lifecen@meta3.net
www.lifeofms.com

Christy Dunaway, Executive Director
Augusta Smith, Assistant Director
Margie Moore, Project Coordinator

The purpose of Living Independence For Everyone is to empower people with significant disabilities to be as independent and as fully involved in their communities as they can and want to be.

3962 **LIFE of South Mississippi**

710 Katie Avenue
Hattiesburg, MS 39401
601-583-2108
800-898-8477
FAX: 601-583-1814
e-mail: lifeofms@aol.com
www.lifeofms.com

Angela Sharp, Regional Coordinator
The purpose of Living Indepdence For Everyone is to empower people with significant disabilities to be as independent and as fully involved in their communities as they can and want to be.

3963 **Life of North Mississippi: Greenville**

638 Main Street
Apt 111
Greenville, MS 38701
601-332-2220
FAX: 601-332-2261
Provides services to consumers with severe disabilities.

3964 **Life of North Mississippi: Tupelo**

201 Jefferson Street
Suite D
Tupelo, MS 38801
662-844-6633
FAX: 662-844-6803
TTY:662-844-6633
e-mail: lifetup@netdoor.com

Michael Sullivan, IL Specialist/Manager
The purpose of Living Independence For Everyone is to empower people with significant disabilities to be as independent and as fully involved in their communities as they can and want to be.

3965 **Life of South Mississippi: Biloxi**

188C Main Street
Biloxi, MS 39530
228-435-5433
FAX: 228-435-1338
e-mail: lifebil@netdoor.com
www.lifeofms.com

Christy Dunaway, Executive Director
Terri Redding, Independent Living Specialist
The purpose of Living Independence For Everyone is to empower people with significant disabilities to be as independent and as fully involved in their communities as they can and want to be.

3966 **Mississippi State Independent Living Center**

300 Capers Avenue
Building 1
Jackson, MS 39203
601-351-1525
FAX: 601-351-1460

Sheila Browning, Director
Offers peer counseling and disability education.

Missouri

3967 **Access II Independent Living Center**

611 W Johnson Street
Gallatin, MO 64640
660-663-2423
FAX: 660-663-2517
TTY:660-663-2663
e-mail: access@accessii.org
www.accessii.org

Debra Hawman, Executive Director
The mission of Access II is to remove architectural and attitudinal barriers that limit the independence of persons with disabilities, promote a positive change in attitudes about disability and persons with disabilities, and encourage greater independence for persons with disabilities within our communities. As a Center for Independent Living, Access II is comitted to the provision of a full range of independent living services.

3968 **Bootheel Area Independent Living Services**

PO Box 326
Kennett, MO 63857
573-888-0002
FAX: 573-888-0708
TTY:573-888-0002
e-mail: tshaw@bails.org
www.bails.org

Tim Shaw, Executive Director
BAILS goal is to foster an open, barrier free society flor all people regardless of their disability. BAILS service area is predominantly rural and includes the Southeast Missouri counties of: Dunklin, New Madrid, Pemiscot and Stoddard.

3969 **Coalition for Independence: Missouri Branch Office**

4911 State Avenue
Kansas City, MO 66102
816-231-7166
FAX: 816-231-7899
e-mail: kolson@cfikc.org
www.cfi-kc.org

Clark Byron, Executive Director
Deborah L Wilmarth, Executive Assistant
Coalition For Independence (CFI) is to facilitate positive and responsible independence for all people with disabilities by acting as an advocate for individuals with disabilities, providing services, and promoting accessibility and acceptance.

3970 **Delta Center for Independent Living**

5933 S Highway 94
Suite 107
St. Charles, MO 63304
636-926-8761
866-727-3245
FAX: 636-447-0341
e-mail: info@dcil.org
www.dcil.org

Nancy Murphy, Executive Director
A non profit corporation which assists people with significant disabilities who want to live more independently.

3971 **Disability Resource Association**

420 S Truman Boulevard
B
Crystal City, MO 63019
636-931-7696
FAX: 636-937-9019
TTY:636-937-9016
e-mail: dra@disabilityresourcesassociation.org
www.disabilityresourceassociation .org

Craig Henning, Executive Director
Nancy Pope, Assistant Director
Suzan Weller, Director/Resource Developer
Independent Living Cener.

3972 **Disabled Citizens Alliance for Independence**

PO Box 675
Viburnum, MO 65566
573-244-5402
FAX: 573-244-5609
TTY:573-244-5402
e-mail: dcitizen@misn.com
www.viburnum.net/dcai

Richard Blakley, Contact
Independent Living Center that supports people with developmental and other disabilities to live and work with dignity in the community.

3973 **Independent Living Center of Southeast Missouri**

511 Cedar Street
Poplar Bluff, MO 63901
573-686-2333
888-890-2333
FAX: 573-686-0733
TTY: 573-686-2333
www.ilcsemo.org

Bruce Lynch, Director
Mission is to make Southeast Missouri barrier free for all persons with disabilities, enabling them to live more independently, extending their rights to control and direct their own lives and empowering them to live more productive lives. To this end we do not do things for the persons with disabilities; we enable them to do for themselves.

3974 Life Skills Foundation
10176 Corporate Square Drive
Suite 100
Saint Louis, MO 63132
314-567-7705
FAX: 314-567-6539
TTY:314-802-5299
e-mail: info@lifeskills-stl.org
www.lifeskills-stl.org

Wendy Buehler, President
Katie Smallen, VP, Programs
Jocelyn Jones, VP, Operations
Supports people with developmental and other disabilities to live and work with dignity in the community.

3975 Midland Empire Resources For Independent Living (MERIL)
4420 S 40th Street
Saint Joseph, MO 64503
816-279-8558
800-242-9326
FAX: 816-279-1550
e-mail: meril@meril.org
www.meril.org

Debbie Merritt, Executive Director
AÆcommunity based, non residential program, designed to promote independent living and to enhance the quality of life for persons with disabilities by empowering them to controll and direct their lives and thus participate actively and independently in society.

3976 Northeast Independent Living Services
142 Jaycee Drive
Hannibal, MO 63401
573-221-8282
877-713-7900
FAX: 573-221-9445
e-mail: neils@neilscenter.org
www.neilscenter.org

Polly Nicholson, Executive Director
NEILS offers afull range of programs for individuals with a disability and any family members, employers, and/or co-workers with disability concerns.

3977 On My Own
111 N Elm Street
Nevada, MO 64772
417-667-7007
FAX: 417-667-6262
e-mail: onmyown@softnet.net

John Klingaman, Executive Director
A non profit independent living center.

3978 Ozark Independent Living
109 Aid Avenue
West Plains, MO 65775
417-257-0038
888-440-7500
FAX: 417-257-2380
TTY: 888-440-7500
e-mail: ozark@townsqr.com
www.ozarkcil.com

Cynthia Moore, Executive Director
OILÆwas created to provide independent living services to persons with disabilities who reside in the following counties in Missouri: Oregon Ozark, Shannon, Wright, Howell, Texas, and Douglas. OIL is non-profit, on-residential supported by grants, donations, and volunteers

3979 Paraquad
5240 Oakland Avenue
Saint Louis, MO 63110
314-289-4200
FAX: 314-289-4201
TTY:314-289-4201
e-mail: contactus@paraquad.org
www.paraquad.org

Robert J Funk, Executive Director
Paraquad looks to empower people with disabilities to increase their independence through choice and opportunity.

3980 Places for People
4130 Lindell Boulevard
Saint Louis, MO 63108
314-535-5600
FAX: 314-535-6037
e-mail: contact@placesforpeople.org
www.placesforpeople.org

Mary Broderick, Executive Director
Places for People provides individualized, high quality and effective services to adults with serious and persistent mental disorders to assist them in living, working and socializing responsibility to serve those individuals who rely on public funding.

3981 RAIL
715 South Baltimore
Kirksville, MO 63501
660-627-7245
888-681-7245
FAX: 660-627-0525
e-mail: center@cableone.net
www.nemr.net~ritt

Theresa Myers, Executive Director
Jean Calhoun, Administrative Assistant
RAIL is an Independent Living Center, one of twenty-two in the State of Missouri, RAIL's Mission is to assist persons with disabilities to live as independently as they choose within the communities of their choice. RAIL offers four core services which are: Advocacy, Peer Support, Information & Referral, and Independent Living Skills Training. RAIL is a Consumer Services Directed Program vendor

3982 Services for Independent Living
1401 Hathman Place
Columbia, MO 65201
573-874-1646
800-766-1968
TTY:573-874-4121
e-mail: sil@computerland.net
www.silcolumbia.org

Mark Stone, Executive Director
Tarzie Hart, Administrative Director
A non-residential, community-based center for independent living. Provides individualized and group services to persons with severe disabilities in the Mid-Missouri area; works to help people with disabilities achieve their highest potential in independent living and community life.

3983 Southeastern Missouri Alliance for Independence (SEMO Alliance)
121 S Broadview Street
Cape Girardeau, MO 63703
573-651-6464
FAX: 573-651-6565
TTY:573-651-6464
e-mail: miki@mail.sadi.org
www.sadi.org

Maryann Gudermuth, Executive Director
SADI is comitted to persons with disabilities to enable them to remain in their own home and community, and not in an institution.

3984 Southwest Center for Independent Living (SWCIL)
2864 S Nettleton Avenue
Springfield, MO 65807
417-886-1188
FAX: 417-886-3619
TTY:417-886-1188
e-mail: scil@swcil.org
www.swcil.org

Ann Morris, Executive Director
Provides services, advocacy, and resources for people with any disability in Southwest Missouri.

3985 Tri-County Center for Independent Living
1420 Highway 72 E
Rolla, MO 65401
573-368-5933
FAX: 573-368-5991
TTY:573-368-5933
e-mail: vevans@fidnet.com
www.tricountycenter.com

Victoria Evans-Heitzler, Executive Director

Mission is to eliminate physical and attitudinal barriers through the power of advocacy, enlightenment, and reformation.

3986 West Central Independent Living Solutions

710d N College Avenue
Warrensburg, MO 64093
660-422-7883
800-236-5175
FAX: 660-422-7895
TTY: 660-422-7894
e-mail: wils@iland.net

Leanne Weakley, Executive Director
Works to empower people with disabilities to become more independent by providing independent living skills training, peer support, information and referral and advocacy.

3987 Whole Person

114 W Gregory Boulevard
Floor 1
Kansas City, MO 64114
816-561-0304
800-878-3037
FAX: 816-753-8163
TTY: 816-627-2201
e-mail: info@thewholeperson.org
www.thewholeperson.org

David Robinson, Executive Director
The Whole Person, assists people with disabilities to live independently and encourages change within the community to expand opportunities for independent living.

Montana

3988 Living Independently for Today and Tomorrow: Glendrive

PO Box 621
Glendrive, MT 59330
406-365-4062
888-502-9700
FAX: 406-365-4064
TTY:406-365-4062
e-mail: liftt@midrivers.org
www.liftt.org

Dave Swanson, Program Director
Sue Davidson, IL Specialist
LIFTT's Independent living program workswith people with disabilities so they can live independently and have access to the community. LIFTT staff, most of whom havge disabilities, serves as mentors to people as they wotk to achieve the goals they have set for themselves.

3989 Living Independently for Today and Tomorrow

914 Wyoming Avenue
Billings, MT 59101
406-259-5181
800-669-6319
FAX: 406-259-5259
e-mail: daves@liftt.org
www.liftt.org

David Swanson, Executive Director
Sue Davidson, IL Specialist
LIFTT's Independent living program works with people with disabilities so they can live independently and have access to the community. LIFTT staff, most of whom have disabilities, serve as mentors to people as they work to achieve the goals they have set for themselves.

3990 Montana Independent Living Project

1820 11th Avenue
Helena, MT 59601
406-442-5755
800-735-6457
FAX: 406-442-1612
TTY: 406-442-5755
e-mail: milbob@qwest.net
www.dphhs.mt.gov

Bob Maffit, Executive Director
Montana Independent Living Center is located in Helena and provides services to southwestern Montana.

3991 North Central Independent Living Services

1120 25th Avenue NE
Black Eagle, MT 59414
406-452-9834
800-823-6245
FAX: 406-453-3940
e-mail: ncils.osborn@sofast.net
www.dphhs.mt.gov

Tom Osborn, Executive Director
North Central Independent Living Services is located in Great Falls and provides services from Glacier County across the Hi-Line to the North Dakota border. A satellite office is set up in Glasgow.

3992 Summit Independent Living Center: Kalipsell

275 Corporate Drive
Suite 901
Kalispell, MT 59901
406-257-0048
800-995-0029
FAX: 406-257-0634
e-mail: flok@summitilc.org
www.summitilc.org

Mike Mayer, Director
Flo Kiewel, County Coordinator/Manager
Advocacy for people with disabilities.

3993 Summit Independent Living Center: Hamilton

316 N 3rd Street
Suite 113
Hamilton, MT 59840
406-363-5242
800-398-9013
FAX: 406-375-9035
e-mail: jverwolf@summitilc.org
www.summitilc.org

Joanne Verwolf, Program Coordinator
Dawn Gauthier, Program Specialist
Mary Millin, People First Advisor
Advocacy and resource center for people with disabilities

3994 Summit Independent Living Center: Missoula

700 SW Higgins Avenue
Suite 101
Missoula, MT 59803
406-728-1630
800-398-9002
FAX: 406-829-3309
e-mail: sbushell@summitilc.org
www.summitilc.org

John Gabe Skibsrude, President
Becky Burke, Peer Advocate Coordinator
Jude Monson, Education Coordinator
Summit ILC helps its consumers continue to live independently in the community through a variety of individual and community services.

Nebraska

3995 Center for Independent Living of Central Nebraska

3204 College Street
Grand Island, NE 68803
308-382-9255
877-400-1004
FAX: 308-384-7832
TTY: 308-382-9255
e-mail: ray.morris@cilne.org
www.cilne.org

Ray Morris, Executive Director
Offers independent living skills training, peer sharing, information and referral, housing counseling and referral, accessibility and barrier removal consultation including ADA training and technical assistance, driver education and training, assistive technology services including demonstration and equipment loan, and a free lending library of adapted toys and ability switches for children with severe disabilities. Serves all diabilities and all ages.

3996 League of Human Dignity: Lincoln
1701 P Street
Lincoln, NE 68508
402-441-7871
888-508-4758
FAX: 402-441-7650
TTY:402-441-7871
e-mail: info@leagueofhumandignity.com
www.leagueofhumandignity.com

Mike Schafer, CEO
The mission of the League of Human Dignity is to actively promote the full integration of individuals with disabilities into society. To this end, we will advocate their needs and rights, and provide quality services to involve these persons in becoming and remaining independent citizens.

3997 League of Human Dignity: Norfolk
400 Elm Street
Norfolk, NE 68701
402-371-4475
800-843-5785
FAX: 402-371-4625
TTY: 402-371-4475
e-mail: ninfo@leagueofhumandignity.com
www.leagueofhumandignity.com

Mike Schafer, CEO
Linda Carey, Executive Director
The mission of the League of Human Dignity is to actively promote the full integration of individuals with disabilities into society. To this end, we will advocate their needs and rights, and provide quality services to involve these persons in becoming and remaining independent citizens.

3998 League of Human Dignity: Omaha
5513 Center Street
Omaha, NE 68106
402-595-1256
800-843-5784
FAX: 402-595-1410
e-mail: oinfo@leagueofhumandignity.com
www.leagueofhumandignity.com

Mike Schafer, CEO
Bob Gomez, Executive Director
The mission of the League of Human Dignity is to actively promote the full integration of individuals with disabilities into society. To this end, we will advocate their needs and rights, and provide quality services to involve these persons in becoming and remaining independent citizens.

3999 Martin Luther Homes of Beatrice
722 S 12th Street
607
Beatrice, NE 68310
402-223-4066
FAX: 402-223-4951
e-mail: jcampbell@mlhs.com

Alan Blakestad, Chief Operating Officer
Jerry Campbell, Program Director
Providing a wide array of services to assist individuals and families in achieving positive life goals. Services to persons with disabilities and other special needs include community living options, training and employment options, spiritual growth and development options, training and counseling support.

4000 Martin Luther Homes of Nebraska
220 W S 21st Street
York, NE 68467
402-362-2180
FAX: 402-362-2961

Jobey King, Executive Director
Jessica Schoepf, Coordinator
Providing a wide array of services to assist individuals and families in achieving positive life goals. Services to persons with disabilities and other special needs include community living options, training and employment options, spiritual growth and development options, training and counseling support.

4001 Panhandle Independent Living Services
PO Box 2454
Scottsbluff, NE 69363
308-635-7901
FAX: 308-635-7676
e-mail: pils@bbc.net

Carolyn Foged, Executive Director
Helps its consumers continue to live independently in the community through a variety of individual and community services.

Nevada

4002 Carson City Center for Independent Living
PO Box 3177
Carson City, NV 89702
775-841-2580

Sandra Coyle, Owner
Helps consumers continue to live independently in the community through a variety of individual and community services.

4003 Northern Nevada Center for Independent Living: Fallon
1919 Grimes Street
Suite B
Fallon, NV 89406
775-423-4900
FAX: 775-423-1399
TTY:775-423-4900
e-mail: nncilf@cccomm.net

Lisa Erquiaga, Director
Independent Living Center.

4004 Northern Nevada Center for Independent Living: Reno
555 Gentry Way
Reno, NV 89502
775-826-2022
800-633-8324
FAX: 775-826-6040
e-mail: info@medtech-services.com
www.medtech-services.com

Paul Gowins, Executive Director
Rick Graver, Owner
Community based, not for profit organizaiton providing quality support services that include: independent living skills training, information and referral, peer counseling, and aggressive advocacy for all people with disabilites and disability issues.

4005 Rural Center for Independent Living
1895 E. Long St.
Carson City, NV 89701
775-841-2580
FAX: 775-267-3969
e-mail: ruralcil@yahoo.com

Dee Dee Foremaster, Executive Director
Advocacy, Benefit Assistance, social security assistance, peer support, housing information and home-less day drop-in center for individuals with disabilities.

4006 Southern Nevada Center for Independent Living: North Las Vegas
3100 E Lake Mead Boulevard
Suite 4A
North Las Vegas, NV 89030
702-649-3822
FAX: 702-649-5022
TTY:702-649-3822
e-mail: sncilnv@aol.com
www.sncil.org

Mary Evilsizer, Director
Rosemarie Meza, Manager
SNCIL is committed to removing barriers preventing indpendent living by providing services designed to empower people with disabilities.

4007 Southern Nevada Center for Independent Living: Las Vegas
6039 Eldora Avenue
Suite H-8
Las Vegas, NV 89146
702-889-4216
800-870-7003
FAX: 702-889-4574
e-mail: info@sncil.org
www.sncil.org

Mary Evilsizer, Executive Director
Alicia Santiago, Administration Assistant

SNCIL is committed to removing barriers preventing Independent Living by providing services designed to empower people with disabilities.

New Hampshire

4008 **Granite State Independent Living Foundation**
267 Main Street
Suite 400
Littleton, NH 03561
603-444-0904
800-588-5772
FAX: 603-444-3128
e-mail: clyde.terry@gsil.org
www.gsil.org

John Irwin, President
Ken Maillous, Second Vice President
GSIL is a statewide non-profit that recognizes the fact that all of us will need some type of support in the course of the lives. GSIL offers tools and resources so that individuals can participate as fully as the choose in their lives, families and communities. Contact the Independent Living Foundation for referrals to living situations.

New Jersey

4009 **Assistive Technology Advocacy Center (ATAC)**
New Jersey Protection and Advocacy
210 S Broad Street
3rd Floor
Trenton, NJ 08608
609-292-9742
800-922-7233
FAX: 609-777-0187
TTY: 609-633-7106
e-mail: advocate@njpanda.org
www.njpanda.org

Ellen Catanese, Executive Director
Sarah Mitchell, Manager
Consumer-driven program whose mission is to increase awareness of and improve access to assistive technology for all people with disabilities in the state. Provides information and referral through its 800 telephone number and Web site regarding all aspects of assistive technology. Also provides advocacy saervices.

4010 **Center for Independent Living: Camden**
2600 Mount Ephraim Avenue
Suite 413
Camden, NJ 08104
856-966-0800
FAX: 856-966-0832
TTY:609-966-0830
e-mail: lorraineccilc@aol.com
www.ilusa.com

Lorraine Culbertson, Executive Director
Provides services designed to empower people with disabilities.

4011 **Center for Independent Living: Edison**
Alliance for Disabled in Action
629 Amboy Avenue
Lower Level
Edison, NJ 08837
732-738-4388
FAX: 732-738-4416
TTY:732-738-9644
e-mail: adacil@adacil.org
www.adacil.org

Richard Ringhof, Executive Director
Alliance for Disabled in Action is a private, not-for-profit center for independent living serving people in Middlesex, Somerset and Union Counties of New Jersey. ADA's mission is to support and promote choice, self-direction and independent living in the lives of people with disabilities, with the right of individuals to inclusion in the community as the primary goal.

4012 **Center for Independent Living: Long Branch**
279 Broadway
Suite 2
Long Branch, NJ 07740
732-571-4884
FAX: 732-571-4003
TTY:732-571-4878
e-mail: moceans@moceans.org
www.moceans.org

Richard Garnger, Chairman
Pat McShane, Executive Director
Stan Soden, Dirirector IL Services
Offers peer support, disability education and personal assistant services. Serving Monmouth and Ocean Counties with information and referrals, advocacy, peer support and independent living instructions.

4013 **Center for Independent Living: South Jersey**
1150 Delsea Drive
Suite 1
Westville, NJ 08093
856-853-6490
800-413-3791
FAX: 856-853-1466
TTY: 856-853-7602
e-mail: cilsj@verizon.net
www.gloucestercountyvolunteers.org

Hazel Lee-Briggs, Executive Director
Danuta Debicki, Program Manager
Dedicated to providing people with disabilities in Gloucester and Camden counties the opportunity to actively participate in society, to provide freedom of choice, to work, to own a home, raise a family and in general, to participate to the fullest extent in day-to-day activities. The center provides information and referrals, advocacy, peer support, and independent living skills training.

4014 **Dial: Disabled Information Awareness & Liv ing**
2 Prospect Village Plaza
Floor 1
Clifton, NJ 07013
973-470-8090
866-277-1733
FAX: 973-470-8171
TTY: 973-470-2521
e-mail: info@dial-cil.org
www.dial-cil.org

John Petix Jr, Executive Director
Ann Anderson Hunt, Administrative Assistant
DIAL is a Center for Independent Living, which is part of a statewide network of non-residential centers designed and operated to provide service to individuals with significant disabilities. Services include information adn referral, advocacy, peer support, and independent living skills training. DIAL serves individuals in Passaic and Essex Counties.

4015 **Disabled Advocates Working for Northwest (DAWN)**
30 Broad Street
Suite 5
Denville, NJ 07834
973-625-1940
888-383-3296
FAX: 973-625-1942
TTY: 973-361-6032
e-mail: info@dawncil.org
www.dawncil.org

Carmela Slivinski, Executive Director
Wanda Kasmedo, Program Assistant
DAWN is the Center for Independent Living serving Morris, Sussex and Warren counties. DAWN empowers people with disabilities to strive for equality and to take control of their own lives by providing the tools that encourage independence and self-advocacy, promoting public awareness of the needs, desires and rights to individuals living with disabilities, and offering community activities that create new experiences and opportunities.

4016 **Family Resource Associates**
35 Haddon Avenue
Shrewsbury, NJ 07702
732-747-5310
FAX: 732-747-1896
e-mail: info@frainc.org
www.frainc.org

Nancy Phalanukorn, Executive Director
Linda Magill, Development Director
FRA is dedicated to helping children, adolescents and people of all ages with disabilities to reach their fullest potential. FRA also connects individuals to independence through modern therapies and advanced technology. FRA provides direct services to those in the greater Nonmouth/Ocean County area.

4017 Heightened Independence and Progress: Hack ensack
131 Main Street
Suite 120
Hackensack, NJ 07601
201-996-9100
FAX: 201-996-9422
TTY:201-966-9424
e-mail: ber@hipcil.org
www.hipcil.org

Eileen Goff, Executive Director
Trish Carney, Finance/Development Director
HIP empowers people with disabilities to achieve independent living through outreach, advocacy and education.

4018 Heightened Independence and Progress: Jers ey City
Hudson County CIL
26 Journal Square
Suite 602
Jersey City, NJ 07306
201-533-4407
FAX: 201-533-4421
TTY:201-413-0521
e-mail: hud@hipcil.org
www.hipcil.org

Patricia Reilly, Executive Director
Trish Carney, Finance/Development Diretor
Empowering People with Disabilities to Achieve Independent Living through Outreach, Advocacy, and Education.

4019 Progressive Center for Independent Living
1262 Whitehorse-Hamilton Road
Building A, Suite 2
Hamilton, NJ 08690
609-581-4500
877-917-4500
FAX: 609-581-4550
TTY: 609-581-4550
e-mail: info@pcil.org
www.pcil.org

Scott Elliot, Executive Director
PCIL advocates for the rights of people with disabilities to achieve and maintain independent lifestyles. Through promotion of choice, self-direction and inclusion, PCIL works with people with disabilities and their families to ensure the same freedoms and civil liberties as everyone else.

4020 Project Freedom
223 Hutchinson Road
Robbinsville, NJ 08691
609-448-2998
FAX: 609-448-5821
e-mail: projectfreedom1@aol.com
www.projectfreedom.org

Norman Smith, Director
Project Freedom is a non-profit organization that develops and operates barrier-free housing to enable individuals with disabilities to live independently. Supportive services such as recreation, training and advocacy are provided. In addition to being a developer of accessible, affordable housing, Project Freedom also provides supportive services, whereby self-directed people with disabilities can live independently in a non-medical environment.

4021 Total Living Center
707 White Horse Pike
The Courtyard, Suite B-8
Absecon, NJ 08201
609-645-9547
FAX: 609-813-2318
TTY:609-645-9593
e-mail: info@tlcenter.org
www.tlcenter.org

Martin T. Carson, President
Jo May Hudson, Vice President
Cathleen Shaner, Secretary
Total Living Center is a non-profit organization whose mission is to empower individuals with significant disabilities to maximize their potential for independence and productivity, to live as fully as possible within the community, taking responsibility for themselves, and sharing this commitment with others.

New Mexico

4022 Ability Center
715 E Idaho Avenue
Building 3E
Las Cruces, NM 88001
505-526-5016
800-376-4372
FAX: 505-526-1202
TTY: 505-526-5016
e-mail: freesom@theabilitycenter.org
www.theabilitycenter.org

Ruth D. Rodriguez, President
Cesar Rodriguez, Vice-President
C. Neil Gibbs, Treasurer
The Ability Center is a private, nonresidential, nonprofit, New Mexico corporation. As a center for independent living (CIL) TACIL provides a variety of services to promote independence, self-reliance, and community integration. Our professional staff and active board of directors are dedicated to helping our consumers maintain their personal freedom at home, in the community, and throughout the state.

4023 CASA Inc.
PO Box 36916
Albuquerque, NM 87176
505-298-7609

Francis Nye, Executive Director
Offers peer counseling and information and referral services.

4024 CHOICES Center for Independent Living
200 E 4th Street
Suite 200
Roswell, NM 88201
505-627-6727
800-387-4572
FAX: 505-627-6754
TTY: 505-627-6727
e-mail: cbailey@ilchoices.com
www.ilchoices.com

Julia Calvert, Executive Director
Offers many core services including independent living skills training, peer support, information and referral, advocacy and transition.

4025 New Mexico Technology Assistance Program
New Mexico State Department Of Education
435 Saint Michaels Drive
Suite D
Santa Fe, NM 87505
505-954-8533
800-866-2253
FAX: 505-954-8608
TTY: 800-659-4915
e-mail: awinnegar@state.nm.us
www.nmtap.com

Andy Winnegar, Director
Caroll Cadena, Public Contact
Examines and works to eliminate barriers to obtaining assistive technology in New Mexico. Has established a statewide program for coordinating assistive technology services; is designed to assist people with disabilities to locate, secure, and maintain assistive technology.

4026 New Vistas
1121 Alto Street
Santa Fe, NM 87501
505-988-3803
FAX: 505-989-8740
e-mail: rgarcia@newvistas.org
www.newvistas.org

Ronald Garcia, Executive Director

The mission of New Vistas is to work in collaboration with individuals with disabilities and families of children with special needs on northern New Mexico to create access to opportunities and to enhance quality of life.

4027 San Juan Center for Independence
3535 E 30th Street
Suite 101
Farmington, NM 87402
505-566-5827
877-484-4500
FAX: 505-566-5842
e-mail: swatson@sjci.org
www.sjci.org

Sherry Watson, Executive Director
Tim Carver, CFO
SJCI is a New Mexico private residential, nonprofit corporation that serves people with disabilities. The purpose of SJCI is to provide a variety of community based, consumer driven service to people with disablities to promote independence, self-residence and intergration into the community.

New York

4028 AIM Independent Living Center: Corning
271 E 1st Street
Corning, NY 14830
607-962-8225
FAX: 607-937-5125
www.aimcil.org

Diane Dimuse, Director
Diane Muth, Executive Director
AIM's goal to enable the consumer to live an independent and comfortable lifestyle in the security of their home environment so they may feel dignity and pride in their achievements while controlig their own care.

4029 AIM Independent Living Center: Elmira
650 Baldwin Street
Elmira, NY 14901
607-733-3718
FAX: 607-733-0180
TTY:607-733-7764
e-mail: dbailey@aimcil.com
www.aimcil.com

Diane Demuth, Executive Director
David Bailey, Site Manager
Kelley Crocker
AIM's goal is to enable the consumer to live an independent and comfortable lifestyle in the security of their home environment so they may feel dignity and pride in their achievements while controling their own care.

4030 ARISE: Center for Independent Living: Syracuse
635 James Street
Syracuse, NY 13203
315-472-3171
FAX: 315-472-9252
TTY:315-479-6363
e-mail: advocate@ariseinc.org
www.ariseinc.org

Thomas McKeown, Executive Director
Ali Stieglitz, Development Director
Offers peer counseling, attendant care registry, referrals and advocacy services, computer recycling, supported employment, career ladders transition program, universal design center.

4031 ARISE: Center for Independent Living: Oswe go
253 E Tenth Street
Oswego, NY 13126
315-342-4088
FAX: 315-342-4107
TTY:315-342-8689
e-mail: info@ariseinc.org
www.ariseinc.org

Tom McKeown, Executive Director
ARISE's mission is to work with people of all abilities to create a fair and just community in which everyone can fully participate. It embrace the guiding principles of independent living-that individuals with disabilities have a right to dignity, personal responsibility, and self-determination. ARISE also offers advocacy and support serivces to people of all ages with all types of disabilities.

4032 Access to Independence of Cortland County
26 N Main Street
Cortland, NY 13045
607-753-7363
FAX: 607-756-4884
e-mail: info@aticortland.org
www.cilcortland.org

Mary Ewing, Executive Director
An independent living center providing resources and advocacy for all people with disabilities. Services include: peer counseling, individual and systems advocacy, independent living skills training, information and referral.

4033 Action Toward Independence: Middletown
130 Dolson Avenue
Suite 35
Middletown, NY 10940
845-343-4284
FAX: 845-343-5269
TTY:845-343-4282
e-mail: ati@warwick.net
www.actiontowardindependence.org

Rachel Bartlow-Pappas, Executive Director
Joann Seligman-Hargabus, Orange County Director
Sarita Castillo-Cuevas, Program Coordinator
Operated as an Independent Living Center. Not only does ATI comply with the laws of both New York State and of the United States of America, but also its commitment to human rights requires a standard that goes above and beyond those rights that are protected by law.

4034 Action Toward Independence: Monticello
33 Lakewood Avenue
Monticello, NY 12701
845-794-4228
FAX: 845-794-4475
e-mail: heaven@warwick.net
www.angelfire.com/ny/advocate

Gilles Malkine, Manager
A not-for-profit, non residential, peer run, referral and advocacy agency for persons with disaiblities in Orange and Sullivan counties. Our services are aimed at promoting, accessibility, community integration and equal opportunity in all aspects of society for persons with all types of challenges.

4035 Bergeron Health Care
15 S 2nd Street
Dolgeville, NY 13329
585-454-5030
800-371-2778
FAX: 315-429-8862
e-mail: info@adaptivemall.com
www.adaptivemall.com

Katie Bergeron PT MS, President/COO
The services at Adaptivemall.com help families find the best equipment to support their children at their highest functioning level. The primary goal is to empower the people with resources that allow you and your child's primary caregivers to make the best decisions to meet your child's unique needs.

4036 Bronx Independent Living Services
3525 Decatur Avenue
Bronx, NY 10467
718-515-2800
FAX: 718-515-2844
e-mail: webmaster@bils.org
www.bils.org

Susan Attzs-Mendoza, Executive Director
BILS is a not-for-profit community agency serving people with all kinds of disabilities. The mission is to empower people with disabilities toward living independent lives. BILS assists individuals by providing advocacy, peer counseling, housing information, and independent living training/counseling.

4037 Brooklyn Center for Independence of the Disabled

2044 Ocean Avenue
Suite B-3
Brooklyn, NY 11230
718-998-3000
FAX: 718-998-3743
TTY:718-998-7406
e-mail: advocate@bcid.org
www.bcid.org

Zainab Jama, Director
Maureen Alexander, Executive Director
Operated by a majority of people with disabilities, BCID is dedicated to guaranteeing the civil rights of people with disabilities. BCID exists to improve the quality of life of brooklyn residents with disabilities thgouh programs that empower them to gain greater control of their lives and achieve full and equal integration into society.

4038 Capital District Center for Independence

875 Central Avenue
Ssouth 4
Albany, NY 12206
518-459-6422
FAX: 518-459-7847
TTY:518-459-6422
e-mail: info@cdciweb.com
www.cdciweb.com

Laurel Kelley, Executive Director
One of 37 Independent Living Centers in New York State, the Center is a non-residential, community based organization, which primarily serves Albany and Schenetady Counties. The Center's mission is to assist people with disabilities to acquire self-advocacy skills and by teaching through example, consumers achieve greater control over the direction of their lives.

4039 Catskill Center for Independence

6104 State Highway 23
Oneonta, NY 13802
607-432-8000
FAX: 607-432-6907
TTY:607-432-8000
e-mail: ccfi@ccfi.us
www.ccfi.us

Chris Zachmeyer, Executive Director
Edward Lynch, Operations Manager
One of 37 community-based independent living centers located throughout the state of New York. As an advocacy agency, we provide a vareity of services to people with disabilities, their friends and family members. In addition, we provide advocacy, training, and technical assistance to our community members, organizations, businesses and state and local governments in a variety of disability related areas. Serves Otsego, Delaware and Schoharie counties.

4040 Center for Independence of the Disabled of New York

841 Broadway
Suite 301
New York, NY 10003
212-674-2300
FAX: 212-254-5953
TTY:212-674-5619
e-mail: info@cidny.org
www.cidny.org

Susan Dooha, Executive Director
CIDNY speaks for everyone who lives with a disability, whether it came at birth, by injury, disease, or during the process of aging. Together, CIDNY works to educate the public, and also advocate for our civil rights and a strong safety net of benefits and services. The staff at CIDNY is also ethnically diverse, with language capacity to assist customers in Spanish, Cantonese, Mandarin, Hindi, Russian, and American Sign Language.

4041 Center for Independent Living: Action Towards Independence

2927 Route 6
Slate Hill, NY 10973
914-355-2030
FAX: 845-355-2060
e-mail: ati@warwick.net

Nancy Horton, Co-Director
Margaret Jeffries, Co-Director
Information, referral, case management, transportation and system and individual advocacy, architectural barrier removal consultations, peer support, independent living skills development and parenting classes.

4042 Center for Independent Living: Amsterdam

2540 Riverfront Center
Amsterdam, NY 12010
518-842-3561
FAX: 518-842-0905
TTY:518-842-3593
e-mail: rcil@link.net
www.rcil.com

Ramon Rodriguez, Program Director
Peer counseling, advocacy, independent living skills training, information and referral services, self-advocacy training, ADA consultation, home and community based services, community education, disability benefits, advisement and more. All programs and services are available in English and Spanish.

4043 Center for Independent Living: Rochester

1641 East Avenue
Rochester, NY 14610
585-442-6470
FAX: 585-271-8558
TTY:585-442-6470
e-mail: bdarling@rcil.org
www.rcil.org

Todd Eggert, Executive Director
Mary Willy, Administrative Assistant
RCIL looks to empower people with disabilities to self-advocate, to live independently and to enhance the quality of community life. The services and programsare primarily of an advocacy nature (both individual and systems). RCIL seeks to overcome the barriers faced by people with disabilities who choose to live independently.

4044 Community Alternatives

115 E Jefferson Street
Suite 300
Syracuse, NY 13202
315-422-5638

Marsha Weissman, Executive Director

4045 DD Center/St Lukes: Roosevelt Hospital Center

St Lukes Roosevelt
1000 10th Avenue
New York, NY 10019
212-523-3179
FAX: 212-523-6241

Steven Wolf, Director
Farooq Chaudry, MD
Independent living center that advocates for people with disabilities by assisting with the application process of housing, benefits, etc.

4046 Finger Lakes Independence Center

215 Fifth Street
Ithaca, NY 14850
607-272-2433
FAX: 607-272-0902
TTY:607-272-2433
e-mail: flic@clarityconnect.com
www.fliconline.org

Lenore Schwager, Executive Director
FLIC assists all people with disabilities, their families and friends to promote independence and make informed decisions in pursuit of their goals. The servides provided are free of charge, and services are primarily served to residents of Tompkins, Schyler counties.

4047 Genesee Region Independent Living Center

61 Swan Street
Batavia, NY 14020
585-343-4524
FAX: 585-343-6656
TTY:716-343-4524
e-mail: grilc@bfn.org
grilc.bfn.org

Ann Bell, Executive Director
GRILC offers a caring environment. GRILC assists in peer counseling, advocacy, benefits advisement, support groups, transportation, architectural barrier consultation, independent living skills instruction, and many other services.

4048 **Glens Falls Independent Living Center**
71 Glenwood Avenue
Queensbury, NY 12804
518-792-3537
FAX: 518-792-0979
TTY:518-792-0505
e-mail: gfilc@adelphia.net
www.gfilc.com

Karen Thayer, Executive Director
Anna Livingston, Assistant Director
The focus at the Glens Falls Independent Living Center is to assist individuals with disabilities to beconme independent empowered self-advocates. GFILC works within the community to remove physical and attitudinal barriers that stand in the way of independence. The Center will promote the comcepts of self-determination and person centered planning for work, leisure and life.

4049 **Harlem Independent Living Center**
289 Saint Nicholas Avenue
Suite 21
New York, NY 10027
212-222-7122
800-673-2371
FAX: 212-222-7199
e-mail: harlemilc@aol.com
www.hilc.org

Christina Curry, Executive Director
Edward Randolph, Intake Coordinator
Marisol Rivera, Receptionist
A non-profit agency that advocates for people with disabilities by assisting with the application process of housing, benefits, etc. Our services are free of charge.
Monthly

4050 **Long Island Center for Independent Living**
3601 Hempstead Turnpike
Suites 208 & 500
Levittown, NY 11756
516-796-0144
FAX: 516-796-0529
TTY:516-796-0135
e-mail: licil@aol.com
www.licil.net

Patricia Moore, Director
Michael Dc, Owner
LICIL is committed to the empowerment of consumers with disabilities. LICIL staff functions as ambassadors to the belief that individuals with disabilities have a responsibility to take an active role in their own lives and self determined view of their futures.

4051 **Massena Center for Independent Living**
156 Center Street
Massena, NY 13662
315-764-9442
FAX: 315-764-9464
TTY:315-764-9442
e-mail: mindepli@twcny.rr.co,

Jeff Reifensnyder, Executive Director
Provides a variety of non-residential direct services as well as educating the public through community awareness campaigns. Also seeks to address the current appropriate unmet needs of persons experiencing a disability - primarily in St Lawrence and Franklin Counties.

4052 **Minority Outreach Project**
200 Hamilton Avenue
White Plains, NY 10601
914-682-3926
FAX: 914-682-8518
www.wilc.org

Joseph Drazo, Executive Director
Programs reflect the requirements of WILC'S consumers and the demands of our evolving society. As people and needs change so do WILC'S Programs and Services in order to fulfil WILC'S mission of supporting self-sufficiency and self-determination

4053 **NYS Independent Living Council, Inc.**
111 Washington Avenue
Suite 101
Albany, NY 12210
518-427-1060
888-469-7452
FAX: 518-427-1139
TTY: 716-373-4602
e-mail: oleanilc@yahoo.com
www.nysilc.org

Leonard Liguori, Executive Director
AÆnot-for-profit, non-governmental consumer controlled organization. The council is composed of 27 appointees from around the state, a majority of whom have disabilities, representing diverse cultures and needs in the state.

4054 **Nassau County Office for the Physically Challenged**
1550 Franklin Avenue
Mineola, NY 11501
516-571-3972
FAX: 516-571-6150

Don Dreyer, Director
This agency serves as the ADA compliance coordinating office for all Nassau County governmental facilities, programs and services. It also serves in an advisory capacity to local, regional and national policy-making organizations, planning committees and legislative bodies and conducts advocacy as well as direct programs and services to enhance inclusion by people with disabilities to employment, consumerism and transportation.

4055 **Newburgh Center for Independent Living**
5 Washington Terrace
Newburgh, NY 12550
845-565-1162
FAX: 845-565-0567
TTY:845-565-0337
e-mail: krivera@myindependentliving.org
www.myindependentliving.org

Kara Dorsey, President
Douglas J Hovey, Executive Director
Arnie Abrams, Assoc Director, Development
A consumer directed, cross-disability organization dedicated to enhancing the quality of life for persons with disabilities

4056 **Niagara Frontier Center for Independent Living**
1522 Main Street
Niagara Falls, NY 14305
716-284-2452
FAX: 716-284-0829
TTY:716-284-2452
e-mail: kpautler@nfcil.org

Kathleen Pautler, Executive Director
Offers peer counseling, referrals and disability education.

4057 **North Country Center for Independent Livin g**
102 Sharron Avenue
Plattsburgh, NY 12901
518-563-9058
FAX: 518-563-0292
TTY:518-563-0292
e-mail: andrew@ncci-online.com
www.ncci-online.com

Andrew Pulrang, Executive Director
Mike Gagnier, Assistant Director
Center for Independent Living serving Clinton and Essex counties, New York. Services include: Information and Referral, Independent Living Skills Training, Advocacy, and Peer Counseling

4058 **Northern Regional Center for Independent Living: Lowville**
7396 Turin Road
Lowville, NY 13367
315-376-8696
800-585-8703
FAX: 315-376-3404
TTY: 315-785-8704
e-mail: aileeng@nrcil.net

Aileen Martin, Executive Director
Karenbolive Martin, Manager
An independent living center that provides services, programs, and advocacy for all people.

4059 Northern Regional Center for Independent Living: Watertown
210 Court Street
Suite 107
Watertown, NY 13601
315-785-8703
800-585-8703
FAX: 315-785-8612
TTY: 315-785-8704
e-mail: brendac@nrcil.net
www.nrcil.net

Brenda Company, Executive Director
An independent living center that offers services, programs and advocacy for all people.

4060 Options for Independence: Auburn
75 Genesee Street
Auburn, NY 13021
315-255-3447
FAX: 315-255-0836
TTY:315-255-3447
e-mail: options@optionsforindependence.org
www.optionsforindependence.org

Guy Thomas Cosentino, Executive Director
Crystal Purcell, Program Director
Options for Independence is and Independent Living Center which assists people with disabilities to gain opportunities, make their own decision, pursue activities and become part of comunity life. also provided is a variety of services to all people with disabilities, their families and friends in Cayuga and Seneca Counties.

4061 Options for Independence: Seneca Falls
55 Fall Street
Seneca Falls, NY 13148
315-568-2724
FAX: 315-568-1844
www.optionsforindependence.org

Guy Thomas Constentino, Executive Director
Crystal Purcell, Program Director
Options for Independence is an independent Living Center which assists people with disabilities to gain opportunities, make their own decisions, pursue activities and become part of community life. Also provided is a variety of services to all people with disabilities, their families and friends in Cayuga and Seneca Counti8es.

4062 Queens Independent Living Center
23-35 Broadway
Astoria, NY 11106
718-204-7114
FAX: 718-393-8575
e-mail: contact@qilc.org
www.qilc.org

Daniel Aliberti, Executive Director
QILC is a consumer directed organization whose mission is to empower people with disabilities to take control of their own lives. QILC provides information and refferal to resources within the community, which persons with disabilities can utilize to achieve their social, vocational, and personal goals. QILC also provides direct assistance to individuals with disabilities in the areas of housing, employment, benefits counseling, group and peer counseling, and voter registration.

4063 Resource Center for Accessible Living
592 Ulster Avenue
Kingston, NY 12401
845-331-0541
FAX: 845-331-2076
TTY:845-331-8680
e-mail: rcal@hvc.rr.com
www.rcal.org

Susan J Hoger, Executive Director
Suzanne de Beaumont, Assistant Executive Director
RCAL is a non-profit, community based service and advocacy run by and for people with any type of disability. RCAL is dedicatd to assisting and empowering individuals, of all ages, to live independently and participate in all aspects of community life.

4064 Rockland Independent Living Center
75 W Route 59
Suite 2130
Nanuet, NY 10954
845-624-1366
FAX: 845-624-1369
TTY:845-426 1180
e-mail: mail@rilc.org
www.rilc.org

Cathrine Oca, Executive Director
Jill Nizen, Vice President
RILC provides services, programs and advocacy for all people in Rockland County, New York who have disabilities so that they may pursue lifestyles of their choice.

4065 SILO: Cental Islip
3180 Express Drive S
Central Islip, NY 11749
516-348-0207
FAX: 516-348-0262

Independent living center.

4066 SILO: Hauppauge
140 Fell Court
Suite 116
Hauppauge, NY 11788
631-348-0207
FAX: 631-348-0262
TTY:631-348-7655
e-mail: eahern@suffolkilc.org

Edward Ahern, Director
Independent living center.

4067 Southern Adirondack Independent Living
418 Geyser Road
Country Club Plaza
Ballston Spa, NY 12020
518-584-8202
FAX: 518-584-1195
TTY:518-584-4752

Teena Willard, Advocate
Dawn Lincoln, Advocate
Karen Thayer, Executive Director
Independent living center

4068 Southern Tier Independence Center
24 Prospect Avenue
Binghamton, NY 13901
607-724-2111
FAX: 607-772-3600
TTY:607-724-2111
e-mail: stic@stic-cil.org
www.stic-cil.org

Maria Dibble, Executive Director
Frank Pennisi, Accessibility Services
STIC provides assistance and services to all people with disabilities of all ages to increase their independence in all aspects of integrated community life. STIC also serves their families and friends, and businesses, agencies, and goverments to enable them to better meet the needs of people with disabilities, and finally STIC educates and influences the community in pursuit of full inclusion of people with disabilities.

4069 Southwestern Independent Living Center
843 N Main Street
Jamestown, NY 14701
716-661-3010
FAX: 716-661-3011
TTY:716-661-3012
e-mail: marie@ilc-jamestown-ny.org
www.ilc-jamestown-ny.org

Marie T Carrubba, Executive Director
Linda Rumbaugh, Independent Living Specialist
Offers disability education, advocacy and information on accessible housing, wheelchair or acessible transportation, interpreting services, brulling, IL skills training, peer support.

4070 Staten Island Center for Independent Living
470 Castleton Ave
Staten Island, NY 10301
718-720-9016
FAX: 718-720-9664
e-mail: dorothy.doran@verizon.net
www.geocities.com/siciliving

Dorothy Doran, Executive Director
Mission is to provide all individuals with the information, life skills training, and facilitative assistance which contributes to independence, individuality, and integration in the community and provides the skills and knowledge necessary to function in the least restrictive, personally fulfilling, most self reliant and productive manner.

4071 Suffolk Independent Living Organization (SILO)
3681 Rte 112
Suite 4
Coram, NY 11727
631-880-7929
FAX: 631-946-6377
TTY:631-654-8076
e-mail: eahern@suffolkilc.org
www.suffolkilc.org

Edward Ahern, Executive Director
A consumer controlled, not-for-profit, non-residential human and civil rights, mentorship and educational organization.

4072 Taconic Resources for Independence
82 Washington Street
Suite 214
Poughkeepsie, NY 12601
845-452-3913
FAX: 845-485-3196
TTY:845-485-8110
e-mail: trionline@taconicresources.net
www.taconicresources.net

Cynthia Siore, Executive Director
Stephanie Jaczko, Assistant Director
A center for independent living, benefits advisement information, and referral, advocacy, independent living skills, peer counseling, parent advocacy, sign language interpreters.

4073 Visions/Services for the Blind & Visually Impaired
500 Greenwich Street
3rd Floor
New York, NY 10013
212-625-1616
888-245-8333
FAX: 212-219-4078
e-mail: info@visionsvcb.org
www.visionsvcb.org

Nancy Miller, Executive Director
Betsy Fabricant, Dir Rec/Residential Programs
Diane Weiss, Dir Rehab/Community Outreach
A vision rehabilitation and social service agency promoting the independence of people of all ages who are blind or visually impaired. Free community center, vision rehabilitation, and camp programs.

4074 Westchester County Independent Living Center
200 Hamilton Avenue
2nd Floor
White Plains, NY 10601
914-682-3926
FAX: 914-682-8518
TTY:914-682-0926
www.wilc.org

Joseph Bravo, Executive Director
Mildred Caballero-Ho, Deputy Executive Director
One of the Independent Living Centers in New York States, the WILC has a long hisotory of providing services designed, directed, and in most cases delivered by individuals with a wide range of disabilities.

4075 Westchester Disabled on the Move
984 N Broadway
Suite L-01
Yonkers, NY 10701
914-968-4717
FAX: 914-968-6137
e-mail: info@wdom.org
www.wdom.org

Melvyn R Tanzman CSW, Executive Director
Scott Smith, Program Director
WDOM empowers people with disabilities to control their own lives; advocates for civil rights and a barrier free society; encourages people with disabilities to participate in the political process; educates government, business, other entities, and a society as a whole to understand, accept, and accommodate people with disabilities; creates an environment that inspires self-respect

4076 Wiswall Center for Independent Living
71 Glenwood Avenue
Queensbury, NY 12804
518-793-5863
FAX: 518-745-7389
e-mail: info@crandalllibrary.org
www.crandalllibrary.org

Christine McDonald, Library Director
Lynn Osterberg, Manager
Independent living center.

North Carolina

4077 Center for Accessible Housing
North Carolina State University
PO Box 8613
Raleigh, NC 27695
919-515-2011
FAX: 919-515-3023
e-mail: cahd@ncsu.edu
www.ncsu.edu

James Oblinger, Manager
Established in 1989, the Center improves the quality and availability of housing for people with disabilities. The center provides assistance and information to individuals and industry through research, collaborative efforts with manufacturers, training and information services.

4078 Disability Awareness Network
609 Country Club Drive
Suite C
Greenville, NC 27834
252-355-5272
FAX: 252-353-5160
e-mail: DAWNpittco@aol.com

Marty Silverthorne, Contact
Information and referral for diabled persons; peer counseling for diabled persons; advocacy on ADA issues; independent living skills and training.

4079 Disability Rights & Resources
5801 Executive Center Drive
Suite 101
Charlotte, NC 28212
704-537-0550
FAX: 704-566-0507
www.disability-rights.org

Niki Stamps, Peer Advocate
Julie Sain, Executive Director
Steve McCallum, Peer Advocate
Offers information and referrals, peer counseling for people with disabilities, advocacy and independent living skills classes. DR&R helps people with disabilities achieve and maintain their independence in the community.

4080 Joy: A Shabazz Center for Independent Living
235 N Greene Street
Greensboro, NC 27401
336-272-0501
FAX: 336-272-0575
TTY:336-272-0501
e-mail: aaron.shabazz@shabazzcenter.org
www.shabazzcenter.org
Benita Williams, Deputy Director
A non-profit, consumer oriented, Center for Independent Living (CIL) providing advocacy, peer counseling and peer support, independent living skills, training, information and referrals, with other related services for persons with disabilites.

4081 Live Independently Networking Center
PO Box 1135
Newton, NC 28658
828-464-0331
FAX: 828-464-7375
TTY:828-464-2838
e-mail: linc@twave.net
www.linconline.org

Donavon Kirby, Deputy Director
Private, nonprofit, federally funded center for independent living located in Western North Carolina.

4082 Live Independently Networking Center: Hickory
2830 16th Street NE
Hickory, NC 28601
828-464-0331
FAX: 828-464-7375
Private, non-profit, federally funded center for independent living

4083 Pathways for the Future
525 Mineral Springs Drive
Sylva, NC 28779
828-631-1167
FAX: 828-631-1169
e-mail: pathways@dnet.net
www.pathwayscil.org

Barbara Davis, Executive Director
Gale Anglin, Assistant Director
Pathways covers the counties of Jackson, Swain, Haywood, Cherokee, Graham, Clay, and Macon. Pathways is dedicated to increasing independence, changing attitudes, promoting equal acess and building a peer support network through the use of community education, independent living services and advocacy.

4084 Western Alliance Center for Independent Living
30-B London Road
Asheville, NC 28803
828-274-0444
FAX: 828-274-4461
e-mail: ashcilnc@bellsouth.net
www.westernalliance.org

Bart Floyd, Site Coordinator
Barbara Davis, Executive Director
Core: Information and Referral, Peer Counseling, Independent Living Skills Training and Advocacy. Counties served: Buncombe, Henderson, Madison, McDowell, Polk, Rutherford and Transylvania.

North Dakota

4085 Center for Independent Living: Fargo
2701 9th Avenue SW
Fargo, ND 58103
701-478-0459
800-450-0459
FAX: 701-478-0510
TTY: 701-478-0459
e-mail: freedom@freedomrc.org
www.freedomrc.org

Nate Aalgaard, Executive Director
Freedom Resource Center is an independent non-profit organization, serving people of all ages and all disabilities. The mission of Freedom Resource Center is to work toward equality and inclusion for people with disabilities through programs of empowerment, community education and systems change.

4086 Dakota Center for Independent Living: Dickinson
40 1st Avenue West
Park Square Mall
Dickinson, ND 58601
701-483-4363
800-489-5013
FAX: 701-483-4361
TTY: 701-483-4363
e-mail: wendydcil@ndsupernet.com
www.dakotacil.org

Wendy Sundheim, Program Coordinator
The Dakota Center for Independent Living advocates for community based services and training opportunities that assist people with disabilities to live more independently. Outreach services are provided in eighteen south west and south central N.D. counties, and on the Standing Rock and the southern part of the Fort Berthold Native American reservations.

4087 Dakota Center for Independent Living: Bism arck
3111 E Broadway Avenue
Bismarck, ND 58501
701-222-3636
800-489-5013
FAX: 701-222-0511
TTY: 701-222-3636
www.dakotacil.org

Royce Schultze, Executive Director
Diana Medicine Stone, Sr Independent Living Counselor
DCIL advocates for community based services and training opportunities that assist people with disabilities to live more independently. Outrech services are provided in eighteen south west and south central N.D. counties, and on the Standing Rock and the southern part of the Fort Berthold Native American reservations

4088 Fraser
2902 University Drive S
Fargo, ND 58103
701-232-3301
FAX: 701-237-5775
e-mail: fraser@fraserltd.org
www.fraserltd.org

Sandra Layland, Executive Director
David Laske, Treasurer
Private non-profit, federally funded center for independent living

4089 Freedom Resource Center for Independent Living: Fargo
2701 9th Avenue SW
Fargo, ND 58103
701-478-0459
800-450-0459
FAX: 701-478-0510
TTY: 218-236-0459
e-mail: freedom@freedomrc.org
www.freedomrc.org

Nate Aalgaard, Executive Director

4090 Resource Center for Independent Living: Minot
300 3rd Avenue SW
Suite F
Minot, ND 58701
701-839-4724
800-377-5114
FAX: 701-838-1677
TTY: 800-839-6561
e-mail: agency@independencecil.org
www.independencecil.org

Stephen Repnow, Executive Director
A resource center for independent living. Mission is to advocate for the freedom of choice for individuals with disabilities to live independently through the removal of all barriers.

Ohio

4091 Ability Center of Defiance
1935 East Second Street
Suite C
Defiance, OH 43512
419-782-5441
877-209-8336
FAX: 419-782-9231
TTY: 419-782-5441
e-mail: knoe@abilitycenter.org
www.abilitycenter.org

Kristina Noe, Executive Director
Mission is to assist people with disabilities to live, work and socialize within a fully accessible community.

4092 Ability Center of Greater Toledo
5605 Monroe Street
Sylvania, OH 43560
419-885-5733
866-885-5733
FAX: 419-882-4813
TTY: 419-885-5733
e-mail: sitemail@abilitycenter.org
www.abilitycenter.org

Tim Harrington, Executive Director
Ability Center is a non-profit independent living center in Northwest Ohio. The Center serves Defiance, Fulton, Henry, Lucas, Ottawa, Williams and Wood, with Satelitte offices in Defiance and Otawa counties. The mission is to assist people with disabilities to live their lives as idependently as possible. Services provided are: advocacy, community living and information, recreation inclusion, and youth and independent living skills.

4093 Access Center for Independent Living
35 S Jefferson Street
Dayton, OH 45402
937-341-5202
FAX: 937-341-5217
TTY:937-341-5218
e-mail: webmaster@acils.com
www.acils.com

Alan Cochrun, Executive Director
Offers peer counseling, disability education and other services to the community.

4094 Fairfield Center for Disabilities and Cerebral Palsy
681 E Sixth Avenue
Lancaster, OH 43130
740-653-5501
FAX: 740-653-6046
e-mail: fcdcp@sbcglobal.net
www.fcdcp.org

Edwin Payne, Board Secretary/Director
Adult Day Program and Transportation. The mission of the Fairfield Center for disabilities and Cerebral Palsy, Inc, is to create a better future for people with a disability by increasing and enhancing their lifestyle opportunities.

4095 Linking Employment Ability Potential: Independent Living Center
2100 N Ridge Road
Elyria, OH 44035
440-324-3444
FAX: 440-324-2112
TTY:440-324-3444
e-mail: edanevich@leapinfo.org
www.leapinfo.org

Elsie Danevich, Program Director
LEAP is consumer directed to ensure a society of equal opportunity for all persons, regardless of disability

4096 Mid-Ohio Board for an Independent Living Environment (MOBILE)
690 S High Street
Columbus, OH 43206
614-443-5936
FAX: 614-443-5954
TTY:614-443-5957
e-mail: bev@mobileonline.org
www.mobileonline.org

Beverly Rackett, Executive Director
A non-profit Center for Independent Living directed by persons with disabilities. MOBILE was founded on principles that affirm the right of persons with disabilities to live their lives with a full measure of liberty and human dignity.

4097 Ohio Statewide Independent Living Council
670 Morrison Road
Suite 200
Gahanna, OH 43230
614-892-0390
800-566-7788
FAX: 614-861-0392
e-mail: info@ohiosilc.org
www.ohiosilc.org

James Schaum, President/CEO
Kay Grier, Office Manager
Committed to promoting a philosophy of consumer control, peer support, self-help, self-determination, equal acess, and individual and systems advocacy, in order to maximize leadership, empowerment, independence, productivity and to support full inclusion and integration of individuals with disabilities into the mainstream of American society.

4098 Rehabilitation Service of North Central Ohio
270 Sterkel Bouleard
Mansfield, OH 44907
419-756-1133
800-589-1133
FAX: 419-756-6544
e-mail: info@therehabcenter.org
www.therehabcenter.org

James Schaum, President/CEO
Linda Williams, VP Medical Rehab
Dan Loguda, VP Vocational Rehab
Private nonprofit organization providing coordinated, team-oriented comprehensive outpatient rehabilitation services to children and adults of all ages. Serves 8 counties in N/C Ohio. Four umbrella areas of service include medical rehabilitation services, vocational rehabilitation services, behavioral health service and drug and alcohol addiction services. Medical rehabilitation services include physical therapy, occupational therapy, speech therapy and audiology.

4099 Samuel W Bell Home for Sightless
3775 Muddy Creek Road
Cincinnati, OH 45238
513-241-0720
FAX: 513-241-1481
e-mail: swbellhome@fuse.net
www.samuelbell.org

Miles Hoff, Executive Director
Holly Hoeffer, Director of Residents
Offers a residential home for the totally blind and legally blind adults, male and female.

4100 Services for Independent Living
25100 Euclid Avenue
Suite 105
Cleveland, OH 44117
216-731-1529
FAX: 216-731-3083
TTY:216-731-1529
e-mail: sil@sil-oh.org
www.sil-oh.org

Linda Hildebrand, Executive Director
Lynn Hildebrand, Manager
Offers support ADA, consultation and education, advocacy, transitional education services, independent living skills training, information and referrals.

4101 Society for Equal Access: Independent Living Center
1458 5th Street NW
New Philiadelphia, OH 44622
330-343-3668
888-213-4452
FAX: 330-343-3721
TTY:330-602-2557
e-mail: ilc@tusco.net
www.seailc.org

Dianne Rennicker, Executive Director
The Society works with individuals to become more independent. Our agency assists with peer support, advocacy, information and referral, independent living skills and transportation. Our goal is to move those with challenges in the direction ofn independence.

Oklahoma

4102 Ability Resources
823 S Detroit
Suite 110
Tulsa, OK 74120
918-592-1235
FAX: 918-592-5651
www.ability-resources.org

Carla Lawson, Executive Director
Debby Newman, Office Manager

Offers disability education, peer counseling and referrals, assistive technology lending library, job readiness training, employment placement, nursing home outreach, ADA training, technical assistance, and benefits counseling.

4103 Green County Independent Living Resource Center

4100 SE Adams Road
Suite C106
Bartlesville, OK 74006
918-335-1314
800-559-0567
FAX: 918-333-1814
TTY: 800-559-0567

Teresa Newton, IL Skills Specialist
Vicki Haws, Executive Director
Carla Potts, IL Skills Specialist/Bookkeeper
Independent living skills training, information and referrals, advocacy, a loan library of adaptive equipment and books. Services available to all individuals with disabilities and their family members who reside in Northeastern Oklahoma.

4104 Oklahomans for Independent Living

321 South 3rd
Suite 2
McAlester, OK 74501
918-426-6220
800-568-6821
FAX: 918-426-3245
e-mail: mikew@tulsaconnect.com
www.oil.cwis.net

Mike Ward, Executive Director
OIL encourages individuals of all ages, with all types of disabilities to increase: personal dependence; empowerment and self determiation; and ful integration and participation in their work, community, school and home activities.

4105 Progressive Independence

121 N Porter Road
Norman, OK 73071
405-321-3203
800-801-3230
FAX: 405-321-7601
TTY: 405-321-2942
e-mail: heathera@progind.org
www.progind.org

Jeff Hughes, Executive Director
Preovides four cores services of Information & Referral, Individaul& Systems Advocacy, Peer Counseling, and Skills Training; in addition, offers accessible computer lab, short term DME loans, ande benefits counseling for SSI/SSDI.

4106 Sandra Beasley Independent Living Center

705 S Oakwood Road
Enid, OK 73703
580-237-8508
800-375-4358
FAX: 580-233-6403
TTY: 508-237-8508
e-mail: sbilcenter@coxinet.net
www.members.tripod.com/lew_3

Frieda Kliewer, Executive Director
An independent living center which offers independent living skills training, peer counseling, attendant care registry, ADA consultation, advocacy services and an equipment Loan Closet.

Oregon

4107 Central Oregon Resources for Independent Living

20436 Clay Pigeon Court
PO Box 9425
Bend, OR 97708
541-388-8103
FAX: 541-388-1226
TTY:541-388-8103
e-mail: coril@coril.org
www.coril.org

Glenn VanCise, Executive Director
CORIL empowers people with disabilities to maximize their independence, productivity and inclusio in community life. CORIL envisions a society where all people have the opportunity to develop their full capabilities with independence, productivity and more meaningful involvment in local community events and activities.

4108 Columbia Gorge Center

2940 Thomsen Road
Hood River, OR 97031
541-386-3520
866-424-2669
FAX: 541-386-7788
e-mail: rrathkey@gorge.net

Patty Elkins, Executive Director
C J Webb, Client Services Coordinator
CGC assists people with disabilities or other barriers to employment or community living to: achieve control of their lives; attain competence in community and employment; an participate in satisfying lifestyles based on the same aspirations as well as citizens.

4109 Eastern Oregon Center for Independent Living

1021 SW 5th Avenue
Ontario, OR 97914
541-889-3119
866-248-8369
FAX: 541-889-4647
e-mail: eocil@eocil.org
www.eocil.org

Kirt Toombs, Chief Executive Officer
EOCIL is a nonprofit community based resource and advocacy center that promotes independent living and equal access for all persons with disabilities. EOCIL serves consumers in the counties of: Baker, Gilliam, Grant, harney, Malheur, Morrow, Umatilla, Union, Wallowa and Wheeler.

4110 HASL Independent Abilities Center

305 NE Street
Grants Pass, OR 97526
541-479-4275
800-758-4275
FAX: 541-479-7261
TTY: 541-479-3588
e-mail: haslstaff@yahoo.com
www.haslonline.org

Randy Samuelson, Executive Director
To promote public awareness of the special needs and legal rights of individuals with cross-disabilities; to facilitate their integration into society and provide support through advocacy, peer counseling, skills training and information and referral to encourage independence.

4111 Independent Living Resources

2410 SE 11th Avenue
Portland, OR 97214
503-232-7411
FAX: 503-232-7480
TTY:503-232-8404
e-mail: ilrpdx@qwest.net
www.ilr.org

Barry Quamee, Executive Director
ILR looks to promote the philosophy of Independent Living by creating opportunities, encouraging choices, advancing equal access, and furthering the level of independence for all people with disabilities

4112 Laurel Hill Center Independent Living Program

2145 Centennial Plaza
Eugene, OR 97401
541-485-6340
FAX: 541-345-9218
e-mail: info@laurel.org
www.laurel.org

Liz Cawood, Member of the Board
Mary Alice Brown, Executive Director
Dee Wirak, Director of Rehabilitation
Laurel Hill Center provides nationally recognized rehabilitation services in Lane County, Oregon for people with severe and persistent mental illness. The Center is committed to providing individuals with mental illness hope and recovery process in rebuilding their lives, developing skills and increasing independence.

4113 **Oregon Commission for the Blind**

535 SE 12th Avenue
Portland, OR 97214

971-673-1588
888-202-5463
FAX: 971-673-1570
TTY: 971-673-1577
e-mail: ocbmail@state.or.us
www.cfb.state.or.us

Frank Armstrong, President
Pat Donell, Executive Director
Oregon Commission for the Blind's mission is to assist blind Oregonians in making informed choices and decisions to achieve full inclusion and integration in society through employment, independent living, and socila self-sufficiency.

4114 **Progressive Options**

657 SW Coast Highway
Newport, OR 97365

541-574-0384
FAX: 541-574-1927
TTY:541-574-1927
e-mail: progop541@yahoo.com
www.progressive-options.org

Dawn Young, Office Manager/Data Entry
Progressive Options seeks to provide free services and support to people with disabilities of all kinds to help them achieve and maintain maximum independence and self-sufficiency in Lincoln County and surrounding areas in Oregon.

4115 **SPOKES Unlimited**

415 Main Street
Klamath Falls, OR 97601

541-883-7547
FAX: 541-885-2469
TTY:541-883-7547
e-mail: info@spokesunlimited.org
www.spokesunlimited.org

Tami Martin, Director
Wendy Howard, Executive Director
Mission is to enhance the ability of people with disabilities to live more independently.

4116 **Umpqua Valley Disabilities Network**

419 NE Winchester Street
PO Box 507
Roseburg, OR 97470

541-672-6336
FAX: 541-672-8606
TTY:541-440-2882
e-mail: uvdn@uvdn.org
www.uvdn.org

David Fricke, Executive Director
Heather Vialpando, Office Manager
UVDN's mission is to promote independent living and community inclusion for people with disabilities.

Pennsylvania

4117 **Abilities in Motion**

416 Blair Aveue
Reading, PA 19601

610-376-0010
888-376-0021
FAX: 610-376-0021
TTY: 610-228-2301
e-mail: staff@abilitiesinmotion.org
www.abilitiesinmotion.org

Ralph Trainer, Executive Director
Michelle Charowsky, Independent Living Specialist
Dedicated to advancing the rights of persons with disabilities in orer to promote a full life in the community through the prevention and elimination of physical, psychological, social and attitudinal barriers which serve to deny them the rights and privileges common to the general public.

4118 **Anthracite Region Center for Independent Living**

Pennsylvania Council on Independent Living
44 W Broad Street
Hazleton, PA 18201

570-455-9800
800-777-9906
FAX: 570-455-1731
TTY: 570-455-9800
e-mail: arcil@intergrafix.net
www.anthracitecil.org

Shirley Ray, Executive Director
Enables individuals with disabilities to attain their highest possible level of independence.

4119 **Brian's House**

1300 South Concord Road
West Chester, PA 19382

610-399-1175
FAX: 610-399-1828
www.brianshouse.org

Lori Plunkett, Executive Director
Nancy Nelson, Director Development
Residential care in a variety of homes and apartments for people with a range of development disabilities. Cost varies with needs. Also year-round recreation programs, vocational training and employment programs.

4120 **Community Resources for Independence**

2222 Filmore Avenue
Erie, PA 16506

814-838-7222
800-530-5541
FAX: 814-838-8491
TTY: 814-838-8115
e-mail: info@crinet.org
www.crinet.org

Timothy Finegan, Executive Director
CRI is committed to preserve, enhance, and enrich the quality of life for all people with disabilities.

4121 **Freedom Valley Disability Center**

3607 Chapel Road
Suite B
Newtown Square, PA 19073

610-353-6640
800-427-4754
FAX: 610-353-6753
TTY: 610-353-8900
www.fvdc.info

Ann Cope, Executive Director
Provides services to people with disabilities in Bucks, Chester, Delaware and Montgomery Counties. Also provided are Independent Living Services of Information and Referral, Peer-Support, Advocacy and Independent Living Skills Training.

4122 **Lehigh Valley Center for Independent Living**

435 Allentown Drive
Allentown, PA 18109

610-770-9781
800-495-8245
FAX: 610-770-9801
TTY: 610-770-9789
e-mail: info@lvcil.org
www.lvcil.org

Amy Beck, Executive Director
Mark Piedmonte, Assistant Director
LVCIL facilitates the empowerment of people with disabilities to reach their full potential, and enhacnes the community's awareness of the assets of its citizens with disabilities through: advocacy, life skills training, information and referral, peer support, housing services, and supported community services.

4123 **Liberty Resources**

714 Market Street
Suite 100
Philadelphia, PA 19106

215-634-2000
888-634-2155
888-634-2155
FAX: 215-634-6628
TTY:215-634-6630
e-mail: lrinc@libertyresources.org
www.libertyresources.org

Thomas Earl, Executive Director/Owner

A non-profit, consumer driven organization that advocates and promotes Independent Living for persons with disabilities.

4124 **Life and Independence for Today**
503 E Arch Street
Saint Marys, PA 15857
814-781-3050
800-341-5438
FAX: 814-781-1917
TTY: 814-781-3050
e-mail: lift@liftcil.org
www.liftcil.org

Robert Mecca, Executive Director
A Center for Independent Living athat provides services to people with disabilities in Cameron, Clearfield, Elk, Jefferson, McKean and Potter counties. The mission is to establish, develop, sponsorm promote or conduct educational programs, research, housing opportunities, human service programs and other charitable activities devoted to improving the health and welfare of individuals with disabilities.

4125 **Northeastern Pennsylvania Center for Independent Living**
431 Wyoming Avenue
Scranton, PA 18503
570-344-7211
800-344-7211
FAX: 570-344-7218
e-mail: nepacilinfo@nepacil.org
www.nepacil.org

Daniel P Loftus, Executive Director
Offers information, referral services, financial management, waiver service coordinator and ASL interpreter referral service.

4126 **Pennsylvania's Initiative on Assistive Technology**
Temple University
1601 N. Broad St.
Suite 610
Philadelphia, PA 19122
800-204-7428
FAX: 215-204-9371
TTY:866-268-0579
e-mail: ATinfo@temple.edu
www.disabilities.temple.edu

Amy S Goldman, Director
Pennsylvania's Initiative on Assistive Technology (PIAT) offers information and referral about assistive Technology (AT), device demonstrations, and awareness-level presentations. PIAT also operates Pennsylvania's AT Lending Library, a free, state-supported program that loans AT devices to Pennsylvanians of all ages. This program allows you to try a device for a limited time to be sure it meets your needs.

4127 **South Central Pennsylvania Center for Inde pendence Living**
1603 9th Avenue
Altoona, PA 16602
814-949-1905
800-237-9009
FAX: 814-949-1909
TTY: 814-949-1912
e-mail: cilscpa@cilscpa.org
www.cilscpa.org

Susan Estep, Executive Director
The missio of the Center for Independent Living of South Central PA is to empower people with disabilities to lead independent lives in their commnuitites. The Center covers Bedford, Blair, cambria, Fulton, Huntingdon, Indiana and Somerset counties.

4128 **Three Rivers Center for Independent Living**
900 Rebecca Avenue
Pittsburgh, PA 15221
412-371-7700
800-633-4588
FAX: 412-371-9430
e-mail: sholbrook@trcil.org
www.trcil.org

Stanley Holbrook, President/CEO
Coleen Vuono, Deputy Director
Offers peer counseling, information and referral services, housing data and referral service, assistive technology program, deinstitutionalization program, consumer-controlled personal assistance program, independent living skills training, advocacy and accessibility consultants.
Sliding Fee

4129 **Tri-County Patriots for Independent Living**
69 E Beau Street
Washington, PA 15301
724-223-5115
FAX: 724-223-5119
TTY:724-228-4028
e-mail: kathleen@tripil.com
www.tripil.com

Kathleen Kleinmann, Executive Director
TRIPIL promotes independent living in Southwestern Pennsylvania for and by individuals with disabilities; to enable them to take control of their lives; to make decisions about themselves and their future; to ensure tgat the necessary support services are available to enable them to be active participants in their communities; and to prevent unncessary institutionalization

4130 **Voices for Independence**
1107 Payne Avenue
Erie, PA 16503
866-407-0064
FAX: 814-874-3497
TTY:814-838-3702
e-mail: vfi@voicesforindependence.org
www.voicesforindependence.org

Shona Eakin, Executive Director
A non-profit advocacy and service organization of and for individuals with disabilities. Voices for Independence was formed by individuals with disabilities who felt that some of the primary disability service providers/organizations in Northwestern Pennsylvania were too paternalistic, laked true consumer direction and consumer control, and thus were not satisfactorily meeting the needs and concerns of individuals with disabilities in our region.

Rhode Island

4131 **Blackstone Valley Center**
115 Manton Street
Pawtucket, RI 02861
401-727-0150
FAX: 401-727-0153
e-mail: contact@bvcriarc.org
www.bvcriarc.org

Peter Holden, Executive Director
Kathy Hunt, Manager
John Padien, President
A private nonprofit organization providing residential, developmental, employment and recreational programs and services to more then 400 individuals with intellectual and related disabilities.

4132 **Franklin Court Assisted Living**
180 Franklin Street
Bristol, RI 02809
401-253-3679
FAX: 401-253-5855
e-mail: jpierce@ebcdc.org

Jean Pierce, Administrator
Offers local seniors an affordable assisted living option with first-rate services and gracious accommodations.

4133 **IN-SIGHT Independent Living**
43 Jefferson Boulevard
Warwick, RI 02888
401-941-3322
FAX: 401-941-3356
e-mail: cbutler@in-sight.org
www.in-sight.org

Judith Smith, President
IN-SIGHT inspires confidence, builds skills, and empowers people who are blind and visually impaired to become fully integrated, equally valued members of society by providing diverse services that produce opportunities and choices.

4134 **Ocean State Center for Independent Living**
1944 Warwick Avenue
Warwick, RI 02889
401-738-1013
866-857-1161
FAX: 401-738-1083
TTY: 401-738-1015
e-mail: oscil@oscil.org
www.oscil.org

Lorna Ricci, Executive Director
OSCIL is a consumer controlled, community based, nonprofit organization established to provide a range of independent living services to enhance, through self direction, the quality of life of Rhode Islander with significant disability and to promote integration into the community.

4135 **Office of Rehabilitation Services**
40 Fountain Street
Providence, RI 02903
401-421-7005
FAX: 401-222-3574
www.ors.ri.gov

Ron Racine, Deputy Administrator For Blind
Steve Brunero, Deputy Administrator-ORS
John Microulis, Deputy Administrator-Disability
Their goal is to help individuals with physical and mental disabilities prepare for and obtain appropriate employment.

4136 **PARI Independent Living Center**
500 Prospet Street
Pawtucket, RI 02860
401-725-1966
FAX: 401-725-2104
TTY:401-725-1966
e-mail: info@pari-ilc.org
www.pari-ilc.org

Leo Canuel, Executive Director
Sue Bilodau, Program Director
Offers information and referral services, personal care attendant services, home modifications, advocacy services and peer counseling, independent living skills training, and recycled equipment.

South Carolina

4137 **Coastal Disability Access**
1021 3rd Avenue
Conway, SC 29526
843-488-1309
FAX: 843-488-0994
e-mail: cdaspecial1@aol.com
www.coastal.edu/carr/srservices

Barbara Cole, IL Specialist
Promotes independent living throughout Horry, Georgetown, and Marion Counties.

4138 **Columbia Disability Action Center**
1115 Belleview Street
Columbia, SC 29201
803-779-5121
800-681-6805
FAX: 803-779-5114
TTY: 803-779-0949
www.dacsc.org

Stephen Maglione, Executive Director
Neyoka Fisher, VP Budget Finance
A non-profit consumer governed Center for Independent Living. Programs and services support persons with disaibilities in taking full advantage of community resources, enhancing personal opportunities, and determining the direction of their lives.

4139 **Graham Street Community Resources**
306 Graham Street
Florence, SC 29501
843-665-6674
FAX: 843-665-6675

Faye Thompson, Manager
Promotes independent living and empowers people with disabilities to reach their highest level of independence.

4140 **Greenville Disability Action Center**
712 Laurens Road
Greenville, SC 29607
864-235-1421
800-681-7715
FAX: 864-235-2056
TTY: 864-235-8798
e-mail: amayne@dacsc.org
www.dacsc.org

Stephen J Maglione, Executive Director
Carl Ennis, ILS
Empowers people with disabilities to reach their highest level of independence.

4141 **SC Independent Living Council**
810 Dutch Square Boulevard
Suite 214
Columbia, SC 29210
803-731-1607
877-217-2331
FAX: 803-731-1439
e-mail: natalie@scilconline.org
www.scilconline.org

Maris Burton, Executive Director
Natalie Derrick, Executive Assistant
The SC Independent Living Council's mission is to jointly (with the DSUs) develop uses for Part B funding throughout the state. These monies can be used to: develop Centers for Independent Living; outreach to unserved and underserved populations; conduct needs assessments and research; make recommendation to policy makers regarding the delivery of IL services and provide resources for direct services.

South Dakota

4142 **Adjustment Training Center**
607 N 4th Street
Aberdeen, SD 57401
605-229-0263
FAX: 605-225-3455

Rob Wanouf, Superintendent/VP
Donna Howard, Business Official
Arlette Keller, Special Education Director
Offers peer counseling, attendant care registry and referrals.

4143 **Black Hills Workshop & Training Center**
Black Hills Workshop
3650 Range Road
Rapid City, SD 57709
605-343-4550
FAX: 605-343-0879
e-mail: wadmin@bhws.com
www.bhws.com

Dennis Popp, Chief Executive Officer
Dince Braun, VP Agency Operations
Offers job placement, housing options, case coordination, supported employment and supported living for all disability groups, as well as specialized services for head trauma victims.

4144 **Communication Service for the Deaf: Yankton**
231 Broadway Avenue
Suite C6
Yankton, SD 57078
605-668-9759
FAX: 605-668-6712
TTY:605-668-9759
e-mail: kmerril@iw.net
Empowers people with disabilities to reach their highest level of independence.

4145 **Communication Service for the Deaf: Rapid City**
150 Knollwood Drive
Rapid City, SD 57701
605-394-6864
FAX: 605-394-6609
TTY:605-394-6864
www.c-s-d.org

Benjamin J Soukup, President/CEO
Scot Atkins, Senior VP, Human Resources
Kevin Barber, Senior VP, Facilities/Technology

A private, nonprofit organization dedicated to providing broad-based services, ensuring public accessibility and increasing public awareness of issues affecting deaf and hard of hearing inividuals.

4146 Native American Advocacy Program for Perso ns with Disabilities

208 S Main Street
PO Box 527
Winner, SD 57580
605-842-3977
800-303-3975
FAX: 605-842-3983
TTY: 605-842-3977
e-mail: admin@sdnaap.org
www.sdnaap.org

Marla Bear, Executive Director
Diane Zephier, Business Manager
Beth Montour, Program Manager
The mission is to encourage a healthy organization that assists Native Americans with disabilities, by providing prevention, education and training, advocacy, support, independent living skills and referrals.

4147 Opportunities for Independent Living

1200 S Main Street
Suite A
Aberdeen, SD 57401
605-626-2976
800-406-2649
FAX: 605-626-2652
TTY: 605-626-2977
e-mail: gary.oil@midconetwork.com
www.oil.org

Gary Wald, Executive Director
Empowers individuals with disabilities who choose to live independently in their own homes and communities.

4148 Prairie Freedom Center for Independent Living of Yankton

413 W 15th Street
Suite 107
Yankton, SD 57078
605-668-2940
800-947-3770
FAX: 605-668-3060
TTY: 605-668-2940
e-mail: p-f-c!@pfcil.org
www.pfcil.org

Joyce Buechler, Manager
Empowers individuals with disabilities who choose to live independently in the communities of their choice and to eliminate barriers of attitude, architecture and communication from the environment. Serves Beadle, Brown, Campbell, Clark, Codington, Day, Deuel, Edmunds, Faulk, Grant, Hamlin, Hand, Hyde, Marshall, McPherson, Roberts, Spink, Sully and Walworth counties.

4149 Prairie Freedom Center for Independent Living

411 Se 10th Street
Suite 102
Madison, SD 57042
605-256-5070
800-947-3770
FAX: 605-256-5071
e-mail: freedom1@hcpd.com

Patty Nelson, Program Coordinator
Empowers individuals with disabilities who choose to live independently in the communities for their choice and to eliminate barriers of attitude, architecture and communication form the environment.

4150 Prairie Freedom Center for Independent Living

301 S Garfiled Avenue
Suite 9
Sioux Falls, SD 57104
605-367-5630
800-947-3770
FAX: 605-367-5639
TTY: 605-367-5630
e-mail: p-f-c@pfcil.org
www.state.sd.us

Charles Anderson, Director
Char Crisp, Executive Director
Empowers individuals with disabilities who choose to live independently in the communities of their choice and to eliminate barriers of attitude, architecture and communication from the environment. Serves Lincoln, McCook, Moody, Minnehaha and Turner counties.

4151 South Dakota Assistive Technology Project

1161 Deadwood Avenue
Suite 5
Rapid City, SD 57702
605-394-6742
800-645-0673
FAX: 605-224-8320
e-mail: info@dakotalink.net
dakotalink.tie.net

Dave Vogel, Project Manager
DakotaLink is a statewide program of resources and supports that enable individuals in South Dakota greater access to assistive technology devices and services, to maintain independence, to explore funding options, and to become educated about assistive technology issues.

4152 Western Resources for dis-ABLED Independence

405 E Omaha Street
Rapid City, SD 57701
605-718-1930
888-434-4943
FAX: 605-718-1933
TTY: 605-718-1930
e-mail: ann@wrdi.org

Ann Van Loan, Executive Director
WRDI advocates for the rights of equal inclusion of people with disabilities in all aspects of community life. WRDI also strives to identify and promote access to existing resources and to advocate for the development of new resources, which may enable people with disabilities to live more independently.

Tennessee

4153 Center for Independent Living of Middle Tennessee

480 Craighead Street
Suite 200
Nashville, TN 37204
615-292-5803
866-992-4568
FAX: 615-383-1176
TTY: 615-292-7790
e-mail: cilmt@tndisability.org
www.cil-mt.org

Tom Hopton, Executive Director
CILMT provides persons with disabilities opportunities to be self advocates and make their own decisions regarding living arrangements, means of transportation, employment, social and recreational activities, as well as other aspects of everyday life. Serves Davidson, Cheatham, Wilson, Robertson, Rutherford, Sumner and Williamson Counties.

4154 DisAbility Resource Center: Knoxville

900 E Hill Avenue
Suite 120
Knoxville, TN 37915
865-637-3666
FAX: 865-637-5616
TTY:865-637-6976
e-mail: drc@drctn.org
www.drctn.org

Lillian Burch, Executive Director
Nicole Craig, Service Coordinator
Thomas Kahler, Independent Living Specialist
DRCTN mission is to empower people with disabilities to fully integrate and participate in the community. DRC is a community-based non-residential program of services designed to assist people with disabilities to gain independence and to assist the community in eliminating barriers of independence.

4155 **Jackson Center for Independent Living**
1981 Hollywood Drive
Suite 200
Jackson, TN 38305
731-668-2211
FAX: 731-668-0406
TTY:731-664-3970
e-mail: jcil05-06@yahoo.com
www.jcilnow.net

Glen Barr, Executive Director
JCIL works with people with significant disabilities and the Deaf Community in achieving their Independent Living Goals while assisting the community in eliminating barriers to Independent Living.

4156 **Memphis Center for Independent Living**
1633 Madison Avenue
Memphis, TN 38104
901-726-6404
FAX: 901-726-6521
TTY:901-726-6404
e-mail: mcil@mcil.org
www.mcil.org

Deborah Cunningham, Executive Director
Sandi Klink, Assistant Director
MCIL is a community based non-profit organization whose primary mission is to facilitate the full integration of persons with disabilities into all aspects of community life.

4157 **Tennessee Technology Access Program (TTAP)**
Citizens Plaza St. Office Building
400 Deadrick Street, 14th Floor
Nashville, TN 37243
615-313-5183
800-732-5059
FAX: 615-532-4685
TTY: 615-313-5695
e-mail: tn.ttap@state.tn.us
www.state.tn.us/humanserv/rehab/ttap.htm

Kevin Wright, Director
TTAP's mission is to maintain a statewide program of technology-rated assistance that is timely, comprehensive and consumer driven to ensure that all Tennesseans with disabilities have the information, services and deices that they need to make choices about where and how they spend their time as independently as possible.

4158 **Tri-State Resource and Advocacy Corporation**
5708 Uptain Road
Suite 350
Chattanooga, TN 37411
423-892-4774
800-868-8724
FAX: 423-892-9866
TTY: 423-892-4774
e-mail: 4trac@bellsouth.net
www.4trac.org

Mark Woofall, Executive Director
TRAC is dedicated to improving opportunities for individuals wuth disabilities.

Texas

4159 **ABLE Center for Independent Living**
3641 N Dixie Boulevard
Odessa, TX 79762
432-580-3439
FAX: 915-580-0280
TTY:915-580-3439
e-mail: abledcil@ablecenter.org
www.able-cil.org

Melvin White, Executive Director
Jacki Campbell, IL Specialist Director
Non-residential, nonprofit organization, guided by the philosophy of consumer choice, to assist people with disabilities achieve and maintain independent lifestyle.

4160 **Austin Resource Center for Independent Living**
825 E Rundberg Lane
Suite A-1
Austin, TX 78753
512-832-6349
FAX: 512-832-1869
TTY:512-832-6349
e-mail: arcil@arcil.com
www.arcil.com

Ronald Roacha, Executive Director
ARCIL of Texas provides independent living services to persons with disabilities, their families and communities throughout Travis and surrounding counties. ARCIL also provides services throughout Hays, Caldwell, Comal and Blanco counties at ARCIL San Marcos, and Williamson, Bell, Burnett and Milan counties at ARCIL Round Rock.

4161 **Austin Resource Center: Round Rock**
100 W. Adams
Suite 304
Temple, TX 76501
512-828-4624
FAX: 512-828-4625
TTY:512-828-4624
e-mail: roundrock@arcil.com
www.arcil.com

Ronald Rocha, Executive Director
Provides independent living services to persons with disabilities, their families and communities throughout the surrounding counties.

4162 **Austin Resource Center: San Marcos**
618 S Guadalupe Street
Suite 103
San Marcos, TX 78666
512-396-5790
FAX: 512-396-5794
TTY:512-396-5790
e-mail: sanmarcos@arcil.com
www.arcil.com

Ronald Rocha, Executive Director
Jack Stratton, Manager
Provides advocacy services, info and refferal, independent living skills and life skills classes. Other services include peer support and social and leisure activities and some community services.

4163 **Brazoria County Center For Independent Living**
1100 D East Mulberry
Angleton, TX 77515
979-849-7060
888-872-7957
FAX: 979-849-8465
TTY: 979-849-7060
e-mail: bccil@neosoft.com
www.coalitionforbarrierfreeliving.com
To promote the full inclusion, equal opportunity and participation of persons with disabilities in every aspect of community life. We believe that people with disabilities have the right to make choices affecting their lives, a right to take risks, a right to fail, and a right to succeed.

4164 **Center Serving Persons with Mental Retardation**
3550 West Dallas
PO Box 130564
Houston, TX 77019
713-525-8400
FAX: 713-525-8444
www.cri-usa.org

C Wayne Johnson, President
Jim Aycock, Vice President
Provides services for more than 600 children and adults with mental retardation and other developmental disabilities. The Center also offers a wide array of programs including education, vocational training and job placement services, three different residential options representing both urban and rural living environments, special programs designed to meet the needs of older adults, and a variety of therapeutic support services.

4165 **Crockett Resource Center for Independent Living**
1020 Loop 304 E
Crockett, TX 75835
936-544-2811
FAX: 936-544-7315
TTY:936-544-2811
e-mail: crcil@consolidated.net

Cynthia Cook, Executive Director
Provides independent living services to cross-disability groups to increase their personal self-determination and minimize dependence on others. Maintain comprehensive information on availability of resources and provides referrals to such resources. Provides instruction to assist people with disabilities to gain skills that would empower them to live independently. Peer counseling, advocacy - both individual and community by assisting to obtain support services to make changes in society.

4166 Houston Center for Independent Living
6201 Bonnhomme Road
Suite 150 South
Houston, TX 77036
713-974-4621
FAX: 713-974-6927
TTY:713-974-2703
e-mail: hcil@neosoft.com
www.coalitionforbarrierfreeliving.com

Sandra Bookman, Executive Director
HCIL promotes the full inclusion, equal opportunity and participation of persons with disabilities in every aspect of community life. HCIL also believes that people with disabilities have the right to make choices affecting their lives, a right to take risks, ad right to fail, and a right to succeed.

4167 Independent Life Styles
PO Box 571874
Houston, TX 77257
713-861-4266
FAX: 713-861-9846
www.independentlifestyles.org

Peter Simmons, Director
Offers peer counseling, advocacy and other services to the community.

4168 Independent Living Research Utilization Project
Institute For Rehabilitation & Research
2323 S Shepherd Drive
Suite 1000
Houston, TX 77019
713-520-0232
FAX: 713-520-5785
TTY:713-520-0232
e-mail: ilru@ilru.org
www.ilru.org

Lex Frieden, Director
Laurie Redd, Executive Director
ILRU is a national center for information, training, research and technical assistance in independent living. Its goal is to expand the body of knowledge in independent living and to improve utilization of results of research programs and demonstration projects in this field. ILRU is a program of The Institute for Rehabilitation and Research, a nationally recognized medical rehabilitation facility for persons with disabilities. TTY phone number: (713) 520-5136.

4169 LIFE/ Run Centers for Independent Living
4902 34th Street
Suite 5
Lubbock, TX 79410
806-795-5433
FAX: 806-795-5607
TTY:806-795-5433
e-mail: wilmacrain@yahoo.com
www.liferun.org

Michelle Crain, Executive Director
Committed to providing individuals with disabilities the information and skills necessary to become independent and to achieve full inclusion in every aspect of their life.

4170 Martin Luther Homes of Texas
520 E Donagun Street
Suite 2
Seguin, TX 78155
830-372-3075
FAX: 830-303-3075

Jerome Boeck, Manager
Providing a wide array of services to assist individuals and families in achieving positive life goals. Services to persons with disabilities and other special needs include community living options, training and employment options, spiritual growth and development options, training and counseling support.

4171 Office for Students with Disabilities, University of Texas at Arlington
PO Box 19510
Arlington, TX 76019
817-272-3364
FAX: 817-272-1447
TTY:817.272.1520
e-mail: dianne@uta.edu
www.uta.edu/disability

Dianne Hengst, Director
Penny Acrey, Assistant Director
Amber Mitchell, Interpreter Coordinator
Offers disability counseling and academic accomodation for UTA community.

4172 Palestine Resource Center for Independent Living
421 Avenue A
Palestine, TX 75801
903-729-7505
888-326-5166
FAX: 903-729-7540
TTY:903-729-7505
e-mail: prcil@earthlink.net

Cynthia Cook, Executive Director
Sara Manton, Manager
Provides independent living services to cross-disability groups to increase their personal self-determination and minimize dependence on others. Maintain comprehensive information on availability of resources and provides referrals to such resources. Provides instruction to assist people with disabilities to gain skills that would empower them to live independently. Peer counseling, advocacy - both individual and community by assisting to obtain support services to make changes in society.

4173 Panhandle Action Center for Independent Living Skills
1118 S Taylor Street
Amarillo, TX 79101
806-374-1400
FAX: 806-374-4550
TTY:806-374-2774
e-mail: advocacy@nts-online.net
www.panhandleilc.org

Carl McMillen, Director
Kevin Oliphant, Manager
PILC is a non profit organization dedicated to the advancement of full participation in all aspects of life. PILC services are developed, directed, delivered, and governed primarily by individuals with disabilities.

4174 REACH of Dallas Resource Center on Independent Living
8625 King George Drive
Suite 210
Dallas, TX 75235
214-630-4796
FAX: 214-630-6390
TTY:214-630-5995
e-mail: reachdallas@reachcils.org
www.reachcils.org

Charlotte Stewart, Executive Director
Susie Reukema, Assistant Director
Information and referral services, peer counseling, independent living skills training, loaner adaptive equipment, advocacy assistance, social, recreational activities and ADA technical assistance.

4175 REACH of Denton Resource Center on Independent Living
405 S Elm Street
Suite 202
Denton, TX 76201
940-383-1062
FAX: 940-383-2742
e-mail: reachden@reachcils.org
www.reachcils.org

Charlotte Stewart, Executive Director
Becky Teal, Manager
REACH is a North Texas based nonprofit organization that provides services to people with disabilities and education to the community on disability-relatd topics.

4176 REACH/Resource Center on Independent Living
1205 Lake Street
Fort Worth, TX 76102
817-870-9082
FAX: 817-877-1622
TTY:817-870-9086
e-mail: reachftw@reachcils.org
www.reachcils.org

Charlotte Stewart, Executive Director
Robin Laffiter, Manager
Information and referral services, peer counseling, independent living skills training, loaner equipment, advocacy assistance, ADA technical assistance and social/recreational activities.

4177 RISE-Resource: Information, Support and Empowerment
755 S 11th Street
Suite 101
Beaumont, TX 77701
409-832-2599
FAX: 409-838-4499
e-mail: cherylbass@risecil.org
www.risecil.org

Cheryl Bass, Executive Director
Provide core services of Individual & Systems Advocacy, Information & Referral, IL Skills, Training, and Peer Support. Also Community Education regarding disability issues.

4178 SAILS
1028 S Alamo St.
San Antonio, TX 78210
210-281-1878
800-474-0295
FAX: 210-281-1759
TTY: 210-281-1878
e-mail: kbrietzke@sailstx.org
www.sailstx.org

Kitty Brietzke JD, Executive Director
Gloria Banik, Assistant Executive Director
SAILS advocates for the rights and empowerment of people with disabilities in San Antonio; as well as surrounding areas. Services are provided to people with disabilities in the following counties: Atacosa, Bandera, Bexar, Calhoun, Comal, DeWitt, Dimmit, Edwards, Frio, Gillespie, Goliad, Gonzalez, Guadalupe, Jackson, Karnes, La Salle, Kendall, Kerr, Kinney, Lavaca, Maverick, Medina, Real, Uvalde, Val Verde, Victoria, Wilson and Zavala.

4179 Texas Rehabilitation Commission Independent Living Services
4900 N Lamar Boulevard
Austin, TX 78751
512-424-4000
800-628-5115
FAX: 512-424-4283
e-mail: drswebfeedback@dars.state.tx.us

Tony Lawrence, Director
Max Arrell, Manager
Provides technical assistance and other support services to the state's Independent Living Council, Independent Living Centers and Independent Living Counseling programs.

4180 VOLAR Center for Independent Living
8929 Viscount
Suite 101
El Paso, TX 79925
915-591-0800
FAX: 915-591-3506
TTY:915-591-0800
e-mail: volar@volarcil.org
www.volarcil.org

Luis Enrique Chew, Executive Director
Dan Monroe, Chief Executive Officer
VOLAR is committed to providing independent living ervices and information and referral, and to developing community options for persons with cross disabilities to empower them to live the kind of lives they choose. VOLAR is an organization of and for people with disabilities, advocating human and civil rights, community options and empowering people to live the lives they choose. Newsletter available.

4181 Valley Association for Independent Living (VAIL)
3012 N McColl Road
Suute B
McAllen, TX 78501
956-668-8245
FAX: 956-631-7914
e-mail: wjohnston@valleyassociation.org
www.valleyassociation.org

Woodie Johnston, Executive Director
Offers information and referral, peer counseling, support groups, independent living skills training, community rehab program, and advocacy.

4182 Valley Association for Independent Living: Harlingen
1824 W. Jefferson
Suite B
Harlingen, TX 78550
956-428-1126
FAX: 956-428-4339
e-mail: tstem@valleyassociation.org
www.valleyassociation.org

Teresa Stem, Independent Living Specialist
Provides information and referral, peer counseling, support groups, independent living skills training, community rehab program and advocacy

Utah

4183 Active Re-Entry
10 S Fairgrounds Road
Price, UT 84501
435-637-4950
FAX: 435-637-4952
TTY:435-637-4950
e-mail: active@arecil.org
www.arecil.org

Nancy Bentley, Executive Director
Active Re-Entry is a community based program which assists individuals with disabilities to acheive or maintain self-sufficient and productive live in their own communities. Active Re-Entry is committed to promoting the rights, dignity, and quality of life for all persons with disabilities.

4184 Active Re-Entry: Vernal
510 E Main Street
Suite 3
Vernal, UT 84078
435-789-4021
FAX: 435-789-1031
TTY:435-789-4021
www.arecil.org

Nancy Bentley, Executive Director
Active Re-Entry is a community based program which assists individuals with disabilities to achieve or maintain self-sufficient and productive lives in their own communities. We are committed to promoting the rights, dignity, and quality of life for all persons with disabilities.

4185 Central Utah Independent Living Center
491 N Freedon Boulevard
Provo, UT 84601
801-373-5044
877-421-4500
FAX: 801-373-5094
TTY: 801-373-5044
e-mail: sandra@cucil.org
www.cucil.org

Sandra Curcio, Executive Director
Bill Peterson, Independent Living Specialist
Central Utah Center for Independent Living (CUCIL) empowers people with disabilities to reach their full potential in community settings through peer support, advocacy, and education.

4186 OPTIONS for Independence
Northern Utah Center for Independent Living
1095 N Main Street
Logan, UT 84341
435-753-5353
FAX: 435-753-5390
TTY:435-753-5353
e-mail: jbiggs@optionind.org
www.optionsind.org

Cheryl Atwood, Executive Director
OPTIONS for Independence, the northern Utah Center for Independent living serves people of all ages with all types of disabilities. OPTIONS is a nonresidential Center that provides services to individuals with disabilities to facilitate their full participation in the community and raise the understanding of disability issues and access to the community. The Independent living philosophy is strictly adhered to: consumer control and choice being the focus.

4187 **OPTIONS for Independence: Brigham Satellit e**
862 S Main Street
Suite 9
Brigham City, UT 84302
435-723-2171
FAX: 435-723-9618
TTY:435-723-2171
e-mail: dcrockettebrigham.net
www.optionsind.org

Cheryl Atwood, Executive Director
Deanna Crockett, Manager
OPTIONS is a nonresidential Independent Living Center where people with disabilities can learn skills to gain more control and independence over their lives. OPTIONS raises the vision and capability of the community at large to the point where people of all abilities will have equal access.

4188 **Red Rock Center for Independence**
515 W 300 N
Suite A
Saint George, UT 84770
435-673-7501
800-649-2340
FAX: 435-673-8808
e-mail: rrci@rrci.org
www.rrci.org

Garry Owens, Executive Director
Mary Light, Assistant Director
Mark Johnson, Independent Living Specialist
Red Rock Center for Independence assists people with disabilities to live and participate independently.

4189 **Red Rock Center for Independence: Fillmore**
PO Box 531
Fillmore, UT 84631
435-619-7724
FAX: 435-619-8808
TTY:435-619-7501
e-mail: rrci@rrci.org
www.rrci.org

Garry Owens, Executive Director
Red Rock Center for Independence assists people with disabilities to live and participate independently.

4190 **Tri-County Independent Living Center**
2726 Washington Boulevard
PO Box 428
Ogden, UT 84401
801-612-3215
866-734-5678
FAX: 801-612-3732
TTY: 801-612-3215
e-mail: vickie@tri-county-ilc.com
www.tri-county-ilc.com

Vickie Brenchley, Deputy Director/Office Manager
Andy Curry, Executive Director
The mission of the Tri-County ILC is to enhance independence for all people with disabilities. Serves Davis, Weber and Morgan Counties.

4191 **Utah Assistive Technology Program (UTAP) Utah State University**
6855 Old Main Hill
Logan, UT 84322
435-797-3824
800-524-5152
FAX: 435-797-2355
e-mail: curtis@cpd2.usu.edu
www.uatpat.org

Martin Blair, Assistant Director
Dan Peterson, Manager
Provides expertise, resources, and a structure to enhance and expand AT services provided by private and public agencies in Utah. Occcurs through monitoring, coordination, information dissemination, empowering individuals, the identification and removal of barriers, and expanding state resources.

4192 **Utah Independent Living Center**
3445 S Main Street
Salt Lake City, UT 84115
801-466-5565
800-355-2195
FAX: 801-466-2363
e-mail: uilc@xmission.com
www.uilc.org

Debra A Mair, Executive Director
Kim Meichle, Program Director
Julie Beckstead, Program Coordinator
Offers information and referral services. To assist persons with disabilities achieve independence by providing services and activities which enhance independent living skillspromote the public's understanding, accomodation, and acceptance of their rights, needs and abilities.

4193 **Utah Independent Living Center: Minersville**
Po Box 168
Minersville, UT 84752
435-691-7724
www.uilcxmission.net
To enhance independence for all people with disaibilities.

4194 **Utah Independent Living Center: Tooele**
33 S Main Street
Tooele, UT 84074
435-843-7353
FAX: 435-843-7359
TTY:435-843-7353
e-mail: uilc@trilobyte.com
www.ilru.org

Angie Slater, Director
Mission is to assist persons with disabilities achieve greater independence by providing services and activities which enhance independent living skills and promote the public's understanding, accomodation, and acceptance of their rights, needs and abilities.

Vermont

4195 **Vermont Assistive Technology Project: Department of Aging & Disabilities**
Department of Aging and Independent Living
103 S Main Street
Waterbury, VT 05671
802-241-2400
800-750-6355
FAX: 802-241-2174
TTY: 802-241-1464
e-mail: jtucker@dad.state.vt.us
www.dad.state.vt.us/atp

Julie Tucker, Project Director
David Tunia, Information/Education Specialist
Patrick Flood, Manager
Encompasses a state coordinating council for assistive technology issues, regional centers for demonstration, trial and technical support with computer and augmentative communication equipment and regional seating and positioning centers.

4196 **Vermont Center for Independent Living: Brattleboro**
28 Vernon Street
Suite 401
Burlington, VT 05401
802-254-6851
800-539-1522
FAX: 802-258-2651
e-mail: vcil@vcil.org
www.vcil.org

Candace Stouman, Peer Advocate Counselor
Missy Boothroyd, Deaf Peer Counselor
Believes that individuals with disabilities have the right to live with dignity and with appropriate support in their own homes, fully participate in their communities, and to control and make decisions about their lives.

4197 **Vermont Center for Independent Living**
11 E State Street
Montpelier, VT 05602
802-229-0501
800-639-1522
FAX: 802-229-0503
TTY: 800-639-1522
e-mail: vcil@vcil.org
www.vcil.org

Deborah Lisi-Baker, Executive Director
VCIL believes that individuals with disabilities have the right to live with dignity and with appropriate support in their own homes, fully participate in their communities, and to control and make decisions about their lives.

4198 **Vermont Center for Independent Living: Bennington**
532 Main Street
Bennington, VT 05201
802-447-0574
FAX: 802-442-4052
TTY:802-447-0574
e-mail: vcilbenn@vcil.org
www.vcil.com

Deborah Lisi-Baker, Executive Director
Rose Rahilly, Manager
VCIL believes that individuals with disabilities have the right to live with dignity and with appropriate support in their own homes, fully participate in their communities, and to control and make decisions about their lives.

Virginia

4199 **Access Independence**
403-B S Loudoun Street
Winchester, VA 22601
540-662-4452
FAX: 540-662-4474
TTY:540-722-9693
e-mail: askai@accessindependence.org
www.accessindependence.org

Kim Shick, Executive Director
Diane Starkey, Programs Manager
Joan Davis, Manager
Offers support services to persons with disabilities to assist in maintaining or increasing their independence and self-determination. Includes housing assistance, independent living skills training, information, referral services, assistance and representative payee and advocacy.

4200 **Appalachian Independence Center**
230 Charwood Drive
Abingdon, VA 24210
276-628-2979
FAX: 276-628-4931
TTY:276-676-0920
e-mail: aicadmin@ntelos.net
wwww.aicadvocates.org

Greg Morrell, Executive Director
Donna Buckland, Assistant Director
Steve Halley, Independent Living Advocate
AIC's mission is to foster a community environment in which people with disabilities will be able to achieve their maximum level of independence. It creates this environment by educating the public and promoting the needs and rights of people with disabilities while working with them to meet their personal potential for independence.

4201 **Blue Ridge Independent Living Center - Troutville**
US Route 11, N Lee Highway
Room 103
Troutville, VA 24175
540-966-4951
FAX: 540-342-9505
TTY:540-966-4951
e-mail: kmichbrilc@aol.com

Leigh Taylor, Executive Director
Empowering individuals with disabilities to become self-sufficient and independent within their communities.

4202 **Blue Ridge Independent Living Center**
1502 B Williamson Road NE
Roanoke, VA 24012
540-342-1231
FAX: 540-342-9505
TTY:540-342-1231
e-mail: kmichalski@brilc.org
www.brilc.org

Karen Michalski, Executive Director
Sara Ingram, Program Services Director
Ava Coles, Independent Living Coordinator
BRILC assists people with disabilities to live independently. The Center also serves the community at large by helping to create an environment that is accessible to all. BRILC offers a variety of servies ranging from referrals to community resources, support services, and direct services. These include peer counseling, support groups, training and seminars, advocacy, education, support services, awareness, aid in obtaining specialized equipment, and much more.

4203 **Blue Ridge Independent Living Center: Christianburg**
210 Pepper Street
Suite D
Christiansburg, VA 24073
540-381-8829
FAX: 540-381-8829
TTY:540-381-8829
e-mail: tlavinder@brilc.org
www.brilc.org

Karen Michalski-Karney, Executive Director
Sara Ingram, Program Services Coordinator
Ava Coles, Independent Living Specialist
Assists people with disabilities to live independently. The center also serves the community at large by helping to create an environment that is accessible to all.

4204 **Blue Ridge Independent Living Center: Low Moor**
PO Box 7
Low Moor, VA 24457
540-862-0252
FAX: 540-862-0252
TTY:540-862-0252
www.brilc.org

Assists to help people with disabilities to live independently. The center also serves the community at large by helping to create an environment that is accessible to all.

4205 **Clinch Independent Living Services**
1139C Plaza Drive
Grundy, VA 24614
276-935-6088
800-597-2322
FAX: 276-935-6342
TTY: 276-935-6088
e-mail: cils@yzavenue.org
www.cils-online.org

Betty Bevins, Executive Director
Nonprofit organization providing information and referral, peer counseling, advocacy and independent living skills training to persons with disabilities.

4206 **Disability Resource Center**
409 Progress Street
Fredericksburg, VA 22401
540-373-2559
800-648-6324
FAX: 540-373-8126
TTY: 540-373-5890
e-mail: rob@drc-fredericksburg.org
www.cildrc.org

Debe Fulps, Executive Director
Mission is to assist people with disabilities, those who support them, and the community, through information, education and resources, to achieve the highest potential and benefit of independent living.

4207 **ENDependence Center of Northern Virginia**
3100 Clarendon Boulevard
Arlington, VA 22201
703-525-3268
FAX: 703-525-3585
TTY:703-525-3553
e-mail: info@ecnv.org
www.ecnv.org

Michael J Cooper, Executive Director

ECNV is a community-based resource and advocacy enter which is managed by and for people with disabilities. ENCV promotes independent living philosophy and equal access for all persons with disabilities and, like the nearly 400 centers for independent living across the country, ECNV grew from local disability rights and self-help movements.

4208 Equal Access Center for Independence
4031 University Drive
Suite 301
Fairfax, VA 22030
703-934-2020
FAX: 703-277-7730
e-mail: drc@patriot.net

David Sharp, Executive Director
Provides information and referral, peer counseling, advocacy and independent living skills training to persons with disabilities.

4209 Independence Empowerment Center
9001 Digges Road
Suite 103
Manassas, VA 20110
703-257-5400
FAX: 703-257-5043
TTY:703-257-5400
e-mail: info@ieccil.org
www.ieccil.org

Mary D. Lopez, Ph.D., Executive Director
A non-profit Center for Independent Living. One of over 500 centers in the United States with roots in civil rights models of the 1960's.

4210 Independence Resource Center
815 Cherry Avenue
Charlottesville, VA 22903
434-971-9629
FAX: 434-497-8242
TTY:434-497-9634
e-mail: tvandever@ntelos.net

Thomas Vandever, Executive Director
Information and referral services.

4211 Independent Living Center Network: Department of the Visually Handicapped
1809 Staples Mill Road
Suite 300
Richmond, VA 23230
804-355-7900
FAX: 804-355-9297

Bob Burton, Director
Robert Kastenbaum, Partner
Information and referral services.

4212 Junction Center for Independent Living
PO Box 1210
Norton, VA 24273
276-679-5988
FAX: 276-679-6569
TTY:276-679-5988
e-mail: jcil1@junctioncenter.org
www.juctioncenter.org

Dennis Horton, Executive Director
JCIL is a non-profit, non-residential program which provides services to persons with disabilities, their families, and their community. JCIL's mission is to assist people who have significant disabilities to live indpenedently in the least restrictive and most integrated environment possible.

4213 Junction Center for Independent Living
4907 Boone Trail Road
PO Box 408
Duffield, VA 24244
276-431-1195
FAX: 276-431-1196
TTY:276-431-1196
e-mail: jcil1@junctioncenter.org
www.junctioncenter.org

Dennis Horton, Executive Director
JCIL is a non-profit, non-residential program which provides services to persons with disabilities, their families, and their community. JCIL's mission is to assist people who have significant disabilities to live independently in the least restrictive and most integrated environment possible.

4214 Lynchburg Area Center for Independent Living
500 Alleghany Avenue
Lynchburg, VA 24501
434-528-4971
FAX: 434-528-4976
TTY:434-528-4972
e-mail: lacil@lacil.org
www.lacil.org

Lindsey Edwards, Community Outreach Director
LACIL is a private non-profit, non-residential consumer driven organization that promotes the efforts of persons with disabilities to live independently in the community and supports the efforts of the community to be open and accessible to all citizens.

4215 Peidmont Independent Living Center
Piedmont Living Center
509 Piney Forest Road
Danville, VA 24541
434-797-2530
FAX: 434-797-2568
TTY:434-797-2530
e-mail: pilc@gamewood.com
www.vhda.com

Clarence Dickerson, Executive Director
Jeanette King, ILS Coordinator/BPAD
Lori Penn, Office Manager
Empowering indiviuals with disabilities to become self-sufficient and independent within their communities.

4216 Peninsula Center for Independent Living
2021-A Cunningham Drive
Suite 2
Hampton, VA 23666
757-827-0275
FAX: 757-827-0655
TTY:757-827-8800
e-mail: iepcil@iepcil.org
www.iepcil.org

Ralph Shelman, Executive Director
IEPCIL is a private non-profit non-residential Agency established to provide services to people with disabilities. The Centers Philosophy is that people with a disability should play a major role in deciding their future.The center provides services to people with disabilities in the cities of Hampton, Newport News, Poquoson, Williamsburg, and counties of James City, York, and Gloucester.

4217 Resources for Independent Living
4009 Fitzhugh Avenue
Suite 100
Richmond, VA 23230
804-353-6503
FAX: 804-358-5606
TTY:804-353-6583
e-mail: woodsonf@cavtel.net
www.ril-va.org

Sandra Wagener, Executive Director
Mission is assisting persons who are severely disabled to live independently in the community and to encourage necessary change within the community so independent living is a possibility.

4218 Valley Associates for Independent Living (VAIL)
Shenandoah Valley Workforce Investment Board
1909 A E Market Street
PO Box 869
Harrisonburg, VA 22803
540-442-7134
FAX: 540-434-0803
e-mail: satterwhite@valleyworkforce.com
www.valleyworkforce.com

Taylor Howell, Manager
Bob Satterwhite, Executive Director
VAIL is a not-for-profit, private Center for Independent Living providing advocacy, information and referral, independent living skills training, supported employment, and peer counseling to individuals with disabilities in our planning district.

4219 Valley Associates for Independent Living: Lexington
25 Northridge Lane
Suite 6
Lexington, VA 24450
540-464-5454
FAX: 540-464-5454
e-mail: vail@govail.org
www.govail.org

Marcia DuBois, Director
Promoting self-direction among people with disabilities and removing barriers to independence in the community.

4220 Woodrow Wilson Rehabilitation Center Training Program
PO Box 1500
Fishersville, VA 22939
540-332-7000
800-345-9972
FAX: 540-332-7132
TTY: 800-811-7893
e-mail: colemawl@wwrc.state.va.us
www.wwrc.net

Richard S Luck EdD, Director
Information & referral services. Six week Virginia residential programs and evaluation services.

Washington

4221 Alliance for People with Disabilities: Sea ttle
4649 Sunnyside Avenue N
Suite 100
Seattle, WA 98103
206-545-7055
866-545-7055
FAX: 206-545-7059
TTY: 206-632-3456
e-mail: info@disabilitypride.org
www.disabilitypride.org

Jeanette Murphy, Executive Director
The Alliance promotes equality and choice for people with disabilities. They provide advocacy, peer support, idependent living skills training, information and referral, transition assistance for youth and civil rights legal aid.

4222 Alliance of People with Disabilities: Redmond
East King County Office
16315 NE 87th Street
Suite B-3
Redmond, WA 98052
425-558-0993
800-216-3335
FAX: 425-558-4773
TTY: 425-861-4773
e-mail: infon@disabilitypride.org
www.disabilitypride.org

Robert Blumenfeld, Manager
Michelle Klekota, Independent Living Program
Charity Ranger, Independent Living Program
Services include: information and referral, independent living skills training, peer groups, disAbility law project (DLP), access reviews, health insurance advising, and systems advocacy.

4223 Coalition of Responsible Disabled
612 N Maple Street
Spokane, WA 99201
509-326-6355
877-606-2680
FAX: 509-327-2420
TTY: 509-326-6355
e-mail: contact@cordwa.info
www.cordwa.info

Linda McClain MSW, Executive Director
Wendi Dunlap MSW, REACH Independent Living Service
Linda Schappals, Executive Director
CORD strives to enhance independent living opportunities and self-determination through advocacy, promoting civil rights, and empowerment. Improves the self-determination and self-reliance of people with disabilities through community and individual advocacy, education and provisions of independent living.

4224 Community Service Center for the Deaf and Hard of Hearing
1609 19th Avenue
Seattle, WA 98122
206-322-4996
877-301-0006
FAX: 206-720-3251
TTY: 206-322-4996
e-mail: cscdhh@cscdhh.org
www.cscdhh.org

Susan Bernick, Interim Executive Director
Angelia Theriault, Advocate Specialist
Community information and referral services; interpreter referral services such as sign language interpreting, real time captioning, relay interpreting, oral interpreting; 9-1-1/TTY eduction program; communication access advocacy; and community education.

4225 Community Services for the Blind and Partially Sighted
9709 3rd Avenue NE
Suite 100
Seattle, WA 98115
206-525-5556
800-458-4888
FAX: 206-525-0422
e-mail: csbps@csbps.com
www.csbps.com

June Mansfield, President/CEO
Founded in 1965 as an independent nonprofit, CSBPS works to restore, maintain, and enhance the independence and well-being of people with impaired vision. Programs include professional counseling and support; safe travel and orientation training; instruction in independent living skills; low vision clinic and low vision rehavilitation; one-on-one volunteer services, education, information and referral, assistive technology center; and an adaptive aids retail, and online store.

4226 DisAbility Resource Connection: Everett
607 SE Everett Mall Way
Suite 6C
Everett, WA 98208
425-347-5768
800-315-3583
FAX: 425-710-0767
TTY: 425-347-5768
e-mail: drcservices@drconline.net
www.drconline.net

Charley Lane, Executive Director
disAbility Resource Connection is all about living your life as you choose. The staff is committed to assisting every individual to connect resources, connect to skills, connect to life.

4227 Independent Living Center of SW Washington
PO Box 2129
Vancouver, WA 98668
FAX: 253-848-0798

Morris Gielser, Director
Offers peer counseling, referral and advocacy services.

4228 Kitsap Community Resources
802 7th Street
Bremerton, WA 98337
360-478-2301
FAX: 360-415-2706
e-mail: info@kcr.org
www.kcr.org

Teri Washburn, President
Heidi Gunter, Vice President
Larry Eyer, Executive Director
Kitsap Community Resources is a local, non-profit organization dedicated to helping people in need. KCR creates hope and opportunity for low-income Kitsap County Residents by providing resources that promote self-sufficiency.

4229 Lilac Blind Foundation
1212 N Howard Street
Spokane, WA 99201
509-328-9116
800-422-7893
FAX: 509-328-8965
e-mail: info@lilacblindfoundation.org
www.lilacblindfoundation.org

Colleen Stevens, President
Al Rubens, Vice President
Cheryl Martin, Executive Director
Lilac Blind Foundation provides adaptive training and equiptment that enables blind and partially sighted individuals to live satisfying lives and pursue vocational or educational opportunities.

4230 National Council on Independent Living
1916 Wilson Boulevard
Suite 209
Arlington, VA 22201
703-525-3406
877-525-3400
FAX: 703-525-3409
TTY: 703-525-4153
e-mail: ncil@ncil.org
www.ncil.org

Anne Marie Hughey, Executive Director
June Sutherland, Project Assistant
Advances the independent living philosophy and advocates for the human rights of and services for people with disabilities to further their full integration and participation in society. The National Council on Independent Living (NCIL) is the oldest cross disability, grassroots organization run by and for people with disabilities.

4231 Resource Center for the Handicapped
20150 45th Avenue NE
Lake Forest Park, WA 98155
206-364-8179
FAX: 425-271-1096

Jeff Sykes, Director
Committed to assisting every individual to connect resources, connect to skills and to connect to life.

4232 Tacoma Area Coalition of Individuals with Disabilities
6315 S 19th Street
Tacoma, WA 98466
253-565-9000
877-538-2243
FAX: 253-565-5578
TTY: 253-565-5445
e-mail: tacid@tacid.org
www.tacid.org

Christopher Ensor, Executive Director
Promotes the independence of individuals with disabilities.

West Virginia

4233 Appalachian Center for Independent Living
4710 Chimney Drive
Suite C
Charleston, WV 25302
304-965-0376
800-642-3003
FAX: 304-965-0377
TTY: 304-965-0377
e-mail: acil@westco.net

Larry E Paxton, Executive Director
Scott Dc, Owner
Provides services and formation to handicapped persons including professional and peer counseling, advocacy, referral, housing, transportation, support groups, build wheelchair ramps, mobility equipment loan, attendant care, older blind services and skills training.

4234 Mountain State Center for Independent Living
329 Prince Street
Beckley, WV 25801
304-255-0122
FAX: 304-255-0157
TTY:304-255-0122
e-mail: kmaynus@mtstcil.org
www.mtstcil.org

Kevin Maynus, Director
Anne Weeks, Chief Executive Officer
This office provides individual and systems advocacy, independent living skills development, information and referral, peer support, personal assistance services, housing referral and training, transportation. Serves Raleigh counties.

4235 Mountain State Center for Independent Living
821 4th Avenue
Huntington, WV 25701
304-525-3324
866-687-8245
FAX: 304-525-3360
TTY: 304-525-3324
e-mail: mtstcil@mtstcil.org
www.mtstcil.org

Anne Weeks, President/CEO
John Gallaher, Manager
Services provided are: individual and systems advocacy, independent living skills development, information and referral, peer support, personal assistance services, supported employment, community integration program, housing referral and training, transportation. Serves Cabell and Wayne counties.

4236 Northern West Virginia Center for Independent Living
601-3 E Brockway Avenue
Suite A&B
Morgantown, WV 26501
304-296-6091
FAX: 304-292-5217
e-mail: nwvcil@nwvcil.org
www.nwvcil.org

Jan Derry, Director
NWVCIL is committed to the philosophy that all persons have equal access and unconditional value, that all individuals shall be respected for their uniqueness and shall have the right to live within the community of their choice, having equal access to participate in and contribute to that community.

Wisconsin

4237 Center for Independent Living of Western Wisconsin
2920 Schneider Avenue E
Menomonie, WI 54751
715-233-1070
800-228-3287
FAX: 715-233-1083
TTY: 715-233-1070
e-mail: info@cilww.com
www.cilww.com

Tim Sheehan, Executive Director
Kay Sommerfeld, Assistant Director
Advocates for the full participation in society of all persons with disabilities. Our goal is empwowering individuals to exercise choices to maintain or increase their indpendence. Our strategy is providing consumer-driven services at no cost to persons with disiabilities in Western Wisconsin

4238 Independence First
600 W Virginia Street
4th Floor
Milwaukee, WI 53204
414-291-7520
FAX: 414-291-7525
e-mail: kavery@independencefirst.org
www.independencefirst.org

Lee Schulz, Executive Director
Serves individuals with disabilities in the metro-Milwaukee four county area. Services include advocacy, independent living skills training, information/referral, peer counseling, youth camp and personal assistance services.

4239 Independence First: West Bend
735 South Main Stret
West Bend, WI 53095
262-306-6717
TTY:262-306-6717
e-mail: lee@independencefirst.org
www.independencefirst.org
Services include advocacy, independent living skills training, information/referral, peer counseling, youth camp and personal assistance services.

4240 Inspiration Ministries
PO Box 948
Walworth, WI 53184
262-275-6131
FAX: 262-275-3355
e-mail: tschnake@inspirationministries.org
www.inspirationministries.org

David Rowland, President
Tim Schnake, VP Resident Services
Formerly known as Christian League for the Handicapped.The ministry is a caring Christian community who enable and encourage people with disabilities. We address physical, mental and spiritual needs through accessible residential accommodations, work opportunities and integration into the local community and its churches. 160 acre campus including residential apartments, a work center, and a retreat center/summer camp (Inspiration Center).

4241 **Mid-state Independent Living Consultants**
10101 Market Street
Suite B20
Mosinee, WI 54455
715-241-6927
877-711-6452
FAX: 715-241-8168
TTY: 877-711-6452
e-mail: jakmilc@charter.net
www.tznet.com/comn/firstcall/database/
Serving people with disabilities.

4242 **Mid-state Independent Living Consultants: Stevens Point**
3262 Church Street
Suite 1
Stevens Point, WI 54481
715-344-4210
800-382-8484
FAX: 715-344-4414
TTY: 800-382-8484
e-mail: milc@milc-inc.org
www.milc-inc.org

Jennifer Fasula, Executive Director
Committed to enhancing personal and community relationships, providing opportunities for growth, and helping people with varying abilities achieve their personal goals.

4243 **North Country Independent Living**
2231 Catlin Avenue
Suite 16
Superior, WI 54880
715-392-9118
800-924-1220
FAX: 715-392-4636
e-mail: ncil@superior-nfp.org
www.northcountryil.com

John Nousaine, Executive Director
Empowers people with disabilities.

4244 **North Country Independent Living: Ashland**
422 3rd Street W.
Suite B114
Ashland, WI 54806
715-682-5676
800-499-5676
FAX: 715-682-3144
TTY: 715-682-5676
e-mail: ncilstew@charterinternet.com
www.northcountryil.com

John Nousaine, Director
Empowers people with disabilities.

4245 **Options for Independent Living: Fond du Lac**
555 Country Club Road
PO Box 11967
Green Bay, WI 54307
920-490-0500
888-465-1515
FAX: 920-490-0700
TTY:920-490-0600
e-mail: info@optionsil.com
www.optionsil.com

Thomas Diedrick, Executive Director
Options for Independent Living, Inc. is a non-profit organization committed to empowering people with disabilities to lead independent and productive lives in their community through advocacy, the provision of information, education, technology and related services.

4246 **Society's Assets: Elkhorn**
615 E Geneva Street
Elkhorn, WI 53121
262-723-8181
FAX: 262-723-8184
TTY:262-723-8181
e-mail: info@sai-inc.org
www.sai-inc.org

Bruce Nelson, Director
Jill Vigueres, Manager
To ensure the rights of all persons with disabilities to live and function as independently as possible in the community of their choice, through supporting individual's efforts to achieve control over their lives and become integrated into community life.

4247 **Society's Assets: Kenosha**
5727 6th Avenue
Kenosha, WI 53140
262-657-3999
888-317-3999
FAX: 262-657-1672
TTY: 262-657-3999
e-mail: info@sai-inc.org
www.sai-inc.org

Joanie May, Manager
Bruce Nelsen, Executive Director
To ensure the rights of all persons with disabilities to live and function as independently as possible in the community of their choice, through supporting individuals efforts to achieve controll over their lives and become integrated into community life.

4248 **Society's Assets: Racine**
5200 Washington Avenue
Suite 225
Racine, WI 53406
262-637-9128
FAX: 262-637-8646
e-mail: info@sai-inc.org
www.sai-inc.org

Bruce Nelsen, Executive Director
Karen Olufs, Director Independent Living
Jean Rumachik, Director Home Care Services
Society's Assets assists people with disabilities to live as independently as possible. A non-profit human services agency, Society's Assets provides information and referal, independent living skills training, peer support, advocacy, and supportive home care. Home health care is provided by SAI Home Health Care. The agency serves 5 counties in southeastern Wisconsin and also provides information about interpreters, employment, benefits, home modifications, assistive equipment and accessibility.
Fees vary

Wyoming

4249 **LifeQuest: Interdisciplinary Rehabilitation**
1969 S. Sheridan Avenue
Sheridan, WY 82801
307-672-7481
888-309-2020
FAX: 307-674-5117
e-mail: mlr@renew-wyo.com
www.renew-wyo.com

Theresa Faulkner
Multi-disciplines organization dedicated to the highest possible economic and social independence for persons with disabilities. Extensive referral service, specialized employment placement, occupational therapy, psychological services, evaluation services, and coordination of external services as needed to meet client plans and objectives.

4250 **Rehabilitation Enterprises of North Easter n Wyoming: Newcastle**
35 Fairgrounds Road
Newcastle, WY 82701
307-746-4733
888-693-9245
888-693-9245
FAX: 307-746-9071
e-mail: ceo@renew-wyo.com
www.renew-wyo.com

Larry Samson, President
Sandy Theil, Vice President
Committed to enhancing personal and community relationships, providing opportunities for growth, and helping people with varying abilities achieve their personal goals.

4251 **Wyoming Services for Independent Living**

1156 S 2nd Street
Lander, WY 82520
307-332-4889
FAX: 307-332-2491
TTY:307-332-7582
e-mail: wsil@wyoming.com

Carol Fontaine, Executive Director
Committed to enhancing personal and community relationships, providing opportunities for growth, and helping people with varying abilities achieve thier personal goals.

Associations & Referral Agencies

4252 AIDS Legal Council of Chicago
180 N. Michigan Ave.
Suite 2110
Chicago, IL 60601 312-427-8990
FAX: 312-427-8419
e-mail: info@aidslegal.com
www.aidslegal.com

Jamal D Edwards, President
Robert F Harris, Vice President
Ann Fisher, Executive Director
Legal advice and services for persons who are HIV positive or have AIDS, and their companions, families, etc., regarding HIV-related legal matters.

4253 AIDSLAW of Louisiana
Greater New Orleans Foundation
PO Box 30203
New Orleans, LA 70190 504-598-4663
FAX: 504-821-8326

Gregory Ben Johnson, President
Linton Carney, Executive Director
Iska Beck, Supervising Attorney
Second year of funding for new legal agency serving persons affected by HIV/AIDS.

4254 Advocacy
7800 Shoal Creek Boulevard
Suite 171-East
Austin, TX 78757 512-454-4816
800-252-9108
FAX: 512-323-0902
e-mail: info@advocacy.org
www.advocacyinc.org

Kathleen D Sheekey, President/CEO
Sharvell Becton, Program Director
Jonas Schwartz, Manager
Advocacy, Inc advocates for, protects and advances the legal, human and service rights of people with disabilities throughout the state of Texas.

4255 Center for Disability and Elder Law
710 N Lake Shore Drive
3rd Floor
Chicago, IL 60611 312-908-4463
FAX: 312-908-0866

Greg Baldwin, President
Greg Price, Executive Officer
Provides legal services at no cost to low income persons with disabilities in Cook County. LCD staff screen applicants to determine if they meet the financial, disability and geographical eligibility requirements for service.

4256 Chicago Lawyers' Committee for Civil Rights Under Law
100 N La Salle Street
Suite 600
Chicago, IL 60602 312-630-9744
FAX: 312-630-1127
e-mail: clccrul@clccrul.com
www.clccrul.org

Clyde Murphy, Executive Director
Alesha Jackson, Office Manager
Provides legal services to individuals and groups with civil rights problems through class action and law reform cases. Also provides technical assistance to community groups. Spanish-speaking staff available. Individual cases and walk-ins are not accepted. Wheelchair accessible.

4257 DNA People's Legal Services
Central Office D NA People Civil Services
PO Box 987
Shiprock, NM 87420 505-368-3200
800-789-8894
FAX: 505-368-3212
www.dnalegalservices.org/dnalegalservices

Loretta Danzuka, Manager
Elsie Shorthair, Office Manager
Offers legal assistance to Native Americans.

4258 Disability Rights Education and Defense Fund
2212 6th Street
Berkeley, CA 94710 510-644-2555
FAX: 510-841-8645
e-mail: dredf@dredf.org
www.dredf.org

Susan Henderson, Managing Director
Beverly Bertaina, Chairperson/President
Nonprofit organization dedicated to advancing the civil rights of individuals with disabilities through legislation, litigation, informal and formal advocacy and education and training of lawyers, advocates and clients with respect to disability issues. DREDF also provides training, advocacy, technical assistance and referrals for parents of disabled children.

4259 Equal Employment Advisory Council
1015 15th Street NW
Suite 1200
Washington, DC 20005 202-789-8650
FAX: 202-789-2291
http://www.eeac.org/

Jeffrey Norris, President
James Poindexter, Office Services Director
A nonprofit association for the purpose of monitoring federal equal employment litigation and filing amicus curiae briefs in precedent-setting cases. Also file comments on equal opportunity employment and affirmative action regulatory proposals and monitors judicial developments.

4260 Guardianship Services Associates
41A South Boulevard
Oak Park, IL 60302 708-386-5398
FAX: 708-386-5970
e-mail: GSAoakpark@aol.com

Robert R Wohlgemuth, Director/Owner
Information and counseling on guardianship issues. Can provide direct assistance in obtaining guardianship for disabled adults. Also provides information and direct assistance on durable powers of attorney. Can assume appointment as guardian in selected cases.

4261 Judge David L Bazelon Center for Mental Health Law
1101 15th Street NW
Suite 1212
Washington, DC 20005 202-467-5730
FAX: 202-223-0409
e-mail: info@bazelon.org
www.bazelon.org

Robert Bernstein, Executive Director
Lee Carty, Communications Director
National litigation and technical assistance center for advocates for people with mental disabilities. Offers a website with advocacy resources and a variety of publications, handbooks, issue papers and manuals to help advocate for, implement, enforce and comply with federal laws and court orders on involuntary outpatient commitment, discrimination based on a label of mental disability, fair housing, criminalization, custody relinquishment for access to children's mental health care.

4262 Legal Action Center
236 Massachusetts Avenue NE
Suite 505
Washington, DC 20002 202-544-5478
FAX: 202-544-5712
e-mail: lacdc@lac.org
www.lac.org

Ellen Weber, Senior VP
Willery Murray, Manager
Provides technical assistance and education programs on ADA issues related to individuals with drug and alcohol abuse and HIV disease and legal assistance to individuals who have faced discrimination on the basis of these disabilities.

4263 Legal Center
455 Sherman Street
Suite 130
Denver, CO 80203
303-722-0300
800-288-1376
FAX: 303-722-0720
e-mail: tlcmail@thelegalcenter.org
www.thelegalcenter.org

Mary Anne Harvey, Executive Director
Mark Ivandick, Manager
The Legal center uses the legal system to protect and promote the rights of people with disabilities and older people in Colorado through direct legal representation, advocacy, education and legislative analysis. We are also the State Ombudsman for nursing homes and assisted living facilities. Call for a free publications and products list.

4264 Legal Center for the Elderly and Disabled
210 W. Truman Road
Independence, MO 64050
816-252-5777
e-mail: jonellison@sbcglobal.net
www.iced.org

Jonathan Ellison, Executive Director
Free civil legal services for low-income people over sixty and permanently disabled persons under sixty, specializing in social security, medical benefits elder law, disability rights and housing in North Central California.

4265 Legislative Handbook for Parents
NAPVI
PO Box 317
Watertown, MA 02471
617-972-7441
800-562-6265
FAX: 617-972-7444
e-mail: napvi@perkins.org
www.napvi.org
Written by parents for parents in dealing with Legislative Processes that ultimately affect their children's lives. *$5.50*
24 pages Paperback

4266 NHeLP
National Health Law Program
2639 S La Cienega Boulevard
Los Angeles, CA 90034
310-204-6010
FAX: 310-204-0891
e-mail: nhelp@healthlaw.org
www.healthlaw.org

Donn Ginoza, Chair
Helps ensure equity and non-discrimination in federal, state, local and private health care programs by assisting local legal service attorneys, paralegal and non-LSC attorneys representing LSC-eligible clients. NHeLP provides advice, co-counsel and other litigation assistance and trainings. *$85.00*
30-32 pages Quarterly

4267 National Center for State Courts
300 Newport Avenue
Williamsburg, VA 23185
757-259-7575
800-616-6164
FAX: 757-564-2022
e-mail: progers@ncsc.dni.us
www.ncsconline.org

Deborah White, HR Director
Toni Engle, Administrative Manager
Mary McQueen, President/Chief Executive Office
Develops a national clearinghouse and resource center for local and state courts to focus on requirements and methods of compliances with ADA.

4268 National Center for Youth Law
405 14th Street
15th Floor
Oakland, CA 94612
510-835-8098
FAX: 510-835-8099
e-mail: info@youthlaw.org
www.youthlaw.org

Peter B Edelman, President
Terrence Lee Hancock, Vice President
John O'Toole, Executive Director
Support services to legal services attorneys and child advocates on SSI (Supplemental Security Income) disability benefits for children.

4269 National Legal Center for the Medically Dependent and Disabled
50 S Meridian Street
Suite 605
Indianapolis, IN 46204
317-632-6245
FAX: 317-632-6245
e-mail: nlcmdd@juno.com
www.tmarzon@aol.com

Howard Howe
Litigation and support center for the disabled specializing in medical treatment lights/attendant care issues. *$49.00*

4270 National Right to Work Legal Defense and Education Foundation
8001 Braddock Road
Springfield, VA 22160
703-321-8510
800-336-3600
FAX: 703-321-9613
e-mail: info@nrtw.org
www.nrtw.org

Reed Larson, President
Raymond LaJeunesse, Vice President
Provides free legal aid to employees whose human and civil rights are being violated by compulsory unionism abuses.

4271 Planning Reasonable Accommodations: A Cost Effective Guide in a Legal Framework
Spina Bifida Association of America
4590 Macarthur Boulevard NW
Suite 250
Washington, DC 20007
202-944-3285
800-621-3141
FAX: 202-944-3295
e-mail: sbaa@sbaa.org
www.sbaa.org

Fritz Rumpel, Editor
Cindy Brownstein, Chief Executive Officer
A 24 page reference guide on the reasonable accomodations process under the ADA. *$9.00*

4272 Pocket Guide to the ADA: Accessibility Gu idelines for Buildings and Facilities
Wiley Publishing
605 3rd Avenue
New York, NY 10158
212-850-6000
FAX: 212-850-6088
Easy-access to the American's with Disabilities Act, which explains the network of federal civil rights laws with which businesses must comply. It includes the scope and technical requirements for accessibility elements and spaces. *$24.95*
144 pages 1997
ISBN 0-471181-37-4

4273 Public Law 101-336
US Department of Justice
950 Pennsylvania Avenue NW Drs
- Nyav
Washington, DC 20530
202-586-5000
800-574-0301
FAX: 202-307-1197
www.ada.gov

Joanne Graham, Manager
Text of the Americans with Disabilities Act, as enacted on July 26, 1990.

4274 **Questions and Answers: The ADA and Hiring Police Officers**
US Department of Justice
950 Pennsylvania Avenue NW Drs
- Nyav
Washington, DC 20530
202-586-5000
800-574-0301
FAX: 202-307-1197
www.ada.gov

Joanne Graham, Manager
A 5-page publication providing information on ADA requirements for interviewing and hiring police officers.

4275 **REACH/Resource Center on Independent Living**
1205 Lake Street
Fort Worth, TX 76102
817-870-9082
FAX: 817-877-1622
TTY:817-870-9086
e-mail: reachfwt@reachcils.org
www.reachcils.org

Charlotte Stewart, Director
Anne Ancy, Case Manager
Robin Laffiter, Manaager
Information and referral services, peer counseling, independent living skills training, loaner equipment, advocacy assistance, ADA technical assistance and social/recreational activities.

4276 **Strengthening the Roles of Independent Living Centers Through Implementing Legal Services**
Independent Living Research Utilization ILRU
2323 S Shepherd Drive
Suite 1000
Houston, TX 77019
713-520-0232
FAX: 713-520-5785
www.ilru.org

Laurie Redd, Executive Director
Featuring the Disability Law Clinic at Community Resources for Independence (CRI) in Northern California.
10 pages

4277 **Summeries of Legal Precedents and Law Review Articles concern Parents with Disabilities**
Through the Looking Glass
2198 6th Street
Suite 100
Berkeley, CA 94710
510-848-1112
800-644-2666
FAX: 510-848-4445
e-mail: TLG@lookingglass.org
www.lookingglass.org

L Baer
D Taube
Megan Kirshbaum, Executive Director
Available in braille, large print or cassette. *$25.00*
24 pages

4278 **TASH Connections**
1025 Vermont Ave.
Floor 7
Washington, DC 20005
202-263-5600
FAX: 202-637-0138
e-mail: info@tash.org
www.tash.org

Nancy Weiss, Executive Director
Priscilla Newton, Director Marketing/Communication
International association of people with disabilities, their family members, other advocates and professionals fighting for a society in which inclusion of all people in all aspects of society is the norm.
November

4279 **Winifred Law Opportunity Center**
106 E 2nd Avenue
PO Box 516
Indianola, IA 50125
515-961-5341
FAX: 515-961-5002
http://www.business-disability.com/

Diane M Griffith MS, Executive Director

Resources for the Disabled

4280 **AACD Legal Series**
American Counseling Association
5999 Stevenson Avenue
Alexandria, VA 22304
703-823-9800
800-347-6647
FAX: 703-823-0252
e-mail: webmaster@counseling.org
www.counseling.org

Sam Gladding, Ace President
Richard Yep, Executive Director
Offering three volumes: Preparing for Court Appearances; Documentation in Counseling Records; and The Counselor and The Law.
3 Volumes

4281 **ABDA/ABMPP Workshop: The Art of Courtroom Testifying**
American Board of Disability Analysts
342 24th Avenue N
Suite 200
Nashville, TN 37203
615-327-2984
FAX: 615-327-9235
e-mail: americanbd@aol.com

Kenneth Anchor, President
February workshop. Workshop leader: Dr. William Tsushima.

4282 **ADA Mandate for Social Change**
Paul H Brookes Publishing Company
PO Box 10624
Baltimore, MD 21285
410-337-9580
800-638-3775
FAX: 410-337-8539

Paul Brooks, Owner
This timely book moves a large step beyond detailing the legislative requirements of the ADA by focusing on the changes the ADA is generating for persons with disabilities. *$32.00*
320 pages Paperback 1993
ISBN 1-557661-17-0

4283 **Americans with Disabilities Act Manual**
American Bar Association
740 15th Street NW
9th Floor
Washington, DC 20005
202-662-1011
800-285-2221
FAX: 202-662-1032
e-mail: hammillj@staff.abanet.org
www.abanet.org/disability

Robert J Grey Jr, President
Robert A Stein, Executive Director
Nancy Scholnick, Manager
An in-depth analysis of the legal and practical implications of the ADA using non-technical language. *$20.00*

4284 **Americans with Disabilities Act: Selected Resources for Deaf**
Gallaudet University Bookstore
800 Florida Avenue NE
Washington, DC 20002
202-651-5271
800-621-2736
FAX: 202-651-5477
e-mail: infotech.services@gallaudet.edu
www.gallaudet.edu

Priscilla O'Donnell, Bookstore Manager
Iva Williams, Bookstore Secretary
Elaine Vance, Human Resources Director
This resource identifies programs and publications specific to the ADA and deafness and also lists ADA materials and programs for people with any disability.

4285 Approaching Equality
T J Publishers
2544 Tarpley Road
Suite 108
Carrollton, TX 75006
972-416-0800
800-999-1168
FAX: 301-585-5930
e-mail: TJPubinc@aol.com

Angela K Thames, President
Jerald A Murphy, Vice President
Public education laws guarantee special education for all deaf children, but may find the special education system confusing, or are unsure of their rights under current laws. For anyone with an interest in education, advocacy and the deaf community, this book reviews dramatic developments in education of deaf children, youth and adults since COED's 1988 report, Toward Equality. *$12.95*
112 pages
ISBN 0-93266 -39-6

4286 Assessment of the Feasibility of Contracting with a Nominee Agency
Mississippi State University
PO Box 6189
Mississippi State, MS 39762
662-325-2001
800-675-7782
FAX: 662-325-8989
www.blind.msstate.edu

Kelly Schaefer, Publications Manager
Elton Moore, Executive Director
Only five State Licensing Agencies currently utilize nominee agreements. This study compared the Pennsylvania program with four states that utilize nominee agencies and four states that do not. Results and recommendations compared state and national data from Federal FY 1991-1993. *$20.00*
152 pages Paperback

4287 Bluebook: Explanation of the Contents of the ADA
Disability Rights Education and Defense Fund
2212 6th Street
Berkeley, CA 94710
510-644-2555
FAX: 510-841-8645
e-mail: dredf@dredf.org
www.dredf.org

Susan Henderson, Managing Director
Written in narrative form for both professionals and lay people, DREDF's bluebook offers detailed, thorough analysis of all of the law's provisions, encompassing ADA legislative history, the statute and regulations. Available in alternative formats. *$100.00*
214 pages

4288 Can America Afford to Grow Old?
Brookings Institution
1775 Massachusetts Avenue NW
Washington, DC 20036
202-797-6000
FAX: 202-797-6004
e-mail: bibooks@brookings.edu
www.brookings.edu

Strobe Talbott, President
Social security laws and regulations. *$8.95*
144 pages Paperback
ISBN 0-815700-43-1

4289 Childcare and the ADA
Eastern Washington University
705 W 1st Avenue
Room 223
Spokane, WA 99201
509-623-4200
FAX: 509-623-4230
e-mail: susan.vanmeter@mail.ewu.edu

Nancy Ashworth, Director Child Development
Allen Barrom, Manager
Provides information on how childcare providers must comply with the ADA. Eight videotapes plus an instructional manual with examples of situations and problems. *$85.00*
Set

4290 Civil Law Handbook on Psychiatric and Psyc hological Evidence and Testimony
ABA Commission on Mental & Physical Disability Law
740 15th Street NW
9th Floor
Washington, DC 20005
202-662-1011
800-285-2221
FAX: 202-662-1032
www.abanet.org/disability

Nanchy Scholnick, Manager

4291 Common ADA Errors and Omissions in New Construction and Alterations
US Department of Justice
950 Pennsylvania Avenue NW Drs
- Nyav
Washington, DC 20530
202-586-5000
800-574-0301
FAX: 202-307-1197
www.ada.gov

Joanne Graham, Manager
This 13-page document lists a sampling of common accessibility errors or omissions that have been identified through the Department of Justice's ongoing enforcement efforts. The significance of the errors is discussed and references are provided to the requirements of the ADA Standards for Accessible Design.

4292 Commonly Asked Questions About Child Care Centers and the Americans with Disabilities Act
US Department of Justice
950 Pennsylvania Avenue NW Drs
- Nyav
Washington, DC 20530
202-586-5000
800-574-0301
FAX: 202-307-1197
www.ada.gov

Joanne Graham, Manager
A 13-page publication explaining how the requirements of the ADA apply to Child Care Centers. The document also describes some of the Department of Justice's ongoing enforcement efforts in the child care area and it provides a resource list on sources of information on the ADA.

4293 Commonly Asked Questions About Title III of the ADA
US Department of Justice
950 Pennsylvania Avenue NW Drs
- Nyav
Washington, DC 20530
202-586-5000
800-574-0301
FAX: 202-307-1197
www.ada.gov

Joanne Graham, Manager
A 6-page publication providing information for state and local governments about ADA requirements for ensuring that people with disabilities receive the same services and benefits as provided to others.

4294 Commonly Asked Questions About the ADA and Law Enforcement
US Department of Justice
950 Pennsylvania Avenue NW Drs
- Nyav
Washington, DC 20530
202-586-5000
800-574-0301
FAX: 202-307-1197
www.ada.gov

Joann Graham, Manager
A 13-page publication explaining ADA requirements for ensuring that people with disabilities receive the same law enforcement services and protections as provided to others.

4295 Complying with the Americans with Disabilities Act
Greenwood Publishing Group
88 Post Road W
Suite 5007
Westport, CT 06880
203-226-3571
FAX: 203-222-1502
www.greenwood.com

Wayne Smith, President
A guidebook for management and people with disabilities. Hardcover.
280 pages $52.95 - $57.95
ISBN 0-899307-14-0

4296 Council for Disability Rights
30 E Adams Street
Suite 1130
Chicago, IL 60603
312-444-9484
FAX: 312-444-1977
TTY:312-444-1967
e-mail: cdr@disabilityrights.org
www.disabilityrights.org

Jo Holzer, Executive Director
Promotes human rights of persons with disabilities and their families. Offers legal referrals, information services and disability awareness training.

4297 Court-Related Needs of the Elderly and Persons with Disabilities
Mental Health Commission
2700 Martin Luther King Jr Ave SE
Washington, DC 20032
202-282-0027
FAX: 202-373-7982
This book features the ground-breaking recommendations from the national Conference on the Court-Related Needs of the Elderly and Persons with Disabilities, funded by the States Justice Institute and co-sponsored by the American Bar Association and National Judicial College. Accompanying the recommendations are detailed commentaries and extensive background research papers organized around issues. *$20.00*
276 pages

4298 Criminal Law Handbook on Psychiatric & Psychological Evidence & Testimony
ABA Commission on Mental & Physical Disability Law
740 15th Street NW
9th Floor
Washington, DC 20005
202-662-1011
800-285-2221
FAX: 202-662-1032
e-mail: hammillj@staff.abanet.org
www.abanet.org/disability

John Hammill, Publications Coordinator
Amy Allbright, Managing Editor
Nancy Scholnick, Manager
Examines the admissibility of psychiatric and psychological evidence and testimony pertaining to key civil mental health standards. *$45.00*
376 pages
ISBN 1-570738-49-1

4299 Department of Justice ADA Mediation Program
US Department of Justice
950 Pennsylvania Avenue NW Drs
- Nyav
Washington, DC 20530
202-586-5000
800-574-0301
FAX: 202-307-1197
www.ada.gov

Joanne Graham, Manager
A 6-page publication describing the Department's ADA mediation program and examples of successful mediation efforts.

4300 Dimensions of State Mental Health Policy
Greenwood Publishing Group
88 Post Road W
Suite 5007
Westport, CT 06880
203-226-3571
FAX: 203-222-1502
www.greenwood.com

Wayne Smith, President
Introduces students to the emerging field of state mental health policy. Hardcover.
320 pages $59.95 - $65
ISBN 0-275932-52-4

4301 Disability Compliance Bulletin
LRP Publications
360 Hiatt Drive
Palm Beach Gardens, FL 33418
561-622-6520
800-341-7874
FAX: 561-622-0757
e-mail: custserve@lrp.com
www.lrp.com

Kenneth Kahn, Founder/CEO
Honora McDowell, Product Group Manager
This biweekly newsletter gives you timely coverage and insightful analyses of the latest developments in disability law. You'll learn the most recent case law dealing with the Americans with Disabilities Act, the Family and Medical Leave Act and more. Disability Compliance Bulletin will help you understand the laws' obligations and show you emerging legal trends. *$165.00*
24 pages BiWeekly

4302 Disability Law in the United States
William Hein & Company
1285 Main Street
Buffalo, NY 14209
716-882-2600
800-828-7571
FAX: 716-883-8100
e-mail: mail@wshein.com
www.wshein.com

Customer Service Department
Kevin Marmion, President
Offers thousands of pages of information on the laws and legislation affecting the disabled in the United States. Its purpose is to provide a clear and comprehensive mandate to end discrimination against individuals with disabilities and to bring disabled persons into the economic and social midstream of American Life. *$650.00*
5750 pages
ISBN 0-899417-97-3

4303 Disability Rights Now
Disability Rights Education and Defense Fund
2212 6th Street
Berkeley, CA 94710
510-644-2555
FAX: 510-841-8645
e-mail: dredf@dredf.org
www.dredf.org

Susan Henderson, Managing Director
Free quarterly publication describing the activities of the Disability Rights Education and Defense Fund, available in alternative formats.
Quarterly

4304 Disability Under the Fair Employment & Housing Act: What You Should Know About the Law
California Department of Fair Employment & Housing
2014 T Street
Suite 210
Sacramento, CA 95814
916-324-4244
800-884-1684
FAX: 916-227-2870
www.dfeh.ca.gov

Dia S Poole, Deputy Director Public Affairs
David Supkofl, Manager
$12.90

ISSN 9311-5126

4305 Discrimination is Against the Law
California Department of Fair Employment & Housing
2014 T Street
Suite 210
Sacramento, CA 95814
916-324-4244
800-884-1684
FAX: 916-227-2870
www.dfeh.ca.gov

Dia S Poole, Deputy Director Public Affairs
David Supkofl, Manager
$12.90

ISSN 9311-5114

4306 Education of the Handicapped: Laws, Legislative Histories and Administrative Documents
William Hein & Company
1285 Main Street
Buffalo, NY 14209
716-882-2600
800-828-7571
FAX: 716-883-8100
e-mail: mail@wshein.com
www.wshein.com

Kevin Marmion, President
Brian Joblonski, Director Marketing/Publications
Focuses upon elementary and secondary Education Act of 1965 and its amendment, Education For All Handicapped Children Act of 1975 and its amendments and acts providing services for the blind, deaf, mentally retarded, etc. Hardcover. *$2850.00*
55 Volume set
ISBN 0-899411-57-6

4307 ElderLawAnswers.com
535 Boylston Street
8th Floor
Boston, MA 02116
866-267-0947
e-mail: support@elderlawanswers.com
www.elderlawanswers.com

Harry Margolis, Founder/President
Mark Miller, Operations Director
Ken Coughlin, Managing Editor
Provides information about legal issues facing senior citizens and a searchable directory of attorneys.

4308 Employment Discrimination Based on Disability
California Department of Fair Employment & Housing
2014 T Street
Suite 210
Sacramento, CA 95814
916-324-4244
800-884-1684
FAX: 916-227-2870
www.dfeh.ca.gov

Dia S Poole, Deputy Director Public Affairs
David Supkofl, Manager
$12.90

ISSN 9311-8413

4309 Employment Standards Administration Department of Labor
200 Constitution Avenue NW
Washington, DC 20210
202-254-8628
877-889-5627
www.dol.gov

Corlis Sellers, Branch Chief
Edie West, Executive Director
Monitors compliance with sub-minimum wage requirements for handicapped workers in sheltered workshops, competitive industry and hospitals and institutions under Section 14 of the Fair Labor Standards Act of 1938.

4310 Enforcing the ADA: A Status Report from th e Department of Justice
US Department of Justice
950 Pennsylvania Avenue NW Drs
- Nyav
Washington, DC 20530
202-586-5000
800-574-0301
FAX: 202-307-1197
www.ada.gov

Joanne Graham, Manager
A quarterly report providing timely information about ADA cases and settlements, building codes that meet ADA accessibility standards, and ADA technical assistance activities. The most current issue of the Status Report is available by Fax.

4311 Ethical and Legal Issues in School Counseling
American Counseling Association
5999 Stevenson Avenue
Alexandria, VA 22304
703-823-9800
800-473-2329
FAX: 703-823-0252
e-mail: webmaster@counseling.org
www.counseling.org

Sam Gladding, Ace President
Richard Yep, Executive Director
This comprehensive text is filled with answers to many of the most controversial and challenging questions faced by the professional every day. This text helps avoid ethical violations and provides thorough information on: confidentiality, privacy, privileged communication, access to school records, using group techniques ethically, computerized record keeping and reporting unethical practices. *$24.95*
341 pages paperback 1988
ISBN 1-556200-55-2

4312 Fedcap News
Fedcap Rehabilitation Services
211 W 14th Street
New York, NY 10011
212-727-4200
FAX: 212-727-4374
e-mail: info@fedcap.org
www.fedcap.org

Jennifer Bertrand, Director Community Relations
Susan Fonsa, Executive Director
A publication from Fedcap Rehabilitation Services.
12 pages

4313 Federal Laws of the Mentally Handicapped: Laws, Legislative Histories and Admin. Documents
William Hein & Company
1285 Main Street
Buffalo, NY 14209
716-882-2600
800-828-7571
FAX: 716-883-8100
e-mail: mail@wshein.com
www.wshein.com

Kevin Marmion, President
Scott Fiddler, Vice President of Production
Chronological compilation of all relevant federal laws dealing with the mentally handicapped along with supporting documentation necessary to create a complete legislative history. *$2200.00*
42 Volume/Set
ISBN 0-899411-06-1

4314 Formed Families: Adoption of Children with Handicaps

Haworth Press
10 Alice Street
Binghamton, NY 13904
607-722-5857
800-429-6784
FAX: 607-722-6362
e-mail: orders@haworthpress.com
www.haworthpress.com

Laraine Masters Glidden Phd, Editor
William Cohen, Owner
Provides broad coverage of the issues relating to the adoption of children with handicaps. Concerned professionals can find here all the answers about clinical programs, legal issues, estimates of frequency, and important factors related to positive and negative outcomes of these adoptions. *$74.95*
242 pages Hardcover 1990
ISBN 0-866569-14-6

4315 Free Appropriate Public Education
Love Publishing Company
9101 E Kenyon Avenue
Denver, CO 80237
303-221-7333
877-240-6396
FAX: 303-221-7444
e-mail: lovepublishing@compuserve.com
www.lovepublishing.com

Laura Banks, Administrative Officer
Stan Love, Owner

Information on significant legislation regarding the handicapped. Laws are discussed with attention to their impact on the child, the parents, the public schools and higher education. *$44.95*

ISBN 0-89108 -11-5

4316 Handbook on Diability Discrimination Law
ABA Commission on Mental & Physical Disability Law
740 15th Street NW
9th Floor
Washington, DC 20005
202-662-1011
800-285-2221
FAX: 202-662-1032
www.abanet.org/disability

Nancy Scholnick, Manager

4317 Handbook on Mental Disability Law
A BA Commission on Mental & Physical Disability La
740 15th Street NW
9th Floor
Washington, DC 20005
202-662-1570
800-285-2221
FAX: 202-662-1032
www.abanet.org/disability

Letty Brown, Publications Coordinator
Amy Allbright, Managing Editor
John Parry, Executive Director
Provides a comprehensive analysis of federal and state statues and case law with a disability discrimination focus. *$45.00*
313 pages

4318 Health Care Quality Improvement Act of 1986
William Hein & Company
1285 Main Street
Buffalo, NY 14209
716-882-2600
800-828-7571
FAX: 716-883-8100
e-mail: mail@wshein.com
www.wshein.com

Kevin Marmion, President
Daniel P Rosati, Senior Vice President
In order to encourage more stringent peer review by doctors and hospitals, and to protect reporting physicians and institutions from retaliatory lawsuits, Congress enacted The Health Care Quality Improvement Act. The Act was also intended to address the increasing incidence of medical malpractice and to prevent the ease with which incompetent practitioners moved from state to state. Hardcover. *$75.00*
730 pages
ISBN 0-899416-93-4

4319 Housing and Transportation of the Handicapped
William Hein & Company
1285 Main Street
Buffalo, NY 14209
716-882-2600
800-828-7571
FAX: 716-883-8100
e-mail: mail@wshein.com
www.wshein.com

Kevin Marmion, President
National laws, recognizing the problems encountered by the handicapped in the areas of housing and transportation and providing assistance in an effort to surmount those problems. Hardcover or microfilm. *$1850.00*
250 documents
ISBN 0-899412-47-5

4320 Human Resource Management and the Americans with Disabilities Act
Greenwood Publishing Group
88 Post Road W
Suite 5007
Westport, CT 06880
203-226-3571
FAX: 203-222-1502
www.greenwood.com

John G Veres Iii, Editor
Ronald R Sims, Editor
Wayne Smith, President
Concrete advice for human resource professionals on how to cope with the vague, often obscure provisions of the Americans with Disabilities Act.
232 pages $59.95 - $62.95
ISBN 0-899308-57-0

4321 International Handbook on Mental Health Policy
Greenwood Publishing Group
88 Post Road W
Suite 5007
Westport, CT 06880
203-226-3571
800-225-5800
FAX: 203-222-1502
e-mail: webmaster@greenwood.com
www.greenwood.com

John G Veres, Author
Ronald R Sims, Author
Wayne Smith, President
The first major reference book for academics and practitioners that provides a systematic survey and analysis of mental health policies in twenty representative countries.
512 pages $110 - $125
ISBN 0-313275-67-X

4322 Issues in Law and Medicine
National Legal Center for the Medically Dependent
3 S 6th Street
Terre Haute, IN 47807
812-232-0103
FAX: 812-232-0103

James Bopp Jr, Editor-in-Chief
Larry Ligget, Subscriptions
A peer-reviewed journal providing technical and informational assistance to attorneys, health care professionals, educators, and administrators concerned with severely disabled persons of all ages who may be subjected to discrimination in the delivery of medical care. *$89.00*
124 pages 3x Year
ISSN 8756-81 0

4323 Knowing Your Rights
A AR P Fulfillment
601 E Street NW
Washington, DC 20049
202-434-2277
800-424-3410
FAX: 202-434-3443
e-mail: member@aarp.org
www.aarp.org

William Novelli, Chief Executive Officer
Lynn Smith, Director of Human Resources
Describes how changes in Medicare's reimbursement policies are designed to reduce health care costs and suggests steps that Medicare beneficiaries, their families and friends can take to assure that they continue to receive quality care under the Prospective Payment System.
19 pages

4324 Law Center Newsletter
Public Interest Law Center of Philadelphia
125 S 9th Street
Philadelphia, PA 19107
215-627-7100

Michael Churchill, Manager
Information on mental health, foster care and public education. Provides all updates concerning the law in these areas.

4325 Legal Center
455 Sherman Street
Suite 130
Denver, CO 80203
303-722-0300
800-288-1376
FAX: 303-722-0720
e-mail: tlcmail@thelegalcenter.org
www.thelegalcenter.org

Mary Anne Harvey, Executive Director
Mark Ivandick, Manager
The Legal center uses the legal system to protect and promote the rights of people with disabilities and older people in Colorado through direct legal representation, advocacy, education and legislative analysis. We are also the State Ombudsman for nursing homes and assisted living facilities. Call for a free publications and products list.

4326 Legal Right: The Guide for Deaf and Hard of Hearing People
Gallaudet University Press
800 Florida Avenue NE
Washington, DC 20002
202-651-5488
800-621-2736
FAX: 202-651-5489
TTY: 800-621-9347
e-mail: gupress@gallaudet.edu
www.gupress.gallaudet.edu

Sy Dubrow, Author
Sarah Geer, Author
Karen Peltz Strauss, Author
This revised fifth edition is in easy-to-understand language, offering the latest state and federal statues and administrative procedures that prohibit discrimination against the deaf, hard of hearing and other physically challenged people. *$24.95*
282 pages Paperback
ISBN 1-563680-00-9

4327 Legal Rights of Persons with Disabilities: An Analysis of Federal Law
LRP Publications
360 Hiatt Drive
Palm Beach Gardens, FL 33418
561-622-6520
800-341-7874
FAX: 561-622-6520
e-mail: custserve@lrp.com
www.lrp.com

Kenneth Khan, Founder/CEO
Gary Bagin, Director of Communications
A comprehensive analysis of the rights accorded individuals with disabilities under federal law covering such issues as: Definitions of individuals with disabilities, reasonable accomidations, architectural barriers, access to transportation and communication services, education and newborns. *$185.00*
1536 pages
ISBN 0-934753-46-6

4328 Legislative Network for Nurses
Business Publishers
2601 University Boulevard W
Suite 200
Silver Spring, MD 20902
301-587-6300
800-274-6737
e-mail: bpinews@bpinews.com
www.bpinews.com

Sarah Spencer, Editor
Adam Goldstein, President
Provides up-to-date information on the nursing shortage, nurse training programs, AIDS and Hepatitis B, unionization, registered care technologies, compensation, child care, home health care staffing and much more. *$286.00*
8 pages Newsl./BiMonth

4329 Loving Justice
Exceptional Parent Library
PO Box 1807
Englewood Cliffs, NJ 07632
201-947-6000
800-535-1910
FAX: 201-947-9376
e-mail: eplibrary@aol.com
www.eplibrary.com
How the Americans with Disabilities Act affects religious institutions, including congregations, hospitals, nursing homes, seminaries, universities and more. *$10.00*

4330 Making News: How to Get News Coverage of Disability Rights Issues
Advocado Press
PO Box 145
Louisville, KY 40201
888-739-1920
FAX: 502-899-9562
e-mail: office@advocadopress.org
www.advocadopress.org

Mary Johnson, Author
Tari Susan Hartman, Author
This book gives examples and tips on how to fight back and get on the front pages, lead the newscasts and influence public debate. *$10.95*
165 pages Paperback
ISBN 0-96270 -43-4

4331 Medicare and Medicaid Patient and Program Protection Act of 1987
William Hein & Company
1285 Main Street
Buffalo, NY 14209
716-882-2600
800-828-7571
FAX: 716-883-8100
e-mail: mail@wshein.com
www.wshein.com

Kevin Marmion, President
This act enables the Department of Health and Human Services to protect Medicare and Medicaid patients and federal health care programs from censured practitioners. Hardcover. *$185.00*
3 Volumes
ISBN 0-899416-95-0

4332 Mental & Physical Disability Law Reporter
American Bar Association
740 15th Street NW
9th Floor
Washington, DC 20005
202-662-1011
800-285-2221
FAX: 202-662-1032
e-mail: hammillj@staff.abanet.org
www.abanet.org/disability

John Hammill, Publications Coordinator
John Parry, Managing Editor
Nancy Scholnick, Manager
Contains over 2,000 summanes per year of federal and state court decisions and legislation that affect persons with mental and physical disabilities. Includes bylined articles by experts in the field regarding disability law developments and trends. *$384.00*
350+ pages BiMonthly

4333 Mental Disabilities and the Americans with Disabilities Act
Greenwood Publishing Group
88 Post Road W
Suite 5007
Westport, CT 06880
203-226-3571
800-225-5800
FAX: 203-222-1502
e-mail: webmaster@greenwood.com
www.greenwood.com

John G Veres III, Author
Ronald R Sims, Author
Wayne Smith, President
A clear, practical compliance guide, written by a psychologist, to help organizations conform to provisions on mental disabilities in the Americans with Disabilities Act. Hardcover.
216 pages $45 - $49.95 1997
ISBN 0-899308-26-0

4334 Mental Disabilities and the Americans with Disabilities Act
A BA Commission on Mental & Physical Disability La
740 15th Street NW
9th Floor
Washington, DC 20005
202-662-1570
FAX: 202-662-1032
e-mail: cmpdl@abanet.org
www.abanet.org/disability

Robert Burgdorf, Director
John Durocher, Director
John Parry, Executive Director
Written for lawyers, advocates, teachers, consumers, employers, and employees, this ADA handbook examines the ADA from the legal and non-legal practitioner's point of view. In six parts, the handbook covers ADA Titles I, II, and III provides case law summaries of ADA court decisions affecting individuals with mental disabilities including mental illness, developmental disabilities, learning disabilities, substance abuse, and organic brain injuries. *$40.00*

4335 Mental Health Law News
Interwood Publications
3 Interwood Place
20241
Cincinnati, OH 45220 513-221-3715

Frank Bardack, Marketing Director/Editor
Mental health case law summaries — malpractice, patient rights, discrimination, alcoholism, guardianship, negligence, professional liability, commitment, drug dependency and conservatorship. *$99.00*
6 pages Monthly Nwslttr
ISSN 0889-01 0

4336 Mental Health Law Reporter
Business Publishers
2601 University Boulevard W
Suite 200
Silver Spring, MD 20902
301-587-6300
800-274-6737
FAX: 301-587-1081
e-mail: custserv@bpinews.com
www.bpinews.com

Leonard A Eiserer, Publisher
Jeremy Bond, Editor MHLR
Bob Grupe, Editor MHLR
MHLR brings you the most timely, focused and thorough information on the legal issues that concern mental health practitioners in mental health litigation. Topics include: malpractice litigation, patient-therapist confidentiality, sexual victimization of patients, the insanity defense, social security administrative case law and much more. *$286.00*
8 pages Monthly

4337 Mental and Physical Disability Law Reporter
ABA Commission on Mental & Physical Disability Law
740 15th Street NW
9th Floor
Washington, DC 20005
202-662-1011
FAX: 202-662-1032
e-mail: hammillj@staff.abanet.org
www.abanet.org/disability

John Hammill, Publications Coordinator
Amy Allbright, Managing Editor
Nancy Scholnick, Manager
Contains over 2,000 summaries of federal and state court decisions and legislation that affect persons with mental and physical disabilities. Includes bylined articles by experts in the field regarding disability law developments and trends. *$374.00*
150+ pages Bimonthly

4338 Mentally Disabled and the Law
William Hein & Company
1285 Main Street
Buffalo, NY 14209
716-882-2600
800-828-7571
FAX: 716-883-8100
e-mail: mail@wshein.com
www.wshein.com

Kevin Marmion, President
Daniel P Rosati, Senior Vice President
Offers information on treatment rights, the provider-patient relationship, and the rights of the mentally disabled persons in the community. *$85.00*
867 pages
ISBN 0-910059-05-5

4339 Myths and Facts
US Department of Justice
950 Pennsylvania Avenue NW Drs
- Nyav
Washington, DC 20530
202-586-5000
800-574-0301
FAX: 202-307-1197
www.ada.gov

Joanne Graham, Manager
A 3-page publication dispelling some common misconceptions about the ADA's requirements and implementation.

4340 NAD Broadcaster
National Association of the Deaf
8630 Fenton Street
Suite 820
Silver Spring, MD 20910
301-587-1788
FAX: 301-587-1791
TTY:301-587-1789
e-mail: NADinfo@nad.org
www.nad.org

Andrew J Lange, President
Mark D Apodaca, Vice President
National newspaper published 11 times a year by the nation's largest organization safeguarding the accessbility and civil rights of 28 million deaf and hard of hearing Americans in education, employment, health care, and telecommunications. Membership: individual $30 per year. *$7.00*

4341 No Longer Disabled: The Federal Courts
Greenwood Publishing Group
88 Post Road W
Suite 5007
Westport, CT 06880
203-226-3571
800-225-5800
FAX: 203-222-1502
e-mail: webmaster@greenwood.com
www.greenwood.com

John G Veres III, Author
Ronald R Sims, Author
Wayne Smith, President
This book is a case study of judicial policy making. It focuses on the role of adjudication in the making and refining of federal policy.
208 pages $45 - $55
ISBN 0-313254-24-9

4342 Nolo's Guide to Social Security Disability
NOLO
950 Parker Street
Berkeley, CA 94710
510-549-1976
800-955-4775
FAX: 510-548-5902
www.nolo.com

Maira Dizgalvis, Trade Customer Service Manager
Susan McConnell, Director Sales
Natasha Kaluza, Sales Assistant
Not many bureaucratic programs are as large- and as confusing- as Social Security disability. This book shows you the ins and outs of the system. *$29.95*
350 pages paperback
ISBN 0-873375-74-2

4343 Opening the Courthouse Door: An ADA Access Guide for State Courts
American Bar Association
740 15th Street NW
9th Floor
Washington, DC 20005
202-662-1000
800-285-2221
FAX: 202-662-1032
e-mail: hammillj@staff.abanet.org
www.abanet.org/disability

Scott Labarre, Chair
John Hammill, Publications Coordinator
Robert Evans, Executive Director
Practical, step-by-step guide explains how to comply with the public access provisions of the ADA in the courthouse. The centerpiece of the guide is a series of action steps. *$12.00*

4344 Operation Help: A Mental Health Advocate's Guide to Medicaid
Nat l Council for Community Behavioral Healthcare
12300 Twinbrook Parkway
Suite 320
Rockville, MD 20852
301-984-6200
FAX: 301-881-7159
www.nccbh.org

Linda Rosenberg, President/Chief Executive Office
Jennie Campbell, Vice President
This book explains the Medicaid entitlement program in easy-to-read language and focuses on the needs of your clients. *$17.00*

4345 **PAL News**
Parent Professional Advocacy League
56 Temple Place
Suite 664
Boston, MA 02111
617-542-7860
800-537-0446
FAX: 617-542-7832
e-mail: pal@fcsn.org
www.ppal.net

Donna Welles, Executive Director
Lisa Lambert, Assistant Director
Offers information on medical and technological updates in the area of research on birth defects, support groups and family resources for persons with disabled children.
Quarterly

4346 **Power of Attorney for Health Care**
Center for Public Representation
PO Box 260049
Madison, WI 53726
608-251-4008
800-369-0388
FAX: 606-251-1263
Discusses Wisconsin law regarding medical decisions, the Cruzan case and ethical considerations in addition to legal implications and advantages of this document. Book tells how to create a personalized Power of Attorney document, including language for the special provisions portion. *$49.95*
132 pages
ISBN 0-93262 -38-0

4347 **Title II & III Regulation Amendment Regarding Detectable Warnings**
U S Department of Justice
950 Pennsylvania Avenue NW
Washington, DC 20530
202-646-5095
800-574-0301
FAX: 202-514-5331
www.ada.gov
This document suspends the requirements for detectable warnings at curb ramps, hazardous vehicular areas, and reflecting pools.

4348 **Title II Complaint Form**
U S Department of Justice
950 Pennsylvania Avenue NW
Washington, DC 20530
202-646-5095
800-514-0301
FAX: 202-307-1197
www.ada.gov

John Wodatch, Chief
Standard form for filing a complaint under Title II of the ADA or Section 504 of the Rehabilitation Act of 1973.

4349 **Title II Highlights**
U S Department of Justice
950 Pennsylvania Avenue NW
Washington, DC 20530
202-646-5095
800-514-0383
FAX: 202-307-1198
www.ada.gov

John L Wodatch, Chief
Allison J Nichol, Deputy Chief
An 8-page outline of the key requirements of the ADA for state and local governments.

4350 **Title III Technical Assistance Manual and Supplement**
U S Department of Justice
950 Pennsylvania Avenue NW
Washington, DC 20530
202-646-5095
800-574-0301
FAX: 202-307-1197
www.ada.gov
A 12-page outline of the key requirements of the ADA for businesses and nonproft service agencies.

4351 **Toward Independence**
National Council on Disability
1331 F Street NW
Suite 850
Washington, DC 20004
202-272-2004
FAX: 202-272-2022
TTY:202-272-2074
www.ncb.gov

Mark Quigley, Communications Director
Ethel Briggs, Executive Director
A 1986 report to the U.S. Congress on the federal laws and programs serving people with disabilities, and recommendations for legislation.

4352 **US Department of Health and Human Services Office for Civil Rights**
200 Independence Avenue SW
Washington, DC 20201
202-690-7650
800-368-1019
FAX: 202-619-3818
www.hhs.gov

Mike Levitt, Secretary
Enforces the Rehabilitation Act of 1973, which prohibits discrimination against handicapped persons by recipients of federal funding.

4353 **US Department of Labor**
200 Constitution Avenue NW
Washington, DC 20210
202-693-5000
866-487-2635
FAX: 202-219-7312

Elaine Chao, Chief Executive Officer
Offers publications to assist employers in determining and achieving workplace accessibility.

4354 **US Department of Labor Office of Federal Contract Compliance Programs**
Kluczynski Federal Building
230 S Dearborn Street, Room 570
Chicago, IL 60604
312-596-7010
FAX: 312-596-7037
e-mail: OFCCP-MW-PreAward@dol.gov
www.dol.gov/esa

Sandra Zeigler, Regional Director
Margaret Kraak, District Director
Administers and enforces three legal authorities that require equal employment opportunity: Executive Order 11246, as amended; Section 503 of the Rehabilitation Act of 1973, as amended; and the Vietnam Era Veterans' Readjustment Assistance Act of 1974, as amended, 38 U.S.C. 4212. These authorities prohibit Federal contractors and subcontractors from discriminating on the basis of race, color, religion, sex, national origin, disability, and protected veteran status.

4355 **University Legal Services AT Program**
220 i Street NE
Suite 130
Washington, DC 20002
202-547-4747
877-221-4638
FAX: 202-547-2662
TTY: 202-547-2657
e-mail: atpdc@uls-dc.org
www.atpdc.org

Jane Brown, Executive Director
Alicia Johns, Program Manager
Designed to empower individuals with disabilities; to promote consumer involvement and advocacy, and provide information, referral and training as they relate to accessing assistive technology services and devices; and to identify and improve access to funding resources.

4356 **Washington Watch**
United Cerebral Palsy Association
3135 8th Street NE
Washington, DC 20017
202-269-1500
FAX: 202-526-0519
TTY:202-973-7197
e-mail: webmaster@ucpdc.org
www.ucpa.org

Ted Bertoron, Director
Dependable, timely information on national legislative and regulatory issues affecting people with disabilities and their families. *$25.00*
4 pages BiWeekly

4357 William S Hein & Company

1285 Main Street
Buffalo, NY 14209
716-882-2600
800-828-7571
FAX: 716-883-8100
e-mail: mail@wshein.com
www.wshein.com

Kevin Marmion, President
Daniel P Rosati, Senior Vice President
Offers a catalog of periodicals, publications and reprints, microforms and government publications on medical, handicapped and health law.

4358 Word from Washington

United Cerebral Palsy
3135 8th Street NE
Washington, DC 20017
202-269-1500
800-USA-5UCP
FAX: 202-526-0519
TTY: 202-973-7197
e-mail: webmaster@ucpdc.org
www.ucpa.org

Stephen Bennett, President/CEO
Duncan Wyeth, Vice Chair
Provides information on national legislation and regulatory affairs, updates on disability and social service fields. *$25.00*
24-36 pages Quarterly

Alabama

4359 **Alabama Institute for Deaf and Blind Library and Resource Center**
295 E South Street
PO Box 698
Talladega, AL 35161
256-761-3237
800-848-4722
FAX: 256-761-3344
e-mail: lacy.teresa@aidb.aidb.state.al.us
www.aidb.org

Dr Terry Graham, President
Teresa Lacy, Director
Book collection includes discs, cassettes, braille and large print. Also closed-circuit TV and magnifiers. Offers braille production and binding.

4360 **Alabama Radio Reading Service Network (ARRS)**
650 11th Street S
Birmingham, AL 35294
205-934-2606
800-444-9246
FAX: 205-934-5075
e-mail: info@wbhm.org
www.wbhm.org

Mike Morgan, General Manager
Phillip Habmeeb, ARRS Program Manager
Services and readings are broadcast over a subcarrier service of public radio WBHM. This is a statewide service devoted to Alabama's blind and handicapped community.

4361 **Alabama Regional Library for the Blind and Physically Handicapped**
Alabama Public Library Service
6030 Monticello Drive
Montgomery, AL 36130
334-213-3906
800-392-5671
FAX: 334-213-3993
e-mail: fzaleski@apls.state.al.us
www.apls.state.al.us

Fara Zaleski, Regional Librarian
Recreational reading in special format for persons unable to use standard print. Reference materials offered include materials on blindness and other handicaps, films, local subjects and authors.

4362 **Houston-Love Memorial Library**
212 West Burdenshaw Street
Dothan, AL 36303
334-793-9767
FAX: 334-793-6645
e-mail: houstonlove@houstonlovelibrary.org
www.houstonlovelibrary.org

Bettye Forbus, Executive Director
Offers magnifiers, summer reading programs and more for the blind and physically handicapped. Scanner, software, jaws for Windows.

4363 **Huntsville Subregional Library for the Blind & Physically Handicapped**
915 Monroe Street
Huntsville, AL 35801
256-532-5940
FAX: 256-532-5994
e-mail: askus@hpl.lib.al.us
www.hpl.lib.al.us

Regina Cooper, Executive Director
Talking books for people who are blind or disabled offering reference materials on the blind and other disabilities, large-print photocopier, thermaform duplicator and more.

4364 **Public Library Of Anniston-Calhoun County**
PO Box 308
Anniston, AL 36202
256-237-8501
FAX: 256-238-0474
e-mail: bandph@anniston.lib.al.us
www.anniston.lib.al.us

Bonnie Seymour, Executive Director
Reference materials on blindness, cassettes, large print books and discs.

4365 **Research for Rett Foundation**
PO Box 50347
Mobile, AL 36605
251-479-8293
800-422-7388
FAX: 251-479-8293

Jack Tillman, Chief Executive Officer
Anna Luce, Executive Director
National, not-for-profit, voluntary organization dedicated to raising funds for critical ongoing medical research into Rett Syndrome, hosting medical research symposia, and funding grant applications. Committed to expanding public awareness of and encouraging Rett Syndrome research within the National Institute of Child Health and Human Development. Provides a variety of educational mateials including brochures and fact sheets.

4366 **Technology Assistance for Special Consumers**
2075 Max Luther Drive
Huntsville, AL 35810
256-852-5600
FAX: 256-532-2355
TTY:205-532-5996
e-mail: tasc@hiwaay.net
www.tasc.ataccess.org

Lisa Synader, Director
Provide individuals with disabilities, their families and/or advocates, and associated professionals access to assistive technology devices and services to increase independence at home, school, and work.

4367 **Tuscaloosa Subregional Library for the Blind & Physically Handicapped**
1801 Jack Warner Parkway
Tuscaloosa, AL 35401
205-345-5820
800-548-2547
FAX: 205-752-8300
TTY: 800-548-2546
e-mail: bjordan@tuscaloosa-library.org
www.tuscaloosa-library.org

Barbara Jordan, Executive Director/Librarian
Provide talking books to patrons who are unable to use standard print because of a visual or physical limitation. Deliver playback equipment to qualified patrons. Provides reference and referral service to this special population also.

Alaska

4368 **Alaska State Library Talking Book Center**
344 W 3rd Avenue
Suite 125
Anchorage, AK 99501
907-269-6575
800-776-6566
FAX: 907-269-6580
e-mail: patience_frederiksen@eed.state.ak.us
www.library.state.ak.us/dev/tbc.htm l

Patience Frederiksen, Librarian
Beverly Griffin, Library Assistant II/Manager
The Talking Book Center circulates fiction and nonfiction books on tape to patrons who are visually handicapped or whose physical handicaps prevent them from reading standard print. The center also has a small collector of large print books available to library patrons statewide.

Arizona

4369 Arizona Braille and Talking Book Library
1030 N 32nd Street
Phoenix, AZ 85008
602-255-5578
800-255-5578
FAX: 602-255-4312
e-mail: btbl@lib.az.us
www.lib.az.us/braille

Linda Montgomery, Executive/Director
Audio and braille books and magazines, summer reading program, volunteer-produced cassette books, braille writer, films, large-print photocopier and more.

4370 Books for the Blind of Arizona
6120 E 5th Street
Unit A107
Tucson, AZ 85711
602-792-9153
FAX: 520-886-9839

Betty Evans, Chairperson
Offers large print photocopier, textbooks, recreational, career, vocational, braille books, talking books, cassettes, large print books and more for the visually impaired K-12, college students and adults.

4371 Children's Center for Neurodevelopmental Studies
5430 W Glenn Drive
Glendale, AZ 85301
623-915-0345
FAX: 623-937-5425
e-mail: info@thechildrenscenteraz.org
www.thechildrenscenteraz.org

Kelli Sullivan, Director
Windy Farr, Special Education Coordinator
Kay King, Executive Director
The Center is a non-profit school and therapy center for children with autism and other developmental delays specializing in the use of sensory integration.

4372 Flagstaff City-Coconino County Public Library
300 W Aspen Avenue
Flagstaff, AZ 86001
928-779-7670
FAX: 928-774-9573
TTY:928-214-2417
e-mail: colguin@fpl.lib.az.us
www.flagstaffpubliclibrary.org

Christina Olguin, Librarian
Kay Whitaker, Executive Director
Reference materials on blindness and other handicaps, braille writer, magnifiers and large-print photocopier. Large-type books, closed captioned videos, adapters and books on tape.

4373 Fountain Hills Lioness Braille Service
PO Box 18332
Fountain Hills, AZ 85269
480-837-3961

Jean Hauck, Chairperson
Braille and large print books on the subjects of recreation, career and vocations, religion, novels and cookbooks for the visually impaired.

4374 Prescott Public Library
215 E Goodwin Street
Prescott, AZ 86303
928-777-1500
FAX: 928-445-1851
www.prescottlibrary.com

Toni Kaus, Director
Roger Faft, Assistant Director
Large print, braille and audio books; magnifiers; text to voice scanner; talking book machine application; toy library for children with special needs; special needs product catalogs; home book delivery; descriptive videos; 43 point PC monitor.

4375 Special Needs Center/Phoenix Public Library
1221 N Central Avenue
Phoenix, AZ 85004
602-262-4636
TTY:602-254-8205
e-mail: specialneeds@phxlib.org
www.phoenixpubliclibrary.org

Mimi Mccain, Supervisor
Toni Grbey, Executive Director
Offers large print books and magazines, print/braille books, amd braille magazines, Descriptive video services videotapes, several video print enlargers and computer workplace for persons with disabilities.

4376 World Research Foundation
41 Bell Rock Plaza
Sedona, AZ 86351
928-284-3300
FAX: 928-284-3530
e-mail: info@wrf.org
www.wrf.org

Steven Ross, President/Co-Founder
LaVerne Boeckmann, Co-Founder
Large research library of alternative medicine; offers a computer search and printout of specific health issues for a nominal fee.

Arkansas

4377 Arkansas Regional Library for the Blind and Physically Handicapped
1 Capitol Mall
Little Rock, AR 72201
501-682-1155
866-660-0885
FAX: 501-682-1529
TTY: 501-682-1002
e-mail: nlsbooks@asl.lib.ar.us
www.asl.lib.ar.us

John D Hall, Director
Public library books in recorded or braille format. Popular fiction and nonfiction books for all ages, books and players are on free loan, sent to patrons by mail and may be returned postage free. Anyone who cannot see well enough to read regular print with glasses on or who has a disability that makes it difficult to hold a book or turn the pages is eligible.

4378 Arkansas School for the Blind
PO Box 668
Little Rock, AR 72203
501-296-1810
800-362-4451
FAX: 501-296-1831
TTY: 501-296-1813
www.arkasasschoolfortheblind.com

Jim Hill, Superintendent
Sharon Berry, Principal
Students at the ASB receive a quality education from specially trained instructors of the Visually Impaired in all academic areas. ASB features a comprehensive Music and Art program, as well as extensive extra-curricular activities. ASB is a proud member of the Arkansas Activities Association and The North Central Association of Schools for the Blind.

4379 Educational Services for the Visually Impaired
2402 Wildwood Avenue
Suite 112
Sherwood, AR 72120
501-835-5448
FAX: 501-835-6840
www.esvi.org

David Beavers, Director
Offers textbooks, braille books and more to the visually impaired grades K-12 in the Arizona area.

4380 Library for the Blind and Physically Handicapped SW Region of Arkansas

PO Box 668
Magnolia, AR 71754
870-234-0399
866-234-8273
FAX: 870-234-5077
e-mail: lbph@hotmail.com
colcnty.lib.ar.us

Sharon Irons, Assistant Director
Sandra Grissom, Manager
A free library service that serves adults and children who meet the eligiblity requirements, offers free loan of cassette machine and recorded books, which meet the reading preferences of a highly diverse clientele.

4381 Northwest Ozarks Regional Library for the Blind and Handicapped

217 E Dickson Street
Fayetteville, AR 72701
501-442-6253
FAX: 501-442-6254
e-mail: arachel@orl.lib.ar.us
www.uark.edu

Rachel Anne Ames, Librarian
Offers a summer reading program, closed-circuit TV, magnifiers, braille writers and large print books.

California

4382 Braille Institute Library

741 N Vermont Avenue
Los Angeles, CA 90029
323-663-1111
800-808-2555
e-mail: bils@braillelibrary.org
www.braillelibrary.org

Leslie Stocker, President
Sally Jameson, Programs/Services VP
Braille Institute provides an environment of hope and encouragement for people who are blind and visually impaired through integrated educational, social and recreational programs and services.

4383 Braille Institute Santa Barbara Center

2031 De La Vina Street
Santa Barbara, CA 93105
805-682-6222
800-272-4553
FAX: 805-962-6331
e-mail: sb@brailleinstitute.org
www.brailleinstitute.org

Leslie E Stocker, President
Thomas Burton, Chairman
Michael Larzarovits, Manager
Offers programs, services and information for persons with visual impairments.

4384 Braille Institute Sight Center

741 N Vermont Avenue
Los Angeles, CA 90029
323-663-1111
800-272-4553
FAX: 323-663-0867
e-mail: la@brailleinstitute.org
www.brailleinstitute.org

Thomas W Burton, Chairman
Leslie E Stocker, President
Offers help, programs, services and information to the blind and visually impaired children and adults.

4385 Braille and Talking Book Library: Californ ia State Library

PO Box 942837
Sacramento, CA 94237
916-654-0261
800-952-5666
FAX: 916-654-1119
e-mail: btbl@library.ca.gov
www.library.ca.gov

Cameron Robertson, Deputy State Librarian
Diane Matsuda, Executive Officer
Aimee Sgourakis, Manager
Provides library services to people in Northern California who are unable to read standard print books because of visual or physical disabilities. Braille and talking books, magazines, machines, catalogs and postage are provided free to qualified appicants. The service is conducted by mail.

4386 Broadcast Services for the Blind

214 Van Ness Avenue
San Francisco, CA 94102
415-431-1481
FAX: 415-863-7568
TTY:415-431-4572
e-mail: dpickering@lighthouse-sf.org
www.lighthouse-sf.org

Chuck Godwin, Executive Support
Anita Aaron, Executive Director
Offers radio broadcasting, braille books, cassettes, records, and more for the visually handicapped in the nine San Francisco Bay Area major cities.

4387 Clearinghouse for Specialized Media and Technology

California Department of Education
1430 N Street
Sacramento, CA 95814
916-319-0800
FAX: 916-323-9732
e-mail: rbrawley@cde.ca.gov
www.cde.ca.gov/re/pn/sm

David Supkofl, Manager
Assists schools and students in the identification and acquisition of textbooks, reference books and study materials in aural media, Braille, large print and electronic media access technology.

4388 Dental Amalgam Syndrome (DAMS) Newsletter

725-9 Tramway Lane NE
Albuquerque, NM 87122
505-291-8239
FAX: 505-294-3339

Dedicated to informing the public about the potential risks of mercury in dental amalgam fillings.

4389 Fresno County Free Library Blind and Handicapped Services

770 N San Pablo Avenue
Fresno, CA 93728
559-488-3217
800-742-1011
FAX: 559-488-1971
TTY: 559-488-1642
e-mail: wendy.eisenberg@fresnolibrary.org
www.fresnolibrary.org/tblb

Wendy Eisenberg, Librarian/Manager
Magnifiers, home visits, volunteer-produced cassette books, discs and cassettes.

4390 Glaucoma Research Foundation

251 Post Street
Suite 600
San Francisco, CA 94108
415-986-3162
800-826-6693
FAX: 415-986-3763
e-mail: info@glaucoma.org
www.glaucoma.org

Thomas M Brunner, President/CEO
Clinical and laboratory studies of glaucoma. We work to prevent vision loss from glaucoma by investing in innovative research, education and support with the ultimate goal of finding a cure.

4391 Herrick Health Sciences Library

Alta Bates Medical Center
2001 Dwight Way
Berkeley, CA 94704
510-204-4444
FAX: 510-204-4091
e-mail: sutterhealth.org
www.altabates.com

Laurie Bagley, Librarian
Carol Hirsch-Butler, Administrator
Information on rehabilitation, psychiatry and psychoanalysis.

4392 **Kuzell Institute for Arthritis and Infectious Diseases**
Medical Research Institute Of San Francisco
2200 Webster Street
San Francisco, CA 94115
415-441-6249
FAX: 415-441-8548

Lowell Young, Director
Edward Byrd, Owner
One of seven units comprising the Medical Research Institute of San Francisco that offers basic and applied research in arthritis and related diseases.

4393 **New Beginnings: The Blind Children's Center**
4120 Marathon Street
Los Angeles, CA 90029
323-664-2153
800-222-3566
FAX: 323-665-3228
www.blindchildrenscenter.org

Midge Horton, Executive Director
Muriel Scharf, Director of Development
The purpose of the Center is to turn initial fears into hope. Helps children and their families become independent by creating a climate of safety and trust. Children learn to develop self confidence and to master a wide range of skills. Services include an infant stimulation program, educational preschool, interdisciplinary assessment services, family services, correspondence program, toll free national hotline and a publication and research service.

4394 **Research & Training Center on Mental Health for Hard of Hearing Persons**
California School of Professional Psychology
6215 Ferris Square
Suite 140
San Diego, CA 92121
619-282-4443
800-HEA-R619
FAX: 800-642-0266

Raymond J Trybus, Director
Thomas J Goulder, Associate Director
Funded by the National Institute on Disability and Rehabilitation Research, this training center aims to address issues of psychological relevance to persons who are hard of hearing or late deafened (as distinct from prelingually, culturally deaf persons). Also serves as information clearinghouse on this topic.

4395 **Rosalind Russell Medical Research Center for Arthritis**
350 Parnassus Avenue
Suite 607
San Francisco, CA 94143
415-476-1192
FAX: 415-476-3526
e-mail: ephraim@itsa.ucsf.edu
www.oarg.ucsf.edu

Ephraim P Engelman M.D., Executive Director
David Wopy M.D., Associate Director
Arthritis research and its probable causes.

4396 **San Francisco Public Library for the Blind and Print Handicapped**
100 Larkin Street
San Francisco, CA 94102
415-557-4400
FAX: 415-557-4375
e-mail: webmail@sfpl.org
www.sfpl.org

Kathy Lawhun, Chief
Martin Maqid, Librarian
Luis Herrera, Manager
Foreign-language books on cassette, children's books on cassettes and more.

4397 **San Jose State University Library**
150 E San Fernando Street
San Jose, CA 95112
408-808-2000
FAX: 408-924-2476
e-mail: office@wahoo.sjsu.edu
www.sjlibrary.org

Patricia Sen Breivik, Dean
Jane Light, Library/Executive Director
Information on physical disabilities, accessibility and learning disabilities.

Colorado

4398 **AMC Cancer Research Center**
1600 Pierce Street
Denver, CO 80214
303-233-6501
800-321-1557
FAX: 303-239-3400
e-mail: contactus@amc.org
www.amc.org

David Silverberg, President
Carolyn Draper, Executive Assistant
Beth Bochniak, Accounting Manager
Provides trained counselors who provide understanding and support for cancer patients; information and referral services; and screening programs.

4399 **Boulder Public Library**
1000 Canyon Boulevard
Boulder, CO 80302
303-441-3100

e-mail: feedback@boulder.lib.co.us
www.boulder.lib.co.us

Liz Abbott, Director
Priscilla Hudson, Manager
Offers braille books, cassettes, talking books, large print photocopier, large print books and more for the visually impaired.

4400 **Colorado Library for the Blind and Physically Handicapped**
Colorado Talking Book Library
180 Sheridan Boulevard
Denver, CO 80226
303-727-9277
800-685-2136
FAX: 303-727-9281
e-mail: ctbl.info@cde.state.co.us
www.cde.state.co.us/ctbl

Debbie MacLeod, Director
Offers reference materials on blindness and other handicaps, children's print/braille books, cassettes, large print books, and volunteer-produced cassette books and magazines.

4401 **National Jewish Medical & Research Center**
1400 Jackson Street
Denver, CO 80206
303-388-4461
800-222-5864
e-mail: allstetterw@njc.org
www.njc.org

Lynn Taussig, President/CEO
Nancy Hafer, Fellowship Coordinator
The only medical center in the country whose research and patient care resources are dedicated to respiratory and immunologic diseases.

Connecticut

4402 **Connecticut Braille Association**
107 Vanderbilt Avenue
West Hartford, CT 06110
203-227-5243
FAX: 860-953-9692

Yolanda Rossi, Manager
Offers textbooks, cassettes, large print books, braille books and more.

4403 **Connecticut State Library**
Connecticut State Government
231 Capitol Avenue
Hartford, CT 06106
860-757-6500
866-866-4478
FAX: 860-757-6677
e-mail: isref@cslib.org
www.cslib.org

Kendall Wiggin, State Librarian/Manager
Mollie Keller, Chairman

Discs, cassettes, braille, reference materials on blindness and other handicaps, closed-circuit TV and large-print photocopier.

4404 **Connecticut Tech Act Project: Connecticut Department of Social Services**
Bureau of Rehabilitations Services
25 Sigourney Street
Hartford, CT 06106
860-424-4881
800-842-4510
FAX: 860-424-4850
TTY: 860-602-4002
e-mail: jficarro@aol.com
www.cttechact.com

John Ficarro, Project Director
Single point of entry, advocacy, information and referral, peer counseling, and access to objective expert advice and consultation for people with disabilities.

4405 **Library for the Blind and Physically Handicapped**
198 W Street
Rocky Hill, CT 06067
860-721-2020
800-842-4516
FAX: 860-721-2056
e-mail: ctaylor@cslib.org
www.cslib.org

Carol Taylor, Executive Director
Braille writer, magnifiers, closed-circuit TV, cassette books and magazines, children's books on cassette, home visits and other reference materials on blindness and other handicaps.

4406 **Prevent Blindness Connecticut**
984 Southford Road
Middlebury, CT 06762
203-598-0529
800-850-2020
FAX: 860-347-0613
e-mail: info@preventblindnesstristate.org
www.preventblindnessct.org

Steven Peterson, President and CEO
Paul Armor, VP
Maria Giarratana, Program Director
The mission of Prevent Blindness Connecticut is to save sight and prevent blindness through eye screenings, education, safety activities and research.

4407 **Yale University: Vision Research Center**
330 Cedar Street
New Haven, CT 06510
203-785-2020
800-395-7949
FAX: 203-785-6123
e-mail: pamela.berkheiser@yale.edu
info.med.yale.edu

Bruce Shields, Chairman
Pam Burkheiser, Manager
Vision including studies on growth and development.

Delaware

4408 **Delaware Assistive Technology Initiative Center for Applied Science and Engineering**
Univ. of Delaware/duPont Hospital for Children
1600 Rockland Road
PO Box 269
Wilmington, DE 19899
302-651-6790
800-870-3284
FAX: 302-651-6793
TTY: 302-651-6794
e-mail: dati@asel.udel.edu
www.dati.org

Beth Mineo Mollica, Director
Sonja Rathel, Project Coordinator
Connects Delawareans who have disabilities with the tools they need in order to learn, work, play and participate in community life safely and independently.

4409 **Delaware Library for the Blind and Physically Handicapped**
Government
43 S Dupont Highway
Dover, DE 19901
302-739-4748
800-282-8676
FAX: 302-739-6787
e-mail: debph@lib.de.us
www.state.lib.de.us

Anne Norman, Director/State Librarian
Books on cassette and playback equipment are provided to patrons who are unable to read regular printed books.

4410 **Elwyn Delaware**
321 E 11th Street
Wilmington, DE 19801
302-658-8860
FAX: 302-657-5658
e-mail: info@elwyn.org
www.elwyn.org

Evangeline E Austin, Director Governmental Relations
Carol Chapin, Executive Director
Provides work training, job placement and supported employment, and elder care services.

District of Columbia

4411 **District of Columbia Public Library: Services to the Deaf Community**
District of Columbia Public Library
901 G Street NW
Washington, DC 20001
202-727-0321
FAX: 202-727-1129
e-mail: library_deaf_dc@yahoo.com
www.dclibrary.org

Marie H Aldridge, President
James Lewis, Vice President
Phillip Long-Cross, Manager
Offers reference services through TTY, signers for library programs, sign language classes, information about deafness, print and non-print materials for persons who have hearing disabilities. Book talks on deaf culture are held once a month

4412 **District of Columbia Regional Library for the Blind and Physically Handicapped**
901 G Street NW
Room 215 (Martin Luther King Lib.)
Washington, DC 20001
202-727-2142
FAX: 202-727-1129
TTY:202-727-2145
e-mail: lbphb_2000@yahoo.com
www.dclibrary.org

Marie H Aldridge, President
James Lewis, Vice President
Phillip Long-Cross, Manager
Regional library/RPH is network library in the Library of Congress, National Library Services for the Blind and Physically Handicapped.

4413 **Georgetown University Center for Child and Human Development**
Box 571485
Washington, DC 20057
202-687-5000
FAX: 202-687-8899
TTY:202-687-5000
e-mail: gucdc@georgetown.edu
gucchd.georgetown.edu

Phillis Magrab, Director
John J DeGioia, President
Established over four decades ago to improve the quality of life for all children and youth, especially those with, or at risk for, special needs and their families. Located in the nation's capital, this center both directly serves vulnerable children and their families, as well as influences local, state, national and international programs and policy.

4414 National Institute on Disability and Rehabilitation Research
U S Department of Education
400 Maryland Avenue SW
Washington, DC 20202
202-401-2000
800-437-0833
FAX: 202-401-0689
TTY: 800-437-0833
e-mail: customerservice@inet.ed.gov
www.ed.gov

Theresa S Shaw, Chief Operating Officer
Grover J Whitehurst, Director Institute of Education
Margaret Spellings, Chief Executive Officer
A national leader in sponsoring research. Mission is to generate, disseminate and promote new knowledge to improve the options available to disabled persons.
1978

Florida

4415 Brevard County Talking Books Library
Brevard County Libraries
308 Forrest Avenue
Cocoa, FL 32922
321-633-1810
FAX: 321-633-1838
e-mail: kbriley@brev.org
www.brev.org

Kay Briley, Librarian
Camille Johnson, Division Supervisor
Catherine J Schweinsburg, Library Services Director
Subregional library for the blind and physically handicapped, assistive reading devices collection, reference materials on blindness and other handicaps, descriptive videos, CCTV, phonic ear, reading edge and LOUD-R assistive listening devices available.

4416 Broward County Talking Book Library
100 S Andrews Avenue
Fort Lauderdale, FL 33301
954-831-4000
FAX: 954-357-7399
www.browardlibrary.org

Robert Cannon, Director
Carolyn Kayne, Manager
Reference materials on blindness and other handicaps, films, closed-circuit TV, discs, cassettes and a book discussion group is offered.

4417 Dade County Talking Book Library
Miami Dade Public Library System
2455 NW 183rd Street
Miami, FL 33056
305-751-8687
800-451-9544
FAX: 305-757-8401
e-mail: talkingbooks@mdpls.org
www.mdpls.org

Raymond Sanpiago, Executive Director
A free Outreach Service of the Miami-Dade Public Library System. A network library, or subregional, of the National Library Service for the Blind and Physically Handicapped, Library of Congress, and of the Florida Bureau of Braille and Talking Books Library Service.

4418 Florida Division of Blind Services
Regional Library
420 Platt Street
Daytona Beach, FL 32114
386-239-6000
FAX: 386-239-6069
TTY:800-226-6075
e-mail: mike-gunde@dbs.doe.state.fl.us
http://dbs.myflorida.com

Linda Hill, Manager
Discs, cassettes, closed-circuit TV, large-print photocopier, films, children's books on cassettes and more.

4419 Florida Instructional Materials Center for the Visually Handicapped
4210 West Bay Villa Avenue
Tampa, FL 33611
813-837-7826
800-282-9193
FAX: 813-837-7979
e-mail: sdalton@fimcvi.org
www.fimcvi.org

Suzanne Dalton, Supervisor
Jeffery Fitterman, Coordinator
John F Cardinale, Coordinator
Operates a clearinghouse depository and production center for braille, large print and recorded texts. Provides assistance in assessment of materials and specialized apparatus, organizes volunteers for material production and more for the visually handicapped.

4420 Hillsborough County Talking Book Library
Tampa-Hillsborough County Public Library
900 N Ashley Drive
Tampa, FL 33602
813-273-3652
FAX: 813-272-5640
TTY:813-273-3610
www.hcplc.org

John F Germany, Public Library
Joe Stines, Executive Director
Serves as the reference hub and resource center for all citzens of Hillsborough County and as the flagship library of the Tampa-Hillsborough County Public Library System.

4421 Lee County Library System: Talking Books Library
13240 N Cleveland Avenue
5-6
North Fort Myers, FL 33903
239-995-2665
800-854-8195
FAX: 239-995-1681
TTY: 239-995-2665
www.lee-county.com/library

Cynthia N Cobb, Director
Terri Crawford, Deputy Director
Debbie Parrott, Manager
Provides free books and magazines to Lee County residents of all ages who have any disability that prevents them from reading printed material. Books are played on special players provided free by the National Library Service. Circulates low tech assistive aids and devices for temporary loan to Lee County Library card holders. Directs people to assistive technology and disability related resources.

4422 Louis de la Parte Florida Mental Health Institute Research Library
University of South Florida
13301 Bruce B Downs Boulevard
Tampa, FL 33612
813-974-4602
FAX: 813-974-7242
e-mail: library@fmhi.usf.edu
http://lib.fmhi.usf.edu

Judy Genshaft, President
David L Shern, Dean
Information offered on mental illness, autism and pervasive development disabilities mental health research and archives management.

4423 Orange County Library System: Audio-Visual Department
101 E Central Boulevard
Orlando, FL 32801
407-835-7323
FAX: 407-835-7646
TTY:407-835-7641
www.ocls.info

Maryann Hodel, Manager
Serves the residents of the Orange County Library District, with headquarters in downtown Orlando.

4424 **Pearlman Biomedical Research Institute**
Mt Sinai Medical Center
1600 NW 10th Avenue
Miami Beach, FL 33140
305-674-2121
FAX: 305-674-2198
e-mail: william-abraham@msmc.com

William Abraham, Director
A 32,000 square feet facility located on the main campus of Mount Sinai. The institute consists of laboratory space, research and administrative offices. The studies conducted within the facility are primarily pre-clinical research.

4425 **Pinellas Talking Book Library for the Blind and Physically Handicapped**
1330 Cleveland Street
Clearwater, FL 33755
727-441-8408
FAX: 727-441-9068
TTY:727-441-3168
e-mail: contactus@pplc.us
www.pplc.us

Marilyn Stevenson, Talking Book Librarian
Harriet Thompson, Assistant Librarian
Marianne Morawetz, Reader Advisor
The Pinellas Public Library Cooperative serves Pinellas County residents in member cities and the unincorporated county. The Cooperative Office provides cooridination of activities and funding as well as marketing services for the the member counties.

4426 **Talking Book Library-Jacksonville Public Libraries**
Jacksonville Public Library
1755 Edgewood Avenue W
Suite 1
Jacksonville, FL 32208
904-768-7404
FAX: 904-768-7404
TTY:904-924-5387
e-mail: jerryr@coj.net

Jerry Reynoods, Department Head
Anthony Jackson, Manager
Offers cassettes, reference materials on blindness and other handicaps, children's braille books, descriptive videos, and some assistive devices.

4427 **Talking Book Service: Mantatee County Central Library**
6081 26th Street W
Bradenton, FL 34207
941-742-5914
FAX: 941-751-7098

Patricia Schobert, Librarian/Manager
Offers children's books on disc and cassette and more reference materials for the blind and physically handicapped.

4428 **Talking Books Library for the Blind and Physically Handicapped**
Palm Beach County Library
3650 Summit Boulevard
West Palm Beach, FL 33406
561-233-2600
888-780-4962
FAX: 561-233-2627
e-mail: webmaster@pbclibrary.org
www.pbclibrary.org

Jerry Brownlee, Librarian Director
Established in 1967, today the County Library system serves Palm Beach County through the Main Library, 2 Regional Libraries, 11 Branch Libraries, a Bookmobile and a library annex. It continues to expand through our involvement with library networks, the Internet, and the World Wide Web.

4429 **Talking Books/Homebound Services**
Brevard County Library System
308 Forrest Avenue
Cocoa, FL 32922
321-635-7845
FAX: 321-633-1838
e-mail: kbriley@brev.org
www.brev.org

Kay Briley, Librarian
Camille Johnson, Executive Director
Offers reference materials on blindness and other handicaps. Subregional library for the blind and physically handicapped, assistive reading devices collection, reference materials on blindness and other handicaps; CCTV, phonic ear, reading edge and LOUD-R assistive listening devices available.

4430 **University of Miami: Bascom Palmer Eye Institute**
Department Of Ophthalmalogy
900 NW 17th Street
Miami, FL 33136
305-326-6000
800-329-7000
FAX: 305-326-7000
www.bascompalmer.org

Carmen Puliafito, Chairman
Teresa Spaulding, Manager
Clinical and basic research into blindness and visual impairments.

4431 **University of Miami: Mailman Center for Child Development**
1601 NW 12th Avenue
Miami, FL 33136
305-243-3985
FAX: 305-326-7594
e-mail: ruben@miami.edu
pediatrics.med.miami.edu

Anna Matias, Staff Associate
Ruben Garcia, Associate Director
Dennis Harris, Manager
Focuses on birth defects and children's illnesses.

4432 **West Florida Regional Library**
200 W Gregory Street
Pensacola, FL 32501
850-436-5060
FAX: 850-436-5039
TTY:850-436-5063
e-mail: hhudson@ci.pensacola.fl.us
www.wfrl.lib.fl.us

Gene Fischer, Library Director
Helen Hudson, Outreach Librarian
Eugene Fischer, Manager
Offers children's print/braille books.

Georgia

4433 **Albany Talking Book Center**
Dougherty County Public Library
300 Pine Avenue
Albany, GA 31701
229-420-3200
800-337-6251
FAX: 229-420-3215
TTY: 912-430-1911
e-mail: katy@docolib.org
www.docolib.org

Michael Dugan, Director
Teresa Cole, Assistant Director
Offers discs, cassettes, reference materials on blindness and other handicaps, large-print photocopiers, summer reading programs, cassette books and more.

4434 **Athens Talking Book Center-Athens-Clarke County Regional Library**
2025 Baxter Street
Athens, GA 30606
706-613-3655
800-531-2063
FAX: 706-613-3660

Stacey Chandler, Manager
Discs, cassettes, large print books, reference materials on blindness, descriptive videos, films, closed-circuit TV, magnifiers, braille writer, summer reading programs, cassette books and magazines and more.

4435 **Augusta Talking Book Center**
902 Green Street
Augusta, GA 30901
706-821-2600
FAX: 706-724-5403
e-mail: talkbook@ecgrl.org
www.ecgrl.public.lib.ga.us

Gary Swint, Director
Audrey Bell, Manager
Discs, cassettes, braille writer, films, large print books, summer reading program, magnifiers and reference materials on blindness and other handicaps.

4436 **Bainbridge Subregional Library for the Blind & Physically Handicapped**
S W Georgia Regional Library
301 S Monroe Street
Bainbridge, GA 39819
229-248-2665
800-795-2680
FAX: 229-248-2670
e-mail: lbph@swgrl.org
www.swgrl.org

Susan Whittle, Librarian/Manager
Kathy Hutchins, Supervisor
Cassettes, large print books, summer reading programs, closed-circuit TV, magnifiers and more.

4437 **Columbus Subregional Library For The Blind And Physically Handicapped**
1120 Bradley Drive
Columbus, GA 31906
706-649-0780
800-652-0782
FAX: 706-649-1914
TTY: 706-649-0974

Dorothy Bowen, Librarian
Braille writer, magnifiers, closed-circuit TV, large-print photocopier, cassette books and magazines, children's books on cassette, home visits and other reference materials on blindness and other handicaps.

4438 **Emory Autism Resource Center**
Emory University
151 Shoup Court
Decatur, GA 30033
404-727-8350
FAX: 404-727-3969
e-mail: tohannon@emory.edu
www.emory.edu/housing/clairmont/autism

Charles Nemeroff, Manager
Offers on-line bulletin boards which are relevant to autism.

4439 **Emory University Laboratory for Ophthalmic Research**

1365b Clifton Road NE
Atlanta, GA 30322
404-778-3381
FAX: 404-778-4143
e-mail: pbennet@emory.edu
www.emory.edu

Henry F Edelhauser, Director
Larry Hagan, Manager
Various studies into the aspects of blindness.

4440 **Georgia Library for the Blind and Physically Handicapped**
Georgia Public Library
1150 Murphy Avenue SW
Atlanta, GA 30310
404-756-4619
800-248-6701
FAX: 404-756-4618
e-mail: dscott@georgialibraries.org
www.georgialibraries.org

Linda Stetson, Director
Deborah Scott, Business Manager
Stella Cone, Executive Director
Discs, cassettes, braille, films, closed-circuit TV, braille writer, large-print photocopier, cassette books and magazines.

4441 **Hall County Library: East Hall Branch and Special Needs Library**
127 Main Street Northwest
Gainesville, GA 30507
770-532-3311
FAX: 770-531-2502
TTY:770-531-2520
e-mail: ehcirc@hallcountylibrary.org
www.hallcountylibrary.org

Barbara Perry, Branch Manager
Adrian Mixson, Manager
Summer reading programs, braille writer, magnifiers, scanners and readers, audio described videos, closed captioned videos, closed-circuit TV, large-print photocopier, cassette books and magazines, large print books, children's books on cassette, home visits and other reference materials on blindness and other handicaps.

4442 **Macon Library for the Blind and Physically Handicapped**
Washington Memorial Library
1180 Washington Avenue
Macon, GA 31201
478-744-0877
800-805-7613
FAX: 478-742-3161
www.co.bibb.ga.us/library

Charles Schmidt, Director
Hoyt Cannon, Finance Officer
Joan Anderson, Executive Director
Summer reading programs, braille writer, magnifiers, closed-circuit TV, large-print photocopier, cassette books and magazines, children's books on cassette, home visits and other reference materials on blindness and other handicaps.

4443 **National Center on Birth Defects and Developmental Disabilities**
Centers for Disease Control and Prevention
1600 Clifton Road
Atlanta, GA 30333
404-639-3311
800-311-3435
FAX: 404-498-3070
www.cdc.gov/ncbddd/

Jose Cordero, Director
Promotes child development, prevents birth defects and developmental disabilities.

4444 **North Georgia Talking Book Center**
LaFayette-Walker Public Library
305 S Duke Street
La Fayette, GA 30728
706-638-2992
888-506-0509
888-506-0509
FAX: 706-638-4028
e-mail: cstubblefield@chrl.org
www.chrl.org

Charles H Stubblefield, Manager
June DeLong, Assistant Manager
We offer books on cassette for the visual and physically disabled induvidual, books in braille, magazines on cassette, zoom text screen magnifier, computer voice program, large-print photocopier, summer reading program, home visits na dother reference materials on blindness and other disabilities.

4445 **Oconee Regional Library**
301 Bellevue Avenue
Dublin, GA 31040
478-272-5710
FAX: 478-275-5381
www.laurens.public.lib.ga.us

Leard Daughety, Director
April Warren, Special Service Manager
Summer reading programs, braille writer, magnifiers, closed-circuit TV, large-print photocopier, cassette books and magazines, children's books on cassette, home visits and other reference materials on blindness and other handicaps.

4446 **Rome Subregional Library for the Blind and Physically Handicapped**
205 Riverside Parkway NE
Rome, GA 30161
706-236-4611
888-263-0769
FAX: 706-236-4631
TTY: 706-236-4618
www.floyd.public.lib.ga.us

Diana Mills, Librarian
Delana Hickman, Manager
The regional library system serves Floyd and Polk counties. System headquarters are located in Rome, Georgia, within the Rome/Floyd County Library Branch.

4447 **South Georgia Regional Library-Valdosta Talking Book Center**
300 Woodrow Wilson Drive
Valdosta, GA 31602
229-333-0086
FAX: 229-333-7669
e-mail: suggestions@sgrl.org
www.sgrl.org

Liza Newsome, Director
Summer reading programs, Braille writer, magnifiers, closed-circuit TV, large print photocopier, cassette books and magazines, children's books on cassette, home visits and other reference materials on blindness and other handicaps.

4448 **Talking Book Center Brunswick-Glynn County Regional Library**
208 Gloucester Street
Brunswick, GA 31520
912-267-1212
FAX: 912-267-9597
e-mail: bransom@trll.org
www.trrl.org/tbc

Betty Ransom, Librarian
Joe Shinnick, Executive Director
The Three Rivers Regional Library system is named for 3 rivers that flow through all 7 counties of the library system. The Three Rivers Regional Library system serves patrons in Brantley, Camden, Charlton, Glynn, Long, McIntosh, and Wayne counties in southeast Georgia.

Hawaii

4449 **Assistive Technology Resource Centers of Hawaii (ATRC)**
414 Kuwili Street
Suite 104
Honolulu, HI 96817
808-532-7110
800-645-3007
FAX: 808-532-7120
TTY: 808-532-7110
e-mail: atrc@atrc.org
www.atrc.org

Barbara Fischlowitz'le, Executive Director
Provides information and training on assistive technology devices, services, and funding resources. Conducts presentations and demonstrations in the community to increase AT awareness and promote self-advocacy among people with disabilities.

4450 **Hawaii State Library for the Blind and Physically Handicapped**
874 Dillingham Blvd.
Honolulu, HI 96817
808-845-9211
800-559-4096
FAX: 808-733-8449
www.hcc.hawaii.edu

Fusako Miyashiro, Manager
Supported by the Hawaii State Public Library System and the National Library Service for the Blind and Physically Handicapped, Library of Congress. Staff with knowledge of sign language; Special interest periodicals; Books on deafness and sign language; captioned media; Special Services: Radio Reading Service, Talking Books Reader's Club, educational and cultural programs, machine lending agency. Braille, cassette and large type. Regional and National service, quarterly newsletter.

Idaho

4451 **Idaho Assistive Technology Project**
University of Idaho
129 W 3rd Street
Moscow, ID 83843
208-885-3557
800-432-8324
FAX: 208-885-3628
TTY: 208-885-3573
e-mail: ywright@uidaho.edu
www.educ.uidaho.edu/idatech

Ron Seiler, Director
Bob Hieronymus, Executive Director
Project engages in systems change activities, training, materials development, information dissemination and advocacy activities directed at increasing the availability of assistive devices and services to Idahoans who have disabilities.

4452 **Idaho State Library: Talking Book Library**
325 W State Street
Boise, ID 83702
208-334-2117
800-458-3271
FAX: 208-334-4016
e-mail: lili@isl.state.id.us
www.lili.org/isl

Sheila Winther, Volunteer Coordinator
Sue Walker, Manager
Offers talking books and magazines, large print materials, braille, equipment and accessories. Available to all residents of Idaho who are visually impaired and/or have disabilities which disallows the use of print material.

Illinois

4453 **Chicago Public Library Talking Book Center**
400 S State Street
Chicago, IL 60605
312-747-4999
800-757-4654
e-mail: dtaylor@chipublib.org
www.chipublib.org

Jayne Carr, President
Cherryl T. Thomas, Vice President
Paul Dykstra, Secretary To The Board
Summer reading programs, braille writer, closed-circuit TV, large print photocopier, cassette books and magazines, children's books on cassette, home visits and other reference materials on blindness and other handicaps. Three assistive technology centers designed and equipped for the blind and visually impaired, funded by the National Library Service for the Blind and Handicapped, a division of the Library of Congress. All services FREE!

4454 **Department of Ophthalmology and Visual Science**
1855 W Taylor Street
Banner Dept: 2-539000
Chicago, IL 60612
312-996-7000
800-786-3937
FAX: 312-996-7770
e-mail: adriadel@uic.edu
www.uic.edu

Dimitri Azar, Professor/Director
Maria Myrianthopolus, Administrator
Adrienne Adelman, Administrative Secretary
Offers help, support, information and research for persons with vision problems, including Retinitis Pigmentosa.

4455 **Guild for the Blind**
180 N Michigan Avenue
Suite 1700
Chicago, IL 60601
312-243-8569
FAX: 312-236-8128
e-mail: info@guildfortheblind.org
www.guildfortheblind.org

David Tabak, Executive Director
Kerry Obrist, Director Of Service

provides worship on vision rehabilitation, training on computers and other adaptive technology, career counseling, and professional development workshops and offers assistive devices for sale.

4456 Horizons for the Blind
2 N Williams Street
Crystal Lake, IL 60014
815-444-8800
FAX: 815-444-8830
e-mail: mail@horizons-blind.org
www.horizons-blind.org
Mission is to improve the quality of life for people who are blind or visually impaired by increasing accessibility to culture, education, recreation and consumer information on a national basis.
1977

4457 Illinois Early Childhood Intervention Clearinghouse
223 South Third St.
Springfield, IL 62704
217-522-4655
800-852-4302
FAX: 217-522-4670
e-mail: clearinghouse@eiclearinghouse.com
www.eiclearinghouse.org

Chet Brandt, Project Director
Patricia Traylor, Project Associate
Free lending library of materials related to early childhood and disability. Books, audiovisuals and articles available. Computerized database with more than 31,000 items available to Illinois residents.

4458 Illinois Regional Library for the Blind and Physically Handicapped
1055 W Roosevelt Road
Chicago, IL 60608
312-746-9210
800-331-2351
FAX: 312-746-9192

Shawn Thomas, Reference Librarian
Barbara Perkins, Acting Director
Summer reading programs, braille writer, magnifiers, closed-circuit TV, large-print photocopier, cassette books and magazines, descriptive videos, children's books on cassette, home visits and other reference materials on blindness and other handicaps.

4459 Mid-Illinois Talking Book Center
600 High Point Lane
East Peoria, IL 61611
800-426-0709
e-mail: info@mitbc.org
www.mitbc.org

Karen Bersche, Director
Valerie Brandon, PR/Outreach Coordinator
Providing a free library service to anyone unable to read regular print because of a visual or physical disability. There are books and magazines on tape and playback equipment; and also in Braille. Books and magazines are mailed free to and from library patrons, wherever they reside.

4460 National Eye Research Foundation (NERF)
910 Skokie Boulevard
Suite 207a
Northbrook, IL 60062
847-205-0002
800-621-2258
FAX: 847-564-0807
e-mail: info@nerf.org
www.nerf.org

Elliot Silber, Owner
Dedicated to improving eye care for the public and meeting the professional nees of eye care practitioners; sponsors eye research projects on contact lens applications and eye care problems. Special study sections in such fields as orthokertology, primary eyecare, pediatrics, and through continuing education programs. Provides eye care information for the public and professionals. Educational materials including pamphlets. Program activities include education and referrals.

4461 National Lekotek Center
3204 W Armitage Avenue
Chicago, IL 60647
773-276-5164
800-366-7529
FAX: 773-276-8644
e-mail: lekotek@lekotek.org
www.ableplay.org

Diana Nielander, Executive Director
Toy library and play-centered programs for children with special needs and their families with branches in 17 states. Sliding fee scale. Lekotek also has a Toy Resource Helpline that provides individualized assistances in the selection of toys and play materials and general resources for families with children with disabilities.

4462 Northwestern University Multipurpose Arthritis & Musculoskeletal Center
303 E Chicago Avenue
Chicago, IL 60611
312-503-8649
FAX: 312-503-1204
e-mail: med-webteam@northwestern.edu
www.fenburg.northwestern.edu/mamdc

James Shedlock, Director
Lewis Landsberg, Administrator
Conducts biomedical, educational and health services research into musculoskeletal diseases.

4463 Skokie Accessible Library Services
Skokie Public Library
5215 Oakton Street
Skokie, IL 60077
847-673-7774
FAX: 847-673-7797
e-mail: info@skokie.libbrary.info
www.skokielibrary.info

Carolyn A Anthony, Executive Director
John J Graham, President
Library services for people with disabilities, including electronic aids, materials in special formats, programs and special services, and access to the North Suburban Library System.

4464 Southern Illinois Talking Book Center
607 S Greenbriar Road
Carterville, IL 62918
618-985-8375
800-455-2665
FAX: 618-985-4211
e-mail: bphdept@shawls.lib.il.us
www.shawls.lib.il.us/talkingbooks

Diana Sussman, Director
Library service, recorded books & magazines for people with difficulty reading print due to visual or physical limitations or reading disability (all ages), reference/referral, descriptive videos, newsline newspaper service, presentations/in-service. Free. Part of the Library of Congress NLS program.

4465 University of Illinois at Chicago: Lions of Illinois Eye Research Institute
University of Illinois at Chicago
957 Lieri
Chicago, IL 60612
312-996-6590
FAX: 312-996-9005
www.uic.edu

John J Denardo, Executive Director
Jingtao Guo, MD
Visual impairments and blindness research, including glaucoma studies.

4466 Voices of Vision Talking Book Center at DuPage Library System
127 S 1st Street
Geneva, IL 60134
630-208-0398
800-227-0625
FAX: 630-208-0399
e-mail: kodean@dupagels.lib.il.us
www.dupagels.lib.il.us

Karen O'Dean, Director

Provides library service to persons who are unable to use standard printed material because of visual or physical disabilities. Part of the Illinois network of Talking Book Libraries. The service is free to those who are eligable. Provides books and magazines on audio-cassettes. Special playback equipment needed to use the books is also loaned. Braille books and magazines are also available. The collection includes popular books, classics and magazines.

Indiana

4467 **Allen County Public Library**
900 Library Plaza
Fort Wayne, IN 46802
260-421-1252
FAX: 260-241-1286
TTY:260-421-1302
e-mail: ncompton@acpl.lib.in.us
www.acpl.lib.in.us

Jeffrey Krull, Director
Steven Fortriede, Associate Director
Mark Allen, Vice President
Summer reading programs, braille writer, magnifiers, closed-circuit TV, large-print photocopier, cassette books and magazines, children's books on cassette, home visits and other reference materials on blindness and other handicaps.

4468 **Bartholomew County Public Library**
536 5th Street
Columbus, IN 47201
812-379-1255
FAX: 812-379-1275
e-mail: library@barth.lib.in.us
www.barth.lib.in.us

Wilma Perry, Librarian
Beth Poor, Executive Director
Summer reading programs, braille writer, magnifiers, closed-circuit TV, large-print photocopier, cassette books and magazines, children's books on cassette, home visits and other reference materials on blindness and other handicaps.

4469 **Elkhart Public Library for the Blind and Physiclly Handicapp**
300 S 2nd Street
Elkhart, IN 46516
574-522-2665
800-622-4970
FAX: 574-293-9213
www.elkhart.lib.in.us/cgi-bin/index

Pat Ciancio, Librarian/Department Supervisor
Connie Ozinga, Executive Director
Summer reading programs, braille writer, magnifiers, closed-circuit TV, large-print photocopier, cassette books and magazines, children's books on cassette, home visits and other reference materials on blindness and other handicaps.

4470 **Indiana Resource Center for Autism**
Indiana Institute on Disability and Community
2853 E 10th Street
Bloomington, IN 47408
812-855-6508
800-825-4733
FAX: 812-855-9630
e-mail: prattc@indiana.edu
www.iidc.indiana.edu/irca

Cathy Pratt, Director
Stott Bellini, Assistant Director
Marilyn Irwin, Executive Director
The Indiana Resource Center for Autism staff conduct outreach training and consultations, engage in research and develop and disseminate information focused on building the capicity of local communities, organizations, agencies and families to support children and adults across the autism spectrum in typical work, school, home and community settings. Please check our website for a complete list of publications.

4471 **Indiana University: Multipurpose Arthritis Center**
School Of Medicine, Rheumatology Division
1110 W Michigan Street
LO 545
Bloomington, IN 47405
317-274-4225
FAX: 317-274-7792
e-mail: dbrandt@iupui.edu
www.research.indiana.edu/centers/mamdc.html

Dr. Kenneth Brandt MD, Director
The mission of the center is to pursue major biomedical research interests relevant to the rheumatic diseases. Current areas of emphasis include; articular cartilage biology, pathogenesis of articular cartilage breakdown in osteoarthritis, causes of pain and disability in QA, the pathogenesis and treatment of various forms of amyloidosis, the pathogenesis of dermatomyositis, and immunologic and biochemical markers of cartilage breakdown and repair.

4472 **Lake County Public Library Talking Books Service**
1919 W 81st Avenue
Merrillville, IN 46410
219-769-3541
FAX: 219-756-9358
e-mail: webmaster@lakeco.lib.in.us
www.lakeco.lib.in.us

Larry Acheff, Manager
Large-print books, descriptive videos, braille writer, magnifiers, closed-circuit TV, large-print photocopier, cassette books and magazines, children's books on cassette, and other reference materials on blindness and other handicaps.

4473 **Special Services Division: Indiana State Library**
140 N Senate Avenue
Indianapolis, IN 46204
317-232-3675
800-622-4970
FAX: 317-232-3728
TTY: 317-232-7763
e-mail: lbph@statelib.lib.in.us
www.statelib.lib.in.us

Lissa Shanahan, Librarian
Barbara Maxwell, State Librarian
C Ewick, Manager
Circulates a collection of braille, recorded, and large print books and magazines and the special equipment needed to play the recorded materials to anyone in Indiana who cannot read regular print due to a visual or physical disability.

4474 **St. Joseph Hospital Rehabilitation Center**
700 Broadway
Fort Wayne, IN 46802
260-425-3000
FAX: 260-425-3741
www.stjoehospital.com

Roberta Archer, Case Manager
Bob Hailes, Vice President
Information offered on rehabilitation.

4475 **Talking Books Service Evansville Vanderburgh County Public Library**
200 SE Martin Luther King Jr Blvd
Evansville, IN 47713
812-428-8200
FAX: 812-428-8397
www.evpl.org

Brenda Scheidler, President
Connie Davis, Vice President
Marcia Au, Executive Director
The Evansville-Vanderburgh County Public Library, an essential provider of shared information and a core community service, promotes reading, lifelong learning, and economic vitality through its resources, services and programs to the residents of Vanderburgh County.

Iowa

4476 **Iowa Department for the Blind Library**
524 4th Street
Des Moines, IA 50309
515-281-1333
800-362-2587
FAX: 515-281-1263
TTY: 515-281-1355
e-mail: information@blind.state.ia.us
www.blind.state.ia.us

Allen Harris, Executive Director
Karen Keninger, Program Manager/Librarian
Summer reading programs, large print, disc, Braille and cassette books and magazines, descriptive videos and reference materials on blindness and other handicaps.

4477 **Iowa Registry for Congenital and Inherited Disorders**
University of Iowa
Department of Epidemiology
M107 Oakdale Hill
Iowa City, IA 52242
319-335-4107
866-274-4237
FAX: 319-335-4030
e-mail: ircid@uiowa.edu
www.public-health.uiowa.edu/ircid/

Paul Romitti, Ph.D, Director
Bradley McDowell, Ph.D, Deputy Director
The mission of the Iowa Registry for Congenital and Inherited Disorders is; maintain statewide surveillance for collecting information on selected congenital and inherited disorders in Iowa, monitor annual trends in occurrence and mortality of these disorders, provide data for research studies and educational activities for the prevention and treatment of these disorders.

4478 **Library Commission for the Blind**
524 4th Street
Des Moines, IA 50309
515-281-1333
800-362-2587
FAX: 515-281-1263
TTY: 515-281-1355
e-mail: library@blind.state.ia.us
www.blind.state.ia.us

Allen Harris, Executive Director
Karen Keninger, Program Director
Summer reading programs, Braille writer, magnifiers, closed-circuit TV, large print photocopier, cassette books and magazines, children's books on cassette and other reference materials on blindness and other handicaps.

Kansas

4479 **CKLS Headquarters**
1409 Williams Street
Great Bend, KS 67530
620-792-4865
800-362-2642
FAX: 620-793-7270
e-mail: jmasden@ckls.org
www.ckls.org

Joaniea Doll-Masden, Dept Head/Consultant
James Swan, Administrator
Summer reading programs, braille writer, magnifiers, closed-circuit TV, large-print photocopier, cassette books and magazines, children's books on cassette, home visits and other reference materials on blindness and other handicaps. Assistive technology available.

4480 **Center for the Improvement of Human Functioning**
3100 N Hillside Street
Wichita, KS 67219
316-682-3100
FAX: 316-682-5054
e-mail: docron@brightspot.org
www.brightspot.org

Hugh D Riordan, President
Olive W Garvey, Chief Medical Officer
Medical, research, and educational facility specializing in the treatment of chronic illness.

4481 **Kansas State Library**
Esu Memorial Union
343 N 300 SW
10th Avenue
Topeka, KS 66612
785-296-3296
800-432-3919
FAX: 620-343-7124
e-mail: tonih@kslib.info
www.kslib.info

Christie Brandau, State Librarian
Jo Kord, Manager
Summer reading programs, braille writer, magnifiers, closed-circuit TV, large-print photocopier, cassette books and magazines, children's books on cassette, home visits and other reference materials on blindness and other handicaps.

4482 **Manhattan Public Library**
629 Poyntz Avenue
Manhattan, KS 66502
785-776-4741
800-432-2796
FAX: 785-776-1545
e-mail: annp@manhattan.lib.ks.us
www.manhattan.lib.ks.us

Ann Pearce, Department Head
Sue Colley, Reader Advisor
Fred Atchison, Manager
Summer reading programs, Braille writer, magnifiers, closed-circuit TV, large-print photocopier, cassette books and magazines, children's books on cassette, home visits and other reference materials on blindness and other disabilities.

4483 **Northwest Kansas Library System Talking Books**
PO Box 446
Norton, KS 67654
785-877-5148
800-432-2858
FAX: 785-877-5697
e-mail: tbook@ruraltel.net
skyways.lib.ks.us

Clarice Howard, Librarian
Leslie Bell, Director
Kimberly Gallentine, Business Manager
Offers books on disc and cassette. Library of Congress talking book and program for qualified individuals. Also offers descriptive videos to eligible persons.

4484 **South Central Kansas Library System**
Talking Bookz/ Sckls
321A N Main Street
South Hutchinson, KS 67505
620-663-5441
800-234-0529
FAX: 620-663-9797
e-mail: ksocha@sckls.org
http://sckls.info

Karen Socha, Librarian
Leroy Gattin, Manager
Summer reading programs, Braille writer, closed-circuit TV, large-print photocopier, cassette books and magazines, children's books on cassette, home visits and other reference materials on blindness and other handicaps.

4485 **Topeka & Shawnee County Public Library Talking Book Service**
1515 SW 10th Avenue
Topeka, KS 66604
785-580-4400
800-432-2925
FAX: 785-231-0579
e-mail: tbooks@tscpl.lib.ks.us
www.tscpl.org

Gina Millsap, Executive Director
Nancy Watkins, Director of Finance
Summer reading programs, braille writer, magnifiers, closed-circuit TV, large-print photocopier, cassette books and magazines, children's books on cassette, home visits and other reference materials on blindness and other handicaps.

4486 **Wichita Public Library**
223 S Main Street
Wichita, KS 67202
316-261-8500
FAX: 316-262-4540
e-mail: friends@wichita.lib.ks.us
www.wichita.lib.ks.us

Donna Aldrich, Director
Barbara Baker, Director
Cynthia Berner-Harris, Executive Director
Summer reading programs, braille writer, magnifiers, closed-circuit TV, large-print photocopier, cassette books and magazines, children's books on cassette, home visits and other reference materials on blindness and other handicaps.

4487 **Wichita Public Library/Talking Book Service**
Wichita Public Library
223 S Main Street
Wichita, KS 67202
316-261-8500
FAX: 316-262-4540
TTY:316-262-3972
e-mail: cnazar@wichita.lib.ks.us
www.wichita.lib.ks.us

Sarah Bagby, Member of the Board
Cynthia Berner-Harris, Executive Director
Eric J Larson, Member of the Board
Furnish recorded reading material (books and magazines) for visually and physically challenged citizens.

Kentucky

4488 **EnTech: Enabling Technologies of Kentuckiana**
Spaulding University
851 S 4th Street
Louisville, KY 40203
502-585-9911
800-896-8941
FAX: 502-585-7158
e-mail: info@spalding.edu
www.spalding.edu

Joy Vessels, Information Contact
Mary Kaye Steinmietz, Outreach Coordinator
Assistive technology resource and demonstration center, serving persons of all ages and disabilities in Kentucky and Southern Indiana. Services include: assistive technology information, demonstration, evaluation, training, technical support and short-term loan of equipment.

4489 **Kentucky Talking Book Library**
PO Box 537
Frankfort, KY 40602
502-564-8300
800-372-2968
FAX: 502-564-5773
e-mail: ktbl.mail@ky.gov
www.kdla.ky.gov

Barbara Penegor, Regional Librarian
Provides library service to those who are physically unable to read print. Cassete and braille books and magazines, descriptive videos, web-braille.

4490 **Louisville Free Public Library**
301 York Street
Louisville, KY 40203
502-574-1611
FAX: 502-574-1657
e-mail: webteam@lfpl.org
www.lfpl.org

Craig Buthod, Director
Summer reading programs, braille writer, magnifiers, closed-circuit TV, large-print photocopier, cassette books and magazines, children's books on cassette, home visits and other reference materials on blindness and other handicaps.

Louisiana

4491 **Central Louisiana State Hospital Medical and Professional Library**
PO Box 5031
Pineville, LA 71361
318-484-6363
FAX: 318-484-6284
www.state.lib.la.us/libdir

Elizabeth Hecker Perkins, Membership Coordinator
Carol Gee, Manager
Information offered on psychiatry, psychology and mental health.

4492 **Louisiana State Library**
701 N 4th Street
Baton Rouge, LA 70802
225-342-4923
800-543-4702
FAX: 225-219-4804
e-mail: admin@state.lib.la.us
www.state.lib.la.us

Rebecca Hamilton, State Librarian/Manager
Diane Brown, Deputy State Librarian
Summer reading programs, braille writer, magnifiers, closed-circuit TV, large-print photocopier, cassette books and magazines, children's books on cassette. Descriptive videoss and other reference materials on blindness and other handicaps.

4493 **Louisiana State University Genetics Section of Pediatrics**
533 Bolivar Street
Room 661
New Orleans, LA 70112
504-568-6117
FAX: 504-568-8500
e-mail: jlabor@lsuhsc.edu
www.medschool.lsuhsc.edu/genetics

Janis Gissel Letourneau, Medical Director
Our goal is to continue building a strong department in which all of the faculty are successful in attracting funding, and committed to establishing productive programs that bring credit to the Department and to the Health Sciences Center as a whole.

4494 **State Library of Louisiana: Services for the Blind and Physically Handicapped**
701 N 4th Street
Baton Rouge, LA 70802
225-342-0035
800-543-4702
FAX: 225-342-6817
e-mail: sbph@state.lib.la.us
www.state.lib.la.us

Margaret C Harrison, Head Svcs For Blind/Handicapped
Emma Schroth, Children's Librarian
Angela Cinquemario, Studio Manager
Summer reading programs, braille publications, cassette books and magazines, children's books on cassette and other reference materials on blindness and other handicaps. Louisiana Hotlines - quarterly newsletter. Affiliated with National Library Service for the Blind and Physically Handicapped, Washington, DC. Louisiana Voices recording program uses volunteers to record books for the blind.

Maine

4495 **Bangor Public Library**
145 Harlow Street
Bangor, ME 04401
207-947-8336
FAX: 207-945-6694
e-mail: bpill@bpl.lib.me.us
www.bpl.lib.me.us

Tanian Erickson, Acquisitions
Anne Murdy, Children's Department Head
Barbara Dade, Manager

Summer reading programs, braille writer, magnifiers, closed-circuit TV, large-print photocopier, cassette books and magazines, children's books on cassette, home visits and other reference materials on blindness and other handicaps.

4496 Cary Library

107 Main Street
Houlton, ME 04730
207-532-1302
FAX: 207-532-4350
e-mail: faucher!@carey.lib.me.us
www.cary.lib.me.us

Betty Fraser, Librarian/Manager
Linda Faucher, Assistant Librarian
Summer reading programs, braille writer, magnifiers, closed-circuit TV, large-print photocopier, cassette books and magazines, children's books on cassette, home visits and other reference materials on blindness and other handicaps.

4497 Lewiston Public Library

200 Lisbon Street
Lewiston, ME 04240
207-784-0135
FAX: 207-784-3011
TTY:207-784-3123
e-mail: lplweb@lplonline.org
www.lplonline.org

Richard Speer, Director
Summer reading programs, braille writer, magnifiers, closed-circuit T.V., large-print photocopier, cassette books and magazines, children's books on cassette, home visits and other reference materials on blindness and other handicaps.

4498 Maine State Library

Maine State
64 State House Station
Augusta, ME 04333
207-287-5600
800-762-7106
FAX: 207-287-5654
TTY: 207-287-5622
e-mail: benitad@ursus3.ursus.maine.edu
www.maine.gov/msl

Linda H Lord, Director Library
J Gary Nichols, State Librarian
Melora Norman, Manager
Summer reading programs, cassette books and magazines, children's books on cassette, home visits and other reference materials on blindness and other handicaps.
Newsl./BiAnnual

4499 New England Regional Genetics Group

PO Box 920288
Needham, MA 02492
781-444-0126
FAX: 781-444-0127
e-mail: mfgnergg@verizon.net
www.nergg.org

Mary Frances Garber, Executive Director
Leah Beukemp, Senior Co-Director
New Englands primary network for collaborative exchange of genetic health information and education.

4500 Portland Public Library

5 Monument Square
Portland, ME 04101
207-871-1700
FAX: 207-871-1703
e-mail: reference@portland.lib.me.us
www.portlandlibrary.com

Steve Podgagiy, Director
Claire Hannan, Business Manager
Summer reading programs, magnifiers, closed-circuit T.V., large-print photocopier, cassette books and magazines, children's books on cassette, home visits and other reference materials on blindness and other handicaps.

4501 Waterville Public Library

73 Elm Street
Waterville, ME 04901
207-872-5433
FAX: 207-873-4779
e-mail: wplhelpdesk@waterville.lib.me.us
www.waterville.lib.me.us

Sarah Sugden, Executive Director
Lee-Anne Folsom, Circulation Coordinator
Summer reading programs, braille writer, magnifiers, closed-circuit T.V., large-print photocopier, cassette books and magazines, children's books on cassette, home visits and other reference materials on blindness and other handicaps.

Maryland

4502 Johns Hopkins University Dana Center for Preventive Ophthalmology

Wilmer Ophthalmology Institute
600 N Wolfe Street
Wilmer Suite 122
Baltimore, MD 21287
410-955-5080
FAX: 410-955-2542
e-mail: hquigley@jhmi.edu
www.hopkinsmedicine.org/wilmer/danacenter

Harry A Quigley, Director
Barbara Lake, Manager
Established in 1979, the Dana Center for Preventive Ophthalmology is dedicated to improving knowlege of risk factors for ocular disease and public health approaches to the prevention of these diseases and their ensuing visual impairment and blindness worldwide.

4503 Johns Hopkins University: Asthma and Allergy Center

5501 Hopkins Bayview Circle
Baltimore, MD 21224
410-550-0545
FAX: 410-550-1733
e-mail: jhuallergy@jhmi.edu
www.hopkinsmedicine.org/allergy

Lawrence Lichtenstein, Director
Studies of allergic diseases and individuals with allergic disease, pulmonary diseases and diseases involving inflammation and immunological processes.

4504 Maryland State Library for the Blind and Physically Handicapped

Maryland State Department of Education
415 Park Avenue
Baltimore, MD 21201
410-230-2424
800-964-9209
FAX: 410-333-2095
e-mail: referenc@lbph.lib.md.us
www.lbph.lib.md.us

Gillian Lewis, Branch Chief
Diana Jarvis, Administrative Specialist
LaTarsha Wilson, Secretary
Provide comprehensive library services to the eligible blind and physically handicapped residents of the State of Maryland. The vision is to provide innovative and quality services to meet the needs and expectations of the patrons of Maryland.

4505 Montgomery County Department of Public Libraries/Special Needs Library

6400 Democracy Boulevard
Bethesda, MD 20817
301-469-7601
TTY:301-897-2217
www.montgomerycountymd.gov/libmpl

Susan F Cohen, Assistant Head Librarian
James Montgomery, Owner
Serves the library information and reading needs of people with disabilities, family members, students and service providers. Some of its services include books, periodicals, and videos on disability issues, adaptive technology, community information; the National Library for the Blind and Physically Handicapped Talking Book program; large print books; and computer room with adaptive technology.

4506 **National Epilepsy Library (NEL)**
Epilepsy Foundation
8301 Professional Place
Landover, MD 20785
301-459-3700
800-332-4050
FAX: 301-577-4941
e-mail: nel@efa.org
www.epilepsyfoundation.org

William E Braulinch, Chairman
Eric Hargis, President
Contains information about epilepsy and seizure disorders and serves physicians and other health professionals. Provides in-house bibliographic database (ESDI), searches and documents delivery and interlibrary loans. Maintains the Albert and Ellen Grass Archives.

4507 **National Rehabilitation Information Center**
4200 Forbes Boulevard
Suite 202
Lanham, MD 20706
301-459-5900
800-346-2742
FAX: 301-459-4263
e-mail: naricinfo@heitechservices.com
www.naric.com

Mark Odum, Director
A national disability and rehabilitation library and information center that collects and disseminates the results of NIDRR-funded research projects. The collection, which also includes commercially published books, journals, articles and audiovisuals, grows at a rate of 300 documents a month. NARIC currently has more than 50,000 documents on all aspects of disability and rehabilitation. Searchable web page includes 5 databases and a calendar of events.

4508 **Red Notebook**
Friends of Libraries for Deaf Action
2930 Craiglawn Road
Silver Spring, MD 20904
301-572-5168
FAX: 301-572-5168
TTY:301-572-5168
e-mail: folda@aol.com
www.folda.net

Alice L Hagemeyer, Founder/President
Merrie Davidson, Webmaster
A binder containing fact sheets, library reprints, announcements and other printed informational materials that are related to both deaf and library issues. It is designed to help build communication among individuals and groups within the deaf community. The focus is on assisting libraries in providing cost-effective and efficient library and information services to these consumers in a unbiased fashion.

4509 **Social Security Library**
U S Social Security Administration
6401 Security Boulevard
Baltimore, MD 21235
410-965-1234
800-772-1213
TTY:800-325-0778
www.socialsecurity.gov

Leo Hollenbeack, Reference Librarian
Jo B Barnhart, Chief Executive Officer
Information on social security and disability insurance.

4510 **Warren Grant Magnuson Clinical Center**
National Institue Health
9000 Rockville Pike
Building 10-Room
Bethesda, MD 20892
301-496-2447
866-411-1010
FAX: 301-480-9793
TTY: 866-411-1010
e-mail: occc@cc.nih.gov
www.cc.nih.gov

John Gallin, Director
Established in 1953 as the research hospital of the National Institutes of Health. Designed so that patient care facilities are close to research laboratories so new findings of basic and clinical scientists can be quickly applied to the treatment of patients. Upon referral by physicians, patients are admitted to NIH clinical studies.

Massachusetts

4511 **Boston University Arthritis Center**
Boston University
715 Albany Street
Boston, MA 02118
617-638-8000
FAX: 617-638-5226
www.bumc.bu.edu

David Felson, Director
Vanesa Vliura, Manager
The Arthritis Center focuses its educational, research and patient care efforts on the diagnosis and treatment of rheumatic diseases. These include the many forms of arthritis; the auto-immune diseases such as Scleroderma, Systemic Lupus, Erythematosus, Rheumatoid Arthritis; localized pain syndromes such as tendonitis, bursitis, and carpal tunnel syndrome; and metabolic bone disorders such as osteoporosis.

4512 **Boston University Center for Human Genetics**
715 Albany Street
W-4th Floor
Boston, MA 02118
617-638-7083
FAX: 617-638-7092
e-mail: amilunsk@bu.edu

Aubrey Milunsky, Director
Jeff Milunsky, Associate Director
Ilga Wohlrab, Manager
Offers research into genetic disorders and growth disorders.

4513 **Boston University Robert Dawson Evans Memorial Dept. of Clinical Research**
75 East Newton Street
Boston, MA 02118
617-638-7250
FAX: 617-638-8728

Norman Levinsky, Director
Jack Ansel, MD
Integral unit of the University Hospital specializing in arthritis and connective tissue studies.

4514 **Braille and Talking Book Library, Perkins School for the Blind**
175 N Beacon Street
Watertown, MA 02472
617-972-7240
800-852-3133
FAX: 617-972-7363
e-mail: library@perkins.org
www.perkinslibrary.org

Kim Johnston, President
Kim Charlson, Executive Director
Provides free books on tape and Braille to persons who cannot read printed material because of a physical disability such as blindness, visual impairment, physical impairment or learning disability. Serves Massachusetts. For Braille, also serves New Hampshire, Rhode Island, Maine and Vermont.

4515 **Brigham and Women's Hospital: Asthma and Allergic Disease Research Center**
75 Francis Street
Boston, MA 02115
617-732-5500
FAX: 617-730-2858
e-mail: arc@partners.org
www.brighhamandwomens.org

K Frank Austen MD, Director
Judith Kennedy, Manager
Integral unit of the hospital focusing research attention on asthma and allergy related disorders.

4516 **Brigham and Women's Hospital: Robert B Brigham Multipurpose Arthritis Center**
Brigham and Women s Hospital
75 Francis Street
Boston, MA 02115
617-732-5500
FAX: 617-432-0979
www.brighamandwomens.org

Matthew Liang MD, Director
Gary Gottlieb, Chief Executive Officer

Research studies into arthritis and rheumatic diseases.

4517 Caption Center
125 Western Avenue
Boston, MA 02134
617-300-3600
FAX: 617-300-1020
e-mail: access@wgbh.org
www.wgbh.org/caption

Tom Apone, Director
Larry Goldberg, Director
Has been pioneering and delivering accessible media to disabled adults, students and their families, teachers and friends for over 30 years. Each year, the Center captions more than 10,000 hours worth of broadcast and cable programs, feature films, large-format and IMAX films, home videos, music videos, DVDs, teleconferences and CD-Roms.

4518 Center for Interdisciplinary Research on Immunologic Diseases
Childrens Hospital Medical Center
300 Longwood Avenue
Boston, MA 02115
617-355-6000
FAX: 617-355-0443
TTY:617-355-0443
e-mail: webteam@tch.harvard.edu
www.tch.harvard.edu

James Mandell, Chief Executive Officer
Sandra Fenwick, Chief Operating Officer
Lynda Scheider, MD
Organizational research unit of the Children's Hospital that focuses on the causes, prevention and treatments of asthma, infections and allergies.

4519 Harvard University Howe Laboratory of Ophthalmology
Massachusetts Eye & Ear Infirmary
243 Charles Street
Boston, MA 02114
617-573-3285
TTY:617-523-5498
e-mail: richard.godfrey@schepens.harvard.edu
www.meei.harvard.edu

George Rabstejnek, Chairman
Joseph W Haley, Vice Chairman
Maryellen Doyle, Manager
Development ophthalmology and eye research.

4520 Laboure College Library
2120 Dorchester Avenue
Dorchester Center, MA 02124
617-296-8300
FAX: 617-296-7947
e-mail: admit@laboure.edu
www.laboure.edu

Mark Ostrem, Director Medical Unit
Andrew Callo, Manager
Offers information on physical disabilities, independent living, peer counseling and advocacy.

4521 Massachusetts Rehabilitation Commission
27 Wormwood Street Fort Point Pl
Suite 600
Boston, MA 02210
617-204-3608
800-245-6543
FAX: 617-727-1354
TTY: 800-245-6543
www.mass.gov/mrc

Elmer C Bartels, Commissioner
Deval Patrick, Governor
Tom Murray, Lieutenant Governor
Vacational Rehabilitation and Independent Living for people with disabilities.

4522 Schepens Eye Research Institute
20 Staniford Street
Boston, MA 02114
617-912-0100
FAX: 617-912-0110
e-mail: geninfo@vision.eri.harvard.edu
www.theschepens.org

Michael Gilmore, President
Kennett Burnes, Chairman
Prominent center for research on eye, vision, and blinding diseases; dedicated to research that improves the understanding, management, and prevention of eye diseases and visual deficiencies; fosters collaboration among its faculty members; trains young scientists and clinicians from around the world; promotes communication with scientists in allied fields; leader in the worldwide dispersion of basic scientific knowledge of vision.

4523 Talking Book Library at Worcester Public Library
3 Salem Square
Worcester, MA 01608
508-799-1730
800-762-0085
FAX: 508-799-1676
e-mail: talkbook@cwmars.org
www.worcpublib.org/talkingbook

James Izatt, Manager
Braille embosser, magnifiers, closed-circuit TV, adapted computers, cassette books and magazines, children's books on cassette, reference materials on blindness and other disabilities.

Michigan

4524 Artificial Language Laboratory
Michigan State University
405 Computer Center
East Lansing, MI 48824
517-353-5399
FAX: 517-353-4766
e-mail: artlang@pilot.msu.edu
www.artlang@pilot.msu.edu

John B Eulenberg, Director
Stephen Blosser, Technical Director
Shawn Miller, Laboratory Manager
Multidisciplinary research center in the Audiology & Speech Science department, Michigan State University. Its basic research program includes speech analysis and synthesis. Applied research is carried out on computer-based systems for persons who are blind and for persons with cerebral palsy and head injury. The laboratory develops physical, cognitive and linguistic assessment technology.

4525 Burger School for the Autistic
30922 Beechwood Street
Garden City, MI 48135
734-762-8420
FAX: 734-793-1831
garden-city.lib.mi.us

Joan Elmouchi, Director
Jan Smith, Assistant Director
Judy Gapp, Director Childrens Unit
Burger school for students with autism is the largest public school in the United States that specializes in the education of students with autism.

4526 Chi Medical Library
Ingham Regional Medical Center
401 W Greenlawn
Lansing, MI 48910
517-334-2121
FAX: 517-334-2939
www.irmc.org

Judith Barnes, Information Resources Coordinato
Consumer health and patient education collection in books, videotapes, pamphlets. Open to the public.

4527 Glaucoma Laser Trial
Sinai Hospital of Detroit: Dept. of Opthalmology
29275 Northwestern Highway
Southfield, MI 48034
248-493-5157
www.nei.nih.gov/neitrials

Hugh Beckman, MD, Chairman
The purpose of the trial is to compare the safety and long-term efficacy of argon laser treatment of the trabecular meshwork with standard medical treatment for primary open-angle glaucoma.

4528 **Grand Traverse Area Library for the Blind and Physically Handicapped**
610 Woodmere Avenue
Traverse City, MI 49686
231-932-8500
877-931-8558
FAX: 231-932-8578
e-mail: webmaster@tadl.tcnet.org
www.tadl.org

Gay Travis, President
Beth Bynum, Vice President
Michael Guire, Executive Director

4529 **Kent District Library for the Blind and Physically Handicapped**
3350 Michael SW
Wyoming, MI 49509
616-647-3980
FAX: 616-336-3256
e-mail: lpbhstaff@kdl.org
www.nlc.lib.mi.us

Claudya Muller, Director
Summer reading programs, braille writer, magnifiers, large-print photocopier, cassette books and magazines, children's books on cassette, and other reference materials on blindness and other handicaps.

4530 **Library of Michigan Service for the Blind**
702 West Kalamazoo Street
Po Box 30638
Lansing, MI 48909
517-241-2236

e-mail: ckrueger@michigan.gov
www.michigan.gov/hal

Mase Sheryl, Director
Christie Brandau, Manager
Braille writer, magnifiers, closed-circuit T.V., large-print photocopier, cassette books and magazines, children's books on cassette, and other reference materials on blindness and other handicaps.

4531 **Macomb Library for the Blind and Physically Handicapped**
16480 Hall Road
Clinton Township, MI 48038
586-286-1580
FAX: 586-286-0634
e-mail: macbld@libcoop.net
www.libcoop.net/macspe

Beverlee Babcock, Division Director
Summer reading programs, braille writer, closed-circuit T.V., large-print books, cassette books and magazines, children's books on cassette, other reference materials on blindness and other handicaps, descriptive videos and bifokal kits. Assistive technology including JAWS, Zoomtext, OpenBook, and Duxbury.

4532 **Michigan's Assistive Technology Resource**
Physically Impaired Association of Michigan
1023 S US 27
St. Johns, MI 48879
989-224-0333
800-274-7426
FAX: 989-224-0330
e-mail: matr@edzone.net
www.cenmi.org/mits

Jeffrey Diedrich, Director
Maryann Jones, Coordinator
Barbara Warren, Information Specialist
Provides information services, support materials, technical assistance, and training to local and intermediate school districts in michigan to increase their capacity to address the needs of students with disabilities for assistive technology.

4533 **Mideastern Michigan Library Co-op**
503 S Saginaw Street
Suite 839
Flint, MI 48502
810-232-7119
800-641-6639
FAX: 810-232-6639
e-mail: rmendel@flint.org
www.mideastern.lib.mi.us

Roger Mendel, Director
Summer reading programs, braille writer, magnifiers, closed-circuit T.V., large-print photocopier, cassette books and magazines, children's books on cassette, home visits and other reference materials on blindness and other handicaps.

4534 **Muskegon County Library for the Blind**
4845 Airline Road
Unit 5
Muskegon, MI 49444
231-737-6248
877-569-4801
FAX: 231-737-6307
TTY: 231-722-4103
e-mail: mclsm@llcoop.org
www.muskcolib.org

Elizabeth Winsche, Chief Executive Officer
Sheila Miller, Librarian
Karla Bates, Assistant Director
Braille typewriter, magnifiers, closed-circuit TV, large-print photocopier, cassette books and magazines, children's books on cassette, home visits and other reference materials on blindness and other handicaps, The Reading Edge, and large print books.

4535 **Northland Library Cooperative**
Library Cooperative/ Library for the blind
316 E Chisholm Street
Alpena, MI 49707
989-356-1622
800-446-1580
FAX: 989-354-3939
e-mail: webmaster@nlc.lib.mi.us
www.nlc.lib.mi.us

Jennifer Dean, Director
Christine Johnston, Executive Director
Summer reading programs, Braille writer, magnifiers, closed-circuit TV, large-print photocopier, cassette books and magazines, children's books on cassette and other reference materials on blindness and other handicaps.

4536 **Oakland County Library for the Visually & Physically Impaired**
1200 N Telegraph Road
Pontiac, MI 48341
248-858-5050
800-774-4542
FAX: 248-858-9313
TTY: 248-452-2247
e-mail: lvpi@.oakgov.com
www.oakgov.com/lvpi

David Conklin, Librarian/Supervisor
The Oakland County Library for the Visually and Physically Impaired was established in 1974 to provide access to free library service for County residents who are unable to read standard printed material because of a visual impairment or physical limitation.

4537 **St. Clair County Library Special Technologies Alternative Resources (S.T.A.R.)**
210 McMorran Boulevard
Port Huron, MI 48060
810-982-3600
800-272-8570
FAX: 810-987-6768
TTY: 810-455-0200
e-mail: star@sccl.lib.mi.us
www.sccl.lib.mi.us/star.html

Mary Jo Koch, Subregional Librarian
James Warwick, Executive Director
Offers library services to the blind, deaf and blind, visually disabled, phsyically disabled, and reading disabled.

4538 **University of Michigan: Orthopaedic Research Laboratories**
University of Michigan
G-161 400 North Ingals
Ann Arbor, MI 48109
734-763-9674
FAX: 734-647-0003
e-mail: svaassen@umich.edu
www.orl.med.umich.edu/orl

Steve Goldstein, Lab Director
Laurence McMahon Jr, MD

Develops and studies the causes and treatments for arthritis including new devices and assistive aids.

4539 **Upper Peninsula Library for the Blind**
1615 Presque Isle Avenue
Marquette, MI 49855
906-228-7697
800-562-8985
FAX: 906-228-5627
TTY: 906-228-7697
e-mail: rruff@uproc.lib.mi.us
www.uproc.lib.mi.us/uplibph

Ruth Ruff, Librarian
Suzanne Dees, Executive Director
Summer reading programs, braille writer, magnifiers, closed-circuit T.V., large-print photocopier, cassette books and magazines, children's books on cassette, home visits and other reference materials on blindness and other handicaps.

4540 **Washtenaw County Library for the Blind & Physically Handicapped**
4135 Washtenaw Avenue
Po Box 8645
Ann Arbor, MI 48107
734-973-4350
FAX: 734-973-4963
e-mail: lbpd@ewashtenaw.org
www.ewashtenaw.org

Mary Udoji, Director
Michigan Subregional Library, Library of Congress National Library Service network. General library service for persons unable to use standard print materials for various physical reasons. Lends audio books and listening equipment, large type books, descriptive videos. Provides reference information and programs. Kurzweil scanner with components which convert standard print to Braille, large type or audio and closed circuit TV magnifier on site.

4541 **Wayne County Regional Library for the Blind**
30555 Michigan Avenue
Westland, MI 48186
734-727-7300
888-968-2737
FAX: 734-727-7333
TTY: 734-727-7330
e-mail: wcrlbph@wayneregional.lib.mi.us
www.wayneregional.lib.mi.us

Reginald Williams, Director
Frederick Howkins, Manager
Summer reading programs, braille writer, magnifiers, closed-circuit T.V., large-print photocopier, cassette books and magazines, children's books on cassette, and other reference materials on blindness and other handicaps.

4542 **Wayne State University: CS Mott Center for Human Genetics and Development**
275 E Hancock Street
Detroit, MI 48201
313-577-1485
FAX: 313-577-8554
e-mail: c.yurkovich@wayne.edu
www.media.wayne.edu

Cheryl Yurkovich, Director Public Relations
Human growth and development disorders.

Minnesota

4543 **Century College**
3300 Century Avenue N
White Bear Lake, MN 55110
651-779-3200
800-228-1978
FAX: 651-779-5779
TTY: 651-773-1715
www.century.cc.mn.us

Larry Litecky, President
Nancy Levingston, Director
Programs of study - Orthotic Practitioner, Orthotic Technician, Prosethetic Practitioner, Prosthetic Technician. In addition, Century College offers more than 50 other programs in liberal arts, career and occupational programs.

4544 **Communication Center/Minnesota State Services for the Blind**
Services for the Blind
2200 University Avenue W
Suite 240
Saint Paul, MN 55114
651-642-0500
800-652-9000
FAX: 651-649-5927
e-mail: chamilto@ssb.state.mn.us
www.mnssb.org/allages/commcenter

Chuck Hamilton, Director
Special library service for the blind and physically handicapped providing tape and Braille transcription of textbooks and vocational materials; Minnesota Radio Talking Book providing current newspaper, magazines and best selling books; Dial-in-News, a touch tone phone accessed newspaper service; Library of Congress cassette and phonograph talking book equipment; repair services for special audio reading equipment, with most services free to Minnesota Residents.

4545 **Duluth Public Library**
520 W Superior Street
Duluth, MN 55802
218-730-4200
FAX: 218-723-3822
e-mail: webmail@duluth.lib.mn.us
www.duluth.lib.mn.us

David Ouse, Interim Library Director
Nancy Eaton, Website
Lucie Holzemer, Special Needs Center
Adapted access to Apple computer, adapted toys and adapted library equipment.

4546 **Minnesota Library for the Blind and Physically Handicapped**
Department of Education
388 SE 6th Avenue
Faribault, MN 55021
507-333-4828
800-722-0550
FAX: 507-333-4832
e-mail: mn.lbph@sate.mn.us
education.state.mn.us

Catherine Durivage, Program Director
Rene Perrance, Librarian
Provides books and magazines in Braille, large print, records, and cassettes to qualified residents of Minnesota who have a visual or physical impairment, including reading disabilities due to an organic cause certified by a medical doctor, that prevents residents from reading standard print or physically handling a book. Equipment for in-house use include magnifiers, braillers, listening equipment, and CCTV. Reference collection for in-house use only on visual impairment topics.

4547 **Special U**
University of Minnesota
PO Box 721-Umhc
Minneapolis, MN 55455
612-625-3846
800-276-8642
FAX: 612-624-0997
e-mail: kdwb-var@umn.edu
Brings together comprehensive sources of information related to youth with chronic or disabling conditions and their families. Topics include psychosocial issues, disability awareness, developmental processes, family, sexuality, education, employment, independent living, cultural issues, gender issues, service delivery, professional issues, advocacy and legal issues, and health issues. Special focus on transition from childhood to adolesecence to adulthood.

Mississippi

4548 **Mississippi Library Commission**
3881 Eastwood Drive
Jackson, MS 39211
601-432-4111
800-647-7542
FAX: 601-354-7007
TTY: 601-354-6411
e-mail: mslib@mlc.lib.ms.us
www.mlc.lib.ms.us

Sharman B Smith, Executive Director
Ewing Ethel, Executive Support Director
Mary Anderson, Manager
Summer reading programs, braille writer, magnifiers, closed-circuit T.V., large-print photocopier, cassette books and magazines, children's books on cassette, home visits and other reference materials on blindness and other handicaps.

4549 **Mississippi Library Commission\Talking Book and Braille Services**
3881 Eastwood Drive
Jackson, MS 39211
601-961-4111
800-446-0892
FAX: 601-354-7007
e-mail: mslib@mlc.lib.ms.us
www.mlc.lib.ms.us

Sharman B Smith, Executive Director
Rey Tuchett, Director for the Blind/Handicapp
Library service for the print handicapped braille, cassette and disc materials (books & periodicals) for children and adults. Large print RG production (copier & printer), braille embosser and other handicaps.

Missouri

4550 **Assemblies of God Center for the Blind**
1445 N Boonville Avenue
Springfield, MO 65802
417-831-1964
FAX: 417-862-5120
e-mail: blind@ag.org
www.blind.ag.org

Paul Weingartner, Director
Caryl Weingartner, Administrative Assistant
Juleen Turnage, Religious Leader
Offers braille and cassette lending library, braille and cassette Sunday School materials for all ages, braille and cassette periodicals, resource assistance, and resources for blind children and children of blind parents.

4551 **Church of the Nazarene**
Nazarene Publishing House
6401 The Paseo
Kansas City, MO 64131
816-333-7000
800-877-0700
FAX: 800-849-9827
e-mail: it@nazarene.org
www.nazarene.org

Hardy Weathers, President
Offers braille and large print books. Also offers a lending library and cassettes for the blind.

4552 **Judevine Center for Autism**
1101 Olivette Executive Parkway
Saint Louis, MO 63132
314-432-6200
FAX: 314-849-2721
e-mail: judevine@judevine.org
www.judevine.org

Becky Blackwell, President
Evaluations and assessments, parent and professional training programs, consultations, workshops, seminars, family support, clinical therapies, adult programs and support, residential services.

4553 **Lutheran Library for the Blind**
7550 Watson Road
Saint Louis, MO 63119
314-918-0415
888-215-2455
FAX: 314-963-0738
e-mail: blind.mission@blindmission.org
www.blindmission.org

Dave Andrus, Executive Director
Gerald Kieschnick, President
Offers Christian books in braille and large print books and cassettes for the blind and visually impaired, on loan, as well as Christian periodicals in braille, large print and cassette tape.

4554 **University of Missouri: Columbia Arthritis Center**
University of Missouri
1 Hospital Drive
Columbia, MO 65212
573-882-4141
FAX: 573-884-3996
e-mail: webeditor@missouri.edu
www.muhealth.org

Jerry C Parker, Director
David Cravens, MD
Research into arthritis and rheumatic diseases. One of the most comprehensive health-care networks in Missouri, our 5 hospitals and numerous clinics, all staffed by University Physicians, offer the finest primary, secondary, and tertiary health-care services. We also provide education for future health-care providers and participate in important research.

4555 **Wolfner Library for the Blind**
Secretary State Office
PO Box 387
Jefferson City, MO 65102
573-751-8720
800-392-2614
FAX: 573-526-2985
TTY: 800-347-1379
e-mail: wolfner@sos.mo.gov
www.sos.mo.gov

Richard J Smith, Division Director
Free library service in alternate formats, braille, recorded, large print. For any Missouri resident who cannot read standard print, due to a physical disability. Summer reading programs, braille writer, magnifiers, closed-circuit T.V., large-print photocopier, cassette books and magazines, children's books on cassette, home visits and other reference materials on blindness and other handicaps.

Montana

4556 **MonTECH**
University of Montana
634 Eddy Avenue
Missoula, MT 59812
406-243-5751
800-732-0323
FAX: 406-243-4730
TTY: 406-243-5676
e-mail: montech@ruralinstitute.umt.edu
http://montech.ruralinstitute.umt.edu

Kathy Laurin, Ph.D, Director
Leslie Mullete, Clinical Coordinator
Mary Swan, Community Relations/Info Liaison
Specializing in Assistive Technology and oversee a variety of AT related grants and contracts. The overall goal is to develop a comprehensive, statewide system of assistive technology related assistance. Striving to ensure that all people in Montana with disabilities have equitable access to assistive technology devices and services in order to enhance their independence, productivity, and quality of life.

4557 **Montana State Library-Talking Book Library**
PO Box 201800
1515 East 6th Avenue
Helena, MT 59620
406-444-2064
800-332-3400
FAX: 406-444-5612
e-mail: mslreference@mt.gov
www.msl.state.mt.us/tbl

Christie Briggs, Supervisor
Darlene Staffeldt, Manager
Over 50,000 titles on 4-track cassette, WebBraille, Web0pac, WebBlud, summer reading programs, braille writer, magnifiers, closed-circuit T.V., large-print photocopier, cassette books and magazines, children's books on cassette, home visits and other reference materials on blindness and other handicaps. Large print and Braille services to blind, low vision, physically handicapped and reading disabled citizens of Montana.

Nebraska

4558 **Martin Luther Home Society Inc.**
650 J Street
Suite 305
Lincoln, NE 68508
402-434-3250
800-443-4899
FAX: 402-434-3253
e-mail: mlhs_MEINTS@compuserve.com

Alice Meints, Resource Center Director
Fred Naumann III, Communications Director
Provides materials and opportunities for consultation with individuals and communities assisting persons with special needs.

4559 **Nebraska Assistive Technology Partnership Nebraska Department of Education**
5143 S 48th Street
Suite C
Lincoln, NE 68516
402-471-0734
888-806-6287
888-806-6287
FAX: 402-471-6052
TTY:402-471-0734
e-mail: atp@atp.state.ne.us
www.nde.state.ne.us/ATP

Mark Schultz, Executive Director
Lilly Blase, Program Coordinator
Provides statewide assistive technology and home modification services for Nebraskans of all ages and disabilities.

4560 **Nebraska Library Commission: Talking Book and Braille Service**
Talking Book and Braille Service
1200 N Street
Suite 120
Lincoln, NE 68508
402-471-4038
800-742-7691
FAX: 402-471-2083
TTY: 402-471-4083
e-mail: talkingbook@nlc.state.ne.us
www.nlc.state.ne.us

Dave Oertli, Director
Kay Goehring, Reader Services Coordinator
Bill Ainsley, Audio Production Studio Manager
Summer reading programs, braille writer, magnifiers, closed-circuit T.V., large-print photocopier, cassette books and magazines, children's books on cassette, home visits and other reference materials on blindness and other handicaps.

Nevada

4561 **Las Vegas-Clark County Library District**
833 Las Vegas Boulevard North
Las Vegas, NV 89101
702-734-7323
FAX: 702-733-1567
www.lvccld.lib.nv.us

Elaine Sanchez, Chairman
Verlia Davis, Vice Chair
Laura Golod, Manager
Summer reading programs, braille writer, magnifiers, closed-circuit T.V., large-print photocopier, cassette books and magazines, children's books on cassette, home visits and other reference materials on blindness and other handicaps.

4562 **Nevada State Library and Archives**
716 N. Carson Street
Suite B
Carson City, NV 89710
775-687-5469
FAX: 775-687-8311
TTY:702-687-8338
e-mail: putnam@equinox.unr.edu
http://dmla.clan.lib.nv.us/docs/nsla

Michael Fischer, Director
Robert Beckley, Computer Systems Technician
Summer reading programs, braille writer, magnifiers, closed-circuit T.V., large-print photocopier, cassette books and magazines, children's books on cassette, home visits and other reference materials on blindness and other handicaps.

New Hampshire

4563 **New Hampshire State Library: Talking Book Services**
117 Pleasant Street
Dolloff Building- 1st Floor
Concord, NH 03301
603-271-3429
FAX: 603-271-8370
e-mail: talking@library.state.nh.us
www.state.nh.us/nhsl/talkbks/index.html

John Barrett, Regional Librarian
Regional Library for National Library Service for the Blind & Physically Handicapped offers cassette books and magazines, children's books on cassette, descriptive videos, large print books, and downloadable digital audio books, and Braille services.

New Jersey

4564 **Children's Specialized Hospital Medical Library - Parent Resource Center**
150 New Providence Road
Mountainside, NJ 07092
908-233-3720
888-244-5373
FAX: 908-301-5509
e-mail: jbrooks@childrens-specialized.org
www.childrens-specialized.org

Mila Lungin, Medical Librarian
Amy Mansue, Chief Executive Officer
Contains some 3,000 books, and journals specializing in nursing, pediatrics, child neurology, and rehabilitation. Also provides a Parent Resource Center, a special collection of books, videos and pamphlets designed to meet the information needs of parents and families, as well as the local community.

4565 **Christopher & Dana Reeve Foundation Resource Center**
636 Morris Tpke
Suite 3a
Short Hills, NJ 07078
973-467-8270
800-539-7309
FAX: 973-467-9845
e-mail: info@paralysis.org
www.paralysis.org

Joe Canose, VP Quality Of Life
Angela Crentillon, Associate Director Operations
A national clearinghouse for information, referral and educational materials on paralysis. Offers a free book "Paralysis Resource Guide" in English or Spanish. Free lending library.

4566 **Eye Institute of New Jersey**
New Jersey Medical School
90 Bergen Street
Newark, NJ 07103
973-972-2111
FAX: 973-972-2068
e-mail: eyereplies@aol.com
www.umdnj.edu/eyeweb

Marco Zarbin, Chairman
Ophthamology, including research into cornea, retina and neuro-ophthamalogy.

4567 **Mycoclonus Research Foundation**
200 Old Palisade Road
Apt 17d
Fort Lee, NJ 07024
201-585-0770
FAX: 201-585-0770
e-mail: research@myoclonus.com

Mark Seiden, VP

Supports clinical and basic research into the cause and treatment of myoclonus; four international workshops facilitated the sharing of information by physicians, scientists, and investigators active in the field, resulted in three publications; supports promising research projects, clinical neurological fellows, with special emphasis on posthypoxic myoclonus and encourages all who are interested in futhering the understanding, treatment, and cure of myoclonus.

4568 New Jersey Center for Outreach and Services for the Autism Community (COSAC)
1450 Parkside Avenue
Suite 22
Ewing, NJ 08638
609-883-8100
800-428-8476
FAX: 609-883-5509
e-mail: information@njcosac.org
www.njcosac.org

Paul A Potito, Executive Director
Purpose is to assist families, individuals and agencies concerned with the welfare and education of children and adults with autism and other pervasive development disorders.

4569 New Jersey Library for the Blind and Handicapped
2300 Stuyvesant Avenue
Po Box 501
Trenton, NJ 08618
609-530-4000
800-792-8322
FAX: 609-530-6384
TTY: 609-530-4000
e-mail: njlbh@njstatelib.org
www.njstatelib.org

Anne McArthur, Outreach & Public Education
Faith Lundgren, Assistant Director
Venetia Demson, Executive Director
Summer reading programs, braille writer, magnifiers, closed-circuit T.V., large-print, cassette, braille books and magazines, children's books on cassette, and other reference materials on blindness and other handicaps. Provides reading material on audio, cassette, large print and braille to eligible NJ residents.

New Mexico

4570 New Mexico State Library for the Blind and Physically Handicapped
325 Don Gaspar Avenue
Santa Fe, NM 87501
505-986-4550
800-456-5515
FAX: 505-827-3888
TTY: 800-659-4915
e-mail: jbrewstr@stlib.state.nm.us
www.stlib.state.nm.us

Glee Wenzel, Librarian
David Abbey, Executive Director
Summer reading programs, braille writer, magnifiers, closed-circuit T.V., large-print photocopier, cassette books and magazines, children's books on cassette, home visits and other reference materials on blindness and other handicaps.

New York

4571 Center on Human Policy: School of Education
Syracuse University
805 S Crouse Avenue
Syracuse, NY 13244
315-443-3851
800-894-0826
FAX: 315-443-4338
e-mail: thechp@syr.edu
www.thechp.syr.edu

Steve Taylor, Director
Rachael Zubal-Ruggieri, Information Coordinator
Raymond Colton, Manager
The Center on Human Policy is a Syracuse University-based policy, research and advocacy organization involved in the national movement to ensure the rights of people with disabilities.

4572 DREAMMS for Kids
273 Ringwood Road
Freeville, NY 13068
607-539-3027
FAX: 607-539-9930
e-mail: janet@dreamms.org
www.dreamms.org

Janet Hosmer, Executive Director
DREAMMS is committed to increasing the use of computers, high quality instructional technology, and assistive technologies for students with special needs in schools, homes and the workplace.

4573 Eastern Paralyzed Veterans Association
75-20 Astoria Boulevard
Jackson Heights, NY 11370
718-803-3782
800-404-2898
FAX: 718-803-0414
e-mail: info@unitedspinal.org
www.unitedspinal.org

Gerard Kelly, Director
Peter Addesso, President
Library offering information on physical disabilities, spinal cord injury and rehabilitation. Also provides literature searches on specific topics. Association news and free publications on architecture and barrier-free designs, legislation and other current events affecting Americans with Disabilities.

4574 Ehrman Medical Library
New York University Medical Center
550 1st Avenue
New York, NY 10016
212-263-5397
FAX: 212-263-6534
library.med.nyu.edu

Karen Brewer, Director
Our mission of the Fredrick L. Ehrman Library is to enhance learning, research and patient care and New York University Medical Center by effectively managing knowledge-based resources, providing client-centered information services and education, and extending access through new initiatives in information technology.

4575 Finger Lakes Developmental Disabilities Service Office
620 Westfall Road
Rochester, NY 14620
585-461-8500
FAX: 585-461-0618
e-mail: folwelbe@nysomr.emi.com

Sue Mann, Director
Carolyn Bassett, Manager
Information on mental retardation and developmental disabilities.

4576 Helen Keller International
352 Park Avenue South
12th Floor
New York, NY 10010
212-532-0544
877-535-5374
FAX: 212-532-6014
e-mail: info@hki.org
www.hki.org

Kathy Spahn, President/CEO
Jennifer Klopp, Dir Development/Communications
Nonprofit international organization whose mission is to combat the causes and consequences of blindness and malnutrition.

4577 Helen Keller National Center for Deaf-Blin d Youths and Adults (HKNC)
141 Middle Neck Road
Sands Point, NY 11050
516-944-8900
FAX: 516-944-7302
e-mail: hkncinfo@hknc.org
www.hknc.org

Nancy O'Donnell, Coordinator Of Special Projects
Joseph McNulty, Executive Director

HKNC is the only national vacational and rehabilitation program providing services exclusively to youth and adults who are deaf-blind.

4578 Institute for Basic Research in Developmental Disabilities

1050 Forest Hill Road
Staten Island, NY 10314
718-494-0600
FAX: 718-494-0833
www.omr.state.ny.us/ws_ibr_resources

W Ted Brown, Director
Peter Piotrkozlowski, Executive Director
Conducts research into neurodegenerative diseases, alzheimer's disease, developmental disabilities, fragile X syndrome, Down's Syndrome, autism, epilepsy and basic science issues underlying all developmental disabilities.

4579 Institute for Visual Sciences

1 E 71st Street
New York, NY 10021
212-249-1140
FAX: 212-472-0295

Francis Lesperance, Chairman
Ophthalmology with emphasis on the development of care for the eye.

4580 JGB Cassette Library International

15 W 65th Street
New York, NY 10023
212-769-6331
FAX: 212-769-6266
e-mail: bemass@aol.com

Peter Williamson, Executive Director
Summer reading programs, braille writer, magnifiers, closed-circuit T.V., large-print photocopier, cassette books and magazines, children's books on cassette, home visits and other reference materials on blindness and other handicaps.

4581 Nassau Library System

900 Jerusalem Avenue
Uniondale, NY 11553
516-292-8920
FAX: 516-481-4777
e-mail: outreach@nassaulibrary.org
www.nassaulibrary.org

Elizabeth Olesh, Manager Outreach Services
Francine Siegel, Sr Connections Project Director
Jackie Thresher, Executive Director
Information about public library services in Nassau County, including services for people with disabilities and the Senior Connections volunteer project (information and referral for seniors and their families).

4582 National Braille Association

National Braille Association
3 Townline Circle
Rochester, NY 14623
585-427-8260
FAX: 585-427-0263
e-mail: nbaoffice@nationalbraille.org
www.nationalbraille.org

Louis Braille, Inventor
Angela Coffaro, Executive Director
Contains over 1800 Braille titles and Braille music scores. Copies produced on demand and sold below cost. Catalog available on request.

4583 New York Public Library: Andrew Heiskell Library for the Blind and Physically Handicapped

New York Public Library
40 W 20th Street
New York, NY 10011
212-206-5400
FAX: 212-206-5418
TTY:212-206-5458
e-mail: ahlbph@nypl.org
www.nypl.org/branch/lb

Robert McBrian, Regional Librarian/Manager
By mail and on-site offers talking books and braille books to eligible patrons in New York City and Long Island. Additional on-site services include large-print books, books on tape, descriptive videos, class visits, programs, and assistive devices such as closed circuit televisions and Karzweil Personal Readers

4584 New York State Talking Book & Braille Library

Empire State Plaza
Albany, NY 12230
518-474-5935
800-342-3688
FAX: 518-486-1957
TTY: 518-474-5935
e-mail: tbbl@mail.nysed.gov
www.nysl.nysed.gov

Jane Somers, Director
Books on audio cassette, cassette players, braille books, summer reading programs, braille writer, magnifiers, closed-circuit T.V., large-print photocopier, cassette books and magazines, children's books on cassette, reference materials on blindness and other handicaps.

4585 Postgraduate Center for Mental Health

124 E 28th Street
New York, NY 10016
212-576-4150
FAX: 212-696-1679
www.dvguide.com/newyork/postgrad.html

Marge Slobetz, Assistant Director
Marie Serrano, Manager
Evaluations and psychotherapy by social workers psychologists for children, adolescents, families and couples. Neuropsychological testing and remedation for learning disabilities.

4586 Rehabilitation Research Library

Human Resources Center
Albertson, NY 11507
516-741-2010
FAX: 516-746-3298

Amnon Tishler, Research Librarian
Susan Feifer, Manager
Information on rehabilitation and occupational rehabilitation.

4587 State University of New York Health Sciences Center

PO Box 32
Brooklyn, NY 11203
718-270-1934
FAX: 718-778-5397

Adolf Christ, Director
James Cottrell, MD
Child psychiatry research programs.

4588 Suffolk Cooperative Library System: Long Island Talking Book Library

Long Island Talking Book Library System
PO Box 9000
Bellport, NY 11713
631-286-1600
866-833-1122
FAX: 631-286-1647
TTY: 631-286-4546
e-mail: lbph@suffolk.lib.ny.us
www.litbl.org

Valerie Lewis, Administrator Of Outreach Srvs.
Kevin Verbesey, Executive Director
Offers a variety of support services to its 55 member libraries and other patrons including, an extensive talking book program, assistive technology and other services for people with disabilities.

4589 Wallace Memorial Library

Rochester Institute Of Technology
90 Lomb Memorial Drive
Rochester, NY 14623
585-475-2562
FAX: 585-475-7007
TTY:585-475-2760
e-mail: circwml@rit.edu
library.rit.edu

Chandra McKenzie, Director
William Destler, President
Information on physical disabilities and deafness.

4590 **Xavier Society for the Blind**
154 E 23rd Street
New York, NY 10010 212-473-7800

Alfred E Ceruana, Director
Kathleen Lynch, Manager
Provides spiritual and inspirational reading material to visually impaired persons in suitable format: braille, large print and cassette, throughout U.S. and Canada. Services are provided both by way of regular periodical publications sent through the mail and non-returnable; and by means of a lending library where books are returned. All services are provided free.

North Carolina

4591 **Genova Diagnostics**
63 Zillicoa Street
Asheville, NC 28801 828-285-0621
800-522-4762
FAX: 828-252-9303
www.gsdl.com

Ted Hull, President/CEO
Patrick J Hanaway, VP/ Chief Medical Officer
Laboratory serves over 8000 primary/specialty physicians and healthcare providers, offering over 125 specialized diagnostic assessments. These innovative tests cover a wide range of physiological areas, including digestive, immune, nutritional, endocrine, and metabolic function. To date, the lab has performed over 2 million individual diagnostic tests.
1986

4592 **North Carolina Library for the Blind and Physically Handicapped**
1811 Capital Boulevard
Raleigh, NC 27635 919-733-4376
888-388-2460
FAX: 919-733-6910
TTY: 919-733-1462
e-mail: nclbph@ncmail.net
statelibrary.dcr.state.nc.us

Francine Martin, Librarian/Manager
Carl Keehn, Assistant Librarian
Free loan of large print, braille, and cassette tape books and magazines and specialized playback equipment to registered eligible North Carolinians. Call for an application form. Collection contains general fiction and nonfiction titles. Registered borrowers may subscribe to receive descriptive videos for a one time fee.

4593 **Pediatric Rheumatology Clinic**
Duke Medical Center
PO Box 3212
Durham, NC 27710 919-477-9292
FAX: 919-684-6575
e-mail: rabin001@mc.duke.edu
www.duke.edu

Egla Rabinovich, Medical Director
Michael Duke, Owner
Clinical and laboratory pediatric rheumatoid studies.

4594 **University of North Carolina at Chapel Hill: Neuroscience Research Building**
Cb 7250
105 Mason Farm Road Bldg 245
Chapel Hill, NC 27599 919-966-4068
FAX: 919-966-1050
www.neuroscience.unc.edu

Eric Schneider, Administrator
An interdepartmental research center on the campus of the UNC-Chapel Hill School of Medicine. Mission is to promote neuroscience research with specific emphasis on developmental , cellular, and disease-related processes.

North Dakota

4595 **North Dakota State Library Talking Book Services**
604 E Boulevard Avenue
Dept 250
Bismarck, ND 58505 701-328-2492
800-472-2104
FAX: 701-328-2040
TTY: 800-892-8622
e-mail: statelib@state.nd.us
ndsl.lib.state.nd.us

Wayne G Sanstead, Superintendent
Doris Ott, State Librarian
Stella B Cone, Talking Manager
The Talking Books Program provides patrons with free access to cassette books and magazines. The Talking Books Program is administered by the National Library Service for the Blind and Physically Handicapped.

Ohio

4596 **Case Western Reserve University**
10900 Euclid Avenue
Cleveland, OH 44106 216-368-2000

e-mail: president@case.edu
www.case.edu

Eric Cottington, Associate VP for Research
Paula Baughn, Director
Edward Hundert, President
Programs which encompass the arts and sciences, engineering, health sciences, law, management, and social work.

4597 **Case Western Reserve University Northeast Ohio Multipurpose Arthritis Center**
11100 Euclid Avenue
Cleveland, OH 44106 216-844-8447
888-844-8447
www.uhhs.com

Fred Rothstein, Executive Director
Basic and clinical research into the causes, diagnosis and treatment of arthritis.

4598 **Cincinnati Children's Hospital Medical Center**
University Of Cincinnati Uap
3333 Burnet Avenue
Cincinnati, OH 45229 513-636-4200
800-344-2462
FAX: 513-636-2837
TTY: 513-636-4900
e-mail: oopes0@chmcc.org
www.cincinattichildren.org

Lee A Carter, Chairman
James M Anderson, Chief Executive Officer
David Schonfeld, Executive Director
Dedicated to providing the highest level of pediatric care. As Greater Cincinnati's only pediatric hospital, Cincinnati Children's is committed to bringing the very best medical care to children in our community.

4599 **Cleveland FES Center**
11000 Cedar Avenue
Cleveland, OH 44106 216-231-3257
FAX: 216-231-3258
TTY:216-231-3257
e-mail: info@fesc.org
http//:fescenter.case.edu

John Chae, Director Stroke Rehab
Peckham P Hunter, Director
Research and development center on functional electrical stimulation. Houses the FES Information Center, a resource center with a library. Publications, newsletters and videotapes for persons with disabilities and others interested in electrical stimulation are offered.

4600 **Cleveland Public Library**
325 Superior Avenue NE
Cleveland, OH 44114
216-623-2800
FAX: 216-623-7015
e-mail: info@library.cpl.org
www.cpl.org

Andrew Venable, Director
Joan Clark, Manager
Summer reading programs, braille writer, magnifiers, closed-circuit T.V., large-print photocopier, cassette books and magazines, children's books on cassette, and other reference materials on blindness and other handicaps.

4601 **Ohio Regional Library for the Blind and Physically Handicapped**
National Library Office
800 Vine Street
Cincinnati, OH 45202
513-369-6900
800-582-0335
FAX: 513-369-3111
TTY: 513-369-6072
e-mail: info@cincinnatilibrary.org
www.cincinnatilibrary.org

Donna Sousg, Director
Summer reading programs, braille writer, magnifiers, closed-circuit T.V., large-print photocopier, cassette books and magazines, children's books on cassette, and other reference materials on blindness and other handicaps.

4602 **State Library of Ohio: Talking Book Program**
National Library Service in Washington
274 E 1st Avenue
Suite 100
Columbus, OH 43201
614-644-6895
800-686-1531
FAX: 614-995-2186
e-mail: jbudler@sloma.state.oh.us
winslo.state.oh.us

Jo Budler, State Librarian
Jim Buchman, Dir Patron & Catalog Services
Peter Bates, Deputy Director
A machine-lending agency for the visually impaired. Provides free recorded books, and magazines to approximately 26,000 eligible blind, visually impaired, physically handicapped, and reading disabled Ohio residents.

Oklahoma

4603 **Oklahoma Library for the Blind & Physically Handicapped**
300 NE 18th Street
Oklahoma City, OK 73105
405-521-3514
800-523-0288
FAX: 405-521-4582
TTY: 405-521-4672
e-mail: library@drs.state.ok.us
www.library.state.ok.us

Vicky Golightly, PR Coordinator
Geraldine Adams, Executive Director
Braille writer, magnifiers, closed-circuit T.V., large-print photocopier, cassette books and magazines, children's books on cassette, home visits and other reference materials on blindness and other handicaps.

4604 **Oklahoma Medical Research Foundation**
825 NE 13th Street
Oklahoma City, OK 73104
405-271-6673
800-522-0211
FAX: 405-271-3980
www.omrf.org

Len Cason, Chairman
James Bass, Chairman/Executive Committee
J Capra, Chief Executive Officer
Focuses on arthritis and muscoloskeletal disease research.

4605 **Tulsa City-County Library System: Outreach Services**
Tulsa City- County Library System
400 Civic Center
1st Floor
Tulsa, OK 74103
918-596-7977
FAX: 918-596-7941
e-mail: os@tulsalibrary.org
www.tulsalibrary.org

Amy Stephens, Program Manager
Linda Saferite, Director
Homebound delivery of library services for the physically disabled.

Oregon

4606 **Oregon Health Sciences University, Elks' Children's Eye Clinic**
Casey Eye Institute
3375 SW Terwilliger Boulevard
Portland, OR 97239
503-494-3000
888-222-6478
FAX: 503-494-4286
e-mail: Roystere@ohsu.edu
www.ohsucasey.com

Earl A Palmer MD, Director
Eleen Reyster, Clinic Manager
James Rosenbaum, Manager
The elks children's eye clinic is the major charitable project of the Oregon State Elks association. The clinic would not be possible without the organization's dedication and commitment to providing eye care for babies and children.

4607 **Oregon Talking Book & Braille Services**
250 Winter Street NE
Salem, OR 97301
503-378-3849
800-452-0292
FAX: 503-588-7119
TTY: 503-378-4276
e-mail: tbabs.info@state.or.us
www.tbabs.org

Evelyn Kimbrell, Quality Coordinator
Eugene Newbill, Machine Program Coordinator
We serve the blind and physically disabled. Cassette books and magazines, Braille books-magazines, for children and adults. Descriptive videos. Audiocassette machines are provided free of charge. Call us for an application.

4608 **Talking Book & Braille Services Oregon State Library**
250 Winter Street NE
Salem, OR 97301
503-378-3849
800-452-0292
FAX: 503-378-4276
e-mail: tbabs@oslmac.osl.state.or.us
www.osl.state.or.us/home/tbabs

Keith Adams, Business Manager
Denise Davis, Program Manager
Jim Scheppke, Manager
Braille writer, magnifiers, large-print photocopier, cassette books and magazines, children's books on cassette and braille books.

Pennsylvania

4609 **Associated Services For The Blind & Visually Impaired**
919 Walnut Street
Philadelphia, PA 19107
215-627-0600
FAX: 215-922-0692
e-mail: asbinfo@asb.org
www.asb.org

Patricia C Johnson, Chief Executive Officer
A service of Associated Services for the Blind. 26 magazines are available on cassette through this subscription service. A magazine list can be sent, in both large print and on audio cassette.
$18.00

4610 **Carnegie Library of Pittsburgh Library for the Blind & Physically Handicapped**
4400 Forbes Avenue
Pittsburgh, PA 15213
412-662-3114
800-242-0586
FAX: 412-687-2442
e-mail: info@carnegielibrary.org
www.clpgh.org

Herb Elish, Director
Sue Murdock, Manager
Jane Dayton, Assistant Director
Loans recorded books/magazines and playback equipment, large print books and described videos to western PA residents unable to use standard printed materials due to a visual, physical, or physically-based reading disability.

4611 **Free Library of Philadelphia: Library for the Blind and Physically Handicapped**
919 Walnut Street
First Floor
Philadelphia, PA 19107
215-683-3213
800-222-1754
FAX: 215-683-3211
e-mail: flpblind@library.phila.gov
www.library.phila.gov

Vickie L Collins, Director
Pat Shotzberger, Technical Services Manager
Jill Gross, GED/Education Coordinator
Summer reading programs for children and teens. Closed-circuit T.V.for enlarging print for low vision; computers with screen readers and large print; cassette books and magazines; braille books and magazines; and descriptive videos for the blind and visually impaired. Unique and acclaimed adult education program for all disabilities. State of the art book recording facilities.

4612 **Pennsylvania College of Optometry Eye Institute**
8360 Old York Road
Elkins Park, PA 19027
215-780-1400
FAX: 215-780-1336
www.pco.edu
Since 1919 the college has led the field in education, in research, and in new approaches to vision diagnosis and correction.

4613 **Reading Rehabilitation Hospital**
Rr 1
Box 250
Reading, PA 19607
610-926-4017
FAX: 610-796-6303

Margaret Hsieh, Librarian
Doug Mehrkam, Owner
Information on physical disabilities, stroke, head injuries, aging and spinal cord injuries.

Rhode Island

4614 **Office Of Library & Information Services for the Blind and Physically Handicapped**
One Capitol Hill
2nd Floor
Providence, RI 02908
401-222-2726
FAX: 401-222-4195
e-mail: webmaster@lori.state.ri.us
www.lori.ri.gov

Anne Parent, Chief Library Services
William J Allen, Member of the Board
Deborah Barchi, Member of the Board
Offers information and services for the visually impaired including reference materials, braille printers, braille writers, large-print books and more.

4615 **Talking Books Plus**
Library for the Blind & Physically Handicapped
1 Capitol Hill
Providence, RI 02908
401-222-5800
FAX: 401-222-4195
e-mail: tbplus@olis.ri.gov
www.lori.state.ri.us/tbp

Andrew Egan, Regional Library Supervisor
Beth Perry, Program Manager
Offers talking book services for the blind and physically handicapped. Collection includes reference materials, braille printer, braille writer, large-print books, adaptive computer workstations and referrals to appropriate agencies/programs for other services.

South Carolina

4616 **Medical University of South Carolina Arthritis Clinical/Research Center**
171 Ashley Avenue
Charleston, SC 29425
843-792-1414
800-424-MUSC
FAX: 843-792-7121
www.muschealth.com

Paula Harper Bethea, Chairman
Morris Kalinsky, Vice Chairman
Offers patient care services and basic and clinical research on various types of arthritis and connective tissue diseases.

4617 **South Carolina State Library**
PO Box 11469
Columbia, SC 29211
803-734-8666
FAX: 803-734-8676
TTY:711-734-4611
e-mail: reference@statelibrary.sc.gov
www.statelibrary.sc.gov

Patti Butcher, Director
James Johnson Jr, Executive Director
Summer reading programs, braille writer, magnifiers, closed-circuit T.V., large-print photocopier, cassette books and magazines, children's books on cassette, home visits and other reference materials on blindness and other handicaps.

South Dakota

4618 **South Dakota State Library**
800 Governors Drive
Pierre, SD 57501
605-773-3131
800-423-6665
FAX: 605-773-4950
TTY: 605-773-4950
e-mail: library@state.sd.us
www.sdstatelibrary.com

Dorothy Liegl, Program Manager Outreach
Summer reading programs, braille writer, magnifiers, closed-circuit T.V., large-print photocopier, cassette books and magazines, children's books on cassette, home visits and other reference materials on blindness and other handicaps.

Tennessee

4619 **Tennessee Library for the Blind and Physically Handicapped**
403 7th Avenue N
Nashville, TN 37243
615-741-3915
800-342-3308
FAX: 615-532-8856
e-mail: tlbph.tsla@state.tn.us
www.tennessee.gov/tsla/lbph

Ruth Hemphill, Director
Donna Cirenza, Assistant Director
Offers free public library services to those unable to hold, read or turn the pages of standard print books and magazines due to physical or visual impairment or reading disabilities. Special library materials are provided by the Library of Congress, and free mailing privileges for these materials is provided through the US Post Office. Playback equipment is provided along with books and magazines on cassette, in Braille and in large print.

Texas

4620 **Baylor College of Medicine Birth Defects Center**
6620 Main Street
Houston, TX 77030
832-822-2229
FAX: 832-825-3141
www.bcm.edu/obgyn/tcfs

Frank Greenberg, Director
One of the few centers in the world that performs fetal surgery. Provides integrated, multidisciplinary care for mothers, carrying babies with genetic or anatomic birth defects requiring therapy before or immediately after birth. This collaboration enables us to efficiently car for both mother and child, providing the full specturm of fetal surgical services.

4621 **Baylor College of Medicine: Cullen Eye Institute**
Baylor College of Medicine
6550 Fannin Street
Suite 1501
Houston, TX 77030
713-798-6100
888-562-3937
FAX: 713-798-1521
www.baylorvision.com

M Bowes Hamill, Director
Al Vaughan, Manager
Michael Cassidy, Plant Manager
Research activities focus on restoring vision and preventing blindness through a better understanding of the disease.

4622 **Brown-Heatly Library**
4900 N Lamar Boulevard
Austin, TX 78756
800-252-5204
800-628-5115
e-mail: dars.inquiries@dars.state.tx.us
www.dars.state.tx.us
Houses a collection of books, audio and video tapes and periodicals focusing on rehabilitation, disabilities, employment skills and practices and management for the Texas Rehabilitation Commission. Houses materials on developmental and other disabilities, assessment and evaluation for the Texas Interagency on Early Childhood Intervention.

4623 **Center for Research on Women with Disabilities**
Baylor College of Medicine
1 Baylor Plaza
Suite B
Houston, TX 77030
713-798-5782
800-443-7693
FAX: 713-798-4688
e-mail: crowd@bcm.tmc.edu
www.bcm.edu/crowd

Margaret Nosek, Executive Director
Rosemary Hughes, Director
Kathy Fire, Administrator
Research organization dedicated to conducting research and promoting, developeing, and disseminating information to expand the life choices of women with disabilities. Conducts research and training activities on issues related to the health, independence and community integration of women and men with physical disabilities. The center has a database of psychosocial behaviors of women with disabilities.

4624 **Christian Education for the Blind**
4200 S Freeway Drive
Suite 702
Fort Worth, TX 76115
817-920-0444
FAX: 817-920-0777
e-mail: ryder@bcebonline.org
www.bcebonline.org

Roger Dyer, Director
Offers braille and large print books and cassettes for the visually impaired.

4625 **Houston Public Library: Access Center**
500 McKinney Street
1st Floor
Houston, TX 77002
832-393-1313
TTY:832-393-1539
e-mail: website@hpl.lib.tx.us
www.hpl.lib.tx.us

Toni Lambert, Director
Offers full library services to the visually and hearing impaired in Houston, TX at no charge. Houses unique and critical services for its users including online access to the Internet in a private and secure area.

4626 **Talking Book Program/Texas State Library**
Talking Book Program
PO Box 12927
Austin, TX 78711
512-463-5458
800-252-9605
FAX: 512-936-0685
e-mail: tbp.services@tsl.state.tx.us
www.texastalkingbooks.org

Ava M Smith, Director
Provides reading materials in special formats to Texas residents who cannot read conventional printed matter because of visual or physical limitations, whether permanent or temporary. The service is free and materials are sent through the mail free. Books and magazines are available in cassette, braille, recorded disk and large print formats. A Disabilities Reference Center can answer questions on topics related to disabilities.

4627 **University of Texas Southwestern Medical Center/Allergy & Immunology**
5323 Harry Hines Boulevard
Dallas, TX 75390
214-648-3111

e-mail: philip.schoch@utsouthwestern.edu
www.utsouthwestern.edu

Philip Schoch, Director
Gail Alexander, MD
Mission is to improve the health care in our community, Texas, our nation, and the world through innovation and education. To educate the next generation of leaders in patient care, biomedical science and disease prevention. To conduct high-impact, internationally recognized research. To deliver patient care that brings UT Southwestern scientific advances to the bedside-focusing on quality, safety and service.

4628 **University of Texas at Austin Library**
1 University Station
Austin, TX 78712
512-471-3434
FAX: 512-495-4347
e-mail: webform@lib.utexas.edu
www.lib.utexas.edu

Curtis Ohlendorf, Director
Sheldon Ekland-Olson, Chief Executive Officer
Provides access to information for all users, including those with disabilities, in accordance with the overall mission of the General Libraries of the University of Texas at Austin.

Utah

4629 Family Resource Library/Center for Persons with Disabilities
6800 Old Main Hill
Logan, UT 84322
435-797-1981
866-284-2821
FAX: 435-797-3944
TTY: 801-753-9750
e-mail: frl@cpd2.usu.edu
www.cpd.usa.edu/frl

Marilyn Hammond, Director
Not-for-profit service organization dedicated to collecting and loaningg materials containing practical information for families of persons with disabilities. Serves persons with disabilities and their famlies in the United States. Educational materials include books, booklets, videotapes and audiotapes.

4630 Utah State Library Division: Program for the Blind and Disabled
250 N 1950 W
Suite A
Salt Lake City, UT 84116
801-715-6777
800-662-5540
FAX: 801-715-6767
e-mail: blind@utah.gov
www.blindlibrary.utah.gov

Bessie Oakes, Program Manager
Michael Sweeny, Readers Advisor Librarian
Sarah Pitkin, Readers Advisor Librarian
Summer reading programs, Braille embosser, cassette books and magazines, children's books on cassette and other reference materials on blindness and other handicaps, descriptive videos, Braille books, large print books and radio reading service.

Vermont

4631 Vermont Department of Libraries/Special Services Unit
578 Paine Tpke N
Berlin, VT 05602
802-828-3273
800-479-1711
FAX: 802-828-2199
e-mail: marianne.kotch@dol.state.vt.us
dol.state.vt.us

Marianne Kotch, Director
Grace W Greene, Program Coordinator
Francis Woods, Manager
Service consists of reading material in large print and in talking book formats. The book collection consists of cassettes and large print. Special collections include: childrens print/braille books, reference materials on blindness, and descriptive videos.

Virginia

4632 Alexandria Library Talking Book Service
5005 Duke Street
Alexandria, VA 22304
703-519-5900
FAX: 703-519-5916
TTY:703-519-5911
e-mail: emccaffrey@alexandria.lib.va.us
www.alexandria.lib.va.us

Loni McCaffrey, Supervisor
Luis Labra, Manager
Summer reading programs, braille writer, magnifiers, closed-circuit T.V., large-print photocopier, cassette books and magazines, children's books on cassette, home visits and other reference materials on blindness and other handicaps.

4633 Arlington County Department of Libraries
Arlington County Library
1015 N Quincy Street
Arlington, VA 22201
703-228-5990
FAX: 703-228-5962
TTY:703-228-6320
e-mail: libraries@arlingtonva.us
www.arlingtonva.us

Chang Liu, Branch Manager
Summer reading programs, braille writer, magnifiers, closed-circuit T.V., large-print photocopier, cassette books and magazines, children's books on cassette, home visits and other reference materials on blindness and other handicaps.

4634 Braille Circulating Library for the Blind
2700 Stuart Avenue
Richmond, VA 23220
804-359-3743
FAX: 804-359-4777

Brian Barton, Executive Director
Offers library materials for the blind and visually impaired on a free-loan basis. Serves the entire USA and 41 foreign countries with cassette tapes, reel to reel tapes, braille books, large print books along with talking book records.

4635 Central Rappahannock Regional Library
1201 Caroline Street
Fredericksburg, VA 22401
540-372-1144
FAX: 540-373-9411
TTY:540-371-9165
www.librarypoint.org

Donna Cote, Director
Alison Heartwell, Librarian
Offers reference materials on blindness and other disabilities.

4636 Council for Exceptional Children
1110 N Glebe Road
Suite 300
Arlington, VA 22201
703-245-0600
888-232-7733
FAX: 703-264-9494
e-mail: president@cec.sped.org
www.cec.sped.org

Janice Burdick, President
Suzanne Martin, Immediate Past President
Bruce Ramirez, Manager
Members are teachers, college faculty members, administrators, supervisors and others concerned with the education and welfare of visually handicapped and blind children and youth. This is a division of the Council For Exceptional Children.

4637 Hampton Subregional Library for the Blind
Hampton Public Library
1 S Mallory Street
Hampton, VA 23663
757-727-1900
800-552-7015
FAX: 757-727-1047
e-mail: mwoolard@city.hampton.va.us

Douglas Peroy, Director
Marsha Knox, Department Head
Merry Woolard, Manager
Summer reading programs, braille writer, magnifiers, closed-circuit T.V., large-print photocopier, cassette books and magazines, children's books on cassette, home visits and other reference materials on blindness and other handicaps.

4638 James Branch Cabell Library
Virginia Commonwealth University
PO Box 842033
Richmond, VA 23284
804-828-1101
866-828-2665
866-828-2665
FAX: 804-828-0151
www.library.vcu.edu

James Branch Cabell, Founder
Gregory Rentz, Manager
Provides individualized orientations and assistance with library research and equipment.

4639 Newport News Public Library System
2400 Washington Avenue
Newport News, VA 23607
757-926-8000
FAX: 757-926-1365
e-mail: icieszyn@ci.newport-news.va.us
www.newport-news.va.us/library

Izabela M Cieszynski, Executive Director Libraries
Summer reading programs, braille writer, magnifiers, closed-circuit T.V., large-print photocopier, cassette books and magazines, children's books on cassette, home visits and other reference materials on blindness and other handicaps.

4640 Northern Virginia Resource Center for Deaf and Hard of Hearing Persons
3951 Pender Drive
Suite 130
Fairfax, VA 22030
703-352-9056
FAX: 703-352-9058
TTY:703-352-9056
e-mail: info@nvrc.org
www.nvrc.org

Cheryl Heppner, Executive Director
Empowering deaf and hard of hearing individuals and their families through education, advocacy and community involvement.

4641 Roanoke City Public Library System
706 S Jefferson Street
Roanoke, VA 24016
540-853-2473
FAX: 540-853-1781
e-mail: main.library@roanokeva.gov
www.roanokegov.com/library

Sheila Umberger, Executive Director
Summer reading programs, braille writer, magnifiers, closed-circuit T.V., large-print photocopier, cassette books and magazines, children's books on cassette, home visits and other reference materials on blindness and other handicaps.

4642 Special Services/Talking Books
Fairfax County Public Library
12000 Government Center Parkway
Suite 123
Fairfax, VA 22035
703-324-3185
FAX: 703-324-8386
TTY:703-324-8365
e-mail: access@fairfaxcounty.gov

E S Clay, Director
Lindsey Culin, Manager
Offers talking books, TDD access, assistive devices such as decoders for three-week loans, support groups for people who are visually impaired, library program interpreters available with four weeks advance notice, adapted computer work station with braille printer and assistive listening devices.

4643 Staunton Public Library Talking Book Center
1 Churchville Avenue
Staunton, VA 24401
540-885-6215
800-995-6215
FAX: 540-332-3906
e-mail: library@ci.staunton.va.us
www.talkingbookcenter.org

Oakley Pearson, Librarian
Offers free library service by circulating recorded books, magazines, and playback equipment to individuals unable to use standard print materials because of visual or physical impairment.

4644 University of Virginia Health System General Clinical Research Group
PO Box 800787
Charlottesville, VA 22908
434-924-2394
FAX: 434-924-9960
e-mail: gcrc@virginia.edu
gcrc.med.virginia.edu

Eugene J Barrett, Program Director
Mary Vance, Associate Director
Cassie Bourne, Manager
Provides investigators with the specialized resources necessary to conduct advanced clinical research. The facility includes ten inpatient beds, skilled research nurses, a core assay laboratory, a metabolic kitchen, outpatient facilities, computing and statistical consultants and facilities, and sleep and exercise physiology laboratories.
1968

4645 Virginia Autism Resource Center
4100 Price Club Boulevard
Midlothian, VA 23112
804-674-8888
877-667-7771
877- -
FAX: 804-276-3970
e-mail: info@varc.org
www.varc.org

Carol Schall, Director
Florence McLeod, Administrative Assistant
Janee Sprinkle, Manager
Provides training, individual case consultation, materials and information to families and professionals working with individuals with autism in Virginia.
1983

4646 Virginia Beach Public Library Special Services Library
936 Independence Boulevard
Virginia Beach, VA 23455
757-464-9175
FAX: 757-464-6741
www.vpgov.com/library

Carolyn Caywood, Director
Allenne Wicher, Manager
A public library for people with visual and physical disabilities, braille writer, magnifiers, closed-circuit T.V., large-print photocopier, cassette books and magazines, children's books on cassette, and other reference materials on blindness and other disabilities.

4647 Virginia Chapter of the Arthtitis Foundation
3805 Cutshaw Avenue
Suite 200
Richmond, VA 23230
804-359-1700
800-456-4687
FAX: 804-359-4900
e-mail: info.va@arthritis.org
www.arthritis.org

W Robert Irby, Medical Director
Provides free information, services and counseling to the public. Services include assistance in locating and accessing government and other health care programs for persons with arthritis, referral to doctors specializing in the treatment of arthritis, free literature about the different types of arthritis and counseling for people with arthritis and their families.

4648 Virginia State Library for the Visually and Physically Handicapped
395 Azalea Avenue
Richmond, VA 23227
804-266-2477
800-552-7015
FAX: 804-371-3508
e-mail: barbara.mccarthy@dbvi.virginia.gov

Nicholas Morgan, Executive Director
Laura Rhodes, Office Manager
Summer reading programs, braille writer, magnifiers, closed-circuit T.V., large-print photocopier, cassette books and magazines, children's books on cassette, home visits and other reference materials on blindness and other handicaps.

Washington

4649 Meridian Valley Clinical Laboratory
801 SW 16th Street
Suite 126
Renton, WA 98055
425-271-8689
FAX: 425-271-8674
e-mail: meridian@meridianvalleylab.com
www.meridianvalleylab.com

Jonathan Wright, Medical Director
Holly Han, Owner
A clinical test facility dedicated to providing the most accurate and informative data for patient diagnosis and therapeutic monitoring. With our current research and up-to-date information and various aspects of clinical nutritional medicine, our methodologies and capabilities include areas of analytical chemistry, heavy metal determination, microbiology, and immunology.

4650 Ophthalmic Research Laboratory Eye Institute/First Hill Campus
747 Broadway
Seattle, WA 98122
206-386-6000
800-793-3474
www.swedish.org

Richard Peterson, Chief Executive Officer
Color vision physiology, vision disorders and blindness research.

4651 Washington Talking Book and Braille Library
2021 9th Avenue
Seattle, WA 98121
206-615-0400
800-542-0866
FAX: 206-464-0247
TTY: 206-615-0418
e-mail: wtbbl@wtbbl.org
www.wtbbl.org

Gloria Leonard, Director
Summer reading programs, braille writer, magnifiers, closed-circuit T.V., large-print photocopier, cassette books and magazines, children's books, and other reference materials on blindness and other handicaps, online catalog, reference station with assistive devices and a radio reading service.

West Virginia

4652 Cabell County Public Library/Talking Book Department/Subregional Library for the Blind
455 9th Street
Huntington, WV 25701
304-528-5700
FAX: 304-528-5701
e-mail: library@cabell.lib.wv.us
www.cabell.lib.wv.us

Lottie Simms, President
Judy Rule, Manager
Summer reading programs, Braille writer, magnifiers, closed-circuit TV, cassette books and magazines, children's books on cassette reference materials on blindness and other handicaps, enlargers and Arkenstone Reader.

4653 Division of Rehabilitation Services: Staff Library
PO Box 1004
Institute, WV 25112
304-766-4644
800-642-8207
e-mail: carolc@mail.drs.state.wv.us

Carol R Johnson, Librarian/Manager
Specialized library with information on disabilities and the rehabilitation there of special collections: deaf and hard of hearing, visually impaired/blind, wellness center, literacy and career. The library has assistive devices such as CCTV, scanner and enhancement software. Also braille magazines, large print, talking books, magazines on cassette, descriptive videos, captioned media program, newspapers, magazines/journals, video, computers with internet access, fax, and a copier.

4654 Kanawha County Public Library
123 Capitol Street
Charleston, WV 25301
304-343-4646
FAX: 304-348-6530
e-mail: webmaster@kanawha.lib.wv.us
/kanawha.lib.wv.us

Pamela D Tarr, President
Linda Wright, Manager
Summer reading programs, large print PC option, magnifiers, large type books, cassette books, and magazines, children's books on cassette, home visits and other reference materials on blindness and other handicaps

4655 Ohio County Public Library Services for the Blind and Physically Handicapped
52 16th Street
Wheeling, WV 26003
304-232-0244
FAX: 304-232-6848
e-mail: ocplweb@weirton.lib.wv.us
wheeling.weirton.lib.wv.us

Lester Hess, Chairman
Dorothy Thomas, Manager
The Ohio Public Library exists to provide books and related materials that will assist the residents of the community in the pursuit of knowledge, information, education, research, and recreation in order to promote an enlightned citizenry and to enrich their quality of life.

4656 Talking Book Department, Parkersburg and Wood County Public Library
3100 Emerson Avenue
Parkersburg, WV 26104
304-420-4587
800-642-8674
FAX: 304-420-4589
e-mail: hickmanm@hp9k.park.lib.wv.us

Michael Hickman, Coordinator Services
Brian Raitz, Manager
Services for the bind and physically handicapped. Library of Congress Talking Book Program.

4657 West Virginia Autism Training Center
Marshall University College Of Educational & Human
1 John Marshall Drive
Suite 316
Huntington, WV 25755
304-696-2332
800-344-5115
www.marshall.edu/coe/atc
Provides education, training, and treatment programs for W Virginians who have autism, pervasive devolopmental disorders or Asperger's disease and have formally been registered with the center.

4658 West Virginia Library Commission
1900 Kanawha Boulevard E
Charleston, WV 25305
304-558-2041
800-642-9021
FAX: 304-558-2044
e-mail: web_one@wvlc.lib.wv.us
http://librarycommision.lib.wv.us

Denise Ash, Director
Joe Manchin, Governor
Sarah Hamrick, Executive Director
Summer reading programs, braille writer, magnifiers, closed-circuit T.V., large-print photocopier, cassette books and magazines, children's books on cassette, home visits and other reference materials on blindness and other handicaps.

4659 West Virginia School for the Blind Library
301 E Main Street
Romney, WV 26757
304-822-4894
FAX: 304-822-4896
e-mail: cjohn@access.mountain.net

Jane McBride, Director
Cynthia Johnson, Librarian
Summer reading programs, braille writer, magnifiers, closed-circuit T.V., large-print photocopier, cassette books and magazines, children's books on cassette, home visits and other reference materials on blindness and other handicaps.

Wisconsin

4660 **Brown County Library**
Central Library Downtown
2255 Main Street
Green Bay, WI 54302
920-391-4600
FAX: 920-391-4601
TTY:920-448-4400
e-mail: bc_library@co.brown.wi.us
www.co.brown.wi.us/library

Bob Bush, President
Mike Aubinger, Vice President
Louanne Crowder, Manager
Summer reading programs, braille writer, magnifiers, closed-circuit TV, large-print photocopier, cassette books and magazines, children's books on cassette, home visits and other reference materials on blindness and other handicaps.

4661 **Eye Institute of the Medical College of Wisconsin and Froedtert Clinic**
925 N 87th Street
Milwaukee, WI 53226
414-456-2020
FAX: 414-456-6300
e-mail: eyecare@mcw.edu
http://doctor.mcw.edu/clinic

Mary Blackwelder, Director
Richard Schultz, MD
A national leader as a full-service academic opthalmology program. Dedicated to the highest quality patient care, education, and vision research, the faculty and staff strive to provide state-of-the-art clinical and surgical patient care in a compassionate and timely way.
1976

4662 **Trace Research and Development Center**
University of Wisconsin-Madison
2107 Engineering Centers Building
1550 Engineering Drive
Madison, WI 53706
608-262-6966
FAX: 608-262-8848
TTY:608-263-5408
e-mail: info@trace.wisc.edu
www.trace.wisc.edu

Gregg Vanderheiden, Center Director
The mission is to prevent the barriers and capitalize on the opportunities presented by current and emerging information and telecommunication technologies, in order to create a world that is as accessible and usable as possible. Currently the center is working on ways to make standard information technologies and telecommunications systems more accessible and usable by people with disabilities.

4663 **Wisconsin Regional Library for the Blind & Physically Handicapped**
813 W Wells Street
Milwaukee, WI 53233
414-286-3045
800-242-8822
FAX: 414-286-3102
TTY: 414-286-3548
e-mail: lbph@mpl.org
http://dpi.state.wi.us/rll/wr;bph/index

Marsha Valance, Regional Librarian/Manager
Circulates recorded materials, playback equipment and braille materials to print-handicapped Wisconsin residents.

Wyoming

4664 **Wyoming Services for the Visually Impaired**
Wyoming Department of Education
2300 Capitol Avenue
Hathaway Building, 2nd Floor
Cheyenne, WY 82002
307-777-7690
FAX: 307-777-6234
e-mail: golson@educ.state.wy.us
www.k12.wy.us/SE/svi.asp

Gary Olson, Supervisor
Services for the Visually Impaired assists people of all ages who have low vision or are blind. The goal is to provide information, education, and support to individuals with low vision in order that they may lead enjoyable and productive lives with maximum degree of independence.

4665 **Wyoming's New Options in Technology (WYNOT) - University of Wyoming**
1000 E University Avenue
Laramie, WY 82072
307-766-2084
800-861-4312
FAX: 307-721-2084
e-mail: wynot.uw@uwyo.edu
http://wind.uwyo.edu/wynot

Kathy Laurin, Executive Director
Britney Alspach, PR Coordinator
Designed to develop and implement a consumer oriented statewide system of technology-related assistance for people with disabilities of all ages.

Children & Young Adults

4666 A Christian Approach to Overcoming Disability: A Doctor's Story
Haworth Press
10 Alice Street
Binghamton, NY 13904
607-722-5857
800-429-6784
FAX: 607-722-6362
e-mail: orders@haworthpress.com
www.haworthpress.com

S Harrington-Miller, Advertising
William Cohen, Owner
This is the personal account of a Christian physician who changed her career specialty from obstetrics and gynecology when she was diagnosed with a genetic disease that would cause her to become blind. Dr. Elaine Eng offers faith-based and psychological techniques for coping with disability. *$29.95*
174 pages Hardcover
ISBN 0-789022-57-5

4667 ABCD Newsletter Volume Reprints
Birth Defect Research for Children
930 Woodcock Road
Suite 225
Orlando, FL 32803
407-895-0802
FAX: 407-895-0824
e-mail: staff@birthdefects.org
www.birthdefects.org

Betty Mekdeci, Executive Director
Offers a variety of reprints from the ABCD newsletter on birth defects
Monthly

4668 AT for Infants and Toddlers with Disabilities
Idaho Assistive Technology Project
129 W 3rd Street
Moscow, ID 83843
208-885-3559
800-432-8324
FAX: 208-885-3628
e-mail: rseiler@uidaho.edu
www.educ.uidaho.edu/idatech

$5.00
68 pages

4669 Assistive Technology for School Age
Idaho Assistive Technology Project
129 W 3rd Street
Moscow, ID 83843
208-885-3559
800-432-8324
FAX: 208-885-3628
e-mail: rseiler@uidaho.edu
www.educ.uidaho.edu/idatech

$5.00
84 pages

4670 Birth Defect News
Birth Defect Research for Children
930 Woodcock Road
Suite 225
Orlando, FL 32803
407-895-0802
FAX: 407-895-0824
e-mail: staff@birthdefects.org
www.birthdefects.org

Betty Mekdeci, Executive Director
Offers updated information on the association activities, events and updates regarding birth defects and environmental exposures.
Monthly

4671 Caring for Children with Chronic Illness
Springer Publishing Company
536 Broadway
New York, NY 10012
212-431-4370
877-687-7476
FAX: 212-941-7842
e-mail: marketing@springerpub.com
www.springerpub.com

Annette Imperati, Marketing/Sales Director
Ursula Springer, President
A critical look at the current medical, social, and psychological framework for providing care to children with chronic illnesses. Emphasizing the need to create integrated, interdisciplinary approaches, it discusses issues such as the roles of families, professionals, and institutions in providing health care, the impact of a child's illness on various family structures, financing care, the special problems of chronically ill children as they become adolescents and more. *$36.95*
320 pages Hardcover
ISBN 0-82615 -00-1

4672 Complete IEP Guide: How to Advocate for Yo ur Special Ed Child
Spina Bifida Association of America
4590 Macarthur Boulevard NW
Suite 250
Washington, DC 20007
202-944-3285
800-621-3141
FAX: 202-944-3295
e-mail: sbaa@sbaa.org
www.sbaa.org

Cindy Brownstein, Chief Executive Officer
This all-in-one guide will help you understand special education law, identify your child's needs, prepare for meetings, develop the IEP and resolve disputes. *$28.95*

4673 Coping with Being Physically Challenged
Rosen Publishing Group
29 E 21st Street
New York, NY 10010
212-777-3017
FAX: 888-436-4643
e-mail: rosenpub@tribeca.ios.com

Roger Rosen, President
Ratto deals with strong emotions, such as general anger and depression, which affect these young adults and their families. The author shows them how to deal and cope on a day-to-day basis. *$15.95*

ISBN 0-82391 -44-9

4674 Delicate Threads
Woodbine House
6510 Bells Mill Road
Bethesda, MD 20817
301-897-3570
800-843-7323
FAX: 301-897-5838
www.woodbinehouse.com

Irv Shapell, Owner
How do friendships between children with and without disabilities develop? How do they compare to friendships between typically developing children? What happens to these friendships over time? In Delicate Threads, author Debbie staub helps to answer these questions through careful observations of friendships between seven pairs of children - each including a child with a moderate to severe disability - who are classmates in an inclusive Pacific Northwest elementary school. *$16.95*
250 pages Paperback
ISBN 0-933149-90-5

4675 Don't Call Me Special: A First Look at Dis ability
Barron's Educational Series

This picture book explores questions and concerns about physical disabilities in a simple and reassuring way. Youger children can find out about individual disabilities, special equipment that is available to help the disabled, and how people of all ages can deal with disabilities and live happy and full lives. *$6.95*

32 pages Paperback 2002
ISBN 0-764121-18-9

4676 Enabling Romance: A Guide to Love, Sex & Relationships for the Disabled
Spina Bifida Association of America
4590 Macarthur Boulevard NW
Suite 250
Washington, DC 20007
202-944-3285
800-621-3141
FAX: 202-944-3295
e-mail: sbaa@sbaa.org
www.sbaa.org

Cindy Brownstein, Chief Executive Officer
An uncensored, illustrated guide to intimacy and sexual expression for persons with physical disabilities. *$15.95*

4677 For Siblings Only
Family Resource Associates
35 Haddon Avenue
Shrewsbury, NJ 07702
732-747-5310
FAX: 732-747-1896

Sue Levine, Social Worker
Nancy Phalanukorn, Manager
A newsletter for brothers and sisters, aged 4 through 10, whose sibling has a disablilty. Includes stories, library resources, activities and discussion of feelings. $12/year for families, $20/year for professionals. *$12.00*
12 pages Quarterly

4678 Helping Children Understand Disabilities
Brookline Books
PO Box 1046
Cambridge, MA 02139
617-868-0360
800-666-2665
FAX: 617-868-1772
e-mail: thestore@brooklinebooks.com
www.brooklinebooks.com
Examines children's literature as a vehicle to help children, parents and teachers understand important issues relating to the effects of disability on children. Using the child as narrator, the author demonstrates how to use popular children's fiction to explore taboo areas and stimulate discussion by children and adults. *$10.95*
Hardcover
ISBN 0-91479 -09-3

4679 Invisible Children
Learning Corporation of America
6493 Kaiser Drive
Fremont, CA 94555
510-490-7311

Oonchia Chia, Owner
Renaldo was blind, Mandy was deaf, and Mark had Cerebral Palsy and used a wheelchair. These child-size puppet characters interacted with non-handicapped puppets.
Film

4680 It isn't Fair!: Siblings of Children with Disabilities
Greenwood Publishing Group
88 Post Road W
Suite 5007
Westport, CT 06880
203-226-3571
FAX: 203-222-1502
www.greenwood.com

Wayne Smith, President
This book presents a wide range of perspectives on the relationship of siblings to children with disabilities. These perspectives are written in the first person by parents, young adult siblings, younger siblings, and professionals.
200 pages $39.95 - $45
ISBN 0-897893-32-8

4681 Kid Kare News
3101 SW Sam Jackson Park Road
Portland, OR 97239
FAX: 503-241-5090
www.shrinershq.org

Barbara Flaherty, New Patient Coordinator
Sonia Bouchard, Rehabilation Services Manager
Kerry Grindeland, Care Coordination Manager
Bi-annual publication from the Shriners Hospital for Children in Portland, Oregon. Free. Produced by the medical staff.

4682 Kidz Korner
Children's Hopes & Dreams Wish Foundation
280 Us Highway 46
Dover, NJ 07801
973-361-7348
800-437-3262
FAX: 973-361-6627
e-mail: chdfdover@juno.com
www.childrenswishes.org

Mariann Oswald, Manager
6 pages Monthly

4683 Laugh with Accent, #3
Accent Books & Products
PO Box 700
Bloomington, IL 61702
309-378-2961
800-787-8444
FAX: 309-378-4420
e-mail: acmtlvng@aol.com

Raymond C Cheever, Publisher
Betty Garee, Editor
These special cartoons prove laughter is the best medicine of all. It's when the laughter stops that we become truly disabled, say readers. *$3.50*
89 pages Paperback
ISBN 0-91570 -16-7

4684 Life Beyond the Classroom: Transition Strategies for Young People
Brookes Publishing
PO Box 10624
Baltimore, MD 21285
410-337-9580
800-638-3775
FAX: 410-337-8539
e-mail: custserv@brookespublishing.com
www.brookespublishing.com

Clary Creighton, Exhibits Coordinator
Tracy Gray, Educational Sales Manager
Paul Brooks, Owner
This textbook is an essential guide to planning, designing, and implementing successful transition programs for students with disabilities. *$44.00*
496 pages
ISBN 1-55766 -05-7

4685 Life Planning Workbook
Exceptional Parent Library
PO Box 1807
Englewood Cliffs, NJ 07632
201-947-6000
800-535-1910
FAX: 201-947-9376
e-mail: eplibrary@aol.com
www.eplibrary.com
A hands-on guide to help parents provide for the future security and happiness of their child with a disability after their death. *$24.95*

4686 Little Children, Big Needs
Exceptional Parent Library
PO Box 1807
Englewood Cliffs, NJ 07632
201-947-6000
800-535-1910
FAX: 201-947-9376
e-mail: eplibrary@aol.com
www.eplibrary.com
Contains candid interviews with fifty families of children with a wide variety of disabilities. *$12.95*

4687 Mandy
William Morrow & Company
1350 Avenue of the Americas
New York, NY 10019
212-974-3100
FAX: 212-261-6595
www.williammorrow.com

Told from the point of view of a deaf child, this warm picture book is neither saccharine nor preachy. Mandy has never heard anyone speak or sing. It is from her close relationship with her grandmother that the small girl learns about the world through lip-reading, facial expression, gesture, touch and sign. *$14.95*
32 pages

4688 Mayor of the West Side
4196 Washington Street
Suite 2
Boston, MA 02131
617-469-4999
800-937-4113
FAX: 617-469-3379
e-mail: info@fanlight.com
www.fanlight.com

Sandy St Louis, Distribution Director
Kelli English, Publicity Coordinator
Ben Achtenberg, Owner
What happens when love gets in the way of letting go? As a teenager with multiple disabilities prepares for his Bar Mitzvah, his family and community consider what Mark's life will be like when they are no longer able to protect him. *$199.00*

ISBN 1-572953-95-0

4689 Me, Too
JB Lippincott
227 E Washington Square
Philadelphia, PA 19106
215-521-8300
800-777-2295
FAX: 215-824-7390

J Lippincott, Chief Executive Officer
Lydia and Lornie were twins. Lydia was a bright twelve year old who vowed to spend her summer vacation teaching her retarded sister, Lornie, how to be normal.
158 pages Hardcover
ISBN 0-39731 -85-X

4690 Miles Away and Still Caring: A Guide for Long Distance Caregivers
AARP Fulfillment
601 E Street NW
Washington, DC 20049
202-434-2277
800-424-3410
FAX: 202-434-3443
e-mail: member@aarp.org
www.aarp.org

William Novelli, Chief Executive Officer
This is one of the most helpful and frequently requested publications. Helps people who must coordinate the care of a loved one from a long distance.
18 pages

4691 My Body is Not Who I Am
Aquarius Health Care Videos
PO Box 1159
Sherborn, MA 01770
508-650-6905
888-440-2963
FAX: 508-650-4216
e-mail: aqvideos@tiac.net
www.aquariusproductions.com

Leslie Kussman, President
This thought-provoking video introduces viewers to people who openly discuss the struggles and triumphs they have experienced living in a body that is physically disabled. They talk honestly about the social stigma of their disability and the problems they face in terms of mobility, health care and family relationships, as well as the challenges of emotional and sexual intimacy. Preview option available. *$195.00*
Video

4692 My Buddy
Exceptional Parent Library
PO Box 1807
Englewood Cliffs, NJ 07632
201-947-6000
800-535-1910
FAX: 201-947-9376
e-mail: eplibrary@aol.com
www.eplibrary.com
Story focuses on the friendship between a boy with a disability and his loyal golden retriever. *$5.95*
Library Binding 1999
ISBN 0-785799-24-9

4693 Negotiating the Disability Maze
Charles C Thomas
2600 S 1st Street
Springfield, IL 62704
217-789-8980
800-258-8980
FAX: 217-789-9130
e-mail: books@ccthomas.com
www.ccthomas.com

Michael Thomas, President
This book has been designed and written to furnish people from diverse backgrounds with important information regarding education of children with disabilities. The authors are as thorough as they are explicit. They analyze the concepts, translate the jargon, and outline the characteristics of various disabilities. Also avalable in cloth edition. *$36.95*
206 pages Paperback
ISBN 0-398066-64-7

4694 Negotiating the Special Education Maze: A Guide for Parents and Teachers
Spina Bifida Association of America
4590 Macarthur Boulevard NW
Suite 250
Washington, DC 20007
202-944-3285
800-621-3141
FAX: 202-944-3295
e-mail: sbaa@sbaa.org
www.sbaa.org

Cindy Brownstein, Chief Executive Officer
An excellent aid for the development of an effective special education program. *$19.00*

4695 New Horizons Independent Living Center
8085 E Manley Drive
Prescott Valley, AZ 86314
928-772-1266
800-406-2377
FAX: 928-772-3808
e-mail: nhilc@cableone.net
www.newhorizonsilc.org

Liz Toone, Executive Director
Zena Taylor, Financial Manager
Jean Lasher, Community Info Coordinator
An advocacy and living center organized by and for people with disabilities, serving Apache, Coconino, Mojave, Navajo and Yavapai counties.

4696 NoBody's Perfect....Educating Children about Disabilities
Aquarius Health Care Videos
PO Box 1159
Sherborn, MA 01770
508-650-6905
FAX: 508-650-4216
e-mail: aqvideos@tiac.net
An upbeat, inclusion-friendly program for kids that profiles three children with disabilties. Viewers discover that accepting differences is an essential part of growing up. We learn how the kids cope and, in the process, are introduced to signing, prosthetics, and assistive technology and Braille. Videocassette, preview option is available. *$ 99.00*

4697 On Our Own Terms: Children Living with Physical Disabilities
Gareth Stevens
1555 N River Center Drive
Milwaukee, WI 53212
414-332-3520
800-542-2595
FAX: 414-225-0377

Bob Famighetti, Publisher
Meet Kicki, a three-year-old with Spina Bifida, battling to walk for the first time. Meet Annelie, nine years old, learning to walk again after a bad car accident. Face the physical challenges with her. *$13.95*

48 pages
ISBN 1-555329-42-X

4698 Recognizing Children with Special Needs
Aquarius Health Care Videos
PO Box 1159
Sherborn, MA 01770
508-650-6905
FAX: 508-650-4216
e-mail: aqvideos@tiac.net
www.aquariusproductions.com

A great overview for caregivers of children on how to recognize special needs. Often-times it is the little things children do everyday to compensate for, or express, a disability that can be observed by their caregiver. All types of disabilities are addressed: emotional, physical, psychological, and chronic illness. A wonderful tool for teachers, childcare staff, and students on how to play a vital role in our children's development. Preview option available. *$125.00*
Video

4699 Reflections on Growing Up Disabled
Council for Exceptional Children
1110 N Glebe Road
Suite 300
Arlington, VA 22201
703-245-0600
FAX: 703-264-9494
www.cec.sped.org

Janice Burdick, President
Bruce Ramirez, Manager
Understand how it feels to be a disabled person in school by tuning in to the first-hand accounts of people who have disabilities. *$10.00*
112 pages

4700 Rolling Along with Goldilocks and the Thre e Bears
Spina Bifida Association of America
4590 Macarthur Boulevard NW
Suite 250
Washington, DC 20007
202-944-3285
800-621-3141
FAX: 202-944-3295
e-mail: sbaa@sbaa.org
www.sbaa.org

Cindy Brownstein, Chief Executive Officer
The familiar fairytale with a special needs twist. Ages 3-7. *$17.00*

4701 Shining Bright: Head Start Inclusion
Brookes Publishing
PO Box 10624
Baltimore, MD 21285
410-337-9580
800-638-3775
FAX: 410-337-8539
e-mail: custserv@brookespublishing.com
www.brookespublishing.com

Paul Brooks, Owner
This documentary depicts the collaborative efforts of a Head Start and a local education agency to include children with severe disabilities in a Head Start program. This video addresses issues such as support for children with severe health impairments, benefits of participating in Head Start, ability of teachers with a general education background to serve children with severe disabilities, and staff relations. Includes a 28-page saddle-stitched booklet. *$45.00*
23 Minutes
ISBN 1-55766 -95-9

4702 Sibling Forum
Family Resource Associates
35 Haddon Avenue
Shrewsbury, NJ 07702
732-747-5310
FAX: 732-747-1896

Susan Levine, Social Worker
Nancy Phalanukorn, Manager
A newsletter for brothers and sisters, aged 10 through teen, whose sibling has a disablilty. Includes input from readers, library resources and discussion of feelings. $12/year for families, $20/year for professionals. *$12.00*
8-12 pages Quarterly

4703 Sibshops: Workshops for Siblings of Children with Special Needs
Brookes Publishing
PO Box 10624
Baltimore, MD 21285
410-337-9580
800-638-3775
FAX: 410-337-8539
e-mail: custserv@brookespublishing.com
www.brookespublishing.com

Paul Brooks, Owner
Sibshops is a program that brings together 8-to 13-year-old brothers and sisters of children with special needs. The siblings receive support and information in a recreational setting, so they have fun while they learn. *$32.00*
256 pages Paperback
ISBN 1-55766 -69-3

4704 Someday's Child
Educational Productions
9000 SW Gemini Drive
Beaverton, OR 97008
503-644-7000
800-950-4949
FAX: 503-350-7000
e-mail: custserv@edpro.com
www.edpro.com

Linda Freedman, President/Co-Owner
Molly Krumm, Marketing Director
This video focuses on three families' search for help and information for their children with disabilities.

4705 Special Children/Special Solutions
Option Indigo Press
2080 S Undermountain Road
Sheffield, MA 01257
413-229-8727
800-562-7171
FAX: 413-229-8727
e-mail: indigo@option.org
www.optionindigo.com

Kate Wilde
This four-tape audio series presents concrete, down-to-earth, no-nonsense alternatives which are full of love and acceptance for the special child while being wholly supportive of parents, professionals and helpers who want to reach out. The accepting (nonjudgmental) attitude presented is the basis of all Samahria's work and is the foundation for the nurturing teaching process that has encouraged and helped parents, children and others to accomplish more than most would have believed. *$55.00*
Audio

4706 Special Education Report
Aspen Publishers
7201 McKinney Circle
Frederick, MD 21704
301-698-7100
800-638-8437
FAX: 301-695-7931
e-mail: customer.service@aspenpubl.com
www.aspenpublishers.com

Judith Ree, Manager
Published biweekly, Special Education Report is the independent news service on law, policy and funding of programs for disabled children. *$16.00*
8-12 pages Newsletter

4707 Special Format Books for Children and Youth Ages 3-19
Cultural Education Center
Albany, NY 12230
518-474-5935
800-342-3688
www.nysl.nysed.gov/tbbl/index.html

Jane Somers, Director

4708 Special Format Books for Children and Youth: Ages 3-19.Serving New York City/Long Island
476 5th Avenue
New York, NY 10018 212-206-5400
e-mail: pleclerc@nypl.org
www.nypl.org

Paul LeClerc, President
Robert Brian, Manager

4709 The Comprehensive Directory: Programs and Services And Special Needs In The Metro NY Area.
Resources for Children with Special Needs
116 E 16th Street
Floor 5
New York, NY 10003 212-677-4650
FAX: 212-254-4070
e-mail: info@resourcesnyc.org
www.resourcesnyc.org

Karen Schlesinger, Executive Director
Dianne Littwin, Director Publishing
The second edition of this publication from resources for children with special needs, inc. covers more than 3000 agencies providing all types of services, education, child care, after school, employment, residential, medical and health care, parenting programs and family support. provides 1500 pages of valuable and timely information. *$ 22.00*
308 pages Yearly
ISBN 0-967836-57-3

4710 Tools for Students
Aquarius Health Care Videos
PO Box 1159
Sherborn, MA 01770 508-650-6905
FAX: 508-650-4216
e-mail: aqvideos@tiac.net
www.aquariusproductions.com
Provides a series of 26 fun occupational therapy sensory processing activities. Designed as an in-home, in-workshop, and in-class exercise leader with students. Activities include: Strenghten the muscles necessary for normal activities, provide the muscles necessary to enhance alertness and concentration, increase the ability to use good posture, help social skills and fitting in and increase coordination; concludes with emphasis on team collaboration between the student, teacher, and parents. *$99.00*
Video

4711 Transition Matters: from School to Independence: A Guide and Directory of Services
Resources for Children with Special Needs
116 E 16th Street
Floor 5
New York, NY 10003 212-677-4650
FAX: 212-254-4070
e-mail: info@resourcesnyc.org
www.resourcesnyc.org

Karen Schlesinger, Executive Director
Dianne Littwin, Director Publications
A guide to the need for transition planning; plus 1000 agencies and organizations that provide post secondary education, vocational services, learning options and family support to children with disabilities transitioning out of high school. *$35.00*
496 pages
ISBN 0-967836-56-5

4712 Understanding Cub Scouts with Disabilities
Boy Scouts of America
1325 W Walnut Hill Lane
Irving, TX 75038 972-580-2000
800-323-0732

Roy Williams, Chief Executive Officer
Manual on how to teach and understand boy scouts with handicaps.
10 pages

4713 Views from Our Shoes
Spina Bifida Association of America
4590 Macarthur Boulevard NW
Washington, DC 20007 202-944-3285
800-621-3141
FAX: 202-944-3295
e-mail: sbaa@sbaa.org
www.sbaa.org

Cindy Brownstein, Chief Executive Officer
Siblings share what it is like to have a brother or sister with a disability. Age 9 and up. *$17.00*
106 pages Paperback

4714 What About Me?
Educational Productions
9000 SW Gemini Drive
Beaverton, OR 97008 503-644-7000
800-950-4949
FAX: 503-350-7000
e-mail: custserve@edpro.com
www.edpro.com

Linda Freedman, President/Co-Owner
Molly Krumm, Marketing Director
This video focuses on two siblings of children with disabilities. The siblings (Brian and Julie) share their perspectives, their worries, concerns and victories about living with a sibling with a disability.

4715 What About Me? Growing Up with a Developme ntally Disabled Sibling
Perseus Publishing

Silverstein, a physician, gives a first-person account of his experiences as the older brother of an autistic sibling. Siegel, a developmental psychologist, presents discussion of family approaches to handicaps based on clinical interviews with some 1,000 families of various ethnic, social, and educational backgrounds. *$24.00*
316 pages Paperback 2001
ISBN 0-738206-30-X

4716 What It's Like to be Me
Friendship Press
PO Box 37844
Cincinnati, OH 45222 513-948-8733
FAX: 513-761-3722
www.ncccusa.org

Nancy Kennedy, Customer Service
Robert Bray, Manager
This was written and illustrated entirely by children with handicapped conditions. These contributions invite the reader to set aside any pity or prejudices and listen. Black and white, and color drawings and photographs make this book visually appealing, enjoyable for all ages. *$10.95*

4717 When Billy Broke His Head...and Other Tales of Wonder
Fanlight Productions
4196 Washington Street
Suite 2
Boston, MA 02131 617-469-4999
800-937-4113
FAX: 617-469-3379
e-mail: info@fanlight.com
www.fanlight.com

Elena Cambio
Ben Achtenberg, Owner
When Billy Golfus, an award-winning journalist, became brain damaged as the result of a motor scooter accident, he joined the ranks of the 43 million Americans with disabilities, this country's largest and most invisible minority. He helped create this video, which blends humor with politics and individual experience with a chorus of voices, to explain what it is really like to live with a disability in America. #136 *$195.00*

ISBN 1-57295 -36-2

4718 When I Grow Up
Britannica Film Company
345 4th Street
San Francisco, CA 94107 415-777-9876

At a costume party each child was to come as what they wanted to be when they grew up. Some of the children had handicaps, and they talked about why their handicaps would not prevent them from fulfilling their desires.
Film

4719 When Parents Can't Fix It
Fanlight Productions
4196 Washington Street
Suite 2
Boston, MA 02131 617-469-4999
800-937-4113
FAX: 617-469-3379
e-mail: fanlight@fanlight.com
www.fanlight.com

Karen McMillen, Marketing Director
Cynthia Conti, Publicity Coordinator
Ben Achtenberg, Owner
This documentary looks at the lives of five families who are raising children with disabilities - the problems they face, how they have learned to cope, and the rewards and stresses of adapting to their child's condition. It explores the medical complexities and financial pressures families encounter, the emotional and physical toll on parents and siblings, and the dangers of child abuse in this population. It offers a very realistic look at different family strengths and coping styles. *$245.00*

4720 Why My Child

800-313-ABDC
www.birthdefects.org
A 9 1/2 minute video that explores the feelings every parent has when their child is born with a birth defect. Emmy-award-winning producer, Karen Dorsett, has created a compelling video that begins with the parents' question, why my child? Follows through to concerns about links between birth defects and environmental exposures to drugs, pesticides, dioxin, radiation, hazardous wastes, etc. *$25.00*

Community

4721 A Commitment to Inclusion: Outreach to Unserved/Underserved Populations
Independent Living Research Utilization ILRU
2323 S Shepherd Drive
Suite 1000
Houston, TX 77019 713-520-0232
FAX: 713-520-5785
www.ilru.org

Laurie Redd, Executive Director
Carol Bradley describes Independent Living Resource Center San Francisco's community organizing/outreach approach to serving under-represented consumers. This organization successfully reaches persons with pychiatric disabilities, environmental illness/multiple chemical sensitivities, chronic fatigue immune deficiency syndrome, learning disabilities, institutionalized persons, Chinese, Latinos, deaf/hard of hearing, and lesbian/bisexual populations.
10 pages

4722 California Community Care News Community Residential Care Association of CA
Charles W Skoien Jr
PO Box 163270
Sacramento, CA 95816 916-455-0723
FAX: 916-455-7201
e-mail: crcac@comcast.net

Charles W Skoien Jr, Editor/Publisher
Forum for the exchange of ideas, information and opinions among clients, families and service providers. Information regarding services and assisted living programs for the elderly, mentally ill and disabled. *$45.00*
24 pages Monthly

4723 Community Recreation and People with Disabilities: Strategies for Inclusion
Brookes Publishing
PO Box 10624
Baltimore, MD 21285 410-337-9580
800-638-3775
FAX: 410-337-8539
e-mail: custserv@brookespublishing.com
www.brookespublishing.com

Paul Brooks, Owner
Offers creative ideas and new techniques for including people with disabilities in community recreation programs. *$39.00*
368 pages Paperback 1997
ISBN 1-55766 -59-2

4724 Crossing the River: Creating a Conceptual Revolution in Community & Disability
Brookline Books
PO Box 1047
Cambridge, MA 02139 617-868-0360
800-666-2665
FAX: 617-868-1772
e-mail: thestore@brooklinebooks.com
www.brooklinebooks.com
For persons with disabilities, a new conception of care is beginning to emerge—a conception seeking to embed these persons in a web of personal relationships, and to involve them in the dynamics of their community. Schwartz explores the promise, potential, and limits of this new direction. *$24.95*
238 pages Paperback
ISBN 0-91479 -82-4

4725 Disablement in the Community
Oxford University Press
2001 Evans Road
Cary, NC 27513 919-677-0977
800-451-7556
FAX: 919-677-1303
www.oup-usa.org

Thomas Carty, Senior Vice President
This book shows how the knowledge of the epidemiology of disablement can help planners, service providers, patients and voluntary organizations choose strategies for community care. *$39.95*
248 pages Illustrated

4726 Getting the Most Out of Consultation Services
Independent Living Research Utilization I LR U
2323 S Shepherd Drive
Suite 1000
Houston, TX 77019 713-520-0232
FAX: 713-520-5785
e-mail: ilru@ilru.org
www.ilru.org

Laurie Redd, Executive Director
A practical, nuts-and-bolts approach to help make working with a consultant a positive, helpful experience for independent living centers.
10 pages

4727 Home and Community Care for Chronically Ill Children
Oxford University Press
2001 Evans Road
Cary, NC 27513 919-677-0977
800-451-7556
FAX: 919-677-1303
www.oup-usa.org

Thomas Carty, Senior Vice President
This book lays common ground for all who have reason and responsibility to enhance the capability of families to care for their ill children over the long term at home. *$32.95*

192 pages

4728 Housing, Support, and Community
Brookes Publishing
PO Box 10624
Baltimore, MD 21285
410-337-9580
800-638-3775
FAX: 410-337-8539
e-mail: custserv@brookespublishing.com
www.brookespublishing.com

Paul Brooks, Owner
Choices and strategies for adults with disabilities. *$32.00*
416 pages Paperback
ISBN 1-55766-90-5

4729 Inclusive Child Care for Infants and Toddlers: Meeting Individual and Special Needs
Brookes Publishing
PO Box 10624
Baltimore, MD 21285
410-337-9580
800-638-3775
FAX: 410-337-8539
e-mail: custserv@brookespublishing.com
www.brookespublishing.com

Paul Brooks, Owner
This book gives child care providers the practical guidance they need to serve infants and toddlers with and without disabilities in inclusive settings. It offers information and helpful advice on handling daily care tasks, teaching responsively, meeting individual needs, developing rapport with parents, understanding toddlers' behavior, working with IFSPs, and maintaining high standards of care. *$34.95*
400 pages Paperback 1997
ISBN 1-55766-96-7

4730 Independence & Transition to Community Living: The Role of Independent Living Centers
Independent Living Research Utilization ILRU
2323 S Shepherd Drive
Suite 1000
Houston, TX 77019
713-520-0232
FAX: 713-520-5785
www.ilru.org

Laurie Redd, Executive Director
This publication covers important information on why we all should make assistance to people living in nursing homes a priority. Just as important, this is an excellent summary of all the facts - quality of life, health, and costs - which support deinstitutionalization.
10 pages

4731 Independent Living Matters
DisAbility Resources of Southwest Washington
5501 NE 109th Court
Suite N
Vancouver, WA 98662
360-694-6790
FAX: 360-694-6910
e-mail: ilrswwa@lqwest.net

Jim Baker, Executive Director
Angela Hartford, Editor/Administrative Technician
Scott Anfinson, Independent Living Specialist
To promote the philosophy of independent living by creating opportunities, encouraging choices, advancing equal access and furthering the level of independence for all people with disabilities.
8-10 pages Quarterly

4732 Keys to Independence
Coalition for Independence
1281 Eisenhower Road
Leavenworth, KS 66048
913-250-0287
FAX: 913-250-0167
e-mail: kolson@cfikc.org
www.cfikc.org

Kathy Cooper, Manager

Bi-Monthly

4733 National Survey Of Americans With Disabilities
National Organization on Disability
910 16th Street NW
Suite 600
Washington, DC 20006
202-293-5960
FAX: 202-293-7999
e-mail: ability@nod.org
www.nod.org

Michael Deland, President
Nancy Starnes, Senior Vice President
John Hershey, Advice and Resource Manager
National cross-disability organization, specializing in employment and emergency preparedness.

4734 Part Two: A Preview of Independence and Transition to Community Living
Independent Living Research Utilization ILRU
2323 S Shepherd Drive
Suite 1000
Houston, TX 77019
713-520-0232
FAX: 713-520-5785
www.ilru.org

Laurie Redd, Executive Director
This publication covers important strategies for helping people leave nursing homes. It includes several important recommendations which CIL leaders and staffs will find useful in organizing transition activities.
10 pages

4735 Resourceful Woman
Rehabilitation Institute of Chicago
345 E Superior Street
Chicago, IL 60611
312-238-1000
FAX: 312-238-1205
TTY:312-908-8523
e-mail: hrcwd@rehabchicago.org
rehabchicago.org

Judy Panko Reis, Director
Kristi Kirchner, MD, Medical Director
Linda E Miller, Domestic Violence Coordinator
National, not-for-profit, general health and service center providing accessible medical services for women with disabilities. Conducts research into health issues concerning disabled women and offers educational resources for healthcare professionals and women with disabilities. Provides materials and educational opportunities through its library and resource center, newsletter, information sheets, brochures, videos and free seminars for women and their healthcare providers.
yearly

4736 Transitioning Exceptional Children and Youth Into the Community
Haworth Press
10 Alice Street
Binghamton, NY 13904
607-722-5857
800-429-6784
FAX: 607-722-6362
e-mail: orders@haworthpress.com
www.haworthpress.com

William Cohen, Owner
Focusing on the dynamic process of mainstreaming exceptional children and youth into the community, experts examine some of the exciting technological advances made to accompany the social changes enacted over the years. *$44.95*
202 pages Hardcover
ISBN 0-866567-33-X

4737 Transitions to Adult Life
Books on Special Children
PO Box 305
Congers, NY 10920
845-638-1236
FAX: 845-638-0847
e-mail: irene@boscbooks.com
Transition programs that can help severely handicapped people become participating, contributing members of the community.
$ 37.00

385 pages Softcover

Employment

4738 A Guide for People with Disabilities Seeking Employment
US Department of Justice
950 Pennsylvania Avenue NW Drs
- Nyav
Washington, DC 20530
202-586-5000
800-574-0301
FAX: 202-307-1197
www.ada.gov

Joanne Graham, Manager
A 2-page pamplet for people with disabilities providing a general explanation of the employment provisions of the ADA and how to file a complaint with the Equal Employment Opportunity Commission.

4739 ADA Questions and Answers
US Department of Justice
950 Pennsylvania Avenue NW Drs
- Nyav
Washington, DC 20530
202-586-5000
800-574-0301
FAX: 202-307-1197
www.ada.gov

Joanne Graham, Manager
A 31-page booklet giving an overview of the ADA's requirements affecting employers, businesses, nonprofit service agencies, and state and local governments programs, including public transportation.

4740 ANCOR Wage and Hour Handbook
American Network of Community Options & Resources
1101 King Street
Suite 380
Alexandria, VA 22314
703-535-7850
FAX: 703-535-7860
e-mail: ancor@ancor.org
www.ancor.org

Renee L Pietrangelo, CEO
Suellen Galbraith, Director Public Policy
This useful publication contains the latest rules and interpretations from the U.S. Department of Labor relative to employment in residential support services for people with disabilities, including copies of enforcement policies and letters of interpretation. It outlines in detail when exemptions from miniimum wage and overtime rules can be applied,a nd when and how employees may be paid on a salary basis. Sample staffing patterns are provided.
121 pages

4741 Ability Magazine
Jobs Information Business Service
1682 Langley Avenue
Irvine, CA 92614
949-622-1040
800-453-JOBS
Provides an electronic classified system which allows employers to recruit qualified individuals with disabilities, and people with disabilities to locate employment opportunities.

4742 Americans with Disabilities
Federal Consumer Information Center
Department 513j
Pueblo, CO 81009
719-948-3334
888-878-3256
FAX: 719-948-9724
e-mail: catalog.pueblo@gsa.gov
www.pueblo.gsa.gov

Alfred Pino, Manager
Explains how civil rights of persons with disabilities are protected at work and in public places.

4743 Americans with Disabilities Act: Questions and Answers
Federal Consumer Information Center
Department 513j
Pueblo, CO 81009
888-878-3256
FAX: 719-948-9724
e-mail: catalog.pueblo@gsa.gov
www.pueblo.gsa.gov

Judi Mahaney, Public Affairs
Explains how the Civil Rights of Persons with disabilities are protected at work and in public places. Free.

4744 Career Education for Handicapped Individuals
McGraw-Hill, School Publishing
220 E Danieldale Road
Desoto, TX 75115
972-224-1111
800-442-9685
FAX: 972-228-1982
mhschool.com

Joseph Gavigan, President
Based on a life-centered career education program that goes beyond elementary school level to include handicapped people of all ages.
454 pages

4745 Earning a Living
Accent Books & Products
PO Box 700
Bloomington, IL 61702
309-378-2961
800-787-8444
FAX: 309-378-4420
e-mail: acmtlvng@aol.com

Raymond C Cheever, Publisher
Betty Garee, Editor
Discusses how to prepare a person for a career, what to say in an interview, and gives examples of both home businesses and jobs away from home. Tells how to modify a worksite and how to be successful on the job. *$9.50*
88 pages Paperback
ISBN 0-91570 -23-0

4746 Employment in the Mainstream
Mainstream
3 Bethesda Metro Center
Suite 830
Bethesda, MD 20814
301-961-9299
800-247-1380
FAX: 301-891-8778
e-mail: info@mainstreaminc.org
www.mainstreaminc.org

David Pichette, Executive Director
Fritz Rumpel, Editor
Charles Moster
Reports on issues, ideas, problems and solutions in employing persons with any kind of physical or mental disability. Quarterly magazine. *$25.00*
32 pages

4747 Encyclopedia of Basic Employment and Daily Living Skills
PO Box 130
Indian Rocks Beach, FL 33785
727-593-2700
800-255-9085
FAX: 727-595-2685

Ruth Bragman PhD, President
Phillip Roy, Manager
$450.00
1200 pages
ISBN 1-568182-25-2

4748 Handbook of Career Planning for Special Needs Students
Pro-Ed Publications
8700 Shoal Creek Boulevard
Austin, TX 78757
512-451-3246
800-897-3202
FAX: 512-451-8542
e-mail: info@proedinc.com
www.proedinc.com

Donald Hammill, Owner
The practitioner's guide will show you how to help special needs adolescents and young adults overcome barriers to employment by identifying goals and problems, assessing interests and aptitudes, involving client families and developing communication skills. *$46.00*
358 pages Hardcover
ISBN 0-890797-06-4

4749 Making News
Avacado Press
PO Box 145
Louisville, KY 40201 502-894-9492
FAX: 502-899-9562
e-mail: office@advocadopress.org
www.advocadopress.org

$8.00
165 pages
ISBN 0-962706-43-4

4750 Making Self-Employment Work for People wit h Disabilities
Brookes Publishing
PO Box 10624
Baltimore, MD 21285 410-337-9580
800-638-3775
FAX: 410-337-8539
e-mail: custserv@brookespublishing.com
www.brookespublishing.com

Paul Brooks, Owner
Practical support for individuals with significant disabilities in starting and maintaining a small business. Covers building a business plan; pinpointing interests, strengths, and goals; and finding helpful information and support *$35.00*
288 pages 2003
ISBN 1-557666-52-0

4751 Making the Workplace Accessible: Guidelines, Costs and Resources
Spina Bifida Association of America
4590 Macarthur Boulevard NW
Suite 250
Washington, DC 20007 202-944-3285
800-621-3141
FAX: 202-944-3295
e-mail: sbaa@sbaa.org
www.sbaa.org

Fritz Rumpel, Editor
Cindy Brownstein, Chief Executive Officer
A 20 page reference guide on how to provide physical access to persons with disabilities in a cost effective manner. *$9.00*

4752 People with Hearing Loss and the Workplace Guide for Employers/ADA Compliances
Hearing Loss Association Of America
7910 Woodmont Avenue
Suite 1200
Bethesda, MD 20814 301-657-2248
FAX: 301-913-9413
e-mail: info@hearingloss.org
www.hearingloss.org

Sharon Christians, Director Of Program Operations
Terry Portis, Executive Director
A guide for both people with hearing loss and their employers to learn about accommodations under the law. Includes employment guidelines, resource list of manufacturers and case studies. *$15.00*
40 pages Paperback

4753 Road Ahead: Transition to Adult Life for Persons with Disabilities
Training Resource Network

Explores transition planning, assessment, instructional strategies, career development and support, social life, quality of life, supported living, and post-secondary education. *$32.95*
223 pages 2002
ISBN 1-883302-46-3

4754 Supported Employment for Disabled People
Human Sciences Press
233 Spring Street
New York, NY 10013 212-229-2859
800-221-9369
FAX: 212-463-0742
Highlights the major features of supported employment. Contributions offer service providers in social work, education and mental health much-needed information. *$38.95*
288 pages Cloth
ISBN 0-89885 -46-6

4755 WORK
64511 Via Real
Suite 9
Carpinteria, CA 93013 805-566-9000
FAX: 805-566-9070

Kathy Webb, Executive Director
Vocational and residential training and support services for adults with developmental disabilities.

General Disabilities

4756 A Guide to Disability Rights Law
US Department of Justice
950 Pennsylvania Avenue NW Drs
- Nyav
Washington, DC 20530 202-586-5000
800-574-0301
FAX: 202-307-1197
www.ada.gov

Joanne Graham, Manager
A 21-page booklet providing a brief description of the ADA, the Telecommunications Act, Fair Housing Act, Air Carrier Access Act, Voting Accessibility for the Elderly and Handicapped Act, National Voter Registration Act, Civil Rights of Institutionalized Persons Act, Individuals with Disabilities in Education Act, Rehabilitation Act, Architectural Barriers Act, and the federal agencies to contact for more information.

4757 A Guidebook on Consumer-Controlled Housing for Minnesotans with Disabilities
Arc Minnesota
770 Transfer Road
Suite 26
Saint Paul, MN 55114 651-523-0823
800-582-5256
FAX: 651-523-0829
e-mail: mikeg@arcmn.org
www.TheArcOfMinnesotta.org

Mike Gude, Administrative Assistant
Steve Larson, Executive Director
$10.00
8 pages
ISBN 0-965040-41-0

4758 A Practical Guide to Art Therapy Groups
Haworth Press
10 Alice Street
Binghamton, NY 13904 607-722-5857
800-429-6784
FAX: 607-722-6362
e-mail: orders@haworthpress.com
www.haworthpress.com

S Harrington-Miller, Advertising
William Cohen, Owner
Unique approaches, materials, and device will inspire you to tap into your own well of creativity to design your own treatment plans. It lays out the ingredients and the skills to get the results you want. *$64.95*

115 pages Hardcover
ISBN 0-789001-36-5

4759 A World Awaits You
Mobility International USA
PO Box 10767
Eugene, OR 97440
541-343-1284
FAX: 541-343-6812
e-mail: info@miusa.org
www.miusa.org

Pamala Houston, Public Relations Coordinator
Tracy Scharn, Project Assstant
Susan Sygall, Executive Director
Free publication from Mobility International USA.
44 pages Yearly

4760 AAPD News
American Association of People with Disabilities
1629 K Street NW
Suite 503
Washington, DC 20006
202-457-0046
800-840-8844
FAX: 202-457-0473
e-mail: aapd@aol.com
www.aapd-dc.org

Anelie Bush, Editor
Quarterly

4761 ADA Guide for Small Businesses
US Department of Justice
950 Pennsylvania Avenue NW Drs
- Nyav
Washington, DC 20530
202-586-5000
800-574-0301
FAX: 202-307-1197
www.ada.gov

Joanne Graham, Manager
A 15-page booklet for businesses that provide goods and services to the public. This publication explains basic ADA requirements, illustrates ways to make facilities accessible, and provides information about tax credits and deductions.

4762 ADA Guide for Small Towns
US Department of Justice
950 Pennsylvania Avenue NW Drs
- Nyav
Washington, DC 20530
202-586-5000
800-574-0301
FAX: 202-307-1197
www.ada.gov

Joanne Graham, Manager
A 21-page guide that presents an informal overview of some basic ADA requirements and provides cost-effective tips on how small towns can comply with the ADA.

4763 ADA Information Services
US Department of Justice
950 Pennsylvania Avenue NW Drs
- Nyav
Washington, DC 20530
202-586-5000
800-574-0301
FAX: 202-307-1197
www.ada.gov

Joanne Graham, Manager
A 2-page list with the telephone numbers and internet addresses of federal agencies and other organizations that provide information and technical assistance to the public about the ADA.

4764 ADA Pipeline
DRTAC: Southeast ADA Center
490 10th Street NW
Atlanta, GA 30318
404-385-0636
800-949-4232
FAX: 404-385-0641
e-mail: sedbtacproject@law.sgr.edu
www.sedbtac.org

Amy Oliveras, Administrative Assistant
Mary Morder, Alternative Format Coordinator
Shelley Kaplan, Director

16 pages Quarterly

4765 ADA Questions and Answers
US Department of Justice
950 Pennsylvania Avenue NW Drs
- Nyav
Washington, DC 20530
202-586-5000
800-574-0301
FAX: 202-307-1197
www.ada.gov

Joanne Graham, Manager
A 31-page booklet giving an overview of the ADA's requirements affecting employers, businesses, nonprofit service agencies, and state and local governments programs, including public transportation.

4766 ADA Tax Incentive Packet for Business
US Department of Justice
950 Pennsylvania Avenue NW Drs
- Nyav
Washington, DC 20530
202-586-5000
800-574-0301
FAX: 202-307-1197
www.ada.gov

Joanne Graham, Manager
A 13-page packet of information to help businesses understand and take advantage of the tax credit and deduction available for complying with the ADA.

4767 ADA and City Governments: Common Problems
US Department of Justice
950 Pennsylvania Avenue NW Drs
- Nyav
Washington, DC 20530
202-586-5000
800-574-0301
FAX: 202-307-1197
www.ada.gov

Joanne Graham, Manager
A 9-page document that contains a sampling of common problems shared by city governments of all sizes, provides examples of common deficiencies and explains how these problems affect persons with disabilities.

4768 ADA-TA: A Technical Assistance Update from the Department of Justice
US Department of Justice
950 Pennsylvania Avenue NW Drs
- Nyav
Washington, DC 20530
202-586-5000
800-574-0301
FAX: 202-307-1197
www.ada.gov

Joanne Graham, Manager
A serial publication that answers Common Questions about ADA requirements and provides Design Details illustrating particular design requirements. The first edition addresses Readily Achievable Barrier Removal and Van Accessible Packing Spaces.

4769 AEPS Family Report: For Children Ages Birth to Three

Brookes Publishing
PO Box 10624
Baltimore, MD 21285
410-337-9580
800-638-3775
FAX: 410-337-8539
e-mail: custserv@brookespublishing.com
www.brookespublishing.com

Clary Creighton, Exhibits Coordinator
Tracy Gray, Educational Sales Manager
Paul Brooks, Owner
This is a 64-item questionnaire that asks parents to rank their child's abilities on specific skills. In packages of 10. *$17.00*

20 pages Saddle-stiched
ISBN 1-557660-99-9

4770 **ARC's Government Report**
Arc of the District of Columbia
817 Varnum Street NE
Washington, DC 20017
202-636-2950
FAX: 202-636-2996
e-mail: arcdc@arcdc.net
www.arcdc.net

Reports on government activities related to individuals with disabilities with a focus on persons with mental retardation. *$ 50.00*

4771 **ARCA Newsletter**
ARCA - Dakota County Technical College
1300 145th Street E
Rosemount, MN 55068
651-423-8000
800-548-5502

Ron Thomas, President
Offers information on support groups, conventions, books, manuscripts and programs for the rehabilitation professional and the disabled.
Monthly

4772 **Able to Laugh**
Fanlight Productions
4196 Washington Street
Suite 2
Boston, MA 02131
617-469-4999
800-937-4113
FAX: 617-469-3379
e-mail: fanlight@fanlight.com
www.fanlight.com

Anthony Sweeny, Marketing Director
Nicole Johnson, Publicity Coordinator
Ben Achtenberg, Owner
An exploration of the world of disability as interpreted by six professional comedians who happen to be disabled. It is also about the awkward ways disabled and able-bodied people relate to one another. *$195.00*

ISBN 1-572951-05-2

4773 **Accent on Living Magazine**
Cheever Publishing
PO Box 700
Bloomington, IL 61702
309-378-2961
800-787-8444
FAX: 309-378-4420

Julie Cheever, Marketing Manager
A magazine published for forty four years, serves physically disabled people, with general interest, travel, and home modification features. *$12.00*
112 pages Quarterly

4774 **Access Design Services: CILs as Experts**
Independent Living Research Utilization ILRU
2323 S Shepherd Drive
Suite 1000
Houston, TX 77019
713-520-0232
FAX: 713-520-5785
www.ilru.org

Laurie Redd, Executive Director
Featuring the Access Design Services of Alpha One in Maine, this month's Readings is another of the winners of the recent competition for innovative CIL programs.
10 pages

4775 **Access Info**
Access to Independence
2345 Atwood Avenue
Madison, WI 53704
608-242-8484
800-362-9877
FAX: 608-242-0383
TTY: 608-242-8485

Tracy Miller, Editor
Covers news, features and resources for people with disabilities living in the Madison, Wisconsin area.

24 pages Semi-Annual

4776 **Access for 911 and Telephone Emergency Services**
US Department of Justice
950 Pennsylvania Avenue NW Drs
- Nyav
Washington, DC 20530
202-586-5000
800-574-0301
FAX: 202-307-1197
www.ada.gov

Joanne Graham, Manager
A 10-page publication explaining the requirements for direct, equal access to 911 for persons who use teletypewriters (TTYs).

4777 **Achieving Diversity and Independence**
Independent Living Research Utilization ILRU
2323 S Shepherd Drive
Suite 1000
Houston, TX 77019
713-520-0232
FAX: 713-520-5785
www.ilru.org

Laurie Redd, Executive Director
10 pages

4778 **Activity-Based Intervention: 2nd Edition**
Brookes Publishing
PO Box 10624
Baltimore, MD 21285
410-337-9580
800-638-3775
FAX: 410-337-8539
e-mail: custserv@brookespublishing.com
www.brookespublishing.com

Paul Brooks, Owner
This 14 minute video illustrates how activity-based intervention can be used to turn everyday events and natural interactions into opportunities to promote learning in young children who are considered at risk for developmental delays or who have mild to significant disabilities. *$39.00*

ISBN 1-55766 -86-3

4779 **Ad Lib Drop-In Center: Consumer Management, Ownership and Empowerment**
Independent Living Research Utilization ILRU
2323 S Shepherd Drive
Suite 1000
Houston, TX 77019
713-520-0232
FAX: 713-520-5785
www.ilru.org

Laurie Redd, Executive Director
Joe describes how Ad Lib ensured consumer control in their Drop-In Center: the DIC came about because of consumer input, and consumers are involved in planning the program; members can choose to become volunteers or paid staff members. All of the staff at the DIC are consumers; and active consumer advisory board helps develop policies and programs and provides input to the Ad Lib board.
10 pages

4780 **Adobe News**
Santa Barbara Foundation
15 E Carrillo Street
Santa Barbara, CA 93101
805-963-1873
805-966-2345

Charles Slosser, Chief Executive Officer
8 pages Bi-Annually

4781 **Advocate**
Arc Massachusetts
217 S Street
Waltham, MA 02453
781-891-6270
FAX: 781-891-6271
e-mail: arcmass@arcmass.org
www.arcmass.org

Leo Sarkissian, Executive Director
$20.00

8-12 pages Quarterly

4782 After School and More
Resources for Children with Special Needs
116 E 16th Street
Floor 5
New York, NY 10003
212-677-4650
FAX: 212-254-4070
e-mail: info@resourcesnyc.org
www.resourcesnyc.org

Karen Schlesinger, Executive Director
Dianne Littwin, Director Publications
More than 450 programs provide a wealth of resources for children in out-of-high school- time program. Information includes contact information, age, disability program capacity, hours, days, transportation, medication administration. *$25.00*
240 pages
ISBN 0-967836-55-7

4783 American Herb Association Newsletter
PO Box 353
Nevada City, CA 95959
530-265-9552
FAX: 530-274-3140
www.ahaherb.com
Information on many different herbs and herb usues. *$ 20.00*

4784 Americans with Disabilities Act Checklist for New Lodging Facilities
US Department of Justice
950 Pennsylvania Avenue NW Drs
- Nyav
Washington, DC 20530
202-586-5000
800-574-0301
FAX: 202-307-1197
www.ada.gov

Joanne Graham, Manager
This 34-page checklist is a self-help survey that owners, franchisors, and managers of lodging facilities can use to identify ADA mistakes at their facilities.

4785 An Interdisciplinary Journal for the Socia l Study of Health, Illness and Medicine
Sage Publications
2455 Teller Road
Thousand Oaks, CA 91320
805-499-0721
800-818-7243
FAX: 805-499-0871
hea.sagepub.com

Alan Radley, Editor
Blaise Simqu, Chief Executive Officer
Quarterly

4786 Annual Report Sarkeys Foundation
530 E Main Street
Norman, OK 73071
405-364-3703
FAX: 405-364-8191

Cheri Cartwright, Manager
Yearly

4787 Applied Kinesiology: Muscle Response in Diagnosis, Therapy and Preventive Medicine
Inner Traditions
1 Park Street
Rochester, VT 05767
802-767-3174
800-246-8648
FAX: 802-767-3726
e-mail: orders@innertraditions.com
www.InnerTraditions.com

Jessica Dudley, Sales Associate
Ehud Sperling, Owner
$12.95
144 pages
ISBN 0-892813-28-8

4788 Arc Connection Newsletter
Arc of Tennessee
151 Athens Way
Suite 100
Nashville, TN 37228
615-248-5878
800-835-7077
FAX: 615-248-5879
e-mail: pcooper@thearctn.org
www.thearctn.org

Walter Rogers, Executive Director
Peggy Cooper, Associate Director
The Arc of Tennessee is a nonprofit organization that offers advocacy, information, referral and support to people with mental retardation or a related developmental disability and their families. This is their publication. It is free to members. *$10.00*
12 pages Quarterly

4789 Aromatherapy Book: Applications and Inhalations
North Atlantic Books
1435a 4th Street
Berkeley, CA 94710
510-559-8277
FAX: 510-559-8279
e-mail: info@northatlanticbooks.com
www.northatlanticbooks.com
Considered a bible for those interested in aromatherapy. *$18.95*
1992
ISBN 1-556430-73-6

4790 Aromatherapy for Common Ailments
Simon & Schuster
100 Front Street
Delran, NJ 08075
800-323-7445
FAX: 800-943-9831
www.simonsays.com
Explains aromatherapy with emphasis on medicinal uses.
96 pages 1991
ISBN 0-671731-34-3

4791 As I Am
Fanlight Productions
4196 Washington Street
Suite 2
Boston, MA 02131
617-469-4999
800-937-4113
FAX: 617-469-3379
e-mail: fanlight@fanlight.com
www.fanlight.com

Anthony Sweeny, Marketing Director
Nicole Johnson, Publicity Coordinator
Ben Achtenberg, Owner
Three young people with developmental disabilities speak for themselves about their lives, the problems they face and their hopes and expectations for the future. *$99.00*

ISBN 1-572950-58-7

4792 Assistive Technology News
South Carolina Assistive Technology Project
University of South Carolina
Columbia, SC 29208
803-779-0343
FAX: 803-935-5342
e-mail: jjendron@usit.net
www.sc.edu/scatp/

Evelyn Evans, Editor
Janet Jendron, Editor
Mary Alice Bechtler, Editor
7-8 pages Bi-annually

4793 Attitudes Toward Persons with Disabilities
Springer Publishing Company
536 Broadway
New York, NY 10012
212-431-4370
877-687-7476
FAX: 212-941-7842
e-mail: marketing@springerpub.com
www.springerpub.com

Annette Imperati, Marketing/Sales Director
Ursula Springer, President
This volume examines what is known of people's complex and multifaceted attitudes toward persons with disabilities. Divided into five areas of concern: theory, origin of attitudes, attitude measurement, attitudes of specific groups and attitude change. *$38.95*
352 pages Hardcover
ISBN 0-82616 -90-1

4794 Authoritative Guide to Self- Help Resource in Mental Health
Guilford Press
72 Spring Street
New York, NY 10012
212-431-9800
800-365-7006
FAX: 212-966-6708
www.guilford.com

Linda F Campbell PhD, Author
Thomas P Smith PsyD, Author
Robert Sommer PhD, Author
Reviews and rates 600+ self-help books, autobiographies, and popular films, and evaluates hundreds of Internet sites. Addresses 28 of the most prevalent clinical disorders and life challenges- from ADHD, Alzheimer's, and anxiety disorders, to marital problems, mood disorders and weight management. Also in cloth at $45.00 (ISBN# 1-57230-506-1) *$25.00*
377 pages Paperback 2000
ISBN 1-572305-80-0

4795 AwareNews
Services for Independent Living
25100 Euclid Avenue
Suite 105
Cleveland, OH 44117
216-731-1529
FAX: 216-731-3083
e-mail: sil@stratos.net

Molly Thomas, Services Coordinator
Lynn Hilderbrand, Manager
12 pages Quarterly

4796 Bach Flower Therapy: Theory and Practice
Inner Traditions
1 Park Street
Rochester, VT 05767
802-767-3174

Ehud Sperling, Owner
Contemporary study of Bach's techniques, intended for practitioners and lay readers alike. Includes lists of symptoms to facilitate diagnosis, ans aims to provide an understanding of psychosomatic elements in relation to physical complaints.
1988
ISBN 0-892812-39-7

4797 Beliefs, Values, and Principles of Self Advocacy
Brookline Books
PO Box 1047
Cambridge, MA 02139
617-868-0360
800-666-2665
FAX: 617-868-1772
e-mail: thestore@brooklinebooks.com
www.brooklinebooks.com
Written by self-advocates around the world, they tell about the beliefs, values, and principles important to them, and the empowerment and personal growth they experience through self-advocacy. *$7.00*
48 pages Paperback
ISBN 0-57129 -22-2

4798 Beliefs: Pathways to Health and Well Being
Metamorphous Press
PO Box 10616
Portland, OR 97296
503-228-4972
FAX: 503-223-9117
www.metamodels.com/meta/bks/hea1.htm

David Balding, Publisher
Explores behavioral technologies and belief change strategies that can alter beliefs that support unhealthy habbits such as smoking, overeating, and drug use. Also covers the changing of thinking processes that create phobias and unreasonable fears, retraining the immune system to eliminate allergies and to deal optinally with cancer, AIDS, and other diseases. Includes strategies to transform unhealthy beliefs into lifelong constructs of wellness.

4799 Bench Marks
Govennor's Council on Developmental Disabilities
1717 W Jefferson Street
Phoenix, AZ 85007
602-542-4049
800-889-5893
FAX: 602-542-5320
e-mail: mward@mail.dc.state.us

Micheal Ward, Executive Director
Susan Madison, Manager
Quarterly

4800 Body Reflexology: Healing at Your Fingertips
Parker Publishing Company
1501 Broadway
Suite 2605
New York, NY 10036
212-354-7100

Valerie Porter
Features step-by-step instructions of how to send healing flows of energy through the body to relieve back pain, headaches, arthritis, and other afflictions. Illustrated.
343 pages Hardcover 1995
ISBN 0-132997-36-3

4801 Body Silent: The Different World of the Disabled
WW Norton & Company
324 State Street
Santa Barbara, CA 93101
800-333-6867
FAX: 805-962-5087
www.specialneeds.com/store/
The author's personal account of his progressive and terminal loss of muscle function caused by a spinal tumor, resulting in quadripilegia. Includes society's fears, myths, and misunderstandings about disability and the damage they inflict. *$9.95*
256 pages 2001
ISBN 0-393320-42-1

4802 Body of Knowledge/Hellerwork
406 Berry Street
Mount Shasta, CA 96067
530-926-2500

Joseph Heller, Owner
Information, referral directory, training and certification.

4803 Bridge Newsletter
Arizona Bridge to Independent Living
1229 E Washington Street
Phoenix, AZ 85034
602-256-2245
800-280-2245
FAX: 602-254-6407
e-mail: azbridge@abil.org
www.abil.org

Phil Pangrazio, Executive Director
12 pages Monthly

4804 Bridging the Gap: A National Directory of Services for Women & Girls with Disabilities
Educational Equity Concepts
114 E 32nd Street
New York, NY 10016
212-725-1803
FAX: 212-725-0947
TTY:212-725-1803
e-mail: infomration@edequity.org
www.edequity.org

Ellen Rubin, Coordinator Disability Programs
Merle Froschl, Editor
Contains a resource section of publications and videos geared specifically to women and girls with disabilities. Available in print, on cassette, and also in braille. *$24.95*

ISBN 0-931629-16-0

4805 **Bulletin of the Association on the Handicapped**
Assoc. on Handicapped Student Service Program
PO Box 21192
Columbus, OH 43221 614-365-5216
FAX: 614-365-6718
Membership journal including Association news, articles and sections such as Literature in Review and Speak Out. *$16.00*

4806 **CDR Reports**
Council for Disability Rights
20 N Wacker Drive
Suite 1540
Chicago, IL 60606 312-444-9484
FAX: 312-444-1977
e-mail: cdrights@interaccess.com
www.disabilityrights.org

Jo Holzer, Executive Director/Editor
Bruce Moore, Employment Specialist
$15.00
8 pages Monthly

4807 **California Financial Power of Attorney**
NOLO
950 Parker Street
Berkeley, CA 94710 510-549-1976
800-955-4775
FAX: 510-548-5902
www.nolo.com

Maira Dizgalvis, Trade Customer Service Manager
Susan McConnell, Director Sales
Natasha Kaluza, Sales Assistant
A plain-English book packed with forms and instructions to give a trusted person the legal authority to handle your financial affairs.
paperback

4808 **Caring for America's Heroes**
Oklahoma City VA Medical Center
921 NE 13th Street
Oklahoma City, OK 73104 405-270-0501
FAX: 405-270-1560
www.va.gov

Steven J Gentling, Director
Kathleen Fogarty, Associate Director
D Robert McCaffree MD, Chief of Staff

4809 **Caring for Persons with Developmental Disabilities**
Research Press
2612 N Mattis Avenue
Champaign, IL 61822 217-352-3273
800-519-2707
FAX: 217-352-1221
e-mail: rp@researchpress.com
www.researchpress.com

Russell Pence, President
A competency-baced video traning program that teaches the skills needed to care for individuals with a wide range of psysical and mental disabilities. Consists of six videotapes that feature demonstrations of respite care procedures. Provides quizzes in which viewers are asked to respond to on-screen situations. *$495.00*
Video

4810 **Center for Health Research: Eastern Washin gton University**
Showalter 209a
Cheney, WA 99004 509-359-2279
800-221-9369
FAX: 509-359-2778
e-mail: sharon.wilson@mail.ewu.edu
iceberg.ewu.edu
Produces eight videotapes, accompanying printed materials, and a videotaped public services announcement to serve as training and resource materials for use by daycare centers.

4811 **Center for Libraries and Educational Improvement**
400 Maryland Avenue SW
Washington, DC 20202 202-260-2226
FAX: 202-401-0689

Malcolm Davis, Acting Director
Administers the Library Services Construction Act, which authorizes grants to the states for library services to the physically handicapped.

4812 **Centers for Disease Control Public Health Service**
US Department of Health and Human Services
Ms C09 1600 Clifton Road NE
Atlanta, GA 30333 404-639-3311

Publishes an annually updated list of infectious and communicable diseases transmitted through the handling of food in accordance with Section 103 of Title I.

4813 **Child With Special Needs: Encouraging Inte llectual and Emotional Growth**
Addison-Wesley Publishing Company
75 Arlington Street
Suite 300
Boston, MA 02116 617-848-6000
800-238-9682
FAX: 617-848-6034
www.awprofessional.com

William Barke, President
Covering all kinds of disabilities — including cerebral palsy, autism, retardation, ADD, and language problems — this guide offers parents specific ways of helping all special needs chidren reach their full intellectual and emotional potential. *$32.00*
496 pages 1998
ISBN 0-201407-26-4

4814 **Chinese Herbal Medicine**
Shambhala Publications
PO Box 308
Boston, MA 02117 617-424-0030
FAX: 617-236-1563
e-mail: editors@shambhala.com
www.shambhala.com

Peter Turner, President
Gives an in-depth look into herbal medicine.
176 pages
ISBN 0-877733-98-8

4815 **Christian Approach to Overcoming Disabilit y: A Doctor's Story**
Haworth Press
10 Alice Street
Binghamton, NY 13904 607-722-5857
800-429-6784
FAX: 607-722-6362
e-mail: orders@haworthpress.com
www.haworthpress.com

William Cohen, Owner
$29.95
128 pages 2003
ISBN 0-789022-57-5

4816 **Close Encounters of the Disabling Kind**
Mainstream
6930 Carroll Avenue
Suite 204
Takoma Park, MD 20912 301-891-8777
FAX: 301-891-8778
e-mail: info@mainstreaminc.org
www.mainstreaminc.org

Lillie Harrison, Information Programs Clerk
Fritz Rumpel, Editor
A training video that provides a hiring manager with information on how to learn the basics of disability etiquette and, by the end of the video, seems much better prepared and willing to interview qualified individuals with disabilities. Includes trainer and trainee guides. *$99.95*

Video

4817 Closing the Gap
PO Box 68
Henderson, MN 56044
507-248-3294
FAX: 507-248-3810
e-mail: info@closingthegap.com
www.closingthegap.com

Megan Turek, Editor
Delores Hagen, President
Explores use of microcomputers as personal and educational tools for persons with disabilities.
36+ pages BiMonthly

4818 Comprehensive Directory of Programs and Services
Resources for Children with Special Needs
116 E 16th Street
Floor 5
New York, NY 10003
212-677-4650
FAX: 212-254-4070
e-mail: info@resourcesnyc.org
www.resourcesnyc.org

Karen Schlesinger, Executive Director
Dianne Littwin, Director Publications
Published every 24-36 months. *$55.00*
1096 pages
ISBN 0-976836-51-4

4819 Constellations
Minnesota STAR Program
50 Sherburne Avenue
Suite 309
Saint Paul, MN 55155
651-296-2771
800-657-3862
FAX: 651-282-6671
e-mail: star.program@state.mn.us
www.admin.state.mn.us/assistivetechnology

Chuck Rassbach, Executive Director
Free quarterly publication from the Minnesota STAR Program.
8 pages Quarterly

4820 Consumer Buyer's Guide for Independent Living
American Occupational Therapy Association (AOTA)
4720 Montgomery Lane
Bethesda, MD 20814
301-652-7590
800-OHE-LP4U
FAX: 301-652-7711

Cheryl Hager, Marketing Director
M Baum, President
A buyer's directory of products and publications for the general public listing suppliers' names, addresses and telephone numbers. This directory lists AOTA publications on numerous topics (back pain, Alzheimers, Carpal Tunnel Syndrome, etc.) and suppliers of equipment to assist in activities of daily living for individuals with disabilities.
60 pages Annual

4821 Coping+Plus: Dimensions of Disability
Greenwood Publishing Group
88 Post Road W
Suite 5007
Westport, CT 06880
203-226-3571
FAX: 203-222-1502
www.greenwood.com

Wayne Smith, President
Everyone can learn new or more effective coping skills and strategies to deal with times of loss, crisis and disability. $55-$59.95
280 pages Hardcover
ISBN 0-275945-44-8

4822 Council News
Northern Nevada Center for Independent Living
999 Pyramid Way
Sparks, NV 89431
775-353-3599
FAX: 775-353-3588
e-mail: nncil@sbcglobal.net

Lee Erquiaga, Executive Director

12 pages Quarterly

4823 Counseling in Terminal Care & Bereavement
Brookes Publishing
PO Box 10624
Baltimore, MD 21285
410-337-9580
800-638-3775
FAX: 410-337-8539
e-mail: custserv@brookespublishing.com
www.brookespublishing.com

Paul Brooks, Owner
Provides practical suggestions for addressing the needs of patients and family members who are anticipating or currently dealing with grief and bereavement, such as hospice care, hospitals, or at home care. *$34.00*
210 pages Paperback
ISBN 1-85433 -78-7

4824 Creating Wholeness: Self-Healing Workbook Using Dynamic Relaxation, Images and Thoughts
Plenum Publishing Corporation
233 Spring Street
Floor 7
New York, NY 10013
212-242-1490
FAX: 212-463-0742

232 pages
ISBN 0-306441-72-1

4825 Creative Care Package Catalog
Centering Corporation
1531 N Saddle Creek Road
Omaha, NE 68104
402-553-1200
FAX: 402-533-0507
e-mail: j1200@aol.com
www.centering.org

Janet Sieff, Editor
Joy Johnson, Executive Director
A full catalog of all our available bereavement resources. We are a small, non-profit organization providing help to families in crisis situations.
32 pages BiAnnually

4826 DRS Connection
Disabled Resource Services
424 Pine Street
Suite 101
Fort Collins, CO 80524
970-482-2700
FAX: 970-407-7072
e-mail: drs@lymis.com
www.drs@fortnet.org

Nancy Jackson, Executive Director
4 pages Quaterly

4827 Demand Response Transportation Through a Rural ILC
Independent Living Research Utilization ILRU
2323 S Shepherd Drive
Suite 1000
Houston, TX 77019
713-520-0232
FAX: 713-520-5785
www.ilru.org

Laurie Redd, Executive Director
Oklahomans for Independent Living's transportation program was selected as exemplary becuase they marketed it by emphasizing people with disabilities as economic constituency.
10 pages

4828 Developing Organized Coalitions and Strategic Plans
Independent Living Research Utilization ILRU
2323 S Shepherd Drive
Suite 1000
Houston, TX 77019
713-520-0232
FAX: 713-520-5785
www.ilru.org

Laurie Redd, Executive Director

10 pages

4829 Dictionary of Congenital Malformations & Disorders
Informa Healthcare
52 Vanderbilt Ave.
16th Floor
New York, NY 10017
212-520-2777
FAX: 212-661-5052
e-mail: orders@crcpress.com
www.informaworld.com

$55.00
193 pages
ISBN 0-850705-77-1

4830 Dictionary of Developmental Disabilities Terminology
Brookes Publishing
PO Box 10624
Baltimore, MD 21285
410-337-9580
800-638-3775
FAX: 410-337-8539
e-mail: custserv@brookesopublishing.com
www.brookespublishing.com

Barbara Y Whitman MSW PhD, Editor
Carla Laszewski MSW
Paul Brooks, Owner
With more than 3,000 easy-to-understand entries, this dictionary provides thorough explanations of terms associated with developmental disabilities and disorders. *$55.95*
368 pages Hardcover 1996
ISBN 1-557662-45-2

4831 Directory of Members
American Network of Community Options & Resources
1101 King Street
Suite 380
Alexandria, VA 22314
703-535-7850
FAX: 703-535-7860
e-mail: ancor@ancor.org
www.ancor.org

Renee L Pietrangelo, CEO
Suellen Galbraith, Director Public Policy
Renee Pietrangelo, Chief Executive Officer
The Directory lists over 600 agencies that provide residential services and supports in 48 states and the District of Columbia. The listings include the name of the Executive Directors, the name, address, and phone number of the agency, describe the types of services that are provided and how many individuals receive services from that agency. *$25.00*
189 pages

4832 Disability Awareness Guide
Central Iowa Center for Independent Living
655 Walnut Street
Suite 131
Des Moines, IA 50309
515-243-1742
FAX: 515-243-5385
e-mail: cicil@raccoon.com
www.raccoon.com/-cicil

Robert Jeppesen, Director
Frank Strong, Assistant Director Programs
Bob Jepson, Manager
The Disability Awareness Guide contains information about our center; who we are and what we do. It also contains the telephone numbers of local and national agencies and resources available for people with disabilities.

4833 Disability Rights Movement
Children's Press
Sherman Tpke
Danbury, CT 06813
800-621-1115
FAX: 800-374-4329

Elena Rockman, Marketing Manager
Author Deborah Kent illuminates both the history of the National Disability Rights Movement and the inspiring personal stories of individuals with various disabilities. *$18.00*
32 pages Hardcover
ISBN 0-53106 -32-3

4834 Disabled People's International Fifth World Assembly as Reported by Two US Participants
Independent Living Research Utilization ILRU
2323 S Shepherd Drive
Suite 1000
Houston, TX 77019
713-520-0232
FAX: 713-520-5785
www.ilru.org

Laurie Redd, Executive Director
This report describes the international conference on independent living held in Mexico City in December 1998 as experienced by staff members from two U.S. centers. Kaye Beneke interviewed Luis Chew and Marco Antonio Coronado for this edition of Readings in Independent Living.
10 pages

4835 Disabled We Stand
Brookline Books
PO Box 1046
Cambridge, MA 02139
617-868-0360
800-666-2665
FAX: 617-868-1772
e-mail: thestore@brooklinebooks.com
www.brooklinebooks.com
This book is impassioned, often angry, but also hopeful and practical, suggesting a series of actions that will lead to constructive change. It is imbued with spirit and energy of disabled people who are determined to take their lives into their own hands. *$ 10.95*
Paperback
ISBN 0-25331 -80-0

4836 Disabled, the Media, and the Information Age
Greenwood Publishing Group
88 Post Road W
Suite 5007
Westport, CT 06880
203-226-3571
FAX: 203-222-1502
www.greenwood.com

Wayne Smith, President
A short and easy-to-read overview of how disabled Americans have been portrayed by the media and how images and the role of the handicapped are changing. *$55.00*
264 pages Hardcover
ISBN 0-313284-72-5

4837 Discovery Newsletter
North Dakota State Library Talking Book Services
604 E Boulevard Avenue
Dept 250
Bismarck, ND 58505
701-328-2000
800-843-9948
FAX: 701-328-2040
e-mail: sbschneider@nd.gov
ndsl.lib.state.nd.us/DisabilityServices.html

Susan Hammer-Schneider, Manager Talking Books
6 pages Bi-Annually

4838 EP Resource Guide
Exceptional Parent Library
PO Box 1807
Englewood Cliffs, NJ 07632
201-947-6000
800-535-1910
FAX: 201-947-9376
e-mail: eplibrary@aol.com
www.eplibrary.com
Lists directories of national organizations, associations, products and services. *$9.95*

4839 ESCIL Update Newsletter
Eastern Shore Center for Independent Living
9 Sunburst Center
Cambridge, MD 21613
410-221-7701
800-705-7944
FAX: 410-221-7714
e-mail: escil@comcast.net
www.escil.org

Shirley Tarbox, Executive Director
Jean Reed, Administrative Assistant
Lisa Morgan, Director IL Services
6 pages Quarterly

4840 Easy Things to Make Things Simple: Do It Yourself Modifications for Disabled Persons
Brookline Books
PO Box 1047
Cambridge, MA 02139
617-495-3682
800-666-2665
FAX: 617-868-1772
e-mail: thestore@brooklinebooks.com
www.brooklinebooks.com

This book aims at older adults and others with physical limitations who require adaptations for safer and easier living in the kitchen, bathroom, bedroom, yard, and garden. The adaptations can be done inexpensively, from common materials. Large print format and detailed diagrams, plus special sections with advice caregivers . *$15.95*
160 pages Paperback
ISBN 1-571290-24-9

4841 Edge Effect: Achieve Total Health and Long evity with the Balanced Brain Advantage
Sterling Press
420 W 1700 S
Salt Lake City, UT 84115
801-486-4641
FAX: 801-467-2221

Dale Parks, Owner
Dr Eric Braverman reveaks the impact that proper brain nourishment can have on the quality of life. He sketches out a program to achieve logevity and well-being by balancing the brain's four important neurotransmitters. *$19.95*
304 pages Hardcover 2004
ISBN 1-402712-05-7

4842 Encyclopedia of Disability
Sage Publications
2455 Teller Road
Thousand Oaks, CA 91320
805-499-0721

e-mail: info@sagepub.com
www.sagepub.com

Gary L Albrecht, Editor
Blaise Simqu, Chief Executive Officer
A five volume set that covers disabilities A-Z *$850.00*
2500 pages 1905
ISBN 0-761925-65-1

4843 EveryBody's Different: Understanding and Changing Our Reactions to Disabilities
Brookes Publishing
PO Box 10624
Baltimore, MD 21285
410-337-9580
800-638-3775
FAX: 410-337-8539
e-mail: custserv@brookespublishing.com
www.brookespublishing.com

Paul Brooks, Owner
This book discusses the emotions, questions, fears, and stereotypes that people without disabilities sometimes experience when they interact with people who do have disabilities. The author teaches readers to become more at ease with the concept of disability and to communicate more effectively with each other. Features activities and exercises that encourage self-examination, helping people to create more enriching personal relationships and work toward a fully inclusive society.
Paperback 1998
ISBN 1-55766 -59-9

4844 Everybody's Guide to Homeopathic Medicines
Jeremy P Tarcher
375 Hudson Street
New York, NY 10014
212-366-2000

Covers alternative treatments in homeopathic medicines.
375 pages 1997
ISBN 0-874778-43-3

4845 Everyday Social Interaction: A Program for People with Disabilities
Brookes Publishing
PO Box 10624
Baltimore, MD 21285
410-337-9580
800-638-3775
FAX: 410-337-8539
e-mail: custserv@brookespublishing.com
www.brookespublishing.com

Paul Brooks, Owner
This source guides teachers and human services professionals in helping people with disabilities acquire social interaction skills and develop satisfying relationships. Included is a checklist and task analyses that shows how complex skills can be broken down into major components for easy performance monitoring accompanied by tips on social courtesies, rewards, praise, and criticism. *$41.95*
342 pages Paperback
ISBN 1-55766 -58-4

4846 Family Challenges: Parenting with a Disability
Aquarius Health Care Videos
PO Box 1159
Sherborn, MA 01770
508-650-6905
888-440-2963
FAX: 508-650-4216
e-mail: aqvideos@tiac.net
www.aquariusproductions.com

Leslie Kussmann, President/Producer
When a parent has a disability, everyone in the family is affected. For children, these experiences may profoundly influence their lives and views of the world. In this sensitive film, you will hear about different roles that all the family members take on at varying times. *$195.00*

4847 Force A Miracle
Writer's Showcase Press

A testament to the inner human strength to overcome extreme adversity, to triumph and continue a worthwhile and self-rewarding life. *$14.95*
244 pages 2002
ISBN 0-595226-88-4

4848 Forum
Coalition for the Education of Disabled Children
165 W Center Street
Marion, OH 43302
740-382-5452
800-374-2806
FAX: 740-383-6421
e-mail: oceed@gte.net
www.oceed.org

Margret Burley, Executive Director
Leeann Derugen, Manager
Forum is a newsletter reporting on legislative and other developments affecting persons with disabilities.
Quarterly

4849 Fosters Botanical and Herb Reviews
B&H Reviews
PO Box 106
Eureka Springs, AR 72632
FAX: 479-253-7442

4850 Foundation Fundamentals for Nonprofit Organizations
Foundation Center
79 5th Avenue
Department Ze
New York, NY 10003
212-620-4230
800-424-9836
FAX: 212-807-3677
www.fdncenter.org

Sara Engelhardt, President

This video is designed to give fundraisers a general overview of the foundation funding process and to introduce them to the many resources available through our libraries and cooperating collections. The video gives clear, step-by-step instructions on how to build a fundraising program. *$24.00*

Video

4851 Four-Ingredient Cookbook

Laurel Designs
1805 Mar West Street
Apt A
Belvedere Tiburon, CA 94920
FAX: 415-435-1451
e-mail: laureld@ncal.verio.com

Janet Sawyer, Owner
Lynn Montoya, Owner

Simple, easy to follow recipes, each containing four ingredients. Particularly suited to persons with limited physical ability. Includes 400 recipes, appetizers to desserts. *$9.00*

4852 Frequently Asked Questions About Multiple Chemical Sensitivity

Independent Living Research Utilization ILRU
2323 S Shepherd Drive
Suite 1000
Houston, TX 77019
713-520-0232
FAX: 713-520-5785
www.ilru.org

Laurie Redd, Executive Director

This FAQ covers important information about multiple chemical sensitivity and environmental illness. The FAQ describes the conditions, recommends strategies for improving access, and lists resources for CILs and other organizations. As the fact sheet states, centers must set an example in assuring that all people can enter their offices.

10 pages

4853 Genetic Disorders Sourcebook

Omnigraphics
615 Griswold Street
Detroit, MI 48226
313-961-1340
800-234-1340
FAX: 800-875-1340
www.omnigraphics.com

Kathy Massimini, Editor
Peter Ruffner, President

Provides information on hereditary diseases and disorders. *$7800.00*

650 pages 2000
ISBN 0-789892-41-1

4854 Genetic Nutritioneering

McGraw-Hill Company
2460 Kerper Boulevard
Dubuque, IA 52001
563-588-1451
800-338-3987
FAX: 614-755-5654
www.mhhe.com/hper/physed

Kurt Strand, Vice President

Describes how to modify the expression of genetic traits, potentially preventing heart disease, cancer, arthritis, and hormone-related problems. Features how to slow biological aging and reduce the risk of age-related diseases. *$16.95*

288 pages 1999
ISBN 0-879839-21-X

4855 Going to School with Facilitated Communication

Syracuse University, School of Education
230 Huntington Hall
Syracuse, NY 13244
315-443-5550

Nancy Mudrick, Manager

A video in which students with autism and/or severe disabilities illustrate the use of facilitated communication focusing on basic principles fostering facilitated communication.

Video

4856 Grief: What it is and What You Can Do

Centering Corporation
1531 N Saddle Creek Road
Omaha, NE 68104
402-553-1200
FAX: 402-533-0507
e-mail: j1200@aol.com
www.centering.org

Joy Johnson, Executive Director

General grief information for all grief issues. *$3.50*

32 pages Paperback

4857 Guidelines on Disability

US Department of Housing & Urban Development
451 7th Street SW
Washington, DC 20410
202-708-1112
TTY:202-708-1455

Contains information on housing and accessibility for persons with disabilities.

4858 Handbook of Services for the Handicapped

Greenwood Publishing Group
88 Post Road W
Suite 5007
Westport, CT 06880
203-226-3571
FAX: 203-222-1502
www.greenwood.com

Wayne Smith, President

A handy reference book offering information and services for disabled individuals. $59.95-$65.00.

291 pages Hardcover
ISBN 0-313213-85-2

4859 Healing Herbs

Rodale Press
33 E Minor Street
Emmaus, PA 18098
610-967-5171
FAX: 610-967-8963
www.rodale.com

Steven Murphy, Chief Executive Officer

Covers everything from growing the herbs to home remedies.

4860 Helen Keller National Center for Deaf-Blin d Youths and Adults (HKNC)

141 Middle Neck Road
Sands Point, NY 11050
516-944-8900
FAX: 516-944-7302
e-mail: hkncinfo@hknc.org
www.hknc.org

Nancy O'Donnell, Coordinator Of Special Projects
Joseph McNulty, Executive Director

HKNC is the only national vacational and rehabilitation program providing services exclusively to youth and adults who are deaf-blind.

4861 Home is in the Heart: Accommodating People with Disabilities in the Homestay Experience

Mobility International USA
PO Box 10767
Eugene, OR 97440
541-343-1284
FAX: 541-343-6812
e-mail: info@miusa.org
www.miusa.org

Susan Sygall, Executive Director
Pamela Houston, Public Relations Coordinator
Tracy Scharn, Project Assistant

Provides information and ideas for exchange organizations. Discusses how to recruit homestay families, meet accessibility needs and accommodate international participants with disabilities. *$49.00*

Video

4862 Hospice Alternative

Harper Collins Publishers/Basic Books
10 E 53rd Street
New York, NY 10022
212-207-7000
800-242-7737
FAX: 212-207-7203

Jane Friedman, Chief Executive Officer
An account of the hospice experience. An innovative and humane way of caring for the terminally ill. *$8.95*
256 pages
ISBN 0-46503 -61-0

4863 How to File a Title III Complaint
US Department of Justice
950 Pennsylvania Avenue NW Drs
- Nyav
Washington, DC 20530
202-586-5000
800-574-0301
FAX: 202-307-1197
www.ada.gov

Joanne Graham, Manager
This publication details the procedure for filing a complaint under Title III of the ADA.

4864 How to Live Longer with a Disability
Accent Books & Products
PO Box 700
Bloomington, IL 61702
309-378-2961
800-787-8444
FAX: 309-378-4420
e-mail: acmtlvng@aol.com

Raymond C Cheever, Publisher
Betty Garee, Editor
Eleven chapters to help you enjoy every aspect of your life, and live easier and happier. Includes sexuality and disability, getting more from the medical community and benefit programs. Co-authored by Robert Mauro, sociologist and Elle Becker, counselor and psychologist, both disabled. *$11.50*
266 pages Paperback
ISBN 0-19570 -38-8

4865 I'm Not Disabled
Landmark Media
3450 Slade Run Drive
Falls Church, VA 22042
703-241-2030
800-342-4336
FAX: 703-536-9540

Michael Hartogs, President
Young people talk about their disabilities and the importance of sports in their lives. The afflictions range from blindness and missing limbs to paralysis. Through physical education and therapy they enjoy freedom of movement and participate in sports such as tennis, basketball, kayaking, skiing, and swimming. *$195.00*
Video

4866 Ideas for Kids on the Go
Accent Books & Products
PO Box 700
Bloomington, IL 61702
309-378-2961
800-787-8444
FAX: 309-378-4420
e-mail: acmtlvng@aol.com

Raymond C Cheever, Publisher
Betty Garee, Editor
This guide shows kids with physical disabilities how to go for it! Lists products and where to get them, and includes tips from others for having fun and getting ahead. Ages 1-18. *$6.95*
69 pages Paperback
ISBN 0-91570 -17-5

4867 If I Only Knew What to Say or Do
AARP Fulfillment
601 E Street NW
Washington, DC 20049
202-434-2277
800-424-3410
FAX: 202-434-3443
e-mail: member@aarp.org
www.aarp.org

William Novelli, Chief Executive Officer
Provides a concise discussion of how to help a friend in crisis. Learn what to say and what not to say.

4868 If it Weren't for the Honor: I'd Rather Have Walked
Accent Books & Products
PO Box 700
Bloomington, IL 61702
309-378-2961
800-787-8444
FAX: 309-378-4420
e-mail: acmtlvng@aol.com

Raymond C Cheever, Publisher
Betty Garee, Editor
Revealing, often humorous, highly interesting and important reading. This book offers an account told by the author who was on the scene and actually saw and participated in many events that paved the way for progress for all those with disabilities. *$14.50*
262 pages Paperback
ISBN 0-91570 -41-8

4869 Imagery Procedures for People with Special Needs
Research Press
PO Box 9177
Champaign, IL 61826
217-352-3273
800-519-2707
FAX: 217-352-1221
e-mail: rp@researchpress.com
www.researchpress.com

Russell Pence, President
This video features numerous training sessions in which clinicians are shown leading individuals through imagery scenes that focus on controlling specific behaviors. *$195.00*
32 Minutes

4870 Imagery in Healing Shamanism and Modern Medicine
Shambhala Publications
PO Box 308
Boston, MA 02117
617-424-0030
FAX: 617-236-1563
e-mail: editors@shambhala.com
www.shambhala.com

Peter Turner, President
Patients use self imagery to fight sickness and pain throughout their lives. *$15.95*
272 pages 2002
ISBN 1-570629-34-x

4871 Include Us
Exceptional Parent Library
PO Box 1807
Englewood Cliffs, NJ 07632
201-947-6000
800-535-1910
FAX: 201-947-9376
e-mail: eplibrary@aol.com
www.eplibrary.com
First children's video to feature a proportionate number of children with disabilities. Inclusion works via eight songs. *$19.95*

4872 Independence
Easter Seals
1219 Dunn Avenue
Daytona Beach, FL 32114
386-255-4568
877-255-4568
FAX: 386-258-7677
e-mail: info@eseals-vf.org
www.easterseals-volusiaflagler.org

Penny Young, Communications Director
Lynn Sinnot, President
4-6 pages Quarterly

4873 Independent Living Centers and Managed Care: Results of an ILRU Study on Involvement
Independent Living Research Utilization ILRU
2323 S Shepherd Drive
Suite 1000
Houston, TX 77019
713-520-0232
FAX: 713-520-5785
www.ilru.org

Laurie Redd, Executive Director

This month's Readings presents findings from an ILRU study of roles centers are taking vis-a-vis managed care. Initiated in spring 1998, we asked Drew Batavia to take the lead in conducting this study for us. We were interested in collecting data on frequency with which centers are contacted by consumers with managed care problems. This is a study that will need to be repeated periodically as our experiences with managed care evolves. Meanwhile, here are the initial findings.

10 pages

4874 Independent Living Challenges the Blues
Independent Living Research Utilization ILRU
2323 S Shepherd Drive
Suite 1000
Houston, TX 77019
713-520-0232
FAX: 713-520-5785
www.ilru.org

Laurie Redd, Executive Director
Patricia's article highlights the Georgia SILC's health care advocacy efforts: the Georgia legislature passed a bill enabling Georgia Bleu to convert to for-profit status without a distribution of assets to similar nonprofit corporations; the Georgia SILC joined other health care advocates in filing a class action law suit to challenge the legality of the conversion; the Georgia SILC continues advocacy efforts to involve people with disabilities in developing and monitoring health care policy.

10 pages

4875 Independent Living Office
Department of Housing & Urban Development (HUD)
451 7th Street SW
Washington, DC 20410
202-863-2800

This office within HUD is charged with encouraging the construction of housing that is accessible to handicapped persons. The Office of Independent Living encourages modifications of apartments and other dwellings so that handicapped persons can enter without assistance.

4876 Independent Newsletter
Easter Seals Nebraska
638 N 109th Plaza
Omaha, NE 68154
402-345-2200
800-650-9880
FAX: 402-345-2500
e-mail: kginder@ne.easterseals.com
www.ne.easterseals.com

Ingra Winkler Anderson, author

4 pages Quarterly

4877 Information Services for People with Developmental Disabilities
Greenwood Publishing Group
88 Post Road W
Suite 5007
Westport, CT 06880
203-226-3571
FAX: 203-222-1502
www.greenwood.com

Linda Lucas Walling, Editor
Marilyn M Irwin, Editor
Wayne Smith, President
Overviews the information needs of people with developmental disabilities and tells librarians how to meet them. $65.oo-$75.00.

368 pages Hardcover
ISBN 0-313287-80-5

4878 Innovative Programs: An Example of How CILs Can Put Their Work in Context
Culture
2323 S Shepherd Drive
Suite 1000
Houston, TX 77019
713-535-2200
FAX: 713-520-5785
www.ilru.org

Jim Alister Sr, President
Another winner in the innovative CIL competition- Steve Brown describes the Talking Books Program of Southeast Alaska Independent Living, discussing their efforts to record the oral history and life experiences of people with disabilities in the larger context of disability culture.

10 pages

4879 Insurance Solutions: Plan Well, Live Better
Demos Medical Publishing
386 Park Avenue S
Suite 201
New York, NY 10016
212-683-0072
800-532-8663
FAX: 212-683-0118
e-mail: orderdep@demospub.com
www.demosmedpub.com

Diana Schneider PhD, President
Phyllis Gold, Owner
Learn how to look at various insurance options from a new perspective — including life, disability, health, and long-term care. Concrete information for dealing with potential problems in your coverage, to secure your financial future. *$24.95*

192 pages 2002
ISBN 1-888799-55-2

4880 Intensive Early Intervention and Beyond School-Based Inclusion Program
Research Press
2612 N Mattis Avenue
Champaign, IL 61822
217-352-3273
800-519-2707
FAX: 217-352-2707
e-mail: rp@researchpress.com
www.researchpress.com

Russell Pence, President
Shows the successful application of a school-based inclusion program. The video focuses on the lives of young children with autism who have shown remarkable progress in personal, social, and academic skills. 22 minutes. *$195.00*

Video

4881 International Directory of Libraries for the Disabled
KG Saur/Division of RR Bowker
121 Chanlon Road
New Providence, NJ 07974
908-286-1090
800-521-8110

Michael Cairns, Chief Executive Officer
An essential resource for improving the quality and quantity of materials available to the print-handicapped audience. Featuring talking books, braille books, large print books as well as production centers for these materials. *$46.00*

257 pages
ISBN 3-59821 -81-1

4882 Issues in Independent Living
Independent Living Research Utilization
2323 S Shepherd Drive
Suite 1000
Houston, TX 77019
713-520-0232
FAX: 713-520-5785

Lex Frieden, Program Director
Laurie Redd, Executive Director
This booklet is a report of the National Study Group on the Implications of Health Care Reform for Americans with Disabilities and Chronic Health Conditions.

30 pages

4883 JAMA: The Journal of the American Medical Association
American Medical Association
515 N State Street
Chicago, IL 60610
312-464-5000
FAX: 312-464-2580
e-mail: ama.jama
jama.ama-assn.org

Roger Rosenberg MD, Editor
Peter Payerli, Publisher
Michael Maves, Chief Executive Officer
Articles cover all aspects of medical research and clinical medicine. *$66.00*

4884 JCIL Advocate Times
Jackson Center for Independent Living
409 Linden Avenue
Jackson, MI 49203
517-784-1723
FAX: 517-784-9921

Perry Stahl, author
Quarterly

4885 Jason & Nordic Publishers
PO Box 441
Hollidaysburg, PA 16648
814-696-2920
FAX: 814-696-4250
e-mail: turtlbks@nb.net
www.jasonandnordic.com

Richard S McPhee, Director
Norma Phee, Owner
Turtle Books for children with disabilities present heroes who look like them, have problems like theirs, have similar doubts and feelings in non-threatening, fun stories. They are motivational, bridge the gap and promote understanding among peers and siblings. 16 children's books (grades preK-3) plus Sensitivity and Awareness Guide containing lesson plans, activities, background information keyed to the series. Disabilities include: Down syndrome, cerebral palsy, blindness, deafness and more.

4886 Journal of Social Work in Disabilty & Rehabilitation
Haworth Press
10 Alice Street
Binghamton, NY 13904
607-722-5857
800-429-6784
FAX: 607-722-6362
e-mail: orders@haworthpress.com
www.haworthpress.com

John T Oardeck PhD, Editor
S Harrington-Miller, Advertising
William Cohen, Owner
Presents and explores issues related to disabilities and social policy, practice, research, and theory. Reflecting the broad scope of social work in disabilty practice, this interdisciplinary journal examines vital issues aspects of the field — from innovative practice methods, legal issues, and literature reviews to program descriptions and cuttinf-edge practice research.
Quarterly

4887 Journal of the Association for Persons with Severe Handicaps
29 W Susquehanna Avenue
Suite 210
Baltimore, MD 21204
410-828-8274
FAX: 410-828-6706
e-mail: info@tash.org
www.tash.org
Provides contemporary articles on specialized topics of interest to TASH members and others in the field of development disabilities. *$25.00*
Quarterly

4888 Just Like Everyone Else
World Institute on Disability
510 16th Street
Suite 100
Oakland, CA 94612
510-763-4100
FAX: 510-763-4109
e-mail: wid@wid.org
www.wid.org
The oversize-format publication, intended for general audiences, provides perspective, inspiration and information about the Independent Living Movement and the Americans with Disabilities Act. *$5.00*
16 pages

4889 Keep the Promise: Managed Care and People with Disabilities
American Network of Community Options & Resource
1101 King Street
Suite 380
Alexandria, VA 22314
703-535-7850
FAX: 703-535-7860
e-mail: ancor@ancor.org
www.ancor.org

Renee L Pietrangelo, CEO
Suellen Galbraith, Director Public Policy
This publication presents a detailed review of the process and the lessons learned. Details a way for all stake holders to work together for a state or local system.
119 pages $18 - $22

4890 Keeping Our Families Together
Through the Looking Glass
2198 6th Street
Suite 100
Berkeley, CA 94710
510-848-1112
800-644-2666
FAX: 510-848-4445
e-mail: TLG@lookingglass.org
www.lookingglass.org

Megan Kirshbaum, Executive Director
Tina Evoyne, Office Manager
Report of the National Task Force on parents with disabilities and their families. Available in braille, large print or cassette. *$2.00*
12 pages

4891 Learn About the ADA in Your Local Library
US Department of Justice
950 Pennsylvania Avenue NW Drs
- Nyav
Washington, DC 20530
202-586-5000
800-574-0301
FAX: 202-307-1197
www.ada.gov

Joanne Graham, Manager
A 10-page annotated list of 95 ADA publications and one videotape that are available in 15,000 public libraries throughout the country.

4892 LifeLines
Disabled & Alone/Life Services for the Handicapped
352 Park Avenue S
11th Floor
New York, NY 10010
212-532-6740
800-995-0066
FAX: 212-532-3588
e-mail: info@disabledandalone.org
www.disabledandalone.org

Roslyn Brilliant, Executive Director
Newsletter providing current and valuable information about lifetime care and planning for persons with disabilities and their families and the organizations serving them. Free upon request.
4-10 pages BiAnnual

4893 Lifelong Leisure Skills and Lifestyles for Persons with Developmental Disabilities
Brookes Publishing
PO Box 10624
Baltimore, MD 21285
410-337-9580
800-638-3775
FAX: 410-337-8539
e-mail: custserv@brookespublishing.com
www.brookespublishing.com

Paul Brooks, Owner
This instructional manual offers ideas and detailed examples that describe how to guide individuals of all ages through popular activities using adaptations that foster skill acquisition and inclusion. Some of the concepts explored are home-school-community collaboration, choice making and the dignity of risk, and leisure skill acquisition for the life span. *$35.00*
352 pages Paperback
ISBN 1-55766 -47-2

4894 Livin'
Lehigh Valley Center for Independent Living
435 Allentown Drive
Allentown, PA 18109
610-770-9781
FAX: 610-770-9801

Amy C Beck, Executive Director

4 pages Quarterly

4895 Living in a State of Stuck
Brookline Books
PO Box 1046
Cambridge, MA 02139
617-868-0360
800-666-2665
FAX: 617-868-1772
e-mail: thestore@brooklinebooks.com
www.brooklinebooks.com

Offers explanations on how adaptive technologies affect the lives of people with disabilities. *$24.95*
3rd ed., paper
ISBN 1-571290-27-3

4896 Living in the Community
Independent Living Research Utilization ILRU
2323 S Shepherd Drive
Suite 1000
Houston, TX 77019
713-520-0232
FAX: 713-520-5785
www.ilru.org

Laurie Redd, Executive Director

James, Lori, and Jamey describe the elements of their successful program to move people out of nursing homes and into the community: providing funding for deposits, first month's rent and other neccessities, including assistive technology; providing training and the other core services before and after consumers leave the nursing home; developing relationships with housing and other service providers.
10 pages

4897 Look Who's Laughing
Aquarius Health Care Videos
PO Box 1159
Sherborn, MA 01770
508-650-6905
FAX: 508-650-4216
e-mail: aqvideos@tiac.net
www.aquariusproductions.com

This video is packed with laugh-out-loud comedic moments, but is also full of intelligent and inspiring messages. Look Who's Laughing introduces viewers to some of today's funniest comedians - who just happen to be physically disabled. We hear them talk openly and honestly about their limitations as well as their abilities and talents. Helpful for those who work with the disabled and motivational to both the disabled and able-bodied. Preview option available. *$95.00*
Video

4898 Loud, Proud and Passionate
Mobility International USA
PO Box 10767
Eugene, OR 97440
541-343-1284
FAX: 541-343-6812
e-mail: info@miusa.org
www.miusa.org

Susan Sygall, Executive Director
Pamela Houston, Public Relations Coordinator
Tracy Scharn, Project Assistant

A resource book for international development and women's organization about including women with disabilities in projects in the community. Informs women sith disabilities about the efforts and successes of their peers worldwide. *$30.00*

4899 Love: Where to Find It, How to Keep It
Accent Books & Products
PO Box 700
Bloomington, IL 61702
309-378-2961
800-787-8444
FAX: 309-378-4420
e-mail: acmtlvng@aol.com

Raymond C Cheever, Publisher
Betty Garee, Editor

Offers ideas such as how to meet other single people, avoid the wrong type; communications skills and much more for the disabled person wanting to date. *$6.95*
104 pages Paperback
ISBN 0-91570 -31-0

4900 MOOSE: A Very Special Person
Brookline Books
PO Box 1046
Cambridge, MA 02139
617-868-0360
800-666-2665
FAX: 617-868-1772
e-mail: thestore@brooklinebooks.com
www.brooklinebooks.com

Moose, which in very human terms, teaches us that each of us is different and that we have our own unique capacity for loving, sharing, enjoying and learning. *$10.95*
Paperback
ISBN 0-91479 -73-5

4901 Mainstream Magazine
2973 Beech Street
San Diego, CA 92102
619-234-3138
FAX: 619-234-3155
e-mail: editor@mainstream.mag.com
www.mainstream-mag.com

Cyndi Jones, Publisher/President

The authoritative, national voice of people with disabilities, publishes in-depth reports on employment, education, new products and technology, legislation and disability rights advocacy, recreation and travel, disability arts and culture, plus personality profiles and challenging commentary. *$24.00*
Monthly

4902 Making Changes: Family Voices on Living Disabilities
Brookline Books
PO Box 1047
Cambridge, MA 02139
800-666-2665
FAX: 617-868-1772
e-mail: thestore@brooklinebooks.com
www.brooklinebooks.com

What are the day to day impacts on the family when a disabled child is born? Or when a child who grows up without a disability becomes disabled through accident or disease? This provocative set of reports illuminates the conditions of those peoples lives, and the way they and those around them adjust to the disabilities. *$16.95*
216 pages Paperback
ISBN 0-91479 -93-

4903 Making Informed Medical Decisions: Where to Look and How to Use What You Find
Patient-Centered Guides
101 Morris Street
Sebastopol, CA 95472
707-829-0515
800-998-9938
FAX: 707-829-0104
www.patientcenters.com

Tim O'Reilly, Chief Executive Officer

Making Informed Medical Decisions acts like a friendly reference librarian, explaining: tips for researching for someone else; medical journal articles; statistics and risk; standard treatment options; clinical trial; making an ally of your doctor; and determining your own best course. Authors Oster, Thomas, and Joseff-a patient advocate, medical librarian, and medical doctor-also share examples and stories. *$17.95*
280 pages Paperback
ISBN 1-565924-59-2

4904 Making Wise Decisions for Long-Term Care
AARP Fulfillment
601 E Street NW
Washington, DC 20049
202-434-2277
800-424-3410
FAX: 202-434-3443
e-mail: member@aarp.org
www.aarp.org

William Novelli, Chief Executive Officer

Here's a comprehensive consumer education effort in the area of long-term care.

28 pages

4905 **Making a Difference**
Government Council on Developmental Disabilities
2 Peachtree Street NW
Atlanta, GA 30303
404-657-2126
888-275-4233
FAX: 404-657-2123
e-mail: eejacobson@dhr.state.ga.us
www.gcdd.org

Eric E Johnson, Executive Director
Beth Spinning, Program Director
Yao Seidu, Public Information Officer

4906 **Making a Difference: A Wise Approach**
Easter Seals
230 W Monroe Street
Chicago, IL 60606
312-726-0653
FAX: 312-726-1494

Janet D Jamieson, Communication Manager
The town of Wise, Virginia, and its leading citizen, Virgil Craft, personify what Making a Difference is all about when a community supports implementing the provisions of the Americans with Disabilities Act. Craft, a person with a disability, has spent his life giving back to the community. The community, in turn, has supported Craft's efforts to improve the environment, education, healthcare and access for disabled persons. A must buy for companies of all sizes, clubs and organizations. *$50.00*

4907 **Managing Your Activities**
Arthritis Foundation
PO Box 7669
Atlanta, GA 30357
404-872-7100
800-283-7800
FAX: 404-872-9559
e-mail: help@arthritis.org
www.arthritis.org

John Klippel, Chief Executive Officer

4908 **Managing Your Health Care**
Arthritis Foundation
PO Box 7669
Atlanta, GA 30357
404-872-7100
800-283-7800
FAX: 404-872-9559
e-mail: help@arthritis.org
www.arthritis.org

John Klippel, Chief Executive Officer

4909 **Medical Aspects of Disability: A Handbook For The Rehabilitation Professional**
Springer Publishing Company
536 Broadway
New York, NY 10012
212-431-4370
877-687-7476
877-687-7976
FAX: 212-941-7842
e-mail: marketing@springerpub.com
www.springerpub.com

Annette Imperati, Marketing/Sales Director
Ursula Springer, President
$62.92
744 pages
ISBN 0-826179-71-1

4910 **Meeting the Needs of Employees with Disabilities**
Resources for Rehabilitation
33 Bedford Street
Suite 19a
Lexington, MA 02420
781-368-9094
FAX: 781-368-9096

Susan Greenblatt
Provides information to help people with disabilities retain or obtain employment. Information on government programs and laws, supported employment, training programs, environmental adaptations and the transition from school to work are included. Chapters on mobility impairment, vision impairment and hearing and speech impairments. *$ 47.95*

167 pages Biennial
ISBN 0-92971 -13-5

4911 **NCD Bulletin**
National Council on Disability
1331 F Street NW
Suite 850
Washington, DC 20004
202-272-2004
FAX: 202-272-2022
www.ncd.gov

Mark Quigley, Communication Director
Ethel Briggs, Executive Director
Reports on the latest issues and news affecting people with disabilities.
2 pages Monthly

4912 **NCDE Survival Strategies for Oversease Liv ing for People with Disabilities**
National Clearinghouse on Disability and Exchange
PO Box 10767
Eugene, OR 97440
541-373-1284
FAX: 541-343-6812
e-mail: info@miusa.org
www.miusa.org

Pamela Houston, Public Relations Coordinator
This book will provide individuals with disablilities information, resources and guidance on pursuing international exchange opportunities. It addresses disability-related aspects of the international exchange process such as choosing a program, applying, preparing for the trip, adjusting to a new country and returning home.

4913 **NOD E-Newsletter**
National Organization on Disability
910 16th Street NW
Suite 600
Washington, DC 20006
202-293-5960
FAX: 202-293-7999
e-mail: ability@nod.org
www.nod.org

Michael Deland, President
Brewster Thackeray, VP Communications
John Hershey, Advice and Resource Manager
Monthly E-Newsletter from the National Organization on Disability. Free.
3 pages Monthly

4914 **National Hookup**
ISC
16 Liberty Street
Larkspur, CA 94939
415-924-3549
FAX: 415-927-9556
e-mail: russbo@microweb.com

Russ Bohlke, Executive Secretary
Newsletter published by ISC, a national organization of people with physical disabilities. *$6.00*
12-16 pages Quarterly

4915 **New Horizons in Sexuality**
Accent Books & Products
PO Box 700
Bloomington, IL 61702
309-378-2961
800-787-8444
FAX: 309-378-4420
e-mail: acmtlvng@aol.com

Raymond C Cheever, Publisher
Betty Garee, Editor
This manual helps both males and females progress toward a satisfying post-injury relationship. *$7.95*
50 pages Paperback
ISBN 0-91570 -42-6

4916 **New Voices: Self Advocacy By People with Disabilities**
Brookline Books
PO Box 1047
Cambridge, MA 02139
617-868-0360
800-666-2665
FAX: 617-868-1772
e-mail: thestore@brooklinebooks.com
www.brooklinebooks.com

A collection of original papers, many by self advocates, that vividly illustrate the dynamic, ever-growing self-advocacy movement — persons with disabilities speaking out and seeking better non-institutional living situations, social and political equality and decent jobs at reasonable pay. *$29.95*

274 pages Paperback
ISBN 1-57129 -04-4

4917 North Star Community Services

3420 University Avenue
Waterloo, IA 50701
319-236-0901
FAX: 319-236-3701
e-mail: info@northstarcs.org
www.northstarcs.org

Mark Witmer, Executive Director
Donna Davis, Dir Development/Public Relations

North Star Community Services is a rehabilitative services organization with home office in Waterloo, IA and several branch offices in Northeast, Northern and Central Iowa. North Star helps indiviuals with disabilities live and work in their communities. Services include: adult day services, supported community living services, employment services, and case management/service coordination.

4918 Nothing is Impossible: Reflections on a N ew Life

Ballantine Books
4958 Main Street
Downers Grove, IL 60515
630-663-1472
www.randomhouse.com/BB/

Reeve offers a uniquely powerful message of hope on topics ranging from the controversial stem cell debate to the mind-body connection he credits with his recent physical improvements. *$6.99*

224 pages 2004
ISBN 0-345470-73-7

4919 Nutritional Desk Reference

Keats Publishing
PO Box 876
New Canaan, CT 06840
203-966-8721
800-323-4900

4920 Nutritional Influences on Illness:

Third Line Press
4751 Viviana Drive
Tarzana, CA 91356
818-996-0076
tlp@third-line.com

Melvyn Werbach, Owner

A comprehensive summary of the world's knowledge concerning the relationship between dietary and nutrtional factors and illness. This book does not try to promote any particular school of thought. Instead of the author telling readers his opinion as to what research says, he makes it easy for them to see data for themselves and then form their own opinions.

504 pages
ISBN 0-879835-31-1

4921 Oregon Clarion

Oregon Developmental Disability Council
540 24th Pl NE
Salem, OR 97301
503-945-9941
800-292-4154
FAX: 503-945-9947
e-mail: ocdd@ocdd.org
www.ocdd.org

Michael T Bailey, Editor
Bill Lynch, Acting Executive Director

A quarterly publication from the Oregon Developmental Disability Council.

4922 Organ Transplants: Making the Most of Your Gift of Life

Patient-Centered Guides
101 Morris Street
Sebastopol, CA 95472
707-829-0515
800-998-9938
FAX: 707-829-0104
www.patientcenters.com

Linda Lamb, Editor
Shawnde Paull, Marketing
Tim O'Reilly, Chief Executive Officer

Over 64,000 people in the US are awaiting an organ transplant. Although transplant surgeries are now fairly routine and can give their recipients the gift of new life, the road to getting a transplant can be long and harrowing. Living with immunosuppressive drugs and strong emotional responses can also be more challenging than families imagine. Medical journalist Robert Finn answers the concerns of these families, with the latest facts about transplantation - as well as the stories behind them. *$19.95*

326 pages Paperback
ISBN 1-565926-34-X

4923 PEAK Parent Center

611 N Weber Street
Suite 200
Colorado Springs, CO 80903
719-531-9400
800-284-0251
FAX: 719-531-9452
e-mail: info@peakparent.org
www.peakparent.org

Barbara Buswell, Executive Director

PEAK Parent Center is a federally-designated Parent Training and Information Center (PTI). As a PTI, PEAK supports and empowers parents, providing them with information and strategies to use when advocating for their children with disabilities. PEAK works one-on-one with families and educators helping them realize new possibilities for children with disabilities by expanding knowledge of special education and offering new strategies for success.

4924 Parallels in Time

MN Governor's Council on Development Disabilities
658 Cedar Street
Saint Paul, MN 55155
651-296-4018
877-348-0505
FAX: 651-297-7200
e-mail: admin.dd@state.mn.us
www.mncdd.org

Colleen Wieck PhD, Executive Director

Parallels in Time traces present attitudes and the treatment of people with disabilities, and supplements the first weekend seesion of Partners in Policymaking. This CD-ROM includes the History of the Parent Movement and the History of the Independent Living Movement, as well as personal stories of self advocates, leaders in the self advocacy movement.

4925 Part of the Team

Easter Seals
230 W Monroe Street
Suite 1800
Chicago, IL 60606
312-726-6800
FAX: 312-726-1494

Janet D Jamieson, Communications Manager
James Williams Jr, Chief Executive Officer

Designed for employers of all sizes, rehabilitation organizations and all others concerned with the employment of people with disabilities. It addresses managers' concerns and questions about supervising persons with disabilities and can be used as a discussion/team-building tool for employees with and without disabilities. The video recognizes people with disabilities as strong contenders for almost any job. *$15.00*

4926 Partnering with Public Health: Funding & Advocacy Opportunities for CILs and SILCs

Independent Living Research Utilization ILRU
2323 S Shepherd Drive
Suite 1000
Houston, TX 77019
713-520-0232
FAX: 713-520-5785
www.ilru.org

Laurie Redd, Executive Director

Laura Rauscher discusses how CILs and SCILs can use funding from the Centers for Disease Control and partnerships with public health agencies to provide innovative programs promoting the health of people with disabilities.

10 pages

4927 Passion for Justice
Fanlight Productions
4196 Washington Street
Suite 2
Boston, MA 02131
617-469-4999
800-937-4113
FAX: 617-469-3379
e-mail: fanlight@fanlight.com
www.fanlight.com

Ben Achtenberg, Owner
An engaging portrait of Bob Perske, the author of Unequal Justice and a crusader for the rights of people with developmental disabilities. The tape focuses on cases in which people with developmental disabilities have been convicted of crimes they didn't commit. The tape asks challenging questions about society's responsibility to this population, and about ways to protect their rights to equality and justice. *$99.00*
29 Minutes

4928 Peer Counseling: Roles, Functions, Boundaries
Independent Living Research Utilization ILRU
2323 S Shepherd Drive
Suite 1000
Houston, TX 77019
713-520-0232
FAX: 713-520-5785
www.ilru.org

Laurie Redd, Executive Director
In this article, the following points were discussed: describing peer support as counseling suggests safeguards and expectations which cannot be provided by nonprofessionals; the purpose of peer counseling is to promote the independent living philosophy and encourage consumers to embrace it; peer counseling cannot and is not intended to help individuals deal with intense emotional stress, whether it is related to their disability or to something else.
10 pages

4929 Peer Mentor Volunteers: Empowering People for Change
Independent Living Research Utilization ILRU
2323 S Shepherd Drive
Suite 1000
Houston, TX 77019
713-520-0232
FAX: 713-520-5785
www.ilru.org

Laurie Redd, Executive Director
Arizona Bridge to Independent Living (ABIL) in Phoenix, featured in this issue, is another winner in the innovative CIL program competition.
10 pages

4930 People and Families
New Jersey Council on Developmental Disabilities
PO Box 700
Trenton, NJ 08625
609-292-3745
800-216-1199
FAX: 609-292-7114
TTY: 609-777-3238
e-mail: njddc@njddc.org
www.njcdd.org

Alison Lozano, Director/Executive
Douglas McGutherz, Deputy Director
Norman Reim, Editor
A free magazine for people with disabilities, their families and the public about disability topics such as personal assistance, deinstitutionalization, health care and community living. Published by the New Jersey council on Developmental Disabilities, a federally funded advocacy and policy advisory body. The council has 25 members - 15 consumer/product volunteers and 10 professionals.
48 pages Quarterly

4931 People with Disabilities & Abuse: Implications for Center for Independent Living
Independent Living Research Utilization ILRU
2323 S Shepherd Drive
Suite 1000
Houston, TX 77019
713-520-0232
FAX: 713-520-5785
www.ilru.org

Laurie Redd, Executive Director
10 pages

4932 People with Disabilities Who Challenge the System
Brookes Publishing
PO Box 10624
Baltimore, MD 21285
410-337-9580
800-638-3775
FAX: 410-337-8539
e-mail: custserv@brookespublishing.com
www.brookespublishing.com

Paul Brooks, Owner
Helpful forms, tables, and case studies plus an emphasis on self-determination point the way to the development of supports so that people who are deaf-blind, have severe to profound physical and cognitive disabilities, or have serious behavior problems can be fully included in the classroom, workplace, and community. *$34.00*
464 pages Paperback
ISBN 1-55766 -29-0

4933 People's Voice
Independence CIL
300 3rd Avenue SW
Suite F
Minot, ND 58701
701-839-4724
800-377-5114
FAX: 701-838-1677

Stephen Repnow, Executive Director
8 pages Quarterly

4934 Personal Perspectives on Personal Assistance Services
World Institute on Disability
510 16th Street
Suite 100
Oakland, CA 94612
510-763-4100
FAX: 510-763-4109
e-mail: wid@wid.org
www.wid.org
This collection of personal essays explores a wide range of perspectives on Personal Assistance Services. Family issues and PAS concerns for people with various different disabilities, of different ages and as members of minority groups are addressed. *$5.00*
80 pages Paperback

4935 Perspectives
National Assoc. of State Directors of DD Services
113 Oronoco Street
Alexandria, VA 22314
703-683-4202
FAX: 703-683-8773
e-mail: klebeau@nasddds.org

Kara Lebeau, State Policy Analyst
Nancy Thaler, Executive Director
Provides a concise summary of national policy developments and initiatives affecting persons with devlopmental disabilities and the programs that serve them. From bills pending before Congress, to the growth in Medicaid-funded services, to changes in federal-state Medicaid policies and the shift of responsibility from Washington to the states, keeps readers in tune with the latest national issues shaping publically funded disability services. *$95.00*
Monthly

4936 Place to Live
Accent Books & Products
PO Box 700
Bloomington, IL 61702
309-378-2961
800-787-8444
FAX: 309-378-4420
e-mail: acmtlvng@aol.com

Raymond C Cheever, Publisher
Betty Garee, Editor
Many disabled people have found that group housing or accessible apartments are the best alternative to living in a nursing home. These articles tell about some of the alternatives people have found so they can live independently. Just one idea might be the answer for better living for you. *$4.95*

64 pages Paperback
ISBN 0-91570 -30-2

4937 Proceedings
AHEAD
PO Box 21192
Columbus, OH 43221
617-287-3880
FAX: 617-287-3881
TTY:617-287-3882
e-mail: aagad@postbox.acs.ohio-state.edu
www.ahead.org
National conferences, innovative programs, research, evaluation services, auxiliary aids, career information and other vital information.

4938 Psychological & Social Impact of Disabilit y
Springer Publishing Company
536 Broadway
New York, NY 10012
212-431-4370
877-687-7476
FAX: 212-941-7842
e-mail: marketing@springerpub.com
www.springerpub.com

Annette Imperati, Marketing/Sales Director
Ursula Springer, President
$49.95
488 pages
ISBN 0-826122-13-2

4939 Psychology and Health
Springer Publishing Company
536 Broadway
New York, NY 10012
212-431-4370
877-687-7476
FAX: 212-941-7842
e-mail: marketing@springerpub.com
www.springerpub.com

Annette Imperati, Marketing/Sales Director
Ursula Springer, President
Content of this book spans a wide range of clinical conditions, including somatization disorders, chronic pain, migraine, anxiety and cancer. *$29.95*
256 pages

4940 Psychology of Disability
Springer Publishing Company
536 Broadway
New York, NY 10012
212-431-4370
877-687-7476
FAX: 212-941-7842
e-mail: marketing@springerpub.com
www.springerpub.com

Annette Imperati, Marketing/Sales Director
Ursula Springer, President
Reactions to the disabled. *$27.95*
288 pages
ISBN 0-82613 -40-1

4941 Quality of Life for Persons with Disabilities
Brookline Books
PO Box 1046
Cambridge, MA 02139
617-868-0360
800-666-2665
FAX: 617-868-1772
e-mail: thestore@brooklinebooks.com
www.brooklinebooks.com
Quality of life generally refers to a person's subjective experience of his or her life and focuses attention on how the individual with a disabling condition experiences the world. This book presents a comprehensive and international view of this concept as applied to a broad range of settings in which persons with disabilities live, work and play. *$35.00*

Paperback
ISBN 0-91479 -92-1

4942 REACHing Out Newsletter
REACH of Dallas Resource on Independent Living
8625 King George Drive
Suite 210
Dallas, TX 75235
214-630-4796
FAX: 214-630-6390
e-mail: reachdallas@reachcils.org
www.reachcils.org

Charlotte Stewart, Executive Director/Owner
Susie Reukema, Assistant Director
Becky Teal, Editor
Quarterly newsletter from REACH of Dallas Resource Center on Independent Living.
16 pages

4943 RTC Connection
Research and Training Center
University of Wisconsin Stout
Menomonie, WI 54751
715-232-2236
FAX: 715-232-2251
e-mail: menz@uwstout.edu
www.rtc.uwstout.edu

Julie Larson, Program Assistant
Bi-annual reports on disability and rehabilitation research and policy topics.
Newsletter

4944 Ragged Edge: The Disability Experience
Advocado Press
PO Box 145
Louisville, KY 40201
502-894-9492
FAX: 502-899-9562
e-mail: office@advocadopress.orgom
www.advocadopress.org

Barrett Shaw, Editor
Anthology of writing from the pages of the first 15 years of The Disability Rag. *$18.95*
245 pages
ISBN 0-96270 -45-0

4945 Rehabilitation Gazette
Gazette International Networking Institute
4207 Lindell Boulevard
Suite 110
Saint Louis, MO 63108
314-534-0475
FAX: 314-534-5070
e-mail: gini_intl@msn.com
www.post-polio.org
International journal of independent living for people with disabilities. *$12.00*
8 pages Bi-Annually

4946 Relaxation Techniques for People with Special Needs
Research Press
2612 N Mattis Avenue
Champaign, IL 61822
217-352-3273
800-519-2707
FAX: 217-352-1221
e-mail: rp@researchpress.com
www.researchpress.com

Gail Salyards, Marketing Services Manager
Russell Pence, President
The developers discuss and demonstrate how to use special relaxation procedures with children and adolescents who have developmental disabilities. They emphasize the need for students to learn relaxation as a means of coping with stress and developing self-control. During the scenes of Dr June Groden conducting relaxation training, viewers will see how to correctly use the training procedures, how to use reinforcement during training and how to use guided imagery. 23 minutes. Includes book. *$195.00*

Video

4947 **Relaxation: A Comprehensive Manual for Adults and Children with Special Needs**
Research Press
2612 N Mattis Avenue
Champaign, IL 61822
217-352-3273
800-519-2707
FAX: 217-352-1221
e-mail: rp@researchpress.com
www.researchpress.com

Gail Salyards, Marketing Services Manager
Russell Pence, President
This unique contribution to the field of relaxation training presents: self relaxation techniques designed for adults, methods for teaching relaxation to adults and older children, and procedures for teaching relaxation to young children and children with developmental disabilities. The clear, concise text is supplemented by over 100 helpful illustrations. *$16.95*
108 pages Paperback
ISBN 0-878221-86-7

4948 **Resources for People with Disabilities and Chronic Conditions**
Resources for Rehabilitation
33 Bedford Street
Suite 19a
Lexington, MA 02420
781-890-6371
FAX: 781-861-7517

Susan Greenblatt
A comprehensive resource directory that helps people with disabilities and chronic conditions achieve their maximum level of independence. Chapters on spinal cord injuries, low back pain, diabetes, hearing and speech impairments, epilepsy, multiple sclerosis. Describes organizations, products and publications. *$49.95*
215 pages Biennial
ISBN 0-92971 -12-7

4949 **Role Portrayal and Stereotyping on Television**
Greenwood Publishing Group
88 Post Road W
Suite 5007
Westport, CT 06880
203-226-3571
FAX: 203-222-1502
www.greenwood.com

Nancy Signorielli, Author
Wayne Smith, President
An annotated bibliography of studies relating to women, minorities, aging, health and handicaps.
214 pages $55 - $59.95
ISBN 0-313248-55-9

4950 **Screening in Chronic Disease**
Oxford University Press
2001 Evans Road
Cary, NC 27513
919-677-0977
800-451-7556
FAX: 919-677-1303
www.oup-usa.org

Thomas Carty, Senior Vice President
Early detection, or screening, is a common strategy for controlling chronic disease, but little information has been available to help determine which screening procedures are worthwhile, until this textbook. *$42.50*
256 pages

4951 **Sexual Adjustment**
Accent Books & Products
PO Box 700
Bloomington, IL 61702
309-378-2961
800-787-8444
FAX: 309-378-4420
e-mail: acmtlvng@aol.com

Raymond C Cheever, Publisher
Betty Garee, Editor
Essential information concerning sexual adjustment for the paraplegic male. *$4.95*
73 pages Paperback
ISBN 0-19570 -00-0

4952 **Sexuality and Disabilities: A Guide for Human Service Practitioners**
Haworth Press
10 Alice Street
Binghamton, NY 13904
607-722-5857
800-429-6784
FAX: 607-722-6362
e-mail: orders@haworthpress.com
www.haworthpress.com

Jackie Blakeslee, Advertising
Romel W Mackelpranf DSW, Editor
Deborah Valentine, Editor
This book addresses persons with physical, sensory, intellectual and cognitive disabilities and their concerns in the areas of intimacy, family issues, sexuality and sexual functioning. *$74.95*
159 pages Hardcover
ISBN 1-560243-75-9

4953 **Sickened: The Memoir of a Muchausen by Pro xy Childhood**
Bantam Books
1540 Broadway
New York, NY 10036
212-782-9000
FAX: 212-302-7985
www.randomhouse.com
From early childhood, Julie Gregory was continually X-rayed, medicated, and operated on — in the vain pursuit of an illness that was created in her mother's mind. Munchausen by proxy (MBP) in which the caretaker — almost always the mother — invents or induces symptoms in her child because she craves the attention of medical professionals. *$24.95*
256 pages Hardcover 2003
ISBN 0-553803-07-7

4954 **Socialization Games for Persons with Disabilities**
Nevalyn F Nevil, Marna L Beatty & David Moxley
2600 S 1st Street
Springfield, IL 62704
217-789-8980
800-258-8980
FAX: 217-789-9130
e-mail: books@ccthomas.com
www.ccthomas.com

Michael Thomas, President
This book is a compilation of practical suggestions and games with easy-to-follow guide lines that provide a solid foundation for the encouragement of positive social behavior. *$47.95*
176 pages Paperback 1997
ISBN 0-398067-46-5

4955 **Sometimes You Just Want to Feel Like a Human Being**
Brookes Publishing
PO Box 10624
Baltimore, MD 21285
410-337-9580
800-638-3775
FAX: 410-337-8539
e-mail: custserv@brookespublishing.com
www.brookespublishing.com

Paul Brooks, Owner
Case studies of empowering psychotherapy with people with disabilities. This text reveals how counseling can be beneficial to individuals with disabilities of all kinds, including autism, mental retardation, sensory impairment, cerebral palsy, or HIV infection. *$ 26.95*
272 pages Paperback
ISBN 1-55766 -96-0

4956 **Space Coast CIL News**
Space Coast Center for Independent Living
331 Ramp Road
Cocoa Beach, FL 32931
321-784-9008
FAX: 321-784-3702
TTY:321-784-9008
e-mail: agrau@bellsouth.net

Anna Grau, Ind. Living Services Coordinator
Donna Taylor, Executive Director
Non-profit organization that provides services which enable people with disabilities to live as independently as possible.

12 pages Quarterly

4957 Special Siblings: Growing Up With Someone with A Disability
Brookes Publishing
PO Box 10624
Baltimore, MD 21285
410-337-9580
800-638-3775
FAX: 410-337-8539
e-mail: custserv@brookespublishing.com
www.brookespublishing.com

Paul Brooks, Owner
The author reveals what she experienced as the sister of a man with cerebral palsy and mental retardation — and shares what others have learned about being and having a special sibling. Weaving a lifetime of memories and reflections with relevant research and interviews with more than 100 other siblings and experts, McHugh explores a spectrum of feelings — from anger and guilt to love and pride — and helps readers understand the issues siblings may encounter. *$21.95*
256 pages Paperback 2002
ISBN 1-557666-07-5

4958 TERI
3225 Roymar Road
Oceanside, CA 92054
760-721-1706

Cheryl Kilmer, Executive Director
A private, nonprofit corporation which has been developing and operating programs for individuals with developmental disabilities since 1980. Offers staff training videos, staff training tools and technique manuals.

4959 Teaching People with Developmental Disabilities
Research Press
PO Box 9177
Champaign, IL 61826
217-352-3273
800-519-2707
FAX: 217-352-1221
e-mail: rp@researchpress.com
www.researchpress.com

Russell Pence, President
Hands-on video training series designed to help teachers, staff, volunteers, or family members master four behavioral techniques vital to teaching functional living skills. The videotapes which provide clear and simple teaching demonstrations, are designed to be stopped and started frequently to allow time for viewer response. Each tape includes numerous scenes of training sessions in which teachers and staff are shown working with individual students. *$595.00*
Video

4960 Technology for the Disabled
Landmark Media
3450 Slade Run Drive
Falls Church, VA 22042
703-241-2030
800-342-4336
FAX: 703-536-9540

Michael Hartogs, President
Physically disabled people cope with the frustrations of a body they cannot control. The computer age has made many disabled more self-reliant; armless feed themselves, the blind read newspapers and the voiceless speak through marvelous technological breakthroughs. *$195.00*
Video

4961 To Live with Grace and Dignity
World Institute on Disability
510 16th Street
Suite 100
Oakland, CA 94612
510-763-4100
FAX: 510-763-4109
e-mail: wid@wid.org
www.wid.org
This unique book combines photographs and essays to allow the reader to enter some of the real day to day relationships that develop between individuals with disabilities and their personal assistants. Looking at and listening to what these relationships are all about is what motivated and inspired this book, says author Lydia Gans. The individuals included in this book represent a wide range of ages, disabilities and cultural backgrounds. *$26.00*

72 pages Paperback

4962 Touch/Ability Connects People with Disabilities & Alternative Health Care Pract.
Independent Living Research Utilization ILRU
2323 S Shepherd Drive
Suite 1000
Houston, TX 77019
713-520-0232
FAX: 713-520-5785
www.ilru.org

Laurie Redd, Executive Director
The people at DIRECT center for Independence and Touch/Ability in Tuscon, Arizona, have collaborated to develop a wellness program that makes alternative health care choices available to people with disabilities. The Touch/Ability Wellness program was selected as one of last year's winners in the Innovative CILs competition because of this outcome of increased options open to people with disabilities.
10 pages

4963 US Role in International Disability Activities: A History

World Institute on Disability
510 16th Street
Suite 100
Oakland, CA 94612
510-763-4100
FAX: 510-763-4109
e-mail: wid@wid.org
www.wid.org
This study was undertaken to present an initial introduction to US involvement in the field of international rehabilitation and disability. *$12.00*
169 pages Paperback

4964 Understanding and Accommodating Physical Disabilities: Desk Reference
Greenwood Publishing Group
88 Post Road W
Suite 5007
Westport, CT 06880
203-226-3571
FAX: 203-222-1502
www.greenwood.com

Wayne Smith, President
Medical conditions that qualify as disabilities under the American's with Disabilities Act are explained in non-medical terminology. Hardcover.
200 pages $52.95 - $55
ISBN 0-899308-14-7

4965 Vestibular Disorders Association
Vestibular Disorders Association
PO Box 13305
Portland, OR 97213
503-229-7705
800-837-8428
FAX: 503-229-8064
e-mail: info@vestibular.org
www.vestibular.org

Lisa Haven, Executive Director
Many books and short publications about inner ear, (vestibular) disorders, dizziness, balance problems, and vertigo. *$ 15.00*
2001
ISBN 0-963261-15-0

4966 Visions & Values
Idaho Council on Developmental Disabilities
802 W Bannock Street
Suite 308
Boise, ID 83702
208-336-8508
800-544-2433
FAX: 208-334-3417
e-mail: msword@icdd.state.id.us
www.state.id.us/icdd

Marilyn B Sword, Executive Director/Editor
Pat Barclay, Manager
A quarterly publication from the Idaho Council on Developmental Disabilities.

4967 Walking Tomorrow
Christopher Reeve Paralysis Foundation
636 Morris Tpke
Suite 3a
Short Hills, NJ 07078
973-379-2690
800-252-0292
FAX: 973-912-9433
e-mail: paralysis@aol.com
www.paralysis.com

Kathy Lewis, President
A newsletter offering medical and technological updates for people with physical disabilities, including paralysis.
Quarterly

4968 Weiner's Herbal
Quantum Books
4 Cambridge Center
Cambridge, MA 02142
617-494-5042
FAX: 617-577-7282
e-mail: orders@quantumbk.com
www.quantumbooks.com

William Szabo, Owner
A-Z index covering all aspects of herbs.
Paperback 1980
ISBN 0-812825-86-1

4969 When the Brain Goes Wrong
Fanlight Productions
4196 Washington Street
Suite 2
Boston, MA 02131
617-469-4999
800-937-4113
FAX: 617-469-3379
e-mail: info@fanlight.com
www.fanlight.com

Elena Cambio, Contact
Ben Achtenberg, Owner
An extraordinary and provocative series of seven short films which profile individuals with a range of brian dysfunctions. The seven brief segments focus on schizophrenia, manic depression, epilepsy, head injury, headaches and addiction. In addition to the personal stories, the segments include interviews with physicians who speak briefly about what is known about the disorders and treatment. #131 *$245.00*

ISBN 1-572951-31-1

4970 Women with Physical Disabilities: Achievin g & Maintaining Health & Well-Being
Spina Bifida Association of America
4590 Macarthur Boulevard NW
Suite 250
Washington, DC 20007
202-944-3285
800-621-3141
FAX: 202-944-3295
e-mail: sbaa@sbaa.org
www.sbaa.org

Cindy Brownstein, Chief Executive Officer
Introduces the critical concept of womens health in the context of physical disabilities. *$42.00*

4971 Work in the Context of Disability Culture
Independent Living Research Utilization ILRU
2323 S Shepherd Drive
Suite 1000
Houston, TX 77019
713-520-0232
FAX: 713-520-5785
www.ilru.org

Laurie Redd, Executive Director
Another winner in the innovative CIL competition-Steve Brown describes the Talking Books Program of Southeast Alaska Independent Living, discussing their efforts to record the oral history and life experiences of people with disabilities in the larger context of the disability culture.
10 pages

Parenting: General

4972 AEPS Family Report: For Children Ages Three to Six
Brookes Publishing
PO Box 10624
Baltimore, MD 21285
410-337-9580
800-638-3775
FAX: 410-337-8539
e-mail: custserv@brookespublishing.com
www.brookespublishing.com

Paul Brooks, Owner
This is a 64-item questionnaire that asks parents to rank their child's abilities on specific skills. In packages of 10 paperback.
$23.00
28 pages Saddle-stiched
ISBN 1-557662-50-9

4973 AT for Parents with Disabilities
Idaho Assistive Technology Project
129 W 3rd Street
Moscow, ID 83843
208-885-3559
800-432-8324
FAX: 208-885-3628
e-mail: rseiler@uidaho.edu
www.educ.uidaho.edu/idatech

$5.00
80 pages

4974 Adapted Physical Activity Programs
Human Kinetics
PO Box 5076
Champaign, IL 61825
800-747-4457
FAX: 217-351-2674
e-mail: orders@hkusa.com
www.humankinetics.com

Patty Lehn, Publicity Manager
Alexis Koontz, Publicity Associate
Human Kinetics produces a variety of resources for adapted physical education practitioners, including books on activities, a research journal and higher education references. *$16.95*
232 pages
ISBN 0-873229-33-9

4975 All of Us: Talking Together, Sex Education for People with Developmental Disabilities
Aquarius Health Care Videos
PO Box 1159
Sherborn, MA 01770
508-650-6905
888-440-2963
FAX: 508-650-4216
e-mail: aqvideos@tiac.net
www.aquariusproductions.com

Leslie Kussmann, President/Producer
For parents, caregivers and young people with developmental disabilities often feel isolated and unsure when approaching sex education with their children. In this video, parents of children with developmental disabilities share their difficulties in talking to their children about the social/sexual arena. Real life conversations between parents and their children demonstrate their discomfort, concerns, thoughts and hopes. *$195.00*
Video

4976 Baby Book for the Developmentally Challenged Child
Exceptional Parent Library
PO Box 1807
Englewood Cliffs, NJ 07632
201-947-6000
800-535-1910
FAX: 201-947-9376
e-mail: eplibrary@aol.com
www.eplibrary.com

This baby book is for parents to write milestones for their developmentally challenged child. It incorporates the usual baby book features with very special sections covering any special needs child. *$25.00*

48 pages Hardcover

4977 Babyface: A Story of Heart and Bones
Spina Bifida Association of America
4590 Macarthur Boulevard NW
Suite 250
Washington, DC 20007
202-944-3285
800-621-3141
FAX: 202-944-3295
e-mail: sbaa@sbaa.org
www.sbaa.org

Cindy Brownstein, Chief Executive Officer
A must read for families that seek insight into coping with a chronic condition. Many useful resources provided. *$32.90*

4978 Backyards and Butterflies
Brookline Books
PO Box 1047
Cambridge, MA 02139
617-868-0360
800-666-2665
FAX: 617-868-1772
e-mail: thestore@brooklinebooks.com
www.brooklinebooks.com
Backyards And Butterflies: Ways to Include Children with Disabilities In Out Door Activites is an illustrated book with dozens of imaginative ways parents can include children with physical disabilities in outdoor activities. Offers clear concise, how-to directions for constructing homemaode toys, utensils, and other items that can be enjoyed outside safely and comfortably *$14.95*
72 pages Paperback
ISBN 1-57129 -11-7

4979 Books on Special Children
BOSC
PO Box 305
Congers, NY 10920
845-638-1236
FAX: 845-638-0847
e-mail: irene@boscbooks.com
www.boscbooks.com

Irene Slovak, Owner
Distributes books by mail to professionals and parents of handicapped children. The BOSC Directory contains facilities for people with learning disabilities (all disabilities, published annually)
300+ pages Hardcover
ISBN O-G61386-08-8

4980 Brothers, Sisters, and Special Needs
Brookes Publishing
PO Box 10624
Baltimore, MD 21285
410-337-9580
800-638-3775
FAX: 410-337-8539
e-mail: custserv@brookespublishing.com
www.brookespublishing.com

Paul Brooks, Owner
Information and activities for helping young siblings of children with chronic illnesses and developmental disabilities. *$30.00*
224 pages Paperback
ISBN 1-55766 -43-3

4981 Building the Healing Partnership: Parents, Professionals and Children
Brookline Books
PO Box 1046
Cambridge, MA 02139
617-868-0360
800-666-2665
FAX: 617-868-1772
e-mail: thestore@brooklinebooks.com
www.brooklinebooks.com
Successful programs understand that the disabled child's needs must be considered in the context of a family. This book was specifically written for practitioner's who must work with families but who have insufficient training in family systems assessment and intervention. It is a valuable blend of theory and practice with pointers for applying the principles. *$24.95*
Paperback
ISBN 0-91479 -63-8

4982 Children with Disabilities
Brookes Publishing
PO Box 10624
Baltimore, MD 21285
410-337-9580
800-638-3775
FAX: 410-337-8539
e-mail: custserv@brookespublishing.com
www.brookespublishing.com

Mark L Batshaw MD, Editor
Paul Brooks, Owner
Extensive coverage of genetics, heredity, pre- and postnatal development, specific disabilities, family roles, and intervention. Features chapters on substance abuse, HIV and AIDS, Down syndrome, fragile X syndrome, behavior management, transitions to adulthood, and health care in the 21st century. Also reveals the causes of many conditions that can lead to developmental disabilities. *$69.95*
912 pages Hardcover
ISBN 1-557665-81-8

4983 Conditional Love: Parents' Attitudes Toward Handicapped Children
Greenwood Publishing Group
88 Post Road W
Suite 5007
Westport, CT 06880
203-226-3571
FAX: 203-222-1502
www.greenwood.com

Wayne Smith, President
Offers parents information on understanding disabled children and mainstreaming them into their normal family life. *$49.95*
312 pages
ISBN 0-89789 -24-7

4984 Coordinacion De Servicios Centrado En La Familia
Brookline Books
PO Box 1047
Cambridge, MA 02139
617-868-0360
800-666-2665
FAX: 617-868-1772
e-mail: thestore@brooklinebooks.com
www.brooklinebooks.com
This book, translated into Spanish from the English original, is designed to orient and educate parents about issues of service coordination, to assist families in caring for an infant or toddler with developmental delays or disabilities. *$7.00*
34 pages Paperback
ISBN 0-91479 -90-5

4985 Developing Personal Safety Skills in Children with Disabilities
Brookes Publishing
PO Box 10624
Baltimore, MD 21285
410-337-9580
800-638-3775
FAX: 410-337-8539
e-mail: custserv@brookespublishing.com
www.brookespublishing.com

Paul Brooks, Owner
A guide for teachers, parents, and caregivers, this volume explores the issue of personal safety for children with disabilities and offers strategies for empowering and protecting them at home and in school. Recognizing that children with disabilities are vulnerable to abuse, this work explores why children with disabilities need personal safety skills, offers, curriculum ideas and exercises, and advocates the development of self-esteem and assertiveness so that children can protect themselves. *$34.00*
220 pages Paperback
ISBN 1-557661-84-7

4986 Developmental Disabilities in Infancy and Childhood
Brookes Publishing
PO Box 10624
Baltimore, MD 21285
410-337-9580
800-638-3775
FAX: 410-337-8539
e-mail: custserv@brookespublishing.com
www.brookespublishing.com

Paul Brooks, Owner
This two volume set explores advances in assessment and treatment, retains a clinical focus, and incorporates recent developments in research and theory. Can be purchased individually or as a set (Vol. 1: Neurodevelopmental Diagnosis and Treatment Vol. 2: The Spectrum of Developmental Disabilities). *$210.00*
Hardcover
ISBN 1-55766O-CA-P

4987 Dictionary of Developmental Disabilities Terminology
Brookes Publishing
PO Box 10624
Baltimore, MD 21285
410-337-9580
800-638-3775
FAX: 410-337-8539
e-mail: custserv@brookespublishing.com
www.brookespublishing.com

Paul Brooks, Owner
Answers thousands of questions for medical or human services professionals, parents or advocates of children with disabilities, or students preparing for their careers. Provides thorough explanations of the most common terms associated with disabilities. *$ 55.95*
368 pages Hardcover
ISBN 1-557662-45-2

4988 Encyclopedia of Genetic Disorders & Birth Defects
Facts on File
132 W 31st Street
Floor 17
New York, NY 10001
212-967-8800
800-322-8755
FAX: 212-967-9196
e-mail: jchambers@factsonfile.com
www.factsonfile.com

Mark Donnell, President
Layperson-accessible entries on genetic terminology and genetically-influenced conditions. *$71.50*
474 pages 2000
ISBN 0-816038-09-0

4989 Exceptional Parent Magazine
Psy-Ed Corp
551 Main Street
Johnstown, PA 15901
877-372-7368
FAX: 740-389-5574
e-mail: EPAR@kable.com
www.eparent.com

Joseph Valenzano Jr, President/CEO
Bob Salluzzo, COO
Kendra Kelly, Ad Traffic Manager
Addresses concerns of raising, treating or teaching children or young adults with disabilities, for parents and professionals. *$4.95*
100 pages Monthly
ISSN 0046-91 7

4990 Face of Inclusion
Special Needs Project
324 State Street
Suite H
Santa Barbara, CA 93101
805-962-8087
800-333-6867
FAX: 805-962-5087
e-mail: eplibrary@aol.com
www.eplibrary.com
A unique and moving parents' perspective of inclusion for administrators, teachers, and parents of children with disabilities. *$99.00*

4991 Families Magazine
New Jersey Developmental Disabilities Council
PO Box 700
Trenton, NJ 08625
609-292-3745
800-216-1199
FAX: 609-292-7114
TTY: 609-777-3238
e-mail: njddc@njddc.org
www.njddc.org

Ethan Ellis, Executive Director/Editor
Norman Reim, Managing Editor
Quarterly magazine for people with disabilities, their families and the public, features family profiles, news, columns and the New Jersey Family support councils newsletter.
Quarterly

4992 Families, Illness & Disability
Through the Looking Glass
2198 6th Street
Suite 100
Berkeley, CA 94710
510-848-1112
800-644-2666
FAX: 510-848-4445
e-mail: TLG@lookingglass.org
www.lookingglass.org

J Rolland
Megan Kirshbaum, Executive Director
$35.00
320 pages

4993 Family Interventions Throughout Disability
Springer Publishing Company
536 Broadway
New York, NY 10012
212-431-4370
877-687-7476
FAX: 212-941-7842
e-mail: marketing@springerpub.com
www.springerpub.com

Annette Imperati, Marketing/Sales Director
Ursula Springer, President
Family attitudes throughout chronic illness and disability. *$31.95*
320 pages
ISBN 0-82615 -80-4

4994 Family-Centered Service Coordination: A Manual for Parents
Brookline Books
PO Box 1047
Cambridge, MA 02139
617-868-0360
800-666-2665
FAX: 617-868-1772
e-mail: thestore@brooklinebooks.com
www.brooklinebooks.com
A manual designed to orient and educate parents about issues of service coordination, to assist families in caring for an infant or toddler with developmental delays or disabilities. *$7.00*
34 pages Paperback
ISBN 0-91479 -90-5

4995 Handbook About Care in the Home
AARP Fulfillment
601 E Street NW
Washington, DC 20049
202-434-2277
800-424-3410
FAX: 202-434-3443
e-mail: member@aarp.org
www.aarp.org

William Novelli, Chief Executive Officer
Offers valuable information for the disabled.
24 pages

4996 LifeLines
Disabled and Alone
352 Park Avenue S
11th Floor
New York, NY 10010
212-532-6740
800-995-0066
FAX: 212-532-3588
e-mail: info@disabledandalone.org
www.disabledandalone.org

Rosyln Brilliant, Executive Director
Disabled and Alone is a national, nonprofit organization whose sole purpose is to assure the well being of disabled individuals, particularly those whose families have died and have engaged Disabled and Alone to provide advocacy and oversight for the lifetime of their disabled children. This newsletter provides information about "future planning" for a person with a disability.

8-16 pages Bi-annual

4997 Loving & Letting Go
Centering Corporation
1531 N Saddle Creek Road
Omaha, NE 68104
402-553-1200
FAX: 402-533-0507
e-mail: j1200@aol.com
www.centering.org

Joy Johnson, Executive Director
For parents who decide to turn away from aggressive medical intervention for their critically ill newborn. *$5.95*
48 pages Paperback

4998 Mobility Training for People with Disabilities
Charles C Thomas
2600 S 1st Street
Springfield, IL 62704
217-789-8980
800-258-8980
FAX: 217-789-9130
e-mail: books@ccthomas.com
www.ccthomas.com

Michael Thomas, President
Children and adults with mental, visual, physical and hearing impairments can learn to travel. Also available in cloth. *$ 28.95*
144 pages Paper
ISBN 0-398063-56-7

4999 Mother to Be
Through the Looking Glass
2198 6th Street
Suite 100
Berkeley, CA 94710
510-848-1112
800-644-2666
FAX: 510-848-4445
e-mail: TLG@lookingglass.org
www.lookingglass.org

J Rogers
M Matsumura
Megan Kirshbaum, Executive Director
Guide to pregnancy and birth for women with disabilities. *$34.00*
410 pages

5000 New Language of Toys: Teaching Communicati on Skills to Children with Special Needs
Spina Bifida Association of America
4590 Macarthur Boulevard NW
Suite 250
Washington, DC 20007
202-944-3285
800-621-3141
FAX: 202-944-3295
e-mail: sbaa@sbaa.org
www.sbaa.org

Cindy Brownstein, Chief Executive Officer
A guide for parents and teachers and a reader-friendly resource guide that provides a wealth of information on how play activities affect a child's language development and where to get the toys and materials to use in these activities. *$19.00*

5001 NewsLine
Federation for Children with Special Needs
56 Temple Place
Suite 664
Boston, MA 02111
617-542-7860
800-537-0446
FAX: 617-542-7832
e-mail: pal@fcsn.org
www.ppal.net

Donna Welles, Executive Director
Lisa Lambert, Asistant Director
Offers information for parents and families on resources, medical updates, activities, fund-raising events and association news for their disabled children.
Quarterly

5002 On the Road to Autonomy: Promoting Self- Competence in Children & Youth with Disabilities
Brookes Publishing
PO Box 10624
Baltimore, MD 21285
410-337-9580
800-638-3775
FAX: 410-337-8539
e-mail: custserv@brookespublishing.com
www.brookespublishing.com

Paul Brooks, Owner
This book provides detailed conceptual, practical, and personal information regarding the promotion of self-esteem, self-determination, and coping skills among children and youth with and without disabilities. *$48.00*
432 pages Paperback
ISBN 1-55766 -35-5

5003 Pain Erasure
M Evans and Company
216 E 49th Street
New York, NY 10017
212-979-0880
FAX: 212-486-4544

Mary Evans, Owner
This book explains Bonnie Prudden's method for pain relief using myotherapy, a method hailed by doctors and patients.
1985
ISBN 0-345331-02-8

5004 Parent Centers and Independent Living Centers: Collectively We're Stronger
Independent Living Research Utilization ILRU
2323 S Shepherd Drive
Suite 1000
Houston, TX 77019
713-520-0232
FAX: 713-520-5785
www.ilru.org

Laurie Redd, Executive Director
This article describes several examples of effective working relationships of PTIs and CILs. The examples highlight how parent and consumer organizations have identified complimentary strengths and formed partnerships to better support children with disabilities and their families. These partnerships can also be a very important way of involving youth in the disability movement so they may become leaders of tomorrow.
10 pages

5005 Parent-Child Interaction and Developmental Disabilities
Greenwood Publishing Group
88 Post Road W
Suite 5007
Westport, CT 06880
203-226-3571
FAX: 203-222-1502
www.greenwood.com

Wayne Smith, President
This volume brings together the original papers by international scholars and practitioners on the question of the effects of parent interaction with developmentally disabled children. $65.00-$69.50.
395 pages Hardcover
ISBN 0-275928-35-7

5006 Parenting
Accent Books & Products
PO Box 700
Bloomington, IL 61702
309-378-2961
800-787-8444
FAX: 309-378-4420
e-mail: acmtlvng@aol.com

Raymond C Cheever, Publisher
Betty Garee, Editor
Experienced parents (who are disabled) discuss: raising children from infant to teens, balancing career and motherhood, discipline methods and more when both parents are disabled. *$7.95*

83 pages
ISBN 0-91570 -26-4

5007 Parenting with a Disability
Through the Looking Glass
2198 6th Street
Suite 100
Berkeley, CA 94710
510-848-1112
800-644-2666
FAX: 510-848-4445
e-mail: TLG@lookingglass.org
www.lookingglass.org

Megan Kirshbaum, Executive Director
International newsletter. Available in braille, large print or cassette.
3 per year

5008 Perspectives on a Parent Movement
Brookline Books
PO Box 1046
Cambridge, MA 02139
617-868-0360
800-666-2665
FAX: 617-868-1772
e-mail: thestore@brooklinebooks.com
www.brooklinebooks.com
This book captures Rosemary Dybwad's truly innovative wisdom and pioneering for people with intellectual limitations in these previously unpublished essays and speeches. *$17.95*
Paperback
ISBN 0-91479 -74-3

5009 Sexuality and the Developmentally Handicapped
Edwin Mellen Press
PO Box 450
Lewiston, NY 14092
716-754-2266
FAX: 716-754-4056
e-mail: mellen@wzrd.com

Herbert Richardson, Owner
Presents the knowledge, attitudes, and skills pertinent to responding to the sexual problems of developmentally handicapped persons, their families and communities. Details fully documented cases, issues concerning the law, and resource materials available. *$89.95*
245 pages Hardcover
ISBN 0-88946 -32-5

5010 Shattered Dreams-Lonely Choices: Birth Parents of Babies with Disabilities
Greenwood Publishing Group
88 Post Road W
Suite 5007
Westport, CT 06880
203-226-3571
FAX: 203-222-1502
www.greenwood.com

Wayne Smith, President
Written by a mother who, without warning, gave birth to a boy with Down Syndrome, this book is meant to help parents through the initial shock and the realization that they are not able to care for their child. $29.95-$35.00. *$29.95*
208 pages Hardcover
ISBN 0-897892-86-0

5011 Since Owen, A Parent-to-Parent Guide for Care of the Disabled Child
Special Needs Project
324 State Street
Suite H
Santa Barbara, CA 93101
805-962-8087
800-333-6867
FAX: 805-962-5087
www.specialneeds.com

Charles Callahan, Editor
Against the background of his experience as the parent of a severely disabled young man, Callahan writes conscientiously to other parents. *$16.95*

486 pages

5012 Sleep Better! A Guide to Improving Sleep for Children with Special Needs
Brookes Publishing
PO Box 10624
Baltimore, MD 21285
410-337-9580
800-638-3775
FAX: 410-337-8539
e-mail: custserv@brookespublishing.com
www.brookespublishing.com

Paul Brooks, Owner
This book offers step-by-step, how to instructions for helping children with disabilities get the rest they need. For problems ranging from bedtime tantrums to night waking, parents and caregivers will find a variety of widely tested and easy-to-implement techniques that have already helped hundreds of children with special needs. *$21.95*
288 pages Paperback 1997
ISBN 1-55766 -15-7

5013 Something's Wrong with My Child
Charles C Thomas
2600 S 1st Street
Springfield, IL 62704
217-789-8980
800-258-8980
FAX: 217-789-9130
e-mail: books@ccthomas.com
www.ccthomas.com

Michael Thomas, President
A straight forward presentation to help professionals and parents to better understand themselves in dealing with the emotionally charged subject of disabled children. Also available in cloth. *$26.95*
210 pages Paperback
ISBN 0-398068-99-2

5014 Sometimes I Get All Scribbly
Exceptional Parent Library
PO Box 1807
Englewood Cliffs, NJ 07632
201-947-6000
800-535-1910
FAX: 201-947-9376
e-mail: eplibrary@aol.com
www.eplibrary.com
Clinical, educational and emotional information from the point of view of a parent. *$16.00*

5015 Son-Rise: The Miracle Continues
2080 S Undermountain Road
Sheffield, MA 01257
413-229-2100
800-714-2779
FAX: 413-229-3202
e-mail: sonrise@option.org
www.son-rise.org
Documents Raun Kaufman's astonishing development from a lifeless, autistic, retarded child into a highly verbal, lovable youngster with no traces of his former condition. Details Raun's extraordinary progress from the age of four into young adulthood, also shares moving accounts of five families that successfully used the Son-Rise Program to reach their own special children.
372 pages 1994
ISBN 0-915811-53-7

5016 Special Kids Need Special Parents: A Resou rce for Parents of Children With Special Needs
Berkley Publishing Group

The author, herself the parent of a child with special needs, draws on interviews with health care professionals, nationally recognized authorities, and other partens to give readers the answers, advice, and comfort they crave. *$13.95*

319 pages Paperback 2001
ISBN 0-425176-62-2

5017 Special Parent, Special Child
Exceptional Parent Library
PO Box 1807
Englewood Cliffs, NJ 07632
201-947-6000
800-535-1910
FAX: 201-947-9376
e-mail: eplibrary@aol.com
www.eplibrary.com

Offers information for facing the challenges of being a special parent. *$21.95*
Hardcover

5018 Strategies for Working with Families of Young Children with Disabilities
Brookes Publishing
PO Box 10624
Baltimore, MD 21285
410-337-9580
800-638-3775
FAX: 410-337-8539
e-mail: custserv@brookespublishing.com
www.brookespublishing.com

Paul Brooks, Owner
This text offers useful techniques for collaborating with and supporting families whose youngest members either have a disability or are at risk for developing a disability. The authors address specific issues such as cultural diversity, transitions to new programs, and disagreements between families and professionals. *$33.00*
272 pages Paperback
ISBN 1-55766 -57-6

5019 That's My Child
Exceptional Parent Library
PO Box 1807
Englewood Cliffs, NJ 07632
201-947-6000
800-535-1910
FAX: 201-947-9376
e-mail: eplibrary@aol.com
www.eplibrary.com

Offers information to help parent successfully navigate the maze of resources and services available for children with special needs. *$12.95*

5020 They Don't Come with Manuals
Fanlight Productions
4196 Washington Street
Suite 2
Boston, MA 02131
617-469-4999
800-937-4113
FAX: 617-469-3379
e-mail: fanlight@fanlight.com
www.fanlight.com

Karen McMillen, Marketing Director
Ben Achtenberg, Owner
The parents and adoptive parents in this video speak candidly of their day to day experiences caring for children with physical and mental disabilities. *$145.00*

5021 They're Just Kids
Aquarius Health Care Videos
PO Box 1159
Sherborn, MA 01770
508-650-6905
888-440-2963
FAX: 508-650-4216
e-mail: aqvideos@tiac.net
www.aquariusproductions.com

Leslie Kussmann, President/Producer
The importance and value of inclusion, excellent for anyone working with kids with disabilities. The documentary explores the advantages of the inclusion of disabled children in the classroom, cub scouts and other extracurricular activities. *$99.00*
Video

5022 To a Different Drumbeat
Alliance for Parental Involvement in Education
PO Box 59
East Chatham, NY 12060
518-392-6900
FAX: 518-392-6900

Parents of special needs children contributed to this book. *$16.95*

5023 Uncommon Fathers
Woodbine House
6510 Bells Mill Road
Bethesda, MD 20817
301-897-3570
800-843-7323
FAX: 301-897-5838
www.woodbinehouse.com

Irv Shapell, Owner
Nineteen fathers talk about the life-altering experience of having a child with special needs and offer a welcome, seldom-heard perspective on raising kids with disabilities, including autism, cerebral palsy, and Down syndrome. Uncommon Fathers is the first book for fathers by fathers, but it is also helpful to partners, family, friends, and service providers. *$14.95*
206 pages Paperback
ISBN 0-933149-68-9

5024 We Can Speak for Ourselves: Self Advocacy by Mentally Handicapped People
Brookline Books
PO Box 1047
Cambridge, MA 02139
617-868-0360
800-666-2665
FAX: 617-868-1772
e-mail: thestore@brooklinebooks.com
www.brooklinebooks.com

Practical advice and support for parents, group resident workers, and others interested in fostering self-advocacy for people with developmental disabilities. *$10.00*
246 pages Paperback
ISBN 0-25336 -65-9

5025 You May Be Able to Adopt
Through the Looking Glass
2198 6th Street
Suite 100
Berkeley, CA 94710
510-848-1112
800-644-2666
FAX: 510-848-4445
e-mail: TLG@lookingglass.org
www.lookingglass.org

L Toms Barker
Megan Kirshbaum, Executive Director
A guide to the adoption process for prospective mothers with disabilities and their partners. Available in braille, large print or cassette. *$10.00*
112 pages

5026 You Will Dream New Dreams
Kensington Publishing

A parent's support group in print. The shared narratives come from those with newly diagnosed children, adult disabled children, and everything in between. *$13.00*
278 pages Paperback 2001
ISBN 1-575665-60-3

5027 Your Child Has a Disability: A Complete So urcebook of Daily and Medical Care
Brookes Publishing
PO Box 10624
Baltimore, MD 21285
410-337-9580
800-638-3775
FAX: 410-337-8539
e-mail: custserv@brookesopublishing.com
www.brookespublishing.com

Paul Brooks, Owner
Offers expert advice on a wide range of issues-from finding the right doctor and investigating the medical aspects of a child's condition to learning care techniques and fulfilling education requirements. *$24.95*

368 pages Paperback 1998
ISBN 1-557663-74-2

Parenting: Specific Disabilities

5028 Cancer Clinical Trials: Experimental Treatments and How They Can Help You
Patient-Centered Guides
101 Morris Street
Sebastopol, CA 95472
707-829-0515
800-998-9938
FAX: 707-829-0104
www.patientcenters.com

Linda Lamb, Editor
Shawnde Paull, Marketing
Tim O'Reilly, Chief Executive Officer
Most cancer patients face treatment options that are less than ideal, whether because of a risk of recurrence or side effects. Finally, however, basic research on cell biology is leading to promising new treatments. If you are not evaluating potential experimental treatments alongside the standard treatment protocols, you aren't considering all the facts you need. Cancer Clinical Trials guide you through understanding your options and finding and considering experimental treatments. *$14.95*
222 pages Paperback
ISBN 1-565925-66-1

5029 Children with Acquired Brain Injury: Education and Supporting Families
Brookes Publishing
PO Box 10624
Baltimore, MD 21285
410-337-9580
800-638-3775
FAX: 410-337-8539
e-mail: custserv@brookespublishing.com
www.brookespublishing.com

Ann Glang PhD, Editor
Janet M Williams MSW, Editor
Paul Brooks, Owner
$28.95
288 pages Paperback 1996
ISBN 1-557662-33-9

5030 Children with Autism
Woodbine House
6510 Bells Mill Road
Bethesda, MD 20817
301-897-3570
800-843-7323
FAX: 301-897-5838
www.woodbinehouse.com

Irv Shapell, Owner
Recommended as the first book parents should read, this volume offers information and a complete introduction to autism, while easing the family's fears and concerns as they adjust and cope with their child's disorder. *$17.95*
368 pages Paperback
ISBN 0-933149-16-6

5031 Final Report: Adapting Through the Looking Glass
Through the Looking Glass
2198 6th Street
Suite 100
Berkeley, CA 94710
510-848-1112
800-644-2666
FAX: 510-848-4445
e-mail: TLG@lookingglass.org
www.lookingglass.org

P Preston
M Lou
Megan Kirshbaum, Executive Director
Adapting Through the Looking Glass intervention model for deaf parents and their children. Available in braille, large print or cassette. *$2.00*
24 pages

5032 Final Report: Challenges and Strategies of Disabled Parents: Findings from a Survey
Through the Looking Glass
2198 6th Street
Suite 100
Berkeley, CA 94710
510-848-1112
800-644-2666
FAX: 510-848-4445
e-mail: TLG@lookingglass.org
www.lookingglass.org

L Toms Barker
V Maralani
Megan Kirshbaum, Executive Director
Available in braille, large print or cassette. *$25.00*
24 pages

5033 Negotiating the Special Education Maze: A Guide for Parents and Teachers
Spina Bifida Association of America
4590 MacArthur Boulevard NW
Suite 250
Washington, DC 20007
202-944-3285
800-621-3141
FAX: 202-944-3295
e-mail: sbaa@sbaa.org
www.sbaa.org

Douglas Soroco, Chairman
Joyce Jones, Vice Chairman
Cindy Brownstein, Chief Executive Officer
An excellent aid for the development of an effective special education program. *$19.00*

5034 Pervasive Developmental Disorders; Finding a Diagnosis and Getting Help
Patient-Centered Guides
101 Morris Street
Sebastopol, CA 95472
707-829-0515
800-998-9938
FAX: 707-829-0104
www.patientcenters.com

Linda Lamb, Editor
Shawnde Paull, Marketing
Tim O'Reilly, Chief Executive Officer
This unique book encompassess both the practical aspects as well as ther personal stories and emotional facets of living with PDD-NOS, the most common pervasive developmental disorder. Parents of an undiagnosed child may suspect many things, from autism to servere allergies. Pervasive Developmental Disorders is for parents (or newly diagnosed adults) who struggle with this neurological condition that profoundly impacts the life of child and family. *$24.95*
580 pages Paperback
ISBN 1-565925-30-0

5035 Raising Kids with Special Needs
Aquarius Health Care Videos
PO Box 1159
Sherborn, MA 01770
508-650-6905
FAX: 508-650-4216
e-mail: aqvideos@tiac.net
www.aquariusproductions.com
An intimate look into the lives of parents of three kids with very different disabilities. The objective of this video is an understanding of paprenting a child with special nees. This outstanding program looks at safety concerns, issues of anger and grief, the importance of a support network and other important issues. Ultimately, this is a narrative about raising and educating a child with disabilities. Preview option is available. *$89.00*
Video

5036 Your Child in the Hospital: A Practical Guide for Parents
Patient-Centered Guides
101 Morris Street
Sebastopol, CA 95472
707-829-0515
800-998-9938
FAX: 707-829-0104
www.patientcenters.com

Linda Lamb, Editor
Shawnde Paull, Marketing
Tim O'Reilly, Chief Executive Officer
This book offers advice from dozens of veteran parents on how to cope with a child's hospitalization, relieving anxious parents so they can help dispel their child's fears and concerns. Parents will find easy-to-read tips on preparing their child, handling procedures without trauma, and preventing insurance snafus. The second edition features a journal to help open communication and give the child a measure of control over the experience. *$11.95*
166 pages Paperback
ISBN 1-565925-73-4

Parenting: School

5037 Allergy and Asthma Network Mothers of Asth matics
2751 Prosperity Avenue
Suite 150
Fairfax, VA 22031
703-641-9595
800-878-4403
FAX: 703-573-7794
e-mail: memserv@aanma.org
www.breatherville.org
Practical, medical,information for school patients, physicians, caregivers and families. *$7.00*

5038 Carolina Curriculum for Infants and Toddlers with Special Needs
Brookes Publishing
PO Box 10624
Baltimore, MD 21285
410-337-9580
800-638-3775
FAX: 410-337-8539
e-mail: custserv@brookespublishing.com
www.brookespublishing.com

Paul Brooks, Owner
This book includes detailed assessment and intervention sequences, daily routine integration strategies, sensorimotor adaptations, and a sample 24-page Assessment Log that shows readers how to chart a child's individual progress. *$41.95*
384 pages Spiral-bound
ISBN 1-557660-74-3

5039 Choosing Outcomes and Accommodations for Children (COACH)
Brookes Publishing
PO Box 10624
Baltimore, MD 21285
410-337-9580
800-638-3775
FAX: 410-337-8539
e-mail: custserv@brookespublishing.com
www.brookespublishing.com

Paul Brooks, Owner
A guide to educational planning for students with disabilities, second edition. Focuses on life outcomes such as social relationships and participation in typical home, school, and community activities. *$37.95*
400 pages Spiral bound 1997
ISBN 1-55766 -23-8

5040 Complete IEP Guide: How to Advocate for Yo ur Special Ed Child
Spina Bifida Association of America
4590 Macarthur Boulevard NW
Suite 250
Washington, DC 20007
202-944-3285
800-621-3141
FAX: 202-944-3295
e-mail: sbaa@sbaa.org
www.sbaa.org

Cindy Brownstein, Chief Executive Officer
This all-in-one guide will help you understand special education law, identify your child's needs, prepare for meetings, develop the IEP and resolve disputes. *$28.95*

5041 Exceptional Student in the Regular Classroom
McGraw-Hill, School Publishing
220 E Danieldale Road
Desoto, TX 75115
972-224-1111
800-442-9685
FAX: 972-228-1982
mhschool.com

Joseph Gavigan, President
Offers good, solid information through a practical understandable presentation unencumbered by specialized jargon. Covers topics associated with special learners.
480 pages

5042 Negotiating the Special Education Maze: A Guide for Parents and Teachers
Spina Bifida Association of America
4590 Macarthur Boulevard NW
Suite 250
Washington, DC 20007
202-944-3285
800-621-3141
FAX: 202-944-3295
e-mail: sbaa@sbaa.org
www.sbaa.org

Cindy Brownstein, Chief Executive Officer
An excellent aid for the development of an effective special education program. *$19.00*

5043 Parent Teacher Packet
Spina Bifida Association of America
4590 Macarthur Boulevard NW
Suite 250
Washington, DC 20007
202-944-3285
800-621-3141
FAX: 202-944-3295
e-mail: sbaa@sbaa.org
www.sbaa.org

Cindy Brownstein, Chief Executive Officer
Includes educational material, learning disabilities literature, children's book, social development and the person with spina bifida and one copy of each fact sheet. *$14.00*

5044 Study Power: Study Skills to Improve Your Learning and Your Grades: A Workbook
Brookline Books
PO Box 1047
Cambridge, MA 02139
617-868-0360
800-666-2665
FAX: 617-868-1772
e-mail: thestore@brooklinebooks.com
www.brooklinebooks.com
The techniques in the easy-to-use, self-teaching manual have yielded remarkable success for students from elementary to medical school, at all levels of intelligence and achievement. Key skills covered include: listening, note taking, concentration, summarizing, reading comprehension, memorization, test taking, preparing papers and reports, time management, and more. These abilities are vital to success throughout every stage of learning; the benefits will last a lifetime. 1999.ISBN 157129067X *$15.95*
Paperback 1998
ISBN 1-57129 -46-X

Parenting: Spiritual

5045 A Miracle to Believe In
Option Indigo Press
2080 S Undermountain Road
Sheffield, MA 01257
413-229-8727
800-562-7171
FAX: 413-229-8727
e-mail: happiness@option.org
www.optionindigo.com
A group of people from all walks of life come together and are transformed as they reach out, under the direction of the Kaufmans, to help a little boy the medical world has given up as hopeless. This heartwarming journey of loving a child back to life will inspire and presents a compelling new way to deal with life's traumas and difficulties. *$7.99*

379 pages Paperback
ISBN 0-44920 -08-2

5046 **After the Tears**
Centering Corporation
1531 N Saddle Creek Road
Omaha, NE 68104
402-553-1200
FAX: 402-533-0507
e-mail: j1200@aol.com
www.centering.org

Joy Johnson, Executive Director
Offers talk, articles on raising a child with a disability. This one book combines feelings and emotions of parents on the subject of raising their disabled child. *$11.00*
87 pages Paperback
ISBN 0-15602 -00-6

5047 **Before and After Zachariah**
Special Needs Project
324 State Street
Suite H
Santa Barbara, CA 93101
805-962-8087
800-333-6867
FAX: 805-962-5087
www.specialneeds.com
This intimate chronicle of one family's life with a severely brain damaged child is recently back in print. *$7.95*
241 pages

5048 **Bethy and the Mouse: A Father Remembers His Children with Disabilities**
Brookline Books
PO Box 1047
Cambridge, MA 02139
617-868-0360
800-666-2665
FAX: 617-868-1772
e-mail: thestore@brooklinebooks.com
www.brooklinebooks.com
A moving collection of poetry, photographs, and prose following a father's experiences with two disabled children—one with Down Syndrome and one with an underdeveloped brain. *$16.95*
184 pages Paperback
ISBN 0-57129 -35-4

5049 **Disabled God: Toward a Liberatory Theology of Disability**
Abingdon Press
201 8th Avenue S
Nashville, TN 37203
615-749-6000
800-251-3320
FAX: 800-836-7802
www.abingdon.org

Dr. Rex Matthews, Senior Editor
Neil Alexander, President
Draws on themes of the disability rights movement to identify people with disabilities as members of a socially disadvantaged minority group rather than as individuals who need to adjust. Highlights the history of people with disabilities in the church and society. *$ 13.95*
27 pages Paperback
ISBN 0-68710 -01-2

5050 **Dying and Disabled Children: Dealing with Loss and Grief**
Haworth Press
10 Alice Street
Binghamton, NY 13904
607-722-5857
800-429-6784
FAX: 607-722-6362
e-mail: orders@haworthpress.com
www.haworthpress.com

Harold M Dick MD, Editor
S Harrington-Miller, Advertising
William Cohen, Owner
In this sensitive and compassionate look at terminally ill and disabled children, professionals from the medical community examine the stresses faced by their parents and siblings. They address the crucial element of communication in dealing with a child's serious illness. Ethical decision making, learning to recognize the child's suffering, and talking to children about death are honestly and clearly discussed. *$ 59.95*

153 pages Hardcover
ISBN 0-866567-59-3

5051 **Hug Just Isn't Enough**
Gallaudet University Bookstore
11030 S Langley Avenue
Chicago, IL 60628
202-651-5488
800-621-2736
FAX: 202-651-5489
Offers valuable information for the disabled. *$15.95*
94 pages Hardcover

5052 **In Time and with Love: Caring for the Special Needs Infant and Toddler**
Newmarket Press
18 E 48th Street
New York, NY 10017
212-832-3575
FAX: 212-832-3629
e-mail: sales@newmarketpress.com
www.newmarketpress.com

Heidi Sachner, Sales Director
Esther Margolis, President
For families and caregivers of preteen and handicapped children in their first three years - more than one hundred tips for adjusting and coping. *$15.95*
208 pages
ISBN 1-557044-45-7

5053 **Journal of Religion, Disability & Health**
Haworth Press
10 Alice Street
Binghamton, NY 13904
607-722-5857
800-429-6784
FAX: 607-722-6362
e-mail: orders@haworthpress.com
www.haworthpress.com

William Gaventa MD, Co-Editor
David Coulter MD, Co-Editor
S Harrington-Miller, Advertising/Journal Liaison
This journal aims to inform religious professionals about developments in the field of disability and rehabilitation in order to facilitate greater contributions on the part of pastors, religious educators and pastoral counselors. *$60.00*
Quarterly

5054 **Nobody's Perfect: Living and Growing with Children Who Have Special Needs**
Brookes Publishing
PO Box 10624
Baltimore, MD 21285
410-337-9580
800-638-3775
FAX: 410-337-8539
e-mail: custserv@brookespublishing.com
www.brookespublishing.com

Paul Brooks, Owner
This book offers parents who have children with special needs a new and positive perspective on the challenges of family life. This book guides parents through the process of adaptation, describing specific strategies for success in balancing one's own life, developing a parenting partnership, and interacting with children, friends, relatives, professionals, and others. *$21.00*
352 pages Paperback
ISBN 1-55766 -43-X

5055 **Special Education Teacher Packet**
LifeWay Christian Resources Southern Baptist Conv.
127 9th Avenue N
Nashville, TN 37234
615-251-2089
800-458-2772
FAX: 615-251-5017
e-mail: SpecialEd@lifeway.com
www.lifeway.com

Ellen Beene, Editor
Wade Stapleton, Manager
Resources to help teachers who lead Sunday School classes for adults and older youth with mental retardation. Includes teaching plans, posters, and one copy of Special Education Bible Study. *$10.00*

Quarterly

5056 **Special Kind of Parenting**
La Leche League International
PO Box 4079
Schaumburg, IL 60168
847-519-7730
FAX: 847-519-0035
e-mail: LLLI@llli.org
www.lalecheleague.org

Schielany Bautista, Marketing Assistant
Judy Torgus, Publications Director
Disabled children have special needs which challenge their parents' emotional and physical resources. This book guides parents through the problems and helps them discover their disabled child as an individual. The author covers both facts and feelings about handicaps, parents' reactions to the initial diagnosis, the grieving process, and effects on the marriage and the rest of the family. They also provide suggestions for choosing the programs and professionals best suited. *$7.50*
172 pages Softcover
ISBN 0-912500-27-1

5057 **That All May Worship**
Exceptional Parent Library
PO Box 1807
Englewood Cliffs, NJ 07632
201-947-6000
800-535-1910
FAX: 201-947-9376
e-mail: mailto:eplibrary@aol.com
www.eplibrary.com
An interfaith handbook to assist congregations in welcoming people with disabilities to promote acceptance and full participation. *$10.00*

5058 **Why Mine?**
Centering Corporation
1531 N Saddle Creek Road
Omaha, NE 68104
402-553-1200
FAX: 402-533-0507
e-mail: j1200@aol.com
www.centering.org

Joy Johnson, Executive Director
Offers quotes from parents all across the country on their fears, feelings, marriage, the ill child and other children. *$3.25*
32 pages Paperback

5059 **Worst Loss: How Families Heal from the Death of a Child**
Exceptional Parent Library
PO Box 1807
Englewood Cliffs, NJ 07632
201-947-6000
800-535-1910
FAX: 201-947-9376
e-mail: mailto:eplibrary@aol.com
www.eplibrary.com
Combines anecdotal case histories and the latest research to help bereaved parents cope with the loss of a child, offering practical and comforting advice on how to overcome the disabling symptoms of grief. *$25.00*

ISBN 0-805032-41-X

Professional

5060 **American Journal of Physical Medicine**
Lippincott, Williams & Wilkins
PO Box 1551
Hagerstown, MD 21741
800-638-3030
FAX: 301-824-7390
www.lww.com
Journal of the Association of Academic Psychiatrists. Articles covering research and clinical studies and applications of new equipment, procedures and therapeutic advances. *$45.00*

5061 **American Journal of Psychiatry**
American Psychiatric Publishing
1000 Wilson Boulevard
Suite 1825
Arlington, VA 22209
703-907-7300
800-368-5777
FAX: 202-789-2648
e-mail: mailto:accessnumber@psych.org
ajp.psychiatryonline.org

Nancy C Andreasen MD PhD, Editor-in-Chief
James Scully, Manager
Peer-reviewed articles focus on developments in biological psychiatry as well as on treatment innovations and forensic, ethical, economic, and social topics. *$56.00*
Monthly

5062 **American Journal of Public Health**
American Public Health Association
1015 15th Street NW
Washington, DC 20005
202-777-2742
FAX: 202-777-2534
e-mail: comments@msmail.apha.org
www.apna.org

Dr. Mervyn Susser, Editor
Georges Benjamin, Executive Director
Association journal containing professional articles and sections such as Notes from the Field and Association News. Single copies are $15.00. $50.00 per year for special consumer membership.
Monthly
ISSN 0090-00 6

5063 **American Rehabilitation**
Rehabilitation Services Administration
3033 Mes
Washington, DC 20202
202-205-8296
FAX: 202-205-9874
e-mail: frank.romano@ed.gov
www.ed.gov/pubs/AmericanRehab

Frank Romano, Editor
Covers medical, social and employment aspects of vocational rehabilitation. *$15.00*
40 pages Quarterly

5064 **Art Therapy**
American Art Therapy Association
5999 Stevenson Avenue
Suite 200
Alexandria, VA 22304
847-949-6064
FAX: 847-556-4580

Nancy Stygar
Publishes articles on the uses of art in the education, enrichment, development and treatment of disabled people. *$10.00*
76+ pages Quarterly
ISSN 0742-16 6

5065 **Bringing Out the Best**
Research Press
PO Box 9177
Champaign, IL 61826
217-352-3273
800-519-2707
FAX: 217-352-1221
e-mail: rp@researchpress.com
www.researchpress.com

Russell Pence, President
This video training program introduces teachers, staff and parents to a variety of techniques for teaching expressive communication skills to children with multiple handicaps. The video illustrates how to assess a child's current levels of expressive ability, build on that ability, then gradually work toward more advanced communication. It shows how to use everyday situations to help children move beyond passive understanding to more active, intentional communication. *$150.00*

Video

5066 Brown University Long Term Care Advisor
Manisses Communications Group
208 Governor Street
Providence, RI 02906
401-831-6020
800-333-7771
FAX: 401-861-6370
e-mail: manisses@manisses.com
www.manisses.com

Fraser Lang, Publisher
Contains practical reports for health care professionals working in long-term care facilities. Published monthly. *$329.00*
8 pages Newsletter
ISSN 1088-92 8

5067 CAREERS & the disABLED Magazine
Equal Opportunity Publications
445 Broadhollow Road
Suite 425
Melville, NY 11747
631-421-9421
FAX: 631-421-0359
e-mail: jschneider@eop.com
www.eop.com

John R Miller III, Publisher
James Schneider, Editorial Director
A career magazine for professional career seekers who have disabilities. Profiles disabled people who have achieved successful careers. Features a career section in Braille, career guide. *$10.00*
64 pages 3X

5068 Clinician's Practical Guide to Attention-Deficit/Hyperactivity Disorder
Brookes Publishing
PO Box 10624
Baltimore, MD 21285
410-337-9580
800-638-3775
FAX: 410-337-8539
www.brookespublishing.com

Paul Brooks, Owner
Quick reference volume with comprehensive data on psychoeducational and neuropsychological assessment, related symptoms, drug and counseling therapies and critical issues. *$39.95*
368 pages 1999
ISBN 1-557663-58-0

5069 Counseling Parents of Children with Chronic Illness or Disability
Brookes Publishing
PO Box 10624
Baltimore, MD 21285
410-337-9580
800-638-3775
FAX: 410-337-8539
e-mail: custserv@brookespublishing.com
www.brookespublishing.com

Paul Brooks, Owner
$23.00
144 pages Paperback
ISBN 1-85433 -91-8

5070 Cystic Fibrosis: Medical Care
Lippincott, Williams & Wilkins
227 E Washington Square
Philadelphia, PA 19106
215-521-8300
800-777-2295
FAX: 301-824-7390
www.lpub.com

J Lippincott, Chief Executive Officer
A guide to the medical community to the principles and practices of cystic fibrosis care. After chapters on the molecular and cellular bases of CF and its diagnosis, they cover the major organ systems affected by CF and deal with surgery for CF patients, transplantation (lung and liver), hospitalization, and terminal care. Also included are chapters on special populations, exercise, and laboratory testing. *$ 47.95*
365 pages 2000
ISBN 0-781717-98-1

5071 Disability Analysis Handbook
American Board of Disability Analysts
345 24th Avenue N
Suite 200
Nashville, TN 37203
615-327-2984
FAX: 615-327-9235
e-mail: americanbd@aol.com

Alex Horwitz MD, Executive Officer
Kenneth Anchor, President
Official newsletter of the American Board of Disability Analysts; features Healthnews Headlines, Meeting Calendar, Application Packet and much more. Free to members; $20 per year for non-members. *$60.00*
396 pages
ISBN 0-787226-70-x

5072 Ethical Conflicts in Management of Home Care
Springer Publishing Company
536 Broadway
New York, NY 10012
212-431-4370
877-687-7476
FAX: 212-941-7842
e-mail: marketing@springerpub.com
www.springerpub.com

Annette Imperati, Marketing/Sales Director
Ursula Springer, President
Offers answers to the questions what is case management and why does it raise ethical issues. *$29.95*
288 pages

5073 Families in Recovery
Brookes Publishing
PO Box 10624
Baltimore, MD 21285
410-337-9580
800-638-3775
FAX: 410-337-8539
e-mail: custserv@brookespublishing.com
www.brookespublishing.com

Paul Brooks, Owner
This book teaches professionals how to use each families strengths to promote recovery. The authors demonstrate effective, family-focused intervention techniques developed in their combined 35 years of practice. Motivational techniques and stress reducers for counselors are also provided. *$34.00*
352 pages Paperback 1997
ISBN 1-55766 -64-9

5074 Family-Guided Activity-Based Intervention for Toddlers & Infants
Brookes Publishing
PO Box 10624
Baltimore, MD 21285
410-337-9580
800-638-3775
FAX: 410-337-8539
e-mail: custserv@brookespublishing.com
www.brookespublishing.com

Paul Brooks, Owner
Early childhood professionals will be able to teach parents and other caregivers how to use daily routines and activities to help young children with special needs gain vital skills. Included on the video are activity-based teaching methods that enhance children's development, accommodate families' daily schedules, address children's IFSP goals, and promote family interactions. *$37.00*
20 Minutes
ISBN 1-55766 -19-3

5075 Journal of Children's Communication Development
CEC Div for Childrens' Communication Development
1920 Association Drive
Reston, VA 20191
703-620-3660
FAX: 703-312-9193

Alexander Brice, Editor
Contains scholarly articles pertaining to the many aspects of communication disorders in children, encompassing speech, language, hearing and learning disabilities. *$16.00*

2x Year

5076 **NHIF Newsletter**
National Head Injury Foundation
1776 Massachusetts Ave NW
Washington, DC 20036
202-452-1999
800-444-6443
FAX: 202-466-4265
www.biausa.org

Christopher Flavin, President
Contains news and articles for families and professionals concerned with head injury. *$25.00*

5077 **National Clearinghouse of Rehabilitation Training Materials**
5202 N Richmond Hill Drive
Stillwater, OK 74078
405-624-7650
800-223-5219
FAX: 405-624-0695
www.nchrtm.okstate.edu

Judy Seefeld, Director
Carolyn Cash, Information Coordinator
Newsletter produced quarterly to provide information and opportunities to learn more about related fields.
Quarterly

5078 **Partners in Everyday Communicative Exchanges**
Brookes Publishing
PO Box 10624
Baltimore, MD 21285
410-337-9580
800-638-3775
FAX: 410-337-8539
e-mail: custserv@brookespublishing.com
www.brookespublishing.com

Paul Brooks, Owner
A Guide to Promoting Intervention Involving people with Severe Intellectual Disability. This book helps improve communication with people with severe disabilities using practical forms, numerous examples, and illustrative case studies. *$43.00*
192 pages Paperback
ISBN 1-55766 -41-X

5079 **Professional Report**
National Rehabilitation Association (NRA)
633 S Washington Street
Alexandria, VA 22314
703-836-0850
FAX: 703-836-0848
TTY:703-836-0849
e-mail: info@nationalrehab.org
www.nationalrehab.org

Linda Winslow, Executive Director
Association newsletter containing news, programs and information of interest to the Association and its members.

5080 **Provider Magazine**
American Health Care Association
1201 L Street NW
Washington, DC 20005
202-842-4444
800-321-0343
FAX: 202-842-3860

Dave Kyllo, Vice President
Magazine for long-term healthcare professionals. *$ 48.00*
72 pages Monthly
ISSN 0888-03 2

5081 **Public Health Reports**
Oxford Journals
Jfk Federal Building
Room 1855
Boston, MA 02203
513-636-0257
FAX: 617-565-4260
e-mail: robert.rinsky@chmcc.org
phr.oupjournals.org

Robert Rinsky PhD, Editor
Scholarly articles on issues that relate to public health and the healthcare system. *$13.00*

BiMonthly

5082 **Public Health/State Capitols**
Wakeman/Walworth
300 N Washington Street
Alexandria, VA 22314
703-768-9600
800-876-2545
FAX: 703-768-9690
e-mail: newsletters@statecapitals.com
www.statecapitals.com

Keyes Walworth, Publisher
Christine Ryan, Editor
Digest of state and municipal health care financing and legislation, including disease control, medicaid, AIDS, abortion, substance abuse programs, cancer prevention such as smoking restrictions, mental health and disability programs, regulation of hospitals & nursing homes, food safety, medical policies, health insurance for children, home regulation, managerial care, public health issues, pest control, and water quality. Issued weekly-52 issues/year. *$245.00*
10 pages

5083 **Ragged Edge Magazine**
Advocado Press
PO Box 145
Louisville, KY 40201
502-894-9492
FAX: 502-899-9562
e-mail: circulation@raggededgemagazine.com
www.raggededgemagazine.com

Mary Johnson, Editor
Ragged Edge magazine is the successor to The Disability Rag, and covers disability in America today: rights, culture, ideas and controversy. Here you'll find new voices speaking out about disability culture and lives; you'll get the newest cutting-edge thinking on headlines in the news today on genetic discrimination, assisted suicide, healthcare policy. *$17.50*
40 pages BiMonthly
ISSN 0749-95 6

5084 **Sexuality and Disability**
Human Sciences Press
233 Spring Street
New York, NY 10013
212-620-8000
800-221-9369
FAX: 212-463-0742
www.wkap.com

Rudiger Gebauer, Owner
A journal devoted to the psychological and medical aspects of sexuality in rehabilitation and community settings. The journal features original scholarly articles that address the psychological and medical aspects of sexuality in the field of rehabilitation, case studies, clinical practice reports, and guidelines for clinical practice. Plenum Publishers is now part of Kluner Academic Publishers. Journal fulfillment in the NYC office as before for HSP and Plenum Journals. *$160.00*
64 pages Quarterly
ISSN 0146-10 4

5085 **Social Perceptions of People with Disabilities in History**
Charles C Thomas
2600 S 1st Street
Springfield, IL 62704
217-789-8980
800-258-8980
FAX: 217-789-9130
e-mail: books@ccthomas.com
www.ccthomas.com

Michael Thomas, President
This book helps to develop a social history on disabilities by providing a multidisciplinary overview of images of people with disabilities in Western history; promotion the exchange of cross-disciplinary information on disabled people from art, literature, original data, and historical works. With the growing interest in people with disabilities and the recent passage of the American Disability Act, this book will be of interest to special educators, humanities students, and social scientists. *$49.95*
324 pages Paperback 1998
ISBN 0-398068-38-0

5086 **Starting and Sustaining Genetic Support Gr oups**
Johns Hopkins University Press

Guide to the establishment and maintenance of genetic support groups for individuals with genetic disorders and their families. For therapists and group leaders. Discusses practical matters including finding a leader, fund-raising, organizing peer support training programs. *$21.95*
152 pages 1996
ISBN 0-801852-64-1

5087 Substance Abuse and Physical Disability
Haworth Press
10 Alice Street
Binghamton, NY 13904
607-722-5857
800-429-6784
FAX: 607-722-6362
e-mail: orders@haworthpress.com
www.haworthpress.com

William Cohen, Owner
This book offers information on alcohol and drug abuse being a contributing factor in traumatic and disabling injuries. *$ 74.95*
289 pages Hardcover
ISBN 1-560242-89-2

5088 TeamRehab Report
PO Box 8987
Malibu, CA 90265
310-317-4522
800-543-4116
FAX: 310-317-9644

Andria Segedy, Publisher
Kim Pfaff, Managing Editor
A magazine for rehab professionals who prescribe, purchase or recommend assistive technology and related services for clients who are permanently disabled. *$24.00*
48 pages Monthly

5089 What Psychotherapists Should Know about Disabilty
Through the Looking Glass
2198 6th Street
Suite 100
Berkeley, CA 94710
510-848-1112
800-644-2666
FAX: 510-848-4445
e-mail: TLG@lookingglass.org
www.lookingglass.org

R Olkin
Mega Kirshbaum, Executive Director
$24.00
368 pages

5090 Women with Visible & Invisible Disabilitie es: Multiple Intersections, Issues, Therapies
Haworth Press
10 Alice Street
Binghamton, NY 13904
607-722-5857
800-429-6784
FAX: 607-722-6362
e-mail: orders@haworthpress.com
www.haworthpress.com

Martha E Banks PhD, Co-Editor
Ellyn Kaschak PhD, Co-Editor
S Harrington-Miller, Advertising
Addesses the issues faced by women with disabilities, examines the social construction of disability, and makes suggestions for the development and modification of culturally relevant therapy to meet the needs fo disabled women. *$69.95*
418 pages Hardcover
ISBN 0-789019-36-1

Vocations

5091 Ability
George J DePontis
PO Box 370788
Miami, FL 33137

Features articles on living, working, playing and entertainment for the disabled. *$12.00*

5092 Case Management in the Vocational Rehabilitation of Disabled Persons
Berkeley Planning Associates
440 Grand Avenue
Suite 500
Oakland, CA 94610
510-465-7884
FAX: 510-465-7885

Linda Toms Barker
Hans Bos, President
Journal examining the effectiveness of case management services in the context of vocational rehabilitation for persons with psychiatric disabilities.

5093 DEP, Disabled Employment Program
Department of Health
PO Box 678
Albany, NY 12201
518-402-7090
FAX: 518-447-4573
e-mail: jcrucetti@albanycounty.com
www.health.state.ny.us

Patricia Hess, Manager

5094 Demystifying Job Development: Field-Based Approaches to Job Development for the Disabled
Training Resource Network

A guide to successful placement of individuals with severe disabilities in quality jobs in the community. *$29.95*
105 pages 2000
ISBN 1-883302-37-4

5095 Economics, Industry and Disability
Paul H Brookes Publishing Company
PO Box 10624
Baltimore, MD 21285
410-337-9580
800-638-3775
FAX: 410-337-8539

Paul Brooks, Owner
An analysis of the movement toward nonsheltered employment, this book addresses the expanding opportunities, future challenges and economic changes surrounding efforts to ensure the development of positive and constructive employment for persons with disabilities. *$42.00*
Hardcover

5096 Life Beyond the Classroom: Transition Str ategies for Young People with Disabilities
Paul H Brookes Publishing Company
PO Box 10624
Baltimore, MD 21285
410-337-9580
800-638-3775
FAX: 410-337-8539
e-mail: custserv@brokespublishing.com
www.brookespublishing.com

Paul Brooks, Owner
Specialists in a variety of disciplines use creative and practical techniques to ensure careful transition planning, to build young people's confidence and competence in work skills, and to foster support from businesses and community organizations for training and employment programs. *$64.95*
543 pages 2001
ISBN 1-557664-76-5

5097 Mentally Retarded Individuals
Mainstream
3 Bethesda Metro Center
Suite 830
Bethesda, MD 20814
301-961-9299
800-247-1380
FAX: 301-654-6714
e-mail: info@mainstreaminc.org

Charles Moster
Mainstreaming mentally retarded individuals into the workplace. *$2.50*

12 pages

5098 OT Practice
American Occupational Therapy Association
164 Rollins Avenue
Suite 301
Rockville, MD 20852
301-951-9070
800-877-1383
FAX: 301-652-7711

Jeanette Bair, Executive Director
Offers information on conferences, books, resources, materials and information and referral services for persons with disabilities.

5099 Options
6610 N Clark Street
Chicago, IL 60626
773-973-7900
FAX: 773-973-5268
e-mail: AskAnixter@Anixter.org
www.anixter.org

Allan Bergman, President
Robert Dolgan, Editor
Anixter Center's quarterly publication. Free.
Quarterly

5100 Preparation and Employment of Students
Paul H Brookes Publishing Company
PO Box 10624
Baltimore, MD 21285
410-337-9580
800-638-3775
FAX: 410-337-8539

Paul Brooks, Owner
A practical guide on vocational training and employment issues for persons with severe multiple and physical disabilities. *$ 213.00*
224 pages Paper

5101 Teaching Chemistry to Students with Disabilities
American Chemical Society
1155 16th Street NW
Washington, DC 20036
202-872-4600
800-227-5558
FAX: 202-776-8299
TTY: 202-872-6355
e-mail: cwd@acs.org
membership.acs.org/C/CWD

Dorothy Miner, Editor
Judith Summers-Gates, Chair, CCD
Anne Swanson, Editor
Promotes the full involvement of individuals with physical and learning disabilities in educational and career opportunities in the chemical and allied sciences. CWD members lead the American Chemical Society's efforts to help: individuals with disabilities who seek education or employment in chemical and allied sciences; employers and educators of persons with disabilities; other committees, offices and members of ACS who are interested in the full involvement of persons with disabilities.
148 pages
ISBN 0-841238-16-2

5102 Transition from School to Work
Paul H Brookes Publishing Company
PO Box 10624
Baltimore, MD 21285
410-337-9580
800-638-3775
FAX: 410-337-8539

Paul Brooks, Owner
A hands-on guide to planning and implementing successful transition programs for adolescents with disabilities. *$25.00*
336 pages Paper 1988

5103 Transition from School to Work for Persons with Disabilities
Longman Publishing Group
10 Bank Street
9th Floor
White Plains, NY 10606
914-993-5000
FAX: 914-421-5598

Joanne Dresner, President
Examines the multidimensional process needed to effectively prepare persons with disabilities for life beyond school and addresses the key issues in the transition process.
251 pages Paper 1989
ISBN 0-801302-28-5

Pamphlets

5104 A Guide for People with Disabilities Seeking Employment
US Department of Justice
950 Pennsylvania Avenue NW Drs
- Nyav
Washington, DC 20530
202-586-5000
800-574-0301
FAX: 202-307-1197
www.ada.gov

Joanne Graham, Manager
A 2-page pamplet for people with disabilities providing a general explanation of the employment provisions of the ADA and how to file a complaint with the Equal Employment Opportunity Commission.

5105 ADA Business Brief: Restriping Parking Lots
US Department of Justice
950 Pennsylvania Avenue NW Drs
- Nyav
Washington, DC 20530
202-586-5000
800-574-0301
FAX: 202-307-1197
www.ada.gov

Joanne Graham, Manager
A 2-page illustrated design guide explaining the number of accessible parking spaces that are required and the restriping requirements for accessible parking spaces for cars and vans.

5106 ADA Business Brief: Service Animals
US Department of Justice
950 Pennsylvania Avenue NW Drs
- Nyav
Washington, DC 20530
202-586-5000
800-574-0301
FAX: 202-307-1197
www.ada.gov

Joanne Graham, Manager
A 1-page publication summarizing the ADA rules on service animals.

5107 Accessible Stadiums
US Department of Justice
950 Pennsylvania Avenue NW Drs
- Nyav
Washington, DC 20530
202-586-5000
800-574-0301
FAX: 202-307-1197
www.ada.gov

Joanne Graham, Manager
A 4-page publication highlighting features that must be accessible in new stadiums including line of sight for wheelchair seating locations.

5108 Arthritis in Children and La Artritis Infantojuvenil
American Juvenile Arthritis Organization
PO Box 7669
Atlanta, GA 30357
404-872-7100
800-283-7800
FAX: 404-872-9559
e-mail: help@arthritis.org
www.arthritis.org

John Klippel, Chief Executive Officer
A medical information booklet about juvenile rheumatoid arthritis. This booklet is written for parents or other adults and includes details about different forms of JRA, medications, therapies and coping issues.

5109 Assistance at Self-Serve Gas Stations
US Department of Justice
950 Pennsylvania Avenue NW Drs
- Nyav
Washington, DC 20530
202-586-5000
800-574-0301
FAX: 202-307-1197
www.ada.gov

Joanne Graham, Manager
A 1-page document providing guidance on the ADA and refueling assistance for customers with disabilities at self-serve gas stations.

5110 Attention Deficit-Hyperactivity Disorder: Is it a Learning Disability?
Georgetown University, School of Medicine
3800 Reservoir Road NW
Washington, DC 20007
202-342-2400

Joy Drass, Chief Executive Officer
Offers information on learning disabilities and related disorders.

5111 BVA Bulletin
Blinded Veterans Association
477 H Street NW
Washington, DC 20001
202-371-8880
800-669-7079
FAX: 303-914-5832
e-mail: bva@bva.org
www.bva.org

Thomas H Miller, Executive Director
John K Williams, Administrative Director
George E Brummell, Nat'l Dir. Field Service Program
Bi-Monthly

5112 Blind and Vision-Impaired Individuals
Mainstream
1030 5th Street NE
Washington, DC 20002
202-898-1400
e-mail: info@mainstreaminc.org
Mainstreaming blind individuals into the workplace. *$ 2.50*
12 pages

5113 Cataracts
National Eye Institute
31 Center Drive
Building 31, Room 6A-32
Bethesda, MD 20892
301-496-0417
FAX: 301-402-1065
e-mail: 2020@nei.nih.gov
www.nei.nih.gov
Provides information about this common condition and its treatment.

5114 Common ADA Problems at Newly Constructed Lodging Facilities
US Department of Justice
950 Pennsylvania Avenue NW Drs
- Nyav
Washington, DC 20530
202-586-5000
800-574-0301
FAX: 202-307-1197
www.ada.gov

Joanne Graham, Manager
This 11-page document lists a sampling of common accessibility problems at newly constructed lodging facilities that have been identified through the Department of Justice's ongoing enforcement efforts.

5115 Commonly Asked Questions About Service Animals in Places of Business
US Department of Justice
950 Pennsylvania Avenue NW Drs
- Nyav
Washington, DC 20530
202-586-5000
800-574-0301
FAX: 202-307-1197
www.ada.gov

Joanne Graham, Manager
A 3-page publication providing information about service animals and ADA requirements.

5116 Connect Information Service
150 S Progress Avenue
Harrisburg, PA 17109
717-657-1798
800-692-7288
Pamphlet offering information on child development, special education programs, resources for parents and local contact persons.

5117 Developing a Functional and Longitudinal Plan
Autism Society of North Carolina Bookstore
505 Oberlin Road
Suite 230
Raleigh, NC 27605
919-743-0204
800-442-2762
FAX: 919-743-0208
e-mail: dcoffey@autismsociety-nc.org
www.autismsociety-nc.org

Darla Coffey, Bookstore Manager
Jill Keel, Executive Director
This booklet examines the importance of planning and possible goals in self-care. *$4.00*

5118 Easy Access Housing
Easter Seals
230 W Monroe Street
Suite 1800
Chicago, IL 60606
312-726-6800
FAX: 312-726-1494

Janet D Jamieson, Communications Manager
James Williams Jr, Chief Executive Officer
Booklet with a checklist for finding homes that are already accessible or structurally adaptable to accommodate changes in physical abilities and needs. Includes suggestions for solving common accessibility problems such as narrow doors, high thresholds and round knob fixtures.
12 pages

5119 Facts: Books for Blind and Physically Handicapped Individuals
National Library Service for the Blind
1291 Taylor Street NW
Washington, DC 20542
202-707-5100
e-mail: nls@loc.gov
www.loc.gov/nls

Frank Cylke, Executive Director
Annual

5120 Heart to Heart
Blind Children's Center
4120 Marathon Street
Los Angeles, CA 90029
323-664-2153
800-222-3567
FAX: 323-665-3828
e-mail: info@blindchildrenscenter.org
www.blindchildrenscenter.org

Midge Horton, Executive Director
Parents of blind and partially sighted children talk about their feelings. *$10.00*
12 pages

5121 How to Find More About Your Child's Birth Defect or Disability
Birth Defect Research for Children
930 Woodcock Road
Suite 225
Orlando, FL 32803
407-895-0802
FAX: 407-895-0824
e-mail: abdc@birthdefects.org
www.birthdefects.org

Betty Mekdeci, Executive Director/Manager
An informational fact sheet that encourages parents who have a child with a birth defect or disability to become the expert on the child's disability with some suggestions on how to educate themselves.

5122 Individuals with Arthritis
Mainstream
1030 5th Street NE
Washington, DC 20002
202-898-1400
e-mail: info@mainstreaminc.org

Mainstreaming individuals with arthritis into the workplace. *$2.50*
12 pages

5123 Learning to Play
Blind Children's Center
4120 Marathon Street
Los Angeles, CA 90029
323-664-2153
800-222-3567
FAX: 323-665-3828
e-mail: info@blindchildrenscenter.org
www.blindchildrenscenter.org

Midge Horton, Executive Director
Discusses how to present play activities to the visually impaired preschool child. *$10.00*
12 pages

5124 Marfan Syndrome Fact Sheet
March of Dimes
1275 Mamaroneck Avenue
White Plains, NY 10605
914-949-7166
FAX: 914-997-4763
e-mail: askus@marchofdimes.com
www.marchofdimes.com

5125 Marriage & Disability
Accent Books & Products
PO Box 700
Bloomington, IL 61702
309-378-2961
800-787-8444
FAX: 309-378-4420
e-mail: acmtlvng@aol.com

Raymond C Cheever, Publisher
Betty Garee, Editor
This guide can help you make the right decision and it can help smooth the way to a happier life. *$7.95*
Paperback
ISBN 0-91570 -34-5

5126 Medical Herbalism
Bergner Communications
PO Box 20512
Boulder, CO 80308
303-541-9552
e-mail: bergner@concentric.com
www.medherb.com

Paul Bergner, Editor
Newsletter written by physicians and published six times a year.

5127 Midtown Sweep: Grassroots Advocacy at its Best
Independent Living Research Utilization ILRU
2323 S Shepherd Drive
Suite 1000
Houston, TX 77019
713-520-0232
FAX: 713-520-5785
www.ilru.org

Laurie Redd, Executive Director
Josie, Janetta, and Linda describe the steps their center's advocacy group have taken to ensure enforcement of the ADA: target one neighborhood; survey and collect information on businesses that are inaccessible; send letters offering to work with the businesses to help them become accessible and providing information on tax incentives; file lawsuits against businesses that do not respond; involve the media.
10 pages

5128 Move With Me
Blind Children's Center
4120 Marathon Street
Los Angeles, CA 90029
323-664-2153
800-222-3567
FAX: 323-665-3828
e-mail: info@blindchildrenscenter.org
www.blindchildrenscenter.org

Midge Horton, Executive Director
A parent's guide to movement development for visually impaired babies. *$10.00*
12 pages

5129 Newsletter of PA's AT Lending Library
Temple University Institute on Disabilities
1301 Cecil B Moore Avenue
Philadelphia, PA 19122
215-204-7331
800-204-7428
FAX: 215-204-9371
TTY: 800-750-7428
e-mail: piat@temple.edu
disabilities.temple.edu

Amy Goldman, Project Director
Sandra McNally, Editor
Newsletter from the Assistive Technology Lending Library in Pennsylvania. It is published quarterly and is free of charge.
4-8 pages Quarterly

5130 Reaching, Crawling, Walking....Let's Get Moving
Blind Children's Center
4120 Marathon Street
Los Angeles, CA 90029
323-664-2153
800-222-3567
FAX: 323-665-3828
e-mail: info@blindchildrenscenter.org
www.blindchildrenscenter.org

Midge Horton, Executive Director
Orientation and mobility for preschool children who are visually imapired. *$10.00*
24 pages

5131 Selecting a Program
Blind Children's Center
4120 Marathon Street
Los Angeles, CA 90029
323-664-2153
800-222-3567
FAX: 323-665-3828
e-mail: info@blindchildrenscenter.org
www.blindchildrenscenter.org

Midge Horton, Executive Director
A guide for parents of infants and preschoolers with visual impairments. *$10.00*
28 pages

5132 Standing On My Own Two Feet
Blind Children's Center
4120 Marathon Street
Los Angeles, CA 90029
323-664-2153
800-222-3567
FAX: 323-665-3828
e-mail: info@blindchildrenscenter.org
www.blindchildrenscenter.org

Midge Horton, Executive Director
A step-by-step guide to designing and constructing simple, individually tailored, adaptive mobility devices for preschool-age children who are visually impaired. *$10.00*
36 pages

5133 Talk to Me
Blind Children's Center
4120 Marathon Street
Los Angeles, CA 90029
323-664-2153
800-222-3567
FAX: 323-665-3828
e-mail: info@blindchildrenscenter.org
www.blindchildrenscenter.org

Midge Horton, Executive Director
A language guide for parents of deaf children. *$10.00*

11 pages

5134 Talk to Me II
Blind Children's Center
4120 Marathon Street
Los Angeles, CA 90029
323-664-2153
800-222-3567
FAX: 323-665-3828
e-mail: info@blindchildrenscenter.org
www.blindchildrenscenter.org

Midge Horton, Executive Director
A sequel to Talk To Me, available in English and Spanish. *$10.00*

15 pages

5135 Teaching Social Skills to Youngsters with Disabilities
Federation for Children with Special Needs
56 Temple Place
Suite 644
Boston, MA 02111
617-542-7860
800-537-0446
FAX: 617-542-7832
e-mail: pal@fcsn.org
www.ppal.net

Donna Welles, Director
Lisa Lambert, Assistant Director
Explains the importance of instruction and training to learn appropriate social behavior.

5136 Understanding
Easter Seals
230 W Monroe Street
Suite 1800
Chicago, IL 60606
312-726-6800
FAX: 312-726-1494

Janet D Jamieson, Communications Manager
James Williams Jr, Chief Executive Officer
A brochure series for use in patient, family and public education programs and in career recruitment and counseling.
10 Brochures

5137 Without Sight and Sound
Helen Keller National Center
111 Middle Neck Road
Sands Point, NY 11050
516-944-8900

e-mail: hkncdir@aol.com
www.helenkeller.org

Joseph McNulty, Executive Director
Pamphlet offering facts, causes, types and descriptions of deaf-blindness.

Audio/Visual

5138 **A Place for Me**
Educational Productions
9000 SW Gemini Drive
Beaverton, OR 97008
503-644-7000
800-950-4949
FAX: 503-350-7000
e-mail: custserve@edpro.com
www.edpro.com

Linda Freedman, President/Owner
Molly Krumm, Marketing Director
In this video, parents discuss the issues they face in planning for their child's future. This program is designed to stimulate discussion of these issues and help increase awareness of the options available in your local community.

5139 **Acting Blind**
Fanlight Productions
4196 Washington Street
Suite 2
Boston, MA 02131
617-469-4999
800-937-4113
FAX: 617-469-3379
e-mail: fanlight@fanlight.com
www.fanlight.com

Nicole Johnson, Publicity Coordinator
Takes audiences behind the scenes as a company of non-professional actors rehearse a play about life without sight. The performers have no problem imagining themselves in these roles: they are blind themselves. *$199.00*

5140 **Adaptive Baby Care Equipment Video and Book**
Through the Looking Glass
2198 6th Street
Suite 100
Berkeley, CA 94710
510-848-1112
800-644-2666
FAX: 510-848-4445
e-mail: TLG@lookingglass.org
www.lookingglass.org

Megan Kirshbaum, Executive Director
Includes Adaptive Baby care Equipment: Guide Lines; Prototypes and Resources, plus a twelve minute video. Available in braille, large print or cassette. *$79.00*

5141 **All About Attention Deficit Disorders, Revised**
Parent Magic
800 Roosevelt Road
Glen Ellyn, IL 60137
630-790-9600
FAX: 630-469-4571
www.parentmagic.com

Nancy Roe, Office Manager
Thomas Phelan, Owner
A psychologist and expert on ADD outlines the symptoms, diagnosis and treatment of this neurological disorder. Video ($49.95 - 2 parts) and audio cassette ($24.95).

5142 **Autism**
Aquarius Health Care Videos
PO Box 1159
Sherborn, MA 01770
508-650-6905
FAX: 508-650-4216
e-mail: aqvideos@tiac.net
www.aquariusproductions.com
This video takes you into the lives of autistic people and their families to understand more about autism. What defines autism and how can we help those living with the disability? Children, teens, and adults are also profiled and we begin to see the varying levels of development and new technology to help these people communicate. Preview Available. *$149.00*

Video

5143 **Basic Course in American Sign Language**
Harris Communications
15155 Technology Drive
Eden Prairie, MN 55344
952-906-1180
800-825-6758
FAX: 952-906-1099
e-mail: mail@harriscomm.com
www.harriscomm.com

Bill Williams, National Sales Manager
Robert Harris, Owner
This series of four one-hour tapes is designed to illustrate the various exercises and dialogues in the text. *$39.95*
Video

5144 **Beginning ASL Video Course**
Harris Communications
15155 Technology Drive
Eden Prairie, MN 55344
952-906-1180
800-825-6758
FAX: 952-906-1099
e-mail: mail@harriscomm.com
www.harriscomm.com

Bill Williams, National Sales Manager
Robert Harris, Owner
You'll watch a family teach you to learn American Sign Language during funny and touching family situations. A total of 15 tapes in the course. *$49.95*
Video

5145 **Blindness**
Landmark Media
3450 Slade Run Drive
Falls Church, VA 22042
703-241-2030
800-342-4336
FAX: 703-536-9540

Michael Hartogs, President
Cataracts are the most common cause of blindness in the 42 million people worldwide defined as blind. 90% live in developing countries. Cataracts are the most common cause but now can be treated cheaply and safely. *$250.00*
Video

5146 **Braille Documents**
Metrolina Association for the Blind
704 Louise Avenue
Charlotte, NC 28204
704-372-3870
800-926-5460
FAX: 704-372-3872

Robert Scheffel, Manager
This production shop creates Braille and large-print documents.

5147 **Business as Usual**
Fanlight Productions
4196 Washington Street
Suite 2
Boston, MA 02131
617-469-4999
800-937-4113
FAX: 617-469-3379
e-mail: fanlight@fanlight.com
www.fanlight.com

Anthony Sweeney, Marketing Director
Nicole Johnson, Publicity Coordinator
Ben Achtenberg, Owner
An enlightening documentary, brings a unique international perspective to this struggle. This film examines five innovative programs which create opportunities for people with mental and physical disabilities to own and operate their own businesses. *$145.00*

5148 **Buying Time: The Media Role in Health Care**
Fanlight Productions
4196 Washington Street
Suite 2
Boston, MA 02131
617-469-4999
800-937-4113
FAX: 617-469-3379
e-mail: fanlight@fanlight.com
www.fanlight.com

Anthony Sweeney, Marketing Director
Nicole Johnson, Publicity Coordinator
Ben Achtenberg, Owner
This video program is a thoughtful and disturbing examination in the role of the media in determining the allocation of health care resources. This program is a powerful tool on ethics, policy, journalism, sociology, medicine and nursing as well as for professional workshops, and continuing education programs. *$99.00*

5149 **Clockworks**
Learning Corporation of America
6493 Kaiser Drive
Fremont, CA 94555 510-490-7311

Oonchia Chia, Owner
Scotty, who has Down Syndrome, is fascinated by clocks. This film follows him on his adventures of employment in the clock shop.
Film

5150 **Deaf Children Signers**
Harris Communications
15155 Technology Drive
Eden Prairie, MN 55344 952-906-1180
800-825-6758
FAX: 952-906-1099
e-mail: mail@harriscomm.com
www.harriscomm.com

Bill Williams, National Sales Manager
Robert Harris, Owner
This three-part collection of children signers is great for children, teachers, parents and interpreters. *$39.95*
Video

5151 **Deaf Culture Series**
Harris Communications
15155 Technology Drive
Eden Prairie, MN 55344 952-906-1180
800-825-6758
FAX: 952-906-1099
e-mail: mail@harriscomm.com
www.harriscomm.com

Bill Williams, National Sales Manager
Robert Harris, Owner
Each video in this five-part series features a topic dealing with the unique culture of deaf people. It is an excellent resource for deaf studies programs, Interpreter Preparation programs and Sign Language programs. *$59.95*
Video

5152 **Deaf Mosaic Series**
Harris Communications
15155 Technology Drive
Eden Prairie, MN 55344 952-906-1180
800-825-6758
FAX: 952-906-1099
e-mail: mail@harriscomm.com
www.harriscomm.com

Bill Williams, National Sales Manager
Robert Harris, Owner
A national magazine show produced monthly by Gallaudet University, this show has been awarded nine Emmys. As the only nation-wide program about the deaf community, these videotapes are the best of the best from the shows programs. *$29.95*
Video

5153 **Do You Hear That?**
Alexander Graham Bell Association
3417 Volta Place NW
Washington, DC 20007 202-337-5220
FAX: 202-337-8314
e-mail: info@agbell.org
www.agbell.org

Todd Houston, Executive Director
This video shows auditory-verbal therapy sessions of a therapist working individually with 11 children who range in age from 7 months to 7 years old and have hearing aids or cochlear implants.
Video

5154 **Doing Things Together**
Britannica Film Company
345 4th Street
San Francisco, CA 94107 415-777-9876

Steve went with his parents to an amusement park. He met another boy named Martin who at first was shocked by Steve's prosthetic hand.
Film

5155 **Dream Catchers**
University of New Hampshire: Inst on Disability
7 Leavitt Lane
Suite 101
Durham, NC 03824 603-862-2110
FAX: 603-862-0555
e-mail: institutedisability@unh.edu
www.iod.unh.edu

Jan Nisbet, Director
Janice Mutschler, Manager
This video tells the stories of three young people with disabilities, and how they each pulled together a network of people called the circle of support.

5156 **Emerging Leaders**
Mobility International USA
PO Box 10767
Eugene, OR 97440 541-343-1284
FAX: 541-343-6812
e-mail: info@miusa.org
www.miusa.org

Susan Sygall, Executive Director
Pamela Houston, Public Relations Coordinator
Tracy Scharn, Project Assistant
Looks at the emergence of people with disabilities as leaders in the world community this video discusses the value of internation exchange programs in fostering leadership skills. Available in English, Spanish and Russian. *$49.00*
Video

5157 **Face First**
Fanlight Productions
4196 Washington Street
Suite 2
Boston, MA 02131 617-469-4999
800-937-4113
FAX: 617-469-3379
e-mail: fanlight@fanlight.com
www.fanlight.com

Karen McMillen, Marketing Director
Cynthia Conti, Publicity Coordinator
Mike Grundmann, Producer
In this documentary, the stories told reflect the reality faced by all those who are seen as different. Despite their difficult experiences, the survival of the profiled individuals affords comic relief &, by adulthood, they possess unusual strengths that shape their careers in pediatrics, disability care, public speaking, and journalism. *$ 195.00*

5158 **Filmakers Library**
124 E 40th Street
New York, NY 10016 212-808-4980
FAX: 212-808-4983
e-mail: info@filmakers.com
www.filmakers.com

Sue Oscar, Owner
A distributor of educational, award-winning videotapes and films on issues relating to disabilities for educators, counsellors and organizations. The films and tapes are available for rental or sale to institutions, schools, hospitals and organizations. Among the topics covered in the videotapes are autism, schizophrenia, and physical disabilties.

$100 - $300

5159 **Films & Videos on Aging and Sensory Change**
Lighthouse International
111 E 59th Street
New York, NY 10022
212-821-9200
800-829-0500
FAX: 212-821-9706
e-mail: info@lighthouse.org

Joanna Mellor, VP Information Services
Tara Cortes, President
An annotated list of over 80 films and videos dealing with age-related sensory change, divided into sections on vision impairment, hearing impairment, and multiple sensory impairments. *$5.00*

5160 **Hear to Listen & Learn: A Language Approach for Children with Ear Infections**
Brookes Publishing
PO Box 10624
Baltimore, MD 21285
410-337-9580
800-638-3775
FAX: 410-337-8539
e-mail: custserv@brookespublishing.com
www.brookespublishing.com

Paul Brooks, Owner
This video describes the behavioral characteristics that signal when middle ear fluid is causing problems for a child. Also provides professionals with ideas for modifying classrooms and incorporating teaching practices that promote learning opportunities and language acquisition for children with middle ear fluid and associated hearing loss. *$42.00*
20-min VHS
ISBN 1-55766 -99-5

5161 **Heart to Heart**
Blind Children's Center
4120 Marathon Street
Los Angeles, CA 90029
323-664-2153
800-222-3567
FAX: 323-665-3828
e-mail: info@blindchildrenscenter.org
www.blindchildrenscenter.org

Midge Horton, Executive Director
Parents of blind and partially sighted children talk about their feelings. *$35.00*
Video

5162 **Helping Hands**
Fanlight Productions
4196 Washington Street
Suite 2
Boston, MA 02131
617-469-4999
800-937-4113
FAX: 617-469-3379
e-mail: fanlight@fanlight.com
www.fanlight.com

Ben Achtenberg, Owner
The ADA mandates equal access and opportunity for the 43 million people with disabilities in the United States. These individuals may have limited speech, sight or mobility; a developmental disability; or a medical condition which limits some life activities. Many, however, are ready, willing and very able to join the workforce. This video demonstrates that many modifications or adaptations can be made simply by using ingenuity or common sense — such as keeping the aisles clear, etc. *$145.00*
37 Minutes

5163 **How Difficult Can This Be ? (Fat City)**
CACLD
25 Van Zant Street
Suite 15-5
Norwalk, CT 06855
203-838-5010
FAX: 203-866-6108
e-mail: cacld@optonline.net
www.CACLD.org

Beryl Kaufman, Executive Director
This informative and entertaining video allows the viewer to see the world through the eyes of a learning disabled child. It features a unique workshop attended by teacher, psychologists, social workers, parents, siblings and a student with LD They participate in a series of classroom activiteis which cause frustration, anxiety and tension; emotions all too familiar to a student with a learning disability.

5164 **How We Play**
Fanlight Productions
4196 Washington Street
Suite 2
Boston, MA 02131
617-469-4999
800-937-4113
FAX: 617-469-3379
e-mail: fanlight@fanlight.com
www.fanlight.com

Karen McMillen, Marketing Director
Ben Achtenberg, Owner
Though most of the people in this new, short documentary are in wheelchairs, and one is blind, they are anything but handicapped. Playing tennis, snorkeling, whitewater canoeing, practicing karate - they are living proof that a disability can be a challenge, not an obstacle. *$99.00*

5165 **My Country**
Aquarius Health Care Videos
PO Box 1159
Sherborn, MA 01770
508-650-6905
888-440-2963
FAX: 508-650-4216
e-mail: aqvideos@tiac.net
www.aquariusproductions.com

Leslie Kussmann, President
By telling the stories of three people with disabilities and their struggle for equal rights under the law, this film draws a powerful parallel between the efforts of disability rights activists and the civil rights struggle of the 1960s. Great for disability awareness programs, and for discussions of disability rights issues. Should be part of every college curriculum on disabilities. Awarded Best of Show Superfest 98. Preview option available. *$195.00*
Video

5166 **No Barriers**
Aquarius Health Care Videos
PO Box 1159
Sherborn, MA 01770
508-650-6905
FAX: 508-650-4216
e-mail: aqvideos@tiac.net
www.aquariusproductions.com
Everyone faces the world with different abilities and disabilities. But everyone has at least one goal in common...to break through their own barriers says Mark Wellman. Mark, a paraplegic, knows this well. No Barriers takes us into Mark's world where he defies the odds for most able bodied individuals by climbing Yosemite's Half Dome and El Capitan. This video is more than inspiring and fun to watch...it helps one make that paradigm shift from can't do to can do! Preview option available *$90.00*
Video

5167 **On The Spectrum**
Fanlight Productions
4196 Washington Street
Suite 2
Boston, MA 02131
617-469-4999
800-937-4113
FAX: 617-469-3379
e-mail: fanlight@fanlight.com
www.fanlight.com

Nicole Johnson, Publicity Coordinator
Adults living with Asperger syndrome describe the ways AS has affected their lives, their work and their relationships. They discuss learning to cope with the disorder and the comfort and reinforcement of participating with others "like them" in an Asperger's support group. 53 min. *$199.00*

5168 Open for Business
Disability Rights Education and Defense Fund
2212 6th Street
Berkeley, CA 94710
510-644-2555
FAX: 510-841-8645
e-mail: dredf@dredf.org
www.dredf.org

Susan Henderson, Managing Director
An award-winning film that depicts the disability and business communities working together in one small town to remove architectural barriers, when readily achievable, as required by the Americans with Disabilities Act. Package includes 15 and 30 minute closed-captioned versions and 15 to 30 minute versions with audio description. *$179.00*

5169 Open to the Public
Aquarius Health Care Videos
PO Box 1159
Sherborn, MA 01770
508-650-6905
FAX: 508-650-4216
e-mail: aqvideos@tiac.net
www.aquariusproductions.com
Provides an overview of the Americans with Disabilities Act as it applies to state and local governments. The ADA doesn't provide recommendations for solving common problems, but this film could provide enough information for governments to solve some common problems without turning to high-priced consultants. Preview option available. *$125.00*
Video

5170 Our Own Road
Aquarius Health Care Videos
PO Box 1159
Sherborn, MA 01770
508-650-6905
FAX: 508-650-4216
e-mail: aqvideos@tiac.net
www.aquariusproductions.com

Leslie Kussmonn, President
This video shows the disabled helping other people who are disabled and portrays the sense of pride they get from helping others. This multicultural program features many different healing techniques, and teaches the importance of helping those who are disabled become independent and productive. *$99.00*

5171 Outsider: The Life and Art of Judith Scott
Fanlight Productions
4196 Washington Street
Suite 2
Boston, MA 02131
617-469-4999
800-937-4113
FAX: 617-469-3379
e-mail: fanlight@fanlight.com
www.fanlight.com

Nicole Johnson, Publicity Coordinator
Judith Scoot has Down Syndrome, is deaf, and does not speak. Yet after 35 years of institutionalization, with the help of a sister who never gave up on her, she emerged to create a series of sculptures that have fascinated and mystified art experts and collectors around the world. 26 minutes. *$199.00*

5172 Phoenix Dance
Fanlight Productions
4196 Washington Street
Suite 2
Boston, MA 02131
617-469-4999
800-937-4113
FAX: 617-469-3379
e-mail: fanlight@fanlight.com
www.fanlight.com

Nicole Johnson, Publicity Coordinator
Reowned dancer Homer Avila lost his right leg and most of his hip to cancer. Following the creation of a pas de deux choreographed by Alonzo King, Phoenix Dance takes us on a journey of transformation and healing, challenging our expectations of what it means to be "disabled". Includes both 16 and 22 minute versions. *$199.00*

5173 Pool Exercise Program
Arthritis Foundation Distribution Center
PO Box 6996
Alpharetta, GA 30023
800-207-8633
FAX: 770-442-9742
www.arthritis.com
This video features water exercises that will help you increase and maintain joint flexibility, strengthen and tone muscles, and increase endurance. All exercises are performed in water at chest level. No swimming skills are necessary. *$19.50*

5174 Potty Learning for Children who Experience Delay
Exceptional Parent Library
PO Box 1807
Englewood Cliffs, NJ 07632
201-947-6000
800-535-1910
FAX: 201-947-9376
e-mail: eplibrary@aol.com
www.eplibrary.com
This video presents a unique developmental approach to supporting the child in learning independence in the management of bathroom skills. *$39.95*

5175 Pushin' Forward
Fanlight Productions
4196 Washington Street
Suite 2
Boston, MA 02131
617-469-4999
800-937-4113
FAX: 617-469-3379
e-mail: fanlight@fanlight.com
www.fanlight.com

Nicole Johnson, Publicity Coordinator
Growing up poor and Latino, James Lilly was a gang member and drug dealer until, at fifteen, he was shot in the back and paralyzed. Today, he shares his story with inner city kids, and tells them about one thing that helped him move on; wheelchair racing. In Pushin' Forward he takes on the world's longest wheelchair race, from Fairbanks to Anchorage, Alaska, in six days! 39 minutes. *$229.00*

5176 Right at Home
Aquarius Health Care Videos
PO Box 1159
Sherborn, MA 01770
508-650-6905
FAX: 508-650-4216
e-mail: aqvideos@tiac.net
www.aquariusproductions.com
Shows simple solutions for complying with the Fair Hoiusing Act amendments. Emphasizes low-cost, practical solutions, and working with people with disabilities to find the best applicable solution. Ideal for people with disabilities and their families, as well as housing providers, university courses, and disability awareness organizations. Preview option is available. *$99.00*
Video

5177 Seat-A-Robics
PO Box 630064
Little Neck, NY 11363
800-484-7046
FAX: EXT- 11-30

Daria Alinovi, President
Offers a variety of safe, affordable and medically approved video exercise programs that are listed in our video chapter. In addition the company offers two resources. The first Healthy Eating & Facts For Kids is geared specifically to health professionals and educators that work with disabled children ($39.95). The second is a recreational resource guide that stimulates children to be creative and get involved. It keeps them actively engaged while having fun and getting fit ($29.95).

5178 Small Differences
Aquarius Health Care Videos
PO Box 1159
Sherborn, MA 01770
508-650-6905
FAX: 508-650-4216
e-mail: aqvideos@tiac.net
www.aquariusproductions.com

What happens when you give children with and without disabilities a camera and ask them to produce a video about disabilities? The result is an uplifting, award-winning disability video that both children and adults can relate to. The kids interviewed adults and children with physical and sensory disabilities. A top-quality production that increases understanding and awareness. Winner, Columbus International Film & Video Festival. Winner, National Education Media Network. Preview option availabe *$110.00*

Video

5179 **Sound & Fury**

Aquarius Health Care Videos
PO Box 1159
Sherborn, MA 01770
508-650-6905
888-440-2963
FAX: 508-650-4216
e-mail: aqvideos@tiac.net
www.aquariusproductions.com

Leslie Kussmann, President/Producer

This film takes viewers inside the seldom seen world of the deaf to witness a painful family struggle over a controversial medical technology called the cochlear implant. Some of the family members celebrate the implant as a long overdue cure for deafness while others fear it will destroy their language and way of life. This documentary explores this seemingly irreconcilable conflict as it illuminates the ongoing struggle for identity among deaf people today. *$195.00*

Video

5180 **The Boy Inside**

Fanlight Productions
4196 Washington Street
Suite 2
Boston, MA 02131
617-469-4999
800-937-4113
FAX: 617-469-3379
e-mail: fanlight@fanlight.com
www.fanlight.com

Nicole Johnson, Publicity Coordinator

The harrowing story of the filmmaker's son Adam, a 12-year-old with Asperger Syndrome, during a tumultuous year in the life of their family. AS makes Adam's life in seventh grade a minefield, where he finds himself isolated and bullied. As he struggles to find a place for himself, his troubles escalate, both at school and at home. *$249.00*

5181 **Three R's for Special Education: Rights, Resources, Results**

Brookes Publishing
PO Box 10624
Baltimore, MD 21285
410-337-9580
800-638-3775
FAX: 410-337-8539
e-mail: custserv@brookespublishing.com
www.brookespublishing.com

Paul Brooks, Owner

This is a guide for parents, and a tool for educators. Through this video parents learn how to work through the steps of the special education system and work toward securing the best education and services for their children. Reviews the laws to protect children with disabilities in easy to understand language. Also provides a list of national organizations that can offer resources, information and advice to parents. *$49.95*

50 Minutes
ISBN 0-96461 -80-7

5182 **Training Module: Adaptive Baby Care Equipment**

Through the Looking Glass
2198 6th Street
Suite 100
Berkeley, CA 94710
510-848-1112
800-644-2666
FAX: 510-848-4445
e-mail: TLG@lookingglass.org
www.lookingglass.org

Megan Kirshbaum, Executive Director

Curriculum for OT programs includes Adaptive Baby Care Equipment Video and Book. *$250.00*

5183 **Video Guide to Disability Awareness**

Aquarius Health Care Videos
PO Box 1159
Sherborn, MA 01770
508-650-6905
FAX: 508-650-4216
e-mail: aqvideos@tiac.net
www.aquariusproductions.com

President Clinton opens and concludes this informative video about disability awareness. A series of candid interviews with people who have a wide range of disabilities provide personal insights into the issues surrounding visual, hearing, physical and mental disabilities. Video comes with written reference guide and is also available with open or closed captioning. Preview option available. *$195.00*

Video

5184 **Video Intensive Parenting**

Systems Unlimited/LIFE Skills
1556 S 1st Avenue
Iowa City, IA 52240
319-338-9212

Ginny Kirschling, Public Information Specialist
Geoffrey Lauer, Program Director
Bill Gorman, President

Parents who have children with special needs share their reactions to their child's diagnosis and how they have learned to cope with their feelings. *$69.95*

5185 **Vital Signs: Crip Culture Talks Back**

Fanlight Productions
4196 Washington Street
Suite 2
Boston, MA 02131
617-469-4999
800-937-4113
FAX: 617-469-3379
e-mail: fanlight@fanlight.com
www.fanlight.com

Karen McMillen, Marketing Director
Cynthia Conti, Publicity Coordinator
Ben Achtenberg, Owner

This edgy, raw video documentary explores the politics of disability through the performances, debates and late-night conversations of artists at a recent national conference of disabilities and the art's. Vital Signs conveys the intensity, variety and vitality of disability culture today. *$225.00*

Video

5186 **White Cane and Wheels**

Fanlight Productions
4196 Washington Street
Suite 2
Boston, MA 02131
617-469-4999
800-937-4113
FAX: 617-469-3379
e-mail: fanlight@fanlight.com
www.fanlight.com

Nicole Johnson, Publicity Coordinator

Carmen and Steve once dreamed of lives on stage and screen, but their plans were cut short by her blindness and his muscular dystrophy. This program is a funny and touching exploration of a relationship filled with frustration, but held together with patience, stubborness, forgiveness, and love. 26 minutes. *$169.00*

Web Sites

5187 **Abledata**

disabilities.about.com/health/disabili

Premier source for information on assistive technology.

5188 **Ablewear Aids for Daily Living**

www.ableware.com

Quality products to achieve independence in performing daily living activities.

5189 Academy for Educational Development

www.aed.org
Committed to addressing human development needs in the United States and throughout the world.

5190 Access Unlimited

accessunlimited.com
Adaptive transportation and mobility equipment for people with disabilities.

5191 Ai Squared

www.aisquared.com
Leaders in low vision software.

5192 Alternatives in Education for the Hearing Impaired (AEHI)

www.aehi.org
AEHI fosters literacy and empowers people with hearing impairments to achieve their full potential through unique educational options.

5193 American Academy of Audiology

www.audiology.org

5194 American Association of People with Disabilities

www.aapd.com
Non-profit, non-partisan, cross-disability, national membership organization whose goals are unity, leadership and impact. AAPD's mission is to advance the economic and political power of all people with disabilities.

5195 American Botanical Council

www.herbalgram.org
Conducts research and provides education on the safe, responsible and scientific uses of medicine herbs to the public, healthcare professionals, government, industry, and the media.

5196 American College of Rheumatology Research and Education Foundation

www.rheumatology.org
Arthritis afflictsone in every seven Americans. Your gift supports research, investigates the causes, improves treatment and works toward the prevention and cure of arthritis.

5197 American Liver Foundation

www.liverfoundation.org
Is the only national voluntary health organization dedicated to preventing, treating, and curing hepatitis and other liver and gall bladder diseases through research and education.

5198 American Mobility: Personal Mobility Solutions

www.americanmobility.com
Source of Pride Scooters, Jazzy Power Chairs, personal mobility vehicles, and lift and recline chairs.

5199 American Speech-Language and Hearing Association

www.asha.org
Exhibits by companies specializing in alternative and augmentative communications products, publishers, software and hardware compinies, and hearing aid testing equipment manufacturers.

5200 Americans with Disabilities Act: ADA Home Page

www.usdoj.gov
Provides facts on the Americans with Disabilities Act and other information relating to disability rights.

5201 Appliance 411

appliance411.com
A guide to remodeling and appliances for people with disabilities.

5202 Arc of the United States

www.thearc.org
National organization of and for people with mental retardation anad thier families.

5203 Assist.com

www.assist.com
Assistive technology web resource.

5204 Assistive Technology Disabilities

www.netins.net
Provides information on assistive technology.

5205 Association for the Cure of Cancer of the Prostate

www.capcure.org.il
CURE is a nonprofit public charity that is dedicated to supporting prostate cancer research and hastening the conversion of research into cures or controls.

5206 Asthma and Allergy Foundation of America

www.aafa.org
Supports research to cure asthma and allergies and helps sufferers through patient education, practical advice, and a nationwide chapter and support group network.

5207 Audiology Foundation of America

www.audfound.org
Commited to fostering the education and training of audiologists to meet the needs of the public, especially those with impaired hearing.

5208 Auditory-Verbal International

www.auditory-verbal.org

5209 Beebe Center

www.beebecenter.org
At the Beebe Center our mission is to help hearing-impaired children to listen and talk.

5210 **Cancer Biotherapy Research Group**

members.aol.com/cancerccsi
Cancer patients receive promising treatments in their communities through a nationwide research network of physicians and hospitals. All contributions are used to fund clinical research.

5211 **Cancer Immunology Research Foundation**

www.cancer-research.org
Immunology research will discover why the immune system fails and cancer develops. Herein lies the cure for cancer, AIDS, and other autoimmune diseases.

5212 **Cancer Immunotherapy and Gene Therapy Institute**

www.skcc.org
Researches effective, non-toxic therapies for cancer. Accelerates taking promising discoveries from the laboratories to clinics to treat people victimized by cancer. Treatments given at no charge.

5213 **Cancer Research Fund of Damon Runyon: Walter Winchell Foundation**

www.cancerresearchfund.org
Goal is to cure cancer. 100% of your gift funds research. With 49 Runyon-Winchell scientists who have won Nobel Prizes, chances are good.

5214 **Center on the Social & Emotional Foundations for Early Learning**

csefel.uiuc.edu
The center will: focus on promoting the social and emotional developmental of children as a means of preventing challenging behaviors; collaborate with existing T/TA providers for the purpose of ensuring the implementation and sustainability of practices at the local level; provide ongoing identification of training needs and preferred delivery formats of local programs and T/TA providers; disseminate evidence-based practices.

5215 **Disability Information and Resources**

www.eskimo.com

5216 **Disability Mall**

www.disabilityproducts.com
Online directory committed to featuring information on disability and medical products, resources and services, with over 2,500 links including over 400 companies for one-stop shopping convenence.

5217 **Disability Net**

www.bargione.co.uk/disabled.htm
The internet resource for disabled people that offers the latest news and events.

5218 **Disability Rights Activist**

www.disrights.org
Provides information to enable anyone intersted in the rights of disabled people to work for those rights.

5219 **DisabilityResources.org**

www.disabilityresources.org
Provides information on disability-related material on the Web.

5220 **Discover Technology**

discovertechnology.com
Provides links to websites that are specifically geared toward persons with disabilities who have special interest in adaptive technology.

5221 **Dynamic Living**

www.dynamic-living.com
Kitchen products, bathroom helpers, and unique daily living products that provide a convienient, comfortable, and safe environment for people with disabilities.

5222 **ElderLawAnswers.com**

www.elderlawanswers.com
Provides information about legal issues facing senior citizens and a searchable directory of attorneys.

5223 **Exploring Autism: A Look at the Genetics of Autism**

www.exploringautism.org
Dedicated to helping families who are living with the challenges of autism stay informed about the exciting breakthroughs involving the genetics of autism. Report and explain new genetic research findings. Explain genetic principles as they relate to autism, provide the latest research news, and seek your imput.

5224 **Federal Resource Center for Special Education**

www.dss.org

5225 **Foundation Fighting Blindness**

www.blindness.org
Largest voluntary, non-government sponsor to cure retinitis pigmentosa (RP), macular degeneration and related inherited disorders—leading causes of blindness and deaf-blindness.

5226 **Freedom Scientific**

www.hj.com
Assistive technology for blind and visually impaired computer users.

5227 **Gallaudet University Press**

www.gallaudet.edu
Source for titles on deafness and deaf related subjects.

5228 **Glaucoma Research Foundation**

www.glaucoma.org
Protecting both sight and independence for those with glaucoma, by providing improved treatments and education today and by leading research towards a cure for tomarrow.

5229 **Herb Research Foundation**

www.herbs.org
Research and public education on the health benefits of medicinal plants. Dedicated to world health through the informed use of herbs.

5230 **Hypokalemic Periodic Paralysis Resource Page**

www.periodicparalysis.org/PPRC/PP
Provides understandable information on HKPP, dynamia linkage to several additional sources of helpful information on the Internet, and offers several online networking opportunities.

5231 **Innovation Management Group**

www.imgpresents.com
US and international onscreen keyboards, Word Prediction, Switch Scanning, Hover and Dwell, Joystick emulation, and Magnification software programs.

5232 **Interstitial Cystitis Association**

www.ichelp.com
Providing information, support and assistance to the patients of Interstitial Cystitis, a highly debilitating bladder disease. We'll find a cure by funding and encouraging research.

5233 **LDOnLine**

www.ldonline.org
The interactive guide to learning disabilities for parents, teachers, and children.

5234 **Lyme Disease Foundation**

www.lyme.org
Provides critical information about tick-borne disease prevention, improves healthcare and funds research for solutions. 500,000 children, adults, and professionals assisted 25 countries.

5235 **Mainstream Online Magazine of the Able-Disabled**

www.mainstream-mag.com
The leading news, advocacy and lifestyle magazine for people with disabilities.

5236 **Med-Sell**

www.kansas.net/~cbaslock/classifi
Helps people buy and sell new and previously owned medical equipment and find accessible housing.

5237 **Medem Network Societies American Academy of Opthamology**

www.medem.com
Physician web site service empowered by the leading medical specialty societies.

5238 **Microsoft Accessibility Technology for Everyone**

microsoft.com/enable/
Information about accessibility features and options included in Microsoft products.

5239 **MossRehab ResourceNet**

www.mossresourcenet.org
Accessible travel, disability fact sheets, ADA, newsgroups, search tools.

5240 **Multiple Sclerosis National Research Institute**

www.ms-national-research.org
Conducts research for development of a vaccine to halt progression of mutiple sclerosis. Initial patient trials show promising results. Help us find a cure soon.

5241 **National Alliance of the Disabled (NAOTD)**

www.naotd.org
Premier source for information on assistive technology.

5242 **National Association for Visually Handicapped**

www.navh.org
Works with millions of people worldwide in dealing with the difficulties of vision impairment.

5243 **National Brain Tumor Foundation**

www.braintumor.org
Brain tumors strike children and adults in the prime of life. Your support gives help and gives hope by funding research and patient support services.

5244 **National Business & Disability Council**

www.business-disability.com
Works toward furthering the intersts of business and people with disabilities.

5245 **National Organization on Disability**

www.nod.org

5246 **National Rehabilitation Center**

www.naric.com
Serves both professionals and the general public intersted in disability and rehabilitation.

5247 **National Women's Health Information Center**

www.4women.gov
Provides information for women with disabilities, health professionals, researchers, and caretakers.

5248 **NeuroControl Corporation**

www.neurocontrol.com
Helps people with spinal cord injuries lead more independent lives.

5249 **Office of Juvenile Justice and Delinquency Prevention**

www.childrenwithdisabilities.ncjrs.org
Offers information and resources to disabled children, their families and service providers. This site is part of a joint effort by several federal agencies to promote a national agenda for children and foster positve youth development, and will provide informatin on learning disabilities, debilitating conditions and physical disabilities. It will include the latest research, programs and events designed specifically for children with disabilities.

5250 **Osteogenesis Imperfecta Foundation**

www.oif.org

Strives to improve the quality of life for indivduals with this brittle bone disorder through research, education, awareness, and mutual support.

5251 Quantum Technology

www.quantech.com
Provides access to information and tools for independence to serve the visually impaired and those with a learning disability.

5252 Research!America

www.researchamerica.org
Builds active public support for more government and private-industry research to find treatments and cures for both physical and mental disorders.

5253 Skin and Dental Dysfunction Foundation

www.nfed.org
Children left toothless from Ectodermal Dysplasia are provided dentures, support services and education. Established by National Foundation for Ectodermal Dysplasias which searches for a cure.

5254 Social Security Online

www.ssa.gov
Official website of the Social Secuirity Administration.

5255 Special Clothes for Special Children

www.special-clothes.com
A catalog of adaptive clothing for children with disabilities - helping boys and girls with special needs meet the world with pride and confidence since 1987.

5256 Standard Search: Oral Health Care for People with Developmental Disabilities

www.nohic.nidcr.hih.gov
Helps meet the information needs of special care patients and health care providers. Staff provides the custom or standardized services on special care topics in oral health, including developmental disabilities. Each record in the search contains a bibliographic citation and abstract including info for the user on how to obtain materials directly.

5257 V Foundation for Cancer Research

www.jimmyv.org
Named for basketball coach and broadcaster, Jim Valvano. The V Foundation funds critical stage research conducted by young researchers at NCI approved cancer research facilities.

5258 ValueOptions

www.valueoptions.com
Serves over 22 million people in behavioral healthcare through publicaly funded, federal, and commercial contracts.

5259 Wardrobe Wagon: The Special Needs Clothing Store

www.wardrobewagon.com
Wearing apparel for individuals with special clothing needs.

5260 We Magazine

www.icdri.org/NEWS/WEMagazine.htm
Lifestyle magazine for people with disabilities.

5261 We Media

www.wemedia.com
Online network for people with disabilities.

5262 WebABLE

www.hisoftware.com/press/webable.html
Provides disability-related internet resources.

5263 WheelchairNet

www.wheelchairnet.org

5264 World Association of Persons with Disabilities

www.wapd.org
Dedicated to improving the quality of life for those with disabilities.

General

5265 Age Appropriate Puzzles

7756 Winding Way
Fair Oaks, CA 95628
916-961-3507
FAX: 916-961-0765
e-mail: miltcher@spcglobal.net

Cheryl Meyers, President
These unique puzzles teach numerous concepts: picture, name, color and shape recognition. Each of the two themes (holidays, and clothing) comes with self-adhesive stickers that name each picture in English, Hmong, Russian, Spanish and Vietnamese. A notch at each puzzle piece makes grasping and lifting the pieces easy to use., They are designed for children from 18 months and up. Special needs children, preschool through high school would also benefit. *$9.95*

5266 All-Turn-It Spinner

AbleNet
2808 Fairview Avenue N
Roseville, MN 55113
651-294-2200
800-322-0956
FAX: 651-294-2222
e-mail: customerservice@ablenetinc.com
www.ablenetinc.com

Rick Osterhaus, Chief Executive Officer
The All-Turn-It Spinner is a random spinner that comes with a dice overlay allowing user's to participate in any commercially-available game that require dice. Activate the spinner with its built-in switch or connect an external switch. Overlays are interchangeable with AbleNet designed spinner games or create your own overlay. A great inclusion tool!. *$89.00*

5267 Anthony Brothers Manufacturing

Convert-O-Bike
1945 South Rancho Santa Fe Road
San Marcos, CA 92069
760-744-4763
FAX: 760-744-2994
e-mail: kids@kidtrikes.com
www.kidtrikes.com

Julia Anthony, President
Sue Coffin, Vice President
Manufacture wheeled toys and goods for disabled children.

5268 Automatic Card Shuffler

Maxi Aids
42 Executive Boulevard
Farmingdale, NY 11735
631-752-0521
800-522-6294
FAX: 631-752-0689
e-mail: sales@maxiaids.com
www.maxiaids.com

Simple to use, perfect for the player with limited hand dexterity. *$14.95*

5269 Backgammon Set: Deluxe

Maxi Aids
42 Executive Boulevard
Farmingdale, NY 11735
631-752-0521
800-522-6294
FAX: 631-752-0689
e-mail: sales@maxiaids.com
www.maxiaids.com

Completely factual with a felt board, raised white dividers and white braille dice for the blind and visually impaired. *$29.95*

5270 Board Games: Snakes and Ladders

Maxi Aids
42 Executive Boulevard
Farmingdale, NY 11735
631-752-0521
800-522-6294
FAX: 631-752-0689
e-mail: sales@maxiaids.com
www.maxiaids.com

A dice game for 2 to 6 players. This children's game is also fun for the whole family. Offers recreation, competition and eye/hand coordination skills. *$34.95*

5271 Board Games: Solitaire

Maxi Aids
42 Executive Boulevard
Farmingdale, NY 11735
631-752-0521
800-522-6294
FAX: 631-752-0689
e-mail: sales@maxiaids.com
www.maxiaids.com

This popular solo board game lends itself to a number of less well-known variations. The board is accompanied by brightly colored pieces that are reversible for the visually impaired player. *$30.95*

5272 Braille Playing Cards: Plastic

Maxi Aids
42 Executive Boulevard
Farmingdale, NY 11735
631-752-0521
800-522-6294
FAX: 631-752-0689
e-mail: sales@maxiaids.com
www.maxiaids.com

Playing cards that offer regular print and braille on plastic cards for the blind or visually impaired player. *$9.95*

5273 Braille: Bingo Cards, Boards and Call Numbers

Maxi Aids
42 Executive Boulevard
Farmingdale, NY 11735
631-752-0521
800-522-6294
FAX: 631-752-0689
e-mail: sales@maxiaids.com
www.maxiaids.com

Bingo products for the visually impaired. Cards, boards and call numbers offer regular print and braille. *$4.99*

5274 Braille: Rook Cards

Maxi Aids
42 Executive Boulevard
Farmingdale, NY 11735
631-752-0521
800-522-6294
FAX: 631-752-0689
e-mail: sales@maxiaids.com
www.maxiaids.com

This set of cards for Rook, the popular bidding card game with 23 variations, has regular size print and braille print for the blind/visually impaired player. *$13.75*

5275 Card Holder Deluxe

Maxi Aids
42 Executive Boulevard
Farmingdale, NY 11735
631-752-0521
800-522-6294
FAX: 631-752-0689
e-mail: sales@maxiaids.com
www.maxiaids.com

A handsome-looking card holder takes the struggle out of holding playing cards in weak or arthritic hands. The two clear plastic tiers hold up to 18 cards. The wooden base has a non-skid bottom to prevent slipping, and is also great for holding recipe cards. *$19.75*

5276 Cards: Musical

Sense-Sations
919 Walnut Street
Philadelphia, PA 19107
215-627-0600
FAX: 215-922-0692
www.asb.org

Patricia Johnson, Chief Executive Officer
These cards, for all occasions, play music when they are opened, for the visually impaired and blind persons. *$2.50*

5277 Cards: UNO

Maxi Aids
42 Executive Boulevard
Farmingdale, NY 11735
631-752-0521
800-522-6294
FAX: 631-752-0689
e-mail: sales@maxiaids.com
www.maxiaids.com

Traditional card game in braille for the blind player recreation. *$10.95*

5278 Checker Set: Deluxe
Maxi Aids
42 Executive Boulevard
Farmingdale, NY 11735
631-752-0521
800-522-6294
FAX: 631-752-0689
e-mail: sales@maxiaids.com
www.maxiaids.com

A wooden board with sunken playing squares. The squares have drilled holes for inserting the checker, offering help with eye/hand coordination for the physically challenged. *$25.95*

5279 Chess Set: Deluxe
Maxi Aids
42 Executive Boulevard
Farmingdale, NY 11735
631-752-0521
800-522-6294
FAX: 631-752-0689
e-mail: sales@maxiaids.com
www.maxiaids.com

Made out of wood material. Boards have raised dark squares and all squares have drilled holes for inserting pegged chessmen, for the physically challenged player with poor eye/hand coordination. *$43.95*

5280 Dice: Jumbo Size
New Vision Store
919 Walnut Street
Philadelphia, PA 19107
215-629-2990
www.thenewvisionstore.com

The large white and black dice are over-sized and have grooved dots to indicate the numbers, for easy reading for the visually handicapped. *$4.95*

5281 Enabling Devices
385 Warburton Avenue
Hastings on Hudson, NY 10706
914-478-0960
800-832-8697
FAX: 914-479-1369
e-mail: info@enablingdevices.com
www.enablingdevices.com

Elizabeth Bell, Marketing Manager
Karen O'Connor, Vice President Operations
Steven Kanor, Owner

For more than 25 years, Enabling Devices has been dedicated to providing affordable learning and assistive devices for the physically challenged. Products include augmentative communicators, adapted toys, capability switches, training and sensory devices and activity centers. Call for a free catalog.

5282 Hands-Free Controller
Nintendo
PO Box 957
Redmond, WA 98073
800-255-3700
www.nintendo.com

Yoshio Tsuboike, Editor-in-Chief

Nintendo controller for the physically disabled.

5283 Let's Count Braille and Tactile Numbers Po ster
Maxi Aids
42 Executive Boulevard
Farmingdale, NY 11735
631-752-0521
800-522-6294
FAX: 631-752-0689
e-mail: sales@maxiaids.com
www.maxiaids.com

Cognitive skills and motor stimulation. *$34.95*

5284 National Lekotek Center
3204 West Armitage Avenue
Chicago, IL 60647
773-276-5164
800-366-PLAY
FAX: 773-276-8644
TTY: 800-573-4446
e-mail: lekotek@lekotek.org
www.lekotek.org

Diana Nielander, Executive Director
Clarice Brown, Programs/Training Asst Director

Maximizes the development of children with special needs through play. Supports families through nationwide family play centers, toy lending libraries and computer play programs. Publishes six-page newsletter three times per year.

5285 New Language of Toys: Teaching Communicati on Skills to Children with Special Needs
Spina Bifida Association of America
4590 Macarthur Boulevard NW
Suite 250
Washington, DC 20007
202-944-3285
800-621-3141
FAX: 202-944-3295
e-mail: sbaa@sbaa.org
www.sbaa.org

Cindy Brownstein, Chief Executive Officer

A guide for parents and teachers and a reader-friendly resource guide that provides a wealth of information on how play activities affect a child's language development and where to get the toys and materials to use in these activities. *$19.00*

5286 Puzzle Games: Cooking, Eating, Community and Grooming
PCI
PO Box 34270
San Antonio, TX 78265
210-670-3866
800-594-4263
FAX: 218-210-3771
www.pci.edu.com

Janie Haugen, Program Director
Jeff McLane, President/CEO
Rebecca Phillips, Executive Director

Each game has 63 pieces which are 2 inches in size. The completed full color puzzle is 19 inch x 15 inch. Step 1 - Work the puzzle. Step 2 - Match picture or word cards to the correct space on the puzzle. These puzzles teach basic life skills. *$19.95*

5287 Single Switch Latch and Timer
AbleNet
1081 10th Avenue SE
Minneapolis, MN 55414
800-322-0956
FAX: 612-379-9143
e-mail: customerservice@ablenetinc.com
www.ablenetinc.com

A Single Switch Latch and Timer allows a user to activate a battery-operated toy or appliance in the latch, timed seconds and timed minutes modes of control. Choose for one user and one device at a time. *$63.00*

5288 Socialization Games for Persons with Disabilities
Charles C Thomas
2600 South 1st Street
Springfield, IL 62704
217-789-8980
800-258-8980
FAX: 217-789-9130
e-mail: books@ccthomas.com
www.ccthomas.com

Michael Thomas, President

This text will assist those who want to teach severely multiple disabled students by providing information on: general principles of intervention and classroom organization; managing the behavior of students; physically managing students and using adaptive equipment; teaching eating skills; teaching toileting, dressing , and hygiene skills; teaching cognition, communication, and socialization skills; teaching independent living skills; and teaching infants and preschool students. *$24.95*

140 pages Paperback
ISBN 0-39806 -73-4

5289 Take a Chance
Speech Bin
1965 25th Avenue
Vero Beach, FL 32960
772-770-0007
800-477-3324
FAX: 772-770-0006
e-mail: info@speechbin.com
www.speechbin.com

Jan J Binney, Senior Editor

Card game for practice of commonly misarticulated speech sounds. *$18.75*

16 pages Book & Cards
ISBN 0-93785 -46-7

5290 Tic Tac Toe

Maxi Aids
42 Executive Boulevard
Farmingdale, NY 11735
631-752-0521
800-522-6294
FAX: 631-752-0689
e-mail: sales@maxiaids.com
www.maxiaids.com

Several versions including tactile large peg and jumbo foam floor tile. *$5.95*

5291 Turnabout Game

Maxi Aids
42 Executive Boulevard
Farmingdale, NY 11735
631-752-0521
800-522-6294
FAX: 631-752-0689
e-mail: sales@maxiaids.com
www.maxiaids.com

A game of strategy for two, with large playing pieces and a bright gameboard for the visually impaired player. *$7.70*

Newsletters & Books

5292 A Guide for the Wheelchair Traveler
Access For Disabled Americans
3685 Mount Diablo Boulevard
Suite 300
Lafayette, CA 94549
925-284-6444
FAX: 925-284-6448
e-mail: psmither@aol.com
www.accessfordisabled.com

Neal Smither, President
Patricia Smither, Editor/Secretary
All you need to know when traveling in a wheelchair. *$30.00*
165 pages Paperback
ISBN 1-928616-00-3

5293 A World Awaits You
Mobility International U SA
132 E. Broadway
Suite 343
Eugene, OR 97401
541-343-1284
FAX: 541-343-6812
e-mail: info@miusa.org
www.miusa.org

Barb Cheshir, Information Services Coordinator
Susan Sygall, Executive Director
A journal of success stories and tips of people with disabilities participating in international exchange programs.
40 pages Yearly

5294 Access Travel: Airports
Consumer Information Center
Department 575a
Pueblo, CO 81009
719-948-3334
e-mail: catalog.pueblo@gsa.gov

Michael Clark, Public Affairs
Alfred Pino, Manager
Tips and suggestions for easier travel for persons with disabilities and the elderly. Lists designs, facilities, and services at 553 airport terminals worldwide.

5295 Architectural Barriers Action League
PO Box 57088
Tucson, AZ 85732
520-628-8118

Martin Floerchinger, Owner
Offers guides to accessible hotels and motels across the country.

5296 Directory of Accessible Van Rentals
Disability Bookshop
PO Box 129
Vancouver, WA 98666
360-694-2462

Designed to help people with disabilities locate rental vans that are accessible throughout the U.S. *$9.95*
30+ pages
ISBN 0-93326 -09-9

5297 Directory of Travel Agencies for the Disabled
Twin Peaks Press
PO Box 129
Vancouver, WA 98666
360-694-2462
800-637-2256
FAX: 360-696-3210
e-mail: twinpeak@pacifier.com
home.pacifier.com

David Lynch, Director
Directory lists more than 360 travel agents specializing in arrangements for people with disabilities. Handbook provides information about accessibility. *$19.95*
40 pages Paperback
ISBN 0-93326 -04-8

5298 Elderly Guide to Budget Travel/Europe
Pilot Books
PO Box 2102
Greenport, NY 11944
631-477-1094
FAX: 631-661-4379
Includes a list of over 250 inexpensive hotels in prime tourist areas. Covers special needs of senior citizens including inexpensive accommodations and fares. *$3.95*

5299 Ideas for Easy Travel
Accent Books & Products
PO Box 700
Bloomington, IL 61702
309-378-2961
800-787-8444
FAX: 309-378-4420
e-mail: acmtlvng@aol.com

Raymond C Cheever, Publisher
Betty Garee, Editor
Ideal for helping the new traveler get started having fun. Points out favorite accessible high-spots as reported by two travel experts (one is disabled), and offers basic ideas to help wherever you go. *$3.25*
55 pages Paperback
ISBN 0-91570 -36-1

5300 Sports n' Spokes Magazine
Paralyzed Veterans of America
801 18th Street NW
Washington, DC 20006
202-872-1300
800-424-8200
888-888-2201
e-mail: info@pva.org
www.pva.org

Joseph L Fox Sr, National President
Tom Wheaton, Senior VP
Gene A Crayton, National VP
Publication of the PVA, a congressionally chartered veterans service organization, with unique expertise on a wide variety of issues involving the special needs of our members— veterans of the armed forces who have experienced spinal cord injury or dysfunction.
1946

5301 Survival Strategies for Going Abroad, A Guide for People with Disabilites
132 E. Broadway
Suite 343
Eugene, OR 97440
541-343-1284
FAX: 541-343-6812
e-mail: info@miusa.org
www.miusa.org

Susan Sygall, Executive Director
Melissa Mitchell, Public Relations
$16.95
225 pages

5302 Travel Information Service/Moss Rehab Hospital
Moss Rehabilitation Hospital
1200 West Tabor Road
Philadelphia, PA 19141
215-456-9900
800-225-5667
e-mail: staff@mossresourcenet.org
www.mossresourcenet.org

Joan Appel, Manager
Alberto Esquenazi, Plant Manager
Offers information and resources, to telephone callers only, for persons with special traveling/accessibility needs.

5303 United States Department of the Interior National Park Service
Superintendent of Documents
1849 C Street NW
Washington, DC 20240
202-208-3100
FAX: 202-619-7302
e-mail: webteam@ios.doi.gov
www.doi.gov

Mainella, Director
Gale Norton, Chief Executive Officer
Offers an informational packet containing books, guides and tours for the disabled and elderly.

5304 **Wheelin Around**
Wheelers Accessible Van Rentals
6614 West Sweetwater Avenue
Glendale, AZ 85304
623-776-8830
800-456-1371
FAX: 623-412-9920
e-mail: info@WheelersVanRentals.com
www.WheelersVanRentals.com

Tammy Smith, President
Ron Smith, Corporate Treasurer

5305 **Where to Stay USA**
Council On International Educational Exchange
633 3rd Avenue
New York, NY 10017
212-822-2600
888-COU-NCIL
FAX: 212-822-2649

Priscilla Tovey, Information Services
A guide to low-cost lodging throughout the United States including information on whether the establishment is accessible. *$ 15.95*
250 pages
ISBN 0-67179 -49-5

Associations & Programs

5306 **Access America**
Northern Cartographic
4050 Williston Road
South Burlington, VT 05403
802-860-2886
FAX: 802-865-4912
e-mail: info@ncarto.com
www.ncarto.com
Offers information on 36 national parks, providing detailed information on accessibility.

5307 **Access Yosemite National Park**
Special Needs Project
324 State Street
Suite H
Santa Barbara, CA 93101
805-962-8087
800-333-6867
FAX: 805-962-5087
e-mail: books@specialneeds.com
www.specialneeds.com

Hod Gray, Executive Director
Laraine Gray, Coordinator
Represents unprecedented combinations of intensive information survey data with high quality cartography. *$7.95*
31 pages

5308 **America West Airlines**
4000 East Sky Harbor Boulevard
Phoenix, AZ 85281
480-693-0800
800-327-7810
FAX: 480-693-3702
www.princetonreview.com

Dan Berkey, Director
W Parket, Chief Executive Officer
This airline trains employees to make sure that passengers with disabilities enjoy convenient, safe and comfortable travel.

5309 **American Hotel and Lodging Foundation**
1201 New York Avenue NW
Suite 600
Washington, DC 20005
202-289-3100
FAX: 202-289-3199
e-mail: comments@ahlaonline.org
www.ahlef.org/

Joseph A McInerney, President/CEO
Joori Jeon, Executive Vice President
Crystal Hammond, Director Of Foundation Programs
Will disseminate information, develop and conduct a series of seminars for the hotel and motel industry at state-level association conferences, and develop and distribute an ADA Compliance handbook for use by the lodging industry.

5310 **Amtrak**
60 Massachusetts Avenue NE
Washington, DC 20002
202-906-3000
800-872-7245
FAX: 202-906-4564
TTY: 202-906-2500
e-mail: access@w0.amtrak.com
www.amtrak.com

Alexander Kummant, President/CEO
Amtrak is committed to making travel for passengers with disabilities more accessible. Anyone interested should contact Amtrak's Special Services Desk at 1-800-USA-RAIL at least 24 hours in advance to arrange for special assistance. The type of equipment and accessibility vary from train to train and station to station.

5311 **Easter Seals Project ACTION**
1425 K Street NW
Suite 200
Washington, DC 20005
202-347-3066
800-659-6428
FAX: 202-737-7914
TTY: 202-347-7385
e-mail: project_action@easterseals.com
www.projectaction.org

Alan Abeson, Director
Donna Zide, Executive Assistant
Lucinda Lefferts, Information Specialist
A national technical assistance program designed to improve access to transportation services for people with disabilities and assist transit providers in implementing the Americans with Disabilities Act. Publishes quarterly newsletter.

5312 **Easy Access to National Parks: The Sierra Club Guide for the Disabled**
Sierra Club Books
85 2nd Street
Floor 2
San Francisco, CA 94105
415-977-5500
FAX: 415-977-5799
www.sierraclub.org

Joan Hamilton, Editor In Chief
Martha Geering, Art Director
Carl Pope, Manager
Includes practical information on planning safe trips to 50 national parks that are designated as best visits for their accessibility. *$16.00*
432 pages
ISBN 0-87156 -20-6

5313 **General Motors Mobility Program for Persons with Disabilities**
GM Mobility Program
PO Box 33170
Detroit, MI 48232
313-665-0746
800-323-9935
www.gm.com

Richard Wagoner, CEO And President
Frederick Henderson, Vice Chairman
GM Mobility Program provides up to $1000 reimbursement toward mobility adaptations for drivers or passengers and/or vehicle alerting devices for drivers who are deaf or hard of hearing. Provided on eligible new Chevrolet, Pontiac, Oldsmobile, Buick, Cadillac, and GMC vehicles. Complete GMC financing available. GM Mobility also offers free resource information, including list of area adaptive equipment installers, plus free resource video.

5314 Kenny Foundation
21700 Northwestern Highway
Suite 730
Southfield, MI 48075
248-552-0202
800-237-3422
FAX: 248-552-0275
e-mail: comnet@uwcs.org
www.comnet.org/kenny

Susan Burstein, Executive Director
Provides education, advocacy & direct services to people with mobility impairments throughout Michigan. Services include Equipment Connection, a database, available online, that connects buyers & sellers of used adaptive equipment; Attitudes is a disability awareness program for 1st & 2nd graders; Information & Referral services; and Accessbility, a program that uses volunteer labor and donated materials to buid ramps for people who can't afford them.

5315 MedEscort International
PO Box 8766
Allentown, PA 18105
610-791-3111
800-255-7182
FAX: 610-791-9189
e-mail: medescort@fast.net
www.medescort.com

David M Stein, Medical Director
Sherrye L Sefcik, Senior Flight Nurse
Craig Poliner, President
MedEscort International was founded over a decade ago with these basic principles and philosophies as its foundation. MedEscort has served the health care community, throughout the world, and has strived to perfect the techniques of moving patients from one place to another. Our medical staff includes registered nurses, respiratory therapists, paramedics, and physicians. MedEscort has developed comprehensive, individual aeromedical services to meet each patient's needs with a personal touch.

5316 Melwood Access Adventures
9035 Ironsides Road
Nanjemoy, MD 20662
301-870-3226
FAX: 301-870-2620
e-mail: accessadventures@melwood.com
www.melwood.com

Earl Copus, CEO and President
Jane Greenweem, Program Manager
Heidi Aldous, Manager
A year round recreation facility that serves mentally and physically disabled individuals, offers a variety of vacations, outdoor recreation, travel and respite care.

5317 Nantahala Outdoor Center
13077 Highway 19 West
Bryson City, NC 28713
828-488-2176
888-905-7238
FAX: 828-488-2498
e-mail: rafting@noc.com
www.noc.com

Cathy Kennedy, Director
Payson Kennedy, Chief Executive Officer
Nantahala Outdoor Center, the leader in outdoor recreation and education for more than 30 years, strongly encourages and supports participants with disabilities. We offer whitewater rafting adventures on six rivers in the Southeast for all skill and thrill levels for groups, also kayak and canoe adaptive instruction. NOC will tailor a whitewater program to your skill and ability level, modify the gear, and pace instruction for you. We also offer a Ropes Challenge Course and team building program

5318 Open Road
102 Brook Lane
Boulder Creek, CA 95006
510-222-6662
FAX: 831-338-3210

Staff, author
Teresa Tucker, Manager
Arts, Music, Sports, and Field Trips for disabled individuals.

2 pages Monthly

5319 Paralysis Society of America
Paralyzed Veterans Of America
801 18th Street NW
Washington, DC 20006
202-872-1300
888-772-1711
FAX: 202-973-8421
TTY: 202-973-8422
e-mail: info@psa.org
www.pva.org/psa

Randy Pleza, President
Trish Armstrong, Membership Coordinator
Joan Winkler, Manager
A national organization whose members are people with spinal cord injury or disease, their family members and caregivers, health-care professionals, and others with an interest in the disciplines of spinal cord medicine and paralsis. One year membership includes NewsWheels, a quarterly newsletter. *$10.00*

5320 Respiratory Health Association
301 Sicomac Avenue
Wyckoff, NJ 07481
201-447-8508

Edward Duffie, President
Offers eight-day cruises for people with respiratory conditions to Bermuda and Alaska at least twice a year.

5321 Shilo Inns & Resorts
11600 SW Shilo Lane
Portland, OR 97225
503-641-6565
800-222-2244
FAX: 503-644-0868
www.shiloinns.com

Mark Hemstreet, President
Ivan McAffee, Director
John Kneeland, Chief Executive Officer
Shilo Inns offers affordable excellence with special assist rooms at many of our locations throughout the western United States. These rooms include larger sized bathrooms equipped with assistance railings and wheelchair access. Special assist dogs are welcome free of charge ar most Shilo Inns. Call 1-800-222-2244 for details or make reservations or check out www.shiloinns.com

5322 Special Assistance Services (SAS)
3 High Street
Helmetta, NJ 08828
FAX: 732-521-9333

James J Muzikowski, President
Steve Rosenel, Assistant Travel Coordinator
The mission of this organization is to empower the quest to travel. They supply this by offering flexible plans and personal assistance. S.A.S. is dedicated to providing various types of assistance to persons with disabilities. The organization serves guests with a variety of special needs, including but not limited to persons with visual and hearing impairments, physical and development disabilities, and the mentally challenged.

5323 Travelers Aid Society
1612 K Street NW
Washington, DC 20006
202-546-1127
FAX: 202-546-9112
e-mail: tadcmichael@aol.com
www.travelersaid.org/ta

Ray Flint, President
Provides crisis intervention and casework services, limited financial assistance, protective travel assistance and information and referrals for travelers, transients and newcomers.

5324 US Servas
1125 16th Street
Suite 201
Arcata, CA 95521
707-825-1714
FAX: 707-825-1762
e-mail: info@usservas.org
www.usservas.org

Julie Schumacher, Program Director
Gilbert Sherr, Manager
Grant Barnes, Board Chair
International network that links travelers with hosts in 130+ countries with the hope of building world peace through understanding and friendship.
Quarterly

5325 **Westin Hotels and Resorts**
1111 Westchester Avenue
White Plains, NY 10604
914-640-8100
FAX: 512-835-4417
www.starwoodhotels.com
Westin Hotels include special parking stalls, wheelchair ramps, wide doors, wheelchairs, braille elevator buttons, recreational facilities for people with disabilities, restaurants and restrooms.

5326 **Wheelers Accessible Van Rentals**
Corporate Office
6614 W Sweetwater Avenue
Glendale, AZ 85304
623-776-8830
800-931-5731
FAX: 623-412-9920
e-mail: info@WheelersVanRentals.com
www.WheelersVanRentals.com
Rental wheelchairs and scooter accessible vans. Technically advanced engineering features bring a world of independence to the user. Locations throughout the U.S. call 800-456-1371 to make reservations at any of our locations nationwide.

5327 **Wilderness Inquiry**
808 14th Avenue SE
Minneapolis, MN 55414
612-676-9400
800-728-0179
FAX: 612-676-9401
TTY: 612-676-9475
e-mail: info@wildernessinquiry.org
www.wildernessinquiry.org

Greg Lais, Executive Director
Steph Schmit, Administration Director
Andy Walz, Program & Technology Director
Allows people of all ages and abilities to share the adventure of wilderness travel. This nonprofit organization was formed in 1978 and conducts tours to some of the most beautiful and remote parts of the world.

Tours

5328 **Accessible Journeys**
35 W Sellers Avenue
Ridley Park, PA 19078
610-521-0339
800-846-4537
FAX: 610-521-6959
e-mail: sales@disabilitytravel.com
www.disabilitytravel.com

Henry Thoreau, President
Howard Coy, Owner
Tour operator for slow walker and wheelchair travelers their families and their friends offering tours to culturally intriguing destinations like Europe, Canada, Alaksa, Great Britain and Hawaii.

5329 **Accesstotheplanet**
Accessible Journeys
35 W Sellers Avenue
Ridley Park, PA 19078
610-521-0339
800-846-4537
FAX: 610-521-6959
e-mail: sales@disabilitytravel.com
www.disabilitytravel.com

Howard Coy, Owner
Kathy Pagliei, Vice President Cruise Operations
Monthly

5330 **Anglo California Travel Service**
4250 Williams Road
San Jose, CA 95129
408-257-2257
FAX: 408-257-2664
www.webtravel.com

Audrey Cooper, President
Plans for one and two week accessible tours.

5331 **Bill Dvorak, Kayak and Rafting Expeditions**
17921 Us Highway 285
Nathrop, CO 81236
719-539-6851
800-824-3795
FAX: 719-539-3378
e-mail: dvorakex@amigo.net
www.dvorakexpeditions.com

Bill Dvorak, President
Jaci Dvorak, Vice President
This organization does river trips for people who are deaf, visually impaired, physically or mentally disabled. Rafting trips with groups and families and whitewater instruction.

5332 **Cunard Line**
6100 Blue Lagoon Drive
Miami, FL 33126
305-463-3000
800-528-6273
FAX: 305-463-3010
www.cunard.co.uk

Debbie Nathanshoan, President
Cunard Line, one of the world's most recognized brand names with a classic British heritage, operated by Cunard Line Limited, has provided the ultimate in deluxe ocean travel experience for the past 158 years. The fleet consists of famed liner Queen Elizabeth 2 and the Caronia, a classic ship formerly identified as Vistafjord. The Cunard Line brand, the epitome of British essence, focuses on recalling the golden age of sea travel for those who missed the first.

5333 **Dell Rapids Sportsmens Club**
PO Box 126
Dell Rapids, SD 57022
605-428-5501
FAX: 605-428-5502
e-mail: ezhealth@sd.cybernex.net
www.rodandgunclub.com

Dan Anderson, Chief Executive Officer

5334 **Diabetic Cruise Desk**
Hartford Holiday Travel
129 Hillside Avenue
PO Box 536
Williston Park, NY 11596
516-746-6670
800-828-4813
FAX: 516-746-6690
e-mail: info@hartfordholidays.com
www.hartfordholidays.com

Les Kertes, President
Offers a seven-day cruise to Alaska for people with diabetes. Includes seminars on diabetes, self management, planning, special guidance for exercise classes and individual dietary advice.

5335 **Dialysis at Sea Cruises**
2504 Merchant Drive
Odessa, FL 33556
813-775-4040
800-544-7604
FAX: 727-372-7396
www.dialysisatsea.com

Steve Debroux, President
Been in the business of providing travel opportunities for persons on hemodialysis and CAPD since 1977. Handle all aspects of their travel and medical requirements. Not Sold Through Travel Agents! Make all reservations and coordinates the total set-up and operation of an onboard ship mobile dialysis clinic. Cruises run from seven days to three weeks and have departures from cities around the world on a variety of cruise lines.

5336 Directions Unlimited Acccessible Tours
Empress Travel
123 Green Lane
Bedford Hills, NY 10507
914-241-1700
800-533-5343
FAX: 914-241-0243

Lois Bonanni, Director
Charles Digiacomo, Manager
Arrange vacations throughout the world for all disabilities including accessible cruises, African safari, rafting and scuba diving, European and Caribbean vacations.

5337 Environmental Traveling Companions
Fort Mason Center
San Francisco, CA 94123
415-474-7662
FAX: 415-474-3919
e-mail: info@etctrips.org
www.etctrips.org

Diane Poslosky, Executive Director
Davido Crow, River Program Manager
Greg Milano, Sea Kayak Program Manager
Aids travelers regardless of physical or financial limitations to experience the beauty and challenge of the wilderness.

5338 Flying Wheels Travel
143 W Bridge Street
PO Box 382
Owatonna, MN 55060
507-451-5005
FAX: 507-451-1685
e-mail: bjacobson@ll.net
www.flyingwheelstravel.com

Barbara Jacobson, President
Arranges worldwide custom independent travel and cruises for the physically challenged.

5339 Golden Eagle Passport
U S Department of the Interior, National Park Serv
1849 C Street NW
Washington, DC 20240
202-208-5815
FAX: 202-208-6956
e-mail: webteam@ios.doi.gov
www.nps.gov

Fran P Mainella, Director
John Sherrod, Executive Director
A free lifetime passport to federally operated parks, monuments, historic sites, recreation areas and wildlife refuges for persons who are blind or permanently disabled.

5340 Guide Service of Washington
733 15th Street NW
Washington, DC 20005
202-628-2842
FAX: 202-638-2812

Neil Amrine, President
A guide service offering tours of Washington DC and vicinity.

5341 Guided Tour for Persons 17 & Over with Developmental and Physical Challenges
7900 Old York Road
Suite 111b
Elkins Park, PA 19027
215-782-1370
800-783-5841
FAX: 215-635-2637
e-mail: gtour400@aol.com
www.guidedtour.com

Irwin Segal DCSW/LSW, Director/Owner
Ari Segal MSW/LSW, Assistant Director
Offers unique travel and vacation programs for individuals with mild to moderate developmental disabilities. We publish a free Rates & Dates brochure twice a year.

5342 Hostelling North America Hostelling International: American Youth Hostels
8401 Colesville Road
Suite 600
Silver Spring, MD 20910
301-495-1240
FAX: 301-495-6697
e-mail: hostels@hiusa.org
www.hiayh.org

Demetria Trent, Executive Director
Hostels are very inexpensive accommodations for travelers of all ages. They provide dorm-style sleeping rooms with separate quarters for males and females, fully equipped self-service kitchens, dining areas and common rooms for relaxing and socializing. HI-AYH has hostels in major cities, in national and state parks, near beaches and in the mountains. Send for a copy of Hostelling North America, a directory of hostels in U.S. and Canada, which lists hostels that are handicap accessible. *$ 3.00*
400 pages Yearly

5343 New Courier Travel
532 Duane Street
Glen Ellyn, IL 60137
630-469-0511
FAX: 630-469-7390

Janice Perkins, Travel Consultant
Ford Mueller, Owner
Offers specialized assistance for independent travel or tours for persons with disabilities including cruises and travel in the USA and abroad. Fee charged for out-of-state clients, long-distance calls and clients who have free air.

5344 New Directions Travel
5276 Hollister Avenue
Suite 207
Santa Barbara, CA 93111
805-967-2841
888-967-2841
FAX: 805-964-7344
e-mail: info@newdirectionstravel.com
www.newdirectionstravel.com

Dee Duncan, Executive Director
David McKeand, Program Director
Jeanne Mohle, Sr Program Manager
A non-profit organization providing high quality local, national, and international travel vacations and holiday programs for people with mild to moderate developmental disabilities. Each year New Directions serves over 600 teenagers, adults and seniors who have brain impairments such as mild to moderate developmental disabilities, mental retardation, cerebral palsy , Down Syndrome and autism.

5345 Norwegian Cruise Line
7665 NW 19th Street
Miami, FL 33126
305-436-4000
FAX: 305-436-4117
www.ncl.com

Colin Veitch, President/CEO
Has accessible cabins but urges mobility impaired passengers to travel in the same cabin with a person who is not mobility impaired. Cruise fares vary.

5346 People and Places
3909 Genesee Street
Cheektowaga, NY 14225
585-937-1813

Joie Budington, Director
Patty Brown Schieder, Assistant Director
Nonprofit organization that provides escorted small group vacation opportunities and outdoor experiences throughout the world for persons with developmental disabilities. Brochure available.

5347 ROW Adventures
314 East Garden Avenue
Coeur D Alene, ID 83814
208-667-1835
800-451-6034
FAX: 208-667-6506
e-mail: info@rowadventures.com
www.rowadventures.com

Peter Grubb, Founder

Offers one to six day rafting trips to physically disadvantaged people. Designs custom itineraries, or trips with a special focus for small groups. For those with special dietary needs, they prepare special meals. So come ride the rapids and enjoy life. They also offer canoe trips aboard 34' voyager canoes along the trail of Lewis and Clark on Montana's upper Missouri River. Free brochure upon request.

5348 **River Odysseys West: ROW**
PO Box 579
Coeur D Alene, ID 83816
208-667-1835

5349 **Sundial Special Vacations**
Sundial Special Vacations
2609 Highway 101 N
Suite 103
Seaside, OR 97138
503-738-3324
800-547-9198
FAX: 503-738-3369
e-mail: ssv@sundial-travel.com
www.sundialtour.com

Bruce Conner, Tour Operations Director/Owner
Patsy Conner, Owner
Cathy Louden, Director of Operations
Provides special vacations for developmentally disabled persons. Provides quality vacations for persons with developmental disabilities. Ratio is 1 for 7 or 1 for 5 depending on tour. Only two people to a room. Exciting destinations. 3 to 4 star properties. Great fun.

5350 **Ventures Travel**
10509 108th Street NW
Annandale, MN 55302
952-852-0101
866-692-7400
FAX: 952-852-0123
e-mail: vt@venturestravel.org
www.venturestravel.org
Ventures Travel a limited liability company is a service of Friendship Ventures-a nonprofit organization that has been enriching the lives of people with mental retardation and related developmental disabilities since 1985. Contact us to learn about our other programs, employment information, volunteer openings or donor opportunities.

5351 **Wheelchair Getaways**
4307 Crittenden Drive
Louisville, KY 40209
502-363-4646
800-458-1115
FAX: 502-363-9756
e-mail: sue@superiorvan.com
www.wheelchairgetaways.com

Rebecca Heim, Manager
Wheelchair Getaways, the largest wheelchair/scooter accessible van rental company in the US, has 50 franchise locations serving major cities and airports throughout the continental US and Hawaii. Rentals by the day, week, month or longer. Delivery/pickup available.

Vehicle Rentals

5352 **ABC Union, ACE, ANLV, Vegas Western Cab**
5010 S Valley View Boulevard
Las Vegas, NV 89118
702-736-8444
FAX: 702-736-5197

George Rodriguez, Manager
Charles Frias, President
Taxi service in Las Vegas that uses vans with wheelchair lifts at regular taxi rates.

5353 **Avis Rent-A-Car**
6 Sylvan Way
Suite 1
Parsippany, NJ 07054
973-496-3500
800-230-4898
FAX: 800-331-2323
www.avis.com

F Salerno, Chief Executive Officer
Requires 24-hour notice for hand control vehicles, available in any location across the US.

5354 **CEH**
4457 63rd Circle
Pinellas Park, FL 33781
727-522-0364
800-677-0364
FAX: 727-522-9024
www.liftsandramps.com

Phillip G Faas, President/Owner
New vans, used vans, rental vans; specializing in quad conversions, all types of handicap equipment. Celebrating 28 years in business.

5355 **Mobile Care**
6201 Riverdale Road
Suite 101
Riverdale, MD 20737
301-649-0564
FAX: 301-699-1865
e-mail: jaklimo@aol.com

Jeffery A Koch, President
Specializing in non-emergency wheelchair service for the elderly and physically challenged.

5356 **National Car Rental System**
600 Terminal Drive
Suite 202
Fort Lauderdale, FL 33315
954-359-8303
FAX: 954-359-8313
www.nationalcar.com

William Decker, Manager
Accommodates special requests subject to availability. Offers hand controls, bench seats, extra mirrors and vans with lifts at many major locations.

5357 **Northwest Limousine Service**
9950 Lawrence Avenue
Schiller Park, IL 60176
847-671-5482
800-376-5466
FAX: 847-671-5482
e-mail: chiohare@aol.com

Kathleen Maloney, Manager
Offers wheelchair accessible mini vans, sedans, stretch and super stretch limousines for hourly or daily rental.

5358 **Over the Rainbow Disabled Travel Services & Wheelers Accessible Van Rentals**
186 Mehani Circle
Kihei, HI 96753
808-879-5521
800-303-3750
FAX: 808-871-7533

David McKown, Vice President
Offers the disabled traveler Hawaii airport arrangements and ticketing accessible accommodations, hotels and condos including roll-in showers, Wheelers' Accessible Van Rentals on Maui and Honolulu or cars with hand controls, personal care attendants, medical or recreational equipment rentals and activities such as: helicopter rides, luau's, whalewatching, boating and more. Airfare varies from departure points and time of the year.

5359 **Public Technology**
US Department of Transportation
Urban Mass Transportation Adm
Washington, DC 20016
202-366-4000

J Rutter, Chief Executive Officer
One of a series of reports concerned with improving transportation for elderly and disabled persons.

28 pages

5360 Rehabiliation Engineering Center for Personal Licensed Transportation

University Of Virginia School Of Engineering
PO Box 400246
Charlottesville, VA 22904 434-924-3072

Tom Connors, Vice President
Mitch Rosen, Director

5361 Wheelchair Getaways Wheelchair/Scooter Accessible Van Rentals

4307 Crittenden Drive
Louisville, KY 40209 502-363-4646
800-458-1115
FAX: 502-363-9756
e-mail: corporate@wheelchairgetaways.com
www.wheelchairgetaways.com

Richard Gatewood, Owner
Moon Ko, Owner
Rebecca Heim, Manager

Rents wheelchair/scooter accessible vans by the day, week, month or longer and offers delivery to major airports and other convenient locations in more than 200 cities in 42 states and Puerto Rico. Also offers full size and mini vans with automatic lifts and ramps. Some vans are equipped with hand controls, six-way power seats and remote controls for powered door operation and lifts.

5362 Wheelers

7101 N 55th Avenue
Glendale, AZ 85301
800-456-1371
FAX: 623-435-9989

Offers delivery to airports in 29 states and Washington, D.C. In about 40 cities, Wheelers works directly with Avis Rent-a-Car. Wheelers offers a variety of van configurations with capacity for up to three wheelchairs, automatic ramps or lifts and nylon tie-downs, hand controls or other modifications.

5363 Wheelers Accessible Van Rentals

6614 W Sweetwater Avenue
Glendale, AZ 85304
800-456-1371
FAX: 623-435-1518
e-mail: info@wheelersvanrentals.com
www.wheelersvanrentals.com

Tammy Smith, President
Ron Smith, Corporate Treasurer

National Administrations

5364 DAV National Service Headquarters
807 Maine Avenue SW
Washington, DC 20024 202-554-3501

e-mail: feedback@davmail.org
www.dav.org

Arthur H Wilson, National Adjutant
David W Gorman, Executive Director
Serves America's disabled veterans and their families. Direct services include legislative advocacy; professional counseling about compensation, pension, educational and job training programs and VA health care; and assistance in applying for those entitlements.

5365 Department of Medicine and Surgery Veterans Administration
810 Vermont Avenue NW
Washington, DC 20420 202-273-8504
FAX: 202-273-9108

Gerald McDonald MD, Senior Consultant
Provides hospital and outpatient treatment as well as nursing home care for eligible veterans in Veterans Administration facilities. Services elsewhere provided on a contract basis in the United States and its territories. Provides non-vocational inpatient residential rehabilitation services to eligible legally blinded veterans of the armed forces of the United States.

5366 Department of Veterans Affairs Regional Office - Vocational Rehab Division
380 Westminster Street
Providence, RI 02903 401-222-2488
800-827-1000
FAX: 401-254-3220
e-mail: dhs.state.ri.us/dhs/dvetsff.htm
www.va.gov

Gerald E Allen, Counseling Officer
Vocational rehabilitation is a program of services administered by the Department of Veterans Affairs for service members and veterans with service-connected physical or mental disabilities. If persons are compensibly disabled and are found in need of rehabilitation services because they have an employment handicap, this program can prepare them for a suitable job; get and keep that job; assist persons to become fully productive and independent.

5367 Department of Veterans Benefits
810 Vermont Avenue NW
Washington, DC 20420 202-273-6763
800-827-1000
www.va.gov

Raymond Vogel, Chief Benefits
Joseph Thompson, Manager
Furnishes compensation and pensions for disability and death to veterans and their dependents. Provides vocational rehabilitation services, including counseling, training, assistance and more towards employment, to blinded veterans disabled as a result of service in the armed forces during World War II, Korea and the Vietnam era; also provides rehabilitation services to certain peace-time veterans.

5368 Disabled American Veterans
PO Box 14301
Cincinnati, OH 45250 859-441-7300
FAX: 859-441-1416
www.dav.org

James E Sursely, National Commander
Advises veterans of their rights and employers of their obligations, under the Rehabilitation Act, the Americans with Disabilities Act, and legislation governing the employment and training of Vietnam era veterans with disabilities.

5369 Federal Benefits for Veterans and Dependents
Government Printing Office
810 Vermont Ave. NW
Washington, DC 20402 202-512-1067
800-827-1000
http://www1.va.gov/opa/vadocs/fedben.pdf

Bill Lewis, President
Offers information on benefits for veterans and their families.
93 pages
ISBN 0-16048 -58-

5370 Hospitalized Veterans Writing Project
5920 Nall Avenue
Room 105
Mission, KS 66202 913-432-1214
FAX: 913-432-1214
http://www.independentcharities.org/

Charlotte Black, Secretary
Priscilla Chansky, Administrator
Individuals and organizations united to encourage hospitalized veterans to write for pleasure and rehabilitation during the hospital stay. Maintains speakers' bureau and audio tape version for the blind. Bestows numerous monetary awards in six areas: article; book review; cartoon and drawing; light verse; poetry and short story. *$ 15.00*
64 pages Magazine
ISSN 0504-07 9

5371 US Department of Veterans Affairs National Headquarters
1120 Vermont Avenue NW
Washington, DC 20420 202-273-5400
800-827-1000
e-mail: washingtondc.query@vba.va.gov
www.va.gov

Togo D West Jr, Secretary Veterans Affairs
Hershel W Gober, Deputy Secretary Vet. Affairs
R Nicholson, Chief Executive Officer
Administers the laws providing benefits and other services to veterans, their dependents, and their beneficiaries. Acts as their principal advocate in ensuring that they recieve medical care, benefits, social support, and lasting memorials promoting the health, welfare, and dignity of all veterans in recognition of their service to this nation. As the DVA heads into the 21st century, they will strive to meet the needs of the Nation's veterans today and tomorrow. Publishes a monthly magazine.
80 pages

5372 US Veteran's Affairs
810 Vermont Avenue NW
Washington, DC 20420 202-273-5400

www.va.gov

Michael J Kussman, Deputy Under Secretary For Healt
Provides a wide range of services for those who have been in the military and their dependents, as well as offering information on driver assessment and education programs.

Alabama

5373 Alabama VA Regional Office
Veterans Benefits Administration, U S Dept. of V A
345 Perry Hill Road
Montgomery, AL 36109
800-827-1000
FAX: 334-213-3461
e-mail: montgomery.query@vba.va.gov
www.va.gov

Joe Morris, Val Representative
William Rumph, Val Representative

5374 Alabama Veterans Facility
809 Green Springs Highway
Homewood, AL 35209 205-916-2700

Robert Herndon, Manager
Veterans medical clinic offering disabled veterans medical treatments.

5375 **Birmingham VA Medical Center**
Veterans Health Administration U S Dept. of V A
700 19th Street S
Birmingham, AL 35233
205-933-8101
800-827-1000
e-mail: g.vhacss@forum.va.gov
www.va.gov

Amos F Bailey, Director of Palliative Care

5376 **Central Alabama Veterans Healthcare System**
Veterans Health Administration, US Dept. of VA
215 Perry Hill Road
Montgomery, AL 36109
334-272-4670
800-827-1000
e-mail: g.vhacss@forum.va.gov
www.va.gov

Kenneth Ruyle, Executive Director

5377 **Tuscaloosa VA Medical Center**
Veterans Health Administration, U S Dept. of V A
3701 Loop Road
Tuscaloosa, AL 35404
205-554-2000
FAX: 205-554-2845
www.va.gov

Todd Hooper, Director
John Goldman, Executive Director

Alaska

5378 **Anchorage Regional Office**
Veterans Benefits Administration, U S Dept. of V A
2925 Debarr Road
Anchorage, AK 99508
907-257-4700
800-827-1000
e-mail: anchorage.query@vba.va.gov
www.va.gov

Claude M Kicklighter, Chief Staff
Alex Spector, Executive Director

5379 **DAV Department of Alaska**
2925 Debarr Road
Room 3101
Anchorage, AK 99508
907-257-4803
FAX: 907-258-9828

George Hausermann, Treasurer
Ian Briggs, Manager

Arizona

5380 **Carl T Hayden VA Medical Center**
Veterans Health Administration, U S Dept. of V A
650 E Indian School Road
Phoenix, AZ 85012
602-277-5551
800-827-1000
e-mail: g.vhacss@forum.va.gov
www.va.gov

D Gregg Gordon, President
Marva Greene, Vice President
John Fears, Chief Executive Officer

5381 **Northern Arizona VA Health Center**
Veterans Health Administration, US Dept. of VA
500 N Us Highway 89
Prescott, AZ 86313
928-445-4860
800-827-1000
FAX: 928-768-6076
e-mail: g.vhacss@forum.va.gov
www.va.gov

Deborah Thompson, Manager

5382 **Southern Arizona VA Healthcare System**
Veterans Health Administration, U S Dept. of V A
3601 S 6th Avenue
Tucson, AZ 85723
520-792-1450
800-827-1000
FAX: 520-629-1818
e-mail: g.vhacss@forum.va.gov
www.va.gov

Patrick F Chorpenning, State Director
Jerry Colye, Manager

Arkansas

5383 **Eugene J Towbin Healthcare Center**
Veterans Health Administration, U S Dept. of V A
2200 Fort Roots Drive
North Little Rock, AR 72114
501-396-4444
800-827-1000
e-mail: g.vhacss@forum.va.gov
www.va.gov

5384 **Fayetteville VA Medical Center**
Veterans Health Administration, US Dept. of VA
1100 N College Avenue
Fayetteville, AR 72703
479-444-4301
800-827-1000
e-mail: g.vhacss@forum.va.gov
www.va.gov

5385 **John L McClellan Memorial Hospital**
Veterans Health Administration, US Dept. of VA
4300 W 7th Street
Little Rock, AR 72205
501-257-1000
800-827-1000
e-mail: g.vhacss@forum.va.gov
www.va.gov

5386 **North Little Rock Regional Office**
Veterans Benefits Administration, U S Dept. of V A
2200 Fort Roots Drive
Building 65
N Little Rock, AR 72114
501-370-3820
800-827-1000
FAX: 501-370-3829
e-mail: littlerock.query@vba.va.gov
www.va.gov

David Fletcher, Director
Doyle Batey, Deputy Director

California

5387 **Jerry L Pettis Memorial VA Medical Center**
Veterans Health Administration, U S Dept. of V A
11201 Benton Street
Loma Linda, CA 92357
909-825-7084
800-741-8387
e-mail: g.vhacss@forum.va.gov
www.lom.med.va.gov

Kevin Dahl, Director
Dean Stordahl, President

5388 **Long Beach VA Medical Center**
Veterans Health Administration, U S Dept. of V A
5901 E 7th Street
Long Beach, CA 90822
562-597-3592
800-827-1000
e-mail: g.vhacss@forum.va.gov
www.va.gov

Stephen Davis, Director
Eric Yamaura, Director
Melinda Pettersen, Executive Director

5389 **Los Angeles Regional Office**
Veterans Benefits Administration, U S Dept. of V A
11000 Wilshire Boulevard
Los Angeles, CA 90024
800-827-1000
e-mail: losangeles.query@vba.va.gov
www.va.gov

Karl Lorenz, Work Group Leader

5390 **Martinez Center for Rehab & Extended Care**
Veterans Health Administration, U S Dept. of V A
150 Muir Road
Martinez, CA 94553
925-372-2665
800-827-1000
e-mail: g.vhacss@forum.va.gov
www.va.gov

John H Simms, Director

5391 **Oakland VA Regional Office**
Veterans Benefits Administration U S Dept. of V A
1301 Clay Street
Room 1300
Oakland, CA 94612
800-827-1000
e-mail: oakland.query@vba.va.gov
www.va.gov

Geri Spearman, Director

5392 **Rehabilitation Research and Development Center**
Department of Veteran s Affairs
3801 Miranda Avenue
Palo Alto, CA 94304
650-493-5000
FAX: 650-493-4919
e-mail: jaffe@roses.stanford.edu
guide.stanford.edu

Loretta V Barrow, Administrator
Louis Fajardo, MD
David L Jaffe MS, Research Biomedical Engineer
The VA Center of Excellence on Mobility in Palo Alto, CA is dedicated to developing innovative clinical treatments and assistive devices for veterans with physical disabilities to increase their independence and improve their quality of life. The clinical emphasis of the center is to improve mobility, either ambulation or manipulation, in individuals with neurologic impairments or orthopaedic impairments. We do not publish any printed books, journals or periodicals.

5393 **Sacramento Medical Center**
Veterans Health Administration U S Department of V
10535 Hospital Way
Mather, CA 95655
916-366-5470
800-827-1000
e-mail: g.vhacss@forum.va.gov
www.va.gov

Gail Crimmins-Wiggins, Director

5394 **San Diego VA Regional Office**
Veterans Benefits Administration, U S Dept. of V A
8810 Rio San Diego Drive
San Diego, CA 92108
858-552-8585
800-827-1000
FAX: 858-552-7436
e-mail: oakland.query@vba.va.gov
www.va.gov

Janet M Peyton, Administrative Officer

5395 **San Francisco VA Medical Center**
Veterans Health Administration, US Dept. of VA
4150 Clement Street
San Francisco, CA 94121
415-221-4810
877-487-2838
FAX: 415-750-2185
www.sf.med.va.gov

Gene Gibson, Public Affairs Officer
Sheila Cullen, Executive Director
The San Francisco VA Medical Center (SFVAMC) serves as a major tertiary care referral center for veterans throughout Northern California. The facility has 124 acute care hospital beds. It is a high acuity medical center with over a third of bed days of care being in intensive care or monitored beds. Long term care programs include a 120 bed nursing home care unit at the San Francisco site and a home-based primary care program.

5396 **VA Central California Health Care Syste**
Veterans Health Administration, U S Dept. of V A
2615 E Clinton Avenue
Fresno, CA 93703
559-225-6100
888-826-2838
FAX: 559-268-6911
e-mail: g.vhacss@forum.va.gov
www.va.gov

Ellen Perry, Director
Susan Shyshka, Associate Director
Alan Perry, Executive Director

5397 **VA Greater Los Angeles Healthcare System**
Veterans Health Administration U S Deptartment of
11301 Wilshire Boulevard
Los Angeles, CA 90073
310-478-3711
800-827-1000
FAX: 310-268-4848
e-mail: g.vhacss@forum.va.gov
www.va.gov

Charles Dorman, Chief Executive Officer

5398 **VA Northern California Healthcare System**
Veterans Health Administration, U S Dept. of V A
150 Muir Road
Martinez, CA 94553
925-372-2000
800-827-1000
e-mail: g.vhacss@forum.va.gov
www.va.gov

Lawrence Sander, Director

5399 **VA San Diego Healthcare System**
Veterans Health Administration, U S Dept. of V A
3350 La Jolla Village Drive
San Diego, CA 92161
858-552-8585
800-827-1000
e-mail: g.vhacss@forum.va.gov
www.va.gov

James R Nicholson, Secretary Veterans Affairs
Claude M Kicklighter, Chief of Staff

Colorado

5400 **Boulder Vet Center**
2336 Canyon Boulevard
Suite 103
Boulder, CO 80302
303-440-7306
FAX: 303-449-3907

Stew Brown PhD, Team Leader
Offers trauma and readjustment from military and civilian life counseling and assistance with disability claims, military benefits and employment are provided.

5401 **Colorado/Wyoming VA Medical Center**
Veterans Benefits Administration U S Dept. of V A
155 Van Gordon Street
Lakewood, CO 80228
800-827-1000
e-mail: denver.query@vba.va.gov
www.va.gov

Forest Farley Jr, Medical Center Director
Thomas E Bowen, Chief of Staff

5402 **Denver VA Medical Center**
Veterans Health Administration, U S Dept. of V A
1055 Clermont Street
Denver, CO 80220
303-399-8020
800-827-1000
e-mail: g.vhacss@forum.va.gov
www.va.gov

Lisa A Brenner, Training Director

5403 **Grand Junction VA Medical Center**
Veterans Health Administration, U S Dept. of V A
2121 North Avenue
Grand Junction, CO 81501
970-242-0731
800-827-1000
FAX: 970-244-1300
e-mail: g.vhacss@forum.va.gov
www.va.gov

Claude M Kicklighter, Chief of Staff
Michael Murphy, Manager

Connecticut

5404 **Hartford Regional Office**
Veterans Benefits Administration U S Department of
555 Willard Avenue
Newington, CT 06111
800-827-1000
e-mail: hartford.query@vba.va.gov
www.va.gov

Jeanette A Chirico Post, Network Director

5405 **Hartford Vet Center**
30 Jordan Lane
Wethersfield, CT 06109
860-240-3543
FAX: 860-563-7246
e-mail: donna.hryb@med.va.gov

Donna Hryb LCSW, Team Leader
Urania Petit BA, Office Manager
A U.S. Department of Veterans Affairs counseling center offering counseling to Vietnam era and combat veterans. Sexual trauma/harassment counseling, medical screening and benefit referral is available to all veterans.

5406 **VA Connecticut Healthcare System: Newington Division**
Veterans Health Administration U S Department. of
555 Willard Avenue
Newington, CT 06111
860-666-6951
800-827-1000
FAX: 860-667-6764
e-mail: g.vhacss@forum.va.gov
www.va.gov

Vincent Ng, Providence Director
The mission of VA Connecticut Healthcare Systems is to fulfill a nation's commitment to its veterans by providing quality healthcare, promoting health through prevention and maintaining excellence in teaching and research. Provides primary, secondary and tertiary care in medicine, geriatrics, neurology, psychiatry and surgery with an operating capacity of 211 hospital beds.

5407 **VA Connecticut Healthcare System: West Haven**
Veterans Health Administration, U S Dept. of V A
950 Campbell Avenue
W Haven, CT 06516
203-932-5711
FAX: 203-937-3868
e-mail: g.vhacss@forum.va.gov
www.va.gov

R James Nicholson, Secretary Veteran Affairs
Claude Kicklighter, Chief of Staff
Roger Johnson, Administrator

Delaware

5408 **Delaware VA Regional Office**
Veterans Benefits Administration U S Dept. of V A
1601 Kirkwood Highway
Wilmington, DE 19805
302-994-2511
800-827-1000
e-mail: wilmington.query@vba.va.gov
www.va.gov

Martin F Konwinski, Research/Development Coordinator
Dexter Dix, Executive Director

5409 **Wilmington VA Medical**
Veterans Health Administration, US Dept. of VA
1601 Kirkwood Highway
Wilmington, DE 19805
302-994-2511
800-827-1000
FAX: 302-633-5516
e-mail: g.vhacss@forum.va.gov
www.va.gov

Dexter Dix, Executive Director

5410 **Wilmington Vet Center**
1601 Kirkwood Highway
Building 3
Wilmington, DE 19805
302-994-1660
866-442-4106
FAX: 302-633-5250

Mark A Kaufki EdD, Team Leader
Veterans counseling program offering individual counseling services, advocacy services and group counseling. The focus is the counseling of all veterans coping with the aftermath of war, sexual abuse/harassment in the military and all veterans of the Vietnam era. The center also has an active outreach program to seek veterans needing services. Hours of operation are between 8:00 AM - 4:30 PM, Monday - Friday and other times by appointment only. Services are free.

District of Columbia

5411 **Disabled American Veterans, National Service & Legislative Headquarters**
807 Maine Avenue SW
Washington, DC 20024
202-554-3501
www.dav.org

Alan W Bowers, Chairman
Paul W Jackson, Vice Chairman

5412 **PVA Sports and Recreation Program**
Paralyzed Veterans of America
801 18th Street NW
Washington, DC 20006
202-872-1300
800-424-8200
FAX: 202-416-7639
e-mail: info@pva.org
www.pva.org

Andy Krieger, Director Sports/Recreation
Randy Pleza, President

5413 **VA Medical Center, Washington DC**
50 Irving Street NW
Washington, DC 20422
202-745-8422
888-553-0242
www.washington.med.va.gov

David J West, Associate Medical Center
Ross D Fletcher, Chief of Staff
Acute general and specialized services in medicine, surgery, neurology, and psychiatry.

5414 **Washington DC VA Medical Center**
Veterans Health Administration, U S Dept. of V A
50 Irving Street NW
Washington, DC 20422
202-745-8000
800-827-1000
FAX: 202-754-8530
e-mail: g.vhacss@forum.va.gov
www.va.gov

James R Nicholson, Secretary of Veterans Affairs
Claude M Kicklighter, Chief of Staff
Bina Lakhanpal, MD

Florida

5415 **Bay Pines VA Medical Center**
Veterans Health Administration, U S Dept. of V A
10000 Bay Pines Boulevard
Bay Pines, FL 33744
727-398-6661
800-827-1000
e-mail: g.vhacss@forum.va.gov
www.va.gov

Wallace M Hopkins, Medical Director
Kaye Green, Assistant Medical Director
Smith Jenkins, Chief Executive Officer

5416 **Gainesville Division, North Florida/South Georgia Veterans Healthcare System**
Veterans Health Administration, U S Dept. of V A
1601 SW Archer Road
Room 165a
Gainesville, FL 32608
352-376-1611
800-324-8387
FAX: 352-379-7445
e-mail: g.vhacss@forum.va.gov
www.va.gov

Claude M Kicklighter, Chief of Staff
Frederick Malphurs, Chief Executive Officer

5417 **James A Haley VA Medical Center**
Veterans Health Administration, U S Dept. of V A
13000 Bruce B Downs Boulevard
Tampa, FL 33612
813-972-2000
800-827-1000
e-mail: g.vhacss@forum.va.gov
www.va.gov

James R Nicholson, Secretary of Veterans Affairs
Claude M Kicklighter, Chief of Staff
Edgar Bueno, MD

5418 **Miami VA Medical Center**
Veterans Health Administration, U S Dept. of V A
1201 NW 16th Street
Miami, FL 33125
305-575-7000
800-827-1000
FAX: 305-575-3266
e-mail: g.vhacss@forum.va.gov
www.va.gov

Stephen M Lucas, Chief Executive Officer

5419 **St. Petersburg Regional Office**
Veterans Benefits Administration, U S Dept. of V A
9500 Bay Pines Boulevard
St Petersburg, FL
727-319-7492
800-827-1000
e-mail: stpete.query@vba.va.gov
www.va.gov

Warren McPherson, Executive Director

5420 **West Palm Beach VA Medical Center**
Veterans Health Administration, U S Dept. of V A
7305 N Military Trail
Riviera Beach, FL 33410
561-882-8262
800-827-1000
FAX: 561-882-6707
e-mail: g.vhacss@forum.va.gov
www.va.gov

Claude M Kicklighter, Chief of Staff
Andre Desgroseillers, MD

Georgia

5421 **Atlanta Regional Office**
Veterans Benefits Administration, U S Dept. of V A
730 Peachtree Street NE
Atlanta, GA 30308
800-827-1000
FAX: 606- -
e-mail: atlanta.query@vba.va.gov
www.va.gov

William J Day

5422 **Atlanta VA Medical Center**
Veterans Health Administration, U S Dept. of V A
1670 Clairmont Road
Decatur, GA 30033
404-321-6111
800-827-1000
FAX: 404-728-7734
e-mail: g.vhacss@forum.va.gov
www.va.gov

James R Nicholson, Secretary of Veterans Affairs
Claude M Kicklighter, Chief of Staff
Thomas Cappello, Chief Executive Officer

5423 **Augusta VA Medical Center**
Veterans Health Administration, U S Dept. of V A
1 Freedom Way
Augusta, GA 30904
706-733-0188
800-827-1000
FAX: 706-823-3934
e-mail: g.vhacss@forum.va.gov
www.va.gov

R James Nicholson, Secretary of Veterans Affairs
Claude Kicklighter, Chief of Staff
James Trustley III, Chief Executive Officer

5424 **Carl Vinson VA Medical Center**
Veterans Health Administration, U S Dept. of V A
1826 Veterans Boulevard
Dublin, GA 31021
478-272-1210
FAX: 478-277-2717
e-mail: dana.doles@med.va.gov
www.va.gov

Claude M Kicklighter, Chief of Staff
Richard Fry, Chief Executive Officer

Hawaii

5425 Hawaii Veterans Centers
Hilo Vet Center
126 Pu'uhonu Way, Ste #2
Hilo, HI 96720
808-969-3833
FAX: 808-969-2025
www.va.gov

Felipe Usales, Director
Richard Talbott, RCS4B Regional Manager
Veterans medical clinic offering disabled veterans medical treatments, readjustment and PTSD counseling to combat veterans

5426 Honolulu VBA Regional Office
Veterans Benefits Administration, U S Dept. of V A
300 Ala Moana Boulevard
Room 1004
Honolulu, HI 96850
808-541-2570
800-827-1000
e-mail: honolulu.query@vba.va.gov
www.va.gov

Claude M Kicklighter, Chief of Staff
Alan Furuno, Manager

5427 Pacific Islands Health Care System
Veterans Health Administration, US Dept. of VA
459 Patterson Road
Honolulu, HI 96819
808-433-0600
800-827-1000
FAX: 808-433-0390
e-mail: g.vhacss@forum.va.gov
www.va.gov

Idaho

5428 Boise Regional Office
Veterans Benefits Administration, U S Dept. of V A
805 W Franklin Street
Boise, ID 83702
208-334-1245
800-827-1000
e-mail: boise.query@vba.va.gov
www.va.gov

Jim Vance, Director
Pat Teague, Service Officer
Tom Ressler, Manager

5429 Boise VA Medical Center
Veterans Health Administration, U S Dept. of V A
500 W Fort Street
Boise, ID 83702
208-422-1000
800-827-1000
FAX: 208-422-1326
e-mail: g.vhacss@forum.va.gov
www.va.gov

Claude M Kicklighter, Chief of Staff

Illinois

5430 Edward Hines Jr Hospital
Veterans Health Administration, U S Dept. of V A
Fifth Avenue & Roosevelt Road
Hines, IL 60141
708-202-5691
800-827-1000
FAX: 708-202-2684
e-mail: g.vhacss@forum.va.gov
www.va.gov/sta/guide/facility.asp?ID=58

Nick Guzzi, Administrative Officer

5431 Marion VA Medical Center
Veterans Health Administration U S Department of V
2401 W Main Street
Marion, IL 62959
618-997-5311
800-827-1000
e-mail: g.vhacss@forum.va.gov
www.va.gov

5432 North Chicago VA Medical Center
Veterans Health Administration, U S Dept. of V A
3001 Green Bay Road
North Chicago, IL 60064
847-688-1900
800-827-1000
e-mail: g.vhacss@forum.va.gov
www.va.gov

Claude M Kicklighter, Chief of Staff
John Avramidis, MD

5433 VA Illiana Health Care System
Veterans Health Administration, U S Dept. of V A
1900 E Main Street
Danville, IL 61832
800-827-1000
FAX: 217-554-4552
e-mail: g.vhacss@forum.va.gov
www.va.gov

Betsy Sleath, Chairman

Indiana

5434 Indianapolis Regional Office
Veterans Benefits Administration U S Department of
575 N Pennsylvania Street
Indianapolis, IN 46204
317-226-7860
800-827-1000
e-mail: indianapolis.query@vba.va.gov
www.va.gov

5435 Richard L Roudebush VA Medical Center
Veterans Health Administration, U S Dept. of V A
1481 W 10th Street
Indianapolis, IN 46202
317-554-0000
800-827-1000
FAX: 317-554-0127
e-mail: g.vhacss@forum.va.gov
www.va.gov

Claude M Kicklighter, Chief of Staff
Becky Hall, Manager

5436 VA North Indiana Health Care System: Fort Wayne Campus
Veterans Health Administration, U S Dept. of V A
2121 Lake Avenue
Fort Wayne, IN 46805
260-426-5431
800-827-1000
e-mail: g.vhacss@forum.va.gov
www.va.gov

Michael W Murphy, Director
Cathi Spivey-Paul, Executive Director

5437 VA Northern Indiana Health Care System: Marion Campus
Veterans Health Administration, U S Dept. of V A
1700 E 38th Street
Marion, IN 46953
765-674-3321
800-827-1000
e-mail: g.vhacss@forum.va.gov
www.va.gov

Claude M Kicklighter, Chief of Staff
Cathi Spivey-Paul, Executive Director

Iowa

5438 Des Moines VA Medical Center
Veterans Health Administration, U S Dept. of V A
3600 30th Street
Des Moines, IA 50310
515-699-5850
800-827-1000
FAX: 515-699-5862
e-mail: g.vhacss@forum.va.gov
www.va.gov

Claudia M Kicklighter, Chief of Staff

5439 Des Moines VA Regional Office
Veterans Benefits Administration, U S Dept. of V A
210 Walnut Street
Room 1033a
Des Moines, IA 50309
515-323-7532
800-944-2039
FAX: 515-323-7405
e-mail: leander@vba.va.gov
www.va.gov

Liz Erickson, Director
Rich Anderson, Service Director

5440 Iowa City VA Medical Center
Veterans Health Administration, U S Dept. of V A
601 Highway, 6 West
Iowa City, IA 52246
319-338-0581
800-827-1000
FAX: 319-339-7171
e-mail: g.vhacss@forum.va.gov
www.va.gov

Kirt A Sickels, Public Affairs Officer
Gary Wilkinson, Administrator
Tertiary care facility, affiliated teaching hospital, and research center seving an aging veteran populatiaon in eastern Iowa and western Illinois. Satellite clinics are located in Bettendord, Dubuque, and Waterloo, Iowa and in Quincy and Galesburg, Illinois.

5441 Knoxville VA Medical Center
Veterans Health Administration, U S Dept. of V A
1515 W Pleasant Street
Knoxville, IA 50138
641-828-5000
800-827-1000
FAX: 641-828-5124
e-mail: g.vhacss@forum.va.gov
www.va.gov

Claudia M Kicklighter

5442 VA Central Iowa Health Care System
3600 30th Street
Des Moines, IA 50310
515-699-5999
FAX: 515-699-5862
www.va.gov

Elaine Brewster, Executive Program Manager
Donald Cooper, Executive Director
Fulfilling the promise is our primary mission.

Kansas

5443 Colmery-O'Neil VA Medical Center
Veterans Health Administration, U S Dept. of V A
2200 SW Gage Boulevard
Topeka, KS 66622
785-350-3111
800-827-1000
e-mail: g.vhacss@forum.va.gov
www.va.gov

Jerry L Calhoun, Chairman

5444 Dwight D Eisenhower VA Medical Center
Veterans Health Administration, U S Dept. of V A
4101 S 4th Street
Leavenworth, KS 66048
913-682-2000
800-827-1000
e-mail: g.vhacss@forum.va.gov
www.va.gov

Donald L Courtney, Research/Development Coordinator
Deborah Fulk, Administrative Officer
Arnulfo Sulit, MD

5445 Kansas VA Regional Office
Veterans Benefits Administration, U S Dept. of V A
5500 E Kellogg Drive
Wichita, KS 67218
800-827-1000
e-mail: wichita.query@vba.va.gov
www.va.gov

Edgar L Tucker, Medical Center Director

5446 Robert J Dole VA Medical Center
Veterans Health Administration, U S Dept. of V A
5500 E Kellogg Drive
Wichita, KS 67218
316-685-2221
888-827-6881
FAX: 316-651-3666
e-mail: g.vhacss@forum.va.gov
www.va.gov

Thomas J. Sanders, Exectuve Director
For over 70 years, the Dole VA Medical and Regional office center has been honored to serve Kansas area veterans. The center provides a full range of primary and specialty acute and extended care services to veterans in 59 counties of Kansas. Special emphasis programs include substance abuse, post traumatic stress disorder (PTSD), women's health, spinal cord injury, visual impairment, prosthetic and sensory aids, and homeless services.

Kentucky

5447 Lexington VA Medical Center
Veterans Health Administration, U S Dept. of V A
1101 Veterans Drive
Lexington, KY 40502
859-233-4511
800-352-4000
e-mail: g.vhacss@forum.va.gov
www.va.gov/sta/guide/facility.asp?ID=72

5448 Louisville VA Medical Center
Veterans Health Administration, U S Dept. of V A
800 Zorn Avenue
Louisville, KY 40206
502-287-4000
800-827-1000
FAX: 502-287-6225
e-mail: g.vhacss@forum.va.gov
www.va.gov

Leslie Beavers, Director

5449 Louisville VA Regional Office
Veterans Benefits Administration, U S Dept. of V A
321 West Main Street
Suite 390
Louisville, KY 40202
502-582-5594
800-827-1000
e-mail: louisville.query@vba.va.gov
www.va.gov

Gene Brainer, Regional Officer

Louisiana

5450 Alexandria VA Medical Center
Veterans Health Administration, U S Dept. of V A
2495 Highway 71 N
Alexandria, LA 71301
318-473-0010
800-827-1000
FAX: 318-483-5029
e-mail: g.vhacss@forum.va.gov
www.va.gov

Hollis T. Reed, MD, Chief Of Staff
Barbara Watkins, Medical Director
Karen James, EEO Program Manager

5451 New Orleans VA Medical Center
Veterans Health Administration, U S Dept. of V A
1601 Perdido Street
New Orleans, LA 70112
504-568-0811
800-935-8387
FAX: 504-589-5210
e-mail: Stacie.Rivera@med.va.gov
www.va.gov

John D Church Jr, Medical Director/President
Fernando Rivera, Association Medical Center Direc
Sam Lucero, Special Assistant to Director
A teaching hospital, providing a full range of patient care services, with state-of-the-art technology as well as education and research. Comprehensive health care is provided through primary care, tetiary care, and long-term care in areas of medicine, surgery, psychiatry, physical medicine and rehabilitation, neurology, oncology, dentistry, geriatrics, and extended care.

5452 Shreveport VA Medical Center
Veterans Health Administration, U S Dept. of V A
510 E Stoner Avenue
Shreveport, LA 71101
318-221-8411
800-827-1000
FAX: 318-424-6156
e-mail: g.vhacss@forum.va.gov
www.va.gov

Dorothy Jarzabek, Administrative Officer
Ali R Mansouri, Acting Acos/R&D
Gracie Specks, Chief Executive Officer

Maine

5453 Maine VA Regional Office
Veterans Benefits Administration, U S Dept. of V A
1 Va Center
Augusta, ME 04330
800-827-1000
FAX: 207-623-5737
e-mail: togus.query@vba.va.gov
www.va.gov

Dale Demers, Director
Scott Karczewski, Manager

5454 Togus VA Medical Center
Veterans Health Administration, U S Dept. of V A
1 Va Center
Augusta, ME 04330
207-623-8411
800-827-1000
e-mail: g.vhacss@forum.va.gov
www.va.gov

Jack Sims, Medical Center Director
John Sims, Executive Director

Maryland

5455 Baltimore Regional Office
Veterans Benefits Administration, U S Dept. of V A
31 Hopkins Plaza
Baltimore, MD 21201
800-827-1000
e-mail: baltimore.query@vba.va.gov
www.va.gov

Jerry L Calhoun

5456 Baltimore VA Medical Center
Veterans Health Administration, U S Dept. of V A
10 N Greene Street
Baltimore, MD 21201
410-605-7000
800-463-6295
FAX: 410-605-7901
e-mail: g.vhacss@forum.va.gov
www.va.gov

David Johnson, Administrative Officer
Peggy Wess, Research Contact
Dennis Smith, Executive Director

5457 Fort Howard VA Medical Center
Veterans Health Administration, U S Dept. of V A
9600 N Point Road
Fort Howard, MD 21052
410-778-0
800-827-1000
FAX: 410-477-7177
e-mail: md.veterans@erols.com
www.mdva.state.md.us

Thomas Hutchins, Secretary

5458 Maryland Veterans Centers
10 N Greene Street
Baltimore, MD 21201
410-605-7000
FAX: 410-605-7901
www.va.gov

James Nocks, Director
Dennis H Smith, Executive Director
Veterans medical clinic offering disabled veterans medical treatments.

5459 Perry Point VA Medical Center
Veterans Health Administration, U S Dept. of V A
Perry Point, MD 21902
410-642-2411
800-827-1000
FAX: 410-642-1161
e-mail: g.vhacss@forum.va.gov
www.va.gov

Dennis H Smith, Executive Director
Allice Krupski, Assistant Director of Operations

5460 VA Maryland Health Care System
10 N Greene Street
Baltimore, MD 21201
410-605-7361
800-827-1000
FAX: 410-605-7900
www.vamhcs.med.va.gov

Christopher Bever, Director
Bruce Kaup, MD
A dynamic and exciting health care organization that is dedicated to providing quality, compassionate and accessible care and service to Maryland's veterans. As a part of one of the largest health care systems in the United States, the VAMHCS has a reputation as a leader in veterans' health care, reserch and education. Provides comprehensive service to veterans including medical, surgical, rehabilitative, nurological and mental health care on both an inpatient and outpatient basis.

Massachusetts

5461 **Boston VA Regional Office**
Veterans Benefits Administration, U S Dept. of V A
1400 Parkway
Boston, MA 02132
617-232-9500
800-827-1000
e-mail: boston.query@vba.va.gov
www.va.gov

Liza Catucci, Administrative Officer
Michael Lawson, President

5462 **Edith Nourse Rogers Memorial Veterans Hospital**
Veterans Health Administration U S Deptartment of
200 Springs Road
Building 61
Bedford, MA 01730
781-687-2926
800-827-1000
FAX: 781-687-3527
e-mail: g.vhacss@forum.va.gov
www.va.gov

Jeannette Chirico Post, Network Director

5463 **Northampton VA Medical Center**
Veterans Health Administration, U S Dept. of V A
421 N Main Street
Leeds, MA 01053
413-584-4040
800-827-1000
FAX: 413-582-3121
e-mail: g.vhacss@forum.va.gov
www.va.gov

Joanne Carney, Manager

5464 **VA Boston Healthcare System: Brockton Division**
Veterans Health Administration, U S Dept. of V A
940 Belmont Street
Brockton, MA 02301
508-583-4500
800-827-1000
FAX: 617-323-7700
e-mail: g.vhacss@forum.va.gov
www.va.gov

Tom Kelly, Commissioner
Richard Spicer, Director of Operations
Christine Croteau, Manager

5465 **VA Boston Healthcare System: Jamaica Plain Campus**
Veterans Health Administration, U S Dept. of V A
150 S Huntington Avenue
Boston, MA 02130
617-232-9500
800-827-1000
FAX: 617-278-4549
e-mail: g.vhacss@forum.va.gov
www.va.gov

Patricia Baker, Research Compliance Officer
Geraldine McGlynn, Director
Michael Lawson, President

5466 **VA Boston Healthcare System: West Roxbury Division**
Veterans Health Administration, U S Dept. of V A
1400 Vfw Parkway
West Roxbury, MA 02132
413-584-4040
800-827-1000
FAX: 413-582-3121
e-mail: g.vhacss@forum.va.gov
www.va.gov

Susan A Mac Kenzie, Associate Director

Michigan

5467 **Aleda E Lutz VA Medical Center**
Veterans Health Administration, U S Dept. of V A
1500 Weiss Street
Saginaw, MI 48602
989-497-2500
800-827-1000
FAX: 989-791-2428
e-mail: g.vhacss@forum.va.gov
www.va.gov

Emily Houle, Research Contact
Menahem Lender, Research/Development Coordinator
Robert Sabin, Executive Director

5468 **Battle Creek VA Medical Center**
Veterans Health Administration, U S Dept. of V A
5500 Armstrong Road
Battle Creek, MI 49015
269-966-5600
800-827-1000
FAX: 269-966-5483
e-mail: g.vhacss@forum.va.gov
www.va.gov

Ronald W Kelley, Research/Development Coordinator
Elinor J Pettee, Research/Development Coordinator
Alice Wood, Manager

5469 **Iron Mountain VA Medical Center**
Veterans Health Administration, U S Dept. of V A
325 E H Street
Iron Mountain, MI 49801
906-774-3300
800-827-1000
FAX: 906-779-3114
e-mail: g.vhacss@forum.va.gov
www.va.gov

C L Holmes MD, Chief Of Staff
Janice Boss, Administrator

5470 **John D Dingell VA Medical Center**
Veterans Health Administration, U S Dept. of V A
4646 John R Street
Detroit, MI 48201
313-576-1000
800-827-1000
FAX: 313-576-1112
e-mail: g.vhacss@forum.va.gov
www.va.gov

Mary J Brady, Administrative Officer

5471 **Michigan VA Regional Office**
Veterans Benefits Administration, U S Dept. of V A
477 Michigan Avenue
Room 1400
Detroit, MI 48226
800-827-1000
e-mail: detroit.query@vba.va.gov
www.va.gov

Keith Thompson, Director
Dennis W Paradowski, Assistant Director

5472 **VA Ann Arbor Healthcare System**
Veterans Health Administration, U S Dept. of V A
2215 Fuller Road
Ann Arbor, MI 48105
734-769-7100
FAX: 734-761-7870
e-mail: g.vhacss@forum.va.gov
www.va.gov

Rodney A Hayward, Director
Susan A Zuk, Administrative Officer
James Roseborough, Executive Director
Accepting eligible veterans.

5473 **Vet Center Readjustment Counseling Service**
1940 Eastern Ave SE
Grand Rapids, MI 49507
616-243-0385
FAX: 616-243-5390
www.va.gov

William Busby PhD, Executive Director
Branden K Lyon, Counselor
Lynn Hall, Clinical Coordinator
Providing a broad range of counseling outreach and referral services to eligible veterans in order to help make readjustments to cilvilian life.

Minnesota

5474 **Minneapolis VA Medical Center**
Veterans Health Administration, U S Dept. of V A
1 Veterans Drive
Minneapolis, MN 55417
612-725-2000
800-827-1000
FAX: 612-725-2049
e-mail: g.vhacss@forum.va.gov
www.va.gov

Hanna E Bloomfield, Director
Dana M Chesness, Project Coordinator

5475 **St. Cloud VA Medical Center**
Veterans Health Administration, U S Dept. of V A
4801 Veterans Drive
Saint Cloud, MN 56303
320-252-6191
800-827-1000
FAX: 320-255-6472
e-mail: g.vhacss@forum.va.gov
www.va.gov

Pat Sohler, Research/Development Coordinator

5476 **St. Paul Regional Office**
Veterans Benefits Administration, U S Dept. of V A
1 Federal Drive
Fort Snelling, MN 55111
800-827-1000
e-mail: stpaul.query@vba.va.gov
www.va.gov

Vincent Crawford, Director

5477 **Vet Center**
405 E Superior Street
Duluth, MN 55802
218-722-8654
FAX: 218-723-8212

Cynthia Macaulay MEd, Counselor
Rob Evanson, Counselor
Debbie Burt, Office Manager
Counseling, social services and benefits assistance for combat veterans and those sexually traumatized in the military.

Mississippi

5478 **Biloxi/Gulfport VA Medical Center**
Veterans Health Administration, U S Dept. of V A
400 Veterans Avenue
Biloxi, MS 39531
228-563-2472
800-827-1000
FAX: 228-563-2898
e-mail: g.vhacss@forum.va.gov
www.va.gov

Kimberly Morgan, Administrative Officer

5479 **Jackson Regional Office**
Veterans Benefits Administration, U S Dept. of V A
1600 E Woodrow Wilson Avenue
Jackson, MS 39216
601-364-7000
800-827-1000
FAX: 601-364-7007
e-mail: jackson.query@vba.va.gov
www.va.gov

Neil Anthony Mcphie, Chairman
Barbara Sapin, Vice Chairman

Missouri

5480 **Harry S Truman Memorial Veterans' Hospital**
Veterans Health Administration, U S Dept. of V A
800 Hospital Drive
Columbia, MO 65201
573-814-6552
800-349-8220
FAX: 573-814-6551
e-mail: g.vhacss@forum.va.gov
www.va.gov

Larry L Propp, Executive Director
Lawrence Propp, Administrative Officer

5481 **John J Pershing VA Medical Center**
Veterans Health Administration, U S Dept. of V A
1500 N Westwood Boulevard
Poplar Bluff, MO 63901
573-778-4721
800-827-1000
FAX: 573-778-4156
e-mail: g.vhacss@forum.va.gov
www.va.gov

Ginny Sartini, Research/Development Coordinator
Linda Haga, Research Contact

5482 **Kansas City VA Medical Center**
Veterans Health Administration, U S Dept. of V A
4801 E Linwood Boulevard
Kansas City, MO 64128
816-861-4700
800-827-1000
e-mail: g.vhacss@forum.va.gov
www.va.gov

Kenneth Grasing, Research/Development
Ram Sharma, Administrative Officer
Kent Hill, Executive Director
The Kansas City VA Medical Center is a modern, well-equipped teriary care inpatient and outpatient center. As the third largest teaching hospital in the metropolitan area, it maintains educational affiliations with the University of Kansas School of Medicine.

5483 **St. Louis Regional Office**
Veterans Benefits Administration, U S Dept. of V A
400 S 18th Street
Saint Louis, MO 63103
800-827-1000
e-mail: stlouis.query@vba.va.gov
www.va.gov

5484 **St. Louis VA Medical Center**
Veterans Health Administration, U S Dept. of V A
915 N Grand Boulevard
Saint Louis, MO 63106
314-589-6333
800-827-1000
FAX: 314-289-7009
e-mail: g.vhacss@forum.va.gov
www.va.gov

Dolores Minor, Administrative Officer

Montana

5485 **Montana VA Regional Office**
3633 Veterans Drive
PO Box 188
Fort Harrison, MT 59636
406-442-7310

5486 **V A Montana Healthcare System**
U S Dept. of V A
3687 Veterans Drive
PO Box 1500
Fort Harrison, MT 59636
406-442-6410
877-468-8387
FAX: 406-447-7916
e-mail: ftharrison.query@vba.va.gov
www.va.gov

Susanne Corbett, Pateint Representative
This is a complete, medically reliable dictionary of congenital malformations and disorders. As the authors explain, "Down syndrome is the only common congenital disorder, the other defects and disorders are rare or very rare, some having been reported fewer than 20 times worlwide." This dictionary covers them all. Examples: Aagenaes syndrome, Acrocallosal syndrome, and Acrodysostosis

5487 **VA Montana Healthcare System**
Veterans Health Administration, U S Dept. of V A
1892 William Street
Fort Harrison, MT 59636
406-442-6410
800-827-1000
FAX: 406-447-7965
e-mail: g.vhacss@forum.va.gov
www.va.gov

Anna Lithgoe, Research/Development Coordinator
Gregory Johnson, MD

5488 **Vet Center**
Readjusment Counciling Service Western Mountain Re
1234 Avenue C
Billings, MT 59102
406-657-6071
FAX: 406-657-6603

Robert Phillips MSW, Team Leader
Luanne Anderson, Office Manager
Barry Osgard MS, Counselor
Readjustment counseling service for counseling veterans who are having difficulty adjusting from military service especially those diagnosed with PTSD.

Nebraska

5489 **Grand Island VA Medical System**
Veterans Health Administration, U S Dept. of V A
2201 N Broadwell Avenue
Grand Island, NE 68803
308-382-3660
800-827-1000
e-mail: g.vhacss@forum.va.gov
www.va.gov

John Hilbert, Executive Director
Daniel L Parker, Deputy Director

5490 **Lincoln Regional Office**
Veterans Benefits Administration, U S Dept. of V A
5631 S 48th Street
Lincoln, NE 68516
800-827-1000
e-mail: lincoln.query@vba.va.gov
www.va.gov

John Hilgert, Executive Director
Daniel Parker, Deputy Director

5491 **Lincoln VA Medical Center**
Veterans Health Administration, U S Dept. of V A
600 S 70th Street
Lincoln, NE 68510
402-486-7825
800-827-1000
FAX: 402-486-7860
e-mail: g.vhacss@forum.va.gov
www.va.gov

Ryon L Adams, Research/Development Coordinator

5492 **VA Nebraska-Western Iowa Health Care System**
Veterans Health Administration, U S Dept. of V A
4101 Woolworth Avenue
Omaha, NE 68105
402-346-8800
FAX: 402-449-0684
www.va.gov

Al Washko, Director
Rowen Zetterman, Chief of Staff

Nevada

5493 **Las Vegas Veterans Center**
1919 S Jones Boulevard
Las Vegas, NV 89146
702-251-7873
FAX: 702-388-6664

Daryl Harding, Resident Counselor LCSW
Matt Watson, Team Leader MSW
Veterans clinical counseling center for veterans and their dependent individual and group counseling, marital and family counseling, alcohol and drug assessment referral or treatment. Community education and consultation, employment counseling.

5494 **Reno Regional Office**
Veterans Benefits Administration U S Deptartment o
1000 Locust Street
Reno, NV 89502
775-328-1486
800-827-1000
FAX: 775-328-1447
e-mail: reno.query@vba.va.gov
www.va.gov

Joseph E Dardillo, Administrative Officer

5495 **VA Sierra Nevada Healthcare System**
Veterans Health Administration, U S Dept. of V A
1000 Locust Street
Reno, NV 89502
775-786-7200
888-838-6256
FAX: 775-328-1816
www.va.gov

Roy F Mackintosh, Acting Aces/Research/Development
Angela Fisher, Manager

5496 **VA Southern Nevada Healthcare System**
Veterans Health Administration, U S Dept. of V A
901 Rancho Lane
Las Vegas, NV 89106
702-636-3000
800-827-1000
FAX: 707-636-3027
e-mail: g.vhacss@forum.va.gov
www.va.gov

Chuck Fulkerson, Executive Director
Steve Long, Deputy Director

New Hampshire

5497 **Manchester Regional Office**
Veterans Benefits Administration, U S Dept. of V A
275 Chestnut Street
Manchester, NH 03101
800-827-1000
e-mail: manchester.query@vba.va.gov
www.va.gov

Jerry Beale, Director

5498 **Manchester VA Medical Center**
Veterans Health Administration, U S Dept. of V A
718 Smyth Road
Manchester, NH 03104
603-624-4366
800-892-8384
e-mail: g.vhacss@forum.va.gov
www.va.gov

Marc Levenson, Executive Director

5499 **New Hampshire Veterans Centers**
103 Liberty Street
Manchester, NH 03104
603-668-7060
800-562-3127
FAX: 603-666-7404

Caryl Ahern Msw, Team Leader
Paulette Landry, Office Manager

Veterans clinic offering combat veterans outpatient counseling

New Jersey

5500 **Disabled American Veterans: Ocean County**
PO Box 1806
Toms River, NJ 08754 732-929-0907
e-mail: bvenga@thecore.com
community.nj.com/cc/dav24

Mary Bencivenga, Contact

5501 **East Orange Campus of the VA New Jersey Healthcare System**
Veterans Health Administration, US Dept. of VA
385 Tremont Avenue
East Orange, NJ 07018 973-676-1000
800-827-1000
FAX: 973-676-4226
e-mail: g.vhacss@forum.va.gov
www.va.gov

Kenneth H Mizrach, Director
Samuel Greene, President

5502 **Lyons Campus of the VA New Jersey Healthcare System**
Veterans Health Administration, U S Dept. of V A
151 Knollcroft Road
Lyons, NJ 07939 908-647-0180
800-827-1000
FAX: 908-647-3452
e-mail: g.vhacss@forum.va.gov
www.va.gov

James J Farsetta, Director
Donna Henderson, Coordinator

5503 **Newark Regional Office**
Veterans Benefits Administration, U S Dept. of V A
20 Washington Place
Newark, NJ 07102
800-827-1000
e-mail: newark.query@vba.va.gov
www.va.gov

Stephen G Abel, Deputy Commissioner for Veterans

New Mexico

5504 **New Mexico VA Healthcare System**
Veterans Health Administration, US Dept. of VA
1501 San Pedro Drive SE
Albuquerque, NM 87108 505-265-1711
800-827-1000
FAX: 505-256-2855
e-mail: g.vhacss@forum.va.gov
www.va.gov

Norman Brownel, Executive Director

5505 **New Mexico Veterans Centers**
PO Box 927
Truth or Consequences, NM 87901 505-894-4200
e-mail: Lori

Montgomery Administrator
Veterans medical clinic offering disabled veterans medical treatments.

New York

5506 **Albany VA Medical Center: Samuel S Stratton**
Veterans Health Administration, U S Dept. of V A
113 Holland Avenue
Albany, NY 12208 518-626-6711
800-823-9656
FAX: 518-626-5500
e-mail: g.vhacss@forum.va.gov
www.va.gov

Linda Blumenstock, Marketing Director
Mary Ellen Piche, Director

5507 **Albany Vet Center**
17 Computer Drive West
Suite 2
Albany, NY 12205 518-626-5130
FAX: 518-458-8613

Maureen Chauvin, Office Manager
Melodie Krahula, Team Leader
Provides readjustment counseling for combat veterans and also provides benefits and job counseling for all veterans.

5508 **Bath VA Medical Center**
Veterans Health Administration U S Deptartment of
76 Veterans Medical Center
Bath, NY 14810 607-664-4000
800-827-1000
FAX: 607-664-4000
e-mail: g.vhacss@forum.va.gov
www.va.gov

Barbara J Mahone, Chairman

5509 **Bronx VA Medical Center**
Veterans Health Administration, U S Dept. of V A
130 W Kingsbridge Road
Bronx, NY 10468 718-584-9000
800-827-1000
FAX: 718-562-9120
e-mail: g.vhacss@forum.va.gov
www.va.gov

Anthony Rotolo, Administrative Officer
Mary Sano, Research/Development Coordinator
Maryann Musumeci, Executive Director

5510 **Brooklyn Campus of the VA NY Harbor Healthcare System**
Veterans Health Administration, U S Dept. of V A
295 Flatbush Avenue Ext
Brooklyn, NY 11201 718-836-6600
800-827-1000
e-mail: g.vhacss@forum.va.gov
www.va.gov

George P Basher, Director
Irving Behr, MD

5511 **Buffalo Regional Office**
Veterans Benefits Administration
3495 Bailey Avenue
Building 20
Buffalo, NY 14215 716-862-6527
800-827-1000
www.va.gov

5512 **Canandiagua VA Medical Center**
Veterans Health Administration, U S Dept. of V A
400 Fort Hill Avenue
Canandaigua, NY 14424 585-394-2000
800-827-1000
e-mail: g.vhacss@forum.va.gov
www.va.gov

Robert W Ratliff, Interim Director
W Smith, Administrator

5513 **Castle Point Campus of the VA Hudson Valley Healthcare System**
Veterans Health Administration, U S Dept. of V A
Castle Point Campus
Castle Point, NY 12511
914-737-4400
800-827-1000
FAX: 914-788-4244
e-mail: g.vhacss@forum.va.gov
www.va.gov

5514 **New York City Campus of the VA NY Harbor Healthcare System**
Veterans Health Administration, U S Dept. of V A
423 E 23rd Street
New York, NY 10010
212-951-7470
800-827-1000
FAX: 212-686-7470
e-mail: g.vhacss@forum.va.gov
www.va.gov

Leslie Dowers, Administrative Officer
Camille R Varacchi, Administrative Officer

5515 **New York Regional Office**
Veterans Benefits Administration, U S Dept. of V A
245 W Houston Street
New York, NY 10014
518-474-6114
800-827-1000
FAX: 518-473-0379
e-mail: newyork.query@vba.va.gov
www.va.gov

George Basher, Director

5516 **Northport VA Medical Center**
Veterans Health Administration, U S Dept. of V A
79 Middleville Road
Northport, NY 11768
631-261-4400
800-827-1000
e-mail: g.vhacss@forum.va.gov
www.va.gov

Martina Parauda, Associate Director

5517 **Syracuse VA Medical Center**
Veterans Health Administration, U S Dept. of V A
800 Irving Avenue
Syracuse, NY 13210
315-476-7461
800-827-1000
e-mail: g.vhacss@forum.va.gov
www.va.gov

George P Basher, Director

5518 **Torah Alliance of Families of Kids with Disabilities**
T AF KI D
1359 Coney Island Avenue
Brooklyn, NY 11230
718-252-2236
FAX: 718-252-2216
e-mail: tafkid@worldnet.att.net
www.tafkid.org

Juby Shapiro, President/Program Director
Serves over 1k families whose children have a variety of disabilities and special needs. Many of these families are large families in the low socioeconomic level. Offers monthly meetings, guest lectures, parent matching, information of new developments in software, technology and techniques, sibling support groups, pen pal lists, audio and video library, alternative medicine and nutrition information and education on legal awareness and rights of disabled citizens.

5519 **VA Hudson Valley Health Care System**
Veterans Health Administration, U S Department of
PO Box 100
Montrose, NY 10548
914-737-4400
FAX: 845-788-4244
www.va.gov

James J Farsette, Network Director
Michael Sabo, Executive Director

5520 **VA Western NY Healthcare System, Batavia**
Veterans Health Administration, U S Dept. of V A
222 Richmond Avenue
Batavia, NY 14020
585-343-7500
800-827-1000
e-mail: g.vhacss@forum.va.gov
www.va.gov

Michael S Finegan, Medical Center Director
Timothy W Liezert, Assistant Director
Mary Olix, Manager

5521 **VA Western NY Healthcare System, Buffalo**
Veterans Health Administration, U S Dept. of V A
3495 Bailey Avenue
Buffalo, NY 14215
716-834-9200
www.va.gov

Michael S Finigan, Director
William Feeley, President

North Carolina

5522 **Asheville VA Medical Center**
Veterans Health Administration, U S Dept. of V A
1100 Tunnel Road
Asheville, NC 28805
828-298-7911
800-827-1000
FAX: 828-299-2502
e-mail: g.vhacss@forum.va.gov
www.va.gov

Joseph Schimansky, Executive Director
Brian Peek, R&D Coordinator

5523 **Charlotte Vet Center**
V A Department Veterans Affairs
223 S Brevard Street
Suite 103
Charlotte, NC 28202
704-333-6107
FAX: 704-344-6470
www.va.gov

Loretta Deaton, Team Leader
Preadjustment Counseling for Combat Veterans with Post Traumatic Stress Disorder (PTSD).

5524 **Durham VA Medical Center**
Veterans Health Administration, U S Dept. of V A
508 Fulton Street
Durham, NC 27705
919-286-0411
800-827-1000
FAX: 919-286-5944
e-mail: leola.jenkins@med.va.gov
www.va.gov

Leola Jenkins, EED Manager

5525 **Fayetteville VA Medical Center**
Veterans Health Administration, U S Dept. of V A
2300 Ramsey Street
Fayetteville, NC 28301
910-488-2120
800-771-6106
FAX: 910-822-7926
e-mail: g.vhacss@forum.va.gov
www.va.gov

Janet Stout, Director

5526 **WG Hefner VA Medical Center**
Vet Health Administration U S Department of VA
1601 Brenner Avenue
Salisbury, NC 28144
704-638-9000
800-827-1000
FAX: 704-638-3395
e-mail: g.vhacss@forum.va.gov
www.va.gov

Nancy Stine, Manager

5527 **Winston-Salem Regional Office**
Veterans Benefits Administration, U S Dept. of V A
251 N Main Street
Winston Salem, NC 27155
919-733-3851
800-827-1000
FAX: 919-733-2834
e-mail: winsalem.query@vba.va.gov
www.va.gov

Charles F Smith, Assistant Secretary

North Dakota

5528 **Fargo VA Medical Center**
Veterans Health Administration, U S Dept. of V A
2101 Elm Street N
Fargo, ND 58102
701-239-7165
800-827-1000
FAX: 701-239-7166
e-mail: g.vhacss@forum.va.gov
www.va.gov

Bob Hanson, Commissioner
Kathy Halgunseth, Manager

5529 **North Dakota VA Regional Office**
Veterans Benefits Administration, U S Dept. of V A
2101 Elm Street N
Fargo, ND 58102
701-239-3700
800-827-1000
FAX: 701-239-3790
e-mail: fargo.query@vba.va.gov
www.va.gov

Thomas Santoro, Director Research Department

Ohio

5530 **Chillicothe VA Medical Center**
Veterans Health Administration, U S Dept. of V A
17273 State Route 104
Chillicothe, OH 45601
740-773-1141
800-827-1000
FAX: 740-772-7023
e-mail: g.vhacss@forum.va.gov
www.va.gov

Douglas Moorman, Executive Director

5531 **Cincinnati VA Medical Center**
Veterans Health Administration, U S Dept. of V A
3200 Vine Street
Cincinnati, OH 45220
513-861-3100
800-827-1000
FAX: 513-475-6500
e-mail: g.vhacss@forum.va.gov
www.va.gov

Ronald D Edwards, Director
Gary Nugent, Executive Director

5532 **Cincinnati Veterans Centers**
801b W 8th Street
Suite 126
Cincinnati, OH 45203
513-741-5600

Veterans medical clinic offering disabled veterans medical treatments.

5533 **Cleveland Regional Office**
Veterans Benefits Administration, U S Dept. of V A
1240 E 9th Street
Cleveland, OH 44199
800-827-1000
e-mail: cleveland.query@vba.va.gov
www.va.gov

P Hunter Peckham, Director
Robert Ruff, Assistant Director

5534 **Dayton VA Medical Center**
Veterans Health Administration U S Department of V
4100 W 3rd Street
Dayton, OH 45428
937-268-6511
800-827-1000
FAX: 937-262-2170
e-mail: g.vhacss@forum.va.gov
www.dayton.med.va.gov

Charlene Ackerman, Director
Kathleen Mannix, Manager

5535 **Louis Stokes VA Medical Center**
Veterans Health Administration, U S Dept. of V A
10701 East Boulevard
Cleveland, OH 44106
440-526-3030
800-827-1000
FAX: 440-838-6017
e-mail: g.vhacss@forum.va.gov
www.va.gov

Anthony J Foster, Interim Director

Oklahoma

5536 **Muskogee VA Medical Center**
Veterans Benefits Administration, U S Dept. of V A
1011 Honor Heights Drive
Muskogee, OK 74401
918-683-3261
800-827-1000
e-mail: muskogee.query@vba.va.gov
www.va.gov

Phillip L Driskill, Director

5537 **Oklahoma City VA Medical Center**
Veterans Health Administration, U S Dept. of V A
921 NE 13th Street
Oklahoma City, OK 73104
405-270-0501
800-827-1000
FAX: 405-270-1560
www.va.gov

Phillip L Driskill, Director
Tom Duchene, Plant Manager
D Robert McCaffree MD, Chief of Staff

5538 **Oklahoma Veterans Centers Vet Center**
3033 N Walnut Avenue
Suite W101
Oklahoma City, OK 73105
405-528-5583

Peter Sharp, Team Leader
Steve Kenzie, Owner
PTSP counseling for all combat Veterans and victims of sexual trauma/sexual harassment.

Oregon

5539 **Oregon Health Sciences University**
3181 SW Sam Jackson Park Road
Portland, OR 97239
503-494-3460

Thomas Talboe
James Morgan, Executive Director
Offers services for the totally blind, legally blind, visually impaired, mentally retarded blind and more with health, counseling, educational, recreational, rehabilitation, computer training and professional training services.

5540 **Portland Regional Office**
Veterans Benefits Administration, U S Dept. of V A
1220 SW 3rd Avenue
Portland, OR 97204 503-373-2388
800-827-1000
e-mail: portland.query@vba.va.gov
www.va.gov

5541 **Portland VA Medical Center**
Veterans Health Administration, U S Dept. of V A
PO Box 1034
Portland, OR 97207 503-220-8262
800-827-1000
FAX: 503-273-5319
e-mail: g.vhacss@forum.va.gov
www.va.gov

Mindy Aisen, Director Rehabilitation Research
Carolyn Tsai, Director of Neurology
Kim Winn, Manager

5542 **Roseburg VA Medical Center**
Veterans Health Administration, U S Dept. of V A
913 NW Garden Valley Boulevard
Roseburg, OR 97470 541-440-1000
800-827-1000
FAX: 541-440-1225
e-mail: g.vhacss@forum.va.gov
www.va.gov

Jim Willis, Director
Mark Traines, MD

5543 **White City VA Domiciliary**
Veterans Health Administration, U S Dept. of V A
8495 Crater Lake Highway
White City, OR 97503 541-826-2111
800-827-1000
FAX: 541-830-3500
e-mail: g.vhacss@forum.va.gov
www.va.gov

George Andries, Executive Director

Pennsylvania

5544 **Butler VA Medical Center**
Veterans Health Administration, U S Dept. of V A
325 New Castle Road
Butler, PA 16001 724-287-4781
800-827-1000
FAX: 724-282-4408
e-mail: g.vhacss@forum.va.gov
www.va.gov

David Wood, Executive Director

5545 **Coatesville VA Medical Center**
Veterans Health Administration, U S Dept. of V A
1400 Blackhorse Hill Road
Coatesville, PA 19320 610-384-7711
800-827-1000
e-mail: g.vhacss@forum.va.gov
www.va.gov

Charlene Ackerman, Director
Gary Devansky, Chief Executive Officer

5546 **Erie VA Medical Center**
Veterans Health Administration, U S Dept. of V A
135 E 38th Street
Erie, PA 16504 814-868-8661
800-274-8387
e-mail: g.vhacss@forum.va.gov
www.va.gov

Michael Adelman, Chief of Staff
Stephen Lucas, Executive Director

5547 **James E Van Zandt VA Medical Center**
Veterans Health Administration, U S Dept. of V A
2907 Pleasant Valley Boulevard
Altoona, PA 16602 814-943-8164
800-827-1000
FAX: 814-940-7898
e-mail: g.vhacss@forum.va.gov
www.va.gov

Cecil B Hengeveld, Director
Gerald Williams, Executive Director

5548 **Lebanon VA Medical Center**
Veterans Health Administration, U S Dept. of V A
1700 S Lincoln Avenue
Lebanon, PA 17042 717-272-6621
800-409-8771
FAX: 717-228-5907
e-mail: g.vhacss@forum.va.gov
www.va.gov

Steven W Young, Associate Director

5549 **Pennsylvania Veterans Centers**
Veterans Health Administration, U S Department of
1000 State Street
Suite 2
Erie, PA 16501 717-861-8901
800-478-8
FAX: 717-861-8589
www.va.gov

Cecil B Hengeveld, Deputy Adjustant General
Veterans medical clinic offering disabled veterans medical treatments.

5550 **Philadelphia Regional Office and Insurance Center**
Veterans Benefits Administration, U S Dept. of V A
5000 Wissahickon Avenue
Philadelphia, PA 19144
800-827-1000
e-mail: phillyro.query@vba.va.gov
www.va.gov

5551 **Philadelphia VA Medical Center**
Veterans Health Administration, U S Dept. of V A
University and Woodland Avenu
Philadelphia, PA 19104 215-823-5800
800-827-1000
e-mail: g.vhacss@forum.va.gov
www.va.gov

Cecil B Hengeveld, Director

5552 **Pittsburgh Regional Office**
Veterans Benefits Administration U S Deparment of
University Drive C
Pittsburgh, PA 15240 412-688-6100
800-827-1000
FAX: 412-688-6121
e-mail: pittsburgh.query@vba.va.gov
www.va.gov

Micahel E Moreland

5553 **VA Pittsburgh Healthcare System, University Drive Division**
Veterans Health Administration, U S Dept. of V A
University Drive
Pittsburgh, PA 15240 412-688-6000
800-827-1000
FAX: 412-688-6901
e-mail: g.vhacss@forum.va.gov
www.va.gov

Michael E Moreland, Chief Executive Officer

5554 VA Pittsburgh Healthcare System, Highland Drive Division
Veterans Health Administration, U S Dept. of V A
7180 Highland Drive
Pittsburgh, PA 15206 412-365-4900
800-827-1000
FAX: 412-365-4213
e-mail: g.vhacss@forum.va.gov
www.va.gov

Cecil Hengeveld, Deputy Adjutant General
Roger Sutton, MD

5555 Wilkes-Barre VA Medical Center
Veterans Health Administration, U S Dept. of V A
1111 E End Boulevard
Wilkes Barre, PA 18711 570-821-7207
800-827-1000
FAX: 570-821-7278
e-mail: g.vhacss@forum.va.gov
www.va.gov

William Grossman MD

Rhode Island

5556 Providence Regional Office
Veterans Benefits Administration, U S Dept. of V A
380 Westminster Street
Providence, RI 02903 401-462-0324
800-827-1000
FAX: 401-254-2320
e-mail: providence.query@vba.va.gov
www.va.gov

Daniel Evangelista, Acting Associate Director

5557 Providence VA Medical Center
Veterans Health Administration, U S Dept. of V A
830 Chalkstone Avenue
Providence, RI 02908 401-273-7100
FAX: 401-457-3360
e-mail: g.vhacss@forum.va.gov
www.va.gov

Vincent Ng, Executive Director

South Carolina

5558 Columbia Regional Office
Veterans Benefits Administration, U S Dept. of V A
1801 Assembly Street
Columbia, SC 29201 803-734-0200
800-827-1000
e-mail: columbia.query@vba.va.gov
www.va.gov

Jimmie Ruff, Executive Director

5559 Ralph H Johnson VA Medical Center
Veterans Health Administration, U S Dept. of V A
109 Bee Street
Charleston, SC 29401 843-789-6710
800-827-1000
FAX: 843-876-5384
e-mail: g.vhacss@forum.va.gov
www.va.gov

Brenda M Synder, Administrative Officer

5560 William Jennings Bryan Dorn VA Medical Center
Veterans Health Administration U S Department of V
6439 Garners Ferry Road
Columbia, SC 29209 803-776-4000
800-827-1000
FAX: 803-695-6739
e-mail: g.vhacss@forum.va.gov
www.va.gov

Cynthia T Boris, Chief of Pharmacy
Julian H Bourn, Program Director
Brian Heckert, Executive Director

South Dakota

5561 Sioux Falls VA Medical Center
Veterans Health Administration, U S Dept. of V A
PO Box 5046
Sioux Falls, SD 57117 605-336-3230
800-827-1000
FAX: 605-333-6878
e-mail: g.vhacss@forum.va.gov
www.va.gov

Joseph Dalpiaz, Director
Gary Million, Assistant Director
R Crawford, Executive Director

5562 South Dakota VA Regional Office
Veterans Benefits Administration, U S Dept. of V A
PO Box 5046
Sioux Falls, SD 57117 605-773-3269
800-827-1000
FAX: 605-773-5380
e-mail: siouxfalls.query@vba.va.gov
www.va.gov

5563 South Dakota Veterans Centers
610 Kansas City Street
Rapid City, SD 57701 605-348-0077
800-743-1070
FAX: 605-348-0878

Gary Johnson, Manager
Veterans medical clinic offering disabled veterans medical treatments.

Tennessee

5564 Alvin C York VA Medical Center
Veterans Health Administration, U S Dept. of V A
3400 Lebanon Road
Murfreesboro, TN 37129 615-867-6000
800-827-1000
FAX: 615-867-5768
e-mail: g.vhacss@forum.va.gov
www.va.gov

David Penninggon, Director

5565 Memphis VA Medical Center
Veterans Health Administration, U S Dept. of V A
1030 Jefferson Avenue
Memphis, TN 38104 901-523-8990
800-636-8262
e-mail: g.vhacss@forum.va.gov
www.va.gov

Peter St Arnold, Administrative Officer
John M Stuart, Research/Development Coordinator
Hardie Phipps, Manager

5566 Mountain Home VA Medical Center
Veterans Health Administration, US Dept. of VA
Mountain Home, TN 37684 423-926-1171
800-827-1000
e-mail: g.vhacss@forum.va.gov
www.va.gov

Nancy Doughtry, Manager

5567 Nasheville Regional Office
Veterans Benefits Administration, U S Dept. of V A
110 9th Avenue S
Nashville, TN 37203
800-827-1000
e-mail: nashville.query@vba.va.gov
www.va.gov

Michael R Walsh, Administrative Officer
Donald H Rubin, Research/Development Coordinator

5568 Nashville VA Medical Center
Veterans Health Administration, US Dept. of VA
1310 24th Avenue S
Nashville, TN 37212
615-327-4751
800-827-1000
FAX: 615-321-6350
e-mail: g.vhacss@forum.va.gov
www.va.gov

David Pennington, President

Texas

5569 Amarillo VA Healthcare System
Veterans Health Administration, U S Dept. of V A
6010 Emerald Boulevard W
Amarillo, TX 79106
806-355-9703
800-827-1000
FAX: 806-354-7869
e-mail: g.vhacss@forum.va.gov
www.va.gov

Wallace N Hopkins, Director

5570 Amarillo Vet Center
Department of Veterans Affairs
3414 Olsen Boulevard
Suite E
Amarillo, TX 79109
806-354-9779
FAX: 806-351-1104

Pedro Garcia Jr, Team Leader
Provides individual, group and family counseling to veterans who served in combat theaters of World War II and Korea, veterans of the Vietnam Era, and veterans of conflicts zones in Lebanon, Grenada, Panama, the Persian Guld and Somalia.

5571 El Paso VA Healthcare Center
Veterans Health Administration, U S Dept. of V A
5001 N Piedras Street
El Paso, TX 79930
915-564-6100
800-827-1000
FAX: 915-564-7920
e-mail: g.vhacss@forum.va.gov
www.va.gov

Stephen Shapiro, R and D Coordinator

5572 Houston Regional Office
Veterans Benefits Administration, U S Dept. of V A
6900 Almeda Road
Houston, TX 77030
713-791-1414
800-827-1000
e-mail: houston.query@vba.va.gov
www.va.gov

Cecil Aultman, Executive Director
Edgar Tucker, Chief Executive Officer

5573 Houston VA Medical Center
Veterans Health Administration, U S Dept. of V A
2002 Holcombe Boulevard
Houston, TX 77030
713-791-1414
800-827-1000
e-mail: g.vhacss@forum.va.gov
www.va.gov

Edgar Tucker, Chief Executive Officer

5574 South Texas Veterans Healthcare System
Veterans Health Administration, U S Dept. of V A
7400 Merton Minter Street
San Antonio, TX 78229
210-617-5300
800-827-1000
e-mail: g.vhacss@forum.va.gov
www.va.gov

Pete Donahoe, Director
Charles Sepich, Chief Executive Officer

5575 VA North Texas Health Veterans Affairs Car e System: Dallas VA Medical Center
Veterans Health Administration, U S Dept. of V A
4500 S Lancaster Road
Dallas, TX 75216
214-742-8387
800-849-3597
FAX: 214-857-1171
www.va.gov

Alan G Harper, Director
Jonnis Hamilton, Manager
Daniel K Heers, Assistant Director
Health care system which serves veterans with medical care and rehabilitation services including spinal cord injury center. For VA benefit inquiries contact 1-800-827-1000. This system has locations in Bonham, Dallas, and Fort Worth.

5576 Waco Regional Office
Veterans Benefits Administration, U S Dept. of V A
701 Clay Avenue
Waco, TX 76799
800-827-1000
e-mail: waco.query@vba.va.gov
www.va.gov

Keith Young, Research/Development Coordinator

5577 West Texas VA Healthcare System
Veterans Health Administration, U S Dept. of V A
300 W Veterans Boulevard
Big Spring, TX 79720
432-264-4810
800-728-7000
FAX: 915-264-4834
e-mail: g.vhacss@forum.va.gov
www.va.gov

Bruce A Gordon, Director
Robert W Ratliff, Deputy Director
Celsa Tiu, MD

Utah

5578 Utah Division of Veterans Affairs
Utah Division of Veterans Affairs
550 Foothill Drive
Suite 202
Salt Lake City, UT 84113
801-524-6048
800-894-9497
FAX: 801-326-2369
e-mail: tandrews@utah.gov
www.ut.ngb.army.mil/veterans

Terry Schow, Director
Todd Andrews, Assistant to the Director
Lavonne Willis, Manager

5579 VA Salt Lake City Healthcare System
Veterans Health Administration, U S Dept. of V A
500 Foothill Drive
Salt Lake City, UT 84148
801-582-1565
800-613-4012
FAX: 801-584-1289
www.va.gov

James R. Floyd, Director
Scott F. Hill, Assistant Director

Vermont

5580 **Vermont VA Regional Office Center**
Veterans Benefits Administration U S Department V
215 N Main Street
White River Junction, VT 05009
802-296-6339
800-827-1000
FAX: 802-290-6354
e-mail: whiteriver.query@vba.va.gov
www.va.gov

Laura Miraldi, Executive Director

5581 **Vermont Veterans Centers**
359 Dorset Street
South Burlington, VT 05403
802-862-1806

Fred Forehand, Manager
Veterans medical clinic offering disabled veterans medical treatments.

Virginia

5582 **Hampton VA Medical Center**
Veterans Health Administration, U S Dept. of V A
100 Emancipation Drive
Hampton, VA 23667
757-722-9961
800-827-1000
FAX: 757-728-3135
e-mail: mike.eisenberg@med.va.gov
www.va.gov

Myron Eisenberg, Aces/ Education & Research
Michelle Fronheiser, Research Contact
Joseph Williams, Executive Director

5583 **Hunter Holmes McGuire VA Medical Center**
Veterans Health Administration, U S Dept. of V A
1201 Broad Rock Boulevard
Richmond, VA 23249
804-675-5151
800-827-1000
FAX: 804-675-5139
e-mail: g.vhacss@forum.va.gov
www.va.gov

Robert C Dresch, Administrative Officer
Lauri A Weiler, Research Contact

5584 **Roanoke Regional Office**
Veterans Benefits Administration, U S Dept. of V A
210 Franklin Road SW
Roanoke, VA 24011
540-857-7104
800-827-1000
e-mail: anne.atkins@vdvs.viginia.gov
www.vdvs.virginia.gov

Vince M Burgess, Commissioner
Bert Boyd, COO/Executive Director

5585 **Salem VA Medical Center**
Veterans Health Administration, U S Dept. of V A
1970 Roanoke Boulevard
Salem, VA 24153
540-982-2463
800-827-1000
FAX: 540-983-1096
e-mail: g.vhacss@forum.va.gov
www.va.gov

Stephen L Lemons, Director

5586 **Virginia Department of Veterans Services**
270 Franklin Road SW
Roanoke, VA 24011
540-857-7104
FAX: 540-857-7573
e-mail: pmigrand131@worldnet.att.net
www.vdva.vipnet.org

Jon A Mangis, Commissioner of Veterans Service
Colbert Boyd, Chief Deputy Commissioner
Colbert Boyd, Executive Director

Washington

5587 **Jonathan M Wainwright Memorial VA Medical Center**
Veterans Health Administration, U S Dept. of V A
77 Wainwright Drive
Walla Walla, WA 99362
509-525-5200
888-687-8863
FAX: 509-946-3062
www.va.gov

Richard D Cornish, R and D Coordinator

5588 **Seattle Regional Office**
Veterans Benefits Administration U S Department of
915 2nd Avenue
Seattle, WA 98174
206-762-1010
800-827-1000
e-mail: seattle.query@vba.va.gov
www.va.gov

Va Ad Harabanim, Executive Director
Timothy Williams, Chief Executive Officer

5589 **Spokane VA Medical Center**
Veterans Health Administration, U S Dept. of V A
4815 N Assembly Street
Spokane, WA 99205
509-434-7000
800-827-1000
FAX: 509-434-7119
e-mail: g.vhacss@forum.va.gov
www.va.gov

Alan Prentiss, Chief of Staff
Dirk Minatre, Coordinator
Joseph Manley, Executive Director

5590 **VA Puget Sound Health Care System**
Veterans Health Administration, U S Dept. of V A
1660 S Columbian Way
Seattle, WA 98108
206-762-1010
800-827-1000
e-mail: g.vhacss@forum.va.gov
www.va.gov

John M King, Director
Timothy Williams, Chief Executive Officer

West Virginia

5591 **Beckley VA Medical Center**
Veterans Health Administration, U S Dept. of V A
200 Veterans Avenue
Beckley, WV 25801
304-255-2121
800-827-1000
FAX: 304-255-2431
e-mail: g.vhacss@forum.va.gov
www.va.gov

Gerard Husson, Director
Karin McGraw, Assistant Director
Debbie Coloski, Manager

5592 **Huntington Regional Office**
Veterans Benefits Administration, U S Dept. of V A
640 4th Avenue
Huntington, WV 25701
304-558-3661
800-827-1000
FAX: 304-558-3662
e-mail: huntington.query@vba.va.gov
www.va.gov

Larry Linch, Director

5593 Huntington VA Medical Center
Veterans Health Administration, U S Dept. of V A
1540 Spring Valley Drive
Huntington, WV 25704
304-429-6755
FAX: 304-429-6713
www.va.gov

Jack E Terry, R and D Coordinator
Richard Manis, MD

5594 Louis A Johnson VA Medical Center
Veterans Health Administration, U S Dept. of V A
1 Med Center Drive
Clarksburg, WV 26301
304-623-7640
800-827-1000
FAX: 304-626-7048
e-mail: g.vhacss@forum.va.gov
www.va.gov

William E Cox, Executive Director
Kathy Keener, Program Assistant
Leilani Sultan-Brown DDS

5595 Martinsburg VA Medical Center
Veterans Health Administration, U S Dept. of V A
Rr 9
Martinsburg, WV 25404
304-263-0811
800-827-1000
FAX: 304-262-7433
e-mail: g.vhacss@forum.va.gov
www.va.gov

Marilyn LaFreniere, Science Coordinator
Fernando Rivera, Director

5596 US Department Veterans Affairs Beckley Vet Center
101 Ellison Avenue
Beckley, WV 25801
304-252-8220
FAX: 304-254-8711
www.va.gov

Melody Friend, Director
Ron Johnson, Manager
Vet Center services includes individual and group readjustment counseling, referral for benefits assistance, liason with community agencies, marital and family counseling, substance abuse counseling, job counseling and referral, sexual trauma counseling, and community education.

Wisconsin

5597 Clement J Zablocki VA Medical Center
Veterans Health Administration U S Department of V
5000 W National Avenue
Milwaukee, WI 53295
414-384-2000
888-827-1000
FAX: 414-382-5319
www.va.gov

Glen W Grippn, Director
Glen Grippen, Chief Executive Officer

5598 Tomah VA Medical Center
Veterans Health Administration, U S Dept. of V A
500 E Veterans Street
Tomah, WI 54660
608-372-3971
800-827-1000
FAX: 608-372-1224
e-mail: g.vhacss@forum.va.gov
www.va.gov

Ronald J Sweeney, R and D Coordinator
Stan Johnson, Executive Director

5599 William S Middleton Memorial VA Hospital Center
Veterans Health Administration, U S Dept. of V A
2500 Overlook Ter
Madison, WI 53705
608-256-1901
800-827-1000
FAX: 608-280-7244
e-mail: g.vhacss@forum.va.gov
www.va.gov

Marvin G Rupp, Administrative Officer
Nathan Geraths, Executive Director

5600 Wisconsin VA Regional Office
Veterans Benefits Administration, U S Dept. of V A
5000 W National Avenue
Building 6
Milwaukee, WI 53295
414-384-2000
800-827-1000
FAX: 414-382-5374
e-mail: milwaukee.query@vba.va.gov
www.va.gov

Philip L Cook, Executive Director
Neil S Mandel, Research/Development Coordinator
Glen Grippen, Chief Executive Officer

Wyoming

5601 Cheyenne VA Medical Center
Veterans Health Administration, U S Dept. of V A
2360 E Pershing Boulevard
Cheyenne, WY 82001
307-778-7322
800-827-1000
FAX: 307-778-7531
e-mail: g.vhacss@forum.va.gov
www.va.gov

William Mcintyre, Research/Development Coordinator

5602 Sheridan VA Medical Center
Veterans Health Administration, U S Dept. of V A
1898 Fort Road
Sheridan, WY 82801
307-672-3473
800-827-1000
FAX: 307-672-1639
e-mail: g.vhacss@forum.va.gov
www.va.gov

Gary Morton, Executive Director

5603 Wyoming Veterans Centers
111 S Jefferson Street
Casper, WY 82601
307-266-3633
FAX: 307-261-5439
Veterans medical clinic offering disabled veterans medical treatments.

5604 Wyoming/Colorado VA Regional Office
Veterans Benefits Administration, U S Dept. of V A
155 Van Gordon Street
Lakewood, CO 80228
303-894-7474
800-827-1000
FAX: 303-894-7442
e-mail: denver.query@vba.va.gov
www.va.gov

E William Belz, Director

Alabama

5605 **Coffee County Training Center**
PO Box 311343
Enterprise, AL 36331
334-393-1732
FAX: 334-347-0252

Vickie Florence, Director
Clients 21 years and up receive training in Independent Living Skills, Self-Care, Language Skills, Learning, Self-Direction and Economic Self-Sufficiency. Transportation is also provided to clients of the center.

5606 **Easter Seal: Opportunity Center**
6300 McClellan Blvd
Anniston, AL 36202
206-820-9960
FAX: 256-820-9592
www.opportunitycenter.com
Work adjustment and remunerative work programs.

5607 **Easter Seals: Achievement Center**
Easter Seals of Alabama
510 W Thomason Circle
Opelika, AL 36801
334-745-3501
FAX: 334-749-5808
e-mail: info@achievement-center.org
www.achievement-center.org

Phil Raley, Administrator
Benita Gunnells, Administratives Services
Job placement programs, remunerative work services and work adjustment training programs. Clients must be at least 16 years old.

5608 **Employment Service Division: Alabama**
Department of Industrial Relations
649 Monroe Street
Room 2813
Montgomery, AL 36131
334-242-8007
FAX: 334-242-3960
e-mail: director@dir.alabama.us
www.dir.alabama.gov

Phyllis Kennedy, Director
Donald K Fisher, Assistant Director
Steve Horton, Director of Employment Services

5609 **Lakeshore Rehabilitation Facility**
3830 Ridgeway Drive
Po Box 59127
Birmingham, AL 35259
205-870-5999
800-441-7609
FAX: 205-879-2685

Paige Hebson, Administrator
Agency with several vocational and employment programs for rehabilitation.

5610 **Montezuma Day Treatment**
402 Academy Drive
Andalusia, AL 36420
334-222-8411

Lillian Dixon, Director
W Underwood, Executive Director
Individuals served in this program must be at least 21 years of age and have a primary diagnosis of mental retardation. Clients receive training in independent living skills, learning, self-direction and economic self-sufficiency. Special Olympic activities are also emphasized.

5611 **Thomasville Rehabilitation Center**
PO Box 1006
Thomasville, AL 36784
334-636-5421
800-335-3237
FAX: 334-636-5421
www.rehab.state.al.us
Offers work adjustment, evaluation and job rediness skills for people with disabilities.

5612 **Vocational Rehabilitation Service Opelika**
520 W Thomason Circle
Opelika, AL 36801
334-749-1259
800-671-6835
FAX: 334-749-8753
www.rehab.state.al.us

Patricia Floyd, Board Chairperson
James Myrick, Supervisor
Available through any of the 21 VRS offices statewide, services can include educational services, vocational assessment, evaluation and counseling, job training, assistive technology, orientation and mobility training and job placement.

5613 **Vocational Rehabilitation Service: Scottsboro**
203 South Market Street
Po Box 296
Scottsboro, AL 35768
256-574-5813
800-418-8823
FAX: 256-574-6033
www.rehab.state.al.us

Steded Shiders, Director
Mark Williams, Manager
Availiable through any of the 21 VRS offices statewide, services can include educational services, vocational assesment, evaluation and counseling, job training, assistive technology, orientation and mobility training and job placement.

5614 **Vocational Rehabilitation Service: Dothan**
795 Ross Clark Circle NE
Dothan, AL 36303
334-699-8600
800-275-0132
FAX: 334-792-1783
www.rehab.state.al.us

Wyndal Adams, Director
Availiable through any of the 21 VRS offices statewide, services can include educational services, vocational assesment, evaluation and counseling, job training, assistive technology, orientation and mobility training, and job placement.

5615 **Vocational Rehabilitation Service: Gadsden**
1100 George Wallace Drive
Gadsden, AL 35903
256-547-6974
800-671-6839
FAX: 256-543-1784
www.rehab.state.al.us

Connie Brechin, Supervisor
Availiable through any of the 21 VRS offices statewide, services can include educational services, vocational assesment, evaluation and counseling, job training, assistive technology, orientation and mobility training, and job placement.

5616 **Vocational Rehabilitation Service: Homewoo d**
236 Goodwin Crest Drive
Birmingham, AL 35209
205-290-4400
800-671-6837
FAX: 205-290-0486
www.rehab.state.al.us

Milton Moats, Building Administrator
Availiable through any of the 21 VRS offices statewide, services can include educational services, vocational assesment, evaluation and counseling, job training, assistive technology, orientation and mobility training, and job placement.

5617 **Vocational Rehabilitation Service: Huntsvi lle**
3000 Johnson Road SW
Huntsville, AL 35805
256-650-1700
800-671-6840
FAX: 256-650-1795
www.rehab.state.al.us

James Odom, Unit Supervisor
Steve Shivers, Commissioner
Available through any of the 21 VRS offices statewide, services can include educational services, vocational assesment, evaluation and counseling, job training, assistive technology, orientation and mobility training, and job placement.

5618 Vocational Rehabilitation Service: Jackson

1401 Forest Avenue
Jackson, AL 36545
334-246-5708
800-671-6836
FAX: 251-246-5224
www.rehab.state.al.us

Jean Stewart, Manager
Available through any of the 21 VRS offices statewide, services can include educational services, vocational assesment, evaluation and counseling, job training, assistive technology, orientation and mobility training, and job placement.

5619 Vocational Rehabilitation Service: Jasper

301 N Walston Bridge Road
Suite 116
Jasper, AL 35504
205-221-7840
800-671-6841
FAX: 205-221-1062
www.rehab.state.al.us

Steve Shivers, Commissioner
Angela Guire, Manager
Available through any of the 21 VRS offices statewide, services can include educational services, vocational assesment, evaluation and counseling, job training, assistive technology, orientation and mobility training, and job placement.

5620 Vocational Rehabilitation Service: Mobile

2419 Gordon Smith Drive
Mobile, AL 36617
251-479-8611
800-671-6842
FAX: 251-478-2197
www.rehab.state.al.us

James Brewer, Manager
Available through any of the 21 VRS offices statewide, services can include educational services, vocational assesment, evaluation and counseling, job training, assistive technology, orientation and mobility training, and job placement.

5621 Vocational Rehabilitation Service: Muscle Shoals

1450 East Avalon Avenue
Muscle Shoals, AL 35661
256-381-1110
800-275-0166
FAX: 256-389-3149
www.rehab.state.al.us

Stece Butler, Director
Available through any of the 21 VRS offices statewide, services can include educational services, vocational assessment, evaluation and counseling, job training, assistive technology, orientation and mobility training and job placement.

5622 Vocational Rehabilitation Service: Selma

2906 Citizens Parkway
Selma, AL 36701
334-872-8422
888-761-5995
FAX: 334-877-3796
www.rehab.state.al.us

Richard Weishaupt, Manager
Available through any of the 21 VRS offices statewide, services can include educational services, vocational assesment, evaluation and counseling, job training, assistive technology, orientation and mobility training, and job placement.

5623 Vocational Rehabilitation Service: Tallade ga

4 Medical Office Park
Talladega, AL 35160
256-362-1300
800-441-7592
FAX: 256-362-6387
www.rehab.state.al.us

Cayla Lackey, Manager
Availiable through any of the 21 VRS offices statewide, services can include educational services, vocational assesment, evaluation and counseling, job training, assistive technology, orientation and mobility training, and job placement.

5624 Vocational Rehabilitation Service: Troy

518 S Brundidge Street
Troy, AL 36081
334-566-2491
800-441-7608
FAX: 334-566-9415
www.rehab.state.al.us

Wendell Adams, Manager
Available through any of the 21 VRS offices statewide, services can include educational services, vocational assessment, evaluation and counseling, job training, assistive technology, orientation and mobility training, and job placement.

5625 Vocational Rehabilitation Service: Tuscalo osa

1305 37th Street East
Tuscaloosa, AL 35403
205-554-1300
800-331-5562
FAX: 205-554-1369
www.rehab.state.al.us

Kathy Reeves, Supervisor
Henry Devasher, Supervisor
Hank Vasher, Manager
Available through any of the 21 VRS offices statewide, services can include educational services, vocational assessment, evaluation and counseling, job training, assistive technology, orientation and mobility training, and job placement.

5626 Vocational Rehabilitation Services: Andalu sa

1082 Village Square Drive
1
Andalusia, AL 36420
334-222-4114
800-671-6833
FAX: 334-427-1216
www.rehab.state.al.us

Steve Shivers, Commissioner
Kathy Wyatt, Manager
Available through any of the 21 VRS offices statewide, services can include educational services, vocational assessment, evaluation and counseling, job training, assistive technology, orientation and mobility training, and job placement.

5627 Vocational Rehabilitation Services: Annist on

1105 Woodstock Avenue
Anniston, AL 36207
256-238-9300
800-671-6834
FAX: 256-231-4852
www.rehab.state.al.us

Robert Watson, Manager
Available through any of the 21 VRS offices statewide, services can include educational services, vocational assessment, evaluation and counseling, job training, assistive technology, orientation and mobility training, and job placement.

5628 Vocational and Rehabilitation Service Columbiana

Community Services Building
PO Box 856
Columbiana, AL 35051
205-669-3829
FAX: 205-669-0605
www.rehab.state.al.us

Available through any of the 21 VRS offices statewide, services can include educational services, vocational assessment, evaluation and counseling, job training, assistive technology, orientation and mobility training, and job placement.

5629 Vocational and Rehabilitation Service: Decatur

621 Cherry Street NE
Decatur, AL 35602
256-353-2754
800-671-6838
FAX: 256-351-2476
e-mail: kate@rehab.state.al.us
www.rehab.state.al.us

Steve Shivers, Director
Jim Harris III, Assistant Director
Available through any of the 21 VRS offices statewide, services can include educational services, vocational assessment, evaluation and counseling, job training, assistive technology, orientation and mobility training and job placement.

5630 **Vocational and Rehabilitation Services: Montgomery**
2129 East South Boulevard
Montgomery, AL 36116
334-288-0220
800-441-7578
FAX: 334-281-1388
TTY: 888-737-2032
e-mail: sshivers@rehab.state.al.us
www.rehab.state.al.us

Steve Shivers, President
Available through any of the 21 VRS offices statewide, services can include educational services, vocational assessment, evaluation and counseling, job training, assistive technology, orientation and mobility training and job placement.

5631 **Wiregrass Rehabilitation Center**
2694 S Park Avenue
Suite 1
Dothan, AL 36301
334-712-2720
FAX: 334-712-7632
www.wrcjobs.com

Hal Edwards, Chairman
Tom West, Vice Chairman
Susan Gilley, Manager
Provides remunerative work.

5632 **Workshops Inc.**
4244 3rd Avenue So.
Birmingham, AL 35222
205-592-9683
888-805-9683
FAX: 205-592-9687
e-mail: mail@workshopsinc.com
www.workshopsinc.com

Jim Crim, Executive Director
Shan Amerman, Director Client Services
Provides vocational training, sheltered employment and other support services to people with disabilities in central Alabama.

Alaska

5633 **Anchorage Job Training Center**
235 E 8th Avenue
Anchorage, AK 99501
907-334-2281
FAX: 907-334-2286
www.ci.anchorage.ak.us

Provides vocational training.

5634 **Employment Service: Alaska**
Alaska Department of Labor
PO Box 115512
Juneau, AK 99811
907-465-2790
FAX: 907-465-2797
labor.state.ak.us

Dan Travis, Executive Director
Providing safe and legal working conditions and advancing opportunities for employment.

5635 **Fair Employment Practice Agency**
Alaska State Commission for Human Rights
800 A Street
Suite 204
Anchorage, AK 99501
907-274-4692
800-478-4692
FAX: 907-276-3177
www.gov.state.ak.us/aschr/aschr.htm

Greg Maxwell, Manager

5636 **Vocational and Rehabilitation Agency**
801 W 10th Street
Suite A
Juneau, AK 99801
907-465-2814
800-478-2815
FAX: 907-465-2856
TTY: 907-465-2856
e-mail: gale_sinnott@labor.state.ak.us
www.labor.state.ak.us

Gale Finnott, Executive Director
Providing safe and legal working conditions and advancing opportunities for employment.

Arizona

5637 **Downtown Neighborhood Learning Center**
1001 W Jefferson Street
Phoenix, AZ 85007
602-256-0784
800-869-8521
FAX: 602-256-2524
e-mail: dnlc@swlink.net
www.swlink.net

Marcia R Newman, Executive Director
Mattie Johnson, Receptionist
Peg Osinski, El Mirage Learning Lab
Adult education agency providing basic skills, GED, ESOL, life skills, computer skills, resume assistance and career testing.

5638 **Fair Employment Practice Agency: Arizona**
Arizona Civil Rights Division
1275 W Washington Street
Phoenix, AZ 85007
602-542-5025
800-352-8431
FAX: 602-542-4085
www.azag.gov

Virginia Gonzales, Director
Bruna Pedrini, Manager
Provides legal advice to most state agencies. The office also investigates and prosecutes consumer fraud, white collar crime, organized crime, public corruption, and civil rights.

5639 **JOBS Administration Job Opportunities & Basic Skills**
1717 W Jefferson Street
Phoenix, AZ 85007
602-542-9596
FAX: 602-542-5171

Gretchen Evans, Program Administrator
Assist applicants and recipients of temporary assistance to needy families to obtain job training and employment that will lead to economic independence.

5640 **TETRA Corporation**
308 W Glenn Street
Tucson, AZ 85705
520-622-4874

Steven King, President
Work hardening and disciplinary programs.

5641 **Vocational and Rehabilitation Agency Rehabilitation Services Administrations**
Division of Employment & Rehabilitation Services
1789 W Jefferson Street
Phoenix, AZ 85007
602-542-4910
800-563-1221
800-563-1221
FAX: 602-542-3778
TTY:602-542-6049
e-mail: tazrsa@azdes.gov
www.azdes.gov/rsa

Jozef De Groot, Manager Program Services
Greg Warren, Administrator
Moises Gallegos, Manager
This program serves individuals with disabilities seeking jobs and job training.

5642 **Yavapai Regional Medical Center-West**
1003 Willow Creek Road
Prescott, AZ 86301
928-445-2700
877-843-9762
FAX: 928-445-0994

Bradley Newman, Executive Director

Widely recognized for the quality and success of the physical, occupational, and speech therapy programs it offers. Provides a wide range of programs and services that enable our patients to reach their maximum level of function and independence- and enjoy the highest possible quality of life.

Arkansas

5643 Arkansas Employment Service Agency and Job Training Program
Arkansas Employment Security Department
PO Box 2981
Little Rock, AR 72203
501-682-2121
FAX: 501-682-2273
www.arkansas.gov/esd

Artee Williams, Director
Wide range of services including employment services, unemployment insurance, and labor market information.

5644 Easter Seal Work Center
11801 Fairview Road
Little Rock, AR 72212
501-221-1063
e-mail: mail@ar.easterseals.com
www.ar.easterseals.com

Lauren Zilk, Administrator
Mission is to provide exceptional services to ensure that all people with disabilities or special needs have equal opportunities to live,learn work and play in their communities.

5645 VCT/A Job Retention Skill Training Program
Arkasas Rehab Services
PO Box 1358
Hot Springs, AR 71902
501-624-4411
FAX: 501-624-0019

Barbara Lewis, Administrator
Mae Robinson, Assistant Administrator
A training program designed for use in rehabilitation and educational settings. Using a social skill training strategy, VCT helps participants learn how to solve on-the-job problems and cope with common supervisory demands.

5646 Vocational and Rehabilitation Agency Division of Services for the Blind
700 Main Street
Little Rock, AR 72201
501-682-5463
800-960-9270
FAX: 501-682-0366
TTY: 501-682-0093
e-mail: jim.hudson@mail.state.ar.us
www.state.ar.us

Lyndel Lybarger, Field Adminstrator
James Hudson, Executive Director

5647 Vocational and Rehabilitation Agency for Persons Who Are Visually Impaired
Arkansas Department of Human Services
PO Box 3237
Little Rock, AR 72203
501-682-5463
800-960-9270
TTY:501-324-9271
e-mail: arkblind@edu.gte.net

James C Hudson, Executive Director
Furnishes a wide variety of services to help people with disabilities return to work.

California

5648 ARC-Adult Vocational Program
1500 Howard Street
San Francisco, CA 94103
415-255-7200
FAX: 415-255-9488
e-mail: info@thearcsanfrancisco.org
www.thearcsanfrancisco.org

Patricia Kemerling, Executive Director
Job placement programs, remunerative work services and work adjustment training programs.

5649 Ability First
3770 E Willow Street
Long Beach, CA 90815
562-426-6161
FAX: 562-426-6148
www.abilityfirst.org

Michael Lande
Barbara Schlosser, Manager
Job placement programs, remunerative work services and work adjustment training programs.

5650 Bakersfield Association for Retarded Citizens
B AR C
2240 S Union Avenue
Bakersfield, CA 93307
661-834-2272
FAX: 661-834-9813
e-mail: barc@barc-inc.org
www.barc-inc.org

Jim Baldwin, President
Employment training & placement.

5651 California Department of Fair Employment & Housing
2000 O Street
Suite 120
Sacramento, CA 95814
916-324-4244
800-884-1684
FAX: 916-323-6092
www.dfeh.ca.gov

Suzanne M Ambrose, Director
David Supkofl, Manager
Mission is to protect the people of California from unlawful discrimination in employment, housing, and public accomodations, and from the perpetration of acts of hate violence.

5652 Career Connection Transition Program
Whittier High School District
9401 Painter Avenue
Whittier, CA 90605
562-698-8121
FAX: 562-693-4414
e-mail: Richard.Rosenberg@wuhsd.k12.ca.us
www.wuhsd.k12.ca.us

Richard L Rosenberg PhD, Vocational Coordinator
Bonnie Bolton, Transition Department Head
Job placement programs, remunerative work services and work adjustment training programs. Transition services.

5653 Career Development Program (CDP)
260 W Grand Avenue
Escondido, CA 92025
760-738-0277
FAX: 760-741-9452

Richard Brady MD
Wendy Hope, Supported Employment
Jill Hennessy, Independent Living
Work hardening and disciplinary programs.

5654 Colton Redlands-Yucaipa Regional Occupational Programs
1214 Indian Court
Redlands, CA 92374
909-793-3115
FAX: 909-793-6901
www.cryrop.org

Stephanie Houston, Superintendent
Sandra Moritensen, Coord. Of Special Needs Services
Kit Alvarez, Director Of Educational Services
Provides quality hands-on training programs in over 40 high demand career fields to assist high school students and adults in acquiring marketable job skills. Works in cooperation with local high schools, adult education colleges, and employers providing a collaborative team of academic and ROP occupational teachers who integrate academic and vocational competencies to provide sequenced paths within career majors. Support services, career guidance and services are provided to disabled people.

5655 Community Outpatient Rehabilitation Center
1925 E Dakota Avenue
Suite 120a
Fresno, CA 93726
559-459-1842
FAX: 559-459-1004
www.communitymedical.org

Andrew Robertson, Chief Medical Officer
Jan-Erik Paris, Manager
Physical, occupational and speech therapy, neuropsychology services available for orthopedic and neurological diagnosis. Lymphedema program.

5656 Desert Haven Enterprises
43437 Copeland Circle
Po Box 2119
Lancaster, CA 93539
661-948-8402
FAX: 661-948-1080
www.deserthaven.org

Roy Williams
Jennie Moran, Manager
Work adjustment and remunerative work programs.

5657 Do-It-Leisure: Work Training Center
3760 Morrow Lane
Suite S
Chico, CA 95928
530-343-6055
FAX: 530-343-4619
e-mail: doitl@ewtc.org
www.wtcinc.org

Carl Ochsner, Executive Director
Ken Steidley, President
Therapeutic recreation programs providing a wide variety of services designed to meet individual needs with specialized, transitional or integrated activities.

5658 ESS Work Center
858 Stanton Road
Burlingame, CA 94010
650-692-3377
FAX: 650-692-9684

Jerry Martin, Executive Director
Work adjustment and remunerative work programs.

5659 Employment Service: California
Employment Development Department
800 Capitol Mall
MIC 83
Sacramento, CA 95814
916-653-0707

Provides job listings and unemployment listings for all.

5660 Feather River Industries
1811 Kusel Road
Oroville, CA 95966
530-534-1112
FAX: 530-534-3137
www.featherriverindustries.com

Randy Guild, Rehabilitation Counselor
Dave Ennes, Manager
Vocational training for persons with developmental disabilities provided through wood products fabrication and assembly tasks. Instructor to trainer rating ranging from 1 to 12, 1 to 8, 1 to 6, and 1 to 4 depending on individual needs and complexity of tasks.

5661 Fit to Work
3581 Palmer Drive
Suite 401
Cameron Park, CA 95682
530-676-7485
FAX: 530-676-9114

Jennifer Roach
Provides remunerative work.

5662 Fresno City College: Disabled Students Programs and Services
Fresno City College
1101 E University Avenue
Fresno, CA 93741
559-442-4600
FAX: 559-485-7304
e-mail: janice.emerzian@fresnocitycollege.edu
www.fresnocitycollege.com

Ned Doffoney, President
Dr Janice Emerzian Ed D, District Director
This program offers services to students with physical, learning and/or psychological disabilities beyond those provided by conventional Fresno City College Programs and enables students to successfully pursue their individual educational, vocational and personal goals.

5663 Heartland Opportunity Center
323 N E Street
Madera, CA 93638
559-674-8828
FAX: 559-674-8857
www.heartlandopportunity.com

Robert J Hand, Director
Job placement programs, remunerative work services and work adjustment training programs.

5664 Hollister Workshop
Hope Rehabilitation Services
2300 Technology Parkway
Suite 7
Hollister, CA 95023
831-637-8283
FAX: 831-637-8726

Kristi Alarid, Executive Director
Work adjustment and remunerative work programs.

5665 Job Training Program Liaison: California
Employment Development Department
800 Capitol Mall
Sacramento, CA 95814
916-654-8210
800-300-5616
FAX: 916-654-9072
www.edd.ca.gov

Patrick Henning, Director
Provides information on filing an Unemployment Insurance or Disability Insurance claim, on-line job and resume bank which boasts thousands of job openings.

5666 King's Rehabilitation Center
PO Box 719
Hanford, CA 93232
559-582-9234
FAX: 559-582-1182
www.kingsrehab.com

Carol A Rogers, Executive Director
Sherrie Martin, Director Human Resources
To enhance the lives of adults with developmental disabilites and other disabilities by providing employment opportunitites, vocational training and recognizing the individuals importance and involvement in our community.

5667 Konocti Industries: People Services
4195 Lakeshore Boulevard
Lakeport, CA 95453
707-263-3810
FAX: 707-263-0552
e-mail: peopleservices@mindspring.com
www.peopleservices.org

Hank Montgomery
Ilene Dumont, Executive Director
Work hardening and disciplinary programs.

5668 **Morongo Basin Work Activity Center**

74325 Joe Davis Drive
Twentynine Palms, CA 92277 760-366-8474

Sheree Fraser
Job placement programs, remunerative work services and work adjustment training programs.

5669 **Mother Lode Rehabilitation Enterprises**

399 Placerville Drive
Placerville, CA 95667 530-622-4848
FAX: 530-622-0204
e-mail: susiedavis@morerehab.org
www.morerehab.org

Susie Davies, Executive Director
A private, non-profit organization dedicated to supporting persons with disabilities. MORE was established by a group of parents, educators, rehabilitation professionals and concerned citizens and first began serving adults with disabilities in 1973.

5670 **NCI Affiliates**

1434 Chestnut Street
Paso Robles, CA 93446 805-238-6630
FAX: 805-239-9073
e-mail: info@nciaffiliates.org
www.nciaffiliates.org

Crystal Nevosh, Executive Director
Provides independent living skills and vocational training to people with disabilities.

5671 **Napa Valley PSI Inc.**

PO Box 600
Napa, CA 94559 707-255-0177
FAX: 707-255-0802

Jeanne Fauquet, President
Work adjustment, work training and educational services for developmentally disabled adults. Emphasis is on manufacture of quality wood products, primarily wooden office furniture.

5672 **Oakland Work Activity Area**

6315 San Leandro Street
Oakland, CA 94621 510-639-9350

Greg Whalley
Dennis Scharssenberg, Manager
Job placement programs, remunerative work services and work adjustment training programs.

5673 **Opportunities for the Handicapped**

3340 Marysville Boulevard
Sacramento, CA 95838 916-925-3522

Kathy Dodd
Work adjustment and remunerative work programs.

5674 **Orange County ARC**

225 W Carl Karcher Way
Anaheim, CA 92801 714-744-5301
FAX: 714-744-5312
e-mail: info@orangecountyarc.org
orangecountyarc.org

Joyce Hearn, Chief Executive Officer
Provides remunerative work through both site and community placements.

5675 **PRIDE Industries**

10030 Foothills Boulevard
Roseville, CA 95747 916-788-2100
800-550-6005
FAX: 916-788-2552
e-mail: info@prideindustries.com
www.prideindustries.com

Michael Ziegler, President
Rosemary Elston, Services Manager
Roxanne Snyder, Employment Services Manager
Vocational rehabilitation and employment services creating jobs for people with disabilites; services include career counseling, vocational assessment, work adjustment, work services, job seeking skills, job development, job placement, on-the-job support (coaching), mentoring, independent living skills, transition services and case management.

5676 **Parents And Friends, Inc**

350 Cypress St.
Fort Bragg, CA 95437 707-964-4940
FAX: 707-964-8536
e-mail: rmoon@parentsand friends.org
www.parentsandfriends.org

Rick Moon, Executive Director
Terry Scott, Controller
Vocational Services provides opportunities for persons with developmental challenges and similar needs to participate fully in our community.

5677 **Pomona Valley Workshop**

4650 Brooks Street
Montclair, CA 91763 909-624-3555
FAX: 909-624-5675
www.pvwonline.org

Karen Jones, Executive Director
Assisting adults with disabilities reach their potential in vocational and socialization skills in order that they may achieve their highest level of employment and comminity integration in work program, supported employment Services, adult devopmental center and senior services.

5678 **Porterville Sheltered Workshop**

187 W Olive Avenue
Porterville, CA 93257 559-784-1399
FAX: 559-781-5651
e-mail: info@pswrehab.com
www.pswrehab.com

Nick Brown
Steve Tree, Executive Director
Work adjustment and remunerative work programs. Mission is to assist disabled individuals achieve a more independent and productive life.

5679 **Project Independence Supported Employment**

3505 Cadillac-Suite P-101
Costa Mesa, CA 92626 714-549-3464
FAX: 714-549-3559
e-mail: pop.mpowercom.net
www.P-I.org

Andrea Erickson, Executive Director
Tim Chervenak, Associate Director
Kristen Cook, Manager
Provides remunerative work. To promote the community integration of adults with developmental disabilities and to create services which expand their opportunities for personal freedom and choice.

5680 **Sacramento Vocational Services**

6950 21st Avenue
Sacramento, CA 95820 916-381-1300
FAX: 916-381-6548

Diane De Rodeff, Director
Work hardening and disciplinary programs.

5681 **San Francisco Vocational Services**

814 Mission Street
Suite 600
San Francisco, CA 94103 415-512-9500
FAX: 415-512-9507
e-mail: sfvs@sfvocational.org
www.sfvocationalservices.org

Robert Campbell, Executive Director
Jeffrey Faircloth, Manager Case Management

Comprehensive vocational rehabilitation center offering vocational evaluation, rehabilitative counseling, business office training, work experience, and job placement.

5682 Shasta County Opportunity Center
1265 Redwood Boulevard
Redding, CA 96003 530-225-5781
FAX: 530-225-5751
e-mail: info@oppcenter.org
www.co.shasta.ca.us

Jane Patterson, Program Manager
An employment training program for people with disabilities in Shasta County. These individuals perform paid work in a number of different work environments and at the same time learn the skills necessary to obtain competetive employment in the local community.

5683 Social Vocational Services
350 Crenshaw Boulevard
Suite A104
Torrance, CA 90503 310-783-0633
FAX: 310-944-3304
e-mail: nto@svsinc.org
www.svsinc.org

Dale Dutton Md, Executive Director
Dan Strohm, Manager
The leading provider of services for people with developmental disabilities in the state of California

5684 South Bay Vocational Center
1526 240th Street
Harbor City, CA 90710 310-784-2032
FAX: 310-539-6342
www.sbvc1.com

Corey Sylve, President/Chief Executive Office
Clare Grey, Vice President/COO
A not-for-profit organization that was founded in 1952. Mission is to provide vocational training, advocacy, counseling, and opportunities for individuals with disabilities.

5685 Tri-County Independent Living Center
955 Myrtle Avenue
Eureka, CA 95501 707-445-8404
877-576-5000
FAX: 707-445-9751
www.tililig.org

Chris Jones, Executive Director
To provide programs, services and information for people with disabilities living in Humboldt, Del Norte and Trinity Counties in northern California in an effort to allow choices for individuals to optimize their independence.

5686 Tulare County Training Center Able Industries
8127 Avenue
Visalia, CA 93291 559-651-8150
FAX: 559-651-0357
www.ableindustries.org

Robert Stephenson
Established in 1962 by parents of individuals with disabilities who joined together to provide paid work and training opportunities for their adult children.

5687 Unyeway
2330 Main Street
Suite E
Ramona, CA 92065 760-789-5960

Hank Newman, Director
Kim Metli, Executive Director
Job placement programs, remunerative work services and work adjustment training programs.

5688 V-Bar Enterprises
720 Gordon Circle
Suisun City, CA 94585 707-864-1334

Lu Brunet
Job placement programs, remunerative work services and work adjustment training programs.

5689 Valley Light Industries
822 N Grand Avenue
Covina, CA 91724 626-331-9966

Gary Miller
Provides remunerative work.

5690 Visalia Workshop
2544 E Valley Oaks Drive
Visalia, CA 93292 559-734-1964

Hortensia Venegas
Work hardening and disciplinary programs.

5691 Westside Opportunity Workshop
9503 Jefferson Boulevard
Culver City, CA 90232 310-838-0521

Edward Oritz
Anthony Vande Wydeven OD, Manager
Job placement programs, remunerative work services and work adjustment training programs.

5692 Work Training Center for the Handicapped
2255 Fair Street
Chico, CA 95928 530-343-7994
FAX: 530-343-4619
www.wtcinc.org

Barrie Dyer
Lee Laney, Manager
A non-profit organization governed by a local Board of Directors, we are dedicated to meeting the training, vocational, and recreational needs of local adults with disabilities.

5693 Work Training Programs
9430 Topanga Canyon Boulevard
Suite 103
Chatsworth, CA 91311 818-773-9570
FAX: 818-885-0816
www.wtpinc.org

Stephen Miller
Established in 1964 to provide job training and job placement services to people who require special assistance. Today, we provide a wide range of residential, day program, and employment services from building social skills, to providing the supports necessary to maintain true independence for a lifetime.

Colorado

5694 Cheyenne Village
6275 Lehman Drive
Colorado Springs, CO 80918 719-592-0200
FAX: 719-548-9947
www.cheyennevillage.org

Ann Turner, Executive Director
Residential and employment programs for adults with developmental disabilities.

5695 Colorado Civil Rights Divsion
1560 Broadway
Suite 1050
Denver, CO 80202 303-894-7855
800-262-4845
FAX: 303-894-7885
e-mail: ccrd@dora.state.co.us
www.dora.state.co.us

Wendell Pryer, Division Director
Virginia Butler, Commissioner
Nancy Snow, Housing Specialist
Fair employment practices agency for Colorado. Accepts and investigates charges of discrimination. Does outreach, alternative dispute resolution and technical training in discrimination laws.

5696 **Colorado Employment Service**
Department of Labor and Employment
600 Grant Street
Suite 900
Denver, CO 80203 303-813-2800

Job placement programs, remunerative work services and work adjustment training programs.

5697 **Developmental Training Services**
1401 Oak Creek Grade Road
Canon City, CO 81212 719-275-4504

Roger Jensen, President
Linda Davis, Administrator
Residential and employment programs for adults with developmental disabilities.

5698 **Dynamic Dimensions**
567th 18 Street
Burlington, CO 80807 719-346-5367
FAX: 719-346-6010

Cheryl Reese, Executive Director
Vocational, evaluation and assessment, training and placement for most disabilities. Group homes and day programs for the developmentally disabled.

5699 **Gray Street Workcenter**
5685 Gray Street
Arvada, CO 80002 303-422-1305
FAX: 303-467-2793

Shelley Richardson, Executive Director
Tammy Drumright, Manager
Residental and employment programs for adults with developmental disabilities.

5700 **Hope Center**
3400 Elizabeth Street
Denver, CO 80205 303-388-4801
FAX: 303-388-0249
e-mail: gghope@qwest.net
www.hopecenterinc.org

George Brantley, Executive Director
A community-based agency dedicated to meeting the needs of individuals with developmental disabilities, developmental delays and persons in need of specialized educational or vocational services.

5701 **Imagine: Innovative Resources for Cognitive & Physical Challenges**
1400 Dixon Street
Lafayette, CO 80026 303-665-7789
FAX: 303-665-2648
e-mail: caroline@imaginecolorado.org
www.imaginecolorado.org

John Taylor, Executive Director
Caroline Siegfried, Executive Assistant
Creating and offering innovative supports to people of all ages with cognitive, developmental, physical and health related needs, so they may live lives of independence and quality in their homes and communities.

5702 **Las Animas County Rehabilitation Center**
1205 Congress Drive
Po Box 781
Trinidad, CO 81082 719-846-3388
FAX: 719-846-4543
www.scdds.com

Duane Roy, Executive Director
Job placement programs, remunerative work services and work adjustment training programs.

5703 **NORESCO Workshop**
903 E Burlington Avenue
Fort Morgan, CO 80701 970-867-5702

Robert Duffield
Nancy Study, Manager
Provides remunerative work.

5704 **Regional Assessment and Training Center**
3520 W Oxford Avenue
Denver, CO 80236 303-866-7253

Russell Porter, Executive Director
Work adjustment and renumerative work programs.

5705 **Sedgwick County Workshop**
113 Elm Street
Julesburg, CO 80737 970-474-2446

Robert Christiansen
Maria Contreras, Manager
Provides remunerative work.

5706 **Valley Industries**
330 State Avenue
Alamosa, CO 81101 719-589-3123

Tim Johnson, Executive Director
Provides remunerative work.

5707 **Vocational and Rehabilitation Agency**
2211 W Evans Avenue
Unit B
Denver, CO 80223 303-866-4150
FAX: 720-884-1213
TTY:720-884-1234
e-mail: diana.huerta@state.co.us
www.cdhs.state.co.us
Purpose is to assist eligible individuals with disabilities to become productive members of the Colorado workforce and to live independently.

5708 **Yuma County Workshop**
710 E 2nd Avenue
Yuma, CO 80759 970-848-3011

Robert Stephens
Andrea Anderson, Manager
Provides remunerative work.

Connecticut

5709 **Area Cooperative Educational Services (ACES)**
350 State Street
North Haven, CT 06473 203-498-6885
FAX: 203-498-6890
e-mail: acesinfo@aces.k12.ct.us
www.aces.k12.ct.us

Craig W Edmondson, Executive Director
Regional Educational Service Center providing high quality educational services in the south central Connecticut region.

5710 **Central Connecticut Association For Retarted Citizens Inc. (CCARC)**
950 Slater Road
New Britain, CT 06053 860-229-6665
FAX: 860-826-6883
www.ccarc.com

Julie Erickson, Day Service Director
Gina Palmieri, Manager
Supported employment, work services, habilitation services, advocacy, recreation and residential services.

5711 **Cheshire Occupational and Career Center**
615 W Johnson Avenue
Suite 3
Cheshire, CT 06410 203-272-5607
FAX: 203-272-4284
www.cocoofcheshire.com

Peter Mason
Linda Fallon, Executive Director
Work adjustment and remunerative work programs.

5712 **Community Enterprises**
29 Bloomfield Avenue
Po Box 176
Windsor, CT 06095 860-688-7918
FAX: 860-688-5599
www.communityenterprises.com

Susan Cauley, VP Operations
Angela Daley, Executive Director
Provide supported education services in a community college setting; supported employment including job training, placement and follow-up; transitional services from group homes and other settings to supported living within the community.

5713 **Connecticut Governor's Committee on Employment of Disabled Persons**
200 Folly Brook Boulevard
Wethersfield, CT 06109 860-566-5505
FAX: 860-263-6039
Work adjustment and remunerative work programs.

5714 **Constructive Workshops**
24 Willow Street
East Hartford, CT 06118 860-569-1410
FAX: 860-895-1168

Sandie Lavoy, Coordinator
Work adjustment and remunerative work programs.

5715 **Fotheringhay Farms**
84 Waterhole Road
Colchester, CT 06415 860-267-4463
FAX: 860-267-7628

Wesley Martins, Executive/Medical Director
Job placement programs, remunerative work services and work adjustment training programs.

5716 **George Hegyi Industrial Training Center**
5 Coon Hollow Road
Derby, CT 06418 203-735-8727

Joan Bucci, Executive Director
Work adjustment and remunerative work programs.

5717 **Greater Enfield Association of Retarded Citizens**
3 Pearson Way
Enfield, CT 06082 860-763-0192

Dean Wem
Work hardening and disciplinary programs.

5718 **Kennedy Center**
2440 Reservoir Avenue
Trumbull, CT 06611 203-365-8522
FAX: 203-365-8533
e-mail: mschwartz@kennedyctr.org
www.thekennedycenterinc.org

Martin D Schwartz, President/CEO
Provides vocational rehabilitation, job training and job placement services to 1,000 adults with disabilities including mental retardation, traumatic brain injury, psychiatric disabilities and more. Residential services, well integrated within the community, serve 97 individuals on a daily basis. Children's programs provide support to 85 children age birth to three, in addition to after hours and recreation programs to appromxately 100 school age children. Staff size is presently 450 employees.

5719 **Quaezar**
2480 Black Rock Tpke
Suite 8
Fairfield, CT 06825 203-339-3476
FAX: 203-377-6144

William J Sedarweck, President
Agency for adult mentally retarded/autistic people providing residential care in a group home or apartment setting. Also provides placement in community employment.

5720 **TEAM Vocational Program**
227 Elm Street
W Haven, CT 06516 203-934-5221
FAX: 203-937-9052

Peter Schwartz, Executive Director
Hannah Carlson, DD Director
Provides remunerative work, vocational training, supported employment, and supportive services. Residential program including group living and supervised apartment, social club.

5721 **Valley Memorial Health Center**
435 E Main Street
Ansonia, CT 06401 203-736-2905

Marilyn Cormack, President
Provides remunerative work.

5722 **Vocational and Rehabilitation Agency**
184 Windsor Avenue
Windsor, CT 06095 860-602-4000
800-842-4510
FAX: 860-602-4020
e-mail: Besb@po.state.ct.us
www.ct.gov/bestb/site/default.asp

Alan Sylvestre, Chairman
Eileen Akers, Requests Correspondence In Brail
Keith Maynard, Plant Manager
Mission is to provide quality educational and rehabilitative services to all people who are legally blind or deaf/blind and children who are visually impaired at no cost to our clients or their families.

5723 **Vocational and Rehabilitation Agency: State Department of Social Services**
Department of Social Services
25 Sigourney Street
Hartford, CT 06106 860-424-4908
800-842-1508
FAX: 860-424-4850
TTY: 8004244839
e-mail: brs.dss@po.state.ct.us
www.dss.state.ct.us

Brenda Moore, Executive Director
Patricia Wilson-Coker, Manager
Provides a broad range of services to the elderly, disabled, families, and individuals who need assistance in maintaining or achieving their full potential for self-direction, self-reliance and independent living.

Delaware

5724 **Delaware Division of Vocational Rehabilitation- Department of Labor**
PO Box 9969
Wilmington, DE 19809 302-761-8275
FAX: 302-761-6611
www.delawareworks.com

Andrea Guest, Director
Cynthia Fairwell, Program Specialist
James Cagle, Manager
Provides opportunities and resources to eligible individuals with disabilities leading to success in employment and independent living.

5725 **Delaware Fair Employment Practice Agency**
Delaware Department of Labor
820 N French Street
Suite 6
Wilmington, DE 19801 302-577-5050

Karen Gimbutas, Vice President
Provides opportunities and resources to eligible individuals with disabilities leading to success in employment and independent living.

5726 **Delaware Job Training Program Liaison**
Division of Employment & Training
PO Box 9828
Wilmington, DE 19809 302-761-8085

Harold Stafford, Manager
Work adjustment and remunerative work programs. Also offers career guidance, supported employment, work readiness and job placement.

5727 **Opportunity Center**
3030 Bowers Street
Wilmington, DE 19802 302-762-0300
800-738-1733
FAX: 302-762-8797
e-mail: csterling@ourpeplework.com
www.ourpeoplework.org

Bob Lennon, Director Community Development
Cindy Sterling, Director Employment Services
Cathie Lloyd, Executive Director
Work adjustment and remunerative work programs. Also offers career guidance, supported employment, work readiness and job placement.

District of Columbia

5728 **Davis Memorial Goodwill Industries**
2200 S Dakota Avenue NE
Washington, DC 20018 202-636-4225
888-817-4323
FAX: 202-526-3994
www.tcgoodwill.org

Catherine Melloy, President/CEO
Offers vocational training, job training, sheltered employment and work experience.

5729 **District of Columbia Department of Employment Services**
609 H Street NE
Washington, DC 20002 202-724-7000
FAX: 202-698-4817
www.does.ci.washington.dc.us

Gottlieb Simon, Executive Director
Linda W Cropp, Chairperson
To foster economic development and growth in the District of Columbia by providing workforce training, bringing together job seekers and employers, compensating unemployed and injured workers and promoting safe and healthy workplaces.

5730 **District of Columbia Dept. of Employment Services: Office of Workforce Development**
64 New York Ave NW
Washington, DC 20001 202-393-5051
877-319-7346
FAX: 202-673-6774
e-mail: diana.johnson@dc.gov
www.does.dc.gov

Diana C Johnson, Public Information Officer
Marianna Lourenco, Specialist/ADA Coordinator
To foster economic development and growth in the District of Columbia by providing workforce training, bringing together job seekers and employers, compensating unemployed and injured workers and promoting safe and healthy workplaces.

5731 **District of Columbia Fair Employment Practice Agencies**
D C Office of Human Rights
441 4th Street NW
Suite 570 N.
Washington, DC 20009 202-727-4559
www.ohr.washingtondc.gov

Elizabeth Noel, Executive Director
Investigations and discrimination complaints.

5732 **Green Door**
1623 16th Street NW
Washington, DC 20009 202-222-0232
FAX: 202-462-7562
e-mail: gdiadmin@aol.com
www.greendoor.org

Judith Johnson, Executive Director
Brenda Randall, Assistant Director
Green Door is a community program which prepares people with a severe and persistent mental illness to live and work independently. Since 1976, Green Door has provided comprehensive services to mentally ill people, including housing, job training, job placement, education, homeless outreach, case management, support for people with substance abuse problems, family support,and specialized help for people who have had repeated hospitalizations.

5733 **Operation Job Match**
National Multiple Sclerosis Society
1800 M Street NW
Suite 750
Washington, DC 20006 202-296-5363
FAX: 202-296-3425
e-mail: swnissen@aol.com
www.operationjobmatch.org

Steven Nissen, Program Director
Jeanne Angulo, Executive Director
Job readiness program for individuals with adult-onset physical disabilities.

5734 **Rehabilitation Services Administration**
810 1st Street NE
10th Floor
Washington, DC 20002 202-442-8400
FAX: 202-442-8742
www.dc.gov

Elizabeth Parker, Administrator
State Rehabilitation Agency providing services to eligible persons with disabilities.

5735 **WAVE Work, Achievement, Value, & Education**
525 School Street SW
Suite 500
Washington, DC 20024 202-484-0103
800-274-2005
FAX: 202-488-7595
e-mail: wave4kids@aol.com
www.waveinc.org

Larry Brown, President
J Taylor, Senior Vice President
Job placement programs, remunerative work services and work adjustment training programs for 18 and 21 years of age in many cities across the country including Drop-Out Recovery Programs and Drop-Out Prevention Programs. Programs also available for youth ages 12-18. Youth Professionals Development and Training and key aspects of WAVE services, as well.

Florida

5736 **Abilities of Florida: An Affiliate of Service Source**
2735 Whitney Road
Clearwater, FL 33760
727-538-7370
FAX: 727-538-7387
e-mail: abilities@ourpeoplework.org
www.ourpeoplework.org

Rhonda Abbott, VP Rehabilitation Services
Lori Simpson, Manager
Provides a full range of employment services including work evaulation, training, job coaching, job placement, advocacy and education. Also provides housing assistance and specialized to adults with cystic fibrosis.

5737 **Career Assessment & Planning Services**
Goodwill Industries- Suncoast Incorporated
10596 Gandy Boulevard
St Petersburg, FL 33702
727-523-1512
FAX: 727-563-9300
e-mail: gw.marketing@goodwillhisuncoast.com
www.goodwill-suncoast.org

Chris Ward, Marketing Manager
Jill Flansburg, Career Assessment/Planning Coord
Career assessment and planning services help determine how prepared an individual is for employment, training, or future education. It is a comprehensive assessment that can predict current and future employment and potential adjustment factors for physically, emotionally or developmentally disabled persons who may be unemployed or underemployed.

5738 **Choices for Work Program**
Goodwill Industries-Suncoast
10596 Gandy Boulevard N
St Petersburg, FL 33702
727-523-1512
888-279-1988
FAX: 727-563-9300
e-mail: gw.marketing@goodwill-suncoast.com
www.goodwill-suncoast.org

Lee Waits, President
Assisting individuals currently eligible for Workman's Compensation, this program allows those recovering from injury on the job to prepare to return to independent employment, either through increasing ability and confidence in using adaptive behaviors and/or equipment to return to related employment, or adjusting to a more compatible employment environment.

5739 **Florida Division of Vocational Rehabilitation**
2002 Old Saint Augustine Road
Building A
Tallahassee, FL 32301
850-245-3399
800-451-4327
FAX: 813-873-4773
www.rehabworks.org

Renee Dominic, Librarian
Rehabilitation services are important when a physical or mental handicap interferes with your ability to work. Our purpose is to help prepare for, and return to, gainful employment.

5740 **Florida Fair Employment Practice Agency**
Florida Commission on Human Relations
2009 Apalachee Parkway
Suite 100
Tallahassee, FL 32301
850-488-7082
FAX: 850-488-5291
e-mail: fchrinfo!fchr.myflorida.com
www.fchr.state.fl.us

The Commission is the state agency charged with enforcing the state's civil rights laws and serves as a resource on human relations for the people of Florida.

5741 **Goodwill Industries-Suncoast Adult Day Training**
10596 Gandy Boulevard
St Petersburg, FL 33702
727-523-1512
888-279-1988
FAX: 727-563-9300
e-mail: gw.marketing@goodwill-suncoast.com
www.goodwill-suncoast.org

Chris Ward, Marketing Manager
Kathy Roegiers, Program Manager
Goodwill's adult day training programs enable people with developmental disabilities to set and achieve personal goals within a work-like setting. Participants work at various jobs throughout Goodwill and engage in a variety of activities that will allow them to become more self-sufficients.

5742 **Goodwill Industries-Suncoast Inc. Adult Day Training**
3033 Drane Field Rd.
Suite 5
Lakeland, FL 33811
863-701-1351
888-279-1988
FAX: 727-563-9300
e-mail: gw.marketing@goodwill-suncoast.com
www.goodwill-suncoast.org

Chris Ward, Marketing Manager
Lori Reed, Site Manager
Goodwill's adult day training programs enable people with developmental disabilities to set and achieve personal goals within a work-like setting. Participants work at various jobs throughout Goodwill and engage in a variety of activities that will allow them to become more self-sufficients.

5743 **Goodwill Industries-Suncoast Inc. Adult Day Training**
7601 Park Blvd
Pinellas Park, FL 33781
727-523-1512
888-279-1988
FAX: 727-563-9300
e-mail: gw.marketing@goodwill-suncoast.com
www.goodwill-suncoast.org

Chris Ward, Marketing Manager
Kathy Roegiers, Program Manager
Goodwill's adult day training programs enable people with developmental disabilities to set and achieve personal goals within a work-like setting. Participants work at various jobs throughout Goodwill and engage in a variety of activities that will allow them to become more self-sufficients.

5744 **Goodwill Industries-Suncoast Non-Residenti al Supports And Services Program**
10596 Gandy Boulevard
St Petersburg, FL 33702
727-523-1512
FAX: 727-563-9300
e-mail: gw.marketing@goodwill-suncoast.com
www.goodwill-suncoast.org

Chris Ward, Marketing Manager
Jean-Marie Moore, Director Of Operations
Provides individualized assistance to help people with disabilities make connections to their community and access the services, facilities, resources and events that are available. This might include recreational activities, safety, transportation, shopping, volunteerism, and civic activities. Emphasis is on building increased independence in individuals lives. Supports are provided one-on-one or in groups of three or less and are tailored to the persons interests, abilities and needs.

5745 **Goodwill Industries-Suncoast Supported Living**
10596 Gandy Boulevard
St Petersburg, FL 33702
727-523-1512
FAX: 727-563-9300
e-mail: gw.marketing@goodwill-suncoast.com
www.goodwill-suncoast.org

Chris Ward, Marketing Manager
Jean-Marie Moore, Director Of Operations

Goodwill's supported living program helps people with developmental disabilities expand their skills so they can lead increasingly independentlives. Individuals receive training and assistance with daily living activities while living in the community. Additional support includes assistance with legal issues, adocacy, community resources, banking, safety procedures, self-medication, household management, meal preparation, interpersonal relationships and parenting training.

5746 Goodwill Industries-Suncoast,Adult Day Training

2920 W. Silver Springs Blvd.
Ocala, FL 34475 352-629-0459
FAX: 727-563-9300
e-mail: gw.marketing@goodwill-suncoast.com
www.goodwill-suncoast.org

Chris Ward, Marketing Manager
Cathy Gray, Site Manager
Goodwill's adult day training programs enable people with developmental disabilities to set and achieve personal goals within a work-like setting. Participants work at various jobs throughout Goodwill and engage in a variety of activities that will allow them to become more self-sufficients.

5747 Goodwill Temporary Services

Goodwill Industries- Suncoast
10596 Gandy Boulevard N
St Petersburg, FL 33702 727-523-1512
888-279-1988
FAX: 727-563-9300
e-mail: gw.marketing@goodwill-suncoast.com
www.goodwill-suncoast.org

R Lee Waits, President/CEO
Martin W Gladysz, Chairman
Provides employment links from potential employees, both disabled and non-disabled alike to employers with immediate employment opportunities seeking qualified candidates. Pre-screening on all applicants include: Employment history, personal references, law enforcement background checks and substance screening.

5748 Impact: Ocala Vocational Services

Goodwill Industries- Suncoast
10596 Gandy Boulevard N
St Petersburg, FL 33702 727-523-1512
888-279-1988
FAX: 727-563-9300
e-mail: gw.marketing@goodwill-suncoast.com
www.goodwill-suncoast.org

R Lee Waits, President/CEO
Designed to enable individuals with disabilities to work in integrated settings in the community, receiving wages and benefits matching those of non-handicapped workers.

5749 Job Works NISH Food Service

Goodwill Industries- Suncoast
10596 Gandy Boulevard N
St Petersburg, FL 33702 727-523-1512
888-279-1988
FAX: 727-563-9300
e-mail: gw.marketing@goodwill-suncoast.com
www.goodwill-suncoast.org

R Lee Waits, President/Chief Executive Office
An enclave style (or group) supported employment program designed to give consumers additional supports that allow and encourage increasingly independent employment opportunities within a food services environment.

5750 Job Works NISH Postal Service

Goodwill Industries- Suncoast
10596 Gandy Boulevard N
St Petersburg, FL 33702 727-523-1512
888-279-1988
FAX: 727-563-9300
e-mail: gw.marketing@goodwill-suncoast.com
www.goodwill-suncoast.org

R Lee Waits, President/CEO
An enclave style (or group) supported employment program designed to give consumers additional supports that allow and encourage increasingly independent employment opportunities within a mailroom environment.

5751 Lighthouse Central Florida (Formerly C.I.T.E)

215 E New Hampshire Street
Orlando, FL 32804 407-898-2483
888-898-2483
FAX: 407-895-5255
www.lighthousecentralflorida.com

Lee Nasehi, Executive Director
Scott Harjn, Resource Development Coordinator
Lee Van Espael, Childrens Services Supervisor
Lighthouse Central Florida (LCF) is the only non-profit organization offering comprehensive, professional, vision rehabilitation services to Central Floridians of all ages with low vision or blindness.

5752 MAClown Vocational Rehabilitation Workshop

6390 NE 2nd Avenue
Miami, FL 33138 305-754-5015

Pat Chavis
Provides remunerative work.

5753 One-Stop Service

Goodwill Industries- Suncoast
10596 Gandy Boulevard N
St Petersburg, FL 33702 727-523-1512
888-279-1988
FAX: 727-563-9300
e-mail: gw.marketing@goodwill-suncoast.com
www.goodwill-suncoast.org

R Lee Waits, President/Chief Executive Office
Provides universal job search and placement related services are available to any person entering the service center. Each One-Stop Services Center provides on-site representation from a variety of employment-related service providers. All One-Stops host and/or facilitate local employment fairs and provides access to computerized job-postings.

5754 Palm Beach Habilitation Center

4522 South Congress Avenue
Lake Worth, FL 33461 561-965-8500
FAX: 561-433-8816
e-mail: postman@pbhab.com
www.pbhab.org

Tina Philips, President/ Chief Executive Offic
Providing work evaluation, work adjustment, job placement, employment, residential and retirement services for mentally, emotionally and physically disabled adults.

5755 Primrose Supported Employment Programs

2733 S Fern Creek Avenue
Orlando, FL 32806 407-898-7201
FAX: 407-898-2120
www.primrosecenter.org

Mary Van Buren, Executive Director
Mission is to transform the lives of people with developmental disabilities by providing opportunities to achieve their fullest potential.

5756 SCARC, Inc Evaluation, Training + Emplomen t Center

213 W McCollum Avenue
Bushnell, FL 33513 352-793-5156
FAX: 352-793-6545
e-mail: marshaperkins@embargmail.com
www.sumtercountyarc.com

Merilyn Johnson, President
Marsha Perkins, Executive Director
Training and employment program for adults with disabilities. SCARC offers vocational evaluation, training, work services, transportation, supported independent living and community based training.

5757 **Seagull Industries for the Disabled**
3879 W Industrial Way
Riviera Beach, FL 33404
561-842-5814
FAX: 561-881-3554
e-mail: main@seagull.org
www.seagull.org

Alfred Elsinger, Executive Director
Dedicated to improving the quality of life of mentally, physically and emotionally challenged adults in Palm Beach County, Florida through advocacy and the provision of a variety of social service, vocational training and residential programs designed to encourage self reliance and independence.

5758 **Supported Employment Program**
Goodwill Industries- Suncoast
10596 Gandy Boulevard N
St Petersburg, FL 33702
727-523-1512
888-279-1988
FAX: 727-563-9300
e-mail: gw.marketing@goodwill-suncoast.com
www.goodwill-suncoast.org

Chris Ward, Marketing Manager
Goodwill's supported employment program enables people with developmental disabilities to work in the community, earning wages and benefits marching those of non-disabled workers. Participants receive intensive on-the-job training at job sites that have been carefully chosen for their suitability. A support facilitator provides follow-up job coaching to ensure success. Serving people in Pinellas, Hillsborough and Pasco counties.

5759 **The Able Trust**
106 E College Avenue
Suite 820
Tallahassee, FL 32301
850-224-4493
888-838-2253
888-838-2253
FAX: 850-224-4496
e-mail: info@abletrust.org
www.abletrust.org

Sharon Griffith, President/CEO
Kristen Knapp, VP Public Relations
Guenevere Crum, VP Grant Programs
Provides grant funds for employment-related programs for non-profit agencies in Florida. Assists families, individuals and agencies through educational conferences, and youth training programs. Provides businesses free resources for hiring people with disabilities.

5760 **Vocational and Rehabilitation Agency Department of Education**
2002 Old Saint Augustine Road
Building A
Tallahassee, FL 32301
850-488-6210
800-451-4327
FAX: 850-488-8062
TTY: 850-488-0867

Linda Parnell, Manager
Work adjustment and remunerative work programs.

5761 **Vocational and Rehabilitation Agency: Division of Blind Services**
2551 W Executive Center Circle
Tallahassee, FL 32301
850-488-1330
800-342-1828
FAX: 850-487-1804
e-mail: craig_kiser@dbe.doe.state.fl.us
www.state.fl.us/dbs

Craig Kiser, Director
Mission is to ensure blind and visually impaired Floridians have the tools, support, and opportunity to achieve success.

5762 **Work Exploration Center**
3000 N West 83rd Street i 40
Gainesville, FL 32606
352-395-5265
FAX: 352-395-5271
http//admin.sfcc.edu/~workex

Karla Wooten, Coordinator
The Work Exploration Center embraces a holistic approach to Comprehensive Vocational Evaluation and Community Employment services, encouraging individual understanding, hope and growth for a productive and fulfilling future.

Georgia

5763 **Employment and Training Division, Region B**
Goodwill Industries of North Georgia
1123 Progress Road
Ellijay, GA 30540
706-276-4722
888-514-8112
FAX: 706-276-4732
e-mail: vti@ellijay.com

Linda Rau, Director Programs/Services
Employment training, assessment and job placement for people who have disabilities and/or are disadvantaged. Serving 15 counties in Northern Georgia.

5764 **Fair Housing and Equal Employment**
Georgia Commission on Equal Opportunity
2 Martin Luther King Jr. Drive S.E.
Suite 1002-West Tower
Atlanta, GA 30334
404-656-1736
800-473-6736
FAX: 404-656-4399
e-mail: gceo@gceo.state.ga.us
www.gceo.state.ga.us

Judith A Harris, Fair Housing Division Manager
Stephanie Randolph, Intake Coordinator/Housing
Abdul Khadeem, Equal Employment Division Man.
To investigate housing and employment discrimination in the state of Georgia.

5765 **Griffin Area Resource Center Griffin Community Workshop Division**
511 Hamilton Boulevard
847
Griffin, GA 30223
770-228-9919
FAX: 770-228-3448
e-mail: griffincomwrkshp@aol.com

Lynn H Leaptrot, Workshop Director
Charles Cary Grubbs, Garc Executive Director
A CARF (The Rehabilitation Accreditation Commission) accredited Employment and Community Support organization providing daily services to participants with disabilities from 16 years of age and up in a 5 county area.

5766 **IBM National Support Center**
Special Needs Systems
PO Box 2150
Atlanta, GA 30301
404-238-3000
800-426-2133
FAX: 561-982-6059
Serves to help health care leaders, agency directors, policy makers, employers, educators, public officials and individuals learn how computers can enhance the quality of life for the disabled person in the school, home and workplace. Also provide information and resource guides on disabilities affecting hearing, learning, speech and language, mobility and vision.

5767 **Kelley Diversified**
PO Box 967
Athens, GA 30603
706-549-4398
FAX: 706-549-4479

Mary Patton, Executive Director
Sherry Burns, Rehabilitation Services Director
Jenny Taylor, Business Operations Manager
Work adjustment and remunerative work programs.

5768 **New Ventures**
306 Fort Drive
Lagrange, GA 30240
706-882-7723
FAX: 706-882-5401
e-mail: customersvc@newventures.org
www.newventures.org

Dave Miller, Executive Director
A rehabilitation and work training facility for individuals with barriers to employability. The program utilizes community based industrial work of varying levels of difficulty. A return to work conditioning program for the industrially injured is offered which features: first-day contact, workers compensation rehabilitation team management, and light-duty work conditioning. A training stipend is paid to defray costs associated with training.

Hawaii

5769 ASSETS School
1 Ohana Nui Way
Honolulu, HI 96818
808-423-1356
FAX: 808-422-1920
e-mail: info@assets-school.net
assets-school.net

Sandi Tadaki, Head of School (Interim)
Jyo Bridegewater Borg, Principal K-8
Patti Jenks, Principal, High School
ASSETS is an independent school for gifted and or dyslexic children that provides an individualized, integrated learning enviroment. ASSETS' enviroment empowers these children to maximize their potential and to find their place as lifelong learners in school and society.

5770 Hawaii Fair Employment Practice Agency
830 Punchbowl Street
Room 411
Honolulu, HI 96813
808-586-8636
800-586-8800
FAX: 808-586-8655
http://hawaii.gov/labor/hcrc

Michael Yamamoto
HCRC enforces state laws prohibiting discrimination in employment.

5771 Hawaii Vocational Rehabilitation Division
601 Kamokila Boulevard
Suite 515
Kapolei, HI 96707
808-692-7715
FAX: 808-692-7727
www.state.hi.us/dhs

John Nolan, Assistant Administrator
Mission is our committed staff strive, day-in day-out, to provide timely efficient and effective programs, services and benefits, for the purpose of achieving the outcome of empowering those who are the most vulnerable in our state to expand thier capacity for self sufficiency , self-determination, independence, healthy choices, quality of life and personal dignity.

5772 Lanakila Rehabilitation Center
1809 Bachelot Street
Honolulu, HI 96817
808-834-2583
FAX: 808-533-7264
e-mail: lanakila@lanakilahawaii.org
www.lanakilahawaii.org

Jim Wakafuji, President/CEO
Lanakila is a private nonprofit organization whose mission is to provide services and supports that assist individuals with physical, mental, or age-related challenges to live as independently as possible within our community. A broad range of services are offered which include meal/senior services, community based adult day programming for individuals with disabilities, work training opportunities, and extended/supported employment for individuals with special needs.

5773 Vocational and Rehabilitation Agency
PO Box 339
Honolulu, HI 96809
808-586-5162
FAX: 808-692-7727
e-mail: nshim@dhs.state.hi.us

Albert Perez, Manager
Work adjustment and remunerative work programs.

5774 Wahiawa Family
330 Walker Avenue
Wahiawa, HI 96786
808-621-7407

Leslie Chinna
Work adjustment and remunerative work programs.

Idaho

5775 Idaho Employment Service and Job Training Program Liaison
Idaho Department of Employment
317 W Main Street
Boise, ID 83735
208-332-3570

Roger Madsen, Manager
Work adjustment and remunerative work programs.

5776 Idaho Fair Employment Practice Agency
Idaho Human Rights Commission
Po Box 83720
Boise, ID 83702
208-334-2873
FAX: 208-334-2664
www2.state.id.us/ihrc/ihrchome.htm

David Rogers, Administrator
Mission is to admininster state and federal anti-discrimination laws in Idaho in a manner that is fair, accurate, and timely; and to work towards ensuring that all people withink the state are treated with dignity and respect in their places of employment, housing, education, and public accomodations.

5777 Idaho Governor's Committee on Employment of People with Disabilities
317 W Main Street
Boise, ID 83735

Work adjustment and remunerative work programs.

5778 Idaho Vocational Rehabilitation Agency
10200 W Emerald Street
Suite 101
Boise, ID 83704
208-327-7411
FAX: 208-327-7411
e-mail: rthomas@vr.idaho.gov
www.vr.idaho.gov

Darrell Quist, Regional Manager
Janet Thaldorf, Supervisor
Vocational Rehabilitation assists many individuals with disabilities to go to work. With VR assistance, these individuals have overcome numerous obstacles and disability related barriers to achieve employment.

5779 Vocational and Rehabilitation Agency
Idaho Commission for the Blind & Visually Impaired
341 West Washington Street
Boise, ID 83702
208-334-3220
800-542-8688
FAX: 208-334-2963
e-mail: aroan@icbvi.state.id.us
www.icbvi.state.id.us

Angela Roan, Administrator
Jackie Bryan, Rehab Services Chief
Maggie Starkovich, Administrative Assistant
Vocational rehabilitation, independent living training, medical intervention, adaptive technology and devices and employer advocacy.

Illinois

5780 Ada S McKinley Vocational Services
725 S Wells Street
1-A
Chicago, IL 60607
312-554-0600
FAX: 312-554-0292
TTY:312-697-9794
e-mail: ksmith@adasmckinley.org
www.adasmckinley.org

Aberra Zewdie, Division Director
George Jones, Executive Director
Mission is to serve those who, because of disabilities or other limiting conditions, need help in finding and pursuing paths leading to healthy, productive, and fulfilling lives.

5781 Anixter Center
6610 N Clark Street
Chicago, IL 60626
773-973-7900
FAX: 773-973-5268
e-mail: AskAnixter@anixter.org
www.anixter.org

Allan Bergman, President/CEO
A Chicago-based human services agency that assists people with disabilities to live and work successfully in the community. Anixter Center provides vocational training, employment services, residences, special education, prevention programs, community services and health care. In addition, Anixter Center offers Illinois' only substance abuse treatment programs specifically for people with disabilities including Addiction Recovery of the Deaf.

5782 C-4 Work Center
5710 N Broadway Street
Chicago, IL 60660
773-728-1000
www.c4chicago.org

Anthony A Kopera, Chief Executive Director
Mark T Hicks, Program Director
Aftercare, case finding, information and referrals, vocational training and work activities offered to mentally ill persons.

5783 Clearbrook
1835 W Central Road
Arlington Heights, IL 60005
847-870-7711
FAX: 847-870-7741
e-mail: info@clearbrook.org
www.clearbrook.org

Carl M La Mell, President
Tracy Martin, Admissions Director
Offers educational, employment and residential services to the developmentally disabled children and adults.

5784 Cornerstone Services
777 Joyce Road
Joliet, IL 60436
815-727-6666
FAX: 815-723-1177
e-mail: jhogan@cornerstoneservices.org
www.cornerstoneservices.org

James A Hogan, President/CEO
Susan Murphy, Coordinator Public Ralations
Cornerstone Services provides progressive, comprehensive services for people with disabilities, promoting choice, dignity and the opportunity to live and work in the community. Established in 1969, the agency provides developmental, vocational, employment, residential and mental health services at various community-based locations. The nonprofit social service agency helps approximately 750 people each day.

5785 Fulton County Rehab Center
500 N Main Street
Canton, IL 61520
309-647-6510
FAX: 309-647-3040

Rex Lewis, Executive Director
Residential rehab center with health care incidental; manufactures wood pallets and skids; job training and vocational rehabilitation services.

5786 Glenkirk
3504 Commercial Avenue
Northbrook, IL 60062
847-272-5111
FAX: 847-272-7350
www.glenkirk.org

Alan Spector, President & CEO
Helps infants, children and adults with developmental disabilities reach higher levels of independence. A non-profit organization serving people in north and northwest Chicago suburbs. Glenkirk's residential, vocational, educational and support programs include services which provide individual evaluation, therapeutic treatment and training.

5787 Illinois Employment Service
Department of Employment Security
401 S State Street
4th Floor
Chicago, IL 60605
312-793-4880
800-247-4984
www.state.il.us/agency/
Work adjustment and remunerative work programs.

5788 Jewish Vocational Services
1 S Franklin Street
Chicago, IL 60606
312-357-4500
FAX: 312-855-3282
www.jvsnj.org/agencycategories.html
Occupational training and job placement for handicapped persons of all religions.

5789 JoDavies Workshop
706 West Street
Po Box 6087
Galena, IL 61036
815-777-2211
FAX: 815-777-3386
e-mail: jdwi@jdwi.org
www.jdwi.org

William Wubben, Treasurer
Tim Zueger, Chairperson
Dale Gereau, Plant Manager
Intake and referral, early intervention for children only, vocational evaluation and work adjustment training services offered.

5790 Kennedy Job Training Center
7361 S Meade Avenue
Bedford Park, IL 60638
708-594-7155
FAX: 708-594-7156

Robin Mertes, Placement Manager
Kandy Stamer, QMRP/Intake Coordinator
Offers vocational evaluation, vocational training work adjustment training, and job placement services for developmentally disabled and hearing impaired persons.

5791 Knox County Council for Developmental Disabilities
2015 Windish Drive
Galesburg, IL 61401
309-344-2600
FAX: 309-344-1754
e-mail: mallen@grics.net
www.kccdd.com

Ned Hippensteel, Executive Director
Developmental training, vocational evaluation, work adjustment training, extended training, placement, supported employment.

5792 Kreider Services
500 Anchor Road
Po Box 366
Dixon, IL 61021
815-288-6691
FAX: 815-288-1636
www.kreiderservices.org

Arlyn McClain, Executive Director

Offers day service programs, vocational training programs, job placement, supported employment, respite care, residential and family support for ages birth to three years.

5793 **Lambs Farm**
14245 W Rockland Road
Libertyville, IL 60048
847-362-4636
FAX: 847-362-0742
e-mail: info@lambsfarm.org
www.lambsfarm.org

Dianne Yaconetti, President/CEO
Barbara Schwarz, Director of Development
Marie Nelso, Asst Dir Vocational Services
Person-centered, comprehensive program of residential, vocational and social support service for adults with developmental disabilities.

5794 **Land of Lincoln Goodwill Industries**
PO Box 8528
Springfield, IL 62791
217-789-0400
FAX: 217-789-0540

Sharon Durbin, Executive Director
Offers a developmental training and community employment programs for persons with disabilities. Workforce development for adults with barriers to employment.

5795 **Orchard Village**
7670 Marmora Avenue
Skokie, IL 60077
847-967-1800
FAX: 847-967-9543
e-mail: info@orchardvillage.org
www.orchardvillage.org

Jim Vail, Executive Director
Vocational program and counseling, respite services and community living group homes for the disabled and cognitively impaired. Orchard village also operates a private hope school especially devoted to teaching young adults independent living and skills necessary to flourish in the community.

5796 **President's Committee on Employment of Employment of the Disabled**
623 E Adams Street
Springfield, IL 62701
217-785-0218
800-ASK-DORI
TTY:217-782-5734

Audrey Mccrimon, Director
Work adjustment and remunerative work programs.

5797 **Sertoma Centre**
4343 W 123rd Street
Alsip, IL 60803
708-371-9700
FAX: 708-371-9747
e-mail: info@sertomacentre.org
www.sertomacentre.org

Gus Van Den Brink, Executive Director
Paula Phillips, Assistant Director
Offers vocational services to promote independence and community integration; day training and residential services provided to individuals. Programs include: vocational evaluation, work adjustment training, janitorial training, job placement, sheltered work, supported employment, developmental training, respite care, residential services.

5798 **Shore Training Center**
Shore Community Services
8035 Austin Avenue
Morton Grove, IL 60053
847-581-0200
FAX: 847-581-0078
e-mail: stcsales@sbcglobal.net
www.shoreinc.org

Lisa Wright, Director
Michael Mack, Plant Manager
Mission is to improve the quality of life for citizens with developmental disabilities through community based services providing education/training.

5799 **Skills Inc.**
1122 5th Avenue
Moline, IL 61265
309-797-3586
FAX: 309-797-4914
www.skills-inc.org

Stuart Olson, President
Accredited through the Commission on Accreditation of Rehabilitation Facilities; offers job training partnership act and vocational evaluation services offered.

5800 **Thresholds AMISS**
12145 Western Avenue
Blue Island, IL 60406
708-597-7997
FAX: 708-597-8073

Julia Rupp, Executive Director
Camille Rucks, Team Leader
Services offered include psychosocial, vocational and residential programs for ages 18 or older with a primary diagnosis of mental illness. Facility is wheelchair accessible.

5801 **Vocational and Rehabilitation Agency**
207 Staehouse
Springfield, IL 62706
217-782-0244
800-843-6154
FAX: 217-524-6262
TTY: 217-782-5734
www.state.il.us

Rod R Blavojevich, Governor
Pat Quinn, Manager
Provides work adjustment and remunerative skills.

5802 **Washington County Vocational Workshop**
781 E Holzhauer Dr.
Nashville, IL 62263
618-327-4461
FAX: 618-327-4477

Keith Curran, Executive Director
Provides job training and related services and vocational rehabilitation services.

5803 **Westside Parents Work Activity Center**
3765 W Ogden Avenue
Chicago, IL 60623
773-522-1200

Offers developmental training programs providing basic skills in self care for multiply and physically handicapped persons.

Indiana

5804 **ADEC Resources for Independence**
Po Box 398
19670 SR 120
Bristol, IN 46507
574-848-7451
877-342-8954
FAX: 574-848-5917
www.adecinc.com

Matt Leachman, Contact
Paula Shively, President
Serves Elkhart County and surrounding area.

5805 **ARC of Allen County**
Arc of U S
2542 Thompson Avenue
Fort Wayne, IN 46807
260-456-4534
800-234-7811
FAX: 260-745-5200
www.easterseals.com

F Gil Perry, Chairperson
Nikki Holm, Senior Vice Chairperson
Steven Hinkle, President
Primary list of services includes:Æcommunity services, intergenerational services, production and work training services, residential services, 24 hour medicaid waiver services and employment services

5806 BI-County Services
425 E Harrison Road
Bluffton, IN 46714
260-824-1253
FAX: 260-824-1892
e-mail: info@adifferentlight.com
www.bi-countyservices.com

Joyce Bussard, Program Director
John Whicker, President
Serves Wells and Adam Counties. Infant services, Medicaid waivers, music therapy, ICF, MR, group homes, sheltered employment, pay program and supported employment services available.

5807 Balance Centers of America
2538 Patricia Street
Portage, IN 46368
219-736-2930

Jane Labar, Contact
Offers developmental training programs providing basic skills in self care for physically handicapped persons.

5808 Bridge Pointe Services & Goodwill of Southern Indiana, Inc
Goodwill International
PO Box 2488
1329 Applegate Lane
Clarksville, IN 47131
812-283-7908
800-660-3355
FAX: 812-283-6248
e-mail: cmarshall@bridepointe.org
www.bridgepionte.org

Caren Marshall, Chief Executive Director
Terry Richards, Director Of Career Services
Gary Purlee, Senior V.P. of Retail Services
Career assesment, job readiness and placement, office skills training. Pediatric family support services. Childrens Academy, a developmental preschool.

5809 Carey Services
2724 S Carey Street
Marion, IN 46953
765-668-8961
FAX: 765-664-6747
www.careyservices.com

Grant Black, Contact
Mark Draves, Chief Executive Officer
The mission of Carey Services is to create pathways towards self-sufficiency with personal satisfaction.

5810 Evansville Association for the Blind
500 2nd Avenue
Po Box 6445
Evansville, IN 47719
812-422-1181
FAX: 812-424-3154
e-mail: eabcdc@evansville.net
www2.evansville.edu/ebaweb

Karla Horrell, Director Rehabilitation
Diane Hagler, Vocational Specialist
Krysti Kite, Orientation/Mobility
An community rehabilitation facility untilizing individual goals to assist persons with disabilities achieve or maintain potenial

5811 Four Rivers Resource Services
PO Box 249
Linton, IN 47441
812-847-2231
FAX: 812-847-8836
e-mail: fourrivers@frrs.org
www.frrs.org

Stephen Sacksteder, Executive Director
Lyna Landis, Marketing Coordinator
Employment, community living, connections, follow-along, early intervention, preschool, healthy families, child care resource and referral and child care voucher program, impact, and transpotation services.

5812 Gateway Services/JCARC
PO Box 216
Franklin, IN 46131
317-738-5500
888-494-8069
FAX: 317-738-5522

Karen Luehmann, Executive Director
Utilizes individual goals to assist persons with disabilities achieve or maintain potential.

5813 Goodwill Industries of Central Indiana
1635 W Michigan Street
Indianapolis, IN 46222
317-524-4313
FAX: 317-524-4336
www.goodwill-indy.org

Irene Mcclesky, Contact
Jim Clelland, President
Goodwill is in the business of helping people find jobs and provides programs and services for people who want to work. Goodwill is a community resource committed to deploying our assets and leveraging our resources with those of others in the community to create more opportunities for people who need assistance to improve their ability to earn a living.

5814 Indiana Employment Services and Job Training Program Liaison
10 N Senate Avenue
Indianapolis, IN 46204
317-232-6702
FAX: 317-233-5499
Offers developmental training programs providing basic skills in self care for physically handicapped persons.

5815 Indiana Fair Employment Practice Agency
100 N Senate Ave.
Room N103
Indianapolis, IN 46204
317-232-2600
800-628-2909
Works to develop public policies that ensure equal opportunity in education to all.

5816 LCAR
2650 W 35th Avenue
Gary, IN 46408
219-884-1138
FAX: 219-980-7315
www.thetimesonline.com/org/lcar

Brian Davis, Contact
Kris Prohl, Executive Director
Mission is to improve the welfare of people with mental retardation and thier families.

5817 Michigan Resources
4315 E Michigan Boulevard
Michigan City, IN 46360
219-874-4288
FAX: 219-874-2689
e-mail: michiana@michianaresources.org

Michael Horton, CEO
Vocational training center for persons 16 and older with disabilities.

5818 New Hope Services
725 Wall Street
Jeffersonville, IN 47130
812-288-8248
800-237-6604
FAX: 812-285-8322
e-mail: info@newhopeservices.org
www.newhopeservices.org

Pat Daily, Chairperson
Charles E Reisert, Vice Chairperson
James Bosley, President
Mission is to provide hope through services which are responsive to individual needs.

5819 New Horizons Rehabilitation
PO Box 98
Batesville, IN 47006
812-934-4528
FAX: 812-934-2522
e-mail: mdausch@venus.net
www.nhrehab.org

Greg Tow, Contact
Marie Dausch, Executive Director
Serves Ripley, Franklin, Ohio, Switzerland Dearborn, and Decatur. Provides training and services to adults with mental/physical disabilities and infants birth to age 3 with developmental delays or conditions of risk which could result in a developmental delay.

5820 **Noble Centers**
7701 East 21st Street
Indianapolis, IN 46219
317-375-2700
FAX: 317-375-2719
www.iidc.indiana.edu

Tom Cain, Contact
Vocational training center for people with disabilities.

5821 **Office of State Coordinator of Vocational Education for Students with Disability**
10 N Senate Avenue
Room 212
Indianapolis, IN 46204
317-232-1829
800-891-6499
e-mail: tfields@dwd.state.in.us
www.state.in.us/dwd/techd
Manages and impliments innovative employment programs, unemployment insurance systems, and facilitates regional economic growth initiatives for Indiana.

5822 **Putnam County Comprehensive Services**
630 Tennessee Street
Greencastle, IN 46135
765-653-4362
877-653-9763
FAX: 765-653-3646
www.pccsinc.org

Tammy Amore
Diana Huff, Manager
A not-for-profit organization serving individuals with disabilities and similar characteristics in Indiana. Our mission is to provide opportunities that lead to a more enjoyable and fulfilling life to those who may have difficulty achieving their goals on their own.

5823 **Southern Indiana Resource Solutions**
1579 S Folsomville Road
Boonville, IN 47601
812-897-4840
FAX: 812-897-0123
e-mail: kelly@sirs.org
www.sirs.org

Kelly Mitchell, CEO/President
Christal Moskos, Chairman of the Board
Adult services including jobs, community connections, and residential, childrens services, including service coordination and all therapies.

5824 **Sycamore Rehabilitation Services**
1001 Sycamore Lane
Danville, IN 46122
317-745-4715
888-298-6617
FAX: 317-745-8271
www.sycamoreservices.com

Bob Gootee, President
Patrick Cockrum, Executive Director
Provides individuals training and services for persons with disabilities that enhance independence in all areas of life.

5825 **Vocational and Rehabilitation Agency**
PO Box 7083
Indianapolis, IN 46207
317-232-1401
800-545-7763
FAX: 317-232-1240
e-mail: peter.bispecos@sssa.in.gov
www.ssa.in.gov

Peter Bispecos, Director
Mike Hedden, Executive Director
Vocational training center for persons with disabilities.

5826 **Wabash/Employability Center**
S C6395 Earl Avenue
Suite 2
Lafayette, IN 47903
765-447-0300
FAX: 765-447-6456

Bill Carmichael, Contact
Serves Tippecanoe County.

Iowa

5827 **ACT Assessment Test Preparation Reference Manual**
American College Testing Program
500 Act Drive
Po Box 168
Iowa City, IA 52243
319-337-1000
FAX: 319-339-3020
www.act.org

Richard L Ferguson, President/CEO
Tom Goedkem, Senior Vice President
This reference manual was developed as a resource for high school teachers and counselors in assisting students with test preparation.

5828 **Franklin County Work Activity Center**
20 5th Street NW
Hampton, IA 50441
641-456-2532
www.accessincorportated.org

Steven Paul Woods, Executive Director
Jim Koenen, Owner
Nonprofit organization providing residential and vocational services in Franklin and Hardin counties in the state of Iowa. Residential Services include RCF/MR services, Supported Community Living Services and Community Supervised Apartment Living Arrangement Services. Vocational Services include Work Services and Supported Employment Services. Accredited by the Commission on Accreditation of rehabilitation Facilities since 1984, and serves individuals with a wide range of needs.

5829 **Innovative Industries**
405 E Madison Street
Winterset, IA 50273
515-462-2926
FAX: 515-462-2870
e-mail: winnind@iowalink.com

Renee Gray, Secretary
Connie Bailey, Program Manager

5830 **Iowa Civil Rights Commission**
400 E 14th Street
Des Moines, IA 50319
515-281-4121
800-457-4516
FAX: 515-242-5840
www.state.ia.us/government/crc

Ralph Rosenberg, Director
Ron Pothast, Executive Director
A neutral, fact-finding administrative agency that enforces the "Iowa Civi Rights Act of 1965," Iowa's anti-discrimination law. The commission doesn not provide legal representation. The commission's vision is a state free of discrimination.

5831 **Iowa Employment Service**
1000 East Grand Avenue
Des Moines, IA 50319
515-282-5823
FAX: 515-288-2184
www.iowacareerconnection.com
Specializes in accounting and human resources talent aquisition in the Upper-Midwest.

5832 **Iowa Job Training Program Liaison**
Iowa Department of Economic Development
200 E Grand Avenue
Des Moines, IA 50309 515-242-4700
FAX: 515-242-4809
e-mail: info@iowalifechanging.com
www.iowalifechanging.com

David Lyons, Executive Director
To engender and promote economic development policies and practices which stimulate and sustain Iowa's economic growth and climate and that integrate efforts across public and private sectors.

5833 **Iowa Valley Community College**
3702 S Center Street
Marshalltown, IA 50158 641-752-4643
FAX: 641-752-5909
www.iavalley.edu

Marge Good, Career Development
Tim Wynes, President
Offers two levels of specialized vocational preparatory programming for adults with disabilities. The Career Development Center serves dependent adults. The goal of the program is to maintain or improve skills to enable persons served to enter sheltered or supported employment. The IRP/CBVT programs are non-credit specialized vocational programs for independent adults served by Vocational Rehabilitation and our programs. The goals are for competitive placements in jobs. CARF accredited.

5834 **Iowa Vocational Rehabilitation Services**
510 E 12th Street
Des Moines, IA 50319 515-281-4211
FAX: 515-281-7645
TTY:515-281-4311
www.ivrs.iowa.gov

Stephen Wooderson, Administrator
Charles Levine, Assistant Chief
The mission is to work for and with individuals who have disabilities to achieve their employment, independence and economic goals.

5835 **New Focus**
102 W Washington Street
Centerville, IA 52544 641-437-1722
FAX: 641-437-1028

Susan Wright, Director Employment Services
Peggy Oden, Executive Director
Provides vocational services for adults with disabilities. Includes work activity, supported employment and supported community living.

5836 **Second Time Around**
110 W Jackson Street
Centerville, IA 52544 641-437-7355

Keith Lindley, Executive Director
Debbie Steen, Store Supervisor
Deana Edwards, Manager
Work training site for adults with disabilities.

Kansas

5837 **Clay Center Adult Training Center**
701 4th Street
Clay Center, KS 67432 785-632-5357
FAX: 785-632-5371

Gail Habluetzel, Executive Director
Work training site for adults with disabilities.

5838 **Kansas Fair Employment Practice Agency**
900 SW Jackson Street
Suite 851-S
Topeka, KS 66612 785-296-3206
FAX: 785-296-0589
www.state.ks.us/public/khrc

Mostafa Kamal, Manager

5839 **Kansas Vocational Rehabilitation Agency**
300 SW Oakley Avenue
Topeka, KS 66606 785-267-5301
FAX: 785-267-0263
TTY:913-296-7029
e-mail: jac@srkspo.wpo.state.ks.us
www.srskansas.org/rehab

Joyce Cussimanio, Director
Helps people with disabilities achieve employment and self-sufficiency. Also links employers with qualified and productive individuals to meet thier work force needs.

Kentucky

5840 **Kentucky Committee on Employment of People with Disabilities**
275 East Main Street
2nd Floor
Frankfort, KY 40601 502-564-7456
FAX: 502-564-7459
www.oet.ky.gov

Dennis Derman, Manager
Provides qualified people for jobs, quality jobs for people, temporary financial support for the unemployed, comprehensive labor market information, and preserve the integrity and viability of the Unemployment Insurance Trust Fund.

5841 **Kentucky Department for Employment Service and Job Training Program Liaison**
275 E Main Street 2-W
Frankfort, KY 40621 502-564-2367
FAX: 502-564-7799
www.desky.org
Provides qualified people for jobs, quality jobs for people, temporary financial support for the unemployed.

5842 **Kentucky Department for the Blind**
PO Box 757
Frankfort, KY 40602 502-564-4754
877-592-5463
FAX: 502-564-2951
TTY: 502-564-2929
e-mail: dbohannon@state.ky.us.dfblind
www.blind.ky.gov

Stephen Johnson, Executive Director
Marcia Egbert, Executive Secretary
Provides career services and assistance to adults with severe visual handicaps who want to become productive in the home or work force. Also provides the Client Assistance Program established to provide advice, assistance and information available from rehabilitation programs to persons with handicaps.

5843 **Kentucky Office For The Blind**
Po Box 757
209 St. Clair Street
Frankfort, KY 40602 502-564-4754
800-321-6668
FAX: 502-564-2951
TTY: 502-564-6817
e-mail: blind@ky.gov
http://blind.ky.gov

Beth Smith, Executive Director
A state government rehabilitation agency that offers assistance to persons who are blind or visually impaired.

5844 Kentucky Vocational Rehabilitation Agency
209 St. Clair
Frankfort, KY 40601
502-564-4400
800-372-7172
FAX: 502-564-6745
http://ovr.ky.gov

Rodney Kelly, Executive Director
Assists eligible individuals with disabilities achieve their employment goals.

5845 Pioneer Vocational/Industrial Services
Po Box 1396
150 Corporate Drive
Danville, KY 40423
859-236-8413
800-527-4198
e-mail: pioneer@pioneerservices.org
www.pioneerservices.org

Jack Goodbey II, Executive Director
Mission is to provide vocational development and extended employment programs to people who are disabled and or disadvantaged to assist them in obtaining employment and maximizing independent living skills.

5846 Work Enhancement Center of Western Kentucky
803 Poplar Street
Murray, KY 42071
270-762-1100
FAX: 502-767-3600

Steve Passmore, Director
John O'Shaughnessy, Chief Executive Officer
The center has been established in order to service industry in the three state area surrounding Kentucky. This service includes job/skill evaluation, job design consultation, pre-employment employee evaluations and economic evaluation.

Louisiana

5847 Community Opportunities of East Ascension
1121 S East Ascension Complex Blvd.
Gonzales, LA 70737
225-621-2000
FAX: 225-621-2022
http://coea.homestead.com

Mark Thomas, Director
Committed to affording individuals the opportunities that reflect and support choices, dignity, individuality, self-determination, community, coherency and commen sense. Programs incloude Respite, Personal Care Attendant, Support Living, Support Environment, Adult Day Training, and Elderly/Adult Waiver Services.

5848 Louisiana Employment Service and Job Training Program Liaison
1001 North 23rd Street
Baton Rouge, LA 70802
225-342-3111
800-259-5154
FAX: 225-342-3030
www.laworks.net

John Smith, Director
Warner Smith, Manager
Provides services for job seekers and job training programs.

5849 Louisiana Vocational Rehabilitation Agency
3500 Canal Street
New Orleans, LA 70119
504-483-4709
800-737-2963
FAX: 504-483-4777
www.dss.state.la.us/departments/lrs

Irby Hornsey, Regional Manager
Ed Barras, Manager
Offers individuals with disabilities a wide range of services designed to provide them with skills, resources, attitudes, and expectations needed to compete in the interview process, get the job, keep the job, and develop a lifetime career.

5850 St. James Association for Retarded Citizens
29150 Health Unit Street
Vacherie, LA 70090
225-265-7910

Jamie Chenier, Executive Director
A private sheltered work program for mentally retarded and developmentally disabled adults.

5851 Westbank Sheltered Workshop
1728 Hermosa Street
New Orleans, LA 70114
504-362-1311

A private non-residential facility serving severely disabled individuals referred through Louisiana Rehabilitation Services.

Maine

5852 Addison Point Specialized Services
PO Box 207
Addison, ME 04606
207-483-6500
FAX: 207-483-2817

Paula Chartrand, Executive Officer
Provides services to individuals who are deaf/blind, mentally retarded, autistic, behaviorally challenged and/or dual diagnosed. Training services to place these individuals in community employment.

5853 Bangor Veteran Center: Veterans Outreach Center
352 Harlow Street
Bangor, ME 04401
207-947-3391
FAX: 207-941-8195
e-mail: bangorvc@aol.com
www.va.gov/visn1/togus/veterans_outreach

Joseph A Degrasse, Team Leader
Robert L Daisey MSW, Clinical Coordinator
Readjustment counseling services for veterans of Vietnam, Vietnam Era, Persian Gulf, Panama, Grenada, Lebanon, Somalia, WWII and Korean conflicts.

5854 Creative Work Systems
443 Congress Street
Portland, ME 04101
207-879-1140
FAX: 207-879-1146
e-mail: kraye@creativeworks.com
www.creativeworksystems.com

Susan Percy, Executive Director
Provides residential, day habilitation and supported emploment in Central and Southern Maine.

5855 Maine Department Of Labor
20 Union Street
Augusta, ME 04330
207-287-3788
FAX: 207-287-5292
e-mail: mdol@maine.gov
www.state.me.us/labor

Valerie Landry, Manager
Provides a wide range of services such as employment, labor market information, rehabilitation/disability and others.

5856 Maine Governor's Committee on Employment of the Disabled
35 Anthony Avenue
Augusta, ME 04330
207-624-5335
800-794-1110
FAX: 207-624-5302
Offers supported employment programs and vocational education.

5857 Maine Human Rights Commission
Maine Human Rights Commission
51 State House Station
Augusta, ME 04333
207-624-6050
FAX: 207-624-6063
www.maine.gov/mhrc

Patricia Ryan, Director
State agency with the responsibility of enforcing Maine's anti-discrimination laws. The commission investigates complaints of unlawful discrimination in employment, housing, education, access to public accommodations, extension of credit and offensive names.

5858 **Northeast Occupational Exchange**
248 Center Street
Bangor, ME 04401
207-942-3816
www.noemaine.org

Dr. Charles Tingley Jr, Executive Director
A fully licensed, comprehensive mental health and substance abuse treatment and rehabilitation facility.

5859 **Vocational and Rehabilitation Agency**
Division for the Blind and Visually Impaired
55 State House Station
Augusta, ME 04333
207-623-7981
800-794-1110
FAX: 207-624-5980
TTY: 207-624-5955
e-mail: paul.e.cote@maine .gov
www.mainecareercenter.com

Jill Busond, Bureau Director

Maryland

5860 **Ardmore Developmental Center**
3000 Lottsford Vista Road
Bowie, MD 20721
FAX: 301-731-4551

Donalda Lovelace, CEO
Offers supported employment programs and vocational education for persons who are mentally retarded as well as residential services and Emergency Respite Care.

5861 **Job Opportunities for the Blind**
National Federation of the Blind
1800 Johnson Street
Baltimore, MD 21230
410-659-9314
FAX: 410-685-5653
e-mail: nfb@iamdigex.net
www.nfb.org

James Geshel, Director Governmental Affairs
Anthony Cobb, Director Job Opportunities
Marc Maurer, President
This free service allows individuals touch-tone telephone access to the thousands of jobs listed in America's Job Bank, and internet service run by the Department of Labor. Any person registered with either a state rehabilitation agency or a state employment service can search across the country for jobs by either type of work or location.

5862 **Mainstream**
3 Bethesda Metro Center
Suite 830
Bethesda, MD 20814
301-961-9299
FAX: 301-891-8778
e-mail: mainstrm@aol.com

Patricia M Jackson, Executive Director
Charles Moster
Nonprofit organization dedicated to improving competitive employment opportunities for persons with disabilities. Provides specialized services and acts as a bridge that links service providers, employers and persons with disabilties. Provides training, educational publications, and videos on disablityemployment issues. Educationa materials include a magazine, brochures, and audio-visual aids.

5863 **Maryland Employment Services and Job Training Program Liaison**
1100 N Eutaw Street
Room 600
Baltimore, MD 21201
410-767-2173

Provides job development and placement and services

5864 **Maryland Fair Employment Practice Agency**
6 St. Paul St. 9th Floor
Baltimore, MD 21202
410-767-8600
800-637-6247
FAX: 410-769-8914
www.mchr.state.md.us

Adrienne Jones, Executive Director
Mission is to ensure equal opportunity to all through the enforcement of Maryland's laws against discrimination in employment, housing, and public accomodations; to provide educational and outreach services related to the provisions of this law: and to promote and improve human relations in Maryland.

5865 **Maryland State Department of Education**
Division of Rehabilitation Services (DI RS)
2301 Argonne Drive
Baltimore, MD 21218
410-554-9100

Robert Burns, Assistant State Supervisor
The Vocational Rehabilitation Program delivers to eligible individuals with physical and/or mental disabilities to enable them to become employed. The Independent Living Program's goal is to assist people in remaining in their homes and communities. The Division operates the Maryland Rehabilitation Center, a comprehensive evaluation and training center that has dormitory space. There are field offices located statewide with counselors to advise and manage the provision of services offered.

5866 **PWI Profile**
Projects W Industry Goodwill Industries of America
9200 Wisconsin Avenue
Bethesda, MD 20814

Newsletter on employment of persons with disabilities.

5867 **Project LINK**
Mainstream
3 Bethesda Metro Center
Suite 830
Bethesda, MD 20814
301-961-9299
800-247-1380
FAX: 301-891-8778
e-mail: info@mainstreaminc.org
www.mainstreaminc.org

Charles Moster
Provides job development and placement in services to dislocated workers with disabilities in the Washington, DC and Dallas, TX areas.

5868 **Treatment and Learning Centers (TLC)**
9975 Medical Center Drive
Rockville, MD 20850
301-424-5200
www.ttlc.org

Richard Pavlin, Executive Director
Helps parents, children and teachers understand and overcome educational difficulties. They offer interdisciplinary diagnostic testing individually tailored to pinpoint the specific strengths and needs of students who may have learning disabilities, Dyslexia or other learning problems.

Massachusetts

5869 Department Of Workforce Development
State of Massachusetts
1 Ashburton Place
Room 2112
Boston, MA 02108 617-626-7122
www.massworkforce.org
Serves as the Governor's principal advisory board on workforce development.

5870 Gateway Arts Program, Crafts Store & Gallery
Vinsen Corporation
62 Harvard Street
Brookline, MA 02445 617-734-1577
FAX: 617-734-3199
e-mail: gateway@vinfen.org
www.gatewayarts.org

Rae T Edelson, Program Director
Ted Lampe, Assistant Program Director
Mona Thaler, Marketing Director
An arts-based vocational service for adults with developmental and other disabilities including mental illness, autism and head injury who can pursue paid work in fine art and crafts with the aid of professional artists/teachers, a professional marketer and a Crafts Store and Gallery. A service of Vinfen.

5871 Massachusetts Fair Employment Practice Agency
1 Ashburton Place
Room 601
Boston, MA 02108 617-727-3990
www.state.ma.us/mcad
The commission works to eliminate discrimination on a variety of bases and areas, and strives to advance the civil rights of the people of commonwealth through law enforcement, outreach and training.

5872 Massachusetts Governor's Commission on Employment of Disabled Persons
19 Staniford Street
3rd Floor
Boston, MA 02114 617-864-2000

Theodore Schipani, Owner
State vocational rehabilitation agency.

5873 Vocational Rehabilitation Agency
27-43 Wormwood Street
Boston, MA 02210 617-204-3600
800-642-0249
FAX: 617-727-1354
TTY: 800-764-0200
e-mail: elmer.bartels@mrc.state.ma.us
www.state.ma.us

Elmer Bartels, Director
Provides residential, day habilitation and supported employment

5874 Vocational and Rehabilitation Agency Massachusetts Commission for the Blind
48 Boyle Street
Boston, MA 02129 617-727-5550
800-392-6450
FAX: 617-727-7685
TTY: 800-392-6556
e-mail: poliver@state.ma.us
www.state.ma.us

David Govostes, Commissioner
Provides residentail, habilitation, and supported employment

5875 Work Inc.
3 Arlington Street
Quincy, MA 02171 617-691-1500
FAX: 617-691-1595
www.workinc.org

James Cassetta, President
Mission is all individuals have the ability to grow, the right to make choices and to participate in community life. It is the mission of WORK inc. to join with others in creating the conditions under which all persons with disablilities will experience.

Michigan

5876 Department Of Human Services
PO Box 30652
Lansing, MI 48909 517-373-2062
800-292-4200
FAX: 517-335-5140
TTY: 5173734025
e-mail: kreinerc@state.mi.us
www.michigan.gov.dhs

Patrick Cannon, Director
The DHS is Michigan's public assistance, child and family welfare agency. DHS directs the operations of public assistance and service programs through a network of over 100 county department of human service offices around the state.

5877 Lamplighter's Work Center
1320 W State Street
Cheboygan, MI 49721 231-627-4319

Robert Spinella, Executive Director
Offers small business conseling and training to individuals with disabilities

5878 Michigan Employment Service
7310 Woodward Avenue
Detroit, MI 48202 313-872-1885
888-605-6722
FAX: 313-876-5760
www.michigan.gov/mdcd
Job development and placement in services to dislocated workers with disabilities

5879 Michigan Fair Employment Practice Agency
Michigan Department of Civil Rights
1200 6th Street
6th Floor
Detroit, MI 48226 313-256-2663
FAX: 313-256-6167
e-mail: MDCR-INFO@michigan.gov
www.mdcr.state.mi.us/mdcr
Investigates and resolves discrimination complaints and works to prevent discrimination through educational programs that promote voluntary compliance with civil rights laws

5880 Michigan Rehabilitation Services: Dept of Labor And Economic Development
PO Box 30010
Lansing, MI 48909 517-373-3390
800-605-6722
FAX: 517-335-7277
e-mail: shamsiddeenj@michigan.gov
www.michigan.gov/mdcd

Jaye Balthazar, Manager
State vocational rehabilitation agency.

5881 Small Business Development Center
Ann Arbor Center for Independent Living
2568 Packard Road
Ann Arbor, MI 48104 313-971-0277
FAX: 313-971-0826

Roseanne Herzog, Director
Phil Zepeda, Manager
Offers small business counseling and training to individuals with disabilities in the state of Michigan.

Minnesota

5882 **Jewish Vocational Service of Jewish Family and Children's Services**
430 First Avenue North
Suite 620
Minneapolis, MN 55401
612-692-8920
FAX: 612-692-8921
e-mail: jvs@jvsmn.org
www.jvsmn.org

Jeremy Waldman, Executive Director
The mission of JVS is to be a recognized leader in delivering employment, training, and career development services that positively impact individuals of all backgrounds, business and society.

5883 **Minnesota Employment Practice Agency**
190 E. 5th Street
Suite 700
Saint Paul, MN 55101
651-296-5663
800-657-3740
www.humanrights.state.mn.us

Velma Korbel, Commissioner
James Kirkpatrick, Deputy Commissioner
Janeen Rosas, Manager
Mission and vision is to make Minnesota discrimination free.

5884 **Minnesota Rehabilitation Services**
332 Minnesota Street
Suite E200
Saint Paul, MN 55101
651-296-5616
800-328-9095
FAX: 651-297-5159
TTY: 800-657-3973
e-mail: Paul.Bridges@state.mn.us
www.deed.state.men.us

Kimberly Pack, Director
Paul Bridges, Manager
Service for people with disabilities who need services to prepare for work, or to find and keep a job.

5885 **PWI Forum**
Multi Resource Centers
1900 Chicago Avenue
Minneapolis, MN 55404
612-752-8138

Newsletter for business, community and government leaders. Focuses on employment of persons with disabilities.

5886 **Vocational and Rehabilitation Agency**
21200 University Ave W
Suite 240
Saint Paul, MN 55114
651-642-0500
800-652-9000
FAX: 651-284-3307
TTY: 612-642-0506
e-mail: info@ngwmail.des.state.mn.us
www.mnwfc.org

Chuck Hamilton, Executive Director
People seeking work, businesses seeking employees, students, and those looking for a first job or returning to the workforce, will find services to meet their needs.

Mississippi

5887 **Allied Enterprises of Tupelo**
Ability Works Incorporated
2701 C R 402
Corinth, MS 38834
662-287-6964
FAX: 662-287-1463

Michael Byrd, Facility Manager
Vocational evaluation, work adjustment and job placement of disabled persons in a rehabilitation workshop.

5888 **Mississippi Department of Rehabilitation Services**
PO Box 1698
Jackson, MS 39215
601-853-5100
800-443-1000
FAX: 601-853-5158
TTY: 800-443-1000
e-mail: bmcmillan@mdrs.state.ms.us
www.mdrs.state.ms.us

Hs Mcmillan, Director
Bob Richards, Manager
Offers low vision aids and appliances, counseling, social work, educational and professional training, residential services, recreational services, computer training and employment opportunities for the handicapped.

5889 **Mississippi Employment Secutity Commission**
1235 Echelon Parkway
Po Box 1699
Jackson, MS 39215
601-321-6000
FAX: 601-961-7405
www.mdes.ms.gov
A federally funded state agency. The programs of MDES, under direction of the governor of Mississippi, report to the federal government.

5890 **Worksight**
Mississippi State University
PO Box 6189
Mississippi State, MS 39762
662-325-2001
800-675-7782
FAX: 662-325-8989
e-mail: jemoor@colled.msstate.edu
www.blind.msstate.edu

Elton Moore, Director
Discusses news, activities, research projects and training programs of the Center.

Missouri

5891 **Missouri Fair Employment Practice Agency**
Missouri Fair Employment Practice Agency
3315 W Truman Boulevard
Jefferson City, MO 65102
573-751-3325
877-781-4236
FAX: 573-751-2905
e-mail: mchr@dolir.mo.gov
www.dolir.state.mo.us/hr

Renell Wynn, Director
Catherine Leapheart, Executive Director

5892 **Missouri Governor's Council on Disability**
301 West High Street Room 250-A
Po Box 1668
Jefferson City, MO 65102
573-751-2600
800-877-8249
FAX: 573-526-4109
TTY: 573-751-2600
e-mail: gcd@oa.mo.gov
www.gcd.oa.mo.gov

Robert Honan, Executive Director
Advocate training, civil rights, community education services, community resource referral, conferences, consumer education, disability awareness program, educational information and resources, information and education services, information and referral, newsletter, policy issues and services, publications, resource directory, seminars, technical assistance, training and seminars.

5893 **Missouri Job Training Program Liaison**
221 Metro Drive
Jefferson City, MO 65109
573-634-2321

Joe Jerkins, Manager
Services for individuals with disabilities who want to become employed.

5894 **Missouri Vocational Rehabilitation Agency**
3024 Dupont Circle
Jefferson Cty, MO 65109
573-751-3251
877-222-8963
FAX: 573-741-1441
TTY: 573-751-3251
www.vr.dese.mo.gov

Don Glann, Assistant Commissioner
Jeanne Loyd, Manager
A team of decicated individuals working for the continuous improvement of education and services for all citizens.

5895 **WX: Work Capacities**
17331 E 40th Highway
Suite 103
Independence, MO 64055
816-478-2333

Carol Lett, Executive Director
Mike Heinz, Manager
Services for individuals with disabilities who want to become employed.

Montana

5896 **Montana Fair Employment Practice Agency**
PO Box 1728
1625 11th Avenue
Helena, MT 59624
406-444-2844
800-542-0807
http://erd.dil.state.mt.us/humanrights/hrhome
Advocate training, civil rights, community education services, community resource referral and conferences

5897 **Montana Governor's Committee on Employment of Disabled People**
Mitchell Building
Po Box 200127
Helena, MT 59620
406-444-3794
800-243-4091
FAX: 406-444-0544
Services for individuals with disabilities who want to become employed.

Nebraska

5898 **Nebraska Employment Services**
Department of Labor
550 S 16th Street
Lincoln, NE 68508
402-471-9000

Services for individuals with disabilities who want to become employed.

5899 **Nebraska Fair Employment Practice Agency**
301 Centennial Mall S
Lincoln, NE 68508
402-471-2024
800-642-6112
www.nol.org/home/neoc

5900 **Nebraska Vocational Rehabilitation Agency**
301 Centennial Mall S
Lincoln, NE 68508
402-471-3644
877-637-3422
FAX: 402-471-0788
e-mail: vr_stateoffice@vocrehab.state.ne.us

Cheryl Ferree, Manager
Services for individuals with disabilities who want to become employed. Services are free to those who qualify.

Nevada

5901 **Nevada Fair Employment Practice Agency**
1455 E Tropicana Avenue
Suite 500
Las Vegas, NV 89119
702-486-7161
FAX: 702-486-7054
http://detr.state.nv.us/nerc

5902 **Nevada Governor's Committee on Employment of Persons with Disabilities**
4600 Kietzke Lane
Suite A108
Reno, NV 89502
775-688-1111
FAX: 775-688-1113
Services for individuals with disabilities who want to become employed.

5903 **Vocational and Rehabilitation Agency**
State of Nevada
505 E King Street
Suite 502
Carson City, NV 89701
775-684-4040
FAX: 775-684-4184
e-mail: mryasmer@nvdetr.org
detr.state.nv.us

Michael Coleman, Administrator
Peter Singleton, Rehabilitation Program Superviso
Bob Nichols, Rehabilitation Manager
The Rehabilitation Division is comprised of four bureaus and the community-based services unit to address prevention, assessment, training, treatment and job placement for Nevadans with functional disabilities. The division places primary emphasis on providing necessary services to help clients work and live independently and substance-free. The division administrator, based in Carson City, oversees programs offered in offices throughout the state.

New Hampshire

5904 **Fit for Work at Exeter Hospital**
10 Buzell Avenue
Exeter, NH 03833
603-778-7311
FAX: 603-778-6671

Kevin Callahan, President
Staffed by a team of allied health professionals, our outpatient rehabilitation program offers functional restoration, work therapy, diagnostic testing and physical therapy.

5905 **New Hampshire Employment Security**
32 S Main Street
Concord, NH 03301
603-224-3311
800-852-3400
FAX: 603-228-4145
TTY: 800-735-2964
e-mail: webmaster@nhes.state.nh.us
www.nhes.state.nh.us

Richard S Brothers, Commissioner
Operates a free public employment service and provides assisted and self directed employment and career related services and labor market information for employers and the general public.

5906 **New Hampshire Fair Employment Practice Agency**
2 Chenell Drive
Concord, NH 03301
603-225-3699
FAX: 603-271-6339

5907 **New Hampshire Job Training Program Liaison**
64 Old Suncook Road
Concord, NH 03301
603-228-3349

5908 **Vocational and Rehabilitation Agency**
Department of Education
21 S Fruit Street
Suite 20
Concord, NH 03301
603-271-3471
TTY:603-271-3471
www.ed.state.nh.us

Paul Leather, Director
Offers services for the totally blind, legally blind, visually impaired, mentally retarded blind and more with health, counseling, educational, recreational, rehabilitation, computer training and professional training services.

New Jersey

5909 **ARC of Gloucester County**
1555 Gateway Boulevard
Woodbury, NJ 08096
856-848-8648
FAX: 856-848-7753
e-mail: webmaster@thearcgloucester.org
www.thearcgloucester.org

Ana Rivera, Executive Director

5910 **ARC of Hunterdon County**
1322 State Route 31
Suite 5
Annandale, NJ 08801
908-735-7775
FAX: 980-730-7726

Barbara Gustassen, Contact
Robin Horne, Manager
Serves Hunterdon County.

5911 **ARC of Mercer County**
180 Ewingville Road
Ewing, NJ 08638
609-406-0181
FAX: 609-406-9258
e-mail: arc@arcmercer.org
www.arcmercer.org

Steven Cook, President
Geoffrey Morris, First Vice President
Dennis Micai, Manager

5912 **ARC of Monmouth**
1158 Wayside Road
Tinton Falls, NJ 07712
732-493-1919
FAX: 732-493-3604
e-mail: info@arcofmonmouth.org
www.arcofmonmouth.org

Philip A. Fina, President, Board
Sherry Blackman, Director Social Services
Mary Scott, Executive Director

5913 **Abilities Center of New Jersey**
1208 Delsea Drive
Westville, NJ 08093
856-848-1025
FAX: 856-848-8429
e-mail: info@abilities2worl.com
www.abilities2work.com

Sharon Knubuehl, President

5914 **Abilities of Northwest New Jersey**
PO Box 251
Washington, NJ 07882
908-689-1118
FAX: 908-689-6363

Richard Lowe, President
Serves northwestern New Jersey.

5915 **Alliance for Disabled in Action New Jersey**
629 Amboy Avenue
Suite Ll
Edison, NJ 08837
732-738-4388
FAX: 732-738-4416
TTY:732-738-9644
e-mail: adacil@adacil.org
www.adacil.org

Richard Ringhof, Executive Director
Serves Somerset, Union and Middlesex Counties in New Jersey.

5916 **Alternatives for Growth: New Jersey**
16-00 208 S
Fair Lawn, NJ 07410
201-797-8330
FAX: 201-797-3586

Donna Flannery, Contact
Serves all New Jersey.

5917 **Arc of Bergen and Passaic Counties**
223 Moore Street
Hackensack, NJ 07601
201-343-0322
FAX: 201-343-0401
e-mail: arcbp@aol.com
www.arcbergenpassaic.org

James E Seath, President/CEO
Kathy Walsh, Vice President
Olga Podolsky, Family Support Supervisor
Serving persons with disabilities and their families in Bergen and Passaic Counties, NJ.

5918 **Career Opportunity Development of New Jersey**
901 Atlantic Avenue
Egg Harbor City, NJ 08215
609-965-6871

Jenine Emil, Contact
Linda Carney, President
Serves Bergen and Passaic Counties.

5919 **Center for Educational Advancement New Jersey**
11 Minneakoning Road
Flemington, NJ 08822
908-782-1480
FAX: 908-782-5370
e-mail: jkunz@ceaemployment.com
www.ceaemployment.com

Joanne Kunz, Vice President
Michael Skoczek, President
Serves Somerset and Hunterdon Counties. Skills training in office technology and food service. Job placement and job coaching services are available. Employer Network for Ticket to Work.

5920 **Cerebral Palsy Association of Middlesex County**
Oak Drive
Edison, NJ 08837
732-549-5580
FAX: 201-603-0284

Dominic Ursino, President
Serves Central New Jersey.

5921 **Easter Seal Hackensack**
171 Atlantic Street
Hackensack, NJ 07601
201-342-5739
FAX: 201-342-4480

Denise Sredeen, Contact
Serves Hackensack.

5922 **Easter Seal Society of New Jersey Highlands Workshop**
Easter Seals
133 Main Street
Franklin, NJ 07416
973-827-9066
FAX: 973-827-3828

Dave Shickle, Contact
Peggy Skipp, Manager
Serves all New Jersey.

5923 **Easter Seal of Ocean County**
150 Oberlin Avenue N
Lakewood, NJ 08701
732-363-8990
FAX: 732-363-7540

Greg Makely, Contact

5924 **Easter Seals New Jersey**
1 Kimberly Road
E Brunswick, NJ 08816
732-257-6662

www.eastersealsnj.org

Brian Fitzgerald, Chief Executive Officer
Serves all New Jersey.

5925 **Eden Acres Administrative Services**
1 Eden Way
Princeton, NJ 08540
609-987-0099
FAX: 609-734-0069

Tom Cool, President
Provides services for the disabilitated.

5926 **Edison Sheltered Workshop**
328 Plainfield Avenue
Edison, NJ 08817
732-985-8834
FAX: 732-985-2216

Ann Marie Stone, Vocational Rehab. Counselor
Veronica Valez, Executive Director
Serves Middlesex County. Vocational training and job placement services.

5927 **First Occupational Center of New Jersey**
391 Lakeside Avenue
Orange, NJ 07050
973-672-5800
800-894-6265
FAX: 973-672-0065
e-mail: ocnj@idt.net
www.ocnj.org

Rocco J Meola, President/CEO
Tanya M. Edghill, VP Of Program Services
A private, nonprofit multi-service community rehabilitation program. Services are offered to all people, such as developmentally disabled, visually impaired, hearing impaired and welfare recipients. Services include vocational evaluation and training, respite care, basic and remedial education and job placement and community support services.

5928 **Goodwill Industries of Southern New Jersey**
2835 Route 735
Maple Shade, NJ 08052
856-439-0174

Mike Shaw, Vice President

5929 **Hausmann Industries**
130 Union Street
Northvale, NJ 07647
201-767-1369
888-428-7626
FAX: 201-767-1369
e-mail: info@hausmann.com
www.hausmann.com

George Batchelor, Director Sales/Marketing
Werner Hausmann, Manager
Wheelchair acessible exam tables, treatment tables and mat platforms.

5930 **Jersey Cape Diagnostic Training & Opportunity Center**

152 Crest Haven Road
Cape May Court House, NJ 08210
609-465-4117
FAX: 609-465-3899

Steve Madzelski, Director
George Plewa, Executive Director
Serves Cape May County.

5931 **New Jersey Commission for the Blind and Visually Impaired**
Department of Human Services
PO Box 47017
Newark, NJ 07101
973-648-3333
877-685-8878
FAX: 973-648-7364
e-mail: Vito.DeSantis@cbvi.nj.us
www.cbvi.nj.gov

Vito J Desantis, Executive Director
Pamela Gaston, Executive Assistant
Khmbrly Howard PhD, Deputy Executive Director
Offers services for the totally blind, legally blind, visually impaired, deaf blind and more with eye health, counseling, educational, recreational, rehabilitation, computer training and vocational services.

5932 **New Jersey Employment Service and Job Training Program Services**
Department of Labor
Trenton, NJ 08625
609-292-1040

Roland Machold, Manager

5933 **Occupational Center of Hudson County**
780 Montgomery Street
Jersey City, NJ 07306
201-432-5959
FAX: 201-432-6227

Christine Remler, Executive Director
Serves Hudson County.

5934 **Occupational Center of Union County**
301 Cox Street
Roselle, NJ 07203
908-241-7200
FAX: 908-241-2025
e-mail: ocuc@OCUCNJ.com

Michele Ford, VP
Provides vocational rehabilitation and mental health service.

5935 **Occupational Training Center of Burlington County**
130 Hancock Lane
Westampton, NJ 08060
609-267-6677
FAX: 609-265-8418

Joseph Bender, President

5936 **Occuptational Training Center of Camden County, New Jersey**
215 W White Horse Pike
Berlin, NJ 08009
856-768-0845
FAX: 856-767-1378

Matt Treihart, President
Serves Camden County.

5937 **Pathways to Independence**
60 Kingsland Avenue
Kearny, NJ 07032
201-997-6155
FAX: 201-991-7530
e-mail: PTI450@aol.com
www.pathwaystoindependencenj.org

Alvin Cox, Executive Director
Tessa Farrell, Program Director
Serves Hudson, South Bergen and Essex counties, providing vocational and pre-vocational services to adults with disabilities.

5938 **Somerset Training and Employment Program**
36 4th Street
Somerville, NJ 08876
732-846-2734

Laurie Falka, Executive Director
Courtney Throckmorton, Owner

5939 **St. John of God Community Services Vocational Rehabilitation**
1145 Delsea Drive
Westville, NJ 08093
856-848-4700
FAX: 856-848-1512

Muncie Buckalew, Executive Director
Serves Gloucester and Camden Counties.

5940 **United Cerebral Palsy Associations of New Jersey**
354 S Broad Street
Trenton, NJ 08608
609-392-4004
888-322-1918
FAX: 609-392-3505
www.cpofnj.org

Jacqueline Stroman, Director of Education
Jack Mudge, Executive Director

5941 **Vocational and Rehabilitation Agency**
PO Box 398
Trenton, NJ 08625
609-292-5987
FAX: 609-292-8347
TTY:609-292-2919
e-mail: tjennings@dol.state.nj.us
www.state.nj.us

Thomas G Jennings, Director

5942 **West Essex Rehab Center**
83 Walnut Street
Montclair, NJ 07042
973-744-7733
FAX: 201-744-3744

Ben Viearisi, Contact
Shannon Williams, Contact
Eugene Stefanelli, Executive Director

New Mexico

5943 **Adelante Development Center**
3900 Osterna NE
Albuquerque, NM 87109
505-341-2000
FAX: 505-341-2001
www.go.adelante.org

Mike Kivitze, Executive Director
Serves Albuquerque and Belin.

5944 **Goodwill Industries of New Mexico**
5000 San Mateo Boulevard NE
Albuquerque, NM 87109
505-881-6612
FAX: 505-884-3157
www.goodwillnm.org

Fred Calkins, President
Richard Thorne, Vice President
Patrick Michaels, Chief Executive Officer
Serves Albuquerque, Santa Fe and Rio Rancho.

5945 **New Mexico Employment Services and Job Training Liaison**
PO Box 1928
Albuquerque, NM 87103
505-827-6827
FAX: 505-827-6812
e-mail: djones2@state.nm.us

Reese Suliten, Director

5946 **RCI**
1023 Stanford Drive NE
Albuquerque, NM 87106
505-247-4936
FAX: 505-255-9971
www.rci-nm.org

Greg Racca, Owner
Serves Bernalillo County.

5947 **Tohatchi Area of Opportunity & Services**
PO Box 49
Tohatchi, NM 87325
505-733-2200
FAX: 505-733-2678

Patrick Keptner, Executive Director
Marcella Franklin, Program Director
Daric Kalleco, Community Living Coordinator
Serves McKinley County, San Jose County and the Havanjo Nation.

5948 **Vocational Rehabilitation Agency**
435 Saint Michaels Drive
Suite D
Santa Fe, NM 87505
505-954-8500
800-224-7005
FAX: 505-954-8556
TTY: 8779548583
e-mail: dvris@state.nm.us
www.dvrgetsjobs.com

Catherine Cross-Maple, Manager

5949 **Vocational and Rehabilitation Agency**
2905 Rodeo Park Drive E
Building 4
Santa Fe, NM 87505
505-954-8500
888-513-7968
FAX: 505-476-4475
e-mail: greg.trapp@state.nm.us
www.state.nm.us/cftb

Greg Trapp, Executive Director
James Salas, Deputy Director
Adelmo Vigil, Deputy Director-IL/OB

New York

5950 **JOBS VI and SAGE**
P ES CO International
21 Paulding Street
Pleasantville, NY 10570
914-769-4266
800-431-2016
FAX: 914-769-2970
e-mail: pesco@pesco.org
www.pesco.org

Charles Kass, Vice President
Joseph Kass, President
A computerized matching system matching people to occupations, training, local jobs, local employers and giving job outlooks for the year 2005. Computerized Sage is online computerized testing with the ability for system to read all questions, and job descriptions. Manual Sage is a hands on-computer scored test battery with various adaptation. Braille, large print, bi-lingual and special devices.

5951 **Just One Break (JOBS)**
120 Wall Street
Fl 20
New York, NY 10005
212-785-7300
FAX: 212-785-4513
e-mail: jobs@justonebreak.com
www.justonebreak.com

Susan S Odiseos, Executive Director
C Jeffrey Knittel, President

5952 **New York State Department of Labor**
State Office Campus
Building 12
Albany, NY 12240
518-485-6800

e-mail: nysdol@labor.state.ny.us
www.labor.state.ny.us

James J Mcgowan, Commissioner
Fredda Peritz, Employment Service Division Dire
Thomas Malone, Unemployment Insur. Div. Dir.

The missin of the New York State Department of Labor is to help New York work by preparing individuals for the jobs of today and tomorrow. Provides direct job search and counseling services to job seekers, and can refer people who have disabilities for training opportunities. Provides unemployment insurance for those out of work through no fault of their own.

5953 Rational Effectiveness Training Systems
IRET Corporate Services Division
45 E 65th Street
New York, NY 10021
212-570-2868

Dr. Dominic DiMattie, Director
Offers advanced training for employee assistance professionals, full service outpatient counseling, consulting services and on-site workshops for the disabled.

5954 Special Education and Vocational Rehabilitation Agency: New York
1 Commerce Plaza
Room 1606
Albany, NY 12234
518-474-2714
800-222-5662
FAX: 518-474-8802
TTY: 518-474-5652
www.vesid.nysed.gov

Rebecca Cort, Director

North Carolina

5955 Division of Employment & Training
4111 N Harrington Street
Raleigh, NC 27603
919-715-6500

Gary Hunt, Executive Director

5956 Iredell Vocational Workshop
200 Clanton Road
Charlotte, NC 28217
704-944-5100
FAX: 704-871-9881
www.lifespanservices.org

Stacey Draison, Director

5957 North Carolina Division of Services for the Blind
Department of Health and Human Services
2601 Mail Service Center
Raleigh, NC 27699
919-733-9822
FAX: 919-733-9769
TTY:919-733-9700
e-mail: debbie.jackson@ncmail.net
www.dhhs.state.nc.us/dsb

Debbie Jackson, Director
Mary Flanagan, Assistant Director

5958 Rowan County Vocational Workshop
2728 Old Concord Road
Salisbury, NC 28146
704-633-6223
FAX: 704-633-6224

Carl Rapsher, Executive Director
Offers vocational assessment and training, adult developmental activities.

5959 Rutherford Vocational Workshop
200 Fairground Road
Spindale, NC 28160
828-286-4352

Larry Brown, Executive Director

5960 Transylvania Vocational Services
PO Box 1115
Brevard, NC 28712
828-884-3195
FAX: 828-884-3102

Nancy Stricker, Executive Director

5961 Vocational and Rehabilitation Agency
2601 Mail Service Center
Raleigh, NC 27699
919-855-3500
FAX: 919-715-7905
TTY:919-733-9700
e-mail: John.DeLuca@ncmail.net
www.dhhs.state.nc.us

Linda Harrington, Manager
Offers services for the totally blind, legally blind, visually impaired, mentally retarded blind and more with health, counseling, educational, recreational, rehabilitation, computer training and professional training services.

5962 Vocational and Rehabilitation Agency: Department of Health and Human Services
2801 Mail Service Center
Raleigh, NC 27699
919-855-3500
FAX: 919-733-7968
TTY:919-733-5924
e-mail: dvr.info@nc.mail.netnet
dvr.dhhs.state.nc.us

Linda Harrington, Director

5963 Webster Enterprises of Jackson County
PO Box 220
Webster, NC 28788
828-586-8981
800-978-2681
FAX: 828-586-8125
www.websterenterprises.org

Darrell Fox, Executive Director
A community based employment and training program for people with disabilities. A full service program which includes a youth transitional program for life beyond high school, job coaching, vocational assessment and job placement.

5964 Western Regional Vocational Rehabilitation Facility Clifford File, Jr.
PO Box 1443
Morganton, NC 28680

Clifford File Jr, Executive Director
Vocational Evaluation, Work Adjustment, Job Placement, On-site Work Services Program. Serves most disability groups including CMI, DD, Deaf and Physically impaired.

North Dakota

5965 North Dakota Department of Labor, Equal Employment Opportunity Division
600 E Boulevard Avenue
Dept 406
Bismarck, ND 58505
701-328-2660
800-582-8032
FAX: 701-328-2031
e-mail: labor@nd.gov
www.state.nd.us/labor

Lisa K Fair McLavers, Comissioner of Labor
Kathy Kulesa, Human Rights Director
Through a work-sharing agreement with the Equal Employment Opportunity Commission (EEOC), the North Dakota Department of Labor enforces the Americans with Disabilities Act (ADA) as related to employment discrimination.

5966 North Dakota Employment Service and Job Training Program Liaison
Job Service North Dakota
PO Box 1537
Bismarck, ND 58502
701-258-6353

Leslie Weiss, Manager

5967 **North Dakota Governor's Committee on Employment of Disabled Persons**
600 S 2nd Street
Suite 1b
Bismarck, ND 58504
701-328-8989
FAX: 701-328-8969

5968 **North Dakota Vocational Rehabilitation Agency**
Prairie Hills Plaza 1237 W Divide
Suite 1b
Bismarck, ND 58501
701-328-8950
800-755-2745
FAX: 701-328-8969
TTY: 701-328-8968

Wanda Byer, Interim Director
Offers services for the totally blind, legally blind, visually impaired, mentally retarded blind and more with health, counseling, educational, recreational, rehabilitation, computer training and professional training services.

Ohio

5969 **Cornucopia**
18120 Sloane Avenue
Lakewood, OH 44107
216-521-4600
FAX: 216-521-9460
www.lkwdpl.org/paths/healingarts/ Nature s

Chris Yurick, Program Manager
Scott Duennes, Executive Director
Provides work adjustment training for people with and developmental disabilities in a unique community based setting; Nature's Bin, a natural fresh foods market. Consumers learn through participation in retail operations in produce, grocery, bakery, deli, maintenance and customer service areas. Retail revenues help offset the cost of the program. Job search skills training and placement assistance available to program graduates.

5970 **Great Oaks Joint Vocational School**
3254 E Kemper Road
Cincinnati, OH 45241
513-772-4603

Harold Carr, Medical Director
Deb Graw, Manager

5971 **Hearth Day Treatment and Vocational Services**
8301 Detroit Avenue
Cleveland, OH 44102
216-281-2660

Ralph Fee, Executive Director

5972 **Highland Unlimited Business Enterprises of CRI**
1322 E McMillan Street
Cincinnati, OH 45206
513-569-4730
FAX: 513-751-2938
e-mail: ddutton@cricincy.com
www.cricincy.com

Tony Datillo, Executive Director
Debbie Dutton Lambert, Director Employment Programs

5973 **Ohio Civil Rights Commission**
1111 E Broad Street
Suite 301
Columbus, OH 43205
614-466-2785
FAX: 614-644-8776

G Payton, Manager

5974 **Ohio Commission On Minority Health**
77 S. High St. eet
7th Floor
Columbus, OH 43215
614-466-4000
FAX: 614-752-9049
e-mail: minhealth@ocinh.state.oh.us
www.mih.ohio.gov

Cheryl Boyce, Executive Director

5975 **Vocational and Rehabilitation Agency**
400 E Campus View Boulevard
Columbus, OH 43235
614-466-9364
800-282-4536
FAX: 614-785-5012
TTY: 614-438-1334
e-mail: john.connellyu@rsc.state.oh.us
www.state.oh.us

John Connelly, Director
Rose Reed, Manager

Oklahoma

5976 **Oklahoma Department of Rehabilitation Services (DRS)**
3535 NW 58th Street
Suite 500
Oklahoma City, OK 73112
405-951-3400
800-845-8476
FAX: 405-951-3529
e-mail: jprice@drs.state.ok.us
www.okrehab.org

Jody Harlem, Public Information Administrator
Linda Parker, Executive Director

5977 **Oklahoma Employment Services and Job Training Program Liaison**
2401 N Lincoln Boulevard
Oklahoma City, OK 73105
405-557-7211
FAX: 405-557-5368

5978 **Oklahoma Governor's Committee on Employment of People with Disabilities**
2712 Villa Prom
Oklahoma City, OK 73107
405-424-8378
FAX: 405-943-7550

Tom Kelly, President

Oregon

5979 **Bend Work Activity Center**
275 NE 2nd Street
Bend, OR 97701
541-389-0129
FAX: 541-389-2084
e-mail: info@ofco.org
www.ofco.org

James Booth, Chairperson
Bill Schertzinger, Vice Chairperson
Cam Chambers, Manager

5980 **Oregon Fair Employment Practice Agency**
Oregon Bureau of Labor & Industry
PO Box 800
Portland, OR 97207
503-229-6601

5981 **State of Oregon Office of Vocational Rehabilitation Service**

3165 10th Street
500
Baker City, OR 97814
541-523-8441
866-752-5235
FAX: 541-524-0441
e-mail: wendy.m.wall@state.or.us

Wendy Wall, Counselor Assistant
Allan McCandless, Voc Rehab Counselor
Samantha McConnell, Voc Rahab Counselor

5982 **Vocational and Rehabilitation Agency**

500 Summer Street NE
E-87
Salem, OR 97301
503-945-5880
877-277-0513
FAX: 503-947-5025
TTY: 503-945-5894
e-mail: bobby.c.simpson@state.or.us
www.oregon.gov/dhs/vr/index.shtml

Stephanie Taylor, Administrator

5983 **Vocational and Rehabilitation Agency: Commision for the Blind**

535 SE 12th Avenue
Portland, OR 97214
503-731-3221
FAX: 503-731-3230
e-mail: linda.mock@state.or.us
www.cfb.state.or.us

Linda Mock, Administrator
Pat Donell, Executive Director

Pennsylvania

5984 **AC-ACLD/An Association for Children and Adults with Learning Disabilities**

4900 Girard Road
Pittsburgh, PA 15227
412-881-2253
FAX: 412-881-2263
e-mail: info@acldonline.org
www.acldonline.org

Thomas Fogarty, President
Offers services to children, adolescents and adults with specific learning disabilities.

5985 **Office of Vocational Rehabilitation**

7th and Forester Street
Harrisburg, PA 17120
717-787-4746
FAX: 717-783-5221

Barry Brandt, Rehabilitation Specialist
Information in vocational counseling and the governor's committee on Employment of People with Disabilities. Also serves persons with disabilities that present a substantial handicap to employment and independence. Services are provided when there is a reasonable expectation that employment is possible as a result of those services.

5986 **Pennsylvania Employment Services and Job Training**

P A Department of Labor and Industry
7th and Forster Street
Room 1700
Harrisburg, PA 17120
717-787-5279
FAX: 717-787-8826
www.dli.state.pa.us

Edward Rendell, Governor
Stephen Schmerin, Manager

5987 **Pennsylvania Governor's Committee on Employment of Disabled Persons**

7th and Forester Street
Harrisburg, PA 17120
717-787-4746

5988 **Pennsylvania Human Relations Commission Agency**

301 Chestnut Street
Suite 300
Harrisburg, PA 17101
717-787-4410
FAX: 717-214-0584
www.phrc.state.pa.us

Homer Floyd, Executive Director

5989 **US Healthworks**

1114 Commons Boulevard
Reading, PA 19605
610-926-0960
FAX: 610-926-6225

Beverly Shaeff, Manager
Helps injured workers overcome injuries or disabilities and return to their jobs.

5990 **Vocational and Rehabilitation Agency**

1521 N 6th Street
Harrisburg, PA 17102
717-787-5244
800-442-6351
FAX: 717-787-3210
TTY: 717-787-5244
e-mail: ovr@dli.state.pa.us
www.dli.state.pa.us

William Gannon, Director
Thomas Washic, Manager

5991 **Vocational and Rehabilitation Agency: Department of Labor and Industry**

909 Green Street
Harrisburg, PA 17102
717-236-6211
800-622-2842
FAX: 717-787-3210
TTY: 717-787-6176
e-mail: cboone@state.pa.us

Thomas Carlock, Chief Executive Officer

Rhode Island

5992 **Goodwill Industries of RI**

100 Houghton Street
Providence, RI 02904
401-861-2080
FAX: 401-454-0889

Laurie Norris, President/CEO
Jeff Machado, Cheif Deputy Officer

5993 **Groden Center**

86 Mount Hope Avenue
Providence, RI 02906
401-274-6310

Michael Smith, Administration
June Groden, Chief Executive Officer

5994 **Newport County Chapter of Retarded Citizens**

PO Box 4390
Middletown, RI 02842
401-846-0340
FAX: 401-847-9459

John Maher, Executive Director

5995 **Office of Rehabilitation Services**

40 Fountain Street
Providence, RI 02903
401-421-7005
FAX: 401-222-3574
www.ors.ri.gov

Ron Racine, Deputy Administrator For Blind
Steve Brunero, Deputy Administrator-ORS
John Microulis, Deputy Administrator-Disability
Their goal is to help individuals with physical and mental disabilities prepare for and obtain appropriate employment.

5996 **Vocational and Rehabilitation Agency: Department of Human Services**
RI Services for the Blind and Visually Impaired
40 Fountain Street
Providence, RI 02903
401-222-2300
FAX: 401-222-1328
TTY:401-222-3010
e-mail: garyw@ors.ri.gov
www.ors.ri.gov

Raymond Carroll, Administrator
Their goal is to help individuals with physical and mental disabilities prepare for and obtain appropriate employment.

South Carolina

5997 **South Carolina Employment Security Commission South Carolina Center**
PO Box 567
Columbia, SC 29202
803-737-9935
800-436-8190
FAX: 803-737-2756
www.sces.org

Camille Fallow, Disability Program Navigator
Regina Ratterros, Program Coordinator/State Office
Public agency taht offers job search assistance. Unemployment Benefits and WIA program. Also offered is Disability Program Navigator who helps persons with disabilities to find needed resources

5998 **South Carolina Governor's Committee on Employment of the Handicapped**
1330 Boston Street
Columbia, SC 29203
803-896-1208
FAX: 803-896-6373

Gayle Brazell, Executive Director

5999 **South Carolina Vocational Rehabilitation Department**
1410 Boston Avenue
PO Box 15
West Columbia, SC 29171
803-896-6500
800-832-7526
TTY:803-896-6553
e-mail: info@scvrd.state.sc.us
www.scvrd.net

Larry C Bryant, Commissioner
The SCVRD's mission is to enable eligible South Carolinians with disabilities to prepare for, achieve and maintain competitive employment.

6000 **Vocational and Rehabilitation Agency: Vocational Rehabilitation Department**
PO Box 15
West Columbia, SC 29171
803-896-6700
800-832-7526
FAX: 803-896-6510
e-mail: kmandeville@scvrd.state.sc.us
www.scvrd.net

Kerry Mandeville, Director Case Services
Dan Parlor, Manager

6001 **Vocational and Rehabilitation Agency: Commission for the Blind**
Vocational and Rehabilitation Agency
PO Box 79
Columbia, SC 29202
803-737-5700
800-922-2222
FAX: 803-898-8852
e-mail: publicinfo@sccb.sc.gov
www.sccbc.sc.us

Nell Carney, Director

South Dakota

6002 **South Dakota Governor's Advisory Committee on Employment of the Disabled**
700 Governors Drive
Pierre, SD 57501
605-773-3423
FAX: 605-773-4236

Patrick Keating, Manager

6003 **South Dakota State Vocational Rehabilitati on**
Department of Human Services
3800 E Highway 34 Hillview Plaza
Pierre, SD 57501
605-773-5990
265-865-9684
FAX: 605-773-5483
TTY: 605-773-3195
e-mail: eric.weiss@state.sd.us
www.state.sd.us

Eric Weiss, Assistant Director
Berrie Grimme, Assistant Director Div of Rehab
Betty Oldenkamp, Manager
South Dakota State Vocational Rehabilitation consists of five agencies; Rehab Services and service to the Blind and Visually Impaired. There mission is the same to provide individualized rehabilitation services that result in optimal employment and independent living outcomes for individuals with disabilities.

6004 **South Dakota Workforce Investment Act Training Programs**
700 Governors Drive
Pierre, SD 57501
605-773-3423
800-952-3216
FAX: 605-773-4211
www.sdjobs.org

Michael Ryan, Director
Patrick Keating, Manager

6005 **Vocational and Rehabilitation Agency: Divi sion of Services to the Blind/Visually Impaired**
3800 E Highway 34 Hillview Plaza
Pierre, SD 57501
605-773-4644
800-265-9684
FAX: 605-773-5483
TTY: 605-773-4644
e-mail: gaye.mattke@state.sd.us
www.state.sd.us

Gaye Mattke, Director

Tennessee

6006 **Division of Rehabilitative Services**
Tennessee Department Human Services
400 Deaderick Street
15th Floor
Nashville, TN 37248
615-313-4714
FAX: 615-741-4165
e-mail: karen.a.wayson@state.tn.us
www.state.tn.us/humanserv/rehabilitation.htm

Andrea Cooper, Assistant Commissioner
Gina Lodge, Commisioner

6007 **Tennessee Department of Labor: Job Training Program Liaison**
501 Union Street
Nashville, TN 37219
615-741-6642

James Neeley, Manager

6008 **Tennessee Fair Employment Practice Agency**
Human Rights Commission
226 Capitol Boulevard
Suite 602
Nashville, TN 37219
615-741-5825

Tricia Crawford, Manager

Texas

6009 **C-CAD Center of United Cerebral Palsy of Metropolitan Dallas**
1950 N Stemmons Freeway
Dallas, TX 75207
214-746-4217
FAX: 214-800-2224
e-mail: info@ucpdallas.org
www.ucp.dallas.org

Debi Jobin, Director Assistive Tech Services
Susan Black, Special Products Coordinator
Offers a wide range of technology opportunities for persons with all types of disabilities, their families and the professionals who serve them. Services include assesments, traiing, technology access showroom, and workshops for rehabilitation and educational personnel.

6010 **Handbook of Career Planning for Students with Special Needs**
Pro- Ed Publications
8700 Shoal Creek Boulevard
Austin, TX 78757
512-451-3246
800-897-3202
FAX: 800-397-7633
e-mail: feedback@proedinc.com
www.proedinc.com

Donald Hammill, Owner
Courtney King, Marketing Coordinator
The practitioner's guide will show you how to help special needs adolescents and young adults overcome barriers to employment by identifying goals and problems, assessing interests and aptitudes, involving client families and developing communication skills. *$42.00*
358 pages

6011 **Texas Employment Services and Job Training Program Liaison**
Texas Workforce Commission
101 E 15th Street
Austin, TX 78778
512-444-7763
800-735-2988
TTY:700-735-2989
www.tec.state.tx.us

6012 **Vocational and Rehabilitation Agency: State Rehabilitation Commission**
Vocational and Rehabilitation Agency
4800 N Lamar Boulevard
Austin, TX 78756
512-424-4060
800-628-5115
FAX: 512-424-4730
TTY: 800-628-5115
e-mail: dars.inquiries@dars.state.tx.us
www.dars.state.tx.us

Sylvia Stacy, Inquiries Staff
Tim Spong, Manager

Utah

6013 **Utah Employment Services**
720 S 200 E
Salt Lake City, UT 84111
801-536-7401
FAX: 801-536-7011

6014 **Utah Governor's Committee on Employment of the Handicapped**
PO Box 45500
Salt Lake City, UT 84145
801-538-4200
FAX: 801-538-4446
www.hsdspd.utah.gov

George Kelner, Executive Director

6015 **Utah Veterans Centers**
750 N 200 W
Suite 105
Provo, UT 84601
801-377-1117
800-246-1197
FAX: 801-377-0227

Dennis Stevens, Executive Director
Brent Price, Manager
Readjustment counseling services to veterans.

6016 **Utah Vocational Rehabilitation Agency**
Utah State Office of Rehabilitation
PO Box 144200
Salt Lake City, UT 84114
801-538-7530
800-473-7530
FAX: 801-538-7522
e-mail: duchida@utah.gov
www.usor.utah.gov

Donald R Uchida, Executive Director
Russell Thelin, Director
Vocational Rehabilitation Services for individuals with disabilities.

6017 **Vocational and Rehabilitation Agency: Division of Services for the Blind/Visually Imp.**
250 N 1950 W
Suite B
Salt Lake City, UT 84116
801-323-4343
800-284-1823
FAX: 801-323-4396
e-mail: wgibson@utah.gov
www.usor.utah.gov

Bill Gibson, Director
Melanie Showell, Assistant Director

Vermont

6018 **State of Vermont Department of Aging and Disabilities**
103 S Main Street
Waterbury, VT 05671
802-241-2210
888-405-5005
FAX: 802-241-2128
e-mail: fredj@dad.state.vt.us
www.dad.state.vt.us/dbvi

Fred Jones, Director

6019 **Vermont Employment Services and Job Training**
5 Green Mountain Drive
PO Box 488
Montpelier, VT 05601
802-828-4000
FAX: 802-828-4022
TTY:802-828-4203
e-mail: tdouse@labor.state.vt.us
www.labor.vermont.gov

Tom Douse, Acting/Deputy Commissioner
Jill Greenwood, Workforce Development Director

6020 **Vermont Governor's Committee on Employment of People with Disabilities**
103 S Main Street
Waterbury, VT 05671
802-241-2186
866-879-6757
FAX: 802-241-3359
www.vocrehad.vermont.org

Diane Dalmasse, Director

6021 **Vocational and Rehabilitation Agency**
103 S Main Street
Waterbury, VT 05671
802-241-2186
866-879-6757
FAX: 802-241-3359
TTY: 802-241-2186
e-mail: diane@dail.state.vt.us
www.vocrehabvermont.org

Diane Dalmasse, Director

Virginia

6022 **Alexandria Community Y Head Start**
418 South Washington Street
Alexandria, VA 22314
703-329-2050
FAX: 703-998-5707

Yvonne Walker
Offers social services, on-the-job-training for parents, play therapy, physical therapy, speech therapy and any other specialized services.

6023 **Didlake**
8641 Breeden Avenue
Manassas, VA 20110
703-361-4195
FAX: 703-369-7141

Rexford Parr Jr, President/CEO
John S Craig, VP Rehabilitation Services
Offers situational assessments, work training, employment and job placement services to people with disabilities.

6024 **Learning Services: Shenandoah**
9524 Fairview Avenue
Manassas, VA 20110
703-335-9771
FAX: 703-335-1064

Peter Patrick, Administrator
Postacute rehabilitation program.

6025 **NISH**
8401 Old Courthouse Road
Vienna, VA 22182
571-226-4660
FAX: 703-849-8916
www.nish.org

E Robert Chamberlin, President/CEO
Lynne Harris, Dir. Corporate Communications
A nonprofit agency desigated by the Committee for Purchase from People Who Are Blind or Severely Disabled to provide technical assistance to rehabilitation programs interested in obtaining federal contracts under Public Law 92-28, the Javits-Wagner-O'Day Act. NISH's primary objective is to assist community rehabilitation programs in providing jobs for people with severe disabilities.

6026 **Richmond Research Training Center**
PO Box 842011
Richmond, VA 23284
804-828-1222

Paul Wehman MD, Director
Dolores Taylor, Executive Director
Research and training center report on the supported employment of persons with developmental and other disabilities.

6027 **ServiceSource**
6295 Edsall Road
Suite 175
Alexandria, VA 22312
703-461-6000
800-244-0817
FAX: 703-461-3906
www.ourpeoplework.org

Janet Samuelson, President
Edie Castner, Assistant Director
Provides training, job placement and employment services in private sector and government contract employment.

6028 **Sheltered Occupational Center of Virginia**
750 23rd Street S
Arlington, VA 22202
703-521-4441
FAX: 703-521-3443
www.socent.org

Charles Richman, President
Virgro Newkirk, Director of Operation
Assists, empowers and supports people with disabilities to achieve employment, independence and integration in the workplace and community. Our services include: printing, copying, hand work, mail shop, fulfillment and distribution.

6029 **Vocational and Rehabilitation Agency**
800 Franklin Darms Drive
Richmond, VA 23229
804-662-7000
800-552-5019
FAX: 804-662-9532
TTY: 800-464-9950
e-mail: drs@drs.virginia.gov
www.vadrs.org

James Rothrock, Commissioner

6030 **Vocational and Rehabilitation Agency: Department for the Blind/Visually Impaired**
397 Azalea Avenue
Richmond, VA 23227
804-371-3140
800-622-2155
FAX: 804-371-3351
e-mail: webmaster@drs.virginia.gov
www.vdbvi.org

Joseph A Bowman, Commissioner
James A Taylor, Chief Deputy

Washington

6031 **Career Connections**
421 N Mullan Road
Spokane Valley, WA 99206
509-928-0423
866-404-5867
FAX: 509-928-0441
e-mail: carconn@mindspring.com
www.peoplelinking.com

Susan Warwick, Executive Director
Teresa Antosyn, Program Coordinator
Dan Moody, CFO

6032 **Department of Services for the Blind National Business & Disability Council**
Department of Services for the Blind
PO Box 40933
Olympia, WA 98504
360-586-1224
800-552-7103
FAX: 360-586-7627
www.dsb.wa.gov

Louana Durand, Executive Director

6033 **Department of Social & Health Services National Business & Disability Council**
Department of Social & Health Services
PO Box 45340
Lacey, WA
360-725-3413
FAX: 360-407-0955
e-mail: dddcoreception@dshs.wa.gov
www1.dshs.wa.gov

Paul Strand, Co-Chair

6034 **SL Stuart and Associates**
25 W Nora Avenue
Spokane, WA 99205
509-328-2740
FAX: 509-326-9207
e-mail: info@slstart.com
www.slstart.com

Ray White, Director Employment Services
Stephen Start, Owner

6035 **School of Piano Technology for the Blind**
2510 E Evergreen Boulevard
Vancouver, WA 98661
360-693-1511
FAX: 360-693-6891
e-mail: info@pianotuningschool.org
www.pianotuningschool.org

Len Leger, Executive Director
Donald Mitchell, Director Instruction
Sharon Mitchell, Registar
Teaches piano tuning and repair to blind and visually impaired menand women, leading to employment and/or self-employment in the piano service industry. Licensed by Washington State and accredited by the Accrediting Commission of Career Schools and Colleges of Technology (ACCSCT). 20-month course.

6036 **Vocational and Rehabilitation Agency: Division of Vocational Rehabilitation**
Department of Social and Health
PO Box 45340
Olympia, WA 98504
360-725-3636
800-637-5627
FAX: 360-438-8007
TTY: 360-438-8000
e-mail: krulik@dshs.wa.gov
www1.dshs.wa.gov/dvr

West Virginia

6037 **West Virginia Division of Rehabilitation Services**
PO Box 50890
Charleston, WV 25305
304-766-4600
800-642-8207
FAX: 304-766-4905
TTY: 304-766-4965
www.wvdrs.org

Deborah Lovely, Acting Director
Donna Ashworth, Assistant Director
Vocational rehabilitation agency.

6038 **West Virginia Employment Services and Job Training Programs Liaison**
112 California Avenue
Charleston, WV 25305
304-558-0342
FAX: 304-558-0349
www.wvbep.org

Valerie Comer, Director
Allan Galloway, Manager

6039 **West Virginia Vocational Rehabilitation**
PO Box 1004
Institute, WV 25112
304-342-9952

Earl Wolfe, Director
Offers services for the totally blind, legally blind, visually impaired, mentally retarded blind and more with health, counseling, educational, recreational, rehabilitation, computer training and professional training services.

Wisconsin

6040 **Vocational and Rehabilitation: Division of Wisconsin**
201 E Washington Avenue
Madison, WI 53702
608-261-0050
FAX: 608-266-1784
TTY:6082435601
www.dwd.state.wi.us/dvr

Roberta Gaßsman, Secretary
Larry Studesville, Administrator
Charlene Dwyer, Manager
Offers services for the totally blind, legally blind, visually impaired, mentally retarded blind and more with health, counseling, educational, recreational, rehabilitation, computer training and professional training services.

6041 **Wisconsin Vocational Rehabilitation Agency**
201 E Washington Avenue
Room A100
Madison, WI 53707
608-243-5600
800-442-3477
FAX: 608-243-5680
TTY: 888-877-5939
e-mail: dwddvr@dwd.state.wi.us
www.dwd.state.wi.us/dvr

Charlene Dwyer, Administrator
Wisconsin's Vocational Rehabilitation is a federal/state program designed to obtain, maintain, and improve employment for people with disabilities by working with VR consumers, employers, and other partners.

Wyoming

6042 **Division of Vocational Rehabilitation of Wyoming**
Wyoming Department of Workforce Services
1100 Herschler Buiding
Cheyenne, WY 82002
307-777-7389
FAX: 307-777-5939
wyomingworkforce.org/how/vr.aspx

Jim Mcintosh, Administrator
Kathy Emmones, Director Workforce Services
Provides only those services which are necessary for eligible individuals to reach the employment goal agreed to in the Individualized Plan for Employment.

6043 **Vocational Rehabilitation, Division of Department of Workforce Services**
1160 Herschler Building
Suite 1e
Cheyenne, WY 82002
307-777-7385
FAX: 307-777-7155
TTY:307-777-7386
e-mail: jmcint@state.wy.us
www.wyomingworkforce.org

Jim McIntosh, Administrator

6044 **Wyoming Department of Employment Unemployment Insurance**
PO Box 2760
Casper, WY 82602
307-235-3288
FAX: 307-235-3278
doe.state.wy.us

Randy Hopper, Administrator

6045 **Wyoming Governor's Committee on Employment of the Handicapped**
Herschler
Room 1102
Cheyenne, WY 82002
307-777-7230
FAX: 307-777-5690

Brenda Oswald, Manager

Alabama

6046 **HealthSouth Rehabilitation Hospital of North Alabama**
107 Governors Drive SW
Huntsville, AL 35801
256-535-2300
FAX: 256-535-2402
www.healthsouth.com

Douglas H. Beverly, Administrator
A comprehensive 50 bed rehabilitation hospital serving the need of patients in the North Alabama area. Guides patients with physically disabling conditions along an individualized treatment pathway so they can reach their highest level of physical, social and emotional well-being. A wide range of medical and theraputic services are delivered by qualified and experienced professionals.

6047 **Lakeshore Rehabilitation Hospital**
3800 Ridgeway Drive
Birmingham, AL 35209
205-868-2098
FAX: 205-868-2007

Terry Brown, Administrator/CEO
Barbie Reedy, Contact
A 100 bed facility whos key services is physical rehabilitation. Also specialized services (inpatient) infection isolation room. In addition, also has outpatient physical rehabilitation and sports medicine. Patient family support services include patient representative, transportation for elderly/handicapped and patient support groups. Imaging services(diagnostic & theraputic) include ct scanner, diagnostic diagnostic radioisotope facility, MRI, and ultrasound.

6048 **Life Skills for Vocational Success**
Workshops
4244 3rd Avenue S
Birmingham, AL 35222
205-592-9683
FAX: 205-592-9687

Jim Crim, Executive Director
$35.00
250 pages

6049 **Marketing Your Abilities: A Guide for the Disabled Job-Seeker**
Mainstream
3 Bethesda Metro Center
Suite 830
Bethesda, MD 20814
301-961-9299
FAX: 301-654-6714
e-mail: info@mainstreaminc.org

Charles Moster
A publication designed to assist the individual with a disability in conducting a successful job search. Major topics include how to write an effective resume and how to give a good interview. *$ 4.95*
24 pages

6050 **Mobile Infirmary Medical Center: Rotary Rehabilitation Division**
5 Mobile Infirmary Circle
Mobile, AL 36607
251-435-2400
800-826-2085
FAX: 251-435-3403
e-mail: resource@mobileinfirmary.org
www.mobileinfirmary.org

E Bramlett, Chief Executive Officer
Our vision is to appreciably enhance in a proactive manner the healthcare status and related quality of life of the residents and communities we serve.

6051 **More Than Just a Job**
Institution on Disability
Morrill Hall
Room 312
Durham, NH 03824

Narrative case studies and interviews with persons with disabilities, their employers, families and experts in the field. *$ 20.00*

6052 **Rocky Mountain Resource & Training Institute**
3630 Sinton Road
Suite 103
Colorado Springs, CO 80907
719-444-0268
800-949-4262
FAX: 719-444-0269
TTY: 800-949-4232
www.adainformation.org

Bob Gattis, Principal Investigator
Randy Dipner, Senior Advisor
Patrick Going, Project Director
Serves people with disabilities and provides training to the agencies that assist them. Facilitates disabled individuals' transition from school to adult life; provides information and resources concerning assistive technology, devices, and services; promotes and ensures compliance with the federal Americans with Disabilities Act (ADA) and other legislation promoting the rights and inclusion of people with disabilities; promotes supported employment, strategic planning and development.

6053 **Work and Disability: Issues and Strategie s in Career Development and Job Placement**
PRO-ED

Textbook. *$60.00*
480 pages 2003
ISBN 0-890799-10-5

Arkansas

6054 **Central Arkansas Rehab Hospital**
2201 Wildwood Avenue
Sherwood, AR 72120
501-835-9919
FAX: 501-834-2227

Randy Harris, Admissions
A nonprofit hospital licensed for 69 acute care beds with all private rooms. Opened in 1999the hospital offers a full range of outpatient diagnostic services, including MRI,CT,PET along with surgical procedures, cardiology, neurology, neurosurgery, othopedic, rehab and a 24 hour emergency department staffed with board certified emergency room physicians. Includes an outpatient surgery center, rehabilitation hospital, senior health program, diabetic program and physician offices.

6055 **HealthSouth Rehabilitation Hospital**
1401 S J Street
Fort Smith, AR 72901
479-785-3300
FAX: 479-785-5203
www.healthsouth.com

Julie Stec, Administrator
Provides physical rehabilitation as its key services. Also provides other services such as end-of-life services, pain management and an infection isolation room.

6056 **Northwest Arkansas Rehabilitation Hospital**
153 E Monte Painter Drive
Fayetteville, AR 72703
479-444-2207
FAX: 479-444-2390

K Hurlbut MD
Denise Wilson, Director Of Clinical Services

6057 **Rebsamen Rehabilitation Center**
1400 West Braden Street NW
Po Box 159
Jacksonville, AR 72076
501-985-7000
FAX: 501-985-7384
www.rebsamenmedicalcenter.com

Mack McAlister, Chairperson
Murice Green, Vice Chairman
Tommy Swaim, Secretary

Mission is to provide personal healthcare for your family. Vision is to develop a family of caregivers to become your community hospital. A 113 bed acute care facility operated by a volunteer Board of Directors made up of community leaders. Rebsamen Medical Center is accredited by the Joint Commission on Accredidation of Healthcare Organizations as well as the Arkansas Department of Health. Through JCAHO we voluntary sumbit to evaluations of our compliance with nationwide hospital standards.

Arizona

6058 Barrow Neurological Institute Rehab Center

350 W Thomas Road
Phoenix, AZ 85013
602-406-3000
FAX: 602-406-4104
www.stjosephs-phx.org

Irwin Altman
Linda Hunt, President
Dedicated resources to delivering compassionate, high-quality, affordable health services; serving and advocating for our sisters and brothers who are poor and disenfranchised; and partnering with others in the community to improve the quality of life. Our vision:a growing and diversified health care ministry distinguished by excellent quality and committed to expanding access to those in need.

6059 HealthSouth Hospital

9630 E Shea Boulevard
Scottsdale, AZ 85260
480-860-3000
FAX: 480-860-3510
www.shc.org

Kathleen Cahill, Admissions
A 343 bed full-service hospital providing medical/surgical, critical care, obstetrics, pediatrics, surgery, cardiovascular, and oncology services, as well as the Sleep Disorder Center. All patient rooms are private. Emergency department is a level II Trauma Center. The Radiology Department offers state-of-the-art diagnostic equipment, including MRI, PET/CT scanning, nuclear medicine and ultrasound. Also located are the Piper Surgery Center, Cancer Center, and several medical office plazas.

6060 HealthSouth Sports Medicine Center

5111 N Scottsdale Road
Suite 100
Scottsdale, AZ 85250
480-941-9232
FAX: 928-772-1276
e-mail: chamine@wiley@healthsouth.com
www.healthsouth.com

Chamine Wiley, Administrator
An out patient facility specialising in sports medicine and treatment of sports injuries.

6061 Healthsouth Rehab Institute of Tucson

2650 N Wyatt Drive
Tucson, AZ 85712
520-325-1300
800-333-8628
FAX: 520-327-4045
www.healthsouth.com

Kelly Silberschlag, Chief Executive Officer
Dave Tupper, Chief Operations Officer
Joan Nelson, Administrator
An accredited member of the Joint Commission On Accreditation of Health Care Organizaions (JCAHO) An 80 bed facility specializing in rehabilitation

6062 St. Joseph Hospital and Medical Center

350 W Thomas Road
Phoenix, AZ 85013
602-406-3000
FAX: 602-406-4190
www.mha.chw.edu/index.asp

Linda Hunt, Manager

Rehabilitation programs offered by the clinic assists clients with rehabilitation health needs in the comfort of their own home. The home care rehabilitation team of professionals focuses on correcting deficiencies in self-care, mobility skills and communication. Services offered include physical therapy, occupational therapy, speech pathology, rehabilitative nursing and restorative nursing assistants.

California

6063 Bakersfield Regional Rehabilitation Hospital

5001 Commerce Drive
Bakersfield, CA 93309
661-323-5500
800-288-9829
FAX: 661-633-5254

Susan Golino, Admissions
Ann Feaver, Chief Executive Officer
A specialty hospital that treats an array of physical disabilities. It has 60 beds and offers physical rehabilitation services including support groups and education classes on illnesses such as arthritis, asthma and strokes. No surgery facilities on site.

6064 Brotman Medical Center: RehabCare Unit

3828 Delmas Ter
Culver City, CA 90232
310-836-7000
FAX: 310-202-4105
e-mail: info@brotmanmed.com
www.brotmanmedicalcenter.com

Ellen Graham, Program Manager
The mission of Brotman Medical Center is to deliver innovative, quality health care to our patients and their families in an environment of compassion, respect, patient saftey, education, and fiscal responsibility.

6065 Casa Colinas Centers for Rehabilitation

255 E Bonita Avenue
Pomona, CA 91767
909-593-0153
800-926-5462
FAX: 909-593-0153
e-mail: rehab@casacolina.org
www.casacolina.org

Stephanie Bradhurst, Director Marketing
Felice Loverso, President/CEO
Casa Colina will provide individuals the opportunity to maximize their medical recovery and rehabilitation potential efficiently in an environment that recognizes their uniqueness, dignity and self esteem. The vision is to strategically reposition themselves at the forefront of the post-acute continuum by becoming the center of excellence in the provision of services to persons who can benefit from rehabilitation care.

6066 Community Hospital of Los Gatos Rehabilitation Services

815 Pollard Road
Los Gatos, CA 95030
408-378-6131
FAX: 408-866-4003
www.communityhospitalLG.com

Modestine Sain, Executive Director
Rehabilitation Services provide individualized treatment programs for inpatient/outpatient care. The team is supervised by a Physiatrist and may include Nurses, Physical Therapists, Occupational Therapists, Speech/Language Therapists, Psychologists, Case Managers, Dietitians, Respiratory Therapists, Recreation Therapists and/or Prosthetists/Orthotists.

6067 Garfield Medical Center

525 N Garfield Avenue
Monterey Park, CA 91754
626-573-2222
FAX: 626-571-8972
www.garfieldmedicalcenter.com

Shelly Hansen, Referrals
Philip Cohen, Chief Executive Officer

Provides quality care to all citizens of all ages. We are foreward looking to meet the changing health care needs of Forsyth and the surrounding area. At the same time, we are a stable organization that is financially sound. We involve all of our medical staff through good communication. We support them by trying to meet their professional needs in training, equipment and services. We emphasize good communication with all county citizens who support us financially and through the use of services

6068 Grossmont Hospital Rehabilition Center

PO Box 158
La Mesa, CA 91944
619-465-0711
800-827-4277
FAX: 619-644-4159
www.sharp.com

Michael Tarbet, CEO
Kari Cornicelli, CFO
It is our mission to improve the health of those we serve with a commitment to excellence in all that we do. Our goal is to offer quality care and programs that set community standards, exceed patients' expectations and are provided in a caring, convenient, cost-effective and accessible manner.

6069 Holy Cross Comprehensive Rehabilitation Center

15031 Rinaldi Street
Mission Hills, CA 91345
818-898-4502
888-432-5464
FAX: 818-898-4472
www.providence.org

Jorilyn Lima, Director
Cindy Damboise, Manager
Known for providing exceptional treatment through its Cancer Centers, Heart Center, Orthopedics, Neurosciences and Rehabilitation Services, as well as Woman's and Children's Services. As a 254-bed, not-for-profit facility, Providence offers a full continuum of health services, from outpatient to inpatient to home health care. Providence operates one of the only round-the-clock trauma centers in the San Fernando Valley and surrounding communities.

6070 Job Hunting Tips for the So-Called Handicapped

Special Needs Project
324 State Street
Suite H
Santa Barbara, CA 93101
805-962-8087
800-333-6867
FAX: 805-962-5087
www.specialneeds.com

Richard Bolles
This nifty booklet from the guru of job hunting himself is sincere, useful and brief. *$4.95*

6071 Kentfield Rehabilitation Hospital & Outpatient Center

1125 Sir Francis Drake Boulevard
Kentfield, CA 94904
415-485-3527
FAX: 415-485-3563
www.kentfieldrehab.com

Susan Jensen, Liaison
Ann Gors, Chief Executive Officer
Provides specialized inpatient and outpatient programs. We provide quality services that are patient centered and family-oriented. Under the medical direction of board-certified hospitalists and other physician specialists, our decicated interdisciplinary teams provide a coordinated, comprehensive treatment approach to a wide range of neurological, orthopedic, pulmonary and complex medical problems.

6072 Laurel Grove Hospital: Rehab Care Unit

19933 Lake Chabot Road
Castro Valley, CA 94546
510-537-1234
FAX: 510-889-6506
e-mail: nissims@sutterhealth.org
www.edenmedcenter.org

George Bischalaney, President & CEO
Ronnie Bayduza, Administrator
Rose Corcoran RN, Vice President
The mission of Eden Medical Center is carried out by our Board of Directors, employees, physicians and volunteers who are committed to providing our patients and their families with the highest quality medical care and customer service. Creating standards of excellence to ensure quality and value for our patients. Maintaining a financially sound organization through effective clinical and administrative support. Encouraging a culture that supports employees and physicians in development.

6073 Lodi Memorial Hospital West

Lodi Memorial Hospital
800 S Lower Sacramento Road
Lodi, CA 95242
209-339-7600
800-876-6750
FAX: 209-339-7652
e-mail: lmh@lodihealth.org
www.lodihealth.org

Joe Harrington, President And CEO
Ron Kreutner, Vice President And CFO
Judy Begley RN, MSN, Chief Nursing Officer
Our vision is to provide a system of health-care services which is clinically effective, quality driven and community focused in an environment that supports and encourages excellence. In partnership with our medical staff, we will assume accountability for the health of our community, be responsible for illness and injury prevention and provide care for the ill and injured. We will measure our success on quality outcomes and customer satisfaction.

6074 Long Beach Memorial Medical Center Memorial Rehabilitation Hospital

2801 Atlantic Avenue
Long Beach, CA 90806
562-933-2000
FAX: 562-933-9018
www.memorialcare.org

Trish Baeseman, Administrator
Barry Arbuckle PhD, President And CEO
The hospital offers rehabilitation after catastrophic injury of disabling disease to give patients the opportunity for maximum recovery. The Hospital offers many of the area's finest rehabilitation specialists and most advanced technology, making it one of Southern California's most respected rehabilitation centers.

6075 North Coast Rehabilitation Center

151 Sotoyome Street
Santa Rosa, CA 95405
707-543-2500
FAX: 707-525-8413
www.santarosamemorial.org

Joyce Cavagnaro, Admissions
Combines state-of-the-art medicine, compassionate care, and the widest array of resources to enhance your health and promote healthy communities. Dedicated to continually introducing new programs and services that help you live life to the fullest.

6076 North Valley Rehabilitation Hospital

1531 Esplanade
Chico, CA 95926
530-332-7300
FAX: 530-894-4139
e-mail: webmaster@enloe.org
www.enloe.org

Darby B. Makel PhD, Chair
Judy Sitton, Vice Chair
Peter Magnusson MD, Secretary/Treasurer
The Mission of Enloe Medical Center is to promote and provide high quality cost-effective care for the people in the communities we serve. Through our best efforts and collaboration with our colleagues, we strive to relieve suffering, cure illness and promote wellness.

6077 Northridge Hospital Medical Center

18300 Roscoe Boulevard
Northridge, CA 91325
818-885-8500
FAX: 818-885-5435
www.northridgehospital.org

Debra Flaherty, Director Rehab Services
Mike Wall, Chief Executive Officer

dedicating resources to delivering compassionate, high-quality, affordable health services; serving and advocating for our sisters and brothers who are poor and disinfranchised; and partnering with others in the community to improve the quality of life.

6078 PEERS Program
8912 W Olympic Boulevard
Beverly Hills, CA 90211
310-553-4833
FAX: 310-553-4833

Paul Berns, Medical Director
Offers a new approach for wheelchair users. PEERS uses a combination of modern physical therapy, the DOUGLAS Reciprocating Gait System and when necessary, functional electrical stimulation to assist selected individuals to walk with recently patented specially made lightweight braces.

6079 PIRS Hotsheet
Placer Independent Resource Services
11768 Atwood Road
Suite 29
Auburn, CA 95603
530-885-6100
FAX: 530-885-3032
e-mail: tmiller@pirs.org
www.pirs.org

Susan Miller, author
Susan Miller, Executive Director
Monthly publication from Placer Independent Resource Services that is provided free of charge to constituents.
6 pages Monthly

6080 Providence Holy Cross Medical Center
Providence Health System
15031 Rinaldi Street
Mission Hills, CA 91345
818-365-8051
818-898-4603
FAX: 818-365-4472
www.providence.org

Derek Brez, Director of Case Management
Kerry Carmody, Chief Executive Officer
Physicains and nurses are among the best and are recoginzed nationally for clinical excellence. We are committed to improving your health and wellness as you journey through life. Our services span beyond the latest advancements in medical procedures, equipment and medication to also include education and wellness services-all provided with compassion and respect. We help our patients understand and use some of the healthiest tools at their disposal, including nutrition & excercise.

6081 Queen of Angels/Hollywood Presbyterian Medical Center
1300 N Vermont Avenue
Los Angeles, CA 90027
213-413-3000
FAX: 213-413-3500
e-mail: info@hollywoodpresbyterian.com
www.hollywoodpresbyterian.com

Lu Hallam, Program Manager
A 434 bed acute-care facility that has been caring for the Hollywood community and surrounding areas since 1924. The hospital is committed to serving local multicultural communities with quality medical and nursing care. With more then 500 physicians representing virtually every speciality. Ready to serve your medical needs and those of your loved ones and strive to distinguish itself as a leading healthcare provider, recognized for providing quality, innovative care in a compassionate manner.

6082 Queen of the Valley Hospital
1000 Trancas Street
Napa, CA 94558
707-252-4411

www.thequeen.org/

Dennis Sisto, President/Chief Executive Office
John Clark, Vice President/CFO
Ned Laubacher, Vice President Strategic Srvcs.
For more then 40 years, Queen of the Valley Hospital has been the premiere medical facility in the Napa Valley. Our long history of providing high quality and caring service is founded on 4 core values:Dignity, Service, Excellence and Justice. These central principals inspire us to reach out to those in need and to help heal the whole person-mind, body and spirit.They are the driving force behind our mission to improve the health and quality of life of people in the community we serve.

6083 Rancho Los Amigos National Rehabilitation Center
7601 E Imperial Highway
Downey, CA 90242
562-401-7111
877-726-2461
888-RAN-CHO
FAX: 562-401-6690
e-mail: webmaster@rancho.org
www.rancho.org

Valerie Orange, Chief Executive Officer
Chris Thomas, Public Relations Director
Anne Potter, Director Business Development
Internationally renowned in the field of medical rehabilitation, consistently ranked in the top Rehabilitation Hospitals in the United States by U.S. News and World Report. It is one of the largest comprehensive rehabilitaion centers in the United States. Licensed for 395 beds, providing service through over 20 centers of excellence.

6084 San Joaquin Valley Rehabilitation Hospital
7173 N Sharon Avenue
Fresno, CA 93720
559-436-3600
FAX: 559-436-3688
e-mail: jpage@svjrehab.com
www.sjvrehab.com

James A Page, Director Marketing
Edward Palacios, Chief Executive Officer
Complete comprehensive rehabilitation services from acute rehab, outpatient and community fitness services.

6085 Santa Clara Valley Medical Center
County of Santa Clara
751 S Bascom Avenue
San Jose, CA 95128
408-885-5000

www.scvmed.org

Susan Murphy, Director
William Jensen MD, Chairman, Department Of Medicine
Thomas Kelsey MD, Program Director
The mission of the medical center is to provide high-quality, cost-effective medical care to all residence of Santa Clara County regardless of their ability to pay. Make availiable a wide range of inpatient, outpatient, emergency services within resource constraints. Maintain an environment within which the needs of our patients are paramount and where patients, their families and all our visitors are treated in a compassionate, supportive, friendly, and dignified manner.

6086 Scripps Memorial Hospital Encinitas
354 Santa Fe Drive
Encinitas, CA 92024
760-633-6501
FAX: 760-633-7348
www.scrippshealth.org/locations.asp?id=3

Chris D Van Gorder, President/CEO
Peter Pieslor, MD
The hospital has 140 acute-care licensed beds and more then 700 employees. Scripps Encinitas offers a full range of clinical and surgical services including 24-hour emergency services, intensive care, cancer/oncology, nuclear medicine, radiology, orthopedics, neurology, urology, ophthalmology and an ambulatory surgery center.

6087 Scripps Memorial Hospital at La Jolla
9888 Genesee Avenue
La Jolla, CA 92037
858-457-4123
800-727-4777
FAX: 858-626-6122
www.scrippshealth.org/locations.asp?id=4

Chris D Van Gorder, President/CEO
Gary Fybel, Executive Director/Administrator
One of the county's 6 designated trauma centers, offers a wide range of clinical and surgical services including 24-hour emergency services; intensive care; interventional cardiology and radiology; radiation oncology; cardiothoracic and orthopedic services; neurology; ophthalmology; and mental health and psychology services.

6088 South Coast Medical Center
31872 Coast Highway
Laguna Beach, CA 92651
149-499-7155
FAX: 949-499-8644
e-mail: info@southcoastmedcenter.com
www.southcoastmedcenter.com

Martha A Farrington, VP/Executive Director
Timothy Mcmahon, Chairman
Bruce Christian, President
A 208 bed acute care hospital. Services include maternity, surgical, subacute care, psychiatric program, eating disorder treatment, chemical dependency treatment, radiology, ICU/CCU, comprehensive rehabilitation services, bariatric surgery and movement disorders program..

6089 St. Joseph Rehabilitation Center
St. Joseph Health System
2200 Harrison Avenue
Eureka, CA 95501
707-441-4414
FAX: 707-441-4429
www.stjosepheureka.org

Michael Purvis, Chief Executive Officer
Sam Fallon, Rehabilitation Director
Mission is to provide physical rehabilitation services in a positive patient-centered environment. This promotes restoration of maximum functional abilities and allows for a dignified quality of life experience. As a staff we are guided by our core values of Dignity, Excellence, Service, and Justice.

6090 St. Jude Brain Injury Network
St. Jude Hospital
251 E Imperial Highway
Suite 440
Fullerton, CA 92835
714-449-4848
866-785-8332
FAX: 714-447-0987
e-mail: bin_tbi@yahoo.com
www.tbioc.org

Jana Gable, Program Coordinator
David Bogdan, Service Coordinator
Lina Marroquin, Servicer Coordinator
Provides comprehensive planning, program referral, assists with funding possibilities, and interagency coordination of services. Areas of emphasis include day treatment, vocational and housing options, and the requirements are adults who have suffered a brain injury from an external force.

6091 St. Jude Medical Center
101 E Valencia Mesa Drive
Fullerton, CA 92835
714-871-3280
800-627-8106
www.stjudemedicalcenter.org

Robert Fraschetti, President/CEO
A 331 bed full-service regional medical center that serves as a major referral hospital attracting rehabilitation patients throughout southern California for over twenty years.

6092 St. Mary Medical Center
1050 Linden Avenue
Long Beach, CA 90813
562-491-9000
FAX: 562-436-6378
www.smmc.com

Joel Yuhas, Chief Executive Officer
A 556-bed hospital owned by the Sisters of Charity of the Incarnate World Healthcare Systems, one of the nation's largest Catholic healthcare networks. Services include a trauma unit, a comprehensive Cancer Care Center, complete older adult services, a Low Vision Center, a Rehabilitation Institute, an outpatient Surgi/Center and the only kidney transplant program in Long Beach. St. Mary's is a teaching hospital affiliated with the UCLA School of Medicine.

6093 Sunnyside Nursing Center
22617 S Vermont Avenue
Torrance, CA 90502
310-320-4130
FAX: 310-320-3232

John Macarthur, Director
Judy Marolda, Administrator
Skilled nursing care facility; residential care facility; intermediate care facility; specialty hospital.

6094 Tustin Rehabilitation Hospital
14851 Yorba Street
Tustin, CA 92780
714-573-5347
FAX: 714-508-4550
www.healthsouth.com

Linda McCaskill, Chief Executive Officer
Scott Rifken, President
Cindi Harrison, Contact

6095 UCLA Medical Center: Department of Anesthesiology, Acute Pain Services
U CL A Medical Center
1245 16th Street Medical Plaza
Suite 225
Santa Monica, CA 90404
310-319-4000
FAX: 310-794-1511
e-mail: access@mednet.ucla.edu
www.medcnt.ucla.edu

Michael Ferrante, Clinical Director
William Parente, MD
A 337-bed acute-care medical center, has been serving the healthcare needs of West Los Angeles and Santa Monica since 1926. Highly regarded for its primary and specialty care, the medical center features many outstanding clinical programs, including its women's and children's services, emergency services, and family medicine programs.

Colorado

6096 Children's Hospital Rehabilitation Center
University of Colorado Health Sciences Center
1056 E 19th Avenue
Denver, CO 80218
303-861-8888
800-624-6553
e-mail: webmaster@tchden.org
www.thechildrenshospital.org

Doris J Biester, Chief Executive Officer
Michael J Farrell, Chief Operating Officer
Helen Martinez, Manager
Private not-for-profit pediatric healthcare network, the hospital is 100 percent dedicated to caring for kids of all ages and stages of growth. That dedication is evident in more then 1000 pediatric specialists and more then 2400 employees. It is also our continual dedication that has placed us at the forefront of research in childhood disease with several nationally and internationally recognized medical programs.

6097 Craig Hospital
3425 S Clarkson Street
Englewood, CO 80113
303-789-8000
FAX: 303-789-8219
e-mail: administration@craighospital.org
www.craighospital.org

Dennis O'Malley MHHC, President
Daniel P. Lammertse M.D., Medical Director
Kelly Johnson RN, MSN, CFNP, Vice President
A 93-bed, private, not-for-profit, free-standing, acute care and rehabilitation hospital that provides a comprehensive system of inpatient and outpatient medical care, rehabilitation, neurosurgical rehabilitative care, an equipment company, and long-term follow up services. Nearly half of Craig's patients come from outside of Colorado, and in 2004 the hospital treated patients from 47 states and several foreign countries. Provides housing for out-of-state families and outpatiients.

6098 Mapleton Center
Boulder Community Hospital
PO Box 9019
1100 Balsam (N Broadway & Balsam
Boulder, CO 80301
303-440-2273
FAX: 303-440-2435
e-mail: pr@bch.org
www.bch.org

David Gehant, President

Comprehensive inpatient and outpatient rehabilitation services for all age groups. Treatment provided by interdisciplinary teams and staff physicians. CARF accredited in brain injury rehabilitation, pediatric rehabilitation, pain management, work hardening and inpatient rehabilitation.

6099 Mediplex Rehab: Denver
Vibra Health Care
8451 Pearl Street
Thornton, CO 80229
303-288-3000
FAX: 303-286-1253
www.northvalleyrehab.com

Walter Sacckett, Chief Executive Officer
Encompasses the broadest mix of professional talent, the finest technology and a total commitment by our people to deliver the highest quality care today, and well into the future. The services can be divided into 4 main categories: long term Acute Care and rehab. Skilled nursing facility and residential ventilator program. Outpatient services and pain management. Adult and Geriatric inpatient psychiatric services.

6100 Rehabilitation Hospital of Colorado Springs
325 Parkside Drive
Colorado Springs, CO 80910
719-630-8000
FAX: 719-636-3772
www.healthsouth.com

Ellen DeAustin, Administrator
A 56 bed rehabilitation hospital, its key services are: cardiology department, physical rehabilitation, and orthopedics department. Accredidted to the Joint Commission on Accreditation of Health Care Organizations (JCAHO)

Connecticut

6101 Mariner Health Care: Connecticut
125 Eugene Oneill Drive
New London, CT 06320
860-701-2000
FAX: 860-701-2202

Arthur W. Stratton Jr. MD, President And CEO
David W. Hanson, Chief Financial Officer
Lawrence R. Deering, Chief Operations Officer/EVP

District of Columbia

6102 National Rehabilitation Hospital
102 Irving Street MW
Washington, DC 20010
202-877-1000
FAX: 202-877-7318
www.nrhrehab.org

Edward B Healton MD, MPH, Medical Director
Robert D. Bunning, Associate Medical Director
A private facility dedicated solely to medical rehabilitation. The hospital offers intensive inpatient programs and full-service outpatient programs.

Florida

6103 Florida Hospital Rehabilitation Center
601 E Rollins Street
Orlando, FL 32803
407-893-8055
FAX: 407-893-9459
e-mail: fh.web@flhosp.org
www.flhosp.org

Diane Lowder, Admissions Director
Florida Hospital Orlando uses the latest technology to treat over 32,000 inpatients and 53,600 outpatients annually. This 881-bed, acute-carecommunity hospital also serves as a major tertiary facility for much of the Southeast, the Caribbean and South America

6104 HealthSouth Regional Rehab Center/Florida
20601 Old Cutler Road
Miami, FL 33189
305-259-6429
FAX: 305-259-0498
www.healthsouth.com

Murray Rolnic, Medical Director
Jackie Arocho, Chief Executive Officer
Martha Madero, Director Clinical Services
HealthSouth Rehabilitation Hospital of Miami is a member of the HealthSouth Corporation, the nation's largest healthcare services provider. The hospital is accredited by the Joint Commission on Accreditation of Healthcare Organizations (JCAHO) and Commission on Accreditaion of Rehabilitation Facilities (CARF). Services offered include dietary services, occupational therapy, and respitory care.

6105 HealthSouth Rehab Hospital: Largo
901 Clearwater Largo Road N
Largo, FL 33770
727-586-2999
FAX: 727-588-3404

Sherri Beasley, Director Marketing Operations
Vicki Yasoua, Manager
A specialty hospital devoted to providing comprehensive medical rehabilitation services. The hospital is licensed as a Comprehensive Medical Rehabilitation Hospital by the state of Florida, and accredited by the Joint Commission on Accreditation of Healthcare Organizations (JCAHO). HealthSouth of Largo is the only free standing Rehabilitation Hospital in the Tampa Bay region, and serves patients of all ages. Provides inpatient medical rehabilitation services as well as outpatient programs.

6106 HealthSouth Sports Medicine & Rehabilitation Center
3280 Ponce De Leon Boulevard
Coral Gables, FL 33134
305-444-0909
FAX: 305-444-5760
www.healthsouth.com

Jay Greeney, President
Ray Jaffet, Administrator
Provides specialized medical and therapeutic services designated to help physically disabled individuals reach their optimum level of independence and function by providing inpatient and outpatient comprehensive medical rehabilitation services.

6107 HealthSouth Sports Medicine and Rehabilitation Center
2141 a S
Lt A1
Jupiter, FL 33477
561-743-8890
FAX: 561-840-8637

Curtis Becker PT, Administrator
Diane Reiley, Manager
Outpatient orthopedic and sports medicine/physical therapy.

6108 HealthSouth Treasure Coast Rehabilitation Hospital
Health South Corporation of Alabama
1600 37th Street
Vero Beach, FL 32960
772-778-2100
FAX: 772-567-6916
www.healthsouth.com

Jason Roebach, Chief Executive Officer
Teresa Hilton, Director Marketing Operations
HealthSouth Treasure Coast Rehabilitation Hospital is a 90-bed inpatient comprehensive rehabilitation hospital serving Indian River, St. Lucie, Martin and Okeechobee counties. Outpatient services are available at the hospital and at four other clinics. Therapies include physical, occupational, speech and psychology services.

6109 Infusion Therapies
7901 SW 36th Street
Suite 206
Davie, FL 33328
800-342-3777
FAX: 954-452-4262

Specializes in fully managed enteral and parenteral therapies. Offers pharmaceuticals, supplies, pumps, equipment and delivery. Infusion cares for pediatrics to geriatrics, patients at home, in extended care facilities, clinics, physician offices, adult congregate living facilities are on site. Provides IV hydration, chemotherapy, gastric/tube feedings, lab/blood work and medical equipment and supplies.

6110 Manatee Springs Care & Rehabilitation Center
5627 9th Street E
Bradenton, FL 34203 941-753-8941
FAX: 941-739-4409
e-mail: cbrooks@seniorcaregroup.com

Cynthia Brooks, Director Adimissions
Donna Steiermann, Administrator
Skilled rehabilitation facility specializing in PT, OT, speech therapy, aquatic therapy and an indoor pool. Piped oxygen bed for specialized respiratory care. Compassionate end of life care. Some Medicare, private insurance, and Medicaid.

6111 Perry Health Facility
207 Forest Drive
Perry, FL 32347 850-584-6334
FAX: 850-838-2370

Jo Ann Gnewuch, Facility Administrator
Michael Brust, Director Rehabilitation
Full rehabilitation team available, Physiatrist, DOR, Psychiatrist, Psychologist, RD, Geriatric Nursing, PT/OT/ST/RT, Orthotiet/Prosthetist. Provider for PPO's & HMO's as well as medicare, private insurance and medicare/medicaid.

6112 Pinecrest Rehabilitation Hospital and Outpatient Centers
Tenet South Florida
5360 Linton Boulevard
Delray Beach, FL 33484 561-495-0400
800-283-8326
FAX: 561-499-6812
www.pinecrestrehab.com

Ruth Stewart, Chief Operating Officer
Migtiala Hernandez, Human Resources Executive
Pinecrest Rehabilitation Hospital is a 90 bed, accredited hospital and is comprised of a Specialty Unit, a Neuro Trauma Unit and Joint Replacement Unit. Additional services at Pincrest include six outpatient rehab centers throughout Palm Beach County. The Outpatient Centers each focus on various specialties such as orthopedic and neurological rehab, pain management, cardiac and pulmonary rehab, occupational medicine, Hearing Institute, dizziness and balance and wellness.

6113 Rehabilitation Institute of Sarasota
3251 Proctor Road
Sarasota, FL 34231 941-921-8796
FAX: 941-922-6228

Stacy Shepherd, Director Clinical Services
a 75-bed hospital that offers individualized medical and theraputic services tailored to patients and clinics for those affected with stroke, multiple sclerosis, Parkinson's, muscular dystrophy and Lou Gehrig's disease (ALS)

6114 Sea Pines Rehabilitation Hospital
101 E Florida Avenue
Melbourne, FL 32901 321-984-4600
FAX: 321-727-7440
e-mail: ellen.lyons-olski@healthsouth.com

Ellen Lyons-Olski, Director
Laura Leitz, Contact
Denise B. McGrath, Administrator
A 90-bed facility specializing in rehabilitation of brain and spinal injuries.

6115 Shriners Hospitals for Children: Tampa
12502 Pine Drive
Tampa, FL 33612 813-972-2250
813-281-0300
FAX: 813-975-7125
www.shrinershq.org/hospitals/tampa

Alice R. Lanford RN, MSN, CHE, Director Patient Care Srvcs.
Cary H. Burcham RN, MBA, CNAA, Chief Of Staff
Recognizing that the family plays a vital role in a child's ability to overcome an illness or injury, Shriners Hospitals helps the family provide the support the child needs by involving the family in all aspects of the child's care and recovery. The purpose of all Shriners Hospitals for Children is to provide care to children with orthopedic problems and burn injuries to help them lead fuller, more productive lives.

6116 South Miami Hospital
6200 SW 73rd Street
South Miami, FL 33143 786-662-4000
www.baptisthealth.net

Hubert Alan Aronson, Medical Director
Wayne Brackin, Chief Executive Officer
The mission is to improve the health and well-being of individuals, and to promote the sanctity and preservation of life, in the communities we serve. We are committed to maintaining the highest standards of clinical and service excellence, rooted in utmost integrity and moral practice.

6117 St. Anne's Nursing Center
11855 Quail Roost Drive
Miami, FL 33177 305-252-4000
FAX: 305-969-6752
www.catholichealthservices.org

Tony Farimello, Executive Director

6118 St. Anthony's Hospital
1200 7th Avenue N
St Petersburg, FL 33705 727-825-1100
www.stanthonys.com

Ian Payne, Director
Ford Kyes, Chief Executive Officer
A not-for-profit, 395-bed hospital established in 1931. St. Anthony's is dedicated to improving the health of the community through community-owned health care that sets the standard for high-quality, compassionate care.

6119 St. Anthony's Rehabilitation Hospital
3075 NW 35th Ave.
Lauderdale Lakes, FL 33311 954-485-4023
954-739-6233
www.catholichealthservices.org

Linda Motte, Hospital Administrator
Kathy Torbertsonn, Dir. Rehab.

6120 St. Catherine's Rehabilitation Hospital and Villa Maria Nursing Center
1050 NE 125th Street
North Miami, FL 33161 305-891-8850
305-891-3361
www.catholichealthservices.org

Virginia Irving, Hospital Administrator
Jim Reiss, Executive Director
Greg Hartley, Dir. Rehab.
St. Catherine's Rehabilitation Hospital is a CARF accredited, 60 bed facility offering inpatient and outpatient rehabilitation and medical clinics; including physical, occupational, and speech therapy, neurology, neurodiagnostics, wound care, and hyperbaric medicine. Villa Maria Nursing center is a JCAHO accredited, 212 bed skilled nursing center providing short term nursing and rehabilitation , as well as long term care.

6121 St. John's Nursing Center
3075 NW 35th Ave.
Lauderdale Lakes, FL 33311 954-739-6233
FAX: 954-733-9579
www.catholichealthservices.org

Diane Dube, Executive Director

6122 **Successful Job Accommodation Strategies**
LRP Publications
PO Box 24668
West Palm Beach, FL 33416
561-622-6520
800-341-7874
FAX: 215-784-9639
e-mail: custserve@lrp.com
www.lrp.com

Honora McDowell, Product Group Manager
Kenneth Kahn, Chief Executive Officer
This monthly newsletter provides you with quick tips, new accommodation ideas and innovative workplace solutions. You learn the outcomes of the latest cases involving workplace accommodations. *$ 140.00*
12 pages Monthly

6123 **Tampa General Rehabilitation Center**
PO Box 1289
Tampa, FL 33601
813-844-7000
FAX: 813-253-4283
e-mail: jstone@tgh.org
www.tgh.org

Sally H. Houston MD, Chief Of Staff
Devanand Mangar MD, Vice Chief Of Staff
Thomas L. Bernasek MD, Secretary/Treasurer
Offers a full range of inpatient and outpatient programs all aimed at helping patients achieve their full potentials. JCAHO and CARF accredited and V.R. designated center. A wide range of inpatient and outpatient programs are available such as Brain and Spinal Cord Injury Programs, Comprehensive Medical Rehabilitation, Pain Management, Cardiac Rehab, Pediatric Therapy Service, Sleep Disorders, Epilepsy, and Wheelchair Seating.Hosts the Florida Alliance for Assistive Services and Technolgy.

6124 **University of Miami: Jackson Memorial Rehabilitation Center**
University of Miami
1611 NW 12th Avenue
Miami, FL 33136
305-585-1111
FAX: 305-585-6092
e-mail: info@jhsmiami.org
www.jhsmiami.org

Mark Brown, Manager
An accredited, non-profit, tertiary care hospital and the major teaching facility for the University of Miami School of Medicine. With more then 1,550 beds, Jackson Memorial is a referral center, a magnet for medical research, and home to the Ryder Trauma Center- the only adult and pediatric level 1 trauma center in Miami-Dade County.

6125 **Winter Park Memorial Hospital**
200 N Lakemont Avenue
Winter Park, FL 32792
407-646-7000
FAX: 407-646-7639
e-mail: healthcare@winterparkhospital.com
www.winterparkhospital.com

Ken Bradley, Chief Executive Officer
Ben Everidge, Developmental Office
Offers Acute Rehabilitation.

Georgia

6126 **Candler General Hospital: Rehabilitation Unit**
5353 Reynolds Street
Savannah, GA 31405
912-819-6176
FAX: 912-819-8829

Virginia Donaldson, Admissions Director
Special Physical Therapy Services at Candler Outpatient Center: Aquatic therapy, pediatric services, outpaitient neurological rehabilitation program, woman's health therapy, orthotics, and spine specialty

6127 **Children's Healthcare of Atlanta at Egleston**
1405 Clifton Road NE
Atlanta, GA 30322
404-785-6000
FAX: 404-315-2158
www.choa.org/default.aspx?id=39

Tricia Easley, Satellite Manager
Rehabilitation Center at Egleston accepts children from birth to age 18 with acute or chronic problems. The length of rehab stay varies for each child according to the determined program of care. The center offers inpatient, outpatient & day rehab programs for comprehensive evaluation & treatment. The program emphasizes the development of the child's abilities & concentrates on helping the family & child compensate for any long-term disabilities. Short term stays require one or two weeks.

6128 **Cobb Hospital and Medical Center: Rehab Ca re Center**
3950 Austell Road
Austell, GA 30106
770-732-4000

e-mail: generalinfo@wellstar.org
www.wellstar.org

Gerald W Bortolazzo, Medical Director
Donald Campbell, Medical Director
Randy Cook, Administrator
To deliver world class healthcare we equip our healthcare facilities and employees with the best technology, resources and education availiable. To deliver world class healthcare we keep seeking ways to improve the way we deliver care knowing each day holds more miracles, more life, more chances, more compassion, and more opportunities.

6129 **HealthSouth Central Georgia Rehabilitation Hospital**
3351 Northside Drive
Macon, GA 31210
478-471-3500
FAX: 478-474-6601
www.healthsouth.com

Vernona L Moseley, Director Market Operations
Beverly Owens, Controller
Elbert T. McQueen, Administrator
HealthSouth Central Georgia rehabilitation hospital is a 55 bed comprehensive medical rehabilitation hospital meeting the medical patients and famloity members in Central Georgia.

6130 **Specialty Hospital**
Floyd Healthcare Resources
304 Turner McCall Boulevard
Rome, GA 30162
706-509-5000
FAX: 706-802-4175
e-mail: contactus@floyd.org
www.floyd.org

Mark Fall, Chief Executive Officer
Susan Stovall, Chief Operations Officer
Jon Dixon, Administrator
Our mission is to be responsive to the communities we serve with a comprehensive and technologically advanced heal care system commited to the delivery of care that is characterized by continually improving quality, accessability, affordability and personal dignity.

Hawaii

6131 **Shriners Hospital for Children: Honolulu**
1310 Punahou Street
Honolulu, HI 96826
808-941-4466
888-888-6314
FAX: 808-942-8573
www.shrinershq.org/hospitals/honolulu

Mike Morris, Interim Administrator
Ellen M. Raney MD, Chief Of Staff (Ortho)
Andi Kubota, Director Of Patient Care Svcs.
One of 22 hospitals across North America that provide excellent, no-cost medical care to children with orthopedic problems and burn industries.

Idaho

6132 Pocatello Regional Medical Center
777 Hospital Way
Pocatello, ID 83201
208-236-6920
FAX: 208-239-3719

Edward Shafer, Manager
Pocatello Regional Medical Center offers 24-hour emergency care, specialized heart services, a dialysis center, a full service rehabilitation unit including transition care, and the Woman's Center For Health including obstetrics.

Illinois

6133 Builders of Skills
515 Busse Highway
Park Ridge, IL 60068
847-292-0870
FAX: 847-292-0873
e-mail: webmaster@avenuesonline.org
www.avenuestoindependence.org

Bob Okavaki, Director
Jay Patel, Manager
Residential setting for hearing-impaired, developmentally disabled adults who are assisted with daily living skills.

6134 Center for Learning
National-Louis University
2840 Sheridan Road
Evanston, IL 60201
847-256-5150
FAX: 845-256-1057
e-mail: kadamle@nl.edu

Jerry Dachs, Manager
Psycho-educational evaluations for children, adolescents, and adults. Individualized remedial academic programs, individual counseling

6135 Institute of Physical Medicine and Rehabilitation
6501 North Sheridan Road
Peoria, IL 61614
309-692-8110
800-957-4767
FAX: 309-692-8673
e-mail: quality@impr.org
www.ipmr.org

Richard Erickson, President
Sue Paul, Manager
Comprehensive CARF accredited programs in outpatient medical rehabilitation services. Eight outpatient locations, specialty programs include adult day services, driving evaluations, balance and visual rehabilitation board certified physiatrists.

6136 LaRabida Children's Hospital and Research Center
E 65th at Lake Michigan
Chicago, IL 60649
773-363-6700
FAX: 773-363-9554
e-mail: pr@larabida.org
www.larabida.org

Paula Jaudas, President
Dedicated to excellence in caring for children with chronic illness, disabilitiesm or who have been abused, allowing them to achieve their fullest potential through expertise and innovation within the health care and academic communities.

6137 Marianjoy Rehabilitation Hospital and Clinics
26 W 171 Roosevelt Road
Wheaton, IL 60187
630-909-8000
800-462-2366
FAX: 630-909-8001
e-mail: dlebloch@marianjoy.org
www.marianjoy.org

Kathleen Yosko, President/CEO
Will Gillett, Chairman
John Oliverio, Vice Chairman
Goal at Marianjoy Rehabilitation Hospital is to help you and your family return to the lifestyle you enjoyed before your illness or injury. To meet this goal, we provide you with a dedicated team of experienced professionals to assist you every step of the way.

6138 Regional ADA Technical Assitance Agency
1640 W Roosevelt Road
Room 405
Chicago, IL 60608
312-413-1407
800-949-4232
FAX: 312-413-1856
e-mail: gldbtac@uic.edu
www.adagreatlakes.org

Robin Jones, Project Director
provides training, technical assistance and consultation on the rights and resposibilities of indiviualsand entities covered by the ADA. Toll free number for technical assistance and materials provided electronically or via mail at no cost.

6139 Rush Copley Medical Center-Rehab Neuro Physical Unit
2000 Ogden Avenue
Aurora, IL 60504
630-978-6200
866-426-7539
FAX: 630-898-4565
e-mail: clord@rsh.net
www.rushcopley.com

John M. Lies, Chairman Of The Board
Ronald Hem, Vice Chairman Of The Board
The mission of the medical center and the medical staff is to work together to serve your healthcare needs through excellence in education, technology and a caring touch. Rush-Copley Medical Center will be the leading healthcare provider of the greater Fox Valley area. At Rush-Copley we pride ourselves on providing everyone with extrodinary service.

6140 Vocational Counseling for Special Populations
Charles G Thomas, Publisher, LTD.
2600 S 1st Street
Springfield, IL 62704
217-789-8980
800-258-8980
FAX: 217-789-9130
e-mail: books@ccthomas.com
www.ccthomas.com

Michael Thomas, President
$36.95
172 pages Paperback
ISBN 0-398056-50-1

6141 Vocational Training and Employment of the Autistic Adolescent
Charles C Thomas
2600 S 1st Street
Springfield, IL 62704
217-789-8980
800-258-8980
FAX: 217-789-9130
e-mail: books@ccthomas.com
www.ccthomas.com

Michael Thomas, President
Professionals and parents are now advocating, demanding and arranging that persons receive vocational training and equal rights for the disabled. Also available in paper edition. *$41.95*
182 pages Cloth
ISBN 0-398058-01-6

Indiana

6142 ATTAIN
U S Department of Education/ NI DR R
32 E Washington Street
Suite 1400
Indianapolis, IN 46204
317-534-0236
800-528-8246
e-mail: attaininfo@attaininc.org
www.attaininc.org

Gary Hand, Executive Director
Mary Duff, Executive Assistant
Kristi Barber, Director, Community Outreach
The mission of Attain is to create solutions that enable people with functional limitations to live, learn, work and play in the community of their choice. All will have access to assistive devices. We will do this in partnership with people with functional limitations, families and members of the community through training, system change, services and support, research, dissemination and consumer advocacy.

6143 Clark Memorial Hospital: RehabCare Unit
1220 Missouri Avenue
Jeffersonville, IN 47130
812-282-6631
FAX: 812-283-2656
e-mail: paula.lamb@clarkmemorial.org
www.clarkmemorial.org

Jan Goldhammer, Program Manager
Carter Brown, MD
Gordon Gutman, Chairman
The mission of Clark Memorial Hospital is to provide superior health services to the people and communities we serve. The vision of Clark Memorial Hospital is to be the best community health care provider in the United States. We value each individual and work together to explore new ways to improve the quality of life of all. We persue excellence in all we do. We treat all individuals with the same compassion, dignity, and privacy that we want in ourselves.

6144 Developmental Disabilities Planning Council
150 W Market Street
Suite 628
Indianapolis, IN 46204
317-232-7770
FAX: 317-233-3712
e-mail: gpcpd@gpcpd.org
www.state.in.us/gpcpd

Suellen Jackson-Boner, Executive Director
Christine Dahlberg, Associate Director
Paul Shankland, Grants Manager
The mission of the Indiana Governor's Council is to promote public policy which leads to the independence, productivity and inclusion of people with disabilities in all aspects of society. This mission is accomplished through planning, evaluation, collaboration, education, research and advocacy. The Council is consumer-driven and is charged with determining how the service delivery system in both the public and private sectors can be most responsible to the people with disabilities.

6145 Easter Seals Wayne/Union Counties
5632 US Highway 40 E
PO Box 86
Centerville, IN 47330
765-855-2482
FAX: 756-855-2482
e-mail: easterseals@juno.com
easterseal swu.tripod.com

Bill Felker, President
Vickey Allen, Vice President
Leslie Mayl Whitney, Secretary
Helps people discover nature and much more at camps equipped to offer physcial, social and emotional support and fun for campers with physical and/or developmental disabilities.

6146 IN Speechl Language-Hearing Association
Po Box 24167
Indianapolis, IN 46224
317-916-4146
FAX: 317-481-1825
e-mail: ann@centraloffice1.com
www.islha.org

Mary Jo Germani, President
Debbie Hartman, President-Elect
Raju Chithala, Treasurer
ISHA is to support its members in the provision of quality services through advocacy, professional development, and public awareness.

6147 IN-SOURCE
Indiana Resource Center for Families with Special
1703 South Ironwood Drive
South Bend, IN 46613
574-234-7101
800-332-4433
FAX: 574-234-7279
e-mail: insource@insource.org
www.insource.org

Richard Burden, Executive Director
Scott Carson, Assistant Director
Dory Lawrence, Project Director
The mission of IN*SOURCE is to provide parents, families and service providers in Indiana the information and training necessary to assure effective educational programs and appropriate services for children and young adults with disabilities.

6148 Indiana Congress of Parent and Teachers
2525 N Shadeland Avenue D4
Indianapolis, IN 46219
317-357-5881
FAX: 317-357-3751
e-mail: indianapta@sbcglobal.net
www.indianapta.org

Marilyn Jones, President
Tina Hartman, Vice President
The mission of the Indiana PTA is three-fold: to support and speak on behalf of children and youth in the schools, community and before governmental agencies and other organizations that make decisions affecting children; to assist parents in developing the skills they need to raise and protect their children; and, to encorage parent and community involvement in the public schools of this state and nation.

6149 Indiana Parent Information Association
7275 Shadeland Avenue
Suite 1
Indianapolis, IN 46250
317-251-7488
800-964-4746
FAX: 317-251-7488
e-mail: FamilyNetw@aboutspecialkids.org
www.ipin.org

Rebecca Kirby, Executive Director
Jane Scott, Director Of Information
Nancy Stone, Project Director
A "Parent to Parent" organization that works throughout the state of Indiana to answer questions and provide support, information and resources. We are parents and family members of children with special needs and we help other families and professionals understand the various systems that are encountered related to special needs. Our central office is where parents from the entire state can access information, resources and support

6150 Job Search Handbook for People with Disabi lities
JIST Publishing
8902 Otis Avenue
Indianapolis, IN 46216
317-613-4200
800-648-5478
FAX: 800-547-8329
e-mail: info@jist.com
www.jist.com

Mike Farr, President
Provides a complete career planning and job search guide identifying the job hunter's strengths and abilities. Explore career options, locate job openings in the hidden job market, when and how to tell a potential employer about a disability, write powerful resumes, cover letters, and follow up correspondence.
$35.00
288 pages 2003
ISBN 1-557666-52-0

6151 Kokomo Rehabilitation Hospital
829 N Dixon Road
Kokomo, IN 46901
765-452-6700
FAX: 765-452-7470

Brenda Harry, Admissions Director
a 60 bed facility specializing in rehabilitation services to the people of Indiana.

6152 **Memorial Regional Rehabilitation Center**

615 N Michigan Street
South Bend, IN 46601
574-647-1000
FAX: 574-647-3195
e-mail: ralexander@memorialsb.org
www.qualityoflife.org

Phil Newbold, Chief Executive Officer
Carl Ellison, Vice President
Sue Wright, Manager
20-bed CARF accredited inpatient rehabilitation, outpatient orthopedic clinic and work performance program, head injury clinic. Outpatient neuro rehab and a driver education and training program are provided.

6153 **Methodist Hospital Rehabilitation Institute**

8701 Broadway
Merrillville, IN 46410
219-738-5500
FAX: 219-738-6636
www.methodisthospitals.org

Andre Artis M.D., President
Adolphus Anekwe M.D., President-Elect
Thomas Golubski, Secretary
The Mission of Methodist Hospitals is to provide compassionate, quality health service to all those in need. Our vision is to provide the best place for employees to work, the best place for patients to receive care and the best place for physicians to practice medicine.

6154 **NAMI Indiana**

PO Box 22697
Indianapolis, IN 46222
317-925-9399
800-677-6442
FAX: 317-925-9398
e-mail: nami-in@nami.org
www.namiindiana.org

Joe Vanable, President
Pamela McConey, Executive Director
NAMI Indiana is a non-profit grassroots organization dedicated to improving the lives of people afflicted by serious and persistant mental illness. We are dedicated to helping families through a network of support, education, advocacy, and promotion of research. NAMI's goal is to help establish a system of care that provides community based services for persons with serious mental illness, as well as support for them and their families.

6155 **Parkview Regional Rehabilitation Center**

2200 Randallia Drive
Fort Wayne, IN 46805
260-373-3601
888-480-5151
FAX: 260-373-3620
www.parkview.com

Elizabeth Williamson, Admissions Coordinator
Sheryl Scott, Executive Director
Provides a full range of inpatient, theraputic services and programs for patients as young as 3 years of age to the very elderly. Our accute care rehabilitation center, is well equipped to care for patients with neurological and orthopedic injuries and diseases.

6156 **Programs for Children with Disabilities: Ages 3 through 5**

Department of Education
229 State House
Indianapolis, IN 46204
317-232-0570
877-851-4106
FAX: 317-232-0589
e-mail: webmaster@doe.state.in.us
www.doe.state.in.us/exceptional

Robert A Marra, Assistant Superintendent
Sheron Cochran, Preschool Coordinator
Suellen Reed, Chief Executive Officer
The division provides leadership and state-level support for public school gifted and talented (grades K-12) programs and for students with disabilities from ages 3-21. The division ensures that Indiana, in its compliance with the federal Individuals With Disabilities Education Act, through monitoring of special education programs, oversight of community and residential programs, provision of mediation and due process rights, and sound fiscal management.

6157 **Programs for Children with Special Health Care Needs**

2 N Meridian Street
Indianapolis, IN 46204
317-233-5578
800-475-1355
e-mail: wgettelf@isdh.state.in.us
www.in.gov/isdh/programs/cshcs

Wendy Gettelfinger, Director
The Children's Special Health Care Services (CSHCS) program provides financial assistance for needed medical treatment to children with serious and chronic medical conditions to reduce complications and promote maximum quality of life.

6158 **Programs for Infants and Toddlers with Disabilities: Ages Birth through 2**

402 West Washington Street
Room W 386
Indianapolis, IN 46204
317-232-1144
800-441-7837
e-mail: firststepsweb@fssa.state.in.us
A family-centered, locally-based, coordinated system that provides early intervention services to infants and young children with disabilities or who are developmentally vulnerable. First Steps brings together families and professionals from education, health and social service agencies. By coordinating locally availiable services, First Steps is working to give Indiana's children and their families the widest possible array of early intervention resources.

6159 **Protection and Advocacy Agency of Indiana**

4701 N Keystone Avenue
Suite 222
Indianapolis, IN 46204
317-722-5555
800-622-4845
FAX: 317-722-5564
e-mail: tgallagher@ipas.state.in.us
www.in.gov/ipas

Thomas Gallagher, Executive Director
IPAS was created in 1977 by state law to protect and advocate the rights of people with disabilities and its Indiana's federally designated Protection (P&A) system and client assist program. It is an independent state agency, with receives no state funding and is independent from all service providers, as required by federal and state law.

6160 **Riley Child Development Center**

702 Barnhill Drive
Room 5837
Indianapolis, IN 46202
317-274-8168
800-248-1199
e-mail: geguthri@iupiu.edu
rileychildrenshospital.com

Steven Viehweg, Manager
Riley Hospital for Children is Indiana's only comprehensive children's hospital, with pediatric specialists in evry field of medicine and surgery. Riley is committed to providing the highest quality health care to children in a compassionate, family-centered environment. Riley is a national leader in cutting edge research and medical education, ensuring health care excellence for children for generations to come. Riley provides medical care to all children, regardless of family's ability to pay.

6161 **St. Anthony Memorial Hospital: Rehab Unit**

301 W Homer Street
Michigan City, IN 46360
219-879-8511
FAX: 219-877-1838
www.saintanthonymemorial.org

Doran Lounsbury, Program Manager
Bruce Rampage, President
Saint Anthony Memorial is an acute care hospital located in Michigan City, primary serving La Porte and Porter Counties in Indiana as well as Berrien County Michigan.

6162 **State Division of Vocational Rehabilitation**

PO Box 7083
Indianapolis, IN 46207
317-232-1401
800-545-7763
e-mail: martin@fssa.state.in.us
www.state.in.us/fssa

Rita Martin, Deputy Director
Mike Hedden, Executive Director

6163 VSA Arts of Indiana
Harrison Center for the Arts
1505 N Delaware Street
Indianapolis, IN 46202
317-974-4123
FAX: 317-974-4124
e-mail: jmcwhirter@vsai.org
www.vsai.org

Gayle Holtman, Director
James Nulty, Executive Director
For over 25 years VSA arts of Indiana has led the movement to make the arts accessable to people with disabilitites. VSA arts of Indiana offers a variety of opportunities for people with disabilities of all ages to engage the power of the arts as a means of education, creative self-expression, and personal and professional growth. As a result, VSA promotes change in public perceptions and raises public awareness, and advocates for increased accessability in providing art experiences for all.

Iowa

6164 Younker Rehabilitation Center of Iowa Methodist Medical Center
1200 Pleasant Street
Des Moines, IA 50308
515-241-4499
FAX: 515-241-8043
www.ihs.org

Fran Wendling, Admissions Coordinator
Sue Knapp, Manager
Robert Rondinelli, Medical Director
Iowa Health System is the state's first and largest integrated healthcare system. We are physicians, hospitals, civic leaders and local volunteers committed to providing the highest possible quality and the lowest possible cost. We serve over 70 communities in Iowa, Western Illinois, and Eastern Nebraska.

Kansas

6165 Kansas Rehabilitation Hospital
1504 SW 8th Avenue
Topeka, KS 66606
785-235-6600
FAX: 785-232-8509
e-mail: leslie.cunningham3@healthsouth.com

Julie DeJean, Administrator
Paul Livingston, Chief Executive Officer
A free standing physical rehabilitation hospital located in Topeka Kansas. Designated to provide a barrier-free access to all treatment and patient service areas. This 79-bed facility offers a total rehabilitation environment in a warm, caring setting that encourages patient, family and staff interaction.

6166 Mid-America Rehabilitation Hospital HealthSouth
Health South Corporation
5701 W 110th Street
Overland Park, KS 66211
913-491-2400
FAX: 913-491-1097
e-mail: tiffany.kiehl@healthsouth.com
www.healthsouth.com

Kristen DeHart, Chief Executive Officer
Tiffany Kiehl, Director Marketing/Operations
Melissa Higgins, Director Clinical Services
80 bed Acute Rehab hospital offering full continuum from in-patient, day treatment and outpatient services for individuals with physical limitations due to CVA, TBI, SCI, other traumas, joint replacement, etc.

Kentucky

6167 Cardinal Hill Rehabilitation Hospital
2050 Versailles Road
Lexington, KY 40504
859-254-5701
800-233-3260
FAX: 859-255-9303
e-mail: webmaster@cardinalhill.org
www.cardinalhill.org

Sandy Shill CRRN, Manager Referral Relations
Beth A Monarch, COO
Kerry Gillihan, Chief Executive Officer
CARF-accredited rehab center provides comprehensive inpatient and outpatient services in two locations to people with physical and cognitive disabilities. We provide diagnosis-specific programs to 100 inpatients, outpatient clinics, outpatient therapies, pain management and therapeutic pool services. The Pediatric Center serves children from birth to age 18 years of age.

6168 HealthSouth Rehabilitation of Louisville
1227 Goss Avenue
Louisville, KY 40217
502-636-1200
FAX: 502-636-0351
www.healthsouth.com

Michele McCoy, Marketing Representative
Regina Durbin, Administrator

6169 Lakeview Rehabilitation Hospital
134 Heartland Drive
Elizabethtown, KY 42701
270-769-3100
FAX: 270-769-6870

Diane Stephens, Assistant Director Marketing
Lorrie Young, Marketing Executive
40-beds, comprehensive physical rehabilitation.

6170 Shriners Hospitals for Children, Lexington
1900 Richmond Road
Lexington, KY 40502
859-266-2101
800-444-8314
FAX: 859-268-5636
www.shrinershq.org/hospitals/lexington

Joan Snowden, Director Family/Cmmty Service
Tony Lewgood, Administrator
A 50-bed, pediatric orthopedic hospital providing FREE, expert orthopedic medical care to children and adolescents in Kentucky, Tennessee, West Virginia, Ohio, and Indiana.

Louisiana

6171 HealthSouth Specialty Hospital Of North Louisiana
1401 Ezelle Street
Ruston, LA 71270
318-251-3126
800-548-9157
FAX: 318-251-5491
www.healthsouth.com

Mark Rice, Executive Director
A 90-bed specialty hospital offering both inpatient and outpatient services. Acute long term care.

6172 Our Lady of Lourdes Rehabilitation Center
611 Saint Landry Street
Lafayette, LA 70506
337-289-2000
FAX: 318-289-2681
e-mail: info@lourdes.net
www.lourdes.net

William Barrow, Chief Executive Officer
Our Lady of Lourdes outpatient physical medicine and rehabilitation department is compprised of a multi-disciplinary team of physical therapists, oppcuptational therapists and speech languare pathologists.

6173 Rehabilitation Center of Lake Charles Memorial Hospital

Lake Charles Memorial Hospital
1701 Oak Park Boulevard
Lake Charles, LA 70601
337-494-3000
FAX: 337-494-2656
e-mail: webmaster@lcmh.com
www.lcmh.com

Candy Marks, Director
Elton Williams Jr, Chief Executive Officer
Rehabilitation center offering intensive physical, occupational, speech, neuropsychology, recreational therapies along with rehabilitation nursing.

6174 Shriners Hospital for Children-Shreveport

3100 Samford Avenue
Shreveport, LA 71103
318-222-5704
FAX: 318-424-7610
www.shrinershc.org

Kim Green MBA, MHA, CHE, Administrator
Charles Penn III, Chairman, Board Of Governors
Richard F McCall MD, Chief Of Staff
An interdisciplinary approach is used in patient care programs to ensure comprehensive care for each patient. The staff includes orthopaedists, pediatricians, nurses, therapists, social workers, child life specialists, and more. The Shreveport Hospital is equipped and staffed to provide care for virtually all pediatric orthopaedic problems, with the exception of acute trauma.

6175 South Louisiana Rehabilitation Hospital

715 W Worthy Street
Gonzales, LA 70737
225-647-8277
FAX: 225-647-2446
e-mail: sober@powerhouseprograms.com
www.powerhouseprograms.com

Tonja S Randolph, President
Mark Broussard, Executive Director
Power House Programs is a male only facility for the treatment of Chemical Dependency/Dual Diagnosis, located in Gonzales, Louisiana. Applicants must have participated in a primary treatment program for substance abuse prior to acceptance. Our program is divided into 3 phases and is staffed by Board Certified Social Workers and Board Certified Substance Abuse Counselors. We provide individual, group and family therapy; plus 12 step meetings in a community setting.

6176 St. Frances Cabrini Hospital: Rehab Unit

St Frances Cabrini Hospital
3330 Masonic Drive
Alexandria, LA 71301
318-487-1122
FAX: 318-448-6822
www.cabrini.org

Stephen Wright, President/CEO
CHRISTUS St. Frances Cabrini Hospital is a 265-bed facility located in Alexandria, Louisiana. Employing approximately 1,400 Associates and with a staff of neary 320 physicians, CHRISTUS St. Frances Cabrini Hospital offers a comprehensive array of services providing the highest quality patient care in a compassionate setting.

6177 St. Patrick Hospital: Rehab Unit

524 S Ryan Street
Lake Charles, LA 70601
337-436-2511
888-722-9355
FAX: 337-491-7157
www.christusstpatrick.org

Ellen Jones, Chief Executive Officer
Committed to providing care and service of the highest quality for children and adults, and to ensuring that the basic human rights of expression, decision making and personal dignity are preseved. We are also committed to treating our patients with respect, understanding and Christian love. We realize that this committment involves much more then attending to your medical needs.

6178 Thibodaux Hospital: Regional Rehabilitatio n Center

602 North Acadia Road
Thibodaux, LA 70301
985-447-5500
800-822-8442
e-mail: info@thibodaux.com
www.thibodaux.com

Jody Plaisance MD, Vice Chairman
Jacob Giardina, Chairman
Mission is to provide the highest quality, most cost effective health care services possible to the people of Thibodaux and surrounding areas. The vision is to be the regional medical center of choice for health care services in the southeast Louisiana by recognizing the value of physicians and employees, committing to quality improvement, partnering with other health care providers, and remaining financially viable in a competitive environment.

Maine

6179 Brewer Rehab And Living Center

74 Parkway South
Brewer, ME 04412
207-989-7300
FAX: 207-989-4240
wwww.brewerrehab.com

Gail Sinclair, Contact
Michael Skirven, Executive Director
Brewer Rehab and Living Center accomodates 106 residents. We are located in Brewer, Maine. We have a 24-hour nursing staff and experienced dedicated on-site physical therapists, occupational therapists and speech language pathologists. We have a specialized inpatient program for individuals with brain injury resulting from a traumatic injury or neurological event such as a stroke. We also have a specialized care unit for individuals with Alzheimer's disease and other dementias.

6180 New England Rehabilitation Hospital of Portland

335 Brighton Avenue
Portland, ME 04102
207-662-8584
FAX: 207-879-8168
e-mail: jaye.sewall@healthsouth.com
www.nerhp.org

Elissa Charbonneau, Medical Director
Victoria Ashton, Associate Medical Director
Mission is to provide individuals with guidance, education, support, and motivation while helping them achieve maximum independence and function. Our professionals work with the patient and family through a team approach, to establish and implement an individualized rehabilitation plan designed to meet specific patient goals.

Maryland

6181 Mt. Washington Pediatric Hospital

1708 W Rogers Avenue
Baltimore, MD 21209
410-578-8600
FAX: 410-466-1715
www.mwph.org

Sheldon J. Stein, President And CEO
Violet Ebbesen RN, Admissions Nurse
Provides inpatient, outpatient and day programs for infants and children with rehabilitation and/or complex medical needs. We are dedicated to maximizing the rehabilitation and development of our patients through the delivery of interdisciplinary services and programs and providing every resource availiable to enable our patients to attain the highest quality of life within their families and their communities.

6182 Project LINK Guidebook

Mainstream
3 Bethesda Metro Center
Suite 830
Bethesda, MD 20814
301-961-9299
800-247-1380
FAX: 301-654-6714
e-mail: info@mainstreaminc.org

Charles Moster
A manual for operating an employment services program for persons with disabilities. *$49.95*
78 pages

6183 Vocational Rehabilitation and Supported Employment
Paul H Brookes Publishing Company
PO Box 10624
Baltimore, MD 21285
410-337-9580
800-638-3775
FAX: 410-337-8539

Paul Brooks, Owner
A timely, comprehensive resource on how vocational rehabilitation can play a major role in facilitating and implementing supported employment programs. *$43.00*
384 pages Paper 1988

Massachusetts

6184 Mediplex Rehabilitation Hospital
4499 Acushnet Avenue
New Bedford, MA 02745
508-995-6900
FAX: 508-998-8131

Albert Loerinc MD

6185 New England Rehabilitation Hospital: Massachusetts
2 Rehabilitation Way
Woburn, MA 01801
781-935-5050
FAX: 781-935-8637
www.newenglandrehab.com

Dr. Deniz Ozel, Medical Director
Grig Murdock, Director Of Therapy Services
Lester Felege, Controller
A 168-bed comprehensive inpatient rehabilitation hospital, which includes 2 off-campus satellite units. Offers an array of area outpatient rehabilitation centers. New England Rehabilitation Hospital remains committed to a personal caring approach. The vision is to provide the communities with a complete continuum of acute rehabilitative programs and services.

6186 Shriners Burns Hospital: Boston
51 Blossom Street
Boston, MA 02114
617-722-3000
800-255-1916
FAX: 617-523-1684
www.shrinershq.org/hospitals/boston

C. Thomas D'Esmond, Hospital Administrator
Ronald G. Thompkins MD, Sc.D., Chief Of Staff/Dir Of Research
Provides treatment for children to their 18th birthday with acute, fresh burns, plastic reconstructive surgery for patients with healed burns, severe scarring and facial deformity. Some non-burn conditions such as Scalded Skin Syndrome, Cleft Lip, Cleft Palate and purpura fulminians are also treated. Call the Hospital for information. All medical treatment is without cost to the patient, parents, or any third party.

6187 Shriners Hospital Springfield Unit Springfield Unit for Crippled Children
516 Carew Street
Springfield, MA 01104
413-787-2000
800-237-5055
FAX: 413-787-2009
www.shrinershq.org/hospitals/springfiled

David M. Drvaric MD, Chief Of Staff
Peter D. Masso MD, Assistant Chief Of Staff
Philip W. Mack MD, Staff Surgeon
Shriners Hospital for Children is fully equipped and staffed to provide care for pediatric orthopaedic conditions and disorders.

6188 Working Together: Workplace Culture, Employment and Disabilities
Brookline Books
PO Box 1046
Cambridge, MA 02139
617-868-0360
800-666-2665
FAX: 617-868-1772
e-mail: thestore@brooklinebooks.com
www.brooklinebooks.com
Presents a new approach to assisting individuals with significant disabilities achieve meaningful careers, the book stresses partnerships between work, service providers and natural support systems to achieve positive employment outcomes. *$27.95*
Paperback
ISBN 0-91479 -88-3

Michigan

6189 Covenant Healthcare Rehabilitation Program
515 N Michigan Avenue
Saginaw, MI 48602
989-583-0000
FAX: 989-583-2843
www.covenanthealthcare.com

Spence Maidlow, President
Offers a broad spectrum of programs and services ranging from obstetrics, neonatal and pediatric care, to acute care including cardiology, oncology, surgery and many other services on the leading edge of medicine. All our programs and services exemplify our commitment to providing quality, compassionate care. As a medical facility with more then 700 beds, and a complete range of medical services, Covenant stands ready to meet the healthcare needs of the 15 counties in Michigan we serve.

6190 Farmington Health Care Center
34225 Grand River Avenue
Farmington, MI 48335
248-477-7373
FAX: 248-477-2888

Michael Mithen, Administrator
Skilled nursing facility specializing in ventilator dependent residents.

6191 Flint Osteopathic Hospital: RehabCare Unit
3921 Beecher Road
Flint, MI 48532
810-762-4682
FAX: 810-762-2153

Susan Malone, Program Manager
Joy Finkenbiner, Executive Director

6192 Integrated Health Services of Michigan at Clarkston
4800 Clintonville Road
Clarkston, MI 48346
248-674-0903
FAX: 248-674-3359

Carol Doll, Admissions Director
Margaret Canny, Administrator
Rose Berg, Admission

6193 St. John Hospital: North Shore
Ascension Health
26755 Ballard Street
Harrison Township, MI 48045
586-465-5501
FAX: 586-466-5397
www.stjohn.org

David Sessions, Chief Executive Officer
Dave Denny, Director for Rehabilitation
A 96-bed specialty hospital that provides comprehensive physical medicine and rehabilitation, along with a wide range of medical and surgical services. St. John North Shores Hospital also provides emergency and urgent care, extensive outpatient rehabilitation services, and most ancillary diagnostic services.

Minnesota

6194 **Sister Kenny Institute**
800 E 28th Street
Minneapolis, MN 55407
612-863-4466
FAX: 612-863-8942
www.allina.com/ahs/ski/nsf

Helen Kettner, Nurse-Liaison
Sister Kenny Rehabilitation Institute can meet your needs with any short-or long-term condition or disability. Sister Kenny specializes in providing individualized patient programs grounded in the most innovative services to give you the hope and tools you need to achieve your personal best.

6195 **Social Skills on the Job**
AGS
PO Box 99
Circle Pines, MN 55014
800-328-2560
FAX: 763-786-9007
www.agsnet.com

Robert Zaske, Market Manager
Gives students a realistic picture of what's expected of them at work and models appropriate behavior on the job through a variety of videos and software. *$259.95*

Missouri

6196 **Columbia Regional Hospital: RehabCare Unit**
404 Keene Street
Columbia, MO 65201
573-875-9000
FAX: 573-875-4417
www.columbiaregional.org

George Gumbert, Program Manager
A medical and physical rehabilitation program serving patients throughout Mid-Missouri with functional deficits due to neurologic, orthopaedic or other medical conditions.

6197 **Jewish Hospital of St. Louis: Department of Rehabilitation**
One Barnes Jewish Hospital Plaza
Saint Louis, MO 63108
314-747-3000
866-867-3627
FAX: 314-454-5277
www.barnesjewish.org

Andrew Ziskind MD, President
Sharon O'Keefe, Chief Operating Officer
John Beatty, Vice President Human Services
We take exceptional care of people by providing world-class healthcare, delivering care in a compassionate, respectful and responsive way. By advancing medical knowledge and continously improving our practices. By educating current and future generations of healthcare professionals.

6198 **St. Mary's Regional Rehabilitation Center**
201 NW R D Mize Road
Blue Springs, MO 64014
816-228-5900
www.carondelethealth.org

Gordon Docking, Chief Executive Officer
Susan Bottmker, Assessment Coordinator
Robin Velaer, Manager
A 143-bed inpatient physical rehabilitation unit offering PT, OT, ST, recreational therapy, psychiatry and all other ancillary services of a full-service hospital. Specialize in orthopedic and neurologic disabilities.

6199 **Three Rivers Health Care**
2620 N Westwood Boulevard
Poplar Bluff, MO 63901
573-785-7721
800-582-9533
FAX: 573-785-9413
e-mail: info@pbrmc.hma-corp.com
www.poplarbluffregional.com

Bruce Eady, Chief Executive Officer
Poplar Bluff Regional Medical Center is a regional medical center with 2 hospital campuses and more then 100 active physicians. The 423-bed facility is the largest medical center in Southeast Missouri and is located in ButlerCounty. With outreach clinics in Bloomfield, Dexter, Malden, Piedmont, and Puxico, Poplar Bluff Regional Medical Center is committed to serving its 6 county region.

Montana

6200 **St. Vincent Hospital and Health Center**
1233 N 30th Street
Billings, MT 59101
406-657-7000
FAX: 406-657-8817

John Brewer, Admission
Mike Bush, MD
Vision is to be recognized for our vitality, best in class performance and providing easy access to compassionate and trust-worthy healthcare. The healthcare we offer is based on community need. We strive to improve the health status of the community, with a special concern for the poor and those who have limited access to healthcare.

Nebraska

6201 **Madonna Rehabilitation Hospital**
5401 South Street
Lincoln, NE 68506
402-489-7102
800-676-5448
FAX: 402-483-9406
e-mail: information@madonna.org
www.madonna.org

Marsha Lommel, President/CEO
Lori Warner, Marketing/PR Manager
Kiranmayi Chilappa, MD
Provides a complete range of inpatient and outpatient rehabilitation for patients of all ages and abilities. Through highly specialized programs and services, Madona offers individualized treatment and support to help every patient.

Nevada

6202 **University Medical Center**
1800 W Charleston Boulevard
Las Vegas, NV 89102
702-383-2000
FAX: 702-383-2536
e-mail: webmaster@umcsn.com
www.umcsn.com

Debbie Gulo, Rehab Evaluator
Lacy Thomas, Chief Executive Officer
Vision is to become the model community healthcare provider and hospital of choice. To provide leadership that ensures safe, high quality, accessable, comprehensive healthcare to the community and visitors while ensuring financial viablilty and social responsiveness.

New Hampshire

6203 **Head Injury Treatment Program at Dover**
307 Plaza Drive
Dover, NH 03820
603-742-2676
FAX: 603-749-5375
www.doverrehab.com

Sue Mills, Program Rep
Jill Bosa, Administrator

A provider of postacute services in the greater New Hampshire Seacost area. We accomodate 112 residents and are licensed by the state of New Hampshire. We employ nearly 150 licensed nurses, therapists, and other healthcare professionals, who strive to provide quality care. The goal of our patient service model is to bridge the gap between hospitalization and home so that recovery and physical functioning are maximized and hospital re-admission is minimized.

6204 Lakeview NeuroRehabilitation Center
101 High Watch Road
Center Ossipee, NH 03814
603-539-7451
800-4R3-H221
FAX: 603-539-8888
www.lakeviewsystem.com

Susan Bartlett Msw Crc, Director Admissions
Tina Trudel PhD, VP Clinical Services
Edward C Morton Jr, Executive Director
Residential treatment center serving individuals with neurologic/behavioral disorders. Lakeview serves both children and adults in functionally based program environment. Transitional programs in various group homes also available to clients as they progress in their treatment.

6205 Northeast Rehabilitation Hospital
70 Butler Street
Salem, NH 03079
603-893-2900
800-825-7292
FAX: 603-893-1628
e-mail: webmaster@northeastrehab.com
www.northeastrehab.com

John Prochilo, President/CEO
NRHN is an organization characterized by the positive and proactive commitment to the delivery of customer centered care. Our employees exemplify our organizational commitment to providing quality rehabilitation services throughout the continuum. NRHN will be prudent with all resources and will take individual and collective responsibility for fiscal health. NRHN will remain a model by which other rehabilitation and post acute networks seek to emulate.

6206 St. Joseph Hospital Rehabilitation
172 Kinsley Street
Nashua, NH 03060
603-595-3175
800-210-9000
FAX: 603-595-3192
www.stjosephhospital.com/rehab

Patti Montyha, Program Director
A comprehensive healthcare system that serves the Greater Nashua area, western New Hampshire and Northern Massachusetts. Our hospital is licensed for 208 beds and includes a Level 2 Trauma Center. In addition to the hospital, St. Joseph Healthcare system also includes a satellite emergency center in Milford, 5 family medical centers, a large network of primary care and specialty physician practices.

New Jersey

6207 Betty Bacharach Rehabilitation Hospital
61 West Jimmie Leeds Road
Pomona, NJ 08240
609-652-7000
FAX: 609-748-3586

Virginia Wells, Admissions
Pat Nalepka, Manager

6208 Children's Specialized Hospital
150 New Providence Road
Mountainside, NJ 07092
908-301-5461
888-344-5373
FAX: 908-301-5509
e-mail: jbrooks@childrens-specialized.org
www.Childrens-specialized.org

Dennis M. Bushe PhD,, Chairman
Amy B. Mansue, President/CEO
Barbara Rothman, First Vice Chairman
New Jersey's largest comprehensive pediatric rehabilitation hospital, treats children and adolescents from birth through 21 years of age. Programs include spinal dysfunction, brain injury, respiratory, burn, Day Hospital, early intervention, preschool, and cognitive rehabilitation. Locations in Fairwood, Roselle Park, Newark, Toms River and Hamilton

6209 HealthSouth Rehabilitation Hospital
14 Hospital Drive
Toms River, NJ 08755
732-244-3100
FAX: 732-244-2542

Dave Coluzzie, Intake Coordinator
Tatty Scewski, Chief Executive Officer
A comprehensive 131-bed medical rehabilitation hospital dedicated to treating individuals with a variety of physical disabilities resulting from injury and illness. We serve all of New Jersey, Manhattan, and Philiadelphia. Accredited by the Joint Commission on Accredidation of Healthcare Organizations (JCAHO). The mission of the hospital is to get people back to work, to play, to living.

6210 JFK Johnson Rehab Institute
65 James Street
Edison, NJ 08820
732-321-7000
FAX: 732-321-0994
e-mail: webmaster@solarishs.org
www.njrehab.org

Norman Batra, Physicians
David Brown, Physicians
The mission of the JFK Johnson Rehabilitation Institute is to provide quality rehabilitation that will assist adults and children living with disabilities to obtain optimal function and independence within an accepting community. The vision is to be the benchmark for the delivery of quality, caring rehabilitative services within a seamless continuum of care.

6211 Kessler Institute for Rehabilitation, Welkind Facility
201 Pleasant Hill Road
Chester, NJ 07930
973-584-7500
800-KES-SLER
FAX: 973-252-6343
e-mail: jkment@kessler-rehab.com
www.kessler-rehab.com

Samuel P Grissom, Associate Medical Director
Steven Kessler
Sue Kida, Vice President, Administration
Set in the rolling hills of Morris County, this 72 bed facility provides specialized services to brain injury patients, including our unique Cognitive Redmediation Program, as well as a full range of stroke, amputee and orthopedic services. Kessler's team of dedicated rehabilitation professionals, including physicians, nurses and therapists, work with each patient to build physical strength, optimize movement, maximize independence, increase cognitive skills and address any other issues.

6212 Mediplex Rehab: Camden
One Cooper Plaza
Camden, NJ 08103
856-342-2000
FAX: 856-342-7979
www.cooperhealth.org/content/locationsCamden

Beth Crawford, Admissions
Celeste Johnson, Administrator
Cooper University Hospital is the leading provider of comprehensive health services, medical education and clinical research in Southern New Jersey and the Delaware Valley. With over 550 physicians in over 75 specialties, Cooper is uniquely equipped to provide an almost unlimited number of medical services. The hospital is committed to excellence in medical education, patient care, and research. Offers training programs to medical students, residents, and nurses in a variety of specialties.

New Mexico

6213 HealthSouth Rehabilitation Center: New Mexico
7000 Jefferson Street NE
Albuquerque, NM 87109
505-344-9478
800-293-7226
FAX: 505-344-2851

Sylia Kelley, Administrator
Serving our community since 1988, and committed to offering the care and support you need to achieve the most complete recovery possible. We will develop and individualized treatment plan based on the needs and goals identified by you, your family and our rehabilitation team. Then we will use that plan as a guide, working together to help you reach the highest level of physical, social and emotional well-being.

6214 St. Joseph Rehabilitation Hospital and Outpatient Center
Ardence
505 Elm Street NE
Albuquerque, NM 87102
505-727-4700
FAX: 505-727-4793
www.sjhs.org

Janelle Raborn, Administrator/CEO
Sherrie Peterson, Director
A member of the four hospital, St. Joseph healthcare system, this facility provides inpatient and outpatient care for those requiring physical medicine and rehabilitation. Specialty programs include brain injury, stroke, spinal cord, orthopedics, occupational and physical therapies, clinical psychology, speech/language pathology, hand clinic and functional capacity evaluations. The only facility in New Mexico accredited in four areas by the commission on accreditation of rehab facilities.

New York

6215 Burke Rehabilitation Hospital
785 Mamaroneck Avenue
White Plains, NY 10605
914-597-2500
888-99B-URKE
FAX: 914-946-0866
e-mail: web@burke.org
www.burke.org

Dr. Mary Walsh, Executive Medical Director/CEO
John J. Ryan, Executive Director/Admin.
A 150 bed rehabilitation hospital providing both in and out patient physical rehabilitation to people with stroke, spinal cord injury, head injury, pulmonary, cardiac, amputee, orthopedic arthritis and other related diagnoses.

6216 No More Job Interviews!: Self-Employment Strategies for People with Disabilities
Training Resource Network

Offers self-employment strategies targeted to people with disabilities, the largest unemployed minority group in the US today. The book reflects recent charges in business, offering Internet tips and business training trends. Also includes four business plans and profiles of individuals with disabilities. *$29.95*
183 pages 2000
ISBN 1-883302-36-6

6217 Occupational Therapy Strategies and Adaptations for Independent Daily Living
Haworth Press
10 Alice Street
Binghamton, NY 13904
607-722-5857
800-429-6784
FAX: 607-722-6362
e-mail: orders@haworthpress.com
www.haworthpress.com

S Harrington-Miller, Advertising
William Cohen, Owner
This contains clinical expertise of some fourteen authors or author teams addressing the issue of occupational therapy to assist in independent daily living. Also available as hardcover. *$74.95*
186 pages Softcover
ISBN 0-866563-50-4

6218 Rusk Institute of Rehabilitation Medicine
400 E 34th Street
New York, NY 10016
212-263-6034
FAX: 212-263-8510
www.med.nyu.edu/rusk

Howard A Rusk, Founder
Jung Hwan, Clinical Professor
Eric Rackow, President
Operates under the auspices of the Dept. Of Rehabilitation Medicine of New York University School of Medicine, one of the nations foremost medical schools. The relationship between Rusk and other clinical and research units within the medical center contributes to an environment which provides the optimal rehabilitation setting for patients.

6219 Silvercrest Center for Nursing & Rehabilitation
14445 87th Avenue
Briarwood, NY 11435
718-480-4000
800-645-9806
FAX: 718-658-2367
e-mail: admissions@silvercrest.org
www.silvercrest.org

Stephen S Mills, President/CEO
Susan Barnett, Director Admissions
Cosmo Costa, Senior Vice President
The Silvercrest Center for Nursing and Rehabilitation has earned a wide-spread reputatiopn for combing the best in clinical care with the best in nursing care and for making available to its communities the broadest menu of services to ease a patients' path to recovery from hospital to home. The Center is for the treatment of medically complex patients beginning their recovery, for the rehabilitation of patients who need restorative therapy before going home and much more.

6220 Vocational Rehabilitation and Employment
Books on Special Children
PO Box 305
Congers, NY 10920
845-638-1236
FAX: 845-638-0847
e-mail: irene@boscbooks.com
Defines kinds of work, expectations, goals and programs. Contributions in general issues of supported employment, training and management and community based programs. *$47.00*
372 pages Hardcover

North Carolina

6221 Horizon Rehabilitation Center
Trans Health Incorporated
3100 Erwin Road
Durham, NC 27705
919-383-1546
800-541-7750
FAX: 919-383-0862
e-mail: michelle.ayers@thicare.com

John Dugan, Administrator
A 125-bed rehabilitation, subacute and long term care facility. HRC is JCAHO and CARF accredited with a physician-directed rehabilitation program, internal case management and a therapy department composed of physical, occupational, speech, recreational and respiratory therapists - pulmonary rehabilitation/ventilator unit.

6222 Integrated Health Services of Durham
Duke University Medical Center
3100 Erwin Road
Durham, NC 27705
919-684-8111
FAX: 919-383-0862
e-mail: webmaster@mcduke.edu
www.mc.duke.edu

Steve Rum, Vice Chancellor for Development
Dottie Williams, Assistant Vice Chancellor for De
Thomas Pafford, Manager

6223 Learning Services Corporation
Corporate Office
10 Speen Street
4th Floor
Framingham, MA 01701
888-419-9955
FAX: 919-419-9966
www.learningservices.com

David Carter, President

A licensed postacute rehabilitation program for adults who have an acquired brain injury. Individuals who are enrolled in the program participate in active, intensive rehabilitation carried out by a team of neuropsychology, speech/language therapy, physical therapy, occupational therapy, vocational services, family services and life skills training. Services include residential rehabilitation, home based treatment, day treatment, subacute rehabilitation and supported living.

Ohio

6224 **Arbors at Columbus**
44 S Souder Avenue
Columbus, OH 43222
614-228-5900
FAX: 614-228-3989

Kelly Fligor, Administrator
Postacute rehabilitation program.

6225 **Franciscan Rehabilitation Center**
601 S Edwin C Moses Boulevard
Dayton, OH 45408
937-229-6081
800-272-8042
FAX: 937-229-6074

Linda Didas, Case Manager
Acute, inpatient rehabilitation, 77 beds. Twenty-plus years serving the Dayton community. Vocational and assistive technology services are available. Extensive outpatient services include: hand therapy, back school, drivers' training. Accredited by JCAHO and CARF. Liaison with community support groups: SCI, BI, stroke, amputee, ALS, chronic pain. On-site clinics: SCI, MDA, amputee and wheelchair/seating.

6226 **Great Lakes Regional Rehabilitation Center**
3700 Kolbe Road
Lorain, OH 44053
440-960-3400
FAX: 440-960-4636
www.ehealthconnection.com/regions/lorain

Roberta Yehman, Admissions Director
Klaus Grm, Owner
Provides excellent, innovative and comprehensive rehabilitation programs to people in our community. Committed to a better quality of life for all individuals, the Rehabilitation Center has grown to become a regional resource for individuals needing all types of rehabilitation services.

6227 **HCR Health Care Services**
1 Seagate
Toledo, OH 43604
419-321-5470
800-736-4427
FAX: 419-252-5543

Charles Norman, CPA
Specialty transitional care and intensive rehabilitation services. Specialized services are focused on patients with catastrophic conditions or whose length of stay at an acute care or rehabilitation hospital can be dramatically reduced by transferring to a subacute level of care.

6228 **Heather Hill Rehabilitation Hospital**
Heather Hill
12340 Bass Lake Road
Chardon, OH 44024
440-285-4040
800-423-2972
FAX: 440-285-0946
e-mail: info@heatherhill.org
www.heatherhill.com

Susan V. Juris, President And CEO
Donald Goddard MD, Chief Medical Officer
Carolyn Lieberman, Administrator
Individualized treatment programs for adults and adolescents can participate in and benefit from three-plus hours a day of active therapy.

6229 **Parma Community General Hospital Acute Rehabilitation Center**
7007 Powers Boulevard
Parma, OH 44129
440-743-4000
FAX: 440-743-4036
www.parmahospital.org

Joseph Coleman, Chairman
Patricia A Ruflin, President/CEO
Terrence Deis, COO
The mission of this CARF accredited unit is to provide the most comprehensive, cost-effective, acute rehabilitation program possible in order for every patient and family to adjust to his/her disability and to achieve the maximum potential of independent functioning when returning to community living.

6230 **Rehabilitation Institute of Ohio at Miami Valley Hospital**
1 Wyoming Street
Dayton, OH 45409
937-208-8000
www.miamivalleyhospital.com

Sharyl Kuhnen RN, Rehab Coordinator
A regional center designed for the treatment of those with disabling conditions. RIO offers physcial, occupational, speech, recreational and pool therapies, as well as the use of a transitional apartment to perpare patients for a return to independent living.

6231 **Retaining At-Risk Students: The Role of Career and Vocational Education**
Center on Education and Training for Employment
1900 Kenny Road
Columbus, OH 43210
614-292-4353
800-848-4815
FAX: 614-292-1260
Reviews the causes of at-risk students and their implications for the U.S. labor force. *$6.00*
48 pages

6232 **Shriners Burn Institute: Cincinnati Unit**
Shriners Hospitals for Children Cincinnati
3229 Burnet Avenue
Cincinnati, OH 45229
513-872-6000
800-875-8580
FAX: 513-872-6999
www.shinners.com/hospitals/cincinnati

Ronald Hitzler, Administrator
All the attention and resources are focused on just one kind of patient-the burn-injured child. Shriners combine excellent clinical skill, compassionate care, and innovative research, providing comprehensive pediatric burn care and reconstructive rehabilitation to achieve the best possible outcome for a child that has suffered a burn injury. There is never a charge to the patient or family for any of the medical care or services provided by the Shriners Hospitals throughout North America.

6233 **St. Francis Health Care Centre**
401 N Broadway Street
Green Springs, OH 44836
419-639-2626
800-248-2552
FAX: 419-639-6222
e-mail: hr@sfhcc.org
www.sfhcc.org

Greg Raubenolt, Director Marketing
Jane Holmer, Admissions Coordinator
Joy Kinnear CRRN, Dir Admissions/Care Coordinator
Provides compassionate care for the elderly and physically challenged. We are a healthcare ministry under the sponsorship of the Franciscan Sisters of Our Lady of Perpetual Help. As a Catholic facility. we respectfully offer those we serve, care hope and dignity in a joyful and compassionate manner.

6234 **St. Rita's Medical Center Rehabilitation Services**
730 W Market Street
Lima, OH 45801
419-226-9772
800-232-7762
FAX: 419-226-9705
www.ehealthconnection.com

Kelly Recker, Administrative Physical Medicine
Sharon Bilopavlovich, Manager
The St. Rita's Inpatient Acute Care Rehabilitation service provides individualized service to you or your family member 7 days a week, wherever you might stay in the hospital. Acute rehabilitation care includes physical, occupational, and speech therapy services. Our goal is to make you as independent as possible before your discarge to home or, when necessary to extended services in other parts of the hospital.

6235 University of Cincinnati Hospital
Health Alliance
234 Goodman Street
Cincinnati, OH 45219
513-584-1000
FAX: 513-584-7712
www.universityhospitalcincinnati/com

James Kingsbury, Executive Director
University Hospital has an international reputation, bringing thousands of people, from the region and around the world to Cincinnati to receive care from world renowned physicians in state-of-the-art medical facilities.

6236 Upper Valley Medical/Rehab Services
3130 N Dixie Highway
Troy, OH 45373
937-440-4000
FAX: 937-440-7337
e-mail: info@uvmc.com
www.uvmc.com

Pam Cornett, Director Rehab Services
A not-for-profit health care system serving the health care needs of Miami County and the surrounding area. The health care system features a state-of-the-art acute care hospital which opened in 1998. Comprehensive inpatient and outpatient services are provided with a full compliment of diagnostic and treatment services and behavioral health care programs.

Oklahoma

6237 HealthSouth Rehab Center: Oklahoma
700 NW 7th Street
Oklahoma City, OK 73102
405-236-3131
FAX: 405-553-1153
www.healthsouth.com

Susan Nelson, Director Business Development
Stacey Smith, Chief Executive Officer
Inpatient Rehab Facility including all therapy services serving people who have been injured and had an illness resulting in a decreased level of independence.

6238 Hilcrest Medical Center: Kaiser Rehab Cent er
1125 S Trenton Avenue
Tulsa, OK 74120
918-579-7100
FAX: 918-579-7110
www.hillcrest.com/kaiser

Kevin Gross, Chief Executive Officer
Kaiser Rehabilitation Center offers a wide range of services to help people regain functionality and independence after a debilitating injury or illness. Our approach to rehabilitation is a team approach, bringing the expertise of physicians, therapists, nurses and other health professionals together with patient family to achieve the best possible outcome. Each patient is given an individualized treatment plan that stimulates and challenges them to achieve their maximum potential.

6239 Jane Phillips Medical Center
Jane Phillips Medical Center
3500 E Frank Phillips Boulevard
Bartlesville, OK 74006
918-331-1857
FAX: 918-331-1360
e-mail: webmaster@jpmc.org
www.jpmc.org

David R. Stire, President/CEO
Mike Moore, CFO
Sharon K. Branham, Vice President/Nursing Servcs.
Jane Phillips Health System is sponsored by St. John Health System. This partnership helps our patients by ensuing access to the most sophisticated levels of care availiable in this area. It offers a wide range of services, including general medicine, surgery, cardiopulmonary care, maternal and infant care, cancer treatment, geriatric care, orthopedics, and physical medicine.

6240 Jim Thorpe Rehabilitation Center at Southwest Medical Center
Southwest Medical Center
4219 Sout Western
Oklahoma City, OK 73109
405-644-5200
800-677-1238
FAX: 405-636-7501
www.integris-health.com

Gary Zook, Unit Director
Denise Uvino, Marketing Director
Stanley Hupfeld, Chief Executive Officer
Provides inpatient rehabilitation for people with head injuries, spinal cord injuries, orthopedic conditions, pain management, neurological diseases, strokes and a variety of diagnoses that stop individuals from being able to take care of themselves independently. Services available include medical direction, physical therapy, social work, occupational therapy, speech therapy, recreational therapy, and aftercare follow-up.

6241 Mercy Memorial Health Center-Rehab Center
1011 14th Avenue NW
Ardmore, OK 73401
580-223-5400
800-572-1182
FAX: 580-220-6681
www.mercyok.net/mmhc/default.asp

Bob Thompson, President/CEO
A full service tertiary hospital with 176 licensed beds, 913 co-workers and 100 physicians. Four primary care clinics

6242 St. Anthony Hospital: Rehabilitation Unit
St. Anthony Hospital
1000 N. Lee Street
Oklahoma City, OK 73102
405-272-7000
800-851-0888
FAX: 405-271-7563
e-mail: st_anthony@ssmhc.com
www.saintsok.com

Joe Hodges, President
18 spacious private rooms, each with bathroom, and furnishings designed with patient safety in mind. Horticulture room where patients can work with plants and flowers as part of their rehabilitation. And a residential-style training apartment with fully equipped kitchen, bathroom, and bedroom to make the patient feel more at home.

Oregon

6243 Shriners Hospitals for Children: Portland
3101 SW Sam Jackson Park Road
Portland, OR 97239
503-241-5090
800-237-5055
FAX: 503-221-3701
www.shrinershq.org/hospitals.org

Bill McMillan, Administrator
Ivan Krajbich MD, Chief Of Staff
William Horton MD, Director Of Research
Pediatric orthopedic and plastic surgery; inpatient and outpatient services. No charge for any services provided at the Hospital. Diagnosis, rehabilitation, surgery, sports and recreation for ages 0-18 for people with physical disabilities involving bones, muscles or joints or in need of plastic surgery for burn scars or cleft lip/palate.

Pennsylvania

6244 Allied Services John Heinz Institute of Rehabilitation Medicine
150 Mundy Street
Wilkes Barre, PA 18702
570-826-3900
FAX: 570-826-3898
e-mail: tpugh@allied-services.org
www.allied-services.org

Thomas E Pugh, VP/CEO
Gregory Basting MD, VP Medical Affairs
Karen Kearney, AVP Inpatient Services
John Heinz Rehab is one of the foremost providers of rehabilitation in the country. Under the supervision of board-certified psychiatrists, a team of highly qualified professionals provides a broad range of specialized services and therapies for inpatients, with speacialized programs in the areas of brain injury, injured worker recovery and pediatrics. John Heinz Rehab is the only CARF accredited program in northeastern Pennsylvania for treatment of brain injury rehabilitation.

6245 Allied Services Rehabilitation Hospital
475 Morgan Highway
Scranton, PA 18508
570-348-2211
FAX: 570-348-1281
www.allied-services.org

Donna Esken, Director Admissions
Susan Lantner, Assistant Director
James Paddock, Executive Director
We are committed to the people of our commuinity, to help them overcome challenges and reach their greatest potential by providing quality care, people-oriented services and comfort. Our approach is a hands-on, people-oriented style which places the physical and emotional needs of those in our care at the center of all we do. Whether in our rehabilitation hospitals, our skilled nursing facilities, or mental health/mental retardation program, we strive to help people reach their potential.

6246 Brighten Place
131 N Main Street
Chalfont, PA 18914
215-997-7746
FAX: 215-997-0403
e-mail: brightenplace@enter.net

Suzann Ditzel, Program Director
William Koffros, Chief Executive Officer
A residential brain injury program with the mission to encourage growth and foster independence on an individual level for each resident. We are CARF accredited and provide additional services which include a day program and respite care.

6247 Chestnut Hill Rehabilitation Hospital
8601 Stenton Avenue
Wyndmoor, PA 19038
215-233-6200
FAX: 215-233-6879
www.chh.org

James Caslin, Administrator
Chestnut Hill Rehab Hospital is dedicated to meeting patients' physical, emotional, social, and vocational goals. Through innovative programs, sophisticated equipment, and support by specially trained staff members committed to the progress of every patient, Chestnut Hill achieves results.

6248 Doylestown Hospital Rehabilitation Center
595 W State Street
Doylestown, PA 18901
215-345-2200
FAX: 215-345-2512
www.dh.org

Donna Seif, Outpatient Rehab Case Manager
Gloria Peterson, Inpatient Rehab Services
Theophila Cemanoff, MD, Owner
The mission of Doylestown Hospital is to provide a responsive healing environment for patients and their families, and to improve the quality of life for all members of our community. We combine the creative energies of Medical Staff, Board, Associates and Volunteers to make Doylestown Hospital a place where each patient and family feels healed and whole, even when disease cannot be cured.

6249 Health Care Solutions
500 B Abbott Drive
Broomall, PA 19008
610-583-3500
800-451-1671
FAX: 610-583-3550
www.lincare.com

John P Byrnes, Chief Executive Officer
Shawn Schabel, Chief Operation Officer
Patty Vitvlli, Manager
Develops unique containment programs, offers equipment set-up, patient instruction, patient assessment and equipment usage. Offers clinical services that include oxygen systems, ventilators, aerosol therapy, suction equipment, T.E.N.S. programs, compression pumps, custom orthotics, enteral feeding.

6250 HealthSouth Harmarville Rehabilitation Hospital
PO Box 11460
Pittsburgh, PA 15238
412-828-1300
FAX: 412-828-7705
www.healthsouth.com

Sharon Noro, Chief Executive Officer
A 202-bed facility providing inpatient and outpatient physical medicine and rehabilitation to adults and adolescents in Pennsylvania, West Virginia, Ohio and Maryland.

6251 HealthSouth Nittany Valley Rehabilitation Hospital
Health South of Nittany Valley
550 W College Avenue
Pleasant Gap, PA 16823
814-359-3421
800-842-6026
FAX: 814-359-5898
www.healthsouth.com

Connie Poisant, Program Director
Susan Hartman, Chief Executive Officer
Comprehensive inpatient and outpatient facilities. Treatment for symptoms relating to: stroke, head injury, pulmonary disease, orthopedic conditions, neurological disorders, cardiac illnesses and spinal cord injuries. Healthsouth Nittany Valley Rehabilitation Hospital is a part of Healthsouth's national network of more than 2,000 facilities in 50 states.

6252 HealthSouth Rehab Hospital Of Erie
143 E 2nd Street
Erie, PA 16507
814-878-1200
800-234-4574
FAX: 814-878-1399
www.healthsouth.com

Kathy Lamb, Admissions
Louis Condrasky, Chief Executive Officer
Sean Maclsaac PT, Contact

6253 HealthSouth Rehabilitation Hospital of Altoona
2005 Valley View Boulevard
Altoona, PA 16602
814-944-3535
800-873-4220
FAX: 814-944-6160

Scott Filler, Administrator/CEO
Paul Sutton, Director Of Clinical Services

6254 Healthsouth Rehabilitation Hospital of Greater Pittsburgh
2380 McGinley Road
Monroeville, PA 15146
412-856-2400
FAX: 412-856-2437

Sharon Noro, Administrator
Rehabilitation and long-term acute care hospital that treats brain injury, stroke, multiple sclerosis, Parkinson's disease, back and spinal cord injuries, cancer, pulmonary disease, cardiac disease, traumatic and work injuries.

6255 Healthsouth Rehabilitation Hospital of Mechanicsburg
175 Lancaster Boulevard
Mechanicsburg, PA 17055
717-691-3831
800-933-3831
FAX: 717-697-6524
www.healthsouthpa.com

Roberta Weaver, Director Admissions
Gregory Toot, Chief Executive Officer
Vicki Harris
HealthSouth provides comprehensive rehabilitation and recovery services to patients with stroke, brain injury, hip fracture, medically complex, pulmonary, wound, spinal cord injury, amputation, and other neuro-muscular, and orthopedic impairments. Our primary goal is to provide individualized treatment programs to people requiring physical rehabilitation and medical recovery in order to help patients get back to work, to play, to living.

6256 **Healthsouth Rehabilitation Hospital of York**
1850 Normandie Drive
York, PA 17408
717-767-6941
FAX: 717-764-1341

Cheryl Fleming, CEO
Susan Hartman, Business Development
Brent Burger, Controller
A 120-bed rehabilitation hospital dedicated to providing advanced, comprehensive services to patients who have suffered head injury, spinal cord injury, stroke, burns, amputation, chronic pain and other neurological and musculoskeletal disorders. HRH of York provides outpatient services in seven locations. Healthsouth is located in York, Pennsylvania, approximately 50 miles north of Baltimore and 25 miles south of Harrisburg.

6257 **Magee Rehabilitation Hospital**
1513 Race Street
Philadelphia, PA 19102
215-587-3000
800-966-2433
FAX: 215-568-3736
e-mail: hskoczen@mageerehab.org
www.mageerehab.org

David Brodar, Director Human Resources
William E Staas, President/CEO
A not-for-profit health organization which is the home to the nation's first brain injury rehabilitation program to be accredited by the Commission on the Accreditation of Rehabilitation Facilities (CARF) and is one of 16 federally designated Regional Spinal Cord Injury Centers. Our staff and management are committed to restoring the highest level of independence possible to individuals with disabilities.

6258 **Moss Rehabilitation Hospital**
1200 W Tabor Road
Philadelphia, PA 19141
215-456-9900
FAX: 215-456-9646
www.einstein.edu/yourhealth/physicalrehab

Mary Stears, Intake Coordinator
Alberto Ezquenazi, Plant Manager
The Philadelphia region's major resource for medical rehabilitation since 1959. This 152 bed facility offers comprehensive care to people with broad ranges of conditions, diagnostic laboratories and a multidisciplinary team of rehabilitation professionals.

6259 **Shriners Hospitals for Children, Philadelphia**
Shrinners Hospitals for Children
3551 N Broad Street
Philadelphia, PA 19140
215-430-4000
800-281-4051
FAX: 215-430-4126
www.shrinershq.org/hospitals/philadelphia

Ernest N. Perilli MBA, Hospital Administrator
Randal R. Betz MD, Chief Of Staff
Dean R. Shacklett, Chairman Of The Board Of Gov's.
The Shriners Hospital in Philadelphia is a 59-bed pediatric orthopaedic hospital providing a complete range of specialized medical and rehabilitation services at no charge to children with orthopaedic problems or spinal injuries. The hospital is one of 22 Shriners Hospitals for Children throughout North america. In addition to treating children with routine and complex orthopaedic problems, the Philadelphia Hospital provides a comprehensive and individualized rehabilitation program.

6260 **Shriners Hospitals for Children, Erie**
1645 W 8th Street
Erie, PA 16505
814-875-8700
FAX: 814-875-8756
www.shrinershq.org/hospitals/erie

Kenneth H. Stafford, Chairman, Board Of Governors
Richard W. Brzuz FACHE, Administrator
Mary Jane Antoon, Director Of Patient Care Srvs.
The Shriners Hospitals for Children, Erie, is a 30-bed pediatric orthopaedic hospital providing comprehensive orthopaedic care to children at no charge. The hospital is one of 22 Shriners Hospitals throughout North America. The Erie Hospital accepts and treats children with routine and complex orthopaedic and neuromuscular problems, utilizing the latest treatments and technology available in pediatric orthopaedics, resulting in early ambulation and reduced length of stay.

6261 **Shriners Hospitals, Philadelphia Unit, for Crippled Children**
3551 N Broad Street
Philadelphia, PA 19140
215-430-4000
FAX: 215-430-4079
www.shrinershq.org/hospitals/philadelphia

Ernest N. Perilli MBA, Hospital Administrator
Randal R. Betz MD, Chief Of Staff
Dean R. Shacklett, Chairman Board Of Governors
Provides comprehensive medical, surgical and rehabilitative care for children with orthopaedic conditions and spinal cord injuries. All services are provided at no charge. The hospital is one of 22 located throughout North America. In addition to treating children with routine and complex orthopaedic problems, the Philadelphia hospital provides a comprehensive and individualized rehabilitation program for children and adolescents who have sustained a traumatic injury to their spine.

South Carolina

6262 **Colleton Regional Hospital: RehabCare Unit**
501 Robertson Boulevard
Walterboro, SC 29488
843-549-2000
FAX: 843-549-0246
www.colletonmedical.com

Johnnie Benson, Program Manager
Rebecca Brewer, Chief Executive Officer
Colleton Medical Center's 8-bed physical and mental rehabilitation department is the oldest in the Lowcountry and has been serving the community for nearly 20 years. Strives to provide patient-centered care in a family atmosphere. The team includes nurses, physical therapists, occupational therapists, speech therapists, and nutritionists. The typical patient requires rehabilitation following a stroke, spinal injury, close head injury, and orthopedic rehabilitation.

6263 **HealthSouth Rehab Hospital: South Carolina**
2935 Colonial Drive
Columbia, SC 29203
803-254-7777
FAX: 803-414-1414
www.healthsouthcolumbia.com

Jackie Kirkwood, Administrator
James Rogers, Contact
Offers a wide range of specialized medical and therapeutic services designed to help physically disabled individuals reach their optimum level of function and independence.

6264 **Rebound Head Injury Recovery Services of the Carolinas**
800 W Meeting Street
Lancaster, SC 29720
803-286-1418
FAX: 803-286-1824

6265 **Shriners Hospitals for Children, Greenville**
Shrinners Hospital sfor Children
950 W Faris Road
Greenville, SC 29605
864-271-3444
866-459-0013
FAX: 864-271-4471
www.shrinershq.org/hospitals/greenville

Gary F. Fraley FACHE, Administrator
Jon R. Davids MD, Chief Of Staff
Ranae M. Thompson RN, MSN, CNA, Director Of Patient Care Srvs.
A 50-bed pediatric orthopaedic hospital providing comprehensive orthopaedic care to children at no charge to their families. The hospital is one of 22 Shriners Hospitals throughout North America. The hospital accepts and treats children with routine and complex orthopaedic problems, utilizing the latest tretments and technology availiable in pediatric orthopaedics, resulting in early ambulatory and reduced length of stay.

Tennessee

6266 Health South Cane Creek Rehabilitation Center
Health South Corporation
180 Mount Pelia Road
Martin, TN 38237
731-587-4231
FAX: 731-588-1454
e-mail: dayle.unger@healthsouth.com

Dayle Unger RN NHN, Administrator
Martha Stephenson RN, Rehab Liaison
Ray Ann Dudley LPN, Rehab Liaison
Offers a wide variety of programs and services for patients in need of acute rehabilitation. Programs and services are availiable through inpatient and outpaitent. Thereapy services availiable are physical, occupational, speech, and respiratory.

6267 HealthSouth Chattanooga Rehabilitation Hospital
2412 McCallie Avenue
Chattanooga, TN 37404
423-697-9160
800-763-5189
FAX: 423-697-9124
www.healthsouth.com

Donna L Bourdon, Administrator/CEO
Scooter Brunson, Marketing Coordinator
Karen Jonakin, Director, Clinical Services
Offers orthopaedic rehabilitation, stroke rehabilitation, amputee rehabilitation, brain injury program, pain management, ventilator weaning, carpal tunnel screening, low intensity program, oncology program, aquatic therapy, day treatment, burn program and outpatient services.

6268 HealthSouth Rehabilitation Cntr/Tennessee
1282 Union Avenue
Memphis, TN 38104
901-722-2000
FAX: 901-722-1968
www.healthsouth.com

Samuel Pieh PT, Contact

6269 Healthsouth Rehabilitation at Sumner
555 Hartsville Pike
Gallatin, TN 37066
615-328-8888
FAX: 615-328-3903

Andrea Sanders, Program Director
Doug Danforth, Director Nurses
Inpatient general rehabilitation programs for orthopedic injury, joint replacements, head injury, arthritis, general weakness and cardio/pulmonary diseases.

6270 James H And Cecile C Quillen Rehabilitation Hospital
2511 Wesley Street
Johnson City, TN 37601
423-952-1700
800-235-1994
FAX: 423-283-0153
www.msha.com

John Turner, Chief Executive Officer
A 60-bed, freestanding comprehensive medical rehabilitation hospital. Full range of outpatient and day treatment, 14-bed traumatic brain injury unit, in ground therapeutic pool, transitional living apartment, outdoor ambulation course. All inpatient and outpatient programs utilize an interdisciplinary team approach designed to improve a patient's physical and cognitive functioning.

6271 Nashville Rehabilitation Hospital
610 Gallatin Road
Nashville, TN 37206
615-226-4330
800-227-3108
FAX: 615-650-2562
www.nrhcares.com

Barton W. Huddleston MD, CEO
Sherry Lawlwer LCSW, Social Services
A free-standing physical rehabilitation facility offering services to patients on an inpatient and outpatient basis. Programs include CVA, orthopedic, neuromuscular, traumatic brain injury, spinal cord injury, general rehabilitation and Bridges - geriatric psychiatric unit. Intra-disciplinary team approach is utilized to assist patients in obtaining their maximum fuctional level.

6272 Patricia Neal Rehab Center : Ft. Sanders R egional Medical Center
Covenant Health
1901 W Clinch Avenue
Knoxville, TN 37916
865-541-1446
800-728-6325
FAX: 865-541-2247
www.patneal.org

Mary Dillon MD, Medical Director
Sharon E. Glass MD, Stroke Program Director
Robert L. Chironna MD, Orthopedic Program Director
A CARF accredited 73-bed facility, it offers a comprehensive team approach to care. Physical, occupational, recreational, behavioral medicine and speech language therapists work with physiatrists to develop individual plans of care designed to return patients to a normal lifestyle as quickly as possible. In addition, rehabilitation nurses collaborate with specialists to teach self-care techniques and provide education to help patients reach optimal functionality.

6273 Rehabilitation Center Baptist Hospital
137 Blount Avenue
Suite 5-A
Knoxville, TN 37901
865-632-5520

Primary focus: Mix of mental health and substance abuse services.

6274 Rehabilitation Center at McFarland Hospital
University Medical Center
500 Park Avenue
Lebanon, TN 37087
615-443-6807
FAX: 615-444-7901
www.universitymedicalcenter.com

Vincent T Cherry Jr, Chief Executive Director
An Acute Inpatient Rehab, located on the hospital's second floor. The center has 26 patient rooms, three therapy treatment rooms, a patient dining area, and an "actuvities of daily living" area which includes a kitchen/laundry area and a patient apartment, for those individuals who will be returning home.

6275 St. Mary's Medical Center: RehabCare Center
900 E. Oak Hill Avenue
Knoxville, TN 37917
865-545-8000
FAX: 865-545-8133

Debra London, Chief Executive Officer
Committed to providing individualized and flexable treatment programs designed for individuals who have been disabled by an injury or illness. The primary mission of the RehabCare Center is to help patients achieve basic skills that may allow independent living and working.

Texas

6276 Bayshore Medical Center: Rehab
4000 Spencer Highway
Pasadena, TX 77504
713-359-2000
FAX: 713-359-1121
www.bayshoremedical.com

Bill Brady, Program Manager
Phillip Robinson, Chief Executive Officer

A 373-bed facility, providing the award-winning care for which we have been nationally recoginzed. Members are here to care for the physical and emotional well-being of those who arrive at Bayshore Medical Center often frightned, in pain and perhaps even alone. We offer patients solace and security through constant communication and compassionate listening in the midst of their medical emergencies and surgical or diagnostic procedures. Kindness, empathy & quality are triats that patients trust.

6277 Cecil R Bomhr Rehabilitation Center of Nacogdoches Memorial Hospital
1204 N Mound Street
Nacogdoches, TX 75961
936-564-4611
FAX: 936-564-4616
e-mail: info@nacmem.org
www.nacmem.org

Bette M Guzman, Director Rehabilitation Services
Tim Hayward, Administrator
The goal of Nacogdoches Memorial Hospital's rehabilitation services is to assist patients in attaining their highest potential activity level for independent daily living, thereby reducing the number of necessary hospitalizations. Keeping folks healthy and in their homes lowers healthcare costs for all of us.

6278 Covenant Health Systems Owens White Outpatient Rehab Center
4010 22nd Street
Lubbock, TX 79410
806-725-5627
FAX: 806-725-4037
www.covenanthealth.org
A comprehensive rehabilitation program designed to help patients attain their maximum level of independence following a debilitating stroke, illness or injury. Our fully accredited program features outpatient physical, occupational and speech language therapies, as well as certified athletic trainers and a certified strength and conditioning specialist.

6279 Gonzales Warm Springs Rehabilitation Hospital
200 Memorial Drive
Luling, TX 78648
830-875-8400
FAX: 830-875-6899
www.warmsprings.org

Brenda Miles, Administrator
Statewide not-for-profit system of inpatient and outpatient rehabilitation speciality centers. Throughout the communities we serve, the Warm Springs Rehabilitation System offers hope and acts as a catalyst for achieving an optimal quality of life by providing comprehensive physical and/or cogenitive care. Investing resources in educational and recreational programs. Supporting research efforts.

6280 Harris Methodist Fort Worth Hospital Mabee Rehabilitation Center
1301 Pennsylvania Avenue
Fort Worth, TX 76104
817-250-2760
866-847-7342
FAX: 814-250-6846
www.texashealth.org
Professionals at the Harris Methodist Fort Worth Hospital's Mabee Rehabilitation Center work closely with each patient to develop a specialzed treatment plan for personal achievement. The center offers highly trained clinical staff members and spacious facilities An incredibly wide range of treatment programs and educational services are provided for both inpatient and outpatient needs.

6281 HealthSouth Plano Rehabilitation Hospital
2800 W 15th Street
Plano, TX 75075
972-612-9000
FAX: 972-423-4293
www.healthsouth.com

Jeanette L. Colson, Administrator
Mary Alexander, Executive Director
A 62-bed medical reahabilitation facility serving inpatient and out patient needs in the Northern Dallas area. The team coordinate all aspects of the patient's rehabilitation to maximize results. The overall effort is directed by board-certified physical medicine and rehabilitation physicians who specialize in medical rehabilitation. Whatever the cause of the disability, our services can benefit patients who have functional limitations in such areas as mobility, communication and self care.

6282 HealthSouth Rehab Hospital Of Arlington
3200 Matlock Road
Arlington, TX 76015
817-468-4000
FAX: 817-468-3055
www.healthsouth.com

Lori Butler PT, Outpatient Lead
A modern 65-bed hospital dedicated to providng inpatient programs in a general rehabilitation setting for persons recovering for a disabling injury or illness. As part of our continuum of care, we also offer outpatient therapy, a day program, and individual therapy services. Our goal is to help our patients resume a productive and more meaningful life through appropriate rehabilitative care and restorative nursing in a wellness-oriented environment that promotes healing and functional recovery.

6283 HealthSouth Rehab Hospital Of Austin
1215 Red River Street
Austin, TX 78701
512-479-3750
FAX: 512-474-2720
www.healthsouth.com

Brian Bowles, Director Of Clinical Services
A comprehensive 83 bed medical rehabilitation hospital serving the needs of patients in the Central Texas area. The mission is to promote recovery for persons with disabling conditions by providing individualized treatment so they can reach the highest level of physical, social and emotional well-being.

6284 HealthSouth Rehabilitation Center of Humble Texas
18903 S Memorial Drive
Humble, TX 77338
281-446-6148
FAX: 281-446-8022
www.healthsouth.com

Katherine Schutz, Administrator
Offers comprehensive rehabilitation services for patients with diverse diagnoses. Rehabilitation can be defined as multidisciplinary therapy designed to increase patient's overall functioning to a level that meets or exceeds where the patient was prior to illness or injury or to maximize current level of ability. The benefits of these services to patients and their families is invaluable.

6285 HealthSouth Rehabilitation Hospital
6701 Oakmont Boulevard
Fort Worth, TX 76132
817-370-4727
FAX: 817-370-4977

Gala Lewis, Admissions
Felipe Garcia, MD

6286 HealthSouth Rehabilitation Hospital of Beaumont
3340 Plaza 10 Drive
Beaumont, TX 77707
409-835-0835
FAX: 409-835-0649
www.healthsouth.com

Bale Clamfoth, Administrator
Sam Coco, Manager
A state of the art freestanding 61-bed comprehensive physical rehabilitation hospital. The hospital is specifically designed to meet the needs of individuals and their families who have experienced a disabling injury or illness or are recovering from a surgery. An experienced team of physicians, nurses, therapists, treat conditions and other disorders.

6287 HealthSouth Rehabilitation Institute Of San Antonio
9119 Cinnamon Hill
San Antonio, TX 78240
210-691-0737
FAX: 210-558-1297
www.healthsouth.com

Aleen Arabit, CEO/Administrator
Larry Spriggs, CFO
HealthSouth Rehabilitation Institute of San Antonio is the largest free-standing physical rehabilitation hospital in San Antonio and is proud to enter our 11th year of delivering quality, comprehensive medical rehabilitation in a pristine environment. HealthSouth annually serves over 1,500 inpatients and more then 20,000 outpatient visits from throughout San Antonio and Mexico. 108-bed hospital has more then 300 personell on staff providing extensive experience.

6288 Hillcrest Baptist Medical Center: Rehab Care Unit

3000 Herring Avenue
Waco, TX 76708
254-202-8155
FAX: 254-202-8975
e-mail: info@hillcrest.net
www.hillcrest.net

J M Dawson, President
Debbie Meurer, Manager
A fully accredited 393-bed acute care facility in Waco including a Level II Trauma Center, Hillcrest Family Health Center, a network of family medicine clinics; and many key services. Hillcrest is a ministry of Texas Baptists and is one of 7 health care institutions affiliated with the Baptist General Convention of Texas.

6289 Institute for Rehabilitation & Research

Tirr System
1333 Moursund Street
Houston, TX 77030
713-942-6159
800-447-3422
FAX: 713-942-5289
e-mail: tirr.referrals@memorialhermann.org
www.tirr.org

Jean Herzog, President
Karen Hart, Vice President Education
A national center for information, training, research, and technical assistance in independent living. The goal is to extend the body of knowledge in independent living and to improve the utilization of results of research programs and demonstration projects in this field. It has developed a variety of strategies for collecting, synthesizing, and disseminating information related to the field of independent living.

6290 Midland Memorial Hospital & Medical Center

2200 W. Illinois Avenue
Midland, TX 79701
432-685-1111
www.midland-memorial.com

Russel Meyers, President/CEO
Dr. Jess H. Parrish, Vice President
Leigh Ann Lane, Secretary
The Occupational and Physical Therapy Center is a specialzed outpatient clinic. The clinic provides a wide variety of rehabilitation services designed to adequately assist you in returning back to your normal duties. Our highly trained professionals are here to help you with all your rehabilitation needs.

6291 Navarro Regional Hospital: RehabCare Unit

Navarro Hospital
3201 West Highway 22
Corsicana, TX 75110
903-654-6895
FAX: 903-872-4627
www.navarrohospital.com

Fredy Woody, Chief Executive Officer
Glenda Teri, Chief Nursing Officer
The rehab unit is located on the 4th floor and is designed for individuals who require intense rehab for an injury or disease process where the goal would be to return home. Our team is committed to helping individuals return to the highest level of functioning. Our team consists of physicians, nurses, physical therapist, occupational therapist, speech therapist, social workers, dieticians and other professionals as needed.

6292 Rebound: Northeast Methodist Hospital

12412 Judson Road
Live Oak, TX 78233
210-757-5065
www.nemh.sahealth.com

Joe Hernandez, Manager
Methodist Healthcare provides quality, comprehensive rehabilitation services for children and adults. Working as a team, rehabilitation professionals help patients define and achieve individual goals in restoring function and productivity.

6293 Rio Vista Rehabilitation Hospital

1740 Curie Drive
El Paso, TX 79902
915-544-3399
800-999-8392
FAX: 915-544-4838

Gene Miller, Administrator

6294 San Antonio Warm Springs Rehabilitation Hospital

5101 Medical Drive
San Antonio, TX 78229
210-595-2380
FAX: 210-614-0649
www.warmsprings.org

Linda Simpson, Administrator
A statewide not-for-profit system of inpatient and outpatient rehabilitation specialty centers. Warm Springs Rehabilitation System offers hope and acts as a catalyst for achieving an optimal quality of life by providing comprehensive physical and/or cognitive rehabilitative care. Invensting resources in educational and recreational programs. Supporting research efforts.

6295 Shannon Medical Center: RehabCare Unit

120 E Harris Avenue
San Angelo, TX 76903
325-657-5617
FAX: 325-657-5706
e-mail: aaronhargett@shannonhealth.org
www.shannonhealth.com

Bryan Horner, President
Committed to improving the health of our community, using the latest technologies available in the spirit of caring and integrity. Strives to create an environment committed to the values of accountability, service, pride, integrity, respect and excellence. We foster growth toward the highest quality care and customer service and strive for excellent financial performance. We hire and develop the best people to accomplish these tasks.

6296 Shriners Burn Institute: Galveston Unit

815 Market Street
Galveston, TX 77550
409-770-6600
FAX: 409-770-6919
www.totalburncare.com

David N. Herndon MD, Chief Of Staff
Art Sanford MD, Professor Of Surgery
Patricia Blakeney PhD, Senior Psychologist
Providing expert, no-cost orthopaedic and burn care to children under 18.

6297 Shriners Hospitals for Children, Houston

6977 Main Street
Houston, TX 77030
713-797-1616
800-853-1240
FAX: 713-797-1029

Steven Reiter, Administrator
Richard J. Haynes MD, Chief Of Staff
Shriners Hospitals provides at no charge quality pediatric orthopedic serivces to children ages newborn to 18 years old. These services include both outpatient and inpatient needs. Specialties include cerebrel palsy, spina bifida, scoliosis, hand, hip and feet problems. An application is required and may be completed by phone.

6298 South Arlington Medical Center: Rehab Care Unit

3301 Matlock Road
Arlington, TX 76015
817-472-4906
FAX: 817-472-4963
www.medicaclcenterarlington.com

Patrice Oliver, Manaager
Above all else, we are committed to the care and improvement of human life. In recognition of this committment, we strive to deliver high-quality, cost-effective healthcare in the communities we serve.

6299 South Texas Rehabilitation Hospital

Ernest Health
425 E Alton Gloor Boulevard
Brownsville, TX 78526
956-554-6000
FAX: 956-350-6150
www.ernesthealth.com

Surya Raguthu MD, Medical Director
Jessie Eason Gonzalez, Chief Executive Officer
Jun Ellorimo, Director Of Therapy Operations

STRH was designed for the provision of specialized rehabilitative care, in the only freestanding acute rehabilitation hospital serving Brownsville and the Rio Grande Valley. The hospital provides rehabilitative services for patients with functional deficits as a result of debilitating illnesses or injuries.

6300 St. David's Rehabilitation Center
St. David s Medical Center
98 San Jacinto Boulevard
Suite 1800
Austin, TX 78701
512-867-5100
FAX: 512-370-4439
www.stdavids.com

Jon M Foster, Chief Executive Officer
Mission is to provide exceptional care to every patient every day with a spirit of warmth, friendliness and personal pride. Values are integrity, compassion, accountability, respect and excellence.

6301 Texas NeuroRehab Center
1106 W Dittmar Road
Austin, TX 78745
512-444-4835
800-252-5151
FAX: 512-462-6749
www.texasneurorehab.com

Nancy Childs, Medical Director
Edgar Prettyman, Administrator
Internationally recognized provider in brain injury/neurobehavioral treatment for children, adolescents, and adults with complex medical, physical and/or behavioral issues. Medical rehabilitation, neurobehavioral, and neuropsychiatric programs combine traditional therapies with education, vocational, substance abuse, and sensory integration services.

6302 Texas Specialty Hospital at Dallas
7955 Harry Hines Boulevard
Dallas, TX 75235
214-637-0000

Waylon Maynard, Director Clinical Services
Cathy Campbell, Chief Executive Officer
66 beds offering active/acute rehabilitation, brain injury day treatment, cognitive rehabilitation, complex care, extended rehabilitation and short term evaluation.

6303 Touchstone Neurorecovery Center
Nexus Health Systems
9297 Wahrenberger Road
Conroe, TX 77304
936-788-7770
800-414-4824
FAX: 936-788-7885
e-mail: tncinfo@nhsltd.com
www.nhsltd.com

John Cassidy, Executive Director
Cindy Mostaffa TRS, Administrator
Judy Bettencourt, Director Of Human Resources
Provides leading edge neurobehavioral rehabilitation. Develops and provides state-of-the-art transitional, residential and vocational rehabilitation services for indivduals with traumatic brain injuries, and other long term ilnesses.

6304 Valley Regional Medical Center: RehabCare Unit
100 E Alton Gloor Boulevard
Brownsville, TX 78526
956-350-7000
FAX: 956-350-7796
www.valleyregionalmedicalcenter.com

David Handley, Chief Executive Officer

Utah

6305 HealthSouth Rehab Hospital Of Utah
8074 S 1300 E
Sandy, UT 84094
801-561-3400
FAX: 801-565-6576
www.healthsouth.com

Vauna Allison, Admissions
Arina Merrill, MD
A full spectrum of services, including inpatient, outpatient, day hospital and home health. Holistic patient care, education and community assimilation are the hallmarks of our programs, and evidence of our leadership in the field of rehabilitation. Working together as a team, we are able to tailor the needs of our patients and provide the highest quality services. We believe that education and involvement of family and friends, will assist them in maintaining independence after discharge.

6306 LDS Hospital Rehabilitation Center
36 So. State Street
Floor 22
Salt Lake City, UT 84111
801-442-2000
800-527-1118
FAX: 801-408-5610
e-mail: contactus@intermountainmail.org
www.intermountainhealthcare.org

Kem C. Gardner, Chairman
Kent H. Murdock, Vice Chairman
Scott Anderson, President/CEO
Located within a Trauma I Center, this facility provides comprehensive inpatient and outpatient rehabilitation to people with physical disabilities. CARF/JCAHO accredited. Low cost family housing is available and Medicaid/Medicare is accepted.

6307 Primary Children's Medical Center
100 N Medical Drive
Salt Lake City, UT 84113
801-662-1000
FAX: 801-588-2318
www.ihc.com

Joseph Horton, CEO
Scott S Parker, President
Primary Children's Medical Center is the pediatric center serving 5 states in the Intermountain West Utah, Idaho, Wyoming, Nevada and Montana. The 235-bed facility is equipped and staffed to treat children with complex illness and injury. PCMC is owned by Intermountain Healthcare, a non-profit health care system. In addition, it is affiliated with the Dept. of Pediatrics, University of Utah, integrating pediatric programs. The hospital is designed to meet the needs of children & their families.

6308 Shriners Hospitals for Children: Intermountain
Fairfax Road @ Virginia Street
Salt Lake City, UT 84103
801-536-3500
800-313-3745
FAX: 801-536-3782
www.shrinershq.org/hospitals/salt_lake_city

J Craig Patchin, Administrator
James W. Roach MD, Chief Of Staff
One of nineteen hospitals in North America specializing in pediatric orthopedics (plus four hospitals providing pediatric burn treatment). This hospital serves the Intermountain region. All services provided in the hospital are at no cost to family, insurance company, nor state/federal agency regardless of ability to pay.

6309 Stewart Rehabilitation Center: McKay Dee Hospital
4401 Harrison Boulevard
Ogden, UT 84403
801-387-2800
FAX: 801-387-7720
e-mail: contactus@intermountainmail.org
intermountainhealthcare.org/xp/public/mc kayde

Bob Martin, Nurse Coordinator
Judy Grover, Manager
With 10 affiliated clinics, McKay-Dee serves northern Utah, and portions of southeast Idaho and western Wyoming. A part of Intermountain Healthcare's system of 21 hospitals, McKay-Dee Hospital Center offers nationally ranked programs such as the Heart & Vascular Institute, the Newborn ICU and a new Cancer Treatment Center.

6310 University Healthcare-Rehabilitation Center
50 N Medical Drive
Salt Lake City, UT 84132
801-587-3422
FAX: 801-585-3778

Sunny Vance-Lauritzen, Director
Trish Jensen, Program Coordinator
Joseph Webster, Executive Director
Provides quality, comprehensive, rehabilitation services to persons with complex rehabilitation needs, including spinal cord injuries, head trauma, stroke, and other disabling conditions. Rehabilitation Services has been serving physicians, their patients, and the community since 1965. Rehabilitation Services has been an established leader in comprehensive inpatient, outpatient and home/community rehabilitation programs. Accredited by CARF and JCAHO.

Vermont

6311 Vermont Achievement Center
88 Park Street
Rutland, VT 05701
802-775-2395
FAX: 802-773-9656
www.vacvt.org

Joanne Mattsson, President/CEO
J. Cortland Jones, Board Chair
Joan F. Gamble, Vice Chair
Vermont Achievement Center is recognized as a catalyst in building a community where all people are capable of change. Individuals flourish because they are nutured, valued and treated with respect. Education is empowering. The family is the primary influence in a person's life. Children belong in a family. Families are enhanced by support of the community. Children and family services are flexible and responsive to changing needs.

Virginia

6312 Inova Mount Vernon Hospital Rehabilitation Program
Inova Rehabilitation Center
2501 Parkers Lane
Alexandria, VA 22306
703-664-7190
800-554-7342
FAX: 703-664-7128
www.inova.com

Toni Jones, Rehab Admissions
Ann Vennell, Executive Director
Inova Rehabilitation Center at Inova Mount Vernon Hospital provides comprehensive inpatient and outpatient programs for patients with brain injuries, stroke and spinal cord, neurological and orthopedic injuries.

6313 Job Placement Digest
National Rehabilitation Association (NRA)
613 S Washington Street
Alexandria, VA 22314
703-836-0850
e-mail: info@nationalrehab.org

Linda Winslow, Executive Director
Newsletter discussing employment options for persons with disabilities.

6314 Journal of Employment Counseling
American Counseling Association
5999 Stevenson Avenue
Alexandria, VA 22304
703-823-9800
800-473-2329
FAX: 703-823-6862
www.counseling.org

Robert Drummond, Editor
Richard Yep, Executive Director
$20.00
Quarterly

6315 Kluge Children's Rehabilitation Center
University of Virginia
2270 Ivy Road
Charlottesville, VA 22903
434-924-5272
800-627-8596
FAX: 434-924-5559
www.healthsystem.virginia.edu

James Blackman MD, MPH, Medical Director
Richard Stevenson MD KCRC, Research Director
Susan Anderson MD
The Kluge Childrens's Rehabilitation Center (KCRC) is a place dedicated to serving children with special needs. Children between the ages of birth and 21 come to the KCRC from all over Virginia, the United States, and even overseas for many reasons. Some need specific therapy or rehabilitation after injuries, accidents, or surgery. Others have chronic illness such as diabetes, and cystic fibrosis. Many families come to find out why their child is experiencing behavior problems.

Washington

6316 Good Samaritan Healthcare Physical Medicine and Rehabilitation
Good Samaritan Hospital
407 14th Ave. SE
Puyallup, WA 98372
253-697-4000
FAX: 253-286-2719
e-mail: info@goodsamhealth.org
www.goodsamhealth.org

Lynn Siedenstrang, Interim Director
Paul Nutter, MD
Good Samaritan is part of the Multi-Care Health System, a non-for-profit medical system serving the growing populations of Pierce and King Counties in the greater Puget Sound region of Washington. Our medical staff includes 1,600 of the regions most respected primary care physicians and specialists.

6317 Northwest Hospital Center for Medical Rehabilitation
1550 N 115th Street
Seattle, WA 98133
206-364-0500
FAX: 206-368-1399
www.nwhospital.org

C Schneider, Chief Executive Officer
Provides complete medical and surgical services in both inpatient and outpatient settings. Services across multiple specialties include: 24hr emergency services, critical care, cardiac care, stroke program, cancer care, childbirth center, rehabilitation center, diagnostic imaging and education and wellness services. Mission is to raise the long-term health status of our community by providing personalized, quality care with compassion dignity, and respect.

6318 Occupational Outlook Quarterly
US Department of Labor/Bureau of Labor Stats
2 Massachusetts Avenue NE
Washington, DC 20212
202-691-5200
FAX: 202-691-7890

Kathleen Utgoff, Chief Executive Officer
Information on new educational and training opportunities, emerging jobs, prospects for change in the work world, and occupational projections. *$9.50*
40 pages Quarterly

6319 Providence Medical Center
500 17th Avenue
Seattle, WA 98124
206-320-2000
FAX: 206-320-3387
www.swedish.org

Paul Casey MD

Swedish offers a complete continuum of rehabilitation services, from acute inpatient care to extensive outpatient therapies, to meet virtually every rehabilitative need for patients of all ages. Nearly 7,000 patients turn to Swedish for these services every year. Through our multidisciplinary team of physical and occupational therapists and speech-language pathologists, Swedish provides the reassurance of a high level of clinical expertise in comfortable, state-of-the-art facilities.

6320 Providence Rehabilitation Services
Providence Rehabilitation Services
1321 Colby Avenue
Everett, WA 98201
425-261-3825
FAX: 425-261-3823
www.providence.org

Elaine Thayer PT, Clinical Director
Leslie Baumgarten, Manager
Continuum of care available: Acute Care, Inpatient Rehabilitation Unit, Transitional Care, Outpatient therapies, and In-home services.

6321 Shriners Hospitals for Children: Spokane
Shriners Hospitals
911 W. 5th Avenue
Spokane, WA 92204
509-455-7844
FAX: 509-623-0474
www.shrinershq.org/hospitals/spokane

Chuck Young, Administrator
Cheri Hollenback, Director Nursing
Ron L Ferguson MD, Chief of Staff
Provides pediatric orthopedic services plus burn scar revision to children birth to 18. All services at no charge to the family.

West Virginia

6322 HealthSouth Mountain View Regional Rehab Hospital
1160 Van Voorhis Road
Morgantown, WV 26505
304-598-1100
800-388-2451
FAX: 304-598-1103
www.healthsouth.com

Carla Stadelman, Assistant Administrator
John Forester, Chief Executive Officer
An 80-bed freestanding rehabilitation hospital serving central WV, southwestern PA, western MD and northwestern VA. Offers specialized programs to serve the patient population. Brain injury, spinal cord injury, stroke, neuromuscular, pulmonary disorders, pediatrics, ventilator dependence, orthopedics, amputee, case management and pain management.

6323 HealthSouth Western Hills Regional Rehab Hospital
3 Western Hills Drive
Parkersburg, WV 26105
304-420-1300
FAX: 304-420-1374
www.healthsouth.com

Dean Hatcher, Chief Executive Officer
A 40-bed medical rehabilitation hospital serving inpatient and outpatient needs in the western West Virginia area. Our hospital is accredited by the Joint Commission on Accreditation of Healthcare Organizations (JCAHO) Our mission is to guide patients whtih physically disabling conditions along an individualized treatment pathway so they can reach the highest level of physical, social and emotional well-being. We strive to provide the highest quality care for you and your family.

Wisconsin

6324 Extendicare Health Services, Inc.
111 W Michigan Street
Milwaukee, WI 53203
414-908-8000
800-395-5000
FAX: 414-908-8143
www.extendicare.com

Frederick B. Ladly, Chairman
Mel Rhinelander, Vice Chairman
Phillip W. Small, President/CEO

6325 St. Catherine's Hospital
9555 76th Street
Kenosha, WI 53140
262-577-8000
FAX: 262-653-5795
www.uhsi.org

Rick Schultz, Program Manager
Committed to living out the healing ministries of the Judeo-Christian faiths by providing exceptional and compassionate healthcare service that promotes the dignity and well-being of the people we serve.

6326 St. Joseph Hospital
611 Saint Joseph Avenue
Marshfield, WI 54449
715-387-1713
FAX: 715-389-3939
e-mail: sjhweb@stjosephs-marshfield.org
www.ministryhealth.org

Raymond Carroll, Head Nurse
Catherine Olson, Director
Michael Schmidt, Chief Executive Officer
A values-driven healthcare delivery network of aligned hospitals, clinics, long-term care facilities, home care agencies, dialysis centers and many other programs and services in Wisconsin and Minnesota.

6327 Vocational Evaluation and Traumatic Brain Injury: A Procedural Manual
Stout Vocational Rehab Institute
University of Wisconsin-Stout
Menomonie, WI 54751
FAX: 715-232-2356

Ronald R Fry, Manager
Darlene Botterbusch, Program Assistant
This is a written guide for rehabilitation professionals interested in effectively developing new or modifying existing evaluation/assessment services for persons with traumatic brain injury. A practical manual for identifying local support services; creating specific processes, tools and techniques; and formulating meaningful outcome information to facilitate the provision or goal-directed services *$ 14.75*
61 pages Softcover

Wyoming

6328 Spalding Rehabilitation Hospital at Memorial Hospital of Laramie
300 E 23rd Street
Cheyenne, WY 82001
307-635-4141

Michael Spaulding MD

Alabama

6329 **Alabama Department of Rehabilitation Services**
2129 E South Boulevard
Montgomery, AL 36116
334-281-8780
800-441-7607
FAX: 334-281-1973
www.rehab.state.al.us

Steve Shivers, President
State agency which provides services and assistance to Alabama's children and adults with disabilities.

6330 **Alabama Goodwill Industries**
2350 Green Springs Highway S
Birmingham, AL 35205
205-323-6331
FAX: 205-324-9059

Don Smith, Director
The mission of Goodwill is to provide rehabilitation services, training, employment, and opportunities for personal growth to the disabled/disadvantaged.

6331 **Association for Retarded Citizens of Jefferson County (The Arc)**
215 21st Avenue S
Birmingham, AL 35205
205-323-6383
FAX: 205-323-0085
netcommunity.thearc.org

William F Hoehle II, Executive Director
Nancy V. Smith, President
The ARC has four primary components. The HOPE Program provides early intervention therapy services to developmentally delayed infants and toddlers up to the age of three years. The ARC also provides services to adults ages 21 and over with mental retardation. Adult services provides education, pre-vocational screening, and socialization skills training. Employment services provides vocational training, a sheltered workshop, off-site job skills training, job coach services and more. Residential s

6332 **Briarcliff Nursing Home & Rehab Facility**
850 9th Street NW
Alabaster, AL 35007
205-663-3859
FAX: 205-663-9791

Michelle Bonner, Director Nursing
Jody McMichen, Administrator
Postacute rehabilitation program.

6333 **Butler Adult Training Center**
680 Hardscramble Road
Greenville, AL 36037
334-382-2353
FAX: 334-382-9518

Nikitin Tayne, Director
Clients 21 years of age and older who are mentally retarded. School age clients are also served at the center and must also be mentally retarded. Clients receive training in Independent Living Skills, Self-Care, Language Skills, Learning, Self Direction and Economic Self-Sufficiency. The clients also participate in Special Olympics activities.

6334 **Cheaha Mental Health**
PO Box 1248
Sylacauga, AL 35150
256-245-1340
FAX: 256-245-1343

Larry Morris, President
Michelle Houston, Business Manager
Offers mental health rehabilitation, respite care, residential facilities and more for the mentally disabled. Serves Talladega, Coosa, Clay and Randolph counties.

6335 **Children's Rehabilitation Service**
2121 E South Boulevard
Montgomery, AL 36116
334-288-0220
800-441-7607
FAX: 334-281-1388
www.rehab.state.al.us/home/services/crs/main

Steve Shivers, Commissioner
Statewide organization of skilled professionals providng quality medical, rehabilitative, coordination and support services for children with special health care needs and their families.

6336 **Chilton-Shelby Mental Health Center/ The Mitchell Center**
67 Highway 67
Calera, AL 35040
205-668-1327
FAX: 205-668-2443
www.chiltonshelby.org/

Melodie Crawford LPC,NCC,NCP, CEO
Kathryn T Crouthers LCSW, COO
Vicki Potts CPA, CFO
Offers mental health rehabilitation services and more for the recovery of mentally disabled adults. Serves Chilton and Shelby counties.

6337 **EL Darden Rehabilitation Center**
1001 East Broad Street
Ste. C
Gadsden, AL 35999
256-547-5751
FAX: 256-547-5761

Tom Strother, Contact
Work hardening and disciplinary programs. Serves the counties of Etawah, Marshall, Dekalb, Clair, and Cherokee

6338 **Easter Seals Central Alabama**
2125 E South Boulevard
Montgomery, AL 36116
334-288-0240
FAX: 334-288-7171
e-mail: easterseals@worldnet.att.net

Larry Johnson, Executive Director
A private, nonprofit organization offering services audiology, physical, occupational, lymphedemia and speech therapy, psychological counseling, vocational evaluation and assessment, person, social and work adjustment training, GED preparation, computer service training, job placement and follow-up, and special learning disabilities service and supported employment service.

6339 **Easter Seals West Alabama**
1110 6th Avenue E
Tuscaloosa, AL 35401
205-759-1211
800-726-1216
FAX: 205-349-1162
e-mail: eswa@dbtech.net
www.alabama.easter-seals.org

Loie Sears Robinson, Administrator
Leading organization in helping children and adults with disabilities to live with equality, dignity and independence. Rehabilitation services are provided in two divisions: outpatient rehabilitation division (physical therapy, occupational therapy, speech therapy, hearing evaluation, sell and service hearind aids) and vocational division (vocational evaulation and vocational development). Services are rendered regardless of age, race, sex, color, creed, national origin, veteran's status.

6340 **Geer Adult Training Center**
PO Box 419
Carrollton, AL 35447
205-367-8032
FAX: 205-367-8032

Yvonne Williams, Program Coordinator

6341 **Goodwill Easter Seals of the Gulf Coast**
2448 Gordon Smith Drive
Mobile, AL 36617
251-471-1581
800-411-0068
FAX: 251-476-4303
alabama.easterseals.com

John McCain, Chief Executive Officer
Stephanie Constantine, VP Marketing
Vocational, medical, pre-school education, day care, recreation and other support services.

6342 **Indian Rivers**
1915 6th Street
2190
Tuscaloosa, AL 35401
205-345-1600
FAX: 205-391-0106

Laurie Prentice-dunn, Director
Jim Moore, Executive Director
Services are available to adults who have serious mental illness resulting in personal, family or work-related problems. Counseling may take place in either individual or group settings, identification, evaluation and treatment services are available to persons who experience problems related to alcohol and drug abuse and counseling services are available for children and adolescents who have a severe emotional disturbance causing discipline problems at home and school.

6343 **Low Vision Clinic/UAB School of Optometry**
1720 University Boulevard
Birmingham, AL 35294
205-956-3276
FAX: 205-934-0911
www.main.uab.edu/optometry

RW Nowakowski, Chief of Staff
Dr. Marsha Swanson, Chief Low Vision Patient Care
Brenda Watkins, Optometric Technician
Multidisciplinary clinic in a major medical center which provides a comprehensive vision evaluation and prescription of low vision aids for those who are visually impaired. Fees are charged for all examination procedures, special diagnostic tests and materials with most insurance plans accepted. Cost depends on services rendered.

6344 **MARC Enterprises**
2424 Gordon Smith Drive
Mobile, AL 36617
251-479-4709
FAX: 251-473-7649
www.mobilearc.org

Andrew Acklen, Executive Director
Serving the mentally retarded of Mobile County both locally and through its state and national affiliations. Their united efforts through this voluntary association assure the availability of services and provide the opportunity for achievement.

6345 **North Central Alabama Mental Retardation Authority**
PO Box 597
Decatur, AL 35602
256-355-7315
FAX: 256-355-7317

Earl E Brightwell, Executive Director
NCA, MRA, Inc. functions as an entrance to the service delivery system for the Alabama Department of Mental Health and Mental Retardation and is responsible for planning, development, implementation of programs, sanction, monitoring, referral, and case management for persons with mental retardation/developmental disabilities in Morgan, Lawrence and Limestone Counties.

6346 **Northwest Alabama Easter Seals Children's Clinic Rehabilitation Center**
1450 E Avalon Avenue
Muscle Shoals, AL 35661
256-391-1110
www.alabama.easter-seals.org

Robert H Nelson, Administrator
Easter Seals has been helping individuals with disabilities and special needs, and their families live better lives for more then 80 years. From child development centers to physical rehabilitation and job training for people with disabilities, Easter Seals offers a variety of services to help people with disabilities address lif's challenges and achieve personal goals.

6347 **Southeastern Blind Rehabilitation Center**
Department of Veterans Affairs Medical Center
700 South 19th Street
Birmingham, AL 35233
205-933-8101
FAX: 205-933-4484
e-mail: george.sands@med.va.gov
www1.va.gov/blindrehab

Frank D Wilkes, Director
Y Parris, Administrator
The Center is a 32-bed inpatient blind rehabilitation program which serves the southeastern region. The majority of client services are for basic adjustment and management to sight loss. Basic services include: low vision, orientation and mobility, manual skills, ADL and communications. Training on electronic mobility aids and adapted computers is also available on a restricted basis. The program maintains graduate education affiliations and an active applied research program.

6348 **Tennessee Valley Rehabilitation**
PO Box 1926
Decatur, AL 35602
256-350-2041
866-350-2041
FAX: 256-350-2806
www.tvrcdecatur.com

Dr. Taylor Byrd, President
Bill Grissim, Vice President
Kathy Cagle, Executive Vice President
Mission is to help persons with disabilities gain and maintain employment in the competitive market. The mission is accomplished by providing quality services for individuals. Being attuned to the needs of each individual served. Respecting the rights of individuals served. Promoting the welfare and dignity of each individual served at all times. Not showing partiality to individuals based on race, color, national origin, gender and religion.

6349 **The Arc Of Alabama Inc.**
300 S Hull Street
Montgomery, AL 36104
334-262-7688
866-243-9557
FAX: 334-834-9737
e-mail: info@thearcofalabama.com
www.thearcofalabama.com

Thomas B Holmes, Executive Director
The Arc of Jefferson County serves children and adults with mental retardation and/or other developmental disabilities. Services are provided through the following programs: the HOPE (Helping Others through Parent Education) Early Intervention Program; Adult Day Services; Residential Services; and Arc-Way Industries, a sheltered and supported employment program.

6350 **Vaughn-Blumberg Services**
PO Box 8646
Dothan, AL 36304
334-793-3102
FAX: 334-793-7740

Ed Dorsey, Executive Director
Child early intervention services for the mentally handicapped adult including diagnosis and evaluation and physical, speech, and occupational therapies. They also offer counseling, day training,employment assistance and residental homes.

6351 **West Central Alabama Easter Seals Rehabilitation Center**
2906 Citizens Parkway
Selma, AL 36701
334-872-8421
800-801-4776
FAX: 334-872-3907
e-mail: wcarcdw@tomnet.com
www.al.easter-seals.org

Larry F Lewis, Administrator
David White, Program Coordinator
Vocational evaluation, job development, employment development, job coaching, counseling, medical services, audiology, pre-school development programs.

Alaska

6352 Alaska Center for the Blind and Visually Impaired
3903 Taft Drive
Anchorage, AK 99517
907-248-7770
800-770-7517
e-mail: info@alaskabvi.org
www.alaskabvi.org

Donna M. Dean, President
Dennis P. Cimmings, Vice President
Christina Y. Dobbins, Treasurer
Services to help the adult residential or community-based student become independent and self-sufficient by offering independent travel, Braille reading and writing, use of assiative technology such as talking computers, manual skills and personal, as well as home management. There is a special program for those 55 years of age and older who are experiencing a vision loss and another program for rural Alaska Native youth who are visually impaired.

6353 Alaska Veterans Facility
4201 Tudor Centre Drive
Suite 115
Anchorage, AK 99508
907-563-6966
FAX: 907-561-7183

Robert Erwin, Team Leader
Robert Nelson, Counselor
Veterans medical clinic offering disabled veterans medical treatments.

Arizona

6354 Arizona Center for the Blind and Visually Impaired
3100 E Roosevelt Street
Phoenix, AZ 85008
602-273-7411
FAX: 602-273-7410
e-mail: jlamay@acbvi.org
www.acbvi.org

James May, Executive Director
Frank Vance, Director
Diana Miladin, Communication/Development Coord.
A private, nonprofit organization that provides comprehensive rehabilitation services and more for the blind and visually handicapped. The staff includes 20 instructional and adminstrative professionals.

6355 Arizona Industries for the Blind
3013 W Lincoln Street
Phoenix, AZ 85009
602-269-5131
FAX: 602-269-9462
www.azdes.gov/aib

Richard Monaco, General Manager
Offers rehabilitation services, vocational/pre-vocational evaluation and training, work adjustment, job development and employment and training opportunities for individuals who are blind.

6356 Banner Good Samaritan Medical Center
1111 E McDowell Road
Phoenix, AZ 85006
602-239-2000
FAX: 602-239-5868
www.bannerhealth.com

Ronald Herrick, Associate Administrator
Annette Bowen, Manager
Nearly 1,700 physicians representing more than 50 specialties work with Banner Good Samaritan staff to care for more then 36,000 inpatients a year. Houses more then 650 licensed patient care beds. A teaching hospital that trains more then 220 physicians annually and a premier medical center in Arizona and the Southwest. Provides a comprehensive foundation of major programs and an equally impressive offering of highly specialized programs not availiable in most hospitals.

6357 Beacon Foundation for the Mentally Retarded
25 E Drachman Street
Tucson, AZ 85705
520-623-3454
FAX: 520-623-3494

Paul Wagler, Chief Executive Director
Wendy Toth, Manager
Committed to effectively assisting adults with disabilities to maximize their personal, social, vocational and educational skills in order to attain a successful and meaningful independence within the Tucson community.

6358 Carondelet Brain Injury Programs and Services (Bridges Now)
350 N Wilmot Road
Tucson, AZ 85711
520-873-3884
FAX: 520-873-3743
e-mail: comments@carondelet.org
www.carondelet.org

Sarah Ascher, Rehab Coordinator
Wes Colvin, Chief Executive Officer
Comprehensive outpatient rehabilitation program. PT, OT, ST, Psychology and Rehab Counseling Services.

6359 Desert Life Rehabilitation & Care Center
1919 W Medical Street
Tucson, AZ 85704
520-297-8311
FAX: 520-544-0930
www.desertlifercc.com

Carolyn Blasi, Executive Director
Accomodates 240 residents. Provides skilled and intermediate nursing with occupational, physical, speech and respiratory therapy services. Offers special programs including an Alzheimer's Unit and a Young Adult program

6360 Freestone Rehabilitation Center
10617 E Oasis Drive
Apache Junction, AZ 85220
480-986-1531
FAX: 480-986-1538

Randy Gray, Executive Director
Cherie Vance, Manager

6361 HealthSouth Valley Of The Sun Rehabilitation Hospital
13460 N 67th Avenue
Glendale, AZ 85304
623-878-8800
FAX: 623-878-5254
www.healthsouth.com

Beth Bacher, Administrator
A 60-bed free-standing hospital that offers acute physical rehabilitation, outpatient therapy services and day hospital treatment. Works in cooperation with local, regional and national managed care organizations and other sources to maximise patient recovery while conserving financial resources.

6362 Institute for Human Development
Northern Arizona University
PO Box 5630
Flagstaff, AZ 86011
928-523-7319
FAX: 928-523-9127
www.nau.edu/ihd

Levi Esguerra, Director
The Institute values and supports the independence, productivity and inclusion of Arizona's citizens with disabilities. Based on the values and beliefs, the Institute conducts training, research and services that further these goals.

6363 John C Lincoln Hospital North Mountain
250 E Dunlap Avenue
Phoenix, AZ 85020
602-943-2381
FAX: 602-944-8062
e-mail: webmaster@jcl.com
www.jcl.com/content/northmountain/default.htm

Daniel Coleman, President/CEO

Mission is to assist each person entrusted to our care to enjoy the fullest gift of health possible, and work with others to build a community where a helping hand is available for our most vulnerable members.

6364 **La Frontera Center**
502 W 29th Street
Tucson, AZ 85713 520-884-9920
www.lafrontera.org

Daniel J. Ranieri PhD, President/CEO
Michael Grassinger, President
Patrick O'Hagin, Vice President
A nonprofit community-based behavioral health agency that has been helping southern Arizona children, adults, and families since 1968.

6365 **Manor Care Nursing and Rehab Center: Tucson**
3705 N Swan Road
Tucson, AZ 85704 520-229-7088
FAX: 520-529-0038
www.hcr-manorcare.com

Mark Bedinger, Administrator
Sheila Powell, Director Admissions/Marketing
A leading provider of short-term post-acute medical care and rehabilitation and long-term skilled nursing care. High quality medical care is provided through registered (RN) and licensed practical (LPN) nurses and certified nursing assistants (CNA) in concert with physical , occupational and speech rehabilitation therapists. Our more then 275 skilled nursing centers are Medicare-and Medicaid-certified.

6366 **Nova Care**
1010 E McDowell Road
Suite 102
Phoenix, AZ 85006 602-256-7232
FAX: 602-256-7292
www.novacare.com

Jeff Sullvin, Manager
NovaCare Rehabilitation's highly respected clinical team provides preventative and rehabilitative services that maximize functionality and promote well-being. NovaCare Rehabilitation also provides physical therapy and athletic training services to more then 20 professional sports teams and 300 universities, colleges, and highschools thoughout the nation.

6367 **Perry Rehabilitation Center**
3146 E Windsor Avenue
Phoenix, AZ 85008 602-956-0400
FAX: 602-957-7610
e-mail: perrycenter@qwest.net

Robin Ratcliff, Director
Jim Musick, President
Provides services for people with disabilities, cognitive disabilities including residential services, day treatment, job training and job placement.

6368 **Phoenix Veterans Center**
141 E Palm Lane
Suite 100
Phoenix, AZ 85004 602-379-4769
FAX: 602-379-4130

John Dooley, Contact Person
Ken Benckwitz, Manager
Veterans medical clinic offering disabled veterans medical treatments.

6369 **Progress Valley: Phoenix**
10830 N 71st Place
Suite 203
Scottsdale, AZ 85254 602-274-5424
FAX: 602-274-5473
e-mail: jlarson@progressvalley.org

Julie Larsson, Associate Director
Joe Brugh, Senior Counselor
Residential aftercare for alcoholism and chemical dependency. Certified chemical dependency counselors provide individual treatment.

6370 **Rehabilitation Services Administration**
1789 W Jefferson 2 NW
Phoenix, AZ 85007 602-542-3332
800-563-1221
FAX: 602-542-3778
TTY: 602-542-6049
e-mail: =azrsa@azdes.gov
www.de.state.az.us/rsa

Craig Warren, Administrator
Provides a variety of specialized services for individuals with physical or mental disabilities that create barriers to employment or independent living. RSA offers 3 major service programs and several specialized programs/services.

6371 **Toyei Industries**
PO Box 55
Ganado, AZ 86505 928-736-2417
888-45T-OYEI
FAX: 928-736-2495

Anthony Lincoln, President & Chairman Of Board
Serves the needs of developmentally disabled and the severely mentally impaired adult citizens of the Navajo Nation and other Indian Nations. Staff of 60+ serves the needs of all the Navajo adults. Services include day treatment programs, home community-based services and residential and group home services.

6372 **Tucson Association for the Blind and Visually Imparied**
3767 E Grant Road
Tucson, AZ 85716 520-795-1331
FAX: 520-795-1336
e-mail: mgordon@saddi.us
www.saavi.us

Robert Heslinga, President
Martina Romero, Vice-President
Richard Chagnon, Treeasurer
Offers health services, counseling, social work, home and personal management, computer training, low vision aids and more for the visually handicapped 18 years or older.

6373 **Yuma Center for the Visually Impaired**
2770 S Avenue B
Yuma, AZ 85364 928-726-1310
FAX: 928-783-3261

Calvin Roberts, Executive Director
A private nonprofit agency offering services for totally blind and legally blind children and adults in the Arizona area.

Arkansas

6374 **Arkansas Lighthouse for the Blind**
69th & Murray Streets
Po Box 192666
Little Rock, AR 72219 501-562-2222
FAX: 501-568-5275

Bill Johnson, Executive Director
Lyn Cossey, Director Of Operations
John McAtee, Accountant-Business Manager
Offers educational industrial evaluation and training to the legally blind and multihandicapped. Funded by workshop sales and contributions, the staff includes ten full time employees

6375 **Beverly Enterprises Network**
1200 S Waldron Road
Fort Smith, AR 72903 479-201-2000
800-666-9996
FAX: 479-452-5131

Randy Churchey, Chief Executive Officer
Offers a progressive approach to subacute care. The goal of this organization is to assist injured and disabled individuals regain the level of independence to which they have been accustomed. Provides support and training programs, patient and family services and specialty programs for patients.

6376 Easter Seals: Arkansas

3920 Woodland Heights Road
Little Rock, AR 72212
501-227-3602
877-533-3600
FAX: 501-227-3658
e-mail: infol@easterseals.com
www.ar.easter-seals.org

Sharon Moone-Jochums, President/CEO
Linda Rogers, VP Programs
Stephanie Smith, VP Finance/Administration
Mission is to provide exceptional services to ensure that all people with disabilities or special needs have equal opportunities to live, learn, work and play in their communitites.

6377 HealthSouth Rehabilitation Hospital Of Fort Smith

1401 S J Street
Fort Smith, AR 72901
479-785-3300
FAX: 479-785-8599
www.healthsouth.com

Julie Stec, Chief Executive Officer
Holli Baker, Director Business Development
A free-standing 80-bed comprehensive physical medicine and rehabilitation hospital offering inpatient and outpatient services. Provides specialized medical and therapy services, designed to assist physically challenged persons to reach their highest level of independent function.

6378 Lions World Services for the Blind

2811 Fair Park Boulevard
Little Rock, AR 72204
501-664-7100
800-248-0754
FAX: 501-664-2743
e-mail: admin@lwsb.org
www.lwsb.org

Ramona Sangalli, Chief Executive Officer
Larry Morgan, Director Of Development
Offers services in the areas of health education, recreation, rehabilitation, counseling, employment, computer training and more for all legally blind residents of the U.S. The staff includes 56 full time employees.

6379 Little Rock Vet Center #0713

Department of Veterans Affairs of Washington DC
201 W Broadway Street
Suite A
North Little Rock, AR 72114
501-324-6395
www.hud.gov/offices/cpd/about/hudvet/state/ar

Jeffrey Geye, Director
Vet Center provides PTSD counseling to veterans of a combat zone. No medical care provided.

6380 Timber Ridge Ranch NeuroRestorative Services

4500 West Commerce Drive
North Little Rock, AR 72116
501-758-8799
800-743-6802
FAX: 501-758-8778
www.neurorestorative.com

Rob Daniels, Executive Director
Comprehensive, individualized services from a transdisciplinary team of licensed professionals assist clients along a course to greater independence. A separate team is dedicated to the needs of children, adolescents, and their families. A clinical team may include professionals from the disciplines of: behavior analysis, neuropsychology, physiatry, psychology, speech-language pathology, occupational therapy, physical therapy, social work, couseling, education, nursing, and case management.

California

6381 ARC Fresno-Kelso Activity Center

4567 N Marty Avenue
Fresno, CA 93722
559-226-6268
FAX: 559-226-6269
www.arcfresno.org

Tami Grinstead
Heather Harrison
Kathleene Moorhead, Manager
Kelso Activity Center was Arc Fresno's first program site in 1963 and remains a vital program serving daily over 100 individuals with moderate to profound mental retardation. Individuality, choice and ability are integral in developing an individual service plan for each person, along with participation in one of the 3 programs at Kelso specific to the individual's needs and personal goals.

6382 ARC Of San-Diego-South Bay

1280 Nolan Avenue
Chula Vista, CA 91911
619-427-7524
FAX: 619-427-4657
e-mail: info@arc-sd.com
www.arc-sd.com/locations

Skit Covell, President
Terri Thorn, Executive Director
Provides remunerative work.

6383 ARC Of Southeast Los Angeles-Southeast Industries

9501 Washburn Road
Downey, CA 90242
562-803-1556
FAX: 562-803-4080
e-mail: info@arcselac.org

Kevin Donald, Executive Director
Provides an offsite extension of your production and warehouse facility. We have reliable and highly trained personnel to meet your needs, including pick-up and delivery service with prompt turn-around times. We offer assembly and packaging at competitive rates while maintaining the highest standards.

6384 ARC: VC Community Connections West

295 Arcade Drive
Ventura, CA 93001
805-652-0541
FAX: 805-652-0542
e-mail: mburke@arcvc.rg
www.arcvc.org

Mary Kay, Program Manager
Larry Rice, Director Community Intergration
Caring and experienced staff is dedicated to serving participants with a variety of physical, mental and social disabilities who require a higher level of support and supervision. Using a person-centered planning approach, Arc Ventura County promotes self-directed services for all clients and families served. Adult development centers serve individuals with physical and mental disabilities, as well as people with challenging behaviors, who require assistance with basic skills such as self care.

6385 ARC: VC Ventura

295 Arcade Drive
Ventura, CA 93003
805-652-0541
FAX: 805-652-0542
e-mail: frobinson@arcvc.org
www.arcvc.org

Mary Kay, Manager
Arc Ventura County is a private, nonprofit organization that provides educational, vocational and residential services for people with developmental disabilities. Informed decisions, positive changes, and integration in the community are fundamental principals in all programs. As evidence of our programming excellence, Arc Ventura County has been accredited by CARF (The Rehabilitation Accreditation Commission.

6386 Ability First L.L. Frank Work Center

1300 E Green Street
Pasadena, CA 91106
626-396-1010
877-768-4600
FAX: 626-396-1010
e-mail: info@abilityfirst.org
www.abilityfirst.org

Lori E. Gangemi, President/CEO
Steve S. Schultz, Vice President Of Development
Mary Beth Perrine, Controller/MIS Manager

Vision is of a society that values each individual and provides the opportunity for all people to lead full and productive lives. For more then 80 years, we have been looking beyond disabilities, focusing on capabilities and expanding possibilities. Offers a broad range of programs & services to help children and adults with physical and developmental disabilities realize their full potential throughout their lives, including employment and socialization programs.

6387 Accentcare

135 Technology Drive
Suite 150
Irvine, CA 92618
949-623-1500
800-834-3059
FAX: 877-766-5250
e-mail: info@accentcare.com
www.accentcare.com

William Comte, Chief Executive Officer
Postacute rehabilitation program: home care aides follow through with rehabilitation instructions given by physical, occupational and speech therapists. Other home care services are available, serving special needs for Alzheimer's, blind, brain injury, MS, ostomies, parkinsonism, spinal injury and stroke.

6388 Anaheim Veterans Center

859 S Harbor Boulevard
Anaheim, CA 92805
714-776-0161
FAX: 714-776-8904
www1.va.gov/directory/guide/facility

Robert Key, Team Leader
Dawn Bankston, Counselor
John Alcantara, Office Manager
Veterans medical clinic offering disabled veterans medical treatments.

6389 Association for Retarded Citizens: Alameda County

575 Independent Road
Oakland, CA 94621
510-639-4680
FAX: 510-639-4684

Ram Sirck, Director
Offers the Right Track program in which selected workers are grouped together on a contract basis to maximize work productivity. Provides a full benefit package, as well as a permanent supervisor. A worker is matched to a job of at least 20 hours per week and then trained by the staff of The Right Track.

6390 Azure Acres Recovery Center

2264 Green Hill Road
Sebastopol, CA 95472
707-823-3385
877-762-3735
FAX: 707-823-8972
e-mail: info@azureacres.com
www.azureacres.com

Shannon Clay, Executive Director
Offers rehabilitation services and residential care for the person with an alcohol or drug abuse related problems.

6391 Back in the Saddle

9775 Mockingbird Avenue
Apple Valley, CA 92308
760-240-3217
FAX: 760-240-3274
www.thesaddle.com

Richard Smith PhD, Owner
Erika Reed, Co-Director
A long term community residential facility for head injured adults. House parents live on-site; and oversee a variety of programs which are individually designed and might include classes in community college, placement in a workshop or on a workstation, volunteer positions and home skills assignments. Recreational outing range from horseback riding to weekend camping. Apartment programs available as set-up. Price: $2800-$3000 per month.

6392 Ballard Rehabilitation Hospital

1760 W 16th Street
San Bernardino, CA 92411
909-473-1200
800-761-1226
FAX: 909-473-1276
www.ballardhospital.com

Robert Herrick, Chief Executive Officer
Mary Hunt, Chief Operating Officer
Patty Meinhardt, Director Marketing/Admissions
Ballard Rehab Hospital is a free standing specialty hospital and provides the complete continuum of acute, subacute and outpatient rehabilitation, dedicated to providing rehab seminars to adults and children. The following inpatient and outpatient programs are available: CNA (Stroke) Rehab; Spinal Cord Injury Rehab; Brain Injury Rehab; Pain Management Rehab; Injured Worker Programs; and Post Amputation Rehab.

6393 Bayview Nursing and Rehabilitation

516 Willow Street
Alameda, CA 94501
510-521-5600
FAX: 510-865-6441
www.bayviewnursing.com

Mary Webster, Administrator
Offers a full range of medical services to meet the individual needs of our residents, including short-term rehabilitative services and long termed skilled care. Working with the resident's physician, our staff-including medical specialists, nurses, nutritionists, dietitians, and social workers-establishes a comprehensive treatment plan intended to restore you or your loved one to the highest practicable potential.

6394 Belden Center

606 Humboldt Street
Santa Rosa, CA 95404
707-579-2735
FAX: 707-579-4145

Wes Killian, Program Director
Pamela Fadden, Owner
Postacute rehabilitation program.

6395 Blind Babies Foundation

1814 Franklin Street
11th Floor
Oakland, CA 94612
510-446-2229
FAX: 510-446-2262
e-mail: bbinfo@blindbabies.org
www.blindbabies.typepad.com

Phillip Hatlen, Executive Director
A private, nonprofit agency offering services in the areas of health, counseling, social work, self help and education to blind and visually impaired infants. The educated staff includes 8 full time and 3 part time employees.

6396 Brotman Medical Center: RehabCare Unit

Brotman Medical Center
3828 Delmas Ter
Culver City, CA 90232
310-836-7000
800-677-1238
FAX: 310-202-4105
e-mail: info@brotmanmed.com
www.brotmanmedicalcenter.com

Jennifer Cortez, Program Manager
Culver City is centrally located within the city of Los Angeles. These are two programs offering inpatient rehabilitation. The acute rehab program is designed for patients who need physical rehabilitation due to injury or medical disability. This program requires patients to participate in 3 hours therapy per day. The sub-acute program is designed especially for patients who need rehab but cannot tolerate the intensity of the acute rehab program.

6397 Build Rehabilitation Industries

1323 Truman Street
San Fernando, CA 91340
818-898-0020
FAX: 818-898-1949
e-mail: jhodgins@buildrehab.org
www.buildindustries.com

Matthew Lynch, President/CEO
Michele A Utley, Vice President
Isabel Boniface, Human Resources Executive

Comprehensive C.A.R.F. Accredited vocational rehabilitation services for adults with disabilities or other barriers to employment. Programs include: Sheltered Workshops, Work Evaluation, Work Hardening and Adjustment, Supported Employment, Job Placement, Independent Living Skills, Behavior Management, Adult Development Center, On-the-Job Training, and One-Stop Workforce Development Career Center.

6398 California Elwyn
18325 Mount Baldy Circle
Fountain Valley, CA 92708
714-557-6313
FAX: 714-963-2961
e-mail: info@caelwyn.org
www.caelwyn.org

Joan McKinney, Executive Director
Provides opportunities for people challenged by physical and mental disabilities who are 18 or older. California Elwyn develops an Individual Rehabilitation Plan for all consumers. Contract work, shrinkwrap, janitorial are just some of the types of jobs done. Supported Employment Services are available and over 100 consumers currently are employed. Funded by the State Department of Rehabilitation and Vocational Rehabilitation.

6399 California Eye Institute
1360 East Herndon
Fresno, CA 93720
209-449-5000
FAX: 209-499-5090

Virgil Snow
Denise Haar, Manager
A private, nonprofit agency offering services such as health, educational, recreational, rehabilitation and employment counseling to the totally blind, legally blind and visually impaired. The staff includes two full time workers.

6400 Camp Recovery Center
3192 Glen Canyon Road
Scotts Valley, CA 95066
877-557-6237
800-924-2879
FAX: 877-438-5833
www.camprecovery.com

Paige Bottom, Executive Director
A free-standing social model recovery center for chemical dependency located on 25 wooded acres in the Santa Cruz Mountains. The services include: medical detoxification, complete medical evaluation, psychiatric evaluation and counseling, psychological testing, individual counseling and more. Helps the recovery from chemical dependency in a easier, warm and caring environment.

6401 Campobello Chemical Dependency Recovery Center
3250 Guerneville Road
Santa Rosa, CA 95401
707-579-4066
800-805-1833
FAX: 707-579-1603
e-mail: campocdrc@aol.com
www.campobello.org

James Cody, Executive Director
Our mission is to provide primary treatment, education, ongoing support and family services for clients seeking a more rewarding, chemically free lifestyle. Our primary goals are: to improve understanding/acceptance of the disease model of addiction. To improve self esteem. To reduce family, job and legal problems. To improve physical/emotional health. To enhance coping and problem solving strategies for recovery.

6402 Casa Colina Centers for Rehabilitation
255 East Bonita Avenue
Po Box 6001
Pomona, CA 91769
909-596-7733
800-926-5462
FAX: 909-593-0153
e-mail: rehab@casacolina.org
www.casacolina.org

Felice Loverso, President/CEO
Casa Colina, has pioneered effective programs to create opportunity for health, productivity and self-esteem for persons with disability since 1936. Through medical rehabilitation, transitional living, residential, community, and prevention and wellness programs. Casa Colina serves more than 7,000 persons annually. Casa Colina, a non-profit organization, offers a unique spectrum of opportunities, achievement and results to patients and their families.

6403 Casa Colina Padua Village
255 East Bonita Avenue
Po Box 6001
Pomona, CA 91769
909-596-7733
800-926-5462
FAX: 909-593-0153
e-mail: rehab@casacolina.org
www.casacolina.org

Chandrahas Agarwal, Medical Director
Felice Loverso, Chief Executive Officer
Long term residential services for adults with developmental disability. Residences include Malmquist House, Woodbend House, and Hillsdale House, all located in Claremont, California.

6404 Casa Colina Residential Services: Rancho Pino Verde
Casa Colina Center for Rehabilitation
11981 Midway Avenue
Lucerne Valley, CA 92356
760-248-6245
FAX: 760-248-2245
e-mail: rehab@casacolina.org
www.casacolina.org

Rodney Peek, Director
Chris Schlanser, Program Director
Long term residential services in rural environment for adults with brain injury.

6405 Casa Colina Transitional Living Center
255 E Bonita Avenue
Pomona, CA 91767
909-596-7733
FAX: 909-593-7541
www.casacolina.org

Barbara Urabe, Program Administrator
Felice Loverso, Chief Executive Officer
Postacute rehabilitation program.

6406 Casa Colina Transitional Living Center: Pomona
PO Box 6001
Pomona, CA 91769
909-596-7733
800-926-5462
FAX: 909-593-0153
e-mail: rehab@casacolina.org
www.casacolina.org

Felice L Loverso, President/CEO
Robert E Duncan, Chairman
Post acute short term residential program for persons with brain injury. In a home-like setting, therapy promotes successful re-entry to home and community living.

6407 Cedars of Marin
PO Box 947
Ross, CA 94957
415-454-5310
FAX: 415-454-0573

Brenda McIvor, Executive Director
Alexa Witter, Executive Assistant
Martin Williamson, Administrator
Provides residential and day programs for adults with developmental disabilities.

6408 Center for Neuro Skills
2658 Mount Vernon Avenue
Bakersfield, CA 93306
661-872-3408
800-922-4994
FAX: 661-872-5150
e-mail: bakersfield@neuroskills.com
www.neuroskills.com

John Schultz, Vice President
Mark J Ashley, President/Owner

A comprehensive, post-acute, community based head-injury rehabilitation program serving over 100 clients per year. Since 1980, CNS has effectively treated the entire spectrum of head-injured clients, including those with severe behavioral disorders, cognitive/perceptual impairments, speech/language problems, physical disabilities and post-concussion syndrome.

6409 Center for the Partially Sighted
12301 Wilshire Boulevard
Suite 600
Los Angeles, CA 90025
310-458-3501
800-481-3937
FAX: 310-458-8179
e-mail: info@low-vision.org
www.low-vision.org

LaDonna Ringering PhD, Executive Director
Pat Jordan, Public Information Manager
Phyllis Amarai PhD, Clinical Director
Services for partially sighted and legally blind people include low vision evaluations, the design and prescription of low vision devices and adaptive technology, as well as counseling and rehabilitation training (independent living skills and orientation/mobility training). Special programs include children's program, diabetes and vision loss program, Technology demonstrations. Store carries low vision aids. Catalog available.

6410 Central Coast Neurobehavioral Center OPTIONS
800 Quintana Road, Suite 2C
PO Box 877
Morro Bay, CA 93443
805-772-6066
FAX: 805-772-6067
e-mail: info@optionsccnbc.org
www.optionsccnbc.org

Michael Mamot, CEO
Ole von Frausing-Borch, COO
Serves adults with developmental disabilities, traumatic head injuries, or other neurological impairments. OPTIONS operates two transitional living centers, eight licensed residential facilities, two licensed community integration day programs and a licensed short term stabilization center. Services offered include: supported and independent living services, group and individual vocational services, neuropsychological assessment, occupational therapy, cognitive therapy, speech therapy and more.

6411 Cerebral Palsy: North County Center
8525 Gibbs Drive #100
San Diego, CA 92123
858-571-7803
888-827-0771
FAX: 858-571-0919
e-mail: ucp@ucpsc.org
www.ucpsd.org

Jim O'Leary, President
Misty Thompson, Vice President
Dave Mulvaney, Secretary
The mission of UCP San Diego County is to advance the independence, productivity and full citizenship of people affected by cerebral palsy and other disabilities. By making solid steps, UCP can build a better community for all in the process.

6412 Children's Hospital Central California Reh abilitation Center
9300 Valley Childrens Place
Madera, CA 93636
559-353-3000
FAX: 559-353-8060
e-mail: webmaster@childrenscentralcal.org
www.valleychildrens.org

Shirleen Fowler, Manager
David Meagher, MD
A 297-bed pediatric medical center on a 50-acre campus. We now have more then 500 doctors practicing in over 40 pediatric subspecialties with clinics and services throughout the state.

6413 Children's Hospital Los Angeles Rehabilitation Program
4650 W Sunset Boulevard
Los Angeles, CA 90027
323-660-2450
FAX: 323-665-4118
e-mail: webmaster@chla.usc.edu
www.childrenshospitalla.org

Luis Montes, Director
Designated as a Level I Pediatric Trauma Center by the Los Angeles County EMS Agency, the hospital treats more then 1,500 pediatric trauma patients per year. Performs more then 13,900 pediatric surgeries a year, including more complex surgical procedures then any other hospital in Southern California

6414 Children's Therapy Center
770 Paseo Camarillo
Suite 120
Camarillo, CA 93010
805-383-1501
FAX: 805-383-1504
e-mail: ctcinc@isle.net

Jo Murphy Hyland, Administrative Director
Provides individual occupational therapy, speech/language therapy, family/child consulting, education services and physical therapy consultation for children. Evaluations and treatment are on an individual basis and special emphasis is placed on a multidisciplinary approach with information sharing, and often team treatment.

6415 Clausen House
88 Vernon Street
Oakland, CA 94610
510-839-0050
FAX: 510-444-5790
e-mail: info@clausenhouse.org
www.clausenhouse.org

Peter Reinke, President
Sue Malick, Vice-President
Jennifer Roloff, Vice-President/Secretary
A private nonprofit organization which emphasizes greater independence for developmentally disabled adults. Programs encompass residential services, adult education, day program training, recreational opportunities, supported employment services, independent living, supported living training and assistance.

6416 Community Gatepath
1764 Marco Polo Way
Burlingame, CA 94010
650-259-8544
FAX: 650-259-0194
e-mail: info@gatepath.com
www.communitygatepath.com

Kirk F Cunningham, President/CEO
Popular center and Peninsula Care merged into a new organization named Community Gatepath. Driving forces behind the merger were to be able to provide expanded and/or better services to indidviduals throughout San Mateo County, using the best practices of both organizations.

6417 Community Hospital and Rehabilitation Center of Los Gatos-Saratoga
815 Pollard Road
Los Gatos, CA 95030
408-378-6131
FAX: 408-866-4003
www.communityhospitalLG.com

Gary Honts, CEO
Offers rehabilitation services, inpatient and outpatient care, physical therapy, occupational therapy and more for the physically challenged adult. We have a commitment to health care excellence. It is in this commitment that we have dedicated ourselves to provide personal and professional service to our patients. Our goal is to work closely with staff, physicians and the community to attain shared goals and positive changes, now and in the future.

6418 Contra Costa ARC
1340 Arnold Drive
Martinez, CA 94553
925-370-1818
FAX: 925-370-2048
e-mail: feedback@arcofcc
www.ContraCostaARC.com

Carol Anne McCrary, Executive Director
Naomi Santos, Program Coordinator
A private nonprofit membership-based organization dedicated to enhancing the quality of life of individuals with mental retardation and other developmental disabilities.

6419 Corona Regional Medical Center- Rehabiltation Center
730 Magnolia Avenue
Corona, CA 92879 951-736-7200

Michael Schultz, President
John Calderone, Chief Executive Officer
Offers inpatient and outpatient rehabilitation services. The Center consists of an acute rehab unit, a subacute rehab unit containing modules for long-term ventilator care, respiratory rehab, coma intervention and orthopedics. In addition to inpatient therapies, the Center's outpatient programs include sports and industrial medicine.

6420 Critical Air Medicine
Montgomery Field
4141 Kearny Villa Road
San Diego, CA 92123 858-514-6060
800-247-8326
FAX: 619-571-0835
Offers emergency medical care by air medical transport carriers. These carriers are fully equipped with medical equipment and supplies for cardiovascular emergencies, respiratory supplies, orthopedic supplies and medications.

6421 Crutcher's Serenity House
Po Box D. 50 Hillcrest Drive
Deer Park, CA 94576 877-274-4968
FAX: 707-963-2309
e-mail: crutcherssh@earthlink.net
www.crutcherssh.com

Robert Crutcher, Owner/CEO
Lu Crutcher, Executive Director
A privately owned and operated facility that introduces to residents a new lifestyle free of all chemicals, and a new awareness of their total being. The length of the program is four weeks and is within five minutes of an acute care hospital. The Center is licensed for 19 beds, male and female located in a home-like setting with an emphasis on maintaining a family atmosphere.

6422 Daniel Freeman Rehabilitation Centers
333 N Prairie Avenue
Inglewood, CA 90301 310-674-7050
FAX: 310-674-3886

Louis Ceppi, Associate Administrator
Comprehensive rehabilitation services which address needs and issues of the physically diabled and their families. We offer accute input rehabilitation, outpatient and short term skilled nursing rehabilitaion. Specialty areas include: brain injury, stroke, spinal chord injury, chronic pain, arthritis.

6423 Delano Regional Medical Center
1401 Garces Highway
Delano, CA 93215 661-725-4800
FAX: 661-721-5211
www.drmc.com

Allan Komarek, Chief Executive Officer
Delano Regional Medical Center (DRMC) is proud to be known throughout California & beyond as an innovative regional hospital, deeply rooted in the local communities and committed to providing an exceptional patient experience. A non-profit acute-care facility serving a region of 10 rural central Californiatowns. With over 100 physicians on our active medical staff and additional courtesy or consulting physicians, patients are assured of receiving high-quality care in multiple specialties.

6424 Desert Regional Medical Center
1156 N Indian Canyon Drive
Palm Springs, CA 92262 760-323-6511
FAX: 760-864-9577
www.desertmedctr.com

Patricia Sandoval, Manager
Our dedicated physicians and caregivers provide a broad array of quality programs and services, including comprehensive cancer care, women's health services, heart care, surgical weight loss reduction and orthopedics.

6425 Devereux Santa Barbara
PO Box 6784
Santa Barbara, CA 93160 805-968-2525
FAX: 805-968-3247
e-mail: amcniff@devereux.org
www.devereux.org

David Dennis, Executive Director
Anna Martinez, Admissions Coordinator
Janis Johnson, Public Relations Coordinator
Serves ages 8-88, who have developmental disabilities, emotional disturbances, neurological impairments, brain injuries, schizophrenia, autism, and dual diagnosis. The Center has a licensed capacity of 188 served in a continuum of services including residential, vocational, educational and more.

6426 Division of Physical Medicine and Rehabilitation
San Joaquin General Hospital
500 W Hospital Road
French Camp, CA 95231 209-468-6280
FAX: 209-468-6281
e-mail: pmradministration@sjgh.hs.co.san-joaquin.ca.u
www.sjphysicalmedicine.com

Carolyn Genschmer, Rehabilitation Coordinator
Ken Cohen, Manager
Offers rehabilitation services, inpatient and outpatient care, speech therapy, physical therapy, occupational therapy and more for the physically challenged individual.

6427 Dr. Karen H Chao Developmental Optometry Karen H. Chao. O.D.
121 S Del Mar Avenue
Suite A
San Gabriel, CA 91776 626-287-0401
FAX: 626-287-1457
e-mail: drkhchao@yahoo.com

James Young, Practice Manager
Karen Chao OD, Owner
Developmental optometrist specializing in the testing and treatment of vision problems and the enhancement of visual performance. Performs visual perceptual testing and training for children and adults. Undetected vision problems interfere with the ability to achieve and are highly correlated with learning difficulties and developmental problems. Provides the opportunity to overcome vision and visual-perceptual dysfunctions.

6428 Early Childhood Services
201 East Ridgecrest Blvd.
Ridgecrest, CA 93555 760-375-9787
FAX: 760-375-1288
e-mail: dart@dartontarget.org
www.dartontarget.org

Deanna Lukens, Coordinator
Provides early intervention services to children who have disabilities or are experiencing delays in development. Provides developmental activities to promote the attainment of developmental milestones so that each child may reach his/her maximum potential. The program also provides therapeutic and educational intervention and offers support and guidance to families.

6429 East Los Angeles Doctors Hospital
4060 Whittier Boulevard
Los Angeles, CA 90023 323-721-2244
FAX: 323-980-9824

Sergio Castilla, Owner
Postacute rehabilitation program.

6430 Easter Seals Disability Svcs: Bay Area
230 W Monroe Street
Suite 1800
Chicago, IL 60606 312-726-6800
800-221-6827
FAX: 312-726-1494
e-mail: info@easterseals.com
www.bayarea.easterseals.com

James Williams Jr, Chief Executive Officer
Johnny Jones, VP

Creates solutions that change the lives of children and adults with disabilities and special needs; and provides support to family members. Through innovative services, Easter Seals Bay Area promotes equality and dignity, providing opportunities for independence, integration, and enhanced health and wellness.

6431 Easter Seals Superior California
Sacramento Center & Regional Offices
3205 Hurley Way
Sacramento, CA 95864
916-485-6711
888-877-3257
FAX: 916-485-2653
e-mail: info@easterseals-superiorca.org
www.superiorca.easterseals.com

Gary Kasai, President/CEO
Terry Colborn, VP Programs/Government Affairs
Jessica Cone, VP Marketing/Development
Provides outpatient rehabilitation services including day training programs for adults with disabilities and traumatic brain injuries, warm water therapy, non-public agency services to children including pediatric OT and PT services, work training/employment services, medical equipment loans, early intervention services for infants and toddlers. Serving the counties of Alpine, Calaveras, El Dorado, Sacramento, San Joaquin, Sutter, Tuolumne, Yolo, Yuba, Amador, Stanislaus, Nevada and Placer, CA.

6432 Exceed: A Division of Valley Resource Cent er
2050 Trumble Road
Po Box 1773
Perris, CA 92572
951-657-0609
800-423-1227
FAX: 909-657-2277
e-mail: vrctwohip@aol.com
www.exceed-aws.com

Pattie Robert, Business Development Specialist
Mary Morse, Marketing Director
Kathy Cooke, Manager
Our vision is an environment where each client is valued as an individual and is provided the opportunity to reach his/her maximum potential. Our mission is to provide service and advocacy, which creates choices and opportunities, for adults with disabilities to reach their maximum potential.

6433 Eye Medical Center of Fresno
Eye Medical Center
1122 S Street
Fresno, CA 93721
559-486-5001
800-606-3937
FAX: 559-439-7854
www.emcfresno.com

Rachel Moring-Garcia, Assistant Administrator
Denise Haar, Administrator
Donald Crumb, Manager
A private, nonprofit agency offering services such as health, educational, recreational, rehabilitation, employment and counseling to the totally blind, legally blind and visually impaired. The staff includes hundreds of full time workers.

6434 Fontana Rehabilitation Workshop
Industrial Support Systems
8333 Almeria Avenue
Fontana, CA 92335
909-428-3883
800-755-4755
FAX: 909-428-3835
e-mail: ceo@industrialsupport.org
www.industrial-support.org

Carole Holt, Executive Director
Antonio Diaz, Owner
The Fontana Rehabilitation Workshop, Inc., through its business divisions is committed to maintaining a stable environment wherein people with disabilities are provided with those services and supports that enable them to overcome barriers to employment and empower them to maximize their employment potential.

6435 Foothill Vocational Opportunities
789 N Fair Oaks Avenue
Pasadena, CA 91103
626-449-0218
FAX: 626-449-4802
e-mail: info@foothillvoc.org
www.foothillvoc.org

John R. Poindexter, President
Harold W. Leavens, Vice-President
Minoru Higa, Treasurer
Foothill Vocational Opportunities maximizes the personal and economic potential of disabled individuals by creating meaningful employment opportunities. Foothill provides our clients and thier families with the tools they need to live fuller, richer lives, bringing a sense of inclusion and dignity to a chronically marginalized and underdeserved group of people.

6436 Fred Finch Youth Center
3800 Coolidge Avenue
Oakland, CA 94602
510-482-2244
FAX: 510-530-2047
e-mail: adamchase@fredfinch.org
www.fredfinch.org

John Steinfirst, Chief Executive Officer
Kathie Jacobson, Chief Operations Officer
Jon D'Alessio, Chief Financial Officer
A structured, psychiatric (JCAH accredited) residential treatment center for emotionally disturbed girls and boys between the ages of 12 and 18. Our treatment incorporates an on-site, non-public, special education school, an extensive activities and recreational program, a strong professional psychotherapy component (providing individual, group, and family therapy) and a parent support group. We provide 24-hour awake staff.

6437 Gateway Center of Monterey County
850 Congress Avenue
Pacific Grove, CA 93950
831-372-8002
FAX: 831-372-2411
e-mail: info@gateway.org
www.gatewaycenter.org

Jim Landman, Chairman
Christopher Panetta, Vice Chair
Bruna Odello, Secretary
Our mission is to be a caring and stimulating environment for the Developmentally Disabled where all people can achieve their individual goals safely and with dignity. Our goal is to continue our programs and to find new and innovative ways of assisting the developmentally disabled to live in our community in surroundings compatable with their ability to live and work at the highest level possible.

6438 Gateway Industries: Castroville
1663 Catalina Street
Sand City, CA 93955
831-393-1575
800-499-6262
e-mail: gwi@redshift.com
www.redshift.com

Mike Sweeney, Executive Director
Anna Foglia, Manager
Located in the Sand City Industrial Park, it provides vocational training and employment to developmentally disabled adults so they can achieve their vocational potential while also providing quality services to bussiness along the Central Coast. The sheltered work environment assists the employees by increasing their income, improving their work skills and habits, and enabling them to participate in the community.

6439 Gilroy Workshop
8855 Murray Avenue
Gilroy, CA 95020
408-842-0334
FAX: 408-842-6770

Cathy Andrade
Sally French, Manager
Work adjustment and remunerative work programs.

6440 Glendale Adventist Medical Center
1509 Wilson Ter
Glendale, CA 91206
818-409-8000
FAX: 818-546-5609
www.glendaleadventist.com/services/rehab

Jan Adduie, Rehabilitation Manager
Rehabilitative team is made up of physician specialists, as well as professional and certified staff nurses, thereapists and others who meet regularly to ensure tht each patients progress is carefully planned and closely monitored.

6441 **Glendale Memorial Hospital and Health Center Rehabilitation Unit**
Glendale Memorial Hospital and Health Center
1420 S Central Avenue
Glendale, CA 91204
818-502-1900
FAX: 818-409-7688
www.glendalememorialhospital.org

Charles Barrett, President
Offers rehabilitation services, occupational therapy, physical therapy, residential services and more for the disabled.

6442 **Goleta Valley Cottage Hospital**
Cottage Health System
351 S Patterson Avenue
Santa Barbara, CA 93111
805-967-3411
800-782-2288
FAX: 805-681-6437
e-mail: cverkiak@cottagehealthsystem.org
www.sbch.org

Diane Wisby, VP Operations
Ron Wreft, Chief Executive Officer
Rob Manchester, Manager
A 122-bed acute care hospital was founded in 1966 to serve the growing community of Goleta Valley. Today, we admit more then 2,000 patients a year, see more then 17,000 emergency visits, and welcome nearly 400 newborns to our designated "Baby Friendly" Birth Center each year. We are also recognized for our Level IV trauma designation. We take great pride in fulfilling our goal of providing each patient with comfortable, personalized care.

6443 **Hacienda La Puente Unified School District**
15959 E. Gala Ave
Po Box 60002
City Of Industry, CA 91746
626-934-2801
FAX: 626-934-2900
e-mail: info@hlpusd.k12.ca.us
www.hlpusd.k12.ca.us

Donald Carmack, Director
Rachelle Wilson, Counselor
Jerry Fenning, Counselor
Provides innovative student-centered learning opportunities and support services to a diverse population that enable individuals to achieve thier goals as lifelong learners, productive workers and effective communicators.

6444 **HealthSouth Tustin Rehabilitation Hospital**
Health South Corporation
14851 Yorba Street
Tustin, CA 92780
714-832-9200
FAX: 714-508-4550
www.healthsouth.com

Roderic Bell, Medical Director
Wilfredo Escober, Neurologist
Cynthia Murphy, Physical Medicine
HealthSouth Tustin Rehabilitation Hospital is part of the HealthSouth Corportation, the nation's largest provider of rehabilitative healthcare services, we are the only facility of its kind in Orange County. Fully accredited by the Joint Commission on Accreditation of Healthcare Organizations (JACHO) we provide inpatient and outpatient care designed to meed individual needs of patients and their families.

6445 **Hi-Desert Medical Center**
6601 White Feather Road
Joshua Tree, CA 92252
760-366-3711
800-782-2288

Larry Kelley, Manager
Postacute rehabilitation program.

6446 **Home of the Guiding Hands**
1825 Gillespie Way
Suite 200
El Cajon, CA 92020
619-938-2850
FAX: 619-448-7208
e-mail: carol@guidinghands.org
www.guidinghands.org

Carol Fitzgibbons, Executive Director
Jane Moore, Development & Marketing
Marcy Blumberg, Events Coordinator
The mission of Guiding Hands is to provide quality services, training and advocacy for people with developmental disabilities, their families, and others who benefit. Our vision is to continue to be a dynamic organization dedicated to serving people with special needs, committed to providing services and care through leadership, innovation and creativity.

6447 **Hospital of the Good Samaritan Acute Rehabilitation Unit**
1225 Wilshire Blvd
Los Angeles, CA 90017
213-977-2121
800-366-8338
FAX: 213-482-2770
www.goodsam.org

Andrew B Leeks, President/CEO
David N Shaw MD, Medical Director Acute Rehab
Physicians, researchers and staff are united by a common mission: to foster growth into one of the most comprehensive medical centers in the West. Services offered include: cardiology and cardiovascular services, neurosciences, movement disorders and Parkinsons disorder, wound care center and transfusion-medicine and surgery center.

6448 **Janus of Santa Cruz**
200 7th Avenue
Suite 150
Santa Cruz, CA 95062
831-462-1060
866-526-8772
FAX: 831-462-4970
e-mail: rtc_mgr@janussc.org
www.janussc.org

Margie Storms, Acting xecutive Director
Kay Owsley, Business Manager
A private not-for-profit corporation, licensed by the state of California. The Janus Clinic has a 3 year accreditation by the Council on Accreditation for Health Care Facilities.

6449 **John Muir Medical Center Rehabilitation Services, Therapy Center**
1601 Ygnacio Valley Road
Walnut Creek, CA 94598
925-930-3000
FAX: 925-947-3262
www.jmmdhs.com

Sandra Reese, Vice President
Patty Haggen, Director
Helen Doughty, Manager
A 324-bed acute care facility that is designated as the only trauma center for Contra Costa County and portions of Solano County. Recognized as one of the region's premier healthcare providers, areas of specialty include high-and low-risk obstetrics, orthopedics, neurosciences, cardiac care and cancer care. The campus is accredited by the Joint Commission on Accreditation of Healthcare Organizations (JCAHO), a national surveyor of quality patient care.

6450 **Kindred Hospital-La Mirada**
14900 E Imperial Highway
La Mirada, CA 90638
562-944-1900
FAX: 562-906-3455
www.kindredlamirada.com

Robin Rapp, Administrator
Adam Darvish, Executive Director
Committed to the delivery of high quality care in a cost-effective manner to enable us to become "a model of excellence" in Long-Term Acute Care. Committed to treat our patients and families with dignity and respect, in the same manner we would want to be treated.

6451 **King's View Work Experience Center- Atwater**
100 Air Park Road
Atwater, CA 95301
209-357-0321
FAX: 209-357-0398
e-mail: kvwec@kingsview.org
www.kingsview.org

Samuel Kalember, Executive Director

The primary mission of the Kings View Work Experience Center (KVWEC) is to serve people who have developmental disabilities. We believe in the dignity and worth of each person and in their right to rehabilitation, education and community integration. It is Kings View's aim to provide quality services to people who need assistance in the development of social, vocational and independent living skills.

6452 LaPalma Intercommunity Hospital

7901 Walker Street
La Palma, CA 90623
714-670-7400
FAX: 714-670-6004
e-mail: debra.culver@wamcoc.com
www.lapalmacommunityhospital.com

Prem Reddy Md, FACC, FCCP, Chairman Of The Board
Sami Shoukair MD, Chief Of Staff
Lapalma Intercommunity Hospital endeavors to provide comprehensive, quality healthcare in a convenient, compassionate and cost effective manner. Lapalma is consistenty at the forefront of evolving national healthcare reform. Our organization provides an innovative and integrated healthcare delivery system. We remain ever cognizant of our patient's needs and desires for high quality affordable healthcare.

6453 Learning Services of Northern California

10855 De Bruin Way
Gilroy, CA 95020
408-848-4379
888-419-9955
www.learningservices.com

Ann Kent, Marketing Manager
Kayree Shreeve, Administrator
Jill Winegardner, Program Director
Located on 10 acres of ranchland in rural Santa Clara Valley, our Gilroy Program offers treatment, structure, and support in a spacious, campus-based living environment. Sharing living residences are complimented by a treatment and recreation facility for individuals who require intensive support.

6454 Learning Services: Morgan Hill

17570 Delmonte Avenue
Suite B
Morgan Hill, CA 95037
408-848-4379
888-419-9955
FAX: 408-848-6509
www.learningservices.com

Jill Winegardner, Program Director
Located in the quaint rural town within walking distance from the old main street of Morgan Hill. Our Morgan Hill program offers the convenience and amenities of small-town living within the supportive community of Morgan Hill.

6455 Learning Services: Supported Living Programs

10855 De Bruin Way
Gilroy, CA 95020
408-848-4379
800-466-4379
FAX: 408-848-6509
www.learningservices.com

Carol Hughes, Admissions Director
Steven P Johnson, Program Director
Kayree Shreeve, Administrator
We offer a variety of diverse and stimulating environments for people with different needs, capabilities and personal goals. Within comfortable, homelike, age-appropriate settings we provide the structure and support necessary to ensure the richest possible quality of life. Program offered in both Northern and Southern facilities of California

6456 Leon S Peters Rehabilitation Center

2823 Fresno Street
Fresno, CA 93715
559-459-3957
800-628-9099
FAX: 559-498-0261
www.communitymedical.org/crmc.htm

Jeff Dimarco RN, Manager
Jenny Lau Rtc Ctrs, Community Liaision Rehab Serv.
Wes Qualls, Finance Executive
Community's flagship hospital that offers world class specialized critical care with the area's only stroke unit with 24-hour vascular neurology and neurosurgery coverage and a team of specially trained stroke nurses. The world's first G4 CyberKnife. The table Mountain Rancheraia Level 1 Trauma Center. The Leon S. Peters burn center. The region's only perinatology program for high rish pregnancies and deliveries. The Da-Vinci robotic surgical system, and 3 helicopeter landing pads.

6457 Lion's Blind Center of Diablo Valley

175 Alvarado Avenue
Pittsburg, CA 94565
925-432-3013
800-750-3937

Phil Sitzman, Director
Peggy Nichols, Executive Director
A private, nonprofit agency offering services such as health, educational, recreational, rehabilitation, employment and counseling to the totally blind, legally blind and visually impaired. The staff includes two full time workers.

6458 Lion's Blind Center of Oakland

3834 Opal Street
Oakland, CA 94609
510-450-1580
FAX: 510-654-3603
e-mail: info@lbcenter.org
www.lbcenter.org

Peggy Nichols, Executive Director
Cathy Manham, Manager
A private nonprofit organization offering services for the totally blind, legally blind, deaf-blind and multihandicapped blind. Services include: professional training, rehabilitation, educational, counseling, social work, self help and more. The staff includes 17 full time and two part time workers.

6459 Living Skills Center for the Visually Impaired

2430 Road 20
B112
San Pablo, CA 94806
510-234-4984
FAX: 510-234-4986
e-mail: patty@livingskillscenter.org
www.livingskillscenter.org

Patricia Williams, Executive Director
A private, nonprofit agency offering services such as independent living skills training, recreational, employment and accessible technology training to the totally blind, legally blind and visually impaired. The staff includes six full time teachers.

6460 Loma Linda University Orthopedic and Rehabilitation Institute

25333 Barton Road
Loma Linda, CA 92354
909-796-0167
FAX: 909-796-4133
www.llu.edu/lluhc/rehabilitation

Todd Nelson, Senior Intake Officer
Offers a full range of clinical programs for both inpatients and outpatient. The specific diagnosis leading to patient admission includes stroke, spinal cord injury, traumatic or anoxic brain damage, amputation, post neurosurgery, chronic neurological disease, Guillain-Barre syndrome, arthritis, multiple trauma or other complex orthopedic problems. The facilities and professional services are comprehensive and ensure that the best care is provided to pediatric and adult patients.

6461 Manor Care Health Services- Citrus Heights

7807 Uplands Way
Citrus Heights, CA 95610
916-967-2929
FAX: 916-965-8439
e-mail: citrusheights@hcr-manorcare.com
www.hcr-manorcare.com

Lisa Schuman, Manager
The nations leader in skilled nursing and rehabilitation care. Our facility has been serving the Sacramento area for more then 12 years. We are known for our beautiful decor, outstanding rehabilitation staff and loving nursing care. We offer short term rehabilitation, long term skilled nursing care, respite care and post hospital surgical care.

6462 Manor Care Health Services- Palm Desert

74-350 Country Club Drive
Palm Desert, CA 92260
760-341-0261
FAX: 760-779-1564
www.hcr-manorcare.com

Debbie Burger, Administrator
Centrally located in the Coachella Valley, specializing in skilled nursing whith an emphasis on rehabilitation, post surgery recovery, hospice, alzheimer's care and long term care. In addition, we offer 2 unique service options for the discriminating consumer. Our Arcadia unit offers a specialized Alzheimer's care program in a dedicated secure wing. ManorCare offers rehabilitation services including physical, occupational and speech therapies for those recovering from illness injury or surgery.

6463 Manor Care Health Services-Fountain Valley

11680 Warner Avenue
Fountain Valley, CA 92708
714-241-9800
FAX: 714-966-1654
e-mail: fountainvelly@hcr-manorcare.com
www.hcr-manorcare.com

Mark Schroepfer, Administrator
Provides 24-hour skilled nursing, rehabilitative therapies and specialized Alzheimer's care. Our in-house therapists provide physical, occupational and speech therapies in our rehabilitation area. Our team is goal oriented and focuses on producing positive outcomes for those recovering from illness, injury or surgery. Our respite care program provides a full range of services for a few days, a week or even a season.

6464 Manor Care Health Services-Hemet

1717 W Stetson Avenue
Hemet, CA 92545
951-925-9171
FAX: 909-925-8186
e-mail: hemet@hcr-manorcare.com
www.hcr-manorcare.com

Ronn Ellenich, Administrator
Provides skilled nursing, Rehabilitation services, and specialized Alzheimer's care. In addition we offer short term respite stays for family caregivers that simply need a break from the stress of daily care. Our Arcadia unit staff is specially trained in the care of residents with Alzheimer's disease. The secured unit is designed to provide a soothing and homelike environment while enhancing each resident's remaining abilities.

6465 Manor Care Health Services-Sunnyvale

1150 Tilton Drive
Sunnyvale, CA 94087
408-735-7200
FAX: 408-736-8619
www.hcr-manorcare.com

John Moreno, Director
Our in-house therapists provide physical, occupational and speech therapies in our rehabilitation area. Our team is goal oriented and focuses on producing positive outcomes for those recovering from illness, injury or surgery. Our skilled nursing staff works with our therapy department and dietary department to provide positive wound care programs for patients requiring skin management care.

6466 Manor Care Health Services-Walnut Creek

1226 Rossmoor Parkway
Walnut Creek, CA 94595
925-975-5000
FAX: 925-947-2149
e-mail: walnutcreek@hcr-manorcare.com
www.hcr-manorcare.com

John Gallick, Executive Director
Provides luxurious long term care and rehabilitation services. In house therapists provide, physical, occupational and speech therapies in our rehabilitation area. Our team is goal oriented and focuses on producing positive outcomes for those recovering from illness, injury or surgery. Our years of combined management experience add value to our resident's quality of life.

6467 Maynord's Chemical Dependency Recovery Centers

PO Box 1657
Tuolumne, CA 95379
209-928-3737
800-228-8208
FAX: 209-928-1152
e-mail: recovery@maynords.com
www.maynords.com

Joan Maynord, Chief Executive Officer
Walter Reed MFT, Clinical Director
Ralph Rutherford MD, Medical Director
Maynord's Recovery Centers has always been dedicated to the recovery of good people whose lives are being destroyed by alcohol and drugs. Since 1978, Maynord's residential program has helped thousands of people put their lives back together after addiction has taken its toll. Today, Maynord's offers a treatment system over much of the San Joaquin Valley and the San Francisco Bay Area.

6468 Maynord's Ranch for Men

PO Box 1657
Tuolumne, CA 95379
209-928-3737
800-228-8208
FAX: 209-928-1152
www.maynords.com

Joan Maynord, Chief Executive Officer
Walter Reed MFT, Clinical Director
Daniel Meador MD, Medical Director
Provides treatment for chemical dependency problems to men. The treatment addresses their recovery through a comprehensive plan created for their individual needs. Also offers a program for women called the Meadows.

6469 Meadowbrook Manor

4600 Woodley Avenue
Encino, CA 91436
818-994-4634

Ayla Zejni, Manager
Postacute rehabilitation program.

6470 Meadowview Manor

19227 South Court
Sonora, CA 95370
209-533-0935

Ron Schoon, Administrator
Bea Schoon, Owner
Provides treatment designed for women that is directed at every important facet of their lives - mentally, physically and spiritually. Clients receive a variety of treatment approaches to facilitate their recovery and a comprehensive treatment plan is created for their individual needs. Issues relating to the cause of addictions are addressed in lectures, one-on-one counseling sessions, group therapy and re entry groups. Also offers a male treatment programs called Maynord's Ranch.

6471 Memorial Hospital of Gardenia

1145 W Redondo Beach Boulevard
Gardena, CA 90247
310-532-4200
800-782-2288

Postacute rehabilitation program.

6472 Mercy Medical Group

Mercy Hospital
406 Sunrise Avenue
Suite 300
Roseville, CA 95661
916-536-2500
FAX: 916-780-5770
www.mymercygroup.org

Margareth Keeling, Director
Lynda Eaton, Client Services Liaison
Located near the Old Rosevill Hospital. There are several primary care physicians, including Family Practice, Internal Medicine and Pediatrics at this location. Specialty services include Diagnostic Imaging, Laboratory and Mental Health Services.

6473 Napa County Mental Health Department
2344 Old Sonoma Road
Bldg D
Napa, CA 94559 707-253-4711
FAX: 707-253-4155

Robin Payne, Manager
Work hardening and disciplinary programs.

6474 Napa Valley Support Systems
650 Imperial Way
Suite 202
Napa, CA 94559 707-253-7490
FAX: 707-253-0115

Beth Atton, Executive Director
Work hardening and disciplinary programs.

6475 North Valley Services
1350 Vista Way
Red Bluff, CA 96080 530-529-2100
FAX: 530-529-4450

Judy Ferrell, Manager
Provides vocational rehabilitation services, such as job counseling, job training, and work experience, to unemployed and underemployed persons, persons with disabilities.

6476 Northridge Hospital Medical Center Rehabiltation Medicine
18300 Roscoe Boulevard
Northridge, CA 91325 818-885-8500
FAX: 818-701-7367
www.northridgehospital.org

Debra Flaherty, Director Rehabilitation Services
A full service, comprehensive rehabilitation program suited to treat patients of all ages who have suffered catastrophic or debilitating injury or illness. The goal of the program is to deliver exceptional patient care to maximise each individual's skills and independence.

6477 Northridge Hospital Medical Center: Center for Rehabilitation Medicine
18300 Roscoe Boulevard
Northridge, CA 91328 818-885-8500
FAX: 818-701-7367
www.northridgehospital.com

Debra Flaherty, Director Rehabilitation Services
Mike Wall, Chief Executive Officer
Committed to serving the health needs of our communities with particular attention to the needs of the poor, the disadvantaged, and vulneralbe, and the comfort of the suffering and dying. Catholic Healthcare West has a commitment to quality-quality healthcare services and the promotion of optimal quality of life for all of life.

6478 Old Adobe Developmental Services
235 Casa Grande Road
Petaluma, CA 94954 707-763-9807
FAX: 707-782-9607
e-mail: webmaster@oadsinc.org

Dennis Orner, Executive Director
Marie Padgett, Controller
Helen Gunderson, Administrative Assistant
The mission of Old Adobe to provide opportunities for individuals with developmental challenges to reach thier fullest potentials. Our job at OADS is to find ways for these individuals to find full expression in all parts of their lives. We have a partnership with the Adult Education Department of the Petaluma School District in providing services to persons with developmental challenges. We are funded by the Dept. of Rehabilitation and the Dept. Of Developmental services.

6479 Old Adobe Developmental Services-Rohnert Park Services (Behavioral)
6920 Commerce Boulevard
Suite 114
Rohnert Park, CA 94928 707-664-8019
FAX: 707-664-8057
e-mail: judy@oadsinc.org
www.oadsinc.org

Dennis Orner, Executive Director
Helen Gunderson, Administrative Assistant
The program services are designed to assist individuals who demonstrate basic work skills, to develop social skills and work habits necessary to succeed in supported or competitive employment. Most often individual program services involve working with the client to replace those behavioral excesses that have been a barrier to vocational placement.

6480 PRIDE Industries
10030 Foothills Boulevard
Roseville, CA 95747 916-788-2100
800-550-6005
FAX: 916-788-2552
e-mail: info@prideindustries.com
www.prideindustries.com

Bob Olsen, Chair
Bob Selvester, Vice Chair
Mike Snegg, Treasurer
To provide opportunities through employment, training, evaluation and placement maximizing community access, independence and quality of life for people with barriers to employment.

6481 Pacific Hospital Of Long Beach-Neuro Care Unit
2776 Pacific Avenue
Long Beach, CA 90806 562-997-2000
FAX: 562-427-0149
e-mail: webmaster@phlb.org
www.phlb.org

Michael D. Drobot, Chief Executive Officer
Tino Bernadett, Chairman Of The Board
Clark Todd, President
Our mission is to heal with compassion and to perform with distinction. Our vision: to improve the hospital's orthopedic and Spine Center of Excellence. Achieve exceptional financial performance to enhance hospital services. Improve the vertically integrated ancillary, outpatient and inpatient surgery system. Develop a professionally challenging work environment that reflects an agile, peak performance culture.

6482 Paradise Vally Hospital-South Bay Rehabilitation Center
2400 E 4th Street
National City, CA 91950 619-470-4321
FAX: 619-470-4126
www.paradisevalleyhospital.org

Fred Harder, President
Jay Flaherty, Executive Director
South Bay Rehabilitation Center, offers a complete range of treatment for patients with physical disabilities. Our specialized inpatient and outpatient programs are designed to meet each person's individual needs or injuries, with the goal of restoring as much independence as possible and significantly improving their lives.

6483 Parents and Friends
350 Cypress Street
Fort Bragg, CA 95437 707-964-4692
800-222-0343
FAX: 707-964-8536
e-mail: moon@parentsandfriends.org
www.parentsandfriends.org

Linda Rosengarten, Executive Director
Teri Scott, Controller
Russ Pals, Vocational Director
Parents and Friends provides opportunities for persons with developmental challenges and similar needs to participate fully in our community.

6484 People Services
4195 Lakeshore Boulevard
Lakeport, CA 95453
707-263-3810
FAX: 707-263-0552
e-mail: peopleservices@mindspring.com
www.peopleservices.org

Dick Lamkin, President
Mike Adams, Vice President
George Lewis, Secretary
Providing an array of services for adults with developmental disabilities and other people with disabilities. Services include supported employment, work services, supported living, personal, social and community training, transportation, specialized individual services and much more.

6485 Petaluma Recycling Center
Old Adobe Developmental Services
315 2nd Street
Petaluma, CA 94952
707-763-4761
FAX: 707-763-4921
e-mail: davide@oadsinc.org
www.oadsinc.org/petarecycle

David Donati, Supervisor
Dennis Orner, Director
Began in 1974; has been one of the major employers of persons with developmental challenges for 26 years; is the primary recycling facility in the growing city of 52,000; accepts over 20 different kinds of recyclables; employs 20-25 persons a day.

6486 Pomerado Rehabilitation Outpatient Service
15615 Pomerado Road
Poway, CA 92064
858-613-4000
FAX: 858-613-4248

Sheila Brown, Director Rehab Services
Jonathan Pee, Manager
A 107-bed acute care hospital. In addition to a round-the-clock Emergency Department, Pomerado offers the area's finest outpaitent surgery center and general medical/surgical services. Pomerado Hospital also is home to a world-class Birth Center and a Level II NICU. Fully JCAHO-accrediidted, Pomerado is well-known for offering only private rooms, each with a scenic view of the North Countryside, which enhances the healing atmosphere.

6487 Pride Industries: Grass Valley
12451 Loma Rica Drive
Grass Valley, CA 95945
530-477-1832
800-550-6005
FAX: 530-477-8038
www.prideindustries.com

Kimberly Jones, Site Manager
Dawn Horwath, Counselor
Craig Hays, Adult Day Program Coordinator
Work adjustment and remunerative work programs. We offer an adult day program as well.

6488 Rancho Adult Day Care Center
Rancho Los Amigos Medical Center
7601 Imperial Highway
Downey, CA 90242
562-401-7111
FAX: 562-401-7991
TTY:562-401-8450
e-mail: radscenter@aol.com
www,rancho.org/ser_adultday

Bryan Kemp, Center Director
Margaret L Campbell, Research Director
Valerie Orange, Chief Executive Officer
Provides personal care, social services and a therapeutic program to older adults in order to improve their quality of life. Offers a Clinical Gerontology Service, an Alzheimer's Disease Diagnostic and Treatment Center and a Geriatric Assessment and Rehabilitation Unit.

6489 Regional Center for Rehabilitation
2288 Auburn Boulevard
Sacramento, CA 95821
916-421-4167
FAX: 916-925-1586

Postacute rehabilitation program.

6490 Rehabilitation Institute of Santa Barbara
2415 De La Vina Street
Santa Barbara, CA 93105
805-687-7444
FAX: 805-683-0381
www.risb.org

Melinda Stavely MS, President/CEO
Scott Silic MBA, Vice President Of Operations
Cheryl Ellis MD, MHA, Vice President Of Medical Srvs.
A regional rehabilitation system with an acute care hospital at the center, the Institute provides specialized inpatient and outpatient programs for brain injury, spinal cord injury, stroke, work-related injury, chronic pain, orthopedic problems and more. Offers a 46-bed acute-care rehabilitation hospital, a free-standing outpatient center, the brain injury continuum, chronic pain program.

6491 Rehabilitation Institute of Southern California
1800 E La Veta Avenue
Orange, CA 92866
714-633-7400
FAX: 714-633-4586
e-mail: rhayes@rio.rehab
www.rio-rehab.com

Priam S. Singh, Executive Director
Carol Reese, Assistant To Executive Director
Gabriela De Leon, Administrative Assistant
Outpatient rehabilitation serving physically and disabled children and adults. Child development programs, adult day care for disabled seniors, child care for disabled and non-disabled children, outpatient therapy, aquatics, adult day healthcare, independent living, vocational services, social services, and housing.

6492 Rubicon Programs
2500 Bissell Avenue
Richmond, CA 94804
510-235-1516
FAX: 510-235-2025
e-mail: rubicon@rubiconpgms.org
www.rubiconprograms.org

Rick Aubry PhD, President
Jane Fischberg MPA, Executive Director
David Samuels MBA CPA, Chief Financial Officer
Rubicon Programs Inc. helps people and communities build assets to achieve greater independence. Since 1973, Rubicon has built and operated affordable housing and provided employment, job training, mental health, and other supportive services to individuals who have disabilities, are homeless, or are otherwise economically disadvantaged.

6493 San Bernardino Valley Lighthouse for the Blind
762 N Sierra Way
San Bernardino, CA 92410
909-884-3121
FAX: 909-884-2964

Robert McBay, Executive Director
Sandra Wood, Administrative Assistant
Provides training in independent living skills - cooking, mobility and orientation, sewing, Braille and typing. Also, we have classes in macrame, ceramics and basket weaving. Weekly support group and Bible study.

6494 Santa Clara Valley Blind Center, Inc.
101 N Bascom Avenue
San Jose, CA 95128
408-295-4016
FAX: 408-295-1398
e-mail: info@visionbeyondsight.org
www.visionbeyondsight.org

Kenneth Frasse, Executive Director
Carolyne Haskin, Program Director
The Santa Clara Valley BlindCenter, Inc. DBA The Lions Blind Center is a social/recreational training facility for any blind or sight impaired person in Santa Clara County over the age of 12. It provides an hospitable atmosphere that utilizes interactive socialization methods and classes to assist the blind and sight-impaired cope with their disability. Staff includes 2 sighted individuals in management positions.

6495 Scripps Memorial Hospital: Pain Center
9888 Genesee Avenue
La Jolla, CA 92037
858-626-4123
FAX: 858-626-7213
www.scrippshealth.org

Corinna Nyquist, Outreach Coordinator
Offers both inpatient and outpatient programs including: physical activity management, individual pain management, group therapy, medication adjustment, pain control classes, occupational therapy, biofeedback training, family counseling, vocational and leisure counseling and recreational therapy.

6496 Sharp Coronado Hospital
250 Prospect Place
Coronado, CA 92118
619-522-3600
FAX: 619-522-3782
www.sharp.com

Marcia Hall, Chief Executive Officer
Providing medical and surgical care, intensive care, sub-acute and long-term care, rehabilitation therapies and emergency services in a peaceful setting is part of our live+heal+grow philosophy. We are one of the county's few community-owned hospitals and are proud of our history of providing convenient , award-winning heath care to Coronado and San Diego.

6497 Shriners Hospitals For Children-Northern California
2425 Stockton Boulevard
Sacramento, CA 95817
916-453-2000
FAX: 916-453-2388
www.shrinershq.org/hospitals

Michelle James MD, Chief Of Staff (Interim) (Ortho)
David G. Greenhalgh MD, Chief Of Staff (Burns)
Craig McDonald MD, Director SCI Unit
The only hospital in the Shriners system that houses facilities for treatment of all 3 Shriner specialties -spinal cord injuries, orthopaedic, and burns. The hospital features 80 patient beds, 9 parent apartments, 5 state-of-the-art operating rooms, a high-tech Motion Analysis lab, and an entire floor devoted to research.

6498 Shriners Hospitals for Children
3160 Geneva Street
Los Angeles, CA 90020
213-388-3151
888-486-5437
888-486-KIDS
FAX: 213-387-7528
e-mail: edever@shrinenet.org
www.shrinershq.org/hospitals/los_angeles

Terence Cunningham FACHE, Administrator
Colin F. Mosley MD, Chief Of Staff
Cecilia Barrios RN, MN, Director Of Patient Care Srvs.
Treats children under the age of 18 with burn scars, orthopedic conditions and limb deficiencies. All medical care is provided completely free of charge for patients and their families. Conditions commonly treated include scoliosis, club feet, leg length discrepancies osteogenesis imperfecta (brittle bone disease), arthrogryposis, orthopedic problems related to cerebral palsy and spina bifida. Also treated are deformities due to burns, scar revision and reconstructive surgery.

6499 Society for the Blind
2750 24th Street
Sacramento, CA 95818
916-452-8271
FAX: 916-452-2622
e-mail: frontdesk@societyfortheblind.org
www.societyfortheblind.org

Alan Frank, Assistant Director of Programs
A private, local nonprofit organization providing blind and visually impaired people with the training supplies and support they need to live independent, productive and fulfilled lives with limited vision. Services include the Low Vision Clinic, Braille classes, computer training, support groups, living skills instruction, mobility training and the Products for Independence Store.

6500 Solutions at Santa Barbara: Transitional Living Center
1135 N Patterson Avenue
Santa Barbara, CA 93111
805-683-1995
FAX: 805-683-4793
e-mail: soludirector@aol.com
www.solutionsatsantabarbara.com

Susan Hannigan, Executive Director
Brandi Fresh, Case Manager
Postacute rehabilitation program. Short-term transitional living program for individuals with traumatic brain injury, stroke, aneurysm and other neurological disorders.

6501 St. John's Pleasant Valley Hospital Neuro Care Unit
2309 Antonio Avenue
Camarillo, CA 93010
805-389-5800
FAX: 805-389-5968
www.chwcareers.org

Rosa Vasquez, Director
Maureen Malone, Administrator
Jerry Conway, President
Houses 82 acute-care beds, a 99-bed extended care unit, and the only hyperbaric medicine unit in Ventura County. Employ's 1,800 people and count 250 active medical staff.

6502 St. John's Regional Medica Center- Industrial Therapy Center
1600 North Rose Ave
Oxnard, CA 93030
805-988-2500
FAX: 805-986-3535
www.stjohnshealth.org

Mark Whitman PT, Manager
A non-profit health care facility offering multi-disciplinary programs for pain management and work hardening, as well as physical and occupational therapy.

6503 Sub-Acute Saratoga Hospital
13425 Sousa Lane
Saratoga, CA 95070
408-378-8875
FAX: 408-378-7419
e-mail: mike@pedisubacute.com
www.subacutesaratoga.com

Michael Zarcone, Pharm, D., MS, President/Ceo
Paul Quintana MD, Medical Director
Milton Wheeler MA, NHA, Administrator
Dedicated to the fulfillment of human needs, desires, and wishes in illness and in health. The cohesiveness of caring in a family community of staff, patients, and their loved ones. The celebration of each unique life through their therapeutic journey, while preserving their individual spirit. The achievement of advanced medical expertise, knowledge, and skill given with the human touch of caring toward the ultimate goal: enhancing the healing process from acute illness to the joy of going home.

6504 Synergos Neurological Center: Hayward
27200 Calaroga Avenue
Hayward, CA 94545
510-264-4000
www.strosehospital.org

Michael Mahoney, President/CEO
Postacute rehabilitation program.

6505 Synergos Neurological Center: Mission Hills
15031 Rinaldi Street
Mission Hills, CA 91345
510-264-4053
www.strosehospital.org
For over 30 years, St. Rose Hospital Rehabilitation Services Department has helped thousands of patients recover from illness and injury through the help of our specially trained therapists. These therapists have been trained in specific rehabilitative areas such as physical, occupational, and speech therapies.

6506 Temple Community Hospital
235 N Hoover Street
Los Angeles, CA 90004
213-382-7252
FAX: 213-389-4559
e-mail: info@templecommunityhospital.com

Herbert Needman, Chief Executive Officer
The mission of Temple Community Hospital is to improve the quality of health in our community and to provide necessary hospital services for those individuals requiring such care.

6507 The ARC Of San Diego-ARROW Center
3035 G Street
San Diego, CA 92102
619-233-8855
FAX: 619-233-4932
www.arc-sd.com

Dorothy Cummings
Melanie McCoy, Area Director
The ARC of San Diego will be the premier provider of services to persons with disabilities. Arc-SD will be an advocate for diversity of opportunities, enhancing individual life choices as a member of the communuity. Our values: Everyone will be be treated equally, without prejudice and with respect. Will provide Quality Services and Supports with a well trained and caring staff. State of the art equipment and methods. A willingness to innovate and collaborate.

6508 The ARC Of San Diego-East County Training Center
1374 E. Lexington Avenue
1865
El Cajon, CA 92019
619-444-9417
FAX: 619-449-7853
www.arc-sd.com/locations

Val Swan
Mike Wasyliw, Executive Director
Work adjustment and remunerative work programs.

6509 The ARC Of San Diego-Rex Industries
9575 Aero Drive
San Diego, CA 92123
760-471-0250
800-748-5575
FAX: 858-715-3788

Gary Luce, Operations Manager
Offers many different programs including: North County Parent/Infant Program which is an educational program for children, birth to three years who are showing delays in development or who are at risk for developmental delays. The Adult Development Center is a program for adults, eighteen and over, with a developmental disability in the severe to profound range. The program focuses on self-help, communication, daily living and pre-vocational skills. Other programs are available.

6510 Tunnell Center for Rehab
1359 Pine Street
San Francisco, CA 94109
415-673-8405
FAX: 415-563-2174

Jan Clements, Administrator
The Tunnell Center for Rehabilitation and Healthcare accomodates 178 residents. We are dedicated to short-term complex medical and rehabilitative care. Using a holistic care management approach we work with residents who have suffered debilitating injury or illness, and who need comprehensive nursing and rehabilitation services to achieve their highest practicable level of functional ability and independence.

6511 Ukiah Valley Association for Habilitation
PO Box 689
Ukiah, CA 95482
707-468-8824
FAX: 707-468-9149
e-mail: pam@uvah.org
www.uvah.org

Pamela Jensen, Executive Director
Kris Vipond, Business Manager
Crystal Anderson, Rural Adult Program Director
Work adjustment and suppoted employment and social and community services.

6512 Valley Center for the Blind
1060 Fulton Mall
Suite 315
Fresno, CA 93721
559-222-4447
FAX: 559-222-4844
e-mail: info@valleycenterblind.org
www.valleycenterblind.org

Russell Hoeltzer, Executive Director
Millie Marshall, Marriage Family Therapist
Roben Asher, Specialist
A private, nonprofit organization that offers educational, health, recreational and professional training services to the totally blind, legally blind or severely visually impaired. Staff numbers one full- time and four part- time employees.

6513 Villa Esperanza Services
2116 E Villa Street
Pasadena, CA 91107
626-449-2919
FAX: 626-449-2850
www.villaesperanzaservices.org

Dottie Cebula Nelson, Chief Executive Officer
Kelly White, Chief Operation Officer
Serving disabled infants to seniors in a school, adult day program, adult work program and residences and adult day health care program and care management program.

6514 Village Square Nursing Center
1586 W San Marcos Boulevard
San Marcos, CA 92078
760-471-2986
800-735-2922
FAX: 760-471-5176
www.villagesquarerehab.com

Melanie Henderson, Director
Ron Caldwell, Executive Director
Accomodates 118 residents offering spacious private and semi-private rooms. We are Medicare and Medi-Cal certified and contracted with most managed care insurance groups.

6515 Vista Center for the Blind & Visually Impaired
2470 El Camino Real
Suite 107
Palo Alto, CA 94306
650-858-0202
800-660-2009
FAX: 650-858-0214
e-mail: info@vistacenter.org
www.pcbvi.org

Pam Brandin, Executive Director
Sharon Hudson, Director of Rehabilitation Servi
Meg Faville, Administrative Assistant
Private nonprofit agency that serves the visually impaired in the San Mateo, Santa Clara and San Benito counties. Offers rehabilitation services, counseling, social work, self support groups, computer training, employment services, orientation and mobility.

6516 Winways
7732 E Santiago Canyon Road
Orange, CA 92869
714-771-5276
FAX: 714-771-1452
e-mail: winways86@aol.com
www.winwaysrehab.com

Pam Kauss, Executive Director
The program offers our clients the safe, relaxed atmosphere of rural living without sacrificing important access to shopping, business, recreational, and educational facilities. Winways at Orange offers highly personalized, comprehensive programs to meet the needs of individuals with traumatic brain injury, stroke, tumors, aneurysm, post concussive syndrome or other neurological disorders.

Colorado

6517 Capron Rehabilitation Center
Penrose Hospital/ St. Francis Healthcare System
2215 N Cascade Avenue
Colorado Springs, CO 80907
719-776-5000
FAX: 719-776-2534
www.penrosestfrancis.org

James O'Connell, Chief Executive Officer
Southern Colorado's most complete inpatient and outpatient rehabilitation center.

6518 **Cerebral Palsy of Colorado**
2200 S Jasmine Street
Denver, CO 80222
303-691-9339
FAX: 303-691-0846
e-mail: info@cpco.org
www.cpco.org

Judith I Ham, President/CEO
Mark Welle, Chairman of the Board
Provides services for children birth-5 years, employment services for adults, information and referral, donation pickup and cell phone/ink cartridge recycling services.

6519 **Cherry Hills Health Care Center**
Kindred
3575 S Washington Street
Englewood, CO 80110
303-789-2265
FAX: 303-781-8808
www.cherryhillshc.com

Michael Speidel, Executive Director
Judy Holmes, Director
Accomodates 92 residents. We serve Medicare, Medicaid, managed-care and private pay clients. Our 2 story facility has a home-like environment with a dining room and a day room one each floor. Our short-term rehab unit was designed for patients who have been in the hospital and need continued intensive nursing care or rehabilitation before returning home.

6520 **Community Hospital Back and Conditioning Clinic**
1060 Orchard Avenue
Grand Junction, CO 81501
970-243-3400
800-621-0926
FAX: 970-856-6510

Amy Hibberd, Executive Director
David Scherman, Manager
Post-accute rehabilitation program

6521 **Laradon Hall Society for Exceptional Children and Adults**
5100 Lincoln Street
Denver, CO 80216
303-296-2400
866-381-2163
FAX: 303-296-4012
e-mail: tim.hall@laradon.org
www.laradon.org

Timothy C Hall, Executive Director
Annie Green, Deputy Director
Corey Kala, Director/Financial Management
Laradon provides educational, vocational and residential services to children and adults with developmental disabilities and other special needs. Laradon was founded in 1948. It is among the largest and most comprehensive service providers in Colorado.

6522 **Learning Services: Bear Creek**
7201 W Hampden Avenue
Lakewood, CO 80227
303-989-6660
FAX: 303-989-2830
Supported living program for persons with acquired brain injury.

6523 **Manor Care Nursing and Rehabilitation Center: Boulder**
Manor Care Ohio
2800 Palo Parkway
Boulder, CO 80301
303-440-9100
FAX: 303-440-9251
e-mail: boulder@hcr.manorcare.com
www.hcrmanorcare.com

Amy Tarrell, Director
Morrine Wise, Administrator
150 bed center offers a full spectrum of nursing care and rehabilitation. This includes our Arcadia Special Care Unit for Alzheimer's patients. Specialized unit for post acute skilled nursing care. Physical and massage therapies. And a 48 bed upscale Heritage unit offering additional amenities and furnishings.

6524 **Manor Care Nursing: Denver**
290 S Monaco Parkway
Denver, CO 80224
303-355-2525
FAX: 303-355-6960
e-mail: denver@hcr-manorcare.com
www.hcrmanorcare.com

Rob Turner, Administrator
Rose Reinhardt, Admissions Director
Our center has delveloped a reputation for its luxurious environment, comprehensive rehabilitation service and focus on quality care. A wide range of individual and group activities and many gracious amenities create the finest combination of elegance and professional skilled nursing care. Arcadia, our special care unit for persons with Alzheimer's disease and related memory impairments, promotes independence and preserves dignity within a safe and secure environment.

6525 **Martin Luther Homes: Colorado Springs**
3707 Parkmoor Village Drive
Suite 1010
Colorado Springs, CO 80917
719-380-0451
FAX: 719-380-7055

Coleen Abeyta, Administrator
Fred Naumann III, Communications
Providing a wide array of services to assist individuals and families in achieving positive life goals. Services to persons with disabilities and other special needs include community living options, training and employment options, spiritual growth and development options, training and counseling support.

6526 **Mediplex of Colorado**
8451 Pearl Street
Thornton, CO 80229
303-288-3000
FAX: 303-286-1253
e-mail: srockley@northvalleyrehab.com
www.northvalleyrehab.com

Ann Marie Zuccarelli, Marketing Director
Wally Sackett, Chief Executive Officer
Our programs and services help each patient along the road to recovery toward our ultimate aim; the greatest possible restoration of the individual's self-esteem, ability to set goals, and self-sufficiency. Also offer specialized acute inpatient rehabilitative services, including special programs in Trauma Rehabilitation.

6527 **Platte River Industries**
490 Bryant Street
Denver, CO 80204
303-825-0041
FAX: 303-825-0564
e-mail: pri01_lil@attglobal.net

Robert Smith, Executive Director
Postacute rehabilitation facility and program.

6528 **Pueblo Diversified Industries**
2828 Granada Boulevard
Pueblo, CO 81005
719-564-0000
800-466-8393
FAX: 719-564-3407
e-mail: pdihs@qwest.net
www.pdipueblo.net

Karen Lillie, President/CEO
Robin Forbes, Director Human Services
Tom Drolshagen, Director Marketing & Operations
A place where people can turn limitations into opportunities. People can experience the independence, pride and self worth of securing and maintaining a job.

6529 **SHALOM Denver**
2498 W 2nd Avenue
Denver, CO 80223
303-623-0251
FAX: 303-620-9584
e-mail: lperez@jewishfamilyservice.org
www.shalomdenver.com

Linda Perez, Sales
Ginger Guiette, Community Worksite Coordinator
Vicky Brittain, Mailing Services

SHALOM Denver provides employment, training, and job placement opportunities to people with disabilities, resettled immigrants, and people moving from welfare to work.

6530 SPIN Early Childhood Care & Education Cntr

1333 Elm Avenue
Canon City, CO 81212 719-275-0550
www.starpointco.com/spin

Paulette Bolton, Deputy Director
SPIN center is a fully inclusive non-discriminating community early childhood program, offering a variety of schedule choices for families. The philosophy of the SPIN program is to promote each child's growth and development. Special attention is given to cognitive, physical, speech language and social-emotional growth. Staff is specifically trained to facilitate and prepare environments that promote exploration, key experiences, creativity and self-expression.

6531 Schaefer Enterprises

500 26th Street
Greeley, CO 80631 970-353-0662
FAX: 970-353-2779
www.schaeferenterprises.com

Richard Kuhn
Valorie Randall, Executive Director
Schaefer Enterprises, Inc., located in Greely, Colorado, is a vaulable community resource that has been fulfilling the outsourcing needs of businesses in Weld County and outlying areas since 1952.

6532 Spalding Rehab Hospital West Unit

150 Spring Street
Morrison, CO 80465 303-697-4334
FAX: 303-697-0570

Postacute rehabilitation program.

Connecticut

6533 ACES/ACCESS Inclusion Program

60 United Drive
North Haven, CT 06473 203-234-1334
FAX: 203-234-1369
e-mail: conukwugha@aces.k12.ct.us
www.aces.k12.ct.us

Cheryl Saloom, Director
Provides a person centered planning approach for integrated employment, volunteer community based opportunities for adults who have developmental disabilities.

6534 Apria Healthcare

40 Sebethe Drive
Cromwell, CT 06416 860-613-4900
800-277-4288
e-mail: contact_us@apria.com
www.apria.com

Mermisa Shaw, Manager
Provides a broad range of high quality and cost effective specialty infusion therapies and related services to patients in their homes throughout the Northeastern United States. Offer home infusion antibiotic therapy, quality pharmacy services, skilled nursing services and related support services.

6535 Arc Of Meriden-Wallingford, Inc.

224-226 Cook Avenue
Meriden, CT 06451 203-237-9975
FAX: 203-639-0946
e-mail: info@mwsinc.net
www.mwsinc.org

Pamela Fields, Executive Director
Barry Sheftel, Board President
Robert Fitzgerald, Financial Director
A membership agency that provides comprehensive, full-service, community-based opportunities for people with disabilities. Guided by over 120 community members and an active Board of Directors, the Arc always has its focus on improving the lives of people with disabilities. The Arc of Meriden-Wallingford offers advocacy and assistance to our members along with advocating for the rights and choices of people with disabilities in our community.

6536 Arc of the Farmington Valley

PO Box 1099
Canton, CT 06019 860-693-6662
FAX: 860-693-8662
e-mail: favarh@favarh.org
www.favarh.org

John Woods, Director Clinical Services
Stephen Morris, Executive Director
Serving over 300 mentally retarded adults through a comprehensive program of residential and support services. These include three group homes, three apartments, competitive and supported employment options, a day program for mentally retarded seniors, community experience day services for severe and profoundly disabled adults, recreation and leisure services, advocacy, transportation, case management, in-home respite and other support services.

6537 Connecticut Subacute Corporation

19 Tuttle Place
Middletown, CT 06457 860-347-6300
FAX: 860-347-2446
www.cpl-usa.com

Evan K Lyle, Managed Care Director
Cheri Kauset, Corporate Rep.
Specializes in subacute medical and rehabilitation programming. The strength of our system is in its' ability to service a broad range of clinical and psychosocial needs which enable each individual to attain his/her optimal potential. Programming includes neurological and orthopedic rehabilitation, post-surgical and wound care management, intravenous therapy, pulmonary rehabilitation including ventilator services, and long term care.

6538 Datahr Rehabilitation Institute

4 Berkshire Boulevard
Bethel, CT 06801 203-775-2418
888-8DA-TAHR
FAX: 203-740-7129
www.datahr.org

Thomas Fanning, President
Providers of comprehensive rehabilitation services with a history of nearly 5 decades of service. This institute is recognized as a leading resource in meeting the needs of those disabled by illness, injury or developmental disorders in Connecticut and New York. A team of rehabilitation and health care professionals offering career development, residential services, supported employment, volunteer services, occupational therapy, day activities and more.

6539 Eastern Blind Rehabilitation Center

950 Campbell Avenue
West Haven, CT 06516 203-937-4850
FAX: 203-937-3806
www1.va.gov/blindrehab

Penny Schuckers, Chief of EBRC
Pamela Redmond, Executive Director Public Affair
James R. Nicholson, Secretary Of Veterans Affiars
Provides residential rehabilitation services to eligible legally blind veterans in the Northeast and Middle Atlantic portions of the country. Referral applications by Veterans Administration Medical Centers and Outpatient Clinics in the geographical area served by the Blind Rehabilitation Center.

6540 FAVRAH Senior Adult Enrichment Program

23 W Avon Road
Avon, CT 06001 860-674-8839
FAX: 860-676-0275

Nancy Ralston, Manager
Provides remunerative work. Post acute rehabilitation programs and facility

6541 Gaylord Hospital
Gaylord Farm Road
Po Box 400
Wallingford, CT 06492
203-284-2800
866-429-5673
FAX: 203-284-2700
e-mail: lcrispino@gaylord.org
www.gaylord.org

James Cullen, President
Works to restore ability and build courage. Offers rehabilitation care with one goal in mind: to help patients return to their homes, communities and jobs.

6542 Hockanum Greenhouse
Hockanum Industry
290 Middle Turnpike (Rte. 44)
Mansfield Depot, CT 06251
860-429-6697
www.hockanumindustries.org

John Cebelius, President
Beth Chaty, Director
Betsy Treiber, Director
A non profit agency that strives to provide gainful employment, training, support and retirement services for developmentally disabled individuals through the dignity of work, community interaction and structured activities.

6543 Kuhn Employment Oppurtunities
1630 N Colony Road
Po Box 941
Meriden, CT 06450
203-235-2583
860-347-5843
FAX: 203-235-0827
e-mail: info@kuhngroup.org
www.kuhnemployment.com

Robert L Stephens, Executive Director/Owner
Kuhn is committed to developing quality skill enhancement programs which provide meaningful employment for persons with disabilities so that they will become independentm gain self-esteem, and be accepted by the community. Our vision is that all individuals have the ability to fully participate in the community through work. Kuhn believes that all participants have a right to integrated community employment.

6544 Norwalk Hospital Section Of Physical Medicine And Rehabilitation
Maple Street
Norwalk, CT 06856
203-852-2000
FAX: 203-852-3597
e-mail: beth.waldman@norwalkhealth.org
www.norwalkhosp.org

Dr. Claudio Petrillo, Director
A 25 bed inpatient Rehabilitation Unit. This CARF and JCAHO accrediidted rehab unit is located on the 8th floor of Norwalk Hospital. The focus of the rehab unit is to restore lost function and assist patients in returning to the community. Who have recently experienced a life changing medical event. The progam is tailored to meet individual therapy needs and address activities of daily living. Family and caregiver participation in the program is welcomed and encouraged.

6545 Rehabilitation Associates
1931 Black Rock Turnpike
Fairfield, CT 06825
203-384-8681
FAX: 203-384-0722
e-mail: info@rehabassoc.com
www.rehabassociatesinc.com

Carol Landsman, Director/Owner
Myra Watnick, Director
A comprehensive outpatient rehabilitation facility offering physical therapy, occupational therapy, speech-language pathology, clinical social work services and nutritional services to all age groups. Facility locations in Fairfield, Stratford, Milford, Shelton and Westport. All facilities are CARF accredited.

6546 Reliance House
40 Broadway
Norwich, CT 06360
860-887-6536
FAX: 860-885-1970
www.reliancehouse.org

David Burnett, Chief Executive Officer
Carrie Dyer, Chief Operating Officer
Susan Shear, Chief Financial Officer
A residential vocational and recreational support network. An active and productive clubhouse where people with mental illness can gain skills, strength and self-esteem.

6547 Yale New Haven Health System-Bridgeport Hospital
267 Grant Street
Bridgeport, CT 06610
203-384-3000
FAX: 203-336-5465
www.yalenewhavenhealth.org

Sally Gammon, President
Medical services are provided by physicians who are specialists in physical medicine and rehabilitation. The physical therapy department provides a variety of services and utilizes sophisticated modalities to restore and reinforce physical abilities.

Delaware

6548 Alfred I DuPont Hospital for Children
Division of Rehabilitation
1600 Rockland Road
Po Box 269
Wilmington, DE 19899
302-651-4000
888-533-3543
FAX: 302-651-4055
e-mail: infodupont@nemours.org
www.nemours.org

Thomas Ferry, VP Hospital Operations/CEO
The hospital is a division of Nemours, which operates one of the nations largest subspecialty group practices devoted to pediatric patient care, teaching, and research. A 180-bed hospital that offers all the specialties of pediatric medicine, surgery, and dentistry in a spacious, comfortable, and family focused facility.

6549 Community Systems Inc.
E.H. Pencadar Corporate Center
250 Corporate Boulevard Suite A
Newark, DE 19702
302-368-2621
FAX: 302-456-5733
e-mail: info@csi-del.org
www.communitysystems.org

George Baer, Executive Director
A 4 state family of non-profit, tax exempt corporations whose mission is helping persons with disabilities to find happiness in their own homes, in their personal relationships, and as contributing members of their community.

6550 DDDS/Georgetown Center
5 Academy Street
Georgetown, DE 19947
302-856-5366
FAX: 302-856-5360
www.dhhs.delaware.gov/dhhs/main

Joyce Oliver, Supervisor
Linda Ragin, Manager
Mission is to improve the quality of life for Delaware's citizens by promoting health and well-being, fostering self-sufficiency, and protecting vulnerable operations. The vision statement is that together we provide quality services as we create a better future for the people of Delaware.

6551 Delaware Association for the Blind
800 N West Street
Wilmington, DE 19801
302-655-2111
888-777-3925
888-777-3925
FAX: 302-655-1442
e-mail: contact@dabdel.org
www.dabdel.org

Linda Lauria, Executive Director
A private, nonprofit organization that offers adjustment to blindness counseling, recreation activities, summer camps and financial assistance for the legally blind. The staff includes five full time, nine part time and twelve seasonal. Operates a store selling items for the blind.

6552 Delaware Veterans Center
1601 Kirkwood Highway
Wilmington, DE 19805
302-994-2511
800-461-8262
FAX: 302-633-5591
www1.va.gov/directory/guide
A 60-bed hospital and 60-bed NHCU, both accredited by the Joint Commission on Accreditation of Healthcare Organizations with a VBA Regional Office and 2 Vet Centers (one on campus) offering veterans the unique opportunity to obtain heathcare, benefits services, and Readjustment Counseling at one location. The center provides a wide spectrum of primary and tertiary acute and extended care inpatient and outpatient activities an an academic setting.

6553 Easter Seals Delaware & Maryland's Eastern Shore
61 Corporate Circle
New Castle, DE 19720
302-324-4444
800-677-3800
FAX: 302-324-4441

Bill Adami, Executive Director
Sandy Tuttle, President
Provides exceptional services to ensure that all people with disabilities or special needs and their families have equal opportunities to live, learn, work and play in their communities.

6554 Edgemoor Day Program
500 Duncan Road
Wilmington, DE 19809
302-762-1391
FAX: 302-762-1652
e-mail: eec@dca.net
www.eec-de.org

Shawn Stevens, Executive Director
Ann Kitchen, Assistant Executive Director
Our mission is providing affordable and accessible services which help improve the quality of life for community members of all ages through a broad range of educational, recreational, self-enrichment, and family support services. ECC is a not-for-profit, community-based, multi-service agency located just north of Wilmington. We provide a broad range of educational, recreational, self-enrichment, and family support services.

6555 Elwyn Delaware
321 E 11th Street
Wilmington, DE 19801
302-658-8860
FAX: 302-654-5815
e-mail: info@elwyn.org
www.elwyn.org

Carol Chapin, Executive Director
A non-profit human services organization recognized nationally and internationally as experts in the education and care of individuals with special challenges and disadvantages. Today Elwyn is a leading provider of services for people with special needs of all ages.

6556 First State Senior Center
291 A Rehoboth Boulevard
Milford, DE 19963
302-422-1510
FAX: 302-422-1354
www.dhss.delaware.gov

Marcella Wilson, Supervisor
Improves the quality of life for Delaware's citizens by promoting health and well-being, fostering self-sufficiency, and protecting vulnerable populations.

6557 Woodside Day Program
941 Walnut Shade Road
Dover, DE 19901
302-739-4494
FAX: 302-697-4490

Connie Grace, Supervisor
Joyce Oliver, Manager

District of Columbia

6558 Barbara Chambers Children's Center
1470 Irving Street NW
Washington, DC 20010
202-387-6755
FAX: 202-319-9066
www.barbarachambers.org

Francisca Torres
Reina Argueta, Administrator
Mission is to provide comprehensive, quality child care services to the community at large, by offering a variety of opportunities for childrens's intellectual, emotional, social and physical development in a clean, safe, and nurturing environment. Our philosophy is to provide a supportive environment in which children can be children..allowing each child to learn at his/her pace and most of all allowing the child to learn through his/her daily play.

6559 District of Columbia General Hospital Physical Medicine & Rehab Services
19th and Mass Avenue
Room 1358
Washington, DC 20003
202-529-6211
FAX: 202-675-7819

Dr. Maribel Bieberach, Chairperson PM&R
Dr. Raman Kapur, Staff Physiatrist
Offers comprehensive physical medicine and rehabilitation services including in and outpatient consultations and electrodiagnostic testing; in and outpatient physical and occupational therapy; inpatient recreational therapy, and a multidisciplinary prosthetic clinic which meets once a month.

6560 George Washington University Medical Center
George Washington University Medical Center
2150 Pennsylvania Avenue NW
Washington, DC 20037
202-715-4000
888-449-4677
FAX: 202-741-2427
www.gwdocs.com

Steven Badger, Director
Offers an Ambulatory Physical Therapy/Sports Medicine Center, a Medical Center Prosthetics/Orthotics Clinic and a Speech and Hearing Center to persons in the District of Columbia, Virginia and Maryland.

6561 HSC Pediatric Center, The
1731 Bunker Hill Road NE
Washington, DC 20017
202-832-4400
800-226-4444
FAX: 202-635-5780
e-mail: nburch@hospsc.org
www.hfscsite.org

Deborah T Zients, COO
Dr Murry M Pollack, VP, Medical Affairs
Provides the highest quality rehabilitative and transitional care for infants, children, adolescents, and young adults with special health care needs and their families in a supportive environment that respects their needs, strengths, vslues and priorities.

6562 Howard University Child Development Center
1911 5th Street NW
Washington, DC 20001
202-865-4620
FAX: 202-865-1483
Offers children with developmental problems diagnosis, treatment, evaluation and follow along visits.

6563 Psychiatric Institute of Washington
4228 Wisconsin Avenue NW
Washington, DC 20016
202-885-5600
800-369-2273
FAX: 202-966-7374
www.psychinstitute.com

Howard Hoffman, Director
Carol Desjuns, Chief Operations Officer
Psychiatric intensive care, crisis intervention, adult day treatment, drug treatment and other services to children and adults who have psychiatric and chemical dependency problems.

6564 Spina Bifida Program of DC Children's Hospital
Department of Physical Medicine and Rehabilitation
111 Michigan Avenue NW
Washington, DC 20010
202-884-5005
800-787-0021
FAX: 202-884-3422
e-mail: tbear@cnmc.org
www.cnmc.org

Sarah Evans, Director
Leslie Phillips, Nurse Practitoner
Offers neurosurgery, orthopedics,physical medicine, social work, urology and nursing. Mission is to improve health outcomes for children regionally, nationally, and internationally. Be a leader in creating innovative solutions to pediatric healthcare problems. Excel in Care, Advocacy, Research, and Education to meet the unique needs of children, adolescents and their families.

Florida

6565 Bayfront Rehabilitation Center
Bayfront Medical Center
701 6th Street S
St Petersburg, FL 33701
727-893-6108
FAX: 727-893-6779
www.bayfront.org

JoAnn W Gardner MA RPT, Director Rehab Services
Daniel Stone, MD
Bayfront Medical Center has an Inpatient Rehabilitation Hospital and two outpatient rehabilitation clinics that each provide progressive, comprehensive, individualized treatment. Specialized care in Physiatry (physical medicine), rehab nursing, occupational therapy, speech language pathology, recreational therapy, patient/family services and psychology is tailored to each patient from admission to community and/or school reintegration.

6566 Brain Injury Rehabilitation Center Dr. P. Phillips Hospital
Brain Injury Rehabilitation Center Dr. P. Phillips
9400 Turkey Lake Road
Orlando, FL 32819
407-351-8580
www.drpphillipshospital.org

Shannon Elswick, President
Dedicated to restoring brain injured patients with rehabilitation potential to their highest level of functioning. This is accomplished through an interdisciplinary team demonstrating personal responsibility to the patient, their family and each other.

6567 Brooks Memorial Hospital Rehabilitation Center
3599 University Boulevard S
Jacksonville, FL 32216
904-858-7600
FAX: 904-858-7619
www.brooksrehab.org

Charles Schauer, President
Douglas Baer, Chief Executive Officer
An entire care facility featuring five day inpatient evaluation, pre-operative evaluation programs, five week pain management program, referral criteria and treatment goals, therapy services, psychological services and more to the physically challenged.

6568 Center for Pain Control and Rehabilitation
2780 Cleveland Avenue
Suite 607
Fort Myers, FL 33901
239-337-4332

Dr. Harris Bonnette, Medical Director

6569 Comprehensive Rehabilitation Center at Lee Memorial Hospital
2776 Cleveland Avenue
Fort Myers, FL 33901
239-334-5200
www.leememorial.org

Jim Nathan, President
Palma Fuson, Director
Lee Memorial hospital has achieved national recognition as one of the top 100 hospitals for stroke, orthopedics, and Intensive Care Unit (ICU) It is a 367 bed hospital that provides 24-hour emergency and trauma care, inpatient rehabilitation, orthopedics, neuroscience, trauma, cancer, diabetes, digestive, general surgery, urology, endocrinology, gastroenterology, opthamology, and many others.

6570 Comprehensive Rehabilitation Center of Naples Community Hospital
350 Seventh St. North
Naples, FL 34102
239-436-5000
FAX: 239-436-5250
www.nchmd.org

William Crone, President
Heather Baker, Administrative Director
Ken Schields, Marketing Coordinator
Offers rehabilitation services, inpatient and outpatient care at 5 locations in the county and more for the benefit of the disabled.

6571 Conklin Center for the Blind
405 White Street
Daytona Beach, FL 32114
386-258-3441
FAX: 386-258-1155
e-mail: info@conklincenter.org
www.conklincenter.org

Robert Kelly, Executive Director
Offers services for the totally blind, legally blind, visually impaired, mentally retarded blind and more with health, counseling, educational, recreational, rehabilitation, through computer training and professional training services. Serves people who are blind and who are challenged by one or more additional disabling conditions. Functional skills training and employment services, including supported employment.

6572 Davis Center for Rehabilitation Baptist Hospital of Miami
8900 North Kendall Drive
Miami, FL 33176
786-596-1960
FAX: 305-270-3640
www.baptisthealth.net/bhs

Elizabeth Matalon, Administrative Director
Bradley Aiken, MD
A full-service, nonprofit community hospital providing a full range of inpatient and outpatient rehabilitation services. The overall commitment to excellence has extended to this specialized field. Access to medical expertise and services ensures that the best in medical resources are available should an unforeseen medical problem arise.

6573 Division of Blind Services
1320 Executive Center Drive
Room 201
Tallahassee, FL 32399
850-245-0370
800-672-7038
FAX: 850-245-0386
e-mail: ana.saint-ford@dbs.fldoe.org
dbs.myflorida.com

Randy Touchton, Director
Craig Kiser, Manager
Serves the totally blind, legally blind, visually impaired, deaf-blind, learning disabled, mentally retarded and other multiply handicapped by offering health, counseling, educational, recreational and computer training services.

6574 Easter Seal Society of Dade County
1475 NW 14th Avenue
Miami, FL 33125
305-325-0470
888-325-0470
FAX: 305-325-0578
e-mail: info@miami.easterseals.com
www.southfloridaeasterseals.com

Joan L Bornstein PhD, Acting President
Hosie Howe, Social Worker
Ronnie Waldman, Principal
Provides services to children and adults with or without disabilities and other special needs. Through our services, we also give support to their families.

6575 Easter Seals Broward County
12701 W. Sunrise Blvd.
Plantation, FL 33323
954-792-8772
FAX: 954-792-8275
e-mail: info@esbc-fl.easterseals.com
www.broward.easterseals.com

Cathy Susskind, Clinic Director
Becky Dausman, Chief Executive Officer
ESBC provides direct services to children and adults with physical, neurological and communications disabilities and their families.

6576 Easter Seals Southwest Flordia
350 Braden Avenue
Sarasota, FL 34243
941-355-7637
800-807-7899
FAX: 941-351-4997
e-mail: info@easterseal.org
swfl.easterseals.org

Mary Hitchcock, President/CEO
Mary Ann Zyla Smith, Director Adult Services
Amy Spears, Director Health/Children Srvcs
Easter Seals Sothwest Florida creates solutions that change lives for children, adults and their families through high quality therapeutic, educational and supportive services.

6577 Easter Seals: Volusia and Flagler Counties , FL
Easter Seals National
1219 Dunn Avenue
Daytona Beach, FL 32114
386-255-4568
877-255-4568
FAX: 386-258-7677
e-mail: info@eseals-vf.org
www.easterseals-volusiaflagler.org

Lynn Sinnot, President
Jane Bronkie, Operations Manager
Provides early intervention services: inclusive pre-school, aquatherapy and sensory processing therapy, OT, PT, ST and parenting programs, audiology services, equipment loan program, assistive technology information and referral. Residential summer camp and respite.

6578 Florida CORF
Columbia Medical Center: Peninsula
264 S Atlantic Avenue
Ormond Beach, FL 32176
386-676-4222
www.memorial-health.com

John Feore, Executive VP
Sandra Trovato, Executive Director
Offers Medicare authorized therapy programs for seniors, disabled and others who need rehabilitation. CORF can provide coordinated and extended services in the home after a hospital stay, or when physical status changes. Patients who are treated at CORF, include amputations, arthritis, chronic/acute pain, depression/anxiety, nerve injury, sports injury, stroke and swallowing problems.

6579 Florida Community College at Jacksonville/ Services for Students with Disabilities
501 W State Street
Jacksonville, FL 32202
904-646-2300
FAX: 904-633-8110
e-mail: info@fccj.edu
www.fccj.org

Cecilia Sumner, Director
Edith Abdullah, President
Florida Community College provides educational support services through the Auxiliary Aids Program within the Office of Services for Students With Disabilities.

6580 Florida Institute Of Rehabilitation Education (FIRE)
1286 Cedar Center Drive
Tallahassee, FL 32301
850-942-3658
888-827-6033
FAX: 850-942-4518
e-mail: fireinformation@earthlink.net
www.firesight.org

Barbara Ross, Executive Director
Provides independent living and vocational rehabilitation services to Florida residents who are legally blind. Services include instruction in orientation and mobility, accessible technology, daily living skills and employability skills. Information, referral and counseling services are also offered. All services are provided without charge.

6581 Florida Institute for Neurologic Rehabilitation, Inc
PO Box 1348
Wauchula, FL 33873
863-773-2857
800-697-5390
FAX: 863-773-0867
e-mail: info@finr.net
www.finr.net

Stephen C Freeley, Director Marketing
Joseph Brennick, President
A residential rehabilitation facility providing a therapeutic environment in which children, adolescents and adults who have survived head-injury can develop the independence and skills necessary to re-enter the community.

6582 Fort Lauderdale Vet Center
713 NE 3rd Avenue
Fort Lauderdale, FL 33304
954-356-7926
FAX: 954-356-7609

Robert White, Executive Director
Veterans medical clinic offering disabled veterans medical treatments.

6583 Halifax Hospital Medical Center Eye Clinic Professional Center
306 N Clyde Morris Boulevard
Daytona Beach, FL 32114
386-254-4000
FAX: 386-274-5889
www.halifax.org

James Clower
Ron Rees, Chief Executive Officer
Offers services for the totally blind, legally blind, visually impaired, mentally retarded blind and more with health, counseling, educational, recreational, rehabilitation, computer training and professional training services.

6584 HealthQuest Subacute and Rehabilitation Programs
Regenta Park
7130 Southside Boulevard
Jacksonville, FL 32256
FAX: 904-641-7896
HealthQuest offers four centers within the state of Florida offering exceptional staff, comfortable surroundings and individually designed, closely monitored programs dedicated to enabling patients to achieve their goals. Each location offers a progressive and cost effective alternative to in-hospital subacute and rehabilitative care. Centers are offered in Jacksonville, Winter Park, Sarasota and Sunrise.

6585 HealthSouth Emeral Coast Sports & Rehabilitation Center
1710 Lisenby Avenue
Panama City, FL 32405
850-784-4878
FAX: 850-769-7566

Jim McGonley MPT/ATC, Director Clinical Services
Michelle Miller, Manager

Outpatient sports medicine and rehabilitation center providing physical therapy, occupational therapy, industrial rehab, work hardening/work simulation, worksite and ergonomic analysis, FCE's, work assessment and pre-employment goals of returning the clients back to work, and returning to all recreational, sports and functional activities safely.

6586 HealthSouth Rehabilitation Hospital of Tallahassee
Healthsouth Corporation
1675 Riggins Road
Tallahassee, FL 32308
850-656-4800
888-476-8849
FAX: 850-656-4809
www.healthsouth.com

Lynn Streetman, Administrator
Paige Mitchell, Director Business Development
Donna Crawford, Director Clinical Services
North Florida's sole acute rehabilitation hospital between Jacksonville \, Panama City, and Gainesville. With 250 employees providing a full continuum of care form its 70 bed facility, the hospital is accredited by JCAHO, CARF and state designated and certified by Vocational Rehabilitation for traumatic brain injury, as well as a wide variety of other diagnoses. With the addition of our outpatients, the facility has served the greater community by touching the lives of over 50,000 patients.

6587 HealthSouth Rehabilitation Hospital Of Miami
20601 Old Cutler Road
Miami, FL 33189
305-251-3800
FAX: 305-251-5978
www.healthsouth.com

Les Alt, Administrator
Jackie Arocho, Chief Executive Officer
A comprehensive source of medical rehabilitation services for Pinellas County, Florida area residents, their families and their physicians. Offers the people of Florida all the clinical, technical and professional resources of the nation's leading provider of comprehensive rehabilitation care.

6588 HealthSouth Rehabilitation Hospital of Sarasota
Health South Corporation in Burmingham Alabama
3251 Proctor Road
Sarasota, FL 34231
941-921-8600
800-873-4222
FAX: 941-925-7526
www.healthsouth.com

Margaret Holloway, Chief Executive Officer
Stacey Shepherd, Director Of Clinical Services

6589 HealthSouth Sea Pines Rehabilitation Hospital
Sea Pines Rehabilitation Hospital
101 E Florida Avenue
Melbourne, FL 32901
321-984-4600
FAX: 321-952-6532

Mark Tellier, Administrator
Denise Grath, Chief Executive Officer

6590 Holy Cross Hospital
Catholic Southwest
4725 N Federal Highway
Fort Lauderdale, FL 33308
954-771-8000
FAX: 954-351-5994
www.holy-cross.com

John C Johnson, President/CEO
Holy Cross Hospital in Fort Lauderdale is a full-service, non-profit Catholic hospital, sponsored by the Sisters of Mercy. Holy Cross is a US News & World Report "Best Hospital" and HealthGrades Distinguished Hospital for Clinical Excellence, 2004 and 2005

6591 Lee Memorial Hospital
2776 Cleveland Ave.
Fort Myers, FL 33901
239-332-1111

Martica Pitt, Director
Catherine Lee, Owner

Offers a complete inpatient program of intensive rehabilitation designed to restore a patient to a more independent level of functioning. The comprehensive care includes medical rehabilitation and training for spinal cord injury, brain injury, stroke and neurological disorders.

6592 Lighthouse for the Blind of Palm Beach
7810 South Dixie Highway
West Palm Beach, FL 33405
561-586-5600
888-299-8881
FAX: 561-586-5604
1218productions.com/lighthouse

William S Thompson, President/CEO
Sandra L Lamb, VP Administration/HR
Dawn M Clemons, VP Development/Services
A private, non-profit rehabilitation and education agency in its 55th year of service. Offers programs to assist persons who areblind or visually impaired, an on-site Industrial Center, a technology training center, an Aids and appliances Store, special equipment grant programs, outreach services for children and adults, Early Intervention and Preschool Services, and a variety of support groups. These programs provide services and education for blind children and their parents.

6593 Lighthouse for the Visually Impaired and Blind
8610 Galen Wilson Boulevard
Port Richey, FL 34668
727-815-0303
FAX: 727-815-0203
e-mail: dgriffin@lighthouse-pasco.org
www.lighthouse-hernando.org

Don Griffin PhD, Executive Director
Nancy Terkeurst, Director Clinical Services
The Lighthouse offers services for visually impaired or blind adults and children ages 0-5 years old. Counseling, educational services, recreational services, rehabilitation, computer training and support groups.

6594 MacDonald Training Center
5420 W Cypress Street
Tampa, FL 33607
813-870-1300
FAX: 813-872-6010
TTY:813-873-7631
e-mail: jfreyvogel@macdonaldcenter.org
www.macdonaldcenter.org

James Freyvogel, President/CEO
Judith DeStasio, MBA, Director Financial Services
Mara Brad, Director Of Services
A private, non-profit, community-based human services organization serving adults with disabilities (since 1953). Persons are provided the opportunity to achieve their highest potential through the Center's various programs that include day training, employment, community living and various support services.

6595 Medicenter of Tampa
4411 N Habana Avenue
Tampa, FL 33614
813-872-2271

Robert Westhoff, Administrator
Postacute rehabilitation program. A 174 bed non-profit facility with postacute reahbilitation programs.

6596 Miami Heart Institute Adams Building
4701 Meridian Avenue
Miami Beach, FL 33140
305-672-1111
www.msmc.com

Steven D. Sonenreich, President/CEO
Lourdes Donikian, Manager
The mission is to provide high quality health care to our diverse community enhanced through teaching, research, charity care and financial responsibility.

6597 Miami Lighthouse for the Blind
601 SW 8th Avenue
Miami, FL 33130
305-856-2288
FAX: 305-285-6967
e-mail: info@miamilighthouse.com
www.miamilighthouse.com

Carol Brady-simmons, Director of Children's Program
Annely Rose, Rehabilitation Teacher
Virginia Jacko, Executive Director
Offers services for the legally blind and severely visually impaired (including those who are developmentally delayed) of all ages in the areas of counseling and educational, recreational, rehabilitation, computer and vocational training services.

6598 Mount Sinai Medical Center Rehabilitation Unit
4300 Alton Road
Miami Beach, FL 33140
305-673-0646
FAX: 305-674-2606
e-mail: webmaster@msmc.com
www.msmc.com

Anne Vale, President
A comprehensive inpatient and outpatient rehabilitation programs have been helping patients recover for more then 20 years. Fully customized treatment plans based on the needs of each patient is 1 reason why our services are among the best in South Florida. Our team approach takes into account the medical, physical, psychological, social, spiritual, cultural and economic needs of patients and their families.

6599 Neuropsychiatric Pain Rehabilitation Clinic
5330 George Street
New Port Richey, FL 34652
727-849-2005
FAX: 727-849-2087

Charlene Evina, Administrative Assistant
Vickie Penick, Administrator
Donna Taylor, Manager
A multidisciplinary outpatient program for the evaluation and treatment of chronic pain. Consultation services for hospitalized patients are also provided upon request.

6600 North Broward Rehab Unit
North Broward Medical Center
201 E Sample Road
Pompano Beach, FL 33064
954-786-6413
FAX: 954-786-6476
www.browardhealth.org

Wendy Burkholder, Regional Manager
Pauline Grant, Chief Executive Officer
CARF accredited, 30-bed inpatient rehabilitation unit treating adults with brain injuries, spinal cord injuries, stroke, orthopedic and neurologic injuries.

6601 Northwest Medical Center
Health Care Corporation of America
2801 N State Road 7
Margate, FL 33063
954-974-0400
866-442-2362
FAX: 954-978-4183
www.northwestmed.com

Richard S. Kennedy, Chief Executive Officer
Michael Bass, Chief Operation Officer
Above all else, we are committed to the care and improvement of human life. In recognition of this commitment, we strive to deliver high quality, cost effective healthcare in the communities we serve. We recognize and affirm the unique and intrinsic work of each individual. We treat all those we serve with compassion and kindness. We act with absolute honesty, integrity, and fairness in the way we conduct our business and the way we live our lives.

6602 Pain Institute of Tampa
4178 N Armenia Avenue
Tampa, FL 33607
813-875-5913
FAX: 813-872-6215

John E. Barsa MD, P.A., Founder
Laszlo Szollas, MD
Offers a comprehensive and multidisciplinary approach to pain controll and management. Most services are provided on-site but other services may require you to be referred elswhere. We will monitor and coordinate your care in a manner to provide optimal recovery potential.

6603 Pain Treatment Center, Baptist Hospital of Miami
8900 N Kendall Drive
Miami, FL 33176
786-596-1960
FAX: 305-273-2406
e-mail: corporatepr@baptisthealth.net
www.baptisthealth.net

Brian Keeley, President
Since 1960, Baptist Hospital of Miami has been one of the most respected medical centers in South Florida. The hospitals full range of medical and technological services is the natural choice for a growing number of people throughout the world.

6604 Pine Castle
4911 Spring Park Road
Jacksonville, FL 32207
904-733-2650
FAX: 904-733-2681
e-mail: info@pinecastle.org
www.pinecastle.org

Jonathan May, Executive Director
Provides remunerative work, training, community employment and community living options for adults with developmental disabilities.

6605 Polk County Association for Handicapped Citizens
1038 Sunshine Drive E
Lakeland, FL 33801
863-665-3846
FAX: 863-665-2330
e-mail: sbaloghweb@pcahc.org
www.pcahc.org

W.H. Wheeler Jr., Chairman
Anthony J. Senzamici Jr., 1st Vice Chairman
Carol N. Asbill, 2nd Vice Chairman
AÆprivate non-profit organization that provides an adult day training program to people with developmental disabilities and is under the direction of a volunteer board of directors. The primary goal for our services is to provide people with knowledge and practical experience to be independent adults so they can become contributing members of their community.

6606 Quest
380 Semorian Commerce Place
Suite B-204
Apopka, FL 32703
407-889-4530
FAX: 407-889-5710
e-mail: WebAdmin@QuestInc.org
www.questinc.org

Katie Porta, President/CEO
Michelle Bellamy, Executive Director
Cheryl Lyng, Associate Exec Dir/Production
A multi-faceted vocational rehabilitation facility. Programs offered are vocational evaluation and assessment, work adjustment, placement, supported employment, community employment, developmental training, long-term sheltered care and residential services.

6607 Rehabilitation Center for Children and Adults
300 Royal Palm Way
Palm Beach, FL 33480
561-655-7266
FAX: 561-655-3269
e-mail: info@rcca.org
www.rcca.org

Pamela Henderson, Executive Director
Ellen O'Bannon, Manager
A private, nonprofit organization whose purpose is to improve physical function, independence and communication of people with physical disabilities. Any child or adult with a physical or speech disability is eligible for services.

6608 Renaissance Center
PO Box 19249
Jacksonville, FL 32245
904-743-1883
FAX: 904-743-5109

Robert Sommers MD, President
Gregory Sikora, Vice President

6609 **Rosomoff Comprehensive Pain Center, The**
5200 NE
2nd Avenue
Miami, FL 33137 305-532-7246
FAX: 309-534-3974
e-mail: painrelief@rosomoffpaincenter.com
www.rosomoffpaincenter.com

Renee Stelle-Rosomoff, Programs Director
Hubert Rossomoff, Owner
A state-of-the-art Center of Excellence offering inpatient, outpatient, outpatient rehabilitation services and seniors programs. The Center became an internationally renowned model for the evalutation and treatment of all persons seeking pain relief.

6610 **Sarasota Memorial Hospital/Comprehensive Rehabilitation Unit**
1700 S Tamiami Trail
Sarasota, FL 34239 941-917-9000
www.smh.com

Phillip Beauchamp, President
G Finlay, Chief Executive Officer
The goal of the 34-bed Comprehensive Rehabilitation Unit (CRU) is to increase patient functional independence, adjust to illness or disability and successfully return to the community. The unit is dedicated to patients who have experienced conditions such as strokes, neurological disease and disorders of the muscles, bones and joints.

6611 **Strive Physical Therapy Centers**
Po Box 4517
Ocala, FL 34478 352-351-8883
888-823-8940
FAX: 352-732-8890
www.striverehab.com

Richard Shutes, President/Owner
Izivan Levinrad, Clinical Director
Certified as an Outpatient Rehabilitation Agency, providing a comprehensive approach to patient evaluation and treatment. Our objective is to return our patients back to a productive life as quickly as possible and safely as possible.

6612 **Sunbridge Care and Rehabilitation**
5627 9th Street E
Bradenton, FL 34203 941-753-8941
FAX: 941-739-4409
www.sunh.com

Donna Steiermann, Administrator
A comprehensive medical rehabilitation facility that is committed to helping individuals with disabilities improve their quality of life. This is a 120-bed facility offering a full range of acute and sub-acute inpatient programs as well as community-based outpatient programs.

6613 **Tampa Bay Academy**
12012 Boyette Road
Riverview, FL 33569 813-677-6700
800-678-3838
FAX: 813-671-3145
e-mail: info@tampayfcs,com
www.tampabay-academy.com

Ted Hoesle, Director
Kenneth Sladkin, Executive Director
A psychiatric residential treatment center and partial hospitalization program for ages 7 to 17.

6614 **Tampa General Rehabilitation Center**
PO Box 1289
Tampa, FL 33601 813-844-7000
FAX: 813-253-4283
e-mail: jstone@tgh.org
www.tgh.org

Sally Houston, Chief Of Staff
Devanand Mangar, Vice Chief Of Staff
Thomas Bernaskek, Secretary-Treasurer
Offers a full range of programs all aimed at helping patients achieve their full potentials. It is one of three centers in the state that provides Driver Training and Evaluation Programs for persons with disabilities, and also an Assisted Reproduction Program for neurologically impaired males. A Community Re-entry Day Treatment Program is available for individuals who have recovered from a brain injury. A wide variety of inpatient and outpatient programs are available.

6615 **Tampa Lighthouse for the Blind**
1106 W Platt Street
Tampa, FL 33606 813-251-2407
FAX: 813-254-4305
e-mail: tlh@templelighthouse.org
www.tampalighthouse.org

Clifford Olstrom, Executive Director
Offers services for the totally blind, legally blind, visually impaired, mentally retarded blind and more with health, counseling, educational, recreational, rehabilitation, computer training and professional training services.

6616 **Upper Pinellas Association for Retarded Citizens**
1501 N Belcher Road
Suite 249
Clearwater, FL 33765 727-799-3330
FAX: 727-799-4632
e-mail: veronica@uparc.com
www.uparc.com

Karen Crown, Executive Director
Offers services to more than 500 persons with mental retardation and other developmental disabilities. Services include two early intervention pre-schools, physical, speech and occupational therapies, homebound education and family support for children, birth to five years and transitional, vocational, habilitation, employment and placement services for adolescents and adults. UPARC operates 31 group homes, a 22 unit apartment complex, and Supported Living options to provide for residential need

6617 **Visually Impaired Persons of Southwest Florida**
35 W Mariana Avenue
North Fort Myers, FL 33903 239-997-7797
FAX: 239-997-8462
e-mail: mmcgrael@vipcenter.org
www.vipcenter.org

Marylou Tuckwiller, Executive Director
Provides training in independent living skills, orientation and mobility, counseling, computer and other communication skills, family support groups, peer counseling, socialization and a low vision clinic. Second location in Charlotte County. Phone: 941-625-8501.

6618 **West Florida Hospital: The Rehabilitation Institute**
8383 N Davis Highway
Pensacola, FL 32514 850-494-4000
FAX: 850-494-4881
www.westfloridahospital.com

Dennis A Taylor, President/CEO
Carol Saxton, Senior VP Patient Care Services
A 58-bed comprehensive rehabilitation facility offering inpatient and outpatient services. JCAHO and CARF accredited and a State designed head and spinal cord injury center. CARF accredited programs include: comprehensive inpatient rehab, spinal cord injury, brain injury and work hardening.

6619 **West Gables Health Care Center**
2525 SW 75th Avenue
Miami, FL 33155 305-262-6800

Frank Jimenez, Executive Director
Charlotte Raymor, Chief Executive Officer
Services provide by West Gables Health Center: activities services are provided onsite to residents. Clinical laboratory services are provided, dental, dietary, housekeeping, mental health services, nursing services, occupational therapy, pharmacy, physical therapy,speech/language pathology services, x-ray services.

6620 **Willough at Naples**
9001 Tamiami Trail E
Naples, FL 34113
239-775-4500
800-722-0100
FAX: 239-775-0534
www.thewilloughatnaples.com

Milton Branham, Director
James O'Shea, President
A licensed psychiatric hospital in Southwest Florida which provides quality management and treatment for eating disorders and chemical dependency in adults.

Georgia

6621 **Annandale at Suwanee**
3500 Annandale Lane
Suwanee, GA 30024
770-945-8381
FAX: 770-945-8693
e-mail: administration@annandale.org
www.annandale.org

Adam Pomeranz, Executive Director
Melissa Burton, Business Office Manager
Creig Turner, Director Of Admissions
Private nonprofit residential facility for adults with developmental disabilities. Located on 124 acres just north of Atlanta. Annandale provides full program and 24 hour residential services, pay program services, respite care and skilled nursing services.

6622 **Atlanta Institute of Medicine and Rehabilitation**
2915 Piedmont Road NE
Suite E
Atlanta, GA 30305
404-365-0160
FAX: 404-365-0751
e-mail: contact@atlantaimr.com
www.atlantaimr.com

Lawrence Eppelbaum MD, PHD, Founder
One of the most famous medical centers in the state of Georgia. The Institute employs more then 40 highly qualified medical professionals and fully equipped with the latest medical equipment. It has gathered recognition and respect from the people of Atlanta because of its solid work ethics and high principals.

6623 **Bobby Dodd Institute (BDI)**
2120 Marietta Boulevard NW
Atlanta, GA 30318
678-365-0071
FAX: 678-365-0098
e-mail: wmcmillan@bdi-atl.org
www.bobbydodd.org

Wayne McMillan, President/CEO
David Turner, Director Finance
Barbara Massey, VP Operations/Marketing
BDI annually serves approximately 400 clients in Atlanta, GA. BDI works primarily with people with developmental disabilities such as autism, down syndrome or mental retardation, but includes clients with physical or acquired disabilities. Client age varies from teenagers to adults.

6624 **Cave Spring Rehabilitation Center**
Georgia Department of Labor
7 Georgia Avenue
Cave Spring, GA 30124
706-777-1770
FAX: 706-777-2366

Joe Holcombe, Director
David Stevenson, Assistant Director

6625 **Center for Assistive Technology and Environmental Access**
GA Institute of Technology
490 10th Street,
Atlanta, GA 30332
404-894-4960
800-726-9119
FAX: 404-894-9320
e-mail: catea@coa.gatech.edu
www.catea.org

Barbara Christopher, Administrative Coordinator
Elizabeth Bryant, Project Director II
The Center for Assistive Technology and Environmental Access (CATEA) promotes maximum function, activity and access of persons with disabilities through the use of technology. The foci of the Center includes the development, evaluation and utilization of Assistive Technology and the design and development of Accessible Environments.

6626 **Center for the Visually Impaired**
739 W Peachtree Street NW
Atlanta, GA 30308
404-875-9011
FAX: 404-607-0062
e-mail: info@cviatlanta.org
www.cviatlanta.org

Susan B Green, Director Development
La Della Holmes-Raddick, Director Client Services
Subie Green, Manager
Offers services to people of all ages who are blind or visually impaired with training in orientation and mobility, computer technology, activities of daily living, communication skills and employment readiness. Aso offers two children's programs, a community-based rehabilitation program for senior citizens, and a low vision clinic.

6627 **Devereux Georgia Treatment Network**
PO Box 1688
Kennesaw, GA 30156
770-427-0147
800-342-3357
FAX: 770-427-4030
e-mail: cfrost@devereux.org
www.devereuxga.org

Mario Bolivar, Executive Director
Serves ages 10 to 17, males and females with a capacity for up to 187. Serves moderate to severe emotional, behavioral and/or learning disabilities. A specialized psychiatric hospital/intensive residential treatment program for below average to superior intelligence. Community programming that serves ages 3 to 21, males and females, providing wraparound, Therapeutic Foster Care and Independent Living Services.

6628 **Easter Seals East Georgia**
1500 Wrightsboro Road
Po Box 2441
Augusta, GA 30903
706-667-9695
FAX: 706-667-8831
e-mail: sthomas@esega.org
www.ga-ea.easter-seals.org

Sheila H Thomas, President/CEO
Easter Seals East Georgia assists people with disabilities and other special needs to maximize opportunities for employment, independence and full inclusion into society.

6629 **Georgia Industries for the Blind**
PO Box 218
Bainbridge, GA 39818
229-248-2666
FAX: 229-248-2669

James Hughes, Executive Director
Offers services for the totally blind, legally blind, visually impaired, mentally retarded blind and more with health, counseling, educational, recreational, rehabilitation, computer training and professional training services.

6630 **Hillhaven Rehabilitation**
26 Tower Road NE
Marietta, GA 30060
770-422-8913
800-526-5782
FAX: 770-425-2085

Leslie Ann Marie Parrish, Case Manager
Valerie Hamilton, Administrator
Routine skilled and subacute medical and rehabilitation care including physical therapy, occupational therapy, speech pathology and therapeutic recreation. Programs include stroke and head injury rehab; orthopedic rehab; complex IV therapy; woundcare; cancer; total parental nutrition and dialysis.

6631 **In-Home Medical Care**
Care Master Medical Services
240 Odell Road
Griffin, GA 30224
770-227-1264
800-542-8889
FAX: 770-412-0014
e-mail: caremaster@accesunited.com
www.caremastermedical.com

Nancy Frederick, VP
Eddie Grogan, Chief Executive Officer
Offers the devoted attention of a professional nurse, the use of I.V. therapies, pain management and provision of medical equipment and supplies right where the patient wants to be.

6632 **Learning Services: Harris House Program**
3914 Sable Drive
Stone Mountain, GA 30083
770-962-4828
888-419-9955
FAX: 770-995-1253
www.learningservices.com

David Carter, President
Situated in the small, historic district of Stone Mountain, just outside of Atlanta, this 6 bed program is designed to encourage independence while providing appropriate support for each individuals needs. Community-based productive activities are customized to accomodate each resident's needs and preferences, using a wide vatiety of supports and programs in teh metro Atlanta area.

6633 **Pain Control & Rehabilitation Institute of Georgia**
2784 N Decatur Road
Suite 120
Decatur, GA 30033
404-297-1400
FAX: 404-297-1427

Shulim Spektor MD, Chief Executive Officer
Anna Britman, Office Manager
Provides pain management for chronic and acute pain resulted from injuries, diseases of muscles and nerve, Reflex Sympathetic Dystrophy, perform disabilities and impairment ratings.

6634 **Savannah Association for the Blind**
214 Drayton Street
Savannah, GA 31401
912-236-4473
FAX: 912-234-4156
www.sabinc.org

W Chandler Simmons, Executive Director
Offers services for the totally blind, legally blind, visually impaired, mentally retarded blind and more with health, counseling, educational, recreational, rehabilitation, computer training and professional training services.

6635 **Shepherd Center for Treatment of Spinal Injuries**
2020 Peachtree Road NW
Atlanta, GA 30309
404-350-7310
FAX: 404-350-7479
e-mail: webmaster@shepherd.org
www.shepherd.org

James Collins, Administrator
Charles Willingham, Manager
David F. Applejr., M.D., Medical Director Emeritus
Dedicated exclusively to the care of patients with spinal cord injuries and other paralyzing spinal disorders. It serves predominately residents of Georgia and neighboring states as one of the only 14 hospitals designated by the U.S. Department of Education as a Model Spinal Cord Injury System Program.

6636 **Transitional Hospitals Corporation**
7000 Central Parkway NE
Suite 1000
Atlanta, GA 30328
770-821-5328
800-683-6868
FAX: 770-913-0015

Dean Rustin, Owner
A national network of intensive care hospitals providing care for patients who suffer from a chronic illness and/or catastrophic accident. The mission is founded on providing quality health care to patients who require highly skilled nursing care and access to technologically advanced therapies.

6637 **Walton Rehabilitation Health System**
1355 Independence Dr.
Augusta, GA 30901
706-724-7746
866-492-5866
FAX: 706-724-5752
e-mail: postmaster@wrh.org
www.wrh.org

Dennis Skelley, President
Frank Lewis, COO
Mike Harrell, CFO
A 58-bed comprehensive physical rehabilitation hospital offering inpatient and outpatient services. Services offered include: stroke recovery, orthopedic injury, pediatrics, head injury, pain management for chronic pain syndrome, TMJ/Craniofacial pain and chronic headache disorders, spinal cord injury, driving instruction, work re-entry, independent living, assistive technology and ADA consulting.

Hawaii

6638 **Rehabilitation Hospital of the Pacific**
226 N Kuakini Street
Honolulu, HI 96817
808-531-3511
FAX: 808-566-3425
e-mail: hr@rehabhospital.org
www.rehabhospital.org

Stuart Ho, President/CEO
Pauline Osborne, Vice President/CFO
Dr Thomas Au, VP Clinical Affairs/Medical Dir
The only acute care medical rehabilitation organization serving both Hawaii and the Pacific. For over 52 years, the hospital and its 7 outpatient clinics on Oahu, and Maui and Hawaii have been dedicated to providing comprehensive, cost effective rehabilitation. Each year, the organization treats nearly 8,000 patients recovering from strokes, brain injury, spinal cord injury, orthopedic injuries, sports injuries and those individuals requiring general rehabilitation.

Idaho

6639 **Ashton Memorial Nursing Home and Chemical Dependency Center**
700 N 2nd
Ashton, ID 83420
208-652-7461
FAX: 208-652-7252
e-mail: ashmem@frtel.com

Sheila Kellogg, Administrator

6640 **Easter Seals-Goodwill Northern Rocky Mountains**
Easter Seals National
1465 S Vinnell Way
Boise, ID 83709
208-378-9924
800-374-1910
FAX: 208-378-9965
www.easterseals.org

Donna Grummer, Executive Director
Provides services for children and adults with disabilities and other special needs, and support to their families

6641 **Idaho Elks Rehabilitation Hospital**
600 North Robbins Road
Boise, ID 83702
208-489-4444
FAX: 208-489-4005
www.idahoelkrehab.org

Joseph Caroselli, Administrator
A nonprofit hospital serving Idaho and the Pacific Northwest. All inpatient and outpatient programs and services are supervised by the hospital's full-time medical directors whose specialty is psychiatry, the profession of physical rehabilitative medicine. Services include: occupational therapy, rehabilitative nursing, social skills, head injury program, physical therapy, speech pathology, audiology and cardiac rehabilitation.

6642 Portneuf Medical Center Rehabilitation
651 Memorial Drive
Pocatello, ID 83201
208-239-1620
FAX: 208-239-1838
e-mail: charlesa@portmed.org
www.portmed.org

Kelly Hirning, Chairman
Carla Wiggins PhD, Vice-Chairman
Gerald Homstad, Treasurer
Provides compassionate, quality health care services needed by the people of eastern Idaho in collaboration with other providers and community resources.

Illinois

6643 Advocate Christ Hospital and Medical Center
4440 W 95th Street
Oak Lawn, IL 60453
708-684-8000
www.advocatehealth.com/christ

Kenneth Lukhard, Chief Executive Officer
A 665-bed, not-for-profit teaching, research and referral medical center in Oak Lawn, Illinois. It also is home to the Advocate Hope Childrens's Hospital, one of the most comprehensive providers of pediatric care in the state. The medical center is a leader in cardiology, pediatrics, surgical services, oncology, women's services and emergency medicine. Christ Medical Center is part of Advocate Health Care, one of the nation's leading integrated health care systems.

6644 Advocate Christ Medical Center & Advocate Hope Children's Hospital
4440 West 95th Street
Oak Lawn, IL 60453
708-684-8000
800-323-8622
FAX: 708-684-4045
www.advocatehealth.com/christ

Kenneth W Lukhard, President
Darcie Brazel, VP/Chief Nurse Executive
The largest fully integrated not-for-profit health care delivery system in metropolitan Chicago and is recognized as one of the top 10 systems in the country. The mission of Advocate Health Care is to serve the health needs of individuals, families and communities through a wholistic philosophy rooted in our fundamental understanding of human beings as created in the image of god.

6645 Advocate Illinois Masonic Medical Center
836 W Wellington Avenue
Chicago, IL 60657
773-975-1600
www.advocatehealth.com/masonic

Susan Lopez, Chief Executive Officer
Otto Aldana-Centeno, MD
Consultation, education, family counseling, parent training in behavior modification techniques offered to developmentally disabled adults.

6646 Alexian Brothers Medical Center
800 Biesterfield Road
Elk Grove Village, IL 60007
847-437-5500
e-mail: costellc@alexian .net
www.alexian.org

Roger Johnson, President/CEO
Caroline Costello, Director/Communications
A threefold mission: Works toward maximizing physical function, enhance independent social skills and optimize communication skills consistent with an individual's ability. The Center helps those disabled by accident or illness achieve a new personal best.

6647 Back in the Saddle Hippotherapy Program
Corcoran Physical Therapy
4200 W Peterson
Chicago, IL 60646
312-286-2266
847-604-4145
FAX: 847-673-8895
e-mail: info@hippotherapychicago.com

Julie Naughton, Program Coordinator
Maureen Corcoran, Physical Therapist
Tom Corcoran, Owner
A direct medical treatment used by licensed physical therapists who have a strong treatment background in posture and movement, neuromotor function and sensory processing. The benefits of Hippotherapy are available to individuals with just about any disability. Two locations: Glen Grove, IL and Morton Grove, IL. Accepts all insurance.

6648 Barbara Olson Center of Hope
3206 N Central Avenue
Rockford, IL 61101
815-964-9275
FAX: 815-964-9607
e-mail: wdovenport@b-olsoncenterofhope.org
www.b-olsoncenterofhope.org

Carm Herman, Executive Director
Nancy Flanagan, President of the Board
Susan Nagy, Accoutant
We provide vocational employment, educational and social opportunities for adults with developmental disabilities.

6649 Bartolucci Center, The- ILC Enterprises
6415 Stanley Avenue
Berwyn, IL 60402
630-789-0511
FAX: 708-788-0831

Cindy Holbrook, Program Director
A nonprofit tax exempt private social service agency serving suburban Chicago offering day treatment and vocational counseling to individuals who encountered a pattern of job loss due to emotional problems.

6650 Baxter Healthcare Corporation
1 Baxter Parkway
Deerfield, IL 60015
847-948-2000
800-422-9837
FAX: 847-948-3642
www.baxter.com

John D Forsyth, Chairman
Gail D Fosler, Executive VP/Chief Economist
Baxter International Inc. is a global healthcare company that, through its subsidiaries assists healthcare professionals and their patients with treatment of complex medical conditions including hemophelia, immune disorders, kidney disease, cancer, trauma and other conditions. Baxter applies its expertise in medical devices, pharmaceuticals, and biotechnology to make a meaningful difference in patient's lives.

6651 Beacon Therapeutic Diagnostic and Treatment Center
10650 S Longwood Drive
Chicago, IL 60643
773-881-1005
FAX: 773-881-1164
www.beacon-diabetic.org

Susan Yna, Executive Director
Cheryl Thompson, Chief Administrator of Office Af
Offers community day treatment, education, diagnostic services, family counseling, learning disabled, speech and hearing and psychiatric services.

6652 Blind Service Association
17 N. State Street
Suite 1050
Chicago, IL 60602
312-236-0808

Debbie Grossman, Executive Director
Louis Bellande Jr, Partner
Offers services for the totally blind, legally blind and visually impaired with reading and recording low vision network, social services, referrals and support groups.

6653 Brandecker Rehabilitation Center
9455 S Hoyne Avenue
Chicago, IL 60620
773-239-2191
FAX: 773-239-6229
www.eastersealschicago.org

Mary COOney, Program Director
Dolores Nickel, Manager
We offer early intervention services for infants and toddlers with developmental delays and disabilities. Our outpatient Medical Rehabilitation Program offers direct therapy services for children from age birth-16.

6654 Brentwood Subacute Healthcare Center
T HI Brentwood
5400 W 87th Street
Burbank, IL 60459
708-423-1200
800-430-0098
FAX: 708-423-8405
www.thicare.com

Audrey Protrowski, Director Business Development
Jill Sattersield, Administrator
John Walton, Chief Executive Officer
Seeks to help patients and their families through what can be a very emotional decision-making process. We provide guidance and consultation on everything from how to properly choose the facility to providing resources that help you cope with the nature of the decision itself.

6655 Caremark Healthcare Services
2211 Sanders Road
Northbrook, IL 60062
847-634-7600
800-423-1411
FAX: 847-634-7624
e-mail: phu@caremark.com
www.caremark.com

Mac Crawford, President
An 80-service-center network providing services anywhere in the U.S. Offers 24 hour access to nursing and pharmacy services, case management resource centers, HIV/AIDS services, women's health services, transplant care services, nutrition support services, infectious disease management and other therapies and programs.

6656 Centegra Northern Illinois Medical Center
4201 W Medical Center Drive
McHenry, IL 60050
815-344-5000
877-236-8347
FAX: 815-759-8062
www.centegra.org

Kathryn Murauskas, Inpatient Rehabilitation Unit
Nora Connors, Director Rehabilitation Network
Lisa Forino, Marketing Coordinator
Providing rehabilitation services in Lake and McHenry Counties, the Rehabilitation Unit is a complete living environment for up to 15 patients after a debilitating illness of trauma. Various locations offering a multitude of services: PT, OT, speech, HT, RT aquatics, work hardening, FCE's, vocational counseling, rehab nursing, physiatry, neuropsychology, case management. Comprehensive Inpatient Rehabilitation Unit, and many more services.

6657 Center for Comprehensive Services
Mentor Network
306 W Mill Street
Po Box 2825
Carbondale, IL 62901
618-529-3060
800-582-4227
FAX: 618-457-5372
e-mail: sandy.boston@thementornetwork.com
www.thementornetwork.com

Sandra Boston, National Director of Admissions
Robin Ray, President
Post-acute rehabilitation services for adults and adolescents with acquired brain injuries. Residential, day-treatment and out-patient services tailored to individual needs.

6658 Center for Rehabilitation at Rush Presbyterian: Johnston R Bowman Health Center
1653 W. Congress Parkway
Chicago, IL 60612
312-942-5000
FAX: 312-942-3601
e-mail: teri_sommerfeld@rush.edu
www.rush.edu

Teri Sommerfeld, Administrator
A 613-bed hospital serving adults and children, the John R. Bowman Health Center and Rush University is home to one of the first medical colleges in the Midwest and one of the nation's top-ranked nursing colleges, as well as graduate programs in allied health, health systems management, and biomedical research. The Medical Center also offers more then 70 highly selective residency and fellowship programs in medical and surgical specialties and subspecialties.

6659 Center for Spine, Sports & Occupational Rehabilitation

345 E Superior Street
Chicago, IL 60611
312-238-1000
FAX: 312-238-7709
e-mail: webmaster@ric.org
www.rehabchicago.org

Wayne Lerner, Executive Director
Sharon Seitz, Manager
Offers evaluation and treatment of patients with acute and subacute musculoskeletal and sports injuries. RIC offers different levels of care, including inpatient, day rehabilitation, and outpatients services, according to the special needs of each patient. At all levels of treatment, specialists from many disciplines are brought together to help patients progress.

6660 Children's Home and Aid Society of Illinois
125 S Wacker Drive
14th Floor
Chicago, IL 60606
312-424-0200

e-mail: contact@chasi.org
www.chasi.org

Nancy B Ronquillo, President/CEO
Private state-wide. Multi-service, racially integrated staff and client populations. Provides educational, placement and community services for children-at-risk and their families. Advocacy, consultation and follow-up services provided according to our philosophy of continuum of care. No one, child or adult, is denied service because of disabilities, if the program services meet their needs. Higher quality in-service training for staff as well as parenting figures.

6661 Clinton County Rehabilitation Center d/b/a CCRC Community Link
1665 North Fourth Street
Breese, IL 62230
618-526-8800
FAX: 618-526-2021
e-mail: marlah@commlink.org
www.commlink.org

Julie Majezel, Service Coordinator
John Sedivy, Executive Director
Provides Adult Day Programs (developmental training, work training, job readiness and job placements); Residentail Programs (CILA Intermittent Care, CILA 24 hour care); Infant Programs (early interventions, early head start); Community Services (specialized services and family support).

6662 Continucare, A Service of the Rehab Institute of Chicago
West Suburban Hospital Medical Center
3 Erie Court
Oak Park, IL 60302
708-383-6200
800-354-7342
FAX: 312-908-1369
www.westsuburbanmedicalcenter.research.org

Heidi Asbury MD
We respond to the needs of the whole person: body, mind and spirit. We foster a climate of care, hospitality and a spirit of community. We develop systems and structures that attend to the needs of those at risk of discrimination because of age, gender, lifestyle, ethnic background, religious beliefs or socioeconomic status.

6663 Delta Center

1400 Commercial Avenue
Cairo, IL 62914
618-734-2665
800-471-7213
FAX: 618-734-1999
e-mail: delta1@midwest.net
www.deltacenter.org

Frederica Garnett, Executive Director
Lisa Tholbert, Assistant Executive Director
The Delta Center is a non-profit mental health center, substance abuse counseling facility, and also provides various community services to Alexander and Pulaski County, Illinois. The purpose and mission is to promote, encourage, foster and engage exclusively in charitable activities and to provide community-based rehabilitation and treatment services to the physically and mentally impaired citizens.

6664 Division of Rehabilitation-Education Services, University of Illinois

1207 S Oak Street
Champaign, IL 61820
217-333-1970
FAX: 217-333-0248
e-mail: disability@uiuc.edu
www.disability.ui.uc.edu

Brad Hedrick, Director
Patrick Davisson, Manager
Offers services for the totally blind, legally blind, visually impaired, mentally retarded blind and more with health, counseling, educational, recreational, rehabilitation, computer training and professional training services.

6665 Easter Seals

Easter Seals in Chicago
212 Barney Drive
Joliet, IL 60435
815-725-2194
FAX: 815-725-5150
www.easterseals.com

Debra Condotti, President
Services for children and adults with disabilities and their families. Pediatric outpatient medical rehabilitation, inclusive childcare, fostercare, residential homes, clinics.

6666 Easter Seals DuPage Dold Center for Children

830 S Addison Avenue
Villa Park, IL 60181
630-620-4433
FAX: 630-620-1148

Mary D'Arcy, Executive Director
Linda Matheson, Program Services
Maximizes independence for infants, children and adults with disabilities by providing physical, occupational and speech therapy, audiology, social work, early intervention, assistive technology, toy lending, equipment loan and special needs day care.

6667 Easter Seals Gilchrist-Marchman Rehab Center

2345 W N Avenue
Chicago, IL 60647
312-939-5115
FAX: 312-939-0283
http://chicago.easterseals.com

Therese O'Shea, Executive Director
Provides comprehensive services for individuals with disabilities or other special needs and their families to improve quality of life and maximize independence.

6668 Easter Seals Jayne Shover Center

799 South McLean Boulevard
Elgin, IL 60123
847-742-3264
FAX: 847-742-9436
e-mail: il-ja.easter-seals.org
www.il-js.easter-seals.org

Larry M Narum, President/CEO
Susan Dilley, Chief Executive Officer
A free-standing, comprehensive outpatient rehabilitation center serving children and adults with physical and developmental disabilities.

6669 El Valor Corporation

Early Intervention Program
1850 W 21th Street
Chicago, IL 60608
312-666-4511
FAX: 312-666-6677
e-mail: info@elvalor.net
www.elvalor.net

Vincent Allocco, Director
Mission is to challenge people with disabilities. It is a center for people with disabilities and their families and serves Chicago and surrounding areas, providing services in English and Spanish to individuals whose lives would be drastically impoverished without them.

6670 Elgin Rehabilitation Center

1485 Davis Road
Elgin, IL 60123
847-888-5540
FAX: 847-888-6079

Robert Borchert, Vice President
Donna Ramsey, Director
Vocational training services to delvelop work habits and attitudes while providing training in small product assembly, sorting, packaging, collating, & material handling. Instuction also offered in job related knowledge & in personal and survival skills. Counseling to assist each individual in building skills on a step-by-step basis in order to help individuals become as independent as possible.

6671 Family Counseling Center

Washington & Market Street
Golconda, IL 62938
618-683-2461
FAX: 618-683-2066
e-mail: fccgolconda@shawneelink.com
//fccinconline.org

Larry Mizell, Executive Director
Beci Gates, Behavioral Health Division Dir.
Donna Perez, Housing Coordinator
Provides counseling, developmental training, evaluations, assisted living services, referrals, psychosocial rehabilitation, and a variety of work services.

6672 Family Matters

A RC Community Support Systems
2502 S Veterans Drive
Effingham, IL 62401
217-347-0880
866-436-7842
FAX: 217-347-5119
e-mail: deinhorn@arc-css.org
www.fmptic.org

Debbie Einhorn, Director Family Support
Nancy Mader, Office Manager
Parent Training and Information Center and family support programs for families of children who have disabilities from the ages of birth through 21. Services include: Parent support and training, school advocacy, home visits, information and referral, parent-to-parent networking, special education rights workshops and other training sessions on special education topics for parents and school personnel throughout Illinois except in the Chicago area.

6673 Five Star Industries

1308 Wells Street Road
Po Box 60
Du Quoin, IL 62832
618-542-5421
FAX: 618-542-5556
e-mail: fivestarinc@5starind.com
www.5starind.com

Susan Engelhardt, Executive Director
Incorporated as a private, non-profit corporation under the laws of the State of Illinois, is an equal opportunity employer and provides equal opportunity in compliance with the Civil Rights Act of 1964 and all other appropriate laws, rules and regulations referring to civil rights.

6674 HSI Austin Center For Development

1819 S Kedzie Avenue
Chicago, IL 60623
773-854-1676
FAX: 773-854-8300

Provides an educational program designed to enhance academic, behavioral and social performance of children 4-14 years of age experiencing emotional disorders that result in exclusion from the public school setting.

6675 Hyde Park-Woodlawn

950 E 61st Street
Chicago, IL 60637
773-493-3400
FAX: 773-533-5521
e-mail: jvshp@jvschicago.org

William Cinwell, Executive Director

6676 Illinois Center for Autism

548 S Ruby Lane
Fairview Heights, IL 62208
618-398-7500
FAX: 618-394-9869
www.illinoiscenterforautism.org

Susan Szekely, Director
Sandra Rodenberg, Principal
A community-based mental health/educational treatment center dedicated to serving autistic clients.

6677 Julius and Betty Levinson Center

332 Harrison Street
Oak Park, IL 60304
708-383-8887
FAX: 708-383-9025
e-mail: info@ucp.net.org
www.ucp.org

Laurie Wisenski, Manager
Houses one of its three adult developmental training programs for substantially physically disabled men and women.

6678 Lake County Health Department

3012 Grand Avenue
Waukegan, IL 60085
847-377-8170
FAX: 847-336-1517
www.co.lake.il.us

Dale Valance, Administrator
Gale Galass, Manager
Includes counseling, crisis intervention, emergency management, psychotherapy and chemotherapy management for individuals and families.

6679 Little Friends

140 N Wright Street
Naperville, IL 60540
630-355-6533
FAX: 630-355-3176
e-mail: chamilton@lilfriends.com
www.littlefriendsinc.com

Tammy Niemeyer, Public Relations Director
Jack Ryan, President
Nonprofit early intervention and special education programs with focus on children with autism or other developmental, emotional or behavioral disabilities. Vocational and residential services for adults with developmental disabilities.

6680 MAP Training Center

7th and Mc Kinley Street
Karnak, IL 62956
618-634-9401
FAX: 618-634-9090

Larry Earnhart, President
Cindy Earnhart, Community Liaison
Training, employment, residential and support services, targeted for adults with developmental disabilities.

6681 Macon Resources

2121 Hubbard Avenue
Po Box 2760
Decatur, IL 62524
217-875-1910
FAX: 217-875-8899
TTY:217-875-8898
e-mail: jpatterson@maconresources.org
www.maconresources.org

Kay Scrogin, Executive Director
Linda Clary, Administrative Assistant
Tommy Nelson, Deputy Director Clinical Svcs.

The purpose is to provide a comprehensive array of habilitative/rehabilitative training programs and support services to assist individuals and/or family units of an individual with a developmental disability, mental illness, or other handicapping condition to live, attend school or day program, and/or work in the least restrictive, most normalized environment possible.

6682 Mary Bryant Home for the Blind

2960 Stanton Street
Springfield, IL 62703
217-529-1611
FAX: 217-529-6975
e-mail: MBHA@springnet1.com
www.marybryanthome.org

Jerry Curry, Administrator
Leonardo Jacobs, Assistant Director
Bobbi Hickey, Office Manager
Supportive living facility for blind or visually impaired adults over the age of 22. A supportive living facility remodeled to foster the move to increased independence for residents. The new apartment style housing combined with personal care and other activities allows residents to live independently and take part in the decision-making. Personal choice, dignity, privacy, and individuality are emphasized.

6683 Northern Illinois Special Recreation Association (NISRA)

820 E Terra Cotta Avenue
Suite 125
Crystal Lake, IL 60014
815-459-0737
FAX: 815-459-0388
e-mail: info@nisra.org
www.NISRA.org

Randy Reopelle, Director
Cindy McCauley, Director
Brian Shahinian, Executive Director
Leisure and recreation services to those with disabilities who are unable to participate successfully in park district and city recreation programs.

6684 Oak Forest Hospital of Cook County

15900 Cicero Avenue
Oak Forest, IL 60452
708-687-7200
FAX: 708-687-7979
TTY:708-687-4794

Cyntjia T Henderson, Interim Hospital Director
Joe Turner, Public Information
Dan Martin, Chief Executive Officer
A 654 bed health care center devoted to the diagnosis, rehabilitation and long-term care of adults suffering from chronic illnesses, diseases and physical impairments.

6685 Peoria Area Blind People's Center

2905 W Garden Street
Peoria, IL 61605
309-637-3693
FAX: 309-673-3699

Mabel Vandeusen, Executive Director
Offers services for the totally blind, legally blind, visually impaired, mentally retarded blind and more with health, counseling, educational, recreational, rehabilitation, computer training and professional training services.

6686 Peoria Association for Retarded Citizens

1913 West Towline Road
Po Box 3418
Peoria, IL 61612
309-691-3800
FAX: 309-689-3613
e-mail: arcpeoria.org
www.parcway.org

Roy Ricketts, Executive Director
Jeannie McAllister, President
Serves all ages that are diagnosed with mental retardation and other developmental and physical disabilities. Programs include early intervention, family support, respite care, vocational training, supported employment, adult day programs and residential services. Serves 1,000 clients with 400 staff members.

6687 Pioneer Center of McHenry County
4001 Dayton Street
McHenry, IL 60050
815-344-1230
FAX: 815-344-3815
e-mail: private@pioneercenter.org
www.pioneercenter.org

Lorraine Kopczynski, President/CEO
Lenard J Duncan, Chairman of the Board
Dan Haligus, VP Programs
Early intervention, sheltered employment, developmental training, employment services, residential services, mental health services, respite care and Voice: Sexual assault services.

6688 Prosthetics and Orthotics Center in Blue Island
2310 York Street
Blue Island, IL 60406
708-597-2611
800-354-7342
FAX: 800-908-1932
www.rehabchicago.org/about/blue_island.php
Provides orthotic and prosthetic fittings and follow-up services to adults and children in the south suburbs of Chicago.

6689 RB King Counseling Center
2300 N Edward Street
Decatur, IL 62526
217-877-8121
FAX: 217-875-0966

Gordon Cross MD
Offers outpatient, individual, group, divorce and meditation, family and re-adjustment counseling.

6690 REHAB Products and Services
3715 N Vermilion Street
Danville, IL 61832
217-446-1146
FAX: 217-446-1191
e-mail: rehab@soltec.net

Frank Drunacci, President
Larry McConkey, Contact
janitorial, lawn care, distribution services.

6691 RIC Northshore
Rehabilitation Institute of Chicago
345 E Superior Street
Chicago, IL 60611
312-238-1000
800-354-7342
e-mail: webmaster@ric.org
www.rehabchicago.org

Wayne Lerner, President/CEO
Provides rehabilitation for sports-related injuries, musculoskeletal conditions, neurological conditions, stroke, arthritis, amputation, burns, and general deconditioning.

6692 RIC Prosthetics and Orthotics Center
1055 175th Street
Suite 101
Homewood, IL 60430
708-597-2611
FAX: 708-957-8353
e-mail: webmaster@rehabchicago.org
www.rehabchicago.org

Wayne Lerner, Executive Director
Offers almost all the prosthetics and orthotics services provided at RIC's main hospital in downtown Chicago, including consultations, fittings and training.

6693 RIC Windermere House
5548 S Hyde Park Boulevard
Chicago, IL 60615
773-256-5050
800-354-7342
FAX: 773-256-5060
www.rehabchicago.org
Evaluation, therapeutic services and patient education are offered in the areas of arthritis, multiple sclerosis, musculoskeletal conditions, orthopedics, stroke, spinal cord injury, brain injury and sports medicine.

6694 RIC and Swedish Covenant Hospital Rehabilitation Services
5145 N California Avenue
Chicago, IL 60625
773-878-8200
FAX: 773-907-3032
e-mail: ask_us@schosp.org
www.schosp.org

Claudia Moorehead, Executive Director
Ketki Modi, Medical Director
Mark Newton, Chief Executive Officer
Provides acute rehabilitation services, subacute care and outpatient services for many types of disabling injuries and conditions, including amputation, arthritis, brain injury, general deconditioning, multiple sclerosis, musculoskeletal injuries, stroke, and joint replacements.

6695 Ray Graham Association for People with Disabilities
2801 Finley Road
Downers Grove, IL 60515
630-620-2222
FAX: 630-628-2350
TTY:630-628-2352
e-mail: cathyfickerterill@yahoo.com
www.ray-graham.org

Cathy Terrill, President/CEO
Ed Bales, Chairperson
Don Buell, Secretary/Treasurer
Provides developmental services at 15 sites to infants, children and adults with disabilities. Services range from 1 hr/wk respite to full-time residential.

6696 Reach Rehabilitation Program: Americana Healthcare
9401 S Kostner Avenue
Oak Lawn, IL 60453
708-423-1505

Jean Roche, Owner
Postacute rehabilitation program.

6697 Rehabilitation Achievement Center
345 E Superior Street
Chicago, IL 60011
312-238-1000

Richard Green, Program Director
Mary Helen Ekstam, Director Clinical Relations
Rehabilitation Institute of Chicago (RIC) has aquired the assets of the Rehabilitation Achievement Center (RAC) On Tuesday, August 5, 2003 RIC, took over the leadership, management and operation of RAC's 3 day rehabilitation centers.

6698 Rehabilitation Institute of Chicago: Alexian Brothers Medical Center
800 Biesterfield Road
Elk Grove Village, IL 60007
847-437-5500
800-354-7342
TTY:847-956-5116
www.alexian.org

Christine Sommerfeldt, Executive Director
A 32-bed rehabilitation unit under the medical direction and supervision of the Rehabilitation Institute of Chicago.

6699 Riverside Medical Center
Mental Health Unit
350 N Wall Street
Kankakee, IL 60901
815-935-7502
FAX: 815-935-7485
e-mail: rhuber@rsh.net
www.riversidehealthcare.org

Rhonda Huber, VP Institutional Advancement
Offers recreation, parenting therapy, emergency services, psychological testing and inpatient treatment programs. Riverside is nationally recognized for its specialty programs in heart care, obstetrics, trauma, oncology, rehabilitation, geriatrics, occupational health, treatment of alcohol and chemical dependency and psychiatric services.

6700 Robert Young Mental Health Center Division of Trinity Regional Haelth System
Trinity Health Foundation
2701 17th Street
Rock Island, IL 61201
309-779-5000
800-322-1431
FAX: 309-779-2027
www.trinityqc.com

Berlinda Tyler-Jamison, President
Services include comprehensive inpatient rehabilitation, chronic pain management programs, outpatient medical rehabilitation, work hardening programs, vocational evaluation, alcohol and other drug dependency rehabilitation programs, Burn Center, and mental health services for inpatient, partial hospitalization, residential treatment, case management, emergency/crisis intervention and outpatient therapy. Licensed for 443 beds, it is the largest health care institution in the Iowa/Illinois area.

6701 Sampson-Katz Center
2020 W Devon Avenue
Chicago, IL 60659
773-761-9000
FAX: 312-553-5523
TTY:773-761-6672
e-mail: jvsskc@jvschicago.org
www.jvschicago.org

Alan Goldstein, Executive Director

6702 Shelby County Community Services
101 East North 12th Street
Shelbyville, IL 62565
217-774-1400
FAX: 217-774-5120

Richard Gloede, Executive Director
Primary focus is substance abuse treatment.

6703 St Elizabeth Hospital Physical Rehabilitation Unit In-Patient/CARFT Certified
211 S 3rd Street
Belleville, IL 62220
618-234-2120
FAX: 618-222-4606

Lucy Beaver, Rehab Services Director
Mike Mecurico, Executive Director
Tom Dibadj, Rehab Therapy Manager
Comprehensive inpatient and outpatient physical rehab services that include the services of a psychiatrist, rehab nursing, OT, PT, Speech, RT, social service, neuro psychologist and other resource and support personnel that support the rehab program.

6704 Streator Unlimited
305 N Sterling Street
Streator, IL 61364
815-673-5574
FAX: 815-673-1714
e-mail: contact@streatorunlimited.org
www.streatorunlimited.com

Jeffrey Dean, Executive Director
Lynn Fukar, Director of Day Services
Julie Caestens, Director Residential Services
Vocational and personal skills training, residential services, client and family support, supported and computerized employment. Serves adults with intellectual disabilities.

6705 TCRC Sight Center
111 W Washington Street
Suite 410
East Peoria, IL 61611
309-698-4001
FAX: 309-698-9227
www.tcrcorg.com

Jeff Turnbull, Administrator/VP
Annecia Payne, Office Manager
Offers services for persons who are totally blind, legally blind, partially sighted or visually impaired along with other disabilities. Have support group, rehabilitation classes, orientation and mobility services, counseling services, low vision clinic, Braille transcription services, technology services and specialized aids and appliances for sale.

6706 Tazewell County Resource Center
Rr 1
Box 12
Tremont, IL 61568
309-477-2272
FAX: 309-925-4241

Gus Van Den Brink, Executive Director
Dale Claus, Administrator
A private, nonprofit agency providing programs for the special needs of infants, adults, children and their families residing in Tazewell County. Services offered include: birth-three infant/parent program, adult day care services, family support, residential, vocational services, sheltered work and activity services programs.

6707 Thresholds Bridge Deaf North
Thresholds Psychiatric Rehabilitation Centers
4101 N Ravenswood Avenue
Chicago, IL 60613
773-880-6260
888-997-3422
FAX: 773-989-1075
TTY: 773-989-1875
www.thresholds.org

Susan Bottum, President
Herminio Cardona Jr, Program Director
Mark Furlong, Administrator
A private, nonprofit psychosocial rehabilitation center that serves the hearing impaired mental health consumers at the highest risk of hospitalization, those with serious and persistent mental illness. The program provides residential and assertive treatment case management services focused on rehabilitation.

6708 Thresholds South Suburbs
12145 Western Avenue
Blue Island, IL 60406
708-597-8073
FAX: 708-597-8053
www.thresholds.org

Natalie Marsh, Program Director
Camille Rucks, Team Leader
Services offered include psychosocial, vocational and residential programs for ages 18 or older with a primary diagnosis of mental illness. Facility is wheelchair accessible.

6709 Trumbull Park
10530 S Oglesby Avenue
Chicago, IL 60617
773-375-7022
FAX: 773-375-5528

Gregory Terry, Director
Diana Moore, Site Supervisor
Ada McKinley, Manager
Offers consultation, education, general counseling, recreation, self-help and social services for children and adults.

6710 University of Illinois Medical Center
1740 W Taylor Street
Chicago, IL 60612
312-355-4000
FAX: 312-996-7770

Timothy McMahon, Chief
Marilyn Plomann, Manager
Offers services for the totally blind, legally blind, visually impaired, mentally retarded blind and more with health, counseling, educational, recreational, rehabilitation, computer training and professional training services.

6711 VanMatre Rehabilitation Center
950 S Mulford Road
Rockford, IL 61108
815-381-8500
866-754-3347
FAX: 815-484-9953
www.healthsouth.com

Dan Woloszyn, Administrator/CEO
Scott Craig, Medical Director
A CARF-accredited comprehensive rehabilitation center based within the Rockford Memorial Hospital providing inpatient and outpatient services for physically and cognitively challenged persons with debilitating illness and injuries.

6712 **Warren Achievement Center**
1220 E 2nd Avenue
Monmouth, IL 61462 309-734-3131
FAX: 309-734-7114
e-mail: info@warrenachievement.com
www.warrenachievement.com

Michael Lewis, President
James Keefe, VP
For developmentally disabled children and adults. Parent-infant education programs are for parents of infants with disabilities or developmental delays; Children's Group Homes which serve children on a fulltime basis and can serve additional children on a respite basis; Vocational training and residential programs assist the handicapped adult and developmental training for adults; adult residential community living; manufacturing, capabilities in workshop includes packaging, and assembly.

Indiana

6713 **Ball Memorial Hospital**
2401 W University Avenue
Muncie, IN 47303 765-747-3111
FAX: 765-747-3313
www.accesschs.org/ball_memorial_hospital

Brent L Batman, President
Robert Curtis, Chief Executive Officer
Offers rehabilitation services, occupational therapy, physical therapy and more for the physically challenged child or adult.

6714 **Community Health Network**
1500 N Ritter Avenue
Indianapolis, IN 46219 317-355-1411
800-775-7775
FAX: 317-351-7723
www.ecommunity.com

Barbara Gebhardt, Executive Director
Anita Harden, President
A leading not-for-profit health system offering convenient access to expert physicians, advanced treatments and leading edge technology, all focused on getting patients well and back to their lives. With caring compassion, Community's 5 hospitals and 70 + sites of care continually strive to improve the health and well being of those individuals in central Indiana who entrust care to us.

6715 **Crossroads Industrial Services**
8320 E 33rd Street
Indianapolis, IN 46205 317-897-7320
FAX: 317-897-9763
www.crossroadsindustrialservices.com

Pamela Leal, Executive Director
Assisting customers with short-term, seasonal, and long-term outsourcing needs. Many consider Crossroads an extension of their company

6716 **Department of Veterans Affairs Vet Center #418**
311 N Weinbach Avenue
Evansville, IN 47711 812-473-5993
FAX: 812-473-4028
e-mail: vcen418@evansville.net
www.in.gov/veteran/sso/fac

Jack Weber, Manager
Provides readjustment counseling to combat veterans of all eras. Onsite assistance for employment problems and Department of Veteran Affairs, Vocational Rehabilitation and Sexual Trauma Counsel.

6717 **Frasier Rehabilitation Center Division of Clark Memorial Hospital**
2201 Greentree N
Clarksville, IN 47129 812-282-4257
FAX: 812-288-1161
www.clarkmemorial.org/subacute.asp

Juanita Love, Manager
Designed to help patients in their adjustment to a physically limiting condition, both psychologically and physically, by helping to maximize each patient's abilities so he or she can function as independently as possible. The program treats patients whose functional impairment may range from temporary to permanent, from partial to total disability.

6718 **HealthSouth Tri-State Rehabilitation Hospital**
4100 Covert Avenue
Evansville, IN 47714 812-476-9983
800-677-3422
FAX: 812-476-4270
www.healthsouth.com

Barbara Butler, President/CEO
Tina Densley, Opperations Director
Dick Ondrey, Clinical Services Director
An 80-bed JCAHO accredited freestanding hospital specializing in comprehensive medical rehabilitation for Brain Injury, Spinal Cord Injury, Orthopedic, Pulmonary, Cardiac, Oncology and disabilities and general disabilities.

6719 **Healthwin Specialized Care**
20531 Darden Road
South Bend, IN 46637 574-272-0100
FAX: 574-277-3233
e-mail: tsmucker@healthwin.org
www.healthwin.org

Teresa Smucker, Administrator
Dawn Long, Director Of Nursing
Judy Morse, Admissions Coordinator
No other facility in the area has a homelike environment like ours. Its simply part of our culture. Rehabilitation therapy that includes physical, occupational, speech, respiratory and a full time in-house therapist. Other services include a wound specialist, nutrition specialist, and restorative therapy 6 times a week.

6720 **Memorial Regional Rehabilitation Center**
615 N Michigan Street.
South Bend, IN 46601 574-647-1000
877-282-0964
FAX: 574-232-1476

Dave Haluta, Director
Judy Smith, Manager
CARF accredited outpatient medical rehabilitation and post acute brain injury program. Serves neurologically impaired adults and young adults.

6721 **Saint Joseph Regional Medical Center- South Bend**
801 E La Salle Avenue
South Bend, IN 46617 574-237-7111
e-mail: sgersp@sjrmc.com
www.sjmed.com

Abraham Marcus, Chairman
Bonnie Raine, Ph.D., Vice Chairman
Charles Viater, Treasurer
Continuum of rehabilitation services offered. Included are: acute rehabilitation, a 26 bed CARF accredited comprehensive inpatient unit, a CARF certified inpatient brain injury program, a CARF outpatient day treatment brain injury program, comprehensive outpatient services, with available case management, and Driver's Training Program, a 30 bed state of the art subacute rehab unit, CARF accredited Industrial Rehabilitation Programs and CARF accredited Pain and Complimentary Medicine Program.

Iowa

6722 **Crossroads of Western Iowa**
One Crossroads Place
Missouri Valley, IA 51555 712-642-4114
FAX: 712-642-4115
e-mail: info@cwiowa.org
www.cwiowa.org

David Lobell, CEO

CWI provides services in Missouri Valley, Onawa and Council Bluffs, Iowa. An array of services for people with mental illness, mental retardation and brain injury are provided in each location.

6723 Des Moines Division-VA Central Iowa Health Care System
3600 30th Street
Des Moines, IA 50310
515-699-5862
800-294-8387
FAX: 515-699-5862
www1.va.gov/directory/guide/facility.
VA Cental Iowa Health Care System is the result of the 1997 merger of the Des Moines and Knoxville, Iowa, VA Medical Centers. This integrated healthcare system brings 2 previously separate organizational structures, located 40 miles apart, into one cohesive entity.

6724 Easter Seals Iowa
Easter Seals National
PO Box 4002
Des Moines, IA 50333
515-289-1933
FAX: 515-289-1281
TTY:515-289-4069
e-mail: infi@eastersealsia.org
www.eastersealsia.org

Tracy Keninzer, Director Marketing
Donna Elbrecht, President
Easter Seals is a leading nonprofit provider of services to Iowans with disabilities. Services include vocational and employment training, camping recreation and respite services, craft training and sales, home and farm adaptations, transportation, scholarships and a club for stroke survivors and their families.

6725 Genesis Regional Rehabilitation Center
Genesis Health System
2720 W Locust Street
Suite B2
Davenport, IA 52804
563-421-3495
FAX: 563-421-3499
www.genesishealth.com

Janet King, Executive Director
Mike Shaw, Supervisor
Serves persons of all ages experiencing a disability, whether acquired at birth or following a serious interdisciplinary service. Rehabilitation programs include acute rehabilitation; adult rehabilitation, pediatric rehabilitation, outpatient orthopaedics. LIFT, a community based, nontraditional approach to the treatment of adolescents and adults with brain injuries is also offered at Genesis. It is designed to facilitate re-entry into the community or return to appropriate employment.

6726 Homelink
Van G Miller & Associates
PO Box 2817
Waterloo, IA 50704
319-235-7100
800-482-1993
FAX: 319-235-7822
www.edm.com

Dave Kazynski, President
A national network of home medical equipment, respiratory therapy, rehabilitation and infusion therapy service providers with over 2,500 locations serving all fifty states.

6727 Iowa Central Industries
127 Avenue M
Fort Dodge, IA 50501
515-576-2126
FAX: 515-576-2251

Quentin Weidner, Director
Tom Eckman, Executive Director
Services include evaluation and training in pre-vocational and vocational skills, personal behavior management, cognitive skills, communication skills, self-care skills and social skills. Services arranged include: independent living training, medical services, psychological services, therapeutic services and social services.

6728 Life Skills Laundry Division
1510 Industrial Road SW
Le Mars, IA 51031
712-546-9554
FAX: 712-546-4985

Don Nore, Executive Director

6729 MIW
909 S 14th Avenue
Marshalltown, IA 50158
641-752-3697
FAX: 641-752-1614
e-mail: jstegmamann@miwi.org

Jack Allen, CEO
Rich Byers, President
Vocational services for adults with disabilities. Includes organizational employment services, supported employment, job placement.

6730 Mercy Dubuque Physical Rehabilitation Unit
250 Mercy Drive
Dubuque, IA 52001
563-589-8000
FAX: 563-589-8193
www.mercydubuque.com

Joan Hentges, Director
Bobbi Schell, Executive Director
Provides services which open the door to improved communication, offering the opportunity to enrich the quality of life. Mercy offers many other branches of services including, rehabilitation services for children, pulmonary rehabilitation program, services for the head-injured patient, back to school, and the disabled driver program.

6731 Mercy Medical Center-Pain Services
1111 6th Avenue
Des Moines, IA 50314
515-247-3121
FAX: 515-248-8867
www.mercydesmoines.org/services/painservices

Dianne Alber, Administrative Director
An outpatient program dedicated to helping people with chronic pain live more productive, satisfying lives. The program is not designed for conditions that are surgically curable, but rather approaches the problem using a comprehensive, holistic treatment.

6732 Nishna Productions-Shenandoah Work Center
902 Day Street
Po Box 70
Shenandoah, IA 51601
712-246-1242
FAX: 712-246-1243
e-mail: nci@nishna.org
www.nishna.org

Sherri Clark, Executive Director
Shelter, workshop and job training for the disabled. Some of the services we provide are Work Activity, Adult Day Activity Program, Personal & Social Adjustment, Residential Services, Home & Community Based Services & Employment Resources.

6733 Northstar Community Services
3420 University Avenue
Waterloo, IA 50701
319-236-0901
800-879-1365
FAX: 319-236-3701
e-mail: info@northdstarcs.org
www.northstarcs.org

Mark Witmer, Executive Director
Denise Hinders, Director, Services
Donna Davis, Director Development/Public Rel
Provides adult day services, employment services and supported community living so people with disabilities can live and work in the community. Populations served include, but are not limited to: senior adults with age-related disabilities, youth with disabilities (age 16+) or withing 2 years of leaving high school, adults with disabilities, including those with mental and physical disabilities. CARF accredited. Serves northeast, north and central Iowa. Head Injury Program serves the whole state

6734 **Options of Linn County**

1019 7th Street SE
Cedar Rapids, IA 52401
319-892-5800
FAX: 319-892-5849
e-mail: optons@linncounty.org
www.linncounty.org/options

Jim Nagel, Director
Reggie Ancelet, Associate Director
Carter Baldwin, Associate Director
Options of Lynn County works with community businesses in providing employment services to adults with disabilities. Options is a publicly operated service provider within the Linn County Community Services department. Options serves over 350 people annually.

6735 **RISE**

106 Rainbow Drive
Elkader, IA 52043
563-245-1868

Edward Josten, Executive Director

6736 **Ragtime Industries**

116 N 2nd Street
Albia, IA 52531
641-932-7813
FAX: 641-932-7814
e-mail: ragtime@cknet.net
www.ragtimeind.com

Diana Shehan, Executive Director
A work-oriented rehabilitation organization which provides training for mentally and physically disabled adults in Monroe County. A variety of programs which help to develop each person's individual potential are offered so that the person may live as normal a life as possible.

6737 **Sunshine Services**

PO Box 225
Spencer, IA 51301
712-262-7805
FAX: 712-262-8369

Ann Vandehar, Executive Director

6738 **Tenco Industries**

710 Gateway Drive
1287
Ottumwa, IA 52501
641-682-8114
FAX: 641-684-4223
e-mail: luehlingtech@lisco.com
www.tenco.org

Lorraine Uhling-Tecagl, Executive Director
Denny Baum, Director Of Vocational Services
To advocate and provide opportunities for people with disabilities, or conditions that limit their abilities, to develop and maintain the skills necessary for personal dignity and independence in all areas of life. Provide a wide array of services to individuals with disabilities. By looking at each person as individuals, we are able to work with them to maximize their skills. Residentials services, including HCBS and CSALA are also provided in all communities.

Kansas

6739 **Arrowhead West**

1100 East Wyatt Earp
Dodge City, KS 67801
620-227-8803
FAX: 620-227-8812
e-mail: web@arrowheadwest.org
www.arrowheadwest.org

Paul Lehmkuhler, Public Relations Coordinator
Janet Heit, Admission Coordinator
Paul Lehmkuhler, Public Relations Coordinator
Services and programs offered include: developmental and therapy services for children birth to age 3. Adult center-based work services and community integrated employment options; adult life skills and retirement programs; adult residential services including supervised living, supported living and independent living services. Staff includes over 200 employees. Services are provided over a 14 county area with service centers in Dodge City, Kinsley, Pratt, Medicine Lodge and Wichita.

6740 **Big Lakes Developmental Center**

1416 Hayes Drive
Manhattan, KS 66502
785-776-9201
FAX: 785-776-9830
e-mail: sfunk@biglakes.org
www.biglakes.org

James Shaver, President
Shawn Funk, Community Education Director
A private nonprofit Community Developmental Disability Organization (CDDO) serving individuals with developmental disabilities in Riley, Geary, Clay and Pottawatome counties in Kansas. Big lakes is supported by county mill levy and federal and state funding.

6741 **Developmental Services of Northwest Kansas**

2703 Hall St.
Suite 10
Hays, KS 67601
785-625-5678
800-637-2229
FAX: 785-625-8204
e-mail: comments@notes1dsnwk.org
www.dsnwk.org

James W Blume, President
Ruth Lang, Administrative Assistant
A private nonprofit organization serving both children and adults with disabilities. Offers services to children ages birth to three years, youth and adults through a network of community-based and outreach programs and inter-agency agreements with other service providers in the eighteen counties of Northwest Kansas.

6742 **ENVISION**

2301 S Water Street
Wichita, KS 67213
316-267-2244
FAX: 316-267-4312
e-mail: envision@envisionus.com
www.envisionus.com

Linda Merrill, President
David Austin, Manager Public Relations
Provides jobs, job training and vision rehabilitation services to people who are blind or low vision. A private not-for-profit agency uniquely combining employment opportunitites with rehabilitation services and public education.

6743 **Heartspring**

8700 E 29th Street N
Wichita, KS 67226
316-634-8700
800-835-1043
FAX: 316-634-0555
www.heartspring.org

Cara Rapp, Admissions Director
Cindy Chapman, Executive Director
Charlene Kuzma LMSW CLP, Life Care Planner
Private, not-for-profit residential school for children from across the country ages five to twenty-one with multiple disabilities. Heartspring serves students with one or more of the following diagnosis: autism, cerebral palsy, maladaptive behaviors, seizures, or other disabilities. Services are provided by an interdisciplinary team of specialists. Assessments and therapies are provided in the areas of speech/language, physical, occupational learning and behavior

6744 **Indian Creek Nursing Center**

6515 W 103rd Street
Overland Park, KS 66212
913-642-5545
FAX: 913-642-3982

Brad Baker, Administrator
Postacute rehabilitation program. A 120-bed nursing home facility.

6745 Johnson County Developmental Supports
10501 Lackman Road
Lenexa, KS 66219
913-826-2626
FAX: 913-492-5171
e-mail: info@jocogov.org
www.jcds.org

Dennis Tucker, President
Shelly Toft, Executive Assistant
JCDS is the community Developmental Disability Organization for Johnson County, Kansas. Provides supports in the form of direct services to people on a daily basis. Through a person-centered process and within availiable resources services are shaped to fit individual needs, preferences, goals, abilities, and interests.

6746 Ketch Industries
1006 E. Waterman
Wichita, KS 67211
316-383-8770
800-766-3777
FAX: 316-383-8715
e-mail: webmaster@ketch.org
www.ketch.org

Ron Pasmore, President/CEO
Carol Wickizer, Ladies Assistant Chairperson
Charles W. Lester, Chairman
The mission of Ketch is to promote independence for persons with disabilities through innovative learning experiences that support individuals choices for working, living and playing in their community.

6747 Lakemary Center
100 Lakemary Drive
Paola, KS 66071
913-557-4000
FAX: 913-294-4361

William R Craig PhD, President
Pauline Hintz, Principal
A private, not-for-profit day and residential training facility which provides for the assessment, education, training, therapy and social development of children and adults, moderate and severe mental retardation. The Center is based 28 miles southwest of Kansas City in Paola, Kansas.

6748 Northview Developmental Services
700 E 14th Street
Newton, KS 67114
316-283-5170
FAX: 316-283-5196
e-mail: nds@northviewdsi.com
www.northviewdsi.org

Stan Zienkewicz, President/CEO
The mission is to provide quality supportive and coordinating services to persons with developmental disabilities, assisting them to grow as they integrate into the community. Further, our mission is to improve the quality of their lives by providing access to person-centered opportunities within the community from which they will be making choices.

Kentucky

6749 Cardinal Hill Rehabilitation Hospital
Cadinal Hill Medical Center
2050 Versailles Road
Lexington, KY 40504
859-254-5701
FAX: 859-254-4612
www.cardinalhill.org

Martin Lautner, Manager Referral Relations
Elizabeth A Monarch, Viec President/coo
Kerry Gillihan, Chief Executive Officer
Provides occupational health services, therapy services and urgent medical treatment of injured workers.

6750 Frazier Rehab Institute
220 Abraham Flexner Way
Louisville, KY 40202
502-587-4011
FAX: 502-582-7477
www.jewishhospital.org

Joanne Berryman, Senior VP/CEO
Cheryl Fugate, VP Frasier Rehab/Neuroscience
Jean Russell, VP Rehab Operations
Frazier Rehab Institute is a regional healthcare system dedicated entirely to rehabilitation. Through an expansive network of inpatient and outpatient facilites in Kentucky and southern Indiana, Frazier offers a wide array of services based on one common goal - helping people with disabilities reach their full potential.

6751 HealthSouth Northern Kentucky Rehabilitation Hospital
201 Medical Village Drive
Edgewood, KY 41017
859-341-2044
800-860-6004
www.healthsouth.com

Brenda Gosney, Chief Executive Officer
Mary Pfeffer, Director Clinical Services
Lynn Bean, Director Nursing
Offers all types of inpatient and outpatient rehabilitation services such as occupational therapy, physical therapy, speech therapy. Respiratory therpay, Psychology, Aquatics, Case Managemenet/Social Work and Nutritional Services.

6752 King's Daughter's Medical Center's Rehab Unit/Work Hardening Program
2201 Lexington Avenue
Ashland, KY 41101
606-327-4000
888-377-5362
FAX: 606-327-7542
e-mail: info@kdmc.net
www.kdmc.com

Harry Bell, Medical Director
Sue Strehle, Service Line Manager
Fred Jackson, Chief Executive Officer
Offers a 27-bed, inpatient rehabilitation services unit treating physical disabilities related to accident or illness. The program provides an interdisciplinary inpatient program designed to restore the individual to the highest level of independence. It is the goal of the staff to provide rehabilitative services that will enable the disabled or injured person to return home and re-enter the community at the maximum level of efficiency.

6753 LifeSkills Industries
992 State Street
Po Box 6499
Bowling Green, KY 42102
270-901-5000
FAX: 270-782-0058
www.lifeskills.com

Joe Miller, Executive Director
Dale Bond, Chief Executive Officer
LifeSkills will be the reliable advocate, dependable safety net and provider of choice, for high quality, accessable services and supports for the citizens of south-central Kentucky whos lives are affected by mental illness, developmental disablilities or substance abuse.

6754 Low Vision Services of Kentucky
120 N Eagle Creek Drive
Suite 501
Lexington, KY 40509
859-263-3900
800-627-2020
FAX: 859-263-3757
e-mail: jwood@retinaky.com
www.lowvisionky.com

William Wood Md, Clinical Director
Jennifer D Wood OD/FAAO, Low Vision Specialist
Helen Wade, Administrator
Offers devices and services for the totally blind, legally blind, visually impaired educational, recreational and rehabilitation.

6755 Muhlenberg County Opportunity Center
615 Opportunity Way
Greenville, KY 42345
270-338-5970
FAX: 270-338-5977

Michael Morgan, Executive Director
Post-acute rehabilitation facility with programs including a workshop with hand packaging of manufactured goods.

6756 New Vision Enterprises
1900 Brownsboro Road
Louisville, KY 40206
502-893-0211
800-405-9135
FAX: 502-893-3885

Robert Jarboe, Chief Executive Officer
Offers employment training and services for the blind and legally blind.

6757 Park DuValle Community Health Center
3015 Wilson Avenue
Louisville, KY 40211
502-774-4401
FAX: 502-775-6195
e-mail: rjones@pdchc.org
www.pdchc.org

Richard Jones, Executive Director
John Howard MD, Medical Director
Dave Gerwig, Chief Financial Officer
Offers services for the totally blind, legally blind, visually impaired, mentally retarded blind and more with health, counseling, educational, recreational, rehabilitation, computer training and professional training services.

Louisiana

6758 Alliance House
2902 Florida Boulevard
Baton Rouge, LA 70802
225-343-5393
FAX: 225-346-0857
A non-residential facility serving male and female chronically mentally ill. Services include: social service, vocational evaluation, pre-vocational training and job placement.

6759 Assumption Activity Center
4201 Highway 1
Napoleonville, LA 70390
985-369-2907
FAX: 985-369-2657
e-mail: arcoa.catbl.net

Warren Gonzales, Executive Director
Reginald Washington, President
A community work center providing prevocational training and extended employment for adults with disabilities. Services include: social services, work activities, specialized training and supported employment.

6760 Bancroft Rehabilitation Living Centers
3434 Canal Street
New Orleans, LA 70119
225-482-3075
FAX: 504-483-2135
www.bancroftneurohealth.org

Dr. Robert Voogt, Owner
Mission is to nurture abilities and independence of people with neurological challenges by providing a broad spectrum of advanced therapeutic and educational programs and by fostering the development of best practices in the field through research and professional education.

6761 Caddo-Bossier Association for Retarded Citizens
4103 Lakeshore Drive
Shreveport, LA 71109
318-425-8888
FAX: 318-221-4262

Janet Parker, Director
A community operated workshop for male and female mentally retarded individuals. It provides work evaluation and transitional and extended employment.

6762 Deaf Action Center of GNO
1000 Howard Avenue
New Orleans, LA 70113
504-523-3755
FAX: 504-523-2789
e-mail: ccano@archdiocese.org
www.ccano.org

Shari Bernius, Administrator
This community service and resource center serves deaf, deaf-blind, hard of hearing and speech-impaired persons in the greater New Orleans area regardless of age, religion, race or secondary disability. DAC provides interpreting services, equipment distribution, sign language classes, case management and advocacy.

6763 Donaldsville Association for Retarded Citizens
1030 Clay Street
Donaldsonville, LA 70346
225-473-4516
FAX: 225-473-4517
e-mail: daarc@eatel.net

Marlene Domingue, Executive Director
A private, nonprofit sheltered work program working with the mentally retarded and developmentally disabled adults.

6764 East Jefferson General Hospital Rehab Center
4200 Houma Boulevard
Metairie, LA 70006
505-454-4000
www.ejgh.org

Cathy Brannon, Director
Tara Fitzpatrick, Supervisor
Provides the highest quality, compassionate healthcare to the people we serve. East Jefferson General Hospital will be the region's healthcare leader providing the highest quality care through innovation and collaboration with our team members, medical staff, and community.

6765 Family Service Society
2515 Canal Street
Suite 201
New Orleans, LA 70119
504-822-0800
FAX: 504-822-0831

Robert Quintana, Executive Director
Ronald Clain, President
Offers services for the totally blind, legally blind, visually impaired, mentally retarded blind and more with health, counseling, educational, recreational, rehabilitation, computer training and professional training services.

6766 Foundation Industries
9995 Highway 64
Zachary, LA 70791
225-654-6283
FAX: 225-654-3988

Jim Lambert-Oswald, President
A private, nonprofit sheltered workshop providing extended employment and work activities for the mentally retarded and developmentally disabled clients. Objectives are to build work skills through supervision, develop social interaction and manifest basic daily living skills.

6767 Handi-Works Productions
2700 Lee Street
Alexandria, LA 71301
318-442-3377
FAX: 318-473-0858
This is a nonprofit workshop for male and female clients who have vocational handicapping conditions. All types of handicapped persons are served in this non-residential workshop.

6768 HealthSouth Rehabilitation Hospital Of Baton Rouge
8595 United Plaza Boulevard
Baton Rouge, LA 70809
225-927-0567
800-264-0567
FAX: 225-926-2357

Jill Root, Admissions Director
Amy Searles, Community Relations
Ken Alexander, Executive Director
Dedicated to one field of medicine - physical rehabilitation medicine - and are committed to one goal, helping patients achieve the highest level of functioning possible after a debilitating injury or illness.

6769 Iberville Association for Retarded Citizens
PO Box 201
Plaquemine, LA 70765
225-687-4062
FAX: 225-687-3272
e-mail: arci@eatel.net

Paul Rhorer, Executive Director
A private sheltered work program operating out of one facility and providing transitional, extended employment and work activities for mentally and developmentally ill adults.

6770 **Lighthouse for the Blind in New Orleans**
123 State Street
New Orleans, LA 70118
504-899-4501
888-792-0163
FAX: 504-895-4162
www.lhb.org

Bill Price, Executive Director
Offers services for the totally blind, legally blind, visually impaired, mentally retarded blind and more with health, counseling, educational, recreational, rehabilitation, computer training and professional training services.

6771 **Louisiana Center for the Blind**
101 S Trenton Street
Ruston, LA 71270
318-251-2891
800-234-4166
FAX: 318-251-0109
e-mail: pallen@lcb-ruston.com
www.lcb-ruston.com

Pam Allen, Executive Director
Neita Ghrigsby, Office Manager
A new kind of orientation and training center for blind persons. The center is privately operated and provides quality instruction in the skills of blindness. Offers employment assistance, computer literacy training, summer training and employment project, special seminars, outreach and referral services.

6772 **Louisiana State University Eye Center**
Lousiana State University
2020 Gravier Street
New Orleans, LA 70112
504-412-1200
FAX: 504-412-1315
www.lsuhsc.edu

Bergs Sma, Director
Mark Graves, Manager
The LSU Eye Center is part of the LSU Medical Center complex in downtown New Orleans. It is in the LSU-Lions Building at 2020 Gravier Street between South Bolivar and South Prieur streets. The Center provides expert eye care at every level, from routine examinations to the most complex surgeries. The LSU Eye Center is committed to the future of eye care and vision science and provides innovative research and an educational program that trains tomorrowo's opthomologists and vision scientists.

6773 **New Orleans Speech and Hearing Center**
1636 Toledano Street
New Orleans, LA 70115
504-897-2606
FAX: 504-891-6048
www.noshc.org

Lesley Jernigan, Executive Director
Patty Connolly, Coordinator Clinical Services
This non-residential facility serves male and female clients for purposes of evaluating speech and hearing problems and providing speech therapy, hearing aids and other assistive technology for speech and hearing.

6774 **Port City Enterprises**
PO Box 113
Port Allen, LA 70767
225-344-1142
FAX: 225-344-1192

Christine Dunlevy, Executive Director
Offers supported employment, sheltered work and supervised programs for the mentally retarded, ages 22 and over.

6775 **Rehabilitation Center at Thibodeaux Regional**
Rehab Care
602 N Acadia Road
Thibodaux, LA 70301
985-447-5500
800-822-8442
FAX: 985-449-4600
e-mail: infoA@thibodaux.com
www.thibodaux.com/rehabilitation.html

Jan Torres, Program Manager
Rose Pipes, Clinical Coordinator
Designed to help patients in their adjustment to a physically limiting condition, both physically and psychologically, by helping to maximize each patients abilities so he or she can function as independently as possible.

6776 **St. Patrick RehabCare Unit**
RehabCare
524 S Ryan Street
Lake Charles, LA 70601
337-436-2511
888-722-9355
FAX: 337-491-7157
www.stpatrichospital.org/serv_rehab_main.htm

Annette Harlow, Program Manager
Ruth Thornton, Admissions
A comprehensive physical and cognitive rehabilitation program designed to help individuals who have experienced a disabling injury or illness. The goal of the Rehabilitation Center is to ensure an optimum level of recovery in a cost-effective way for each patient.

6777 **Touro Rehabilitation Center**
1401 Foucher Street
New Orleans, LA 70115
504-897-7011
FAX: 504-897-8393
e-mail: info@touro.com
www.touro.com

Gary Glynn, Medical Director
Suzy Laborde, Director Inpatient Service
Keith Randazzo, Neuro Rehab Coordinator
Located in New Orleans' Garden District, Touro Rehabilitation is a comprehensive rehabilitation facility dedicated to the restoration of function and independence for individuals with disabilities. The scope of rehabilitation services is broad, with 4 CARF accreditations for Brain Injury, Spinal Cord Injury, Chronic Pain and General Rehabilitation. TRC opened in 1984 and offers 69 rehab beds. TRC is part of Touro Infirmary which has a proud 150 year history as a nonprofit teaching hospital.

6778 **Training, Resource & Assistive-Technology**
Lakefront Campus
PO Box 1051
New Orleans, LA 70148
504-280-5700
FAX: 504-280-5707
e-mail: ggaglian@uno.edu
www.uno.edu/trac

Gayle Gagliano, Director
Rose Angelocci, Rehab Training Specialist
Barbara Connors, Case Manager
Provides quality services to persons with disabilities, rehabilitation professionals, educators and employers. Built a solid reputation for its innovative training programs and community outreach efforts. The Center is recognized as a valuable resource statewide, nationally and internationally on disability issues.

Maine

6779 **Charlotte White Center**
PO Box 380
Dover Foxcroft, ME 04426
207-564-2464
888-440-4158
FAX: 207-564-2404
www.charlottewhitecenter

Pam Jacobson, Executive Director
Anthony Zambrono, Director Operations
A nonprofit agency, devoted to assisting adults and children with mental retardation, mental health, physical handicaps, and elder age related issues. With headquarters in Dover-Foxcroft Maine, the agency provides multiple levels of social services, including: residential, day treatment, clinical counseling, vocational, and in-home supports.

6780 **Iris Network for the Blind**
189 Park Avenue
Portland, ME 04102
207-774-6273
800-715-0097
FAX: 207-774-0679
e-mail: sobremski@theiris.org
www.theiris.org

Steven Obremski, President/CEO
Offers services to persons who are blind, visually impaired or multi-disabled blind with rehabilitation, counseling, educational, recreational, computer training and professional training services.

6781 **Roger Randall Center**
45 School Street
Houlton, ME 04730
207-532-9446
FAX: 207-532-1359
www.cla-maine.org

Tom Moakler, President
Lloyd Chase, Vice President
Rob Faulkner, Treasurer
The Roger Randall Cneter is one of five Day Habilitation Programs adminsitered by Community Living Association, a private, non-profit agency. These programs may provide a supportive environment that allows the individual to achieve their maximum growth potential. Individualized services address but are not limtied to the following areas: fine/gross motor skills, communication, community awareness and involvement, appropriate social skills, and independent living skills.

6782 **Sebasticook Farms-Great Bay Foundation**
PO Box 65
Saint Albans, ME 04971
207-938-4615
FAX: 207-938-5670
e-mail: tad@tdstelme.net
www.greatbayfoundation.org

Tom Davis, Executive Director
Pam Erskin, Program Coordinator
Provides residential, educational and vocational services to adults who are developmentally disabled in order to maximize independent living and to provide assistance in obtaining an earned income.

6783 **Social Learning Center**
984 Sabattus Street
Lewiston, ME 04240
207-783-4672
FAX: 207-783-4673

Deborah Beam, Unit Manager
Post accute rehabilitation program.

Maryland

6784 **Blind Industries and Services of Maryland**
3345 Washington Boulevard
Baltimore, MD 21227
410-737-2600
888-322-4567
FAX: 410-737-2665
www.bism.com

Rosemary Lerdahl, Rehab Director
Fred Puente, President
Offers a comprehensive residential rehabilitation training program for people who are blind. Areas of instruction: braille, cane travel, independent living, computer, adjustment and blindness seminars.

6785 **Center for Neuro-Rehabilitation**
2340238 N Cary Street
Annapolis, MD 21223
410-263-1704
410-462-4711
e-mail: cnrnhq@erols.com

Jeanne Fryer
Laurent Pierre-Philippe
Provide community-based inpatient and outpatient acute rehabilitation, vocational services and long-term care. Specializing in treating complex neurological conditions including spinal cord injuries, multiple sclerosis, strokes, and other brain injuries resulting from trauma, anoxia, tumors, genetic malformations and other related conditions. Locations in Annapolis, Bethesda, Frederick, Towson, MD and Fairfax, Va. CNR is licensed, a Medicare provider and CARF accredited.

6786 **Child Find/Early Childhood Disabilities Unit Montgomery County Public Schools**
10731 Saint Margarets Way
Suite A4
Kensington, MD 20895
301-929-2224
FAX: 301-929-2223

Julie Bader, Supervisor
Offers free developmental screening for children ages 3 years until eligible for kindergarten, evaluation and placement services.

6787 **Greater Baltimore Medical Center**
6701 N Charles Street
Baltimore, MD 21204
443-849-2000
800-597-9142
FAX: 443-849-2631
www.gbmc.org/medicine/hoover

Janet Sunness, Director Hoover Services
Trenitta Brady, Office Manager
Offers services for the visually impaired and blind with low vision exams. Rehabilitation teaching and orientation and mobility in the home or workplace. Also offers a bimonthly newsletter for $12/yr for Hoover patients and monthly share group.

6788 **Greenery Extended Care Center: Baltimore**
1300 S Ellwood Avenue
Baltimore, MD 21224
410-342-6644
FAX: 301-327-3949

Shane Duffy, Administrator
150 beds offering complex care treatment, extended rehabilitation and neurological restorative care.

6789 **James Lawrence Kernan Hospital**
2200 Kernan Drive
Baltimore, MD 21207
410-285-6566
888-453-7626
FAX: 410-448-6854
www.kernan.org

Dennis Grote, Executive Director
James Lawrence III, MD
Kernan reigns as Maryland's origional orthopaedic hospital with a staff which consists of a support team of orthopaedic physician assistants and dedicated nurses in the Post Anesthesia Care Unit and on the Medical/Surgical Unit, guaranteeing the highest quality care in the acute hospital setting.

6790 **Levindale Hebrew Geriatric Center**
2434 W Belvedere Avenue
Baltimore, MD 21215
410-601-2400
FAX: 410-367-9066
www.lifebridgehealth.org

Ronald Rothstein, President/CEO
a 292-licensed bed facility, which includes 172-comprehensive care beds, 20 subacute beds, and a 26-bed dementia care unit. Levindale's 120-bed specialty hospital consists of 20 gerospychiatric beds, 80 complex medical beds, some with ventilator capacity and 20 acute rehabilitation beds.

6791 **Meridan Medical Center For Subacute Care**
770 York Road
Towson, MD 21204
410-821-5500
FAX: 410-337-7233

Yvette Caldwell, Administrator

Patients receive around-the-clock professional nursing care; physical and occupational, speech and respiratory therapists also assist patients. Each patient's individualized plan of care is reviewed and updated as patient needs change. Careful discharge planning prepares patients and their families for success at home by teaching them how to avoid complications that might lead to rehospitalization.

6792 Rehabilitation Opportunities

5100 Philadelphia Way
Lanham, MD 20706 301-731-4242
FAX: 301-322-5891
www.roiworks.org

Rory Brett, Executive Director
Organization offering day programs, evaluation, work adjustments and sheltered workshops for persons who are mentally retarded or developmentally disabled.

6793 Rosewood Center

200 Rosewood Lane
Owings Mills, MD 21117 410-951-5000
888-300-7071
FAX: 410-581-6157
www.dhmh.state.md.us/dda/rosewood

Leslie Smith, Program Director
James Anzalone, Director
Rosewood Center is a State residential Center that supports adults with mental retardation from the central Maryland region. Rosewood will provide comprehensive supports to Maryland citizens with developmental disabilities and their families in a setting that is supportive of community integration. Community inclusion will be enhanced through opportunities for exposure and experience in the community at large.

6794 TLC: Treatment and Learning Centers

9975 Medical Center Drive
Rockville, MD 20850 301-424-5200
FAX: 301-424-8063
e-mail: dpaton@ttlc.org
www.ttlc.org

Patricia A Ritter PhD, Assistant Executive Director
Richard Pavlin, Executive Director
Provides audiological evaluations, testing and hearing aids, physical and occupational therapy and evaluation; speech-language evaluation and therapy, psycho-educational testing and tutoring services for learning disabled students, head injury services and infant and early childhood services including child care, summer therapeutic camp and a special education preschool-8th grade.

6795 Workforce and Technology Center

Division of Rehabilitation Services
2301 Argonne Drive
Baltimore, MD 21218 410-554-9385
888-554-0334
FAX: 410-554-9112
www.dors.state.md.us

Jean Jackson, Program Director
Kathi Santora, Public Information/Planning
Robert Burns, Manager
Is one of nine state operated comprehensive rehabilitation facilities in the country providing a wide range of services to individuals with disabilities. The Maryland Division of Rehabilitation Services operates the Workforce and Technology Program. Available services include medical functional evaluation, career training, mobility training, placement assistance, career assessment, rehab. technology assessments, driver's education and independent living skills training.

Massachusetts

6796 Baroco Corporation

17 New South Street
Northampton, MA 01060 413-584-9978
FAX: 413-585-9010
www.baroco.com

Richard Barnard, President/Owner
Gail Rollins, Treasurer
Provides training and therapeutic support for its recipients with developmental disabilities in order to aid them in securing and maintaining placement in a less-restrictive setting.

6797 Berkshire Meadows

249 N Plain Road
Housatonic, MA 01236 413-528-2523
FAX: 413-528-0293
e-mail: berkshiremeadows@jri.org
www.berkshiremeadows.org

Lisa Kelly, Program Director
Gail Charpentier, Administrator
Private, non profit school for children, adolescents, young adults who are severely, developmentally disabled. approved special education learning center, work site program and foster care. Physical therapy, speech and language development, behavioral programming, occupational therapy, aquatic therapy, round-the-clock nursing. Also included is our state of the art equipment. *$8200.00*

6798 Blueberry Hill Healthcare

75 Brimbal Avenue
Beverly, MA 01915 978-927-2020
FAX: 978-922-4643
www.blueberryhillrehab.com

Phil Sher, Administrator
Sharon Spittle, Executive Director
Accomodates 146 residents. We are centrally located close to Route 128 and Route 1A in Beverly Massachusetts. We offer short-term rehab care, long term care and Alzheimer's Special Care Programs. Our interdisciplinary team designs individual care plans for each resident. For some Blueberry Hill is the gap between hospital and home when a short-term stay is needed. For others we strive to provide the care and peace of mind that only 24 hour supervision can provide.

6799 Boston University Hospital Vision Rehabilitation Services

720 Harrison Avenue
Boston, MA 02118 617-638-8340
FAX: 617-638-8321
Offers services for the totally blind, legally blind, visually impaired, mentally retarded blind and more with health, counseling, educational, recreational, rehabilitation, computer training and professional training services.

6800 Burbank Rehabilitation Center

275 Nichols Road
Fitchburg, MA 01420 978-343-5110
FAX: 978-343-5342
www.umassmemorial.org

Diane O'Brien, Program Director
Jim Lillie, Manager
The largest community hospital and regional referral center in the area. Offers the most extensive high quality, cost-effective healthcare services in the region. The hospital provides outstanding hospital-based services such as case management of high risk elderly and the region's only comprehensive geriatric evaluation service. Also offers patients access to a complete continuum of healthcare, skilled nursing homes, and adult day care. This range of services affords patients prompt care.

6801 CPB/WGBH National Center for Access Media

W GB H Educational Foundation
125 Western Avenue
Boston, MA 02134 617-300-3400
FAX: 617-300-1035
TTY:617-300-2489
e-mail: ncam@wgbh.org
www.wgbh.org/ncam

Larry Goldberg, Director

Dedicated to the issues of media and information technology for people with disabilities in their homes, schools, workplaces, and communities. NCAM's mission is to expand access to present and future media for people with disabilities; explore how existing access technologies may benefit other populations; present its constituents in industry, policy and legislative circles; and to provide access to educational and media technologies for special needs students.

6802 Carroll Center for the Blind
770 Centre Street
Newton, MA 02458
617-969-6200
800-852-3131
FAX: 617-969-6204
e-mail: rrosenbaum@carroll.org
www.carroll.org

Rachel Rosenbaum, President
Arthur O'Neill, Public Relations Director
Offers services for the totally blind, legally blind, visually impaired, mentally retarded blind and more with health, counseling, educational, in dependent living, tronell skills, computer traing, recreational, rehabilitation, computer training and professional training services.

6803 Center for Psychiatric Rehabilitation
Boston University
940 Commonwealth Avenue
Boston, MA 02215
617-353-3549
FAX: 617-353-7700
www.bu.edu/cpr

William A Anthony PhD, Executive Director
Linda Getgen, Publications Manager
Kathy Furlong-Norman, Director Resource Information
The mission of the Center is to increase knowledge, to train treatment personnel, to develop effective rehabilitation programs and to assist in organizing both personnel and programs into efficient and coordinated service delivery systems for people with mental illness.

6804 Clark House Nursing Center At Foxhill Village
Kindred Healthcare
30 Longwood Drive
Westwood, MA 02090
781-326-5652
FAX: 781-326-4034
www.clarkhousefhv.com

Chris Wasel, Administrator
Clark House At Fox Hill Village accomodates 70 residents. We are part of the Fox Hill Village Assisted Living and Retirement Center campus. Clark House Nursing center has been named a recipient of a 2005 step II quality Award from the American Health Care Association. Last year, Clark House Nursing Center received a Step I Quality Award.

6805 College Internship Program at the Berkshire Center
18 Park Street
Lee, MA 01238
413-243-2576
FAX: 413-243-3351
e-mail: admissions@berkshirecenter.org
www.berkshirecenter.org

Gary Shaw, Program Director
Margaret Katz, Admissions Director
Michael McManmon, Executive Director
A highly individualized postsecondary program for learning disabled young adults 18-30. Provides job placement services and follow-ups; college support; money management and social skills. Residential students share an apartment and have their own room. They learn independent living skills and leisure skills. Clinically, each student has individual and group therapy. Psychiatric consultation is available as well as medication supervision if necessary.

6806 Eagle Pond Rehabilitation And Living Center
PO Box 208
South Dennis, MA 02660
508-385-6034
FAX: 508-385-7064
www.eaglepond.com

Paul Marchwat, Administrator
Ellen Reil, Marketing Director
Michael Gallagher, Executive Director
Eagle Pond accomodates 142 residents. Medicare and Medicaid certified as well as being accredited by the Joint Comission (formerly (JCAHO) which enables us to contract with many insurance companies.

6807 FOR Community Services
75 Litwin Lane
Chicopee, MA 01020
413-592-6142
FAX: 413-598-0478
e-mail: ggolash1@aol.com

Gina M Golash, Executive Director/President
Providing a world of meaning for individuals with developmental disabilities throughout Western Massachusetts since 1967.

6808 Fairlawn Rehabilitation Hospital
189 May Street
Worcester, MA 01602
508-791-6351
FAX: 508-753-2087
www.fairlawnrehab.org

Peter Mantegazza, President/CEO
Arthur Pappas, Chairman Of The Board Of Direct.
Offers comprehensive rehabilitation on both an inpatient and outpatient basis. Specialty programs include: head injury, spinal cord injury, young/senior stroke, oncology, geriatrics and orthopedics.

6809 Greenery Extended Care Center: Worcester
59 Acton Street
Worcester, MA 01604
508-791-3147
800-633-0887
FAX: 508-753-6267

Joel Stevens, Administrator
173 beds offering complex care, extended rehabilitation and neurobehavioral intervention. Offering life care homes and Nursing home services. Specialties include life events and physical care, long term and home health care, and nursing homes and nursing care communities.

6810 Greenery Rehabilitation & Skilled Nursing Center
23 Issac Street
Po Box 1330
Middleboro, MA 02346
508-947-9295
FAX: 508-947-7974
201 beds offering programs of active/acute rehabilitation, cognitive rehabilitation, respiratory care and short-term evaluations.

6811 Harrington House Nursing And Rehabilitation Center
160 Main Street
Walpole, MA 02081
508-660-3080
FAX: 508-660-1634
www.harringtonrehab.com

Anthony Lacke, Administrator
Accomodates 90 residents. Our state-of-the-art center offers post-accute services including rehabilitation and medical management. Our center also provides a long term care program including hospice services.

6812 HealthSouth Rehabilitation Hospital Of Western Massachusetts
14 Chestnut Plaza
Ludlow, MA 01056
413-589-7581
FAX: 413-589-1688
www.healthsouthrehab.org

Bonnie Breit, Outpatient Services
A 53-bed acute Rehabilitation Hospital. The facility has been operating for 14 years and has provided rehabilitative care to patients and families in the greater Springfield area with an outstanding reputation for attention to detail and compassion. Because rehabilitation is HeathSouth's primary focus, our expert staff dedicates all their skills and knowledge to a single goal-improving each patient's functional abilities through intensive, individualized theraputic services.

6813 Holiday Inn Boxborough Woods

242 Adams Place
Boxborough, MA 01719
978-263-8701
800-465-4329
FAX: 978-263-0518
e-mail: box_sales@fine-hotels.com
www.holiday-inn.com

Kathleen Kelly, Director Sales
Marcel Girard, Manager
Located on 35 acres of wooded countryside just off I-495 at exit #28. Minutes from the Mass Turnpike, Route 2, 290 and 9. Conference center located on main level with 30,000 square feet of meeting space. Guest rooms feature two-line telephones, voice mail and dataports, irons and ironing boards, hair dryers and coffemakers. $129-$159.
$129 - $159

6814 Kolburne School

343 NM Southfield Road
New Marlborough, MA 01230
413-229-8787
FAX: 413-229-7708
e-mail: kgreco@kolburne.net

Jeane K Weinstein, MA, Executive Director
Neil Berger, PhD, MS, Administrative Director
John DeAngelo MEd, Director Of Human Resources
A family owned residential treatment center offering psychiatric clinics and retirement therapeutic services, special education and vocational programs iwth campuses and community based group homes.

6815 Lifeworks Employment Services

588 Pleasant Street
Norwood, MA 02062
781-769-1212
FAX: 781-551-0045
e-mail: able@lifeworksma.org
www.lifeworksma.org

Bill Abel, President
Dan Burke, Vice President
Providing homes, jobs, education and supportive living for people with developmental disabilities.

6816 Massachusetts Eye and Ear Infirmary & Vision Rehabilitation Center

243 Charles Street
Boston, MA 02114
617-523-7900
FAX: 617-573-4178
TTY:617-523-5498
www.meei.harvard.edu

Joel Kraut MD FACS, Medical Director
Pat McCabe MPH, Director
Paulette Demors-Turco, Associate Director
Visual rehabilitation encompasses a low vision rehabilitation evaluation, occupational therapy evaluation (with home visit if necessary), and social service evaluation.

6817 New England Center for Children

33 Turnpike Road
Southborough, MA 01772
508-481-1015
FAX: 508-485-3421
e-mail: cwelch@necc.org
www.necc.org

Vincent Strully, Executive Director
Catherine Welch, Director Admissions
A comprehensive year-round program for students with autism and PDD who require a highly specialized educational and behavior management program. Students are from all over the country and receive intensive, positive, behavioral counseling and social skills training free of aversive treatment and excessive medication.

6818 New Medico Rehabilitation and Skilled Nursing Center at Lewis Bay

89 Lewis Bay Road
Hyannis, MA 02601
508-775-7601
FAX: 508-790-4239

Edmund Steinle, Executive Director
Post acute rehabilitation services.

6819 Protestant Guild Learning Center

411 Waverly Oaks Road
Waltham, MA 02452
781-893-6000
FAX: 781-893-1171
e-mail: admin@protestantguild.org
www.protestantguild.org

Deborah Rossery, Executive Director
Marc De Chabert, Admissions Director
Pam Grath, Religious Leader
Offers services for the diagnostically disabled children and adolescents with ages 6-22 years with health, counseling, educational, recreational, rehabilitation, computer training and professional training services.

6820 Shaughnessy-Kaplan Rehabilitation Hospital

Dove Avenue
Salem, MA 01970
978-745-9003
FAX: 978-740-4730
e-mail: skrhinfo@partners.org
www.shaughnessy-kaplan.org

Anthony Sciola, President/CEO
A 160-bed private, non-profit hospital. We have been providing care for residents of greater North Shore communities since 1975. Shaughnessy has 120 long-term care hospital beds and a 40-bed transitional care unit sometimes referred to as a skilled nursing facility.

6821 Son-Rise Program

2080 S Undermountain Road
Sheffield, MA 01257
413-229-2100
FAX: 413-229-3202
e-mail: correspondence@option.org
www.autismtreatmentcenter.org

Glenna Klein, Publicist
THe Son-Rise Program is a powerful, effective and totally unique treatment for children and adults challengedby Autism, Autuism Spectrum Disorders, Pervasive Developmental Disorder (PDD), Asperger's Syndrome and other developmental difficulties.

6822 Southern Worcester County Rehabilitation Inc.

44 Morris Street
Webster, MA 01570
508-943-0700
FAX: 508-949-6129
e-mail: swcrc@swcrcinc.org
www.swcrcinc.org

J Thomas Amick, Executive Director
Provides day habilitation services, residential services, evaluation and personal adjustment training, sheltered employment, supported employment services, supported work services for individuals with mental health problems. Serves the physically disabled, developmentally disabled, mental health and mental retardation. Vocational services and job placement programs are available as well.

6823 Tufts-New England Medical Center

Vision Rehabilitation Service
750 Washington Street
Boston, MA 02111
617-636-5000
800-231-3316
FAX: 617-636-4658
e-mail: eli@vision.eri.harvard.edu
www.nemc.org

Eli Peli Od, Director Vision Rehabilitation
Maria Mercuri OD, Optometrist
Offers services for the legally blind, visually impaired, mentally retarded blind and more with health, counseling, educational, recreational, rehabilitation, computer training and professional training services.

6824 Vinfen Corporation

950 Cambridge Street
Cambridge, MA 02141
617-441-1800
877-284-6336
FAX: 617-441-1858
www.vinfen.org

Gary W Lamson, President/CEO

A private, nonprofit company, Vinfen Corporation is the largest human services provider in Massachusetts. Vinfen offers clinical, educational, residential and support services to individuals of all ages with mental illness and or mental retardation, who also may have another disability (e.g. substance abuse, homelessness, AIDS). The company also trains professionals in the mental health field and helps consumers to learn to live in community-based settings at the highest levels.

6825 Visiting Nurse Association of North Shore

5 Federal Street
Danvers, MA 01923
978-777-6100
800-728-1862
FAX: 978-777-6517
www.vnacarenetwork.org

Susan Comparone, President
Elaine Kahigian, Manager
Home health services including nurses, physical, occupational and speech therapy, home health aides and more. Special programs include nutrition counseling, IV care, pediatric therapy, HIV/AIDS services and wound management. Provides services 7 days a week, 365 days a year and we accept Medicare, Medicaid and most HMO's and health insurers.

6826 Weldon Center for Rehabilitation

233 Carew Street
Springfield, MA 01104
413-748-6800
FAX: 413-748-6806
www.mercycares.com

Dr. James Lomastro, Vice President
One of the most vital, necessary health resources in the region by helping thousands of people toward restored health and independence. A comprehensive, integrated, non-profit facility offering inpatient, outpatient, day rehabilitation and pediatric services on one site.

6827 Youville Hospital & Rehab Center

1575 Cambridge Street
Cambridge, MA 02138
617-876-4344
FAX: 617-547-5501

T Richard Quigley, President
Daniel Leahey, Chief Executive Officer
Meets the long and short term health care and rehabilitation needs of patients who are physically disabled and chronically ill. Strives to develop and maintain health as a human right on physical, social, vocational and spiritual levels. The ultimate goal of the hospital is to treat and assist each individual patient in reaching his or her optimal level of living. Services include: stroke, brain injury, spinal cord trauma, orthopedic disabilities and more.

Michigan

6828 Botsford Center For Rehabilitation & Health Improvement-Redford

26905 Grand River Avenue
Redford, MI 48240
313-537-1100
877-442-7900
FAX: 313-537-1695
e-mail: info@botsfordsystem.org
www.botsfordsystem.org

Allen Zieger, Executive Director
A 20 bed inpatient physical rehabilitation unit, servicing individuals who have experienced a stroke, amputation, orthopedic fracture, or other neurological impairment.

6829 Chelsea Community Hospital Rehabilitation Unit

775 S Main Street
Chelsea, MI 48118
734-475-4040
FAX: 734-475-4102
www.cch.org

Sally Flack, Rehab Program Coordinator
Jackie Dalton, Neuro Rehab Services
A private, non-profit, acute care facility that combines the best of small town values with national standards of healthcare excellance. The hospital has a 19-bed acute care inpatient rehabilitation unit with comprehensive outpatient programs, including a coordinated brain injury program.

6830 Clare Branch

790 Industrial Drive
Clare, MI 48617
989-386-7707
888-773-7664
FAX: 989-386-2199
e-mail: mail@mmionline.com
www.mmionline.org

Cris Zeigler, Executive Director
MMI will strive to be the premier provider of person-centered services to people with barriers to employment. We will connect individuals with community resources that provide mutual benefit to them and to the community. MMI will be known for excellence in service provision, ethical business practices, a quality work environment, and for providing services that enhance the dignity and value of the people we serve.

6831 Clarkston Spec Healthcare Center

4800 Clintonville Road
Clarkston, MI 48346
248-674-0903
800-837-1913
FAX: 248-674-3431

Margaret Canny, Administrator
120 beds offering active/acute rehabilitation, complex care, day treatment, extended rehabilitation, neurobehavioral intervention and short-term evaluation.

6832 DMC Health Care Center-Novi

42005 W 12 Mile Road
Novi, MI 48377
248-305-7575
FAX: 248-347-4578
www.dmc.org

Helene Rimer, Intake Coordinator
James Cole, Executive Director
The Detroit Medical Center's record of service has provided medical excellence throughout the history of the Metropolitan Detroit area. From the founding of the Children's Hospital in 1886, to the creation of the first mechanical heart at Harpers Hospital 50 years ago, to our compassion for the underdeserved, our legacy of caring is unmatched.

6833 Eight CAP, Inc. Head Start

904 Oak Drive
Turk Lake
Greenville, MI 48838
616-754-9315
FAX: 616-754-9310

Ralph Loeschner, Executive Director
Nancy Secor, Contact
Post accute rehabilitation programs.

6834 Greater Detroit Agency for the Blind and Visually Impaired

16625 Grand River Avenue
Detroit, MI 48227
313-272-3900
FAX: 313-272-6893
e-mail: info@gdabvi.org
www.gdabvi.org

Gail L McEntee, Executive Director
Offers services for seniors 60 and over who are legally blind. Also provides eye health information, counseling, education and rehabilitation services.

6835 Hope Network Rehabilitation Services

Hope Network
1490 E Beltline Avenue SE
Grand Rapids, MI 49506
616-940-0040
FAX: 616-940-8151
e-mail: jbaker@hopenetwork.org
www.hopenetworkrehab.org

Margaret Kroese, Executive Director
Mary Baily, Admissions Manager
Amanda Lake, Admissions Manager

An office of Hope Network, one of the largest, private, nonprofit organizations of its kind in Michigan. The purpose is to assist people with brain injuries and/or physical disabilities in achieving an optimal level of self-determination, dignity, and independence as they develop and attain goals to overcome environmental barriers and mobilize adaptive skills.

6836 Lakeland Center
26900 Franklin Road
Southfield, MI 48033
248-350-8070
FAX: 248-350-8078
e-mail: peggys@thelakelandcenter.net
www.thelakelandcenter.net

Harold Rodner, Medical Director
Santhosh Madhavan, Director Physical Medicine
Gary Yashinsky, Associate Medical Director
Subacute rehabilitation program directed toward those with severe neurologic diagnoses, ie: TBI, cerebral aneurysm, anoxic encephalopathy, CVA and cerebral hemorrhage, orthopedic injuries, and spinal cord injury. Subacute rehabilitation is provided for those who recover slowly and require individualized treatment plans. Residential program available as well.

6837 Mary Free Bed Rehabilitation Hospital
235 Wealthy Street SE
Grand Rapids, MI 49503
616-242-0481
800-528-8989
FAX: 616-493-9666
e-mail: info@maryfreebed.com
www.maryfreebed.com

Meg Derrer, Marketing Director/Webmaster
Bill Blessing, President
Mary Free Bed Rehabilitation Hospital exists to restore independence, hope, and freedom through rehabilitation to people with disabilities. Mary Free Bed will be the dominant, high-value provider of an integrated system of rehabilitation services in Michigan for children and adults with the following conditions: spinal injuries, brain injuries, strokes, orthopedic injuries, neurological conditions, congenital abnormalities, pain and amputation.

6838 Michigan Career And Technical Institute
11611 Pine Lake Road
Plainwell, MI 49080
269-664-4461
877-901-7360
FAX: 269-664-9850

Dennis Hart, Executive Director
A residential vocational training center for adults with physical, mental or emotional disabilities.

6839 Michigan Commission for the Blind Training Center
1541 Oakland Drive
Kalamazoo, MI 49008
269-337-3875
FAX: 269-337-3872
www.mcb1.gov

Melody Lindsey, Director
Residential facility that provides instruction to legally blind adults in Braille, computers, handwriting, keyboarding, cane travel, adaptive kitchen skills, daily living, industrial arts and also crafts. Clients may also learn to use a variety of adaptive devices such as raised dot timers and watches, hand tools, talking calculators, tape recorders, reading machines and computers. Special training is also offered in vending stand operation, college preparation and job seeking skills.

6840 Mid-Michigan Industries
2426 Parkway Drive
Mt Pleasant, MI 48858
989-773-6918
888-773-7664
888-773-7664
FAX: 989-773-1317
e-mail: mail@mmionline.com
www.mmionline.com

Alan Schilling, President
Andrea Christopher, Director Admissions
Chris Zeigler, VP Operations
Providing jobs and training for persons with barriers to employment. Services include vocational evaluation, job placement, supported employment, work services, prevocational training and case management

6841 New Medico Community Re-Entry Service
216 St Marys Lake Road
Battle Creek, MI 49017
FAX: 269-962-2241

James Rekshan, Executive Director

6842 Sanilac County Community Mental Health
171 Dawson Street
Sandusky, MI 48471
810-648-0330
888-225-4447
888-225-4447
FAX: 810-648-0319
e-mail: deanr@sanilacmentalhealth.org

Roger Dean MD, Executive Director
Post-acute rehabilitation facility and programs.

6843 Special Tree Rehabilitation System
1640 Axtell Drive
Troy, MI 48084
248-649-0101
800-649-5011
FAX: 248-649-5445
e-mail: info@specialtree.com
www.specialtree.com

Joseph Richert, Founder
Margo Riza, Manager
Special Tree exists to provide hope, encouragement, and expertise for people who have experienced life-altering changes. Our team approach to rehabilitation, custom designed for each person's needs and goals, offers these individuals the best opportunity for healing and recovery.

6844 Thumb Industries
1263 Sand Beach Road
Bad Axe, MI 48413
989-269-9229
FAX: 989-269-2587

Rhonda Wisenbaugh, Executive Director
Provides job training and employment for disabled persons. Vocational rehabilitation agency, manufactures household furnishings, direct mail advertising service.

6845 Visually Impaired Center
1422 W Court Street
Flint, MI 48503
810-235-2544
FAX: 810-235-2597
e-mail: info@vicflint.org
www.vicflint.org

Jared D. Whittey, Board President
Aaron Whitson, Board Vice President
Ethel Mason, Board Treasurer
Committed to developing resources and collaborative programs as well as providing services that enable independent life for people with vision loss. Services include: Information and referals, assessments of needs, peer support groups, training by a Rehabilitation teacher of the blind and visually impaired, independent living skills, computer skills, training by an Orientation and Mobility Specialist, safe traveling skills, Diabetes management/education.
a pages

6846 Welcome Homes Retirement Community for the Visually Impaired
1953 Monroe Avenue NW
Grand Rapids, MI 49505
616-363-9088
888-939-9292
888-939-9292
FAX: 616-363-3099
e-mail: info@welcomehomes.org

Kathy Higgins, CEO
Offers services for the totally blind, legally blind, visually impaired, mentally retarded blind and more with health, counseling, educational, recreational, rehabilitation, computer training and professional training services.

6847 William H Honor Rehabilitation Center Henry Ford Wyanclotte Hospital
Henry Ford Health System
2333 Biddle Street
Wyandotte, MI 48192 734-246-6000
FAX: 734-246-6926
www.henryfordwyandotte.com

Denise Dailing, Administration Leader/rehabilita
James Sexton, Chief Executive Officer
Henry Ford, Owner
Henry Ford Wyandotte Hospital offers an array of educational programs, health screenings, and support groups.

Minnesota

6848 Industries
500 Walnut Street S
Mora, MN 55051 320-679-2354
FAX: 320-679-2355
e-mail: lmorrison@industriesinc.org

Lee Morrison, Executive Director
Nonprofit organization that does vocational assessment and training for people with disabilities.

6849 Shriners Hospitals for Children: Twin Cities
2025 E River Parkway
Minneapolis, MN 55414 612-596-6100
888-293-2832
888-293-2832
FAX: 612-339-5954
www.shrinershq.org

Lynn Shelander, Public Relations Specialist
Charles Lobeck, Director
Shriners Hospital for Children-Twin Cities offers quality orthopedic medical care at no cost. Shriners Hospitals provide inpatient and outpatient services, surgery, casts, braces, artificial limbs, X-rays and physical and occupational therapy to any child under 18 who may benefit from treatment. To obtain an application, call toll free at (888)293-2832.

6850 Vision Loss Resources
1936 Lyndale Avenue S
Minneapolis, MN 55403 612-871-2222
FAX: 612-872-0189
www.visionlossresources.com

Steven Fischer, Executive Director
Frank Alden, Low Vision Specialist
Offers services for the totally blind, legally blind, visually impaired, and more with health, counseling, educational, recreational, rehabilitation, computer training and professional training services.

Mississippi

6851 Addie McBryde Rehabilitation Center for the Blind
PO Box 5314
Jackson, MS 39296 601-364-2700
FAX: 601-364-2677
e-mail: kbrown@mdrs.ms.us
www.mdrs.state.ms.us/client/addie_2.asp

Karen Brown, Director
Karen Wallace, Assistant Director
Rosie Gibson, Assistant Director
Offers services for the totally blind, legally blind, visually impaired, mentally retarded blind and more with health, counseling, educational, recreational, rehabilitation, computer training services and orientation and mobility.

6852 Mississippi Methodist Rehabilitation Center
1350 E Woodrow Wilson Avenue
Jackson, MS 39216 601-981-2611
800-223-6672
FAX: 601-364-3465
www.mmrcrehab.org

Mark A Adams, President/CEO
Rebuild lives that have been broken by disabilities and impairments from serious illness or severe injury. The challenge is to help patients regain abilities, restore function and movement, and renew emotionally. It features personal rehabilitation treatment plans administered by specialized teams of health care professionals through a variety of outpatient programs, treatments and other services.

Missouri

6853 Alpine North Nursing and Rehabilitation Center
4700 NW Cliff View Drive
Kansas City, MO 64150 816-741-5105
FAX: 816-746-1301

Sharon Garcia, Clinical Director
Bob Richard, Administrator
Postacute rehabilitation program.

6854 Christian Hospital Northeast
11133 Dunn Road
Saint Louis, MO 63136 314-653-5000
FAX: 314-653-4130
www.christianhospital.org

Paul Macek, Chief Executive Officer
Ron McMullen, President
A non-profit organization, a 493 bed acute care facility on 28 acres. Christian Hospital has more then 600 physicians on staff and a diverse workforce of more then 2,5000 health-care professionals who are dedicated to providing the absolute best care with the latest technology and medical advances.

6855 Integrated Health Services of St. Louis at Gravois
10954 Kennerly Road
Saint Louis, MO 63128 314-843-4242
FAX: 314-843-4031

Lisa Niehaus, Administrator
Subacute, skilled and intermediate care; ventilator/tracheostomy management program; wound management program and complex rehabilitation program.

6856 Metropolitan Employment & Rehabilitation Service
M ER S Goodwill
1727 Locust Street
Saint Louis, MO 63103 314-241-3464
FAX: 314-241-9348
e-mail: info@mersgoodwill.org
www.mersgoodwill.org

Joan Newman, Chiarperson
Paul Kravitz, 1st Vice Chairperson
Jack Minner, 2nd Vice Chairperson
Vocational rehabilitation, primarily with the disabled, skills training and placement services.

6857 Missouri Easter Seal Society: Southeast Region
13975 Manchester Road
Manchester, MO 63011 636-227-6030
800-664-5025
FAX: 636-779-2270
www.mo.easter-seals.org
The mission of the Easter Seal Society is to work with individuals, their families and the community to enhance the independence and quality of life for persons with disabilities.

6858 Poplar Bluff RehabCare Program
Lucy Lee Hospital
2620 Westwood Boulevard
Poplar Bluff, MO 63901 573-785-7721
FAX: 573-686-5987

Jim Martin, Program Manager
Chris Murray, Care Coordinator
Darlene Hill, Care Admissions Coordinator
Provides physical medicine and rehabilitation to individuals with a physically limiting condition. The program is designed to help individuals function as independently as possible by maximizing their strength and abilities.

6859 Service Club for the Blind
3719 Watson Road
Saint Louis, MO 63109
314-647-3306
FAX: 314-644-2806

Kathleen Demsky, President
Joann Hall, Office Assistant
Kathleen Demsky, Office Assistant
Offers services for the totally blind, legally blind, visually impaired, mentally retarded blind and more with health, counseling, educational, recreational, rehabilitation, computer training and professional training services.

6860 Shriners Hospitals for Children St. Louis
2001 S Lindbergh Boulevard
Saint Louis, MO 63131
314-432-3600
800-850-2960
FAX: 314-432-2930
www.shrinershq.org/hospitals/st.louis

Carolyn P Golden, Administrator
Tammy M Dugan, Director Community Relations
Alice Woodruff, Executive Assistant
Medical care is provided free of charge for children 18 and under with orthopaedic conditions.

6861 St. Louis Society for the Blind and Visually Impaired
8770 Manchester Road
Saint Louis, MO 63144
314-968-9000
FAX: 314-968-9003
e-mail: socscrv@slsbvi.org
www.slsbvi.org

David C Ekin, President
Brenda Dunn, Client Services Coordinator
Offers vision rehabilitation services for the totally blind, legally blind, visually impaired, including counseling, educational, recreational, rehabilitation, computer training and professional training services. Low vision aids and appliance available through low vision clinic by appointment.

6862 Truman Neurological Center
15600 Woods Chapel Road
Kansas City, MO 64139
816-373-5060
FAX: 816-373-5787
e-mail: info@tnccommunity.com
www.tnccommunity.com

James Landrum, Executive Director
A licensed habilitation center established for the purpose of assisting persons with developmental disabilities and/or mental retardation. The minimum age is 18. Residential care is provided in four group homes in the community licensed by the DMH and CARF accredited.

6863 Visual Independence Program
Eye Foundation of Kansas City
2300 Holmes Street
Kansas City, MO 64108
816-404-1780
FAX: 816-404-1786
www.umkc-efkc.org

Camille Matta MD, Medical Director
Brendan Smith OTR, Program Director
Program offers in home rehabilitation services to older adults with visual impairments including training in use of magnifying devices for reading and other activities of daily living. Specialized rehabilitation program for persons with visual impairment secondary to stroke or head trauma.

Montana

6864 Benefis Healthcare
1101 26th Street S
Great Falls, MT 59405
406-455-5000
FAX: 406-455-2110
e-mail: benefis@benefis.org
www.benefis.org

John Goodnow, President/CEO
Laura Goldhahn-Konen, Chief Operation Officer
Benefis Healthcare is a not-for-profit community asses governed by a 15-member local board of directors. Benefis is locally owned and controlled. Benefis is a Level II trauma center- one of only 4 in the state and 107 in the country.

6865 Disability Services Division Of Montana Department Of Public Health
111 North Sanders Street
Helena, MT 59604
406-444-2590
FAX: 406-444-0230
e-mail: dphhs@mt.gov
www.dphhs.state.mt.us/dsd

Joe A Mathews, Administrator
Sandi Gory, Administrative Assistant
Janice Frisch, Chief Management Operations
Responsible for coordinating, developing and implementing comprehensive programs to assist Montanans with disabilities with activities of daily living, community base services and coordinated programs of habilitation, rehabilitation and independent living.

Nebraska

6866 Career Achievement Center
PO Box 83589
Lincoln, NE 68501
402-467-5097
800-742-7653
FAX: 402-476-5180
www.careerachievement.com

Susie Feistner, Executive Director
Richard Peters, Owner
Post accute rehabilitation services.

6867 Las Vegas Healthcare And Rehabilitation Center
2832 S Maryland Parkway
Las Vegas, NV 89109
702-735-5848
800-326-6888
FAX: 702-735-0383
www.lasvegaskindred.com

Rick Eddins, Manager
Accomodates 79 residents. Serving the community for approximately 40 years. Located in close proximity to local hospitals and surrounded by medical complexes, out center offers both short-term rehabilitation and long term.care.

6868 Sierra Pain Institute
265 Golden Lane
Reno, NV 89502
775-323-7092
FAX: 775-323-5259

Lyle Smith, Owner
The program consists of a medically supervised outpatient program managed by an interdisciplinary team with input from specialties of Pain Medicine, Physical Therapy and Occupational Science. The format insures that each patient receives the full range of behavioral techniques in a well-integrated, individually tailored therapeutic regimen.

New Hampshire

6869 Crotched Mountain Adult Brain Injury Center
Crotched Mountain Foundation
1 Verney Drive
Greenfield, NH 03047
603-547-3311
800-966-2672
FAX: 603-547-3232
e-mail: admissions@crotchedmountain.org
www.crotchedmountain.org

Brant A Elkind, Director
Rita Phinney, Admissions Director
John Young, Registrar
Adult Brain Injury Center provides sub-acute rehabilitative services and individualized care to survivors of acquired (including traumatic) brain injury. Ambulatory and non-ambulatory adults are served. Ages range from 18-59, the staff to client ratio is 3:1 and services are provided by experienced interdisciplinary clinical and therapeutic teams. Crotched Mountain is a licensed Special Hospital providing 24 hour medical coverage and skilled nursing. Clients reside in semi-private rooms w/superv

6870 Department of Physical Medicine and Rehabilitation
Exeter Hospital
5 Alumni Drive
Exeter, NH 03833
603-778-7311
FAX: 603-778-6671
www.foreveryday.com

Kevin Callahan, President/CEO
Offers patient treatment, committed to enhancing the lives of individuals with short and long term physically disabling conditions.

6871 Farnum Rehabilitation Center
580 Court Street
Keene, NH 03431
603-354-6630
FAX: 603-355-2078

Susan Loughrey, Program Director
Judy Bell, Manager
Offers rehabilitation services, occupational therapy, physical therapy and more for the physically challenged individual.

6872 Hackett Hill Nursing Center and Integrated Care
191 Hackett Hill Road
Manchester, NH 03102
603-668-8161
FAX: 603-622-2584

Claudia Gallo, Case Manager
Brett Lennerton, Administrator
A 68-bed certified nursing home.Postacute rehabilitation program.

6873 New Hampshire Rehabilitation and Sports Medicine
Catholic Medical Center
769 South Main Street
Suite 201
Manchester, NH 03102
603-641-6700
800-437-9666
FAX: 603-668-5348

Heidi George, Director
Victor Carbone, Manager
A specialized facility for comprehensive rehabilitation for individuals who have been injured or have a disability.

6874 New Medico, Highwatch Rehabilitation Center
Highwatch Road
Center Ossipee, NH 03814
FAX: 603-539-8888

William Burke, Executive Director
Post-acute rehabilitation service.

6875 Northern New Hampshire Mental Health and Developmental Services
87 Washington Street
Conway, NH 03818
603-447-3347
FAX: 603-447-8893
www.nnhmhds.org

Stanley Marsden, Director
Provides mental health and developmental services to northern New Hampshire, including early intervention, elderly services, residential program, outpatient services, employee assistance programs, inpatient services, etc.

6876 The Mental Health Center: Riverside Courtyard
3 12th Street
Berlin, NH 03570
603-752-7404
FAX: 603-752-5194

Charles Cotton, Executive Director
A center to help people that have mental disabilities.

New Jersey

6877 All Garden State Physical Therapy
750 Broadway
Paterson, NJ 07514
973-345-1312
FAX: 973-742-0669
e-mail: agspt750@yahoo.com

Carlos Chaparro, General Manager
Maria Maval, Manager
Post-acute rehabilitation program.

6878 Bancroft NeuroHealth
425 Kings Hwyighway
Haddonfield, NJ 08033
856-429-0010
800-774-5516
FAX: 856-429-1613
e-mail: inquiry@bancroft.org
www.bancroft.org

Tom Pergolin, President
Kathy M. Ross, Vice President
Michelle Stewart, Director Communciations
Private, not-for-profit organization serving people with disabilities since 1883. Based in Haddonfield, New Jersey, help more than 1000 children and adults with autism, developmental disabilities, brain injuries, and other neurological impairments. Operates more than 140 sites throughout the U.S. and abroad.

6879 Daughters of Miriam Center/The Gallen Institute
Po Box 2698
155 Hazel Street
Clifton, NJ 07015
973-772-3700
FAX: 973-253-5389
e-mail: administration@daughtersofmiriamcenter.org
www.daughtersofmiriamcenter.o rg

Fred Feinstein, Executive Director
Dedicated to providing the highest quality care, the Center has far exceeded a stereotypical nursing home by offering a continuum of care environment, making us a leader in Jewish eldercare.

6880 Devereux Center in New Jersey
286 Mantua Grove Road
Bldg, #4
West Depford, NJ 08096
856-384-9680
FAX: 856-384-6742
www.devereux.org

Vincent Winterling, Director
Maureen Walsh, Executive Director
Carol Poirier, Admissions Assistant

Serves emotionally disturbed females, ages 5-21, who have affective disorders, bi-polar disorders, adjustment reactions, behavioral disorders, specific developmental disorders, identity disorders, attention deficit disorders, schizoid disorders, anxiety disorders, enuresis, runaway behavior, substance abuse, in remission and personality disturbances. The center offers 95-100 full-time staff including, teachers, administrators, counselors, therapists, recreation staff and support services.

6881 Integrated Health Services of New Jersey at Somerset Valley
1621 Route 22 West
Bound Brook, NJ 08805 732-469-2000
FAX: 732-469-8917

Carolyn Allen, Executive Director
Janice Vyzas, Social Work Director
Subacute rehabilitation program, long term care, respite care.

6882 Ladacain Network
Schroth School & Technical Education Center
1701 Kneeley Boulevard
Wanamassa, NJ 07712 732-493-5900
FAX: 732-493-5980
www.ladacin.org

Patricia Carlesimo, Executive Director
Provides an array of services and programs specifically for children and adults with developmental and physical disabilities. Services include approved Department of Education school programs; adult education and training; vocational training, personal care assistance services, in-home and Saturday respite; child care programs, housing opportunities, and more.

6883 Lourdes Regional Rehabilitation Center
Our Lady of Lourdes Medical Center
1600 Haddon Avenue
Camden, NJ 08103 856-757-3548
FAX: 856-968-2522
e-mail: info@lourdesnet.org
www.lourdesmed.org

Mark T Bateman, Chief Administrative Officer
Susan Cleveland, Manager
Bernadette Summer, Outpatient Scheduling Coord.
We serve the healthcare needs of the South Jersey community with compassion, integrity, and a commitment to those who are in need.

6884 Mt. Carmel Guild
1160 Raymond Boulevard
Newark, NJ 07102 973-596-3854

Edda Stewart, Coordinator
Anita Holland, Religious Leader
Offers services for the totally blind, legally blind, visually impaired, mentally retarded blind and more with health, counseling, educational, recreational, rehabilitation, computer training and professional training services.

6885 Pediatric Rehabilitation Department, JFK Medical Center
65 James Street
Edison, NJ 08818 732-321-7000
FAX: 732-548-7751
www.jfkmc.org

Patricia Munday MD, Director Pediatric Rehab
Comprehensive interdisciplinary, family focused outpatient pediatric rehabilitation services including evaluation and individual and group treatment programs for children birth-21.

6886 REACH Rehabilitation Program: Leader Nursing and Rehabilitation Center
550 Jessup Road
Paulsboro, NJ 08066 856-848-9551

Karen Fattore, Case Manager
Anthony Stenson, Administrator
Postacute rehabilitation program.

6887 REACH Rehabilitation and Catastrophic Long-Term Care
1180 Route 22
Mountainside, NJ 07092 908-654-0020

Linda Sweeney, Program Director
Archie Ordana, Manager
Postacute rehabilitation program.

6888 Rehabilitation Specialists
18-01 Pollitt Drive
Suite 1A
Fairlawn, NJ 07410 973-636-9366
800-441-7488
FAX: 201-478-4201
e-mail: pres@rehab-specialist.com
www.rehab-specialist.com

Carol Sloman, Admissions Coordinator
Dawn Thomas, Executive Director
Rehabilitation Specialists, founded in 1983, is a quality, cost effective community re-entry center treating individuals with acquired brain injury. A non clinical environment based in the community is utilized that offers professional services enabling participants to learn skills they need to return to a productive life. Both our Day and Residential programming emphases focus on Functional Life Skills, Work Skills and Learning Skills. Each participant's program is tailored to meet their needs.

6889 Summit Ridge Center
20 Summit Street
West Orange, NJ 07052 973-736-2000
FAX: 973-731-4582

Charlene Harn, Admissions/Marketing Director
Chad Murin, Administrator
Offers rehabilitation services, occupational therapy, physical therapy and more for the physically challenged. A 152-bed nursing home.

New Mexico

6890 Lifecourse Rehabilitation Services
525 S Schwartz Drive
Farmington, NM 87401 505-327-3422
FAX: 505-327-6562

Bobi Logsdon RN, Case Manager
Uses a team of professionals to provide a comprehensive rehabilitation program. Accomplishing the best possible physical and cognitive improvement is the aim of the following treatment members: nurses, physical therapists, physicians, speech and occupational therapists, therapeutic recreation specialist. Providing inpatient and out patient services.

6891 Southwest Communication Resource
PO Box 788
Bernalillo, NM 87004 505-867-3396
FAX: 505-867-3398
e-mail: info@abrazosnm.org
www.abrazosnm.org

Norman Segel, Executive Director
Services for infants, children and adults with developmental disabilities in Sandoval County New Mexico.

New York

6892 Bronx Continuing Treatment Day Program
1527 Southern Boulevard
Bronx, NY 10460 718-893-1414
FAX: 718-893-0707

Hermina Torres, Executive Director
Post-acute rehabilitation program.

6893 **Brooklyn Bureau of Community Service**
285 Schermerhorn Street
Brooklyn, NY 11217
718-310-5600
FAX: 718-855-1517
e-mail: info@bbcs.org
www.bbcs.org

Leslie Klein, Director Adult Rehabilitation
Maryclare Scerbo, Director Volunteer Services
Sonea Smith, Executive Director
Offers independent living skills, counseling, work readiness, vocational triening, job placement and job follow-up services to individuals with disabilities (to include individuals with psychiatric, physical, and developmental disabilities). Special programs to move disabled welfare recipients from welfare to work. Publishes a bi-annual newsletter.

6894 **Buffalo Hearing and Speech Center**
50 E North Street
Buffalo, NY 14203
716-885-8318
FAX: 716-885-4229
www.askbhsc.org

Janet Maher, President
Assists individuals with speech, language and/or hearing impairments to achieve maximum communication potential.

6895 **Cora Hoffman Center Day Program**
2324 Forest Avenue
Staten Island, NY 10303
718-815-2182
FAX: 718-815-2182

Kevin Kenney, Executive Director
Post-acute rehabilitation program specializing in Cerebral Palsy. Part of the Cerebral Palsey Association of New York State

6896 **Elmhurst Hospital Center**
79-01 Broadway
Elmhurst, NY 11373
718-334-4000

www.nyc.gov/html/hhc/html/facilities/elmhurst

Chris Constantino, Administrator
Benjamin Chu, Chief Executive Officer
Hospital is comprised of 525 beds and is a Level I Trauma Center, and Emergency Heart Care Stattion and a 911 recieving hospital. It is the premiere health care organization for key areas such as Surgery, Cardiology, Women's health, Pediatrics, Rehabilitation Medicine, Renal and Mental Health Services.

6897 **Federation Employment And Guidance Service (F-E-G-S)**
315 Hudson Street
New York, NY 10013
212-366-8400
FAX: 212-366-8441
e-mail: info@fegs.org
www.fegs.org

Jill Colon-Regus, Rehabilitation Services Director
Loel Tayler, Treatment Programs Director
Rena Moore, Intensive Psychiatric Rehab Prgm
The largest and most diversified private, not-for-profit health related and human service organization in the United States. With operations in over 258 facilities, residences, and off-site locations, F-E-G-S has served more then 2 million people since its inception.

6898 **Flushing Hospital**
4500 Parsons Boulevard
Flushing, NY 11355
718-670-5000
FAX: 718-670-3082
www.flushinghospital.org

David P. Rosen, President And CEO
Bruce J. Flanz, Executive Vice President/COO
Mounir Doss, Executive Vice President/CFO
Offers services for the totally blind, legally blind, visually impaired, mentally retarded blind and more with health, counseling, educational, recreational, rehabilitation, computer training and professional training services.

6899 **Gateway Community Industries Inc.,**
One Amy Kay Parkway
Kingston, NY 12401
845-331-1261
800-454-9295
FAX: 845-331-2112
e-mail: info@gatewayindustries.org
www.gatewayindustries.org

Francoise Dunalsky, President/CEO
Mary Anne Hildebrandt, Rehabilitation Services Director
Darcy McCourt, Residential Services Director
Gateway Community Industries, Inc., founded in 1957, is one of the leading independent not-for-profit vocational rehabilitation and training centers for people with mental and/or physical disabilities. The agency provides comprehensive services in vocational evaluation, job training, job placement, vocational work center employment, supported employment, psychiatric rehabilitation, continuing day treatment, and residential habilitation/rehabilitation.

6900 **Henkind Eye Institute Division of Montefiore Hospital**
3400 Bainbridge Avenue
Bronx, NY 10467
718-920-6244
FAX: 718-920-6244
www.montefiore.org

Lanny M Binstock
Jonathan Hoenig, MD
Offers services for the totally blind, legally blind, visually impaired, mentally retarded blind and more with health, counseling, educational, recreational, rehabilitation, computer training and professional training services. Low vision services offered.

6901 **Industries for the Blind of New York State**
296 Washington Avenue Extension
Albany, NY 12203
518-456-8671
800-421-9010
FAX: 518-456-3587
www.ibnys.org

Richard Healey, President/CEO
Offers services for the totally blind, legally blind, visually impaired, mentally retarded blind and more with health, counseling, educational, recreational, rehabilitation, computer training and professional training services.

6902 **Inpatient Pain Rehabilitation Program**
301 E 17th Street
New York, NY 10003
212-598-6745
FAX: 212-598-6468

William Pinter Phd, Administrative Director
The Inpatient Rehabilitation Program, established in 1983 specializes in the treatment of chronic pain. Our inpatient program is one of the oldest and well established pain programs in the country. It is the only interdisciplinary inpatient pain program in the tri-state area and one of only 20 pain programs in the entire US to have CARF accreditation. Upon completion of an extensive evaluation, patients are admitted for an 18-day inpatient stay.

6903 **Koicheff Health Care Center**
2324 Forest Avenue
Staten Island, NY 10303
718-447-0200
FAX: 718-981-1431

Paul Castello, Clinic Director
Post-accute rehabilitation programs.

6904 **New York-Presbyterian Hospital**
622 W 168th Street
New York, NY 10032
212-305-2500
FAX: 212-305-1017
www.nyp.org

Michael Bradley, Executive Director
Herbert Pardes, Chief Executive Officer
New York Presbyterian Hospital is internationally recognized for its outstanding comprehensive services. Its medical, surgical, and emergency care services provide each patient with the highest possible level of care. In addition, as part of the Hospital's commitment to the total well-being of each patient, it offers a range of specialized services, as well as special healthcare programs for neighboring communities.

6905 **Norman Marcus Pain Institute**
30 E 40th Street
New York, NY 10016
212-532-7999
FAX: 212-532-5957
e-mail: info@nmpi.com
www.nmpi.com

Norman Marcus MD, Medical Director
Brooke Johnson, Manager
We focus on muscles as the cause of most common pains, i.e. back, neck, shoulders, and headaches. We make specific muscle diagnoses and have specific treatments that in many cases will eliminate the need for surgery or relieve the pain. Patients diagnosed with herniated disc, spinal stenosis, rotator cuff tear, impingement syndrome, sciatica, fibromyalgia and headache will generally find relief.

6906 **Pain Alleviation Center**
Comprehensive Pain Management Associates
125 South Service Road
Jericho, NY 11753
516-997-7246
FAX: 516-997-7281
www.paincenter.com

Alex Weingarten, Director
Phillip Fyman, Director
Marisa French, Manager
One of the first pain clinics to gain national accreditation from the Commission on Accreditation of Rehabilitation Facilities. This is due largely to a patient-centered program based on the latest research.

6907 **Pathfinder Village**
3 Chenango Road
Edmeston, NY 13335
607-965-8377
FAX: 607-965-8655
e-mail: info@pathfindervillage.org
www.pathfindervillage.org

Edward Shafer, Chief Executive Officer
Pathfinder Village is a warm, friendly community in the rolling hills of Central New York. Here children and adults with Down Syndrome gain independence, build lasting friendships, become partners in the world and take in all that life has to offer.

6908 **Pilot Industries: Ellenville**
845-331-4300
48 Canal Street
Ellenville, NY 12428
845-647-7711
FAX: 845-647-7711

Peter Pierri, Executive Director
Betty Marks, Plant Manager
Post-accute rehabilitation services.

6909 **Skills Unlimited**
405 Locust Avenue
Oakdale, NY 11769
631-567-3320
FAX: 516-567-3285
e-mail: info@skillsunlimited.org
www.skillsunlimited.org

Richard Kassnove, Executive Director
Our basic goals is to offer persons with disabilities the opportunity to explore and develop their full vocational potential. Our programs are unique in that by offering comprehensive services, individuals are able to deal with many different issues that could potentially affect their vocational success. Any individual that has an impairment that interferes with their ability to work is entitles to the services that we offer.

6910 **United Cerebral Palsy of Western New York**
7 Community Drive
Buffalo, NY 14225
716-894-5399
FAX: 716-894-8257

Virginia C Purcell, Executive Director
Provides comprehensive services, to individuals with disabilities from infancy through adulthood. Also serves people with all types of developmental disabilities as well as providing clinical services to persons with other types of disabilities such as: spinal cord injury, multiple sclerosis, head trauma and others. The center employs over 750 people.

North Carolina

6911 **Center for Vision Rehabilitation**
Academy Eye Associates
3115 Academy Road
Durham, NC 27707
919-493-7456
800-942-1499
FAX: 919-493-1718
e-mail: henry.greene@academyeye.com
www.academyeye.com

Henry A Greene OD, President/Owner
Vision rehabilitation and low-vision care for the visually impaired, post-stroke, head trauma and for neuro-oncology vision complications.

6912 **Diversified Opportunities**
1010 Herring Avenue E
Wilson, NC 27893
252-291-0378
FAX: 252-291-1402
www.diversifiedopportunities.com

Mike Petty, Executive Director
Vocational rehabilitation agency, better outcomes, lower cost, guaranteed performance standards.

6913 **Forsyth Medical Center**
3333 Silas Creek Parkway
Winston Salem, NC 27103
336-718-5000
FAX: 336-718-9250
www.forsythmedicalcenter.org

Mary Jo Weavil, Director
Provides care that is state-of-the-art and second to none, both because of advanced treatments availiable through our clinical research and technology to the academic excellence-and caring nature-of our doctors and nurses.

6914 **Industries of the Blind**
920 W Lee Street
Greensboro, NC 27403
336-274-1591
800-909-7086
FAX: 336-544-3739
www.industriesoftheblind.com

Mark Durge, Director
Glenn Rainey, President
Offers services for the totally blind, legally blind, visually impaired, mentally retarded blind and more with health, counseling, educational, recreational, rehabilitation, computer training and professional training services.

6915 **Johnston County Industries**
912 N Brightleaf Boulevard
Po Box 1688
Smithfield, NC 27577
919-934-0677
FAX: 919-934-1288
www.jcindustries.com

Vicki Shore, Executive Director
JCI is an entrepreneurial not-for-profit corporation dedicated to empowering people with disabilities or disadvantages to succeed through training and employment

6916 **Learning Services: Carolina**
707 Morehead Avenue
Durham, NC 27707
919-688-4444
FAX: 919-419-9951
www.learningservices.com

Brian Preston, Executive Director
Located in an historic neighborhood in the heart of Durham, this campus-style setting offers easy access to resources at 3 outstanding facilities: Duke University, The University of North Carolina at Chapel Hill, and Research Triangle Park. This program provides a range of services and activities that draw upon the many resources availiable in the community.

6917 **LifeSpan**
940 Beaumont Avenue
High Point, NC 27260
336-883-0111
FAX: 336-883-0031
e-mail: lifespanhp@hotmail.com
www.lifespanhp.org

Patti Huggins, Program Director
Provide vocational and enrichment program for adults with developmental disabilities.

6918 **Lions Club Industries for the Blind**
1810 E Main Street
Durham, NC 27703
919-596-8277
FAX: 919-598-1179

William Hudson, Executive Director
Offers services for the totally blind, legally blind, visually impaired, mentally retarded blind and more with health, counseling, educational, recreational, rehabilitation, computer training and professional training services.

6919 **Lions Services Inc.**
4600 N Tryon Street
Charlotte, NC 28213
704-921-1527
FAX: 704-921-1577
e-mail: lsisale@aol.com
www.thomasnet.com

Charles Lamb, Administrator
Jimmy Cranford, President
Offers services for the totally blind, legally blind, visually impaired, mentally retarded blind and more with health, counseling, educational, recreational, rehabilitation, computer training and professional training services.

6920 **Regional Rehabilitation Center Pitt County Memorial Hospital**
2100 Stantonsburg Road
Greenville, NC 27834
252-847-4448
FAX: 252-816-7552
e-mail: mdixon@pcmh.com
www.uhseast.com/rehab

Martha M Dixon, VP General Services
An accredited, comprehensive rehabilitation center-part of a statewide network- and we're the largest such facility in eastern North Carolina. Our service area covers 29 counties, and we offer a complete array of rehabilitation services for patients of all ages. Because the Regional Rehabilitation Center is associated with both Pitt County Memorial Hospital And the Brody School of Medicine at East Carolina University, patients have access to a full range of state of the art medical services.

6921 **Rehab Home Care**
2660 Yonkers Road
Raleigh, NC 27604
800-447-8692
FAX: 919-831-2211

Alan Silver, Chief Executive Officer
Janis Hansen, Chief Operating Officer
A Medicare/Medicaid certified, state-licensed home health agency with emphasis on rehabilitation.

6922 **Thoms Rehabilitation Hospital**
Thoms Rehabilitation Hospital
68 Sweeten Creek Road
Asheville, NC 28803
828-277-4800
FAX: 828-277-4812
www.carepartners.org

Kathi Petersen, Director Planning/Communications
Edgardo Diez MD, Medical Director of Brain Injury
Kathy Price, Director Admissions
Freestanding physical rehabilitation hospital, founded 1938 - 100 beds, including 90 acute and 10 transitional - JCAHO accredited.

6923 **Winston-Salem Industries for the Blind**
7730 N Point Boulevard
Winston Salem, NC 27106
336-759-0551
800-242-7726
FAX: 336-759-0990
e-mail: info@wsifb.com
www.wsifb.com

Daniel Boucher, President
John Googe, Chairman of the Board
Offers services for the totally blind, legally blind, visually impaired, mentally retarded blind and more with health, counseling, educational, recreational, rehabilitation, computer training and professional training services.

Ohio

6924 **Bellefaire Jewish Children's Bureau**
22001 Fairmount Boulevard
Shaker Heights, OH 44118
216-932-2800
800-879-2522
FAX: 216-932-8520
e-mail: yulishj@bellefairejcb.org
www.bellefairejcb.org

Larry Pollock, President
Adam G. Jacobs PhD, Executive Vice President
Residential treatment for ages 12 to 17 1/2 at time of admission offering individualized psychotherapy, special education, and group living for severaly emotionally disturbed children and adolescents. Also offers a variety of other programs including specialized and therapuetic foster care, partial hospitilization, outpatient counseling, home-based intensive counseling and adoption services.

6925 **Christ Hospital Rehabilitation Unit**
2139 Auburn Avenue
Cincinnati, OH 45219
513-585-2000
FAX: 513-585-3300
wwwchristhospitalcincinnati.com

Richard Seim, Senior VP
Regina Hartman, Manager
Patients of this 555-bed, not-for-profit acute care facility receive personalized health care provided by trained specialists using the most sophisticated medical technology available, including state-of-the-art intensive care units, surgical facilities, cardiac catheterization labs, three new electrophysiology labs, and the tristates first positron emission tomography (PET) scanning capabilities.

6926 **Cleveland Society for the Blind**
Cleveland Sight Center
1909 East 101st Street
Po Box 1988
Cleveland, OH 44106
216-791-8118
FAX: 216-791-1101
e-mail: jcarey@clevelandsightcenter.org
www.clevelandsightcenter.org

John David Sidley, Manager Public Education
Michael E Grady, Executive Director
Social, rehabilitation, education and support services for blind and visually impaired children and adults, early intervention program for children birth to age 6, low vision clinic, aid and appliance shop, Braille and taping transcription, training for rehabilitation, orientation, mobility and computer access, employment services and job placement, recreation program, resident camping, talking books, radio reading services, food service training and snack bar employment. Free screening.

6927 **Columbus Speech and Hearing Center**
510 E N Broadway Street
Columbus, OH 43214
614-263-5151
FAX: 614-263-5365
www.columbusspeech.org

Dawn Gleason, President/CEO
Joanne Shannon, Director Vocational Services
Serves persons who have speech-language and hearing challenges. Provides vocational rehabilitation services for individuals who are deaf, hard-of-hearing or deaf-blind.

6928 CommuniCare of Clifton Nursing and Rehabilitation Center
Communi Care Health Services
625 Probasco Street
Cincinnati, OH 45220
513-281-2464
FAX: 513-281-2559

Lisa Renaker, Director of Nursing
Cindy Phillips
Sylvia Salvado, Owner
A long term care facility which specializes in rehabilitation. Offers a full range of rehabilitative services including physical therapy, occupational therapy and speech therapy.

6929 Doctors Hospital
5100 W Broad Street
Columbus, OH 43228
614-544-1000
800-837-7555
FAX: 614-870-9639
www.ohiohealth.com/homedoctors

Janet Hymiak, Executive Director
Kreg Gruber, Chief Executive Officer
We believe our first responsibility is to the patients we serve. We respect the physical, emotional and spiritual needs of our patients and find that compassion is essential to fostering healing and wholeness.

6930 Dodd Hall at the Ohio State University Hospitals
410 W 10th Avenue
Columbus, OH 43210
614-293-3300
800-293-5123
www.medicalcenter.osu.edu

Fred Sanfilippo, Senior Vice President
Peter E Geier, Associate VP
Dennis Smith, Administrator
Dodd Hall is a full service medical rehabilitation hospital offering comprehensive inpatient and outpatient rehabilitation.

6931 Easter Seal Society of Mahoning
National Easter Seals Chicago
299 Edwards Street
Youngstown, OH 44502
330-743-1168
FAX: 330-743-1616
www.mtc.easterseals.com

Kenan J Sklenar, President/CEO
Outpatient medical rehabilitation - physical therapy, speech therapy, occupational therapy, warm-water therapy and adult day services.

6932 Four Oaks Center
623 Dayton Xenia Road
Xenia, OH 45385
937-222-7474

Margareth Conrad, School Administrator
Starts children on the road to discovery by providing a learning environment rich in opportunities and encouragement. The program was designed to give children with delays or disabilities, or those at-risk the extra help needed to develop fully. Any child under the age of six who exhibits developmental delays, handicapping conditions, or is considered at risk may qualify to participate.

6933 Genesis Healthcare System
Rehabilitation Services
800 Forest Avenue
Zanesville, OH 43701
740-454-5000
800-322-4762
FAX: 740-455-7527
e-mail: llynn@genesishcs.org
www.genesishcs.org

Keela Barker, Outpatient Manager
Kim Gates, Manager
Karen Eyberger, Rehab Development Manager
A CARF and JACHO accredited 19-bed rehabilitation facility located within Genesis Healthcare System, a 732 bed, non-profit hospital system, located in Zanesville, Ohio. Freestanding outpatient services, including work hardening, pain management, vocational services, audiology, lymphedema, vestibular rehab, off-the-road driving evals, aquatic therpay, womens health and sports enhancement.

6934 George A Martin Center
3603 Washington Avenue
Cincinnati, OH 45229
513-961-0144
FAX: 513-221-3514

William Poole, Administrator
Offers services for the totally blind, legally blind, visually impaired, mentally retarded blind and more with health, counseling, educational, recreational, rehabilitation, computer training and professional training services.

6935 Grady Memorial Hospital
561 W Central Avenue
Delaware, OH 43015
740-369-8711
800-487-1115
FAX: 740-363-3175
www.gradyhospital.com

Everett Weber, Executive Director
Steve Garlock, Chief Executive Officer
As a progressive healthcare leader, Grady Memorial Hospital is committed to excellence while providing the Deleware community with comprehensive quality service delivered with compassionate, personal care. Our membership in Ohio's largest healthcare system, Ohio Health, enables us to improve access to a broader range of healthcare services, enhance development of new programs and services, and provide a complete continuum of care for patients in the deleware area.

6936 Hamilton Adult Center
3400 Symmes Road
Hamilton, OH 45015
513-867-5970
FAX: 513-874-2977

Donald Musnuff, Executive Director

6937 Holzer Clinic
90 Jackson Pike
Gallipolis, OH 45631
740-446-5411
FAX: 740-446-5532
e-mail: webmaster@holzerclinic.com
www.holzerclinic.com

Wayne Munro, President
John Sullivan, Vice President
Serves medical needs of patients in an 8 county area, including counties in Ohio and West Virginia.

6938 Holzer Clinic Sycamore
Holzer Medical Center
4th Avenue & Sycamore Street
Gallipolis, OH 45631
740-446-5244
FAX: 740-446-5100
www.holzer.org

Johanna Lampert, Program Manager
Lori Cremans, Director
Lamar Wyse, President
Offers an individualized quality comprehensive rehabilitation program for people with disabilities by an interdisciplinary team including physical therapy, occupational, speech, nursing and social services to restore the patient to the highest degree of rehab outcomes attainable.

6939 IKRON Institute for Rehabilitative and Psychological Services
2347 Vine Street
Cincinnati, OH 45219
513-621-1117
FAX: 513-621-2350
www.ikron.org

Randy E Strunk, Executive Director
Ken Carbonell, Fiscal Officer
Ann Webb, Program Director
An accredited mental health facility and a certified rehabilitation center. Through a variety of creative treatment and rehabilitation services, IKRON assists adults with mental health and/or substance abuse problems to attain greater independence, to lead lives of sobriety, to obtain competitive work and live more satisfying lives. IKRON places a strong emphasis on respect and support for persons with problems of adjustment. Special contracts to persons desiring job placement.

6940 Integrated Health Services at Waterford Commons
955 Garden Lake Parkway
Toledo, OH 43614
419-382-2200
FAX: 419-381-0188

Elaine Heatherwick, Administrator
A subacute and rehabilitation program specializing in ventilator weaning and management, I.V. therapeutics and pain management, wound management and subacute rehabilitation.

6941 Lester H Higgins Adult Center
3041 Cleveland Avenue S
Canton, OH 44707
330-484-4814
FAX: 330-484-9416

Dr. Joseph James, Superintendent
Ed Allar, Manager
Post-accute rehabilitation service

6942 Live Oaks Career Development Campus
5936 Buckwheat Road
Milford, OH 45150
513-575-1906
FAX: 513-575-0805

Harold Carr MD, Superintendent
Robin White, President/CEO
Jim Dixon, Principal
Post-accute rehabilitation facility and services.

6943 Metro Health: St. Luke's Medical Center Pain Management Program
2500 Metrohealth Drive
Cleveland, OH 44109
216-778-4428
FAX: 216-368-7140
www.metrohealth.org

Thomas McCafferty, Health Center Director
J Glen Smith, Health Center Director
Ceil Lewandowski, Manager
CARF accredited comprehensive multidisciplinary pain management program.

6944 MetroHealth Medical Center
3395 Scranton Road
Cleveland, OH 44109
216-778-4982
FAX: 216-778-8376
www.metrohealth.org

Henry Manning, Executive Director
Located on the near west side of Cleveland, is a leader in trauma, emergency, and critical care; women's and childrens's services, including high risk obstetrical care and neonatal intensive care; comprehensive medical and surgical subspecialties.

6945 Middletown Regional Hospital: Inpatient Rehabilitation Unit
105 McKnight Drive
Middletown, OH 45044
513-424-2111
800-338-4057
FAX: 513-420-5718
www.middletownhospital.org

Bob Gauder, Program Manager
Douglas McNeill, Chief Executive Officer
Our mission is to serve and help people, improving the status of their health and the quality of thier lives. Our vision is to be the premier integrated delivery system in Southwest Ohio. Our Values are quality, respect, service and teamwork

6946 Newark Healthcare Center
75 McMillen Drive
Newark, OH 43055
740-344-0357
FAX: 740-344-8621
www.newarkhealthcare.com.

Joanne Whiteman, Administrator
Brian Newman, Executive Director
Accomodates 300 residents. We are located in the heart of Newark, Ohio. Newark Healthcare is a 2004 recipient of the American Health Care Association's Quality Award.

6947 Parma Community General Hospital Acute Rehabilitation Center
7007 Powers Boulevard
Parma, OH 44129
440-743-4041
FAX: 440-743-4036
e-mail: pat.ruflin@parmahospital
www.parmahospital.org

Dale Winsberg, Administrative Director
Patricia Ruflin, Chief Executive Officer
The mission of this CARF accredited unit is to provide the most comprehensive, cost-effective, acute rehabilitation program possible in order for every patient and family to adjust to his/her disability and to achieve the maximum potential of independent functioning when returning to community living.

6948 Peter A Towne Physical Therapy Center
447 Nilles Road
Suite 10
Fairfield, OH 45014
513-829-6100
FAX: 513-829-7726
www.townept.com/fairfield

Debbie Wilkerson, Office Manager
Outpatient, private practice physical and occupational therapy. Three other offices in Hamilton, Monroe and West Chester.

6949 Philomatheon Society of the Blind
2701 Tuscarawas St W
Canton, OH 44708
330-453-9157
www.my.raex.com/~philo

Shirley Beckner, President
Offers services for the totally blind, legally blind, visually impaired, mentally retarded blind and more with health, counseling, educational, recreational, rehabilitation, computer training and professional training services.

6950 Providence Hospital Work
2270 Banning Road
Cincinnati, OH 45239
513-853-5261
FAX: 513-853-5910

Christopher West, Executive Director
Post-acute rehabilitation services.

6951 SCI: Six County
2845 Bell Street
Zanesville, OH 43701
740-454-9766
FAX: 740-588-6452
e-mail: info@sixcounty.org
www.sixcounty.org

David O Wesner, Program Research
SCI has been meeting community mental health needs for over 40 years. Today, in addition to the traditional treatment services, specialized services have been developed to reach people with ever changing needs. Employee assistance, sheltered employment, intensive outpatient, and residential services are only a few of these innovative programs.

6952 Society for Rehabilitation
9521 Lake Shore Boulevard
Mentor, OH 44060
440-352-8993
800-344-3159
FAX: 440-352-6632
e-mail: info@societyhelps.org
www.societyhelps.org

Richard Kessler, Executive Director
Vision is to provide individuals with comprehensive services to improve their quality of life. Our mission is to meet the needs of individuals and their families by delivering a wide range of affordable accessible and personalized services, providing treatment by a team of highly qualified, caring professionals. Collaborating with other agencies to meet community needs.

6953 Southeast Ohio Sight Center
358A Lincoln Avenue
Lancaster, OH 43130
740-687-4785
800-969-3490
FAX: 740-689-9753
e-mail: sosc@seohiosightcenter.org
www.charityadvantage.com

John Sterba, Executive Director
Offers services for the blind and visually impaired to include functional low vision evaluations, community rehabilitation trading, counseling, educational, recreational, rehabilitation and vocational services.

6954 St. Francis Rehabilitation Hospital
401 N Broadway Street
Green Springs, OH 44836
419-639-2626
800-248-2552
FAX: 419-639-6222
www.sfhcc.org

Martha Stevens, Marketing Coordinator
Dan Schwanke, Chief Executive Officer
Program offers specialized treatment for patients who have suffered a head injury, spinal cord injury, or stroke, or who have an orthopedic injury. The Head Injury Program provides a continuum of care from coma stimulation through transitional living. Their physicians, nurses, counselors and therapists are dedicated to helping our patients develop the motivation, strength and skills needed to overcome or adapt to their disability.

6955 TAC Industries
2160 Old Selma Road
Springfield, OH 45505
937-527-7400
FAX: 937-525-7401
www.tacind.com

Mary Brandstetter, Executive Director
TAC Industries, Inc., provides employment opportunities for individuals to develop marketable skills by completing contract work in partnership with other industries. Work and self-help skills, social adjustment, and a variety of daily living experiences are offered to the workers by our specialized staff.

Oklahoma

6956 Dean A McGee Eye Institute
608 Stanton L Young
Oklahoma City, OK 73104
405-271-6060
FAX: 405-271-4442
www.dmei.org

David W. Parke II, M.D., President/CEO
Matthew D. Brown, Executive Vice President
Penny Mills Voss, CFRE, Vice President Of Development
Offers services for the totally blind, legally blind, visually impaired, mentally retarded blind and more with health, counseling, educational, recreational, rehabilitation, computer training and professional training services.

6957 Jane Phillips Medical Center
Rehab Care
3500 SE Frank Phillips Boulevard
Bartlesville, OK 74006
918-333-7200
FAX: 918-333-7801
e-mail: webmaster@ipmc.org
www.sjmc.org

Jim Fram, President
Evan O Zorn, Executive Vice President
James Carver, MD
Comprehensive inpatient rehabilitation services are provided to patients with orthopedic, neurologic, and other medical conditions of recent onset or regression, who have experienced a loss of function in activities of daily living, mobility, cognition and communication.

6958 McAlester Regional Health Center RehabCare Unit
1 E Clark Bass Boulevard
McAlester, OK 74501
918-426-1800
FAX: 918-421-6832
e-mail: nbrinlee@mrhcok.com
www.mrhcok.com

Shawn Bedds, Administrator
Joel Tate, Chief Executive Officer
A 19-bed inpatient physical rehabilitation unit serving the Southeast Oklahoma area. Offers physical therapy, occupational therapy, social work, speech and psychological services in an interdisciplinary framework.

6959 Oklahoma League for the Blind
501 N. Douglas Ave.
Oklahoma City, OK 73106
405-232-4644
FAX: 405-236-5438
e-mail: info@olb.org
www.olb.org

Lauren White, President/CEO
Carol Campbell, Executive Assistant
Bob Allen, President
Offers services for the blind and visually impaired, counseling, educational, recreational, rehabilitation, computer training and professional training services.

6960 Valley View Regional Hospital-RehabCare Unit
430 N Monte Vista Street
Ada, OK 74820
580-332-2323
FAX: 580-421-1395
e-mail: valleyview@wrh.com
www.valleyviewregional.org

Ronand Webb, Chief Executive Officer
Comprehensive physical medicine and rehabilitation services designed to help patients in their adjustment to a physically limiting condition.

Oregon

6961 Garten Services
3334 Industrial Way NE
Salem, OR 97301
503-581-4472
FAX: 503-581-4497
e-mail: garten@garten.org
www.garten.org

Tim Rocak, Executive Director
Garten's mission is to support people with disabilities in their effort to contribute to the community through employment, career, and retirement opportunities. Our actions increase society's awareness of human potential. Garten's vision is to be recognized as an organization positively demonstrating to the community that people with disabilities can be contributing and valued employees of a thriving business.

6962 Legacy Emanuel Rehabilitation Center
3025 N Vancouver Avenue
Portland, OR 97227
503-335-2000
FAX: 503-413-1501
www.legacyhealth.org

Gary Guidetta, Executive Director
Gail Weisgerber, Manager
A non-profit tax-exempt corporation that includes 5 full-service hospitals and a children's hospital. The Legacy system provides an integrated network of healthcare services, including acute and critical care, inpatient and outpatient treatment, community health education and a variety of specialty services.

6963 Oakcrest Care Center
2933 Center Street NE
Salem, OR 97301
503-585-5850
FAX: 503-585-8781

Postacute rehabilitation program.

6964 Oakhill-Senior Program
1190 Oakhill Avenue SE
Salem, OR 97302
503-364-9086
FAX: 503-365-2879

Jan Dillon, Senior Services Manager
Garten Senior Services provides an adult day service program to seniors with and without developmental disabilities. The program will provide community opportunities, college classes and a wide variety of leisure activities in group and individual settings.

6965 Pacific Spine and Pain Center
1801 Highway 99 N
Ashland, OR 97520
541-488-0170
866-482-5515
FAX: 541-482-2433

Christine Gorrin, Manager

6966 Vision Northwest
9225 SW Hall Boulevard
Portland, OR 97223
503-684-8389
800-448-2232
FAX: 503-684-9359
e-mail: marthaz@visionnw.com
www.visionnw.com

Evelyn Maizels, Executive Director
Offers services for the totally blind, legally blind, visually impaired, mentally retarded blind and more with health, counseling, educational, recreational, rehabilitation, computer training and professional training services.

6967 Willamette Valley Rehabilitation Center
1853 W Airway Road
Lebanon, OR 97355
541-258-8121
FAX: 541-451-1762
www.wvrc.org

Martin Buckman, Executive Director
Provides the best professional vocational services to those adults in the community who, by virtue of their physical or mental limitations, are negatively impacted by their ability to attain or maintain employment.

Pennsylvania

6968 Alpine Nursing and Rehabilitation Center of Hershey
Pennstate
405 Marion Place
State College, PA 16801
814-865-1710
FAX: 814-863-9423
e-mail: geron@psu.edu
geron.psu.edu

Melissa A Hardy, Director
Anna Shuey, Administrative Assistant
Postacute rehabilitation program.

6969 Alpine Ridge and Brandywood
Devereux Foundation
600 Boot Road
Downingtown, PA 19335
610-873-4900
800-345-1292
FAX: 610-430-0567
www.devereus.org

MaryAnn Fullam, Director
Sam Ewing, Owner
Offers a continuum of services for residents requiring services ranging from minimal care and supervision to total physical and medical care.

6970 Amity Lodge
Devereux Foundation
600 Boot Road
Downingtown, PA 19335
610-873-4900
800-345-1292
FAX: 610-524-3000

Kim Nash, Director
Sam Ewing, Owner
Offers residents a continuum of services ranging from minimal care and supervision to total physical and medical care.

6971 Beechwood Rehabilitation Services A Community Integrated Brain Injury Program
469 E Maple Avenue
Langhorne, PA 19047
215-750-4299
800-782-3299
FAX: 215-750-4327
e-mail: dcerra-tyl@wood.org
www.beechwoodrehab.com

Deborah Cerra-Tyl, Director Program Development
Thomas Felicetti, President
Services include residential, day treatment and community based support services. Individuals with brain injury are served. The facility is Care Accredited.

6972 Blind & Vision Rehabilitation Services Of Pittsburgh
1800 West Street
Homestead, PA 15120
412-368-4400
800-706-5050
FAX: 412-368-4090
www.pghvis.org

Leroy Bectwy, Director
Linda Hill, Manager
Offers services for the totally blind, legally blind, visually impaired, mentally retarded blind and more with health, counseling, educational, recreational, rehabilitation, computer training and professional training services.

6973 Bradford Regional Medical Center
116 Interstate Parkway
Bradford, PA 16701
814-368-4143
FAX: 814-362-3202
www.brmc.org

Carma Horner, Supervisor
Andrew Lehman, Executive Director
Offers rehabilitation services to individuals with an alcohol or drug related problem.

6974 Bryn Mawr Rehabilitation Hospital
414 Paoli Pike
Malvern, PA 19355
610-251-5400
888-734-2241
888-734-2241
FAX: 610-647-3648
www.brynmawrrehab.org

Donna Phillips, President
We are dedicated to serving individuals and their families whose lives can be enhanced through physical or cognitive rehabilitation. We continually strive for excellence by providing care and services which are valued by those we serve and by contributing to the community through education, research and prevention of disability.

6975 Clara Burke Nursing Home
251 Stenton Avenue
Plymouth Meeting, PA 19462
610-828-2272
FAX: 610-828-7939

Terri Herd, Admissions
Jim Foulke, Administrator
Postacute rehabilitation program.

6976 Daman Villa
Devereux Foundation
600 Boot Road
Downingtown, PA 19335
610-873-4900
800-345-1292
FAX: 610-430-0567
www.devereux.org

Robert Kreider, President & CEO
Sam Ewing, Owner
Offers residents a continuum of services ranging from minimal care and supervision to total physical and medical care.

6977 Devereux
444 Devereux Dr
Villanova, PA 19085
610-520-3000
800-345-1292
FAX: 610-542-3100
e-mail: knash@devereux.org
www.devereux.org

Kimberleigh Nash, Director Corporate Communication
Robert Kreider, Chief Executive Officer
Nationwide network of residential, day, and community-based services for children and adults who have special emotional and/or developmental needs.

6978 Devereux Foundation Health Services Center
600 Boot Road
Downingtown, PA 19335
610-873-4900
800-345-1292
FAX: 610-430-0567
www.devereux.org

MaryAnn Fullam, Director
Sam Ewing, Owner
Provides a continuum of residential services for adults with developmental disabilities. active treatment is offered in a safe and therapeutic environment which allows on-going assessment and individual growth that will enhance the quality of life for each of its residents. Candidates could have needs that range from minimal care and supervision to those requiring medical and behavioral assistance with an intensive support system. $145-$161.00 per day.

6979 Devereux's Kanner Center
620 E Boot Road
West Chester, PA 19380
610-873-4930
FAX: 610-873-4969
e-mail: kanner@devereux.org
www.devereuxcares.org

Steve Silverman, Admissions Director
Kelly McCool, Admissions Coordinator
Carol Leeson, Director Network Relations
A private nonprofit nationwide network of treatment services for individuals of all ages with emotional and/or developmental disabilities. Located in twelve states and the District of Columbia, Devereux's continuum includes inpatient and partial hospitalization, residential treatment, community based programs and outpatient services. Provides a continuum of care to children, adolescents and young adults who have developmental disabilities, mental retardation, autism and emotional disturbances.

6980 Fox Subacute Center
2644 Bristol Road
Warrington, PA 18976
215-343-2700
FAX: 215-343-8023
e-mail: jfoulke@foxsubacute.com
www.foxsubacute.com

James Foulke, CEO
Vic Costenko, COO
Walter Dunsmore, CFO
Fox subacute recognizes the great need for alternative programs for today's medically compromised patients. Fox has developed Models of Care and offers subacute programs fore the management of ventilator-dependent patients. We recognize that the best road to recovery for these patients is an environment with special care in an alternative setting. We believe that setting should be outside the hospital, in facilities where the focus is on the management of individual patients.

6981 Good Samaritan Health System
Po Box 1281
Lebanon, PA 17042
717-270-7500
866-276-3082
FAX: 215-238-0804
www.gshleb.org

John Jeffers, Director
Frederick Davis, VP Clinical Services
Offers services for the totally blind, legally blind, visually impaired, mentally retarded blind and more with health, counseling, educational, recreational, rehabilitation, computer training and professional training services.

6982 Good Samaritan Hospital-Health System Center
Good Samaritan Hospital
4th & Walnut Streets
Lebanon, PA 17042
717-270-7500
FAX: 717-270-7840
www.gshleb.org

Joanne Ebert, Rehab Coordinator
Stuart Hartman, Medical Director
Comprehensive inpatient rehab unit for adults regarding general physical rehabilitation. Specific programs include orthopedic, neurological, stroke, amputee, etc.

6983 IHS of Greater Pittsburgh
890 Weatherwood Lane
Greensburg, PA 15601
724-837-8076
FAX: 724-837-7456
e-mail: pattim@tri-state-health.com
www.ihsgreaterpittsburgh.com

Patti Mikosky RN CRRN, Provider Relations Specialist
Laurie Tamasy, Administrator
Marhsa Echard, Admissions Coordinator
Subacate care, ventilator and pulmonary managment, comprehensive rehabilitation.

6984 Pediatric Center at Plymouth Meeting Integrated Health Services
491 Allendale Road
King of Prussia, PA 19406
610-265-9290
800-220-7337

Fran Currick, Manager
Subacute programs such as intensive respiratory care, stressing ventilator dependent children, pre and post transplant care, total parenteral nutrition, IV therapy, intensive/behavioral oral feeding programs. Provides extensive discharge planning including teaching or review for all the above programs with an emphasis on development and accessing community resources.

6985 Penn State Milton S. Hershey Medical Center College Of Medicine
500 University Drive
Hershey, PA 17033
717-531-8070
800-243-1455
FAX: 717-531-4558
www.hmc.psu.edu

Lori Benner, Director
a non-sectarian, not-for-profit community hospital whose purpose is to provide high quality acute, rehabilitative and preventive health services for the entire community, regardless of creed, race, nationality, or ability to pay.

6986 Pennsylvania Pain Rehabilitation Center
252 W Swamp Road
Suite 2
Doylestown, PA 18901
215-348-5106
FAX: 215-348-5106

Reza Azar MD
Post acute rehabilitation facility and programs.

Rhode Island

6987 In-Sight
43 Jefferson Boulevard
Warwick, RI 02888
401-941-3322
FAX: 401-941-3356
e-mail: cbutler@in-sight.org
www.in-sight.org

Judith Smith, President
Offers services for the totally blind, legally blind, visually impaired, mentally retarded blind and more with health, counseling, educational, recreational, rehabilitation, computer training and professional training services.

6988 Vanderbilt Rehabilitation Center
Newport Hospital
Friendship Street
Newport, RI 02840
401-845-1605
FAX: 401-845-1087
www.lifespan.org/newport/services/vrc

Robert Healey, Executive Director
Arthur Sampson, Chief Executive Officer
The Vanderbilt Rehabilitation Center at Newport Hospital has been providing comprehensive rehabilitation sercices for more then a century and is known throughout the region for its unique programs and high-quality, patient focused care.

South Carolina

6989 Association for the Blind
1071 Morrison Drive
Charleston, SC 29403
843-723-6915
e-mail: aftb@aerolina.com

Cornelia Pelzer, Executive Director
Offers services for people who are blind, or are visually impaired with health, counseling, educational, recreational, rehabilitation, computer training and professional training services.

6990 Hitchcock Rehabilitation Center
690 Medical Park Drive
Aiken, SC 29801
803-643-0001
800-207-6924
FAX: 803-649-4639
e-mail: mail@hitchcockhealthcare.org

Pat Samuel, Executive Director
Dan Hillman, Case Manager
Carrie Morgan, Finance Director
Comprehensive outpatient rehabilitation for adults, children, geriatrics, pediatric therapy, special needs preschool, sports medicine, home health and hospice.

6991 The Mentor Network
3200 Devine Street
Columbia, SC 29205
803-799-9025
800-297-8043
FAX: 803-931-8962
www.thementornetwork.com

Lynn Epps, Executive Director
Mentor provides a full network of individually tailored services for people with development disabilities and their families. Individuals may be served in their homes, shared living home, or in a host home.

Tennessee

6992 Humana Hospital: Morristown RehabCare
726 McFarland Street
Morristown, TN 37814
423-586-2930
FAX: 423-587-4417

James Perry, Program Director
Designed to help patients in their adjustment to a physically limiting condition by helping to maximize each patient's abilities so he or she can function as independently as possible.

6993 Opportunity East Rehabilitation Services for the Blind
758 West Morris Blvd.
Morristown, TN 37813
423-586-3998
800-278-6274
FAX: 423-586-2004
e-mail: bandit75@charter.net
www.opportunityeast.org

Fred Overbay, Executive Director
Vic Mende, Director Rehabilitation Services
Offers services for the totally blind, legally blind, visually impaired, mentally retarded blind and more with health, counseling, educational, recreational, rehabilitation, computer training and professional training services.

6994 Patrick Rehab Wellness Center
Lincoln County Health System
106 Medical Center Boulevard
Fayetteville, TN 37334
931-138-1100
FAX: 931-438-7456
www.ichealthsystem.com

Denning Harter, Director Rehab
Gloria Meadows, Administrator
Jim Stewart, Principal
Provides rehabilitation services of physical, occupational, and speech therapy. Also, wellness memberships are available to the public.

6995 PharmaThera
1785 Nonconnah Boulevard
Memphis, TN 38132
901-348-8100
800-767-6714
FAX: 901-348-8200
Offers 10 locations serving patients throughout the southern United States, each with an in-house, expertly trained staff. All locations use the latest technologies and techniques in infusion care to provide a broad range of individualized home infusion therapies.

6996 Siskin Hospital For Physical Rehabilitation
1 Siskin Plaza
Chattanooga, TN 37403
423-634-1200
www.siskinrehab.org

Debby Barker, VP Development
Robert Siskin, Owner
Dedicated exclusively to physical rehabilitation and offers specialized treatment programs in brain injury, amputation, stroke, spinal cord injury, orthopedics, and major multiple trauma. The hospital also provides treatment for neurological disorders and loss of muscle strength and controll following illness or surgery.

6997 St. Mary's RehabCare Center
900 E Oak Hill Avenue
Knoxville, TN 37917
865-545-7793
FAX: 865-545-8133

Debbie Keeton, Director
Beth Greco, Executive Director
Provides comprehensive rehabilitation services for patients experiencing CVA, head trauma, orthopedic conditions, spinal cord injury or neurological impairment.

Texas

6998 Baylor Institute for Rehabilitation
3505 Gaston Avenue
Dallas, TX 75246
214-820-9300
888-7BA-YLOR
FAX: 214-841-2679

Alice Douden, Admissions Manager
Luci Neumann, President
A 92-bed specialty hospital offering comprehensive rehabilitation services for persons with spinal cord injury, traumatic brain injury, stroke, amputation, and other orthopedic and neurological disorders.

6999 Brown-Karhan Health Care
400 Old Highway 290
Dripping Springs, TX 78620
512-894-0801
FAX: 512-858-4627
e-mail: info@brown-karhan.com
www.brown-karhan.com

James R Karhan, Chief Executive Officer
Eric Makowski, President

Postacute rehabilitation program, long-term neuropsychiatric program, apartment living and full compliment of therapies, including cognitive rehabilitation. $225-$800/day.

7000 Center for Neuro Skills

1320 W. Walnut Hill
Irving, TX 75038
972-580-8500
800-544-5448
FAX: 972-255-3162
e-mail: texas@neuroskills.com
www.neuroskills.com

Rocky Brogdon, Admissions
John Schultz, Administrator
Centre for Neuro Skills (CNS) seeks to provide medical rehabilitation programs, lifecare programs, advocacy, and research for people with brain injury in order to achieve a maximum quality of life.

7001 Dallas Services for Visually Impaired Children

4242 Office Parkway
Dallas, TX 75204
214-828-9900
FAX: 214-828-9901
www.dallasservices.org

Jim Gibson, Executive Director
Offers services for the totally blind, legally blind, visually impaired, mentally retarded blind and more with health, counseling, educational, recreational, rehabilitation, computer training and professional training services.

7002 Devereux Texas Treatment Network Adult Community

PO Box 2666
Victoria, TX 77902
361-575-8271
800-383-5000
FAX: 361-575-6520
www.devereux.org

Fred Williams, Executive Director
April Krus, Admissions Coordinator
Provides a permanent home for individuals with chronic psychiatric and/or developmental disabilities who require long term or lifelong care, support or a transitional home for individuals who progress to a less structured setting. Located on a beautiful 400+ acre campus in sunny south Texas, the primary focus is to offer, in keeping with the philosophies of least restrictive alternatives and normalization, active treatment which will facilitate growth.

7003 El Paso Lighthouse for the Blind

200 Washington Street
El Paso, TX 79905
915-532-4495
FAX: 915-532-6338
www.lighthouse-elpaso.com

Lea Cochran, President
John McCain, Vice President
Lola Dawkins, Secretary
Enables people of all ages to embody blindness and vision impairment through training, rehabilitation, employment opportunity, advocacy and research. Provides access to opportunities and quality of life so that the blind and visually impaired can reach their fullest potential for self-sufficiency and independence.

7004 Harris Methodist Fort Worth/Mabee Rehabilitation Center

1301 Pennsylvania Avenue
Fort Worth, TX 76104
817-882-2760
FAX: 817-882-2753
www.texashealth.org

Michelle Wilson, Speciality Program Manager
Peggyo Ehrlich, Rehab Manager
Karen Mallett, Executive Director
A hospital based inpatient rehab program and outpatient day programs in chronic pain management, work hardening and brain injury transitional services.

7005 HealthSouth Hospital Of Houston

17506 Red Oak Drive
Houston, TX 77090
281-580-1212
FAX: 281-580-6714
www.healthsouth.com

Jerome Lengel, Executive Officer
Dewitt Hilton, Owner
Offers an individualized approach to the process of rehabilitation for severely injured or disabled individuals. The process begins with a pre-admissions assessment of each referred patient. The Center combines state-of-the-art technology and equipment with multi-disciplinary therapy and education in a cheerful, secure environment.

7006 Heights Hospital Rehab Unit

1917 Ashland Street
Houston, TX 77008
713-861-6161
FAX: 713-802-8537

Theresa Davis, Administrator
This program is designed to assist patients with physical disabilities achieve their maximum functional abilities.

7007 Hillcrest Baptist Medical Center

3000 Herring Avenue
Waco, TX 76708
254-202-2000
FAX: 254-202-5105
www.hillcrest.net

Carl Lutz MSW, Program Director
Ann Gammel, Nurse Manager
Debbie Meurer, Manager
Designed to assist patients in adjustment to a physically limiting condition, utilizing interdisciplinary strategies to maximize each patient's ability and capability.

7008 Institute for Rehabilitation & Research

1333 Moursund Street
Houston, TX 77030
713-799-5000
800-447-3422
FAX: 713-797-5289
www.tirr.org

John Kajander, Chief Executive Officer
Jean Herzog, President
A national center for information, training, research, and technical assistance in independent living. The goal is to extend the body of knowledge in independent living and to improve the utilization of results of research programs and demonstration projects in this field. It has developed a variety of strategies for collecting, synthesizing, and disseminating information related to the field of independent living.

7009 Integrated Health Services of Amarillo

5601 Plum Creek Drive
Amarillo, TX 79124
806-351-1000
FAX: 806-355-9650
www.medcenter.org

Jayton McCoy, Case Manager
Neal Duncan, Executive Director
Roger Alexander, Administrator
Provides acute, post acute, residential and outpatient health care services. IHS of Amarillo is a 153-bed facility with 120 beds licensed by The Texas Department of Health and Human Services, and is accredited by JCAHO. We serve urban and rural populations of over 500,000, drawing from a 5-state region.

7010 Lighthouse of Houston

3602 W Dallas Street
Houston, TX 77019
713-527-9561
FAX: 713-284-8451
e-mail: tgarza@houstonlighthouse.org
www.houstonlighthouse.org

Gibson M Terroil, President
Shelagh Moran, VP/COO
Teresa Gaiza, Director Education
Serves the blind, visually impaired, deaf-blind and multihandicapped blind. Provides workshops, vocational training and placement, low vision clinic, orientation and mobility, housing, Braille, volunteer services, senior center, visual aid sales, counseling and support, diabetic education and day health activity services and day summer camp, Summer Transition for Youth.

7011 **Mainland Center Hospital RehabCare Unit**
6801 Emmet F. Lowry Expwy
Texas City, TX 77592
409-938-5000
FAX: 409-938-5501
www.mainlandmedical.com

David Roberts, Program Manager
The RehabCare program is designed and staffed to assist functionally impaired patients improve to their maximum potential. The opportunities for improvement and adjustments are provided in a pleasant, supportive inpatient environment by therapists from the occupational, physical, recreational and speech therapy disciplines.

7012 **North Texas Rehabilitation Center**
1005 Midwestern Parkway
Wichita Falls, TX 76302
940-322-0771
FAX: 940-766-4943
www.ntrehab.org

Lesa Enlow, Director Programs
Cindy Duncan, Human Resource
Mike Castles, President
Provides outpatient rehabilitation services to maximize independence or promote development to children and adults with disabilities. Programs include: physical, occupational, speech therapy, closed head injury, infant/child development, support groups, aquatics and wellness program and a child achievement program.

7013 **South Texas Lighthouse for the Blind**
PO Box 9697
Corpus Christi, TX 78469
361-883-6553
888-255-8011
FAX: 361-883-1041
www.stlb.net

Regis Barber, President/CEO
Nicky Ooi, Vp Mfg. & New Business
Offers services for the totally blind, legally blind, visually impaired, mentally retarded blind and more with health, counseling, educational, recreational, rehabilitation, computer training and professional training services.

7014 **Texas Specialty Hospital at Dallas**
7955 Harry Hines Boulevard
Dallas, TX 75235
214-637-0000
FAX: 214-637-6512
www.fundltc.com

Waylon Maynard, Director Clinical Services
Cathy Campbell, Chief Executive Officer
66 beds offering active/acute rehabilitation, brain injury day treatment, cognitive rehabilitation, complex care, extended rehabilitation and short term evaluation.

7015 **Transitional Learning Center at Galveston**
1528 Post Office Street
Galveston, TX 77550
409-762-6661
800-852-4769
FAX: 409-763-3930
www.tlcrehab.org

Lee Kinard, Managed Care/Account Manager
Jim McCurdy, Director Business Development
The Transitional Learning Center at Galveston has specialized in post-acute brain injury since 1982. TLC is a leader who offers comprehensive therapies in a residential setting, 24-hour monitoring, outcome focused pathways, superior staff credentials - including physician and nursing staff on-site to address medical issues, innovative clinical research integrated into treatment plans, discharge lifecare planning, and long-term living at Tideway Lodge.

7016 **Treemont Nursing And Rehabilitation Center**
5550 Harvest Hill Road
Dallas, TX 75230
972-661-1862
FAX: 972-715-5550

Craig Hodges, Administrator
Postacute rehabilitation program.

7017 **West Texas Lighthouse for the Blind**
2001 Austin Street
San Angelo, TX 76903
325-653-4231
FAX: 325-657-9367
e-mail: wtlb@wcc.net
www.lighthousefortheblind.org

Robert Porter, Executive Director
Ron Beard, Operations Manager
Margene Hale, Office Manager
Offers services for the totally blind, legally blind, visually impaired, mentally retarded blind and more with health, counseling, educational, recreational, rehabilitation, computer training and professional training services.

Utah

7018 **Quincy Rehabilitation Institute of Holy Cross Hospital**
1050 E South Temple
Salt Lake City, UT 84102
801-350-8140
FAX: 801-350-4483

Dave Jenson, President
Postacute rehabilitation program.

7019 **Wasatch Vision Clinic**
849 E 400 S
Salt Lake City, UT 84102
801-328-2020
FAX: 801-363-2201
e-mail: craig@wasatchvision.com
www.wasatchvision.com

Craig Kellar OD, Owner
Postacute rehabilitation program.

Vermont

7020 **Rutland Mental Health Services**
78 S Main Street
Rutland, VT 05701
802-775-2381
FAX: 802-747-7699
www.rmhsccn.org

Mark G Monson, President/CEO
A private, non-profit comprehensive community mental health center. It provides services to individuals and families for mental health and substance abuse related problems and also to persons who are mentally retarded.

Virginia

7021 **Bay Pine-Virginia Beach**
1148 First Colonial Road
Virginia Beach, VA 23454
757-481-3321
FAX: 757-481-4413

David Vevoda, Administrator
Postacute rehabilitation program.

7022 **Carilion Rehabilitation: New River Valley**
PO Box 5
Radford, VA 24143
540-731-2992
FAX: 540-731-2011
e-mail: info@carilion.com
www.carilion.com

Jennie Smith, Clinical Team Leader
Rhonda Fanning, Department Secretary/Referrals
Robin Sutphin, Rehabilitation Assistant

CARF-accredited pain management program, work hardening program and comprehensive outpatient therapy clinic, massage therapy, outpatient programs and more. Program emphasis is on interdisiplinary behavioral rehab based pain management and functional restoration in conjunction with medical treatment. Work hardening is a transdisciplinary work simulation program taylored to the individual. Comprehensive outpatient program is multi-disciplinary with emphasis on manual treatment.

7023 Faith Mission Home
3540 Mission Home Lane
Free Union, VA 22940
434-985-2294
FAX: 434-985-7633
www.beachyam.org

Merle Miller, Administrator
Reuben Yoder, Director
A Christian residential center that serves 60 mentally retarded children, including individuals with Down Syndrome, Cerebral palsy and other similar conditions. Children may be admitted from the time they are ambulatory until they reach 15 years of age. He or she may stay as long as it is in the child's best interests. The training program stresses the following areas: self-care, social, academic, vocational, crafts, speech and physical development.

7024 ManorCare Health Services-Arlington
550 S Carlin Springs Road
Arlington, VA 22204
703-379-7200
FAX: 703-578-5524
e-mail: arlington@hcr-manorcare.com
www.hcr-manorcare.com

Marcia K Jarrell, Administrator
Ric Birch, Marketing Director
ManorCare-Arlington offers residents a full Continuum of Care in a caring environment. ManorCare's wide range of services includes subacute medical and rehabilitation programs for short term patients transitioning from hospital to home and Skilled Nursing Care.

7025 Pines Residential Treatment Center
825 Crawford Parkway
Portsmouth, VA 23704
757-393-0061
FAX: 757-393-1029

Dr. Leonard Lexier MD, Medical Director
Judy Kemp, Admissions Director
A 310-bed residential treatment center in Portsmouth Virginia, providing a therapeutic environment for severely emotionally disturbed children and youth. Five unique programs meet behavioral, educational and emotional needs of males and females, five to twenty-two years of age. Multi-disciplinary teams devise individual service plans to enhance strengths and reverse self-defeating behavior. A highly effective positive reinforcement program with a proven track record.

7026 Resurrection Children's Center
2280 N Beauregard Street
Alexandria, VA 22311
703-998-0888
FAX: 703-820-2912
e-mail: office@welcometoresurrection.org
www.welcometoresurrection.org

Anne Gavin Ritchie, Rector
Robert A. Becker, Assistant To The Rector
H. Vance Johnson, Adjunct Priest
Offers children ages 2-5 with varying disabilities academic education, parent education, opportunities including classes, workshops, support groups and individual counseling.

7027 Roanoke Memorial Hospital
Carilion Health System
PO Box 13367
Roanoke, VA 24033
540-772-1736
FAX: 540-981-8233
e-mail: direct@carilion.com
www.carilion.com

Beth Lindille, Director
Eric Carlen, President
Carilion Health System exists to improve the health of the communities it serves. The vision is to assure accessible, affordable, high quality healthcare that meets the needs of the community. Motivate and educate individuals to improve their health. Champion community initiatives to reduce health risk

7028 Southside Virginia Training Center
Po Box 4030
Petersburg, VA 23803
804-524-7284
FAX: 804-524-7228
www.svtc.dmhmrsas.virginia.gov

John Holland, Director
Beverly Garnes, Client Advocate
Theolette Ledbetter, Director Public Relations
Offers residential, vocational, occupational, physical, and speech therapies.

7029 Woodrow Wilson Rehabilitation Center
PO Box 1500
Fishersville, VA 22939
540-332-7000
800-345-9972
FAX: 540-332-7132
e-mail: colemawl@wwrc.state.va.lls
www.wwrc.net

Greta Hodberg, Admissions Director
Wendell L Coleman, Volunteer Services Director
Comprehensive residential rehabilitation center offering complete medical and vocational rehabilitation services including: vocation evaluation, vocational training, transition from school to work, occupational therapy, physical therapy, speech, language and audiology, assistive technology, rehabilitation engineering, counseling/case management, behavioral health services, nursing and physician services, etc.

Washington

7030 Arden Rehabilitation And Healthcare Center
16357 Aurora Avenue N
Seattle, WA 98133
206-542-3103
FAX: 206-542-4562
www.ardenrehab.com

Gail Brockway, Administrator
Arden can accomodate 90 residents- post-acute/rehabilitation patients as well as long term residents. Medicare certified, the center also takes most managed healthcare insurance plans, as well as VA, respite and hospice patients.

7031 Bellingham Care Center
1200 Birchwood Avenue
Bellingham, WA 98225
360-734-9295
FAX: 360-671-4368

Sheila Oberg, Administrator
Postacute rehabilitation program.

7032 Division of Vocational Rehabilitation Department of Social and Health Services
PO Box 45130
Olympia, WA 98504
360-725-3636
800-737-0617
FAX: 360-438-8007
e-mail: krulik@dshs.wa.gov
www1.dshs.wa.gov/dvr

Mike O Brien, Director
Lynnea Ruttledge, Manager
Information on computers, supported employment, marketing rehabilitation facilities and transition.

7033 First Hill Care Center
1334 Terry Avenue
Seattle, WA 98101
206-624-1484
FAX: 206-624-0188

Postacute rehabilitation program.

7034 Harborview Medical Center, Low Vision Aid Clinic
Harborview Medical Center
325 9th Avenue
Seattle, WA 98104 206-731-3000
www.uwmedicine.org

Thomas Gillette, Director
Susan Worden, Manager
Offers services for the totally blind, legally blind, visually impaired, mentally retarded blind and more with health, counseling, educational, recreational, rehabilitation, computer training and professional training services.

7035 Integrated Health Services of Seattle
820 NW 95th Street
Seattle, WA 98117 206-783-7649
FAX: 206-781-1448

Jerry Harvey, Administrator
Marlette Basada, Director Nursing
Flavia Lagrange, Director Admissions
Postacute rehabilitation program. IHS provides 24 hour subacute and long-term care. We can handle vent/trach/hemo andritoneal dialysis and provide a full scope of rehabilitation services.

7036 Lakeside Milam Recovery Centers (LMRC)
535 Dock Street
Tacoma, WA 98402 253-272-2242
800-231-4303
FAX: 253-272-0171
www.lakesidemilam.com/locationtacoma.htm

Michael Kinder, Administrator
LMRC was established in 1983 with a single mission, to help victims and families recover from the pain of drug/alcohol addiction. Enlightned by the work of Dr. James Milam in the 1960's and 70's, the founders of LMRC created a treatment system based on a bedrock set of principals.

7037 Lakewood Health Care Center
11411 Bridgeport Way SW
Lakewood, WA 98499 253-581-9002
FAX: 253-581-7016
www.lakewoodhc.com

Janice Olson, Admissions Coordinator
Patty Wood, Administrator
Linda Doll, Social Services
Accomodates 80 residents. We offer 24 hour skilled nursing services, long-term care and rehab services which include Physical, Occupational and Speech Therapy.

7038 Manor Care Health Services-Tacoma
5601 S Orchard Street
Tacoma, WA 98409 253-474-8421
FAX: 253-474-8172
e-mail: tacoma@hcr-manorcare.com
www.hcr-manorcare.com

Robin Leitch, Administrator
124-bed skilled nursing and rehabilitation center provides services for those seeking long term Skilled Nursing Care, short term subacute care, hospice services, Alzheimer's and respite care. Our Acadia Wing, a specialized Alzheimer's care unit, provides specialized programming and trained staff that truly makes us the leader in Alzheimers Services.

7039 ManorCare Health Services-Lynnwood
3701 188th Street SW
Lynnwood, WA 98037 425-775-9222
FAX: 425-744-1602
e-mail: lynnwood@hcr-manorcare.com
www.hcr-manorcare.com

Irene Dondo, Director
Liza Loyet, Administrator
Our in-house therapists provide physical, occupational and speech therapies in our state-of-the-art therapy gym. Our team is goal oriented and focuses on producing positive outcomes for those recovering from illness, injury or surgery.

7040 ManorCare Health Services-Spokane
6025 N Assembly Street
Spokane, WA 99205 509-326-8282
FAX: 509-326-4790
e-mail: spokane@hcr-manorcare.com
www.hcrmanorcare.com

Susan Cooper, Admissions Director
Sandra Hayes, Administrator
Provides skilled nursing and respite stays for those needing a break from care giving. We specialize in Rehabilitation Services provided by our in-house occupational, physical and speech therapists.

7041 Northwest Continuum Care Center
Kindred Health Care
128 Beacon Hill
Longview, WA 98632 360-423-4060
FAX: 360-636-0958
www.nwcontinuum.com

Steve Ross, Administrator
Tami Wilson, Director of Nursing
Accomodates 69 residents. Employs the Angel Care Program designed to address any special needs that may arise during a resident's stay in our facility. The program focuses extra attention on residents and, in some cases, family members. The goal is to meet the special needs of the people we provide care to every day.

7042 Park Manor Convalescent Center
1710 Plaza Way
Walla Walla, WA 99362 509-529-4218
FAX: 509-522-1729
www.parkmanorcare.com

Chris Bohnsack, Administrator
Krista Maiuri, Directr Of Nursing
Kris Spears, Business Office Manager
Residents of Park Manor enjoy a range of activities, developed to meet their needs, inculding excercise programs, social and recreational activities, arts and crafts, shopping trips and other excursions. We also offer religious services.

7043 Queen Anne Health Care
Queen Anne Health Care
2717 Dexter Avenue N
Seattle, WA 98109 206-284-7012
FAX: 206-283-3936
www.queenannehealthcare.com

Heather Eacker, Administrator
Our goal is to provide quality, compassionate care. Our cozy building accomodates 120 residents. We offer semi private rooms with space to add items from home for a special personalized touch

7044 Rainier Vista Care Center
920 12th Avenue SE
Puyallup, WA 98372 253-841-3422
FAX: 253-848-3937
www.rainiervistacc.com

Debi Thompson, Administrator
Accomodates 120 residents. We are certified for Medicare and Medicaid and we offer a continuum of healthcare services from short-term or outpatient rehabilitation to long-term care. We offer semi-private and private rooms as well as rehabilitation and hospice suites. Rainier Vista Care Center is a 2005 recipient of the American Health Care Association Quality Award.

7045 Rehabilitation Enterprises of Washington
430 E Lauridsen Boulevard
Port Angeles, WA 98362 360-452-9789
FAX: 360-452-9700

Brett White, President
REW is the professional trade association representing community rehabilitation programs before government and other publics. These organizations provide a wide array of employment and training services for people with disabilities. The goal is to assist member organizations to provide the highest quality rehabilitative and employment services to their customers.

7046 **Seattle Medical and Rehabilitation Center**
Evergreen Healthcare
12040 NE 128th Street
Kirkland, WA 98034 425-899-1000

e-mail: comment@evergreenhealthcare.org
www.evergreenhealthcare.org

Steven E Brown, Chief Executive Officer
Louis Filhour, Senior Vice President
Matt Murray, Director Admissions
103 beds offering subacute rehabilitation, complex care, subacute treatment and short-term evaluation. Pulmonary unit offering long and short term care for ventilator dependent patients.

7047 **Slingerland Institute for Literacy**
Educators Publishing Service
1 Bellevue Center
411 108th Avenue NE
Bellevue, WA 98004 425-453-1190
FAX: 425-635-7762
e-mail: mail@slingerland.org
www.slingerland.org

Susan Heinz MD, Executive Director
Elyce Newton, Program Support
A nonprofit public corporation founded in 1977 to carry on the work of Beth H. Slingerland in providing classroom teachers with the techniques, knowledge and understanding necessary for identifying and teaching children with Specific Language Disability. The main objective is to educate teachers in successful methods of identifying, diagnosing and instructing children and adults with SLD and to promote literacy through reading, writing and oral expression.

7048 **Timberland Opportunities Association**
400 W Curtis Street
Aberdeen, WA 98520 360-533-5823
FAX: 360-533-5848
e-mail: jimeddy@techline.com
www.users.olynet.com/timberlandopp

Jim Eddy, Executive Director
Provides training and employment for disabled people.

7049 **Vancouver Health and Rehabilitation Center**
400 E 33rd Street
Vancouver, WA 98663 360-696-2561
FAX: 360-750-0665

Kevin Bowen, Manager
Postacute rehabilitation program.

West Virginia

7050 **West Virginia Rehabilitation Center**
Barron Drive
Institute, WV 25112 304-766-4600
800-642-8207
FAX: 304-766-4989
www.wvdrs.org

Michael Meadows, Assistant Director Client
Bill Tanzey, Manager Center Services
Tracy Carr, Mgr State and Federal Relations
The West Virginia Rehabilitation Center has been called West Virginia's best kept secret. Set on a 33-acre campus near Charleston, WV, the Center complex houses a school with 9 training areas, dormitories, a full-service rehabilitation hospital, a recreation program, a state-of-the-art assistive technology program and extension services statewide.

Wisconsin

7051 **Colonial Manor Medical And Rehabilitation Center**
1010 E Wausau Avenue
Wausau, WI 54403 715-842-2028
FAX: 715-848-0510
www.colonialmanormrc.com

Terry Mantia, Administrator
Colonial Manor Medical and Rehabilitation Center is part of the Kindred Community and is located in Wausau, Wisconsin. The corporate headquarters are based in Louisville Kentucky. Our facility accomodates 150 residents.

7052 **Waushers Industries**
210 East Chicago Road
Wautoma, WI 54982 920-787-4696
FAX: 920-787-4698

Richard King, Executive Director
Provides various programming for individuals with disabilities in waushara county.

7053 **Woodstock Health and Rehabilitation Center**
3415 Sheridan Road
Kenosha, WI 53140 262-657-6175
FAX: 262-657-5756
www.woodstockheath.com

Steven Spencer, Executive Director
Offers a full range of medical services to meet the individual needs of our residents, including short term rehabilitative services and long-tern skilled care.

Alabama

7054 **Rehabilitation & Healthcare Center Of Birmingham**
2728 10th Avenue S
Birmingham, AL 35205
205-933-7010
FAX: 205-933-8720
www.birminghamrehab.com

Mary Edmonds, Administrator
Rehabilitation and Healthcare Center of Birmingham is conveniently located on Birmingham's beautiful and historic Southside. We accomodate 114 residents and we are Medicare and Medicaid certified. Saint Vincent's Hospital, University of Alabama in Birmingham Hospital, and Baptist Medical Center Montclair are either within walking distance or just minutes away. We have caring professionals who strive to meet the needs of our residents.

Alaska

7055 **Fairbanks Memorial Hospital/Denali Center**
1650 Cowles Street
Fairbanks, AK 99701
907-452-8181
FAX: 907-458-5324
www.bannerhealth.com/locations/alaska

Linda Smith, Assistant Administrator
Mike Powers, Chief Executive Officer
Offers the following rehabilitation services: Physical Therapy, Occupational Therapy, Speech Therapy, Sub-Acute Rehab.

Arizona

7056 **Desert Life Rehabilitation & Care Center**
Kindred Healthcare
1919 W Medical Street
Tucson, AZ 85704
520-297-8311
FAX: 520-544-0930
www.desertlifercc.com

Susan Rice, Director
Jane Olmstead, Director of Nursing
Carolyn Blasi, Executive Director
Accomodates 240 residents. We provide skilled and intermediate nursing with occupational, physical, speech and respiratory therapy services. We offer special programs including an Alzheimer's Unit and a Young Adult Program, and are located in beautiful Southern Arizona where there is plenty of sunshine, mountains and desert views. Desert Life is a 2005 recipient of the American Health Care Association Quality Award.

7057 **Hacienda Rehabilitation and Care Center**
660 S Coronado Drive
Sierra Vista, AZ 85635
520-459-4900
FAX: 520-458-4082
www.haciendarcc.com

Maria Ritter, Administrator
Accomodates 100 residents. We are located in Sierra Vista, near Kartchner Caverns, Fort Huachuca, Coronado National Forest and historic Tombstone. Serving the medical needs of the community since 1983, we strive to provide care with quality, compassion and integrity.

7058 **Kachina Point Health Care & Rehabilitation Center**
505 Jacks Canyon Road
Sedona, AZ 86351
928-284-1000
FAX: 928-284-0626
www.kachinapointrehab.com

Christine Walker, Administrator
Accomodates 120 residents. We have met the healthcare needs of the community since 1984. Kachina Point is a 2004 recipient of the American Health Care Association's Quality Award.

7059 **Mayo Clinic Scottsdale**
13400 East Shea Blvd.
Scottsdale, AZ 85259
480-301-8000
FAX: 480-301-4391
www.mayoclinic.org/scottsdale

Pasquale Palumbo MD
Mayo clinic is a not-for-profit medical practice dedicated to the diagnosis and treatment of virtually every type of complex illness. Mayo clinic staff members work together to meet your needs. You will see as many doctors, specialists, and other health care professionals as needed to provide comprehensive diagnosis, understandable answers and effective treatment.

7060 **Sonoran Rehabilitation and Care Center**
Kindred
4202 N 20th Avenue
Phoenix, AZ 85015
602-264-3824
FAX: 602-279-6234
www.sonoranrehab.com

Jeffrey Barrett, Executive Director
Offers the following rehabilitation services: Respiratory Therapy, Physical Therapy, Speech Therapy, Occupational Therapy, Restorative Therapy, Sub-Acute Rehabilitation, Wound Care.

7061 **Valley Health Care and Rehabilitation Cent er**
Kindred Health Care Center
5545 E Lee Street
Tucson, AZ 85712
520-296-2306
FAX: 520-296-4072
www.valleyhcr.com

Stephanie Boatman, Executive Director
Sandra Lewis, Administrator
Offers the following rehabilitation services: Physical Therapy, Occupational Therapy, Speech Therapy, Sub-Acute Rehab.

California

7062 **Alamitos-Belmont Rehab Hospital**
3901 E 4th Street
Long Beach, CA 90814
562-434-8421
FAX: 562-433-6732

Darien Dahl, Administrator
Offers the following rehabilitation services: Speech Therapy, Occupational Therapy, Physical Therapy, Sub-Acute Rehab.

7063 **Bay View Nursing and Rehabilitation Center**
Kindred Health Care
516 Willow Street
Alameda, CA 94501
510-521-5600
FAX: 510-865-6441
www.bayviewnursing.com

Lauren Atkinson, Executive Director
Say Silva, Assistant Executive Director
Mary Webster, Administrator
Accomodates 180 residents. Bay View is a 2004 recipient of the American Health Care Association's Quality Award. We provide short-term rehabilitative care, traditional long-term skilled care and Alzheimer's/dementia special care. Our combination of clinical skill and comprehensive rehabilitation services enables us to care for a variety of complex medical conditions.

7064 **Foothill Nursing and Rehab Center**
401 W Ada Avenue
Glendora, CA 91741
626-335-9810
FAX: 626-963-0720
www.foothillsnursing.com

Yolanda Wilson, Chief Operating Officer
Marianne Schultz, Administrator
Offers the following rehabilitation services: Physical Therapy, Occupational Therapy, Speech Therapy, In and Out Patient Rehab.

7065 **Long Beach Memorial Medical Center Memorial Rehabilitation Hospital**
2801 Atlantic Avenue
Long Beach, CA 90806 562-933-2000
www.memorialcare.org/long_beach

Trish Baeseman, Administrator
The hospital offers rehabilitation after catastrophic injury of disabling disease to give patients the opportunity for maximum recovery. The Hospital offers many of the area's finest rehabilitation specialists and most advanced technology, making it one of Southern California's most respected rehabilitation centers.

7066 **Mercy Medical Center Mt. Shasta**
914 Pine Street
Mount Shasta, CA 96067 530-926-6111
FAX: 530-926-0517
www.mercymtshasta.org

Gary Blebins, Director
Susan Vrh, Manager
Mercy Medical Center is committed to furthering the healing ministry of Jesus, and to provide high-quality, affordable healthcare to the communities we serve.

7067 **Northridge Hospital Medical Center**
18300 Roscoe Boulevard
Northridge, CA 91328 818-885-8500
www.northridgehospital.org

Debra Flaherty, Director Rehab Administration
Mike Wall, Chief Executive Officer
Offers the following rehabilitation services: Physical Therapy, Occupational Therapy, Speech Therapy, Sub-Acute Rehab. As a member of the Catholic Heathcare West Northridge Hospital Medical Center is committed to serving the health needs of our communities with particular attention to the needs of the poor, the disadvantaged and vulnerable, and the comfort of the suffering and dying.

7068 **Riverside Community Hospital**
445 Magnolia Avenue
Riverside, CA 92501 951-788-3000
FAX: 909-788-3616
www.riversidecommunityhospital.org

Jaime Wesolowski, Chief Executive Officer
At Riverside Community Hospital, we are able to provide the healthcare services that you and your family will need through the many stages of your life. Services like Emergency/Trauma, Labor and Delivery, Cardiac Care, Orthopedics and Transplant are among our many Centers of Excellence.

7069 **Saint Jude Medical Center**
101 E Valencia Mesa Drive
Fullerton, CA 92835 714-871-3280
800-870-7537
FAX: 714-992-3029
www.stjudemedicalcenter.org

Winkie Sonnefield, Director for Physical Therapy
Robert Fraschetti, Chief Executive Officer
Offers the following rehabilitation services: Out-patient Rehab, Sub-Acute Rehab, Occupational Therapy, Physical Therapy, Speech and Audiology Therapy, Pain Management Program.

7070 **South Coast Medical Center**
31872 Coast Highway
Laguna Beach, CA 92651 949-499-1311
FAX: 949-499-8644
e-mail: info@southcoastmedcenter.com
www.southcoastmedcenter.com

Nancy Boerner, Director
Bruce Christian, President
Offers the following services: physical therapy, occupational therapy, speech therapy, cardica rehabilitation, incontinence program, sub-acute rehabilitation.

7071 **Valley Garden Health Care and Rehabilitati on Center**
1517 Knickerbocker Drive
Stockton, CA 95210 209-957-4539
FAX: 209-957-5831
www.valleygardenshealth.com

Keith Braley, Administrator
Accomodates 120 residents. Our center provides short-term nursing and rehabilitative care as well as traditional long-term skilled care. Our combination of clinical skill and comprehensive rehabilitation services enables us to care for a variety of complex medical conditions. Rehabilitative therapies are provided as needed by physical, occupational and speech therapists.

Colorado

7072 **Boulder Community Hospital Mapleton Center**
Po Box 9019
1100 Balsam (N Broadway & Balsam)
Boulder, CO 80301 303-440-2273
e-mail: pr@bch.org
www.bch.org

Ron Secrist, President
Offers comprehensive rehabilitation services for individuals of all ages on both an inpatient and outpatient basis. Specialty programs include brain injury, chronic pain management, and pediatric rehabilitation.

7073 **Fairacres Manor**
1700 18th Avenue
Greeley, CO 80631 970-353-3370
FAX: 970-353-9347
www.fairacresmanor.com

Kathy Mekelburg, Administrator
Offers the following rehabilitation services: Physical Therapy, Occupational Therapy, Speech Therapy, Restorative Therapy, Skilled Nursing, and Sub-Acute Rehabilitation.

7074 **Rowan Community**
4601 E Asbury Circle
Denver, CO 80222 303-757-1228
FAX: 303-759-3390
e-mail: tgleisner@pinonmgt.com
www.pinonmgt.com

Tammy Gleisner, Admissions/Marketing Director
Sixty bed skilled nursing facility in southwest Denver, serving younger residents with multiple sclerosis traumatic brain injury, chronic mental illness, 24 hour care need behavior.

Connecticut

7075 **Hamilton Rehabilitation and Healthcare Cen ter**
89 Viets Street
New London, CT 06320 860-889-8358
FAX: 860-889-0395

Jim Christofori, Administrator
Offers the following rehabilitation services: Sub-Acute, Occupational Therapy, Speech Therapy, Physical Therapy.

7076 **Hospital For Special Care (HSC)**
2150 Corbin Avenue
New Britain, CT 06053 860-223-2761
FAX: 860-832-6236
e-mail: info@hfsc.org
www.hfsc.org

John Votto, President/CEO

HSC is a private, not-for-profit 200-bed rehabilitation long-term acute and chronic care hospital, widely-known and respected for its expertise in physical rehabilitation, respiratory care, and medically-complex pediatrics. Special programs for spinal cord injuries, pulmonary rehabilitation, acquired brain injuries, stroke, ventilator management and geriatrics, make HSC an important regional resource for patients with special healthcare needs.

7077 Masonic Healthcare Center
MasoniCare Corporation
22 Masonic Avenue
Wallingford, CT 06492
203-679-5900
877-424-3537
FAX: 203-679-6427
e-mail: info@masonicare.org
www.masonicare.org

William Piper, Vice President
Arthur Santilli, President
The states leading provider of healthcare and retirement living communities for seniors. We are not-for-profit and have more then 100 years of experience behind us. We're recognized for the quality, compassionate care and steadfast support we provide to our residents and patients.

7078 Stamford Hospital
30 Shelburne Road
Stamford, CT 06902
203-276-1000
FAX: 203-325-7905
e-mail: cmurphy@stamhealth.org
www.stamfordhospital.org

Dorothy Turnbull MD
A not-for-profit, community teaching hospital that has been serving Stamford and surrounding communities for more then 100 years. We have 305 inpatient beds in medicine, surgery, obstetrics/gynecology, psychiatry, and medical and surgical critical care units and maintain an educational partnership with Columbia University College of Physicians and Surgeons for its teaching program in the internal medicine, family practice, obstetrics/gynecology and surgery

7079 Windsor Rehabilitation and Healthcare Cent er
581 Poquonock Avenue
Windsor, CT 06095
860-688-7211
FAX: 860-688-6715
www.windsorrehab.com

Laurie Tillestie, Director
Melissa Romano, Admissions
Jim Fidanza, Administrator
Accomodates 116 residents. We offer private and semi-private rooms with access to private telephones and cable television. Our goal is to be a comprehensive, leading care center viewed by our community as an excellent resource for patients, families, and professionals.

Delaware

7080 Arbors at New Castle
32 Buena Vista Drive
New Castle, DE 19720
302-328-2580
FAX: 302-328-2036
e-mail: leighweber@extendicare.com

Leigh Weber, Administrator
A subacute and rehabilitation center offering skilled medical services, infusion therapies, cardiac recovery services, renal disease services, cancer services and digestive disease services. Skilled rehabilitation services include physical therapy, occupational therapy and speech therapy. Also provides case management and discharge planning, general nursing and restorative care and respite care.

Florida

7081 Boca Raton Rehabilitation Center
755 Meadows Road
Boca Raton, FL 33486
561-391-5200
FAX: 561-391-0685

Diana Buck LPN, Admissions Director
Tracey Dougherty, Administrator
Offers the following rehabilitation services: Occupational Therapy, Speech Therapy, Physical Therapy, Sub-Acute Rehabilitation

7082 Cape Coral Hospital
2629 Del Prado Boulevard S
Cape Coral, FL 33990
239-574-2323
FAX: 239-574-6968
www.leememorial.org

Joann Hodges, Administrator
We are a progressive, financially sound health care provider with more then 8,000 employees, 3000 volunteers and auxilians, and 1,200 physicians on staff, and 1,600 licensed beds. The System is a member of Voluntary Hospitals of America, Florida Partnership

7083 Evergreen Woods Health and Rehabilitation Center
7045 Evergreen Woods Trail
Spring Hill, FL 34608
352-596-8371
FAX: 352-596-8032

Maria Seger, Administrator
Offers the following rehabilitation services: Sub-Acute rehabilitation, Occupational therapy, Speech pathology therapy, Physical therapy.

7084 Healthcare and Rehabilitation Center of Sanford
950 S Mellonville Avenue
Sanford, FL 32771
407-322-8566
FAX: 407-322-0121

David Hunt, Administrator
Vicky Smith, Director Admissions
Offers the following rehabilitation services: Sub-Acute rehab, Stroke rehab, Cardiac rehab, Orthopedic rehab, Occupational therapy, Speech therapy, Physical therapy for long term care.

7085 Highland Pines Rehabilitation Center
1111 S Highland Avenue
Clearwater, FL 33756
727-446-0581
FAX: 727-442-9425

Jena Carpenter, Administrator
Offers the following rehabilitation services: Sub-Acute rehabilitation, Occupational Therapy, Speech Therapy, Physical Therapy.

7086 Jupiter Medical Center-Pavilion
1210 S Old Dixie Highway
Jupiter, FL 33458
561-774-4444
FAX: 561-743-5042
e-mail: pr@jupitermed.com
www.jupitermed.com/pavilion/pavilion.htm

Jay Mikosch, Administrator
R Barry, Chief Executive Officer
Offers the following rehabilitation services: Sub-Acute Rehabilitation, Occupational Therapy, Speech Therapy, Physical Therapy.

7087 North Broward Medical Center
401 E Sample Road
Pompano Beach, FL 33064
954-941-4100
FAX: 954-941-4233
www.browardhealth.org

Jeff Naubaum, Administrator
Offers the following rehabilitation services: Sub-Acute rehabilitation, Physical Therapy, Occupational Therapy, Speech Therapy, Respiratory Therapy.

7088 Oaks at Avon Nursing and Rehabilitation Ce nter
1010 US 27 North
Avon Park, FL 33825 863-453-5200
FAX: 863-453-5308
www.seniorhm.com/properties/518.html

Juanita Ullman, Administrator
Oaks at Avon provides a full range of skilled nursing services including infusion therapy, enteral therapy, wound care, tracheotomy care, and portable diagnostics.

7089 Pompano Rehabilitation and Nursing Center
Senior Health Care Management
51 W Sample Road
Pompano Beach, FL 33064 954-942-5530
FAX: 954-942-0941

Teggy Jarmolych, Administrator
Elaine Daniels, Director of Nursing
Offers the following rehabilitation services: Sub-Acute Rehabilitation, Physical Therapy, Occupational Therapy, Speech Therapy

7090 Rehabilitation Center of Palm Beach
301 Northpoint Parkway
West Palm Beach, FL 33407 561-712-1717
FAX: 561-712-1118

Amy Roberts, Administrator
Offers the following rehabilitation services: Sub-Acute Rehabilitation, Physical Therapy, Occupational Therapy, Speech Therapy

7091 Rehabilitation and Healthcare Center of Ta mpa
4411 N Habana Avenue
Tampa, FL 33614 813-872-2771
FAX: 813-871-2831

Kate Hawk, Administrator
Melanie Cloud, Manager
Offers the following rehabilitation services: Sub-Acute Rehabilitation, Physical Therapy, Occupational Therapy, Speech Therapy, Respiratory Therapy.

7092 Shands Rehab Hospital
4101 NW 89th Boulevard
Gainesville, FL 32606 352-265-5491
FAX: 352-265-5430
www.shands.org

Marina Cecchini, Director
Linda Brown, Director Marketing
Offers the following rehabilitation services: Sub-acute rehabilitation, traumatic brain injury, spinal cord injury, stroke, degenerative neurological conditions, amputations, burns, organ transplantation.

7093 St. Anthony's Hospital
1200 7th Avenue N
St Petersburg, FL 33705 727-825-1040
www.stanthonys.com

Angelo Cappelli, Chairman
Bill Kent, Director
Offers the following rehabilitation services: Sub-Acute rehabilitation, Occupational Therapy, Speech/Language Pathology services, Physical Therapy.

7094 Winkler Court
3250 Winkler Avenue Ext
Fort Myers, FL 33916 239-939-4993
FAX: 239-939-1743

Ed Shoman, Administrator
Offers the following rehabilitation services: Sub-Acute Rehabilitation, Physical Therapy, Speech Therapy, Occupational Therapy.

7095 Winter Park Memorial Hospital
200 N Lakemont Avenue
Winter Park, FL 32792 407-646-7000
FAX: 407-646-7639
e-mail: healthcare@winterparkhospital.com
www.winterparkhospital.com

Terry Barter, Director Rehabilitation
Ken Bradley, Chief Executive Officer
Offers the following rehabilitation services: Sub-Acute Rehabilitation, Occupational Therapy, Speech Pathology, Physical Therapy.

Georgia

7096 Athena Rehab of Clayton
2055 Rex Road
Lake City, GA 30260 404-361-5144
FAX: 404-363-6366

Reginald Washington, Administrator
Offers the following rehabilitation services: Sub-Acute rehabilitation, Occupational therapy, Speech therapy, Physical therapy, Restorative care.

7097 Lafayette Nursing and Rehabilitation Center
110 Brandywine Boulevard
Fayetteville, GA 30214 770-461-2928
FAX: 770-461-8507
www.lafayetterehab.com

Jo Brooks, Executive Director
Virginia Tarr, Assistant Director
Lafayette Nursing and Rehab Center accomodates 179 residents. We are Medicare certified and our center also features a 25-bed postacute rehab unit and a 24-bed dementia unit. We have RN's LPN's and CNA's 24 hours a day. We also have physician services availiable seven days a week.

7098 Savannah Rehabilitation and Nursing Center
815 E 63rd Street
Savannah, GA 31405 912-352-8615
FAX: 912-355-4642
www.savannahrehab.com

Lettie Wilson, Administrator
Offers the following rehabilitation services: Sub-Acute rehabilitation, Physical Therapy, Occupational Therapy, Speech Therapy

7099 Specialty Hospital
304 Turner McCall Blvd.
Po Box 1566
Rome, GA 30162 706-509-4100
FAX: 706-509-4159
www.thespecialtyhospital.com

Jon Dixon, Chief Executive Officer
Kurt Stuenkel, President
A 34-bed acute long-term care hospital located in Rome, Georgia, designed for those patients who require treatment for extended periods of time. The patients of The Specialty Hospital are those who do not need the medical resources of a general hospital but whose conditions are too severe for a lower level of care. Patients are admitted to TSH through physician and case manager referrals.

7100 Walton Rehabilitation Health System
1355 Independence Drive
Augusta, GA 30901 706-724-7746
866-492-5866
FAX: 706-724-5752
e-mail: postmaster@wrh.org
www.wrh.org

Dennis Skelley, President
Frank Lewis, Chief Operating Officer
Mike Harrell, CFO
Has Centers of Excellence in Stroke Brain Injury, Complex Orthopedics, Spinal Cord Injury and Pain Management. 58-bed nonprofit facility.

7101 Warner Robins Rehabilitation and Nursing C enter
1601 Elberta Road
Warner Robins, GA 31093 478-922-2241
FAX: 478-328-1984

David Thorton, Administrator
Offers the following rehabilitation services: Sub-Acute rehabilitation, Physical Therapy, Occupational Therapy, Speech Therapy.

Hawaii

7102 Aloha Nursing and Rehab Center
45-545 Kamehameha Highway
Kaneohe, HI 96744 808-247-2220
FAX: 808-235-3676
www.alohanursing.com

Charles Harris, Executive Director
Donna Wong, Administrator
Our unique nursing care facility is nestled in the picturesque town of Kaneohe, Oahu, amid the towering Koolau Mountains and the panoramic vistas of Kaneohe Bay. In this tranquil setting, our 141-bed facility offers both long and short term care to residents who meet intermediate or skilled level of care criteria.

Idaho

7103 Boise Health And Rehabilitation Center
1001 S Hilton Street
Boise, ID 83705 208-345-4464
FAX: 208-345-2998
www.boiserehab.com

Nolan Hoffer, Administrator
Offers the following rehabilitation services: Sub-acute rehabilitation, occupational therapy, speech therapy, physical therapy.

7104 Eastern Idaho Regional Medical Center
3100 Channing Way
Idaho Falls, ID 83404 208-529-6111
FAX: 208-529-7021
www.eirmc.com

Doug Crabtree, Chief Executive Officer
The largest medical facility in the region, Eastern Idaho Regional Medical Center (EIRMC) is a modern, JCAHO-accredidted, full-service hospital. EIRMC serves as the region's healthcare hub, offering specialty services including open-heart surgery, leading-edge cancer treatment, trauma, neurosurgery, intensive care for adults and infants, and a helicopeter service.

7105 Emmett Rehabilitation and Healthcare
Kindred Healthcare
714 N Butte
Emmett, ID 83617 208-365-4425
FAX: 208-365-6989
www.emmettrehab.com

John Schulikn, Executive Director
Emmett Rehab & healthcare accomodates 95 residents. We are located in Emmett, Idaho, a rural community located an easy 30 minute drive from Boise. Emmett Rehab &Æhealthcare has served the area for more then 40 years by providing healthcare for residents of Gem County.

7106 Lewiston Rehabilitation and Care Center
3315 8th Street
Lewiston, ID 83501 208-743-9543
FAX: 208-743-3945
www.lewistonrehab.com

Debbie Freeze, Director
Lewiston Rehabilitation and Care Center has years of experience providing diversified healthcare services. We have our own staff of physical, occupational and speech therapists. Our therapy gym and rehab kitchen are a lovely atmosphere in which to work toward your therapy goals. We are an Eden Alternative Certified facility.

7107 Mountain Valley Care and Rehabilitation Ce nter
Box 689, 601 West Cameron Avenue
Kellogg, ID 83837 208-784-1283
FAX: 208-784-0151
www.mountainvalleycare.com

Maryruth Butler, Administrator
Mountain Valley Care and Rehabilitation Center accomodates 68 residents. We are conveniently located in the heart of Kellogg Idaho. We strive to offer quality care and superior customer service in a home-like environment. Upon admission, you or your loved one is looked after by an assigned staff member. We call this our "Angel Care" program. Our rehabilitation program focuses on meething the individual needs of the resident so you or your loved one can see how they are going to progress.

Illinois

7108 Chevy Chase Nursing and Rehabilitation Cen ter
3400 S Indiana Avenue
Chicago, IL 60616 312-842-5000
FAX: 312-842-3790
www.carepath.com/chevy.cfm

Barbara Casey, Administrator
Our approach to care is multidisciplinary; our medical staff members work together as a team in a proactive fashion, challenging residents each and every day, in order to motivate them to rehabilitate and achieve their ultimate potential.

7109 Glenview Terrace Nursing Center
1511 Greenwood Road
Glenview, IL 60026 847-729-9090
FAX: 847-729-9135
e-mail: bwilz@glenviewterrace.com
www.glenviewterrace.com

Amy Salzman, Administrator
Comfortable private and semi-private rooms and suites. A stylish day spa. Private dining in lavish surroundings to spend a special occasion. And, of course, compassionate skilled nursing, rehabilitative, Alzheimer's and respite care that's unsurpassed in the Chicago area.

7110 Halsted Terrace Nursing Center
10935 S Halsted Street
Chicago, IL 60628 773-928-2000
FAX: 773-928-9154
e-mail: admissions@halstedterrace.com
www.halstedterrace.com

Bonnie Williams, Administrator
Offers the following rehabilitation services: Sub-acute rehabilitation, physical therapy, occupational therapy, speech therapy, cardiac rehabilitation.

7111 Harmony Nursing and Rehabilitation Center
3919 W Foster Avenue
Chicago, IL 60625 773-588-9500
FAX: 773-588-9533
e-mail: jpatino@harmonychicago.com
www.harmonychicago.com

John Sianghio, Administrator
Offers a friendly healthcare experience. You'll find compassionate experts who provide short-term rehabilitation and therapy, wound care, Alzheimer's and memory loss care, long-term nursing care and more.

7112 Imperial
1366 W Fullerton Avenue
Chicago, IL 60614 773-248-9300
FAX: 773-935-0036
www.carepath.com/imperial.cfm

David Hartman, Administrator
Offers the following rehabilitation services: Sub-acute rehabilitation, physical therapy, occupational therapy, speech therapy.

7113 Jackson Square Nursing and Rehabilitation Center
5130 W Jackson Boulevard
Chicago, IL 60644
773-921-8000
FAX: 773-921-3980
www.carepath.com/jackson.cfm

Farhat Sharif, Administrator
Offers the following rehabilitation services: Sub-acute rehabilitation, physical therapy, occupational therapy, speech therapy.

7114 Renaissance at 87th Street
2940 W 87th Street
Chicago, IL 60652
773-434-8787
FAX: 773-434-8717
www.carepath.com/ren87.cfm

Tom Smith, Administrator
Offers the following rehabilitation services: Sub-acute rehabilitation, occupational therapy, physical therapy, speech therapy.

7115 Renaissance at Hillside
4600 Frontage Road
Hillside, IL 60162
708-544-9933
FAX: 708-544-9966
www.carepath.com/renhillside.cfm

Colleen Kamin, Administrator
Offers the following rehabilitation services: Sub-acute rehabilitation, physical therapy, occupational therapy, speech therapy.

7116 Renaissance at Midway
4437 S Cicero Avenue
Chicago, IL 60632
773-884-0484
FAX: 773-884-0485
www.carepath.com/renmidway.cfm

Robin Harris, VP Marketing
Debra Kroner, Director Admissions
Mark Berger, Executive Director
Offers extensive rehabilitation services, designed to aggressively assist individuals to return to thier prior levels of functioning after suffering unexpected truamas such as strokes or bone fractures. In addition, the Renaissance provides Physician Directed Complex Medical Services, Respiratory Care, Cardiac Care, Pain Management, IV therapies, and Wound Care.

7117 Renaissance at South Shore
2425 E 71st Street
Chicago, IL 60649
773-721-5000
FAX: 773-721-6850
www.carepath.com/rensshore.cfm

David Schecter, Administrator
Benitta Harris, Human Resources Executive
Offers the following rehabilitation services: Sub-acute rehabilitation, physical therapy, occupational therapy, speech therapy.

7118 Schwab Rehabilitation Hospital
Mt. Sinai
1401 S California Avenue
Chicago, IL 60608
773-522-2010

e-mail: schwabinquiries@sini.org
www.sinai.org/rehabilitation/

Suzan Rayner MD, Medical Director
Judith Waterston, Chief Executive Officer
Treats medically stable patients who require nursing and medical care that cannot be supplied at home, in an outpatient facility or in a nursing home. Treats stroke patients, amputees, individuals with brain injuries, burns, diabets and spinal cord injuries.

Indiana

7119 Angel River Health and Rehabilitation
5233 Rosebud Lane
Newburgh, IN 47630
812-473-4761
FAX: 812-473-5190
www.angelriverhc.com

Kay Congleton, Administrator
Offers the following rehabilitation services: Sub-acute rehabilitation, speech therapy, occupational therapy, physical therapy.

7120 Chalet Village Health and Rehabilitation C enter
1065 Parkway Street
Berne, IN 46711
260-589-2127
FAX: 260-589-3521

Steven Schaaf, Administrator
Offers the following rehabilitation services: Sub-acute rehabilitation, physical therapy, occupational therapy, speech therapy, respiratory therapy.

7121 Columbus Health and Rehabilitation Center
2100 Midway Street
Columbus, IN 47201
812-372-8447
FAX: 812-375-5117
www.columbushrc.com

Mike Spencer, Executive Director
Accomodates 235 residents. We offer a continuum of healthcare services. Our center also provides a Special Care Alzheimer's Unit. We are licensed by the Stat of Indiana and are Medicare and Medicaid approved provider. We are proud to offer a friendly home-like atmosphere while providing comprehensive healthcare services. These services include short-term medical and rehabilitation treatment, which is designed to address the individual needs of our residents and patients.

7122 Harrison Health and Rehabilitation Centre
150 Beechmont Drive NE
Corydon, IN 47112
812-738-0550
FAX: 812-738-6273
www.harrisonrehab.com

Inez Voyles, Administrator
Offers the following rehabilitation services: Sub-Acute rehabilitation, speech therapy, physical therapy, occupational therapy.

7123 Indian Creek Health and Rehabilitation Center
240 Beechmont Drive NE
Corydon, IN 47112
812-738-8127
877-380-7211
FAX: 812-738-2917
e-mail: sherry.leclair@kindredhealthcare.com
www.indiancreekhealthcare.com

Marianne Keller, Administrator
Sherry LeClair, Admissions Director
Bonnie Fallin, Executive Director
140 bed facility offering the following rehabilitation services: Sub-Acute rehabilitation, Physical therapy, Occupational Therapy, Speech Therapy, pain management, Wound rehabilitation. Short and long term skilled nursing care certified for Medicare, Medicaid, Private Pay and Private Insurance. Hospice and respite care rated #1 in clinical care in southern Indiana district for 2002.

7124 Meadowvale Health and Rehabilitation Cente r
Kindred Health Care
1529 Lancaster Street
Bluffton, IN 46714
260-824-4320
800-743-3333
FAX: 260-824-4689
e-mail: meadowvalehealth@kindredhealthcare.com
www.meadowvalerehab.com

Sally Sharp, Executive Director
Offers the following rehabilitation services: Sub-acute rehabilitation, physical therapy, occupational therapy, speech therapy.

7125 Muncie Health Care and Rehabilitation
4301 N Walnut Street
Muncie, IN 47303
765-282-0053
800-743-3333
FAX: 765-282-3290
www.muncierehab.com

Debbie Anderson, Administrator
Offers the following rehabilitation services: Sub-Acute rehabilitation, physical therapy, occupational therapy, speech therapy.

7126 Rehabilitation Hospital of Indiana
4141 Shore Drive
Indianapolis, IN 46254
317-329-2000
FAX: 317-329-2104
www.rhin.com

Dennis Armington, CEO
Nancy Stover, Director Operations
Offers the following rehabilitation services: Sub-acute rehabilitation, brain injury, spinal cord injury programs.

7127 Sellersburg Health and Rehabilitation Cent re
7823 Old State Road 60
Sellersburg, IN 47172
812-246-4272
FAX: 812-246-8160
www.sellersburghrehab.com

Donna Thomas, Director of Nursing
Chris Hansen, Executive Director
Sellersburg is a modern healthcare center conveniently located on the edge of the community. Our center accomodates 110 residents and includes a rehabilitative program with a goal of returning residents home as quickly as possible. Sellersburg is a 2006 recipient of the American Health Care Association Quality Award.

7128 Westpark Rehabilitation Center
1316 North Tibbs Avenue
Indianapolis, IN 46222
317-634-8330
FAX: 317-263-9442
www.westparkhealthcare.com

Lara Beck, Administrator
Offers the following rehabilitation services: Sub-acute rehabilitation, occupational therapy, physical therapy, speech therapy, respiratory therapy.

7129 Westview Nursing and Rehabilitation Center
1510 Clinic Drive
Bedford, IN 47421
812-279-4494
FAX: 812-275-8313
www.westviewhealthcare.com

Sandi Harpe
Mike Spencer, Executive Director
Offers the following rehabilitation services: Sub-acute rehabilitation, physical therapy, occupational therapy, speech therapy.

7130 Windsor Estates Health and Rehab Center
429 W Lincoln Road
Kokomo, IN 46902
765-453-5600
FAX: 765-455-0110
www.windsorestateshrc.com

Jeff Hayne, Administrator
We offer a full range of medical services to meet the individual needs of our residents, physician, our staff-including medical specialists, nurses, nutritionists, dietitians, and social workers-establishes a comprehensive treatment plan intended to restore you or your loved one to the highest practicable potential.

Iowa

7131 Madison County Rehab Services
Madison County Hospital
300 W Hutchings Street
Winterset, IA 50273
515-462-2373
FAX: 515-462-5108

Marcia Jones, Utilization Review Nurse
Panndee Stebbins, Director
Andrea Miner, Manager
Offers the following rehabilitation services: Sub-acute rehabilitation, occupational therapy, physical therapy, speech therapy, home health rehab, wellness programs.

7132 Mercy Subacute Care
603 E 12th Street
Des Moines, IA 50309
515-247-4400
FAX: 515-643-8871

Bonnie McCoy, Administrator
Pam Nelson, Intake Coordinator
Offers the following rehabilitation services: Sub-acute rehabilitation, physical therapy, speech therapy, occupational therapy.

Kentucky

7133 Danville Centre for Health and Rehabilitat ion
642 N 3rd Street
Danville, KY 40422
859-236-3972
FAX: 859-236-0033

Jennifer Phillips, Administrator
Offers the following rehabilitation services: Sub-acute rehabilitation, physical therapy, occupational therapy, speech therapy.

7134 Lexington Center for Health and Rehabilita tion
353 Waller Avenue
Lexington, KY 40504
859-252-3558
FAX: 859-233-0192

Melissa Lammoore, Administrator
Offers the following rehabilitation services: Sub-acute rehabilitation, speech therapy, occupational therapy, physical therapy.

7135 Paducah Centre For Health and Rehabilitati on
Wellsouth Health Systems
501 N 3rd Street
Paducah, KY 42001
270-444-9661
FAX: 270-443-9407

Terri Humes, Director
Offers the following rehabilitation services: subacute rehabilitation, speech therapy, occupational therapy, physical therapy.

7136 Pathways Brain Injury Program
4200 Browns Lane
Louisville, KY 40220
502-459-8900
FAX: 502-459-5026

Pam Pearson, Program Director
Offers the following rehabilitation services: Sub-acute rehabilitation, speech therapy, occupational therapy, physical therapy, recreational therapy.

7137 Winchester Centre For Health & Rehabilitation
200 Glenway Road
Winchester, KY 40391
859-744-1800
800-648-6057
FAX: 859-744-0285
www.winchestercentre.com

Robert Hollins, Administrator
Offers the following rehabilitation services: Sub-acute rehabilitation, speech therapy, physical therapy, occupational therapy.

Louisiana

7138 Guest House of Slidell Sub-Acute and Rehab Center
1051 Robert Boulevard
Slidell, LA 70458
985-643-5630
800-303-9872
FAX: 985-649-6065
e-mail: jburch@ghslidell.com

Linda Rogers, Administrator
116 bed healthcare center offering the following subacute services within the skilled nursing setting: physical, occupational, and speech therapies, infusion therapy, respiratory care, wound care, neurological rehabilitation, cardiac reconditioning, pain management, post surgical recovery, orthopedic rehabilitation.

7139 Irving Place Rehabilitation and Nursing Ce nter
1736 Irving Place
Shreveport, LA 71101
318-221-1983
FAX: 318-222-2095

Linda Johnson, Administrator
Offers the following rehabilitation services: sub-acute rehabilitation, speech therapy, occupational therapy, physical therapy

Maine

7140 Augusta Rehabilitation Center
188 Eastern Avenue
Augusta, ME 04330
207-622-3121
800-457-1220
FAX: 207-623-7666
www.augustarehabcenter.com

Carolyn Deblasi, Acting Administrator
Beth Whitcomb, Finance Executive
Accomodates 72 residents. Augusta Rehabilitation Center offers a continuum of healthcare services including respite, short-term rehabilitation and long-term care. We are proud to have a dedicated team of veteran healthcare professionals on hand. This group establishes a plan of care upon admission that includes the resident and family. Our goal is to care for the medical, psychosocial, and emotional needs of your loved one, addressing all aspects of his or her care and well being.

7141 Brentwood Rehabilitation and Nursing Cente r
370 Portland Street
Yarmouth, ME 04096
207-846-9021
800-457-1220
FAX: 207-846-1497
www.brentwoodrnc.com

Laurie Farren, Executive Director
Brentwood accomodates 82 residents. We are located at 370 Portland Street in Yarmouth, Maine. We strive to meet the healthcare needs of the greater Yarmouth community, including Portland and Brunswick, which are located within 10 miles of the center. In addition to Brentwood's rehabilitation and skilled nursing services, we also offer Alzheimer's specialty care in a comfortable setting.

7142 Den-Mar Rehabilitation and Nursing Center
44 South Street
Rockport, MA 01966
978-546-6311
800-439-2370
www.denmarrnc.com

Tricia Shaw, Executive Director
Den-Mar nursing and Rehab center accomodates 80 residents. We provide skilled nursing and rehabilitation services as well as long term care. We are certified for Medicare and Medicaid as well as many insurance carriers. We offer semi-private and private rooms, with many common areas for socializing.

7143 Eastside Rehabilitation and Living Center
516 Mount Hope Avenue
Bangor, ME 04401
207-947-6131
800-457-1220
FAX: 207-942-0884
www.eastsiderehab.com

Michael Speidel, Executive Director
Accomodates 67 residents. We offer short-term rehabilitation, complex medical care, skilled nursing services, respite, and traditional long-term care. We specialize in the treatment of respiratory or breathing diseases and/or disorders. Utilizing a team approach, we develop individualized plans of care for each patient or resident with a goal of restoring health and function to the fullest extent possible.

7144 Kennebunk Nursing & Rehabilitation Center
158 Ross Road
Kennebunk, ME 04043
207-985-7141
800-457-1220
FAX: 207-985-0961
www.kenebunknursing.com

Thomas Foran, Administrator
Kennebunk Nursing and Rehabilitation Center accomodates 76 residents. We offer short-term rehabilitation, complex medical care, skilled nursing services, traditional long-term care, and adult day care. Utilizing an interdisciplinary approach, we develop individualized plans of care for each resident.

7145 Norway Rehabilitation and Living Center
29 Marion Avenue
Norway, ME 04268
207-743-7075
800-457-1220
FAX: 207-743-9269
www.norwayrehab.com

Carolyn Farley, Administrator
Norway Rehabilitation and Living center accomodates 70 residents. We offer short-term rehabilitation, complex medical care, skilled nursing services and long-term care, plus a residential care unit for a more independent resident population. A compassionate staff dedicated to serving the physical and emotional needs of patients strives to provide high quality treatment. Utilizing an interdisciplinary team approach, we develop individualized plans of care for each patient.

7146 Shore Village Rehabilitation & Nursing Center
201 Camden Street
Rockland, ME 04841
207-596-6423
800-457-1220
FAX: 207-596-7235
www.shorevillagerehab.com

Phyllis Nickerson, Administrator
Shore Village accomodates 60 residents and is located in the mid-coast region of the state of Maine. We have a cozy size and a primary goal for the staff is to ensure a home-like atmosphere for all the residents. Shore Village provides skilled nursing and rehabilitation, respite care, and long term care. The facility is dually certified for Medicare and Medicaid and accepts many commercial insurance plans.

Maryland

7147 Greater Baltimore Medical Center
6701 N Charles Street
Baltimore, MD 21204
443-849-2000
FAX: 443-849-3024
www.gbmc.org

Laurence Merlis, Chief Executive Officer
GBMC includes Greater Baltimore Medical Center (GBMC), Central Maryland's leading community hospital; Hospice of Baltimore, which provides comfort and care to patients with life-limiting illnesses; and the GBMC Foundation, which supports the GBMC mission by managing fundraising efforts. The 292-bed Medical Center, located on a beautiful suburban campus serves nearly 22,000 inpatients annually as well as providing some 50,000 emergency room visits.

Massachusetts

7148 Bolton Manor Nursing Home
400 Bolton Street
Marlborough, MA 01752
508-481-6123
800-439-2370
FAX: 508-481-6130
www.boltonmanor.com

Scott Bullock, Administrator
Bolton Manor accomodates 157 residents. We are located in Marlboro, Massachusetts. We provide medical management and long-term care through comprehensive skilled and post-acute nursing services. We also provide physical, occupational, and speech therapy services from an onsite dedicated staff of therapists. The facility is Joint Commission (formerly JCAHO) accredited and has an excellent survey history with the State Department of Public Health.

7149 Brigham Manor Nursing and Rehabilitation Center
77 High Street
Newburyport, MA 01950
978-462-4221
800-439-2370
FAX: 978-463-3297
www.brighammanor.com

Christine Rich, Administrator
Brigham Manor accomodates 64 residents. We are a Medicare-certified facility offering private, semi-private and multi-bed suites. Our bright, formal dining room, with French doors that open to a shaded courtyard, provides a warm atmosphere for entertaining family and friends. Each resident's personal tastes and medical needs are considered in the planning of our weekly menus.

7150 Country Gardens Skilled Nursing and Rehabilitation Center
2045 Grand Army Highway
Swansea, MA 02777
508-379-9700
800-439-2370
FAX: 508-379-0723
www.cntrygrdns.com

John Corliss, Administrator
Country Gardens Skilled Nursing and Rehabilitation Center accomodates 86 residents. We are located in a beautiful rural setting conveniently located about 15 minutes east of Providence and 10 minutes west of Fall River. We have provided healthcare service to the greater Swansea area for over 34 years.

7151 Country Manor Rehabilitation and Nursing C enter
180 Low Street
Newburyport, MA 01950
978-465-5361
800-439-2370
FAX: 978-463-9366
www.countryrehab.com

Shari Laroche, Administrator
Country Rehabilitation and Nursing Center accomodates 123 residents. We are located in the quaint seaport town of Newburyport, Massachusetts. We provide medical management and long-term care through comprehensive skilled and intermediate nursing services. We also provide physical, occupational, and speech therapy services from an onsite dedicated staff of therapists. The center offers an Alzheimer's special care unit with staff trained in dimentia care and dementia specific programs.

7152 Franklin Skilled Nursing and Rehabilitation Center
130 Chestnut Street
Franklin, MA 02038
508-528-4600
800-439-2370
FAX: 508-528-7976
www.franklinskilled.com

Karen Wadlow, Administrator
Kevin Diehl, Executive Director
Franklin Skilled Nursing and Rehabilitation Center accomodates 82 residents. Each program and department is designed and operated to give you quality care. From our compassionate nursing staff to our helpful and friendly housekeepers, we strive to lend a listning ear, a gentle hug, and a thoroughly trained, competent staff member to assist you and your family members. We understand the necessity of working together to make our center feel a bit more like home, and we appreciate suggestions.

7153 Great Barrington Rehabilitation and Nursing Center
148 Maple Avenue
Great Barrington, MA 01230
413-528-3320
800-439-2370
FAX: 413-528-2302
www.greatbarringtonrnc.com

Katie Coburn, Executive Director
Great Barrington Rehabilitation and Nursing Center accomodates 106 residents. As part of a national network of long-term healthcare centers, we have the expertise and resources to provide care appropriate to the individual needs of each and every one of our residents. We provide personal care with minimal daily living assistance to the most skilled treatment for medically complex patients.

7154 Ledgewood Rehabilitation and Skilled Nursing Center
87 Herrick Street
Beverly, MA 01915
978-921-1392
800-439-2370
FAX: 978-927-8627
www.ledgewoodrehab.com

Laurie Roberto, Executive Director
Ledgewood accomodates 123 residents. We are located on the campus of Beverly Hospital, with acute care services close by. The leadership and staff at Ledgewood continue to strive for excellence through thier ongoing performance inprovement mentality. We are proud that our facility has achieved outstanding survey results including eight deficiency-free Department of Public Health Surveys and a score of 96 on the 2002 Joint Commission survey.

7155 Leo P La Chance Center for Rehabilitation and Nursing
59 Eastwood Circle
Gardner, MA 01440
978-632-8776
FAX: 978-632-5048
www.lachancecenter.com

Dennis Lopata, Administrator
A privately owned facility, combines the best of medical technology with the ultimate in healing, compassionate rehabilitation and nursing care. Our goal is to help each client reach that ultimate goal of living life to the fullest.

7156 Oakwood Rehabilitation and Nursing Center
11 Pontiac Avenue
Webster, MA 01570
508-943-3889
800-439-2370
FAX: 508-949-6125
www.oakwoodrehab.com

Daniel O'Neil, Administrator
George Mercier, Executive Director
Oakwood Rehabilitation and Nursing Center accomodates 81 residents. We offer 24-hour skilled nursing, inpatient rehabilitation, respite care, and hospice services. Our center has been successfully serving the greater Webster, Massachusetts, community for 35 years. We have a dedicated and caring staff and our common goal is to promote recovery and enhance quality of live whether your needs are short or long term.

7157 Walden Rehabilitation and Nursing Center
785 Main Street
Concord, MA 01742
978-369-6889
800-439-2370
FAX: 978-369-8392
www.waldenrehab.com

Dan Burns, Administrator

Walden Rehabilitation and Nursing Center accomodates 123 residents. We are located in the quaint town of Concord, Massachusetts, across the street from Emerson Hospital and a short drive from the town center. Walden provides medical management and long-term care through comprehensive skilled and intermediate nursing services. We also provide physical, occupational, and speech therapy services from an onsite dedicated staff of therapists.

Michigan

7158 **Boulder Park Terrace**
14676 W Upright Street
Charlevoix, MI 49720
231-547-1005
FAX: 231-547-1039
www.northernhealth.org

Saur Mackenzie, Director
Deb Saur-Macenzie, Administrator
A partnership formed with Charlevoix Area Hospital, Boulder Park Terrace is a long-term care facility and Sub-acute Rehabilitation Center located in Chalrevoix near the shores of Lake Michigan. The Sub-acute Rehabilitation Center was created as a transition between an acute care hospital and home. Patients enter into the program to increase their strength, endurance and over-all functioning before returning home.

Minnesota

7159 **Park Health And Rehabilitation Center**
4415 W 36 1/2 Street
St Louis Park, MN 55416
952-927-9717
FAX: 952-927-7687

Jennifer Kuhn, Administrator

Missouri

7160 **Barnes-Jewish Hospital Washington University Medical Center**
1 Barnes Jewish Hospital Plaza
Saint Louis, MO 63110
314-747-3000
866-867-3627
FAX: 314-286-0305
www.barnesjewish.org

Steven Lipstein, President
Barnes-Jewish Hospital at Washington University Medical Center is the largest hospital in Missouri and the largest private employer in the St. Louis region. An affiliated teaching hospital of Washington University School of Medicine, Barnes-Jewish Hospital has a 1,700 member medical staff with many who are recognized in the "Best Doctors in America".

Montana

7161 **Parkview Acres Care and Rehabilitation Cen ter**
200 N Oregon Street
Dillon, MT 59725
406-683-5105
866-253-4090
FAX: 406-683-6388
www.parkviewacres.com

Jake Bowen, Administrator
William Harlow, Executive Director
We are Medicare and Medicaid certified skilled nursing facility which accomodates 108 residents serving scenic Dillon and surrounding Montana communities.

Nebraska

7162 **Homestead Healthcare and Rehabilitation Ce nter**
4735 S 54th Street
Lincoln, NE 68516
402-488-0977
800-833-0920
FAX: 402-488-4507
www.homesteadrehab.com

Connie Crawford, Director
David Pettijohn, Administrator
Matt Romshek, Executive Director
Homestead Healthcare and Rehabilitation Center is one of the area's oldest providers of skilled nursing and rehabilitation services. We are a 163-bed skilled nursing and rehabilitation center nestled in a lovely, quiet established neighborhood in South Lincoln.

7163 **Madonna Rehabilitation Hospital**
5401 South Street
Lincoln, NE 68506
402-489-7102
FAX: 402-486-5448
www.madonna.org

Marsha Lommel, President/CEO
Kiranmayi Chilappa, MD
Patients who need only one or two types of therapy for a specific condition are served in the subacute program. Patients who have a diagnosis suggesting a positive course of recovery are typical for the subacute level of care.

7164 **Mary Lanning Memorial Hospital**
715 N Saint Joseph Avenue
Hastings, NE 68901
402-463-4521
866-460-5884
e-mail: tanderson@mlmh.org
www.mlmh.org

Michael Kearney, President
Mark Vincent, Vice President
W Kearney, Chief Executive Officer
Mary Lanning Memorial Hospital, A regional health system, is committed to a tradition of excellence through leadership in the provision of quality medical services and health education for the people of Central Nebraska. Our mission is achieved through a dedicated, caring staff, using advanced technology within a healthy and pleasant environment, in a cost effective manner.

Nevada

7165 **Las Vegas Healthcare and Rehabilitation Ce nter**
2832 S Maryland Parkway
Las Vegas, NV 89109
702-735-5848
800-326-6888
FAX: 702-735-0383
www.lasvegaskindred.com

Randy Fuller, Executive Director
Las Vegas Healthcare accomodates 79 residents. We have been serving the community for approximately 40 years. Located in close proximity to local hospitals and surrounded by medical complexes, our center offers both short-term rehabilitation and long-term care.

New Hampshire

7166 **Dover Rehabilitation and Living Center**
307 Plaza Drive
Dover, NH 03820
603-742-2676
800-735-2964
FAX: 603-749-5375
www.doverrehab.com

Jill Bosa, Administrator

Dover Rehab is a provider of postacute services in the greater New Hampshire Seacost area. We accomodate 112 residents and are licensed by the state of New Hampshire. We employ nearly 150 licensed nurses, therapists and other healthcare professionals, who strive to provide quality care. The goal of our patient service model is to bridge the gap between hospitalization and home so that recovery and physical functioning are maximized and hospital readmission is minimized.

7167 **Northeast Rehabilitation Clinic**
70 Butler Street
Salem, NH 03079
603-893-2900
800-825-7292
FAX: 603-893-1628
e-mail: webmaster@northeastrehab.com
www.northeastrehab.com

John Prochilo, Executive Director
Tom Prince, Administrator Officer
Subacute rehabilitation at NRH was designed for people who have experienced an acutely disabling orthopedic, medical, or neurologic condition but who either do not require or are unable to participate in a full acute inpatient program. Impairment groups pertinent to this level of care include brain injury, spinal cord injury (traumatic/non-traumatic), stroke, orthopedic injury, amputation, and neurologic disorder.

New Jersey

7168 **Atlantic Coast Rehabilitation & Healthcare Center**
485 River Avenue
Lakewood, NJ 08701
732-364-7100
FAX: 732-364-2442
e-mail: contact@atlanticcoastrehab.com
www.atlanticcoastrehab.com

Simon Shain, Administrator
Sharon Sckbower, Director of Nursing
Offers the following rehabilitation services: Sub-acute rehab, physical therapy, occupational therapy, speech therapy.

7169 **Crestwood Nursing & Rehabilitation Center**
101 Whippany Road
Whippany, NJ 07981
973-887-0311
FAX: 973-887-8355

Carol Shepard, Administrator
Sub-acute rehabilitation facility.

7170 **Lakeview Subacute Care Center**
130 Terhune Drive
Wayne, NJ 07470
973-839-4501
FAX: 973-616-3409
www.lakeviewsubacute.com

Richard Grosso, Executive Director
Susan R Ahlers, Director of Admission
Offers physical therapy, occupational therapy, speech therapy, recreational therapy, respiratory therapy, aqua therapy. 68-bed subacute unit.

7171 **Merwick Rehabilitation and Sub-Acute Care**
79 Bayard Lane
Princeton, NJ 08540
609-497-3000
FAX: 609-497-3024
www.mcp.org

Kathy Ales, Medical Director
Ryan Wismer, Administrator
76-bed skilled nursing and residential center as well as a separate 17-bed comprehensive rehabilitation center. Offers rehabilitation, physiatry, occupational therapy, respite care, speech/hearing therapy, sub-acute care.

7172 **Seacrest Village Nursing Center**
1001 Center Street
Little Egg Harbor Twp, NJ 08087
609-296-9292
FAX: 609-296-0508
e-mail: info@seacrestvillagenj.com
www.seacrestvillagenj.com

Brian T Holloway, Administrator
Seacrest Village Nursing and Rehabilitation Center has specialized in quality rehabilitation, transitional and restorative care for more then a decade and is a perfect alternative for bridging the gap between hospital and home.

7173 **St. Lawrence Rehabilitation Center**
2381 Lawrenceville Road
Lawrenceville, NJ 08648
609-896-9500
FAX: 609-895-0242
www.slrc.org

Charles Brennan, Chief Executive Officer
St. Lawrence Rehabilitation Center, a non-profit facility sponsored by the Roman Catholic Diocese of Trenton, is committed to maximizing the quality of human life by providing comprehensive physical rehabilitation and related programs to meet the healthcare needs of our communities.

7174 **Summit Ridge Center Genesis Eldercare**
20 Summit Street
West Orange, NJ 07052
973-736-2000
800-699-1520
FAX: 973-731-4582
www.ghv.com

Chad Murin, Administrator
Elizabeth Martin, Customer Relations Manager
Skilled nursing facility with a total of 152 beds. 40 bed sub-acute unit and 24 bed secure dementia unit. Able to care for a wide variety of rehab and medical cases from orthopedics to TPN and tracheostomies.

New York

7175 **Beth Abraham Health Services**
612 Allerton Avenue
Bronx, NY 10467
718-519-4000
888-238-4223
FAX: 718-519-4010
e-mail: info@bethabe.org
www.bethabe.org

Michael Fassler, Chief Executive Officer
Offers the following rehabilitation services: Sub-Acute rehabilitation, brain injury rehabilitation, pain management, post-operative recovery. Home visits and a network of community-based programs help patients and their families with a successful transition home.

7176 **Central Island Healthcare**
825 Old Country Road
Plainview, NY 11803
516-868-6097
FAX: 516-868-7251
www.centralislandhealthcare.net

Dominic D. Sclafani, Administrator
Michael Ostreicher, Assistant Administrator
Moshe Shirazi, Medical Director
Serving the community for over 33 years, Central Island Healthcare is Long Island's largest and most active sub-acute care provider. We offer comprehensive programs focused on restoring our patients to their maximum potential and returning home. Central Island's 202-bed facility provides top notch professionals and the latest in rehabilitation and therapeutic equipment in a beautiful and comfortable setting.

7177 **Clove Lakes Health Care and Rehabilitation Center**
25 Fanning Street
Staten Island, NY 10314
718-289-7900
FAX: 718-761-8701
www.clovelakes.com

Helen Demisay, Chief Executive Officer
M Gemisay, Executive Director
CLove Lakes provides a full range of services to individuals who are in need of skilled nursing, therapeutic and/or rehabilitation care. Our success in providing compassionate quality care is evidenced by the excellent reputation we enjoy in our areas of specialization.

7178 **Dr. William O Benenson Rehabilitation Pavilion**
3617 Parsons Boulevard
Flushing, NY 11354
718-445-3539
FAX: 718-939-5032
www.flushingmanors.com

Richard Sherman, Administrator
The Dr. William O Benson Reahbilitation Pavilion is a subacute short-term rehabilitation center committed to the excellence of elevated health care for our patients. Through the use of the most comprehensive and specialized services available, our staff of dedicated professionals are devoted to putting patients back to the road to full recovery 24 hours a day.

7179 **Flushing Manor Nursing and Rehab**
35-15 Parsons Boulevard
Flushing, NY 11354
718-961-3500
FAX: 718-461-1784
e-mail: jenella.nh@flushingmanors.com
www.flushingmanors.com

Jerry Enella, Administrator
Esther Benenson, Owner
At the Flusing Manor Nursing and Rehabilitation, we stress the importance of family involvement because it is the true source of strength and stability in ones life...a tie that brings us all together as a team, enhancing the quality of life of the patients in our care.

7180 **Glengariff Health Care Center**
Dosoris Lane
Glen Cove, NY 11542
516-676-1100
FAX: 516-759-0216
e-mail: info@glenhaven.org
www.glenhaven.org

Jean Campo, Director Admissions
Michael Miness, President
Licensed skilled nursing and subacute medical and rehabilitation facility.

7181 **Haym Salomon Home for The Aged**
2340 Cropsey Avenue
Brooklyn, NY 11214
718-373-1700
FAX: 718-449-9028

Haym Lipschupv, Administrator
Religious nonmedical health care institution.

7182 **Kings Harbor Multicare Center**
2000 E Gun Hill Road
Bronx, NY 10469
718-320-0400
FAX: 718-320-0557
e-mail: info@kingsharbor.com
www.kingsharbor.com

Morris Tenenbaum, Owner
Kings Harbor Multicare Center provides long-term and short-term skilled nursing care for more then 700 residents. Kings Harbor is located in the Pelham Gardens neighborhood of Northeast Bronx, easily accessible to major highways and near public transportation. A 3 building campus facility with surrounding gardens ensures that residents with similar capabilities are grouped together.

7183 **Northwoods of Cortland**
28 Kellogg Road
Cortland, NY 13045
607-753-9631
FAX: 607-756-2968

Amy Simrell, Yucca Executive Director
Dorothy Zegarelli, Administrator
Subacute rehabilitation facility.

7184 **Port Jefferson Health Care Facility**
Dark Hollow Road
Port Jefferson, NY 11777
631-473-5400
FAX: 631-474-5402
e-mail: info@glenhaven.org
www.glenhaven.org

Anne Kohlmann, Director Admissions
Kathy Peets, VP Corporate/External Affairs
Ellen Harte, Administrator
Subacute medical and rehabilitative care and long term residential skilled nursing care.

7185 **Rehab Institute at Florence Nightingale He alth Center**
1760 3rd Avenue
New York, NY 10029
212-410-8760
800-786-8968
FAX: 212-410-8792
e-mail: info@rehabinstitute.org
Sub-acute rehabilitation facility.

7186 **Schnurmacher Center for Rehabilitation and Nursing**
Beth Abraham of Family Health Services
12 Tibbits Avenue
White Plains, NY 10606
914-287-7200
888-238-4223
FAX: 914-428-1216
e-mail: info@bethabe.org
www.bethabe.org/schnurmacher93

Karen Nodiff, Director Admissions
Diane McKillop, Director Nursing
Karen Kaplan Blick, Director Social Services
The environment at Schnurmacher is tailored to the needs of patients who require medical and nursing services but who do not need the complexity of services associated with an acute-care hospital. And Schnurmacher Subacute Medical patients are out of bed more quickly and as often as possible, which helps them maintain functional status while recovery progresses.

7187 **South Shore Healthcare**
275 W Merrick Road
Freeport, NY 11520
516-868-6097
FAX: 516-868-7251
www.southshorehealthcare.net

Cathie Geraghty, Administrator
Serving the community for over 45 years, South Shore Healthcare is Long Island's first sub-acute care provider. We offer comprehensive programs focused on restoring our patients to their maximum potential and returning home. Our facility offers top notch professionals and the latest in rehabilitation and therapeutic equipment in a beautiful and comfortable setting.

7188 **St. Camillus Health and Rehabilitation Cen ter**
813 Fay Road
Syracuse, NY 13219
315-488-2951
FAX: 315-488-3255
www.st-camillus.org

Aileen Balitz, President
Since our founding in 1969, St. Camillus' mission has been to provide high-quality services and facilities emphasizing the rehabilitation of individuals to their maximum potential. The importance of the human spirit drives all we do. We are dedicated to caring for life and helping individuals achieve their highest possible level of independence.

North Carolina

7189 **Chapel Hill Rehabilitation and Healthcare Center**
1602 E Franklin Street
Chapel Hill, NC 27514
919-967-1418
800-735-8262
FAX: 919-967-1457
www.chapelhillhc.com

Robert Park, Administrator
John R. Jarrell, Executive Director
Chapel Hill Rehabilitation and Healthcare Center accomodates 120 residents. We are located in downtown Chapel Hill on Franklin Street and we provide roud the clock nursing care 365 days a year. Intensive rehabilitation services are administered by our licensed speech, occupational and physical therapists. Our staff is trained to care for medically complex patients such as those requiring intensive wound care, dialysis, and artificial nutrition.

7190 Cypress Pointe Rehabilitation and Healthca re Center
2006 S 16th Street
Wilmington, NC 28401
910-763-6271
800-735-8262
FAX: 910-251-9803
www.cypresspointehc.com

Dan Daly, Administrator
Cypress Pointe offers comprehensive physical, occupational, speech and respiratory therapy services. Following a physician's referral, patients are evaluated to determine their needs. Recommendations are then made for the appropriate interventions and rehabilitation. If therapy is required, a personalized care plan is developed.

7191 Pettigrew Rehabilitation and Healthcare Center
1551 W Pettigrew Street
Durham, NC 27705
919-286-0751
800-735-8262
FAX: 919-286-5992
www.pettigrewghc.com

Mark Anthony, Administrator
Pettigrew Rehabilitation and Healthcare Center accomodates 107 residents. Our healthcare center is certified by Medicare and Medicaid. We have experienced staff members who care for our residents. We strive to improve the quality of life our residents experience as a result of the services they receive from our nursing and therapy departments.

7192 Raleigh Rehabilitation and Healthcare Cent er
616 Wade Avenue
Raleigh, NC 27605
919-828-6251
800-735-8262
FAX: 919-828-3294
www.raleighrehabhc.com

Steve Harrison, Administrator
Raleigh Rehabilitation and Healthcare Center accomodates 172 residents. We provide short-term rehabilitation-including, physical, occupational, and speech therapies-as well as long-term nursing services. We specialize in neurological disorders, complex diabetes treatment, amputation recovery and pain management. We welcome short stays (respite care). Transportation services are availiable for physician appointments and dialysis treatments.

7193 Rehabilitation and Healthcare Center of Almanace
779 Woody Drive
Graham, NC 27253
336-228-8394
800-735-8262
FAX: 336-228-8574
www.almanacehc.com

Cassandra Smith, Executive Director
Our center houses ambulatory as well as bedfast residents and our goal is to offer quality nursing and rehabilitation care at a reasonable price. We are approved by the State Board of Health and employ only trained personnel to cater to resident needs. Our staff is supervised by licensed RN's and there is a physician on call 24 hours a day.

7194 Rehabilitation and Healthcare Center of Mo nroe
1212 Sunset Drive
Monroe, NC 28112
704-283-8548
800-735-8262
FAX: 704-283-4664
www.monroehc.com

Judy Olson, Administrator
We accomodate 159 residents and are certified for Medicare and Medicaid. We specialize in short-term rehabilitation as well as long-term care. Our therapists, wound nurse and dietician work closely to administer wound care. We hav 2 dialysis centers within a 10-block radius and gladly accpet their patients. We have an on-staff medical director as well as a psychiatrist.

7195 Winston-Salem Rehabilitation and Healthcar e Center
1900 W 1st Street
Winston Salem, NC 27104
336-724-2821
800-735-8262
FAX: 336-725-8314
www.winstonsalemhc.com

Leah Gage, Administrator
We accommodate 230 residents and we have approximately 250 employees. Our staffing ratio averages 1 licensed nurse for every 20 residents and 1 Certified Nursing Assistant for every 10 residents. We offer a wide range of services including but not limited to respiratory care, tracheotomy care and gastric tube feeding and we also feature an in house licensed therapy program.

Ohio

7196 Arbors East Subacute and Rehabilitation Center
5500 E Broad Street
Columbus, OH 43213
614-575-9003
FAX: 614-575-9101
Subacute rehabilitation facility.

7197 Arbors at Canton Subacute And Rehabilitation Center
2714 13th Street NW
Canton, OH 44708
330-456-2842
FAX: 330-456-5343

Kim Joye, Administrator
Subacute rehabilitation programs and facility.

7198 Arbors at Dayton
320 Albany Street
Dayton, OH 45408
937-496-6200
FAX: 937-496-1990

Ed Roberts, Administrator
Subacute rehabilitation facility with with 106 certified beds. Rehabilitation programs.

7199 Arbors at Marietta
400 N 7th Street
Marietta, OH 45750
740-373-3597
FAX: 740-373-3915
Subacute rehabilitation services and facility.

7200 Arbors at Milford
5900 Meadowcreek Drive
Milford, OH 45150
513-248-1655
FAX: 513-248-0466

Jennifer Fehn, Administrator
A nursing center hospital in search of giving the joy and fulfillment to the elderly.

7201 Arbors at Sylvania
7120 Port Sylvania Drive
Toledo, OH 43617
419-841-2200
FAX: 419-841-2822

Steve Arthur, Administrator
Subacute rehabilitation programs and facility.

7202 Arbors at Toledo Subacute and Rehab Centre
2920 Cherry Street
Toledo, OH 43608
419-242-7458
FAX: 419-242-6514

Michelle Hoff, Administrator
Subacute rehabilitation services and facility.

7203 Bridgepark Center for Rehabilitation and Nursing Services
145 Olive Street
Akron, OH 44310
330-762-0901
800-750-0750
FAX: 330-762-0905
www.bridgeparkrehab.com

Jim Kallevig, Executive Director

A skilled nursing and rehabilitation center located in Akron, Ohio, across the street from St. Thomas Hospital with a beautiful view of the Akron skyline. Access to Interstate 77 and State Route 8 is just minutes away. Our entire staff is committed to providing caring, customer-focused skilled nursing and rehabilitation. For your convenience, we accept Medicare, Medicaid and most managed care and private insurance.

7204 **Broadview Multi-Care Center**
5520 Broadview Road
Parma, OH 44134
216-749-4010
FAX: 216-778-6860
e-mail: info@broadviewmulticare.com
www.broadviewmulticare.com

Debra Cerr, Administrator
Harold Shachter, Owner
Broadview Multi-Care Center's Comprehensive Medical Rehabilitation Program has been developed to maximize the functional, psychological and social capabilities of its residents, using a Transdisciplinary Approach. Our multidisciplinary team asses each resident and individualizes a plan to attain the highest practicable functioning of each person under our care.

7205 **Caprice Care Center**
9184 Market Street
North Lima, OH 44452
330-965-9200
FAX: 330-726-6097
e-mail: capriceadm@chcccompanies.com

Alison Alvino, Manager
A 106-bed skilled nursing, subacute and rehabilitation facility. Our goal is to provide comfortable living to all who are in our care. Caprice Health Care Center is a contemporary Medicare and Medicaid approved facility specializing in short-term rehabilitation services. The inpatient/outpatient rehab department includes physical, occupational, speech therapies, indoor aquatic therapy pool, as well as complimentary van transportation for outpatient services.

7206 **Cleveland Clinic**
9500 Euclid Avenue
Cleveland, OH 44195
216-444-2200
800-223-2273
FAX: 216-444-7021
www.ccf.com

Floyd Loop, Chief Executive Officer
A not-for-profit, multispecialty academic medical center that integrates clinical and hospital care with research and education. Cleveland clinic was founded in 1921 by 4 renowned physicians with a vision of providing outstanding patient care based upon the principals of cooperation, compassion and innovation. Today, Cleveland Clinic is one of the largest and most respected hospitals in the country.

7207 **Columbus Rehabilitation And Subacute Institute**
44 S Souder Avenue
Columbus, OH 43222
614-228-5900
FAX: 614-228-3989

Kelly Fligor, Administrator
Subacute rehabilitation programs and facility.

7208 **LakeMed Nursing and Rehabilitation Center**
70 Normandy Drive
Painesville, OH 44077
440-357-1311
800-750-0750
FAX: 440-357-1299
www.lakemednursing.com

Chad Strong, Executive Director
Our goal is to provide you with quality care and we are known for our successful short-term rehab and care of the clinically complex. We also offer respite services to give caregivers a rest, and hospice services through our local hospice care provider. Our interdisciplinary team works together as they strive to deliver quality care and responsive service to our residents.

7209 **Oregon Nursing And Rehabilitation Center**
904 Isaac Streets Drive
Oregon, OH 43616
419-691-2483
FAX: 419-697-5401

Jill Schlievert, Administrator
Subacute rehabilitation facility and services.

7210 **Sunset View Castle Nursing Homes Castle Nursing Homes**
434 N Washington Street
Millersburg, OH 44654
330-674-0015
FAX: 330-763-2238
e-mail: info@castlenursinghomes.com
www.castlenursinghomes.com

Becky Snyder, Admissions Coordinator
Kathy Edwards, Admissions And Marketing
310 licensed, certified beds. Subacute rehabilitation facility and programs.

Oregon

7211 **Care Center East Health & Specialty Care Center**
Expendicare
11325 NE Weidler Street
Portland, OR 97220
503-253-1181
FAX: 503-253-1871

Phyllis Radzom, Director
Subacute rehabilitation facility and programs

7212 **Medford Rehabilitation and Healthcare Cent er**
Kindred Healthcare
625 Stevens Street
Medford, OR 97504
541-779-3551
800-735-1232
FAX: 541-779-3658
www.medfordrehab.com

Grant Gloor, Executive Director
We strive to provide quality, compassionate care. Our cozy building accomodates 110 residents. Our smaller size creates an inviting and homelike environment. We offer semi-private rooms with space to add items from home for a special personalized touch.

Pennsylvania

7213 **Dresher Hill Health and Rehabilitation Cen ter**
1390 Camp Hill Road
Dresher, PA 19034
215-643-0600
FAX: 215-641-0628

Gary Heinrich, Administrator
Subacute rehabilitation facility and programs: physical/speech.

7214 **Good Shepherd Rehabilitation**
850 South 5th Street
Allentown, PA 18103
610-776-3100
888-447-3422
FAX: 610-776-3552
e-mail: info@goodshepherdrehab.org
www.goodshepherdrehab.org

Sally Gammon, President/CEO
Maryellen Dickey, Vice President
A world class rehabilitation network, Good Shepherd provides comprehensive inpatient and outpatient services throughout Pennsylvania's Lehigh Valley. Founded in 1908, Good Shepherd has steadily expanded over last 95 years. Good Shepherd is one of the most comprehensive rehabilitation institutes in the worlld.

7215 **Statesman Health and Rehabilitation Center**
2629 Trenton Road
Levittown, PA 19056
215-943-7777
FAX: 215-943-1240

Patricia Keyes, Administrator
Subacute rehabilitation facility and programs.

7216 **UPMC Braddock**
400 Holland Avenue
Braddock, PA 15104
412-636-5000
FAX: 412-636-5398
http://braddock.upmc.com

Mark Sevco, President
Rodney Jones, Vice President
With a team of more then 43,000 employees, UPMC serves the health needs of more then 4 million people each year, improving lives in western Pennsylvania-and beyond-through redefined models of health care delivery and superb clinical outcomes.

7217 **UPMC McKeesport**
Presby
1500 Fifth Avenue
McKeesport, PA 15132
412-664-2000
FAX: 412-664-2318
http://mckeesport.upmc.com

Ronald Ott, Chief Executive Officer
Offers 56 beds for patients who need skilled nursing care. Offers ongoing rehabilitation and educational programs to patients with cardiac, neurologic, and orthopaedic diagnosis.

7218 **UPMC Passavant**
9100 Babcock Boulevard
Pittsburgh, PA 15237
412-367-6700
800-533-8762
http://passavant.upmc.com

Cynthia Tomazich, Dir Inpatient Physical Therapy
Teresa Petrick, Chief Executive Officer
Patients who have had an acute illness, injury, or exacerbation of a disease and no longer need the intensity of services in the acute care setting, but still require some complex medical care or supervision and rehabilitation services, may be appropriate to be transferred into the Subacute Unit.

Rhode Island

7219 **Kindred Heights Nursing & Rehabilitation Center**
Kindred Healthcare
100 Wampanoag Trail
East Providence, RI 02915
401-438-4275
800-745-6575
FAX: 401-438-8093
www.kindredheights.com

Sandy Sarza, Executive Director
Jean Aubin, Director
Kindred Heights Nursing and Rehabilitation Center accomodates 58 residents and serves the needs of elders in the greater East Bay and Providence area. We are conveniently located on Wampanoag Trail in East Providence. Kindred Heights provides skilled nursing, short-term rehab and long-term care in a family environment, but we are large enough to manage the complex nursing and rehab care needs our residents may have.

7220 **Oak Hill Nursing and Rehabilitation Center**
Kindered Health Care
544 Pleasant Street
Pawtucket, RI 02860
401-725-8888
800-745-6575
FAX: 401-725-8926
www.oakhillrehab.com

Scott Sanborn, Executive Director
Heidi Capela, Director Nursing
Amybeth Almeida, Director Admissions
Accomodates 143 residents. Throughout our 40 year history, Oak Hill has developed a reputation as one of the finest healthcare centers in Rhode Island. Our center consists of 3 separate units. A 34-bed post-acute unit provides care to the medically complex and those in need of extensive rehabilitative services. A 20-bed Alzheimer's Special Care Unit provides a unique style of care utilizing habilitative therapy in comfortable, home-like surroundings.

7221 **Southern New England Rehab Center**
21 Peace Street
Providence, RI 02907
401-456-4500
888-456-4501
FAX: 401-456-4550
www.snerc.com

Sylvia Procaccini, Manager
The Center's skilled staff of over 100 professionals provides a full range of coordinated rehabilitative care. Our clinical expertise and compassion make a big difference as we develop first-rate plans of care for the unique needs of each patient. Our medical staff is comprised of physicians board-certified in rehabilitation medicine and internal medicine.

South Carolina

7222 **Tuomey Healthcare System**
129 N Washington Street
Sumter, SC 29150
803-774-9000
FAX: 803-774-9489
www.tuomey.com

Jay Cox, Chief Executive Officer
Here to anticipte the needs of the communities we serve, responding with proactive healthcare initiatives, providing expert rehabilitative services and delivering life-saving acute care.

Tennessee

7223 **Camden Healthcare and Rehabilitation Center**
197 Hospital Drive
Camden, TN 38320
731-584-3500
FAX: 731-584-2753

Mark Walker, Administrator
Subacute rehabilitation products and services, nursing and life care homes.

7224 **Centennial Medical Center Tri Star Health System**
2300 Patterson Street
Nashville, TN 37203
615-342-1000
FAX: 615-342-1045
www.centennialmedicalcenter.com

Larry Kloess, Chief Executive Officer
Above all else we are committed to the care and improvement of human life by caring for those we serve with integrity, compassion, a positive attitude, respect and exceptional quality.

7225 **Cordova Rehabilitation and Nursing Center**
955 Germantown Road
Cordova, TN 38018
901-754-1393
800-848-0299
FAX: 901-754-3332
www.cordovahealthcare.com

John Palmer, Administrator
Renee Tutor, Executive Director
Our professional staff can help you make an informed decision. Upon admission, our interdisciplinary team develops a comprehensive care plan to meet not only physical and rehabilitative goals, but also social and emotional needs. We understand the importance of family and resident involvement and encourage participation in the development of a personalized plan of care.

7226 **Erlanger Medical Center Baronness Campus**
975 E 3rd Street
Chattanooga, TN 37403
423-778-7000
FAX: 423-778-7615
www.erlanger.org

Jim Brexler, Chief Executive Officer
Our mission is to improve the health of the people we touch. Our vision is to be recognized locally, regionally, and and nationally, as a premiere healthcare system.

7227 **Huntington Health and Rehabilitation Cente r**
635 High Street
Huntingdon, TN 38344
731-986-8943
FAX: 731-986-3188

Anthony Mays, Administrator
Subacute rehabilitation facility and programs.

7228 **Madison Healthcare and Rehabilitation Cent er**
431 Larkin Springs Road
Madison, TN 37115
615-865-8520
800-848-0299
FAX: 615-868-4455
www.madisonrehab.com

Melissa Hansen, Executive Director
Madison Healthcare and Rehabilitation Center accomodates 102 residents. We are certified for Medicare and located near 2 major hospitals in the Madison area. We provide inpatient and outpatient therapies with a concentration on inpatient treatments. We have a proven success rate- we discharge approximately one third of our patients home or to an increased level of care (IE assisted living).

7229 **Mariner Health of Nashville**
3939 Hillsboro Circle
Nashville, TN 37215
615-297-2100
FAX: 615-297-2197

Molly Mitchell, Administrator
Amy Artrip, Director of Nursing
Religious nonmedical health care institution. 150-bed subacute rehabilitation facility

7230 **Pine Meadows Healthcare and Rehabilitation Center**
700 Nuckolls Road
Bolivar, TN 38008
731-658-4707
FAX: 731-658-1824
www.pinemeadowsrehab.net

Larry Shrader, Administrator
Our goal is to take care of your loved ones. Our professional team works with skilled hands, is directed by creative minds and is guided by compassionate hearts. Upon your admission, our interdisciplinary team develops a comprehensive care plan designed with a goal of meeting not only physical and rehabilitative objectives, but also social and emotional needs. We understand the importance of family and resident involvement and encourage participation in the development of a plan of care.

7231 **Primacy Healthcare and Rehabilitation Cent er**
Kindred Health Care
6025 Primacy Parkway
Memphis, TN 38119
901-767-1040
800-848-0299
FAX: 901-685-7362
www.primacyrehab.com

George Munchow, Executive Director
Donni Dubert, Administrator
Upon a resident's admission, our interdisciplinary team develops a comprehensive care plan with a goal of meeting not only physical and rehabilitative objectives but also social and emotional needs. We understand the importance of family and resident involvement and encourage participation in the development of a personalized plan of care.

7232 **Ripley Healthcare and Rehabilitation Cente r**
118 Halliburton Street
Ripley, TN 38063
731-635-5180
FAX: 731-635-0663
www.ripleyhealthcare.org

Jonathan Owens, Administrator
Brandon Whiteside, Executive Director
Upon admission, our interdisciplinary team develops a comprehensive care plan to meet not only physical and rehabilitative goals, but also social and emotional needs. We understand the importance of family and resident involvement and encourage participation in the development of a personalized care plan. Our goal is to take care of your loved ones.

7233 **Shelby Pines Rehabilitation and Healthcare Center**
3909 Covington Pike
Memphis, TN 38135
901-377-1011
FAX: 901-377-0032

Jeff Adams, Executive Director
Subacute rehabiltation facility and programs.

7234 **Siskin Hospital for Physical Rehabilitation**
1 Siskin Plaza
Chattanooga, TN 37403
423-634-1200
FAX: 423-634-4538
e-mail: info@siskinrehab.org
www.siskinrehab.org

Teresa Dinger, Director Marketing/Communication
Dedicated exclusively to physical rehabilitation and offers specialized treatment programs in brain injury, amputation, stroke, spinal cord injury, orthopeadics, and major multiple trauma.

Texas

7235 **North Hills Hospital**
4401 Booth Calloway Road
North Richland Hills, TX 76180
817-255-1000
FAX: 817-255-1967
www.northhillshospital.com

Randy Moresi, Chief Executive Officer
North Hills Hospital's services include a wide range of cardiovascular services, surgical services, emergency services, radiology, a rehabilitation unit, a senior health center, therapy services, and women's services.

7236 **Valley Regional Medical Center**
100 E Alton Gloor Boulevard
Brownsville, TX 78526
956-350-7000
FAX: 956-350-7999
www.valleyregionalmedicalcenter.com

David Handley, Administrator
Above all else, we are committed to the care and improvement of human life. In recognition of this committment, we strive to deliver high quality, cost effective healthcare in the communities we serve. In persuit of our mission, we recognize and affirm the unique and intrinsic worth of each individual. We treat all those we serve with compassion and kindness. We act with absolute honesty and integrity and fairness in the way we conduct our business and the way we live our lives.

Utah

7237 **Crosslands Rehabilitation and Healthcare Center**
575 E 11000 S
Sandy, UT 84070
801-571-7600
800-346-4128
FAX: 801-571-4875
www.crosslandsrehab.com

Wayne Barney, Executive Director
Lyle Black, Manager
Crossroads Rehabilitation and Healthcare accomodates 120 residents. We are fully Medicare and Medicaid certified. We are proud of our reputation for providing quality, compassionate care. Services availiable include in-house physical, occupational and speech therapies, as well as 24-hour licensed nursing staff coverage. We offer therapeutic recreation, in-house social services and registered dietician services, among many other professional services.

7238 **Federal Heights Rehabilitation and Nursing Center**
41 South Ninth East
Salt Lake City, UT 84102
801-532-3539
800-346-4128
FAX: 801-328-3926
www.federalheightsrehab.com

Terry Parker, Executive Director
Federal Heights accomodates 120 residents. We are located near three major hospitals in the Salt Lake Valley. We specialize in providing nursing services for complex medical and rehabilitation conditions. Our discharge planning works jointly with the family and resident in determining the future needs and goals upon discharge.

7239 **St. George Care and Rehabilitation Center**
Kindred Health Care Publications
1032 E 100th S
Saint George, UT 84770
435-628-0488
800-346-4128
FAX: 435-628-7362
www.stgeorgecare.com

Jeff Christensen, Executive Director
Erin Hammon, Director of Nursing
St. George Care and Rehabilitation accomodates 95 residents. We offer a 4,000 square foot rehabilitation gym with an indoor therapy pool for inpatient and outpatient services. Therapy is provided to meet specific needs seven days a week. There is a dietitian on staff for individualized nutritional needs. We offer an Alzheimer's unit with specialized staff. We provide compassionate health services including physicians, nurses, physical therapists, and occupational therapist and licensed aides.

7240 **St. Mark's Hospital**
1200 E 3900 South
Salt Lake City, UT 84124
801-268-7111
FAX: 801-268-7779
www.stmarkshospital.com

John Hanshaw, Chief Executive Officer
Above all else we are committed to the care and improvement of human life. In recognition of this commitment, we strive to deliver high quality, cost effective healthcare in the communities we serve. We define quality as "caring people with the commitment to a continuous process of improvement in the services provided, that will better enable the hospital to meet or exceed our customer's needs and expectations."

7241 **Wasatch Valley Rehabilitation**
Kindred Healthcare
2200 E 3300 S
Salt Lake City, UT 84109
801-486-2096
800-346-4128
FAX: 801-484-3443
www.wasatchvalleyrehab.com

Jamie Anderson, Admissions
Ric Toomer, Executive Director
Wasatch Valley accomodates 110 residents. We are licensed for Medicare and Medicaid and we are conveniently located in the heart of Salt Lake City with easy access from I-15 and I-215. We are known by the area hospitals as a specialist in wound care and for the care we provide to those with complex medical conditions.

Virginia

7242 **Nansemond Pointe Rehabilitation and Health care Center**
200 Constance Road
Suffolk, VA 23434
757-539-8744
800-828-1140
FAX: 757-539-6128
www.nansemondhc.com

David O'Brien, Executive Director
Nansemond Pointe Rehabilitation and Healthcare Center accomodates 160 residents in private and semi-private rooms. We have been serving the needs of Suffolk, Virginia and the surrounding areas for over 38 years. We offer an entire continuum of care from assisted living apartments to skilled nursing to long-term care. Our licensed therapists, working with our dedicated nursing staff, share a common goal- to help our residents improve their level of recovery and independence.

7243 **Rehabilitation and Research Center Virginia Commonwealth University**
PO Box 980661
Richmond, VA 23298
804-828-2156
FAX: 804-828-5074
e-mail: beagle@hsc.vcu.edu
www.rrc.pmr.vcu.edu

Richard Sicemore, Executive Director
The Rehabilitation and Research Center is a collaborative effort between the Department of Physical Medicine and Rehabilitation and the Medical College of Virginia Hospitals. The goals of the Rehabilitation and Research Center at the Medical College of Virginia Hospitals (MCVH) are to provide highly-skilled, interdisciplinary, inpatient rehabilitative care to adults with complex needs; to be an advocate and educator for patients and people with disabilities.

7244 **Warren Memorial Hospital**
1000 N Shenandoah Avenue
Front Royal, VA 22630
540-636-0300
FAX: 540-636-0475
www.ivalleyhealth.com

Patrick Noland, Administrator
A nonprofit organization of health care providers, Valley Health offers a full spectrum of services in acute care, rehabilitation and extended care facilities, and outpatient and community settings to help the people of the region manage their health and enjoy a high quality of life. Valley Health has the resources to diagnose, treat and help patients manage virtually any medical problem that may be encountered.

7245 **Winchester Rehabilitation Center**
333 West Cork Street
Winchester, VA 22601
540-536-5114
800-382-0772
FAX: 540-536-1122
e-mail: wwilliam@valleyhealthlink.com
www.ivalleyhealthlink.com

Micheal J Halseth, President/CEO
Dena Kent, Executive Director
Offers the following rehabilitation services: Sub-Acute inpatient rehabilitation, Speech therapy, Physical therapy, Occupational therapy, Disability evaluations. 30-bed inpatient center.

Washington

7246 **Aldercrest Health and Rehabilitation Center**
21400 72nd Avenue W
Edmonds, WA 98026
425-775-1961
FAX: 425-771-0116

Sandy Wilkenson, Administrator
Subacute rehabilitation facility and programs.

7247 **Arden Rehabilitation and Healthcare Center**
16357 Aurora Avenue N
Shoreline, WA 98133
206-542-3103
800-833-6384
FAX: 206-542-4562
www.ardenrehab.com

Gail Brockway, Executive Director
Arden Rehabilitation has been an integral part of the Shoreline community since 1953. It is a one-level building set on mature grounds with several beautiful courtyards for the residents to enjoy. Arden can accomodate 90 residents-post acute/rehabilitation patients as well as long-term residents. Medicare certified, the center also takes most managed healthcare insurance plans, as well as VA, respite and hospice patients. Arden is well known for its rehabilitative and nursing care and wound care

7248 **Bellingham Health Care and Rehabilitation Services**
1200 Birchwood Avenue
Bellingham, WA 98225
360-734-9295
800-833-6384
FAX: 360-671-4368
www.bellinghamhc.com

Sheila Oberg, Administrator
At Bellingham Health Care and Rehab, we strive to provide quality, compassionate care. Our cozy building accomodates 84 residents. Our smaller size creates an inviting and homelike environment for your loved one. We offer semi-private rooms with space to add items from home for a special personalized touch. Provides meals served restaurant style in our dinning room overlooking our beautiful grounds.

7249 Bremerton Convalescent and Rehabilitation Center
2701 Clare Avenue
Bremerton, WA 98310
360-377-3951
FAX: 360-377-5443

Stephanie Bonanzino, Administrator
Subacute rehabilitation facility and programs.

7250 Edmonds Rehabilitation & Healthcare Center er
Kindred Healthcare
21008 76th Avenue W
Edmonds, WA 98026
425-778-0107
800-833-6384
FAX: 425-776-9532
www.edmondsrehab.com

Jane Davis, Executive Director
At Edmonds Rehabilitation and Healthcare, we strive to provide quality, compassionate care. Our center accomodates 91 residents. Our smaller size creates an inviting and homelike environment. We offer semi-private rooms with space to add items from home for a special personalized touch. Edmonds Rehabilitation and Healthcare provides delicious meals served restaurant style in our dinning room.

7251 Heritage Health and Rehabilitation Center
Kindred Health Care
3605 Y Street
Vancouver, WA 98663
360-693-5839
800-833-6384
FAX: 360-693-3991
www.heritagerehab.com

Michael Moses, Executive Director
Su Patchett, Director of Nursing
Heritage Health & Rehabilitation Center is the smallest free-standing healthcare center in southwest Washington with accomodations of 49, enabling more personal care and a more home-like environment. Heritage has licensed nursing staff, restorative aides, and certified nurses assistants, trained and experienced in providing Alzheimer's care, end of life/hospice care, psychiatric care, rehabilitative care, and respite care.

7252 North Auburn Rehabilitation And Health Center
2830 I Street NE
Auburn, WA 98002
253-833-1260
800-395-5000
FAX: 253-735-5159

Terri Thornberg, Manager
Subacute rehabilitation facility and programs.

7253 Northwoods Lodge
2321 NW Schold Place
Silverdale, WA 98383
360-698-3930
FAX: 360-613-9520
www.encorecommunities.com

Leslie Krueger, Owner
Provides you with a full-range of services from weekly housekeeping and laudry services, to grounds keeping and maintenance. Our monthy fee inculdes utilities and hot, delicious, nutritious meals served table side every day. We offer transportation services, full-time activities directors, and numerous amenities to add to your comfort and enjoyment.

7254 Pacific Specialty & Rehabilitation Center r
1015 N Garrison Road
Vancouver, WA 98664
360-694-7501
FAX: 360-694-8148

Michael Coy, Manager
Subacute rehabilitation facility and programs.

7255 Puget Sound Healthcare Center
4001 Capitol Mall Drive SW
Olympia, WA 98502
360-754-9792
FAX: 360-754-2455
www.puget-sound.med.va.gov

Dan Murray, Administrator
Our goal is to provide excellence in patient care, veteran's benefits and customer satisfaction. We have reformed our department internally and are striving for high quality, prompt and seamless service to veterans. Our department employees continue to offer their dedication and commitment to help veterans get the services they have earned.

7256 Vancouver Health & Rhabilitation Center
400 E 33rd Street
Vancouver, WA 98663
360-696-2561
800-833-6384
FAX: 360-750-0665
www.vancouverhealthcare.com

Kevin Bowen, Manager
At Vancouver Health and Rehab Center we strive to provide quality, compassionate care. Our cozy building accomodates 98 residents. Our smaller size creates an inviting and homelike environment. We offer semi-private rooms with space to add items from home for a special personalized touch. Provides delicious meals served restaurant style in our dining room.

West Virginia

7257 War Memorial Hospital
109 War Memorial Drive
Berkeley Springs, WV 25411
304-258-1234
www.warmemorialhospital.com

William C Locke, President
John H Borg, Administrator
Offers physical therapy, occupational therapy, speech therapy, social services, and patient/family education for individuals who have experienced a recent physical disability due to disease, dysfunction, or general debilitation. Helps patients to maximize their abilities through activities of daily living, mobility, self-medication, and self-care and restore their ability to return to their previous lifestyle.

Wisconsin

7258 Cedar Spring Health and Rehabilitation Cen ter
N27 W5707 Lincoln Boulevard
Cedarburg, WI 53012
262-376-7676
FAX: 262-376-7808

Mary Wirth, Executive Director
Subacute rehabilitation facility and programs.

7259 Clearview-Brain Injury Center
199 Home Road
Juneau, WI 53039
920-386-3400
877-386-3400
FAX: 920-386-3800
www.dodgecountywi.com

Jane Goyer, Administrator
A 30-bed, state certified, subacute neuro-rehabilitation program in Juneau, WI. We are located just 45 minutes northeast of Madison WI and 10 minutes east of Beaver Dam, WI. We are the first and longest standing of only 2 community re-entry programs in the state of Wisconsin providing subacute neuro-rehabilitation to teens and adults who have experienced a brain injury.

7260 Colonial Manor Medical and Rehabilitation Center
1010 East Wausau Avenue
Wausau, WI 54403
715-842-2028
800-947-6644
FAX: 715-845-5810
www.colonialmanormrc.com

Terry LaMantia, Executive Director
Colonial Manor Medical and Rehabilitation Center is part of the Kindred Community and is located in Wausau, Wisconsin. The corporate headquarters are based in Louisville Kentucky. Our facility accomodates 150 residents.

7261 Eastview Medical and Rehabilitation Center
729 Park Street
Antigo, WI 54409
715-623-2356
800-947-6644
FAX: 715-623-6345
www.eastviewmedrehab.com

Wanda Hose RN NHA, Executive Director
Eastview Medical Center and Rehabilitation Center accomodates 165 residents. We are Medicare and Medicaid certified, as well as being Joint Commission accredited. Our "TEAM" approach means specially trained staff work around the clock to assist in meeting rehabilitative goals established by our team of professionals. We encourage family involvement in our rehabilitative process. The support of loved ones is a major key to a speedy recovery.

7262 Family Heritage Medical and Rehabilitation Center
130 Strawberry Lane
Wisconsin Rapids, WI 54494
715-424-1600
FAX: 715-424-4817

Art Schmitz, Administrator
Subacute rehabilitation facility and programs.

7263 Hospitality Nursing Rehabilitation Center
8633 32nd Avenue
Kenosha, WI 53142
262-694-8300
FAX: 262-694-3622

Georgette Miller, Administrator
Subacute rehabilitation facility and programs.

7264 Kennedy Park Medical Rehabilitation Center
Kindred Healthcare
6001 Alderson Street
Schofield, WI 54476
715-359-4257
800-947-6644
FAX: 715-355-4867
www.kpmrc.com

Lori Koppel, Executive Director
Judy Kowalski, Plant Manager
Kennedy Park Medical & Rehabilitation Center accomodates 154 residents. We are located in Schofield, WI. At Kennedy Park, we specialize in dementia care, with our Reflections and Passages Units. Short-term rehabilitation and sub-acute care are provided in a setting conducive to meeting the individual needs of our residents and patients. We also provide general nursing care for persons with long-term care needs.

7265 Middleton Village Nursing & Rehabilitation
Kindred
6201 Elmwood Avenue
Middleton, WI 53562
608-831-8300
800-947-6644
FAX: 608-831-4253
www.middletonvillage.com

David Johnston, Interim Administrator
Middleton Village accomodates 97 residents. We specialize in post-surgical and post-acute rehabilitation and long-term care services.

7266 Mount Carmel Health & Rehabilitation Center
5700 W Layton Avenue
Milwaukee, WI 53220
414-281-7200
FAX: 414-281-7183

Mike Berry, Administrator
Subacute rehabilitation facility and programs.

7267 Mount Carmel Medical and Rehabilitation Center
677 E State Street
Burlington, WI 53105
262-763-9531
800-947-6644
FAX: 262-763-7579
www.mtcarmelrehab.com

Kathlene Walker, Administrator
Jeanne Piccioni, Executive Director
Mount Carmel Medical and Rehabilitation Center accomodates 155 residents. We are located in Burlington Wisconsin. Mount Carmel Medical and Rehabilitation center is a 2005 recipient of the American Health Care Association Quality Award.

7268 North Ridge Medical and Rehabilitation Cen ter
1445 N 7th Street
Manitowoc, WI 54220
920-682-0314
800-947-6644
FAX: 920-682-0553
www.nmrc.com

Jane P. Conway NHA, Executive Director
North Ridge Medical and Rehabilitation Center accomodates 110 residents. We have been serving the Manitowoc, Wisconsin area for over 25 years. Our goal is to provide services in a warm, homey environment. Many of our staff in all departments have a long history with North Ridge and have worked here for more then 20 years. We also take pride in the fact that we have all in-house staff. Our therapy team is availiable to provide physical, occupational and speech therapy 7 days a week.

7269 Oshkosh Medical and Rehabilitation Center
1580 Bowen Street
Oshkosh, WI 54901
920-233-4011
FAX: 920-233-5177

Tom Wagner, Administrator
Subacute rehabilitation facility and programs.

7270 San Luis Medical and Rehabilitation Center
2305 San Luis Place
Green Bay, WI 54304
920-494-5231
800-947-6644
FAX: 920-494-2964
www.sanluismedrehab.com

Jennifer Smith NHA, Executive Director
San Luis Medical and Rehabilitation Center accomodates 126 residents. We are located in Green bay, WI. At San Luis, we strive to meet the needs of our residents and we specialize in dementia care, with our Reflections Unit. Our goal is to provide short-term rehabilitation and sub-acute care in a setting conducive to assisting the needs of our residents.

Wyoming

7271 Mountain Towers Healthcare & Rehabilitation Center
3128 Boxelder Drive
Cheyenne, WY 82001
307-634-7901
800-877-9975
FAX: 307-634-7910
www.mttowersrehab.com

Licrecia Patterson, Administrator
Toni Wyenn, Director of Nursing
Mountain Towers Healthcare and Rehabilitation Center accomodates 170 residents, including a 16-bed acute secure unit. We offer a full range of nursing and medical care to meet individual needs. We have a full staff to meet the needs of our residents.

7272 South Central Wyoming Healthcare and Rehabilitation
Kindred Healthcare
542 16th Street
Rawlins, WY 82301
307-324-2759
800-877-9975
FAX: 307-324-7579

Mickey Hanser, Administrator
Chris Tanner, Executive Director
South Central Wyoming Healthcare and Rehabilitation accomodates 52 residents. We are located in Rawlings, in south central Wyoming. We are Medicare and Medicaid certified by the State of Wyoming. We strive to provide quality personal services, long-term care or short-term rehabilitation to our residents in a comfortable home-like environment.

7273 **Wind River Healthcare and Rehabilitation Center**
Kindred Health Care
1002 Forest Drive
Riverton, WY 82501
307-856-9471
800-877-9975
FAX: 307-856-1665
www.kindredhealthcare.com

Bonnie Deyo, Executive Director
Sandy Morton, Director
Offers a full range of medical services to meet the individual needs of our residents, including short-term rehabilitative services and long-term skilled care. Working with the residents physician, our staff-including medical specialists, nurses, nutritionists, dietitians and social workers-establishes a comprehensive treatment plan intended to restore you or your loved one to the highest practicable potential.

Glossary of Disability-Related Terms

Accessible: In the case of a facility, readily usable by a particular individual; in the case of a program or activity, presented or provided in such a way that a particular individual can participate, with or without auxiliary aid(s); in the case of electronic resources, accessible with or without adaptive computer technology.

Access barriers: Any obstruction that prevents people with disabilities from using standard facilities, equipment and resources.

Accessible Web design: Creating World Wide Web pages according to universal design principles to eliminate or reduce barriers, including those that affect people with disabilities.

Accommodation: An adjustment to make a program, facility, or resource accessible to a person with a disability.

Adaptive technology: Hardware or software products that provide access to a computer that is otherwise inaccessible to an individual with a disability.

ALT attribute: HTML code that works in combination with graphical tags to provide alternative text for graphical elements.

Alternative keyboard: A keyboard that is different from a standard computer keyboard in its size or layout of keys.

Americans with Disabilities Act of 1990 (ADA): A comprehensive federal law that prohibits discrimination on the basis of disability in employment, public services, public accommodations and services operated by private entities, and telecommunications .

American Standard Code for Information Interchange (ASCII): Standard for unformatted plain text which enables transfer of data between platforms and computer systems.

Applet: Computer program that runs from within another application.

Assistive technology: Technology used to assist a person with a disability, e.g., wheelchair, handsplints, computer-based equipment.

Binary files: Electronic files with formatting information that is software dependent.

Braille: System of embossed characters formed by using a Braille cell, a combination of six dots consisting of two vertical columns of three dots each. Each simple Braille character is formed by one or more of these dots and occupies a full cell or space. Some Braille may use eight dots.

Browser: Software designed to access and display information available on the World Wide Web. Browsers may be graphical or text-based. Text-only browsers cannot display images, sound clips, video and plug-in features that graphical browsers can. Talking browsers are also available for use by people who have difficulty reading text due to a learning disability or visual impairment.

Captioned film or videos: Transcription of the verbal portion of films or videos displayed to make them accessible to people who are deaf.

Captioning: Text that is included with video presentations or broadcasts that enables people with hearing impairments to have access to the audio portion of the material.

Closed Circuit TV Magnifier (CCTV): Camera used to magnify books or other materials to a monitor or television.

Communication device: Hardware that allows a person who has difficulty using their voice clearly to use words or symbols for communication. May range in complexity from a simple picture board to complex electronic devices that allow personalized, unique construction of ideas.

Compensatory tools: Adaptive computing systems that allow people with disabilities to use computers to complete tasks that they would have difficulty doing without a computer, e.g., reading, writing, communicating, accessing information.

Digital: Computer formatted data or information.

Disability: Physical or mental impairment that substantially limits one or more major life activities; a record of such an impairment; or being regarded as having such an impairment (Americans with Disabilities Act of 1990).

Discrimination: Act of making a difference in treatment or favor on a basis other than individual merit.

Electronic information: Any digital data for use with computers or computer networks including disks, CD-ROMs, World Wide Web resources.

Facility: All or any portion of a physical complex, including buildings, structures, equipment, grounds, roads, and parking lots.

FM Sound Amplification System: Electronic amplification system consisting of three components: a microphone / transmitter, monaural FM receiver and a combination charger / carrying case. It provides wireless FM broadcast from a speaker to a listener who has a hearing impairment.

Graphical User Interface (GUI): Program interface that presents digital information and software programs in an image-based format as compared to a character-based format.

Hardware: Physical equipment related to computers.

Hearing impairments: Complete or partial loss of ability to hear caused by a variety of injuries or diseases including congenital defects.

Helper: An external program that can be called up by a Web browser to display specially formatted material, such as word processed documents, spreadsheet documents or video / sound pieces. The Helper program is launched by the Web browser as a separate application to view or play the file.

Host: Any computer which holds Internet resources for access by others, or the computer that maintains your Internet access and electronic mail account.

HTML validation: Process that analyzes HTML documents identifies HTML errors and non-standard codes.

HyperText Transfer Protocol (HTTP): Communication protocol used by the World Wide Web to transfer text, graphics, audio, and video.

Hyperlink, hypertext: Highlighted word or graphic on a Web page that when selected allows the user to jump to another part of the document or another Web page.

Hypertext Markup Language (HTML): Programming language or code used to create World Wide Web pages.

Image map: Picture or graphic on a Web page in which hyperlinks are embedded.

Input: Any method by which information is entered into a computer.

Internet: Computer network connecting government, education, commercial, other organization and individual computer systems.

Interpreter: Professional person who assists a deaf person in communicating with hearing people.

Java: Programming language used to create programs or applets that work with some World Wide Web browsers to include features with animation or other characteristics not available through standard HTML.

Joystick: A device consisting of a lever that allows a pointer to move up, right, left, or down and serves as an alternative to a mouse. It usually includes buttons to enable mouse clicks.

Keyboard emulation: A method of having an alternative device and/or software, such as a switch-based system, serve the role of a keyboard.

Keyguard: A plastic or metal shield that covers a keyboard with holes over the keys. It allows use of a keyboard without undesired activation of surrounding keys.

Large print books: Most ordinary print is six to ten points in height (about 1/16 to 1/8 of an inch). Large type is 14 to 18 points (about 1/8 to 1/4 of an inch) and sometimes larger. The format of large print books is also proportionately larger (usually 8 1/2 x 11 inches).

Lynx: Text-based World Wide Web browser.

Mainstreaming, inclusion: The inclusion of people with disabilities, with or without special accommodations, in programs, activities, and facilities with their non-disabled peers.

Major life activities: Functions such as caring for oneself, performing manual tasks, walking, seeing, hearing, speaking, breathing, learning, working, and participating in community activities (Americans with Disabilities Act of 1990).

Mobility impairment: Disability that affects movement ranging from gross motor skills such as walking to fine motor movement involving manipulation of objects by hand.

Mouse emulation: A method of having an alternative device and/or software, such a switch based system, serve the role of a mouse.

Multimedia: In terms of electronic information, any data which is presented through several formats including text, graphics, moving pictures and sound.

Onscreen keyboard: See *Virtual Keyboard.*

Optical character recognition (OCR): Technology system that scans and converts printed materials into electronic text.

Output: Any method of displaying or presenting electronic information to the user through a computer monitor or other device.

Peripheral Neuropathy: A condition caused by damage to the nerves in the peripheral nervous system which includes nerves that run from the brain and spinal cord to the rest of the body.

Physical or mental impairment: Any physiological disorder or condition, cosmetic disfigurement, or anatomical loss affecting one or more of the following body systems: neurological; musculoskeletal; special sense organs; respiratory, including speech organs; cardiovascular; reproductive; digestive; genitourinary; hemic and lymphatic; skin; and endocrine; or any mental or psychological disorder, such as mental retardation, organic brain syndrome, emotional or mental illness, and specific learning disabilities (Americans with Disabilities Act of 1990).

Plug-in: Separate program written to be launched by a specific Web browser to display or run special elements in Web pages, such as animation, video, or audio.

Qualified individual with a disability: An individual with a disability who, with or without reasonable modification to rules, policies, or practices, the removal of architectural, communication, or transportation barriers, or the provision of auxiliary aids and services, meets the essential eligibility requirements for the receipt of services or the participation in programs or activities provided by a public entity (Americans with Disabilities Act of 1990).

Reader: Volunteer or employee of an individual with a disability (e.g., visual impairment, learning disability) who reads printed material in person or records to audio-tape.

Reading system: Hardware and software designed to provide access to printed text for people with visual impairments, mobility impairments, or learning disabilities. Character recognition software controls a scanner that takes an image of a printed page, converts it to computer text using recognition software and then reads the text using a synthesized voice.

Refreshable Braille Display: Hardware connected to a computer that echoes screen text on a box that has cells consisting of pins that move up and down to create Braille characters.

Repetitive Stress Injury (RSI): This disability may be chronic or acute and usually is described as pain caused by overuse of extremities, usually hands and wrists.

Scanning input: A switch-based method of controlling a computer. Activations of a switch will, in order, bring up a control panel that upon subsequent switch activations, allow a user to focus in on a desired control or keystroke. Custom scanning layouts can be created for a variety of purposes and programs and may also be used in a communication device.

Screen enlargement: Hardware and/or software that increases the size of characters and text on a computer screen.

Screen reader: Software used to echo text on a computer screen to audio output, often used by people who are blind, with visual impairments, or with learning disabilities.

Screen resolution: Refers to the clarity or sharpness of an image. For computer monitors, this term indicates the number of dots on the screen used to create text and graphics. Higher resolution means more dots, indicating increased sharpness and potentially smaller text.

Section 508 of the Rehabilitation Act: Legislation that requires Federal Agencies to develop, procure, and use accessible electronic and information technology.

Sensory impairment: A disability that affects touch, sight and/or hearing.

Server: Any computer that stores information that is available to other users, often over the Internet.

Sign language: Manual communication commonly used by deaf. The gestures or symbols in sign language are organized in a linguistic way. Each individual gesture is called a sign. Each sign has three distinct parts; the handshape, the position of the hands, and the movement of the hands. American Sign Language (ASL) is the most commonly used sign language in the United States. Deaf people from different countries speak different sign languages.

Specific Learning Disability: Disorder in one or more of the basic psychological processes involved in understanding or in using language, spoken or written, which may manifest itself in difficulties listening, thinking, speaking, reading, writing, spelling, or doing mathematical calculations. Frequent limitations include hyperactivity, distractibility, emotional instability, visual and/or auditory perception difficulties and/or motor limitations, depending on the type(s) of learning disability.

Speech impairment: Problems in communication and related areas such as oral motor function, ranging from simple sound substitutions to the inability to understand or use language or use the oral-motor mechanism for functional speech.

Speech input or speech recognition: A method of controlling a computer and creating text by dictation. Speech input software is combined with a microphone.

Standard HTML: Version of HTML accessible by all browsers.

Streaming multimedia: A method of transferring audio and/or video via a network from a server to an end user's computer. During the transmission, the material is displayed or played on the target computer.

Switch input: A method of controlling a computer or communication device. It is most often used with Morse code or scanning methods, but may also be used for controlling household appliances and related controls. Switches are available in a nearly endless array of sizes, shapes, and activation methods.

Tag: HTML code that prescribes the structure and formatting of Web pages.

Telecommunications Device for the Deaf (TDD) or Teletypewriter (TTY): A device which enables someone who has a speech or hearing impairment to use a telephone when communicating with someone else who has a TDD/TTY. TDD/TTYs can be used with any telephone, and one needs only a basic typing ability to use them.

Trackball: A mouse alternative that is basically an upside-down mouse. Useful for some people with mobility impairments because it isolates pointer movement from button clicking.

Traumatic Brain Injury (TBI): Open and closed head injuries resulting in impairments in one or more areas, including cognition; language; memory; attention; reasoning; abstract thinking; judgment; problem-solving; sensory, perceptual, and motor abilities; psychosocial behavior; physical functions; information processing; and speech. The term does not apply to brain injuries that are congenital, degenerative, or induced by birth trauma.

Universal design: Designing programs, services, tools, and facilities so that they are useable, without modification, by the widest range of users possible, taking into account a variety of abilities and disabilities.

Universal design of instruction: The design of instructional materials and activities that make learning achievable by students with a wide variety of abilities and disabilities.

Universal Resource Locator (URL): Address used to locate a specific resource on the Internet. DO-IT's URL is *http://www.washington.edu/doit/*.

Vocational Rehabilitation Act of 1973: Act prohibiting discrimination on the basis of disability which applies to any program that receives federal financial support. Section 504 of the Act is aimed at making educational programs and facilities accessible to all students. Section 508 of the Act requires that electronic office equipment purchased through federal procurement meets disability access guidelines.

Virtual keyboard: Software used to emulate a keyboard. A picture of a keyboard is displayed on a computer screen and the user points and clicks on the pictures of keys to enter text.

Vision impairments: Complete or partial loss of ability to see, caused by a variety of injuries or diseases including congenital defects. Legal blindness is defined as visual acuity of 20/200 or less in the better eye with correcting lenses, or widest diameter of visual field subtending an angular distance no greater than 20 degrees.

Word prediction: Software that reduces the number of keystrokes needed to type words and sentences. As characters are entered on either a standard, alternative or virtual keyboard, suggested completions of the word that has been started are provided to the user.

World Wide Web (WWW, W3, or Web): Hypertext and multimedia gateway to the Internet.

Grants and gifts funds DO-IT publications, videotapes, and programs to support the academic and career success of people with disabilities. Contribute today by sending a check to DO-IT, Box 355670, University of Washington, Seattle, WA 98195-5670.

Your gift is tax deductible as specified in IRS regulations. Pursuant to RCW 19.09, the University of Washington is registered as a charitable organization with the Secretary of State, State of Washington. For more information, call the Office of the Secretary of State, 800-322-4483.

About DO-IT

DO-IT (Disabilities, Opportunities, Internetworking, and Technology) helps individuals with disabilities transition to college and careers. Primary funding for DO-IT is provided by the National Science Foundation, the U.S. Department of Education, and the State of Washington. For more information, to be placed on the mailing list, or to request materials in an alternate format, contact:

DO-IT
University of Washington
Box 355670
Seattle, WA 98195-5670
doit@u.washington.edu
http://www.washington.edu/doit/
206-221-4171 (FAX)
206-685-DOIT (voice/TTY)
888-972-DOIT (voice/TTY) WA, outside Seattle
509-328-9331 (voice/TTY) Spokane
Director: Sheryl Burgstahler, Ph.D.

DO·IT

University of Washington
College of Engineering
Computing & Communications
College of Education

Resources by Disability Category

Blind & Deaf

Cognitive

Dexterity

Aging

Hearing

Mobility

Specific Disabilities
Cancer, Cerebral Palsy, Diabetes, Epilespy,
Respiratory Ailments, Spina Bifida, etc.

Speech & Language

Visual

This section includes all or some of the following: *Associations; Camps; Print & Non-Print Resources; Sports; Support Groups*

Associations

7274 American Association of the Deaf-Blind
8630 Fenton Street
Suite 121
Silver Spring, MD 20910
301-495-4403
800-735-2258
FAX: 301-495-4404
TTY: 301-495-4402
e-mail: aadb-info@aadb.org
www.aadb.org

Jamie Pope, Executive Director
Arthur Roehrig, President
Elizabeth Spiers, Director Of Programs/Services
A national consumer organization of, by and for deaf-blind americans. The mission of this association is to endeavor to enable deaf-blind persons to achieve their maximum potential through increased independence, productivity and integration into the community. *$15.00*
Membership dues

7275 Arena Stage
11101 Sixth Street
Washington, DC 20024
202-554-9066
FAX: 202-484-6279
e-mail: info@arenastage.org
www.arenastage.org

Thomas C Fichandler, Founding Executive Director
Stephen Richard, Chief Executive Officer
A pioneer in providing access to theater for people with disabilities and the birthplace of Audio Description. Offers infrared assistive listening devices (both loop and headset), program books in Braille, large print and wheelchair accessible seating with adjacent companion seating. Audio cassette format available upon request. Sign Interpretation and Audio Description are offered at selected performances. Cafe menus and shop lists in Braille. Wheelchair-accessible with lifts and ramps.

7276 National Family Association for Deaf-Blind
141 Middle Neck Road
Sands Point, NY 11050
516-944-8900
800-225-0411
FAX: 516-883-9060
e-mail: nfadb@aol.com
www.nfadb.org

Linda Syler, President
Pearl Veesart, Vice President
Debbie Ethridge, Secretary
A membership organization which provides resources, education, advocacy, referrals and support for families with children who are deaf-blind; professionals in the field and individuals who are deaf-blind.

7277 National Information Center for Children and Youth with Disabilities (NICHCY)
PO Box 1492
Washington, DC 20013
202-884-8200
800-695-0285
FAX: 202-884-8441
e-mail: nichcy@aed.org
www.nichcy.org

Susan Ripley, Manager
Provides fact sheets, state resource sheets and general information to assist parents, educators, caregivers, advocates and others in helping children and youth with disabilities participate as fully as possible in their communities.

7278 National Information Clearinghouse on Children who are Deaf-Blind
Teaching Research
345 N. Monmouth Avenue
Monmouth, OR 97361
503-838-8391
800-438-9376
FAX: 503-838-8150
TTY: 800-854-7013
e-mail: dblink@tr.wou.edu
www.tr.wou.edu/dblink

John Reiman, Project Director
Betsy McGinnity, Information Specialist
Nancy O'Donnell, Information Specialist
Collects, organizes, and disseminates information related to children and youth of ages 0 to 21 who are deaf-blind and connects consumers of deaf-blind information to the appropriate resources. Publishes a number of topical papers and publishes Deaf-Blind Perspective.

Camps

7279 Florida School for the Deaf and Blind
207 North San Marco Avenue
Saint Augustine, FL 32084
904-827-2200
800-344-3732
FAX: 904-827-2222
e-mail: dillinghame@fsdb.k12.fl.us
www.fsdb.k12.fl.us

Elmer Dillingham, President/Administrator
Kathy Gillespie, Director Public Information
Margaret W Van Ormer, Director Instructional Services
There is no cost to families for tuition for eligible Florida residents to enroll their children in this program which includes such activities as swimming, walking club, yoga, in addition to arts/crafts, game nights and much more.

Print & Non-Print Resources

7280 Beam
1850 W Roosevelt Road
Chicago, IL 60608
312-666-1331
FAX: 312-243-8539
www.thechicagolighthouse.org

James Kesteloot, Executive Director
Terrence Longo, Assistant Director
Quarterly newsletter of the organization offering progressive programs for the blind, visually impaired, deaf-blind and multi-disabled children and adults, including vocational programs, computer and office skills training, job placement, independent living skills, orientation and mobility training, counseling and a low vision clinic.

7281 Communicating with People Who Have Trouble Hearing & Seeing: A Primer
National Association for Visually Handicapped
22 W 21st Street
Floor 6
New York, NY 10010
212-889-3141
FAX: 212-727-2931
e-mail: staff@navh.org
www.navh.org

Lorianie Marchi, Chief Executive Officer
Line drawings that depict problems for those with both deficiencies. *$2.00*

7282 Deaf-Blind Perspective
Teaching Research
345 Monmouth Avenue
Monmouth, OR 97361
503-838-8391
800-438-9376
FAX: 503-838-8150
e-mail: dblink@tr.wou.edu
www.tr.wou.edu/dblink

John Reiman PhD, Director
Meredith Brodsky, Executive Director

7283 Getting in Touch
Research Press
PO Box 9177
Champaign, IL 61826
217-352-3273
800-519-2707
FAX: 217-352-1221
e-mail: rp@researchpress.com
www.researchpress.com

Russell Pence, President
When communicating with a child who is deaf/blind, there are certain basic procedures that can be used to help the child understand. This video introduces these procedures to teachers, staff, parents and others who work with children who have sensory impairments. The video demonstrates techniques that involve the use of two types of tactile cues - Touch Cues (signals made by actually touching the child) and Object Cues (signals made by presenting an object to the child). *$150.00*
19 Minutes

7284 Helen and Teacher: The Story of Helen & Anne Sullivan Macy
American Foundation for the Blind/AFB Press
PO Box 1020
Sewickley, PA 15143
412-741-1142
800-232-3044
FAX: 412-741-0609
e-mail: afborders@abdintl.com
www.afb.org

Stephanie Biagioli, Marketing Coordinator
A pictorial biography emphasizing Hellen Keller's accomplishments in public life over a period of more than 60 years. Traces Anne Sullivan's early years and her meeting with Helen Keller, and goes on to recount the joint events of their lives. A definitive biography. $29.95.
Paperback
ISBN 0-891282-89-0

7285 Independence Without Sight and Sound: Suggestions for Practitioners
American Foundation for the Blind/AFB Press
PO Box 1020
Sewickley, PA 15143
412-741-1142
800-232-3044
FAX: 412-741-0609
e-mail: afborders@abdintl.com
www.afb.org
This practical guidebook covers the essential aspects of communicating and working with deaf-blind persons. Includes useful information on how to talk with deaf-blind people, and adapt orientation and mobility techniques for deaf-blind travelers. *$39.95*
193 pages Paperback
ISBN 0-891282-46-7

7286 Journey
Landmark Media
3450 Slade Run Drive
Falls Church, VA 22042
703-241-2030
800-342-4336
FAX: 703-536-9540

Michael Hartogs, President
A moving portrayal of the extraordinary journey to Japan of 74-year-old Billie Sinclair, who is deaf, blind and mute. He funds his travels by weaving and selling baskets. In Japan he rides a roller coaster, tries judo and visits a deaf and blind acupuncturist. He demonstrates how it is possible to communicate by touch alone. *$195.00*
Video

7287 News from Advocates for Deaf-Blind
National Family Association for Deaf-Blind
111 Middle Neck Road
Sands Point, NY 11050
516-944-8900
800-225-0411
FAX: 516-944-7302
e-mail: NFADB@aol.com
www.NFADB.org

Mary Fox, Administrative Assistant
Joseph Nulty, Executive Director
A membership organization which provide resources, education, advocacy, referrals and support for families with children who are deaf-blind; professionals in the field; and individuals who are deaf-blind.
20 pages TriAnnual

7288 Supporting Young Adults Who are Deaf-Blind in Their Communities
Brookes Publishing
PO Box 10624
Baltimore, MD 21285
410-337-9580
800-638-3775
FAX: 410-337-8539
e-mail: custserv@brookespublishing.com
www.brookespublishing.com

Paul Brooks, Owner
A Transition Planning Guide for Service Providers, Families, and Friends. This handbook stresses the importance of person-centered planning in helping individuals who are deaf-blind make the transition from school to adult life. *$39.95*
384 pages Paperback
ISBN 1-55766 -61-8

7289 The Deaf-Blind American
American Association of the Deaf-Blind (AADB)
8630 Fenton Street
Suite 121
Silver Spring, MD 20910
301-495-4403
FAX: 301-495-4404
e-mail: aadb-info@aadb.org
www.aadb.org

Elizabeth Spears, Director Of Information Services
We are a consumer membership organization of, by and for people who have dual vision and hearing loss. Services we provide include an information clearinghouse on deaf blindness, a quarterly magazine (The Deaf Blind American), a newsletter, AADB news, a task force to improve interpreting for deaf-blind people, a listen for members, a partnership with the American Red Cross, and national conferences. *$5.00*
Quartlery

Support Groups

7290 Aurora of Central New York
518 James Street
Suite 100
Syracuse, NY 13203
315-422-7263
FAX: 315-422-4792
TTY:3154229746
e-mail: auroracny@auroracny.org
www.auroraofcny.org

Debra Chaiken, Executive Director
Professional counseling services to assist individuals and their families deal with the trauma of hearing or vision loss.

Associations

7291 ARC
1010 Wayne Avenue
Suite 650
Silver Spring, MD 20910
301-565-3842
800-433-5255
FAX: 301-565-3843
e-mail: info@thearc.org
www.thearc.org

Martha Hulse, CFO
Steven M Eidelman, Chief Executive Officer
Chris Privett, Director Communications
National organization of people and for people with mental retardation and related developmental disabilities and their families. Devoted to promoting supports and services for people with mental retardation and their families. Also fosters research and education regarding the prevention of mental retardation in infants and young children.

7292 ARRISE
Oak Leyden Developmental
9238 Park lane Avenue
Franklin Park, IL 60131
847-451-2740
FAX: 847-451-4008

Jayna Sullivan, Manager
Provides information about adult autism. Referrals from Department of Mental Health and schools. Vocational in home program, and adult living arrangement's for small groups. Group homes, Housing-transitional and vocational training.

7293 Autism Services Center
PO Box 507
Huntington, WV 25710
304-525-8014
FAX: 304-525-8026
e-mail: candy@autismwv.org
www.autismservicescenter.org

Ruth C Sullivan, Executive Director
Mark Gravy, Director
Provides developmental disabilities services with a specialty in autism. Services include case management, residential, personal care, assessments and evaluations, supported employment, independent living and family support.
1979

7294 Autism Treatment Center of America
615 Westfield Avenue West
Roselle Park, NJ 07204
908-241-8500
FAX: 908-241-4008
e-mail: information@son-rise.org
www.son-rise.org
Since 1983, the Autism Treatment Center of America has provided innovative training programs for parents and professionals caring for children challenged by Autism, Autism Spectrum Disorders, Pervasive Developmental Disorders (PDD) and other development difficulties. The Son-Rise Program teaches a specific yet comprehensive system of treatment and education designed to help families and caregivers enable their children to dramatically improve in all areas of learning.

7295 Best Buddies
2333 Dundas Street W
Suite 204
Toronto, Ontario, ZZ M6R
416-531-0003
888-779-0061
FAX: 416-531-0325
e-mail: info@bestbuddies.ca
www.bestbuddies.ca

Steven Pinnock, Executive Director
Anna Nelson, National Program Director
Our program gives people with intellectual disabilities the chance to have experiences which most people take for granted.

7296 Brain Injury Association of America
8201 Greensboro Drive
Suite 611
McLean, VA 22102
703-761-0750
800-444-6443
FAX: 703-761-0755
e-mail: shconnors@biausa.org
www.biausa.org

Susan H Connors, President/CEO
Mark J. Ashley ScD, CCC-SLP, Chairperson
Wayne Gordon PhdD, Vice Chairperson
Founded in 1980, the Brain Injury Association of America (BIAA) is the leading national organization serving and representing individuals, families and professionals who are touched by a life-altering, often devistating, traumatic brain injury (TBI) Together with its network of more then 40 charted state affiliates, as well as hundreds of local chapters and support groups across the country, the BIAA provides information, education and support to assist the 5.3 million living with brain injuries

7297 Brain Injury Association of New York State
10 Colvin Avenue
Albany, NY 12206
518-459-7911
800-228-8201
FAX: 518-482-5285
e-mail: info@bianys.org
www.bianys.org

Michael Kaplen Esq., President
Judith Avner, Executive Director
Judith Sandman, Director Membership and Developm
(BIANYS) is a statewide non-profit membership organization that advocates on behalf of individuals with brain injury and their families, and promotes prevention. Established in 1982, BIANYS provides education, advocac, and community support services that lead to improved outcomes for children and adults with brain injuries and their families. BIANYS also offers chapters and support groups throughout the state, prevention programs, mentoring programs, speakers bureau and publications library.
1982

7298 Brain Injury Association of Texas
316 W. 12th Street
Suite 405
Austin, TX 78701
512-326-1212
800-392-0040
512-326-8088
FAX: 512-478-3370
e-mail: info@biatx.org
www.biatx.org

Eric Makowski, President
Jonas Schwartz, Treasurer
Rose Pelzel, Secretary
The Brain Injury Association of Texas is an organization which arose from the mutual frustration and sense of helplessness experienced by families in their search for appropriate facilities and support to return loved ones who had sustained brain injuries to maximum functioning potential. It was organized in 1982 as the Texas Head Injury Association by a group of family members and health care professionals in an effort to meet the needs of the survivors of brain injury.
1982

7299 Center Academy
6710 86th Avenue N
Pinellas Park, FL 33782
727-541-5716
FAX: 727-544-8186
e-mail: infopp@centerccademy.com
www.centeracademy.com

Mack Hicks, Founder
Andrew P. Hicks, PhD, CEO
Eric V. Larson PhD, President/COO
Since 1968, Center Academy has been specifically designed for the learning disabled child and other children with difficulties in concentration, social skills, impulsivity, distractibility and study strategies. Programs offered include: academic day school and 5 week remedial summer program. 11 locations throughout Florida.

7300 Dynamic Learning Center

PO Box 112
Ben Lomond, CA 95005
831-336-3457
FAX: 831-336-5854
e-mail: teresanlp@aol.com
www.nlpu.com

Robert B. Dilts, Co Founder
The vision of NLP (neuro-lingusitic programming)University is to create a context in which professionals of different backgrounds can develop fundamental and advanced NLP skills for applications relevant to their profession. The mission of NLP University is to provide the organizational structure through which the necessary guidance, training, culture, and community support can be brought to the people who are interested in exploring the global potential of Systemic NLP.

7301 Focus Alternative Learning Center

126 Dowd Avenue
Po Box 452
Canton, CT 06019
860-693-8809
FAX: 860-693-0141
e-mail: info@focus-alternative.org
www.focus-alternative.org

Donna Swanson MSN, CS, APRN, Executive Director
Jen Haggerty MA, Clinical Coordinator
Sandy Kissel RN, BSN, MSN, Nurse Clinician
A private non profit, licensed clinical and learning center specialized in the treatment of creatively wired and socially challenged kids. We treat kids on the autism spectrum who suffer from high anxiety, experience processing difficulties and learning problems.

7302 Life Development Institute

18001 N 79th Avenue
Suite E71
Glendale, AZ 85308
623-773-2774
FAX: 623-773-2788
e-mail: rcrawford@life-development-inst,org
www.life-development-inst.org

Veronica Crawford, President
Robert Crawford, Chief Executive Officer
Serves older adolescents and adults with learning disabilities, ADD and related disorders. The purpose of the training is to enable program participants to pursue responsible independent living, enhance academic/workplace literacy skills and facilitate placement in educational/employment opportunities, commensurate with individual capabilities. Includes a stand alone, regionally accredited 2-year college.

7303 NLP Comprehensive

Po Box 648
Indian Hills, CO 80454
303-987-2224
800-233-1657
FAX: 303-987-2228
e-mail: learn@nlpco.com
www.nlpco.com

Tom Dotz, President
Tom Hoobyar, Director of Planning
Charles Faulkner, Director of Programs
NLP, or Neuro-Linguistic Programming, is the science of how the brain codes learning and experience. This coding affects all communication and behavior. NLP Comprehensive helps individuals and businesses make the fullest use of their talents and resources. We teach the thought processes and communication strategies of exceptional performers through workshops, books, and tapes.

7304 National Alliance on Mental Illness (NAMI)

Colonial Place Three
2107 Wilson Boulevard, Suite 300
Arlington, VA 22201
703-524-7600
800-950-6264
FAX: 703-524-9094
TTY: 703-516-7227
www.nami.org

Suzanne Vogel-Scibilia MD, President
Fredrick R Sandoval, First Vice President
Anand Pandya MD, Second Vice President
NAMI is a nonprofit, grassroots, self-help, support and advocacy organization of consumers, families, and friends of people with severe mental illnesses, such as schizophrenia, schizoaffective disorder, bipolar disorder, major depressive disorder, obsessive-compulsive disorder, panic and other severe anxiety disorders, autism and pervasive developmental disorders, attention deficit/hyperactivity disorder, and other severe and persistent mental illnesses that affect the brain.

7305 National Association for Down Syndrome

PO Box 206
Wilmette, IL 60091
630-325-9112
FAX: 630-325-8842
e-mail: info@nads.org
www.nads.org

Diane Gomboz, President
Jackie Rotondi, First VP
M Sheila Hebein, Executive Director
Works for a strong network of support systems within their own organization and with medical, educational and school service professionals who work with children and adults with Down Syndrome. NADS serves the Chicago Metropolitan area.

7306 National Down Syndrome Congress

1307 Center Drive
Suite 102
Atlanta, GA 30338
770-604-9500
800-232-6372
FAX: 770-604-9898
e-mail: info@ndsccenter.org
www.ndsccenter.org

David Tolleson, Executive Director
Betty Totten, Manager
provides information, advocacy and support concerning all aspects of life for individuals with Down syndrome. A world with equal rights and opportunitites for people with Down syndrome. It is the purpose of the NDSC to create a national climate in which all people will recognize and embrace the value and dignity of people with Down syndrome. That purpose is enhanced by the commitment of the NDSC to promote the accessability to a full range of opportunities that meet the needs of the individual.

7307 National Down Syndrome Society

666 Broadway
New York, NY 10012
212-460-9330
800-221-4602
FAX: 212-979-2873
e-mail: info@ndss.org
www.ndss.org

Alan P Brownstein, President
Not-for-profit organization increases public awareness about Down syndrome and works to discover its underlying causes through research, education and advocacy. Distributes timely and informative materials, encourages and supports the activities of local parent support groups, sponsors sonferences and scientific symposia and undertakes major advocacy efforts—all to increase awareness and acceptance of people with Down syndrome.
1979

7308 St. John Valley Associates

10c 11th Avenue
Madawaska, ME 04756
207-728-7197
FAX: 207-728-7550
e-mail: sjva@nci1.net

Stephen Richard, Administrator
A nonprofit association with the mission of empowering adult citizens with mental retardation to dignify themselves. Three broad-based programs and services (Independence Plus, Job Involvements, People Now) are designed to allow each individual to upgrade learning skills, assert rights, increase independence and accept new responsibilities. *$75.00*

7309 TEACCH

University of North Carolina at Chapel Hill
100 Renee Lynne Court
Chapel Hill, NC 27599
919-966-4127
FAX: 919-966-2174
e-mail: teacch@unc.edu
www.teacch.com

Gary Mesibov, Director
Ricky Bass, Manager
Focus on the person with autism and the development of a program around this person's skills, interests and needs.

Camps

7310 **Adventure Learning Center at Eagle Village**
4507 170th Avenue
Hersey, MI 49639
231-832-2234
800-748-0061
FAX: 231-832-1729
e-mail: info@eaglevillage.org
www.eaglevillage.org

Jon Lauderbach, Chairman
Gary Bennett, President/CEO
Anne Soczawa, Director of Finance
This program accepts youth, ages 5-17, who are high risk or special needs - behavioral problems, emotionally unstable or Attention Deficit. The camping experience includes canoeing, hiking, swimming and high adventure activities. Half-week, one-week, and two-week sessions June-August. Coed.

7311 **CNS Camp New Connections**
Mclean Hospital
115 Mill Street
Belmont, MA 02478
617-855-2000
800-333-0338
FAX: 617-855-3691
e-mail: info@mclean.harvard.edu
www.mcleanhospital.org

Roya Ostovar PhD, Center Director
Brandi Henson PsyD, Camp Coordinator
Joseph Gold MD, Clinical Director
Six-week sessions June-August for children with autism. Coed, ages 6-14.

7312 **Camp Baker**
Greater Richmond ARC
7600 Beach Road
Chesterfield, VA 23838
804-748-4789
FAX: 804-496-9657
e-mail: campbaker@RichmondARC.org
www.richmondarc.org

Marshall Butler Jr., President
Thom Horsey, Chair
Supports children from age 6 through adulthood with mental retardation and similar developmental disabilities.

7313 **Camp Betsey Cox**
140 Betsey Cox Lane
Pittsford, VT 05763
802-483-6611

e-mail: betcoxvt@aol.com
www.campbetseycox.com

Lorrie Byrom, Camp Director
Devri Byrom, Winter Office Director
Camp is located in Pittsford, Vermont. Summer sessions for girls aged 9-15 with ADD.

7314 **Camp Buckskin**
PO Box 389
Ely, MN 55731
218-365-2121
FAX: 218-365-2880
e-mail: buckskin@spacestar.net
www.campbuckskin.com

Thomas R Bauer CCD, Camp Director
Camp is located in Ely, Minnesota. Buckskin assists LD and ADD/ADHD individuals to realize and develop the potentials and abilities which they possess. Teaches a combination of traditional camp, academic activities and social skills so the campers experience success in many areas. 1:3 staff ratio ensures the program is individualized to meet each camper's needs.

7315 **Camp Horizons**
PO Box 323
South Windham, CT 06266
860-456-1032
FAX: 860-456-4721
e-mail: lauren.perrotti@camphorizons.org
www.camphorizons.org

Lauren Perrotti, Director Operations
Chris Naboe, Executive Director
Janice Chamberlain, Associate Executive Director
Two, four, six and eight-week sessions June-August for campers with developmental disabilities and autism. Coed, ages 8-40.

7316 **Camp Huntington**
56 Bruceville Road
High Falls, NY 12440
845-687-7840
FAX: 845-687-7211
e-mail: dfalk@camphuntington.com
www.camphuntington.com

Bruria Bodek Falik, Executive Director
Daniel Falk, Director
Harvey Goodman, Operation/Program Supervisor
A co-ed residential camp for the learning disabled, ADD, neurologically impaired and mild-moderate mental retardation.

7317 **Camp Kaleidoscope**
City of Lebanon New Hampshire
51 North Park Street
Lebanon, NH 03766
603-448-4220

e-mail: recreation@lebcity.com
www.lebcity.com

Cindy Heath, Executive Director
Kevin Talcott, Assistant Director
Paul Coats, Program Coordinator
Summer sessions for campers with ADD. Coed, ages 5-12.

7318 **Camp Nissokone**
YMCA Camping Services
7300 Hickory Ridge Road
Holly, MI 48442
248-887-4533
FAX: 248-887-5203
e-mail: office@ycampingservices.org
www.ycampingservices.org/

Jennifer Buckelew, Director
David Marks, Director
A six week summer resident camp program for boys and girls whose learning and behavior styles have made successful participation in the traditional camp program difficult. All camp activities have a special emphasis on building self-esteem and peer relationships. Strong in waterfront, nature, campcrafts and a special arts program.

7319 **Camp Northwood**
132 State Route 365
Remsen, NY 13438
315-831-3621
FAX: 315-831-5867
e-mail: campinfo@nwood.com
www.nwood.com

Gordon W Felt, Camp Director
Donna Felt, International Counselor
Summer sessions for children with ADD. Coed, ages 8-18.

7320 **Camp Nuhop**
404 Hillcrest Drive
Ashland, OH 44805
419-289-2227
FAX: 419-289-2227
e-mail: campnuhop@zoominternet.net
www.campnuhop.org

Jerry Dunlap, Executive Director
Ann Bell, Co-Director Summer Program
Mark Sommer, Director Support Services
A summer residential program for any youngster from 6 to 18 with a learning disability, behavior disorder or Attention Deficit Disorder. 84 campers and 41 staff members live on site in groups of to seven campers to every three counselors. Activities focus on positive self-concept and behaviors and teaches children to learn how to find their strengths, abilities and talents from a positive, yet realistic viewpoint.

7321 Camp Ramapo
Route 52 Salisbury Turnpike
PO Box 266
Rhinebeck, NY 12572
845-876-8403
FAX: 845-876-8414
e-mail: office@ramapoforchildren.org
www.ramapoforchildren.org

Bernie Kosberg, Executive Director
Mike Kunin, Associate Director
Residential program which serves children, ages 4-16, with a wide range of emotional, behavioral and learning problems. A one-to-one ratio of counselors-to-campers enables children to build healthy relationships, increase self-esteem and improve learning skills. Character values such as honesty, concern for others, responsibility and the courage to do one's best are encouraged. Campers demonstrate significant gains in their ability to maintain relationships, control impulses and adjust.

7322 Camp Royall
Autism Society of North Carolina
505 Oberlin Road
Suite 230
Raleigh, NC 27605
919-743-0204
FAX: 919-542-1033
e-mail: info@autismsociety-nc.org
www.autismsociety-nc.org

Ann Palmer, President
Jill Hinton-Keel, Executive Director
Nancy Huber, Events Manager
Camping sessions for children and adults with autism. Coed, ages 4-99.

7323 Camp Ruggles
113 Stone Dam Road
North Scituate, RI 02857
401-647-5508
e-mail: info@ricamps.org
www.ricamps.org

John Jacques, President
Camp Ruggles is located in Glocester, RI, and is a summer day camp for emotionally handicapped children. The Camp offers a 6 week co-ed summer session for 60 children ages 6-12.

7324 Camp Sisol
Jewish Community Center of Greater Rochester/JCC
1200 Edgewood Avenue
Rochester, NY 14618
585-461-2000
FAX: 585-461-0805
TTY:585-461-2000
e-mail: rrosner@jccrochester.org
www.jccrochester.org

Jane Glazer, President
Leslie Berkowitz, Director
Camp is located in Honeoye Falls, New York. Summer sessions for children with autism. Coed, ages 5-16.

7325 Camp World Light
Florida Baptist Convention
1230 Hendricks Avenue
Jacksonville, FL 32207
904-396-2351
800-226-8584
FAX: 904-396-6470
e-mail: bluesprings@flbaptist.org.
www.flbaptist.org

John Sullivan, Executive Director
Bob Bumgarner, Director Leadership Development
Camp is located in Marianna, Florida. One-week sessions June-July for girls with ADD. Ages 8-18. Activities include arts/crafts, challenge/rope courses, clowning, community service, dance, drama, drawing/painting, leadership development, performing arts and sailing.

7326 Camp-A-Lot
Arc Of San Diego
9575 Aero Drive
San Diego, CA 92123
858-715-3780
FAX: 858-715-3788
e-mail: info@arc-sd.com
www.arc-sd.com

Lin Taylor, Camp Director
Offers one-week sessions for children and adults with attention deficit disorder, autism, mobility limitation and developmental disabilities.

7327 Carroll School Summer Programs
25 Baker Bridge Road
Lincoln, MA 01773
781-259-8342
FAX: 781-259-8852
e-mail: info@carrollscholl.org
www.carrollschool.org

Philip Burling, Chairman
Stephen Wilkins, Principal
Academic and recreational programs designed to improve learning skills and build self-confidence. The school is a tutorial program for students not achieving their potential due to poor skills in reading, writing and math. The summer camp complements the summer school offering outdoor activities in a supportive, non-competitive environment.

7328 Casowasco Camp, Conference and Retreat Center
158 Casowasco Drive
Moravia, NY 13118
315-364-8756
FAX: 315-364-7636
e-mail: info@casowasco.org
www.casowasco.org

Michael D Huber, Executive Director
Roger Marshall, Property Manager
Robbin Hunsberger, Food Service Manager
Camp is located in Moravia, New York. Summer sessions for children with ADD. Coed, ages 6-18 and families.

7329 Center Academy at Pinellas Park
6710 86th Avenue North
Pinellas Park, FL 33782
727-541-5716
FAX: 727-544-8186
e-mail: infopp@centeracademy.com
www.centeracademy.com/PinellasPark.htm

John Porter MD, Academy Director
Mack R Hicks PhD, Founder/Chairman of the Board
Andrew P Hicks PhD, CEO/Clinical Director
Specifically designed for the learning disabled child and other children with difficulties in concentration, strategy, social skills, impulsivity, distractibility and study strategies. Programs offered include: attention training, visual-motor remediation, socialization skills training, relaxation training, horseback riding and more. The day camp meets weekdays from 9-3 for 3,4 or 5 week sessions.

7330 Council for Extended Care of Mentally Retarded Citizens
5257 Shaw Avenue
Suite 305
Saint Louis, MO 63110
314-781-4950
FAX: 314-771-8880
e-mail: cecmrc@aol.com
cecstl.org

Vicky Presnell, Executive Director
Marge Lindhorst, Supported Living Director
Services are provided to adults and children with developmental disabilities. Supported living arrangements are located in St. Louis city, St. Louis county and St. Charles County. Group home and camp services are located in Dittmer, MO. Travel program also available.

7331 Dallas Academy
950 Tiffany Way
Dallas, TX 75218
214-324-1481
FAX: 214-327-8537
e-mail: mail@dallas-academy.com
www.dallas-academy.com

Jim Richardson, Executive Director
Miscy Stockton, Director of the Lower School
7-week summer session for students who are having difficulty in regular school classes.

7332 **Eagle Hill School: Summer Program**
242 Old Petersham Road
Hardwick, MA 01037
413-477-6000
FAX: 413-477-6837
e-mail: admission@ehs1.org
www.ehs1.org

Peter J Donald, Headmaster
For children ages 9-19 with specific learning (dis)abilities and/or Attention Deficit Disorder, this summer program is designed to remediate academic and social deficits while maintaining progress achieved during the school year. Electives and sports activities are combined with the academic courses to address the needs of the whole person in a camp-like atmosphere.

7333 **Easter Seals Oklahoma**
Easter Seals America
701 Northeast 13th Street
Oklahoma City, OK 73104
405-239-2525
FAX: 405-239-2278
e-mail: esok1@coxinet.net
www.eastersealsoklahoma.org

Patricia Filer, Executive Director
Providing services such as adult day services, child development center, OTIPT, speech therapy, reading/tutoring, vision and hearing screening.

7334 **Elling Camps**
Rr 1
Box 54
Thompson, PA 18465
717-756-2706
FAX: 717-756-3306

Lloyd E Elling, Director
For youth ages 6-21 with learning disabilities and accompanying difficulties. This camp allows them to learn to adjust socially in a community atmosphere. The structured camp program includes land and water sports, nature and forestry, industrial arts, construction and work programs, and arts and crafts.

7335 **Englishton Park Academic Remediation**
Englishton Park Presbyterian
PO Box 228
Lexington, IN 47138
812-889-2046
e-mail: tbarnet@venus.net
www.englishtonpark.org

Lisa Barnett, Co-Director
Thomas Barnett, Co-Director
Camp is located in Lexington, Indiana. Two-week sessions for children with ADD. Boys and girls, ages 7-12.

7336 **Florida Sheriffs Caruth Camp**
Florida Sheriffs Youth Ranches
PO Box 2000
Boys Ranch, FL 32064
386-842-5501
800-765-3797
FAX: 386-842-2429
e-mail: fsyr@youthranches.org
www.youthranches.org

Sheriff Bill Farmer, Chairman of the Board
Roger Bouchard, President
Dan Hager, Vice Chairman
Camp is located in Inglis, Florida. One-week sessions for children with ADD. Coed, ages 10-15.

7337 **Gow School Summer Programs**
2491 Emery Road
PO Box 85
South Wales, NY 14139
716-652-3450
FAX: 716-652-3457
e-mail: webmaster@gow.org
www.gow.org

David Mendlewski, Director of Summer Program
Bradley Rogers, Principal/Headmaster
Gayle Hutton, Development Director
Co-ed summer programs for students ages 8-16 with dyslexia or similar learning disabilities offer a balanced blend of morning academics, afternoon/evening traditional camp activities and weekend overnights. The primary purpose of these programs is to provide a positive experience while balancing these three elements. Committed to the creation of a positive and enjoyable experience for each participant by defining and merging the goals of the camp and the school, with those of camper students.

7338 **Hill School of Fort Worth**
4817 Odessa Avenue
Fort Worth, TX 76133
817-923-9482
FAX: 817-923-4894
e-mail: hillschool@hillschool.org
www.hillschool.org

David Bucher, Chairman
Mark Jackson, Senior Vice President
Greg Owens, Principal
Provides an alternative learning environment for students having average or above-average intelligence with learning differences. Hill school is an established leader in North Texas with a 25 year history of effectively serving LD children. Beginning in 1961 as a tutorial service, Hill became a formal school in 1973. Our mission is to help those who learn differently develop skills and strategies to succeed. We do this by developing academic/study skills, and self-discipline.

7339 **Indian Acres Camp for Boys**
1712 Main Street
Fryeburg,, ME 04037
207-935-2300
FAX: 954-349-7812
e-mail: geoff@indianacres.com
www.indianacres.com

Lisa Newman, Director/Co-Owner
Jeffrey Newman, Director/Co-Owner
Michael Burness, Asistant Director
Camp is located in Fryeburg, Florida. Four and seven-week sessions June-August for boys with ADD ages 7-16.

7340 **Lab School of Washington**
4759 Reservoir Road Northwest
Washington, DC 20007
202-965-6600
FAX: 202-965-5106
e-mail: labschool@webmail.org
www.labschool.org

Sally Smith, Founder/Manager
The Lab School six week summer session includes individualized reading, spelling, writing, study skills and math programs. A multisensory approach addresses the needs of bright learning disabled children. Related services such as speech/language therapy and occupational therapy are integrated into the curriculum. Elementary/Intermediate; Junior High/High School.

7341 **Lions Den Outdoor Learning Center**
600 Kiwanis Drive
Eureka, MO 63025
636-938-5245
FAX: 636-938-5289
e-mail: info@wymancenter.org
www.wymancenter.org

Mia Olmer, Director
Varied programs for mentally retarded children, ages 6 and up, includes daily living, socialization and language skills. Sports, tent camping, crafts, and nature study are also offered. Sliding scale tuition for 2 weeks.

7342 **Maplebrook School**
5142 Route 22
Amenia, NY 12501
845-373-9511
FAX: 845-373-7029
e-mail: admin@maplebrookschool.org
www.maplebrookschool.org

Donna Konkolics, Headmaster
Mark Metzger, President
Priscilla Buckley, Vice President
A coeductional boarding school which offers a six week camp for children with learning differences and ADD.

7343 Marvelwood Summer
Marvelwood School
PO Box 3001
Kent, CT 06757
860-927-0047
FAX: 860-927-5325
e-mail: summerschool@marvelwood.org
www.themarvelwoodschool.net

Scott E Pottbecker, Headmaster of School
Anne Scott, Principal
The emphasis in this summer program is on diagnosis and remediation of individual reading, spelling, writing, mathematics and study problems. Offered to ages 12-16.

7344 New Jersey YMHA/YWHA Camps Milford
21 Plymouth Street
Fairfield, NJ 07004
973-575-3333
800-776-5657
FAX: 973-575-4188
e-mail: info@njycamps.org
www.njycamps.org

Leonard M Robinson, Camp Director
Bruce Nussman, President
Camp is located in Milford, Pennsylvania. Summer sessions for children with ADD. Coed, ages 6-17 and families.

7345 Oakland School & Camp
Boyd Tavern
Keswick, VA 22947
434-293-9059
FAX: 434-296-8930
e-mail: oaklandschool@earthlink.net
www.oaklandschool.net

Joanne Dondero, President
Carol Smieciuch, Executive Director
A highly individualized program stresses improving reading ability. Subjects taught are reading, English composition, math and word analysis. Recreational activities include horseback riding, sports, swimming, tennis, crafts, archery and camping. For girls and boys, ages 8-14.

7346 Outside in School
PO Box 639
Greensburg, PA 15601
724-837-1518
FAX: 724-837-0801
e-mail: outside@icubed.com
www.outsideinschool.com

Michael C Henkel, Executive Director
Camp is located in Bolivar, Pennsylvania. Sessions for children with ADD and substance abuse problems. Boys 11-18 and girls 13-18.

7347 Phelps School Summer School
583 Sugartown Road
Malvern, PA 19355
610-644-1754
FAX: 610-644-6679
e-mail: admis@thephelpsschool.org
www.thephelpsschool.org

Mike Reardon, Director of Admissions
Emily Shaker, Admissions Representative
Norman Phelps Jr, Principal
Open for grades 7-11 to make up academic deficiencies or complete studies in English, math and reading. Sports include riding, tennis and swimming. A program is also available to a limited number of international students in English as a Second Language.

7348 Quest Camp
2333 San Ramon Valley Boulevard
Suite 125
San Ramon, CA 94583
925-743-1370
FAX: 925-743-1937
e-mail: bfield12@aol.com
www.questcamps.com

Robert Field Phd, Director
Camp is located in Alamo, California. Day camp offering three to eight-week sessions including psychological treatment for children with ADD and other mild to moderate psychological disorders. Coed, ages 6-15.

7349 Raven Rock Lutheran Camp
17912 Harbaugh Valley Road
PO Box 136
Sabillasville, MD 21780
410-303-2108
800-321-5824
e-mail: ravenrock@innernet.net
www.ravenrock.org

Brenda Minnich, Executive Director
Stephen Demik, Program Director
John Corkal, Director
Christ-centered program for youth and mentally retarded adults.

7350 Rimland Services for Autistic Citizens
1265 Harney Avenue
Evanston, IL 60202
847-328-4090
877-395-6937
FAX: 847-328-8364
e-mail: dwork@rimland.org
www.rimland.org

Pamela Watson, Chief Executive Officer
Edna Adams, Operations Assoc Exec Director
Dave Work, Programs Assoc Exec Director
An accessible camp facility that can be utilized by groups for day use or overnight camping experiences. Six winterized cabins, a meeting facility, indoor pool, full food service, and an excellent staff are available. Educational programs can be arranged or you can utilize the facility to manage your own programs.

7351 Rolling Hills Country Day Camp
14 Dittmar Road
PO Box 6623
Freehold, NJ 07728
732-308-0405
FAX: 732-780-4726
e-mail: info@rollinghillsdaycamp.com
www.rollinghillsdaycamp.com

Billy Breitner, Director/Owner
Stan Breitner, Director/Owner
Dustin Breitner, Director/Owner
Summer sessions for children with ADD. Coed, ages 3-12.

7352 SOAR Summer Adventures
PO Box 388
Balsam, NC 28707
828-456-3435
FAX: 828-456-3449
e-mail: jonathan@soarnc.org
www.mysummercamps.com/

Jonathan Jones, Executive Director
John Willson, LD and AD/HD Services Director
Ed Parker, Admissions Director
A nonprofit adventure program working with disadvantaged youth diagnosed with learning disabilities in an outdoor, challenge based environment. Focuses on esteem building and social skills development through rock climbing, backpacking, whitewater rafting, mountaineering, sailing, snorkeling, and much more. Offers two week, one month, and semester programs available. SOAR programs utilize North Carolina, Florida, Colorado, American Southwest, Alaska, and Jamaica as program areas.

7353 Sherman Lake YMCA Outdoor Center
6225 North 39th Street
Augusta, MI 49012
269-731-3000
FAX: 269-731-3020
e-mail: shermanlakeymca@ymcasl.org
www.shermanlakeymca.org

Luke Austenfeld, Executive Director
Jeff Brown, Program Manager
Lorrie Syverson, Director Camping Services
Summer camping sessions for campers with ADD and spina bifida. Coed, ages 6-15 and families, seniors.

7354 Squirrel Hollow Summer Camp
The Bedford School
5665 Milam Road
Fairburn, GA 30213
770-774-8001
FAX: 770-774-8005
e-mail: bbox@thebedfordschool.org
www.thebedfordschool.org

Betsy Box, Founder/Executive Director
Anne Miller, Development Director
Jim Pridmore, Facilities Director
A remedial summer program for children with academic needs held on the campus of The Bedford School in Fairburn, Georgia. It is a five week day camp held from June 19 to July 21 and serves ages 6-16. For mor information contact Betsy Box at (770) 774-8001.

7355 **Summer Day Camp**
Yorba Linda Placentia Farm YMCA
13821 Newport Avenue
Suite 200
Tustin, CA 92780
714-549-9622
FAX: 714-777-1903
www.ymcaoc.org

Clare Kenna, Executive Director
Alfred Herzing, Board Chair
Dave Gruchow, Board of Governors
One-week sessions for children with ADD and speech/communication impairment. Coed, ages 5-14.

7356 **Summit Camp**
18 East 41st Street
Suite 402
New York, NY 10017
212-689-3880
800-323-9908
FAX: 212-689-3880
e-mail: info@summitcamp.com
www.summitcamp.com

Mayer and Ninette Stiskin, Executive Directors/Co-Founders
Regina Skyer, Clinical Social Worker
Tim Kedge, Head Counselor/Program Director
Camp is located in Honesdale, Pennsylvania. Summer sessions for children with ADD. Coed, ages 8-17.

7357 **Sunnyhill Adventure Center**
Council for Extended Care
6555 Sunlit Way
Dittmer, MO 63023
636-274-9044
314-781-4950
FAX: 636-285-1305
e-mail: cecmrc@aol.com
www.sunnyhilladventures.org

Rob Darroch, Executive Director
Kim Smallacombe, Program Director
Camp is located in Dittmer, Missouri. Summer sessions for campers with developmental disabilities and autism. Coed, ages 8-99. Sunnyhill Adventures is program that offers campers fun, exciting, educational experiences in a beautiful outdoor setting. Our residential summer camp combines traditional camping activities plus specially selected and adapted events to meet the needs of each camper group.

7358 **Talisman Summer Camp**
64 Gap Creek Road
Zirconia, NC 28790
888-458-8826
e-mail: summer@stonemountainschool.com
www.talismansummercamp.com

Linda Tatsapaugh, Director
Charlie Talley, Executive Director
Emily Darby, Sight Program Manager
Camp is located in Black Mountain, North Carolina. Offers a program of hiking, rafting, climbing, and caving for learning disabled ADD/ADHD and autistic young people. Coed, ages 9-18.

7359 **Timbertop Nature Adventure Camp**
YMCA Camp Glacier Hollow
1000 Division Street
Stevens Point, WI 54481
715-342-2980
FAX: 715-342-2987
e-mail: pmatthai@spymca.org
www.spymca.org

Peter Matthai, Camp Director
Dave Morgan, Executive Director
For children who can benefit from an individualized program of learning in a non-competitive outdoor setting under the skilled leadership of people who understand the environment and the unique potential of these children.

7360 **Tower Program at Regis College**
Regis College
235 Wellesley Street
Weston, MA 02493
781-768-7000
FAX: 781-768-8339
e-mail: admission@regiscollege.edu
www.regiscollege.edu

Mary England, President
Pamela Menke, Vice Prsident
Helps average and above average college-bound students, ages 16-17, having a diagnosed dyslexic learning disability, to adjust to a college setting. Emphasis is on instruction and academic reinforcement, affective support, awareness of support services available on most college campuses and strategy training.

7361 **Triangle Y Ranch YMCA**
Y MC A of Tri- County mtero mil
161 West Wisconsin Ave
Suite 4000
Milwaukee, WI 53203
262-675-9622
FAX: 414-224-0151
e-mail: kwilliams@ymcamke.org
www.ymcamke.org

Cathy Palmer, Executive Director
Cliss Clauer, Executive Director
Camp is located in West Bend, Wisconsin. Summer camping for children with ADD. Coed, ages 5-14.

7362 **University of Iowa: Wendell Johnson Speech and Hearing Clinic**
250 Hawkins Drive
Iowa City, IA 52242
319-335-1845
FAX: 319-335-8851
e-mail: wendy-fick@uiowa.edu
www.shc.uiowa.edu

Linda Louko, Clinic Director
Marlea O'Brien, Child Language Research Center
Dorothy Albright, Department Administration
The clinic offers assessment and remediation for communication disorders in adults and children. The clinic also offers a Intensive Summer Residential Clinic for school age children needing intervention services because of speech, language, hearing and/or reading problems.

Print & Non-Print Resources

7363 **A Miracle to Believe In**
Option Indigo Press
2080 S Undermountain Road
Sheffield, MA 01257
413-229-8727
800-714-2779
FAX: 413-229-8727
e-mail: indigo@bcn.net
www.optionindigo.com
A group of people from all walks of life come together and are transformed as they reach out, under the direction of the Kaufmans, to help a little boy the medical world had given up as hopeless. This heartwarming journey of loving a child back to life will not only inspire you, the reader, but presents a compelling new way to deal with life's traumas and difficulties.
379 pages 1981
ISBN 0-449201-08-2

7364 **ADD, Stepping Out of the Dark**
ADD Videos
PO Box 622
New Paltz, NY 12561
845-255-3612
FAX: 845-883-6452

Lenae Madonna, Producer

A powerful, effective video, ideal for health professionals, educators and parents providing a visual montage designed to promote an understanding and awareness of attention deficit disorder. Based on actual accounts of those who have ADD, including a neurologist, an office worker, and parents of children with ADD. The video allows the viewer to feel the frustration and lack of attention that ADD brings to many. *$52.95*
Video

7365 ADD/ADHD Behavior-Change Resource Kit
Jossey-Bass

For teachers, couselors and parents, this resource offers information and practical strategies to help kids with attention deficits learn to control and change their own behaviors and build the academic, social, and personal skills necessary for success iun scholl and in life. The kit first explains ADD/ADHD behavior, its biological bases and basic characteristics and describes procedures used for diagnosis and various treatment options. *$29.95*
416 pages 2002
ISBN 0-876281-44-7

7366 ADD/ADHD Checklist
Jossey-Bass

This resource supplies up-to-date facts, findings, and proven strategies and techniques for understanding and helping children and adolescents with attention deficit problems and hyperactivity. *$ 12.95*
272 pages 2002
ISBN 0-137623-95-X

7367 ADD: Helping Your Child
Warner Books
1271 Avenue of the Americas
New York, NY 10020
212-522-7200
FAX: 212-522-7989

Laurence Krishbaum, Chief Executive Officer
$12.95
224 pages Paperback
ISBN 0-446670-13-8

7368 ADHD
Learning Disabilities Association of America
4156 Library Road
Pittsburgh, PA 15234
412-341-1515
FAX: 412-344-0224
e-mail: info@ldaamerica.org
www.ldaamerica.org
A booklet for parents offering information on Attention Deficit-Hyperactivity Disorders and learning disabilities. *$3.00*

7369 ADHD Book of Lists: A Practical Guide for Helping Children and Teens with ADDs
Jossey-Bass

Current information about Atention Deficit/Hyperactivity Disorder including strategies, supports, and interventions that have been found to be the most effective. For teachers, parents, and counselors. *$29.95*
320 pages 2003
ISBN 0-787965-91-X

7370 ADHD Report
Guilford Press
72 Spring Street
New York, NY 10012
212-431-9800
800-365-7006
FAX: 212-966-6708
e-mail: info@guilford.com

Bob Matloff, President
Presents the most up-to-date information on the evaluation, diagnosis and management of ADHD in children, adolescents and adults. This important newsletter is an invaluable resource for all professionals interested in ADHD. *$49.95*
BiMonthly
ISSN 1065-8025

7371 ADHD in Adults
Guilford Press
72 Spring Street
New York, NY 10012
212-431-9800
800-365-7006
FAX: 212-966-6708
e-mail: info@guilford.com
www.guilford.com

Bob Matloff, President
This program integrates information on ADHD with the actual experiences of four adults who suffer from the disorder. Representing a range of professions, from a lawyer to a mother working at home, each candidly discusses the impact of ADHD on his or her daily life. These interviews are augmented by comments from family members and other clinicians who treat adults with ADHD. *$95.00*
Video
ISBN 0-898629-86-1

7372 ADHD in Schools: Assessment and Intervention Strategies
Guilford Press
72 Spring Street
New York, NY 10012
212-431-9800
800-365-7006
FAX: 212-966-6708
e-mail: info@guilford.com

Bob Matloff, President
This landmark volume emphasizes the need for a team effort among parents, community-based professionals, and educators. Provides practical information for educators that is based on empirical findings. Chapters focus on: how to identify and assess students who might have ADHD; the relationship between ADHD and learning disabilities; how to develop and implement classroom-based programs; communication strategies to assist physicians; and the need for community-based treatments. *$ 36.00*
269 pages Hardcover
ISBN 0-898622-45-X

7373 ADHD with Comorbid Disorders: Clinical Assessment and Management
Guilford Press
72 Spring Street
New York, NY 10012
212-431-9800
800-365-7006
FAX: 212-966-6708
www.guilford.com

James M Swanson, Author
Bob Matloff, President
$44.00
Cloth
ISBN 1-572304-78-2

7374 ADHD: Handbook for Diagnosis & Treatment
Western Psychological Services
12031 Wilshire Boulevard
Los Angeles, CA 90025
310-478-2061
800-648-8857
FAX: 310-478-7838

Gregg Gillmar, Vice President
This second edition helps clinicians diagnose and treat Attention Deficit Hyperactivity Disorder. Written by an internationally recognized authority in the field, it covers the history of ADHD, its primary symptoms, associated conditions, developmental course and outcome, and family context. A workbook companion manual is also available. *$ 68.00*
700 pages

7375 ADHD: What Can We Do?
Guilford Press
72 Spring Street
New York, NY 10012
212-431-9800
800-365-7006
FAX: 212-966-6708
e-mail: info@guilford.com

Bob Matloff, President

A video program that introduces teachers and parents to a variety of the most effective technologies for managing ADHD in the classroom, at home, and on family outings. *$95.00*
Video
ISBN 0-898629-72-1

7376 ADHD: What Do We Know?
Guilford Press
72 Spring Street
New York, NY 10012
212-431-9800
800-365-7006
FAX: 212-966-6708
e-mail: info@guilford.com

Bob Matloff, President
An introduction for teachers and special education practitioners, school psychologists and parents of ADHD children. Topics outlined in this video include the causes and prevalence of ADHD, ways children with ADHD behave, other conditions that may accompany ADHD and long-term prospects for children with ADHD. *$95.00*
Video
ISBN 0-898629-71-3

7377 About Attention Disorder
CACLD
25 Van Zant Street
Suite 15-5
Norwalk, CT 06855
203-838-5010
FAX: 203-866-6108
e-mail: CACLD@optonline.net
www.CACLD.org

Beryl Kaufman, Executive Director
Introduction to ADHD for the child with the disorder, parents, professionals, family and friends. Brief description as well as causes, challenges involved, treatment options, ways for parents and teachers to help and how children can help themselves. Published by Connecticut Association for Children & Adults with Learning Disabilities (CACLD). *$2.00*
14 pages

7378 Adolescents with Down Syndrome: Toward a More Fulfilling Life
Brookes Publishing
PO Box 10624
Baltimore, MD 21285
410-337-9580
800-638-3775
FAX: 410-337-8539
e-mail: custserv@brookespublishing.com
www.brookespublishing.com

Paul Brooks, Owner
Written for health care professionals, psychologists, other developmental disabilities practitioners, educators, and parents, it covers biomedical concerns; behavioral, psychological, and psychiatric challenges; and education, employment, recreation, community, and legal concerns. *$35.95*
416 pages Paperback 1997
ISBN 1-55766 -81-9

7379 Adult ADD: The Complete Handbook: Everyt hing You Need to Know About How to Cope with ADD
Prima Publishing
PO Box 1260
Rocklin, CA 95677
916-787-7000
800-632-8676
FAX: 916-787-7001
e-mail: websupportlife@primapub.com
www.primapublishing.com
In simple and friendly terms, the authors offer help to those leading frustrating lives. They provide coping mechanisms, both psychological and an up-to-date guide to the latest technology *$14.95*
272 pages 1997
ISBN 0-761507-96-5

7380 All About Attention Deficit Disorders, Revised
Parent Magic
800 Roosevelt Road
Glen Ellyn, IL 60137
630-790-9600
FAX: 630-469-4571
www.parentmagic.com

Nancy Roe, Office Manager
Thomas Phelan, Owner
A psychologist and expert on ADD outlines the symptoms, diagnosis and treatment of this neurological disorder. *$12.95*
248 pages Paperback
ISBN 1-889140-11-2

7381 American Journal on Mental Retardation
American Association on Mental Retardation
444 N Capitol Street NW
Washington, DC 20001
202-387-1968
800-424-3688
FAX: 202-387-2193
e-mail: aamr@access.digex.net
www.aamr.org

Bruce Appelgen, Director Publications
Doreen Croser, Executive Director
Articles cover biological, behavioral, and educational research: theory papers; and reviews of research literature on specific aspects of mental retardation. *$142.00*
112 pages BiMonthly

7382 Annals of Dyslexia
International Dyslexia Association
382 S Chester Street
Baltimore, MD 21231
800-ABC-D123
FAX: 410-296-0232
www.interdys.org
Offers information on auditory discrimination, dyslexia, attitudes, advocacy and more on people with learning disabilities. *$ 15.00*
Paper

7383 Arc Connection Newsletter
Arc of Tennessee
151 Athens Way
Suite 100
Nashville, TN 37228
615-248-5878
800-835-7077
FAX: 615-248-5879
e-mail: pcooper@thearctn.org
www.thearctn.org

Walter Rogers, Executive Director
Quarterly publication from the ARC of Tennessee. *$ 10.00*
12 pages Quarterly

7384 Arc Light
Arc of Arizona
5610 S Central Avenue
Phoenix, AZ 85040
602-268-6101
800-252-9054
FAX: 602-268-7483
e-mail: Arcofarizona@aol.com
www.arcofarizona.org

Cindy Waymire, Manager
Quarterly

7385 Around the Clock: Parenting the Delayed AD HD Child

Guilford Press
72 Spring Street
New York, NY 10012
212-431-9800
800-365-7006
FAX: 212-966-6708
e-mail: info@guilford.com

Bob Matloff, President
This videotape provides both professionals and parents a helpful look at how the difficulties facing parents of ADHD children can be handled. Video. *$150.00*

ISBN 0-898629-68-3

7386 Attention
Children & Adults with ADHD
8181 Professional Place
Suite 150
Landover, MD 20785
301-306-7070
800-233-4050
FAX: 301-306-6788
www.chadd.org

Clarke Ross, CEO
Karen White, Director Natl Resource Center
Marsha Bokamn, Manager
A bi-monthly publication from CHADD. Free with membership.

bi-monthly

7387 **Attention Deficit Disorder**
Pro-Ed
8700 Shoal Creek Boulevard
Austin, TX 78757
512-451-3246
800-897-3202
FAX: 512-451-8542
e-mail: info@proedinc.com
www.proedinc.com

Donald Hammill, Owner
A book providing helpful suggestions for both home and classroom management of students with attention deficit disorder.

7388 **Attention Deficit Disorder and Learning Disabilities**
Books on Special Children
PO Box 305
Congers, NY 10920
845-638-1236
FAX: 845-638-0847
e-mail: irene@boscbooks.com
Introduces ADD and learning disabilities. This is an easy reading book. Gives definitions and discusses some effective and controverial medication, dietary, biofeedback, cognitive therapy, and many more issues. *$15.95*
246 pages Softcover
ISBN 0-385469-31-4

7389 **Attention Deficit Disorder in Adults Workbook**
Taylor Publishing Company
1550 W Mockingbird Lane
Dallas, TX 75235
214-637-2800
FAX: 214-819-8580

Don Percenti, Chief Executive Officer
$17.99
192 pages Paperback
ISBN 0-878338-50-0

7390 **Attention Deficit Disorder: A Different Perception**
Underwood-Miller
708 Westover Drive
Lancaster, PA 17601
717-285-2255
FAX: 717-285-2255
$9.95
180 pages Paperback
ISBN 0-887331-56-4

7391 **Attention Deficit Disorder: Adults**
Aquarius Health Care Videos
PO Box 1159
Sherborn, MA 01770
508-650-6905
FAX: 508-650-4216
e-mail: aqvideos@tiac.net
www.aquariusproductions.com
Adults with ADD talk about how the disorder that went undiagnosed for so many years has affected their choice of spouses and work, and what they have found to help them. Biofeedback, which is growing as a treatment, is explained and demonstrated by its founder, Dr. Joel Lubar. Medical treatments like antidepressants and stimulants are also discussed, along with behavioral changes that can help the person with ADD and his or her spouse and family. *$149.00*
Video

7392 **Attention Deficit Disorder: Children**
Aquarius Health Care Videos
PO Box 1159
Sherborn, MA 01770
508-650-6905
888-440-2963
FAX: 508-650-4216
e-mail: aqvideos@tiac.net
www.aquariusproductions.com

Leslie Kussmann, President/Producer
Everyone has been impulsive or easily distracted for different periods of time, so these symptoms that are hallmarks of Attention Deficit Disorder (ADD) have also led to criticism that too many people are being diagnosed with this biochemical brain disorder. This program examines who is being diagnosed, and what treatments are working. An innovative private school specializing in alternative education is profiled, and tips on structuring the school and home environment are included. *$149.00*
Video

7393 **Attention Deficit Disorders: Assessment & Teaching**
Brooks/Cole Publishing Company
511 Forest Lodge Road
Pacific Grove, CA 93950
831-333-1175
FAX: 408-375-6414
e-mail: bc-info@brookscole.com
www.brookscole.com

Theresa Brooks, President
A handy resource that offers teachers, school psychologists, councelors, social workers, administrators, and parents practical advice for working with children who have attention deficit disorders. *$18.95*
258 pages Paperback
ISBN 0-534250-44-0

7394 **Attention-Deficit Hyperactivity Disorder: Symptoms and Suggestons for Treatment**
Slosson Educational Publications
PO Box 280
East Aurora, NY 14052
716-652-0930
FAX: 800-655-3840
e-mail: slosson@slosson.com
www.slosson.com

Leslie Foote, Office Personnel
Peggy Meyer, Office Personnel
Steven Slosson, President
An exhaustive review of current research and decades of experience as practicing school-based professionals, as well as being a parent of an ADHD child, have culminated in this brief, to-the-point, and yet informed ADHD package which has recieved tremendous reviews. Well-grounded answers and suggestions which would facillitate behavior, learning, social-emotional functioning, and other factors in preschool and adolesence are discussed. Answers most commonly asked questions about ADHD/ADD. *$60.00*
61 pages

7395 **Attention-Deficit/Hyperactivity Disorder, What Every Parent Wants to Know**
Brookes Publishing
PO Box 10624
Baltimore, MD 21285
410-337-9580
800-638-3775
FAX: 410-337-8539
e-mail: custserv@brookespublishing.com
www.brookespublishing.com

Paul Brooks, Owner
New easy-to-understand, non-technical edition helps teachers and parents get accessible answers to their ADHD. *$21.95*
304 pages Paperback 2000
ISBN 1-557663-98-X

7396 **Augmenting Basic Communciation in Natural Contexts**
Brookes Publishing
PO Box 10624
Baltimore, MD 21285
410-337-9580
800-638-3775
FAX: 410-337-8539
e-mail: custserv@brookespublishing.com
www.brookespublishing.com

Paul Brooks, Owner
Here you will find the techniques needed to establish a basic communication system for people of all ages with cognitive disabilities or motor sensory impairments. *$41.95*

304 pages Paperback
ISBN 1-55766 -43-6

7397 Autism
Autism Society of North Carolina Bookstore
505 Oberlin Road
Suite 230
Raleigh, NC 27605
919-743-0204
800-442-2762
FAX: 919-743-0208
e-mail: dcoffey@autismsociety-nc.org
www.autismsociety-nc.org

Darla Coffey, Bookstore Manager
Jill Keel, Executive Director
Everything there is to know about autism research book. *$17.95*

7398 Autism Handbook: Understanding & Treating Autism & Prevention Development
Oxford University Press
2001 Evans Road
Cary, NC 27513
919-677-0977
800-451-7556
FAX: 919-677-1303
www.oup-usa.org

Thomas Carty, Senior Vice President
$25.00
320 pages
ISBN 0-195076-67-2

7399 Autism Research Institute
4182 Adams Avenue
San Diego, CA 92116
619-281-7165
FAX: 619-563-6840
www.autismresearchinstitute.com

Bernard Rimland Phd, Executive Director
Matt Kabler, Assistant Director
Conducts research on the causes, diagnosis, and treatment of autism and publishes a quarterly newsletter that reviews worldwide research. Literature on causes and treatment available. Refers patients and families to health care professionals and clinics. Request publication list and sample newsletter, Autism Research Review.

7400 Autism Research Review International
Autism Research Institute
4182 Adams Avenue
San Diego, CA 92116
619-281-7165
FAX: 619-563-6840
e-mail: br@autismresearchinstitute.com
www.autismresearchinstitute.com

Bernard Rimland PhD, Director
$18.00
8 pages Quarterly

7401 Autism Society of North Carolina
Autism Society Of North Carolina Bookstore
505 Oberlin Road
Suite 230
Raleigh, NC 27605
919-743-0204
800-442-2762
FAX: 919-743-0208
e-mail: info@autismsociety-nc.org
www.autismsociety-nc.org

Jill Keel, Executive Director
Tracey Sheriff, Director Operations
David Laxton, Director Communications
One of the largest autism-specific bookstores in the US. All proceeds are used to provide services to people with autism and their families.

7402 Autism Treatment Guide
Autism Society of North Carolina Bookstore
505 Oberlin Road
Suite 230
Raleigh, NC 27605
919-743-0204
800-442-2762
FAX: 919-743-0208
e-mail: dcoffey@autismsociety-nc.org
www.autismsociety-nc.org

Darla Coffey, Bookstore Manager
Jill Keel, Executive Director
A comprehensive book covering treatments and methods used to help individuals with autism. *$12.95*

7403 Autism and Asperger Syndrome
Autism Society of North Carolina Bookstore
505 Oberlin Road
Suite 230
Raleigh, NC 27605
919-743-0204
800-442-2762
FAX: 919-743-0208
e-mail: dcoffey@autismsociety-nc.org
www.autismsociety-nc.org

Darla Coffey, Bookstore Manager
Jill Keel, Executive Director
Chapters include topics such as the relationship of autism and asperger syndrome, living with the syndrome and asperger syndrome in adulthood. *$23.95*

7404 Autism and Learning
David Fulton Publishers
2 Barbon Close Great Ormond Street
London, WCIN
171-405-5606
FAX: 171-831-4840
This book is about how a cognitive perception on the way in which individuals with autism think and learn may be applied to particular curriculum areas.
160 pages Paperback
ISBN 1-853464-21-X

7405 Autism in Adolescents and Adults
Plenum Publishing Corporation
233 Spring Street
New York, NY 10013
212-242-1490
FAX: 212-463-0742
e-mail: info@plenum.com

$63.00
456 pages
ISBN 0-306410-57-5

7406 Autism...Nature, Diagnosis and Treatment
Autism Society of North Carolina Bookstore
505 Oberlin Road
Suite 230
Raleigh, NC 27605
919-743-0204
800-442-2762
FAX: 919-743-0208
e-mail: dcoffey@autismsociety-nc.org
www.autismsociety-nc.org

Darla Coffey, Bookstore Manager
Jill Keel, Executive Director
Covers perspectives, issues, neurobiological issues and new directions in diagnosis and treatment. *$49.00*

7407 Autism: A Strange, Silent World
Filmakers Library
124 E 40th Street
New York, NY 10016
212-808-4980
FAX: 212-808-4983
e-mail: info@filmakers.com
www.filmakers.com

Sue Oscar, Co-President/Owner
British educators and medical personnel offer insight into autism's characteristics and treatment approaches through the cameos of three children.

7408 Autism: A World Apart
Fanlight Productions
4196 Washington Street
Suite 2
Boston, MA 02131
617-469-4999
800-937-4113
FAX: 617-469-3379
e-mail: fanlight@fanlight.com
www.fanlight.com

Anthony Sweeny, Marketing Director
Nicole Johnson, Publicity Coordinator
Ben Achtenberg, Owner

Autism's cause is unknown. There is no cure, and it strikes each victim differently. In this documentary, three families show us what the textbooks and studies cannot - what it is like to live with autism day after day - to love and raise children who may be withdrawn and violent, and unable to make personal connections with their families. *$195.00*

7409 Autism: Explaining the Enigma
Autism Society of North Carolina Bookstore
505 Oberlin Road
Suite 230
Raleigh, NC 27605
919-743-0204
800-442-2762
FAX: 919-743-0208
e-mail: dcoffey@autismsociety-nc.org
www.autismsociety-nc.org

Darla Coffey, Bookstore Manager
Jill Keel, Executive Director
Explains the nature of autism. *$27.95*

7410 Autism: From Tragedy to Triumph
Branden Publishing Company
17 Station Street
Brookline, MA 02445
617-734-2045
FAX: 781-790-1056
e-mail: branden@branden.com
www.branden.com
A new book that deals with the Lovaas method and includes a foreward by Dr. Ivar Lovaas. The book is broken down into two parts — the long road to diagnosis and then treatment. *$12.95*

7411 Autism: Identification, Education and Treatment
Autism Society of North Carolina Bookstore
505 Oberlin Road
Suite 230
Raleigh, NC 27605
919-743-0204
800-442-2762
FAX: 919-743-0208
e-mail: dcoffey@autismsociety-nc.org
www.autismsociety-nc.org

Darla Coffey, Bookstore Manager
Jill Keel, Executive Director
Chapters include medical treatments, early intervention and communication development in autism. *$36.00*

7412 Autism: The Facts
Oxford University Press
2001 Evans Road
Cary, NC 27513
919-677-0977
800-451-7556
FAX: 919-677-1303
www.oup-usa.org

Thomas Carty, Senior Vice President
$19.95
128 pages
ISBN 0-192623-28-1

7413 Autistic Adults at Bittersweet Farms
Haworth Press
10 Alice Street
Binghamton, NY 13904
607-722-5857
800-429-6784
FAX: 607-722-6362
e-mail: orders@haworthpress.com
www.haworthpress.com

Norman Giddan PhD, Editor
Jane Giddan MA, Editor
William Cohen, Owner
A touching view of an inspirational residential care program for autistic adolescents and adults. Also available in softcover. *$94.95*
Hardcover
ISBN 1-560240-42-3

7414 Avoiding Unfortunate Situations
Autism Society of North Carolina Bookstore
505 Oberlin Road
Suite 230
Raleigh, NC 27605
919-743-0204
800-442-2762
FAX: 919-743-0208
e-mail: dcoffey@autismsociety-nc.org
www.autismsociety-nc.org

Darla Coffey, Bookstore Manager
Jill Keel, Executive Director
A collection of tips and information from and about people with autism and other developmental disabilities. *$5.00*

7415 Be Quiet, Marina!
Star Bright Books

A noisy little girl with cerebral palsy and a quiet little girl with Down Syndrome learn to play together and eventually become best friends. *$16.95*
40 pages Hardcover 2001
ISBN 1-887734-79-1

7416 Biology Concepts Through Discovery
Educational Activities Software
PO Box 754
Baldwin, NY 11510
516-867-7878
800-645-2796
FAX: 516-379-7429
e-mail: achieve@ea-software.com

Alan Stern, Manager
These videos, available in English and Spanish versions, encourage learning by presenting interactive problem solving in an effective VISUAL/AUDITORY style. *$89.00*
Video

7417 Biology of the Autistic Syndromes
Autism Society of North Carolina Bookstore
505 Oberlin Road
Suite 230
Raleigh, NC 27605
919-743-0204
800-442-2762
FAX: 919-743-0208
e-mail: dcoffey@autismsociety-nc.org
www.autismsociety-nc.org

Darla Coffey, Bookstore Manager
Jill Keel, Executive Director
A revision of the original classic text in the light of new developments and current knowledge. This book covers the epidemiological, genetic, biochemical, immunological and neuropsychological literature on autism. *$74.95*

7418 Breakthroughs: How to Reach Students with Autism
Aquarius Health Care Videos
PO Box 1159
Sherborn, MA 01770
508-650-6905
FAX: 508-650-4216
e-mail: aqvideos@tiac.net
www.aquariusproductions.com
A hands-on, how-to program for reaching students with autism, featuring Karen Sewell, Autism Society of America's teacher of the year. Here Sewell demonstrates the successful techniques she's developed over a 20-year career. A separate 250 page manual ($59) is also available which covers math, reading, fine motor, self help, social adaptive, vocational and self help skills as well as providing numerous plan reproducibles and an exhaustive listing of equipment and materials resources. Video. *$99.00*

7419 Bus Girl: Selected Poems
Brookline Books
34 University Road
Brookline, MA 02445
617-558-8010
800-666-2665
FAX: 617-558-8011
e-mail: brbooks@yahoo.com
www.brooklinebooks.com
Poems written over several decades by a young woman with Down Syndrome. *$14.95*

144 pages Paperback
ISBN 1-57129 -41-9

7420 **But I'm Ready to Go**
Bradbury Press
8306 Aurora Avenue N
Seattle, WA 98103
206-524-4910
800-257-5755

Jack Bradbury, Owner
Judy always had a problem learning math and performing skills that required good motor control.
230 pages Hardcover
ISBN 0-87888 -07-7

7421 **Chadder**
Children & Adults with Attention Deficit Disorder
499 NW 70th Avenue
Suite 101
Plantation, FL 33317
954-587-3700
800-233-4050
FAX: 954-587-4599

Quarterly

7422 **Change Your Brain, Change Your Life: The Breakthrough Program for Conquering Depression**
Three Rivers Press

Clinical neuroscientist and psychiatrist Amen uses nuclear brain imaging to diagnose and treat behavioral problems. He explains how the brain works, what happens when things go wrong, and how to optimize brain function. Five sections of the brain are discussed, and case studies clearly illustrate possible problems. *$15.00*
352 pages 2000
ISBN 0-812929-98-5

7423 **Child Who Never Grew Up**
Exceptional Parent Library
PO Box 1807
Englewood Cliffs, NJ 07632
201-947-6000
800-535-1910
FAX: 201-947-9376
e-mail: eplibrary@aol.com
www.eplibrary.com
Offers Pearl Buck's inspiring account of her struggle to understand and help her daughter with mental retardation. *$14.95*
112 pages 1992
ISBN 0-933149-49-2

7424 **Child and Adolescent Therapy: Cognitive-Be havioral Procedures, Second Edition**
Guilford Press
72 Spring Street
New York, NY 10012
212-431-9800
800-365-7006
FAX: 212-966-6708
www.guilford.com

Bob Matloff, President
Incorporating significant developments in treatment procedures, theory and clinical research, new chapters in this second edition examine the current status of empirically supported interventions and developmental issues specific to work with adolescents. *$45.00*
432 pages Cloth 2000
ISBN 1-572305-56-8

7425 **Children with Mental Retardation**
Woodbine House
6510 Bells Mill Road
Bethesda, MD 20817
301-897-3570
800-843-7323
FAX: 301-897-5838
www.woodbinehouse.com

Irv Shapell, Owner
A book for parents of children with mild to moderate mental retardation, whether or not they have a diagnosed syndrome or condition. It provides a complete and compassionate introduction to their child's medical, therapeutic, and educational needs, and discusses the emotional impact on the family. New parents can rely on Children with Mental Retardation to provide that solid foundation and confidence they need to help their child reach his or her highest potential. *$14.95*
437 pages Paperback
ISBN 0-933149-39-5

7426 **Cogrehab**
Life Science Associates
1 Fenimore Road
Bayport, NY 11705
631-472-2111

Divided into six groups for diagnosis and treatment of attention, memory and perceptual disorders to be used by and under the guidance of a professional. $95.-$1,950

7427 **Come Back Jack: The Revealing Story of a Child Diagnosed with Autism**
Aquarius Health Care Videos
PO Box 1159
Sherborn, MA 01770
508-650-6905
FAX: 508-650-4216
e-mail: aqvideos@tiac.net
www.aquariusproductions.com
Persistent ear infections, medically misguided over-treatment with antibiotics, and other mysterious physiological factors sent Jack's mind spinning. By the time Jack reached the age of two, his intellectual and emothional development had come to a schreeching halt. Terrified by the prospect of losing their youngest son, Jack's parents began searching for answers. Chronicles the ups and downs. *$ 99.00*

7428 **Communication Development in Children with Down Syndrome**
Brookes Publishing
PO Box 10624
Baltimore, MD 21285
410-337-9580
800-638-3775
FAX: 410-337-8539
e-mail: custserv@brookespublishing.com
www.brookespublishing.com

Paul Brooks, Owner
This book offers an extensive, detailed explanation of communication development in children with Down syndrome relative to their advancing cognitive skills. It introduces a critical framework for assessing and treating hearing, speech, and language problems and provides explicit intervention methods and tested clinical protocols.
Paperback 1998
ISBN 1-55766 -50-5

7429 **Communication in Autism**
Federal Government
31 Center Drive Msc2320
Bethesda, MD 20892
800-241-1044
FAX: 301-402-0018
e-mail: nidcdinfo@nidcd.nih.gov
www.nidcd.nih.org
Describes what is autism, who is affected by autism, the communication problems with autism, how are the speech and language problems of autism treated, and what research is being conducted to improve the communication of individuals with autism.

7430 **Comprehensive Guide to ADD in Adults: Research, Diagnosis & Treatment**
Taylor & Francis
7625 Empire Drive
Florence, KY 41042
859-371-9571
800-634-7064
FAX: 800-248-4724

Jeff Taylor, Owner
$50.95

426 pages
ISBN 0-876307-60-8

7431 Concentration Cockpit: Explaining Attention Deficits
Educators Publishing Service
PO Box 9031
Cambridge, MA 02139
617-367-2700
800-225-5750
FAX: 617-547-0412
www.epsbooks.com

This eight-page pamphlet explains the administration of The Concentration Cockpit, a newly revised poster that helps children with attention deficits gain insight into their problems and monitor their progress in grappling with these problems. *$64.50*

ISBN 0-838820-59-X

7432 Concentration Video
Learning disAbilities Resources
PO Box 716
Bryn Mawr, PA 19010
610-525-8336
800-869-8336
FAX: 610-525-8337

An instructional video which provides a perspective about attention problems, possible causes and solutions. *$19.95*
Video

7433 Coping with ADD/ADHD
Rosen Publishing Group
29 E 21st Street
New York, NY 10010
212-777-3017
800-237-9932
FAX: 888-436-4643
e-mail: rosenpub@tribeca.ios.com

Roger Rosen, President
At least 3.5 million American youngsters suffer from attention deficit disorder. This book defines the syndrome and provides specific information about treatment and counseling. *$16.95*

ISBN 0-823920-70-4

7434 Count Us In
Exceptional Parent Library
PO Box 1807
Englewood Cliffs, NJ 07632
201-947-6000
800-535-1910
FAX: 201-947-9376
e-mail: eplibrary@aol.com
www.eplibrary.com

Offers information on growing up with Downs Syndrome. *$9.95*

7435 Culture and the Restructuring of Community Mental Health
Greenwood Publishing Group
88 Post Road W
Suite 5007
Westport, CT 06880
203-226-3571
FAX: 203-222-1502
www.greenwood.com

Wayne Smith, President
Examines treatment, organizational planning and research issues and offers a critique of the theoretical and programmatic aspects of providing mental health services to traditionally underserved populations. $45.00-$52.95.
168 pages Hardcover
ISBN 0-313268-87-8

7436 Diagnosis and Treatment of Autism
Autism Society of North Carolina Bookstore
505 Oberlin Road
Suite 230
Raleigh, NC 27605
919-743-0204
800-442-2762
FAX: 919-743-0208
e-mail: dcoffey@autismsociety-nc.org
www.autismsociety-nc.org

Darla Coffey, Bookstore Manager
Jill Keel, Executive Director
Various chapters written by professionals working with autistic children and adults. *$150.00*

7437 Difficult Child
Bantam Books
1540 Broadway
New York, NY 10036
212-782-9000
FAX: 212-302-7985
www.randomhouse.com

The classic and definitive work on parenting hard-to-raise children with new sections on ADHD and the latest medications for childhood disorders. *$15.95*
302 pages Paperback 2000
ISBN 0-553380-36-2

7438 Disability Culture Perspective on Early Intervention
Through the Looking Glass
2198 6th Street
Suite 100
Berkeley, CA 94710
510-848-1112
800-644-2666
FAX: 510-848-4445
e-mail: TLG@lookingglass.org
www.lookingglass.org

Megan Kirshbaum
For parents with physical or cognitive disabilities and their families. Available in braille, large print or cassette. *$2.00*
12 pages

7439 Down Syndrome
Aquarius Health Care Videos
PO Box 1159
Sherborn, MA 01770
508-650-6905
FAX: 508-650-4216
e-mail: aqvideos@tiac.net
www.aquariusproductions.com

This is an excellent video for families who have just had a baby with Down Syndrome as well as professionals in the field of genetics and nursing. Through honest and open discussion, parents of children with Down Syndrome express the feelings and concerns they had during the early years of their child's life. Preview option available. *$150.00*
Video

7440 Driven to Distraction
National Alliance for the Mentally Ill
2107 Wilson Boulevard
Suite 300
Arlington, VA 22201
703-524-7600
800-950-6264

Suzanne Vogel-Scibilia, President
A practical book discussing adult as well as child attention deficit disorder (ADD). Non-technical, realistic and optimistic, it is an informative how-to manual for parents and consumers. *$23.00*

7441 Dyslexia over the Lifespan
Educators Publishing Service
PO Box 9031
Cambridge, MA 02139
617-367-2700
800-225-5750
FAX: 617-547-0412
www.epsbooks.com

Discusses the educational and career development of 56 dyslexic boys from a private school that was one of the first to have a program to detect and treat developmental language disabilities. *$ 18.00*
224 pages
ISBN 0-838816-70-3

7442 Educating Inattentive Children
Western Psychological Services
12031 Wilshire Boulevard
Los Angeles, CA 90025
310-478-2061
800-648-8857
FAX: 310-478-7838

Gregg Gillmar, Vice President
An excellent resources for teachers who encounter inattention and hyperactivity in the classroom. It helps teachers distinguish deliberate misbehavior from the incompetent, nonpurposeful behavior of the inattentive child. *$120.00*

Video

7443 **Embracing the Monster: Overcoming the Cha llenges of Hidden Disabilities**
Paul H Brookes Publishing Company
PO Box 10624
Baltimore, MD 21285
410-337-9580
800-638-3775
FAX: 410-337-8539
e-mail: custserv@brokespublishing.com
www.brookespublishing.com

Paul Brooks, Owner
The author shares her experience of living with LD, ADHD and bipolar disorder to give readers an awareness of the challenges of living with hidden disabilities and what can be done to help
$21.95
192 pages 2002
ISBN 1-557665-22-2

7444 **Encounters with Autistic States**
Jason Aronson
400 Keystone Industrial Park
Dunmore, PA 18512
800-782-0015
FAX: 201-840-7242
www.aronson.com

$50.00
Hardcover
ISBN 0-765700-62-

7445 **Enhancing Communication in Individuals with Autism Through Pictures/Words**
Autism Society of North Carolina Bookstore
505 Oberlin Road
Suite 230
Raleigh, NC 27605
919-743-0204
800-442-2762
FAX: 919-743-0208
e-mail: dcoffey@autismsociety-nc.org
www.autismsociety-nc.org

Darla Coffey, Bookstore Manager
Jill Keel, Executive Director
Booklet addressing the description and implementation of visually aided communication. *$4.00*

7446 **Equal Treatment for People With Mental Ret ardation: Having and Raising Children**
Harvard University Press

A Harvard law professor and civil liberties practitioner provide a comprehensive examination of the reproductive and parental rights of mentally retarded citizens. *$19.95*
464 pages Paperback 2001
ISBN 0-674006-97-6

7447 **Fact Sheet: Attention Deficit-Hyperactivit y Disorder**
Learning Disabilities Association of America
4156 Library Road
Pittsburgh, PA 15234
412-341-1515
FAX: 412-344-0224
e-mail: info@ldaamerica.org
www.ldaamerica.org
A pamphlet offering factual information on ADHD.

7448 **Fact Sheet: Autism Spectrum Disorders**
Autism Society of America
7910 Woodmont Avenue
Suite 300
Bethesda, MD 20814
301-657-0881
800-3AU-TISM
FAX: 301-657-0869
e-mail: info@autism-society.org
www.autism-society.org

Ann Pulley, Manager
Offers information on autism spectrum disorders. What it is, symptoms, causes, diagnosis, treatments and research. Also provides Autism Source, a free online referral database of autism services and support at www.autismsource.org.

7449 **Family Therapy for ADHD: Treating Children , Adolescents and Adults**
Guilford Press
72 Spring Street
New York, NY 10012
212-431-9800
800-365-7006
FAX: 212-966-6708
www.guilford.com

Bob Matloff, President
$40.00
Cloth
ISBN 1-572304-38-3

7450 **Farmington Valley ARC**
10 Tower Lane
Avon, CT 06001
860-693-6662
FAX: 860-693-8662

Lynn Flerri, President
Tom Thompson, Executive Director
The official newsletter containing information, new ideas, progress and more on the Farmington Valley Association for Retarded and Handicapped Citizens.

7451 **Fighting for Darla: Challenges for Family Care & Professional Responsibility**
Baker & Taylor, International
1200 Us Highway 22
Bridgewater, NJ 08807
908-541-7000
FAX: 908-541-7862
e-mail: intsale@bakertaylor.com

D Sopko, Manager
Follows the story of Darla, a pregnant adolescent with autism.
$18.95
176 pages
ISBN 0-807733-56-3

7452 **Fragile Success: Nine Autistic Children, Childhood to Adulthood**
Autism Society of North Carolina Bookstore
505 Oberlin Road
Suite 230
Raleigh, NC 27605
919-743-0204
800-442-2762
FAX: 919-743-0208
e-mail: dcoffey@autismsociety-nc.org
www.autismsociety-nc.org

Darla Coffey, Bookstore Manager
Jill Keel, Executive Director
A book about the lives of autistic children, whom the author has followed from their early years at the Elizabeth Ives School in New Haven, CT, through to adulthood. *$27.50*

7453 **Getting Our Heads Together**
Thoms Rehabilitation Hospital
68 Sweeten Creek Road
Asheville, NC 28803
828-274-2400
FAX: 828-274-9452

Kathi Petersen, Director Planning/Communication
Edgardo Diez MD, Medical Director Brain Injury
Kathy Price, Director Admissions
A handbook for families of head injured patients - available in Spanish as well as English. *$4.00*
40 pages Paperback

7454 **Getting Started with Facilitated Communication**
Syracuse University, Institute on Communication
805 S Krouse
Syracuse, NY 13244
315-443-4485

Raymond Colton, Manager
Describes in detail how to help individuals with autism and/or severe communication difficulties to get started with facilitated communication.

Video

7455 Getting Together: A Head Start/School District Collaboration
Brookes Publishing
PO Box 10624
Baltimore, MD 21285
410-337-9580
800-638-3775
FAX: 410-337-8539
e-mail: custserv@brookespublishing.com
www.brookespublishing.com

Paul Brooks, Owner
This video describes how to include children with disabilities in the Head Start classrooms. Addresses such issues as leadership, staff support, and policy development. Comes with a 24-page saddle-stitched booklet. *$34.95*
25 Minutes
ISBN 1-55766 -97-5

7456 Getting a Grip on ADD: A Kid's Guide to Understanding & Coping with ADD
Educational Media Corporation
PO Box 21311
Minneapolis, MN 55421
763-781-0088
800-966-3382
FAX: 763-781-7753
educationalmedia.com

Earl Sorenson, President/Owner
Free catalog of resources.
64 pages Yearly

7457 Guide to Successful Employment for Individuals with Autism
Brookes Publishing
PO Box 10624
Baltimore, MD 21285
410-337-9585
800-638-3775
FAX: 410-337-8539
e-mail: custserv@brookespublishing.com
www.brookespublishing.com

Melissa Behm, President
Describing all aspects of job placement, this book details strategies for assessing workers, networking for job opportunities, and tailoring job supports to each individual. Also illustrates how to help individuals with autism become productive workers, and with detailed descriptions of specific jobs help provide ideas for employment. *$ 32.95*
336 pages Paperback
ISBN 1-55766 -71-5

7458 Handbook of Autism and Pervasive Developmental Disorders
Autism Society of North Carolina Bookstore
505 Oberlin Road
Suite 230
Raleigh, NC 27605
919-743-0204
800-442-2762
FAX: 919-743-0208
e-mail: dcoffey@autismsociety-nc.org
www.autismsociety-nc.org

Darla Coffey, Bookstore Manager
Jill Keel, Executive Director
A list of contributors address such topics as characteristics of autistic syndromes and interventions. *$125.00*

7459 Helping People with Autism Manage Their Behavior
Autism Society of North Carolina Bookstore
505 Oberlin Road
Suite 230
Raleigh, NC 27605
919-743-0204
800-442-2762
FAX: 919-743-0208
e-mail: dcoffey@autismsociety-nc.org
www.autismsociety-nc.org

Darla Coffey, Bookstore Manager
Jill Keel, Executive Director
Covers the broad topic of helping people with autism manage their behavior. *$7.00*

7460 Helping Your Child with Attention-Deficit Hyperactivity Disorder
Learning Disabilities Association of America
4156 Library Road
Pittsburgh, PA 15234
412-341-1515
FAX: 412-344-0224
e-mail: info@ldaamerica.org
www.ldaamerica.org

7461 Helping Your Hyperactive: Attention Deficit Child
Prima Publishing
PO Box 1260
Rocklin, CA 95677
916-787-7000
800-632-8676
FAX: 916-787-7001
e-mail: websupportlife@primapub.com
www.primapublishing.com

$19.95

ISBN 1-559584-23-8

7462 Hidden Child: The Linwood Method for Reaching the Autistic Child
Woodbine House
6510 Bells Mill Road
Bethesda, MD 20817
301-897-3570
800-843-7323
FAX: 301-897-5838
www.woodbinehouse.com

Irv Shapell, Owner
Chronicle of the Linwood Children's Center's successful treatment program for autistic children. *$17.95*
286 pages Paperback
ISBN 0-933149-06-9

7463 How To Reach and Teach Children and Teens with Dyslexia
Jossey-Bass

This practical resource gives educators at all levels essential information, techniques, and tolls for understanding dyslexia and adapting teaching methods in all subject areas to meet the learning style, social, and emotional needs of students who have dyslexia. *$ 22.95*
340 pages 2002
ISBN 0-130320-18-8

7464 How to Own and Operate an Attention Deficit Disorder
Learning Disabilities Association of America
4156 Library Road
Pittsburgh, PA 15234
412-341-1515
FAX: 412-344-0224
e-mail: info@ldaamerica.org
www.ldaamerica.org
Clear, informative and sensitive introduction to ADHD. Packed with practical things to do at home and school, from a professional and mother of a son with ADHD. *$8.95*
43 pages

7465 Hyperactive Child, Adolescent, and Adult: ADD Through the Lifespan
CACLD
25 Van Zant Street
Suite 15-5
Norwalk, CT 06855
203-838-5010
FAX: 203-866-6108
e-mail: CACLD@optonline.net
www.CACLD.org

Beryl Kaufman, Executive Director
Comprehensive general review. Update on previous research by the author, offering a basic text. Published by Ccnnecticut Association for Children & Adults with Learning Disabilities (CACLD). *$8.75*

162 pages

7466 Hyperactivity, Attention Deficits, and School Failure: Better Ways
Learning Disabilities Association of America
4156 Library Road
Pittsburgh, PA 15234
412-341-1515
FAX: 412-344-0224
e-mail: info@ldaamerica.org
www.ldaamerica.org

7467 I Want My Little Boy Back
A Britsh Broadcasting Corporation Documentary
2080 S Undermountain Road
Sheffield, MA 01257
413-229-2100
800-714-2779
FAX: 413-229-8931
e-mail: happiness@option.org
www.option.org

A great video for parents and professionals caring for children with special needs. Join one British family and their autistic son before, during and after their journey to America to attend The Son-Rise Program at The Autism Treatment Center of America. This informative, inspirational and deeply moving story not only captures the joy, tears, challenges and triumps of this amazing little boy and his family, but also serves as a powerful introduction to the attitude and principles of the program. *$25.00*

7468 Imagine!
Imagine!
1400 Dixon Avenue
Lafayette, CO 80026
303-665-7789
FAX: 303-665-2648
e-mail: gstebick@imaginecolorado.org
www.imaginecolorado.org

Gary Stebick, Communication Coordinator
Fred Hobbs, Director Marketing
For people of all ages with cognitive, developmental, physical & health related needs, so they may live lives of independence & quality in their homes and communities.
12-16 pages quarterly

7469 In Search of Wings: A Journey Back from T raumatic Brain Injury
Wings Press

The true story of one woman coping with traumatic brain injury after a car accident that affected her cognitive skills and memory *$14.95*
233 pages 1992
ISBN 1-882332-00-8

7470 In Their Own Way
Alliance for Parental Involvement in Education
PO Box 59
East Chatham, NY 12060
518-392-6900
FAX: 518-392-6900

For the parents whose children are not thriving in school, Armstrong offers insight into individual learning styles. *$11.95*

7471 Increasing Behaviors of Persons with Severe Retardation and Autism
Research Press
2612 N Mattis Avenue
Champaign, IL 61822
217-352-3273
800-519-2707
FAX: 217-352-1221
e-mail: rp@researchpress.com
www.researchpress.com

Russell Pence, President
Shows how to increase desirable behaviors by using techniques such as shaping, prompting, fading, modeling, backward chaining, and graduated guidance. Includes exercises, review questions, and numerous examples. *$15.95*

230 pages Paperback
ISBN 0-878222-63-4

7472 It's Just Attention Disorder
Western Psychological Services
12031 Wilshire Boulevard
Los Angeles, CA 90025
310-478-2061
800-648-8857
FAX: 310-478-7838

Gregg Gillmar, Vice President
This ground-breaking videotape takes the critical first steps in treating attention-deficit disorder: it enlists the inattentive or hyperactive child as an active participant in his or her treatment. *$99.50*
Video

7473 Journal of Cognitive Rehabilitation
Neuroscience Publishers
6555 Carrollton Avenue
Indianapolis, IN 46220
317-257-9672
FAX: 317-257-9674
e-mail: nsc@netdirect.net
www.jofcr.com

Odie L Bracy III PhD, Editor/Executive Director
Andrea Oakes, Production Manager
Nancy Bracy, Managing Editor & Subscriptions
Publication for therapists, family and patient, designed to provide information relevant to the rehabilitation of impairment resulting from brain injury. *$50.00*
36-48 pages Quarterly

7474 Jumpin' Johnny Get Back to Work, A Child's Guide to ADHD/Hyperactivity
25 Van Zant Street
Suite 15-5
Norwalk, CT 06855
203-838-5010
FAX: 203-866-6108
e-mail: CACLD@optonline.net
www.CACLD.org

Beryl Kaufman, Executive Director
Written primarily for elementary age youngsters with ADHD to help them understand their disability. Also valuable as an educational tool for parents, siblings, friends and classmates. Includes two pages on medication. *$12.50*
24 pages

7475 Keys to Parenting a Child with Attention Deficit Disorder
Barron's Educational Series
250 Wireless Boulevard
Hauppauge, NY 11788
631-434-3311
800-645-3476
FAX: 631-434-3723
e-mail: info@barronseduc.com
www.barronseduc.com
Lonny Stein , Director Marketing
Manuel Barron, Chief Executive Officer
This book shows how to work with the child's school, effectively manage the child's behavior and act as the child's advocate. *$6.95*
160 pages Paperback
ISBN 0-812014-59-6

7476 Keys to Parenting a Child with Downs Syndrome
Barron's Educational Series
250 Wireless Boulevard
Hauppauge, NY 11788
631-434-3311
800-645-3476
FAX: 631-434-3723
e-mail: info@barronsedu.com
www.barronseduc.com

Lonny Stein, Director Marketing
Manuel Barron, Chief Executive Officer
Down Syndrome poses many challenges for children and their families. This book prepares parents and guardians to raise a child with Down Syndrome by discussing adjustment, advocacy, health and behavior, education and planning for greater independence. *$5.95*

160 pages Paperback
ISBN 0-812014-58-8

7477 Keys to Parenting the Child with Autism
Barron's Educational Series
250 Wireless Boulevard
Hauppauge, NY 11788
631-434-3311
800-645-3476
FAX: 631-434-3723
e-mail: barrons@barronseduc.com
www.barronseduc.com

Manuel Barron, Chief Executive Officer
Parents of children with autism will find a solid balance between home and practical information in this book. It explains what autism is and how it is diagnosed, then advises parents on how to adjust to their child and give the best care. *$6.95*
208 pages Paperback
ISBN 0-812016-79-3

7478 LD Child and the ADHD Child: Ways Parents & Professionals Can Help
1406 Plaza Drive
Winston Salem, NC 27103
336-768-1374
800-222-9796
FAX: 336-768-9194
e-mail: southern@blairpub.com
www.blairpub.com

Carolyn Sakowski, President
John F Blair, Publisher
Book about learning disabilities available to parents. Stevens cuts through the jargon and complex theories which usually characterize books on the subject to present effective and practical techniques that parents can employ to help their child succeed at home and at school. New edition adds information about ADHD children. *$12.95*
201 pages Paperback
ISBN 0-895871-42-4

7479 Labeling the Mentally Retarded
University of California Press
2120 Berkeley Way
Berkeley, CA 94720
510-642-4247
FAX: 510-643-7127
www.ucpress.edu

Lynne Whity, Executive Director
Clinical and social system perspectives on mental retardation. *$12.95*
333 pages Paper

7480 Learning a Living: A Guide to Planning Yo ur Career and Finding a Job for People with ADD
Woodbine House
6510 Bells Mill Road
Bethesda, MD 20817
301-897-3570
800-843-7323
FAX: 301-897-5838
e-mail: info@woodbinehouse.com
www.woodbinehouse.com

Irv Shapell, Owner
Focuses on helping people with learning disabilities, dyslexia, and ADD. The author has worked with thousands of people with these disabilities and shares her personal experiences. Provides a wide array of vital information, tips, insights, and advice for anyone seeking to overcome learning disabilities and pursue a successful career. *$ 18.95*
340 pages 2000
ISBN 0-933149-87-5

7481 Let Community Employment be the Goal for Individuals with Autism
Autism Society of North Carolina Bookstore
505 Oberlin Road
Suite 230
Raleigh, NC 27605
919-743-0204
800-442-2762
FAX: 919-743-0208
e-mail: dcoffey@autismsociety-nc.org
www.autismsociety-nc.org

Darla Coffey, Bookstore Manager
Jill Keel, Executive Director
A guide designed for people who are responsible for preparing individuals with autism to enter the work force. *$7.00*

7482 Making the Writing Process Work
Brookline Books
PO Box 1047
Cambridge, MA 02139
617-868-0360
800-666-2665
FAX: 617-868-1772
e-mail: thestore@brooklinebooks.com
www.brooklinebooks.com
Making the Writing Process Work: Strategies for Composition and Self-Regulation is geared toward students who have difficulty organizing their thoughts and developing their writing. The specific strategies teach students how to approach, organize, and produce a final written product. *$24.95*
240 pages Paperback
ISBN 1-57129 -10-9

7483 Management of Autistic Behavior
Pro-Ed Publications
8700 Shoal Creek Boulevard
Austin, TX 78757
512-451-3246
800-897-3202
FAX: 800-397-7633
e-mail: feedback@proedinc.com
www.proedinc.com

Donald Hammill, Owner
Courtney King, Marketing Coordinator
This excellent reference is a comprehensive and practical book that tells what works best with specific problems. *$41.00*
450 pages

7484 Management of Children and Adolescents with AD-HD
Learning Disabilities Association of America
4156 Library Road
Pittsburgh, PA 15234
412-341-1515
FAX: 412-344-0224
e-mail: info@ldaamerica.org
www.ldaamerica.org

7485 Managing Attention Disorders in Children: A Guide for Practitioners
Books on Special Children
PO Box 305
Congers, NY 10920
845-638-1236
FAX: 845-638-0847
e-mail: irene@boscbooks.com
Offers information about human personality, structure and dynamics, assessment and adjustment. *$27.50*
214 pages

7486 Mental Retardation
McGraw-Hill, School Publishing
220 E Danieldale Road
Desoto, TX 75115
972-224-1111
800-442-9685
FAX: 972-228-1982
mhschool.com

Joseph Gavigan, President
Combines significant findings from the most current research, focusing on a unique relationship between the special educator and the learner with mental retardation.
656 pages Casebound

7487 Mental Retardation: A Life-Cycle Approach
McGraw-Hill, School Publishing
220 E Danieldale Road
Desoto, TX 75115
972-224-1111
800-442-9685
FAX: 972-228-1982
mhschool.com

Joseph Gavigan, President
This text considers the needs of the retarded individual at every stage of life.

512 pages

7488 **Mentally Retarded Individuals**
Mainstream
3 Bethesda Metro Center
Suite 830
Bethesda, MD 20814
301-961-9299
800-247-1380
FAX: 301-654-6714
e-mail: info@mainstreaminc.org

Charles Moster
Mainstreaming mentally retarded individuals into the workplace. *$2.50*
12 pages

7489 **NADS News**
PO Box 4542
Oak Brook, IL 60522
630-325-9112
FAX: 630-325-8842
www.nads.org

Kim Xidas, Family Support Coordinator
A bi-monthly publication from the National Association for Down Syndrome. Subscription prices: $20 for parents; $25 for professionals.
12 pages Bi-monthly

7490 **Neurobiology of Autism**
Johns Hopkins University Press
2715 N Charles Street
Baltimore, MD 21218
410-516-6900
FAX: 410-516-6998

William Brody, President
This book discusses recent advances in scientific research that point to a neurobiological basis for autism and examines the clinical implications of this research. *$28.00*
272 pages
ISBN 0-801856-80-9

7491 **New York Families for Autistic Children**
9516 Pitkin Avenue
Ozone Park, NY 11417
718-641-3441
FAX: 718-641-4452
e-mail: help@nyfac.org
www.nyfac.org

Andrew Baumann, Chief Executive Officer
Education, recreation and support services for families and children with developmental disabilities.

7492 **Out of Darkness**
CACLD
25 Van Zant Street
Suite 15-5
Norwalk, CT 06855
203-838-5010
FAX: 203-866-6108
e-mail: CACLD@optonline.net
www.CACLD.org

Beryl Kaufman, Executive Director
Article by an adult who discovers at age 30 that he has ADD. *$1.00*
4 pages

7493 **Out of the Fog: Treatment Options and Cop ing Strategies for ADD**
Hyperion

Discusses the recent recognition of attention deficit disorder as a problem that is not outgrown in adolescence, and cogently summarizes the stumbling blocks this affliction creates in the pursuit of a career or attainment of a healthy family life *$14.95*
300 pages 1995
ISBN 0-786880-87-2

7494 **Out-Of-Sync Child: Recognizing and Coping With Sensory Integration Dysfunction**
Perigee Books

This guide explains how SI Dysfunction can be confused with ADD, learning disabilities, and other problems, tells how parents can recognize the problem and offers a drug-free treatment approach for children who need help. *$14.95*
322 pages 1998
ISBN 0-399523-86-3

7495 **Overcoming Dyslexia**
Vintage

Yale neuroscientist Shaywitz demystifies the roots of dyslexia (a neurologically based reading difficulty affecting one in five children) and offers parents and educators hope that children with reading problems can be helped. *$15.00*
432 pages 1905
ISBN 0-679781-59-5

7496 **Parent Survival Manual**
Exceptional Parent Library
PO Box 1807
Englewood Cliffs, NJ 07632
201-947-6000
800-535-1910
FAX: 201-947-9376
e-mail: eplibrary@aol.com
www.eplibrary.com
A guide to crises resolution in autism and related developmental disorders. *$39.95*

7497 **Parent's Guide to Autism**
Autism Society of North Carolina Bookstore
505 Oberlin Road
Suite 230
Raleigh, NC 27605
919-743-0204
800-442-2762
FAX: 919-743-0208
e-mail: dcoffey@autismsociety-nc.org
www.autismsociety-nc.org

Darla Coffey, Bookstore Manager
Jill Keel, Executive Director
An essential handbook for anyone facing autism. *$14.00*

7498 **Parent's Guide to Down Syndrome: Toward a Brighter Future**
Brookes Publishing
PO Box 10624
Baltimore, MD 21285
410-337-9580
800-638-3775
FAX: 410-337-8539
e-mail: custserv@brookespublishing.com
www.brookespublishing.com

Paul Brooks, Owner
Highlights developmental stages and shows the advances that improve a child's quality of life. Includes discussions on easing the transition from home to school and choosing integration and curricular priorities, as well as guidelines for confronting adolescent and adult issues such as social and sexual needs and independent living and vocational options. *$21.95*
352 pages 2000
ISBN 1-557664-52-8

7499 **Parenting Attention Deficit Disordered Teens**
CACLD
25 Van Zant Street
Suite 15-5
Norwalk, CT 06855
203-838-5010
FAX: 203-866-6108
e-mail: CACLD@optonline.net
www.CACLD.org

Beryl Kaufman, Executive Director
Detailed outline of the various problems of adolescents with ADHD. Published by Connecticut Association for Children & Adults with Learning Disabilities (CACLD). *$3.25*
14 pages

7500 **Parents Helping Parents: A Directory of Support Groups for ADD**
Novartis Pharmaceuticals Division
59 State Route 10
East Hanover, NJ 07936
862-778-7500
800-742-2422

Paulo Costa, Chief Executive Officer

7501 Please Don't Say Hello
Human Sciences Press
233 Spring Street
New York, NY 10013
212-229-2859
800-221-9369
FAX: 212-463-0742

Paul and his family moved into a new neighborhood. Paul's brother was autistic. The children thought that Eddie was retarded until they learned that there were skills that he could do better than they could. *$10.95*
47 pages Paperback
ISBN 0-89885 -99-8

7502 Preventable Brain Damage
Springer Publishing Company
536 Broadway
New York, NY 10012
212-431-4370
877-687-7476
FAX: 212-941-7842
e-mail: marketing@springerpub.com
www.springerpub.com

Annette Imperati, Marketing/Sales Director
Ursula Springer, President
Offers information on brain injuries from motor vehicle accidents, contact sports and injuries of children. *$35.95*
256 pages

7503 Pure Facts
Feingold Association of the US
554 E Main Street
Suite 301
Riverhead, NY 11901
631-369-9340
800-321-3287
FAX: 631-369-2988
e-mail: help@feingold.org
www.feingold.org

Jane Hersey, Editor
Debbie Lehner, Manager
Relationship between foods, food additives and behavior/learning problems, including Attention Deficit Disorder (ADD) and hyperactivity. *$38.00*
10+ pages Monthly

7504 Reading, Writing and Speech Problems in Children
International Dyslexia Association
382 S Chester Street
Baltimore, MD 21231
800-ABC-D123
FAX: 410-296-0232
www.interdys.org
A tribute to the man who more than any other aroused the attention of the scientific community and who provided the sound educational principles on which much teaching of dyslexics today is based. *$27.00*

ISBN 0-89079 -79-1

7505 Reality of Dyslexia
Brookline Books
PO Box 1047
Cambridge, MA 02139
617-868-0360
800-666-2665
FAX: 617-868-1772
e-mail: thestore@brooklinebooks.com
www.brooklinebooks.com
An informative and sensitive study of living with dyslexia which affects one in 25. He introduces the reader to the subject by sharing the difficulties of his dyslexic son. He then uses the personal accounts of other children and adult dyslexics, even entire dyslexic families, to illuminate the problems they encounter. *$14.95*
150 pages Paperback
ISBN 1-57129 -17-6

7506 Record Book for Individuals with Autism
Autism Society of North Carolina Bookstore
505 Oberlin Road
Suite 230
Raleigh, NC 27605
919-743-0204
800-442-2762
FAX: 919-743-0208
e-mail: dcoffey@autismsociety-nc.org
www.autismsociety-nc.org

Darla Coffey, Bookstore Manager
Jill Keel, Executive Director
Developed with parent input to provide one place to keep information about an autistic child. *$7.00*

7507 Relationship Development Intervention with Young Children
Taylor & Francis Group

Social and emotional development activities for Asperger Syndrome, Autism, PDD and NLD. Comprehensive set of activities emphasizes foundation skills for younger children between the ages of two and eight. Covers skills such as social referencing, regulating behvior, conversational reciprocity, and synchronized actions. For use in therapeutic settings as well as schools and parents. *$22.95*
256 pages 2002
ISBN 1-843107-14-7

7508 Retarded Isn't Stupid, Mom!
Brookes Publishing
PO Box 10624
Baltimore, MD 21285
410-337-9580
800-638-3775
FAX: 410-337-8539
e-mail: custserv@brookespublishing.com
www.pbrookescom/store/books/kaufman-3785

Paul Brooks, Owner
Sandra Kaufman reveals the feelings of denial, guilt, frustration and eventual acceptance that resulted in a determination to help her daughter, Nicole, live an independent life. This edition, revised on the 10th anniversary of the book's original publication, adds a progress report that updates readers on Nicole's adult years and reflects on the revolutionary changes in society's attitudes toward people with disabilities since Nicole's birth. *$22.95*
272 pages Paperback 1999
ISBN 1-557663-78-5

7509 Rethinking Attention Deficit Disorder
Brookline Books
PO Box 1047
Cambridge, MA 02139
617-868-0360
800-666-2665
FAX: 617-868-1772
e-mail: thestore@brooklinebooks.com
www.brooklinebooks.com
In contrast to the common focus on behavioral symptoms of attention disorders, this book emphasizes internal factors that make attention regulation difficult. In-depth discussions of social, emotional, and academic consequences and appropriate interventions are provided. *$27.95*
250 pages Paperback
ISBN 1-57129 -37-0

7510 Riddle of Autism: A Psychological Analysis
Jason Aronson
400 Keystone Industrial Park
Dunmore, PA 18512
800-782-0015
FAX: 201-840-7242
www.aronson.com
Dr. Victor examines the myths that cloud an understanding of this disorder and describes the meanings of its specific behavioral symptoms. *$30.00*

356 pages Softcover
ISBN 1-568215-73-8

7511 School Based Assessment of Attention Deficit Disorders
National Clearinghouse of Rehabilitation Materials
5202 N Richmond Hill Drive
Stillwater, OK 74078
405-624-7650
800-223-5219
FAX: 405-624-0695
Presents an overview of current thoughts concerning ADD from an educational perspective, contrast traditional assessment strategies with an alternative model, and describe phases of evaluation.Paperback *$6.10*
61 pages

7512 Schools for Children with Autism Spectrum Disorders
Resources for Children with Special Needs
116 E 16th Street
Floor 5
New York, NY 10003
212-677-4650
FAX: 212-254-4070
e-mail: info@resourcesnyc.org
www.resourcesnyc.org

Karen Schlesinger, Executive Director
Dianne Littwin, Director Publications
Published every 24-36 months. *$20.00*
160 pages
ISBN 0-967836-53-0

7513 Serving Adults with Cognitive Disabilities
Independent Living Research Utilization ILRU
2323 S Shepherd Drive
Suite 1000
Houston, TX 77019
713-520-0232
FAX: 713-520-5785
www.ilru.org

Laurie Redd, Executive Director
Darrel, Tyrone and Susan of Arizona Bridge to Independent Living (ABIL) describe the success of their Community Living Options Program for adults with developmental disabilities in this months readings.
10 pages

7514 Sex Education: Issues for the Person with Autism
Autism Society of North Carolina Bookstore
505 Oberlin Road
Suite 230
Raleigh, NC 27605
919-743-0204
800-442-2762
FAX: 919-743-0208
e-mail: dcoffey@autismsociety-nc.org
www.autismsociety-nc.org

Darla Coffey, Bookstore Manager
Jill Keel, Executive Director
Discusses issues of sexuality and provides methods of instruction for people with autism. *$4.00*

7515 Shoebox Tasks: Work Activities
Autism Society of North Carolina Bookstore
505 Oberlin Road
Suite 230
Raleigh, NC 27605
919-743-0204
800-442-2762
FAX: 919-743-0208
e-mail: dcoffey@autismsociety-nc.org
www.autismsociety-nc.org

Darla Coffey, Bookstore Manager
Jill Keel, Executive Director
$250.00

7516 Son-Rise: The Miracle Continues
2080 S Undermountain Road
Sheffield, MA 01257
413-229-2100
800-562-7171
FAX: 413-229-3202
e-mail: sonrise@option.org
www.son-rise.org

Part One is the astonishing record of Raun Kaufman's development from an autistic and retarded child into a loving, brilliant youngster who shows no traces of his former condition. Part Two follows Raun's development after the age of four, teaching the limitless possibilities of the Son-Rise Program. Part Three shares moving accounts of five other ordinary families who became extraordinary when they used the Son-Rise Program to reach their own unreachable children. *$12.95*
343 pages
ISBN 0-915811-53-7

7517 Soon Will Come the Light
Autism Society of North Carolina Bookstore
505 Oberlin Road
Suite 230
Raleigh, NC 27605
919-743-0204
800-442-2762
FAX: 919-743-0208
e-mail: dcoffey@autismsociety-nc.org
www.autismsociety-nc.org

Darla Coffey, Bookstore Manager
Jill Keel, Executive Director
Offers new perspectives on the perplexing disability of autism. *$19.95*

7518 Spectrum
Autism Society of North Carolina
505 Oberlin Road
Suite 230
Raleigh, NC 27605
919-743-0204
800-442-2762
FAX: 919-743-0208
e-mail: dcoffey@autismsociety-nc.org
www.autismsociety-nc.org

David Laxton, Editor
Jill Keel, Executive Director
Quarterly publication from the Autism Society of North Carolina. *$30.00*
Quarterly

7519 Successful Job Search Strategies for the D sabled: Understanding the ADA
Wiley Publishing
605 3rd Avenue
New York, NY 10158
212-850-6000
FAX: 212-850-6088
Following a concise overview of the Americans with Disabilities Act (ADA), covers such topics as job identification, self-assessment, job leads, resumes, disability disclosure, interviewing, and accommodating specific disabilities. Includes dozen of relevant and instructive situation analyses, case examples, and answers to commonly asked questions. *$165.00*
229 pages 1994

7520 Taking Charge of ADHD Complete Authoritative Guide for Parents
Guilford Press
72 Spring Street
New York, NY 10012
212-431-9800
800-365-7006
FAX: 212-966-6708
www.guilford.com

Bob Matloff, President
Revised and updated to incorporate the most current information on ADHD and its treatment. Provides parents with the knowledge, guidance and confidence they need to ensure that their child receives the best care possible. Also in cloth at $40.00 (ISBN# 1-57230-600-9 *$18.95*
321 pages Paperback 2000
ISBN 1-572305-60-6

7521 Teach and Reach Students with Attention Deficit Disorders
MultiGrowth Resources
12345 Jones Road
Suite 101
Houston, TX 77070
281-890-5334
FAX: 281-894-8611

Nancy Eisenberg, Owner
Handbook and resource guide for parents and educators of ADD students. *$19.95*

200 pages
ISBN 0-963084-70-4

7522 Teaching Children with Autism: Strategies for Initiating Positive Interactions

Brookes Publishing
PO Box 10624
Baltimore, MD 21285
410-337-9580
800-638-3775
FAX: 410-337-8539
e-mail: custserv@brookespublishing.com
www.brookespublishing.com

Clary Creighton, Exhibits Coordinator
Tracy Gray, Educational Sales Manager
Paul Brooks, Owner

Stategies for initiating positive interactions and improving learning opportunities. This guide begins with an overview of characteristics and long-term strategies and proceeds through discussions that detail specific techniques for normalizing environments, reducing disruptive behavior, improving language and social skills, and enhancing generalization. *$32.95*

256 pages Paperback
ISBN 1-55766 -80-4

7523 Teaching and Mainstreaming Autistic Children

Love Publishing Company
9101 East Kenyon Avenue
Suite 2200
Denver, CO 80237
303-221-7333
FAX: 303-221-7444
e-mail: lpc@lovepublishing.com
www.lovepublishing.com

Stan Love, Owner

Dr. Knoblock advocates a highly organized, structured environment for autistic children, with teachers and parents working together. His premise is that the learning and social needs of autistic children must be analyzed and a daily program designed with interventions that respond to this functional analysis of their behavior. *$24.95*

ISBN 0-89108 -11-9

7524 Techniques for Aphasia Rehab: (TARGET) Generating Effective Treatment

Speech Bin
1965 25th Avenue
Vero Beach, FL 32960
772-770-0007
800-477-3324
FAX: 772-770-0006
www.speechbin.com

Practical treatment manual for use by aphasia clinicians. *$45.00*

384 pages
ISBN 0-93785 -50-5

7525 Teenagers with ADD

Woodbine House
6510 Bells Mill Road
Bethesda, MD 20817
301-897-3570
800-843-7323
FAX: 301-897-5838
www.woodbinehouse.com

Irv Shapell, Owner

This best selling guide to understanding and coping with teenagers with attention deficit disorder (ADD) provides complete coverage of the special issues and challenges faced by these teens. Based on current diagnostic criteria and the latest literature and research in the field, the book discusses diagnosis, medical treatment, family and school life, intervention, advocacy, legal rights, and options after high school. Parents find strategies for dealing with their teen's difficult behaviors. *$18.95*

370 pages Paperback
ISBN 0-933149-69-7

7526 Traumatic Brain Injury: Cognitive & Communication Disorders

Federal Government
31 Center Drive Msc2320
Bethesda, MD 20892
800-241-1044
FAX: 301-402-0018
e-mail: nidcdinfo@nidcd.nih.gov
www.nidcd.nih.org

Explains what is traumatic brain injury, who suffer from head trauma, what are the cognitive and communication problems that result from traumatic brain injury, how cognitive and communication probles assessed and how they are treated, and what research is being done for the cognitive and communication prblems caused by traumatic brain injury.

7527 Traumatic Brain Injury: Mechanisms of Damage, Assessment & Intervention

Pro-Ed Publications
8700 Shoal Creek Boulevard
Austin, TX 78757
512-451-3246
800-897-3202
FAX: 800-397-7633
e-mail: feedback@proedinc.com
www.proedinc.com

Donald Hammill, Owner
Courtney King, Marketing Coordinator

Traumatic Brain Injury ranks as one of the most prevalent disorders with estimates ranging in hundreds of thousands of new cases each year. This book focuses on the mechanisms of acquired brain injury and the methods of assessment, along with treatment and outcome variables. *$41.00*

458 pages Hardcover

7528 Understanding ADHD

Aquarius Health Care Videos
PO Box 1159
Sherborn, MA 01770
508-650-6905
FAX: 508-650-4216
e-mail: aqvideos@tiac.net
www.aquariusproductions.com

A look at some of the controversies surrounding Attention Deficit Hyperactivity Disorder. This video shows how the disorder is diagnosed and presents strategies for living with a child with the disorder. Diverse and candid opinions from teachers, social workers, a behavior specialist, a pediatrician and a parent with ADHD twins. Recommended for child development students, social workers, and caregivers. Preview option available. *$120.00*

Video

7529 Understanding Attention Deficit Disorder

CACLD
25 Van Zant Street
Suite 15-5
Norwalk, CT 06855
203-838-5010
FAX: 203-866-6108
e-mail: CACLD@optonline.net
www.CACLD.org

Beryl Kaufman, Executive Director

A video in an interview format for parents and professionals providing the history, symptoms, methods of diagnosis and three approaches used to ease the effects of attention deficit disorder. Published by Connecticut Association for Children & Adults with Learning Disabilities (CACLD). *$20.00*

45 Minutes

7530 Understanding Autism

Fanlight Productions
4196 Washington Street
Suite 2
Boston, MA 02131
617-469-4999
800-937-4113
FAX: 617-469-3379
e-mail: fanlight@fanlight.com
www.fanlight.com

Karen McMillen, Marketing Director
Ben Achtenberg, Owner

This program explores some basic components of a behavioral analysis approach to educating individuals with autism. After giving an introduction to the disability, the program goes on to illustrate the principles of reinforcement, teaching methods and data collection and analysis, as well as outlining the philosophy behind using behavior modification techniques with children with autism. *$195.00*

7531 **Understanding Down Syndrome: An Introduction for Parents**
Brookline Books
PO Box 1046
Cambridge, MA 02139 617-868-0360
800-666-2665
FAX: 617-868-1772
e-mail: thestore@brooklinebooks.com
www.brooklinebooks.com

Using positive and readable language, this book helps parents understand Down Syndrome. Medical details are explained in lay terms, and advice is given on working with professionals, obtaining services, and treatment techniques that help the child. Cunningham alerts families to potential problems, the prospects for the child in schooling and the passage to adulthood. Revised 1996. *$14.95*

Softcover
ISBN 1-57129 -09-5

7532 **Understanding the Nature of Autism**
Autism Society of North Carolina Bookstore
505 Oberlin Road
Suite 230
Raleigh, NC 27605 919-743-0204
800-442-2762
FAX: 919-743-0208
e-mail: dcoffey@autismsociety-nc.org
www.autismsociety-nc.org

Darla Coffey, Bookstore Manager
Jill Keel, Executive Director
$54.00

7533 **Unlocking Potenial: College and Other Choi ces for People with LD and AD/HD**
Spina Bifida Association of America
4590 Macarthur Boulevard NW
Suite 250
Washington, DC 20007 202-944-3285
800-621-3141
FAX: 202-944-3295
e-mail: sbaa@sbaa.org
www.sbaa.org

Cindy Brownstein, Chief Executive Officer
An indispensible look for high school students with learning disabilities and AD/HD. Includes comprehensive listing of resources. *$22.95*

7534 **Until Tomorrow: A Family Lives with Autism**
Autism Society of North Carolina Bookstore
505 Oberlin Road
Suite 230
Raleigh, NC 27605 919-743-0204
800-442-2762
FAX: 919-743-0208
e-mail: dcoffey@autismsociety-nc.org
www.autismsociety-nc.org

Darla Coffey, Bookstore Manager
Jill Keel, Executive Director
The central theme of this book is an effort to show what it is like to live with a child who cannot communicate. *$10.00*

7535 **We're Not Stupid**
Aquarius Health Care Videos
PO Box 1159
Sherborn, MA 01770 508-650-6905
FAX: 508-650-4216
e-mail: aqvideos@tiac.net
www.aquariusproductions.com

The U.S. Department of Education has estimated that up to five percent of students have problems in school because of attention deficit disorders. These kids often are impulsive and angry. They hear throughout their schooling what not to do, but not what to do. I know because I was diagnosed in high school with mild dyslexia and ADD. This film is about people discussing what their lives were like having learning problems. $125.00

Video

7536 **Why Won't My Child Pay Attention?**
Western Psychological Services
12031 Wilshire Boulevard
Los Angeles, CA 90025 310-478-2061
800-648-8857
FAX: 310-478-7838

Gregg Gillman, Vice President
Practical and reassuring videotape, noted child psychologist tells parents about two of the most common and complex problems of childhood: inattention and hyperactivity. *$49.50*

Video

7537 **Without Reason: A Family Copes with Autism**
Books on Special Children
PO Box 305
Congers, NY 10920 845-638-1236
FAX: 845-638-0847
e-mail: irene@boscbooks.com

The author discovers his son has autism. He delves into problems of the autistic person and explains reasons for their actions. *$20.95*

292 pages Hardcover

7538 **Women with Attention Deficit Disorder: Em bracing Disorganization at Home and Work**
Underwood-Miller
708 Westover Drive
Lancaster, PA 17601 717-285-2255
FAX: 717-285-2255

Addresses the millions of withdrawn little girls and chronically overwhelmed women with ADD who go undiagnosed because they don't fit the stereotypical notion of people with ADD. *$11.95*

288 pages 1995
ISBN 1-887424-05-9

7539 **World Without AIDS: The Controvertial Holistic Health**
HarperCollins
1350 Avenue of the Americas
New York, NY 10019 212-261-6500

Erin Gorman, Sales Executive
A convincing argument that conventional medicine approaches do not 'cure' disease, which outlines how AIDS can be treated using methods of naturopathic medicine. Also includes an appendix outlining 21 ways to strengthen the immune system.

288 pages Paperback 1988
ISBN 0-722516-32-0

7540 **You Mean I'm Not Lazy, Stupid or Crazy?!: A Self-Help Book for Adults with ADD**
Scribner

Practical advice on controlling adult ADD, a straightforward guide explains how to get along in groups, become organized, improve memory, and pursue professional help. *$15.00*

464 pages 1996
ISBN 0-684815-31-1

7541 **You and Your ADD Child**
Nelson Publications
1 Gateway Plaza
Port Chester, NY 10573 914-937-8400
FAX: 914-937-8950

$12.99

252 pages Paperback
ISBN 0-785278-95-8

Support Groups

7542 Autism Society of America
7910 Woodmont Avenue
Suite 300
Bethesda, MD 20814
301-657-0881
800-3AU-TISM
www.autism-society.org

Ann Pulley, Manager
ASA is the largest and oldest grassroots organization within the autism community, with more than 200 chapters and over 20,000 members and supporters nationwide. ASA is the leading source of education, information and referral about autism and has been the leader in advocacy and legislative initiatives for more than three decades.

7543 National Autism Hotline
Autism Services Center
929 4th Avenue
Huntington, WV 25701
304-525-8014
FAX: 304-525-8026
www.autismservicescenter.com

Ruth C Sullivan PhD, Executive Director
Jodi Fields, Director of Office Administratio
Service agency for individuals with autism and developmental disabilities, and their families. Assists families and agencies attempting to meet the needs of individuals with autism and other developmental disabilities. Makes available technical assistance in designing treatment programs and more. The hotline provides informational packets to callers and assists via telephone when possible.

7544 National Health Information Center
U S Department of Health
PO Box 1133
Washington, DC 20013
301-565-4167
800-336-4797
301-468-7394
FAX: 301-984-4256
e-mail: info@nhic.org
Identifies health information resources, channels requests for information to these resources and develops publications available for small handling fees.

Associations

7545 **American Amputee Foundation**
PO Box 250218
Little Rock, AR 72225
501-666-2523
FAX: 501-666-8367
e-mail: info@americanamputee.org
www.americanamputee.org

Catherine J Walden LSW,MPA,CLCP, Executive Director
Jack M. East LSW,MA, Rehabilitation Counseling
Serenity Tinkle, Office and Finance Manager
Serves primarily as a national information clearinghouse and referral center assisting mainly amputees and their families. AAF researches and gathers information including studies, product information, services, self-help publications and review articles written within the field. AAF has helped with claims, justification letters to payers, testimony and life care planning. Free information packet for phone or letter inquiries.
1975

7546 **American Board for Certification in Orthotics & Prosthetics**
330 John Carlyle Street
Suite 210
Alexandria, VA 22314
703-836-7114
FAX: 703-836-0838
e-mail: info@abcop.org
www.abcop.org

Catherine Carter, Executive Director
Heather Harris, Director
Scott Williamson, Director
The American Board for Certification in Orthotics and Prosthetics (ABC) is the national certifying and accrediting body for the orthotic and prosthetic professions. The public requires and deserves assurance that the persons providing orthotic and prosthetic services and care are qualified to provide the appropriate services, and it was on this basis that the ABC was established as a credentialing organization.

7547 **American Stroke Association**
American Heart Association
7272 Greenville Avenue
Dallas, TX 75231
214-373-6300
888-478-7653
FAX: 214-706-5231
e-mail: strokeconnection@heart.org
www.strokeassociation.org

M Wheeler, Chief Executive Officer
Fifty-five state affiliates monitoring local chapters offering educational materials, seminars, conferences and transportation for members nationwide. Maintains a listing of over 1,000 stroke support groups across the nation for referral to stroke survivors, their families, caregivers and interested professionals.

7548 **Epilepsy Foundation**
4351 Garden City Drive
Landover, MD 20785
301-459-3700
800-332-1000
FAX: 301-459-3700
e-mail: epilepsy@peaknet.net
www.epilepsyfoundation.org

Tony Coelho, Chair of Board of Directors
Bruce P. Hermann PhD, Chair of Advisory Board
Eric R. Hargis, President/CEO
The Epilepsy Foundation is the national voluntary agency solely dedicated to the welfare of the 2.7 million people with epilepsy in the U.S. and their families. The organization works to ensure that people with seizures are able to participate in all life experiences; and to prevent, control and cure epilepsy through research, education, advocacy and services.
1968

7549 **National Amputation Foundation**
40 Church Street
Malverne, NY 11565
516-887-3600
FAX: 516-887-3667
e-mail: amps76@aol.com
www.nationalamputation.org

Alfred Pennacchia, President
John Devine, First Vice President
Al Pennacchia, Second Vice President
Helps people who have had amputations to adjust to society. Members are military veterans with service connected amputations, as well as civilian amputees, who help show new amputees how to cope. Publishes a veteran newsletter for amputees. Donated medical equipment give-a-way program to anyone in need. Items must be picked up.
Quarterly 1919

7550 **National Stroke Association**
9707 E Easter Lane
Buliding B
Centennial, CO 80112
303-649-9299
800-878-6537
FAX: 303-649-1328
e-mail: info@stroke.org
www.stroke.org

George L Davis, Chairman of the Board
James Baranski, Chief Executive Officer
Dr. Maya Angelou, Board Of Directors
The only national health organization solely committed to stroke prevention, treatment, rehabilitation and community reintegration. Provides packaged training programs, on-site assistance, physician, patient and family education materials to acute and rehab hospitals. Develops workshops; operates the Stroke Information & Referral Center and produces professional publications such as Stroke: Clinical Updates and the Journal of Stroke and Cerebrovascular Diseases.

7551 **World Chiropractic Alliance**
2950 N Dobson Road
Suite 1
Chandler, AZ 85224
480-786-9235
800-347-1011
FAX: 480-732-9313
e-mail: comments@worldchiropracticalliance.org
www.worldchiropracticalliance.org

Jack Masche, Chief Operating Officer
Linda Bevel, Executive Assistant
Barbara J. Bigham, Director Of Communication
Dedicated to protecting and strengthening chiropractic around the world. Serving as a watchdog and advocacy organization, we place our emphasis on education and political action.
1989

Print & Non-Print Resources

7552 **Carpal Tunnel Syndrome**
Arthritis Foundation
PO Box 7669
Atlanta, GA 30357
404-872-7100
800-283-7800
FAX: 404-872-9559
e-mail: help@arthritis.org
www.arthritis.org

John Klippel, Chief Executive Officer
Offers an introduction to Carpal Tunnel, causes, symptoms, diagnosis and resources.

7553 **Don't Feel Sorry for Paul**
JB Lippincott
E Washington Square
Philadelphia, PA 19105
215-521-8300
FAX: 215-824-7390

J Lippincott, Chief Executive Officer

Paul is seven but was born with deformities of both hands and feet. Paul must wear a prosthesis on both feet so that he can walk. He has a third prosthesis for his right hand. The third prosthesis has a pair of hooks Paul uses as fingers.

94 pages Hardcover
ISBN 0-39731 -88-0

7554 Functional Restoration of Adults and Child ren with Upper Extremity Amputation

Demos Medical Publishing
386 Park Avenue S
Suite 201
New York, NY 10016
212-683-0072
800-532-8663
FAX: 212-683-0118
e-mail: orderdep@demospub.com
www.demosmedpub.com

Phyllis Gold, Owner

Provides a comprehensive reference to the surgery, prosthetic fitting, and rehabilitation of individuals sustaining an arm amputation. Covers the recent advancements in prosthetics and rehabilitation. *$150.00*

384 pages 2004
ISBN 1-888799-73-0

7555 Progress in Research

Christopher Reeve Paralysis Foundation
636 Morris Tpke
Suite 3a
Short Hills, NJ 07078
973-379-2690
800-225-0292
FAX: 973-912-9433
e-mail: paralysis@aol.com
www.paralysis.org

Kathy Lewis, President

Summarizes research on paralysis and spinal cord injury, emphasizing neural regeneration.

7556 Single-Handed: A Book for Persons with the Use of Only One Hand

Accent Books & Products
PO Box 700
Bloomington, IL 61702
309-378-2961
800-787-8444
FAX: 309-378-4420
e-mail: acmtlvng@aol.com

Raymond C Cheever, Publisher
Betty Garee, Editor

Includes information on devices and aids; special techniques; tips on how-to; illustrations; other helpful publications and more. *$4.25*

25 pages Paperback
ISBN 0-91570 -06-0

7557 Stroke Connection

American Heart Association
7272 Greenville Avenue
Dallas, TX 75231
214-373-6300
800-553-6321
FAX: 214-369-3685

M Wheeler, Chief Executive Officer

A forum for stroke survivors and their families to share information about coping with stroke. Provides information and referrals, and carries stroke related books, videos and literature available for purchase.

7558 Teaching Dressing Skills: Buttons, Bows and More

Therapro
225 Arlington Street
Framingham, MA 01702
508-872-9494
800-257-5376
FAX: 508-875-2062
e-mail: info@theraproducts.com
www.theraproducts.com

Karen Conrad, Owner

Teaches us how to teach children and adults of varying abilities how to tie shoes, button buttons, use zippers and put on/remove clothing. Developed by an experienced occupational therapist, these methods have been successfully used with many children. Each task is broken down with each step clearly illustrated and specific verbal directions given to avoid confusion and to eliminate verbalization that can distract the learner. *$9.95*

5 pages Pamphlets

Associations

7559 Aging in America
1500 Pelham Parkway S
Bronx, NY 10461
718-419-8200
877-244-6469
FAX: 718-409-8281
e-mail: pointofentry@aiamsh.org
www.aiamsh.org

William T. Smith, President/CEO
Julie Dalton, Vice President
Research and services organization for professionals in gerontology. Objectives are: to produce, implement and share effective and affordable programs and services that improve the quality of life for the elderly community; to better prepare professionals and students interested in or currently involved with, aging and the aged. Conducts research projects, educational and training seminars, and in-service curricula for long-term and acute care facilities.

7560 Alabama Association of Homes and Services for the Aging
1520 Cooper Hill Road
Birmingham, AL 35210
205-951-2442
FAX: 205-956-5001
e-mail: info@methodist-homes.org
www.methodist-homes.org

Wray Tomlin, President
Provides a retirement community environment of abundant life combined with the care of qualified professionals. Currently serves more than 1600 residents and employs more then 800 persons. 6 leves of care offered: independent cottage living, retirement apartments, assisted living, special needs units, nursing beds, and alzheimer's units.

7561 Alzheimer's Disease Education and Referral Center (ADEAR)
PO Box 8250
Silver Spring, MD 20907
800-438-4380
FAX: 301-495-3334
e-mail: adear@nia.nih.gov
www.alzheimers.nia.nih.gov

Jennifer Watson, Project Director
The Alzheimer's Disease Education and Referral (ADEAR) center provides information about Alzheimer's disease and related disorders to health professionals, patients and their families and the public. Most of the publications are provided at no charge as a service of the National Institute on Aging (NIA), one of the Federal Government's National Institutes of Health.
1990

7562 American Association of Homes and Services for the Aging
2519 Connecticut Avenue NW
Washington, DC 20008
202-783-2242
FAX: 202-783-2255
e-mail: info@aahsa.org
www.aahsa.org

William Minnix Jr. D.Min., President And CEO
Margaret M. Mullan, Chairwoman, Board Of Directors
The American Association of Homes and Services for the Aging (AAHS) represents not-for-profit organizations dedicated to providing high-quality health care, housing and services to the nation's elderly. AAHSA organizations serve more than one million older persons af all income levels, creeds and races.

7563 Arizona Association of Homes and Housing for the Aging
3839 N 3rd Street
Suite 201
Phoenix, AZ 85012
602-230-0026
FAX: 602-230-0563
e-mail: azaha@azaha.org
www.azaha.org

Genny Rose, Executive Director
Edwina Camplin MA, Office Manager
The Arizona Association of Homes and Houses for the Aging is a not-for-profit trade association representing more than 100 facilities dedicated to providing quality health care, housing and services to over 12,000 elderly Arizona citizens. AzAHA is the only association in Arizona representing the full continuum of long term care, housing and services including: retirement communities, HUD subsidized senior housing, assisted living and nursing facilities.

7564 Association of Ohio Philanthropic Homes and Housing for Aging
855 S Wall Street
Columbus, OH 43206
614-444-2882
FAX: 614-444-2974
e-mail: info@aopha.org
www.aopha.org

R. Douglas Spitler, Chair
Richard S. Lamden, Chair Elect
Founded in 1937, AOPHA, the advocate of not-for-profit services for older Ohioans, is a statewide nonprofit trade association representing over 335 not-for-profit senior housing apartments, home and community-based service providers, assisted living facilities, nursing homes and continuing care retirement communities (CCRCs).

7565 California Association of Homes and Services for the Aging
1315 i Street
Suite 100
Sacramento, CA 95814
916-392-5111
FAX: 916-428-4250
e-mail: aburnsjohnson@aging.org
www.aging.org

Anne Burns Johnson, CEO and President
Stuart Greenbaum, Director Of Communications
The California Association of Homes and Services for the Aging (CAHSA) is the primary statewide association for not-for-profit organizations providing health care, housing and community services to older adults.

7566 Center for Assistive Technology
University at Buffalo
322 Stockton Kimball Tower
Buffalo, NY 14214
716-829-3141
800-628-2281
FAX: 716-829-3217
TTY: 716-829-3141
e-mail: cat-webmaster@buffalo.edu
www.cat.buffalo.edu

Sue Arnold, Business Manager For CAT
Stephen Bauer, Ph.D., Co Director
Katie Beaver, MS, Associate Director, CAT
The Center for Assistive Technology (CAT) was established within the School of Health Related Professions in 1988. CAT conducts research, education and service programs in assistive technology for persons with disabilities and the elderly, in four related areas: Research, development and communications, education programs, client assessment and training services and dissemination.

7567 Children of Aging Parents
PO Box 167
Richboro, PA 18954
215-945-6900
800-227-7294
FAX: 215-945-8720
e-mail: info@caps4caregivers.org
www.caps4caregivers.org
A national clearinghouse for caregivers of the elderly. It provides information and referral, educational programs and materials and caregiver support groups. CAPS also produces a quarterly newsletter which is available through the organization. Individuals: $25.00. Organizational/Professional: $100.00.

7568 Colorado Association of Homes and Services for the Aging (CAHSA)
1888 Sherman Street
Suite 610
Denver, CO 80203
303-837-8834
FAX: 303-837-8836
www.cahsa.org

Laura Landwirth, Executive Director
Karen Simmering, Director Of Operations
Carol Hull, Assisted Living Consultant
The American Association of Homes and Services for the Aging (AAHS) represents nonprofit organizations dedicated to providing high quality health care, housing and services to the nation's elderly. AAHSA organizations serve more than one million older persons af all income levels, creeds and races.

7569 Connecticut Association of Not-for-Profit Providers for the Aging
1340 Worthington Ridge
Berlin, CT 06037
860-828-2903
FAX: 860-828-8694
e-mail: canpfa@canpfa.org
www.canpfa.org
CANPFA promotes a vision of the world in which every community offers an integrated and coordinated continuum of high quality, affordable health care, housing and community based services. CANPFA members are all mission-driven, not-for-profits. Not-for-profits focus on caring and providing services for their residents and clients. They re-invest their income into their facilities, resident programs and staff development. They are rooted in their communities.

7570 Georgia Association of Homes and Services for the Aging
607 Peachtree Street NE
Atlanta, GA 30308
404-872-9191
FAX: 404-872-1737
e-mail: gahsa@gahsa.org
www.gahsa.org

Tom Rockenbach, Chair
Joyce O. Wilson, Chair-Elect
Bob Rees, Treasurer
The Georgia Association of Homes and Services for the Aging (GAHSA) is an affiliated partner of the American Association of Homes and Services of the Aging (AASHA), which represents over 5,600 nonprofit facilities, over one million older adults in the United States and maintains an impressive staff of 80 professionals at its headquarters in Washington, D.C.

7571 Indiana Association of Homes for the Aging
PO Box 68829
Indianapolis, IN 46268
317-733-2380
FAX: 317-733-2385
e-mail: jimleich@iahsa.com
www.iahsa.com

Jim Leich, President
Susan Darwent, VP of Operations
Linda Woolley, VP of Health Policy
Indiana Association of Homes and Services for the Aging (IAHSA) members are non-profit organizations, providing hgh quality health care, services and housing for over 25,000 seniors in Indiana.

7572 Iowa Association of Homes and Services for the Aging
1701 48th Street
Suite 203
West Des Moines, IA 50266
515-440-4630
888-440-4630
FAX: 515-440-4631
e-mail: iahsa@ageiowa.org
www.ageiowa.org

Dana Petrowsky, President/CEO
Mark Tiegland, VP Member Services
Kristie Oliver, VP Government Relations
IAHSA inspires leadership and benevolence in its members through networking education, information and advocacy.

7573 Kansas Association of Homes for the Aging
217 SE 8th Avenue
Topeka, KS 66603
785-233-7443
800-264-5242
FAX: 785-233-9471
e-mail: kahsainfo@kahsa.org
www.kahsa.org

John Grace, President and CEO
Kevin McFarland, Executive VP
Debra Harmon Zehr, Executive VP
KAHSA represents 160 not-for-profit nursing homes, retirement communities, hospital long-term care units, assisted living facilities, senior housing and community based service programs for the elderly.

7574 Kentucky Association of Not-for-Profit Homes and Services for the Aging
2501 Nelson Miller Parkway
Louisville, KY 40223
502-992-4380
FAX: 502-992-4390
e-mail: info@kahsa.com
www.kahsa.com

Timothy L Veno, President
Founded in 1977, the association represents not-for-profit community, church, proprietary and govt. sponsored health care facilities, retirement communities, assisted living, housing and service programs for the elderly and disabled. The mission of the (KAHSA)is to provide services to the members that will enchance the quality of life of those they serve.

7575 Life Service Network of Illinois: Springfi eld
2 Lawrence Square
Springfield, IL 62704
217-789-1677
FAX: 217-789-1778
e-mail: info@lsni.org
www.lsni.org

Kirk Riva, Vice President
Jennifer Pickett, Director Marketing
Jen Frink, Manager Of Sales
The American Association of Homes and Services for the Aging (AAHS) represents not-for-profit organizations dedicated to providing high-quality health care, housing and services to the nation's elderly. AAHSA organizations serve more than one million older persons af all income levels, creeds and races.

7576 Life Services Network of Illinois
911 N Elm Street
Suite 228
Hinsdale, IL 60521
630-325-6170
FAX: 630-325-0749
e-mail: info@lsni.org
www.lsni.org

Dennis Bozzi, President
For nearly 75 years, Life Services Network of Illinois, a statewide trade association, has represented providers of the complete contiuum of services for older adults, including nursing facilities, assisted living, senior housing and home and community based services. Our success as an association is founded in our commitment to helping our members overcome obstacles while identifying future opportunities for their success.

7577 Louisiana Association of Homes and Service for the Aging
PO Box 1748
Marrero, LA 70072
225-757-1350
FAX: 504-689-3982
e-mail: gulfstatesahsa@aol.com
www.gulfstatesahsa.org

Karen Contrenchis, President
Along term care system which offers accessable, affordable, high-quality and innovative healthcare, housing and comminuty services. Provides value to the the senior population and their families through personal and professional commitment, in a compassionate manner, supported by benevolence and integrity. Socially resposible and accountable for promoting excellence in long-term care and support services.

7578 Massachusetts Aging Services Association

60 Seminary Avenue
Auburndale, MA 02466
617-224-2999
FAX: 617-663-7046
e-mail: office@MassAging.org
www.massaging.org

Elissa Sherman PhD, President
Susan Gershenfeld MSW NBA, Vice President/Member Services
The Massachusetts Aging Services Association (MassAging) is the only Massachusetts membership association representing the full continuum of not-for-profit providers of aging services. MassAging works to achieve a system of healthy, affordable, and ethical aging services for older persons in Massachusetts. MassAging is proudly affiliated with the American Association of Homes and Services for the Aging (AAHSA), a national associaton of not-for-profit homes and services for he aging.

7579 Michigan Association of Homes and Serivces for the Aging

6512 Centurion Drive
Suite 380
Lansing, MI 48917
517-323-3687
FAX: 517-323-4569
e-mail: dherbel@mahsahome.org
www.mahsahome.org

David E Herbel, CEO and President
Karlene Ketola, VP of Member Services
Deanna L. Mitchell, VP System Design and Evaluation
The Michigan Association of Homes and Services for the Aging represents and promotes the common interests of its members through leadership, advocacy, education and other services in order to enhance members' ability to serve their constituencies.

7580 Mid-Atlantic LifeSpan

2 Uite 220
Columbia, MD 21046
410-381-1176
FAX: 410-381-0240
e-mail: admin@manpha.org
www.manpha.org

Isabella Firth, President
LifeSpan is the newest, largest and most powerful senior care provider association in the Mid-Atlantic, representing more than 300 senior care provider organizations in Maryland and the District of Columbia. LifeSpan's members include non-profits and proprietary assisted living, contiuing care retirement communities, nursing facilities, subsidized senior housing and community and hospital based programs.

7581 Minnesota Health and Housing Alliance

2550 University Avenue West
Suite 350S
Saint Paul, MN 55114
651-645-4545
800-462-5368
FAX: 651-645-0002
e-mail: info@mhha.com
www.mhha.com

Gayle Kvenvold, President/CEO
Elizabeth Sether, Nurse Consultant/Policy Analyst
Nancy Garrett, Executive Assistant
Minnesota's largest statewide trade association for providers of older adult services, MHHA represents the complete continuum of care, including nursing home care, senior housing with supportive services, independent senior housing and community-based services.

7582 Mississippi Association of Homes and Services for the Aging

Po Box 1748
Marrero, LA 70072
225-757-1350
FAX: 504-689-3982
www.gulfstatesahsa.org

Karen Contrenchis, President
Wayne Plaisance, Vice Chair
Cindy Ladnier, Secretary/Treasurer
a long term care system which offers accessible, affordable, high-quality and innovative healthcare, housing and community services. Provides value to the senior population and their families through personal and professional commitment, in a compassionate manner, supported by benevolence and integrity. Socially responsible and accountable for promoting excellence in long-term care and support services.

7583 Missouri Association of Homes for the Aging

515 East High Street
Suite 101W
Jefferson City, MO 65101
573-635-6244
FAX: 573-635-6618
e-mail: info@moah.org
www.moaha.org

Denise Clemonds, Executive Director
Founded in 1969 and devoted to furthering the interests of the continuum of long term care, including skilled nursing facilities, health related facilities, residential care facilities, independent housing facilities, HUD facilities and other community based services.

7584 National Organization of the Senior Blind

111 Marquette Avenue
Apt 503
Minneapolis, MN 55401
612-375-1625
e-mail: judysanders@usfamily.net
www.nfb.org

Judy Sanders, President
Membership organization of elderly blind persons providing support and information to other blind seniors. Issues include concerns such as remaining active in community and social life, maintaining private homes or living in retirement communities or nursing homes, learning the techniques used by the blind, independently caring for oneself and maintaining a positive apporach to vision loss.

7585 National Voluntary Organizations for Independent Living for the Aging

1901 L Street, NW,
4th Floor
Washington, DC 20036
202-479-1200
FAX: 202-479-0735
e-mail: info@ncoa.org
www.ncoa.org

James Firman, President and CEO
The National Council on the Aging is a national network of organizations and individuals dedicated to improving the health and independence of older persons and increasing their continuing contributions to communities, society and future generations.

7586 Nebraska Association of Homes for the Aging

625 S 14th Street
Suite A
Lincoln, NE 68508
402-436-2165
FAX: 402-434-5685
e-mail: ron@nebahsa.org
www.nebahsa.org

Julie Kaminski, President
Kevin Moriarty, Vice President
Dottie Brown, Secretary
serves the needs of the Nebraska's not-for-profit facilities and services for our state's elderly with representation and advocacy, educational and professional development, shared services and programs, and statewide leadership.

7587 New Jersey Association of Nonprofit Homes for the Aging

13 Roszel Road
Suite A-104
Princeton, NJ 08540
609-452-1161
FAX: 609-452-2907
e-mail: jduggan@njanpha.org
www.njanpha.org

June Duggan, CEO and President
Francis Byrne, VP
Fred Brand, Director Of Membership Services

The New Jersey Association of Non-Profit Homes for the Aging (NJANPHA) is the statewide association of not-for-profit organizations which are dedicated to providing and enhancing quality of life services to the diverse aging population. The Association encourages cooperaton with communities and ther entities, both public and private, interested in aging.

7588 New York Association of Homes and Services for the Aging
150 State Street
Suite 301
Albany, NY 12207
518-449-2707
FAX: 518-455-8908
www.nyahsa.org

Carl S Young, President
Nancy Caban, Executive Assistant
Joan Twiss, Receptionist/Office Assistant
NYAHSA is a statewide organization of socially responsible, community-benefit organizations dedicated to providing high quality health care, housing, and community services to the elderly and people with special needs.

7589 North Carolina Association of Nonprofits for the Aging
3700 National Drive
Suite 218
Raleigh, NC 27609
919-571-8333
FAX: 919-571-1297
e-mail: swilliamson@ncanpha.org
www.ncanpha.org

Susan Williamson, President/CEO
Leslie Rosenboro, Member Services Manager
The North Carolina Association of Non-Profit Homes for the Aging (NCANPHA) is the state association of not-for-profit providers dedicated to providing quality health care, housing, health, community and related services to the elderly.

7590 Northern New England Association of Homes and Services for the Aging
75 Pearl Street
Portland, ME 04101
207-773-4822
FAX: 207-773-0101
e-mail: sderingis@nneahsa.org
www.nneahsa.org

Denise Vachon, Chairman
Thomas Argue, Chair Elect
Peter Warecki, Treasurer
NNEAHSA's mission is to promote the interests of its not-for-profit members in Maine, New Hampshire, and Vermont which provide healthy, affordable and ethical long-term care to our older citizens through education, advocacy, representation and collaboration.

7591 Oklahoma Association of Homes and Services for the Aging
PO Box 1383
El Reno, OK 73036
405-640-8040
FAX: 405-640-8040
e-mail: info@okahsa.org
www.okahsa.org

Karen Stanhope, President
Mary Brinkley, Executive Director
The Oklahoma Association of Homes and Services for the Aging is the Oklahoma state association of not-for-profit organizations dedicated to establishing the highest standards of excellence for services to the aging in Oklanhoma. OKAHSA's purpose is to be supportive of each member organization's quest for excellence.

7592 Oregon Association of Homes for the Aging
7340 SW Hunziker Street
Suite 104
Tigard, OR 97223
503-684-3788
FAX: 503-624-0870
e-mail: rgulyas@oashs.org
www.oashs.org

Cathleen Sullivan, President/AAHSA Delegate
David Parrett, President Elect
Chet Patterson, Treasurer
The Oregon Alliance of Senior & Health Services is the state association of not-for-profit, mission-directed organizations dedicated to providing quality housing, health, community and related services to the elderly and disabled.

7593 Pennsylvania Association of Nonprofit Homes for the Aging
1100 Bent Creek Boulevard
Mechanicsburg, PA 17050
717-763-5724
800-545-2270
FAX: 717-763-1057
e-mail: info@panpha.org
www.panpha.org

Ron Barth, President and CEO
W M Russ McDaid, VP Chief Public Policy Officer
Karen E. Ryan, Public Policy Assistant
PANPHA represents over 320 nonprofit providers of long-term care and housing services for 65,000 elderly residents across Pennsylvania. The Association is committed to helping its members provide quality care efficiently and effectively for the individuals and families they serve. In the age of impersonal care, PANPHA members put people before profits.

7594 Quality Health Care Foundation of Wyoming
716 Randall Avenue
Cheyenne, WY 82001
307-637-7575
FAX: 307-638-8472

Dan J. Lex, Executive Director
The American Association of Homes and Services for the Aging (AAHS) represents not-for-profit organizations dedicated to providing high-quality health care, housing and services to the nation's elderly. AAHSA organizations serve more than one million older persons af all income levels, creeds and races.

7595 Rhode Island Association of Facilities for the Aging
225 Chapman Street
Box 7
Providence, RI 02905
401-490-7612
866-883-1631
FAX: 401-490-7614
TTY: 401-490-4597
e-mail: info@riafsa.org
www.riafsa.org

Julie Richard, President
Paul Barrette, Secretary
Christopher Novak, Manager
RIAFSA was formally organized in 1989 as an associaton of non-profit facilities and services primarily for the elderly. RIAFSA members include senior housing, assisted living, nursing homes and home and community based services.

7596 Senior Citizens and the Law
Center for Public Representation
PO Box 260049
Madison, WI 53726
608-251-4008
800-369-0388
FAX: 606-251-1263
e-mail: cpr@lawmail.law.wisc.edu
www.law.wisc.edu
An introduction to legal problems facing the elderly in Wisconsin. This edition discusses legal problems associated with Social Security, Medicare, SSI, guardianship and its alternatives, community-based services, probate, taxes, private health insurance and consumer protection. *$5.00*

ISBN 0-936226-15-1

7597 Shiloh Senior Citizens Center
1510 9th Street NW
Washington, DC 20001
202-232-1425
FAX: 202-232-1425

Jacqueline Thompkins, Executive Director
Offers daily programs, activities, counseling, noon meals, and transportation for deaf and hard of hearing seniors, 60 and older, living in the District of Columbia.

7598 South Carolina Association of Nonprofit Homes for the Aging
1110 Marshall Road
Greenwood, SC 29646
803-227-7231
FAX: 803-227-7161

Danny Satterfield, Manager
The American Association of Homes and Services for the Aging (AAHS) represents not-for-profit organizations dedicated to providing high-quality health care, housing and services to the nation's elderly. AAHSA organizations serve more than one million older persons af all income levels, creeds and races.

7599 Tennessee Association of Homes for the Aging
500 Interstate Boulevard S
Suite 325
Nashville, TN 37210
615-256-1800
FAX: 615-726-3082
e-mail: cermshar@tha.com
www.tha.com/tnahsa/

Carrie Ermshar, President
TNAHSA is an association of faclities and professionals providing quality housing, health, community and related services for the elderly. TNAHSA represents and promotes the common interest of its members through leadership, advocacy, education, communication and other services in order to enhance members' ability to serve their constituencies.

7600 Texas Association of Homes and Services for the Aging
2205 Hancock Drive
Austin, TX 78756
512-467-2242
FAX: 512-467-2275
e-mail: cassandra@tahsa.org
www.tahsa.org

George Linial, CEO and President
Donna Loflin, VP of Education
The American Association of Homes and Services for the Aging (AAHS) represents not-for-profit organizations dedicated to providing high-quality health care, housing and services to the nation's elderly. AAHSA organizations serve more than one million older persons af all income levels, creeds and races.

7601 Washington Association of Housing and Services for the Aging
1570 Wilmington Drive
Suite 220
Dupont, WA 98327
253-964-8870
FAX: 253-964-8876
e-mail: wahsa@wahsa.com
www.wahsa.com

Deb Murphy, Chief Executive Officer
Heather Skinner, Chief Operating Officer
Paul Montgomery, Director Of Financial Services
Washington Association of Housing and Services for the Aging (WASHA) is the state association serving primarily not-for-profit organizations dedicated to providing quality housing, health, community and related services to older persons.

7602 Wisconsin Association of Homes & Services for the Aging
204 S Hamilton Street
Madison, WI 53703
608-255-7060
FAX: 608-255-7064
e-mail: jsauer@wahsa.org
www.wahsa.org

Miriam Ownby, President
Mike Christensen, Director
Mary Ann Dreschler, Director
The Wisconsin Association of Homes and Services for the Aging (WAHSA) is a statewide membership organization of not-for-profit corporations principally serving the elderly and disabled.

Print & Non-Print Resources

7603 Abstracts in Social Gerontology: Current Literature on Aging
National Council on the Aging
600 Maryland Avenue SW
Washington, DC 20024
202-479-1200
FAX: 202-479-0735

James Firman, Chief Executive Officer
Detailed abstracts are provided for recent major journal articles, books, reports and other materials on many facets of aging, including: adult education, demography, family relations, institutional care and work attitudes.

7604 Activities in Action
Haworth Press
10 Alice Street
Binghamton, NY 13904
607-722-5857
800-429-6784
FAX: 607-722-6362
e-mail: orders@haworthpress.com
www.haworthpress.com

William Cohen, Owner
An invaluable resource which serves as a catalyst for professional and personal growth and provides a national forum on geriatric and activity issues. *$74.95*
98 pages Hardcover
ISBN 1-560241-32-2

7605 Activities with Developmentally Disabled Elderly and Older Adults
Haworth Press
10 Alice Street
Binghamton, NY 13904
607-722-5857
800-429-6784
FAX: 607-722-6362
e-mail: orders@haworthpress.com
www.haworthpress.com

William Cohen, Owner
Learn how to effectively plan and deliver activities for a growing number of older people with developmental disabilities. It aims to stimulate interest and continued support for recreation program development and implementation among developmental disability and aging service systems. *$59.95*
156 pages Hardcover
ISBN 1-560240-92-X

7606 Aging & Vision News
Lighthouse International
111 E 59th Street
New York, NY 10022
212-821-9200
800-829-0500
FAX: 212-821-9706
e-mail: info@lighthouse.org
www.lighthouse.org

Joanna Mellor, VP Information Services
Tara Cortes, President
Intended for professionals engaged in research, education or service delivery in the field of vision and aging.
6-12 pages BiAnnually

7607 Aging Eye and Low Vision
Lighthouse International
111 E 59th Street
New York, NY 10022
212-821-9200
800-829-0500
FAX: 212-821-9706
e-mail: info@lighthouse.org

Joanna Mellor, VP Information Services
Tara Cortes, President
A study guide for physicians on common age-related vision disorders.

7608 **Aging News Alert**
CD Publications
8204 Fenton Street
Silver Spring, MD 20910
301-588-2280
800-666-6380
FAX: 301-588-6385
e-mail: cdpubs@clark.net
www.cdpublications.com/seniors/ana.htm
Publishes short articles on legislation and other federal action affecting elderly people. *$237.00*
16-18 pages Weekly
ISSN 1050-31 8

7609 **Aging Process: Therapeutic Implications**
Lippincott, Williams & Wilkins
227 E Washington Square
Philadelphia, PA 19106
215-521-8300
800-777-2295
FAX: 301-824-7390
www.lpub.com

J Lippincott, Chief Executive Officer
Experts examine the physiological and biological aspects of aging that impinge upon drug disposition and medical therapeutics.
352 pages

7610 **Aging Research & Training News**
Business Publishers
2601 University Boulevard W
Suite 200
Silver Spring, MD 20902
301-587-6300
800-274-6737
FAX: 301-587-4530
e-mail: bpinews@bpinews.com
www.bpinews.com

Leonard A Eiserer, Publisher
Nancy Aldrich, Editor
Katie Johnson, Marketing Manager
Essential information on aging education and staff training, funding and grant oppurtunities, the National Institute on Aging, medical and scientific research, ans statistical measures in geveontology and genetics. *$282.00*
10 pages Monthly

7611 **Aging and Developmental Disability: Current Research, Programming, and Practice**
Haworth Press
10 Alice Street
Binghamton, NY 13904
607-722-5857
800-429-6784
FAX: 607-722-6362
e-mail: orders@haworthpress.com
www.haworthpress.com

Joy Hammel PhD OTR/L, Co-Editor
Susan M Nochajski PhD OTR, Co-Editor
S Harrington-Miller, Advertising
Explores research findings and their implications for practice in relation to normative and disability-related aging experiences and issues. It discusses the effectiveness of specific intervention targeted toward aging adults with developmental disabilities such as Down's Syndrome, cerebral palsy, autism, and epilepsy, and offers suggestions for practice and future research in this area. *$39.95*
100 pages Hardcover
ISBN 0-789010-39-9

7612 **Aging and Family Therapy: Practitioner Perspectives on Golden Pond**
Haworth Press
10 Alice Street
Binghamton, NY 13904
607-722-5857
800-429-6784
FAX: 607-722-6362
e-mail: orders@haworthpress.com
www.haworthpress.com

William Cohen, Owner
Here are creative strategies for use in therapy with older adults and their families. This significant new book provides practitioners with information, insight, reference tools, and other sources that will contribute to more effective intervention with the elderly and their families. *$74.95*
244 pages Hardcover
ISBN 0-866567-78-X

7613 **Aging and Our Families**
Human Sciences Press
233 Spring Street
New York, NY 10013
212-229-2859
800-221-9369
FAX: 212-463-0742

Handbook for family caregivers. *$18.95*
132 pages Paperback
ISBN 0-89885 -41-5

7614 **Aging and Vision News**
National Center for Vision and Aging
111 E 59th Street
New York, NY 10022
212-821-9200
800-829-0500
FAX: 212-821-9707
TTY: 212-821-9713

Tara Cortes, President
3x Year

7615 **Aging in Stride**
CAREsource Program Development
2200 6th Avenue
Suite 833
Seattle, WA 98121
206-625-9128
800-448-5213
FAX: 206-682-2901
e-mail: service@caresource.com
www.caresource.com

Connie Parsons, VP Marketing
Dennis Kenny, Owner
Guide to aging, the special needs of older adults, and the demands of providing care and support. Experts explain potential conflicts, planning opportunities and strategies for success. Six guides. *$49.95*
475 pages Paperback
ISBN 1-87886 -12-5

7616 **Aging in the Designed Environment**
Haworth Press
10 Alice Street
Binghamton, NY 13904
607-722-5857
800-429-6784
FAX: 607-722-6362
e-mail: orders@haworthpress.com
www.haworthpress.com

William Cohen, Owner
The key sourcebook for physical and occupational therapists developing and implementing environmental designs for the aging. *$74.95*
133 pages
ISBN 1-560240-31-8

7617 **Aging with a Disability**
Special Needs Project
324 State Street
Suite H
Santa Barbara, CA 93101
805-962-8087
800-333-6867
FAX: 805-962-5087
www.specialneeds.com
This unique and recent book discusses the role of family, financial resources and the American health care system in the life of aging adults with developmental disabilities. $32.95

7618 **Assistive Technology for Older Persons**
Idaho Assistive Technology Project
129 W 3rd Street
Moscow, ID 83843
208-885-3559
800-432-8324
FAX: 208-885-3628
e-mail: rseiler@uidaho.edu
www.educ.uidaho.edu/idatech

$5.00

60 pages

7619 California Financial Power of Attorney
NOLO
950 Parker Street
Berkeley, CA 94710
510-549-1976
800-955-4775
FAX: 510-548-5902
www.nolo.com

Maira Dizgalvis, Trade Customer Service Manager
Susan McConnell, Director Sales
Natasha Kaluza, Sales Assistant
A plain-English book packed with forms and instructions to give a trusted person the legal authority to handle your financial affairs.
paperback

7620 Caring for Alzheimer's Patients
Plenum Publishing Corporation
233 Spring Street
New York, NY 10013
212-242-1490
800-221-9369
FAX: 212-463-0742
e-mail: info@plenum.com
This handbook is designed for families, friends, and health-care professionals coping with the myriad of problems encountered by those afflicted with Alzheimer's disease. *$22.95*
308 pages Cloth
ISBN 3-06431 -98-

7621 Caring for Those You Love: A Guide to Compassionate Care for the Aged
Horizon Publishers
191 N 650 E
Bountiful, UT 84010
801-295-9451
800-453-0812
FAX: 801-295-0196

Duane Crowther, Owner
This book is a practical guide to coping with special problems of the aged and infirm, and examines the many challenges of caring for the elderly on a personal and family level. *$12.98*

ISBN 0-88290 -70-9

7622 Caring for the Disabled Elderly
Brookings Institution
1775 Massachusetts Avenue NW
Washington, DC 20036
202-797-6000
FAX: 202-797-6004
e-mail: bibooks@brookings.edu
www.brookings.edu

Strobe Talbott, President
Financial information for the elderly. *$31.95*
318 pages Cloth
ISBN 0-815774-97-4

7623 Choose the Right Long Term Care: Home Care Assisted Living and Nursing Homes
NOLO
950 Parker Street
Berkeley, CA 94710
510-549-1976
800-955-4775
FAX: 510-548-5902
www.nolo.com

Maira Dizgalvis, Trade Customer Service Manager
Susan McConnell, Director Sales
Natasha Kaluza, Sales Assistant
This book helps you choose a nursing home, or find a viable alternative. Covers how to get the most out of Medicare and other benefit programs. *$21.95*
336 pages paperback
ISBN 0-873375-15-7

7624 Chronically Disabled Elderly in Society
Greenwood Publishing Group
88 Post Road W
Suite 5007
Westport, CT 06880
203-226-3571
FAX: 203-222-1502
www.greenwood.com

Wayne Smith, President
This timely work increases awareness of and knowledge about problems of societal living among the chronically disabled elderly, with implications for policy makers, educational institutions, advocacy groups, families and individuals. Hardcover.
160 pages $52.95 - $55
ISBN 0-313291-09-8

7625 Communication Disorders in Aging
Gallaudet University Press
800 Florida Avenue NE
Washington, DC 20002
202-651-5000
800-451-1073
FAX: 202-651-5489

Erving Jordan, President
This text presents contemporary practices in the medical and clinical assessment of the aged, reviews clinical evaluation techniques, and provides a comprehensive discussion of neurological imaging techniques. *$39.95*
528 pages Hardcover

7626 Coping and Caring: Living with Alzheimer's Disease
AARP Fulfillment
601 E Street NW
Washington, DC 20049
202-434-2277
800-424-3410
FAX: 202-434-3443
e-mail: member@aarp.org
www.aarp.org

William Novelli, Chief Executive Officer
Addresses the questions: What is Alzheimer's? How does the disease progress? How long does it last? How can families cope?

24 pages

7627 Directory of Self-Help/Mutual Aid Support Groups for Older People
Lighthouse International
111 E 59th Street
New York, NY 10022
212-821-9200
800-829-0500
FAX: 212-821-9706
e-mail: info@lighthouse.org

Joanna Mellor, VP Information Services
Tara Cortes, President
State-by-state listings of over 650 support groups for older people with impaired vision, plus listings of state commissions for the blind, self-help clearinghouses, vision rehabilitation agencies, and national resource organizations. *$10.00*

7628 Domestic Mistreatment of the Elderly: Towards Prevention
AARP Fulfillment
601 E Street NW
Washington, DC 20049
202-434-2277
800-424-3410
FAX: 202-434-3443
e-mail: member@aarp.org
www.aarp.org

William Novelli, Chief Executive Officer
This comprehensive publication addresses the problem of mistreatment or neglect in the home.
39 pages

7629 Early Story of Alzheimer's Disease
Lippincott, Williams & Wilkins
227 E Washington Square
Philadelphia, PA 19106
215-521-8300
800-777-2295
FAX: 301-824-7390
www.lpub.com

J Lipppincott, Chief Executive Officer
Translation of the historical papers by Alos Alzheimer. *$58.50*

160 pages Illustrated
ISBN 0-88167 -68-4

7630 Elder Abuse
Human Sciences Press
233 Spring Street
New York, NY 10013
212-229-2859
800-221-9369
FAX: 212-463-0742
Practice, policy and laws for abuse on the aging.
232 pages Cloth
ISBN 0-89885 -15-6

7631 Elder Care
Center for Public Representation
PO Box 260049
Madison, WI 53726
608-251-4008
800-369-0388
FAX: 608-251-1263
www.law.wisc.edu/pal
A compendium of alternatives for providing and financing long-term care. This practical guide provides the most comprehensive and comforting information to help navigate a number of consumer mine fields. *$16.95*
224 pages
ISBN 0-87337 -13-5

7632 Enabling News
Access II Independent Living Centers
611 W Johnson Street
Gallatin, MO 64640
660-663-2423
FAX: 660-663-2517
e-mail: access@accessii.org
www.accessii.org

Debra Hawman, Executive Director
Charlotte Hamilton, Program Manager
8 pages Quarterly

7633 Exercise Activities for the Elderly
Springer Publishing Company
11 W 42nd Street
15th Floor
New York, NY 10036
212-431-4370
877-687-7476
FAX: 212-941-7842
e-mail: contactus@springerpub.com
www.springerpub.com

Sheri Sussman, Vice President
Annette Imperati, Marketing/Sales Director
Ursula Springer, President
A variety of exercises geared to clients with such conditions as arthritis, diabetes and Parkinson's disease, and others which are designed to build up muscular strength and maintain flexibility. *$39.95*
224 pages Softcover
ISBN 0-826187-03-X

7634 Exercise and the Older Adult
Kendall/Hunt Publishing Company
1900 Association Drive
Reston, VA 20191
703-476-3400
800-213-7193
FAX: 703-476-9527
e-mail: aaalf@aahperd.org
www.aahperd.org

Jan A Seaman MBA PED, Executive Director
Michael Davis, Manager
The latest information on physical activity for the older adults is in this textbook. Biomechanics, exercise physiology, health issues, sensory-motor function and measurement are covered by leading experts in the field. Other topics addressed include low-impact aerobics, strength development, exercise and activities for the frail elderly. *$35.00*
202 pages
ISBN 0-787210-04-8

7635 Explore Your Options
Kansas Department on Aging
503 S Kansas Avenue
Topeka, KS 66603
785-296-4986
800-432-3535
FAX: 785-296-0256
www.agingKansas.org
Yearly

7636 Falling in Old Age
Springer Publishing Company
536 Broadway
New York, NY 10012
212-431-4370
877-687-7476
FAX: 212-941-7842
e-mail: marketing@springerpub.com
www.springerpub.com

Annette Imperati, Marketing/Sales Director
Ursula Springer, President
Presented are practical techniques for the prevention of falls and for determining and correcting the causes.

7637 Family Intervention Guide To Mental Illness
New Harbinger Publications
5674 Shattuck Avenue
Oakland, CA 94609
510-652-0215
800-748-6273
FAX: 510-652-5472
e-mail: customerservice@newharbinger.com

Matthew McKay, Owner
This book helps readers understand, identify, and assist family members or close loved ones who suffer from the early signs of mental illness. It offers nine fundamental techniques for recognizing, managing, and recovering from mental illness. *$12.95*
300 pages
ISBN 1-87923 -10-5

7638 Functional Fitness Assessment for Adults
American Alliance for Health, Phys. Ed. & Dance
1900 Association Drive
Reston, VA 20191
703-476-3400
FAX: 703-476-9527
e-mail: aaalf@aahperd.org

Michael Davis, Manager
This field test assesses the functional fitness of adults over 60 years of age. It is designed to serve the larger population through field based measurement techniques that can be used in a facility where older persons live and can be conducted by personnel not necessarily trained for clinical responsibilities. *$7.50*
24 pages
ISBN 0-88314 -47-6

7639 Handbook of Assistive Devices for the Handicapped Elderly
Haworth Press
10 Alice Street
Binghamton, NY 13904
607-722-5857
800-429-6784
FAX: 607-722-6362
e-mail: orders@haworthpress.com
www.haworthpress.com

William Cohen, Owner
Concise yet comprehensive reference of assistive devices for handicapped elders. *$34.95*
77 pages Hardcover
ISBN 0-866561-52-8

7640 Handbook on Ethnicity, Aging and Mental Health
Greenwood Publishing Group
88 Post Road W
Suite 5007
Westport, CT 06880
203-226-3571
FAX: 203-222-1502
www.greenwood.com

Wayne Smith, President

State-of-the-art reference by leading experts and first book-length appraisal of research, practices and policies concerning mental health needs of the ethnic elderly in America. $95-$99.50.

376 pages Hardcover
ISBN 0-313282-04-8

7641 Health Care of the Aged
Haworth Press
10 Alice Street
Binghamton, NY 13904
607-722-5857
800-429-6784
FAX: 607-722-6362
e-mail: orders@haworthpress.com
www.haworthpress.com

William Cohen, Owner
Focusing on the need for developing new service delivery models for the aged, this book examines fiscal, political, and social criteria influencing this challenge of the 1990's. The aged are caught in the sweeping changes currently occurring in the financing, organizing and delivery of human health care services. *$74.95*

183 pages Hardcover
ISBN 1-560240-65-2

7642 Health Promotion and Disease Prevention
Lippincott, Williams & Wilkins
227 E Washington Square
Philadelphia, PA 19106
215-521-8300
800-777-2295
FAX: 301-824-7390
www.lpub.com

J Lippincott, Chief Executive Officer
Professional directory offering information on health care and rehabilitation for the elderly. *$87.00*

218 pages
ISBN 0-88167 -90-0

7643 International Health Guide for Senior Citizen Travelers
Pilot Books
PO Box 2102
Greenport, NY 11944
631-477-1094
FAX: 631-477-0978

Covers essential pre-departure health planning; advice on specific health concerns; disease prevention and more. *$4.95*

7644 Life Planning for Adults with Developmental Disabilities
New Harbinger Publications
5674 Shattuck Avenue
Oakland, CA 94609
510-652-0215
800-748-6273
FAX: 510-652-5472
e-mail: customerservice@newharbinger.com

Matthew McKay, Owner
A much-needed resource for parents, family, and caregivers of adults with developmental disabilities like downs syndrome, fragile x, and autism, this book offers resources and planning tools for helping developmentally disabled adults build skills in employment, education, relationships, independant living, and finances. *$12.95*

300 pages
ISBN 1-87923 -10-5

7645 Managing Aging and Human Services Agencies
Springer Publishing Company
536 Broadway
New York, NY 10012
212-431-4370
877-687-7476
FAX: 212-941-7842
e-mail: marketing@springerpub.com
www.springerpub.com

Annette Imperati, Marketing/Sales Director
Ursula Springer, President
Offers specialized information for the human resources professional who works with the elderly. *$27.95*

160 pages

7646 Mastering the Medicare Maze
Center for Public Representation
PO Box 260049
Madison, WI 53726
608-251-4008
800-369-0388
FAX: 606-251-1263

This book provides simple explanations of how to appeal denied Medicare claims. Less than 3% of Medicare claims are ever appealed. But of those that are, over 60% are successful in returning dollars to beneficiaries. With simple instructions, this book tells you how to do it and includes all the necessary forms. *$9.95*

128 pages
ISBN 0-93262 -40-2

7647 Medicare Maximization
Center for Public Representation
PO Box 260049
Madison, WI 53726
608-251-4008
800-369-0388
FAX: 606-251-1263
e-mail: cpr@lawmail.law.wisc.edu
www.law.wisc.edu/pal

This manual for nursing homes provides information on Medicare billing procedures, Medicare coverage guidelines - Part A and Part B as well as Medicare Bed Certification for nursing homes. Chapters with examples and exercises give you the knowledge to maximize Medicare reimbursements. *$39.95*

150 pages
ISBN 0-93262 -34-8

7648 Mentally Impaired Elderly: Strategies and Interventions to Maintain Function
Haworth Press
10 Alice Street
Binghamton, NY 13904
607-722-5857
800-429-6784
FAX: 607-722-6362
e-mail: orders@haworthpress.com
www.haworthpress.com

S Harrington-Miller, Advertising
William Cohen, Owner
Provides effective support and sensitive care for the most vulnerable segment of the elderly population, those with mental impairment. *$74.95*

171 pages Hardcover
ISBN 1-560241-68-3

7649 Mirrored Lives: Aging Children and Elderly Parents
Greenwood Publishing Group
88 Post Road W
Suite 5007
Westport, CT 06880
203-226-3571
FAX: 203-222-1502
www.greenwood.com

Wayne Smith, President
Discusses geriatric decline connected to nonterminal illness in old age. Koch takes a sensitive but thorough look at the declining years of his father. $19.95-$21.95.

240 pages Hardcover
ISBN 0-275936-71-6

7650 Now Where Did I Put My Keys?
AARP Fulfillment
601 E Street NW
Washington, DC 20049
202-434-2277
800-424-3410
FAX: 202-434-3443
e-mail: member@aarp.org
www.aarp.org

William Novelli, Chief Executive Officer
Your copies of this brochure won't last long on your information counter.

7651 Older Adults with Developmental Disabilities: Optimizing Choice and Change
Brookes Publishing
PO Box 10624
Baltimore, MD 21285
410-337-9580
800-638-3775
FAX: 410-337-8539
e-mail: custserv@brookespublishing.com
www.brookespublishing.com

Paul Brooks, Owner
$37.00
416 pages Paperback
ISBN 1-55766 -20-0

7652 On Your Behalf
CAREsource Program Development
505 Seattle Tower
Seattle, WA 98101
206-625-9128
800-448-5213
FAX: 206-682-2901
e-mail: service@caresource.com
www.caresource.com

Dennis Kenny, Owner
This book takes the mystery out of very important sets of legal options. It gives lay people as well as advisors, service providers, and caregivers the information they need to understand their options and the importance of individual choice.
16 pages Books & Video
ISBN 1-87886 -14-1

7653 Operation Help: A Mental Health Advocate Guide to Medicaid
Nat'l Council for Community Behavioral Healthcare
12300 Twinbrook Parkway
Suite 320
Rockville, MD 20852
301-984-6200
FAX: 301-881-7159
www.nccbh.org

Linda Rosenberg, Chief Executive Officer
Explains the Medicaid entitlement program in easy-to-understand language and focuses on the needs of adults with serious mental illness, children with serious emotional disturbance and elderly persons who need mental health care. *$17.00*

7654 Part B News
United Communications Group
11300 Rockville Pike
Rockville, MD 20852
301-816-8950
FAX: 301-816-8945
www.ucg.com
Washington news practical strategies for maximizing Medicare Part B.

7655 Perspective on Aging
National Council on the Aging
600 Maryland Avenue SW
Washington, DC 20024
202-479-1200
FAX: 202-479-0735

James Firman, Chief Executive Officer
Explores significant developments in the field of aging, including disabilities, through opinion articles, profiles and book reviews. *$4.00*

7656 Perspectives on Prevention and Treatment of Cancer in the Elderly
Lippincott, Williams & Wilkins
227 E Washington Square
Philadelphia, PA 19106
215-521-8300
800-777-2295
FAX: 301-824-7390
www.lpub.com

J Lippincott, Chief Executive Officer
This book presents an exchange of ideas and information on the complexities of cancer and aging. Clinicians and investigators from a wide range of pertinent disciplines highlight the issues unique to the elderly patient in cancer prevention, diagnosis and treatment. *$113.00*
360 pages

7657 Physical & Occupational Therapy in Geriatrics...Current Trends in Geriatrics Rehab
Haworth Press
10 Alice Street
Binghamton, NY 13904
607-722-5857
800-429-6784
FAX: 607-722-6362
e-mail: orders@haworthpress.com
www.haworthpress.com

Ellen Dunievey Taira OTR/L, Editor
Jodi Carison MS, OTR/L, Assistant Editor
S Harrington-Miller, Advertising
Focuses on current practices and emerging issues in the care of the older client, including long-term care in institutional and community settings, crisis intervention, and innovative programming; the entire range of problems experienced by the elderly; and the current skills needed for working with older clients.
Quarterly

7658 Prescriptions for Independence
American Foundation for the Blind/AFB Press
PO Box 1020
Sewickley, PA 15143
412-741-1142
800-232-3044
FAX: 412-741-0609
e-mail: afborders@abdintl.com
www.afb.org
Easy-to-read manual on how older visually impaired persons can pursue their interests and activities in community residences, senior centers, long-term care facilities and other community settings. Paperback. *$29.95*

ISBN 0-891282-44-0

7659 Rehabilitation in the Aging
Lippincott, Williams & Wilkins
227 E Washington Square
Philadelphia, PA 19106
215-521-8300
800-777-2295
FAX: 301-824-7390
www.lpub.com

J Lippincott, Chief Executive Officer
This volume provides the physician with a comprehensive approach to the medical and rehabilitative management of geriatric patients. *$82.50*
390 pages

7660 Senior Citizens and the Law
Center for Public Representation
PO Box 260049
Madison, WI 53726
608-251-4008
800-369-0388
FAX: 606-251-1263
e-mail: cpr@lawmail.law.wisc.edu
www.law.wisc.edu
An introduction to legal problems facing the elderly in Wisconsin. This edition discusses legal problems associated with Social Security, Medicare, SSI, guardianship and its alternatives, community-based services, probate, taxes, private health insurance and consumer protection. *$5.00*

ISBN 0-936226-15-1

7661 So Many of My Friends Have Moved Away or Died
AARP Fulfillment
601 E Street NW
Washington, DC 20049
202-434-2277
800-424-3410
FAX: 202-434-3443
e-mail: member@aarp.org
www.aarp.org

William Novelli, Chief Executive Officer
A typical problem faced by older persons, discussion focuses on coping with the loss of old friends and finding new ones.

7662 Social Security Bulletin
US Social Security Administration
4301 Connecticut Avenue NW
Room 209
Washington, DC 20008
202-523-0588
800-772-1213
FAX: 202-282-7219
www.ssa.gov/policy

Reports on results of research and analysis pertinent to the Social Security and SSI programs. *$16.00*

Monthly

7663 Social Security, Medicare, and Pensions
NOLO
950 Parker Street
Berkeley, CA 94710
510-549-1976
800-955-4775
FAX: 510-548-5902
www.nolo.com

Maira Dizgalvis, Trade Customer Service Manager
Susan McConnell, Director Sales
Natasha Kaluza, Sales Assistant

A plain-speaking guide explaining the ins and outs of the Social Security system; retirement, disability and benefits for dependents and survivors. *$24.95*

320 pages paperback
ISBN 0-873374-87-8

7664 Successful Models of Community Long Term Care Services for the Elderly
Haworth Press
10 Alice Street
Binghamton, NY 13904
607-722-5857
800-429-6784
FAX: 607-722-6362
e-mail: orders@haworthpress.com
www.haworthpress.com

S Harroington-Miller, Advertising
William Cohen, Owner

Experienced practitioners provide examples of successful community-based long term care service programs for the elderly. *$ 74.95*

174 pages
ISBN 0-866569-87-1

7665 Therapeutic Interventions in Alzheimer's
Aspen Publishers
200 Orchard Ridge Drive
Gaithersburg, MD 20878
301-698-7100
800-234-1660
FAX: 301-695-7931
www.aspenpublishers.com

A program of functional skills for activities of daily living. Hardcover. *$65.00*

256 pages
ISBN 0-834209-30-6

7666 Topics in Geriatric Rehabilitation
Aspen Publishers
200 Orchard Ridge Drive
Gaithersburg, MD 20878
301-698-7100
800-638-8437
FAX: 301-695-7931
www.aspenpublishers.com

Peer-review journal presenting clinical, basic and applied research as well as theoretical information. Published quarterly. *$ 86.00*

90 pages

7667 Unloving Care
Harper Collins Publishers/Basic Books
10 E 53rd Street
New York, NY 10022
212-207-7000
800-242-7737
FAX: 212-207-7203

Jane Friedman, Chief Executive Officer

A leading public health expert gives a definitive account of what nursing homes are really like. *$9.95*

305 pages
ISBN 0-46508 -81-3

7668 Victims of Dementia: Services, Support and Care
Haworth Press
10 Alice Street
Binghamton, NY 13904
607-722-5857
800-429-6784
FAX: 607-722-6362
e-mail: orders@haworthpress.com
www.haworthpress.com

S Harrington-Miller, Advertising
William Cohen, Owner

Provides an in-depth look at the concept, construction and operation of Wesley Hall, a special living area at the Chelsea United Methodist retirement home in Michigan. *$74.95*

155 pages Hardcover
ISBN 1-560242-64-7

7669 Vision and Aging: Issues in Social Work Practice
Haworth Press
10 Alice Street
Binghamton, NY 13904
607-722-5857
800-429-6784
FAX: 607-722-6362
e-mail: orders@haworthpress.com
www.haworthpress.com

S Harrington-Miller, Advertising
William Cohen, Owner

Responds to the needs of the growing population of blind or severely disabled elderly. *$74.95*

196 pages Hardcover
ISBN 1-560241-99-3

7670 Visually Impaired Seniors as Senior Companions: A Reference Guide
American Foundation for the Blind/AFB Press
PO Box 1020
Sewickley, PA 15143
412-741-1142
800-232-3044
FAX: 412-741-0609
e-mail: afborders@abdintl.com
www.afb.org

This useful guide describes the Senior Companion Program that is intended to broaden opportunities for older persons with disabilities. Appendix includes training materials, evaluation forms, recruitment and public relations information. *$15.00*

108 pages Paperback
ISBN 0-891282-38-6

7671 Work, Health and Income Among the Elderly
Brookings Institution
1775 Massachusetts Avenue NW
Washington, DC 20036
202-797-6000
FAX: 202-797-6004
e-mail: bibooks@brookings.edu
www.brookings.edu

Strobe Talbott, President

Employment, health and financial information for the elderly. *$26.95*

318 pages Cloth
ISBN 0-815774-97-4

Associations

7672 Academy of Dispensing Audiologists
401 N Michigan Avenue
Suite 2200
Chicago, IL 60611
866-493-5544
FAX: 312-673-6725
e-mail: info@audiologist.org
www.audiologist.org

Larry Engelmann, President
David Berkey, President Elect
Susan Williamson, Secretary
The ADA is dedicated to leadership in advancing practitioner excellence, high ethical standards, professional autonomy, hearing technology, and sound business practices in the provision of quality audiological care.

7673 Academy of Rehabilitative Audiology
PO Box 26532
Minneapolis, MN 55426
952-920-0484
FAX: 952-920-6098
e-mail: ara@incnet.com
www.audrehab.org

Gabrielle Saunders, President
Patricia B. Kricos, President Elect
Jan Moore, Treasurer
Provides professional education, research and interest in programs for hearing handicapped persons. The primary purpose of the ARAÆis to promote excellence in hearing care through the provision of comprehensive rehabilitative and habilitative services.

7674 Alexander Graham Bell Association for the Deaf and Hard of Hearing
3417 Volta Place NW
Washington, DC 20007
202-337-5220
FAX: 202-337-8314
TTY:202-337-5221
e-mail: info@agbell.org
www.agbell.org

Karen Youdelman, President
John R. Wyant, President Elect/Treasurer
Jessica Ripper, Sr. Dir Marketing/Communications
The Alexander Graham Bell Association for the Deaf and Hard of Hearing (AG Bell) is the world's oldest and largest membership organization promoting the use of spoken language by children and adults who are hearing impaired. Members include parents of children with hearing loss, adults who are deaf or hard of hearing, educators, audiologists, speech-language pathologists, physicians and other professionals in fields related to hearing loss and deafness.

7675 American Society for Deaf Children
3820 Hartzdale Drive
Camp Hill, PA 17011
717-703-0073
800-942-2732
FAX: 717-909-5599
TTY: 916-641-6084
e-mail: ascd@deafchildren.org
www.deafchildren.org

Natalie Long, President
ASDC was founded in 1967 as a parent-helping-parents organization. Today, ASDC is a national, independent non-profit organization whose purpose is providing support, encouragement, and information to families raising children who are deaf or hard of hearing.
1967

7676 American Speech-Language-Hearing Association
10801 Rockville Pike
Rockville, MD 20852
240-638-8255
888-498-6699
FAX: 240-333-4705
e-mail: actioncenter@asha.org
www.asha.org

Lawrence W Higdon, President
Arlene Pietranton, Executive Director
Roberta B Aungst, VP
Provides information for both the general public and physicians in an easy-to-access manner, on speech, hearing and language disorders. Exhibits by companies specializing in alternative and augmentative communications products, publishers, software and hardware companies, and hearing aid testing equipment manufacturers.

7677 American Tinnitus Association
PO Box 5
Portland, OR 97207
503-248-9985
800-634-8978
FAX: 503-248-0024
e-mail: tinnitus@ata.org
www.ata.org

David P. Fagerlie, Chief Executive Officer
Terri Baltus, Chief Development Officer
Helen Connor, Director Of Marketing
The American Tinnitus Association (ATA) is the national champion of tinnitus awareness, prevention, and treatment. Under its guiding principles—Education, Advocacy, Research and Support—the ATA offers prevention programs in schools, urges governmental and private organizations to support hearing conservation, funds the nation's brightest researchers, and facilitates self-help groups around the country.

7678 Arena Stage
11101 Sixth Street
Washington, DC 20024
202-554-9066
FAX: 202-484-6279
e-mail: info@arenastage.org
www.arenastage.org

Thomas C Fichandler, Founding Executive Director
Stephen Richard, Chief Executive Officer
A pioneer in providing access to theater for people with disabilities and the birthplace of Audio Description. Offers infrared assistive listening devices (both loop and headset), program books in Braille, large print and wheelchair accessible seating with adjacent companion seating. Audio cassette format available upon request. Sign Interpretation and Audio Description are offered at selected performances. Cafe menus and shop lists in Braille. Wheelchair-accessible with lifts and ramps.

7679 Arkansas Rehabilitation Research and Training Center for the Deaf and Hard of Hearing
University Of Arkansas
26 Corporate Hill Drive
Little Rock, AR 72205
501-686-9691
FAX: 501-686-9698
TTY:501-686-9691
e-mail: rehabres@cavern.uark.edu
www.uark.edu/deafrtc

Douglas Watson, Prof. & Project Director
Glenn Anderson, Prof. & Director Of Training
Steven Boone, Prof. & Director Of Research
Focuses on issues affecting the employability of deaf and hard of hearing rehabilitation clients; career assessment, career mobility, and advancement. Provides information and/or databases related to the rehabilitation of deaf and hard of hearing people served by the Federal/State Vocational Rehabilitation Program.

7680 Association of Late-Deafened Adults
8038 MacIntosh Lane
Rockford, IL 61107
815-332-1515
866-402-2532
e-mail: alda@alda.org
www.alda.org

Bernie Palmer, President
Christine Seymour, President Elect
Matt Ferrara, Treasurer
Provides resources, information, and advocacy of the needs of deafened adults. Publishes ALDA News.

7681 Better Hearing Institute
515 King Street
Suite 420
Alexandria, VA 22314
703-684-3391
888-432-7453
FAX: 703-684-6048
e-mail: mail@betterhearing.org
www.betterhearing.org

Sergei Kochkin PhD, Executive Director
Sasha Ward, Administrative Director
The BHI is a not-for-profit corporation that educates the public about the neglected problem of hearing loss and what can be done about it. Founded in 1973 we are working to erase the stigma and end the embarassment that prevents millions of people from seeking help for hearing loss and show the negative consequences of untreated hearing loss for millions of Americans. And to promote treatment and demonstrate that this is a national problem that can be solved.

7682 Boys Town National Research Hospital
555 N 30th Street
Omaha, NE 68131
402-498-6520
FAX: 402-498-6638
e-mail: peb@boystown.org
www.boystownhospital.org

Patricia G. Stelmachowicz, Director, Audiological Services
Michael P. Gorga PhD, Director. Human Sensory Physiol.
Kathryn Beauchaine M.S., Coordinator Audiological Serv.
The Audiology Center provides comprehensive audiological services to patients both young and old. Close ties between research and clinical programs at the research hospital have resulted in state-of-the-art services. The hospital is designed as a child-friendly environment, with specialized techniques to test infants and young children. A wide range of services is availiable for adults as well. Regardless of age, a hearing evaluation is essential to determine the best course of treatment.

7683 Caption Center
125 Western Avenue
Boston, MA 02134
617-300-3600
FAX: 617-300-1020
e-mail: access@wgbh.org
www.wgbh.org/caption

Larry Goldberg, Director
Tom Apone, Director Of Operations
Mary Alice Holmes, Director Of Finance
Has been pioneering and delivering accessible media to disabled adults, students and their families, teachers and friends for over 30 years. Each year, the Center captions more than 10,000 hours worth of broadcast and cable programs, feature films, large-format and IMAX films, home videos, music videos, DVDs, teleconferences and CD-Roms.

7684 Captioned Media Program
National Association of the Deaf
1447 E Main Street
Spartanburg, SC 29307
864-585-1778
800-237-6819
FAX: 864-585-2611
TTY:864 585 2617
e-mail: info@dcmp.org
www.cfv.org

Bill Stark, Project Director
Provides open-captioned media on a free-loan basis to deaf and hard of hearing persons, parents and teachers of hard of hearing children and groups/organizations that serve deaf and hard of hearing persons. Over 4,000 titles in our collection and media is available via mail (postage paid both ways) and through Internet streaming via our website.

7685 Center on Employment
National Technical Institute For The Deaf (NTID)
52 Lomb Memorial Drive
Rochester, NY 14623
585-475-6219
FAX: 585-475-7570
e-mail: ntidcoe@rit.edu
www.rit.edu/ntid/coop/jobs

Allen Vaala, Director
Donna Becker
Kathy Dollinger
The NTID Center on Employment is a resource for employers seeking qualified, technically trained college graduates and coops/interns who are deaf. Some 1,100 students from all over the U.S. study at NTID, and the seven other colleges of Rochester Institute of Technology, in programs at various degree levels in Business. Computing and Information Sciences, the Graphic Arts and Science and Engineering.

7686 Cochlear Implant Club International
5335 Wisconsin Avenue NW
Suite 440
Washington, DC 20015
202-895-2781
FAX: 202-895-2782
e-mail: info@cici.org

John McCelland, President
Not-for-profit voluntary organization dedicated to serving implant users, candidates, their families and professional supporters. Purposes are to promote opportunities afforded by the use of cochlear implants through mutual sharing of ideas and personal experiences; enhance community awareness of hearing impairment and to promote better understanding of implants; and to promote improved financial support. Publishes educational materials including a newsletter, brochures, and audiovisual aids.

7687 Communication Service for the Deaf (CSD)
102 N Krohn Place
Sioux Falls, SD 57103
605-367-5760
800-642-6410
FAX: 605-367-5958
TTY: 605-367-5761
e-mail: rnorris@c-s-d.org
www.c-s-d.org

Barbara Forinash, Director Human Resources
Rick Postl, Director National Programs
Since 1975, CSD has provided a variety of services to deaf and hard of hearing individuals. From relay services to community interpreting, advocacy to education, CSD promotes self-actualization, professional growth, independence and greater access for our consumers across the country.
1975

7688 Conference of Educational Administrators Serving the Deaf
PO Box 1778
St Augustine, FL 32085
904-810-5200
FAX: 904-810-5525
e-mail: email@ceasd.org
www.ceasd.org

James E. Tucker, President
Ed Bosso, President-Elect
Michael J. Bello, Treasurer
CEASD provides an opportunity for professional educators to work together for the improvement of schools and educational programs for individuals who are deaf or hard of hearing. The organization brings together a rich composite of resources and reaches out to both enhance educational programs and influence educational policy makers.

7689 Council of American Instructors of the Deaf
PO Box 377
Bedford, TX 76095
817-354-8414
FAX: 817-354-8414
e-mail: caid@swbell.net
www.caid.org

Kathy Obenhaus, President
Larry Quinsland, Vice President
Joseph Stanslow, Treasurer
The mission of the Council of the American Instructors of the Deaf, Incorporated is to focus on an organizaion of teachers and other education related personnel to promote student learning and development by bringing together local, state, regional, and national interest organizations.

7690 Davis Center for Hearing, Speech and Learning: Hearing Therapy
200 Valley Road
Suite 205
Mt. Arlington, NJ 07856
973-398-2710
FAX: 973-398-2721
e-mail: info@daviscenter.net
www.thedaviscenter.com

Dorinne S Davis MA, CCC-A, FAAA, Director
Laura Darby, Sound Therapist
Janine Ruth MA, Child Development Specialist
The Davis Center's Sound Therapy Programs make positive changes for children and adults with Autism, ADD/ADHD, Auditory Processing Issues, Dyslexia, Learning Disabilities and other learning challenges. Our programs adress issues such as: phonics, spelling, writing, reading comprehension, hearing only parts of words, following directions, discriminating between sounds, sound sensitivity, behavioral responses, focus, attention and more.

7691 **Deaf REACH**
3521 12th Street NE
Washington, DC 20017
202-832-6681
FAX: 202-832-8454
e-mail: info@deaf-reach.org
www.deaf-reach.org

Rudy Gawlik, President
Peter Goodman, VP
Mary Jane Tyler, Secretary
The psychosocial rehabilitation approach, ulitzed by all Deaf-REACH programs, provides the solid foundation to member's success. Participants are activly involved in establishing the format and level of highly individualized service delivery that they receive. The concept, which has achieved national acclaim, involves teaching members necessary life skills, thus minimizing the need for assistance from a service professional. This is part of what distinguishes the approach at Deaf-REACH.

7692 **Deafness Research Foundation**
280 Park Avenue
Fl 35
New York, NY 10017
617-426-7080
FAX: 212-672-7080
e-mail: info@drf.org
www.drf.org

Angelo Damante, Founder And President
Richard A. Uzuanis, Vice President
Collette Baker, Founder
Founded in 1958, the Deafness Research Foundation is the leading source of private funding for basic and clinical research in the hearing science. The DRF is committed to making lifelong hearing health a national priority by funding research and implementing education projects in both the government and private sectors.
1958

7693 **Deafness and Communicative Disorders Branch of Rehab Services Administration Office**
Special Education And Rehab Services
400 Maryland Avenue SW
Washington, DC 20202
202-245-7489
800-872-5327
FAX: 202-205-9340
TTY: 800-437-0833
e-mail: customerservice@inet.ed.gov
www.ed.gov

Clare Cotton, Chairperson
Promotes improved rehabilitation services for deaf and hard of hearing people and individuals with speech or language impairments. Provides technical assistance to public and private agencies and individuals.

7694 **Dogs for the Deaf**
10175 Wheeler Road
Central Point, OR 97502
541-826-9220
FAX: 541-826-6696
TTY:541-826-9220
e-mail: info@dogsforthedeaf.org
www.dogsforthedeaf.org

Robin Dickson, CEO and President
Trains hearing dogs to alert deaf persons to certain sounds. Dogs are chosen from pet adoption shelters and assigned on the basis of a prioritized waiting list. Five to six months of training teaches them to alert their masters to the sounds of alarm clocks, smoke alarms, doorbells, oven timers, telephones, etc.

7695 **Ear Foundation**
Po Box 330867
Nashville, TN 37203
615-627-2724
800-545-4327
FAX: 615-627-2728
TTY: 615-284-7807
e-mail: amy@earfoundation.org
www.earfoundation.org

Michael E. Glasscock, President Emeritus/Founder
Steve Masie, Chair
Vic Alexander, Treasurer
National, nonprofit organization committed to integrating the hearing and balance impaired into the mainstream of society through public awareness and medical education. Also administers The Meniere's Network, a national network of patient support groups providing people with the opportunity to share experiences and coping strategies.

7696 **Episcopal Conference of the Deaf**
475 N 5th Street
Philadelphia, PA 19123
215-247-1059
FAX: 215-247-1059
TTY:610-408-9747
e-mail: bmose@aol.com
www.ecdeaf.com

Rev Dcn Bill Moiser, President
Rev Barbara Allen, First Vice President
Rev Carla McCook, Second Vice President
Promotes ministry for deaf people throughout the Episcopal Church. Affiliated with approximately 65 congregations in the United States. Publishes The Deaf Episcopalian. *$10.00*
8-12 pages Quarterly

7697 **Gallaudet University Alumni Association**
Gallaudet University
800 Florida Avenue NE
Washington, DC 20002
202-651-5300
FAX: 202-651-5477
TTY:202-651-5000
e-mail: infotech.services@gallaudet.edu
www.gallaudet.edu

Erving Jordan, President
Represents more than 14,000 alumni of Gallaudet University across the United States and around the world. A liberal arts university for students who are deaf or hard of hearing. Publishes Gallaudet Today.

7698 **Georgiana Institute**
PO Box 10
Roxbury, CT 06783
860-355-1545
FAX: 860-355-1560
e-mail: georgianainstitute@snet.net
www.georgianainstitute.org

Annabel Stehli
Peter Stehli, Manager
Organization promoting Auditory Integration Training in the USA.

7699 **HEAR Center**
301 E Del Mar Boulevard
Pasadena, CA 91101
626-796-2016
FAX: 626-796-2320
e-mail: auditory@hearcenter.org
www.hearcenter.org

Josephine Wilson, Executive Director
Auditory and verbal program designed to help hearing impaired children, infants and adults lead normal and productive lives. Seeks to develop auditory techniques to aid people who have communication problems due to deafness. Offers diagnostic evaluations for speech and hearing. Individual auditory, verbal training and speech-language therapy.

7700 **Health Resource Center**
American Council On Education
1 Dupont Circle NW
Washington, DC 20036
202-939-9300
800-544-3284
FAX: 202-833-4760
e-mail: comments@ace.nche.edu
www.acenet.edu

David Ward, President
Terry Hartle, Senior Vice President
Brian Jenkins, Director
Offers publications and a telephone service of use to administrators, service providers, teachers, instructors, rehabilitation counselors, health professionals and individuals with disabilities and their families.

7701 Hear Now
9745 E Hampden Avenue
Suite 300
Denver, CO 80231
303-695-7797
800-648-4327
Committed to making technology accessible to deaf and hard of hearing individuals throughout the United States. Provides hearing aids and cochlear implants for very low income, hard of hearing and deaf individuals.

7702 Hearing Education and Awareness for Rockers
PO Box 760847
San Francisco, CA 94146
415-409-3277
FAX: 415-409-5683
e-mail: orders@hearnet.com
www.hearnet.com

Kathy Peck, Executive Director/Co Founder
Flash Gordon MD, Co-Founder
Jerome Goldstein Dr., Senior Executive Vice President
H.E.A.R. is a non-profit volunteer organization dedicated to raising awarensss of the real dangers of repeated exposure to excessive noise levels from music which can lead to permanent, and sometimes debilitating, hearing loss and tinnitus.

7703 House Ear Institute
2100 W 3rd Street
Los Angeles, CA 90057
213-483-4431
800-388-8612
FAX: 213-484-2642
e-mail: webmaster@hei.org
www.hei.org

Jim Boswell, CEO
Howard House, MD
Offers pediatric hearing tests, otologic and audiologic evaluation and treatment, rehabilitation, hearing aid dispensing, and cochlear implant services. Outreach programs focus on families with hearing impaired children.

7704 International Catholic Deaf Association
7202 Buchanan Street
Landover Hills, MD 20784
301-429-0697
FAX: 301-429-0698
e-mail: homeoffice@icda-us.org
www.icda-us.org

James Kelly, Treasurer
Peter Un, President
Brian Swatek, VP
Responds to spiritual-related requests worldwide from deaf or hard of hearing Catholics.

7705 International Hearing Dog
5901 E 89th Avenue
Henderson, CO 80640
303-287-3277
FAX: 303-287-3425
TTY:303-287-3277
e-mail: ihdi@aol.com
www.ihdi.org

Martha Foss-Brugger, President and Director
Trains dogs to assist deaf and hearing impaired persons by alerting to smoke alarms, alarm clocks, telephones, doorbells, babies, etc.

7706 International Hearing Society
16880 Middlebelt Road
Suite 4
Livonia, MI 48154
734-522-7200
800-521-5247
FAX: 734-522-0200
www.ihsinfo.org

James Ogurek, President
Chris Gustafson, President Elect
Larry Farris, Secretary
The IHSis the professional association that represents Hearing Instrument Specialists worldwide. IHS members are engaged in the practice of testing human hearing and selecting, fitting and dispensing hearing instruments. Founded in 1951, the Society continues to recognize the need for promoting and maintaining the highest possible standards for its members in the best interestof the hearing impaired it serves.

7707 International Lutheran Deaf Association
1333 S Kirkwood Road
Saint Louis, MO 63122
314-965-9917
800-433-3954
FAX: 314-965-9000
www.lcmsdeaf.org/ilda

Pam Kane, President
Greg Desrosiers, President-Elect
Jennifer Bonura, Secretary
An organization that is committed to spreading the gospel of Jesus Christ among deaf and hard of hearing people through mission work in the United States and around the world. The main focus of ILDA is to support Lutheran mission work with deaf people in other countries.
1971

7708 John Tracy Clinic
806 W Adams Boulevard
Los Angeles, CA 90007
213-748-5481
800-522-4582
FAX: 213-749-1651
TTY: 213-747-2924
e-mail: mmartindale@jtc.org
www.jtc.org

Barbara Hecht PhD, President
Kevin Matthews, VP, Finance And Administration
Mary Ann Bell, Vp, Developmant & Communications
Educational facility for infants and preschool-aged children who have hearing losses and their families. In addition to on-site services, worldwide correspondence courses in English and Spanish are offered to parents whose children are preschool age and are hard of hearing, deaf, or deaf-blind. All services of JTC are free of charge to the families. The Clinic also offers on site and online Master's Degrees in Deaf Education with USC.

7709 Junior National Association of the Deaf
8630 Fenton Street
Suite 820
Silver Spring, MD 20910
301-587-1788
FAX: 301-587-1791
TTY:301-587-1789
e-mail: nadinfo@nad.org
www.nad.org

Rosaline H. Crawford, Director
Anita B Farb, Director of Outreach
Marc P. Charmatz, Attorney
Develops and promotes citizenship, scholarship, and leadership skills in deaf and hard of hearing students of grades 7 through 12.

7710 League for the Hard of Hearing
50 Broadway
Floor 6
New York, NY 10004
917-305-7700
FAX: 917-305-7888
e-mail: appointments@lhh.org
www.lhh.org

Laurie Hanin PhD, CCC-A, Executive Director
Ellen Lafargue AuD., CCC-A, Director, Audiology
Anita Myers AuD, CCC-A, Assistant Director, Audiology
National diagnostic rehabilitation, human services agency founded in 1910. Offers comprehensive services for infants, children and adults with hearing loss regardless of age or mode of communication. Clinical programs iclude Tinnitus Center and Cochlear Implant evaluation, consultation, auditory training. LHH also offers extensive public education programs, advocacy, support and publications.

1910

7711 **Lexington School for the Deaf: Center for the Deaf**
30th Avenue and 75th Street
Jackson Heights, NY 11370
718-350-3300
FAX: 718-899-1621
e-mail: generalinfo@lexnyc.org
www.lexnyc.org

Regina Carroll PhD, Superintendent/CEO
Adele Agin, C.S.W, Executive Director
Joanna Roufous M.A. CCC-A, Executive Director
Offers a comprehensive range of services to deaf, hard of hearing and speech impaired persons from infancy to elderly through its affiliate agencies: The Center for Mental Health Services; The Lexington Hearing and Speech Center, Lexington Vocational Services, and the Lexington School for the Deaf. The Lexington Center also provides services through its research division which houses the only federally funded Rehabilitation Engineering Center.

7712 **Michigan Association for Deaf and Hard of Hearing**
2929 Covington Court
Suite 200
Lansing, MI 48912
517-487-0066
800-968-7327
FAX: 517-487-0202
TTY: 517-487-2586
e-mail: yourear@madhh.org
www.madhh.org

Nancy Asher, Executive Director
Dave Coyne, Program Coordinator
SaDonna White, Interpreter/Project Coordinator
Substance abuse and anti violence prevention videos for deaf and hard of hearing students (alcohol, marijuana, inhalants) acted in sign language, voicing and captioning. HIV/AIDS prevention and information for the deaf and hard of hearing. Lending library books, videos and audio tapes. Accessibility to courts video and information. TTY distribution program.

7713 **National Association of the Deaf**
814 Thayer Avenue
Suite 250
Silver Spring, MD 20910
301-587-1788
FAX: 301-587-1791
TTY:301-587-1789
e-mail: NADinfo@nad.org
www.nad.org

Nancy J Bloch, CEO
Kelby Brick, Director Law and Advocacy
Anita B Farb, Director Communications
Nation's largest organization safeguarding the accessability and civil rights of 28 million deaf and hard of hearing Americans in education, employment, health care, and telecommunications. Focuses on grassroots advocacy and empowerment, captioned media deafness-related information and publications, legal assistance, and policy development.

7714 **National Black Deaf Advocates**
PO Box 22846
Rochester, NY 14692
585-475-2411
800-421-1220
FAX: 585-475-6500
e-mail: president@nbda.org
www.nbda.org

Albert Simone, President
Claudia Gordon, VP
The Mission of the National Black Deaf Advocate is to promote the leadership development, economic and educational opportunities, social equality, and to safeguard the general health and welfare of Black deaf and hard of hearing people.

7715 **National Captioning Institute**
1900 Gallows Road
Suite 3000
Vienna, VA 22182
703-917-7600
FAX: 703-917-9853
TTY:703-917-7600
e-mail: mail@ncicap.org
www.ncicap.org

Gene Chao, President & CEO
Mary Presswood, Corporate Secretary
Tina Cooper, Director Of Finance & Accounting
Formed in 1979, the nonprofit National Captioning Institute is the global captioning leader, supplying the highest quality closed-captioning services to the television, cable, and home video industries.
1979

7716 **National Catholic Office of the Deaf**
7202 Buchanan Street
Landover Hills, MD 20784
301-577-1684
FAX: 301-577-1684
TTY:301-577-4184
e-mail: info@ncod.org
www.ncod.org

Arvilla Rank, Executive Director
Helps coordinate efforts of deaf or hard of hearing people who are involved in the ministry, acts as a resource center, assists bishops and pastors become available to the deaf and hard of hearing.

7717 **National Deaf Education Network and Clearinghouse**
Gallaudet University
800 Florida Avenue NE
Washington, DC 20002
202-651-5051
FAX: 202-651-5044
TTY:202-651-5052
e-mail: clearinghouse@infotogo@gallaudet.edu
www.clerccenter.gallaudet.edu

Katherine A. Jankowsi Dr., Dean
Ms. Janne M. Harrelson, Director
Margaret Hallau Dr., Director
Committed to developing the full potential of deaf and hard of hearing students from diverse linguistic and cultural backgrounds who have a variety of abilities, skills, and experiences. Our goal is to provide an education that is academically challenging and fully accessable, where students develop a positive sense of self-worth and broad-based literacy. This includes the knowledge, skills and attitudes necessary to function as successful, independent, contributing members of society.

7718 **National Fraternal Society of the Deaf**
1118 S 6th Street
Springfield, IL 62703
217-789-7429
FAX: 217-789-7489
TTY:217-789-7438
e-mail: thefrat@nfsd.com
www.nfsd.com

Al Nevel, President
Christopher McQuaid, Chairman
Work in the area of life insurance and advocacy for deaf people. Has 75 divisions across the country.

7719 **National Institute on Deafness and Other Communication Disorders (NIDCD)**
31 Center Drive
MSC 2320
Bethesda, MD 20892
301-496-7243
800-241-1044
FAX: 301-402-0018
TTY: 301-402-0252
e-mail: wengeri@nidcd.nih.gov
www.nidcd.nih.gov

Patricia Blessing, Chief OHCPL/NIDCD
James F. Battey Jr., Director
The NIDCD Information Clearinghouse is a national resource center for health information about hearing, balance, smell, taste, voice, speech and language for health professionals, patients, industry and the public.

7720 **National Rehabilitation Information Center (NARIC)**
4200 Forbes Boulevard
Suite 202
Lanham, MD 20706
301-459-5900
800-346-2742
FAX: 301-459-4263
TTY: 301-459-5984
e-mail: naricinfo@heitechservices.com
www.naric.com

Mark Odum, Director
Provides information and referral services on disability and rehabilitation, including quick information and referral, database searches of the bibliographic database REHABDATA, and document delivery.

7721 National Technical Institute for the Deaf
52 Lomb Memorial Drive
Rochester, NY 14623
585-475-6700
866-644-6843
FAX: 585-475-2696
TTY: 585-475-6400
e-mail: ntidmc@rit.edu
www.rit.edu/ntid

T Alan Hurwitz, VP and Dean
Linda L. Hoke, Assistant To Vice President
Donald H. Bell, Executive Assistant To VP
Provides technological postsecondary education to deaf and hard-of-hearing students. One of eight colleges of Rochester Institute of Technology.

7722 National Theatre of the Deaf
139 North Main Street
West Hartford, CT 06107
860-236-4193
FAX: 860-236-4163
TTY:860-236-4193
e-mail: ntd-info@ntd.org
www.ntd.org

Paul Winters, Executive Director
Professional development of deaf actors, national theatrical touring company of deaf and hearing actors.

7723 Registry of Interpreters for the Deaf
333 Commerce Street
Alexandria, VA 22314
703-838-0030
FAX: 703-838-0454
TTY:703-838-0459
e-mail: info@rid.org
www.rid.org

Clay Nettles, Executive Director
Matthew O'Hara, Director Of Finance & Administ.
Caroline Kemper, Accountant
A membership organization with over 7,000 members, including professional interpreters and translators, individuals who are deaf or hard of hearing, and professionals in related fields.

7724 Rehabilitation Engineering Research Center on Hearing Enhancement and Assistive Devices
Lexington School for the Deaf/Center for the Deaf
800 Florida Avenue NE
Washington, DC 20002
202-651-5335
FAX: 202-651-5324
TTY:202-651-5335
e-mail: rerc.he@gmail.com
www.hearingresearch.org

Matthew Bakke Ph.D, Director
Arlene C. Neuman Ph.D, Director
Stephanie Adamovich, M.S., Staff
The Rehabilitation Engineering Center (RERC) on Hearing Enhancement is a national project funded by the United States Department of Education, National Institute on Disability and Rehabilitation Research (NIDRR) in the Office of Special Education and Rehabilitation Services (OSERS). The objective of the project is to conduct research programs that promote technological solutions to problems confronting people who are hard of hearing.

7725 Rehabilitation Research & Training Center for Persons Who Are Hard of Hearing or Deafened
California School Of Professional Psychology
6160 Cornerstone Ct E
San Diego, CA 92121
858-623-2777
800-432-7619
FAX: 858-642-0266
e-mail: ckrirschner@allient.edu
www.hknc.org

Focuses on conducting research and developing training programs related to employment and personal adjustment of individuals who are hard of hearing or late deafened.

7726 SEE Center for the Advancement of Deaf Children
PO Box 1181
Los Alamitos, CA 90720
562-430-1467
FAX: 562-795-6614
e-mail: seecenter@seecenter.org
www.seecenter.org

Esther Zawolkow, Executive Director
Information and referral for parents and educators of deafness-related topics and Signing Exact English (SEE).

7727 Self Help for Hard of Hearing People
7910 Woodmont Avenue
Suite 1200
Bethesda, MD 20814
301-657-2248
FAX: 301-913-9413
TTY:301-657-2249
e-mail: info@hearingloss.org
www.hearingloss.org

Terry Portis Ed.D, Executive Director
Barbara Kelley, Editor-In-Chief
Toni Barrient, Director Of Member Services
A nonprofit, educational organization that is dedicated to the well-being of people of all ages and communication styles who do not hear well. SHHH is the largest international consumer organization of its kind.

7728 Sound, Listening, and Learning Center
1635 E. Seldon Lane
Suite A107
Phoenix, AZ 85012
602-381-0086
FAX: 602-957-6741
e-mail: soundlisten@soundlistening.com
www.soundlistening.com

Billie M. Thompson, Ph.D, President
Kirk D. Thompson Ph.D., P.E, Vice President
Sound Listening & Learning Center provides the Tomatis Method, a truly transformative program of sound stimulation, audio-vocal activities, and consultation using patented equipment. The Method focuses on our most basic skill—listening. How we listen to ourselves and others profoundly affects our learning, speech/language, communication, thoughts, feelings, and relationships.

7729 Telecommunications for the Deaf (TDI)
8630 Fenton Street
Suite 604
Silver Spring, MD 20910
301-589-3786
FAX: 301-589-3797
TTY:301-589-3006
e-mail: info@tdi-online.org
www.tdi-online.org

Roy Miller, President
Joseph Duarte, Vice President
Tom Driscoll, Secretary
Promoting equal access to telecommunications and media for people who are deaf, late-deafened, hard of hearing or deaf-blind through consumer education and involvement; technical assistance and consulting; applications of exisiting and emerging technologies; networking and collaboration; uniformity of standards; and national policy development and advocacy.

7730 Vestibular Disorders Association
Vestibular Disorders Association
PO Box 13305
Portland, OR 97213
503-229-7705
800-837-8428
FAX: 503-229-8064
e-mail: veda@vestibular.org
www.vestibular.org

Elizabeth A Commerford MSW, President
Al Bowman DPT, Vice President
Claire Haddad CFA, Treasurer
Provides information and support for people with inner-ear vestibular disorders and the professionals who treat them, and develops awareness of the issues surrounding these disorders.

1987

7731 WRAD
PO Box 3211
Quartz Hill, CA 93586
FAX: 805-943-6112
TTY:805-943-8879
e-mail: wradceo@aol.com

Bruce Gross, President/CEO
WRAD represents the community of persons that are deaf or hard of hearing and all of its subgroups. People who were formerly greatly restricted by deafness, and who believed there was no possible remediation for deafness or way for inclusion into general society, now have laws, technologies, and better opportunities for success and achievement. WRAD provides the needed advocacy and resources for this community.

Camps

7732 Bishopswood
Diocese of Maine Episcopal
143 State Street
Portland, ME 04101
207-772-1953
FAX: 207-773-0095
e-mail: gkoch@diomaine.org
www.diomaine.org

Georgia L Koch, Director
Heidi Shott, Press Officer/Communications
Elizabeth Ring, Director Resource Center
Camp is located in Hope, Maine. One to seven-week sessions for hearing impaired children June-August. Coed, ages 7-16.

7733 CHAMP Camp
St Vincent Children s Specialty Hospital
700 N. High School Rd
Indianapolis, IN 46240
317-679-1860
FAX: 317-536-8860
e-mail: admin@champcamp.org
www.champcamp.org

David Carter, Co-Founder
Brian Burhenn, Camp Director
Deb Wagner, Manager
Camp in Cleveland, Ohio for children with hearing impairment, developmental disabilities, speech/communication impairment and visual impairment/blindness.

7734 Camp Capella
United Cerebral Palsy of Maine
700 Mount Hope Avenue
Suite 320
Bangor, ME 04401
207-941-2952
FAX: 207-941-2955
e-mail: ucp2@midmaine.org
www.ucp.org

Tricia Kail, Director of Services
Bobbi Jo Yeager, Executive Director
Stephanie Cote, Public Relations/Development
Provides an opportunity for children with disabilities to engage in various recreational and social experiences.

7735 Camp Comeca
Overlook Lodge
75670 Road 417
Cozad, NE 69130
308-784-2808
FAX: 308-784-4208
e-mail: comeca@cozadtel.net
www.campcomeca.com

Mary Garner, Director
Chic Garner, Directors
Charles Garner, Manager
Camp is located in Cozad, Nebraska. Summer sessions for campers with diabetes and hearing impairment. Coed, ages 6-19, families, seniors, single adults.

7736 Camp El Camino Pines
Lutheran Retreats
PO Box 3288
Camarillo, CA 93011
818-243-8700
800-464-2417
FAX: 818-243-2700
e-mail: anthony@lrcchome.com
www.lrccsca.org

Anthony Briggs, Executive Director
Glen Egertson, Camp Director
Chris Smith, Program Director
Camp is located in Frazier Park, California. Christian camp offering half-week and one-week sessions for hearing impaired campers. Coed, ages 8-18. Also families.

7737 Camp Emanuel
P O Box 2146
Dayton, OH 45401
937-278-2928
e-mail: Info@CampEmanuel.org
www.campemanuel.org/

Nan Crawford, Executive Director
Douglas Lehrer, MD, President
James Brink, Vice President/Treasurer
Camp for hearing impaired and normal hearing youth.

7738 Camp Isola Bella
American School for the Deaf
139 North Main Street
West Hartford, CT 06107
860-570-2300
FAX: 860-824-4276
TTY:860-570-2222
e-mail: Steve.Borsotti@asd-1817.org
www.asd-1817.org

Harvey J Corson, Executive Director
Steve Borsotti, Director
Carleton Mowell, President
Hearing-impaired children, ages 6-19, blend educational instruction in communications with recreational activities. Qualified deaf and hearing staff members with experience in education, child care and counseling are employed at the camp.

7739 Camp Joy
3325 Swamp Creek Road
Schwenksville, PA 19473
610-754-6878
FAX: 610-754-7880
e-mail: campjoy@fast.net
www.campjoy.com

Angus Murray, Camp Director
A special needs camp for kids and adults (ages 4-80+) with developmental disabilities such as: mental retardation, autism, brain injury, neurological disorder, visual and/or hearing impairments, Angelman and Down syndromes, and other developmental disabilities.

7740 Camp Mark Seven
Mark Seven Deaf Foundation
144 Mohawk Hotel Road
Old Forge, NY 13420
315-357-6089
FAX: 315-357-6403
e-mail: execdir@campmark7.org
www.campmark7.org

Dave Staehle, Executive Director
Jane Fluman, Program Director
Ursula Smith, Deaf Youth Program Director
Adirondack Mountain camp for hard-of-hearing, deaf and hearing people. Coed, ages 1-99, families, seniors and single adults.

7741 Camp Taloali
D Sipp
15934 N Santiam Highway
Stayton, OR 97383
503-769-6415
TTY:503-769-6415
e-mail: info@taloali.org
www.taloali.org

Georgia Ortiz, Camp Director
Rolland Hart, Executive Director
Summer sessions for children with hearing impairment. Coed, ages 9-17.

7742 Camp Tekoa UMC
Western NC Conference/United Methodist Church
211 Thomas Road
PO Box 211
Hendersonville, NC 28739
828-692-6516
828-696-3699
FAX: 828-697-3288
e-mail: director@camptekoa.org
www.camptekoa.org

Karen Rohrer, Business Manager
James S Johnson, Director
Mike Pruett, Program Manager
Camping for children with asthma/respiratory ailments, hearing impairment and developmental disabilities. Coed, ages 6-17.

7743 Central Michigan University Summer Clinics
Health Professions, Building 1165
Central Michigan University
Mount Pleasant, MI 48859
989-774-4000
FAX: 989-744-1891
e-mail: churc1g@cmich.edu
www.chp.cmich.edu

Dan Konkle, Director
Gerald Church, Audiology Division Director
Laurie Bahlke, Speech/Language Supervisor
Designed for children, ages 6 and up, with speech, language and hearing disorders who can benefit from intensive clinical work. A wide range of recreational and social activities form part of the clinical program and promote the social use of skills learned in class.

7744 Childrens Beach House
100 W 10th Street
Suite 411
Wilmington, DE 19801
302-655-4288
FAX: 302-655-4216
e-mail: inquiry@cbhinc.org
www.cbhinc.org

Teresa Tipton, Program Coordinator
Richard Garrett, Director
Rick Deale, Camp Director
Camp is located in Lewes, Delaware. Four-week sessions June-August for Delaware children with hearing impairment or speech/communication impairment. Coed, ages 6-12.

7745 Deaf or Hard of Hearing Services New York State Education Department
Vocational-Educational Services for Individuals with Disabilities
1 Commerce Plaza, Room 1601
Albany, NY 12234
518-474-5652
800-222-5627
FAX: 518-473-5769
TTY: 518-474-5652
e-mail: dsteele@mail.nysed.gov
www.vesid.nysed.gov

Dorothy Steele, Program Coordinator
Rebecca Cort, Deputy Commisioner
Richard Mills, Commisioner
A non-profit community that has a mission to empower clients to overcome barriers facing individuals experiencing deafness and hearing loss and to give them full access to opportunities that are readily available to persons who hear.

7746 Easter Seals Oklahoma
Easter Seals America
701 Northeast 13th Street
Oklahoma City, OK 73104
405-239-2525
FAX: 405-239-2278
e-mail: esok1@coxinet.net
www.eastersealsoklahoma.org

Patricia Filer, Executive Director
Providing services such as adult day services, child development center, OTIPT, speech therapy, reading/tutoring, vision and hearing screening.

7747 Father Drumgoole Connelly Summer Camp
Catholic Youth Organization
6581 Hylan Boulevard
Staten Island, NY 10309
718-317-2600
FAX: 718-317-2830
www.mountloretto.org

Frank Minotti, Camp Director
Summer sessions for children with epilepsy, hearing impairment and developmental disabilities. Coed, ages 5-13.

7748 Lions Camp Merrick
PO Box 375
Waldorf, MD 20604
301-645-5616
FAX: 301-374-2282
e-mail: cmpmerrick@aol.com
www.lionscampmerrick.org

Gregory V Floberg, Executive Director
Kevin V Rupert, Camp Administrator
Pat Moffat, Administrative Assistant
This recreational camp for special needs children offers a complete waterfront program including swimming, canoeing and fishing for ages 6-16. Designed for children who are deaf and hard of hearing, children of deaf parents, and children with diabetes. Also helps children to learn to deal with their special conditions.

7749 Meadowood Springs Speech and Hearing Camp
Institute for Rehabilitation Research
PO Box 1025
Pendleton, OR 97801
541-276-2752
FAX: 541-276-7227
e-mail: meadowoodcamp@uci.net
www.meadowoodsprings.com

Irene Willard, Administrator
Marie Story, Assistant
On 143 acres in the Blue Mountains of Eastern Oregon, this camp is designed to help young people who have diagnosed clinical disorders of speech, hearing or language. A full range of activities in recreational and clinical areas is available.

7750 Ramah in the Poconos
261 Old York Road
Suite 734
Jenkintown, PA 19046
215-885-8556
FAX: 215-885-8905
e-mail: info@ramahpoconos.org
www.ramahpoconos.org &campramah.org

Marla Berkowits, Kesher Director
Todd Zeff, Executive Director
Camp is located in Lake Como, Pennsylvania. Summer sessions for children and adults with hearing impairment. Coed, ages 10-16, families and seniors.

7751 Summer Enrichment Camp
Alabama School for Deaf
P O Box 698
205 East South Street
Talladega, AL 35160
205-761-3328
FAX: 205-761-3378
e-mail: graham.terry@aidb.aidb.state.al.us
www.aidb.state.al.us/aidb

Terry Graham Ed.D, President
Teresa Caudle, Director Audiology
Walter Ripley, Director Athletic Programs
The Alabama School for the Deaf Summer Enrichment Camp is designed especially for deaf and hard of hearing children ages 6-15. Recreation activities include swimming, skating, outdoor games, horseback riding, field trips, arts and craft. Tuition is free.

7752 Texas Lions Camp
PO Box 290247
Kerrville, TX 78029
830-896-8500
FAX: 830-896-3666
e-mail: tlc@ktc.com
www.lionscamp.com

Stephen S Mabry, Executive Director

The primary purpose of the League shall be to provide, without charge, a camp for physically disabled, hearing/vision impaired and diabetic children from the State of Texas, regardless of race, religion, or national origin. Our goal is to create an atmosphere wherein campers will learn the can do philosophy and be allowed to achieve maximum personal growth and self-esteem. The camp welcomes boys and girls ages 7-16.

7753 **University of Iowa: Wendell Johnson Speech and Hearing Clinic**
250 Hawkins Drive
Iowa City, IA 52242
319-335-1845
FAX: 319-335-8851
e-mail: wendy-fick@uiowa.edu
www.shc.uiowa.edu

Linda Louko, Clinic Director
Marlea O'Brien, Child Language Research Center
Dorothy Albright, Department Administration
The clinic offers assessment and remediation for communication disorders in adults and children. The clinic also offers a Intensive Summer Residential Clinic for school age children needing intervention services because of speech, language, hearing and/or reading problems.

7754 **YMCA Camp Fitch**
Youngstown YMCA
17 North Champion Street
Youngstown, OH 44503
330-744-8411
FAX: 330-744-8416
www.campfitch.com

Mike Shaffer, Executive Director
Kathy Portman, Assistant Director
Camp is located in North Springfield, Pennsylvania. Camping sessions for children and adults with diabetes, hearing impairment, developmental disabilities, mobility limitation and speech/communication impairment. Ages 8-16, families and seniors.

7755 **YWCA Camp Westwind**
Y WC A of Greater Portland
1111 SW 10th Avenue
Portland, OR 97205
503-294-7400
FAX: 503-294-7399
e-mail: LindaD@ymca-pox.org
www.ywca-pdx.org

Adella MacDonald, Executive Director
Kathryn Cooney, Associate Executive Director
Camp is located in Neotsu, Oregon. Sessions for children with hearing impairment. Coed, ages 7-17 and families.

7756 **Youth Leadership Camp**
National Association of the Deaf
8630 Fenton Street
Suite 820
Silver Spring, MD 20910
301-587-1788
FAX: 301-587-1791
TTY:301-587-1789
e-mail: infor@nad.org
www.nad.org

Bill Stark, Camp Director
Jennifer Yost Ortiz, Youth Programs Coordinator
Sponsored by the National Association of the Deaf, this camp emphasizes leadership training for deaf teenagers and young adults. In addition to many recreational activities and sports, there are academic offerings and camp projects.

Print & Non-Print Resources

7757 **ABC Sign with Me**
TJ Publishers
2544 Tarpley Road
Suite 108
Carrollton, TX 75006
972-416-0800
800-999-1168
FAX: 301-585-5930
e-mail: TJPubinc@aol.com

Angela K Thames, President
Jerald A Murphy, VP
Offers bright pictures of familiar objects, lower case alphabet and corresponding manual alphabet hand shapes. *$3.95*
32 pages Softcover
ISBN 0-93984 -00-3

7758 **ASHA Leader**
American Speech-Language-Hearing Association
10801 Rockville Pike
Rockville, MD 20852
301-897-5700
800-638-8255
FAX: 301-897-7348
e-mail: actioncenter@asha.org
www.asha.org

Joanne K Jessen, Publications Director
John E Bernthal, President
Arlene Pietranton, Executive Director
Association publication containing news, notices of events and activities and information for members on issues facing the profession of audiology and speech-language pathology. *$80.00*
35 pages 2 x month

7759 **Access for All: Integrating Deaf, Hard of Hearing and Hearing Preschoolers**
Gallaudet University Bookstore
800 Florida Avenue NE
Washington, DC 20002
202-651-5000
800-451-1073
FAX: 202-651-5489

Erving Jordan, President
This exciting new 90 minute videotape and manual describes a model program for integrating deaf and hard of hearing children in early education. *$24.95*
150 pages

7760 **Adult Bible Lessons for the Deaf**
LifeWay Christian Resources Southern Baptist Conv.
127 9th Avenue N
Nashville, TN 37234
615-251-2089
800-458-2772
FAX: 651-251-5764
e-mail: specialed@lifeway.com
www.lifeway.com

Wade Stapleton, Manager
Bible study lessons for every three months written by and for persons who are deaf. Based on the Family Bible Series (International Sunday School Lessons).
Quarterly

7761 **Advanced Sign Language Vocabulary: A Resource Text for Educators**
2600 S 1st Street
Springfield, IL 62704
217-789-8980
800-258-8980
FAX: 217-789-9130
e-mail: books@ccthomas.com
www.ccthomas.com

Michael Thomas, President
A resource text for educators, interpreters, parents and sign language instructors. *$46.95*
202 pages Paperback
ISBN 0-398057-22-2

7762 **American Annals of the Deaf**
PO Box 1778
St Augustine, FL 32085
904-810-5200
FAX: 904-810-5525
e-mail: email@ceasd.org
www.ceasd.org

Joe Finnegan, Executive Director
Barbara Raimondo, Government Relations Liaison
Mike Bello, Treasurer
Quarterly publication from the Conference of Educational Administrators Serving the Deaf.

Quarterly

7763 **American Journal of Audiology**
American Speech-Language-Hearing Association
10801 Rockville Pike
Rockville, MD 20852
301-897-5700
800-638-8255
FAX: 301-897-7348
e-mail: info@asha.org
www.asha.org

John E Bernthal, President
Arlene Peitranton, Executive Director
Joanne Jessen, Publications Director
Articles concern screening, assesment, and treatment techniques; prevention; professional issues; supervision; administration. Includes clinical forums, clinical reviews, letters to the editor, or research reports that emphasize clinical practice.

7764 **American Sign Language (ASL): Quick Facts**
Federal Government
31 Center Drive Msc2320
Bethesda, MD 20892
800-241-1044
FAX: 301-402-0018
e-mail: nidcdinfo@nidcd.nih.gov
www.nidcd.nih.gov
Ouick facts on what is ASL, where did it orginate, how it compares with spoken language, and why has ASL become a first language for many deaf people.

7765 **American Sign Language Handshape Dictionary**
Gallaudet University Press
11030 S Langley Avenue
Chicago, IL 60628
800-621-2736
FAX: 800-621-8476
TTY:800-621-9347
gupress.gallaudet.edu

Richard A Tennant, Co-Author
Marianne Gluszak Brown, Co-Author
More than 1,600 sign illustrations arranged by handshape for easy identification. Allows readers to look up signs they have seen without needing to know their English meaning beforehand, complemented by a complete English index cross-referenced to every sign. *$45.00*
408 pages Hardcover

7766 **American Sign Language Phrase Book**
TJ Publishers
2544 Tarpley Road
Suite 108
Carrollton, TX 75006
972-416-0800
800-999-1168
FAX: 301-585-5930
e-mail: TJPubinc@aol.com

Angela K Thames, President
Jerald A Murphy, VP
The author provides interesting, realistic and meaningful situations. Sign language is learned through novel remarks cleverly organized around everyday topics. *$18.95*
362 pages Softcover
ISBN 0-80923 -00-5

7767 **American Sign Language: A Look at Its Structure & Community**
TJ Publishers
2544 Tarpley Road
Suite 108
Carrollton, TX 75006
972-416-0800
800-999-1168
FAX: 301-585-5930
e-mail: TJPubinc@aol.com

Angela K Thames, President
Jerald A Murphy, VP
Answers basic questions about American Sign Language. What is it? What is its history? Who uses it? What is the deaf community? *$3.95*
22 pages Softcover
ISBN 0-93266 -01-9

7768 **Anna's Silent World**
JB Lippincott
227 E Washington Square
Philadelphia, PA 19106
215-521-8300
800-777-2295
FAX: 215-824-7390

J Lippincott, Chief Executive Officer
Anna was a hearing impaired child who lived in New York City with her family. The text followed Anna through a hearing evaluation, speech therapy, and her participation in a class for hearing impaired children.
48 pages Hardcover
ISBN 0-39731 -39-5

7769 **At Home Among Strangers**
Gallaudet University Press
2544 Tarpley Road
Suite 108
Carrollton, TX 75006
972-416-0800
800-999-1168
FAX: 301-585-5930
e-mail: TJPubinc@aol.com

Angela K Thames, President
Jerald A Murphy, Executive Assistant
Discusses deaf culture and its uniqueness in two sections: the first describes the deaf community - its development, structure and culture; the second explains Schein's theory of deaf community development. *$34.50*
256 pages Hardcover
ISBN 1-563681-41-2

7770 **Auditory Processing Disorders in Children: What Does It Mean?**
Federal Government
31 Center Drive Msc2320
Bethesda, MD 20892
800-241-1044
FAX: 301-402-0018
e-mail: nidcdinfo@nidcd.nih.gov
www.nidcd.nih.gov
This fact sheet describes what is auditory processing disorder, what causes APD diffculty, what are the symtoms, how is it diagnosed, what treatments are available, and current research into the rehabilitation of child language disorders which will help us better understand the nature of auditory processing disorders.

7771 **Auricle**
Auditory-Verbal International
1390 Chain Bridge Road
100
Mc Lean, VA 22101
703-739-1049
FAX: 703-739-0395
TTY:703-739-0874
e-mail: audiverb@aol.com
www.auditory-verbal.org

Sara Blair Lake, Executive Director/CEO
Tom Lucches, President
To provide the choice of listening and speaking as the way of life for children and adults who are deaf or hard of hearing.
Quarterly

7772 **BPPV**
Vestibular Disorder Association
PO Box 4467
Portland, OR 97208
503-229-7705
800-837-8428
FAX: 503-229-8064
e-mail: veda@vestibular.org
www.vestibular.org

Lisa Haven, Editor
Connie Pilcher, Outreach Coordinator

2000

7773 Basic Course in American Sign Language Package
T J Publishers
2544 Tarpley Road
Suite 108
Carrollton, TX 75006
972-416-0800
800-999-1168
FAX: 301-585-5930
e-mail: TJPubinc@aol.com

Angela K Thames, President
Jerald A Murphy, VP
Accompanying videotapes and textbooks will include voice translations. Hearing students can analyze sound for initial instruction, or opt to turn off the sound to sharpen visual acuity. Package includes the A Basic Course in American Sign Language text, Student Study Guide, the original four 1-hour videotapes plus the ABCASL Vocabulary Videotape. *$139.95*
280 pages

7774 Basic Course in Manual Communication
Gallaudet University Bookstore
11030 S Langley Avenue
Chicago, IL 60628
202-651-5488
800-621-2736
FAX: 202-651-5489
Teach your students manual communication - that living, changing, growing language of signs. *$11.95*
158 pages Softcover

7775 Basic Vocabulary: ASL for Parents and Children
TJ Publishers
2544 Tarpley Road
Suite 108
Carrollton, TX 75006
972-416-0800
800-999-1168
FAX: 301-585-5930
e-mail: TJPubinc@aol.com

Angela K Thames, President
Jerald A Murphy, VP
Carefully selected words and signs include those that children use every day. Alphabetically organized vocabulary incorporates developmental lists helpful to both deaf and hearing children and over 1000 clear sign language illustrations. *$8.95*
240 pages Softcover
ISBN 0-93266 -00-0

7776 Beginning Reading and Sign Language
Harris Communications
15155 Technology Drive
Eden Prairie, MN 55344
952-906-1180
800-825-6758
FAX: 952-906-1099
e-mail: mail@harriscomm.com
www.harriscomm.com

Bill Williams, National Sales Manager
Robert Harris, Owner
Features a deaf performer signing more than 120 words while standing in front of the object she is signing. Appropriate for children eighteen months to eight years. *$21.95*
Video

7777 Ben's Story: A Deaf Child's Right to Sign
TJ Publishers
2544 Tarpley Road
Suite 108
Carrollton, TX 75006
972-416-0800
800-999-1168
FAX: 301-585-5930
e-mail: TJPubinc@aol.com

Angela K Thames, President
Jerald A Murphy, Executive Assistant
This is a mother's story of how she responded to the diagnosis of her son's deafness and how she struggled to have her son educated using sign language. *$7.95*
267 pages Softcover
ISBN 0-930323-47-5

7778 Between Friends
Beltone Electronics Corporation
4201 W Victoria Street
Chicago, IL 60646
773-583-3600
FAX: 773-583-1361

Renee Rockoff, Editor
Dave McKissack
For hearing aid wearers: quizzes, jokes, health, recipes and financial items.
6 pages

7779 Book of Name Signs
Gallaudet University Bookstore
11030 S Langley Avenue
Chicago, IL 60628
202-651-5488
800-621-2736
FAX: 202-651-5489
Discusses the rules for American Sign Language name sign formation and their appropriate use. *$12.95*
112 pages

7780 Bridges Beyond Sound
Brookes Publishing
PO Box 10624
Baltimore, MD 21285
410-337-9580
800-638-3775
FAX: 410-337-8539
e-mail: custserv@brookespublishing.com
www.brookespublishing.com

Paul Brooks, Owner
An instructional workbook on understanding and including students with a hearing loss. Supplement to the Bridges Beyond Sound videotape. Besides the videotape script, background information on hearing loss, discussion questions, activities, and reproducible worksheets are included. *$33.00*
176 pages Spiral-bound
ISBN 1-55766 -26-6

7781 Bulletin Newsletter
806 W Adams Boulevard
Los Angeles, CA 90007
213-748-5481
800-522-4582
FAX: 213-749-1651
e-mail: mmartindale@jtc.org
www.jtc.org

Barbara F Hecht PhD, Executive Director
Mary Ann Bell, VP Development & Communications
Jack Cooper, Editor
Bi-annual publication from the John Tracy Clinic.
8 pages Bi-annually

7782 CSD Spectrum
Communication Service for the Deaf (CSD)
102 N Krohn Place
Sioux Falls, SD 57103
605-367-5760
800-642-6410
FAX: 605-367-5958
e-mail: info@c-s-d.org
www.c-s-d.org

Marvin Miller, Author/Editor
A free quarterly publication from CSD.
Quarterly

7783 Captions for Deaf and Hard-of-Hearing View ers
Federal Government
31 Center Drive Msc2320
Bethesda, MD 20892
800-241-1044
FAX: 301-402-0018
e-mail: nidcdinfo@nidcdnih.gov
www.nidcd.nih.gov
This fact sheet explains what are the captions, current research studying caption features, speeds, and the effects od visula impairments on reading captions, ans offers additional resources.

7784 Changing the Rules
TJ Publishers
2544 Tarpley Road
Suite 108
Carrollton, TX 75006
972-416-0800
800-999-1168
FAX: 301-585-5930
e-mail: TJPubinc@aol.com

Angela K Thames, President
Jerald A Murphy, VP
Like many deaf adults, Frank Bowe was mainstreamed in the small Pennsylvania town where he was raised. This is a humorous and poignant account of the obstacles that shaped this leading disability rights activist. Bowe's account of coming of age and personal growth, the discovery of signed language and an insider's view of the equal rights movement is a compelling record of one man's struggle with the challenges of profound deafness. *$8.95*
204 pages Hardcover
ISBN 0-93266 -31-0

7785 Chelsea: The Story of a Signal Dog
Gallaudet University Bookstore
800 Florida Avenue NE
Washington, DC 20002
202-651-5000
800-451-1073
FAX: 202-651-5489

Erving Jordan, President
This is a story of a young deaf couple and their Belgian sheepdog, who acts as their ears. It explains how these dogs are trained and paired with their new owners. *$18.95*
169 pages

7786 Children of a Lesser God
Gallaudet University Bookstore
11030 S Langley Avenue
Chicago, IL 60628
202-651-5488
800-621-2736
FAX: 202-651-5489
The movie that won the hearts of thousands. This is a story of a deaf woman who refuses to succumb to the hearing people's image of what a deaf person should be. *$4.50*
91 pages Softcover

7787 Choices in Deafness
Woodbine House
6510 Bells Mill Road
Bethesda, MD 20817
301-897-3570
800-843-7323
FAX: 301-897-5838
www.woodbinehouse.com

Irv Shapell, Owner
A useful aid in choosing the appropriate communication option for a child with a hearing loss. Experts present the following communication options: Auditory-Verbal Approach, Bilingual-Bicultural Approach, Cued Speech, Oral Approach, and Total Communication. This new edition explains medical causes of hearing loss, the diagnostic process, audiological assessment, and cochlear implants. Children and parents also offer their personal experiences. *$16.95*
275 pages Paperback
ISBN 0-933149-85-9

7788 Christmas Stories
Gallaudet University Bookstore
11030 S Langley Avenue
Chicago, IL 60628
202-651-5488
800-621-2736
FAX: 202-651-5489
The unique talents of Bobby Giles and Doris Wilding present these great stories in American Sign Language. *$29.95*
Video

7789 Clerc: The Story of His Early Years
Gallaudet University Press
2544 Tarpley Road
Suite 108
Carrollton, TX 75006
972-416-0800
800-999-1168
FAX: 301-585-5930
e-mail: TJPubinc@aol.com

Angela K Thames, President
Jerald A Murphy, VP
This imaginative tale recounts the youthful history of Laurent Clerc, the deaf teacher who helped Thomas Gallaudet establish schools for the deaf in the 19th century. Early experiences influenced the teaching methods Clerc developed in later life and young adults will relish identifying with the hero of this entertaining story. *$13.95*
208 pages paperback
ISBN 0-93032 -23-8

7790 Closer Look: The English Program at the Model Secondary School for the Deaf
Gallaudet University Bookstore
800 Florida Avenue NE
Washington, DC 20002
202-651-5000
800-451-1073
FAX: 202-651-5489

Erving Jordan, President
Job placement programs, remunerative work services and work adjustment training programs incorporating the whole language philosophy into classroom routines. *$8.50*
67 pages

7791 Cochlear Implants
Federal Government
31 Center Dirve Msc2320
Bethesda, MD 20892
800-241-1044
FAX: 301-402-0018
e-mail: nidcdinfo@nidcd.nih.gov
www.nidcd.nih.gov
This fact sheet explains what is a cochlear implant, how it works, who gets cochlear implants, how someone receives a cochlear impant and what the future holds for cochlear impants.

7792 Cochlear Implants and Children
Alexander Graham Bell Association
3417 Volta Place NW
Washington, DC 20007
202-337-5220
FAX: 202-337-8314
e-mail: info@agbell.org
www.agbell.org

Todd Houston, Executive Director
Designed to educate readers about cochlear implants, including surgery, the importance of rehabilitation and the significance of parents' and professionals' roles. *$42.95*
189 pages Paperback

7793 Cochlear Implants for Kids
Alexander Graham Bell Association
3417 Volta Place NW
Washington, DC 20007
202-337-5220
FAX: 202-337-8314
e-mail: info@agbell.org
www.agbell.org

Todd Houston, Executive Director
Designed to educate readers about cochlear implants, including surgery, the importance of rehabilitation and the significance of parents' and professionals' roles. *$42.95*
404 pages Paperback

7794 Cognition, Education and Deafness
Gallaudet University Press
800 Florida Avenue NE
Washington, DC 20002
202-651-5000
800-451-1073
FAX: 202-651-5489

Erving Jordan, President
The work of 54 authors is gathered in this definitive collection of current research on deafness and cognition. The articles are grouped into seven sections: cognition, problem solving, thinking processes, language development, reading methodologies, measurement of potential, and intervention programs. *$21.95*

260 pages Hardcover

7795 College and Career Programs for the Deaf
Gallaudet University Bookstore
11030 S Langley Avenue
Chicago, IL 60628
202-651-5488
800-621-2736
FAX: 202-651-5489

Which college is the right one for you? This is a guide to colleges in the United States and Canada that offer special programs for deaf students. *$12.95*
108 pages Softcover

7796 Come Sign with Us
Gallaudet University Press
11030 S Langley Avenue
Chicago, IL 60628
800-621-2736
FAX: 800-621-8476
TTY:800-621-9347
gupress.gallaudet.edu

Jan C Hafer, Co-Author
Robert M Wilson, Co-Author
This fun guide for parents and educators on teaching hearing children how to sign has been thoroughly revised with completely new activities that provide contexts for practice. *$29.95*
160 pages Softcover

7797 Communicating with Deaf People: An Introduction
Gallaudet University Bookstore
800 Florida Avenue NE
Washington, DC 20002
202-651-5000
800-451-1073
FAX: 202-651-5489

Erving Jordan, President
This illustrated publication introduces the various ways deaf people can communicate, including gesture and facial expression, speech-reading, fingerspelling and other manual communication systems. *$2.00*
20 pages

7798 Communication Options for Children Who are Deaf or Hard-of-Hearing
Federal Government
31 Center Drive McS2320
Bethesda, MD 20892
800-241-1044
FAX: 301-402-0018
e-mail: midcdinfo@nidcd.nih.gov
www.nidcd.nih.gov

Explains how hearing loss or deafness is identified in newborns, how later onset of hearing loss is identified in young children, what causes hearing loss or deafness in newborns, what communication options are available to deaf and har-of-hearing children, and how your family can particiapte in research related hereditary deafness, hearing impairment, or intervention strategies.

7799 Communique
Michigan Association for Deaf Hard Of Hearing
2929 Covington Court
Unit 200
Lansing, MI 48912
517-487-0066
800-968-7327
FAX: 517-487-2586
e-mail: yourear@madhh.org
www.madhh.org

Nancy Asher, Executive Director
4-8 pages Bi-annually

7800 Comprehensive Reference Manual for Signers and Interpreters
Charles C Thomas
2600 S 1st Street
Springfield, IL 62704
217-789-8980
800-258-8980
FAX: 217-789-9130
e-mail: books@ccthomas.com
www.ccthomas.com

Michael Thomas, President
Manual for signers. *$47.95*
314 pages Paperback
ISBN 0-398059-19-5

7801 Comprehensive Signed English Dictionary
Gallaudet University Press
11030 S Langley Avenue
Chicago, IL 60628
800-621-2736
FAX: 800-621-8476
TTY:800-621-9347
gupress.gallaudet.edu

Harry Bornstein, Co-Author
Karen L Saulnier, Co-Author
Lillian B Hamilton, Co-Author
This complete dictionary has over 3,100 signs, including signs reflecting lively and contemporary vocabulary. *$45.00*
464 pages Hardcover

7802 Connect
Hearing, Speech & Deafness Center (HSDC)
1625 19th Avenue
Seattle, WA 98122
206-323-5770
FAX: 206-328-6871
e-mail: hsdc@hsdc.org
www.hsdc.org

David Delmar, Editor
Susie Burdick, Executive Director
A not-for-profit United Way Agency building community through communications since 1937. Call V/TTY. The mission of HSDC is to strengthen community by promoting effective communication
8 pages Quarterly

7803 Connect Newsletter
Hearing, Speech & Deafness Center (HSDC)
1625 19th Avenue
Seattle, WA 98122
206-323-5770
FAX: 206-328-6871
e-mail: hsdc@hsdc.org
www.hsdc.org

Susie Burdick, Executive Director
8 pages Bi-annually

7804 Conversational Sign Language II
Gallaudet University Press
15155 Technology Drive
Eden Prairie, MN 55344
952-906-1180
800-825-6758
FAX: 952-906-1099
e-mail: mail@harriscomm.com
www.harriscomm.com

Bill Williams, National Sales Manager
Robert Harris, Owner
This book presents English words and their American Sign Language equivalents. *$17.95*
218 pages Paperback
ISBN 0-913580-00-7

7805 Coping with the Multi-Handicapped Hearing Impaired: A Practical Approach
Charles C Thomas
2600 S 1st Street
Springfield, IL 62704
217-789-8980
800-258-8980
FAX: 217-789-9130
e-mail: books@ccthomas.com
www.ccthomas.com

Michael Thomas, President
Professional text offers suggestions on how to deal with the multi-handicapped deaf person. Also available in cloth.

90 pages $20.95
ISBN 0-398063-33-8

7806 **Deaf Catholic**
International Catholic Deaf Association
1030 S La Grange Road
Suite 9
La Grange, IL 60525
FAX: 708-579-5847
TTY:708-579-5817
e-mail: icdaus@ameritech.com

Richard Kush, Editor
Quarterly publication from the International Catholic Deaf Association. *$15.00*
16 pages Quarterly

7807 **Deaf Empowerment: Emergence, Struggle and Rhetoric**

Gallaudet University Press
11030 S Langley Avenue
Chicago, IL 60628
800-621-2736
FAX: 800-621-8476
TTY:800-621-9347
gupress.gallaudet.edu
The story of the Deaf social movement, from its beginnings in the mid 1800s through its growth and strengthening in the late 20th century, much of it due to rhetoric and tactics adopted from other social movements. *$45.95*
192 pages Hardcover
ISBN 1-563680-61-0

7808 **Deaf Heritage: A Narrative History**
Gallaudet University Bookstore
11030 S Langley Avenue
Chicago, IL 60628
202-651-5488
800-621-2736
FAX: 202-651-5489
This in-depth history of deaf America contains pictures, illustrations, vignettes, and biographical profiles. *$21.95*
500 pages Paperback

7809 **Deaf History Unveiled: Interpretations from the New Scholarship**
Gallaudet University Press
11030 S Langley Avenue
Chicago, IL 60628
800-621-2736
FAX: 800-621-8476
TTY:800-621-9347
gupress.gallaudet.edu

John Vickrey Van Cleve, Editor
An all-star cast of historians explores the new themes driving Deaf History, including comparisons with other minority cultures and the social paternalism that affects deaf communities around the globe. *$36.95*
316 pages Softcover
ISBN 1-563680-87-4

7810 **Deaf Like Me**
Gallaudet University Press
800 Florida Avenue NE
Washington, DC 20002
202-651-5000
800-451-1073
FAX: 202-651-5489

Irving Jordan, President
Written by the uncle and father of a deaf girl, this is an account of parents coming to terms with deafness. This paperback edition contains a special epilogue by Lynn Spradley, grown and in her twenties, as she reflects on her growing-up years with the advantage of hindsight. *$16.95*

292 pages Softcover
ISBN 0-930323-11-4

7811 **Deaf Parents and Their Hearing Children**
Through the Looking Glass
2198 6th Street
Suite 100
Berkeley, CA 94710
510-848-1112
800-644-2666
FAX: 510-848-4445
e-mail: TLG@lookingglass.org
www.lookingglass.org

J L Singleton
M D Tittle
Megan Kirshbaum, Executive Director
$2.00
8 pages

7812 **Deaf in America: Voices from a Culture**
TJ Publishers
2544 Tarpley Road
Suite 108
Carrollton, TX 75006
972-416-0800
800-999-1168
FAX: 301-585-5930
e-mail: TJPubinc@aol.com

Angela K Thames, President
Jerald A Murphy, VP
Now available in paperback, this book opens deaf culture to outsiders, inviting readers to imagine and understand a world of silence. This book shares the joy and satisfaction many people have with their lives and shows that deafness may not be the handicap most hearing people think. *$12.95*
134 pages Softcover
ISBN 0-67419 -24-1

7813 **EASE**
Telecommunications for the Deaf (TDI)
8630 Fenton Street
Suite 604
Silver Spring, MD 20910
301-589-3786
FAX: 301-589-3797
e-mail: info@tdi-online.org
www.tdi-online.org

Claude L Stout, Executive Director
James D House, Member Service/Public Rel. Dir.
Training package for 911 professionals.
48 pages

7814 **Effectiveness of Cochlear Implants and Tactile Aids for Deaf Children**
Alexander Graham Bell Association
3417 Volta Place NW
Washington, DC 20007
202-337-5220
FAX: 202-337-8314
e-mail: info@agbell.org
www.agbell.org

Todd Houston, Executive Director
This monograph presents a fascinating study to evaluate differences in the rate of change in speech perception, speech production and spoken language skills among children using the Nucleus 22-channel cochlear implant, tactile aids and conventional hearing aids. This monograph also offers teaching strategies in perception, lipreading and spoken language. *$13.95*
232 pages Paperback

7815 **Encyclopedia of Deafness and Hearing Disorders**
Gallaudet University Bookstore
800 Florida Avenue NE
Washington, DC 20002
202-651-5000
800-451-1073
FAX: 202-651-5489

Erving Jordan, President
Presents the most current information on deafness and hearing disorders in an authoritative A-to-Z compendium. *$45.00*

278 pages

7816 Exploring the Bible: Bible Studies for the DEAF
Lifeway Church Resources
127 9th Avenue N
Nashville, TN 37234
615-251-2089
800-458-2772
FAX: 615-251-2710
e-mail: lifewaynews@lifeway.com
www.lifeway.com/lwc

Rob Phillips, Director
Wade Stapleton, Manager
Bible study lessons for every three months written by and for persons who are deaf. Based on the Family Bible Series (International Sunday School Lessons).

7817 Expressive and Receptive Fingerspelling
Gallaudet University Bookstore
800 Florida Avenue NE
Washington, DC 20002
202-651-5000
800-451-1073
FAX: 202-651-5489

Erving Jordan, President
Here is a new and meaningful way for adults to increase their comfort with fingerspelling. The system is based on the principles of phonetics rather than letters of the English alphabet. *$2.50*
42 pages Softcover

7818 Eye-Centered: A Study of Spirituality of Deaf People
NCOD
7202 Buchanan Street
Landover Hills, MD 20784
301-577-1684
FAX: 301-577-1690
e-mail: ncod@erols.com
www.ncod.org

Arvilla Rank, Executive Director
The findings of the five-year De Sales Project conducted by The National Catholic Office for the Deaf. *$12.00*
167 pages

7819 Fairy Tales & Christmas Stories
Harris Communications
15155 Technology Drive
Eden Prairie, MN 55344
952-906-1180
800-825-6758
FAX: 952-906-1099
e-mail: mail@harriscomm.com
www.harriscomm.com

Bill Williams, National Sales Manager
Robert Harris, Owner
A collection of videotapes featuring classic fairytales and Christmas stories signed by deaf storytellers. *$29.95*
Video

7820 Fantastic Series
Harris Communications
15155 Technology Drive
Eden Prairie, MN 55344
952-906-1180
800-825-6758
FAX: 952-906-1099
e-mail: mail@harriscomm.com
www.harriscomm.com

Bill Williams, National Sales Manager
Robert Harris, Owner
These videotapes offer a blend of entertainment and information to both deaf and hearing children ages 6-10. A total of eight tapes in the series. *$29.95*

7821 Fingerspelling: Expressive and Receptive Fluency
Gallaudet University Bookstore
11030 S Langley Avenue
Chicago, IL 60628
202-651-5488
800-621-2736
FAX: 202-651-5489
Improve your fingerspelling with this new video guide. A 24-page instructional booklet is included with fingerspelling practice suggestions. *$39.95*

120 Minutes

7822 Flute Song Magic
TJ Publishers
2544 Tarpley Road
Suite 108
Carrollton, TX 75006
972-416-0800
800-999-1168
FAX: 301-585-5930
e-mail: TJPubinc@aol.com

Angela K Thames, President
Jerald A Murphy, Executive Assistant
Gallaudet student Andrea Shettle created a memorable fantasy world, Nevlin, where it is forbidden to talk with people below one's class. An improbable friendship leads the High Noble Flutir to discover that friendship and individuality defy class limitations. *$ 2.95*
218 pages Softcover
ISBN 0-380762-25-0

7823 For Hearing People Only
Harris Communications
15155 Technology Drive
Eden Prairie, MN 55344
952-906-1180
800-825-6758
FAX: 952-906-1099
e-mail: mail@harriscomm.com
www.harriscomm.com

Bill Williams, National Sales Manager
Robert Harris, Owner
A book that answers some of the questions hearing people ask about deaf culture. Also availible in hardcover. *$19.95*
336 pages Paperback
ISBN 0-963401-61-0

7824 From Gesture to Language in Hearing and Deaf Children
Gallaudet University Press
11030 S Langley Avenue
Chicago, IL 60628
800-621-2736
FAX: 800-621-8476
TTY:800-621-9347
gupress.gallaudet.edu

Virginia Volterra, Editor
Carol J Erting, Editor
In 21 essays on communicative gesturing in the first two years of life, this vital collection demonstrates the importance of gesture in a child's transition to a linguistic system. *$45.95*
358 pages Softcover
ISBN 1-563680-78-5

7825 From Mime to Sign Package
TJ Publishers
2544 Tarpley Road
Suite 108
Carrollton, TX 75006
972-416-0800
800-999-1168
FAX: 301-585-5930
e-mail: TJPubinc@aol.com

Angela K Thames, President
Jerald A Murphy, VP
As a drama professor, television personality, performer and storyteller, multiple Emmy winner Gil Eastman has developed a unique presentation style. Now, he shares his expressive communication approach in a highly illustrated American Sign Language text and videotape series. A text and three videotapes. *$139.95*
183 pages

7826 GA and SK Etiquette
Gallaudet University Bookstore
800 Florida Avenue NE
Washington, DC 20002
202-651-5000
800-451-1073
FAX: 202-651-5489

Erving Jordan, President
This booklet presents guidelines for proper usage of the TDD. It includes everything you wanted to know about sending and receiving TDD calls. *$8.95*

53 pages

7827 GA-SK
Telecommunications for the Deaf
8630 Fenton Street
Suite 604
Silver Spring, MD 20910
301-589-3786
FAX: 301-589-3797
e-mail: info@tdi-online.org
www.tdi-online.org

Claude L Stout, Executive Director
James D House, Member Service/Public Rel. Dir.
Promoting equal access to telecommunications and media for people who are deaf, late-deafened, hard-of-hearing or deaf-blind through consumer education and involvement; technical assistance and consulting; applications of exisiting and emerging technologies; networking and collaboration; uniformity of standards; and national policy development and advocacy.
48 pages Quarterly

7828 Gallaudet Survival Guide to Signing
Gallaudet University Press
15155 Technology Drive
Eden Prairie, MN 55344
952-906-1180
800-825-6758
FAX: 952-906-1099
e-mail: mail@harriscomm.com
www.harriscomm.com

Bill Williams, National Sales Manager
Robert Harris, Owner
Features 500 of the most frequently used signs with clear illustrations and descriptions for each one. *$9.95*
203 pages Paperback
ISBN 0-930323-67-x

7829 Gallaudet University Press Journal: Sign Language Studies
Gallaudet University Press
800 Florida Avenue NE
Washington, DC 20002
202-651-5000
800-451-1073
FAX: 202-651-5489

7830 Getting Better
Vestibular Disorders Association
PO Box 4467
Portland, OR 97208
503-229-7705
800-837-8428
FAX: 503-229-8064
e-mail: veda@vestibular.org
www.vestibular.org

Dr. Lisa Haven, Executive Director
Connie Pilcher, Outreach Coordinator
A non-profit organization dedicated to providing education and support to people with inner ear balance/dizziness disorder and their families and people who help them. *$25.00*
Quarterly
ISBN 0-963261-17-7

7831 Goldilocks and the Three Bears in Signed English
Gallaudet University Press
11030 S Langley Avenue
Chicago, IL 60628
800-621-2736
FAX: 800-621-8476
TTY:800-621-9347
gupress.gallaudet.edu

Harry Bornstein, Co-Author
Karen L Saulnier, Co-Author
The classic story is told again but with a twist. Full color illustrations show the Bears, Goldilocks and the text. Includes line drawings that show the story in Signed English. *$15.95*
48 pages Hardcover

7832 Granny Good's Signs of Christmas
Gallaudet University Bookstore
11030 S Langley Avenue
Chicago, IL 60628
202-651-5488
800-621-2736
FAX: 202-651-5489

Come join the folks at Granny's cottage where Hans Signer, from the silent forest, interprets his favorite story, Twas The Night Before Christmas. *$29.95*
Video

7833 Growing Together: Information for Parents of Deaf Children
Gallaudet University Bookstore
800 Florida Avenue NE
Washington, DC 20002
202-651-5000
800-451-1073
FAX: 202-651-5489

Erving Jordan, President
This publication answers questions often asked by parents of children with a hearing loss. *$8.00*
92 pages

7834 Guidelines for Helping Deaf-Blind Persons
Helen Keller National Center
111 Middle Neck Road
Sands Point, NY 11050
516-944-8900
800-225-0411
FAX: 516-944-7302
e-mail: hkncdir@aol.com
www.helenkeller.org

Joseph McNulty, Executive Director
Pamphlet offering information on how persons should interact with deaf-blind individuals. Includes drawings of the one hand manual alphabet.

7835 Handtalk Zoo
MacMillan Publishing Company
135 S Mount Zion Road
Lebanon, IN 46052
800-257-5755
FAX: 800-882-8583
Wonderful photographs are used to show children at the zoo communicating with sign language.
28 pages Hardcover
ISBN 0-02700 -01-0

7836 Hearing Aids
Federal Government
31 Center Drive Msc2320
Bethesda, MD 20892
800-241-1044
FAX: 301-402-0018
e-mail: nidcdinfo@nidcd.nih.gov
www.nidcd.nih.gov
Explains what is a hearing aid, how can hearing aids help, what to expect from hearing aids, what questions to ask before buying hearing aids, tips for taking care of hearing aids, and what research is being done on hearing aids.

7837 Hearing Impaired Employee
Allyn & Bacon
75 Arlington Street
Suite 300
Boston, MA 02116
617-848-6000
FAX: 617-848-7490
www.ablongman.com
An invaluable aid for both large and small firms for employment agencies and counselors and for all firms, schools and associations providing equipment or services for the hearing impaired.
1991
ISBN 0-887441-08-4

7838 Hearing Loss: The Journal of Self Help for Hard of Hearing People
Hearing Loss Association Of America
7910 Woodmont Avenue
Suite 1200
Bethesda, MD 20814
301-657-2248
FAX: 301-913-9413
TTY:301-657-2249
e-mail: info@hearingloss.org
www.hearingloss.org

Sharon Christians, Director Of Program Operations
Terry Portis, Executive Director

SHHH, a non-profit, educational organization is dedicated to the well-being of people of all ages and communication styles who do not hear well. SHHH is the largest international consumer organization of its kind. SHHH offers a nationwide support network of chapters and groups, a bi-monthly magazine, discounted publications and resource materials for members, an annual convention, state and regional conferences and more. *$25.00*
40 pages BiMonthly

7839 **Hearing, Speech & Deafness Center (HSDC)**
1625 19th Avenue
Seattle, WA 98122
206-323-5770
FAX: 206-328-6871
e-mail: hsdc@hsdc.org
www.hsdc.org

Susie Burdick, Development/Marketing Director
David Stoner, Editor
Mission is to enrich the lives of all adults and children who experience hearing loss, speech and language impairments, or who are deaf, by providing professional services and technology, and by promoting community awareness and accessibility. A not-for-profit United Way Agency.
16 pages Yearly 1937

7840 **Hearing, Speech and Deafness Center (HSDC)**
Hearing, Speech & Deafness Center (HSDC)
1625 19th Avenue
Seattle, WA 98122
206-323-5770
FAX: 206-328-6871
e-mail: hsdc@hsdc.org
www.hsdc.org

Susie Burdick, Executive Director
Our mission is to enrich lives of all adults and children who experience hearing loss, speech and language impairments or who are deaf, by providing professional services and by promoting community awareness and accessibility.

7841 **Hearing-Impaired Children and Youth with Developmental Disabilities**
Gallaudet University Bookstore
800 Florida Avenue NE
Washington, DC 20002
202-651-5000
800-451-1073
FAX: 202-651-5489

Erving Jordan, President
The insights of 24 experts help clarify relationships between hearing impairment and developmental difficulties and propose interdisciplinary cooperation as an approach to the problems created. *$29.95*
416 pages

7842 **Helping the Family Understand**
Vestibular Disorders Association
PO Box 4467
Portland, OR 97208
503-229-7705
800-837-8428
FAX: 503-229-8064
e-mail: veda@vestibular.org
www.vestibular.org

Lisa Haven, Editor
Connie Pilcher, Editor
2002

7843 **Hollywood Speaks**
Gallaudet University Bookstore
800 Florida Avenue NE
Washington, DC 20002
202-651-5000
800-451-1073
FAX: 202-651-5489

Erving Jordan, President
How deafness has been treated in movies and how it provides yet another window onto social history in addition to a fresh angle from which to view Hollywood. *$24.95*
167 pages Hardcover

7844 **How You Gonna Get to Heaven if You Can't Talk with Jesus?**
TJ Publishers
2544 Tarpley Road
Suite 108
Carrollton, TX 75006
972-416-0800
800-999-1168
FAX: 301-585-5930
e-mail: TJPubinc@aol.com

Angela K Thames, President
Jerald A Murphy, VP
This collection of articles examines deaf culture and its relationship, profiling sociolinguistic and anthropological perspectives in research on American deaf society and culture. *$4.50*
78 pages Softcover
ISBN 0-93266 -15-9

7845 **I Have a Sister, My Sister is Deaf**
TJ Publishers
2544 Tarpley Road
Suite 108
Carrollton, TX 75006
972-416-0800
800-999-1168
FAX: 301-585-5930
e-mail: TJPubinc@aol.com

Angela K Thames, President
Jerald A Murphy, VP
An emphatic, affirmative look at the relationship between siblings, as a young deaf child is affectionately described by her older sister. This Coretta Scott King Honor Award winner helps young children develop an understanding that deaf children share the same interests as hearing children. *$5.95*
32 pages Softcover
ISBN 0-06443 -59-6

7846 **In This Sign**
Gallaudet University Bookstore
800 Florida Avenue NE
Washington, DC 20002
202-651-5000
800-451-1073
FAX: 202-651-5489

Erving Jordan, President
This modern classic follows a family of deaf parents and their hearing child through several decades of growth and pain, tragedy and triumph. *$10.95*
275 pages Softcover

7847 **Innovative Practices for Teaching Sign Language Interpreters**
Gallaudet University Press
11030 S Langley Avenue
Chicago, IL 60628
800-621-2736
FAX: 800-621-8476
TTY:800-621-9347
gupress.gallaudet.edu

Cynthia B Roy, Editor
Six experts draw upon the new understanding of sign language interpreting as a discourse between two languages and cultures. Develops bold, original techniques for training interpreters. *$34.95*
200 pages Hardcover

7848 **Intermediate Conversational Sign Language**
Gallaudet University Press
2544 Tarpley Road
Suite 108
Carrollton, TX 75006
972-416-0800
800-999-1168
FAX: 301-585-5930
e-mail: TJPubinc@aol.com

Angela K Thames, President
Jerald A Murphy, VP
Unique approach to using American Sign Language and English in a bilingual setting. Each of the 25 lessons includes an introductory paragraph, glossed vocabulary review, translation exercises, grammatical notes, substitution drills and activities. *$21.95*

400 pages Softcover
ISBN 7-91358 -79-1

7849 **International Directory of Periodicals Related to Deafness**
Gallaudet University Bookstore
800 Florida Avenue NE
Washington, DC 20002
202-651-5000
800-451-1073
FAX: 202-651-5489

Erving Jordan, President
This one-of-a-kind directory has useful information on more than 500 magazines and journals related to deafness. The entries come from all over the world. *$10.00*
150 pages

7850 **International Telephone Directory**
Gallaudet University Bookstore
800 Florida Avenue NE
Washington, DC 20002
202-651-5000
800-451-1073
FAX: 202-651-5489

Erving Jordan, President
Almost 12,000 TDD numbers for Telecommunications for the Deaf, members and organizations serving deaf people. *$20.00*
190 pages Softcover

7851 **Interpretation: A Sociolinguistic Model**
Gallaudet University Bookstore
800 Florida Avenue NE
Washington, DC 20002
202-651-5000
800-451-1073
FAX: 202-651-5489

Erving Jordan, President
This text presents a sociolinguistically sensitive model of the interpretation process. The model applies to interpretation in any two languages although this one focuses on ASL and English. *$16.95*
199 pages

7852 **Interpretations**
Fanlight Productions
4196 Washington Street
Suite 2
Boston, MA 02131
617-469-4999
800-937-4113
FAX: 617-469-3379
e-mail: fanlight@fanlight.com
www.fanlight.com

Karen McMillen, Marketing Director
Ben Achtenberg, Owner
This new film uses humor and drama to explore the interaction between the deaf and hearing communities. Janice, a freelance photographer who is deaf, has been given her first assignment by an advertising agency. She hires her hearing friend Maureen to interpret for her. When conflicts arise between Janice and the client, Maureen changes Janice words. The film looks at the interplay of dependence and responsibility in the relationship of communicator and interpreter. $145.00.

7853 **Interpreting: An Introduction, Revised Edition**
TJ Publishers
2544 Tarpley Road
Suite 108
Carrollton, TX 75006
972-416-0800
800-999-1168
FAX: 301-585-5930
e-mail: TJPubinc@aol.com

Angela K Thames, President
Jerald A Murphy, VP
This text is written by a practicing interpreter and includes information on history, terminology, research, competence, setting and a comprehensive bibliography. *$22.50*

244 pages Softcover
ISBN 0-91688 -01-9

7854 **Journal**
Academy of Rehabilitative Audiology
PO Box 26532
Minneapolis, MN 55426
952-920-0484
FAX: 952-920-6098
e-mail: ara@incnet.com
www.audrehab.org

Frances Laven, Assistant Director
Yearly publication from the Academy of Rehabilitative Audiology.
Yearly

7855 **Journal of Speech, Language and Hearing Re search**
American Speech-Language-Hearing Association
10801 Rockville Pike
Rockville, MD 20852
301-897-5700
800-638-8255
FAX: 301-897-7348
e-mail: irc@asha.org
www.asha.org

John E Berntah;, President
Arlene Pietranton, Executive Director
Joanne Jessen, Publications Director
Pertains broadly to studies of the processess and disorders of hearing, language, and speech diagnosis and treatment of such disorders.

7856 **Journal of the American Deafness and Rehabilitation Association**
JADARA
6212 Ferris Square
San Diego, CA 92121
619-558-7444

Articles of interest to professionals providing services to deaf people, with special emphasis on research-practice interactions and on mental health issues.

7857 **Joy of Signing**
Gallaudet University Bookstore
800 Florida Avenue NE
Washington, DC 20002
202-651-5000
800-451-1073
FAX: 202-651-5489

Erving Jordan, President
This manual on signing includes illustrations, information on sign origins, practice sentences, and step-by-step descriptions of hand positions and movements. *$16.95*
336 pages Hardcover

7858 **Joy of Signing Puzzle Book**
Harris Communications
15155 Technology Drive
Eden Prairie, MN 55344
952-906-1180
800-825-6758
FAX: 952-906-1099
e-mail: mail@harriscomm.com
www.harriscomm.com

Bill Williams, National Sales Manager
Robert Harris, Owner
Whether you are learning sign language to communicate with a family member, co-worker, student or friend, this puzzle book makes the learning fun and interesting. *$3.95*
57 pages Paperback
ISBN 0-882435-38-8

7859 **Kid-Friendly Parenting with Deaf and Hard of Hearing Children: A Treasury of Fun Activities**
Gallaudet University Press
11030 S Langley Avenue
Chicago, IL 60628
800-621-2736
FAX: 800-621-8476
TTY:800-621-9347
gupress.gallaudet.edu

Denise Chapman, Co-Author
Daria Medwid, Co-Author

Scores of activities, parenting techniques and insights by experts, both hearing and deaf, to help parents of deaf and hard of hearing children. Activities are designed to promote better behavior and educate. *$24.95*
382 pages Softcover

7860 LSDC News
DC Public Library, Services to the Deaf
901 G Street NW
Room 215
Washington, DC 20001
202-727-1101
FAX: 202-727-1129
e-mail: library_deaf_dc@yahoo.com
www.dclibrary.org

Janice Rosen, Librarian
Francis Buckley Jr, Manager
Newsletter
5-6 pages Quarterly

7861 Let's be Friends
Britannica Film Company
345 4th Street
San Francisco, CA 94107
415-777-9876

The teacher left the room and asked Shelly, a hearing impaired child to be the mother. Margaret, an emotionally disturbed child, became frightened and verbally attacked Shelly. The teacher worked to get them to become friends and understand each other's problems.
Film

7862 Linguistics of ASL: An Introduction
Gallaudet University Press
11030 S Langley Avenue
Chicago, IL 60628
800-621-2736
FAX: 800-621-8476
TTY:800-621-9347
gupress.gallaudet.edu

Clayton Valli, Co-Author
Ceil Lucas, Co-Author
An introduction to the struture of American Sign Language, featuring all the linguistic disciplines plus practice exercises. *$ 75.00*
460 pages Hardcover/CD

7863 Lisa and Her Soundless World
Human Sciences Press
233 Spring Street
New York, NY 10013
212-229-2859
800-221-9369
FAX: 212-463-0742
Describes the impact deafness has on communication and functioning in a hearing world. Lisa, born with a severe hearing loss, was not diagnosed as hearing impaired until her parents were worried about her lack of speech and other children had rejected her. *$18.95*
30 pages Hardcover
ISBN 0-87705 -04-6

7864 Listen to Me
Alexander Graham Bell Association
3417 Volta Place NW
Washington, DC 20007
202-337-5220
FAX: 202-337-8314
e-mail: info@agbell.org
www.agbell.org

Todd Houston, Executive Director
Entertaining wookbook contains exercises that help adults who are hard of hearing learn to listen and concentrate. *$9.95*
65 pages Paperback

7865 Listening and Talking
Alexander Graham Bell Association
3417 Volta Place NW
Washington, DC 20007
202-337-5220
FAX: 202-337-8314
e-mail: info@agbell.org
www.agbell.org

Todd Houston, Executive Director

This research-based text for professionals promotes communication by developing language, audition and speech in early intervention programs for young children with hearing loss. *$25.95*
191 pages Paperback

7866 Literacy & Your Deaf Child: What Every Pa rent Should Know
Gallaudet University Press
11030 S Langley Avenue
Chicago, IL 60628
202-651-5488
800-621-2736
FAX: 202-651-5489
www.gallaudet.edu
David A Stewart, Bryan R Clarke, author
An instructional guide specifically appropriate for parents of deaf and hard-of-hearing children who want to do everything they can to insure their hearing-impaired child learns to read and write with fluency and competence. *$21.95*
208 pages 2003
ISBN 1-563681-36-6

7867 Literature Journal
Gallaudet University Bookstore
800 Florida Avenue NE
Washington, DC 20002
202-651-5000
800-451-1073
FAX: 202-651-5489

Erving Jordan, President
This book includes extensive examples of student and teacher entries taken from actual journals of deaf high school students. *$7.95*
44 pages

7868 Loss for Words
Gallaudet University Bookstore
11030 S Langley Avenue
Chicago, IL 60628
202-651-5488
800-621-2736
FAX: 202-651-5489
She was an interpreter for her parents at four, a virtual head of household at eight, teacher and helper for her little sisters, buffer between her family and the world. Here is a daughter's account of growing up with loving parents, both of whom are deaf. *$11.00*
208 pages Paperback

7869 Managing Your Symptoms
Vestibular Disorders Association
PO Box 4467
Portland, OR 97208
503-229-7705
800-837-8428
FAX: 503-229-8064
e-mail: veda@vestibular.org
www.vestibular.org

$25.00

ISBN 0-963261-16-9

7870 Mask of Benevolence: Disabling the Deaf Community
Gallaudet University Bookstore
800 Florida Avenue NE
Washington, DC 20002
202-651-5000
800-451-1073
FAX: 202-651-5489

Erving Jordan, President
Dr. Harlan Lane does not view deafness as a handicap but rather a different state from hearing. Deaf people are a societal minority and should be treasured, not eradicated. *$23.00*
310 pages

7871 Mother Father Deaf: Living between Sound and Silence

Through the Looking Glass
2198 6th Street
Suite 100
Berkeley, CA 94710
510-848-1112
800-644-2666
FAX: 510-848-4445
e-mail: TLG@lookingglass.org
www.lookingglass.org

P Preston
Megan Kirshbaum, Executive Director
$18.00
278 pages

7872 My First Book of Sign
TJ Publishers
2544 Tarpley Road
Suite 108
Carrollton, TX 75006
972-416-0800
800-999-1168
FAX: 301-585-5930
e-mail: TJPubinc@aol.com

Angela K Thames, President
Jerald A Murphy, VP
Full-color book gives alphabetically grouped signs for 150 words most frequently used by young children. *$14.95*
76 pages Hardcover
ISBN 0-93032 -20-3

7873 My Signing Book of Numbers
Gallaudet University Press
800 Florida Avenue NE
Washington, DC 20002
202-651-5000
800-621-2736
FAX: 202-651-5489
TTY: 888-630-9347

Dan Wallace, Marketing Manager
Erving Jordan, President
This full-color book helps children learn their numbers in sign language. Each two-page spread of this delightfully illustrated book has the appropriate number of things or creatures for the numbers 0 through 20. *$14.95*
56 pages Hardcover
ISBN 0-93032 -37-8

7874 National Deaf Bowling Association
9244 E Mansfield Avenue
Denver, CO 80237
303-771-9018

Van K Scheppach, President
Russell Stecker, VP
Keith Thompson, Publishing Director
Holds world Deaf Bowling Torunament annually in July. Also holds Las Vegas Scratch Classic annually in October.

7875 Newsletter of American Hearing Research Foundation
American Hearing Research Foundation
8 S Michigan Avenue
Suite 814
Chicago, IL 60603
312-726-9670
FAX: 312-726-9695
e-mail: ahrf@american-hearing.org
www.american-hearing.org

William L Lederer, Executive Director
Sharon Parmet, Development/Communication Assoc.
The purposes of the Foundation are to promote, conduct and furnish financial assistance for medical research into the cause, prevention and cure of deafness, impaired hearing and balance disorders; encourage the collaboration of clinical and laboratory research; encourage and improve teaching in the medical aspects of hearing problems; and disseminate the most reliable scientific knowledge to physicians, hearing professionals and the public.

7876 Not Deaf Enough: Raising a Child Who is Hard of Hearing
Alexander Graham Bell Association
3417 Volta Place NW
Washington, DC 20007
202-337-5220
FAX: 202-337-8314
e-mail: info@agbell.org
www.agbell.org

Todd Houston, Executive Director
This sensitive book portrays a family's struggle to identify, accept and support their youngest child through his diagnosis of mild to moderate hearing loss. This book provides a much needed overview of this under-diagnosed and under-served disability. *$24.95*
242 pages Paperback

7877 Nursery Rhymes from Mother Goose
Gallaudet University Press
800 Florida Avenue NE
Washington, DC 20002
202-651-5000
FAX: 202-651-5704
TTY:888-630-8347

Dan Wallace, Marketing Manager
Erving Jordan, President
Each complete nursery rhyme is presented in Signed English and delightfully illustrated in full color. *$14.95*
64 pages
ISBN 0-93032 -99-8

7878 On the Edge of Deaf Culture: An Annotated Bibliography of Hearing Children/Deaf Parents
Through the Looking Glass
2198 6th Street
Suite 100
Berkeley, CA 94710
510-848-1112
800-644-2666
FAX: 510-848-4445
e-mail: TLG@lookingglass.org
www.lookingglass.org

Megan Kirshbaum, Executive Director
$35.00
360 pages

7879 On the Level
Vestibular Disorders Association
PO Box 4467
Portland, OR 97208
503-229-7705
800-837-8428
FAX: 503-229-8064
e-mail: veda@vestibular.org
www.vestibular.org

Lisa Haven, Editor
Connie Pilcher, Outreach Coordinator
$25.00
12 pages Quarterly

7880 Once Upon a Time...Children's Classics Retold in American Sign Language
Harris Communications
15155 Technology Drive
Eden Prairie, MN 55344
952-906-1180
800-825-6758
FAX: 952-906-1099
e-mail: mail@harriscomm.com
www.harriscomm.com

Bill Williams, National Sales Manager
Robert Harris, Owner
Children's classics come alive on videotapes. Six tapes are available, each telling a favorite fairy tale. *$29.95*

7881 Otitos Media in Young Children: Medical, Developmental, & Educational Considerations
Brookes Publishing
PO Box 10624
Baltimore, MD 21285
410-337-9580
800-638-3775
FAX: 410-337-8539
e-mail: custserv@brookespublishing.com
www.brookespublishing.com

Ina F Wallace PhD, Editor
Frederick W Henderson, Editor
Paul Brooks, Owner
This book reviews the current literature on the epidemiology, diagnosis, and medical management of otitis media; its secondary audiologic and communicative effects; and its impact on children and families. *$48.95*

352 pages Hardcover 1997
ISBN 1-557662-78-9

7882 Outsiders in a Hearing World
Gallaudet University Bookstore
800 Florida Avenue NE
Washington, DC 20002
202-651-5000
800-451-1073
FAX: 202-651-5489

Erving Jordan, President
An introduction to the social world of deaf people. The author gives a sociologists view of what it's like to be deaf. *$19.95*
240 pages Softcover

7883 Paws for Silence
International Hearing Dog
5901 E 89th Avenue
Henderson, CO 80640
303-287-3277
FAX: 303-287-3425
e-mail: ihdi@aol.com
www.ihdi.org

Valerie Foss-Brugger, President/Director
Publication from International hearing dog.
4-8 pages Quarterly

7884 Perigee Visual Dictionary of Signing
Harris Communications
15155 Technology Drive
Eden Prairie, MN 55344
952-906-1180
800-825-6758
FAX: 952-906-1099
e-mail: mail@harriscomm.com
www.harriscomm.com

Bill Williams, National Sales Manager
Robert Harris, Owner
An A-to-Z guide to American Sign Language vocabulary. *$15.95*
450 pages Paperback
ISBN 0-399519-52-1

7885 Perspective: Parent-Child Folio
Gallaudet University Bookstore
800 Florida Avenue NE
Washington, DC 20002
202-651-5000
800-451-1073
FAX: 202-651-5489

Erving Jordan, President
Ranging from table conversation to bedtime reading, the seven articles collected here emphasize family communications while providing important information for parents about deafness and deaf culture. *$5.95*
29 pages

7886 Phone of Our Own: The Deaf Insurrection Against Ma Bell
Gallaudet University Press
11030 S Langley Avenue
Chicago, IL 60628
202-651-5488
800-621-2736
FAX: 202-651-5489
TTY: 800-621-9347
gupress.gallaudet.edu
A recount of the history of the teletypewriter, from the three deaf engineers who developed the acoustic coupler that made mass communication on TTY's feasible, through the deaf community's twenty-year struggle against the government and AT&T to have TTY's produced and distributed. *$34.50*
304 pages Hardcover
ISBN 1-563680-90-4

7887 Place of Their Own: Creating the Deaf Community in America
Gallaudet University Press
2544 Tarpley Road
Suite 108
Carrollton, TX 75006
972-416-0800
800-999-1168
FAX: 301-585-5930
e-mail: TJPubinc@aol.com

Angela K Thames, President
Jerald A Murphy, VP
Traces development of American deaf society to show how deaf people developed a common language and sense of community. Views deafness as the distinguishing characteristic of a distinct culture. *$22.95*
212 pages Paperback
ISBN 0-930323-49-1

7888 PreReading Strategies
Gallaudet University Bookstore
800 Florida Avenue NE
Washington, DC 20002
202-651-5000
800-451-1073
FAX: 202-651-5489

Erving Jordan, President
Here is a wealth of good advice for preparing students to understand what they read, building comprehension and enjoyment. *$8.95*
65 pages

7889 Psychoeducational Assessment of Hearing-Impaired Students
Pro-Ed Publications
8700 Shoal Creek Boulevard
Austin, TX 78757
512-451-3246
800-897-3202
FAX: 800-397-7633
e-mail: feedback@proedinc.com
www.proedinc.com

Donald Hammill, Owner
Courtney King, Marketing Coordinator
This book includes a comprehensive presentation of issues and procedures related to the assessment of hearing-impaired students. *$29.00*
251 pages Paperback

7890 Psychology of Deafness
Longman Publishing Group
10 Bank Street
9th Floor
White Plains, NY 10606
914-993-5000
FAX: 914-421-5598

Roth Wilkofsky, Systems Contact
Joanne Dresner, President
Portrays hearing impairments as a psychological variable causing life experiences of the deaf to consistently differ from those of the non-deaf. Covers all levels of hearing loss, from prelingual and profound deafness to partial and mild hearing loss. Demonstrates how and why a hearing loss creates psychological stress no matter what its degree.
292 pages Hardcover
ISBN 0-801303-22-2

7891 Quad City Deaf & Hard of Hearing Youth Group: Tomorrow's Leaders for our Community
Independent Living Research Utilization ILRU
2323 S Shepherd Drive
Suite 1000
Houston, TX 77019
713-520-0232
FAX: 713-520-5785
www.ilru.org

Laurie Redd, Executive Director
IICIL staff see this program as a way to develop young leaders for themovement. Emphasis is given to providing oppportunities for members of the youth group to develop skills in planning and organizing activities.
10 pages

7892 Registry of Interpreters for the Deaf
8630 Fenton Street
Suite 324
Silver Spring, MD 20910
301-608-0050
FAX: 301-608-0508
e-mail: pr@rid.org
www.rid.org
Membership association for sign language interpreters; promoting national certification, professional development and training, and quality assurance through ethical practices system.

Monthly

7893 Religious Signing: A Comprehensive Guide for All Faiths
TJ Publishers
2544 Tarpley Road
Suite 108
Carrollton, TX 75006
972-416-0800
800-999-1168
FAX: 301-585-5930
e-mail: TJPubinc@aol.com
www.agbell.org

Angela K Thames, President
Jerald A Murphy, VP
Contains over 500 religious signs for all denominations and their meanings illustrated by clear upper torso illustrations that show movements of hand, body and face. Includes a section on signing favorite verses, prayers and blessings. *$17.95*
219 pages Paperback
ISBN 0-553344-44-

7894 Seeing Voices: A Journey into the World of the Deaf
TJ Publishers
2544 Tarpley Road
Suite 108
Carrollton, TX 75006
972-416-0800
800-999-1168
FAX: 301-585-5930
e-mail: TJPubinc@aol.com

Angela K Thames, President
Jerald A Murphy, VP
Well known for his exploration of how people respond to neurological impairments, Dr Sacks explores the world of the deaf and discovers how deaf people respond to their loss of hearing and how they develop language. A highly readable introduction to deaf people, deaf culture and American Sign Language. *$11.00*
186 pages Softcover
ISBN 0-06097 -47-1

7895 Sign Language Coloring Books
Gallaudet University Bookstore
800 Florida Avenue NE
Washington, DC 20002
202-651-5000
800-451-1073
FAX: 202-651-5489

Erving Jordan, President
A mischievous mouse and a spinning top, a doll on the sofa, a hobo clown with this friend the elephant: these coloring books are a FUNtastic way for children to learn to sign, fingerspell, read and write. *$4.50*

7896 Sign Language Feelings
Gallaudet University Bookstore
800 Florida Avenue NE
Washington, DC 20002
202-651-5000
800-451-1073
FAX: 202-651-5489

Erving Jordan, President
Worksheets teach signs for happy, sad and all of the feelings in between. *$4.50*

7897 Sign Language Interpreters and Interpreting
Gallaudet University Bookstore
800 Florida Avenue NE
Washington, DC 20002
202-651-5000
800-451-1073
FAX: 202-651-5489

Erving Jordan, President
This monograph presents articles about personal characteristics and abilities of interpreters, the effects of lag time on interpreter errors, and the interpretation of register. *$15.95*
161 pages

7898 Sign with Me Books
Gallaudet University Bookstore
11030 S Langley Avenue
Chicago, IL 60628
202-651-5488
800-621-2736
FAX: 202-651-5489

Bold, colorful pictures and accurate diagrams make it fun for beginners to learn everyday signs. Titles in this series include ABC Sign With Me; Colors Sign With Me; Weather Sign With Me; and 1,2,3 Sign With Me. *$3.95*
Per Title

7899 Signed English Starter
Gallaudet University Press
15155 Technology Drive
Eden Prairie, MN 55344
952-906-1180
800-825-6758
FAX: 952-906-1099
e-mail: mail@harriscomm.com
www.harriscomm.com

Bill Williams, National Sales Manager
Robert Harris, Owner
The first book to use when learning Signed English. *$ 13.95*
208 pages Paperback
ISBN 0-913580-82-1

7900 Signing Family: What Every Parent Should Know About Sign Communication
Gallaudet University Press
11030 S Langley Avenue
Chicago, IL 60628
800-621-2736
FAX: 800-621-8476
TTY:800-621-9347
gupress.gallaudet.edu

David A Stewart, Co-Author
Barbara Luetke-Stahlman, Co-Author
This reader-friendly book shows parents how to create a set of goals around the communication needs of their deaf child. Describes in even-handed terms the major signing options available, from American Sign Language to Signed English. *$24.95*
192 pages Softcover

7901 Signing for Reading Success
Gallaudet University Press
800 Florida Avenue NE
Washington, DC 20002
202-651-5000
800-451-1073
FAX: 202-651-5489

Erving Jordan, President
This booklet provides summaries of four research students on the usefulness of signing for reading achievement. *$7.95*
24 pages Softcover
ISBN 0-930323-18-1

7902 Signing: How to Speak with Your Hands
TJ Publishers
2544 Tarpley Road
Suite 108
Carrollton, TX 75006
972-416-0800
800-999-1168
FAX: 301-585-5930
e-mail: TJPubinc@aol.com

Angela K Thames, President
Jerald A Murphy, VP
Presents 1,200 basic signs with clear illustrations in logical topical groupings. Linguistic principles are described at the beginning of each chapter, giving insight into the rules which govern American Sign Language. *$17.95*
248 pages Paperback
ISBN 0-553375-39-3

7903 Signs Across America
Gallaudet University Press
2544 Tarpley Road
Suite 108
Carrollton, TX 75006
972-416-0800
800-999-1168
FAX: 301-585-5930
e-mail: TJPubinc@aol.com

Angela K Thames, President
Jerald A Murphy, VP
A look at regional variations in ASL. Signs for selected words collected from 25 different states. More than 1,200 signs illustrated in the text. *$28.95*

285 pages Paperback
ISBN 0-913580-96-1

7904 Signs Everywhere
Harris Communications
15155 Technology Drive
Eden Prairie, MN 55344
952-906-1180
800-825-6758
FAX: 952-906-1099
e-mail: mail@harriscomm.com
www.harriscomm.com

Bill Williams, National Sales Manager
Robert Harris, Owner
This books includes signs for towns, cities, states and provinces. *$14.95*
254 pages Paperback
ISBN 0-916708-05-5

7905 Signs for Computing Terminology
Gallaudet University Bookstore
11030 S Langley Avenue
Chicago, IL 60628
202-651-5488
800-621-2736
FAX: 202-651-5489
This sign reference will facilitate communication among deaf persons involved with computers by providing a significant vocabulary base for the computing field of today and tomorrow. *$12.95*
182 pages Softcover

7906 Signs for Me: Basic Sign Vocabulary for Children, Parents & Teachers
TJ Publishers
2544 Tarpley Road
Suite 108
Carrollton, TX 75006
972-416-0800
800-999-1168
FAX: 301-585-5930
e-mail: TJPubinc@aol.com

Angela K Thames, President
Jerald A Murphy, VP
Sign language vocabulary for preschool and elementary school children introduces household items, animals, family members, actions, emotions, safety concerns and other concepts. *$12.95*
112 pages Softcover
ISBN 0-91503 -27-8

7907 Signs for Sexuality: A Resource Manual
Gallaudet University Bookstore
800 Florida Avenue NE
Washington, DC 20002
202-651-5000
800-451-1073
FAX: 202-651-5489

Erving Jordan, President
An important book for those who want to listen to and talk with other people about feelings, loving and caring. *$24.95*
122 pages Softcover

7908 Signs of the Times
Gallaudet University Press
11030 S Langley Avenue
Chicago, IL 60628
800-621-2736
FAX: 800-621-8476
TTY:800-621-9347
gupress.gallaudet.edu
An excellent beginner's contact signing book that fills the gap between sign language dictionaries and American Sign Language text. Designed for use as a classroom text. *$34.95*
448 pages Softcover
ISBN 0-913580-76-7

7909 Silent Garden: Raising Your Deaf Child
Gallaudet University Press
11030 S Langley Avenue
Chicago, IL 60628
202-651-5488
800-621-2736
FAX: 202-651-5489
www.gallaudet.edu

Paul W Ogden, author
The author explain the broad range of hearing loss types, from minor to profound. Parents also are advised about what type of school their child should attend and what kinds of professional help will be best for the entire family. The book describes all forms of communication, including choices in signing from American Sign Language to the various manual systems based upon English. Technological alternatives are presented also, including when and when not to consider cochler implants. *$34.95*
313 pages 1996
ISBN 1-563680-58-0

7910 Simultaneous Communication, ASL, and Other Communication Modes
Gallaudet University Bookstore
800 Florida Avenue NE
Washington, DC 20002
202-651-5000
800-451-1073
FAX: 202-651-5489

Erving Jordan, President
This monograph presents four major articles that examine issues surrounding communications in an educational environment. *$ 15.95*
236 pages

7911 Sing Praise Hymnal
Broadman and Holman
127 9th Avenue S
Nashville, TN 37203
615-251-5005
800-458-2772
FAX: 651-251-5764
www.bssb.com/lwc

Ken Stephens, President
A song book for the deaf. *$6.95*

7912 Sleeping Beauty
Gallaudet University Press
800 Florida Avenue NE
Washington, DC 20002
202-651-5000
800-621-2736
FAX: 800-660-8476
TTY: 888-630-9347

Dan Wallace, Marketing Manager
Erving Jordan, President
The popular fairytale of the princess put to sleep for a hundred years is presented with beautiful full color illustrations and selected sentences in American Sign Language. *$14.95*
64 pages
ISBN 0-93032 -97-1

7913 Sleeping Beauty Videotape
Gallaudet University Bookstore
11030 S Langley Avenue
Chicago, IL 60628
202-651-5488
800-621-2736
FAX: 202-651-5489
Presents the entire story of Sleeping Beauty told in American Sign Language. Includes voice over. *$29.95*
30 Minutes

7914 Spring Dell Center
6040 Radio Station Road
La Plata, MD 20646
301-870-2474

Melissa Tyner, Transportation Director
Donna Retzlaff, Executive Director
Since 1967, Spring Dell center has been, bridging the gap to enhance the lives of developmentally disabled people. Spring Dell's goal is to empower people in every aspect of their lives through the implementation of two programs, employment/vocational services and residential services including transportation. Spring Dell offers transportation door-to-door for persons with developmental disabilities, including day care programs, supportive environment, residential and any other transportation.

7915 **TDI National Directory & Resource Guide: Blue Book**
Telecommunications for the Deaf
8630 Fenton Street
Suite 604
Silver Spring, MD 20910
301-589-3786
FAX: 301-589-3797
e-mail: info@tdi-online.org
www.tdi-online.org

Claude L Stout, Executive Director
James D House, Member Service/Public Rel. Dir.
$27.00
639 pages Annual

7916 **Talk with Me**
Alexander Graham Bell Association
3417 Volta Place NW
Washington, DC 20007
202-337-5220
FAX: 202-337-8314
e-mail: info@agbell.org
www.agbell.org

Todd Houston, Executive Director
This book addresses the urgent need to enlighten parents and professionals responsible for the crucial early decisions that affect the speech, language, social, emotional and intellectual development of children who are deaf and hard of hearing. *$22.95*
222 pages Paperback

7917 **Teaching Social Skills to Hearing-Impaired Students**
Alexander Graham Bell Association
3417 Volta Place NW
Washington, DC 20007
202-337-5220
FAX: 202-337-8314
e-mail: info@agbell.org
www.agbell.org

Todd Houston, Executive Director
This book provides teachers and parents with a comprehensive, clearly presented hands-on program to develop social skills in children and young adults who are deaf or hard of hearing. *$21.95*
203 pages

7918 **Telecommunication Relay Services**
Ferderal Government
31 Center Drive Msc2320
Bethesda, MD 20832
800-241-1044
FAX: 301-402-0018
e-mail: nidcdinfo@nidcd.nih.gov
www.nidcd.nih.gov
This telecommunication relay services fact sheet explains what the service is, how the relay service allows people who are deaf, har-of-hearing or speech impaired to communicate through a communications assiatnt with people who use a standard telephone.

7919 **Telephone Communication and Hearing Impaired**
Taylor & Francis
47 Runway Drive
Suite G
Levittown, PA 19057
215-625-8900
FAX: 215-625-2940
This is a practical book containing valuable information for audiologists, teachers and others concerned with rehabilitation of the hearing impaired.
200 pages Illustrated
ISBN 0-85066 -18-3

7920 **Telling Stories**
Harris Communications
15155 Technology Drive
Eden Prairie, MN 55344
952-906-1180
800-825-6758
FAX: 952-906-1099
e-mail: mail@harriscomm.com
www.harriscomm.com

Bill Williams, National Sales Manager
Robert Harris, Owner
This international award winning play, now on video, uses the symbols and myths drawn from the struggles between the world of the deaf and the world of the hearing. *$59.95*
Video

7921 **The Mask of Benevolence: Disabling the De af Community**
Dawnsign Press

A look at the gulf that seperates the deaf minority from the hearing world, this book sheds light on the mistreatment of the deaf community by a hearing establishment that resists understanding and awareness. *$11.95*
334 pages 1999
ISBN 1-581210-09-4

7922 **Theoretical Issues in Sign Language Research**
Gallaudet University Bookstore
11030 S Langley Avenue
Chicago, IL 60628
202-651-5488
800-621-2736
FAX: 202-651-5489
These volumes are an outgrowth of a conference held at the University of Rochester in 1986, dealing with the four traditional core areas of phonology, morphology, syntax and semantics. *$29.95*
338 pages

7923 **They Grow in Silence**
Taylor & Francis
47 Runway Drive
Suite G
Levittown, PA 19057
FAX: 215-785-5515
Gives a comprehensive picture of the deaf child in society, not only looking at the individual but also, at the related problems for the family, community and the professional. Only by the examination of such a broad perspective can questions on the position and circumstances of the deaf child be fully considered.
223 pages Paper
ISBN 0-85066 -54-6

7924 **Tinnitus Today**
American Tinnitus Association
PO Box 5
Portland, OR 97207
503-248-9985
800-634-8978
FAX: 503-248-0024
e-mail: tinnitus@ata.org
www.ata.org
Published quarterly by the American Tinnitus Association. Also available online. Online ISSN# is 1530-6569. *$25.00*
28 pages Quarterly

7925 **US Government TTY Directory**
Consumer Information Center
Department 627f
Pueblo, CO 81009

e-mail: catalog.pueblo@gsa.gov

Judi Mahoney, Public Affairs
Gives details on how to use the Federal Relay Service and which agencies and congressional offices have text telephone devices.

7926 **Understanding Deafness Socially**
Charles C Thomas
2600 S 1st Street
Springfield, IL 62704
217-789-8980
800-258-8980
FAX: 217-789-9130
e-mail: books@ccthomas.com
www.ccthomas.com

Michael Thomas, President
A look at the social difficulties of being hearing impaired in a hearing society. Also available in cloth. *$29.95*
168 pages Softcover
ISBN 0-398065-70-5

7927 **Vision**
National Catholic Office of the Deaf
7202 Buchanan Street
Landover Hills, MD 20784
301-577-1684
FAX: 301-577-1690
e-mail: ncod@erols.com

Arvilla Rank, Executive Director/Editor
Published as a pastoral service for the deaf and hard of hearing. Provides information to members and others working in ministry. Prepares an annual gathering called Pastoral Week meeting in January. Price: $15.00 per year, $25 for 2 years; Foreign: $17 per year; $27 for 2 years. *$15.00*
16 pages quarterly

7928 Volta Review
Alexander Graham Bell Association
3417 Volta Place NW
Washington, DC 20007
202-337-5220
FAX: 202-337-8314
e-mail: info@agbell.org
www.agbell.org

Todd Houston, Executive Director
Professionally refereed journal that publishes articles and research on education, rehabilitation and communicative development of people who have hearing impairments. Also includes subscription to Volta Voices, up-to-date magazine, bimonthly. *$62.00*
Quarterly

7929 Volta Voices
Alexander Graham Bell Association
3417 Volta Place NW
Washington, DC 20007
202-337-5220
FAX: 202-337-8314
e-mail: info@agbell.org
www.agbell.org

Todd Houston, Executive Director
Contains Association news and educates readers on the abilities and needs of children and adults who are deaf or hard of hearing. Includes subscription to The Volta Review, published four times a year. *$62.00*

7930 We CAN Hear and Speak
Alexander Graham Bell Association
3417 Volta Place NW
Washington, DC 20007
202-337-5220
FAX: 202-337-8314
e-mail: info@agbell.org
www.agbell.org

Todd Houston, Executive Director
Written by parents for families of children who are deaf or hard of hearing, this work describes auditory-verbal terminology and approaches and contains personal narratives written by parents and their children who are deaf or hard of hearing. *$24.95*
171 pages Paperback

7931 Week the World Heard Gallaudet
Gallaudet University Press
800 Florida Avenue NE
Washington, DC 20002
202-651-5220
800-451-1073
FAX: 202-651-5489
e-mail: gupress@gallaudet.edu
gupress.gallaudet.edu/homeSLSorder.html
This day-to-day description of the events surrounding the Deaf President Now movement at Gallaudet University includes full color and black and white photographs and interviews with people involved in the events of that week. *$34.50*
192 pages
ISBN 0-930323-54-8

7932 What Can Baby Hear?: Auditory Tests and Interventions for Infants with Multiple Disabilities
Brookes Publishing
PO Box 10624
Baltimore, MD 21285
410-337-9580
800-638-3775
FAX: 410-337-8539
e-mail: custserv@brookespublishing.com
www.brookespublishing.com

Paul Brooks, Owner
This video and accompanying booklet explain the principles and methods of various auditory tests designed for early detection and teach viewers how to assess infants' auditory needs to begin appropriate intervention. *$45.00*
30 Minutes 1997
ISBN 1-557662-88-6

7933 What You Need To Know
Vestibular Disorders Association
PO Box 4467
Portland, OR 97208
503-229-7705
800-837-8428
FAX: 503-229-8064

$24.95
Quarterly
ISBN 0-963261-13-4

7934 What is Auditory Processing?
Speech Bin
1965 25th Avenue
Vero Beach, FL 32960
772-770-0007
800-477-3324
FAX: 772-770-0006
www.speechbin.com

Jan J Binney, Senior Editor
Booklet for parents and teachers explaining children's difficulties in listening and auditory skills. Set of ten copies. *$ 14.95*
16 pages
ISBN 0-93785 -45-9

7935 When the Mind Hears
Gallaudet University Bookstore
800 Florida Avenue NE
Washington, DC 20002
202-651-5000
800-451-1073
FAX: 202-651-5489

Erving Jordan, President
Comprehensive history of the deaf and their relationship with hearing academic communities. *$19.95*
414 pages Paperback

7936 Without Sight and Sound
Helen Keller National Center
111 Middle Neck Road
Sands Point, NY 11050
516-944-8900

e-mail: hkncdir@aol.com
www.helenkeller.org

Joseph McNulty, Executive Director
Pamphlet offering facts, causes, types and descriptions of deaf-blindness.

7937 You And Your Deaf Child
TJ Publishers
2544 Tarpley Road
Suite 108
Carrollton, TX 75006
972-416-0800
800-999-1168
FAX: 301-585-5930
e-mail: TJPubinc@aol.com

Angela K Thames, President
Jerald A Murphy, VP
Designed specifically for parents who have children newly diagnosed as hearing impaired. Provides vital information on hearing impairment, setting limits, behavior management, nonverbal behavior and much more. *$28.95*
142 pages Softcover
ISBN 1-563680-60-2

7938 You and Your Deaf Child: A Self-Help Guide for Parents of Deaf and Hard of Hearing Children
Gallaudet University Press
11030 S Langley Avenue
Chicago, IL 60628
800-621-2736
FAX: 800-621-8476
TTY:800-621-9347
gupress.gallaudet.edu
The classic self-instructional guide has been completely written with more information dealing with feelings, communication and other issues. Includes worksheets and practice exercises. *$19.95*

224 pages Softcover

Sports

7939 American Hearing Impaired Hockey Association
1143 W Lake Street
Chicago, IL 60607
312-226-5880
FAX: 312-829-2098
TTY:773-767-3130
e-mail: cheryl_hager@ahiha.org
www.ahiha.org

Stan Mikita, Co Founder/President
Irv Tiahnybik, Manager
Supports hockey for hearing-impaired youths.

7940 USA Deaf Sports Federation
102 N Krohn Place
Sioux Falls, SD 57103
605-367-5760
FAX: 605-977-6625
TTY:6053675761
e-mail: homeoffice@usadeafsports.org
www.usdeafsports.org

Dr. Lawrence Fleischer, President
John J. Knetzger, Vice President Of Member Service
Robert C. Steele, Vice President Of Financial Aff.
The USA Deaf Sports Federation's purpose was to foster and regulate uniform rules of competition and provide social outlets for deaf members and their friends; serve as a parent organization for regional sports organizations; conduct annual athletic competitions; and assist in the participation of U.S. teams in international competition.

Support Groups

7941 Dial-a-Hearing Screening Test
300 S Chester Road
Swarthmore, PA 19081
800-222-EARS
FAX: 610-543-2802
e-mail: dahst@aol.com

George Biddle, Executive Director
Hearing help information center. Provides toll free phone number for accurate telephone hearing screening test. Provides referral to audiologist or ear, nose and throat doctor. All services are free. Hours are 9 AM to 5 PM ET Monday to Friday.

7942 Stay Tuned
Fanlight Productions
4196 Washington Street
Suite 2
Boston, MA 02131
617-469-4999
800-937-4113
FAX: 617-469-3379
e-mail: fanlight@fanlight.com
www.fanlight.com

Karen McMillen, Marketing Director
Ben Achtenberg, Owner
This program looks at ways of coping with hearing loss. The program introduces us to one woman who, after suffering a mid-life hearing loss, confronts her situation and regains her ability to function and enjoy her life through taking advantage of hearing aids, speech reading instruction, assistive listening devices and the support of other hearing impaired people. *$99.00*

Associations

7943 **Access Unlimited**
570 Hance Road
Binghamton, NY 13903
607-669-4822
800-849-2143
FAX: 607-669-4595
www.accessunlimited.com

Sherry Sinai, Administrative Coordinator
Sherry Lowry, Director
Thomas Egan, Owner
At Access Unlimited, we believe that mobility, like people, comes in all shapes and colors. We celebrate the rich diversity of our customers' needs by creating products that alow easy access to any vehicle, from cars and vans to trucks and SUVs. We believe that adaptive equipment should be unobtrusive and should meet the needs of its user with a minimum of modifications to vehicle and lifestyle.

7944 **American Association of Spinal Cord Injury Psychologists & Social Workers**
7520 Astoria Boulevard
East Elmhurst, NY 11370
718-803-3782
FAX: 718-803-0414
e-mail: aascipsw@unitedspinal.org
www.aascipsw.org

Vivian Beyda DrPH, Associate Executive Director
Sarah Lerman MPH, Program Manager
Marion Smith, Administrative Assistant
Organized and operated for scientific and educational purposes to advance and improve the psychosocial care of persons with spinal cord impairment, develop and promote education and research related to the psychosocial care of persons with spinal cord injury, recognize psychologists and social workers whose careers are devoted to the problems of spinal cord impairment.

7945 **American Back Society**
2647 International Boulevard
Suite 401
Oakland, CA 94601
510-536-9929
FAX: 510-536-1812
e-mail: info@americanbacksoc.org
www.americanbacksoc.org

Scott Haldeman D.C., M.D.PhD, President
Ronald Donelson M.D., M.S., Vice President
Thomas E. Dreisenger PhD, Secretary
The American Back Society was founded in Oakland, California in 1982 as a nonprofit organization dedicated to providing an interdisciplinary forum for health care professionals and scientists interested in relieving pain and diminishing impairment through proper diagnosis and treatment of patients suffering from spinal pathology.
1982

7946 **American Juvenile Arthritis Organization (AJAO)**
Arthritis Foundation
PO Box 7669
Atlanta, GA 30357
404-872-7100
800-283-7800
www.arthritis.org

L. Brunson White, Chair
John H Klippel, CEO/President
Gin Bell, Board of Trustees
Arthritis Foundation efforts center on the three-fold mission of the organization: research, prevention and quality of life. The Arthritis Foundation currently provides nearly $20 million in grants to nearly 300 researchers to help find a cure, prevention or better treatment for arthritis. The Arthritis Foundation's sponsorship of research for more than 50 years has resulted in major treatment advances for most arthritis diseases.

7947 **American Paraplegia Society**
Journal Of Spinal Cord Medicine
75-20 Astoria Boulevard
Jackson Heights, NY 11370
718-803-3782
FAX: 718-803-0414
e-mail: aps@unitedspinal.org
www.apssci.org

Vivian Beyda Dr.PhD, Associate Executive Director
Sara Lerman MPH, Program Manager
Marion Smith, Administrative Assistant
Organized and operated for scientific and educational purposes to advance and improve health care of persons with spinal cord impairment, develop and promote education and research related to spinal cord impairment, recognize physicians and doctoral level researchers whose careers are devoted to the problems of spinal cord impairment.

7948 **American Spinal Injury Association**
2020 Peachtree Road NW
Atlanta, GA 30309
404-355-1826
FAX: 404-355-1826
e-mail: asiaoffice@shepherd.org
www.asia-spinalinjury.org

Marcalee Alexander MD, President and Director
Glenn Rechtine MD, President Elect & Director
Amie Jackson, MD, Secretary-Treasurer & Director
The mission of the American Spinal Injury Association is to promote and establish standards of excellence for all aspects of health care of individuals with spinal cord injury from the onset throughout life. To educate members, other healthcare professionals, patients and their families on all aspects of spinal cord injury and its consequences in order to improve care, increase availability of services and maximize the injured individuals potential for full participation in community life.
1973

7949 **American Stroke Association**
American Heart Association
7272 Greenville Avenue
Dallas, TX 75231
214-373-6300
888-478-7653
FAX: 214-706-5231
e-mail: strokeconnection@heart.org
www.strokeassociation.org

M Wheeler, Chief Executive Officer
Fifty-five state affiliates monitoring local chapters offering educational materials, seminars, conferences and transportation for members nationwide. Maintains a listing of over 1,000 stroke support groups across the nation for referral to stroke survivors, their families, caregivers and interested professionals.

7950 **Amytrophic Lateral Sclerosis Association**
27001 Agoura Road
Suite 150
Calabasas Hills, CA 91301
818-880-9007
800-782-4747
FAX: 818-880-9006
e-mail: alsinfo@alsa-national.org
www.alsa.org

Gary A. Leo, CEO and President
Rick Ventura, Chief Operating Officer
John Applegate, Vice President Finance
The ALS association is the only national not-for-profit health organization dedicated soley to lead the fight against ALS. The Association covers all the bases-research, patient and community services, public education, and advocacy-in providing help and hope to those facing the disease. The mission is to lead the fight to cure and treat ALS through global cutting edge research, and to empower people with Lou Gehrig's disease to live fuller lives & provide them with compassion care and support.

7951 **Arthritis Consulting Services**
2787 E Oakland Park Boulevard
Suite 204
Fort Lauderdale, FL 33306
954-739-3202
800-327-3027
FAX: 954-337-2887
e-mail: acs@stoparthritis.com
www.stoparthritis.com

Donna K Pinorsky RN BA, Administrator
Pat Rothblatt, Office Manager

For over 40 years Arthritis Consulting Services has been committed to the treatment and elimination of symptoms commonly associated with arthritis. Through the use of natural hormones/compounds and ingredients we have successfully alleviated arthritic symptoms in our patients.

7952 Arthritis Foundation

1330 W Peachtree Street NW
Suite 100
Atlanta, GA 30309
404-872-7100
800-283-7800
FAX: 404-872-9559
e-mail: help@arthritis.org
www.arthritis.org

John H Klippel, CEO/President
Offers information and referrals regarding educational materials and programs, fund-raising, support groups, seminars and conferences offered by 55 local chapters across the United States.

7953 Association for Network Care

444 Main Street
Longmont, CO 80501
303-678-8101
FAX: 303-678-8089
e-mail: info@associationfornetworkcare.com
www.associationfornetworkcare.com

Donald Epstein D.C., Board Of Directors
Richard Kaye D.C., Board Of Directors
Jackie Knowles D.C., Board Of Directors
Supports the consciousness, advances the practice of, and promotes the public availability of Network Spinal Analysis. Supports the advancement and understanding of the relationship of the spine and nervous system to consciousness, the expression of innate intelligence, self-organization, and healing. Encourages the support of the science, art, and philosophically similar and compatible models in various healing arts through workshops, seminars, journals, newsletters and research projects.

7954 Association for Neurologically Impaired Brain Injured Children

21212 26th Avenue
Bayside, NY 11360
718-423-9550
FAX: 718-423-9838
e-mail: info@anibic.org
caresdb.uwnyc.org/cares/detail_45.cfm?detrec

Alvin Clotkin, President
Gerard Smith, Executive Director
Christine Fisher, Intake Coordinator
ANIBIc is a voluntary, multi-service organization that is dedicated to serving individuals with severe learning disabilities, neurological impairments and other developmental disabilities. Services include: residential, vocational, family support services, recreation (children and adults), respite (adult), in home support services, counseling and tramatic brain injury services (adults).

7955 Association of Children's Prosthetic/Orthotic Clinics

6300 N River Road
Suite 727
Rosemont, IL 60018
847-698-1637
FAX: 847-823-0536
e-mail: raymond@aaos.org
www.acpoc.org

Sheril King, Executive Director
Established for the purpose of supporting clinical teams that treat children with prosthetic or orthotic devices. Goals are achieved through programs of professional education and clinical research.

7956 Christopher Reeve Paralysis Foundation

636 Morris Tpke
Suite 3a
Short Hills, NJ 07078
973-379-2690
800-225-0292
FAX: 973-912-9433
e-mail: info@paralysis.org
www.christopherreeve.org , www.paralysis.org

Peter Kiernan III, Chairman Of The Board
Henry G. Stifel III, Vice Chairman
Robert Guyett, Treasurer

Committed to funding research that develops treatments and cures for paralysis caused by spinal cord injury and other central nervous system disorders. The Foundation also vigorously works to improve the quality of life for people living with disabilities through its grants program, paralysis resource center and advocacy efforts.

7957 Epilepsy Foundation

4351 Garden City Drive
Landover, MD 20785
301-459-3700
800-332-1000
FAX: 301-459-3700
e-mail: epilepsy@peaknet.net
www.epilepsyfoundation.org

Tony Coelho, Chair of Board of Directors
Bruce P. Hermann PhD, Chair of Advisory Board
Eric R. Hargis, President/CEO
The Epilepsy Foundation is the national voluntary agency solely dedicated to the welfare of the 2.7 million people with epilepsy in the U.S. and their families. The organization works to ensure that people with seizures are able to participate in all life experiences; and to prevent, control and cure epilepsy through research, education, advocacy and services.
1968

7958 Friends of Disabled Adults and Children

4900 Lewis Road
Stone Mountain, GA 30083
770-491-9014
FAX: 770-491-0026
e-mail: chrisbrand@fodac.org
www.fodac.org

Chris Brand, CEO and President
Pam Holleyrt, Director Of Admininstration
Mile Maijala, Director Of Operations
Not-for-profit organization dedicated to providing necessary services and support to physically and mobility impaired people of all ages. Provides free mobility impairment, rehabilitative, and home healthcare equipment. Provides variety of brochures and pamphlets. Community reentering program.

7959 Kessler Institute for Rehabilitation

1199 Pleasant Valley Way
West Orange, NJ 07052
973-731-3600
800-721-3214
FAX: 973-243-6819
www.kessler-rehab.com

Robert Brehm, President
Bonnie Evans, Manager
Kessler Institute for Rehabilitation is world renowned for treating individuals with physical disabilities, resulting from spinal cord and brain injuries, stroke and amputee, sports and work-related, and other illnesses and injuries. Kessler offers comprehensive programs designed to meet each person's individual needs.

7960 Matheny School and Hospital

PO Box 339
Peapack, NJ 07977
908-234-0011
FAX: 908-719-2137
e-mail: info@matheny.org
www.matheny.org

Steven Proctor, President
A residential and outpatient facility for children and adults with physical disabilities such as Cerebral Palsy, Spina Bifida, Muscular Dystrophy and Lesch-Nyhan disease. Matheny offers medical and dental care, therapies, augmentative communication, and other allied health services as well as special education, respite care and adult medical day care.

7961 Mobility International USA

132 E Broadway
Suite 343
Eugene, OR 97401
541-343-1284
FAX: 541-343-6812
e-mail: info@miusa.org
www.miusa.org

Susan Sygall, Executive Director
Cerise Roth-Vinson, Director of Administration
Cindy Lewis, Director Programs

A US based national nonprofit organization dedicated to empowering people with disabilities around the world through leadership development, training and international exchange to ensure inclusion of people with disabilities in international exchange and development programs. The National Clearinghouse on Disability & Exchange, a joint project managed by MIUSA provides free information and referrals.

7962 NIH Osteoporosis and Related Bone Diseases National Resource Center

2 AMS Circle
Bethesda, MD 20892
202-223-0344
800-624-2663
FAX: 202-293-2356
TTY: 202-466-4315
e-mail: naimsboneinfo@mail.nih.gov
www.naims.nih.gov/bone

Doug Boyer, Administrative Technician
Marsha Hennings, Contractor
Mary Junious, Lead Purchasing Agent
Distributes information to patients, health professionals and the public on osteoporosis, Paget's disease of bone, osteogenesis imperfecta, and other metabolic bone diseases. Information on prevention, early detection and treatment of these diseases is available.

7963 National Institute of Arthritis and Musculoskeletal and Skin Diseases

31 Center Drive MSC 2350
Bldg. 31, Room 4CO2
Bethesda, MD 20892
301-496-8190
877-226-4267
FAX: 301-480-2814
TTY: 301-565-2966
e-mail: niamsinfo@mail.nih.gov
www.nih.gov/niams

Dr Stephen I Katz, Director
Kelly Collins, Manager
Mission is to support research into the causes, treatment and prevention of arthritis and musculoskeletal and skin diseases, the training of basic and clinical scientists to carry out this research, and the dissemination of information on research progress in these diseases.

7964 National Institute of Neurological Disorders and Stroke

PO Box 5801
Bethesda, MD 20824
301-496-5751
800-352-9424
FAX: 301-402-2186
TTY: 301-468-5981
www.ninds.nih.gov

Story C. Landis, PH.D, Director
Walter J. Koroshetz M.D., Deputy Director
Audrey S. Penn M.D., Special Advisor To Director
America's focal point for support of research on brain and nervous system disorders. Its active public information program provides physicians, patients and the public with educational materials and research highlights. Materials provided by the public information program include brochures, fact sheets, information packets and special reports. All publications are free of charge.

7965 National Mobility Equipment Dealers Association

3327 W Bearss Avenue
Tampa, FL 33618
813-264-2697
800-833-0427
FAX: 813-962-8970
e-mail: nmeda@aol.com
www.nmeda.org

Dana Roeling, Executive Director
Marilyn Myers, Administrative Assistant
Doris Cruzado, Mebership Coordinator
NMEDA is a non-profit trade association of mobility equipment dealers, driver rehabilitation specialists, and other professionals dedicated to broadening the opportunities for people with disabilities to drive or be transported in vehicles modified with mobility equipment. All members work together to improve transportation options of people with disabilities.

7966 National Multiple Sclerosis Society

733 3rd Avenue
New York, NY 10017
212-986-3240
800-344-4867
FAX: 314-781-1440
e-mail: info@gatewaymssociety.org
www.nationalmssociety.org

Joyce M. Nelson, President/CEO
Weyman T. Johnson Jr., Chairman Of The Board
Craig T. Lynch, Secretary
Mission is to end the devastating effects of MS. Provides professional and public education; information and referral; and supports research. One hundred and forty local chapters and branches offer counseling services, advocacy, discount prescription and health care products program, and assistance in obtaining adaptive equipment.

7967 National Parkinson Foundation

1501 NW 9th Avenue Bob Hope Road
Miami, FL 33136
305-243-6666
800-327-4545
FAX: 305-243-5595
e-mail: contact@parkinson.org
www.parkinson.org

Jose Garcia- Pedrosa, Chief Operating Officer
Ruth Hagestuen, Director Of Field Services
Pamela Olmo, Controller
The purpose of this Foundation is to find the cause and cure for Parkinson's Disease and related neurodegenerative disorders through research, to educate general medical practitioners to detect the early warning signs of Parkinson's Disease and to improve the quality of life for both patients and their caregivers. Provides current information to patients, caregivers and families. Publishes quarterly newsletter.
1957

7968 Paralyzed Veterans of America

801 18th Street NW
Washington, DC 20006
202-872-1300
800-424-8200
FAX: 202-872-2564
e-mail: info@pva.org
www.pva.org

Randy Pleva Sr., President
Gene A. Crayton, Senior Vice President
Jack Franklin, Vice President
A congressionally chartered veterans service organization, has developed a unique expertise on a wide variety of issues involving the special needs of our members— veterans of the armed forces who have experienced spinal cord injury or dysfunction.
1946

7969 Polio Health International

4207 Lindell Boulevard
Suite 110
Saint Louis, MO 63108
314-534-0475
FAX: 314-534-5070
e-mail: info@post-polio.org
www.post-polio.org

Lawrence C. Becker PhD, President/Chairperson
William G. Strothers, Vice President
Marny K. Eulberg MD, Secretary
Enhances the lives and independence of polio survivors and home ventilator users through education, advocacy, research and networking.

7970 Polio Society

4200 Wisconsin Avenue
#106273
Washington, DC 20016
301-897-8180
FAX: 202-994-3153

Jessica Scheer, Executive Director
The Polio Society was created for the purpose of providing educational resources and support group services to people who had polio and are now experiencing the late effects of polio. We are a chartered non profit organization governed by a board of directors composed primarily of polio survivors and family members of polio survivors. Our programs and services are funded by membership dues, gifts and private contributions.

7971 **Post-Polio Health International**
4207 Lindell Boulevard
Suite 110
Saint Louis, MO 63108
314-534-0475
FAX: 314-534-5070
e-mail: info@post-polio.org
www.post-polio.org

Lawrence C. Becker PhD, President and Chairperson
William Strothers, Vice President
Marny K. Eulberg MD, Secretary
Post-Polio Health International's mission is to enhance the lives and independence of polio survivors and home ventilator users through education, advocacy, research and networking.

7972 **Society for Progressive Supranuclear Palsy (SPSP)**
11350 McCormick Road
Suite 906
Hunt Valley, MD 21031
410-785-7004
800-457-4777
FAX: 410-785-7009
e-mail: info@curepsp.org
www.psp.org

Kenneth A. McKusick MD, Chairman
Jim Barron Ph.D., Vice Chairman
James E. Koehnlein, Treasurer
The Society for PSP is dedicated to increasing awareness of Progressive Supranuclear Palsy, advancing research towards a cure, and providing hope, support and education for persons with PSP, their families and healthcare professionals.

7973 **Spinal Cord Society (SCS)**
19051 County Highway 1
Fergus Falls, MN 56537
218-739-5252
FAX: 218-739-5262
www.members.aol.com/scsweb

Chas E. Carson, President
Richard A. Stonestrom, Secretary
Norman Gronwold, Treasurer
SCS is a large grass roots organization linked by over 200 chapters, a monthly Newsletter, and thousands of members throughout North America and 24 other countries. Its goal is cure of spinal cord injury paralysis. It is an organization of the spinal cord injured, their families and friends, and dedicated scientists and physicians who are aiming at the ultimate goal of cure through improved treatment and research.
1978

7974 **Vermont Back Research Center**
1 S Prospect Street
Burlington, VT 05401
802-656-4582
800-527-7320
FAX: 802-660-9243

Rebecca Mueller, Information Specialist
Conducts research aimed at reducing back-related disability following injury or acute pain episodes. Current research includes studies of posture, seating, vibration, materials handling, and exercise. The Center develops and tests assistive devices, and promotes employment of people with back disorders and rapid return to work after injury. The staff provides a variety of information services, including bibliographic searches and fact finding.

7975 **Walking Tomorrow**
Christopher & Dana Reeve Paralysis Resource Center
636 Morris Tpke
Suite 3a
Short Hills, NJ 07078
800-539-7309
FAX: 973-912-9433
e-mail: info@paralysis.org
www.paralysis.org

Christopher Reeve, Founder
Dana Reeve, Founder

7976 **Wheelchair Access**
PO Box 12
Glenmoore, PA 19343
610-942-0282
FAX: 610-942-0282
e-mail: frankgomez@waccess.org
www.waccess.org

Frank Gomez, Contact
Dedicated to providing comprehensive information to individuals with disabilities concerning wheelchair accessible homes for sale or rent, vans, wheelchairs, and any other equipment they require. Produces a variety of educational materials including a regular newsletter.

7977 **World Chiropractic Alliance**
2950 N Dobson Road
Suite 1
Chandler, AZ 85224
480-786-9235
800-347-1011
FAX: 480-732-9313
e-mail: comments@worldchiropracticalliance.org
www.worldchiropracticalliance.org

Jack Masche, Chief Operating Officer
Linda Bevel, Executive Assistant
Barbara J. Bigham, Director Of Communication
Dedicated to protecting and strengthening chiropractic around the world. Serving as a watchdog and advocacy organization, we place our emphasis on education and political action.
1989

Camps

7978 **Camp Esperanza Arthritis Foundation**
Southern California Chapter
4311 Wilshire Boulevard
Suite 530
Los Angeles, CA 90010
323-954-5760
FAX: 323-954-5790
e-mail: jziegler@arthritis.org
www.arthritis.org/communities/

Kristie Quinn, Camp Director
John H Klippel MD, President/CEO
Laura Robbins, Chair
A one-week camp in August that allows children suffering from arthritis to participate in such activities as horseback riding, swimming, etc. in a fun-filled environment.

7979 **Camp Oakhurst**
New York Service for the Handicapped
853 Broadway
Suite 605
New York, NY 10003
212-533-4020
FAX: 212-533-4023
e-mail: oakhurst06@aol.com
www.campchannel.com/campoakhurst/

Marvin A Raps, Executive Director
Camp is located in Oakhurst, New Jersey. Summer sessions for campers with cerebral palsy, mobility limitation and spina bifida. Coed, age 8-18.

7980 **Easter Seals Camp Stand by Me**
Easter Seal Society of Washington
17809 S Vaughan Road
Vaughn, WA 98394
253-884-2722
FAX: 253-884-0200
e-mail: camp@wa.easterseals.com
www.seals.org

Cathy Bisaillon, Chief Executive Officer
Camp is located in Vaughn, Washington. Summer camping for adults and children with developmental disabilities and mobility limitation. Coed, ages 7-65, seniors. Respite weekends October thru May.

7981 Hughen Center
2849 9th Avenue
Port Arthur, TX 77642
409-983-6659
FAX: 409-983-6408
e-mail: hughencenter@yahoo.com
http://hughencenter.org/home.html

Rita Morston, Administrator
The Center provides a therapeutic, educational, and recreational program for children with physical disabilities. Physical and occupational therapy are featured. Day and residential.

7982 Oak Spring Program
Girl Scouts of Delaware-Raritan
108 Church Lane
East Brunswick, NJ 08816
732-821-9090
800-572-2656
FAX: 732-821-4211
e-mail: info@gsofdr.org
www.gsofdr.org

Allen Vicky, Facilities Director
Ginger Haithcox, Oak Spring Daycamp Director
Mark Timari, Oak Spring Camp Ranger
Camp is located in Somerset, New Jersey. Sessions for girls with mobility limitation, ages 6-16.

7983 Summer Wheelchair Sports Camp
University of Illinois/Division of Rehab Education
1207 S Oak Street
Champaign, IL 61820
217-333-4607
FAX: 217-333-0248
TTY:217-333-1970
e-mail: sportscamp@uiuc.edu
www.disability.uiuc.edu/athletics/

Maureen Gilbert, Coordinator
Karen Wold, Learning Disability Specialist
Theresa Rear, Hearing Impaired Interpreter
Rigorous camps designed for individuals with lower extremity physical disabilities. Camp attendees will spend an average of 8-9 hours a day, focusing on development and refinement of fitness, techniques and strategies. Strength training, nutrition and mental training sessions will also be included in all camps. The camp staff is comprised of athletic staff and faculty front, the Division of Rehabilitation Education Services and local wheelchair athletes with coaching experience.

7984 Twin Lakes Camp
1451 East Twin Lakes Road
Hillsboro, IN 47949
765-798-4000
FAX: 765-798-4010
e-mail: outdoors@twinlakescamp.com
www.twinlakescamp.com

Jon Beight, Executive Director
Brad Carter, Director
Walter Payne, Director
Provides a summer camp program for special needs children and young adults. Campers suffer from a wide range of maladies including crippling accidents, Spina Bifida, epilepsy, Cerebral Palsy, Muscular Dystrophy, Quadriplegia, Paraplegia, and other disabling diseases. Campers range in age from 8 to 27.

7985 YMCA Camp Fitch
Youngstown YMCA
17 North Champion Street
Youngstown, OH 44503
330-744-8411
FAX: 330-744-8416
www.campfitch.com

Mike Shaffer, Executive Director
Kathy Portman, Assistant Director
Camp is located in North Springfield, Pennsylvania. Camping sessions for children and adults with diabetes, hearing impairment, developmental disabilities, mobility limitation and speech/communication impairment. Ages 8-16, families and seniors.

Print & Non-Print Resources

7986 A Wheelchair for Petronilia
Fanlight Productions
4196 Washington Street
Suite 2
Boston, MA 02131
617-469-4999
800-937-4113
FAX: 617-469-3379
e-mail: info@fanlight.com
www.fanlight.com

Anthony Sweeny, Marketing Director
Nicole Johnson, Publicity Coordinator
Ben Achtenberg, Owner
Profiles a program, organized and run by Guatemalans with disabilities, which trains them to manufacture and repair cheap, sturdy wheelchairs designed for conditions in developing countries. 28 Minutes. *$199.00*

ISBN 1-572953-98-5

7987 A World Awaits You
Mobility International USA
PO Box 10767
Eugene, OR 97440
541-343-1284
FAX: 541-343-6812
e-mail: info@miusa.org
www.miusa.org

Misty Gren, Information Services Coordinator
Pamela Houston, Public Relations Coordinator
Susan Sygall, Executive Director
A yearly publication from Mobility International USA. Free.
44 pages Yearly

7988 AJAO Newsletter
American Juvenile Arthritis Organization
PO Box 7669
Atlanta, GA 30357
404-872-7100
800-283-7800
FAX: 404-872-9559
e-mail: help@arthritis.org
www.arthritis.org

Janet Austin MEd, Editor
John Klippel, Chief Executive Officer
Offers information and updates about the organization's activities and events. Legislative information, medical updates, camp information and more for children living with arthritis.
Quarterly

7989 Alerter
San Diego Area Chapter of the Arthritis Foundation
9089 Clairemont Mesa Boulevard
Suite 104
San Diego, CA 92123
858-492-1090
800-422-8885
FAX: 858-492-9248
e-mail: cchase@arthritis.org
www.arthritis.org

Chris Chase, Programs & Services Coordinator
Veronica Braun, President
Offers chapter updates, information on activities and events, resources and medical research for members.

7990 Arthritis 101: Questions You Have Answers You Need
Arthritis Foundation Distribution Center
PO Box 6996
Alpharetta, GA 30023
800-207-8633
FAX: 770-442-9742
www.arthritis.com
Expert reviewers answer questions about basic arthritis facts, treatments, research, surgery and more. Also, specific information about six common conditions: rheumatoid arthritis, osteoarthritis, osteoporosis, fibromyalgia, lupus and gout. *$11.95*

144 pages

7991 Arthritis Accent
Arthritis Foundation Southern N.E. Chapter
35 Cold Spring Road
Suite 411
Rocky Hill, CT 06067
860-563-1177
800-541-8350
FAX: 860-563-6018
e-mail: inpubne@arthritis.org
www.arthritis.org

Susan Nesci, Program Director - CT
Stephen Evangelista, President
Offers information on chapter events and activities.
Quarterly

7992 Arthritis Answers: Basic Information About Arthritis
Arthritis Foundation
PO Box 7669
Atlanta, GA 30357
404-872-7100
800-283-7800
FAX: 404-872-9559
e-mail: help@arthritis.org
www.arthritis.org

John Klippel, Chief Executive Officer

7993 Arthritis Bible
Healing Arts Press
1 Park Street
Rochester, VT 05767
802-767-3174
800-246-8648
FAX: 802-767-3726
e-mail: orders@innertraditions.com
www.InnerTraditions.com

Jessica Dudley, Sales Associate
Ehud Sperling, Owner
A comprehensive guide to the alternative therapies and conventional treatments for Arthritic diseases including Osteoarthritis, Rheumatoid Arthritis, Gout, Fibromyalgia and more. *$14.95*
272 pages
ISBN 0-892818-25-5

7994 Arthritis Foundation of Illinois News
2621 N Knoxville Avenue
Peoria, IL 61604
309-682-6600
800-795-9115
FAX: 309-682-6732
e-mail: greaterillinois@arthritis.org

Marilynn J Cason, Chairman
Gary Dutro, President
A publication offering information about the activities of the chapter. Program news, legislative information, workshops and resources are also included.
Quarterly

7995 Arthritis Foundation: Greater Southwest Chapter
1313 E Osborn Road
Suite 200
Phoenix, AZ 85014
602-264-7679
800-477-7679
FAX: 602-264-0563
e-mail: info.caz@arthritis.org
www.arthritis.org

Sherry Ladd, Administration
Vikki Scarafiotti, President
Provides information, programs and services for people affected by arthritis.
Quarterly

7996 Arthritis Helpbook
Addison-Wesley Publishing Company
75 Arlington Street
Suite 300
Boston, MA 02116
617-848-6000
617-848-6034
www.awprofessional.com

William Barke, President
A self-care program for coping with arthritis that includes diet, nutrition, exercise, and mind/body techniques such as guided imagery and meditation.

7997 Arthritis Helpbook: A Tested Self-Management Program for Coping
Addison-Wesley Publishing Company
75 Arlington Street
Suite 300
Boston, MA 02116
617-848-6000
800-238-9682
FAX: 617-848-6034
www.awprofessional.com

William Barke, President
$13.50
288 pages 4th Edition
ISBN 0-201409-63-1

7998 Arthritis Information: Children
Arthritis Foundation
PO Box 7669
Atlanta, GA 30357
404-872-7100
800-283-7800
FAX: 404-872-9559
e-mail: help@arthritis.org
www.arthritis.org

John Klippel, Chief Executive Officer
List of materials for children with arthritis, their families and the health professionals who care for them.

7999 Arthritis News
Wisconsin Chapter of the Arthritis Foundation
1650 S 108th Street
Milwaukee, WI 53214
414-321-3933
FAX: 262-872-0457
e-mail: info@wi@arthritis.org
www.arthritis.org

Dana Motley, Public Relations Coordinator
Kim Wilbur, Administrator
Offers information on activities, events, medical research, information and referrals to persons living in the Wisconsin area that are afflicted with arthritis.
8 pages Quarterly

8000 Arthritis Observer
Rocky Mountain Chapter of the Arthritis Foundation
2280 S Albion Street
Denver, CO 80222
303-756-8622
800-475-6647
e-mail: sturman@arthritis.org

Susan Turman, VP Operations
James Goddard, President
Offers chapter information and updates on fund-raising events and activities, resources and publications and medical updates for the arthritis community.
Quarterly

8001 Arthritis Relief at Your Fingertips
Warner Books
1271 Avenue of the Americas
New York, NY 10020
212-522-7200
FAX: 212-522-7989
www.twbookmark.com

Laurence Kirshbaum, Chief Executive Officer
A self-help guide for relieving arthritis pain through exercise and acupressure massage by a leader in the field.

8002 Arthritis Reporter
New York Chapter of the Arthritis Foundation
122 E 42nd Street
Floor 18
New York, NY 10168
212-984-8700
FAX: 212-878-5960
e-mail: info.ny@arthritis.org
www.arthritis.org

Phyllis Geraghty, Editor
Theresa Davis, Program Director
Ross Alfieri, President

Chapter newsletter offering information on upcoming events, activities and groups for the arthritis community.
Quarterly

8003 **Arthritis Self Help Products**
Aids for Arthritis Inc.
35 Wakefield Drive
Medford, NJ 08055
609-654-6918
800-654-0707
FAX: 609-654-8631
e-mail: aidsforar@aol.com
www.aidsforarthritis.com
More than 200 arthritis self-help products for kitchen, resting, dressing, bathroom, driving, therapy and foot care. Available online or through catalog. Low prices, quick shipping, since 1979.
24 pages Quarterly

8004 **Arthritis Self-Help Book**
Addison-Wesley Publishing Company
75 Arlington Street
Suite 300
Boston, MA 02116
617-848-6000
800-238-9682
FAX: 617-848-6034
www.awprofessional.com

William Barke, President
A useful and informative book used in conjunction with the Arthritis Foundation's Self-Help Course. *$12.00*

8005 **Arthritis Today**
Arthritis Foundation
1330 W Peachtree Street NW
Atlanta, GA 30309
404-872-7100
FAX: 404-872-9559
www.arthritis.org

John Klippel, Chief Executive Officer
Magazine for patients, physicians, public authorities and others with an interest in the field of arthritis. (Price noted paid for yearly subscription) *$20.00*

8006 **Arthritis and Diet**
National Institute of Arthritis
1 Ams Circle
Bethesda, MD 20892
301-495-4484
877-226-4267
FAX: 301-881-2731
e-mail: niamsinfo@mail.nih.gov
www.nih.gov/niams

Kelly Collins, Manager
Offers information on nutrition and diet pertaining to the arthritis community. *$2.00*
16 pages

8007 **Arthritis and Employment: You Can Get the Job You Want**
Arthritis Foundation
PO Box 7669
Atlanta, GA 30357
404-872-7100
800-283-7800
FAX: 404-872-9559
e-mail: help@arthritis.org
www.arthritis.org

John Klippel, Chief Executive Officer

8008 **Arthritis and Pregnancy**
Arthritis Foundation
PO Box 7669
Atlanta, GA 30357
404-872-7100
800-283-7800
FAX: 404-872-9559
e-mail: help@arthritis.org
www.arthritis.org

John Klippel, Chief Executive Officer
How arthritis affects pregnancy, managing pregnancy and a new baby.

8009 **Arthritis in Children**
National Institute of Arthritis
1 Ams Circle
Bethesda, MD 20892
301-495-4484
877-226-4267
FAX: 301-881-2731
e-mail: niamsinfo@mail.nih.gov
www.nih.gov/niams

Kelly Collins, Manager

8010 **Arthritis in Children: Resources for Children, Parents and Teachers**
National Institute of Arthritis
9000 Rockville Pike
Bethesda, MD 20892
301-495-4484
877-226-4267
FAX: 301-881-2731
e-mail: niamsinfo@mail.nih.gov
www.nih.gov/niams

Kelly Collins, Manager
A resource offering information on juvenile arthritis, causes, treatments and prevention.
38 pages

8011 **Arthritis on the Job: You Can Work with It**
Arthritis Foundation
PO Box 7669
Atlanta, GA 30357
404-872-7100
800-283-7800
FAX: 404-872-9559
e-mail: help@arthritis.org
www.arthritis.org

John Klippel, Chief Executive Officer

8012 **Arthritis, Rheumatic Diseases and Related Disorders**
National Institute of Arthritis
9000 Rockville Pike
Bethesda, MD 20892
301-495-4484
877-226-4267
FAX: 301-881-2731
e-mail: niamsinfo@mail.nih.gov
www.nih.gov/niams

Kelly Collins, Manager
This pamphlet offers information, technical articles and research on arthritis and related disorders. Also included are referral organizations to help patients uncover more information.

8013 **Arthritis: A Comprehensive Guide**
Addison-Wesley Publishing Company
75 Arlington Street
Suite 300
Boston, MA 02116
617-848-6000
800-238-9682
FAX: 617-848-6034
www.awprofessional.com

William Barke, President
Reviews types of arthritis, different aspects of treatment including exercise, medications, surgery, the role of diet and an extensive section on challenges of daily living. *$12.00*

8014 **Arthritis: Do You Know?**
Arthritis Foundation
PO Box 7669
Atlanta, GA 30357
404-872-7100
800-283-7800
FAX: 404-872-9559
e-mail: help@arthritis.org
www.arthritis.org

John Klippel, Chief Executive Officer
A brief overview of arthritis and the services of the Arthritis Foundation.

8015 Arthritis: Stop Suffering, Start Moving
Walker Publishing Company
104 5th Avenue
New York, NY 10011
212-727-8300
800-289-2553
FAX: 212-727-0984
e-mail: orders@walkerbooks.com
www.walkerbooks.com

Ramsey Walker, Vice President
$22.95
160 pages
ISBN 0-802713-08-4

8016 Arthritis: Taking Care of Yourself Health Guide for Understanding Your Arthritis
Addison-Wesley Publishing Company
75 Arlington Street
Suite 300
Boston, MA 02116
617-848-6000
FAX: 617-848-6034
www.awprofessional.com

William Barke, President
$13.50
4th Edition
ISBN 0-201409-17-8

8017 Arthritis: What Exercises Work
St. Martin's Press
175 5th Avenue
New York, NY 10010
212-674-5151
800-221-7945
FAX: 212-420-9314

John Sargent, Chief Executive Officer
$19.95
160 pages
ISBN 0-312097-43-3

8018 Arthritis: Your Complete Exercise Guide
Human Kinetics Press
PO Box 5076
Champaign, IL 61825
217-351-5076
FAX: 217-351-2674
e-mail: orders@hkusa.com
www.humankinetics.com

Rainer Martens, President
The Cooper Clinic and Research Institute Fitness Series provides an exercise rehabilitation alternative for people with chronic medical conditions. *$13.95*
152 pages Paperback
ISBN 0-873223-92-6

8019 Away with Arthritis
Vantage Press
516 W 34th Street
New York, NY 10001
212-736-1767
FAX: 212-736-2273

Martin Kleinwald, President
$12.50

ISBN 0-533108-14-4

8020 Beyond the Barriers
Aquarius Health Care Videos
PO Box 1159
Sherborn, MA 01770
508-650-6905
888-440-2963
FAX: 508-650-4216
e-mail: aqvideos@tiac.net
www.aquariusproductions.com

Leslie Kussmann, Presdient
For too many years, paraplegics, amputees, quadraplegics and the blind have felt trapped by their disabilities. No more! Mark Wellman and other disabled adventurers, rock climb the desert towers of Utah, sail in British Columbia, body-board the big waves of Pipeline and Waimea Bay, scuba dive with sea lions in Mexico and hand glide the California coast. This film delivers the simple message: Don't give up, and never give in. If you can't ever lose, then you can't ever win. Preview option. *$90.00*
Video

8021 Bone Up on Arthritis
Arthritis Foundation
PO Box 6996
Alpharetta, GA 30023
800-207-8633
FAX: 770-442-9742
www.arthritis.com
A self-help education packet designed for home-study use, this program can improve your pain and function levels by teaching proven self-help techniques. *$19.50*
w/Audio Tapes

8022 Breathing Lessons: The Life and Work of Mark O'Brien
Fanlight Productions
4196 Washington Street
Suite 2
Boston, MA 02131
617-469-4999
800-937-4113
FAX: 617-469-3379
e-mail: fanlight@fanlight.com
www.fanlight.com

Anthony Sweeny, Marketing Director
Nicole Johnson, Publicity Coordinator
Ben Achtenberg, Owner
A new documentary which focuses on poet-journalist Mark O'Brien. Crippled by polio in childhood, and later forced to rely on an iron lung as a result of post-polio syndrome, for more than forty years he has fought against illness and bureaucracy in his determination to lead an independent life. According to Mark O'Brien, the two mythologies of disabled people break down to one: we can't do anything or two; we can do everything. But the truth is we're just human. *$195.00*
35 Minutes

8023 Bursitis, Tendonitis and Other Soft Tissue Rheumatic Syndromes
Arthritis Foundation
PO Box 7669
Atlanta, GA 30357
404-872-7100
800-283-7800
FAX: 404-872-9559
e-mail: help@arthritis.org
www.arthritis.org

John Klippel, Chief Executive Officer

8024 CC-M Productions
7755 16th Street NW
Washington, DC 20012
202-882-7430
800-453-6280
FAX: 202-882-7432
e-mail: info@managementwisdom.com
www.armchairfitness.com

Jon Abel, Marketing Manager
Robert Mason, Executive Director
Armchair Fitness video series. 4 cassettes: Armchair Fitness Aerobic, Armchair Fitness Gentle, Armchair Fitness Strength and Armchair Fitness Yoga. $29.95-$39.95.
$29.95 - $39.95

8025 Diet and Arthritis
Arthritis Foundation
PO Box 7669
Atlanta, GA 30357
404-872-7100
800-283-7800
FAX: 404-872-9559
e-mail: help@arthritis.org
www.arthritis.org

John Klippel, Chief Executive Officer

8026 Don't Feel Sorry for Paul
JB Lippincott
E Washington Square
Philadelphia, PA 19105
215-521-8300
FAX: 215-824-7390

J Lippincott, Chief Executive Officer

Paul is seven but was born with deformities of both hands and feet. Paul must wear a prosthesis on both feet so that he can walk. He has a third prosthesis for his right hand. The third prosthesis has a pair of hooks Paul uses as fingers.
94 pages Hardcover
ISBN 0-39731 -88-0

8027 Exercise and Your Arthritis
Arthritis Foundation
PO Box 7669
Atlanta, GA 30357
404-872-7100
800-283-7800
FAX: 404-872-9559
e-mail: help@arthritis.org
www.arthritis.org

John Klippel, Chief Executive Officer
Types of exercise for people with arthritis and how to do them.

8028 Focus
Arthritis Foundation
3740 Ridge Mill Drive
Hilliard, OH 43026
614-876-8200
888-382-4673
FAX: 614-876-8363
www.arthritis.org

Irene Baird, President
Offers updated information on arthritis as well as news of the services and activities of the Chapter.
Quarterly

8029 Fourth and Long
Kent Walderep National Paralysis Foundation
16415 Addison Road
Suite 550
Addison, TX 75001
972-248-7100
877-724-2873
FAX: 972-248-7313
e-mail: lkoen@spinalvictory.org
www.spinalvictory.org

Lisa Koen, Office Manager/Media Coordinator
$19.95
207 pages
ISBN 0-824515-08-0

8030 Freedom from Arthritis Through Nutrition & Help for Allergies
Tree of Life Publications
PO Box 126
Joshua Tree, CA 92252
760-366-2395
FAX: 760-228-9081

Michael Tree, Manager
$14.95
256 pages Paperback
ISBN 0-930852-15-X

8031 Freedom of Movement: IL History and Philosophy
Independent Living Research Utilization ILRU
2323 S Shepherd Drive
Suite 1000
Houston, TX 77019
713-520-0232
FAX: 713-520-5785
www.ilru.org

Laurie Redd, Executive Director
10 pages

8032 Functional Electrical Stimulation for Ambulation by Paraplegics
Krieger Publishing Company
PO Box 9542
Melbourne, FL 32902
321-724-9542
800-724-0025
FAX: 321-951-3671
e-mail: info@krieger-publishing.com
www.krieger-publishing.com

R Krieger, Owner
FES is employed to enable spinal cord injury patients who are complete paraplegics to stand and ambulate without bracing. The text covers 12 years of amulation experience. Also available in hardcover, ISBN #0-89464-845-4, selling for $42.50. *$32.50*
210 pages Paper
ISBN 1-575240-28-9

8033 How Come You Walk Funny?
4196 Washington Street
Suite 2
Boston, MA 02131
617-469-4999
800-937-4113
FAX: 617-469-3379
e-mail: info@fanlight.com
www.fanlight.com

Sandy St Louis, Distribution Director
Kelli English, Publicity Coordinator
Ben Achtenberg, Owner
Profiles a unique experiment in reverse integration: a school where non disabled kids attend a kindergarten designed for children with physical disabilities. The kids and families tackle their differences and discover common ground through finding a way that all can play. *$ 179.00*
2004
ISBN 1-572954-18-3

8034 How to Deal with Back Pain and Rheumatoid Joint Pain
Global Health Solutions
2146 Kings Garden Way
Falls Church, VA 22043
703-848-2333
800-759-3999
FAX: 703-848-0028
e-mail: shipping@watercure.com
www.watercure.com

Kristin Swan, Secretary
Joy Barber, Secretary
Xiaopo Batmanghelidj, President
The physiology of pain production and its direct relationship to chronic regional dehydration of some joint spaces is explained: Special movements that would create vacuum in the disc spaces and draw water and the displaced discs into the vertebral joints are demonstrated.

8035 I Can Do It
Britannica Film Company
345 4th Street
San Francisco, CA 94107
415-777-9876

Tommy's parents took him shopping. Although he had trouble moving around with his braces he wanted to go shopping alone. In the pet shop he had some trouble moving around, but he was able to solve his problems and even help other customers. A teacher's guide is available with this video.
Film

8036 In Control
Arthritis Foundation
PO Box 7669
Atlanta, GA 30357
404-872-7100
800-283-7800
FAX: 404-872-9559
e-mail: help@arthritis.org
www.arthritis.org

John Klippel, Chief Executive Officer
An excellent at-home program which includes video, audio cassettes and the Arthritis Helpbook. Provides tools to help meet the challenges of arthritis.

8037 Individuals with Arthritis
Mainstream
3 Bethesda Metro Center
Suite 830
Bethesda, MD 20814
301-961-9299
800-247-1380
FAX: 301-654-6714
e-mail: info@mainstreaminc.org

Charles Moster
Mainstreaming individuals with arthritis into the workplace.
$2.50

12 pages

8038 Inside The Halo and Beyond: The Anatomy o f a Recovery
WW Norton & Company
324 State Street
Santa Barbara, CA 93101
800-333-6867
FAX: 805-962-5087
www.specialneeds.com/store/

A skilled horsewoman and lifelong athlete, poet Kumin was 73 when a riding accident left her with two broken vertebrae in her neck. Kumin survived in the face of overwhelming odds that she would be paralyzed for the rest of her life. Miraculously, however, she was walking again within weeks of the accident; now, though one hand and an arm remain partially immobilized, her life has largely resumed its normal course. Here is the journal of her first nine months of recovery. *$ 13.95*

208 pages 2001
ISBN 0-393322-61-0

8039 JRA and Me
American Juvenile Arthritis Organization
PO Box 7669
Atlanta, GA 30357
404-872-7100
800-283-7800
FAX: 404-872-9559
e-mail: help@arthritis.org
www.arthritis.org

John Klippel, Chief Executive Officer

A workbook for school-aged children who have juvenile arthritis. This book offers a variety of educational games, puzzles and worksheets to teach children about their illness and how to take care of themselves. *$7.85*

57 pages

8040 Key Changes: A Portrait of Lisa Thorson
Fanlight Productions
4196 Washington Street
Suite 2
Boston, MA 02131
617-469-4999
800-937-4113
FAX: 617-469-3379
e-mail: fanlight@fanlight.com
www.fanlight.com

Karen McMillen, Marketing Director
Ben Achtenberg, Owner

A documentary profiling Lisa Thorson, a gifted vocalist who uses a wheelchair. Ms. Thorson defines herself as a performer first, a person with a disability second, and this thoughtful portrait respects that distinction. Her work as a jazz singer is at the heart of the film, reflecting her philosophy that the biggest contribution that she can make to the struggle for the rights of people with disabilities is doing her art the best way she can. *$145.00*

8041 Kids Get Arthiritis Too!
American Juvenile Athritis Organization (AJAO)
PO Box 7669
Atlanta, GA 30357
404-872-7100
800-283-7800
FAX: 404-872-9559
e-mail: help@arthritis.org
www.arthritis.org

John Klippel, Chief Executive Officer
8 pages Quarterly

8042 Life on Wheels: For the Active Wheelchair User
Patient-Centered Guides
101 Morris Street
Sebastopol, CA 95472
707-829-0515
800-294-4747
FAX: 800-997-9901
e-mail: order@oreilly.com
www.patientcenters.com

Linda Lamb, Editor
Shawnde Paull, Marketing
Tim O'Reilly, Chief Executive Officer

For 1.5 million Americans, life includes a wheelchair for mobility. Life on Wheels is for people who want to take charge of their life experience. Author Gary Karp describes medical issues (paralysis, circulation, rehab, cure research); day-to-day living (exercise, skin, bowel and bladder, sexuality, home access, maintaining a wheelchair); and social issues (self-image, adjustment, friends, family, cultural attitudes, activism). *$24.95*

573 pages Paperback
ISBN 1-565922-53-0

8043 Living with Rheumatoid Arthritis
Johns Hopkins University Press
2715 North Charles Street
Baltimore, MD 21218
410-516-6900
800-537-5487
FAX: 410-516-6998
www.jhupbooks.com

William Brody, President

This book offers practical and usable answers to the questions of everyday life. The authors provide clear explanations of the causes, diagnosis, and treatment of the disease, and why medication, joint protection, physical activity, and good nutrition are essential components of care. *$18.95*

312 pages Paperback
ISBN 0-801851-85-8

8044 Loop the Loop
William Morrow & Company
1350 Avenue of the Americas
New York, NY 10019
212-974-3100
FAX: 212-974-3188
www.williammorrow.com

Anne has never met anyone like Mrs. Simpson. She travels in a wheelchair and performs fabulous yo-yo tricks. *$14.00*

32 pages

8045 Managing Your Fatigue
Arthritis Foundation
PO Box 7669
Atlanta, GA 30357
404-872-7100
800-283-7800
FAX: 404-872-9559
e-mail: help@arthritis.org
www.arthritis.org

John Klippel, Chief Executive Officer

8046 Managing Your Pain
Arthritis Foundation
PO Box 7669
Atlanta, GA 30357
404-872-7100
800-283-7800
FAX: 404-872-9559
e-mail: help@arthritis.org
www.arthritis.org

John Klippel, Chief Executive Officer

8047 Nancy's Special Workout for the Physically Challenged
Laurel Designs
1805 Mar West Street
Apt A
Belvedere Tiburon, CA 94920
FAX: 415-435-1451
e-mail: laureld@ncal.verio.com

Janet Sawyer, Owner
Lynn Montoya, Owner

Aerobic exercise video with syncopated music for seated people with disabilities from minimal to severe. *$42.00*

45 Minutes

8048 New Mobility
23815 Stuart Ranch Road
Malibu, CA 90265
310-317-4522
800-543-4116
FAX: 310-317-9644
www.newmobility.com

Sam Maddox, Publisher
Barry Corbet, Editor

The full-service, full-color lifestyle magazine for the disability community. The award-winning magazine is contemporary, witty and candid. Produced by professional journalists and visual artists, the magazine's voice is uncompromising and unsentimental, yet practical, knowing and friendly. The magazine covers issues that matter to readers: medical news, and cure research; jobs, benefits and civil rights; sports, recreation and travel; product news, technology and innovation.

ISSN 1065-21 4

8049 Nobody is Burning Wheelchairs
Easter Seals
230 W Monroe Street
Chicago, IL 60606
312-726-0653
FAX: 312-726-1494

Janet D Jamieson, Communications Manager
Explains the employment, public accommodations, transportation and telecommunications provisions of the Americans with Disabilities Act and what this law means to people with disabilities and business and industry. The video can be used for training and information seminars, awareness training and for groups interested in learning more about people with disabilities. *$35.00*

8050 Osteoarthritis
Arthritis Foundation
PO Box 7669
Atlanta, GA 30357
404-872-7100
800-283-7800
FAX: 404-872-9559
e-mail: help@arthritis.org
www.arthritis.org

John Klippel, Chief Executive Officer
Offers introductions, examples, explanations and research pertaining to this type of arthritis.

8051 Overcoming Rheumatoid Arthritis
Arthritis Foundation - Michigan Chapter
17117 W 9 Mile Road
Suite 960
Southfield, MI 48075
248-424-9001
800-968-3030
www.arthritis.org

Anthony Zambraus, Owner
Provides extensive information about the disease and treatment, with an emphasis on what you can do for yourself. *$5.00*

8052 PACE II
Arthritis Foundation
PO Box 6996
Alpharetta, GA 30023
800-207-8633
FAX: 770-442-9742
www.arthritis.com

$19.50

8053 Pacing Yourself
Accent Books & Products
PO Box 700
Bloomington, IL 61702
309-378-2961
800-787-8444
FAX: 309-378-4420
e-mail: acmtlvng@aol.com

Raymond C Cheever, Publisher
Betty Garee, Editor
A guide loaded with ideas and tips on starting the day, housekeeping, meal preparation, parenting and socializing. Also includes information on how to group errands and manage household chores, improve posture to make movement easier, and much more. *$10.95*
141 pages Paperback
ISBN 0-91570 -31-0

8054 Paraplegics and Quadriplegics
Mainstream
3 Bethesda Metro Center
Suite 830
Bethesda, MD 20814
301-961-9299
800-247-1380
FAX: 301-654-6714
e-mail: info@mainstreaminc.org

Charles Moster
Mainstreaming paraplegics and quadriplegics into the workplace. *$2.50*
12 pages

8055 Pathways to Better Living
Arthritis Foundation
PO Box 6996
Alpharetta, GA 30023
800-207-8633
FAX: 770-442-9742
www.arthritis.com

$29.95

8056 Primer on the Rheumatic Diseases
Arthritis Foundation
PO Box 6996
Alpharetta, GA 30023
800-207-8633
FAX: 404-872-0457
www.arthritis.com
Written to educate medical students and family physicians, this is the authoritative guide on the rheumatic diseases. *$39.95*
513 pages

8057 Progress in Research
Christopher Reeve Paralysis Foundation
636 Morris Tpke
Suite 3a
Short Hills, NJ 07078
973-379-2690
800-225-0292
FAX: 973-912-9433
e-mail: paralysis@aol.com
www.paralysis.org

Kathy Lewis, President
Summarizes research on paralysis and spinal cord injury, emphasizing neural regeneration.

8058 Psoriatic Arthritis
National Institute of Arthritis
1 Ams Circle
Bethesda, MD 20892
301-495-4484
877-226-4267
FAX: 301-881-2731
e-mail: niamsinfo@mail.nih.gov
www.nih.gov/niams/

Kelly Collins, Manager

8059 Rajesh
Atheneum
135 S Mount Zion Road
Lebanon, IN 46052
FAX: 800-882-8583
Rajesh, a student in a headstart program, was born without complete legs and must wear two prostheses to walk. When Rajesh first attended school he found that older children teased him. After he explained about his legs to the class, his classmates began to accept him.
32 pages Hardcover
ISBN 0-68931 -74-9

8060 Rheumatoid Arthritis
National Institute of Arthritis
1 Ams Circle
Bethesda, MD 20892
301-495-4484
877-226-4267
FAX: 301-881-2731
e-mail: niamsinfo@mail.nih.gov
www.nih.gov/niams/

Kelly Collins, Manager
Offers an introduction and definition of Rheumatoid Arthritis, treatments, causes, objectives, daily living, resources and medical information.

8061 Source of Help and Hope Newsletter
Arthritis Foundation
3544 N Progress Avenue
Suite 204
Harrisburg, PA 17110
717-763-0900
800-776-0746
FAX: 717-763-0903
www.arthritis.org

Catherine Penrod, President
Offers information on activities and events of the Chapter.
3x Year

8062 Still Me
Ballantine Books
4958 Main Street
Downers Grove, IL 60515
630-663-1472
www.randomhouse.com/BB/
The man who was Superman begins with his debilitating riding accident, then weaves back and forth between past and present, creating a thorough biography of Reeve's life. *$7.99*
324 pages 1999
ISBN 0-345432-41-X

8063 Superkids
Superkids
60 Clyde Street
Newton, MA 02460
www.super-kids.org
Non-profit organization and newsletter for families and friends of children with limb differences. It is published twice a year and is free to interested families and professionals. Offers timely information and support to those affected by limb differences.

8064 Thinking About Tomorrow: A Career Guide for Teens with Arthritis
Arthritis Foundation
PO Box 7669
Atlanta, GA 30357
404-872-7100
800-283-7800
FAX: 404-872-9559
e-mail: help@arthritis.org
www.arthritis.org

John Klippel, Chief Executive Officer

8065 Two Hundred Fifty Tips for Making Life with Arthritis Easier
Arthritis Foundation Distribution Center
PO Box 6996
Alpharetta, GA 30023
800-207-8633
FAX: 770-442-9742
www.arthritis.com
What do aerosol cooking spray and snow-shoveling have in common? Learn the answer to this question, and other clever and handy tips to make your life with-or without-arthritis easier. Plus learn about helpful serviced you didn't know were available through you bank, post office, phone company, grocery store, and other businesses you frequent. *$9.95*
88 pages

8066 Understanding Juvenile Rheumatoid Arthritis
American Juvenile Arthritis Organization
PO Box 7669
Atlanta, GA 30357
404-872-7100
800-283-7800
FAX: 404-872-9559
e-mail: help@arthritis.org
www.arthritis.org

John Klippel, Chief Executive Officer
A manual for health professionals to use in teaching children with JRA and their families about disease management and self-care. *$61.20*
372 pages

8067 Volunteer Voice
Kentucky Chapter of the Arthritis Foundation
2908 Brownsboro Road
Suite 100
Louisville, KY 40206
502-585-1866
FAX: 502-585-1657
www.kecc.org

Barbara Perez, Chief Executive Officer
Newsletter offering information and updates on chapter activities, events, camps, juvenile programs and government/legislative information.

8068 WA & NEWS
Wheelchair Access
PO Box 12
Glenmoore, PA 19343
610-942-3266
FAX: 610-942-0282
e-mail: info@waccess.org
www.waccess.org

Frank Gomez, Publisher
Features wheelchair accessible houses and apartments for rent or for sale. Currently the newsletter includes ads from all states. Ads received from any State will be accepted free of charge. Featured also are ads of wheelchairs, vans, equipment, etc., for sale. Complete ad information and more is listed in the Web site. A free copy of WA & NEWS sent upon request. *$12.00*
20 pages Monthly

8069 Wheelchair Batteries
Accent Books & Products
PO Box 700
Bloomington, IL 61702
309-378-2961
800-787-8444
FAX: 309-378-4420
e-mail: acmtlvng@aol.com

Raymond C Cheever, Publisher
Betty Garee, Editor
Offers valuable tips for trouble-free travel at minimum cost: selecting the right battery the first time and how to use and re-charge your battery to make it last longer. *$3.50*
32 pages Paperback
ISBN 0-91570 -22-1

8070 Wheelin' Around
6614 W Sweetwater Avenue
Glendale, AZ 85304
623-776-8830
800-456-1371
FAX: 623-412-9920
e-mail: info@WheelersVanRentals.com
www.WheelersVanRentals.com

Tammy Smith, Manager
A quarterly publication. Free.
Quarterly

8071 When Your Student Has Arthritis: A Guide for Teachers
Arthritis Foundation
PO Box 7669
Atlanta, GA 30357
404-872-7100
800-283-7800
FAX: 404-872-9559
e-mail: help@arthritis.org
www.arthritis.org

John Klippel, Chief Executive Officer
A medical information booklet written for teachers or other adults who have arthritis. The booklet describes different forms of juvenile arthritis, how arthritis might affect the child at school, and how to help the child work around these problems.

8072 With Standing Ovation
Aquarius Health Care Videos
PO Box 1159
Sherborn, MA 01770
508-650-6905
FAX: 508-650-4216
e-mail: aqvideos@tiac.net
www.aquariusproductions.com

Profiles two dynamic young people, Peaches and Daniel, who were born with severe congenital limb deformities; spent much of their time as children in hospitals learning to use mechanical prostheses to aid them in their daily activities. Despite the training however, both shed the devices and mastered active and creative lives with only a minimal reliance on their prostheses. Encourages health care providers to view their occupational therapy and rehabilitation patients as people with abilities. *$195.00*

Video

8073 Without Pity
Aquarius Health Care Videos
PO Box 1159
Sherborn, MA 01770
508-650-6905
FAX: 508-650-4216
e-mail: aqvideos@tiac.net
www.aquariusproductions.com

This HBO documentary, narrated by Christopher Reeve, celebrates the efforts of the disabled to live full, productive lives. We meet a cross section of Americans. A young woman with cerebral palsy cares for her baby, while a man with cerebral palsy lives successfully on his own after forty years in an institution. We go to tschool with a remarkable 6-year-old without arms or legs, visit the workplace of a blind computer expert and meet a professor with polio. Preview option is available. *$129.00*

Video

Sports

8074 Access to Sailing
6475 E Pacific Coast Highway
Long Beach, CA 90803
562-433-0561
FAX: 562-437-7655
e-mail: info@accesstosailing.org
www.access2sailing.org

Duncan Milne, Founder
John Martineau, Boating Supervisor
Peter Martineau, Assistant Director
Sports association.

8075 Achilles Track Club
42 W 38th Street
Suite 400
New York, NY 10018
212-354-0300
FAX: 212-354-3978
e-mail: achillestc@aol.com
http://www.achillestrackclub.org/

Mary Bryant, Executive Director
Organization whose goal is to guide disabled athletes into the able-bodied community. Quarterly newsletter has affiliate chapters in various cities overseas.

8 pages

8076 Adapted Aquatics: Swimming for Persons with Physical or Mental Impairments
American Red Cross
2025 E Street NW
Washington, DC 20006
202-639-3685
800-435-7669
FAX: 202-303-0047
e-mail: ncctech@usa.redcross.org
www.redcross.org

Jack McGuire, President/CEO
Magazine for disabled swimmers.

8077 Adapted Physical Education and Sport
Human Kinetics
PO Box 5076
Champaign, IL 61825
800-747-4457
800-747-4457
FAX: 217-351-1549
e-mail: info@hkusa.com
www.humankinetics.com

Colin Higgs, Director
Designed as a resource for both present and future physical education leaders, this book is an exceptional book for teaching exceptional children. It emphasizes the physical education of young people with disabilities. *$47.00*

472 pages
ISBN 0-873225-78-1

8078 Adaptive Sports Center
PO Box 1639
Crested Butte, CO 81224
970-349-2296
866-349-2296
FAX: 970-349-2077
e-mail: info@adaptivesports.org
www.adaptivesports.org

Christopher Hensley, Executive Director
Karen Render, Summer Program Director
Year round adaptive, adventure recreation program located at the base of Crested Butte Mountain Resort, Crested Butte ,CO. The Adaptive Sports Centers provides adaptive downhill and cross country ski lessons, ski rentals and snowboarding lessons in the winter. Offers a variety of wilderness based programs in the summer including multi-day trips into the back country, extensive cycling programs, canoeing, and white water rafting.

8079 American Wheelchair Bowling Association
PO Box 69
Clover, VA 24534
434-454-2269
FAX: 434-454-6276
TTY:954-630-2566
e-mail: bowlawba@aol.com
http://www.ncpad.org/

Gary Robb, Executive Director
Sports association.

8080 Basketball School
PO Box 698
Talladega, AL 35161
256-761-3259
FAX: 256-761-3362

Carl Ponder, Principal

8081 Bold Tracks: Skiing for the Disabled
Johnson Books: A Cordillera Press Guide
1880 57th Court S
Boulder, CO 80301
303-443-1576
800-258-5830
FAX: 303-443-1106
e-mail: books@jpcolorado.com
www.amazon.com

Richard Croog, Sales/Promotion
Jerry Johnson, President
The first complete teaching and learning guide to skiing for the disabled. The guide is essential for instructor and student alike. Beginning with the basic American Teaching System and continuing through three-track and four-track methods, the manual covers skiing for the visually and hearing impaired as well as the physically and developmentally disabled. It includes glossaries of skiing and medical terms and tips for skin program development. *$807.20*

U60 pages Paperback 19I
ISBN 1-555661-14-9

8082 Bowling: Ball Ramp
Cleo Of New York
S Buckout Street
Irvington, NY 10533
914-591-4900
800-321-0595

Elliott Goldberg, President
Bowling devices for wheelchair occupants. *$109.00*

8083 Center for Health and Fitness
Rehabilitation Institute of Chicago
710 N Lake Shore Drive
Chicago, IL 60611
312-238-1149
FAX: 312-238-5017
e-mail: trichey@ric.org
www.richealthfit.org

Tom Richey, Director
Pam Redding, Business Support Manager
Deborah Gaebler-Spira, MD

Provides free sports and programs to individuals with physical disabilities in the greater Chicago area. Programs in 16 different sports including center for health and fitness which provides exercise opportunities seven days a week.

8084 Challenge Golf
Motivation Media
1245 Milwaukee Avenue
Glenview, IL 60025
847-827-9057
FAX: 847-297-6829

Dorothy Bauer, Coordinator
A plain-language video, Challenge Golf is packed with information for beginners or veterans. Peter Longo covers 5 handicaps (one-arm, one-leg, in a seated position, blind, and arthritis) clearly and concisely, on how to play golf with a physical disability. In color, complete with special effects, graphs and real handicapped golfers at play. *$38.95*
Home Edition

8085 Chesapeake Region Accessible Boating
PO Box 6564
Annapolis, MD 21401
410-626-0273
FAX: 410-626-0273
e-mail: info@crab-sailing.org
www.crab-sailing.org

Donald Backe, Executive Director
Howard Baker, Program Director
CRAB provides opportunities for the disabled and their friends to sail the Chesapeake Bay. Day sails, lessons, organized races. Call for charter information. Sail for free on the fourth Sunday of each month, May through October.

8086 Conditioning with Physical Disabilities
Human Kinetics
PO Box 5076
Champaign, IL 61825
800-747-4457
FAX: 217-351-2674
e-mail: info@hkusa.com
www.humankinetics.com
The first practical, authoritative exercise guide for people with all classifications and levels of physical disabilities. The authors share the successful strength and conditioning program they created at the highly regarded Rehabilitation Institute of Chicago - a pioneering program that is now the leading exercise approach for people with physical disabilities. *$22.95*
288 pages
ISBN 0-873226-14-3

8087 Disability and Sport
Human Kinetics
PO Box 5076
Champaign, IL 61825
800-747-4457
FAX: 217-351-1549
e-mail: info@hkusa.com
www.humankinetics.com

Rainer Martens, President
This new book, written by leading experts in adapted physical education and disability sport, is intended to serve as a comprehensive reference about the disability sport world. Topics include adapted equipment, event management, women and disability sport, medical management of disabled athletes and research highlights. This book should serve as a valuable reference for disabled individuals and their families interested in sport, physical educators and medical personnel who work with disabled. *$40.00*
312 pages
ISBN 0-873228-48-0

8088 Disabled Sports USA
451 Hungerford Drive
Suite 100
Rockville, MD 20850
301-217-0960
FAX: 301-217-0968
e-mail: information@dusa.org
www.dsusa.org

Kirk Bauer, Executive Director
Cherly Collins, Administrative Services Manager
Patty Cornelius, Program Service Coordinator
Provides year-round sports and recreation opportunities for people with physical disabilities, veterans and non-veterans alike, such as sanctioned regional and national events in alpine and Nordic skiing, cycling, shooting swimming, table tennis, track and field, volleyball, and weightlifiting. The organization handles physical disabilities which restrict mobility, including amputations paraplegia, quadriplegia, cerebral palsy, head injury, mulitple sclerosis, muscular dystrophy, and more.

8089 Disabled Sports USA, Far West
Tahoe Adaptive Ski School
PO Box 9780
Truckee, CA 96162
530-581-4161
FAX: 530-581-3127
e-mail: info@dsusafw.org
www.dsusafw.org

Katherine Rodriguez, Vice President
Doug Pringle, President
John Chase, Director
Snow ski and snowboard lessons for people with disabilities. December through April. Two and a half hour lesson, adaptive equipment and beginner lift ticket: $50 midweek. Summer programs include: Water Skiing, Whitewater Rafting, Cycling, 4WD Backcountry Access and Kayaking.

8090 Disabled Watersports Program Mission Bay Aquatic Center
PO Box 250218
Little Rock, AR 72225
501-666-2523
FAX: 501-666-8367
www.americanamputee.org

Peter K Ballantyne, Program Manager
Marci Honstead, Program Coordinator
Catherine Walden, Executive Director
A cooperative, collegiate waterfront facility which is intended and designed to provide water-oriented programs and equipment and to be a resource center for water oriented sports and activities of all types, instructional and recreational. Since 1980, the center has offered aquatic activities for disabled individuals. This program serves hundreds of people yearly throughout the southwest United States and particularly San Diego, and serves as a model for similar programs.

8091 FORE! Future Opportunity for Recreation and Employment for the Handicapped
Southern California Golf Association
3740 Cahuenga Boulevard
North Hollywood, CA 91604
818-980-3630
800-554-7242
FAX: 818-980-2709
e-mail: info@scga.org
www.scga.org

Bill Cunnerty, President
Errol Shaw, Vice President
Tom Morgan, Executive Director
Golfing association for the physically handicapped.

8092 Fitness Programming for Physical Disabilities
Human Kinetics
PO Box 5076
Champaign, IL 61825
217-351-2674
800-747-4457
FAX: 217-351-2674
e-mail: info@hkusa.com
www.humankinetics.com

Rainer Martens, President
Julie Martens, Vice President
A book offering information for developing and conducting exercise programs for groups that included people with physical disabilities. A dozen authorities in exercise science and adapted exercise programming explain how to effectively and safely modify existing programs for individuals with physical disabilities. *$32.00*

208 pages
ISBN 0-873224-34-5

8093 Guide to Wheelchair Sports and Recreation
Paralyzed Veterans of America
801 18th Street NW
Washington, DC 20006
202-872-1300
800-424-8200
888-860-7244
FAX: 202-416-7639
e-mail: info@pva.org
www.pva.org

Randy Pleza, President
PVA's new booklet has been produced in part through a generous grant from Everest & Jennings, Inc., to serve individuals as a resource guide to sports and recreation activities and equipment suppliers.
28 pages

8094 Handicapped Scuba Association International
Handicapped Scuba Association
1104 El Prado
San Clemente, CA 92672
949-498-4540
FAX: 949-498-6128
e-mail: hsa@hsascuba.com
www.hsascuba.com

Jim Gatacre, Founder
Patricia Derk, Vice President
A nonprofit volunteer organization dedicated to improving the physical and social well being of those with special needs through the exhilarating sport of scuba diving. An educational program for able bodied scuba instructors to learn to teach and certify people with special needs. Accessible travel opportunities. Publishes quarterly newsletter.

8095 Hang Gliding and Paragliding Mag
U S Hang Gliding Association
PO Box 1330
Colorado Springs, CO 80901
719-632-8300
800-616-6888
719-632-6417
FAX: 719-632-6417
e-mail: ushga@ushga.org
www.ushga.org

Jayne Depanfilif, Executive Director

8096 High Adventure Hang Gliding
4231 Sepulveda Avenue
San Bernardino, CA 92404
909-882-1880
FAX: 909-883-8488
e-mail: robndi@flytandem.com
www.flytandem.com

Rob McKenzie, Founder
Dianne McKenzie, Founder
Susan Haugh
Tandem adventures.

8097 ISC: National Organization of People with Physical Disabilities
16 Liberty Street
Larkspur, CA 94939
415-924-3549
FAX: 415-927-9556
e-mail: russab@earthlink.net
www.localcommunities.org

Ellen Lieber, President
Providing opportunities for the handicapped to participate in accessible community activities is the objective of this service organization which has regional chapters in many states.

8098 Inclusive Games
Human Kinetics
PO Box 5076
Champaign, IL 61825
217-351-2674
800-747-4457
FAX: 217-351-1549
e-mail: info@hkusa.com
www.humankinetics.com

Rainer Martens, President
Julie Martens, Vice President
Features more than 50 games, helpful illustrations, and hundreds of game variations. The book shows how to adapt games so that children of every ability level can practice, play and improve their movement skills together. The game finder makes it easy to locate an appropriate game according to its name, approximate grade level, difficulty within the grade level, skills required/developed, and number of players. *$14.95*
120 pages Paperback
ISBN 0-873226-39-9

8099 Lakeshore Foundation
4000 Ridgeway Drive
Birmingham, AL 35209
205-313-7400
FAX: 205-313-7475
e-mail: information@lakeshore.org
www.lakeshore.org

Norman B Davis Jr, Vice President
Jeffery Underwood, President
Offers fitness, recreation and competitive sports programs for persons with physical disabilities.

8100 Leaning Tower YMCA: Conquerors Gym and Swim Program
Leaning Tower Y MC A
1979 Marcus Ave.
Suite 210
Lake Success, NY 11042
516-622-2340
FAX: 801-457-8291
e-mail: leaningtower@ymcacommunity.net
www.campdepot.com

Samantha Vircol, Director
Chris Bertana, Director
Mission to support the spiritual, mental and physical well being of inviduals and families in order to improve their quality of life. Provides quality programs to meet the need of the individuals with and without disabilities.

8101 National Disability Sports Alliance
25 W Independence Way
Kingston, RI 02881
401-792-7130
FAX: 401-792-7132
e-mail: info@ndsaonline.org
www.ndsaonline.org

Jerry McCole, Executive Director
Serves to present disabled athletes with the opportunity to perform in many different sports. Participants range from the beginning athlete to the elite, international caliber athlete.

8102 National Skeet Shooting Association
5931 Roft Road
San Antonio, TX 78253
210-688-3371
800-877-5338
FAX: 210-688-3014
e-mail: nssa@nssa-nsca.com
http://www.mynssa.com/

Don Snyder, Executive Director
Carl Hensch, Director
Louise Terry, President
Offers information on sporting clay targets for the disabled hunter.

8103 National Sports Center for the Disabled
PO Box 1290
Winter Park, CO 80482
970-726-1540
FAX: 970-726-4112
e-mail: info@nscd.org
www.nscd.org

Craig Pollitt, President
Hal O'Leary, Founder
Free newsletter with information and tips for adaptive skiing and other mountain sports for people with disabilities.
6-8 pages Quarterly

8104 National Wheelchair Poolplayers Association
9651 Halekulani Drive
Garden Grove, CA 92841
866-636-3371
FAX: 714-636-3371
e-mail: KenForce@nwpainc.org
www.nwpainc.org

Ken Force, CEO
Works together with other groups, organizations, and tournaments to update rules to include wheelchair players.

8105 PALAESTRA: Forum of Sport/PE/Recreation for Those with Disabilities
Challenge Publications Limited
PO Box 508
Macomb, IL 61455
309-833-1902
FAX: 309-833-1902
e-mail: challpub@macomb.com
www.palaestra.com

Julian Stein, Associate Editor
David Beaver, Editor-in-Chief
David Beaver, Owner
The most comprehensive resource on sport, physical education and recreation for individuals with disabilities, their parents and professionals in the field of adapted physical activity. Published in cooperation with US Paralympics and AAHPERD's Adapted Physical Activity Council. Informative yet entertaining and delivers valuable insights for consumers, families and professionals in the field. Published quarterly.

8106 Recreation & Sports
Accent Books & Products
PO Box 700
Bloomington, IL 61702
309-378-2961
800-787-8444
FAX: 309-378-4420
e-mail: acmtlvng@aol.com

Raymond C Cheever, Publisher
Betty Garee, Editor
A guide to fun, excitement and travel offering options for disabled persons. Includes photos and sources of some special products. *$4.95*
65 pages Paperback
ISBN 0-91570 -18-3

8107 Rehabilitation Institute of Chicago Learning Resource Center
345 E Superior Street
Chicago, IL 60611
312-238-1000
800-354-7342
FAX: 312-908-1369
e-mail: education@ric.org
www.ric.org

Wayne M Lerner, President/Chief Executive Office
Laura Ferrio, Vice President
Henry Betts, Chairman
Offers information on rehabilitation and physical disabilities.

8108 Sailing Fascination
4010 Park Newport
Apt 224
Newport Beach, CA 92660
949-760-8650
800-735-2922
FAX: 949-760-8650
TTY: 949-760-2646
e-mail: feedback@socalsail.com
www.socalsail.com

Jack W Hester, President
Tom Tolbert, Vice President
Sailing Fascination provides sailing programs for anyone who is disabled. A non profit educational and charitable California State Corp. with an all volunteer staff, officers, and directors. Year round sailing classes are held on a 24 foot sailboat that is equipped to be accessible to the disabled student sailor.

8109 Slow Motion/Sea Legs
Aquarius Health Care Videos
18 North Main Street
Sherborn, MA 01770
508-650-6905
FAX: 508-650-4216
e-mail: aqvideos@tiac.net
www.aquariusproductions.com

Leslie Kussmonn, President

Probably the last place you would expect to find a disabled person is flying down a mountain in a bucket...attached to a board. Mario Solis and Carla toll introduce a community where physical limitations need no longer stand in the way of strenuous physical performance... the community of disabled snow skiing. *$79.00*

8110 Special Olympics
1133 19th Street NW
Washington, DC 20036
202-628-3630
FAX: 202-824-0200
e-mail: info@specialolympics.org
www.specialolympics.org

Jay Emmett, President
Andrew Robertson, Chief Executive Officer
Jimmy Carnes, Executive Director
A year-round worldwide program that promotes physical fitness, sports training and athletic competition for children and adults with intellectual disabilities.

8111 Special Olympics International
1133 19th Street NW
Washington, DC 20036
202-628-3630
FAX: 202-824-0200
e-mail: info@specialolympics.org
www.specialolympics.org

Timothy Shriver, President/CEO
Nadia Comaneci, Chief Administrative Officer
Drake Turrentine, Chief Legal Officer/Secretary
Provides year-round training and athletic competition in a variety of well-coached, Olympic-type sparts for persons with mental retardation. Offers opportunities to develop physical fitness, prepare for entry into school and community sports programs. Athletes express courage, experience joy and participate in gifts, skills and friendship with their families and other Special Olympics athletes. Local information can be provided by regional offices.

8112 Sport Science Review: Adapted Physical Activity
Human Kinetics
PO Box 5076
Champaign, IL 61825
217-351-2674
800-747-4457
FAX: 217-351-1549
e-mail: info@hkusa.com
www.humankinetics.com

Rainer Martens, President
Julie Martens, Vice President
This special issue addresses disability and sport. Researchers from diverse academic backgrounds and parts of the world review the issues and controversies surrounding inclusion in physical education and sport. The papers explore inclusion in school settings, the history of disability sport, psychological and sociological aspects of adapted physical activity, and the need to identify reliable classification systems. *$15.00*
96 pages
ISBN 0-736029-88-5

8113 Sports & Recreation for the Disabled
Exceptional Parent Library
PO Box 1807
Englewood Cliffs, NJ 07632
201-947-6000
800-535-1910
FAX: 201-489-0074
e-mail: eplibrary@aol.com
www.eplibrary.com
A book designed to make dreams come true. *$32.00*

8114 Sports Market Place Directory
Grey House Publishing
185 Millerton Road
Millerton, NY 12546
518-789-8700
800-562-2139
FAX: 518-789-0545
e-mail: books@greyhouse.com
www.greyhouse.com

Leslie Mackenzie, Publisher
Richard Gottlieb, President
This annual directory lists over 13,000 organizations and their key executives. This comprehensive directory has offered direct access to the Who, What, When & Where of the Sports Industry, including hundreds of resources for disabled individuals.

8115 Sports and Exercise for Children with Chronic Health Conditions
Human Kinetics
PO Box 5076
Champaign, IL 61825
800-747-4457
FAX: 217-351-1549
e-mail: info@hkusa.com
www.humankinetics.com

Brian R Holding, Chief Executive Officer
Adrian C Hutber, Division Director
Written by leading pediatric authorities, the practical guidelines in Sports and Exercise for Children with Chronic Health Conditions address these twenty common medical conditions: spina bifida, epilepsy, childhood progressive neuromuscular disease, cerebral palsy, childhood arthritis, asthma, cystic fibrosis, AIDS, hepatitis, hypertension, congenital heart disease-shunt lesions, congenital obstructive valvular heart disease, carditis, anemia, hemophilia and more. *$49.00*
392 pages Hardcover

8116 Strides Magazine
North America Riding for the Handicapped Associati
PO Box 33150
Denver, CO 80233
303-452-1212
800-369-7433
FAX: 303-252-4610
e-mail: narha@narha.org
www.narha.org

Sheila Kemperdietrich, Chief Executive Officer
Andrea Spridgen, Editor
NARHA's monthly publication. *$35.00*
42 pages Quarterly

8117 Tennis in a Wheelchair
United States Tennis Association
707 Alexander Road
Princeton, NJ 08540
609-987-2300
FAX: 985-641-2267

John Babcock, Manager
A practical manual of tennis playing techniques for the wheelchair athlete. Included are sections on basic strokes from a wheelchair, wheelchair mobility, singles and doubles strategy, and more. Readers will discover how enjoyable and challenging the game of wheelchair tennis can be. *$3.75*
40 pages Illustrated

8118 US Hang Gliding Association Jayne Defanfils
PO Box 1330
Colorado Springs, CO 80901
719-632-8300
800-616-6888
FAX: 719-632-6417
e-mail: ushga@ushga.org
www.ushga.org

Jayne Depanfilif, Executive Director
Offers information for the disabled about how they may discover to hang glide or paraglide in an tandem with a instructor.

8119 United Foundation for Disabled Archers
PO Box 251
20 NE 9th Ave.
Glenwood, MN 65334
320-634-3660

e-mail: bowtwang@charter.net
www.uffdaclub.com

Daniel Hendricks, President/Founder
Promotes and provides access to the sport of archery for any physically challenged person. Arranges Archery hunts throughout the United States.

8120 Wheelchair Motorcycle Association
101 Torrey Street
Brockton, MA 02301
508-583-8614

http://www.uchsc.edu/

Eli Factor DDS, President
Founded in 1975, after Scott Factor sustained injury resulting in paraplegia, this association offers information on all types of off-road vehicles for use by people with disabilities, also offers a newsletter.

8121 Wheelchair Sports, USA
PO Box 5266
Kendall Park, NJ 08824
732-422-4546
FAX: 732-422-4546
e-mail: wsusa@aol.com
www.wsusa.org

Barbara Chambers, Chairperson
Initiates, stimulates and promotes the growth and development of wheelchair sports.

Support Groups

8122 Arthritis Foundation Information Hotline
PO Box 7669
Atlanta, GA 30357
404-872-7100
800-283-7800
FAX: 404-872-9559
e-mail: help@arthritis.org
www.arthritis.org

John Klippel, Chief Executive Officer
Offers information and referrals, counseling, physicians information and more to persons living with arthritis.

8123 Kids on the Block Arthritis Programs
Arthritis Foundation
PO Box 7669
Atlanta, GA 30357
404-872-7100
800-283-7800
FAX: 404-872-9559
e-mail: help@arthritis.org
www.arthritis.org

Dawnn Johnson, Employment Manager
John Klippel, Chief Executive Officer
State and local programs that use puppetry to help children understand what it is like for children and adults who have arthritis.

Associations

8124 **Academy of Dentistry for Persons with Disabilities**

401 N Michigan Avenue
Suite 2200
Chicago, IL 60611
312-527-6764
FAX: 312-673-6663
e-mail: scda@scdonline.org
www.scdonline.org

Roseann Mulligan DDS MS, VP
Kristen Smith, Executive Director
Special Care Dentistry (SCD) is headquartered in Chicago and has a wide ranging membership that includes: dentists, dental hygienists; dental assistants; non-dental health care providers; health program administrators; and others who share our mission. There is also a participating membership category for hospitals, agencies that serve people with special needs and other advocacy and heath care organizations.

8125 **Acid Maltase Deficiency Association (AMDA)**

PO Box 700248
San Antonio, TX 78270
210-494-6144
FAX: 210-490-7161
e-mail: tianrama@aol.com
www.amda-pompe.org

Randall House, IPA, Chairman
Offers a newletter, informational materials, networking, referrals to local resources, national advocacy efforts, and also maintains a research registry.
1994

8126 **American Academy of Child and Adolescent Psychiatry**

3615 Wisconsin Avenue NW
Washington, DC 20016
202-966-7300
FAX: 202-966-2891
e-mail: webthing@aacap.org
www.aacap.org

Thomas F. Anders M.D, President
Gregory Fritz M.D, Secretary
James C. MacIntyre II, M.D., Treasurer
A 501 (C)(3) nonprofit membership organization composed of over 6,500 child and adolescent psychiatrists. Members actively research, evaluate, diagnose and treat psychiatric disorders and pride themselves on giving direction to and responding quickly to new developments in addressing the health care needs of children and their families.
53 pages

8127 **American Academy of Osteopathy**

3500 Depauw Boulevard
Suite 1080
Indianapolis, IN 46268
317-879-1881
FAX: 317-879-0563
e-mail: snoone@academyofosteopathy.org
www.academyofosteopathy.org

Claudia L. McCarthy DO, FAAO, President
Mark S. Cantieri DO, FAOO, Secretary/Treasurer
Guy A. DeFeo, DO, President/Elect
The mission of the American Academy of Osteopathy is to teach, advocate, and research the science, art and philosophy of osteopathic medicine, emphasizing the integration of osteopathic principles, practice and manipulative treatment in patient care.

8128 **American Academy of Otolaryngology: Head and Neck Surgery**

1 Prince Street
Alexandria, VA 22314
703-836-4444
FAX: 703-683-5100
TTY:703-519-1585
www.entnet.org

Jennifer Derebery, President
Tom Harlow, Finance Executive
Promotes the art and science of medicine related to otolaryngology-head and neck surgery, including providing continuing medical education courses and publications.

8129 **American Academy of Physical Medicine and Rehabilitation**

330 North Wabash Avenue
Suite 2500
Chicago, IL 60611
312-464-9700
FAX: 312-464-0227
e-mail: info@aapmr.org
www.aapmr.org

Joel M. Press, President
William F. Micheo, MD, Vice President
Kurt Hoppe, MD, Secretary
This national medical specialty society represents more than 6,500 physical medicine and rehabilitation physicians, whose patients include people with physical disabilities and chronic, disabling illnesses. The academy's mission is to maximize quality of life, minimize the incidence and prevalence of impairments and disability, promote societal health and enhance the understanding and development of the specialty. The organization offers information, referrals, and patient materials.

8130 **American Group Psychotherapy Association**

25 E 21st Street
6th Floor
New York, NY 10010
212-477-2677
877-668-2472
FAX: 212-979-6627
e-mail: info@agpa.org
www.agpa.org

Elizabeth B. Knight MSW, CGP, FAGPA, President
Barry Helfmann PsyD,CGP, Secretary
Kathleen H. Ulman PhD,CGP,FAGPA, Treasurer
AGPA serves as the national voice specific to the interests of group psychotherapy. Its 4,100 members and 31 affiliate societies provide a wealth of professional, educational and social support for group psychotherapists in the United States and around the world.

8131 **American Psychiatric Association**

Psychiatric Services
1000 Wilson Boulevard
Suite 1825
Arlington, VA 22209
703-907-7300
800-368-5777
FAX: 703-907-1095
e-mail: psjournal@psych.org
www.ps.psychiatryonline.org

Constance Gartner, Managing Editor
Andrew Prugar, Editorial Assistant
James Scully, Manager
The American Psychiatric Association is a medical specialty society recognized worldwide. Its over 35,000 U.S. and international member physicians work together to ensure humane care and effective treatment for all persons with mental disorder, including mental retardation and substance-related disorders. It is the voice and conscience of modern psychiatry. Its vision is a society that has avaliable, accessible quality psychiatric diagnosis and treatment.

8132 **American Social Health Association**

PO Box 13827
Research Triangle Park, NC 27709
919-361-8400
800-227-8922
FAX: 919-361-8425
www.ashastd.org

Jim Allen, President
The American Social Health Association is recognized by the public, patients, providers and policy makers for developing and delivering accurate, medically reliable information about STDs. Public and college health clinics across the US order ASHA educational pamphlets and books to give to clients and students. Community-based organizations depend on ASHA, too, to help communicate about risk, transmission, prevention, testing, and treatment.

8133 **Behavior Therapy and Research Society**

Temple University Medical School
3420 N Broad Street
Philadelphia, PA 19140
215-707-7000
800-331-2839
FAX: 215-707-4086
www.medschool.temple.edu

John M Daly MD, Dean
Judith Russo, Manager
This organization promotes behavior therapy by conducting and facilitating research in behavioral interventions and providing information through consultations, conferences and publications, about the use of these methods.

8134 Cerebral Palsy Associations of New York State Annual Conference
90 State Street
Suite 929
Albany, NY 12207
518-436-0178
FAX: 518-436-8619
e-mail: information@cpofnys.org
www.cpofnys.org

Susan Constantino, President/CEO
Michael Alvaro, Executive Vice President
Marie Colbert, Administrative Assistant
Offers 50 sessions and features many outstanding presenters in areas such as assitive technology, education, health care, clinical services, public relations and development, and finance and management.
October

8135 Child Neurology Service
Inova Fairfax Hospital For Children
3300 Gallows Road
Falls Church, VA 22042
703-776-4001
FAX: 703-776-4010
www.inova.org

John Singleton, President
Offers infants and children to age 21 with neurological problems diagnosis, consultation, recommendations for therapy and more services. We also care for adults with cerebral palsy.

8136 Division for Physical and Health Disabilities
1110 N Glebe Road
Suite 300
Arlington, VA 22201
888-232-7733
800-224-6830
FAX: 703-264-9494
www.cec.sped.org

Bruce Ramirez, Executive Director
Elizabeth Turnbull, Senior Executive Assistant
Maggie Sullivan, Executive Assistant
Advocates for quality education for individuals with physical disabilities, multiple disabilities, and special health care needs served in schools, hospitals, or home settings. DPHD's members include classroom teachers, administrators, related service personnel, hospital/homebound teachers, and parents.

8137 Environmental Health Center: Dallas
8345 Walnut Hill Lane
Suite 220
Dallas, TX 75231
214-368-4132
FAX: 214-691-8432
e-mail: contact@ehcd.com
www.ehcd.com

William J Rea, Director
David Hicks, Manager
Clinic providing patient care in the areas of Immunotherapy, Nutrition, Physical Therapy, Chemical Depuration, Energy Balancing, Electromagnetic Sensitivity Testing, Psychological Support Services, Family Practice Medicine and Internal Medicine.

8138 Epilepsy Foundation
4351 Garden City Drive
Landover, MD 20785
301-459-3700
800-332-1000
FAX: 301-459-3700
e-mail: epilepsy@peaknet.net
www.epilepsyfoundation.org

Tony Coelho, Chair of Board of Directors
Bruce P. Hermann PhD, Chair of Advisory Board
Eric R. Hargis, President/CEO
The Epilepsy Foundation is the national voluntary agency solely dedicated to the welfare of the 2.7 million people with epilepsy in the U.S. and their families. The organization works to ensure that people with seizures are able to participate in all life experiences; and to prevent, control and cure epilepsy through research, education, advocacy and services.
1968

8139 Families of Spinal Muscular Atrophy
PO Box 196
Libertyville, IL 60048
847-367-7620
800-886-1762
FAX: 847-367-7623
e-mail: sma@fsma.org
www.fsma.org

Jill Jarecki PhD FSMA, Research Director
Arthur H. Burghes PhD, Advisory Board
Tom Crawford M.D., Advisory Board
Families of Spinal Muscular Atrophy is the largest international organization dedicated solely to: eradicating spinal muscular atrophy (SMA) by promoting and supporting research, helping families cope with SMA through informational programs and support, and educating the public and professional community about SMA.
1984

8140 Health Education AIDS Liason (HEAL)
PO Box 1103
New York, NY 10113
212-873-0780
FAX: 212-873-0891
www.healaids.com

Michael Ellner, President
Roberto Giraldo, Member of the Board
Barnett J Weiss, Member of the Board
Nonprofit, community-based educational organization providing information, hope, and support to people who are HIV positive or living with AIDS. The men and women at HEAL are health professionals, people living with life threatening diseases, and concerned volunteers.

8141 Herpes Resource Center
American Social Health Association
PO Box 13827
Research Triangle Park, NC 27709
919-361-8400
800-227-8922
FAX: 919-361-8425
e-mail: info@ashastd.org
www.ashastd.org

Lynn Barclay, President/CEO
Deborah Arrindell, VP, Health Policy
Lisa K. Gilbert PhD, Senior Researcher
The Herpes Resource Center (HRC) focuses on increasing education, public awareness, and support to anyone concerned about herpes. Since its formation in 1979, the HRC has helped over five million people. The work of the HRC is funded primarily through individual gifts, subscriptions and product sales, with additional support in the form of corporate contributions. Today, people continue to depend on ASHA and the HRC for educational information about herpes.

8142 International Academy of Biological Dentistry and Medicine
17222 Red Oak Drive
Suite 101
Houston, TX 77090
281-651-1745
FAX: 281-440-1258
e-mail: drdawn@drdawn.et
www.biologicaldentistry.org

Edward Arana D.D.S, President/Executive Director
Gary Verigni, Co-Founder
Promotes non-toxic diagnostic and therapeutic approaches in dentistry; hosts seminars on biological diagnosis and therapy.

8143 International Academy of Oral Medicine and Toxicology
8297 Champions Gate Boulevard
193
Champions Gate, FL 33896
863-420-6373
FAX: 863-419-8136
e-mail: info@iaomt.org
www.iaomt.org

Kim Smith, Executive Director
Boyd Haley, PhD, FIAOMT, Chairman
Thomas Burbacher PhD, Associate Professor
Nonprofit organization dedicated to funding solid peer-reviewed scientific research in the area of toxic substances used in dentistry as well as providing continuing education and carefully reviewed procedures, protocols, and methodologies to reduce the risk for patients and professionals.

8144 **International Association for Cancer Victors: Northern California Chapter**
5336 Harwood Road
San Jose, CA 95124
408-249-4516
FAX: 408-264-9659
e-mail: cavictor@ix.netcom.com
www.cancervictors.org
Volunteer community service organization to inform and support interested persons who want to learn more about natural, nontoxic remedies and practices.
1962

8145 **International Association of Professional Natural Hygientists**
2000 S Ocean Drive
Hallandale Beach, FL 33009
954-454-2220

Nick Jnega, Owner
Members are physicians who specialize in therapeutic fasting.

8146 **International Medical and Dental Hypnotherapy Association**
Rural Route #2
Box 2468
Laceyville, PA 18623
570-869-1021
800-553-6886
FAX: 570-869-1249
e-mail: info@imdha.com
www\.imdha.com

Robert Otto, CEO
Linda Otto, Executive Director
provides and encourages education programs to further the knowledge, understanding and application of hypnosis in complimentary health care; to encourage research and scientific publications in the field of hypnosis; to promote the further recognition and acceptance of hypnosis as an important tool in health care and focus for scientific research; to cooperate with other professional organizations that share mutual goals, ethics, and interests and provide professional community who use hypnosis.

8147 **International Ozone Association**
PO Box 28873
Scottsdale, AZ 85255
480-529-3787
FAX: 480-473-9068
e-mail: infO3zone@io3a.org
www.int-ozone-assoc.org
The IOA is a not-for-profit educational association which performs its information-sharing functions through sponsorship of international symposia, seminars, publications, and the development of personal relationships among ozone specialists throughout the world.

8148 **International Rett Syndrome Association**
9121 Piscataway Road
#2B
Clinton, MD 20735
301-856-3334
800-818-7388
FAX: 301-856-3336
e-mail: admin@rettsyndrome.org
www.rettsyndrome.org

Kathy Hunter, Founder/President
Barry Rinehart, CEO
Michelle McLean, COO/CFO
Nonprofit voluntary organization dedicated to serving as an information and referral center for physicians and families of children with Rett Syndrome. The Association's mission includes supporting and promoting research into the prevention, control, and cure of the disorder; increasing public awareness; and providing emotional support for affected families. Engages in patient advocacy; promotes family and professional education; and provides referrals to support groups.
1985

8149 **Leukemia & Lymphoma Society**
1311 Mamaroneck Avenue
White Plains, NY 10605
914-949-5213
800-955-4572
FAX: 914-949-6691
www.leukemia.org

Dwayne Howell, CEO and President
Cynthia Gardner, Executive VP
Richard Geswell, Executive VP
The Leukemia and Lymphoma Society is the world's largest voluntary health organization dedicated to funding blood cancer research, education and patient services. Thier mission: cure leukemia, lymphoma, Hodgkin's disease and myeloma, and improve the quality of life of patients and their families. Since its founding in 1949, the Society has invested more then $483 million for research specifically targeting blood cancers.
1949

8150 **Leukemia Society of America**
600 3rd Avenue
4th Floor
New York, NY 10016
212-573-8484
800-955-4572
FAX: 212-681-3615
www.leukemia.org

Dwayne Howell PhD, President/CEO
Cynthia Gardner, Executive Vice President
Richard Geswell, Executive Vice President
National voluntary health agency dedicated to curing leukemia, lymphoma, Hodkin's disease and myeloma and to improving the quality of life and their families. Provides mutual support for people and family members with leukemia and its related diseases. Meetings, financial assistance, treatment, transportation, referrals, information and education.

8151 **Little People of America**
5289 NE Elam Young Parkway
Suite F-100
Hillsboro, OR 97124
503-846-1562
888-572-2001
888-572-2001
FAX: 503-846-1590
e-mail: info@lpaonline.org
www.lpaonline.org

Lois Gerage-Lamb, President
Jeff Simms, Senior Vice President
Craig Holloway, Vice President Of Finance
Assists dwarfs with their physical and developmental concerns resulting from short stature, usually no taller then 4' 10". Provides medical, environmental, educational, vocational, and parental guidance, so that short-statured individuals and their families may enhance their lives and lifestyles with minimal limitations.
1957

8152 **Multiple Sclerosis Center of Oregon**
Oregon Health & Sciences University
3181 SW Sam Jackson Park Road
Portland, OR 97239
503-494-3460
FAX: 503-494-3480
www.ohsu.edu

Peter O Kohler MD, President
Steven D Stadum JD, Chief Administrative Officer
James Morgan, Executive Director
OHSU's fundamental purpose is to improve the well-being of people in Oregon and beyond. As part of its multifaceted public mission, OHSU strives for excellence in education, research, clinical practice, scholarship and community service. Through its dynamic interdisciplinary environment, OHSU stimulates the spirit of inquiry, initiative and cooperation among students, faculty and staff.

8153 Multiple Sclerosis Foundation
6350 N Andrews Avenue
Fort Lauderdale, FL 33309
954-776-6805
800-225-6495
FAX: 954-938-8708
e-mail: admin@msfocus.org
www.msfocus.org

Eric Schenck, President, Director
Michael Austin, Vice President, Director
Dr. Traci Seidman, Secretary, Director
Contemporary national, nonprofit organization that provides free support services and public education for persons with Multiple Sclerosis, newsletters, toll-free phone support, information, referrals, home care, assitive technology, and support groups.

8154 Myositis Association
1233 20th Street NW
Suite 402
Washington, DC 20035
202-887-0088
800-821-7356
FAX: 202-466-8940
e-mail: tma@myositis.org
www.myositis.org

Bob Goldberg, Executive Director
Theresa Reynolds Curry, Communications Manager
Katheryn A. Spooner, Programs Manager
The Myositis Association is dedicated to finding a cure for inflammatory and other related myopathies, while serving those affected by these diseases. The aim of TMA's programs and services is to provide information, support, advocacy and research for those concerned about myositis. Support groups offer members the chance to share their feelings and discuss their concerns with people in similar situations. These groups encourage an atmosphere of communication and compassion.
1993

8155 National AIDS Fund
729 15th Street NW
Floor 9
Washington, DC 20005
202-408-4848
888-234-2437
FAX: 202-408-1818
e-mail: info@aidsfund.org
www.aidsfund.org

Kandy Ferree, President and CEO
Krista Bradley, Program Officer
Lissa Gilden, Development Officer
The National AIDS Fund was founded in 1988 to reduce the incidence and impact of HIV/AIDS by promoting leadership and generating resources for effective community responses to the epidemic. Through its unique expanding network of Community Partnerships, NAF supports over 400 grassroots organizations annually which in turn provide HIV prevention, care and support services to underserved individuals and populations most impacted by HIV/AIDS including communities of color, youth and women.

8156 National Association for Continence
PO Box 1019
Charleston, SC 29402
843-377-0900
800-252-3337
FAX: 843-377-0905
e-mail: memberservices@nafc.org
www.nafc.org

Nancy Muller, Executive Director
Katherine F. Jeter EdD, Founder
Melissa Ross, Membership And Fund Development
NAFC's mission is to educate the public about the causes, diagnosis, categories, treatment options and management alternatives for incontinence, voiding disfunction and related pelvic floor disorders. To network with other organizations and agencies to elevate the visibility and priority given to these areas; and to advocate on behalf of consumers who suffer from such symptoms as a result of disease or other illness.

8157 National Association to Advance Fat Acceptance
PO Box 188620
Sacramento, CA 95818
916-558-6880
FAX: 916-558-6881
www.naafa.org

Carole Cullum, Co-Chair
Jason Docherty, Co-Chair
Frances White, Treasurer/Finance Chair
A non-profit human rights organization dedicated to improving the quality of life for fat people. NAAFA works to eliminate discrimination based on body size and provide fat people with the tools for self-empowerment through public education, advocacy, and member support.

8158 National Ataxia Foundation
2600 Fernbrook Lane N
Suite 119
Minneapolis, MN 55447
763-553-0020
FAX: 763-553-0167
e-mail: naf@ataxia.org
www.ataxia.org

DeNiece Roach, President
Charlene Danielson, Vice President
Michael Parent, Executive Director
The National Ataxia Foundation is a nonprofit, membership-supported organization established in 1957 to help ataxia families. The Foundation is dedicated to improving the lives of persons affected by ataxia through support, education, and research.
1957

8159 National Brachial Plexus/Erb's Palsy Association
PO Box 23
Larsen, WI 54947
920-836-2151
FAX: 920-836-5813
e-mail: info@nbpepa.org
www.nbpepa.org

Brenda Copeland-Moore, President
Kris Kiesow, Treasurer
Cheryl Pratt, VP
To educate, inform, and assist those affected by Brachial Plexus Palsy by offering information, contacts, resources, parent matching, and assistance developing chapters or support groups throughout the United States. National Brachial Plexus/Erb's Palsy Association, Inc. Programs include parent matching services, assistance forming chapters, or support groups, provide support to families dealing with children with diagnosis of Brachial Plexus Injury & Erb's Palsy as well as other conditions.

8160 National Diabetes Information Clearinghouse
1 Information Way
Bethesda, MD 20892
301-654-3327
800-860-8747
FAX: 703-738-4929
e-mail: ndic@info.niddk.nih.gov
www.diabetes.niddk.nih.gov

Judith Franklin M.D., Executive Director
An information and referral service of the National Institute of Diabetes and Digestive and Kidney Diseases, one of the National Institutes of Health. The clearinghouse responds to written inquiries, develops and distributes publications about diabetes, and provides referrals to diabetes organizations, including support groups. The NDIC maintains a database of patient and professional education materials, from which literature searches are generated.
1978

8161 National Digestive Diseases Information Clearinghouse
2 Information Way
Bethesda, MD 20892
301-654-3810
800-891-5389
FAX: 703-738-4929
e-mail: nddic@info.niddk.nih.gov
www.digestive.niddk.nih.gov

Stephen P. James M.D., Executive Editor
Information and referral service of the National Institute of Diabetes and Digestive and Kidney Diseases. A central information resource on the prevention and management of digestive diseases, the clearinghouse responds to written inquiries, develops and distributes publications about digestive diseases, provides referrals to digestive disease organizations and support groups, and maintains a database of patient and professional education materials from which literature searches are generated.

1980

8162 National Fragile X Foundation
PO Box 190488
San Francisco, CA 94119
925-938-9300
800-688-8765
FAX: 925-938-9315
e-mail: NATLFX@FragileX.org
www.fragilex.org

Robert Miller, Executive Director
Unites the fragile X community to enrich lives through educational and emotional support, promote public and professional awareness and advance research toward improvement treatments and cure for fragile X syndrome.

8163 National Hemophilia Foundation
116 W 32nd Street
Floor 11
New York, NY 10001
212-328-3700
800-424-2634
FAX: 212-328-3777
e-mail: info@hemophilia.org
www.hemophilia.org

Dr. Allan Kinniburgh, Chief Executive Officer
Ray Stanhope, Chair Of The Board
Michael O'Connor, Vice Chair Of The Board
The National Hemophilia Foundation is dedicated to finding better treatments and cures for bleeding and clotting disorders and to preventing the complications of these disorders through education,advocacy and research. Established in 1948, The National Hemophilia Foundation has chapters throughout the country. Its programs and initiatives are made possible through the generosity of individuals, corporations, and foundations as well as through the Centers for Disease Controll and Prevention (CDC)

8164 National Kidney and Urologic Diseases Information Clearinghouse
3 Information Way
Bethesda, MD 20892
301-654-4415
800-891-5390
FAX: 703-738-4929
e-mail: nkudic@info.niddk.nih.org
www.kidney.niddk.nih.gov

Mel Eagle, Manager
Griffin P. Rogers M.D., Director
NKUDIC was established in 1987 to increase knowledge and understanding about diseases of the kidneys and urologic system among people with these conditions and their families, health care professionals, and the general public.
1987

8165 National Mental Health Association
2001 N Beauregard Street
12th Floor
Alexandria, VA 22311
703-684-7722
800-969-6642
FAX: 703-684-5968
TTY: 800-433-5959
e-mail: infoctr@nmha.org
www.nmha.org

Michael Faenza, President and CEO
Sergio Gaxiola MD, Chair Of The Board
Ann Boughtin, Senior Vice President
Nonprofit organization addressing all issues related to mental health and mental illness. With more than 340 affiliates nationwide, NMHA works to improve the mental health of all Americans, especially the 54 million individuals with mental disorders, through advocacy, education, research and service.
1909

8166 Okada Specialty Guide Dogs
7509 E Saviors Path
Floral City, FL 34436
352-344-2212
FAX: 352-344-0210
e-mail: okada@okadadogs.com
www.okadadogs.com

Pat Putnam, Director
Trains dogs to aid deaf, hearing-impaired, Alzheimer's, seizure, amnesia and residential companion guide dogs.

8167 Overeaters Anonymous World Service Office
PO Box 44020
Rio Rancho, NM 87174
505-891-2664
FAX: 505-891-4320
e-mail: info@oa.org
www.oa.org

Naomi Lippel, Executive Director
OA is not just about weight loss, obesity or diets; it addresses physical, emotional and spiritual well-being. It is not a religious organization and does not promote any particular diet. To address weight loss, OA encourages members to develop a food plan with a health care professional and a sponsor.

8168 People Against Cancer
PO Box 10
Otho, IA 50569
515-972-4444
FAX: 515-972-4415
e-mail: info@PeopleAgainstCancer.net
www.peopleagainstcancer.com

Frank Wiewel, Executive Director
Publication of People Against Cancer, a nonprofit, grassroots, public benefit organization dedicated to 'New Directions in the War on Cancer.' We are a democratic organization of people with cancer, their loved ones and citizens working together to protect and enhance medical freedom of choice.
8 pages

8169 Prader-Willi Alliance of New York
PO Box 1114
Niagara Falls, NY 14304
716-276-2211
800-442-1655
FAX: 716-271-2782
e-mail: alliance@prader-willi.org
www.prader-willi.org

Barbara McManus, President
Harry Persanis, Vice President
Henry Singer, Vice President
To provide information to the general public about Prader-Willi syndrome (PWS):Æto promote awareness of PWS among the general public and medical professionals; to provide forms for discussion and professional interchange on the subject of PWS. To provide assistance, information, referral, and advocacy services to families and friends of persons suffering from PWS. To encourage and support research into the causes, cure and treatment of PWS.

8170 Prader-Willi Syndrome Association USA
5700 Midnight Pass Road
Suite 6
Sarasota, FL 34242
941-312-0400
800-926-4797
FAX: 941-312-0142
e-mail: national@pwsausa.org
www.pwsausa.org

Janalee Heinemann, Executive Director
Daniel J Driscol PhD, MD, Chair
Moris Angulo MD, Chair
National, nonprofit public charity that works for the benefit of individuals with Prader-Willi syndrome and their families. An organization of parents and others who are making a difference in the lives of those with Prader-Willi syndrome. Dedicated to serving individuals affected by Prader-Willi syndrome (PWS) their families, and interested professionals. To provide information, education, and support services to its members.

8171 Rasmussen's Syndrome and Hemispherectomy Support Network
8235 Lethbridge Road
Millersville, MD 21108
410-987-5221
FAX: 410-987-521
e-mail: rssnlynn@aol.com

Al & Lynn Miller, Founders
National not-for-profit organization dedicated to providing information and support to individuals affected by Rasmussen's Syndrome and Hemispherectomy. Publishes a periodic newsletter and disseminates reprints of medical journal articles concerning Rasmussen's Syndrome and its treatments. Maintains a support network that provides encouragement and information to individuals affected by Rasmussen's Syndrome and their families.

8172 **Scientific Health Solutions**

1621 N Circle Drive
Colorado Springs, CO 80909
719-548-1600
800-331-2303
FAX: 719-572-8081
www.tomlevymd.com/serumtest.htm

Thomas Levy, Founder
SHS seeks to help those who are looking to avoid new dental toxicity by offering serum biocompatibility testing to help guide the choice of replacement dental materials. Every attempt is also made to help these people find dentists who are familiar with the testing, as well as with the general concepts of dental toxicity that are addressed on TomLevyMD.com

8173 **Simonton Cancer Center**

PO Box 6607
Malibu, CA 90264
818-879-7904
800-459-3424
FAX: 310-457-0421
e-mail: simontoncancercenter@msn.com
www.simontoncenter.com

O Carl Simonton, Medical Director/Founder
The Simonton Cancer Center offers a "New Patient Program" for cancer patients and their support person. In these sessions, Dr. Simonton presents the refined specific information for increasing survival, decreasing tumor growth and most important, improving the quality of life of the individual.

8174 **Spina Bifida Association of America**

4590 Macarthur Boulevard NW
Suite 250
Washington, DC 20007
202-944-3285
800-621-3141
FAX: 202-944-3295
e-mail: sbaa@sbaa.org
www.sbaa.org

Douglas Sorocco, President
Cindy Brownstein, Chief Executive Officer
Nonprofit organization. Mission is to promote the prevention of spina bifida and to enhance the lives of all affected. Addresses the specific needs of the spina bifida community and serves as the national representative of almost 60 chapters. Toll free 800 information and referral service. Legislative updates.
1973

8175 **Support Group for Brachial Plexus Injury**

18 Staci Lane
Webster, NY 14580
716-787-0197
FAX: 716-787-2458
e-mail: jdebryne@aol.com
The Support Group for Brachial Plexus Injury was established to provide resources and emotional support to families impacted by Erb's Palsy and other brachial plexus injuries by advising on how best to receive and obtain insurance and treatment for this disorder.

8176 **Tourette Syndrome Association**

4240 Bell Boulevard
Bayside, NY 11361
718-224-2999
888-486-8738
FAX: 718-224-9596
e-mail: ts@tsa-usa.org
www.tsa-usa.org

Fred Cook, Director
Judit Ungar, President
National, nonprofit membership organization. Mission is to identify the cause of, find the cure for, and control the effects of this disorder. A growing number of local chapters nationwide provide educational materials, seminars, conferences and support groups for over 35,000 members. Publishes brochures, flyers, educational materials and papers on treatment and research. Offers videos for purchase through a catalog of publications.
1972

8177 **United Cerebral Palsy Association**

1660 L Street NW
Suite 700
Washington, DC 20036
202-776-0406
800-872-5827
FAX: 202-776-0414
TTY: 202-973-7197
e-mail: info@ucp.org
www.ucpa.org

Stephen Bennett, President & CEO
Chris Thomson, Director Corporate Affairs
Anita Porco, Vice President
National not-for-profit self-help organization dedicated to providing information and support to individuals with Cerebral Palsy and other disabilities, and their families. Supports more than 160 local affiliates; these affiliates provide a variety of programs and services for affected families, including support groups. Offers several educational and support materials, including a quarterly magazine, regular newsletters, and research reports.

8178 **United Cerebral Palsy Association of New York State**

80 Maiden Lane
8th Floor
New York, NY 10038
212-683-6700
FAX: 212-685-8394
e-mail: info@cerebralpalsynys.org
www.ucpnyc.org

Martin Hausman, President, Board Of Directors
Edward R. Matthews, Executive Director
Mission is to advocate and provide direct services with and for individuals with cerebral palsy and other significant disabilities, and their families, throughout New York State, in order to promote lifelong opportunities and choices for independence, inclusion and enhanced quality of life. Provides services and programs for more than 40,000 individuals with cerebral palsy and developmental disabilities and their families.

8179 **Universal Institute: Rehab & Fitness Center**

15-17 Microlab Road
Suite 101
Livingston, NJ 07039
973-992-8181
FAX: 973-992-9797
e-mail: chesney12@comcast.net

Scott Chesney, Director
Jaymee Bernstein, Executive Director
Universal institute is a 15,000 square foot, state of the art rehabilitation facility that specializes in neurological disorders such as brain injuries, spinal cord injury, strokes, etc. We offer PT, OT, speech patholgy, cognitive remediation, aqua therapy and EMG biofeedback.

Camps

8180 **ADA Camp for Kids**

American Diabetes Association
2625 Pennsylvania Street Northeast
Suite 225
Albuquerque, NM 87110
505-266-5716
888-342-2383
FAX: 505-268-4533
e-mail: askada@diabetes.org
www.diabetes.org

Cyndy Ankiewicz, Executive Director
One-week camping session for children with diabetes. Coed, ages 8-13. Camp will be held at Manzano Mountain Retreat, one hour from Albuquerque, New Mexico. Please call for exact dates.

8181 ADA Teen Camp at Covenant Point
American Diabetes Association
30 North Michigan Avenue
Suite 2015
Chicago, IL 60602
312-346-1805
888-342-2383
FAX: 312-346-5342
e-mail: sapsey@diabetes.org
www.diabetes.org/

Loynn Nicholas, CEO
Nancy Harris, Executive Director
Suzanne Aspey, Program Director
One-week sessions for children and teenagers with diabetes. Coed, ages 4 to 9. Camp season runs from June through August and is located in Iron River, Michigan. Featured activities include: arts and crafts, nature/environmental studies, recreational swimming and team building.

8182 ADA Triangle D Camp
American Diabetes Association
30 North Michigan Avenue
Suite 2015
Chicago, IL 60602
312-346-1805
888-342-2383
FAX: 312-346-5342
e-mail: sapsey@diabetes.org

Suzanne Apsey, Program Director
Sara Wichman, Program Assistant
Nancy Harris, Executive Director
A special camp program combining summer activities, diabetes education and medical supervision with one week sessions during July. Coed, ages from 9 to 13. Featured activities include: archery, arts and crafts, baseball/softball, boating, challenge/rope courses, soccer and recreational swimming.

8183 AH! Asthma Camp
YMCA Camp of Maine
305 Winthrop Center Road
Winthrop, ME 04364
207-395-4200
207-395-7230
FAX: 207-395-7230
e-mail: info@maineycamp.org
www.maineycamp.org/htm/

Rhonda Vosmus RRT-AE-C, Camp Director
Jon Musmand MD, Medical Director
AH! Asthma camp is an overnight camp. It is held at the State YMCA Camp in Winthrop, Maine, for one week during the month of August. Children participate in canoeing, swimming, arts and crafts, and other activities alongside Y-Campers. Asthma Camp is a great way for kids to have fun while learning more about their asthma and how to keep it under control. Doctors, Nurses, and Respiratory Therapists provide medical care around the clock to AH! Campers. Coed, ages of 8 and 13.

8184 ASCCA
Alabama Easter Seal Society
PO Box 21
5278 Camp ASCCA Drive
Jacksons Gap, AL 36861
256-825-9226
FAX: 256-825-8332
e-mail: info@campascca.org
www.campascca.org

Matt Rickman, Camp Director
Geni Payne, Program Director
John Stephenson, Administrator
Programs for campers with asthma/respiratory ailments, blood disorders, diabetes, epilepsy and spina bifida. Coed, ages 6-99. One-week sessions June-August.

8185 Adventure Day Camp
Lake Ridge Campus
3480 Commission Ct.
Lake Ridge, VA 22192
703-491-1444
www.princewilliamacademy.com

Samia Harris, Principal
Camping for children with asthma/respiratory ailments and cancer. Coed, ages 2-13.

8186 Agassiz Village
238 Bedford Street
Suite 8
Lexington, MA 02420
781-860-0200
FAX: 781-860-0352
www.agassizvillage.com

Lisa M Gillis, Executive Director/Camp Director
Sarah Dodd, Program Director
Denise Donellan, Health Director
Camp is located in Poland, Maine. Camp is located in Poland, Maine. Offers two and three-week sessions June-August for children with cerebral palsy, mobility limitation and spina bifida. Coed, ages 7-14.

8187 American Diabetes Association
1323 23rd Street S
Suite C
Fargo, ND 58103
701-234-0123
888-342-2383
FAX: 701-235-3080
e-mail: schristensen@diabetes.org
www.diabetes.org

Sheila Christensen, Executive Director

8188 American Diabetes Association Summer Camp
American Diabetes Association
PO Box 385
Huntsville, AL 35804
902-479-0857
FAX: 902-431-0680
e-mail: labramson@eastlink.ca
www.diabetescamps.org

Lorne Abramson, Executive Director
Kathy Latimer, Administrative Assistant
Rocky Wilson, President
Camp is located in Rush, New York. Sessions for children with diabetes. Coed, ages 8-16.

8189 American Diabetes Association: Camp Grenada
American Diabetes Association
30 N. Michigan Ave Ste 2015
Chicago, IL 60602
312-346-1805
312-346-6567
e-mail: dscott@diabetes.org
www.diabetes.org

Donna Scott, Executive Director
Camp is located in Monticello, Illinois. One-week sessions for children with diabetes. Boys and girls 8-17.

8190 American Diabetes Summer Camp
American Diabetes Association
801 W Fireweed Lane
Suite 103
Anchorage, AK 99503
907-272-1424
800-342-2383
FAX: 907-272-1428
e-mail: askada@diabetes.org
www.diabetes.org

Eileen Stankavich, Program Director
Michelle Cassano, Executive Director
A residential camp for children with diabetes, ages 7 to 17.

8191 Arizona Camp Sunrise
American Cancer Society
2929 E Thomas Road
Phoenix, AZ 85016
602-224-0524
800-865-1582
FAX: 602-381-1582
e-mail: tina@azcampsunrise.org
www.azcampsunrise.org/prog_sunrise.htmL

Barbara Nicholas, Program Director
Steve Slaughter, President
Melissa Lee, Camp Director
Camp is in Payson, Arizona. Provides one-week summer camping sessions at no charge to children aged 8-18 who have had, or currently have, cancer.

8192 Bar 717 Ranch/Camp Trinity

PO Box 150
Hayfork, CA 96041 530-628-5992

e-mail: camptrinity@bar717.com
www.bar717.com

Kent Collard, Director
Offers two, three and four-week camping sessions May-September. Accepts campers with diabetes and mobility limitation. Coed, ages 8-16. Also families, single adults and seniors.

8193 Becket Chimney Corners YMCA Outdoor Center

748 Hamilton Road
Becket, MA 01223 413-623-8991
FAX: 413-623-5890
e-mail: bccymca@bccymca.org
www.bccymca.org

Philip Connor, Executive Director
Steve Hammil, Outdoor Camp Director
Sasha Armstrong, Officer Manager
Half-week and one-week sessions for campers with asthma/respiratory ailments. Coed, ages 1-99, families, seniors, single adults.

8194 Boggy Creek Gang Camp

30500 Brantley Branch Road
Eustis, FL 32736 352-483-4200
866-468-6443
FAX: 352-483-0589
e-mail: info@boggycreek.org
www.boggycreek.org

Dorcas Tomasek, Camp Director
June Clark, President/COO
James R Ellis Lt General, CEO/Chairman
Year-round sessions for children with a variety of chronic or life-threatening illnesses including cancer, hemophila, epilepsy, heart defects, HIV, spina bifida and asthma/respiratory ailments. Coed, ages 7-16.

8195 Bright Horizons Summer Camp

Sickle Cell Disease Association of Illinois
200 North Michigan Avenue
Suite 605
Chicago, IL 60601 312-345-1100
866-798-1097
FAX: 312-803-1953
e-mail: support@sicklecelldisease-il.org
www.sicklecelldisease-il.org

Howard Anderson, President
Valeria C Beckley, Director
Dorothy C Moore MD, Chief Medical Officer
Camp is located in Williams Bay, Wisconsin. Camping for children with blood disorders, ages 7-13.

8196 Camp Alpine

Alpine Alternatives
2518 E Tudor Road
Suite 105
Anchorage, AK 99507 907-561-6655
800-361-4174
FAX: 907-563-9232
e-mail: info@alpinealternatives.org
www.alpinealternatives.org/getinvolved.HTML

Gayla Valle, President
Kris Johnston, Vice President
Margaret Webber, Director
Our programs are designed to help people expand their horizons, master new skills, make new friends, and increase motor coordination. Most importantly, participants experience growth in self-confidence and independence that affects all aspects of an individual's life. Our services are open to all, regardless of type of disability or age. Activities include canoeing, hiking, swimming, outdoor games, sports, nature identification and much more.

8197 Camp Birchwood

Muscular Dystrophy Association (MDA)
PO Box 670049
Chugiak, AK 99567 907-688-2734
FAX: 907-688-2734
e-mail: campinfo@birchwoodcamp.org
www.birchwoodcamp.org

Sara Gaar, Director
Chris Robinson, Director
Ramona Jobe, Health Care Services Director
A summer camp at Birchwood Camp in Chugiak, Alaska for individuals ages 6-21 who are affected by any of the 40-plus neuromuscular diseases in MDA's program. Common activities include: swimming, hockey, baseball, soccer, football, boating, horseback riding, fishing, music, cooking, arts and crafts, movies, dancing, talent shows, Harley-Davidson motorcycle sidecar or three-wheeled cycle rides, a visit from fire fighters and time for socializing and laughing.

8198 Camp Bon Coeur

The Heart Camp
PO Box 53765
Lafayette, LA 70505 337-233-8437
FAX: 337-233-4160
e-mail: info@heartcamp.com
www.heartcamp.com

Calvin Guidry, President
Claire Foret, Vice President
Susannah Craig, Executive Director
Two-week sessions June-July for children with heart defects. Coed, ages 8-16.

8199 Camp Breathe Easy

American Lung Association
2452 Spring Road
Smyrna, GA 30080 770-434-5864
800-LUN- USA
FAX: 770-319-0349
e-mail: cmobley@alaga.org
www.alaga.org/CBE1.html

Chanda Mobley PhD, Executive Director
Starla Hairston, Program Director
Donna Brazzell, Director Special Projects
Camp Breathe Easy is a seven-day, six-night overnight camp for children, ages 7-13, with asthma who need medication and are limited in summer camping opportunities. The children learn asthma self-management techniques and coping strategies to better handle their illness. Campers swim, repel off trees, fish, canoe, play soccer, basketball and miniature golf, and participate in ceramics and arts and crafts.

8200 Camp Carefree

The American Diabetes Association
1846 West Seventh Street
Piscataway, NJ 08850 732-752-5847
603-859-0410
e-mail: carefreecamp@aol
www.campcarefreekids.org

Phyllis Woestemeyer, Camp Director
Camp is located in Wolfeboro, New Hampshire. Sessions for campers with diabetes.

8201 Camp Carolina Trails for Children

American Diabetes Association
1701 N Beauregard Street
Alexandria, VA 22311
800-342-2383
888-342-2383
e-mail: AskADA@diabetes.org
www.diabetes.org/

Emily Nivens, Director
Mona Tucker, Principal
Richard Kahn PhD, Chief Scientific/Medical Officer
The American Diabetes Association Camp Carolina Trails is an exciting week of summer fun for boys and girls entering grades 4 through 11. Camp includes many sports and activities such as swimming, hiking, canoeing and arts and crafts. It is held at YMCA Camp Hanes on 400 acres next to hanging Rock State Park which is located at the base of Sauratown Mountain, just 30 minutes north of Winston-Salem, North Carolina. Camp for ages 10-17. Use address given in Virginia for more information.

8202 Camp Catch-a-Rainbow
American Cancer Society
1755 Abbey Road East
Lansing, MI 48823
517-332-2222
800-ACS-2345
FAX: 517-664-1497
e-mail: deb.dillingham@cancer.org
www.cancer.org

Debra Dillingham, Director
Greg Bontrager, Chief Executive Officer
Camp is located in Montague, Michigan. One-week sessions for children with cancer. Co-ed ages 7-15.

8203 Camp Cheerful
Achievement Centers For Children
15000 Cheerful Lane
Strongsville, OH 44136
440-238-6200
FAX: 440-238-1858
e-mail: tim.fox@achievementctrs.org
www.achievementcenters.org

Patricia W Nobili, Executive Director
Tim Fox, Director Camp Services
Susan Hyman, Manager Rehabilitation Services
Sessions for campers with developmental disabilities, mobility limitation and speech/communication impairment. Coed, ages 7-99.

8204 Camp Christmas Seal
American Lung Association of Oregon
7420 Southwest Bridgeport Road
Suite 200
Tigard, OR 97224
503-924-4094
800-LUN- USA
FAX: 503-924-4120
e-mail: info@lungoregon.org
www.lungoregon.org

Beverly Stewart, Camp Director
Scott Hill, Chairman
Jennifer Baldwin, Development/Communications
Camp is located in Sisterhood, Oregon. Sessions for children with asthma/respiratory ailments. Coed, ages 8-15.

8205 Camp Classen YMCA
YMCA of Greater Oklahoma City
Rt1 Box 47
Davis, OK 73030
580-369-2272
FAX: 580-369-2284
e-mail: amcwhort@ymcaokc.org
www.campclassenymca.org

Albert P McWhorter, Executive Director
Rick Burris, Associate Executive Director
Camp is located in Davis, Oklahoma. Sessions for children and adults with diabetes. Coed, ages 8-17, families, seniors and single adults.

8206 Camp Conrad Chinnock
Diabetic Youth Services
501 W Walnut Street
Compton, CA 90220
310-604-2473
888-800-4010
FAX: 888-800-4010
e-mail: programs@dys.org
www.dys.org

Rocky Wilson, Executive Director
Ryan Martz, Program Director
Tom Jenkins, Chief Administrator
Offers one and two-week sessions for campers with diabetes. Coed, ages 7-16. Also families.

8207 Camp Courage North
PO Box 1626
Lake George, MN 56458
218-266-3658
FAX: 231-826-6345
e-mail: camping@courage.org
www.couragecamps.org

Tom Fogarty, Director
Mary Jensen, Manager
Camp is located in Lake George, Minnesota. Summer sessions for campers who have blood disorders, hearing impairment, mobility limitation or are blind/visually impaired. Coed, ages 7-70.

8208 Camp Crosley YMCA
Muncie Family YMCA
165 EMS T2 Lane
North Webster, IN 46555
574-834-2331
877-811-6189
FAX: 574-834-3313
e-mail: info@campcrosley.org
www.campcrosley.org

Richard Armstrong, Executive Director
Larry McCullin, Program Director
Randle Cassady, Summer Camp Director
Camp is located in North Webster, Indiana. Half-week, one, two and three-week sessions for campers with asthma/respiratory ailments and diabetes. Coed, ages 7-17. Also families and seniors.

8209 Camp Del Corazon
11615 Hesby Street
North Hollywood, CA 91601
818-754-0312
888-621-4800
FAX: 818-754-0842
e-mail: information@campdelcorazon.org
www.campdelcorazon.org

Lisa Knight RN, Executive Director/Co-Founder
Kevin Shannon MD, Medical Director/Co-Founder
Glenn Knight, CEO/Board Member
Active program for campers with heart disease, Camp del Corazon provides summer activities free of charge that include hiking and archery, arts and crafts, court and field games, waterfront activities and a beach barbecue.

8210 Camp Discovery
American Diabetes Association
837 S Hillside Street
Wichita, KS 67211
316-684-6091
800-362-1355
888-342-2838
FAX: 316-684-5675
e-mail: askada@diabetes.org
www.diabetes.org

Crystal Walter, Camp Director
Lawrence T Smith, Chair
Lynn B Nicholas FACHE, Chief Executive Officer
Camp is located in Junction City, Kansas. Offers young people with diabetes a week of fun at rock springs 4-H Center. Special attention to diabetes makes Camp Discovery a safe environment for active youth while providing valuable diabetes managment education. Call the American Diabetes Association Kansas area office for more information. Coed, ages 8-17.

8211 Camp Eden Wood
Friendship Ventures
6350 Indian Chief Road
Eden Prairie, MN 55346
952-852-0101
800-450-8376
FAX: 952-852-0123
e-mail: fv@friendshipventures.org
www.friendshipventures.org

Georgann Rumsey, President/CEO
Laurie Tschetter, Program Director
Camp is located in Eden Prairie, Minnesota. Offers resident camp programs for children, teenagers and adults with developmental, physical or multiple disabilities, Down Syndrome, special medical conditions, Williams Syndrome, autism and/or other conditions. Fishing, creative arts, golf, sports and other activities are available. Respite care weekend camps year round for children, teenagers and adults. Guided vacations for teens and adults with developmental disabilities or other unique needs.

8212 **Camp Enchantment**
American Cancer Society
10501 Montgomery Boulevard NE
Suite 300
Albuquerque, NM 87111
505-559-9423
FAX: 505-559-9423
e-mail: gesquive@cancer.org
www.cancer.org

Geraldine Esquivel, Director
Camp Enchantment offers an exciting opportunity for children with cancer to have fun and celebrate life through friendships and discoveries in a safe and respectful atmosphere. Held in June of each year, this one-week camp session is designed especially for kids with cancer and provides opportunities to celebrate life, enhance one's emotional well-being, increase decision-making and coping skills, and to deal with the impact of cancer. Coed, ages 7-17.

8213 **Camp Fatima**
32 Fatima Road
PO Box 206
Gilmanton Iron Works, NH 03837
603-569-5851
FAX: 603-569-5038
e-mail: info@ diocamps.org
www.diocamps.org

Gus Planchett, Executive Director
Michael Drumm, Marketing Director
Joanne Towle, Business Manager/Registrar
Summer sessions for children with developmental disabilities, mobility limitation and speech/communication impairment.

8214 **Camp Floyd Rogers**
Floyd Rogers Foundation
PO Box 31536
Omaha, NE 68131
402-341-0866
FAX: 402-341-0866
www.campfloydrogers.com

Kelly Krambeck, Camp Director
A camp for diabetic children. Coed, ages 8-18. 100 children come to Camp Floyd Rogers each summer. They come to enjoy activities, participate in special events, engage in innovative evening programs, and they meet other children their own age with diabetes. Camp Floyd Rogers offers young people an opportunity to share some of life's adventures with others who also happen to have diabetes.

8215 **Camp Fun in the Sun**
Inland North West Health Services
PO Box 469
Spokane, WA 99210
509-232-8135
FAX: 509-232-8151
e-mail: randalll@cherspokane.org
www.campfuninthesun.org

Lisa Randall, Director
Diane Lenier, Executive Director
Summer camping for children with diabetes. Coed, ages 6-18.

8216 **Camp Glengarra**
Girl Scouts - Foothills Council
33 Jewett Place
Utica, NY 13501
315-733-2391
FAX: 315-733-1909
e-mail: nbrown@girlscoutsfoothills.org
www.girlscoutsfoothills.org

Natalie Brown, Executive Director
Karen Lubecki, Camp Director
Kristi Brennan, Development/Communications Mgr
Camp Glengarra is located on 500+ acres of fields and forests, about eight miles west of Camden. This Girl Scout Camp hosts a myriad of programs throughout the year as well as summer day and resident camp. Summer sessions for girls 5-17 with ADD or asthma/respiratory ailments.

8217 **Camp Glyndon**
American Diabetes Association
800 Wyman Park Drive
Suite 110
Baltimore, MD 21211
410-265-0075
800-342-2383
FAX: 410-235-4048
e-mail: askada@diabetes.org
www.diabetes.org

Larry K Ellingson, Chairman
Lynn B Nicholas, Chief Executive Officer
Alan D Cherrington, President
Camp is located in Nanjemoy, Maryland. One and two-week sessions July-August for children with diabetes and their families. Coed, ages 8-16.

8218 **Camp Harkness**
301 Great Neck Road
Route 213
Waterford, CT 06385
860-443-7818
866-284-1595
FAX: 860-236-6205
TTY: 860-859-5493
e-mail: info@ciboakhill.org
www.campharkness.com/Default.htm

Vicki Severin, Camp Director
Scott Walls, Program Manager
Trish Hesslein, Director Community Relations
In 1991 a group of parents and adults with spina bifida, were brought together with the mission to educate the public about spina bifida and issues affecting people who have this disability in addition To providing support and information and promoting programs that will help people with spina bifida. Since then SBAC has worked hard to support parents, adults with spina bifida and families

8219 **Camp Hertko Hollow**
101 Locust Street
Des Moines, IA 50309
515-276-2237
800-DIA-ETES
888-437-8652
FAX: 515-251-5831
e-mail: a.wolf@camphertkohollow.com
www.CampHertkoHollow.com

Ann Wolf, Exeuctive Director
Vivian Murry, Camp Director
Camp Hertko Hollow is a resident camp held at the Des Moines YMCA Camp site, located along the Des Moines River north of Boone, Iowa. Activities include horseback riding, swimming, canoeing, rappelling, crafts, ropes course, archery and riflery to name a few, plus special activities for different ages. Half-week and one-week sessions for children with diabetes. Coed, ages 6-16.

8220 **Camp Hickory Hill**
Central Missouri Diabetic Childrens Camp
PO Box 1942
Columbia, MO 65205
573-445-9146
FAX: 573-445-5196
e-mail: camphickoryhill@yahoo.com
www.camphickoryhill.com

Pamela Marquis, Camp Director
Educates diabetic children concerning diabetes and its care. In addition to daily educational sessions on some aspects of diabetes, campers participate in swimming, sailing, arts and crafts and overnight camping. Coed, ages 8-17.

8221 **Camp Ho Mita Koda**
Diabetes Association Of Greater Cleveland
3601 Green Road
Suite 100
Cleveland, OH 44122
216-591-0800
FAX: 216-591-0320
e-mail: camp@dagc.org
www.camphomitakoda.org

Liberty A Wright, Camp Administrator
Jackquie Dickinson, President
Camp is located in Newbury, Ohio. Summer sessions for children with type 1 diabetes. Coed, ages 6-15. Type 2 diabetes, coed, ages 12-17. Bicycle adventure, coed, ages 13-19. Mini-day camp, ages 4-7, coed.

8222 Camp Hodia
1701 North 12th Avenue
Boise, ID 83702
208-336-6829
FAX: 208-322-0402
e-mail: info@hodia.com
www.hodia.com

Don Scott RN, Summer Camp Director
Lynn Wilson RN, Assistant Camp Director
Barb Scott RN, Secretary
Camp is located in Alturas Lake, Idaho. One-week sessions for children with diabetes. Coed, ages 8-18. Ski Camp in Sun Valley in January, ages 12-18.

8223 Camp Honor
Hemophilia Association
Inc. 818 East Osborn
Suite 105
Phoenix, AZ 85014
602-955-3947
FAX: 602-955-1962
e-mail: cindy@hemophiliaz.org
www.hemophiliaz.org

Richard Traulsen, President
Neil Frick MS, VP Medical/Research Information
Cindy Komar, Interim Executive Director
Camp is located in Payson, Arizona at the Whispering Hope Ranch. One-week sessions for children with hemophilia or HIV and their siblings, as well as children of hemophiliacs. Coed, ages 7-17. Activities include swimming, canoeing, sports, archery and arts and crafts (to name a few fun things).

8224 Camp Independence
2951 Flowers Road South
Suite 211
Atlanta, GA 30341
770-452-1539
800-633-2339
e-mail: tracy@kidneyga.org
www.nkfg.org/services/campind.htm

Tracy Jenny, Camp Director
Christopher Starr, Executive Director
Charles C Starr, Chief Executive Officer
Camp Independence is Georgia's a overnight, week-long summer camp providing essential medical care, treatment & fun for kids with kidney disease and transplants. Camp Independence recognizes that campers are normal children but have special needs providing these children with opportunities for development & individual growth, peer support & normal life experiences. Activities include swimming, arts & crafts, fishing and horsebackriding, in addition to archery, games and sports, and ceramics.

8225 Camp Jened
United Cerebral Palsy Association New York
Adams Road
PO Box 483
Rock Hill, NY 12775
845-434-2220
FAX: 845-434-2253
e-mail: jened@catskill.net
www.campjened.org

Michael Branam, Executive Director
Camp is located in Rock Hill, New York. Sessions for adults with severe developmental and physical disabilities. Coed, ages 18-99.

8226 Camp Jewell YMCA Outdoor Center
YMCA of Greater Hartford
6 Prock Hill Road
PO Box 8
Colebrook, CT 06021
860-379-4679
888-412-2267
FAX: 860-397-8715
TTY: 888-412-2267
e-mail: camp.jewell@ghymca.org
www.ghymca.org

Brian Rupe, Executive Director
Eric Tucker, Associate Executive
Jodi Gove, Ranch Program Coordinator
Camp is located in Colebrook, Connecticut. Two-week sessions for children with cancer. Coed, ages 8-16. Also families.

8227 Camp John Warvel
American Diabetes Association
6415 Castleway West Drive
Suite 114
Indianapolis, IN 46250
317-352-9226
888-342-2383
FAX: 317-594-0748
www.diabetes.com

Elaine McClane, Director Programs
Renea Marsh, Executive Director
Camp is located in North Webster, Indiana. Provides an enjoyable, safe and educational out-of-doors experience for children with insulin-dependent diabetes. A unique learning atmosphere for children to acquire new skills in caring for their disease. The camp experience instills confidence for the child's self-management of diabetes. Offers one-week sessions and can accommodate 200 campers, boys and girls aged 7-16.

8228 Camp Joslin
One Joslin Place
Boston, MA 02215
617-732-2400
FAX: 617-735-1925
e-mail: camp@joslin.harvard.edu
www.joslin.org

C Ronald Kahn, President/Director
Stephanie Holloway, Camp Coordinator
Martin J Abrahamson MD, SVP Medical Director
Camp is located in Charlton, Massachusetts. For boys, ages 7-16, with diabetes. This program offers active summer sports and activities, supplemented by medical treatment and diabetes education. Coed Winter Camp and Coed Weekend Retreats are offered during the school year.

8229 Camp Joy
3325 Swamp Creek Road
Schwenksville, PA 19473
610-754-6878
FAX: 610-754-7880
e-mail: campjoy@fast.net
www.campjoy.com

Angus Murray, Camp Director
A special needs camp for kids and adults (ages 4-80+) with developmental disabilities such as: mental retardation, autism, brain injury, neurological disorder, visual and/or hearing impairments, Angelman and Down syndromes, and other developmental disabilities.

8230 Camp L-Kee-Ta
Girl Scouts of Shining Trail
1308 Broadway Street
PO Box 190
West Burlington, IA 52655
319-752-3639
FAX: 319-753-1410
e-mail: info@girlscoutsofstc.org
www.girlscoutsofstc.org

Donna Logan, Chief Executive Officer
Becky Godfrey, Camp Director
Kim Hull, Associate Executive Director
Camp is located in Danville, Iowa. Half-week and one-week sessions June-August for children with asthma/respiratory ailments. Girls, ages 7-18 and families.

8231 Camp Libbey
Maumee Valley GSC
28325 State Route 281
Defiance, OH 43512
419-243-8216
800-860-4516
FAX: 419-245-5357
e-mail: lbowerman@mvgsc.org
www.gsmvc.org/contact.htm

Bowerman Laura, Executive Director
Jeff Baldwin, Camp Ranger
Christine Gustin, Camp Manager
Camp for girls 7-18 with asthma/respiratory ailments, diabetes, epilepsy and muscular dystrophy is located in Defiance, Ohio.

8232 Camp MITIOG
Share
10015 Northwest Ambassador Drive
Kansas City, MO 64153
816-221-6268
FAX: 816-221-1420

Brenda O'Dell, Director
Camp is located in Excelsior Springs, Missouri. One-week summer sessions for children with spina bifida. Coed, ages 6-16.

8233 Camp Magruder
Conference of United Methodists
17450 Old Pacific Highway
Rockaway Beach, OR 97136
503-355-2310
FAX: 503-355-8701
e-mail: magruder@gocamping.org
www.campmagruder.org/

Miranda Lovegren, Camp Director
Nicole Robbins, Program Director
Pat Ryan, Facilities Manager
Camp is located in Rockaway Beach, Oregon. Sessions for children and adults with cancer and developmental disabilities. Coed, ages 9-18, families, seniors and single adults.

8234 Camp Mokuleia
Episcopal Church Of Hawaii
68-729 Farrington Highway
Waialua, HI 96791
808-637-6241
FAX: 808-637-5505
e-mail: info@campmokuleia.com
www.campmokuleia.com/main.php

Laurie Schlegel, General Manager
Mandy McMahan, Camp Director
Nani Lowery, Business Manager
One and two-week sessions for children with cancer. Boys and girls, ages 7-17.

8235 Camp Not-A-Wheeze American Lung Association
102 West McDowell Road
Phoenix, AZ 85003
602-258-7507
FAX: 602-258-7507
e-mail: infophoenix@lungaz.org
http://www.azasthma.org/aac-su-camp.htm

Rhonda Follman, Health Services/Camp Director
John Kirkwood, ALA President/CEO
Joseph Bergen, Chief Operating Officer/EVP
Camp Not-A-Wheeze is designed especially for kids ages 7-14 with moderate to severe asthma and was created to provide a traditional residential camp experience and teach children how to manage their asthma.

8236 Camp Okizu
Okizu Foundation
16 Digital Drive
Novato, CA 94949
415-382-9083
FAX: 415-382-8384
e-mail: info@okizu.org
www.okizu.org

Suzanne Randall, Executive Director
Camp is located in Berry Creek, California. Offers one-week sessions June-August for children who have cancer. Coed, ages 6-17. Also siblings.

8237 Camp Rainbow
Phoenix Childrens Hospital (PCH)
1919 E Thomas Road
Phoenix, AZ 85016
602-546-1000
888-908-5437
FAX: 602-546-0276
www.phxchildrens.com/about/services/

Kathy Nord, Director
Robert Meyer, President/CEO PCH
David Notrica MD, President Medical Staff PCH
Camp is located in Prescott, Arizona. Offers one-week sessions for children who have had, or currently have, cancer. Boys and girls ages 7-17. Camp activities include swimming, horseback riding, arts and crafts, canoeing, performing arts, archery, rollerskating, fishing, an overnight camping trip and much more! It's a week filled with laughter, new experiences and new friends.

8238 Camp Rap-A-Hope Medical Society and the Alliance to the Medical
Society State of Alabama
2701 Airport Boulevard
Mobile, AL 36606
251-476-9880
FAX: 251-476-9495
e-mail: rapahope@earthlink.net
www.camprapahope.org

Kathy Simpson, President
Melissa McNichol, Camp Director
Nell Gustavson, Administrative Assisant
Camp Rap-A-Hope is a one-week summer camp for children and teenagers who are battling cancer or have ever been diagnosed with cancer and are 7 to 17 years of age. It is free of charge. Camp Rap-A-Hope strives to make sure every camper gets the opportunity to develop new skills and self-confidence. Camp activities are appropriate for our campers' ages and abilities and include, but are not limited to: swimming, music, arts and crafts, archery, fishing, canoeing and horseback riding.

8239 Camp Ronald McDonald for Good Times
Ronald McDonald House of California
1954 Cotner Avenue
Los Angeles, CA 90025
310-268-8488
800-625-7295
FAX: 310-473-3338
e-mail: info@campronaldmcdonald.org
www.campronaldmcdonald.org

Carol Horvitz, Executive Director
Chadwick Edwards, Program Director
Ken Mortensen, Facilities Director
Camp is located in Mountain Center, California. Year-round camping sessions at no charge for children who have cancer. Coed, ages 7-18. Also families.

8240 Camp Setebaid
Setebaid Services
PO Box 196
Winfield, PA 17889
570-524-9090
FAX: 570-523-0769
e-mail: info@setebaidservices.org
www.setebaidservices.org

Mark Moyer, Executive Director
Diane Facer, Office Assistant
Camping sessions for children with diabetes. Coed, ages 3-13 years. Family retreat for children with diabetes and their families.

8241 Camp Shady Brook
YMCA of the Pikes Peak Region (PPYMCA)
207 North Nevada Avenue
Colorado Springs, CO 80903
719-473-9622
FAX: 719-471-1723
e-mail: campinfo@ppymca.org
www.ppymca.org

Clint Knox, Executive Director
Tish Johnston, Program Director
Karstin Knutson, Officer Manager
Camp is located in Sedalia, Colorado. One-week sessions for campers with HIV. Boys and girls 7-16. Also families, seniors and single adults.

8242 Camp Sioux
American Diabetes Association
Box 5234
101 North Third Street
Grand Forks, ND 58206
701-746-4427
800-666-6709
FAX: 701-235-3080
e-mail: AskADA@diabetes.org
www.diabetes.org/

Becky Martin, Camp Director
Camp Sioux, located in Park River, ND, is a week-long residential summer camp for children ages 8-14 who are living with diabetes. Programs encourage independence and self management with appropriate medical supervision to ensure the best possible experience for every camper. Nutrition activities, blood glucose monitoring, and injections/medications are integrated into the camp program.

8243 Camp Smile-A-Mile
PO Box 550155
Birmingham, AL 35255
205-323-8427
888-500-7920
FAX: 205-323-6220
e-mail: campsam@mindspring.com
www.campsam.org

Jennifer Queen, Program Director
Lynn Thompson, Executive Director
Stephanie C Wilkins, Community Relations Manager
Camp Smile-A-Mile is a non-profit organization for children who have or had cancer in Alabama. Camp Smile-A-Mile's mission is to provide challenging, unforgettable recreational and educational experiences for young cancer patients from across Alabama at no cost to their families. Our purpose is to provide these children with avenues for fellowship, to help them cope with their disease, and to prepare them for life.

8244 Camp Sunrise
American Cancer Society Maryland
8219 Town Center Drive
Baltimore, MD 21236
410-931-6850
888-670-0472
FAX: 410-931-6875
e-mail: sherryce.robinson@cancer.org
www.cancer.org

Sherryce Robinson, Mission Delivery Manager
Kira Elring, Regional Mission Director
Gloria Jetter, Regional Executive Director
Camp is located in Whitehall, Maryland. One-week sessions free of charge to children who have had, or currently have, cancer. Coed, ages 4-18.

8245 Camp Sweeney
Southwestern Diabetic Fund
PO Box 918
Gainesville, TX 76241
940-665-2011
FAX: 940-665-9467
e-mail: info@campsweeney.org
www.campsweeney.org

Milton Dixon, Chairman
Ernie Fernandez, Executive Director
Teaches self-care and self-reliance to children ages 7-18 with diabetes. Campers participate in such activities such as swimming, fishing, horseback riding and arts and crafts while learning about how to self manage their diabetes.

8246 Camp Tall Turf
Christian Camps and Inner City Youth
935 Baxter Street Southeast
Grand Rapids, MI 49506
616-459-7206
FAX: 616-988-4596
e-mail: tallturf@iserv.net
www.tallturf.org

Steve Farber, Chairman
Jack Kooyman, President
Denise Fase, Program Administrator
Camp is located in Walkerville, Michigan. Summer camping sessions for youth with asthma/respiratory ailments and ADD. Coed, ages 8-16.

8247 Camp Vacamas
Vacamas Program for Youth
256 Macopin Road
West Milford, NJ 07480
973-838-1394
877-428-8222
FAX: 973-838-7534
e-mail: info@vacamas.org
www.vacamas.com

Michael Friedman, Executive Director
Sandi Friedman, Associate Executive Director
William Stein, President
Disadvantaged children with asthma or sickle cell anemia, ages 8-16, are offered special programs in canoeing, backpacking, camping, music and leadership training. Sliding scale tuition. Year round programs for youth at risk groups. Conference center facility open for group rentals.

8248 Camp Waziyatah
19 Vose Lane
East Walpole, MA 02032
508-668-9758
FAX: 508-668-2665
e-mail: info@wazi.com
www.wazi.com

Penny Kerns, Director
Camp is located in Waterford, Massachusetts. Three, four and seven-week sessions June-August for campers with cancer and diabetes. Coed, ages 8-15 and families, single adults.

8249 Camp Wheezeaway American Lung Association of Alabama
3125 Independence Drive
Suite 325
Birmingham, AL 35209
205-933-8821
251-456-1115
FAX: 251-456-1116
e-mail: Lungcs1@aol.com
www.alabamalung.org

Connie Sullivan, Camp Director
Margaret Jakes MD, Medical Director
Joseph LaRussa MD, Co-Medical Director
Camp WheezeAway is a 5 day overnight camp for 8-12 with moderate to severe asthma in Alabama held at Camp ASCCA in Jackson's Gap, AL and is sponsored by the American Lung Association. Children are monitered while enjoying all the normal camp activities including ropes courses, canoeing, swimming, arts & crafts, horseback riding, fishing, tubing & more and above all learn to manage their asthma.

8250 Camps for Children & Teens with Diabetes
Diabetes Society of Santa Clara Valley
1165 Lincoln Avenue
Suite 300
San Jose, CA 95125
408-287-3785
800-989-1165
FAX: 408-287-2701
e-mail: camp@diabetesscv.org
www.diabetesscv.org

Dougles Metz, Executive Director
Glen Wong, Development Director
Thomas Smith, Director Of Programs/Camps
Since 1974, sponsors up to 20 day camps, family camps and resident camps for children 4 through 17. These camps provide an opportunity for children with diabetes to go to camp, meet other children and gain a better understanding of their diabetes. The total experience can help campers develop more confidence in their abilities to control their diabetes effectively while enjoying the traditional camp experience. Camps are located throughout CA and parts of Nevada.

8251 Cedar Ridge Camp
4010 Routt Road
Louisville, KY 40299
502-267-5848
FAX: 502-267-0116
e-mail: andrew@cedarridgecamp.com
www.cedarridgecamp.com/

Andrew Hartmans, Executive Director
Half-week, one and two-week sessions for children with diabetes, developmental disabilities and muscular dystrophy. Coed, ages 6-17.

8252 Champ Camp American Lung Association of Alaska
500 W. Int'l Airport Road
Suite A
Anchorage, AK 99518
317-679-1860

e-mail: mferreira@aklung.org
www.aklung.org/asthma/champcamp/

Michelle Ferreira, Lung Health Progam Coordinator
Kathy Case MD, Medical Director
Marge Larson, Chief Executive Officer

Champ Camp is a week long summer recreation and asthma education program at Camp Kushtaka on the beautiful shores of Kenai Lake. Campers are able to explore their skills in outdoor activities including canoeing, hiking, swimming, archery, and arts and crafts. More importantly, Champ Camp boosts self-confidence and instills a sense of responsibility. It teaches preventive measures to improve asthma management, and avoid asthmatic episodes as well as increases a camper's sense of independence.

8253 Clara Barton Diabetes Camp
Clara Barton For Girls With Diabetes
30 Enis Road
PO Box 356
North Oxford, MA 01537
508-987-2056
FAX: 508-987-2002
e-mail: info@bartoncenter.org
www.bartoncenter.org

John Maconga, President
Kerry Packard, Program Coordinator
Martha Houlihan, Finance/Technology Coordinator
Girls, ages 3-17, with diabetes participate in a well-rounded camp program with special education in diabetes, health and safety. Activities include swimming, boating, sports, dance, music and arts and crafts. Two week adventure camp for high school girls offering camping, hiking, canoeing, etc. Also a minicamp (one week) for girls 6-12. Day camps are offered in Worcester, Boston, and New York City.

8254 Crestfield Camp
Pittsburgh Presbytery
195 Taggert Road
Slippery Rock, PA 16057
724-794-4022
800-794-1948
FAX: 724-794-1665
e-mail: programs@crestfield.net
www.childrenwithdiabetes.com/camps

Ida Eckstein, Executive Director
Kevin Starchaer, Program Director
Camp is located at 195 Taggart Road, Slippery Rock, Pennsylvania. Summer sessions for children with diabetes. Coed, ages 9-18 and families.

8255 Des Moines YMCA Camp
YMCA Of Greater Des Moines
1192 166th Drive
Boone, IA 50036
515-432-7558
866-902-9622
FAX: 515-432-5414
e-mail: ycamp@dmymca.org
www.y-camp.org

David Sherry, Director
Tom Hamilton, Chief Volunteer Officer
Vernon Delpesce, President/CEO
Camp is located in Boone, Iowa. Year-round one and two-week sessions for boys and girls with cancer, diabetes, asthma, cystic fibrosis, hearing impaired and other disabilities. Coed, ages 6-16 and families.

8256 Diabetic Youth Foundation
5167 Clayton Road
Suite F
Concord, CA 94521
925-680-4994
FAX: 925-680-4863
e-mail: info@dyf.org
www.dyf.org

Mats Wallin, Executive Director
Pip Pipkins, Camp Director
Janet Kramschuster, Program Director
We offer summer residential camp programs (Bearskin Meadow Camp) and year-round educational and recreational programs for children, teens and families affected by diabetes.

8257 EDI Camp
Wyman Center
600 Kiwanis Drive
Eureka, MO 63025
636-938-5245
FAX: 636-938-5289
e-mail: info@wymancenter.org
www.wymancenter.org

David Hilliard, President
Kristine Ramsey, Chief Development Officer
Carl Hill, Chief Operating Officer
Youngsters with diabetes learn how to care for themselves while participating in a wide variety of outdoor activities and trips. The camp, managed and financed by the American Diabetes Association Greater St. Louis Affiliate, offers camperships to children from the Greater St. Louis area, ages 7-16, but nonresidents may also apply.

8258 Echoing Hills
36272 CR 79
Warsaw, OH 43844
740-327-2311
800-419-6513
FAX: 740-327-6371
e-mail: info@campechoinghills.org
www.campechoinghillsvillages.org

Christy Kuhns, Camp Program Director
Larry Stitt, Camp Administrator
Jimmy McNutt, Camp Activities Coordinator
Summer camp for children and adults with cerebral palsy. Coed, ages 7-70.

8259 FCYD Camp
Foundation for Children and Youth
1995 W 9000 S
West Jordan, UT 84088
801-566-6913
e-mail: fcydwebstaff@networld.com
www.fcyd-inc.org

Dave Okubo, President
Elizabeth Elmer, Vice President
Sherrie Hardy, Director
Camping for children with diabetes. Coed, ages 1-18 and families.

8260 Father Drumgoole Connelly Summer Camp
Catholic Youth Organization
6581 Hylan Boulevard
Staten Island, NY 10309
718-317-2600
FAX: 718-317-2830
www.mountloretto.org

Frank Minotti, Camp Director
Summer sessions for children with epilepsy, hearing impairment and developmental disabilities. Coed, ages 5-13.

8261 Florida Diabetes Camp
PO Box 14136
Gainesville, FL 32604
352-334-1323
FAX: 352-334-1325
e-mail: fccyd@hotmail.com
www.floridadiabetescamp.org

Rosalie Bandyopadhyay, Executive Director
Al Avendano, Program Director
Gary Cornwell, Volunteer Program Director
Camp is located in De Leon Springs, Florida. One and two-week sessions June-August for children with diabetes. Coed, ages 6-18 and families.

8262 Friends Academy Summer Camps
270 Duck Pond Road
Locust Valley, NY 11560
516-676-0393
FAX: 516-393-4276
e-mail: info@fa.org
www.fa.org

Patty Ziplow, Director of Admissions
Richard Mack, Executive Director
Carl Pozzi, Development Director
Summer sessions for children with diabetes. Coed, ages 3-14, families.

8263 Growing Together Diabetes Camp
PO Box 6400
Tyler, TX 75711
903-596-3645
800-648-8141
FAX: 903-535-6783
www.etmc.org

Marie Taylor, Director
Marty Wiggins, Director
A summer camp for youths ages 6 to 15 with Type 1 or Type 2 diabetes.

8264 Guide to ACA Accredited Camps
American Camping Association
5000 State Road 67 N
Martinsville, IN 46151
765-342-8456
800-428-2267
FAX: 765-349-6357
e-mail: bookstore@ACAcamps.org
www.acacamps.org

Melody Snider, Director Bookstore/Distribution
Peg Smith, Chief Executive Officer
A national listing of accredited camping programs. Listed by: special clientele, specific disabilities, camp name, activities.
$10.95
Quarterly

8265 Happiness is Camping
2169 Grand Concourse
Bronx, NY 10453
718-295-3100
FAX: 718-295-0406
e-mail: hicoffice@happinessiscamping.org
www.happinessiscamping.org

Murray Struver, Founder/CEO
Kurt Struver, Director
Louis Agostino, President of the Board
Camp is located in Blairstown, New Jersey. Camping sessions for children with cancer. Coed, ages 7-15.

8266 Hole in the Wall Gang Camp
565 Ashford Center Road
Ashford, CT 06278
860-429-3444
FAX: 860-429-7295
e-mail: ashford@holeinthewallgang.org
www.holeinthewallgang.org

James Canton, Executive Director
Padraig Barry, Assistant Camp Director
Matthew Cook, Manager
Low-cost eight-week sessions June-August for children with cancer and HIV. Coed, ages 7-15.

8267 Kansas Jaycees Cerebral Palsy Ranch
PO Box 267
Augusta, KS 67207
316-775-2421
FAX: 316-775-2421
e-mail: execdirector@cpranch.org
www.cpranch.org

Cheryl Schmeidler, Executive Director
Jana Allar, Program Coordinator
Sarah Walker, Camp Director
Our mission is to provide a program which will allow individuals to enjoy their highest level of functioning and independence, consistant with their abilities, in a summer camp setting.

8268 Kiwanis Camp Wyman
Wyman Center
600 Kiwanis Drive
Eureka, MO 63025
636-938-5245
FAX: 636-938-5289
e-mail: info@wymancenter.org
www.wymancenter.org

David A Hilliard, President
Claire Wyneken, Chief Programs Officer
Kristine Ramsey, Chief Development Officer
Summer sessions for youth with diabetes. Coed, ages 8-16, run in conjunction with the American Diabetes Association. Call for program description.

8269 Ko-Man-She
American Diabetes Association
2555 South Dixie Drive
Suite 112
Kettering, OH 45409
937-220-6611
FAX: 937-224-0240
e-mail: info@diabetesdayton.org
www.diabetesdayton.org

Mike Robinette, Executive Director
Susan McGovern, Program Director
Sally Kattau, President
Camp is located in Bellefontaine, Ohio. Summer sessions for children with diabetes. Coed, ages 8-17. Held in July.

8270 Kweebec
PO Box 511
Penn Valley, PA 19072
610-667-2123
800-543-9830
FAX: 610-667-6376
e-mail: ckweebec@aol.com
www.kweebec.com

Les Weiser, Director
Camp is located in Schwenksville, Pennsylvania. Sessions for children and adults with diabetes. Coed, ages 6-16, families, seniors and single adults.

8271 LA Lions LPDCI Camp Pelican
1835 Saint Roch Avenue
New Orleans, LA 70117
504-944-0166
FAX: 504-948-9555
e-mail: mlandry@tulane.edu
www.lionscamp.org/

R Tony Ricard, President/CEO
Cathy Allain, Assistant Camp Director
Michael Landry MD, Medical Director
Camp Pelican is an overnight residential camp for children with moderate to severe asthma or other pulmonary problems. Founded in 1977, Camp Pelican is jointly sponsored by the Louisiana Pulmonary Disease Camp Inc and the Louisiana Lions Camp. Over 100 children attend annually and participate in education, sports, arts and crafts, swimming and other camping activities. Medical staff including physicians, nurses, respiratory therapists and social workers participate in camp. Coed, ages 5-17.

8272 Madden Open Hearts Camp
250 Monument Valley Road
Great Barrington, MA 01230
413-528-2229
888-611-1113
FAX: 413-528-6553
e-mail: info@openheartscamp.org
www.openheartscamp.org

David Zaleon, Camp Director
Eight week program for children who have had and are fully recovered from open heart surgery or a heart transplant. Four two week sessions by age group. Small camp - 25 campers per session.

8273 Makemie Woods Camp
Presbytery of Eastern Virginia
PO Box 39
Barhamsville, VA 23011
757-566-1496
800-566-1496
FAX: 757-566-8803
e-mail: makwoods@makwoods.org
www.makwoods.org

Mike Burcher, Director
Jenny Mcdevitt, Program Director
Michelle Burcher, Administrator
Residential Christian camp that tailors each group and individual goals. Counselors serve as teachers, friends and activity leaders. For children 8-18 with diabetes.

8274 Makemie Woods Camp/Conference Retreat
Presbytery of Eastern Virginia
PO Box 39
Barhamsville, VA 23011
757-566-1496
800-566-1496
FAX: 757-566-8803
e-mail: info@pcusa-peva.org
www.makwoods.org

Jenny McDevitt, Program Director
Richard J Short, Religious Leader
Counselors serve as teachers, friends and activity leaders. The individual is important within the small group. No camper is lost in the crowd, but is an integral partner in the group process. Residential Christian Camp and conference center. Summer camp for children 8-18 and special camp for children with diabetes.

8275 Marist Brothers Mid-Hudson Valley Camp
PO Box 197
Esopus, NY 12501
845-384-6620
FAX: 845-384-6479
www.esopuscamps.com

Bro Don Nugent, Administrator
Bro Damian Novello, Director
Michelle Fleming, Director Special Children
Serves special people: children who have cancer or who are HIV positive, deaf or mentally retarded.

8276 Med-Camps of Louisiana
102 Thomas Road
Suite 615
West Monroe, LA 71291
318-329-8405
877-282-0802
FAX: 318-329-8407
e-mail: medcamps@hotmail.com
www.medcamps.com

Mike Epler, President
Caleb Seney, Executive Director
Serves children with severe asthma and allergies and many more.

8277 Mountaineer Spina Bifida Camp
350 Capitol Street
Suite 427
Charleston, WV 25301
304-558-7098
800-642-9704
FAX: 304-558-2866
www2.kidscamps.com

Nancy Dunst, Camp Director
Tonya Brown-Stobble, RN
Is a non profit organization which pursues education and training and focuses on activities that promote independence and those that facilitate everyday life. The objectives are to build self esteem, promote independence and enhance the development of social skills.

8278 Muscular Dystrophy Association Free Camp
121 W Fireweed Ln
Anchorage, AK 99503
907-276-2131

Chris Robinson, Executive Director

8279 NeSoDak Bible Camp/Klein Ranch
Lutherans Outdoors South Dakota
2001 S. Summit Ave
Sioux Falls, SD 57197
605-274-5326
800-888-1464
FAX: 605-274-5024
e-mail: nesodak@lutheransoutdoors.org
www.lutheransoutdoors.org

Karen Kraus, Development Director
Layne Nelson, Director Of Operations Beginning
Neil Sorensen, Executive Director
Camp is located in Waubay, South Dakota. Sessions for children with diabetes. Coed, ages 8-18.

8280 Needlepoint Daypoint
American Diabetes Association
715 Florida Avenue South
Florida West Bldg, Suite 307
Minneapolis, MN 54426
763-593-5333
FAX: 763-593-1520
e-mail: rmartin@diabetes.org
www.diabetes.org

Becky Martin, Program Director
Carol Holten, Program Assistant
Diane Fave, Manager
Camping for children who have type 1 diabetes. Coed, ages 5-16.

8281 Nejeda
Camp Nejeda Foundation
PO Box 156
910 Saddleback Road
Stillwater, NJ 07875
973-383-2611
FAX: 973-383-9891
e-mail: info@campnejeda.org
www.campnejeda.org

James Daschbach, Director
Philip Rea, Executive Director
For children with diabetes, ages 7-15. Provides an active and safe camping experience which enables the children to learn about and understand diabetes. Activities include boating, swimming, fishing, archery, as well as camping skills.

8282 Northwest Kiwanis Camp
PO Box 1227
Port Hadlock, WA 98339
360-732-7222

e-mail: nwkc@earthlink.net
kiwaniscamp.com

Brianna McNamara, Program Director
Jim Ott, Board President
Sharron Sherfick, Camp Administrator
Campers range from 6-60 in age, and includes those with developmental disabilities, cerebral palsy, autism, downs syndrome, and other physical and/or mental handicaps.

8283 Phantom Lake YMCA Camp
S110w30240 Ymca Camp Road
Mukwonago, WI 53149
262-363-4386
FAX: 262-363-4351
e-mail: office@phantomlakeymca.com
www.phantomlakeymca.com

Ted Anderson, Member of the Board
Riley Cooper, Member of the Board
Kathy Jensen, Member of the Board
Summer camping for children with epilepsy, ages 7-15.

8284 Shady Oaks Camp
16300 South Parker Road
Homer Glen, IL 60491
708-301-0816
FAX: 708-301-5091
e-mail: soc16300@aol.com
www.shadyoakscamp.org

Scott Steele, Executive Director
Shady Oaks Camp provides outdoor fun and recreation for children and adults with cerebral palsy and similar disabilities. Our camp is organized with the goal of providing stimulating life experiences that our campers may not have the opportunity to engage in elsewhere.

8285 Sherman Lake YMCA Outdoor Center
6225 North 39th Street
Augusta, MI 49012
269-731-3000
FAX: 269-731-3020
e-mail: shermanlakeymca@ymcasl.org
www.shermanlakeymca.org

Luke Austenfeld, Executive Director
Jeff Brown, Program Manager
Lorrie Syverson, Director Camping Services
Summer camping sessions for campers with ADD and spina bifida. Coed, ages 6-15 and families, seniors.

8286 Strength for the Journey
OR/ID Conference of United Methodist Church
1505 S W 18th Avenue
Portland, OR 97201
503-226-7931
800-593-7539
FAX: 503-228-3196
e-mail: info@gocamping.org
www.gocamping.org

Lisa Hoefner, Executive Director
Camp is located near Sisters, Oregon. For adults living with HIV/AIDS.

8287 Summer Camp for Children with Muscular Dystrophy
Muscular Dystrophy Association
3300 E. Sunrise Drive
Tucsongham, AZ 85718
205-823-8191
800-344-4863
FAX: 205-823-1057
e-mail: birminghamdistrict@mdausa.org
www.mdausa.org

Robert Ross, President/CEO
Debbie Sutton, Manager
Michael A Blishak, Director Community Programs
Offers a wide range of activities specially designed for young people who have limited mobility or use wheelchairs.

8288 Suttle Lake United Methodist Camp
Conference of United Methodists
29551 SW Suttle Lake Road
Sisters, OR 97759
541-595-6663
FAX: 541-595-2818
e-mail: camping@gocamping.org
www.gocamping.org

Lisa Jean Hoefner, Director
Jane Petke, Program Director
Bob Meyers, Religious Leader
Camp is located in Sisters, Oregon. Camping sessions for children and adults with HIV. Coed, ages 6-18, families, seniors and single adults.

8289 TSA CT Kid's Summer Event
Tourette Syndrome Association of Connecticut (TSA)
915 Brickyard Road
Woodstock, CT 06281
203-912-7310
e-mail: ts@tsact.org
www.tsact.org

Donna Blain, President/Chairperson
Andrew Vogel, Executive Director
Stefanie Fuller, Director
TSA of Connecticut sponsors summer events for children with TS/Tourette Syndrome activities of which include minature golf in addition to an Annual Conference. The kids' program at this annual conference provides children who have TS a unique opportunity to meet other children like them who also struggle with TS. Entertainment includes puppeteers, magicians, learning karate from the experts, getting face paintings and more.
uniqu pages

8290 Texas Lions Camp
PO Box 290247
Kerrville, TX 78029
830-896-8500
FAX: 830-896-3666
e-mail: tlc@ktc.com
www.lionscamp.com

Stephen S Mabry, Executive Director
The primary purpose of the League shall be to provide, without charge, a camp for physically disabled, hearing/vision impaired and diabetic children from the State of Texas, regardless of race, religion, or national origin. Our goal is to create an atmosphere wherein campers will learn the can do philosophy and be allowed to achieve maximum personal growth and self-esteem. The camp welcomes boys and girls ages 7-16.

8291 Twin Lakes Camp
1451 East Twin Lakes Road
Hillsboro, IN 47949
765-798-4000
FAX: 765-798-4010
e-mail: outdoors@twinlakescamp.com
www.twinlakescamp.com

Jon Beight, Executive Director
Brad Carter, Director
Walter Payne, Director
Provides a summer camp program for special needs children and young adults. Campers suffer from a wide range of maladies including crippling accidents, Spina Bifida, epilepsy, Cerebral Palsy, Muscular Dystrophy, Quadriplegia, Paraplegia, and other disabling diseases. Campers range in age from 8 to 27.

8292 VACC Camp
Miami Childrens Hospital
3200 SW 60th Court
Suite 203
Miami, FL 33155
305-662-8222
FAX: 305-663-8417
e-mail: bela.florentin@mch.com
www.vacccamp.com

Moises Simpser MD, Director
Bela Florentin, VACC Camp Coordinator
Free week-long overnight camp for ventilation assisted children and their families.

8293 Wisconsin Lions Camp
Wisconsin Lions Foundation
3834 County Road A
Rosholt, WI 54473
715-677-4969
877-463-6953
FAX: 715-677-3297
TTY: 715-677-6999
e-mail: ifno@wisconsinlionscamp.com
www.wisconsinlionscamp.com

Andrea Yenter, Camp Operations Manager
Evett Hartvig, Executive Director
Kris Kutschera, President
Serves children who have either a visual, hearing or mild cognitive disability, as well as diabetes types I and II. Program activities include sailing, ropes course, hiking and canoe trips, environmental education, swimming, camping, canoeing, outdoor living skills and handicrafts. ACA accredited, located in central Wisconsin, near Stevens Point.

8294 YMCA Camp Fitch
Youngstown YMCA
17 North Champion Street
Youngstown, OH 44503
330-744-8411
FAX: 330-744-8416
www.campfitch.com

Mike Shaffer, Executive Director
Kathy Portman, Assistant Director
Camp is located in North Springfield, Pennsylvania. Camping sessions for children and adults with diabetes, hearing impairment, developmental disabilities, mobility limitation and speech/communication impairment. Ages 8-16, families and seniors.

8295 YMCA Camp Horseshoe
Ohio and W Virginia Y MC A
Rr 2
Box 138
Saint George, WV 26287
304-478-2481
FAX: 304-478-4446
e-mail: horseshoe@hi-y.org
www.hi-y.org

David King, Executive Director
Sharon Cassidy, Camp Horseshoe Secretary
Summer camping for children with cancer, ages 7-18.

8296 YMCA Camp Ihduhapi
Minneapolis YMCA Camping Services
3425 Ihduhapi Road
Loretto, MN 55357
612-822-2267
FAX: 612-823-2482
e-mail: info@campicaghowan.org
www.campicaghowan.org

Bryan Burns, Executive Director
Matt Saari, Assistant Executive Director
Camp is located in Loretto, Minnesota. Summer sessions for campers with asthma/respiratory ailments and epilepsy. Coed, ages 7-16.

8297 YMCA Camp Kitaki
Lincoln YMCA
216 North 11th Street
Suite 400
Lincoln, NE 68508
402-434-9205
FAX: 402-434-9208
www.ymcalincoln.org

Ron Navratil, Chief Voltuneer Officer
Chris Klingenberg, Branch Excutive Director
Barbara A Bettin, President/CEO
Camp is located in Louisville, Nebraska. Summer sessions for children with cystic fibrosis. Coed, ages 7-17 and families.

8298 YMCA Camp Orkila
Y MC A of Greater Seattle
909 4th Avenue
Seattle, WA 98104
206-382-5003
FAX: 206-382-4920
www.seattleymca.org

Dimitri Stankevich, Program Director
Camping for children with blood disorders and diabetes, ages 8-18.

8299 YMCA Camp Weona
YMCA of Greater Buffalo
280 Cayuga Road
Buffalo, NY 14225
716-565-6008
FAX: 716-565-6007
e-mail: dschaefer@buffaloymca.org
www.wnybiz.com.campweona/

Jennifer Schubert, Executive Director
Shauna Parkinson, Program Director
Camp is located in Gainesville, New York. Camping sessions for children and adults with epilepsy. Coed, ages 7-16, families and single adults. Nestled in 1,000 acres of hardwood and pine forests, Weona has miles of picturesque hiking trails, brooks, a heated outdoor pool and a world class adventure ropes course. Our indoor facilities include arts and crafts studios, environmental classrooms and a challenging rock climbing wall. It is the ideal setting for hands-on fun, adventure and learning.

8300 YMCA Outdoor Center Campbell Gard
4803 Augspurger Road
Hamilton, OH 45011
513-867-0600
877-224-9622
e-mail: pruby@gmvymca.org
www.ccgymca.org

Rick Taylor, Executive Director
Vicky Williams, Senior Program Director
Curt Wright, Program Director
Camp is located in Hamilton, Ohio. Camping sessions for children with ADD, autism, developmental disabilities and blindness/visual impairment. Coed, ages 6-17 and families.

Print & Non-Print Resources

8301 A Woman's Guide To Living With HIV Infecti on
Johns Hopkins University Press

A resource for women with HIV that discusses coping with the diagnosis, finding a physician, recognizing symptoms, and preventing complications. Explains the latest treatment options and advice on coping with gynecologic infections. *$15.95*
288 pages 2004
ISBN 0-801879-14-0

8302 ABC of Asthma, Allergies & Lupus
Global Health Solutions
2146 Kings Garden Way
Falls Church, VA 22043
703-848-2333
800-759-3999
FAX: 703-848-0028
e-mail: shipping@watercure.com
www.watercure.com

Kristin Swan, Secretary
Joy Barber, Secretary
Xiaopo Batmanghelidj, President
$17.00
240 pages 2000
ISBN 0-962994-26-x

8303 ABC's of Latex Allergy
Asthma and Allergy Foundation of America
1125 15th Street NW
Suite 502
Washington, DC 20005
202-466-7643
FAX: 202-466-8940
e-mail: info@aafa.org
www.aafa.org

Bill Lin, Executive Director
Brochure provides excellent coverage of this topic including symptoms, diagnosis, causes, and treatments.

8304 ACPOC News
6300 N River Road
Suite 727
Rosemont, IL 60018
847-698-1637
FAX: 847-823-0536
e-mail: raymond@aaos.org
www.acpoc.org

Sheril King, Executive Director
Quarterly publication from the Association of Children's Prosthetic/Orthotic Clinics. Included with membership.
35-40 pages Quarterly

8305 AID Bulletin
Project AID Resource Center
PO Box 5190
Kent, OH 44242
330-672-2672
FAX: 330-672-4724

Alex Boros PhD, Director AID
J Sue Adams, Senior Counselor
Peter Mueller, Executive Director
Has the latest news on upcoming conferences, literature, developments in programs and/or services for disabled persons who are substance abusers. Offers articles on their experiences, ideas and questions of others in this field which includes providers and consumers. *$7.50*

8306 AIDS 2nd Edition
JB Lippincott
227 E Washington Square
Philadelphia, PA 19106
215-521-8300
800-777-2295
FAX: 301-824-7390

J Lippincott, Chief Executive Officer
Gives the latest information on AIDS covering basic science considerations, clinical aspects and public health issues. *$ 55.00*

474 pages

8307 AIDS Alert
American Health Consultants
3525 Piedmont Road
Building 6
Atlanta, GA 30305
404-262-7436
800-688-2421
FAX: 800-850-1232
e-mail: customerservice@ahcpub.com
www.ahcpub.com

Glen Harris, Managing Editor
Jeff MacDonald, Executive Vice Presidet
Source of AIDS news and advice for health care professionals. Covers up-to-the-minute developments and guidance on the entire spectrum of AIDS challenges, including treatment, education, precautions, screening, diagnosis and policy. *$467.00*
12 pages Monthly
ISSN 0887-02 2

8308 AIDS Disease State Management Resource
PO Box 740056
Atlanta, GA 30374
404-262-7436
FAX: 800-284-3291
e-mail: customerservices@ahcpub.com
www.ahcpub.com

Milo Falcon, Managing Editor
Jeff MacDonald, Executive Vice President

Provides staff and patient education materials on HIV/AIDS. *$299.00*
Paperback

8309 **AIDS and Other Manifestations of HIV Infec tion**
Academic Press

A comprehensive overview of the biological properties of this etiologic viral agent, its clinicopathological manifestations, the epidemiology of its infection, and present and future therapeutic options. *$249.95*
1000 pages 2004
ISBN 0-127640-51-7

8310 **AIDS in the Twenty-First Century: Disease and Globalization**
Palgrav Macmillan

The authors — exprets in the field for over 15 years — argue that it is vital to not only look at AIDS in terms of prevention and treatment, but to also consider consequences which affect households, communities, companies, governments, and countries. This is a major contribution toward understanding the global public health crisis, as well as the relationship between poverty, inequality, and infectious diseases. *$19.95*
432 pages 2003
ISBN 1-403900-06-X

8311 **AIDS, What Does it Mean to You?**
Walker Publishing Company
104 5th Avenue
New York, NY 10011 212-727-8300
800-289-2553
FAX: 212-727-0984
e-mail: orders@walkerbooks.com

Ramsey Walker, Vice President
Researchers have been working frantically to solve the puzzle of AIDS - a disease that has taken the lives of thousands of men and women during the past ten years. *$13.95*
128 pages Cloth/Hardcover
ISBN 0-802782-02-7

8312 **AIDS: The HIV Myth**
St. Martin's Press
175 5th Avenue
New York, NY 10010 212-674-5151
www.stmartins.com

John Sargent, Chief Executive Officer
Challenges the theory that AIDS is caused by a virus called HIV. Puts forward the view that in the rush to identify the cause of an apparently new disease, a harmless passenger virus was leapt upon as the sole culprit.
1989
ISBN 0-333489-30-6

8313 **AIDS: The Official Journal of the Internat ional AIDS Society**
Lippincott Williams & Wilkins
590 Walnut Street
Philadelphia, PA 19106 215-521-8300
www.aidsonline.com

J Lippincott, Chief Executive Officer
The latest groundbreaking research on HIV and AIDS. *$433.00*
18 per year

8314 **APLA Update**
AIDS Project Los Angeles
550 N Larchmont Boulevard
Suite 202
Los Angeles, CA 90004 323-993-1600
FAX: 323-993-1392
Presents news about AIDS and programs of AIDS Project Los Angeles to people affected by the disease.
20 pages

8315 **About Asthma**
American Lung Association
61 Broadway
New York, NY 10006 212-315-8700
FAX: 212-315-8870
e-mail: info@lungusa.org
www.lungusa.org

John Kirkwood, Chief Executive Officer
A popular style pamphlet explaining symptoms, treatment and more for persons with asthma.
16 pages

8316 **Adaptive Tracks**
Adaptive Sports Center
PO Box 1639
Crested Butte, CO 81224 970-349-2296
866-349-2296
FAX: 970-349-4950
e-mail: info@adaptivesports.org
www.adaptivesports.org

Christopher Hensley, Executive Director
The Adaptive Sports Center (ASC) of Crested Butte, Colorado is a non-profit organization that provides year-round recreation activities for people with disabilities and their families. The ASC provides adaptive snowboarding downhill skiing, cross country skiing as well as backcountry trips. Summer activities include a variety of wilderness-based programs, multi-day trips into the back country, extensive cycling programs, canoeing, and white water rafting.
6 pages Quarterly

8317 **Adult Leukemia: A Comprehensive Guide for Patients and Families**
Patients-Centered Guides
101 Morris Street
Sebastopol, CA 95472 707-829-0515
800-998-9938
FAX: 707-829-0104
www.patientcenters.com

Linda Lamb, Editor
Shawnde Paull, Marketing
Tim O'Reilly, Chief Executive Officer
For the tens of thousands of Americans with adult leukemia, Adult Leukemia: A Comprehensive Guide for Patients and Families addresses diagnosis, medical tests, finding a good oncologist, treatments, side effects, getting emotional and other support, resources for further study, and much more. The book includes real-life stories from those who have battled leukemia themselves. *$29.95*
536 pages Paperback
ISBN 0-596500-01-7

8318 **Advanced Breast Cancer: A Guide to Living with Metastic Disease**
Patients-Centered Guides
101 Morris Street
Sebastopol, CA 95472 707-829-0515
800-998-9938
FAX: 707-829-0104
www.patientcenters.com

Linda Lamb, Editor
Shawnde Paull, Marketing
Tim O'Reilly, Chief Executive Officer
This is the only book on breast cancer that deals honestly with the realities of living with metastic disease, yet offers hope and comfort. All aspects of facing the disease are covered, including: coping with the shock of recurrence, seeking information and making treatment decisions, communicating effectively with medical personnel finding support, and handling disease progression and end-of-life issues. A comprehensive guide, it also provides updated resources and treatment developments. *$24.95*

532 pages Paperback
ISBN 1-565925-22-X

8319 **Advanced Diagnosis and Treatment for Neck and Back Pain**
American Back Society
2647 International Boulevard
Suite 401
Oakland, CA 94601
510-536-9929
FAX: 510-536-1812
e-mail: info@americanbacksoc.org
www.americanbacksoc.org

Nedra Swartz, Manager
A membership organization dedicated to relieving the pain and impairment caused by back problems. Sponsors symposia for presenting research findings.

8320 **Adventures in Fast Forward: Life, Love, a nd Work for the ADD Adult**
Taylor & Francis
47 Runway Drive
Suite G
Levittown, PA 19057
215-269-0400
FAX: 215-625-2940

Harold Stecker, President
The Q&A format provides access to the following queries: do I have ADD? What are the symptoms? Would I be taking medication? How can I manage the condition? How do I explain ADD to the significant people in my life? Why can't my spouse understand me? Is this the right job for me? Are there techniques to increase my memory? Can I go back to college and do well? Does ADD affect men and women differently? What should I consider when choosing a doctor or therapist? *$23.95*
210 pages 1996
ISBN 0-876308-00-0

8321 **Agent Orange & Spina Bifida**
Spina Bifida Association of America
4590 Macarthur Boulevard NW
Suite 250
Washington, DC 20007
202-944-3285
800-321-6141
FAX: 202-944-3295
e-mail: sbaa@sbaa.org
www.sbaa.org

Cindy Brownstein, Chief Executive Officer

8322 **Alex: The Life of a Child**
Rutledge Hill Press

Alexandra Deford was just eight years old when she died in 1980 following a battle against cystic fibrosis. In a new Introduction, her father summarizes some of the developments made in combating the disease and tells how the family has come to terms with her loss. *$ 13.98*
228 pages 1997
ISBN 1-558535-52-7

8323 **Alive at 25: How I'm Beating Cystic Fibro sis**
Longstreet Press
325 N Milledge Avenue
Athens, GA 30601
706-543-5999
FAX: 404-254-0016
e-mail: info@longstreetpress.com
www.longstreetpress.com
The author's personal journey of dealing with a deadly disease. *$24.95*
256 pages
ISBN 1-563526-81-6

8324 **All the Way Up There**
Britannica Film Company
345 4th Street
San Francisco, CA 94107
415-777-9876

This is the story of Bruce Burgess who has Cerebral Palsy but wants to climb a mountain. Bruce makes his dreams come true with the help of Grame Dingle, a New Zealand mountain climber.
Film

8325 **Allergies Sourcebook, 2nd Edition**
Omnigraphics
615 Griswold Street
Detroit, MI 48226
313-961-1340
800-234-1340
FAX: 800-875-1340
www.omnigraphics.com

Peter Ruffner, President
Includes information on the causes of allergies, identification, treatments and statistics. *$78.00*
650 pages 2000
ISBN 0-780803-76-0

8326 **Alternative Approach to Allergies**
Harper Perennial
10 E 53rd Street
New York, NY 10022
212-207-7000
FAX: 212-207-7145
www.harpercollins.com

Abigail Kunath, Marketing Executive
A comprehensive guide to staying well and allergy-free by a pioneer in the field of environmental medicine.

8327 **Alternative Medicine and Multiple Sclerosis**
Demos Medical Publishing
386 Park Avenue S
Suite 201
New York, NY 10016
212-683-0072
800-532-8663
FAX: 212-683-0118
e-mail: orderdep@demospub.com
www.demosmedpub.com

Diana Schneider PhD, President
Phyllis Gold, Owner
Offers reliable information on the relevance, safety, and effectiveness of various alternative therapies that are not typically considered in discussions of MS management, yet are in widespread use. *$24.95*
272 pages 2001
ISBN 1-888799-52-8

8328 **American Academy of Allergy, Asthma and Immunology**
555 E Wells Street
Suite 1100
Milwaukee, WI 53202
414-272-6071
800-822-2762
FAX: 414-272-6070
e-mail: info@aaaai.org
www.aaaai.org

David P. Huston MD, FAAAAI, Leadership Chair
Amal Assa'ad MD, FAAAAI, Chair Elect
Nonprofit association representing allergists, clinical immunologists, asthma specialists, allied health professionals, and others with a special interest in allergy and asthma. The AAAAI's mission is to advance the knowledge, education and practice of allergy, asthma and immunology.

8329 **American Academy of Pediatrics Guide to Yo ur Child's Alleriges And Asthma**
Villard Books

Consumer resource for parents who need answers and information about their children's allergies and asthma. Current advice on identifying allergies and asthma, preventing attacks, minimizing triggers, understanding medications, explaining allergies to young children, and helping children manage symptoms. *$15.00*
191 pages 2000
ISBN 0-679769-82-X

8330 **American Association of Spinal Cord Injury Nurses**
American Association of Spinal Cord Injury Nurses
7520 Astoria Boulevard
Jackson Heights, NY 11370
718-803-3782
FAX: 718-803-0414
www.aascin.org

Sara Lerman MPH, Program Manager
Disseminates information to nurses and others caring for spinal cord injured individuals. Membership in AASCIN represents registered and licensed practical and vocational nurses in the US and Canada who practice in the diverse SCI settings such as intensive care, acute care and long-term care; rehabilitation; home care; and outpatient care. Annual educational conference.

8331 American Heart Association Guide to Stroke Treatment, Recovery & Prevention
Random House
1540 Broadway
New York, NY 10036
212-782-9000
800-726-0600
FAX: 212-302-7985
e-mail: customerservice@randonhouse.com
www.randomhouse.com

Peter Olson, Chief Executive Officer
From the nation's premier authority on heart disease and stroke, the definitive book on stroke prevention, treatment and recovery. *$29.00*
304 pages

8332 American Journal of Orthopsychiatry
American Orthopsychiatric Association
330 7th Avenue
18th Floor
New York, NY 10001
212-564-5930
FAX: 212-564-6180
e-mail: amerortho@aol.com

Joan Adler, Managing Editor
Ellen L Bassuk, Editor
Mental health issues from multidisciplinary and interprofessionals perspectives: clinical, research and expository approaches. *$45.00*
160 pages Quarterly

8333 Amyotrophic Lateral Sclerosis: A Guide for Patients and Families
Demos Medical Publishing
386 Park Avenue S
Suite 201
New York, NY 10016
212-683-0072
800-532-8663
FAX: 212-683-0118
e-mail: orderdep@demospub.com
www.demosmedpub.com

Diana Schneider PhD, President
Phyllis Gold, Owner
This comprehensive guide covers every aspect of the management of ALS. Beginning with discussions of its clinical features of the disease, diagnosis, and an overview of symptom management, major sections deal with medical and rehabilitative management, living with ALS, managing advanced disease and end-of-life issues, and reources that can provide support and assistance. *$34.95*
350 pages 2000
ISBN 1-888799-28-5

8334 Ankylosing Spondylitis
Arthritis Foundation
PO Box 7669
Atlanta, GA 30357
404-872-7100
800-283-7800
FAX: 404-872-9559
e-mail: help@arthritis.org
www.arthritis.org

John Klippel, Chief Executive Officer

8335 Annals of Otology, Rhinology and Laryncology
Annals Publishing Company
4507 Laclede Avenue
Saint Louis, MO 63108
314-367-4987
FAX: 314-367-4988
e-mail: manager@annals.com
www.annals.com

Kenneth A Cooper Jr, Business Manager
Ken Cooper, Owner
Original, peer-reviewed articles in the fields of otolaryngology - head and neck medicine and surgery, broncho-esophagology, audiology, speech, pathology, allery, and maxillofacial surgery. Official journal of the American Laryngological Association/American Broncho-Esophagological Association. *$170.00*
112 pages Monthly

8336 Answering Your Questions About Spina Bifid a
Spina Bifida Association of America
4590 Macarthur Boulevard NW
Suite 250
Washington, DC 20007
202-944-3285
800-621-3141
FAX: 202-944-3295
e-mail: sbaa@sbaa.org
www.sbaa.org

Cindy Brownstein, Chief Executive Officer
Provides information to help you understand the basic medical, educational and socail issues which commonly affect people with spina bifida. *$8.00*

8337 Archives of Neurology
American Medical Association
515 N State Street
Chicago, IL 60610
312-464-5000
FAX: 312-464-4184
e-mail: ama-subs@ama-assn.org
www.archneurol.com

Roger Rosenberg MD, Editor
Robert Musacchio, Publisher
Michael Maves, Chief Executive Officer
Mission is to publish scientific information primarily important to those physicians caring for people with neurologic disorders, but also for those interested in the structure and function of the normal and diseased nervous system. *$235.00*
198 pages Monthly

8338 Ask the Doctor: Asthma
Andrews McMeel Publishing
4520 Main Street
Kansas City, MO 64111
816-932-6700
800-826-4216
FAX: 800-437-8683

Kathleen Andrews, Chief Executive Officer
$8.95
128 pages Soft Cover
ISBN 0-836270-23-1

8339 Asperger's Syndrome: A Guide for Parents a nd Professionals
Taylor & Francis Group

A guide to the most relevant and useful information on Asperger's Syndrome, incorporating case studies from the author's own practical experience as a Clinical Psychologist, with examples of, and numerous quotations from people with Asperger's. *$22.95*
256 pages 2002
ISBN 1-843107-14-7

8340 Asthma Alert
American Lung Association
61 Broadway
New York, NY 10006
212-315-8700
FAX: 212-315-8870
e-mail: info@lungusa.org
www.lungusa.org

John Kirkwood, Chief Executive Officer
Quick reference folders with information on asthma, the symptoms and what to do in an emergency.

8341 Asthma Challenge
Asthma and Allergy Foundation of America
1125 15th Street NW
Suite 502
Washington, DC 20005
202-466-7643
FAX: 202-466-8940
e-mail: info@aafa.org
www.aafa.org

Bill Lin, Executive Director
Fun and engaging activity to assess asthma knowledge. This custom designed, full colored stand up board comes with two sets of pre-tested question cards and can be used with large or small groups. Players test their knowledge in categories like Sneezes and Wheezes, and Nuts and Bolts. *$50.00*

8342 Asthma Handbook
American Lung Association
61 Broadway
New York, NY 10006
212-315-8700
FAX: 212-315-8870
e-mail: info@lungusa.org
www.lungusa.org

John Kirkwood, Chief Executive Officer
Explains asthma, gives self-care methods for handling it and helps patients work more effectively with their doctor.
28 pages

8343 Asthma Handbook Slides
American Lung Association
61 Broadway
New York, NY 10006
212-315-8700
FAX: 212-315-8700
e-mail: info@lungusa.org
www.lungusa.org

John Kirkwood, Chief Executive Officer
Slides and script based on The Asthma Handbook for asthma patients and others.
Film

8344 Asthma Lifelines
American Lung Association
61 Broadway
New York, NY 10006
212-315-8700
FAX: 212-315-8700
e-mail: info@lungusa.org
www.lungusa.org

John Kirkwood, Chief Executive Officer
Promotional brochure providing descriptions of ALA asthma education materials.
12 pages

8345 Asthma Resource Directory
National Allergy and Asthma Network
3554 Chain Bridge Road
Suite 200
Fairfax, VA 22030
703-385-4403
FAX: 703-352-4354
Valuable reference tool with over 2,500 listings of resources and products nationwide including suppliers, camps, research centers and support groups.

8346 Asthma Sourcebook
Omnigraphics
615 Griswold Street
Detroit, MI 48226
313-961-1340
800-234-1340
FAX: 800-875-1340
www.omnigraphics.com

Annemarie S Muth, Editor
Peter Ruffner, President
Provides information about asthma, including symptoms, remidies and research updates. *$78.00*
650 pages 2000
ISBN 0-780803-81-7

8347 Asthma and Allergy Answers: A Patient Education Library
Asthma and Allergy Foundation of America
1125 15th Street NW
Suite 502
Washington, DC 20005
202-466-7643
FAX: 202-466-8940
e-mail: info@aafa.org
www.aafa.org

Bill Lin, Executive Director
A resource tool has information on more than 40 topics of interest to patients. These reproducible camera ready Answers are written in a patient friendly questions and answer format. There is space to personalize these handy patient education materials with your practice or facility information. *$50.00*

8348 Asthma and Exercise
Henry Holt and Company
3554 Chain Bridge Road
Suite 200
Fairfax, VA 22030
703-385-4403
FAX: 703-352-4354
This book offers clear and detailed advice on how adults and children with asthma can participate in exercise and sports activities. *$10.00*

8349 Asthma in the School: Improving Control with Peak Flow Monitoring
National Allergy and Asthma Network
3554 Chain Bridge Road
Suite 200
Fairfax, VA 22030
703-385-4403
FAX: 703-352-4354
Comprehensive and practical guide to help the school nurse monitor and assist students with asthma. *$7.00*

8350 Asthma in the Workplace
John H Dekker & Sons
2941 Clydon Avenue SW
Grand Rapids, MI 49519
616-538-5160
FAX: 616-538-0720

John Dekker, President
$199.00
664 pages
ISBN 0-824787-99-4

8351 Awareness Posters
Spina Bifida Association of America
4590 Macarthur Boulevard NW
Suite 250
Washington, DC 20007
202-944-3285
800-621-3141
FAX: 202-944-3295
e-mail: sbaa@sbaa.org
www.sbaa.org

Cindy Brownstein, Chief Executive Officer
An aid for building community awareness of Spina Bifida and the need for adequate amounts of folic acid in pregnant women. *$ 7.00*

8352 Being Close
National Jewish Center for Immunology
1400 Jackson Street
Denver, CO 80206
303-388-4461
e-mail: allstetterw@njc.org
www.njc.org

William Allstetter, Media Relations Manager
Lynn Taussig, Chief Executive Officer
A booklet offering information to patients suffering from a respiratory disorder such as emphysema, asthma or tuberculosis, that discusses sexual problems and feelings.

8353 Bittersweet Chances: A Personal Journey o f Living and Learning in the Face of Illness
PublishAmerica

Recounts Doug and Dana Broehl's journey of growth through the darkness of cystic fibrosis and the renewed hope of a double lung transplant. *$19.95*
192 pages 2004
ISBN 1-413713-24-6

8354 Blooming Where You're Planted
Meeting Life's Challenges
9042 Aspen Grove Lane
Madison, WI 53717
608-824-0402
FAX: 608-824-0403
e-mail: help@MeetingLifesChallenges.com
www.MeetingLifesChallenges.com

Author Shelley Peterman Schwarz takes you on her journey of self-discovery and change following her diagnosis of multiple sclerosis in 1979. Her personal stories are warm and humorous, and insightful. This 138-page book will motivate and inspire you to rise above life's challenges and live life to its fullest. *$12.95*

138 pages
ISBN 0-891854-01-1

8355 Bowel Cancer
Oxford University Press
2001 Evans Road
Cary, NC 27513
919-677-0977
800-451-7556
FAX: 919-677-1303
www.oup-usa.org

Thomas Carty, Senior Vice President
Offers information and public awareness on the disease of bowel cancer. *$18.95*
152 pages

8356 Bowel Continence & Spina Bifida
Spina Bifida Association of America
4590 Macarthur Boulevard NW
Suite 250
Washington, DC 20007
202-944-3285
800-621-3141
FAX: 202-944-3295
e-mail: sbaa@sbaa.org
www.sbaa.org

Cindy Brownstein, Chief Executive Officer
An excellent book aimed at anyone trying to attain bowel continence with sample menus, bowel tracking charts and glossary of terms. *$8.00*

8357 Bowel Management: A Manual of Ideas and Techniques

Accent Books & Products
PO Box 700
Bloomington, IL 61702
309-378-2961
800-787-8444
FAX: 309-378-4420
e-mail: acmtlvng@aol.com

Raymond C Cheever, Publisher
Betty Garee, Editor
Paras and quads can gain much greater freedom. Includes considerations as frequency, timing, water intake, exercise and successful programs from three rehab centers. *$3.50*
25 pages Paperback
ISBN 0-91570 -02-7

8358 Brain Allergies: The Psychonutrient
Keats Publishing
PO Box 876
New Canaan, CT 06840
203-966-8721
800-323-4900
A comprehensive look at the role nutrition and orthomolecular medicine can play in treating brain allergies, including a self-help protocol and a special appendix for physicians.

8359 Breaking Ground
Tennessee Council on Developmental Disabilities
500 Deaderick Street
13th Floor
Nashville, TN 37243
615-313-9980
FAX: 615-532-6964
e-mail: tnddc@state.tn.us
www.state.tn.us/cdd

Linda Moynihan, Executive Director
20 pages 6 A Year

8360 Breaking New Ground News Note
Purdue University
1146 Abe Building
W Lafayette, IN 47907
765-494-4600
800-825-4264
FAX: 765-496-1356
e-mail: bng@ecn.purdue.edu
engineering.purdue.edu/CEM/News/2002/cem_news

Paul Jones, Coordinator
Martin Jischke, Chief Executive Officer
News, practical ideas and success stories of and for farmers with physical disabilities.
12-16 pages Quarterly

8361 Breast Cancer Sourcebook
Omnigraphics
615 Griswold Street
Detroit, MI 48226
313-961-1340
800-234-1340
FAX: 800-875-1340
www.omnigraphics.com

Edward J Prucha, Editor
Peter Ruffner, President
Provides information on the prevention of Breast Cancer, self care, treatment options, alternative therapies and diagnostic methods. *$78.00*
600 pages 2000
ISBN 0-780802-44-6

8362 Breathe Easy Young People's Guide to Asthma
Magination Press
2751 Prosperity Avenue
Suite 150
Fairfax, VA 22031
703-385-4403
800-878-4403
FAX: 703-573-7794
www.aanma.org
Practical, personal guide for those up to age 13 with asthma. They will learn how to control their asthma with techniques that will bring increased self-confidence. *$9.95*
Video

8363 Breathe Free
Lotus Press
PO Box 325
Twin Lakes, WI 53181
262-889-8561
800-824-6396
FAX: 262-889-2461
e-mail: lotuspress@lotuspress.com
www.lotuspress.com

Santosh Krinsky, President
A nutritional and herbal medicine self-help guide to treating a full range of respiratory conditions, including colds and flu.
179 pages 1998
ISBN 0-914955-07-1

8364 Breathing Disorders: Your Complete Exercise Guide
Human Kinetics
PO Box 5076
Champaign, IL 61825
217-351-5076
800-747-4457
FAX: 217-351-1549
e-mail: orders@hkusa.com
www.humankinetics.com

Rainer Martens, President
$11.95
144 pages Paperback
ISBN 0-873224-26-4

8365 Bronchial Asthma: Principles of Diagnosis and Treatment
Humana Press
999 Riverview Drive
Suite 208
Totowa, NJ 07512
973-256-1699
FAX: 973-256-8341

Thomas Lanigan, Owner
$125.00
784 pages
ISBN 0-896032-53-1

8366 Cancer Sourcebook
Omnigraphics
615 Griswold Street
Detroit, MI 48226
313-961-1340
800-234-1340
FAX: 800-875-1340
www.omnigraphics.com

Edward J Prucha, Editor
Peter Ruffner, President

Includes information on the major forms and stages of cancer. *$78.00*

1100 pages 2000
ISBN 0-780802-27-6

8367 Cancer Victors Journal
International Association for Cancer Victors
5336 Harwood Road
San Jose, CA 95124
408-448-4094
FAX: 408-264-9659
www.cancervictors.org

Published by the volunteer community service organization to inform and support interested persons who want to learn more about natural, nontoxic remedies and practices.

8368 Caring for Children with Cerebral Palsy: A Team Approach
Brookes Publishing
PO Box 10624
Baltimore, MD 21285
410-337-9580
800-638-3775
FAX: 410-337-8539
e-mail: custserv@brookespublishing.com
www.brookespublishing.com

Paul Brooks, Owner
A guide to the interdisciplinary care of children with cerebral palsy. Delivers detailed information on a multitude of issues relevant to treatment and supports. *$38.95*
496 pages Paperback 1998
ISBN 1-55766 -22-X

8369 Cerebral Palsy: A Complete Guide for Care giving
Johns Hopkins University Press

A guide for parents and caregivers of children and adults with cerebral palsy, as well as for adolescents and adults with the condition. *$19.95*
465 pages 1998
ISBN 0-801859-49-2

8370 Challenge
Spina Bifida Association of America
4590 Macarthur Boulevard NW
Suite 250
Washington, DC 20007
202-944-3285
800-621-3141
FAX: 202-944-3295
e-mail: sbaa@sbaa.org
www.sbaa.org

Cindy Brownstein, Chief Executive Officer
Fourteen minute video tape. An excellent introduction to the physical and social challenges faced by individuals with spina bifida. *$20.00*

8371 Chesity
Spina Bifida Association of America
4590 Macarthur Boulevard NW
Suite 250
Washington, DC 20007
202-944-3285
800-621-3141
FAX: 202-944-3295
e-mail: sbaa@sbaa.org
www.sbaa.org

Cindy Brownstein, Chief Executive Officer

8372 Childhood Asthma: A Matter of Control
American Lung Association
61 Broadway
New York, NY 10006
212-315-8700
FAX: 212-315-8700
e-mail: info@lungusa.org
www.lungusa.org

John Kirkwood, Chief Executive Officer
A guide for parents of children with asthma, this booklet covers topics such as identifying asthma signs and symptoms as well as controlling the condition.

28 pages

8373 Childhood Cancer Survivors: A Practical Guide to Your Future
Patient-Centered Guides
101 Morris Street
Sebastopol, CA 95472
707-829-0515
800-998-9938
FAX: 707-829-0104
www.patientcenters.com

Linda Lamb, Editor
Shawnde Paull, Marketing
Tim O'Reilly, Chief Executive Officer
More than 250,000 people have survived childhood cancer - a cause for celebration. Authors Keene, Hobbie, and Ruccione chart the territory of long-term survivorship: relationships; overcoming employment or insurance discrimination; maximizing health; follow-up schedules; medical late effects. The stories of over sixty survivors - their challenges and triumphs - are told. Includes medical history record-keeper. *$27.95*
510 pages Paperback
ISBN 1-565924-60-6

8374 Childhood Cancer: A Parent's Guide to Solid Tumor Cancers
Patient-Centered Guides
101 Morris Street
Sebastopol, CA 95472
707-829-0515
800-998-9938
FAX: 707-829-0104
www.patientcenters.com

Linda Lamb, Editor
Shawnde Paull, Marketing
Tim O'Reilly, Chief Executive Officer
Childhood Cancer: A Parent's Guide to Solid Tumor Cancers features a wealth of resources for parents of children with solid tumor cancers, plus many stories of veteran parents. Parents will encounter medical facts simply explained, practical advice to ease their daily lives, and tools to be strong advocates for their child. Includes a passport to record patient's medical history. *$24.95*
537 pages Paperback
ISBN 1-565925-31-9

8375 Childhood Leukemia: A Guide for Families, Friends & Caregivers
Patient-Centered Guides
101 Morris Street
Sebastopol, CA 95472
707-829-0515
800-998-9938
FAX: 707-829-0104
www.patientcenters.com

Linda Lamb, Editor
Shawnde Paull, Marketing
Tim O'Reilly, Chief Executive Officer
The second edition of this comprehensive guide offers detailed and precise medical information for parents that includes day-to-day practical advice on how to cope with procedures, hospitalization, family and friends, school, and social, emotional, and financial issues. It features a wealth of tools for prents and contains significant updates on treatments and procedures. *$24.95*
513 pages Paperback
ISBN 1-565926-32-3

8376 Children With Cerebral Palsy: A Manual for Therapists, Parents and Community Workers
ITDG Publishing

The book provides sets of principles by which to observe and analyze a child's problems and then plan treatment. *$24.95*
204 pages 2003
ISBN 1-853395-65-X

8377 Children With Cerebral Palsy: A Parents' G uide
Woodbine House

A classic primer for parents that provides a complete spetrum of information and compassionate advice about cerebral palsy and its effect on their child's development and education. *$16.95*

481 pages 1998
ISBN 0-933149-82-4

8378 Children with Asthma: A Manual for Parents
Allergy Control Products
PO Box 793
Ridgefield, CT 06877
203-438-9580
800-422-3878
FAX: 203-431-8963
www.allergycontrol.com

Edward Steube, President
Known as the asthma bible, this second edition is sprinkled with anecdotes by patients and their parents. *$10.00*
296 pages Paperback

8379 Children with Cerebral Palsy
Woodbine House
6510 Bells Mill Road
Bethesda, MD 20817
301-897-3570
800-843-7323
FAX: 301-897-5838
www.woodbinehouse.com

Irv Shapell, Owner
It provides a complete spectrum of information and compassionate advice about cerebral palsy and its effect on their child's development and education. Covers these areas: diagnosis, medical issues, family life, legal rights, early intervention, coping, therapies, treatment, development, advocacy, special ed., and daily care. *$16.95*
470 pages Paperback
ISBN 0-933149-82-4

8380 Children with Facial Difference: A Parent' s Guide
Woodbine House
6510 Bells Mill Road
Bethesda, MD 20817
301-897-3570
800-843-7323
FAX: 301-897-5838
www.woodbinehouse.com

Irv Shapell, Owner
The first guide for parents about their child's congenital craniofacial anomaly - a condition that affects the appearance and function of the head and face. This accessible book discusses conditions such as cleft lip, cleft palate, and Teacher Collins, Apert, and Crouzon syndromes, and more. Parents learn about the diagnostic process, interdisciplinary treatment approach, education, speech and language issues, and how to help their child and family adjust emotionally. *$ 16.95*
361 pages Paperback 1996
ISBN 0-933149-61-1

8381 Children with Spina Bifida: A Parents Guide
Spina Bifida Association of America
4590 Macarthur Boulevard NW
Suite 250
Washington, DC 20007
202-944-3285
800-621-3141
FAX: 202-944-3295
e-mail: sbaa@sbaa.org
www.sbaa.org

Cindy Brownstein, Chief Executive Officer
Provides parents with information, guidance and support to help meet the child's needs through childhood. *$16.95*

8382 Children with Tourette Syndrome
Exceptional Parent Library
PO Box 1807
Englewood Cliffs, NJ 07632
201-947-6000
800-535-1910
FAX: 201-947-9376
e-mail: eplibrary@aol.com
www.eplibrary.com
Written by a team of professionals and parents, this book covers medical, educational, legal, family life, daily care, and emotional issues. *$14.95*

8383 Chronic Fatigue Syndrome: Your Natural Gu ide To Healing with Diet, Herbs and Other Methods
Prima Publishing
PO Box 1260
Rocklin, CA 95677
916-787-7000
800-632-8676
FAX: 916-787-7001
e-mail: websupportlife@primapub.com
www.primapublishing.com
Explains specific measures sufferers can take to improve stamina, mental energy, and physical abilities. *$12.95*
196 pages 1994
ISBN 1-559584-90-4

8384 Cleft Palate-Craniofacial Journal
American Cleft Palate-Cranifacial Association
1504 E Franklin Street
Suite 102
Chapel Hill, NC 27514
919-933-9044
FAX: 919-933-9604
e-mail: cleftpalj@aol.com
www.acpa-cpf.org

Jerald Moon PhD, Editor
Debbie Ogle, Editorial Assistant
Nancy Smythe, Executive Director
A peer revived international multidisciplinary journal dedicated to current research on the care and treatment of children born with cleft lip and palate and other craniofacial anomalies. 6 issues/year

8385 Clinical Care in Rheumatic Disease
Arthritis Foundation Distribution Center
PO Box 6996
Alpharetta, GA 30023
800-207-8633
FAX: 770-442-9742
www.arthritis.com
This book was written for all health professionals caring for people with rheumatic diseases and for students in these disciplines. *$35.00*
224 pages

8386 Club Foot & Other Foot Deformities Fact Sheet
March of Dimes
1275 Mamaroneck Avenue
White Plains, NY 10605
914-949-7166
FAX: 914-997-4763
e-mail: askus@marchofdimes.com
www.marchofdimes.com
Provides information about pregnancy, birth defects, genetics, drug use, environmental hazzards and related topics. The Resource Center's health information specialists provide acccurate and up-to-date information via e-mail and Web site. One copy of this fact sheet can be obtained free of charge by visiting our website.

8387 Coffee in the Cereal: The First Year with Multiple Sclerosis
Pathfinder Publishing

Moorhead recounts the experience of her first year with multiple sclerosis with a vitality unique in the often gloomy world of personal medical histories. *$14.95*
96 pages 2003
ISBN 0-934793-07-7

8388 Colon & Rectal Cancer: A Comprehensive Guide for Patients & Families
Patient-Centered Guides
101 Morris Street
Sebastopol, CA 95472
707-829-0515
800-998-9938
FAX: 707-829-0104
www.patientcenters.com

Linda Lamb, Editor
Shawnde Paull, Marketing
Tim O'Reilly, Chief Executive Officer

The fourth most common cancer, colon and rectal cancer is diagnosed in 130,000 new cases in the United States each year. Patients and families need uo-to-date and in-depth information to participate wisely in treatment decisions (e.g., knowing what sexual and fertility issues to discuss with the doctor before surgery). This book covers coping with tests and treatment side effects, caring for ostomies, finding supportt, and other practical issues. *$24.95*

544 pages Paperback

ISBN 1-565926-33-1

8389 Colon Health: Key to a Vibrant Life

Norwalk Press
Prescott, AZ
928-445-5567
FAX: 928-445-5567

Includes complete glossary of terms and index of referrals.

8390 Complete Guide To Mercury Toxicity from De ntal Fillings

Environmental Dental Association
285 N El Camino Real
Suite 102
Encinitas, CA 92024
858-586-1208
800-388-2184
FAX: 858-756-7843
e-mail: info@enviormentaldental.com
www.enviormentaldental.com

191 pages

ISBN 0-944796-36-2

8391 Complete Kid's Allergy and Asthma Guide: T he Parent's Handbook for Children of All Ages

Robert Rose

For a child who has not yet received a medical diagnosis, The Complete Kid's Allergey & Asthma Guide provides parents with vital information on how to read the signs of allergy and asthma — from keeping a food diary, to monitoring asthma symptoms, to tracking allergic reactions. *$17.95*

288 pages 2003

ISBN 0-778800-78-4

8392 Confronting the Challenges of Spina Bifida

Spina Bifida Association of America
4590 Macarthur Boulevard NW
Suite 250
Washington, DC 20007
202-944-3285
800-621-3141
FAX: 202-944-3295
e-mail: sbaa@sbaa.org
www.sbaa.org

Cindy Brownstein, Chief Executive Officer

A group curriculum addressing self care, self esteem and social skills in eight to 13 year olds. *$19.00*

8393 Connections Newsletter

Kessler Institute for Rehabilitation
1199 Pleasant Valley Way
West Orange, NJ 07052
973-731-3600
888-KES-SLER
FAX: 973-243-6992

Maura Bergen, Editor/Public Relations Coordin.
Maria Anan, Editor/N. NJSCI System Coord.
Karen Hwang, Editor

Quarterly newsletter for individuals with a spinal cord injury. Funded by the Northern New Jersey Spinal Cord Injury System.

Quarterly-Free

8394 Conquering the Darkness: One Story of Reco vering from a Brain Injury

Paragon House
1925 Oakcrest Avenue
Suite 7
Saint Paul, MN 55113
651-644-3087
800-447-3709
FAX: 800-494-0997
e-mail: info@paragonhouse.com
www.paragonhouse.com

Rosemary Yokoi, Publicity Department
Gordon Anderson, Executive Director

The course of recovery from a brain injury by a woman who lived through it. *$15.95*

420 pages 1999

ISBN 1-557787-63-8

8395 Control Your Child's Asthma

Owl Publishing

Offers parents of children with asthma ways to create an asthma-management plan geared specifically toward the child's needs, incorporating medical, social and emotional needs into one system. Includes a detailed resource section of organizations dealing with asthma management. *$14.00*

256 pages 2001

ISBN 0-805064-55-9

8396 Controlling Asthma

American Lung Association
61 Broadway
New York, NY 10006
212-315-8700
FAX: 212-315-8870
e-mail: info@lungusa.org
www.lungusa.org

Cindy Kirkwood, Chief Executive Officer

For parents of children with asthma, this news magazine tells how parents can help their child deal with the many problems presented by asthma.

16 pages

8397 Coping When a Parent Has Multiple Sclerosis

Rosen Publishing Group
29 E 21st Street
New York, NY 10010
212-777-3017
800-237-9932
FAX: 888-436-4643
e-mail: triciab@rosenpub.com
www.rosenpub.com

Tricia Bauer, Director Special Markets
Roger Rosen, President

Explains to young people how living with a parent who has Multiple Sclerosis will affect their lives. Hardcover. *$19.95*

128 pages

ISBN 0-823914-06-2

8398 Coping and Prevailing with Multipe Scleros is and Other Life Struggles

J&T Corp

A journey of victorious self-discovery. *$14.95*

102 pages 2002

ISBN 0-971761-40-X

8399 Coping with Asthma

Rosen Publishing Group
29 E 21st Street
New York, NY 10010
212-777-3017
800-237-9932
FAX: 888-436-4643
e-mail: rosenpub@tribeca.ios.com

Roger Rosen, President

This book prepares students by explaining to them the dangers of asthma, a condition which, when properly treated, is completely manageable. *$16.95*

ISBN 0-823920-69-0

8400 Coping with Cerebral Palsy

Pro-Ed Publications
8700 Shoal Creek Boulevard
Austin, TX 78757
512-451-3246
800-897-3202
FAX: 512-451-8542
e-mail: info@proedinc.com
www.proedinc.com

Donald Hammill, Owner

This second edition book provides parents of children and adults with cerebral palsy the answers to more than 300 questions that have been carefully researched. It represents 40 years of experience by the author and is presented in a highly readable, jargon-free manner. *$26.00*

252 pages

8401 Coping with Mild Traumatic Brain Surgery

Avery Publishing Group
375 Hudson Street
New York, NY 10014
212-366-2000

Explains what is involved in the diagnosis, treatment, and rehabilitation of brain-injured people *$15.95*

334 pages 1998
ISBN 0-895297-91-4

8402 Coping with Special Needs Classmates

Rosen Publishing Group
29 E 21st Street
New York, NY 10010
212-777-3017
800-237-9932
FAX: 888-436-4643
e-mail: rosenpub@tribeca.ios.com

Tricia Bauer, Director Special Markets
Roger Rosen, President

Special needs classmates include people who are physically different, disfigured or challenged, emotionally disturbed, or those who have learning disabilities. The author offers guidance on how to get past discomfort or fear of confrontation with someone who seems very different, but is, in reality, not so different after all. Hardcover. *$17.95*

128 pages
ISBN 0-823915-98-0

8403 Coping with a Physically Challenged Brother or Sister

Rosen Publishing Group
29 E 21st Street
New York, NY 10010
212-777-3017
800-237-9932
FAX: 888-436-4643
e-mail: rosenpub@tribeca.ios.com

Tricia Bauer, Director Special Needs
Roger Rosen, President

Dealing with a relative who is born physically challenged or who suffers a personal tragedy is one of the biggest adjustments in life. This book shows step-by-step methods of coping with these emotions so the reader may learn how to have a happy life once again. Hardcover. *$17.95*

ISBN 0-823914-92-5

8404 Counseling People with Diabetes

Brookes Publishing
PO Box 10624
Baltimore, MD 21285
410-337-9580
800-638-3775
FAX: 410-337-8539
e-mail: custserv@brookespublishing.com
www.brookespublishing.com

Paul Brooks, Owner
$29.00

158 pages Paperback
ISBN 1-85433 -36-1

8405 Counseling for Heart Disease

Brookes Publishing
PO Box 10624
Baltimore, MD 21285
410-337-9580
800-638-3775
FAX: 410-337-8539
e-mail: custserv@brookespublishing.com
www.brookespublishing.com

Paul Brooks, Owner
$25.00

144 pages Paperback
ISBN 1-85433 -96-9

8406 Curing MS: How Science is Solving the Mys teries of Multiple Sclerosis

Crown Publishing Group
1540 Broadway
New York, NY 10036
212-782-9000
FAX: 212-302-7985

Founder-director of the Multiple Sclerosis Center at Mass General Hospital discusses what ends up as a deconstruction of the last 30 years of his own and general MS research and of experience in treating patients with the puzzling disorder. Weiner summarizes what is currently known about treatments and the potential for a cure. *$24.95*

320 pages 2004
ISBN 0-609609-00-9

8407 Cystic Fibrosis in the 20th Century: Peop le, Events, and Progress

AM Publishing

A blend of science, clinical concerns, and personal accounts of those touched by Cystic Fibrosis. It tells the story of the efforts of investigators, clinicians, and members of the CF community, documenting the rapid progress of research and treatment and improvement in survival rates since the first description of the disease in 1938. *$35.95*

417 pages 2002
ISBN 0-971706-40-9

8408 Cystic Fibrosis: A Guide for Patient and F amily

Lippincott Williams & Wilkins

Text is designed specifically for patients with cystic fibrosis and their families. Explains the disease process, outlines the fundamentals of diagnosing and screening, and addresses the challenges of treatment for those living with CF. Includes new material on carrier testing, infection control, and more. *$29.95*

448 pages 2003
ISBN 0-781741-52-1

8409 Deenie

Bradbury Press
135 S Mount Zion Road
Lebanon, IN 46052
800-257-5755
FAX: 800-882-8583

Deenie, a beautiful thirteen-year-old girl, had a mother who was pushing her to become a model. The agency representatives told Deenie she had the looks but walked differently. Deenie's main wish was to become a cheerleader. Her close friend, Janet, made the cheerleading squad but Deenie didn't make the final list. After this her gym teacher noticed her posture and called her family. After seeing therapists, the diagnosis of adolescent idiopathic scoliosis was made.

159 pages Hardcover
ISBN 0-02711 -20-6

8410 Detecting Your Hidden Allergies

Professional Books/Future Health
211 N Sycamore Street
Newtown, PA 18940
215-504-1700
FAX: 215-860-5374

Gives specific instructions on how to use an elimination diet to determine food allergies.

8411 Determined to Win The Inspirational Story of Paradymic Athlete Jean Driscoll

Spina Bifida Association of America
4590 Macarthur Boulevard NW
Suite 250
Washington, DC 20007
202-944-3285
800-621-3141
FAX: 202-944-3295
e-mail: sbaa@sbaa.org
www.sbaa.org

Cindy Brownstein, Chief Executive Officer
$21.00

8412 Determined to Win: Children Living with Allergies and Asthma
Gareth Stevens
1555 N Rivercenter Drive
Milwaukee, WI 53212
414-332-3520
800-542-2595
FAX: 414-332-3567
www.gsinc.com

Claire Messier, Marketing Associate
Bob Famighetti, Publisher
Isabell, a six year old girl, has been living with allergies and asthma almost her entire life. With proper medical care and a determined attitude, she leads an active life. *$15.95*
48 pages
ISBN 0-83681 -75-9

8413 Diabetes 101
Chronimed Publishing
13911 Ridgedale Drive
Minnetonka, MN 55305
612-916-2500
800-848-2793
FAX: 952-513-6170

Sandra A Hintz, Marketing Coordinator
A pure and simple guide for people who use insulin. *$ 10.95*
208 pages Paperback
ISBN 1-56561 -24-5

8414 Diabetes Self-Management
RA Rapaport Publishing
150 W 22nd Street
New York, NY 10011
212-989-0200
FAX: 212-989-4786

James Hazlett, Editor
Jim Moorehead, Circulation Director
Publishes practical how-to information, focusing on the day-to-day and long-term aspects of diabetes in a positive and upbeat style. Gives subscribers up-to-date news, facts and advice to help them maintain their wellness and make informed decisions regarding their health. *$18.00*
BiMonthly

8415 Different Heart
Fanlight Productions
4196 Washington Street
Suite 2
Boston, MA 02131
617-469-4999
800-937-4113
FAX: 617-469-3379
e-mail: fanlight@fanlight.com

Karen McMillen, Marketing Director
Ben Achtenberg, Owner
Though hundreds of children are born each year with potentially fatal heart disease, their parents may feel isolated from those facing similar crises. This sensitive video profiles three such families. *$99.00*

8416 Directions
Families of Spinal Muscular Dystrophy
PO Box 196
Libertyville, IL 60048
847-367-7620
800-886-1762
FAX: 847-367-7623
e-mail: sma@fsma.org
www.fsma.org

Audrey Lewis, Executive Director
Colleen McCarthy
Audrey Lewis, Manager
$35.00
60-70 pages Quarterly

8417 Duchenne Muscular Dystrophy
Oxford University Press
198 Madison Avenue
New York, NY 10016
212-726-6000
800-451-7556
FAX: 919-677-1303
www.oup-usa.org

Laura Brown, Chief Executive Officer
Identification of the genetic defect responsible for Duchenne Muscular Dystrophy and isolation of the protein dystrophin have led to the development of new theories for the disease's pathogenesis. This title incorporates these advances from the field of molecular biology, and describes the resultant opportunities for screening, prenatal diagnosis, genetic counselling and management. *$125.00*
272 pages 2003
ISBN 0-198515-31-6

8418 Eating Disorders Sourcebook
Omnigraphics
615 Griswold Street
Detroit, MI 48226
313-961-1340
800-234-1340
FAX: 800-875-1340
www.omnigraphics.com

Dawn D Mattews, Editor
Peter Ruffner, President
Provides general imformation, causes and treatments of eating disorders. *$78.00*
600 pages 2000
ISBN 0-780803-35-3

8419 Eating Out: Your Guide to More Enjoyable Dining
Plume
375 Hudson Street
New York, NY 10014
212-366-2000

In this book, a nationally recognized expert on diabetes nutrition, shows you how eating out can be fun, without fear of weight gain or an uncontrolled rise in blood sugar. *$4.95*
272 pages Paperback 2000
ISBN 0-452279-76-3

8420 Educational Issues Among Children with Spi na Bifida
Spina Bifida Association of America
4590 Macarthur Boulevard NW
Suite 250
Washington, DC 20007
202-944-3285
800-321-6141
FAX: 202-944-3295
e-mail: sbaa@sbaa.org
www.sbaa.org

Cindy Brownstein, Chief Executive Officer

8421 Efficacy of Asthma Education, Selected Abstracts
American Lung Association
61 Broadway
New York, NY 10006
212-315-8700
FAX: 212-315-8700
e-mail: info@lungusa.org
www.lungusa.org

John Kirkwood, Chief Executive Officer
Abstracts documenting the efficacy of asthma education programs for physicians and other health professionals.

8422 Encyclopedia of AIDS: Social, Political, C ultural, and Scientific Record of the HIV Epidemic
Penguin Books

A reference on Autoimmune Deficiency Syndrome as a historical phenomenon, focusing on the period from 1981 when the first cases began to be identified among gay men in the US and 1996 with the introduction of the class of potent antiviral medications called protease inhibitors. *$25.00*
782 pages 2001
ISBN 0-140514-86-4

8423 Epilepsy, 199 Answers: A Doctor Responds t o His Patients' Questions

An epilepsy specialist answers questions about the causes, diagnosis, and treatments, and how to live and work with this brain disorder. Includes an epilepsy history timeline, patient health record form, resources, and a glossary. *$19.95*

8424 Epilepsy: Patient and Family Guide
FA Davis Company

A guide for adults with epilepsy and for parents of children with the disorder explains the nature and diversity of seizures, the risks and benefits of the various antiepileptic drugs, and medical and surgical therapies. *$26.95*
434 pages 2001
ISBN 0-803604-98-X

8425 EpilepsyUSA
Epilepsy Foundation
4351 Garden City Drive
Landover, MD 20785
301-459-3700
800-332-1000
FAX: 301-577-2684
e-mail: postmaster@efa.org
www.epilepsyfoundation.org

Judith O'Toole, Editor
Eric Hargis, President
Magazine reporting on issues of interest to people with epilepsy and their families. *$15.00*
22 pages Quartlery

8426 Facts About Asthma
American Lung Association
61 Broadway
New York, NY 10006
212-315-8700
FAX: 212-315-8700
e-mail: info@lungusa.org
www.lungusa.org

John Kirkwood, Chief Executive Officer
Primary public information leaflet on asthma.
12 pages

8427 Fall Down, Laughing: How Squiggy Caught M ultiple Sclerosis and Didn't Tell Nobody
Jeremy P Tarcher
375 Hudson Street
New York, NY 10014
212-366-2000

Diagnosed with the illness after filming the last episode of Laverne & Shirley, Lander continued to develop his film and television career while hiding his illness. His success was an astonishing testament to his physical and emotional strength and his determination to prove that those with MS can still enjoy fulfilling and challenging lives. *$22.95*
200 pages 2000
ISBN 1-585420-52-2

8428 Family Urology
American Foundation for Urologic Disease
1100 Corporate Boulevard
Linthicum, MD 21090
800-242-2383
FAX: 410-468-1808
e-mail: admin@afud.org
www.afud.org

Jodi L Miller, Director Education
Dedicated to the prevention of urologic diseases through the expansion of patient education, research, public awareness and advocacy. Available with annual membership dues.
Quarterly

8429 Fibromyalgia Interval Training
Arthritis Foundation Distribution Center
PO Box 6996
Alpharetta, GA 30023
800-207-8633
FAX: 770-442-9742
www.arthritis.com
This video was designed for people with fibromyalgia. The video features warm water exercises in shallow and deep water, including warmup, stretching, upper and lower body exercises, aerobics, strengthing, cool-down and relaxation. Designed to help you manage the pain, stiffness and fatigue of fibromyalgia. *$29.99*

8430 Focus Newsletter
Attention Deficit Disorder Association
PO Box 543
Pottstown, PA 19464
847-432-2332
FAX: 847-432-5874
e-mail: michelenovotni@yahoo.com
www.add.org

Michele Novotni PhD, President/Editor
ADDA's mission is to help people with AD/HD lead happier, more successful lives through education, research and public advocacy. Whether you have AD/HD yourself, someone special in your life does, or you treat, counsel or teach those who do, ADDA is an organization for you. ADDA focuses especially on the needs of AD/HD adults and young adults with AD/HD. Parents of children with AD/HD are also welcome.

8431 Folic Acid Counseling Pocket Card
Spina Bifida Association of America
4590 Macarthur Boulevard NW
Suite 250
Washington, DC 20007
202-944-3285
800-621-3141
FAX: 202-944-3295
e-mail: sbaa@sbaa.org
www.sbaa.org

Cindy Brownstein, Chief Executive Officer
For health care professionals. Quick reference card that fits in the white coat pocket. *$18.00*

8432 Fragile X Family
4196 Washington Street
Suite 2
Boston, MA 02131
617-469-4999
800-937-4113
FAX: 617-469-3379
e-mail: info@fanlight.com
www.fanlight.com

Sandy St Louis, Distribution Director
Kelli English, Publicity Coordinator
Ben Achtenberg, Owner
Fragile X Family takes viewers inside the lives of a developmentally disabled family who are affected by Fragile X Syndrome, an inherited chromosomal disorder which is the second most common cause of mental retardation. *$149.00*
2004
ISBN 1-572954-14-0

8433 Free to Breathe
Allergy and Asthma Network/Mothers of Asthmatics
2751 Prosperity Avenue
Suite 150
Fairfax, VA 22031
703-641-9595
800-878-4403
FAX: 703-573-7794
www.aanma.org
Characters rap, joke, and learn different ways to use inhalers. Kids are encouraged to talk to their parents and doctor about their choices. 8 minutes. *$10.00*
Video

8434 From Where I Sit: Making My Way wih Cereb ral Palsy
Scholastic

An autobiographical account of a young woman explores how it feels to live with cerebral palsy while struggling to have a full life despite the challenges facing her every day. *$13.00*
136 pages 1999
ISBN 0-590395-84-X

8435 Genetics and Spina Bifida
Spina Bifida Association of America
4590 Macarthur Boulevard NW
Suite 250
Washington, DC 20007
202-944-3285
800-621-3141
FAX: 202-944-3295
e-mail: sbaa@sbaa.org
www.sbaa.org

Cindy Brownstein, Chief Executive Officer

8436 **Going Places, Children Living with Cerebral Palsy**
Gareth Stevens
1555 N River Center Drive
Milwaukee, WI 53212
414-332-3520
800-542-2595
FAX: 414-225-0377

Bob Famighetti, Publisher
Mathias is a charming six-year-old with cerebral palsy. He needs special exercises to help him learn to control his muscles. He is also almost completely deaf. But with the love and encouragement of his family, Mathias is developing an interesting and busy life. Every morning finds him eager to start the day's activities. *$13.95*
48 pages
ISBN 0-836801-99-7

8437 **Growing Up with Epilepsy: A Pratical Guide for Parents**
Demos Medical Publishing
386 Park Avenue S
Suite 201
New York, NY 10016
212-683-0072
800-532-8663
FAX: 212-683-0118
e-mail: orderdep@demospub.com
www.demosmedpub.com

Diana Schneider PhD, President
Phyllis Gold, Owner
Developed to help parents with the uniques challenges that this disorder presents *$19.95*
156 pages 2003
ISBN 1-888799-74-9

8438 **Guide to Hydrocephalus**
Spina Bifida Association of America
4590 Macarthur Boulevard NW
Suite 250
Washington, DC 20007
202-944-3285
800-621-3141
FAX: 202-944-3295
e-mail: sbaa@sbaa.org
www.sbaa.org

Cindy Brownstein, Chief Executive Officer
Information to help you understand the circumstances that surround you and facilitate job advocacy. *$8.00*

8439 **Guide to Living With HIV Infection: Develo ped at the Johns Hoplins AIDS Clinic**
Johns Hopkins Press Health Book

A handbook and reference for people living with HIV infection and their families, friends, and caregivers. *$18.95*
428 pages 2001
ISBN 0-801867-44-4

8440 **Guidelines for Spina Bifida & Health Care Services Throughout Life**
Spina Bifida Association of America
4590 Macarthur Boulevard NW
Suite 250
Washington, DC 20007
202-944-3285
800-621-3141
FAX: 202-944-3295
e-mail: sbaa@sbaa.org
www.sbaa.org

Cindy Brownstein, Chief Executive Officer
These guidelines are designed to help people who have spina bifida expirence a greater sense of purpose and place in society. *$19.00*

8441 **HIV Drug Book Revised**
Pocket

From a community-based AIDS treatment information and advocacy organization comes a comprehensive guide to the drugs and experimental treatments most used by those who are HIV-positive or suffering from AIDS. *$30.95*
704 pages 1998
ISBN 0-671014-90-0

8442 **Handbook of Chronic Fatigue Syndrome**
Wiley Publishing
605 3rd Avenue
New York, NY 10158
212-850-6000
FAX: 212-850-6088

Discusses diagnosis and treatment as well as the history, phenomenology, symptomatology, assessment, and pediatric and community issues. Introduces phase-based therapy and nutritional approaches. *$ 90.00*
794 pages 2003
ISBN 0-471415-12-X

8443 **Handbook of Epilepsy**
Lippincott, Williams & Wilkins
227 E Washington Square
Philadelphia, PA 19106
215-521-8300
800-777-2295
FAX: 301-824-7390
www.lpub.com

J Lippincott, Chief Executive Officer
Pocket-sized reference provides concise, up-to-date, clinically oriented reviews of each of the major areas of diagnosis and management of epilepsy. *$42.95*
272 pages 2003
ISBN 0-781743-52-4

8444 **Head Injury: The Facts: A Guide for Fami lies and Care-Givers**
Oxford University Press
198 Madison Avenue
New York, NY 10016
212-726-6000
800-451-7556
FAX: 919-677-1303
www.oup-usa.org

Laura Brown, Chief Executive Officer
A pocket-sized explanation of head injuries for patients. *$19.95*
167 pages
ISBN 0-192627-13-9

8445 **Headache Newsletter**
19 Mantua Road
Mount Royal, NJ 08061
856-423-0043
800-255-2243
FAX: 856-423-0082
e-mail: achehq@talley.com
www.achenet.org

Linda Gillicuddy, Executive Director
$20.00
Quarterly

8446 **Healing HIV: How To Rebuild Your Immune Sy stem**
Healthfirst Press

Practical advice that focuses on overall health for HIV sufferers. *$19.95*
362 pages 1998
ISBN 0-966637-30-5

8447 **Healthcare Guidelines for Spina Bifida and Healthcare Services Throughout Life**
Spina Bifida Association of America
4590 Macarthur Boulevard NW
Suite 250
Washington, DC 20007
202-944-3285
800-621-3141
FAX: 202-944-3295
e-mail: sbaa@sbaa.org
www.sbaa.org

Cindy Brownstein, Chief Executive Officer
$19.00

8448 Healthy Breathing
National Jewish Center for Immunology
1400 Jackson Street
Denver, CO 80206 303-388-4461
e-mail: allstetterw@njc.org
www.njc.org

William Allstetter, Media Relations Manager
Lynn Taussig, Chief Executive Officer
Offers patients with lung or respiratory disorders information on exercise and healthy breathing.

8449 Heart Disease in Persons with Down Syndrome
Brookes Publishing
PO Box 10624
Baltimore, MD 21285 410-337-9580
800-638-3775
FAX: 410-337-8539
e-mail: custserv@brookespublishing.com
www.brookespublishing.com

Susie Burdick, Executive Director
Offers access to findings from state-of-the-art research on congenital heart disease in children and adults with Down syndrome. Information on cardiac malformations and anomalies, heart and lung pathology, hemodynamic evaluations, and surgical intervention. *$62.00*
240 pages Hardcover
ISBN 1-55766 -24-X

8450 Heart of the Mind
Real People Press
PO Box F
Moab, UT 84532 435-259-7578
FAX: 435-259-4042
e-mail: realpoep@lasal.net
www.realpeoplepress.com

Susan Ossana, Office Manager
Provides common NLP problems and several new techniques.

8451 Help Yourself Cookbook
Arthritis Foundation
PO Box 6996
Alpharetta, GA 30023
800-207-0633
FAX: 770-442-9742
www.arthritis.com

$12.95
158 pages

8452 Helping Others Breathe Easier
National Allergy and Asthma Network
3554 Chain Bridge Road
Suite 200
Fairfax, VA 22030 703-385-4403
FAX: 703-352-4354
Offers information on educational resources, support groups and the Network for persons afflicted with asthma or allergic disorders.

8453 Hip Function & Ambulation
Spina Bifida Association of America
4590 Macarthur Boulevard NW
Suite 250
Washington, DC 20007 202-944-3285
800-621-3141
FAX: 202-944-3295
e-mail: sbaa@sbaa.org
www.sbaa.org

Cindy Brownstein, Chief Executive Officer

8454 Home Control of Allergies and Asthma
American Lung Association
61 Broadway
New York, NY 10006 212-315-8700
FAX: 212-315-8700
e-mail: info@lungusa.org
www.lungusa.org

John Kirkwood, Chief Executive Officer
Discusses substances in the home that may trigger asthma and allergy problems and offers suggestions for controlling them.

12 pages

8455 How to Live with a Spinal Cord Injury
Accent Books & Products
PO Box 700
Bloomington, IL 61702 309-378-2961
800-787-8444
FAX: 309-378-4420
e-mail: acmtlvng@aol.com

Raymond C Cheever, Publisher
Betty Garee, Editor
A guide packed with realistic information about how this disability affects your life and what you can do about it. Answers lots of questions and gives you positive information providing hope and plenty of encouragement. *$6.95*
58 pages Paperback
ISBN 0-91570 -27-2

8456 How to Outsmart Your Allergies
Asthma and Allergy Foundation of America
1125 15th Street NW
Suite 502
Washington, DC 20005 202-466-7643
FAX: 202-466-8940
e-mail: info@aafa.org
www.aafa.org

Bill Lin, Executive Director
Colorful poster that will enhance any office or waiting room while educating patients. Contains innovative and factual tips for avoiding allergens and reducing or eliminating allergic symptoms. The poster depicts common allergens in an appealing format. *$1.00*

8457 Hydrocephalus: A Guide for Patients, Families & Friends
Patient-Centered Guides
101 Morris Street
Sebastopol, CA 95472 707-829-0515
800-998-9938
FAX: 707-829-0104
www.patientcenters.com

Linda Lamb, Editor
Shawnde Paull, Marketing
Tim O'Reilly, Chief Executive Officer
Hydrocephalus is a life-threatening condition often referred to as, water on the brain, that is treated by surgical placement of a shunt system. Hydrocephalus: A Guide for Patients, Families and Friends educates families so they can select a skilled neurosurgeon, understand treatments, participate in care, know what symptoms need attention, discover where to turn for support, keep records needed for follow-up treatments, and make wise lifestyle choices. *$19.95*
379 pages Paperback
ISBN 1-565924-10-X

8458 I Just Found Out I Have HIV... Now What?
1stBooks Library

Issues surrounding living with HIV. *$15.50*
144 pages 2002
ISBN 1-403321-65-5

8459 IAL News
International Association of Laryngectomees
8900 Thornton Road
Stockton, CA 95209 209-472-0516
866-425-3678
FAX: 209-472-0516
e-mail: ial@larynxlink.com

Jack Henslee, Executive Director
Focuses on rehabilitation and well-being of persons who have had laryngectomy surgery.

8460 If Your Child Has Diabetes: An Answer Book for Parents
Putnam Publishing Group
200 Madison Avenue
New York, NY 10016 212-889-6330

Alex Luchars, Owner
Provides information and recommendations for parents of children with diabetes on subjects such as school, recreation, medical and life insurance and employment as well as general information about diabetes. *$9.95*

8461 Immune Deficiency Foundation Newsletter
Immune Deficiency Foundation
40 W Chesapeake Avenue
Suite 308
Towson, MD 21204
410-321-6647
800-296-4433
FAX: 410-321-9165
e-mail: idf@primaryimmune.org
www.primaryimmune.org

Marcia Boyle, President/Founder/CEO
C Belser, Marketing
Offers information on immune deficiencies. How to treat them, what they are and more.
4-6 pages

8462 In the Middle
Fanlight Productions
4196 Washington Street
Suite 2
Boston, MA 02131
617-469-4999
800-937-4113
FAX: 617-469-3379
e-mail: fanlight@fanlight.com
www.fanlight.com

Karen McMillen, Marketing Director
Ben Achtenberg, Owner
Documents the problems and joys shared by Ryanna, who has Spina Bifida, and her parents, teachers and classmates during her first year of being mainstreamed in a Head Start Program. *$99.00*

8463 Individuals with Cerebral Palsy
Mainstream
3 Bethesda Metro Center
Suite 830
Bethesda, MD 20814
301-961-9299
800-247-1380
FAX: 301-654-6714
e-mail: info@mainstreaminc.org

Charles Moster
Mainstreaming individuals with cerebral palsy into the workplace. *$2.50*
12 pages

8464 Informed Touch
Healing Arts Press
1 Park Street
Rochester, VT 05767
802-767-3174
800-246-8648
FAX: 802-767-3726
e-mail: orders@innertraditions.com
www.InnerTraditions.com

Jessica Dudley, Sales Associate
Ehud Sperling, Owner
A Clinician's guide to the evaluation and treatment of myofascial disorders. *$30.00*
224 pages
ISBN 0-892817-40-2

8465 Informer
Simon Foundation
PO Box 835
Wilmette, IL 60091
847-864-3913
800-237-4666
FAX: 847-864-9758
www.simonfoundation.org

Cheryle B Gartley, President
Publishes items of interest to people with bladder or bowel incontinence, including medical articles, helpful devices, publications and a pen pal list. Quarterly newsletter.

8466 Injured Mind, Shattered Dreams: Brian's Survival from a Severe Head Injury
Brookline Books
PO Box 1046
Cambridge, MA 02139
617-868-0360
800-666-2665
FAX: 617-868-1772
e-mail: thestore@brooklinebooks.com
www.brooklinebooks.com
Brian, headed for normal adulthood, crashes his car and suffers a severe head injury. This book speaks to the issues in his recovery and the victory a family can achieve through caring advocacy and faith. *$17.95*
Paperback
ISBN 0-91479 -95-6

8467 Inside MS
National Multiple Sclerosis Society
421 New Karner Road
Suite 6
Albany, NY 12205
518-464-0630
800-344-4867
FAX: 518-464-1232
e-mail: chapter@msupstateny.org
www.nationalmssociety.org

Jim Ahearn, President
News and information on research progress, medical treatments, patient services, therapeutic claims and activities.

8468 Interdisciplinary Clinical Assessment of Young Children with Developmental Disabilities
Brookes Publishing
PO Box 10624
Baltimore, MD 21285
410-337-9580
800-638-3775
FAX: 410-337-8539
e-mail: custserv@brookespublishing.com
www.brookespublishing.com

Paul Brooks, Owner
Offers insight from veteran team members on interdisciplinary team assessments. Professionals organizing a team as well as students preparing for practice will find advice on how practitioners gather information, approach assessment, make decisions, and face the challenges of their individual fields. Includes case studies and appendix of photocopiable questionnaires for clinicians and parents. *$42.00*
432 pages Hardcover 2000
ISBN 1-557664-50-1

8469 International Ventilator Users Network
Gazette International Networking Institute
4207 Lindell Boulevard
Suite 110
Saint Louis, MO 63108
314-534-0475
FAX: 314-534-5070
e-mail: gini_intl@msn.com
www.post-polio.org/ivun

Joan L Headley, Executive Director
Judith R Fischer, Editor
IVUN is a worldwide network of ventilator users and health professionals experienced in and committed to home care and long term mechanical ventilation. IVUN News, a quarterly newsletter, offers articles on family adjustments, equipment, techniques, travel, ethical issues, medical topics, and resources. Also publishes the annual iVUN resource directory, listing ventilator users, health professionals, equipment manufacturers and vendors, as well as other related organizations. *$ 17.00*
8 pages Quarterly

8470 Introduction to Spina Bifida
Spina Bifida Association of America
4590 Macarthur Boulevard NW
Suite 250
Washington, DC 20007
202-944-3285
800-621-3141
FAX: 202-944-3295
e-mail: sbaa@sbaa.org
www.sbaa.org

Cindy Brownstein, Chief Executive Officer
An aid for parents, family and nonmedical people who care for a child with spina bifida. *$7.00*

8471 It's All in Your Head
Avery Publishing Group
375 Hudson Street
New York, NY 10014 212-366-2000

Dr. Higgins's critique of the use of mercury, a toxic element and environmental hazard, in dentistry. For those suffering mercury poisoning, the book examines a number of conventional and alternative treatments.

8472 Joslin Guide to Diabetes
Joslin Diabetes Center
1 Joslin Place
Boston, MA 02215 617-732-2400
FAX: 617-732-2452
www.joslin.harvard.edu

Discusses the causes of diabetes, the role of diet and exercise, meal planning and complications. Also provide information on drawing blood, mixing and injecting insulin, special challenges, living with diabetes. *$20.00*
352 pages

8473 Journal of Head Trauma Rehabilitation
Aspen Publishers
200 Orchard Ridge Drive
Gaithersburg, MD 20878 301-698-7100
800-234-1660
FAX: 301-695-7931
www.aspenpublishers.com

Scholarly journal designed to provide information on clinical management and rehabilitation of the head-injured for the practicing professional. Published bimonthly. *$119.00*
128 pages

8474 Journey to Well: Learning to Live After S pinal Cord Injury
Altarfire Publishing

The author's close-up view of what life is like during and after such an incident, including her experience with institutional medicine and insurance companies (for better and for worse), and her determined - and ultimately successful - effort to rehabilitate herself and reconstruct her life. *$15.95*
251 pages 1997
ISBN 0-965555-82-8

8475 Keeping the Balance
Fanlight Productions
4196 Washington Street
Suite 2
Boston, MA 02131 617-469-4999
800-937-4113
FAX: 617-469-3379
e-mail: fanlight@fanlight.com
www.fanlight.com

Karen McMillen, Marketing Director
Ben Achtenberg, Owner

Brothers and sisters of children with serious lung diseases share their experiences of being the normal child. Insightful and articulate, they explore the frequent conflict between their feelings of love and concern, and their resentment over the attention denied to them because of the sibling's illness. *$99.00*

8476 Ketogenic Diet: A Treatment for Epilepsy
Demos Medical Publishing

Patient education reference on the use of the ketogenic diet to conrol epilepsy in children. *$24.95*
224 pages Paperback 2000
ISBN 1-888799-39-0

8477 Keys to Parenting a Child with Cerebral Palsy
Barron's Educational Series
250 Wireless Boulevard
Hauppauge, NY 11788 631-434-3311
800-645-3476
FAX: 631-434-3723
e-mail: info@barronsedu.com
www.barronseduc.com

Margaret E Myers, Author
Manuel Barron, Chief Executive Officer

This volume helps parents adjust to the challenge of having a child with cerebral palsy. It stresses the child's potential and encourages independence. Facets of the child's total well-being are discussed, including common health problems, physical, mental and social development, therapy, and new trends in medical management. *$6.95*
Paperback
ISBN 0-764100-91-2

8478 Know Your Diabetes, Know Yourself
Joslin Diabetes Center
1 Joslin Place
Boston, MA 02215 617-732-2400

An hour-long videotape in which Joslin patients talk about daily issues of diabetes management - meal planning, exercise, monitoring, injections, foot and eye care, and managing the disease when sick or traveling. *$3.00*

8479 Latex Allergy in Spina Bifida Patients
Spina Bifida Association of America
4590 Macarthur Boulevard NW
Suite 250
Washington, DC 20007 202-944-3285
800-621-3141
FAX: 202-944-3295
e-mail: sbaa@sbaa.org
www.sbaa.org

Cindy Brownstein, Chief Executive Officer

8480 Lead Poisoning in Childhood
Brookes Publishing
PO Box 10624
Baltimore, MD 21285 410-337-9580
800-638-3775
FAX: 410-337-8539
e-mail: custserv@brookespublishing.com
www.brookespublishing.com

Paul Brooks, Owner

This book examines the epidemiology, etiology, and pathophysiology of lead poisoning - the most prevalent preventable childhood health problem today. Also provides practical prevention strategies that are cost-effective and easy to implement. *$31.95*
256 pages Paperback
ISBN 1-55766 -32-0

8481 Learning Among Children with Spina Bifida
Spina Bifida Association of America
4590 Macarthur Boulevard NW
Suite 250
Washington, DC 20007 202-944-3285
800-621-3141
FAX: 202-944-3295
e-mail: sbaa@sbaa.org
www.sbaa.org

Cindy Brownstein, Chief Executive Officer

8482 Let's Talk About Having Asthma
Rosen Publishing Group's PowerKids Press
29 E 21st Street
New York, NY 10010 212-777-3017
800-237-9932
FAX: 888-436-4643
e-mail: rosenpub@tribeca.ios.com

Roger Rosen, President

This book talks about the cause and treatments for asthma as well as the precautions sufferers should take. Recommended for grades K-4. *$13.95*

ISBN 0-823950-32-8

8483 Life After Trauma: A Workbook for Healing
Guilford Press
72 Spring Street
New York, NY 10012 212-431-9800
800-365-7006
FAX: 212-966-6708
www.guilford.com

Bob Matloff, President

$18.95
352 pages Paperback 1999
ISBN 1-572302-39-9

8484 Life Line
National Hydrocephalus Foundation
12413 Centralia Street
Lakewood, CA 90715
562-402-3523
888-857-3434
888-260-1789
FAX: 562-924-6666
e-mail: debbifields@nhfonline.org
www.nhfonline.org

Debbi Fields, Executive Director
A national and worldwide organization established in order to provide information and education on the conditions of hydrocephalus. We also offer video/DVD on the subject, offer contacts for peer support, quarterly meetings that help individuals state and maintain a support group in their area and offer a quarterly newsletter to our membership. *$35.00*
12 pages Quarterly

8485 Lipomas & Lipomyelomeningocele
Spina Bifida Association of America
4590 Macarthur Boulevard NW
Suite 250
Washington, DC 20007
202-944-3285
800-621-3141
FAX: 202-944-3295
e-mail: sbaa@sbaa.org
www.sbaa.org

Cindy Brownstein, Chief Executive Officer

8486 Living Beyond Multiple Sclerosis: A Woman 's Guide
Hunter House Publishers
PO Box 2914
Alameda, CA 94501
510-865-5282
800-266-5592
FAX: 510-865-4295
e-mail: sales@hunterhouse.com
www.hunterhouse.com

Tim O'Reilly, Chief Executive Officer
This collection of e-mail conversations provides anecdotal and personal information contributed by women with multiple sclerosis. *$14.95*
256 pages 2000
ISBN 0-897932-93-5

8487 Living Well With HIV and AIDS
Bull Publishing

New drugs and drug combinations have turned HIV/AIDS into a long-term illness rather than a death sentence. Practical advice on mental adjustments and physical vigilance is outlined. *$18.95*
245 pages 2000
ISBN 0-923521-52-6

8488 Living Well with Asthma
Guilford Press
72 Spring Street
New York, NY 10012
212-431-9800
800-365-7006
FAX: 212-966-6708
www.guilford.com

Cynthia L Divino PhD, Author
Bob Matloff, President
$15.95
213 pages Paperback 1998
ISBN 1-572300-51-5

8489 Living Well with Chronic Fatigue Syndrome and Fibromyalgia
HarperCollins
1350 Avenue of the Americas
New York, NY 10019
212-261-6500
virusmyth.net/aids/books/mcbsurv.htm

Erin Gorman, Sales Executive
A comprehensive guide to the diagnosis and treatment of chronic fatigue syndrome and fibromyalgia. *$14.95*
416 pages 2004
ISBN 0-060521-25-2

8490 Living with Asthma and Allergies Brochure Series
Asthma and Allergy Foundation of America
1125 15th Street NW
Suite 502
Washington, DC 20005
202-466-7643
FAX: 202-466-8940
e-mail: info@aafa.org
www.aafa.org

Bill Lin, Executive Director
Informative series was developed to provide up-to-date, accurate information on common topics. Written in easy to understand language, with helpful illustrations, cover some of the most commonly asked questions about asthma and allergies.

8491 Living with Brain Injury: A Guide for Fam ilies
Delmar Learning

A consumer text to aid people living with brain-injured survivors, includes facts on neuroplasticity, experimental rehabilitation research, and the process of rehabilitation itself. *$16.95*
225 pages 2001
ISBN 1-891525-09-3

8492 Living with Spina Bifida: A Guide for Fam ilies and Professionals
University of North Carolina at Chapel Hill
Cb
Wing E # 7180
Chapel Hill, NC 27599
919-962-2211
FAX: 919-966-4127
www.teacch.com

James Moeser, Chief Executive Officer
A handbook that addresses patients' biopsychosocial and developmental needs from birth through adolescence and into adulthood. Sandler's holistic approach encourages families to focus more on the child and less on the disability while providing abundant information about this condition. *$19.95*
296 pages 2004
ISBN 0-807855-47-2

8493 Lung Cancer: Making Sense of Diagnosis, Treatment, & Option
Patient-Centered Guides
101 Morris Street
Sebastopol, CA 95472
707-829-0515
800-998-9938
FAX: 707-829-0104
www.patientcenters.com

Linda Lamb, Editor
Shawnde Paull, Marketing
Tim O'Reilly, Chief Executive Officer
Straightforward language and the words of patients and their families are the hallmarks of this book on the number one cancer killer in the US. Written by a widely respected author and patient advocate, Lung Cancer: Making Sense of Diagnosis, Treatment, & Options has been meticulously reviewed by top medical experts and physicians. Readers will find medical facts simply explained, advice to ease their daily life, and tools to be strong advocates for themselves or a family member. *$ 27.95*
530 pages Paperback
ISBN 0-596500-02-5

8494 Lupus: Alternative Therapies That Work
Healing Arts Press
1 Park Street
Rochester, VT 05767
802-767-3174
800-246-8648
FAX: 802-767-3726
e-mail: orders@innertraditions.com
www.InnerTraditions.com

Jessica Dudley, Sales Associate
Ehud Sperling, Owner
$14.95

256 pages
ISBN 0-892818-89-1

8495 **MAGIC Touch**
MAGIC Foundation for Children's Growth
6645 North Avenue
Oak Park, IL 60302
708-383-0808
800-362-4423
FAX: 708-383-0899
e-mail: mary@magicfoundation.org
www.magicfoundation.org

Dianne Andrews, Executive Director
Provides support and education regarding growth disorders in children and related adult disorders, including adult GHD. Dedicated to helping children whose physical growth is affected be a medical problem by assisting families of afflicted children through local support groups, public education/awareness, newsletters, specialty divisions and programs for the children.
36-40 pages Quarterly

8496 **MSFOCUS Magazine**
Multiple Sclerosis Foundation
6350 N Andrews Avenue
Fort Lauderdale, FL 33309
954-776-6805
888-673-6287
FAX: 954-351-0630
e-mail: support@msfocus.org
www.msfocus.org

Kathleen Truax, Case Worker
Jules Kuperberg, Administrator
Contemporary national, nonprofit organization that provides free support services and public education for persons with Multiple Sclerosis, newsletters, toll-free phone support, information, referrals, home care, assitive technology and support groups.
48 pages Quarterly

8497 **Management of Autistic Behavior**
Pro-Ed
8700 Shoal Creek Boulevard
Austin, TX 78757
512-451-3246
800-897-3202
FAX: 512-451-8542
e-mail: info@proedinc.com
www.proedinc.com

Donald Hammill, Owner
Comprehensive and practical book that tells what works best with specific problems. *$41.00*
450 pages Paperback
ISBN 0-890791-96-1

8498 **Management of Genetic Syndromes**
Wiley-Liss

Clinical information on 30 of the most common genetic syndromes. *$157.00*
554 pages 2001
ISBN 0-471312-86-X

8499 **Managing Post-Polio Syndrome**
Polio Connection of America
PO Box 182
Howard Beach, NY 11414
718-835-5536
FAX: 718-738-1509
e-mail: w1066@msn.com
www.geocities.com/w1066w

240 pages

8500 **Managing the Symptoms of Multiple Sclerosis**
Demos Medical Publishing
386 Park Avenue S
Suite 201
New York, NY 10016
212-683-0072
800-532-8663
FAX: 212-683-0118
e-mail: orderdep@demospub.com
www.demosmedpub.com

Diana Schneider PhD, President
Phyllis Gold, Owner
Guide for the management of MS symptoms, providing both up-to-date pathophysiological explanation and carefully weighed clinical advice. *$19.95*
192 pages 2003
ISBN 1-888799-78-1

8501 **Many Faces of Asthma**
American Lung Association
61 Broadway
New York, NY 10006
212-315-8700
FAX: 212-315-8700
e-mail: info@lungusa.org
www.lungusa.org

John Kirkwood, Chief Executive Officer
Provides an overview of asthma as a major public health problem, describes what happens during asthma attacks and explains how asthma is treated and managed.
12 pages

8502 **Meeting the Challenge of Progressive Multiple Sclerosis**

Demos Medical Publishing
386 Park Avenue S
Suite 201
New York, NY 10016
212-683-0072
800-532-8663
FAX: 212-683-0118
e-mail: orderdep@demospub.com
www.demosmedpub.com

Diana Schneider PhD, President
Phyllis Gold, Owner
A concise, practical and useful overview of worsening MS and the dilemma faced when progression presents its challenges to patients and those who care about them. *$21.95*
136 pages 2001
ISBN 1-888799-46-3

8503 **Meniere's Disease**
Vestibular Disorders Association
PO Box 4467
Portland, OR 97208
503-229-7705
800-837-8428
FAX: 503-229-8064
e-mail: veda@vestibular.org
www.vestibular.org

Lisa Haven, Editor
Connie Pilcher, Editor
1998

8504 **Menopause without Medicine**
Hunter House
PO Box 2914
Alameda, CA 94501
510-865-5282
800-266-5592
FAX: 510-865-4295
e-mail: sales@hunterhouse.com
www.hunterhouse.com

JoAnne Retzlaff, Sales/Marketing Associate
Christina Sverdrup, Customer Service Manager
Kiran Rana, Publisher
Research on nutrition, exercise, and osteoporosis, including good news about the body's ability to rebuild bone later in life; describes how women can best prepare their minds and bodies for the transition of menopause, and explains how women can prevent osteoporosis and control the disturbing symptoms of hot flashes, insomnia, fatigue, and weight gain. *$15.95*
368 pages
ISBN 0-897932-81-1

8505 **Moisture Seekers**
Sjogren's Syndrome Foundation
366 N Broadway
Suite Ph
Jericho, NY 11753
301-718-0300
800-475-6473
FAX: 301-718-0322
e-mail: ssf@sjogrens.org
www.sjogrens.org

Alexis Stegemann, Executive Director

Newsletter of the organization for lay people and professionals interested in Sjogren's Syndrome. Contains medical news, current research, and essential tips for daily living. *$25.00*
15-16 pages Monthly

8506 Moonrise: One Family, Genetic Identity, a nd Muscular Dystrophy
St. Martin's Press
175 5th Avenue
New York, NY 10010
212-674-5151
www.stmartins.com

John Sargent, Chief Executive Officer
A first-person account of the author's family, her son Ansel, and his progressive disability, caused by genetic disease, Duchenne muscular dystrophy. The journey begins when he is born and deemed a particularly beautiful baby, continues with the alarming possibility, at the age of two, of wrongness, through the diagnosis of disease and prognosis of early death, and to his adolescence, where his parents are never sure if the moon is rising or setting over his life. *$23.95*
256 pages 2003
ISBN 0-312289-08-

8507 Multiple Sclerosis
Demos Medical Publishing
386 Park Avenue S
Suite 201
New York, NY 10016
212-683-0072
800-532-8663
FAX: 212-683-0118
e-mail: orderdep@demospub.com
www.demosmedpub.com

Diana Schneider PhD, President
Phyllis Gold, Owner
Guide for living and coping with multiple sclerosis. *$39.95*
615 pages 2000
ISBN 1-888799-43-9

8508 Multiple Sclerosis and Having A Baby
Healing Arts Press
1 Park Street
Rochester, VT 05767
802-767-3174
800-246-8648
FAX: 802-767-3726
e-mail: orders@innertraditions.com
www.InnerTraditions.com

Jessica Dudley, Sales Associate
Ehud Sperling, Owner
Everything you need to know about conception, pregnancy and parenthood. *$12.95*
160 pages
ISBN 0-892817-88-7

8509 Multiple Sclerosis: The Guide to Treatmen t and Management
Demos Medical Publishing
386 Park Avenue S
Suite 201
New York, NY 10016
212-683-0072
800-532-8663
FAX: 212-683-0118
e-mail: orderdep@demospub.com
www.demosmedpub.com

Phyllis Gold, Owner
A current guide to modern therapies. *$24.95*
152 pages 2001
ISBN 1-888799-54-4

8510 Multiple Sclerosis: A Guide for Patients and Their Families
Lippincott, Williams & Wilkins
227 E Washington Square
Philadelphia, PA 19106
215-521-8300
800-777-2295
FAX: 301-824-7390
www.lpub.com

J Lippincott, Chief Executive Officer
$16.00
288 pages

8511 Multiple Sclerosis: A Guide for the Newly Diagnosed
Demos Medical Publishing
386 Park Avenue S
Suite 201
New York, NY 10016
212-683-0072
800-532-8663
FAX: 212-683-0118
e-mail: orderdep@demospub.com
www.demosmedpub.com

Diana Schneider PhD, President
Phyllis Gold, Owner
A must-have title for anyone who has recently been diagnosed with MS and a good idea for family members and friends. *$ 21.95*
160 pages 2002
ISBN 1-888799-60-9

8512 Muscular Dystrophies
Oxford University Press
198 Madison Avenue
New York, NY 10016
212-726-6000
800-451-7556
FAX: 919-677-1303
www.oup-usa.org

Laura Brown, Chief Executive Officer
Describes the opportunities for management of more than 30 types of MD through respiratory care, physiotherapy and surgical correction of contractures, and examines the potential for effective treatment utilizing the new techniques of gene and cell therapy *$ 106.00*
316 pages 2002
ISBN 0-192632-91-4

8513 Muscular Dystrophy and Other Neuromuscular Diseases
Haworth Press
10 Alice Street
Binghamton, NY 13904
607-722-5857
800-429-6784
FAX: 607-722-6362
e-mail: orders@haworthpress.com
www.haworthpress.com

S Harrington-Miller, Advertising
William Cohen, Owner
A thoughtful new book from professionals who assist persons afflicted with neuromuscular disorders to help them and their families adapt to lifestyle changes accompanying the onset of these disorders. *$74.95*
250 pages Hardcover
ISBN 1-560240-77-6

8514 Muscular Dystrophy in Children: A Guide fo r Families
Demos Medical Publishing
386 Park Avenue S
Suite 201
New York, NY 10016
212-683-0072
800-532-8663
FAX: 212-683-0118
e-mail: orderdep@demospub.com
www.demosmedpub.com

Phyllis Gold, Owner
Defines the available medical options at every stage of the disease and offers guidance even when it may seem that little or nothing can be done. Includes a glossary and suggestions for furhter reading. *$19.95*
130 pages Paperback 1999
ISBN 1-888799-33-1

8515 Muscular Dystrophy: The Facts
Oxford University Press
198 Madison Avenue
New York, NY 10016
212-726-6000
800-451-7556
FAX: 919-677-1303
www.oup-usa.org

Laura Brown, Chief Executive Officer
A good first book for individuals and families faced with the likelihood or reality of a muscular dystrophy diagnosis. *$19.95*

166 pages 2000
ISBN 0-192632-17-5

8516 My House Is Killing Me! The Home Guide for Families With Allergies and Asthma
Johns Hopkins University Press

Chemical consultant May describes where and how the various parts of a residence can cause temporary or chronic illness for those with allergies or other sensitivities. *$17.95*
338 pages 2001
ISBN 0-801867-30-4

8517 Myositis
Arthritis Foundation
PO Box 7669
Atlanta, GA 30357
404-872-7100
800-283-7800
FAX: 404-872-9559
e-mail: help@arthritis.org
www.arthritis.org

John Klippel, Chief Executive Officer

8518 Narcolepsy
Fanlight Productions
4196 Washington Street
Suite 2
Boston, MA 02131
617-469-4999
FAX: 617-469-3379
e-mail: fanlight@fanlight.com
www.fanlight.com

Ben Achtenberg, Owner
Presents the experiences of three individuals who lives and relationships have been disrupted by narcolepsy. Rental $50/day. *$195.00*
25 Minutes

8519 Neuropsychiatry of Epilepsy
Cambridge University Press

Covers the practical implications of ongoing research, and offers a diagnostic and management perspective. Topics include cognitive aspects, nonepileptic attacks, and clinical aspects. For professionals treating epileptic patients. *$70.00*
360 pages 2002
ISBN 0-521005-16-7

8520 Nick Joins In
Spina Bifida Association of America
4590 Macarthur Boulevard NW
Suite 250
Washington, DC 20007
202-944-3285
800-621-3141
FAX: 202-944-3295
e-mail: sbaa@sbaa.org
www.sbaa.org

Cindy Brownstein, Chief Executive Officer
When Nick, who is in a wheelchair, enters a regular classroom for the first time, he realizes that he has much to contribute. *$17.00*

8521 No More Allergies
Villiard Books
1540 Broadway
New York, NY 10036
212-782-9000
FAX: 212-302-7985

Carol Schneider, Marketing Executive
A detailed investigation into the causes of allergies related both to food and the environment, as well as their link to other illnesses, such as asthma, arthritis, chrinic fatigue syndrome, and diabetes. Also outlines testing methods, treatments, and a diet plan to restore immune function.

8522 No Time for Jello: One Family's Experience
Brookline Books
PO Box 1046
Cambridge, MA 02139
617-868-0360
800-666-2665
FAX: 617-868-1772
e-mail: thestore@brooklinebooks.com
www.brooklinebooks.com
One family's story of their attempts to remediate and cure the effects of a cerebral palsied condition the oldest son was born with. The Bratts traveled traditional routes, through distinguished medical centers in Boston, and nontraditional routes in a search for treatments that would help their son. *$17.95*
Softcover
ISBN 0-91479 -56-5

8523 Nocturnal Asthma
National Jewish Center for Immunology
1400 Jackson Street
Denver, CO 80206
303-388-4461

e-mail: allstetterw@njc.org
www.njc.org

William Allstetter, Media Relations Manager
Lynn Taussig, Chief Executive Officer
Offers information to patients about how to understand and manage asthma at night.

8524 Non-Hodgkin's Lymphomas: Making Sense of Diagnosis, Treatment & Options
O'Reilly
101 Morris Street
Sebastopol, CA 95472
707-829-0515
800-294-4747
FAX: 800-997-9901
e-mail: order@oreilly.com
www.patientcenters.com

Tim O'Reilly, Chief Executive Officer
$24.95
580 pages Paperback
ISBN 1-565924-44-4

8525 Obesity
Spina Bifida Association of America
4590 Macarthur Boulevard NW
Suite 250
Washington, DC 20007
202-944-3285
800-621-3141
FAX: 202-944-3295
e-mail: sbaa@sbaa.org
www.sbaa.org

Cindy Brownstein, Chief Executive Officer
$8.00

8526 Obesity Sourcebook
Omnigraphics
615 Griswold Street
Detroit, MI 48226
313-961-1340
800-234-1340
FAX: 800-875-1340
www.omnigraphics.com

Wilma Caldwell, Editor
Peter Ruffner, President
Discusses diseases and other problems associated with obesity. *$48.00*
400 pages 2000
ISBN 0-780803-33-7

8527 Occulta
Spina Bifida Association of America
4590 Macarthur Boulevard NW
Suite 250
Washington, DC 20007
202-944-3285
800-621-3141
FAX: 202-944-3295
e-mail: sbaa@sbaa.org
www.sbaa.org

Cindy Brownstein, Chief Executive Officer
$8.00

8528 Occupational Asthma: Lung Hazards on the Job
American Lung Association
61 Broadway
New York, NY 10006
212-315-8700
FAX: 212-315-8700
e-mail: info@lungusa.org
www.lungusa.org

John Kirkwood, Chief Executive Officer
Discusses occupational asthma, a form of asthma in which airways overreact to various irritants in the workplace.

8529 Official Patient's Sourcebook on Cystic Fi brosis
Icon Health

For parents who have decided to make education and research an integral part of the treatment process. Although it also gives information useful to doctors, caregivers and other health professionals, it tells paretns where and how to look for information covering virtually all topics related to cystic fibrosis (also fbrocystic disease of pancreas; mucosis; mucoviscidosis; pancreatic fibrosis), from the essentials to the most advanced areas of research. *$28.95*
356 pages 2002
ISBN 0-597831-46-7

8530 Official Patient's Sourcebook on Muscular Dystrophy
Icon Health

Created for patients who have decided to make education and research an integral part of the treatment process. Although it also gives information useful to doctors, caregivers and other health professionals, it tells patients where and how to look for information covering virtually all topics related to muscular dystrophy. *$24.95*
268 pages 2002
ISBN 0-597832-10-2

8531 Official Patient's Sourcebook on Post-Poli o Syndrome: A Revised and Updated Directory
Icon Health

A sourcebook created for patients who have decided to make education and Internet-based research an integral part of the treatment process. Although it gives information useful to doctors, caregivers and other health professionals, it also tells patients where and how to look for information covering virtually all topics related to post-polio syndrome, from the essentials to the most advanced areas of research. *$28.95*
124 pages 2003
ISBN 0-597835-31-4

8532 One Day at a Time: Children Living with Leukemia
Gareth Stevens
1555 N Rivercenter Drive
Milwaukee, WI 53212
414-332-3520
800-542-2595
FAX: 414-225-0377
beta.healthlinkusa.com/bookpage/184_27.html

Claire Messier, Marketing Associate
Bob Famighetti, Publisher
Focus on Hanna, two years old, and 3 year old Frederick. Both diagnosed with Leukemia and follows them as they are treated for their illness. Includes such daily routines as eating breakfast, washing and playing. *$16.95*
56 pages Hardcover
ISBN 1-55532 -13-6

8533 Options
People Against Cancer
PO Box 10
Otho, IA 50569
515-972-4444
FAX: 515-972-4415
e-mail: info@PeopleAgainstCAncer.com
www.peopleagainstcancer.com

Frank Wiewel, Executive Director
8 pages Quarterly

8534 Options: Revolutionary Ideas in the War on Cancer
People Against Cancer
PO Box 10
Otho, IA 50569
515-972-4444
FAX: 515-972-4415
e-mail: info@PeopleAgainstCancer.net
www.peopleagainstcancer.com
Publication of People Against Cancer, a nonprofit, grassroots public benefit organization dedicated to 'New Directions in the War on Cancer.' We are a democratic organization of people with cancer, their loved ones and citizens working together to protect and enhance medical freedom of choice.

8535 Oral/Facial Clefts Fact Sheet
March of Dimes
1275 Mamaroneck Avenue
White Plains, NY 10605
914-949-7166
FAX: 914-997-4763
e-mail: askus@marchofdimes.com
www.marchofdimes.com
The March of Dimes Resource Center provides information about pregnancy, drug use, environmental hazards and other related topics. The Resource Center's health information specialists provide accurate and up-to-date information via e-mail and Web site.

8536 Orthotics and Prosthetics Almanac
Orthotics and Prosthetics National Office
1650 King Street
Suite 500
Alexandria, VA 22314
703-836-7114
FAX: 703-836-0838
e-mail: opalmanac@aol.com
www.aopanet.org

Stacey L Bell, Editor-in-Chief
Kathy Carter, Executive Director
Features articles covering current professional, patient care, government, business and National Office activities affecting the orthotics and prosthetics profession and industry. *$40.00*
80 pages Monthly
ISSN 1061-46 1

8537 Osteoporosis Sourcebook
Omnigraphics
615 Griswold Street
Detroit, MI 48226
313-961-1340
800-234-1340
FAX: 800-875-1340
www.omnigraphics.com

Allan R Cook, Editor
Peter Ruffner, President
Discusses causes, risk factors, treatments and traditional and non-traditional pain management issues concerning osteoporosis. *$ 78.00*
600 pages 2000
ISBN 0-780802-39-X

8538 PDF News
Parkinson's Disease Foundation
833 W Washington Boulevard
Chicago, IL 60607
312-733-1893
800-457-6676
FAX: 312-733-1896
e-mail: info@pdf.org
www.pdf.org

Lewis P Rowland MD, President
Jeanne Rosner, Executive Director
8-12 pages Quarterly

8539 PDF Newsletter
Parkinson's Disease Foundation
1359 Broadway
Suite 1509
New York, NY 10018
212-923-4700
800-457-6676
FAX: 212-923-4778
e-mail: info@pdf.org
www.pdf.org

Christiana Evers, Director Of Communications
Yasnahia Cortorreal, Manager Of Administration
12-16 pages Quarterly

8540 PDP Products
14524 61st Street Court N
Stillwater, MN 55082
651-439-8865
FAX: 651-439-0421
e-mail: products@pdppro.com
www.pdppro.com

Alexis Richter, Administrator
PDP Products acquires books and therapy materials recommended or developed by therapists and makes those materials available at PDP courses and through mail order.

8541 POZ Magazine
Smart + Strong
1 Little West 12th Street
6th Floor
New York, NY 10014
212-242-2163
www.poz.com

Sean Strub, Owner
A health title written for individuals who are HIV+, their friends and families. POZ provides the latest treatment information, investigative journalism and survivor profiles.

8542 PSP Advocate
Society for Progressive Supranuclear Palsy
1838 Greene Tree Road
Baltimore, MD 21208
410-486-3330
800-457-4777
FAX: 410-486-4283
e-mail: spsp@psp.org
www.psp.org

Elizabeth Brisson, President
Stephen Hamer, VP
Kelley Harrison PhD, Secretary
Quarterly newsletter. The society's mission is to promote and fund research into finding the cause and cure for progressive supranuclear palsy (PSP). Provides information, support and advocacy to persons diagnosed with PSP, their families and caregivers. Educates physicians and allied health professionals on PSP and how to improve patient care.

8543 Parent Teacher Packet
Spina Bifida Association of America
4590 Macarthur Boulevard NW
Suite 250
Washington, DC 20007
202-944-3285
800-621-3141
FAX: 202-944-3295
e-mail: sbaa@sbaa.org
www.sbaa.org

Cindy Brownstein, Chief Executive Officer
Includes educational material, learning disabilities literature, children's book, social development and the person with spina bifida and one copy of each fact sheet. *$14.00*

8544 Parent's Guide to Allergies and Asthma
National Allergy and Asthma Network
3554 Chain Bridge Road
Suite 200
Fairfax, VA 22030
703-385-4403
FAX: 703-352-4354
A up-to-date, easy-to-read resource offering essential information on asthma and allergies.

8545 Parkinsons Report
National Parkinson Foundation
1501 NW 9th Avenue
Miami, FL 33136
305-547-6666
800-327-4545
FAX: 305-243-4403
e-mail: mailbox@parkinson.org
www.parkinson.org

Julian Pearson, Administrator
Jose Garcia-Pedrosa, Executive Director
Articles, reports and news on Parkinson's disease and the activities of the National Parkinson Foundation.
32 pages Qarterly

8546 Partial Seizure Disorders: Help for Patients and Families
Patient-Centered Guides
101 Morris Street
Sebastopol, CA 95472
707-829-0515
800-998-9938
FAX: 707-829-0104
www.patientcenters.com

Linda Lamb, Editor
Shawnde Paull, Marketing
Tim O'Reilly, Chief Executive Officer
Partial Seizure Disorders helps patients and families get an accurate diagnosis of this condition, understand medications and their side effects, and learn coping skills and other adjuncts to medication. It walks readers through developmental and school issues for young children; adult issues such as employment and driving; working with an existing health plan; and getting further help through advocacy and support organizations, articles, and online resources. *$19.95*
288 pages Paperback
ISBN 0-596500-03-3

8547 Penitent, With Poses: An HIV+ Mother Refle cts
Middlebury College Press

Peterson, a married, middle-class, Jewish mother, was diagnosed with full-blown AIDS four years into her marriage and 11 months after her son was born. In seven poignant autobiographical essays and a collection of letters to her uninfected, four-year-old son, the author maintains an upbeat tone and describes her unsuccessful attempts to find the source of her infection (her husband tested negative), her relationships with her doctors, and her work as an HIV activist. *$ 26.95*
256 pages 2001
ISBN 1-584651-28-8

8548 People Against Cancer
604 East Street
P.O. Box 10
Otho, IA 50569
515-972-4444
FAX: 515-972-4415
e-mail: info@peopleagainstcancer.net
www.peopleagainstcancer.com

Frank Wiewel, Executive Director
A nonprofit, grassroots public benefit organization dedicated to 'New Directions in the War on Cancer.' We are a democratic organization of people with cancer, their loved ones and citizens working together to protect and enhance medical freedom of choice. Through our Alternative Therapy Program we find our members the best cancer treatment.

8549 Personal Guide to Living Well with Fibromyalgia
Arthritis Foundation Distribution Center
PO Box 6996
Alpharetta, GA 30023
800-207-8633
FAX: 770-442-9742
www.arthritis.com
With this guide you'll learn the latest information about fibromyalgia, what researchers have uncovered about its causes, and an overview of the best treatment options available. Helpful worksheets and tables allow you to manage your condition and document your progress. *$14.95*
224 pages

8550 Pharmacologic Therapy of Pediatric Asthma
American Lung Association
61 Broadway
New York, NY 10006
212-315-8700
FAX: 212-315-8700
e-mail: info@lungusa.org
www.lungusa.org

John Kirkwood, Chief Executive Officer
A Learning Resource Program developed by a joint committee of the American Thoracic Society and the ALA.

Film

8551 Plan Ahead: Do What You Can
Spina Bifida Association of America
4590 Macarthur Boulevard NW
Suite 250
Washington, DC 20007
202-944-3285
800-621-3141
FAX: 202-944-3295
e-mail: sbaa@sbaa.org
www.sbaa.org

Cindy Brownstein, Chief Executive Officer
Folic aciid information for women at risk for recurrence. *$15.00*

8552 Polio Network News
Gazette International Networking Institute
4207 Lindell Boulevard
Suite 110
Saint Louis, MO 63108
314-534-0475
FAX: 314-534-5070
e-mail: gini_intl@msn.com
www.post-polio.org
International newsletter for polio survivors, support groups and health professionals concerned about the late effects of polio. *$20.00*
12 pages Quarterly

8553 Polymyalgia Rheumatica and Giant Cell Arthritis
Arthritis Foundation
PO Box 7669
Atlanta, GA 30357
404-872-7100
800-283-7800
FAX: 404-872-9559
e-mail: help@arthritis.org
www.arthritis.org

John Klippel, Chief Executive Officer

8554 Post Polio
Accent Books & Products
PO Box 700
Bloomington, IL 61702
309-378-2961
800-787-8444
FAX: 309-378-4420
e-mail: acmtlvng@aol.com

Raymond C Cheever, Publisher
Betty Garee, Editor
What does post-polio syndrome mean? What can make a difference in a persons future mobility? These questions and more are answered in this great guide. *$3.95*
47 pages Paperback
ISBN 0-91570 -21-3

8555 Post-Polio Health
Post-Polio Health International
4207 Lindell Boulevard
Suite 110
Saint Louis, MO 63108
314-534-0475
FAX: 314-534-5070
TTY:800-735-2966
e-mail: info@post-polio.org
www.post-polio.org

John L Headly, Editor
To enhance the lives and independence of polio survivors by promoting education, networking, and advocacy among these individuals and healthcare providers. Post-Polio Health supports Post-Polio Health International's educational, research, and advocacy efforts. Offers information about relevant events.
12 pages quarterly

8556 Post-Polio Syndrome Information Book
PO Box 182
Howard Beach, NY 11414
718-835-5536
FAX: 718-738-1509
e-mail: w1066@msn.com
www.geocities.com/w1066w

100 pages

8557 Post-Polio Syndrome: A Guide for Polio Su rvivors and Their Families
Yale University Press

A guide for polio survivors, their families, and their health care providers offers expert advice on all aspects of post-polio syndrome. Based on the author's experience treating post-polio patients, Silver discusses issues of critical importance, including how to find the best medical care, deal with symptoms, sustain mobility, manage pain, approach insurance issues, and arrange a safe living environment. *$ 16.95*
304 pages 2002
ISBN 0-300088-08-6

8558 Prader-Willi Alliance of New York Monthly Newsletter
267 Oxford Street
Rochester, NY 14607
585-442-1655
800-442-1655
FAX: 716-271-2782
e-mail: balleregballer@aol.com
www.prader-willi.org

Elinor G Baller, Secretary
Volena How, Owner
The Prader-Willi Foundation is a national, nonprofit public charity that works for the benefit of individuals with Prader-Willi syndrome and their families.

8559 Prader-Willi Syndrome: Development and Ma nifestations
Cambridge University Press

Seeks to identify and provide the latest findings about how best to manage the complex medical, nutritional, psychological, educational, social and therapeutic needs of people with PWS. *$100.00*
230 pages 2004
ISBN 0-521840-29-5

8560 Preventing Secondary Conditions Associated with Spina Bifida or Cerebral Palsy
Spina Bifida Association of America
4590 Macarthur Boulevard NW
Suite 250
Washington, DC 20007
202-944-3285
800-621-3141
FAX: 202-944-3295
e-mail: sbaa@sbaa.org
www.sbaa.org

Cindy Brownstein, Chief Executive Officer
This report is for health professionals, parents and teachers. *$3.00*

8561 Protecting Against Latex Allergy
Spina Bifida Association of America
4590 Macarthur Boulevard NW
Suite 250
Washington, DC 20007
202-944-3285
800-621-3141
FAX: 202-944-3295
e-mail: sbaa@sbaa.org
www.sbaa.org

Cindy Brownstein, Chief Executive Officer
Because awareness and proper action may help prevent an allergic reation, learning about latex allergy is especially important for parents, health care workers and anyone who is exposed to latex regulary. *$20.00*

8562 Quality Care Newsletter
National Association for Continence
PO Box 1019
Charleston, SC 29402
843-377-0900
800-252-3337
FAX: 843-377-0905
e-mail: memberservices@nafc.org
www.nafc.org

Rachel Leukowicz, Health Educator
Nancy Muller, Executive Director
Caryn Antos, Publicity + Publications
Newsletter from NAFC. *$25.00*
14-16 pages Quarterly

8563 Questions and Answers: The ADA and Persons with HIV/AIDS
US Department of Justice
950 Pennsylvania Avenue NW Drs
- Nyav
Washington, DC 20530
202-586-5000
800-574-0301
FAX: 202-307-1197
www.ada.gov

Joanne Graham, Manager
A 16-page publication explaining the requirements for employers, businesses and nonprofit agencies that serve the public, and state and local governments to avoid discriminating against persons with HIV/AIDS.

8564 Rasmussen's Syndrome and Hemispherectomy Support Network Newsletter
8235 Lethbridge Road
Millersville, MD 21108
410-987-5221
FAX: 410-987-521
e-mail: rssnlynn@aol.com

Al & Lynn Miller, Founders
National, not-for-profit organization dedicated to providing information and support to individuals affected by Rasmussen's Syndrome and hemispherectomy. Publishes a periodic newsletter and disseminates reprints of medical journal articles concerning Rasmussen's Syndrome and its treatments. Maintains a support network that provides encouragement and information to individuals affected by Rasmussen's Syndrome and their families.

8565 Raynaud's Phenomenon
Arthritis Foundation
PO Box 7669
Atlanta, GA 30357
404-872-7100
800-283-7800
FAX: 404-872-9559
e-mail: help@arthritis.org
www.arthritis.org

John Klippel, Chief Executive Officer

8566 Reaching the Autistic Child: A Parent Trai ning Program
Brookline Books/Lumen Editions
PO Box 1047
Cambridge, MA 02139
617-868-0360
800-666-2665
FAX: 617-868-1772
e-mail: thestore@brooklinebooks.com
Detailed case studies of social and behavioral change in autistic children and their families show parents how to implement the principles for improved socialization and behavior. *$15.95*
Softcover
ISBN 1-571290-56-7

8567 Regular Kid
American Lung Association
61 Broadway
New York, NY 10006
212-315-8700
FAX: 212-315-8700
e-mail: info@lungusa.org
www.lungusa.org

John Kirkwood, Chief Executive Officer
This film shows how families and children cope with asthma problems. Proven asthma management strategies are presented through the experiences of four children with asthma, ranging in age from toddler to teenager.
Film

8568 Reiter's Syndrome
Arthritis Foundation
PO Box 7669
Atlanta, GA 30357
404-872-7100
800-283-7800
FAX: 404-872-9559
e-mail: help@arthritis.org
www.arthritis.org

John Klippel, Chief Executive Officer

8569 Ride the Red Cycle
Houghton Mifflin
222 Berkeley Street
Boston, MA 02116
617-351-5000
800-225-3362
www.hmco.com

Tony Lucki, Chief Executive Officer
Jerome Johnson is nine, but due to brain damage he can't walk and his speech is hard to understand. Jerome gets around in a wheelchair, but he knows that if he could get a tricycle he could go where and when he wanted. His parents not only agreed to buy him the cycle, but his dad built up the pedals and added a seat with a back and a seatbelt to hold Jerome.
34 pages Hardcover
ISBN 0-39529 -83-6

8570 Rights of People Who Are HIV Positive
America Civil Liberites Union

The authors tackle the subject in four parts: the disease itself and the related testing, public health, and confidentiality issues; day-to-day issues involving insurance, family law, and healthcare decision-making; discrimination in housing and work; and AIDS in prisons, schools, as a factor in immigration, and among IV drug users. The topics are broached using a question-and-answer format, and each chapter is documented with citations to source material. *$19.95*
448 pages 1996
ISBN 0-809319-92-6

8571 SCI Psychosocial Process
Amer. Assn. of Spinal Cord Injury Psych./Soc. Wks.
7520 Astoria Boulevard
East Elmhurst, NY 11370
718-803-3782
FAX: 718-803-0414
e-mail: ssofer@epua.org
www.aascipsw.org

E Jason Mask LCSW, Editor
Peter Addesso, President
Quarterly newsletter.

8572 SCI/LIFE
National Spinal Cord Injury Association
6701 Democracy Boulevard
Suite 300-9
Bethesda, MD 20817
301-214-4006
800-962-9629
FAX: 301-588-9414
e-mail: Info@spinalcord.org
www.spinalcord.org

Charles W Haynes, Publisher
J Charles Haynes JD, Publisher
Thomas H Countee Jr, Esq, Editor-in-Chief
SCI/LIFE is dedicated to the presentation of news concerning people with spinal cord injuries caused by trauma or disease. *$38.00*
39 pages Quarterly

8573 SPINabilities: A Young Person's Guide to Spina Bifida
Spina Bifida Association of America
4590 Macarthur Boulevard NW
Suite 250
Washington, DC 20007
202-944-3285
800-621-3141
FAX: 202-944-3295
e-mail: sbaa@sbaa.org
www.sbaa.org

Cindy Brownstein, Chief Executive Officer
A cool and practical book for young adults becoming independent. *$19.00*

8574 Screening in Chronic Disease
Oxford University Press
2001 Evans Road
Cary, NC 27513
919-677-0977
800-451-7556
FAX: 919-677-2673
e-mail: humaneres@oup-usa.org
www.oup-usa.org

Henry Reece, Chief Executive Officer
Thomas Carty, Senior Vice President
Early detection, or screening, is a common strategy for controlling chronic disease, but little information has been available to help determine which screening procedures are worthwhile. *$42.50*
256 pages

8575 Seizures and Epilepsy in Childhood: A Guid e
John Hopkins University Pres

A resources for parents of a child with epilepsy. Information allows parents to have informed discussions with physician and treatment teams. Also provides information for parents to become participants in treatment plans. *$19.95*
360 pages 2002
ISBN 0-801870-51-8

8576 Sexuality After Spinal Cord Injury: Answers to Your Questions
Brookes Publishing
PO Box 10624
Baltimore, MD 21285
410-337-9580
800-638-3775
FAX: 410-337-8539
e-mail: custserv@brookespublishing.com
www.brookespublishing.com

Paul Brooks, Owner
Anatomy, fertility, sexually transmitted diseases, self-esteem, sexual satisfaction, and parenting are among the many physical and emotional issues discussed in this guide. Question-and-answer format. *$24.95*
272 pages Paperback 1997
ISBN 1-557662-65-7

8577 Sexuality and the Person with Spina Bifida
Spina Bifida Association of America
4590 Macarthur Boulevard NW
Suite 250
Washington, DC 20007
202-944-3285
800-621-3141
FAX: 202-944-3295
e-mail: sbaa@sbaa.org
www.sbaa.org

Cindy Brownstein, Chief Executive Officer
Dr Sloan foucuses on sexual development, sexual activity and other important issues. *$11.00*

8578 Simon Foundation for Continence
PO Box 815
Wilmette, IL 60091
847-864-3913
800-23S-IMON
FAX: 847-864-9758
www.simonfoundation.org

Cheryle B Gartley, President
Publishes items of interest to people with bladder or bowel incontinence, including medical articles, helpful devices, publications and a pen pal list.

8579 Sinus Survival
Jeremy P Tarcher
8552 E Dry Creek Place
Centennial, CO 80112
888-434-0033
FAX: 303-221-5320
Self-help manual for sufferers of bronchitis, sinusitis, allergies, and colds.

8580 Social Development and the Person with Spi na Bifida
Spina Bifida Association of America
4590 Macarthur Boulevard NW
Suite 250
Washington, DC 20007
202-944-3285
800-621-3141
FAX: 202-944-3295
e-mail: sbaa@sbaa.org
www.sbaa.org

Cindy Brownstein, Chief Executive Officer
Examines how spina bifida and hydrocephalus may influence development and learning social skills.

8581 Solving the Puzzle of Chronic Fatigue
Life Sciences Press
1216 S 1580 W
Suite A
Orem, UT 84058
801-224-6228
800-336-6308
e-mail: info@essentialscience.net
www.insight-books.com/new/0943685117.html
Although primarily a book about CFS, this comprehensive study also provides a detailed overview of candidiasis, including its causes and best approaches for treatment. *$14.95*
190 pages 1992
ISBN 0-943685-11-7

8582 Son-Rise: The Miracle Continues
2080 S Undermountain Road
Sheffield, MA 01257
413-229-2100
800-714-2779
FAX: 413-229-3202
e-mail: sonrise@option.org
www.son-rise.org
Documents Raun Kaufman's astonishing development from a lifeless, autistic, retarded child into a highly verbal, lovable youngster with no traces of his former condition. Details Raun's extraordinary progress from the age of four into young adulthood, also shares moving accounts of five families that successfully used the Son-Rise Program to reach their own special children.
372 pages 1994
ISBN 0-915811-53-7

8583 Special Care in Dentistry
Academy of Dentistry for Persons with Disabilities
211 E Chicago Avenue
Floor 5
Chicago, IL 60611
312-337-2169
FAX: 312-440-2824
e-mail: fosccdzz@worldnet.att.net
www.specialdentistry.org

John Rutkauskaf, Executive Director
$125.00
48 pages BiMonthly

8584 Spina Bifida
Spina Bifida Association of America
4590 Macarthur Boulevard NW
Suite 250
Washington, DC 20007
202-944-3285
800-621-3141
FAX: 202-944-3295
e-mail: sbaa@sbaa.org
www.sbaa.org

Cindy Brownstein, Chief Executive Officer

8585 Spinabilities: A Young Person's Guide to Spina Bifida
Woodbine House
6510 Bells Mill Road
Bethesda, MD 20817
301-897-3570
800-843-7323
FAX: 301-897-5838
e-mail: info@woodbinehouse.com
www.woodbinehouse.com

Irv Shapell, Owner
Advice for teenagers on managing daily and long-term healthcare, tips on sex and relationships, and strategies for success at school and on the job. *$16.95*

138 pages 1997
ISBN 0-933149-86-7

8586 Spinal Cord Injury Life
National Spinal Cord Injury Association
8701 Georgia Avenue
Suite 500
Silver Spring, MD 20910
617-469-0004
800-962-9629
FAX: 301-588-9414
e-mail: nscia2@aol.com
www.spinalcord.org

Thomas H Countee Jr, Executive Director
Includes sections such as Legislative Action, Information Resources and Research Notes. *$30.00*
45-60 pages Quarterly

8587 Spinal Cord Injury Series
Fanlight Productions
4196 Washington Street
Suite 2
Boston, MA 02131
617-469-4999
800-937-4113
FAX: 617-469-3379
e-mail: fanlight@fanlight.com
www.fanlight.com

Karen McMillen, Marketing Director
Ben Achtenberg, Owner
A series of three videos produced by an individual who has experienced spinal cord injury himself. Changes: is about the consequences of spinal cord injury and the process of rehabilitation. Outside: emphasizes the life-long aspect of rehabilitation for people with spinal cord injury. Survivors: interviews 23 men and women who have lived at least 24 years with spinal cord injury. *$200.00*

8588 Spine
JB Lippincott
E Washington Square
Philadelphia, PA 19105
215-521-8300
FAX: 215-824-7390

J Lippincott, Chief Executive Officer
Publishes original papers on theoretical issues and research concerning the spine and spinal cord injuries. *$9.00*
Monthly

8589 Spirit of Lo: An Ordinary Family's Extraor dinary Journey
Mind Matters

An ordinary family is faced with an extraordinary challenge, a child with cystic fibrosis. Their love, faith and commitment to each other carry them through battles with depression, anger, despair and the ravages of the disease as they join a race with death for a cure. *$14.95*
280 pages 2000
ISBN 0-970193-40-8

8590 Standards for the Diagnosis and Care of Patients with Asthma
American Lung Association
61 Broadway
New York, NY 10006
212-315-8700
FAX: 212-315-8700
e-mail: info@lungusa.org
www.lungusa.org

John Kirkwood, Chief Executive Officer
Standards developed by the American Thoracic Society, the medical section of the ALA. For physicians.

24 pages

8591 Steps to Independence: Teaching Everyday S kills to Children with Special Needs
Spina Bifida Association of America
4590 Macarthur Boulevard NW
Suite 250
Washington, DC 20007
202-944-3285
800-621-3141
FAX: 202-944-3295
e-mail: sbaa@sbaa.org
www.sbaa.org

Cindy Brownstein, Chief Executive Officer
A guide to help parents teach life skills to their disabled child. *$28.00*

8592 Stricken: Voices from the Hidden Epidemic of Chronic Fatigue Syndrome
Haworth Press
10 Alice Street
Binghamton, NY 13904
607-722-5857
800-429-6784
FAX: 607-722-6362
e-mail: orders@haworthpress.com
www.haworthpress.com

William Cohen, Owner
A collection of personal accounts from sufferers of chronic fatigue immune dysfunction syndrome. The contributions come from patients from all walks of life, from a former marathon runner to a public health activist living in the margins of race and gender. An exploration of the complex social and political dynamics surrounding the disorder. *$24.95*
270 pages 2000
ISBN 0-789008-95-5

8593 Symptomatic Chiari Malformation
Spina Bifida Association of America
4590 Macarthur Boulevard NW
Suite 250
Washington, DC 20007
202-944-3285
800-621-3141
FAX: 202-944-3295
e-mail: sbaa@sbaa.org
www.sbaa.org

Cindy Brownstein, Chief Executive Officer

8594 TSA Newsletter
Tourette Syndrome Association
4240 Bell Boulevard
Bayside, NY 11361
718-224-2999
800-237-0717
FAX: 718-279-9596
e-mail: ts@tsa-usa.org
www.tsa-usa.org

Fred Cook, Editor
Judit Ungar, Editor
Tracy Colletti-Flynn, Editor
Quarterly

8595 Taking Charge
Spina Bifida Association of America
4590 Macarthur Boulevard NW
Suite 250
Washington, DC 20007
202-944-3285
800-621-3141
FAX: 202-944-3295
e-mail: sbaa@sbaa.org
www.sbaa.org

Cindy Brownstein, Chief Executive Officer
Teenagers talk about life and physical disabilities. *$7.95*

8596 Teens Talk to Teens about Asthma
Asthma and Allergy Foundation of America
1125 15th Street NW
Suite 502
Washington, DC 20005
202-466-7643
FAX: 202-466-8940
e-mail: info@aafa.org
www.aafa.org

Bill Lin, Executive Director
Brochure provides support to a teen you care about. Includes quotes and thoughts from teens that capture the essence of what it feels like to live with asthma.

8597 Tempered Wind
Atheneum
135 S Mount Zion Road
Lebanon, IN 46052
FAX: 800-882-8583
Gabrielle was a dwarf and was never out of her house until her parents died and she was sent from one aunt to the next. At age thirteen she was enrolled in school for the first time. The children teased her about being a dwarf, and although she excelled academically, she failed socially. After three years in school an illness forced her aunt to take Gabrielle to the doctor. The doctor's prognosis was grim and led Gabrielle's aunt to tell her that she would have to find a job.
210 pages Hardcover
ISBN 0-68931 -39-X

8598 Ten Things I Learned from Bill Porter
New World Library

Bill Porter worked for the Watkins Corp, selling household products door-to-door in one of Portland's worst neighborhoods. Afflicted with cerebral palsy and burdened with continual pain, Porter was determined not to live on government disability and went on to become Watkin's top-grossing salesman in Portland, the Northwest, and the US. This book was written by the woman who worked as Porter's typist and driver and later became his friend and cospeaker. *$20.00*
160 pages 2002
ISBN 1-577312-03-1

8599 Tethering Cord
Spina Bifida Association of America
4590 Macarthur Boulevard NW
Suite 250
Washington, DC 20007
202-944-3285
800-621-3141
FAX: 202-944-3295
e-mail: sba@sbaa.org
www.sbaa.org

Cindy Brownstein, Chief Executive Officer

8600 The River: A Journey to the Source of HIV and AIDS
Back Bay Books

The author's thesis, that HIV made the jump from simians to humans via the administration of oral polio vaccine in Africa in the 1950s, is still controversial, all that is lacking is conclusive proof. *$24.95*
1168 pages 2000
ISBN 0-316371-67-8

8601 There are Solutions for the Student with Asthma
American Lung Association
61 Broadway
New York, NY 10006
212-315-8700
FAX: 212-315-8700
e-mail: info@lungusa.org
www.lungusa.org

John Kirkwood, Chief Executive Officer
Leaflet telling how parents and school personnel can work together to make life easier for children with asthma.
4 pages

8602 Thinking Big
William Morrow & Company
1350 Avenue of the Americas
New York, NY 10019
212-974-3100
FAX: 212-261-6595
www.williammorrow.com
Eight-year-old Jaime's lively personality shines through in this perceptive photo essay which explains what being a dwarf means physically and then presents Jaime's world at home and at school from her viewpoint. *$15.95*
48 pages

8603 Three Hundred Tips for Making Life with Multiple Sclerosis Easier
Demos Medical Publishing
386 Park Ave S
Suite 201
New York, NY 10016
212-683-0072
800-532-8663
FAX: 212-683-0118
e-mail: orderdep@demosmedpub.com
www.demosmedpub.com

Diana Schneider PhD, President
Phyllis Gold, Owner
This latest book in the Making Life Easier series features tip, techniques and shortcuts for conserving time and energy so you can do more of the things you want to do. These tips should help increase the number of good days you have while encouraging you to develop your own techniques for making life easier. *$18.95*
109 pages 1999
ISBN 1-888799-23-4

8604 Tourette Syndrome Association Annual Medical Letter
4240 Bell Boulevard
Bayside, NY 11361
718-224-2999
800-237-0717
FAX: 718-279-9596
e-mail: ts@tsa-usa.org
www.tsa-usa.org

Fred Cook, Chair
Judit Ungar, President
National, nonprofit membership organization. Mission is to identify the cause of, find the cure for, and control the effects of this disorder. A growing number of local chapters nationwide provide educational materials, seminars, conferences and support groups for over 35,000 members.

8605 Tourette Syndrome Association Children's Newsletter
4240 Bell Boulevard
Bayside, NY 11361
718-224-2999
800-237-0717
FAX: 718-279-9596
e-mail: ts@tsa-usa.org
www.tsa-usa.org

Fred Cook, Chair
Judit Ungar, President
National, nonprofit membership organization. Mission is to identify the cause of, find the cure for, and control the effects of this disorder. A growing number of local chapters nationwide provide educational materials, seminars, conferences and support groups for over 35,000 members.

8606 Tourette Syndrome Association Newsletter
4240 Bell Boulevard
Bayside, NY 11361
718-224-2999
800-237-0717
FAX: 718-279-9596
e-mail: ts@tsa-usa.org
www.tsa-usa.org

Fred Cook, Chair
Judit Ungar, President
National, nonprofit membership organization. Mission is to identify the cause of, find the cure for, and control the effects of this disorder. A growing number of local chapters nationwide provide educational materials, seminars, conferences and support groups for over 35,000 members.
Quarterly

8607 Tourette Syndrome: The Facts
Oxford University Press
198 Madison Avenue
New York, NY 10016
212-726-6000
800-451-7556
FAX: 919-677-1303
www.oup-usa.org

Laura Brown, Chief Executive Officer
The causes of the syndrome, how it is diagnosed, and the ways in which it can be treated. *$19.95*

110 pages 1998
ISBN 0-198523-98-X

8608 Tourette's Syndrome - Tics, Obsessions, Co mpulsions: Developmental Psychopathology
Wiley Publishing
605 3rd Avenue
New York, NY 10158 212-850-6000
FAX: 212-850-6088
Contains 21 contributions compromising the work of researchers associated with the Yale Child Study Center, which has been at the forefront of research on Tourette's syndrome and associated disorders. *$65.00*
600 pages 2001
ISBN 0-471113-75-1

8609 Tourette's Syndrome: Finding Answers and Getting Help
Patient-Centered Guides
101 Morris Street
Sebastopol, CA 95472 707-829-0515
800-998-9938
FAX: 707-829-0104
www.patientcenters.com

Linda Lamb, Editor
Shawnde Paull, Marketing
Tim O'Reilly, Chief Executive Officer
Tourette's Syndrome is a neurological disorder usually diagnosed in childhood and characterized by tics, physical jerks, and involuntary vocalizations. Tourette's can be a devastating disability. The good news is that it's very treatable. Tourette's Syndrome helps you secure a diagnosis, understand medical interventions, get healthcare coverage, and manage Tourette's in family life, school, community, and workplace. *$24.95*
356 pages Paperback
ISBN 0-596500-07-6

8610 Transition in Adolescence
Spina Bifida Association of America
4590 Macarthur Boulevard NW
Suite 250
Washington, DC 20007 202-944-3285
800-621-3141
FAX: 202-944-3295
e-mail: sbaa@sbaa.org
www.sbaa.org

Cindy Brownstein, Chief Executive Officer

8611 Treating Epilepsy Naturally: A Guide to A lternative and Adjunct Therapies
McGraw-Hill Company
2460 Kerper Boulevard
Dubuque, IA 52001 563-588-1451
800-338-3987
FAX: 614-755-5654
www.mhhe.com/hper/physed

Kurt Strand, Vice President
Offers alternative treatments to replace and to complement traditional therapies and sound advice to find the right health practitioner. *$16.95*
288 pages 2001
ISBN 0-658013-79-3

8612 Twitch and Shout
Fanlight Productions
4196 Washington Street
Suite 2
Boston, MA 02131 617-469-4999
800-937-4113
FAX: 617-469-3379
e-mail: fanlight@fanlight.com
www.fanlight.com

Karen McMillen, Marketing Director
Cynthia Conti, Publicity Coordinator
Laurel Chiten, Producer
This documentary provides an intimate journey into the startling world of Tourette Syndrome (TS), a genetic disorder that can cause a bizarre range of involuntary movements, vocalizations, and compulsions. Through the eyes of a photojournalist with TS, the film introduces viewers to others who have this puzzling disorder. This is an emotionally absorbing, sometimes, unsettling, and finally uplifting program about people who must contend with a society that often sees them as crazy or bad. *$275.00*

8613 Understanding Asthma
National Jewish Center for Immunology
1400 Astackson Street
Denver, CO 80206 303-388-4461

e-mail: allstetterw@njc.org
www.njc.org

William Allstetter, Media Relations Manager
Lynn Taussig, Chief Executive Officer
Offers a brief introduction to asthma and then goes into the physiology of asthma, the triggers of asthma, and diagnosis and monitoring of asthma.
27 pages

8614 Understanding Asthma: The Blueprint for Breathing
National Allergy and Asthma Network
3554 Chain Bridge Road
Suite 200
Fairfax, VA 22030 703-385-4403
FAX: 703-352-4354
A layman's guide to asthma facts based on a presentation from the first national asthma patient conference.

8615 Understanding Cystic Fibrosis
University Press of Mississippi

A reference for CF patients and their families. *$12.00*
133 pages 1998
ISBN 0-878059-67-9

8616 Understanding Multiple Sclerosis
MacMillan Publishing Company
135 S Mount Zion Road
Lebanon, IN 46052
FAX: 800-882-8583
Two psychologists discuss their roles with a member who has multiple sclerosis. Includes chapters on adolescents with multiple sclerosis, employment, and research.

8617 Understanding and Coping with Achromatopsia
PO Box 214
Berkeley, CA 94701 510-540-4700
FAX: 510-540-4767
e-mail: futterman@achromat.org
www.achromat.org

8618 Urologic Care of the Child with Spina Bifida
Spina Bifida Association of America
4590 Macarthur Boulevard NW
Suite 250
Washington, DC 20007 202-944-3285
800-621-3141
FAX: 202-944-3295
e-mail: sbaa@sbaa.org
www.sbaa.org

Cindy Brownstein, Chief Executive Officer

8619 Usher Syndrome
Federal Government
31 Center Drive Msc2320
Bethesda, MD 20892
800-241-1044
FAX: 301-402-0018
e-mail: nidcdinfo@nidcd.nih.gov
www.nidcd.nih.gov
Explains what is Usher Syndrome, who is affected by Usher syndrome, what causes Usher syndrome, how is Usher syndrome treated, and what research is being conducted on Usher syndrome.

8620 **Ventilator-Assisted Living**
Post-Polio Health International
4207 Lindell Boulevard
Suite 110
Saint Louis, MO 63108
314-534-0475
FAX: 314-534-5070
TTY:800-735-2966
e-mail: info@post-polio.org
www.post-polio.org

To enhance the lives and independence of ventilator-assisted living by promoting education, networking, and advocacy among these individuals and healthcare providers. Ventilator-Assisted Living supports Post-Polio Health International's educational, research, and advocacy efforts. Offers information about relevant events.
12 pages quarterly

8621 **Voice of the Diabetic**
Diabetes Action Network of the NFB
1412 i 70 Drive SW
Suite C
Columbia, MO 65203
573-875-8911
FAX: 573-875-8902
e-mail: ebrnant@socvet.net
www.nfb.org/voice.htm

Ed Bryant, Editor
Newsletters containing personal stories and practical guidelines by blind diabetics and medical professionals, medical news, resource column and a recipe corner. We are a support and information network for all diabetics.
28 pages Quarterly

8622 **What Everyone Needs to Know About Asthma**
National Allergy and Asthma Network
3554 Chain Bridge Road
Suite 200
Fairfax, VA 22030
703-385-4403
FAX: 703-352-4354
Offers information and facts on gaining control of asthma, asthma triggers and monitoring asthma disorders.

8623 **What School Personnel Should Know About Asthma**
American Lung Association
61 Broadway
New York, NY 10006
212-315-8700
FAX: 212-315-8700
e-mail: info@lungusa.org
www.lungusa.org

John Kirkwood, Chief Executive Officer
Professionally produced videotape discussing the triggers, symptoms and management of childhood asthma.
Video

8624 **What Your Doctor May Not Tell You About Ch ildren's Allergies and Asthma**
Warner Books

The authors explain to parents: why children with allergies are sometimes misdiagnosed as having other ailments; how to use alternative treatments and holistic remedies; simple methods to allergy-proof their homes and pets; the 10 things parents do that make their children's allergy symptoms worse. *$14.95*
336 pages 2003
ISBN 0-446679-88-7

8625 **What's a Virus, Anyway? The Kid's Book About AIDS**
Waterfront Books
85 Crescent Road
Burlington, VT 05401
802-658-7477

A simple introduction to help adults talk with children about the subject of AIDS. Includes children's drawings and questions and provides basic information in a manner appropriate for 4-10 years old. *$8.95*
67 pages

8626 **When the Road Turns: Inspirational Storie s About People with MS**
Health Care Communications
11 Heritage Lane
Rye, NY 10580
845-687-2328

An inspiring collection of stories written by people living with multiple sclerosis. *$12.95*
300 pages 2001
ISBN 1-558749-07-1

8627 **World's Best Books from the Diabetes Experts: Publications Catalog**
American Diabetes Association
1701 N Beauregard Street
Alexandria, VA 22311
703-549-1500
800-232-6733
FAX: 770-442-9742
e-mail: bookorders@diabetes.org
www.diabetes.org

John Fedor, Associate Director
Janel Chrobot, Marketing Specialist
Lynn Nicholas, Chief Executive Officer
A 24 page, full-color catalog of more than 80 books and products for people with diabetes. Titles of categories of books include: cookbooks, meal planning and nutrition, new books and self-care.

8628 **Young Person's Guide to Spina Bifida**
Spina Bifida Association of America
4590 Macarthur Boulevard NW
Suite 250
Washington, DC 20007
202-944-3285
800-621-3141
FAX: 202-944-3295
e-mail: sbaa@sbaa.org
www.sbaa.org

Cindy Brownstein, Chief Executive Officer
Gives practical tips and suggestions for becoming independent and managing your health. *$19.00*

8629 **Your Child and Asthma**
National Jewish Center for Immunology
1400 Jackson Street
Denver, CO 80206
303-388-4461

e-mail: allstetterw@njc.org
www.njc.org

William Allstetter, Media Relations Manager
Lynn Taussig, Chief Executive Officer
A booklet offerring information to parents and family about their child with asthma. Offers information on diagnosis, treatments, triggers and family concerns.

8630 **Your Cleft-Affected Child**
Publishers Group West

Pocket-sized consumer text covers causes of cleft palate and how it can be fixed. Includes advice on feeding, dental and speech-related issues. *$15.95*
288 pages Paperback\ 2001
ISBN 0-897931-85-8

Sports

8631 **National Sports Center for the Disabled**
PO Box 1290
Winter Park, CO 80482
970-726-1540
FAX: 970-726-4112
e-mail: info@nscd.org
www.nscd.org

Craig Politt, President/CEO
Hal O'Leary, Founder
Beth Fox, Operations Manager

Innovative non-profit organization that provides year-round recreation for children and adults with disabilities. The world's largest adaptive ski program, teaching 25,000 lessons per winter at Winter Park Resort, Colorado. Also snowboarding, ski racing, showshoeing, cross-country skiing. Summer sports: rafting, sailing, camping, hiking, hand cycling, mountain biking, tandem biking, in-line skating, horseback riding, fishing, rock climbing. Sports symposium and clinics.

8632 Rehabilitation Institute of Chicago's Virginia Wadsworth Sports Program

710 N Lake Shore Drive
3rd Floor
Chicago, IL 60611
312-238-5002
FAX: 312-238-5017
e-mail: mcarr1@ric.org
www.richealthfit.org

Susan Barclay, President
Laura Davis, VP
Mitch Carr, Fitness Coordinator

RIC's Center for Health and Fitness is a full service fitness center for individuals with disablilties and the administrative offices for RIC's Wirtz Sports Program. Eighteen different sport and recreation programs are offered free of charge. The facility is adjacent to RIC's main building and also is the location of a branch of The National Center for Physical Activity and Disability (NCPAD), a joint project operated by the University of Illinois-Chigcago.

8633 US Paralympics

1 Olympic Plaza
Colorado Springs, CO 80909
719-866-2030
FAX: 719-866-2029
www.usparalympics.org

A division of the US Olympic Committee focused on enhancing programs, funding and opportunities for persons with physical disabilities to participate in Paralymic sports.

Support Groups

8634 AAN's Toll-Free Hotline

Allergy and Asthma Network Mothers of Asthmatics
2751 Prosperity Avenue
Suite 150
Fairfax, VA 22031
703-641-9595
800-878-4403
FAX: 703-573-7794
www.aanma.org

Grace Gerzian, Executive Director

Offers answers to questions regarding allergies and asthma, provides referrals and support to assist the patient and his or her family.

8635 American SIDS Institute

509 Augusta Drive
Marietta, GA 30067
770-426-8746
800-232-7437
FAX: 770-426-1369
www.sids.org

Betty McEntire PhD, Executive Director

American SIDS Institute is a national nonprofit health care organization that is dedicated to the prevention of sudden infant death and the promotion of infant health through an aggressive, comprehensive nationwide program of: research, clinical services, education and family support.

8636 Breaking New Ground Resource Center

Purdue University
1146 Abe Building
W Lafayette, IN 47907
765-494-4600
800-825-4264
FAX: 765-496-1356
e-mail: bng@ecn.purdue.edu
www.agrability.org

William Field, Director
Paul Jones, Information Specialist
Martin Jischke, Chief Executive Officer

A resource center devoted to helping farmers and ranchers with physical disabilities. Several resource materials and a free newsletter are available to anyone.

8637 Camp Candlelight

Eplilepsy Foundation North and Central Alabama
1900 Crestwood Blvd
Birmingham, AL 35210
205-324-4222
800-950-6662
FAX: 205-324-4338
e-mail: epilepsy@aol.com
www.epilepsyfoundation.org/ncalabama/

Joyce Bender, Executive Officer
Heather Hill, Program Director
Angel Burgett, Program Assistant

Every summer, the Epilepsy Foundation offers a week-long camp for children ages 6 to 18. Activities are held on the 230 wooded acres of Camp ASCCA. Trained counselors, program staff and three registered nurses supervise the campers.

8638 Cancer Information Service

National Cancer Institute
6116 Executive Boulevard
Suite 3036a
Bethesda, MD 20892
301-496-2481
800-422-6237
www.cancer.gov

Andrew C Von Eschenback, Director
Sallie Baird, Manager

A nationwide network of 19 regional field offices supported by the National Cancer Institute which provides accurate, up-to-date information on cancer to patients and their families, health professionals and the general public. The CIS can provide specific information in understandable language about particular types of cancer, as well as information on second opinions and the availability of clinical trials.

8639 Clearinghouse on Disability Information: Office of Special Education & Rehab

U S Department of Education
330 C Street SW
Room 3132
Washington, DC 20202
202-208-5815
FAX: 202-401-2608
www.ed.gov/OFFICE/OSERS

Carolyn Corlett, Director
John Sherrod, Executive Director

Provides information to people with disabilities or anyone requesting information, by doing research and providing documents in response to inquiries. The information provided includes areas of federal funding for disability-related programs. Information provided may be useful to disabled individuals and their families, schools and universities, teacher's and/or school administrators, and organizations who have persons with disabilities as clients.

8640 Compassionate Friends

PO Box 3696
Oak Brook, IL 60522
630-990-0010
877-969-0010
FAX: 630-990-0246
e-mail: nationaloffice@compassionatefriends.org
www.compassionatefriends.org

Patricia Loder, Executive Director

Peer support for bereaved parents, grandparents and siblings, offering 600 chapters in the United States. The organization also offers a quarterly magazine, We Need Not Walk Alone, and TCF resources of booklets, tapes and brochures for the bereaved parent, grandparent and sibling.

8641 Cornerstone Services Inc.

777 Joyce Road
Joliet, IL 60436
815-727-6666
FAX: 815-723-1177
e-mail: jhogan@cornerstoneservices.org
www.cornerstoneservices.org

James Hogan, President/CEO

Cornerstone Services provides progressive, comprehensive services for people with disabilities, promoting choice, dignity and the opportunity to live and work in the community. Established in 1969, the agency provides developmental, vocational, residential and behavior health services.

8642 Disability Network
3600 S Dort Highway
Suite 54
Flint, MI 48507
810-742-1800
FAX: 810-742-2400
TTY:810-742-7647
e-mail: tdn@disnetwork.org
www.disnetwork.org

Mike Zelley, President/CEO
The Disability Network's mission is to realize consumer empowerment, self determination, full inclusion and participation of all people in the communities through independent living philosophy and the unequivocal implementation of the Americans with Disabilities Act

8643 Disability and Health, National Center for Birth Defects and Developmental Disabilities
4770 Buford Highway
F-35
Atlanta, GA 30341
770-488-7080
FAX: 770-488-7075
TTY:770-488-7083
e-mail: ncehinfo@cdc.gov
www.cdc.gov/ncbddd/dh

Lisa Sinclair, Health Policy Analyst
Located within the new CDC, National Center for Birth Defects and Developmental Disabilities, the Disability and Health section, operates a ralatively small program that primarily supports: data collection on the prevalence of people with disabilities & their health status and risk factors for poor health and well-being; research on measures of disability, functioning and health; health promotion intervention studies; and dissemination of health information.

8644 Easter Seals
230 W Monroe Street
Suite 1800
Chicago, IL 60606
312-726-6200
800-221-6827
FAX: 312-726-1494
TTY: 312-726-4258
www.easterseals.com

James Williams Jr, Chief Executive Officer
Easter Seals has been helping individuals with disabilities and special needs, and their families, live better lives for over 80 years. From child development centers to physical rehabilitation and job training for people with disabilities, Easter Seals offers a variety of services to help people with disabilities address life's challenges and achieve personal goals.

8645 Epilepsy Foundation for the National Capitol Area
4224 6th Street SE
Washington, DC 20032
202-561-6114

Offers information and referrals, support groups for dually diagnosed persons.

8646 Family Support Project for the Developmentally Disabled
3424 Kossuth Avenue
Room 15a10
Bronx, NY 10467
718-519-5000

Monica Sanabria, Project Coordinator

8647 Head Injury Hotline
PO Box 84151
Seattle, WA 98124
206-329-1371
FAX: 206-329-0912
e-mail: brain@headinjury.com
www.headinjury.com

Disseminates head injury information and provides referrals to facilitate adjustment to life following head injury. Organizes seminars for professionals, head injury survivors, and their families.

8648 Headlines Support Group
Center for Community Re-entry
313 N Main Street
Rockford, IL 61101
815-964-9555
FAX: 815-484-9035

Pamela Solberg, Office Manager
A local support group reaching northern Illinois and southern Wisconsin, for survivors and families of brain injury. The group helps survivors and families cope with awareness difficulties, social adjustment, and leisure awareness. The group shares information regarding head injuries and provides updates from the state and national associations. Headlines continually searches for new ideas, information and services which can help survivors fulfill their maximum potential.

8649 Human Policy Press
Center on Human Policy
PO Box 35127
Syracuse, NY 13235
315-443-2761
800-894-0826
FAX: 315-443-4338
e-mail: thechp@sued.syr.edu
thechp.syr.edu/humanpolicypress/

Rachael Zubal-Ruggieri, Information Coordinator
Independent press started by the Center on Human Policy in 1974 to promote positive attitudes towards people with disabilities.

8650 International Braille and Technology Center for the Blind
National Federation of the Blind
1800 Johnson Street
Baltimore, MD 21230
410-659-9314
FAX: 410-685-5653
e-mail: nfb@nfb.org
www.nfb.org

Marc Maurer, President
Joyce Scanlan, Program Director
World's largest and most complete evaluation and demonstration center of all assistive technology used by the blind from around the world. Includes all braille, synthetic speech, print-to-speech scanning, internet and portable devices and programs. Available for tours by appointment to blind persons, employers, technology manufacturers, teachers, parents and those working in the assistive technology field.

8651 Kaleidoscope Network
1777 NE Loop 410
Suite 300
San Antonio, TX 78217
210-436-2611
FAX: 210-829-1388
www.kALIVE.com

Phyllis Nichols, Chief Operating Officer
Ron Dixon, President Programming Production
KALEIDOSCOPE Network, inc. (KNI) is a broadband, multimedia health and lifestyle company which produces and distributes television and on-line programming and content emphasizing health and wellness. KNI airs its programming on PAX Television with a reach to 73% of the country or 74 million households. KNI's interactive web site provides authoritative health content, with links to its more than 240 health and disability-related National Advisory Board organizations.

8652 Lung Line Information Service
National Jewish Center for Immunology
1400 Jackson Street
Denver, CO 80206
303-697-5095
800-222-LUNG
www.nationaljewish.org

Lynn Taussig, President
Kris Frederickson, Owner
A free information service answering questions, sending literature and giving advice to patients with immunologic or respiratory illnesses. The Line is an educational service and not a substitute for medical care. Diagnosis or suggested treatment will not be provided for a caller's specific condition.

8653 Medic Alert Foundation, International
2323 Colorado Avenue
Turlock, CA 95382
209-668-3333
800-432-5378
FAX: 209-669-2495
e-mail: customer_service@medicalert.org
www.medicalert.org

Paul Kortschak, Chief Executive Officer
Emergency medallions and bracelets containing emergency medical information and 24-hour emergency information telephone services.

8654 Medicaid Information
7500 Security Boulevard
Baltimore, MD 21244
410-786-3000
877-267-2323
www.cms.hhs.gov

Michelle Snyder, Executive Director
Information about eligibility and benefits for needy citizens who require health care is available by contacting the Health Care Financing administration or by contacting the local public welfare office.

8655 Medicare Information
200 Independence Avenue SE
Washington, DC 20201
202-690-6726
www.medicare.gov

Thomas Scully, President
Eligibility and benefits for the health care of the older american is available by contacting the health care financing office.

8656 National AIDS Hotline
Centers for Disease Control and Prevention
1600 Clifton Road NE
Atlanta, GA 30329
404-639-3533
800-342-2437
www.cdc.gov

Julie Gerberding, Director
Elizabeth Unger PhD
Offers free confidential information and publications on HIV infection and AIDS.

8657 National Association for Home Care
Val J Halomandaris
228 7th Street SE
Washington, DC 20003
202-547-7424
FAX: 202-547-3540
e-mail: webmaster@nahc.org
www.nahc.org

Val J Halamandaris, President
Kristy Wright, Vice Chairman
This is a non-profit trade association representing various home care, hospice and health aid organizations. Website contains a section with information on how to choose a home care provider and a zip code driven locator for home care and hospice. Publishes monthly newsletter.

8658 National Institute of Child Health and Human Development
PO Box 3006
Rockville, MD 20847
301-496-7339
800-370-2943
FAX: 301-984-1473
e-mail: NICHDInformationResourceCenter@mail.nih.gov
www.nichd.nih.gov

Duane Alexander, Director
Yvonne Thompson Maddox, Deputy Director
Sandra Ott, Manager
Government agency that supports and conducts research on topics related to the health of children, adults, families and communities; offers free materials and information.

8659 National Service Dog Center
Delta Society
875 124th Avenue NE
Suite 101
Bellevue, WA 98005
425-226-7357
FAX: 425-235-1076
e-mail: info@deltasociety.org
www.deltasociety.org

Robert T Franklin, Chairman
Alex Bolen, Chairman
Lawrence Norvell, Chief Executive Officer
A service of the Delta Society, provides information about the selection, training, stewardship, and roles of service dogs; referral to service dog training programs and related resources; education to businesses and health care professionals regarding service dog issues; research assistance through a resource library and network of professional experts and advocacy on behalf of people with service dogs.

8660 PALS Support Groups
Parent Professional Advocacy League
45 Bromfield Street
10th Floor
Boston, MA 02108
617-542-7860
866-815-8122
FAX: 617-542-7832
e-mail: info@ppal.net
http://ppal.net/default/

Andy Pond, Chair
Lisa Lambert, Executive Director
Offers emotional support to parents and families of disabled children.

8661 PXE International
4301 Connecticut Avenue NW
Suite 404
Washington, DC 20008
202-362-9599
FAX: 202-966-8553
e-mail: info@pxe.org
www.pxe.org

Sharon Terry, Executive Director/Owner
Offers vital services to those with pseudoxanthoma elasticum, a connective tissue disorder causing calcification of connective tissue in various places throughout the body, often affecting the membrane behind the eye.

8662 Parent Assistance Network
Good Samaritan Health Systems
PO Box 1810
Kearney, NE 68848
308-865-2009
FAX: 308-865-2933
e-mail: sheilameyer@catholichealth.net
www.gshs.org

Sheila Meyer, Parent Assistance Service Coordi
Laura Meyer, Director
Provides information and emotional support to all parents and especially to parents of children with disabilities in the central Nebraska area. Ongoing activities include parent support group meetings, parent-to-parent networking and referrals and Respite Care provider trainings.

8663 Parent as Parnters in Education of Alabama
576 Azalea Rd. Suite 105
PO Box 161274
Mobile, AL 36616
251-478-1208
800-222-7322
FAX: 251-473-7877
e-mail: seacofmobile@seacpac.com
www.parentsaspartnersineducation.com

Dr Barbara Wheat, Director

8664 Post-Polio Support Group
Hinsdale Hospital
120 N Oak Street
Hinsdale, IL 60521
630-856-9000
FAX: 630-856-7524
www.ahsmidwest.org

Todd Werner, Chief Executive Officer

Information and support for polio patients and their families; meets the fourth Wednesday of each month.

8665 Prevent Child Abuse of Metropolitan Washington
7404 Salford Court
Alexandria, VA 22315
202-223-0020
FAX: 202-296-4046
e-mail: pcamw@juno.com
www.pcamw.org

Kendra Dunn, Executive Director
Through public education, community partnerships and support services, PCAMW helps everyone play a role in prevention. We share information on prevention stategies and effective parenting at community forums and events and advocate for policies and services that keep children safe. We operate PhoneFriend, a telephone support line for children at home without adult supervision and conduct personal safety workshops in schools, camps and libraries. PhoneFriend support line: 202-223-2244.

8666 RET Project: (Rehabilitation Engineering Technology San Francisco State University
1600 Holloway Avenue
San Francisco, CA 94132
415-338-1333
FAX: 415-338-1501
e-mail: rgrott@sfsu.edu

Ray Grott, Director
RET Training Project is designed as a one-year Graduate Certificate program for people interested in the field of assistive technology used by people with disabilities.

8667 Son-Rise Program
2080 S Undermountain Road
Sheffield, MA 01257
413-229-2100
800-714-2779
FAX: 413-229-3202
e-mail: sonrise@option.org
www.autismtreatmentcenter.org

Glenna Klein, Publicist
Internationally renowned and highly effective method for working with children challenged by autism, autism spectrum disorders, PDD and all other developmental difficulties. The program teaches parents, relatives, volunteers and professionals how to design and implement a child-centered, home-based educational program. Modality comprises an innovative and comprehensive system for learning and growth with specific impact in areas including eye contact, speech and communication and more.

8668 Special Children
1306 Wabash Avenue
Belleville, IL 62220
618-234-6876
FAX: 618-234-6150
e-mail: kcullan@peaknet.net
www.specialchildren.net

Kathleen Cullen, Executive Director
John Hill, Controller/Accountant
A nonprofit agency serving children with developmental disabilities ages birth to 6 years

8669 Special Education Action Commette
PO Box 161274
Mobile, AL 36616
251-478-1208

Mavis Smith, Executive Director

8670 Support Works
1018 East Boulevard
Suite 5
Charlotte, NC 28203
704-331-9500

www.supportworks.org

Joel Fisher, Owner
SupportWorks helps people find and form support groups. An 8 page publication Power Tools, clearly walks new group leaders through steps of putting together a healthy self-help group. SupportWorks also has a telephone conference program which allows people with similar diseases or other nonprofit issues to meet by phone conference for free or at very low cost.

8671 Teratogen and Birth Defects Information Project
University of South Dakota
414 E Clark Street
Vermillion, SD 57069
605-677-5306
FAX: 605-677-5778

Jim Abbott, President
For South Dakota residents only.

8672 Toll-Free Information Line
Asthma and Allergy Foundation of America
1233 20th Street NW
Suite 402
Washington, DC 20036
202-466-7643
800-7AS-THMA
FAX: 202-466-8940
e-mail: Unfo@aafa.org
www.aafa.org

08082007, author
Bill Lin, Executive Director
I
AG pages

8673 Visiting Nurse Association of America
99 Summer Street
Suite 1700
Boston, MA 02110
617-737-3200
888-866-8773
FAX: 617-737-1144
e-mail: vnaa@vnaa.org
www.vnaa.org

Andy Carter, President
Judy Duhl, Director
Scott Gardner, Director
The VNAA is the official national association for not-for-profit, community based home health organizations known as the Visiting Nurse Associations (VNA's). They created the profession of home health care more then 100 years ag. They have a united mission to bring compassionate, high-quality and cost-effective home care to individuals in their communities.

Associations

8674 American Speech-Language-Hearing Association
10801 Rockville Pike
Rockville, MD 20852
240-638-8255
888-498-6699
FAX: 240-333-4705
e-mail: actioncenter@asha.org
www.asha.org

Lawrence W Higdon, President
Arlene Pietranton, Executive Director
Roberta B Aungst, VP
Provides information for both the general public and physicians in an easy-to-access manner, on speech, hearing and language disorders. Exhibits by companies specializing in alternative and augmentative communications products, publishers, software and hardware companies, and hearing aid testing equipment manufacturers.

8675 Davis Center for Hearing, Speech and Learning: Hearing Therapy
200 Valley Road
Suite 205
Mt. Arlington, NJ 07856
973-398-2710
FAX: 973-398-2721
e-mail: info@daviscenter.net
www.thedaviscenter.com

Dorinne S Davis MA, CCC-A, FAAA, Director
Laura Darby, Sound Therapist
Janine Ruth MA, Child Development Specialist
The Davis Center's Sound Therapy Programs make positive changes for children and adults with Autism, ADD/ADHD, Auditory Processing Issues, Dyslexia, Learning Disabilities and other learning challenges. Our programs adress issues such as: phonics, spelling, writing, reading comprehension, hearing only parts of words, following directions, discriminating between sounds, sound sensitivity, behavioral responses, focus, attention and more.

8676 Deafness and Communicative Disorders Branch of Rehab Services Administration Office
Special Education And Rehab Services
400 Maryland Avenue SW
Washington, DC 20202
202-245-7489
800-872-5327
FAX: 202-205-9340
TTY: 800-437-0833
e-mail: customerservice@inet.ed.gov
www.ed.gov

Clare Cotton, Chairperson
Promotes improved rehabilitation services for deaf and hard of hearing people and individuals with speech or language impairments. Provides technical assistance to public and private agencies and individuals.

8677 National Center for Accessible Media
Wgbh Educational Foundation
125 Western Avenue
Boston, MA 02134
617-300-3400
FAX: 617-300-1035
TTY:617-300-2489
e-mail: ncam@wgbh.org
ncam.wgbh.org

Larry Goldberg, Director
Brad Botkin, Director
Marcia Brooks, Project Director
Aims to increase access to public mass media (television, radio, print, movies, multimedia) for unserved customers, such as disabled people or speakers of other languages.

8678 National Cued Speech Association
Information Service
5619 McClean Drive
Bethesda, MD 20814
301-915-8009
800-459-3529
FAX: 301-915-8009
TTY: 800-459-3529
www.cuedspeech.org

Sarina Roffe, President
Susan Coffer, Vice President
Polly Earl, Secretary
The NCSA champions effective communication, language development and literacy through the use of cued speech. The NCSA envisions that individuals communicate effectively in the languageof their family and society. Families are informed about Cued Speech along with other communication options. Their rights are respected and instruction is provided to facilitate the use of cued languages. Students achieve literacy through full access to language and education.

8679 Providence Speech and Hearing Center
1301 W Providence Avenue
Orange, CA 92868
714-639-4990
FAX: 714-744-3841
e-mail: pshc@pshc.org
www.pshc.org

Raul Lopez, COO/Director Of Finance
Elaine Brewster, Director Of Rehibilitation
Bobbi Dickinson, Co-Director
Mission is to provide the highest quality services available in the identification, diagnosis, treatment and prevention of speech, language and hearing disorders for persons of all ages.

8680 Scottish Rite Center for Childhood Language Disorders
Childrens Hospital
3227 N.E. 125th Street
Seattle, WA 98125
206-324-6293
FAX: 206-324-3332
www.srccld.org

T Robinson, Executive Director
Offers speech-language evaluations and treatment, hearing screening and consultations to children ages birth through adolescence. Bilingual services are also available.

8681 Stuttering Foundation of America
3100 Walnut Grove Road
Memphis, TN 38111
901-452-7343
800-992-9392
FAX: 901-452-3931
e-mail: info@stutteringhelp.org
www.stutteringhelp.org

Jane Fraser, President
Anne Edwards, Coordinator
Toll-free hotline, brochures, books and videotapes on stuttering.

8682 Texas Speech-Language-Hearing Association
918 Congress Avenue
Suite 200
Austin, TX 78701
512-494-1127
888-729-8742
FAX: 512-494-1129
e-mail: tsha@assnmgmt.com
www.txsha.org

Don Canada, Executive Director
Traci Miller, Associate Manager
Krista Richter, Meeting And Event Manager
Mission is to encourage and promote the role of the speech-language pathologist and audiologist as a professional in the delivery of clinical services to persons with communications disorders. Encourages basic scientific study of processes of individual human communication with reference to speech, hearing and language.

Camps

8683 Camp Chatterbox
150 New Providence Road
Mountainside, NJ 07092 908-301-5451
e-mail: campchatterbox@earthlink.net
www.campchatterbox.org

Joan Bruno, Director
Is an intensive therapy camp for children ages 5-16, who use augmentative and alternative communications (AAC) devices and a training program for their parents. A unique feature of Camp Chatterbox is that a parent attends the program with his or her child. This not only widens the scope of training opportunities for the parents, but it helps siblings become an integral part of the training program. Parents, siblings and campers stay together in the cabins with campers of similar ages.

8684 Childrens Beach House
100 W 10th Street
Suite 411
Wilmington, DE 19801 302-655-4288
FAX: 302-655-4216
e-mail: inquiry@cbhinc.org
www.cbhinc.org

Teresa Tipton, Program Coordinator
Richard Garrett, Director
Rick Deale, Camp Director
Camp is located in Lewes, Delaware. Four-week sessions June-August for Delaware children with hearing impairment or speech/communication impairment. Coed, ages 6-12.

8685 Easter Seals Oklahoma
Easter Seals America
701 Northeast 13th Street
Oklahoma City, OK 73104 405-239-2525
FAX: 405-239-2278
e-mail: esok1@coxinet.net
www.eastersealsoklahoma.org

Patricia Filer, Executive Director
Providing services such as adult day services, child development center, OTIPT, speech therapy, reading/tutoring, vision and hearing screening.

8686 Meadowood Springs Speech and Hearing Camp
Institute for Rehabilitation Research
PO Box 1025
Pendleton, OR 97801 541-276-2752
FAX: 541-276-7227
e-mail: meadowoodcamp@uci.net
www.meadowoodsprings.com

Irene Willard, Administrator
Marie Story, Assistant
On 143 acres in the Blue Mountains of Eastern Oregon, this camp is designed to help young people who have diagnosed clinical disorders of speech, hearing or language. A full range of activities in recreational and clinical areas is available.

8687 Multiple Sclerosis Q&A: Reassuring Answer s to Frequently Asked Questions
Avery Publishing Group
375 Hudson Street
New York, NY 10014 212-366-2000

Answers to many questions that overwhelm those undergoing testing and treatment for multiple sclerosis. It discusses traditional and complementary therapies for MS; explains medical terminology and diagnostics; and compassionately addresses the lifestyle changes many patients face while learning to manage this chronic and potentially debilitating disorder. *$14.95*
208 pages 2003
ISBN 1-583331-74-3

8688 Sequanota
PO Box 245
Jennerstown, PA 15547 814-629-6627
FAX: 814-629-0128
e-mail: campsequanota@foodcity.net
www.sequanota.net

Heather Dungey, Program Director
George Mason, Interim-Executive Director
Summer sessions for adults with developmental disabilities and speech/communication impairment.

8689 University of Iowa: Wendell Johnson Speech and Hearing Clinic
250 Hawkins Drive
Iowa City, IA 52242 319-335-1845
FAX: 319-335-8851
e-mail: wendy-fick@uiowa.edu
www.shc.uiowa.edu

Linda Louko, Clinic Director
Marlea O'Brien, Child Language Research Center
Dorothy Albright, Department Administration
The clinic offers assessment and remediation for communication disorders in adults and children. The clinic also offers a Intensive Summer Residential Clinic for school age children needing intervention services because of speech, language, hearing and/or reading problems.

8690 YMCA Camp Fitch
Youngstown YMCA
17 North Champion Street
Youngstown, OH 44503 330-744-8411
FAX: 330-744-8416
www.campfitch.com

Mike Shaffer, Executive Director
Kathy Portman, Assistant Director
Camp is located in North Springfield, Pennsylvania. Camping sessions for children and adults with diabetes, hearing impairment, developmental disabilities, mobility limitation and speech/communication impairment. Ages 8-16, families and seniors.

Print & Non-Print Resources

8691 ASHA Leader
American Speech-Language-Hearing Association
10801 Rockville Pike
Rockville, MD 20852 301-897-5700
800-638-8255
FAX: 301-897-7348
e-mail: actioncenter@asha.org
www.asha.org

Joanne K Jessen, Publications Director
John E Bernthal, President
Arlene Pietranton, Executive Director
Association publication containing news, notices of events and activities and information for members on issues facing the profession of audiology and speech-language pathology. *$80.00*
35 pages 2 x month

8692 American Forensic Association Journal
American Forensic Association
University of Wisconsin River Fls
River Falls, WI 54022 715-425-3198
FAX: 715-425-9533
e-mail: james.wpratt@uwrf.edu

James Pratt, Manager
Communication disorders newsletter. *$25.00*

8693 American Journal of Speech-Language Pathology
American Speech-Language-Hearing Association
10801 Rockville Pike
Rockville, MD 20852 301-897-5700
800-638-8255
FAX: 301-897-7348
e-mail: info@asha.org
www.asha.org

John E Bernthal, President
Arlene Pietranton, Executive Director
Joanne Jessen, Publications Director

8694 Aphasia
Federal Government
31 Center Drive Msc2320
Bethesda, MD 20892
800-241-1044
FAX: 301-402-0018
e-mail: nidcdinfo@nidcd.nih.gov
www.aphasia.org/NAAfactsheet.html

This fact sheet explains who has aphasia, the causes of aphasia, how aphasia is diagnosed and treated, and what research is being conducted on aphasia.

8695 Aphasia: What is It?
Speech Bin
1965 25th Avenue
Vero Beach, FL 32960
772-770-0007
800-477-3324
FAX: 772-770-0006
www.speechbin.com

Brochures for families and caregivers of persons who have suffered aphasic language disorders secondary to strokes. Set of ten copies. *$14.95*

16 pages Package of 10
ISBN 0-93785 -56-4

8696 Augmentative and Alternative Communication International Society For (ISAAC)
Suite 308
49 The Donway West
Toronto, Ontario, Canada, M3C-3
416-385-0351
FAX: 416-385-0352
e-mail: info@issaconline.org
www.isaac-online.org

This 2nd edition contains the most recent information available on implementing augmentative and alternative communication (AAC), explaining principles and procedures of AAC assessment and offering intervention techniques. *$59.95*

592 pages Hardcover 1998
ISBN 1-55766 -33-5

8697 Beyond Baby Talk: From Sounds to Sentence s, a Parent's Guide to Language Development
Prima Publishing
PO Box 1260
Rocklin, CA 95677
916-787-7000
800-632-8676
FAX: 916-787-7001
e-mail: websupportlife@primapub.com
www.primapublishing.com

The authors discuss the best ways to help your child develop the all-important skill of communication and to recognize the signs of language development problems. *$15.00*

224 pages 2001
ISBN 0-761526-47-1

8698 Breaking the Speech Barrier: Language Develpment Through Augmented Means
Brookes Publishing
PO Box 10624
Baltimore, MD 21285
410-337-9580
800-638-3775
FAX: 410-337-8539
e-mail: custserv@brookespublishing.com
www.brookespublishing.com

Paul Brooks, Owner

This resource describes the creation of the System for Augmenting Language (SAL) for school-age youth with mental retardation and offers important insights into the language development of children who are not learning to communicate typically. *$37.00*

224 pages Paperback
ISBN 1-557663-90-4

8699 Building Communicative Competence with Indiv. Who Use Augmentative & Alternative Commun.
Brookes Publishing
PO Box 10624
Baltimore, MD 21285
410-337-9580
800-638-3775
FAX: 410-337-8539
e-mail: custserv@brookespublishing.com
www.brookespublishing.com

Paul Brooks, Owner

This is a hands-on instructional program offering goal-setting, teaching, and coaching methods for improving the communicative skills of people who depend on AAC systems. Appropriate for children, adolescents, and adults at any state of communicative development. *$36.95*

336 pages Spiral-bound 1997
ISBN 1-55766 -24-6

8700 Burnish Me Bright
Pantheon Books
1540 Broadway
New York, NY 10036
212-782-9000
800-638-6460
FAX: 212-302-7985
www.randomhouse.com/pantheon/

Carol Schneider, Marketing Executive

Hilaire, a famous mime, had retired to a small village to live out his life. He met frail Auguste, who was unable to speak, and immediately he saw the potential for this agile and physically expressive youth to become a mime.

80 pages Hardcover 1970

8701 Childhood Speech, Language & Listening Pro blems
Wiley Publishing
605 3rd Avenue
New York, NY 10158
212-850-6000
FAX: 212-850-6088

Language pathologist Hamaguchi employs her 15 years of experience to show parents how to recognize the most common speech, language, and listening problems. *$16.95*

224 pages Paperback 2001
ISBN 0-471387-53-3

8702 Communication Coloring Book
Speech Bin
1965 25th Avenue
Vero Beach, FL 32960
772-770-0007
800-477-3324
FAX: 772-770-0006
www.speechbin.com

Jan J Binney, VP

Publisher and distributor of books and materials for professionals in rehabilitation, speech-language pathology, special education and related fields and persons interested in communication disorders and related disabilities. Major product lines include professional and children's books, computer software, diagnostic tests, instructional games and materials for children and adults and specialty items. *$14.95*

48 pages
ISBN 0-93785 -53-0

8703 Communication Development and Disorders in African American Children
Brookes Publishing
PO Box 10624
Baltimore, MD 21285
410-337-9580
800-638-3775
FAX: 410-337-8539
e-mail: custserv@brookespublishing.com
www.brookespublishing.com

Paul Brooks, Owner

Research, Assessment, and Intervention. This text presents research on communication disorders and language development in African American children. Also addresses multicultural aspects of service delivery and intervention and discusses issues in assessing, diagnosing, and treating communication disorders. *$39.00*

400 pages Paperback
ISBN 1-55766 -53-3

8704 Communication Development in Children with Down Syndrome
Brookes Publishing
PO Box 10624
Baltimore, MD 21285
410-337-9580
800-638-3775
FAX: 410-337-8539
e-mail: custserv@brookespublishing.com
www.brookespublishing.com

Paul Brooks, Owner

This book offers an extensive, detailed explanation of communication development in children with Down syndrome relative to their advancing cognitive skills. It introduces a critical framework for assessing and treating hearing, speech, and language problems and provides explicit intervention methods and tested clinical protocols.

Paperback 1998
ISBN 1-55766 -50-5

8705 Communication Outlook
Artificial Language Laboratory
405 Computer Center
East Lansing, MI 48824
517-353-0870
FAX: 517-353-4766
e-mail: artling@msu.edu
www.msu.edu/~artlang

Caroline Watt, Editor
Katie Smith, Editor
Communication Outlook (CO) is an international quarterly magazine, which focuses on the techniques and technology of augmentative and alternative communication. CO provides information on technological developments for persons experiencing communication handicaps due to neurological, sensory or neuromuscular conditions. *$18.00*

32 pages Quarterly

8706 Connect
Hearing, Speech & Deafness Center (HSDC)
1625 19th Avenue
Seattle, WA 98122
206-323-5770
FAX: 206-328-6871
e-mail: hsdc@hsdc.org
www.hsdc.org

David Delmar, Editor
Susie Burdick, Executive Director
A not-for-profit United Way Agency building community through communications since 1937. Call V/TTY. The mission of HSDC is to strengthen community by promoting effective communication

8 pages Quarterly

8707 Coping for Kids Who Stutter
Speech Bin
1965 25th Avenue
Vero Beach, FL 32960
772-770-0007
800-477-3324
FAX: 772-770-0006
www.speechbin.com

Jan J Binney, Senior Editor
Informative book for children and adults about stuttering and how to manage it. *$15.95*

32 pages
ISBN 0-93785 -43-2

8708 Disorders of Motor Speech: Assessment, Treatment, and Clinical Characterization
Brookes Publishing
PO Box 10624
Baltimore, MD 21285
410-337-9580
800-638-3775
FAX: 410-337-8539
e-mail: custserv@brookespublishing.com
www.brookespublishing.com

Paul Brooks, Owner
This book provides a probing examination of normal, dysarthric, and apraxic speech. Great for speech-language pathologists, neurologists, physical or occupational therapists, and physiatrists. *$47.00*

400 pages Hardcover
ISBN 1-55766 -23-1

8709 Employment for Individuals with Asperger S yndrome or Non-Verbal Learning Disability
Taylor & Francis
47 Runway Drive
Suite G
Levittown, PA 19057
215-269-0400
FAX: 215-625-2940

Harold Stecker, President
With practical and technical advice on everything from job-hunting to interview techniques, from fitting in in the workplace to whether or not to disclose diagnosis, this book guides people with NLD or AS successfully through the employment field. *$22.95*

272 pages 2004
ISBN 1-843107-66-X

8710 Enhancing Communication in Individuals with Autism Through Pictures/Words
Autism Society of North Carolina Bookstore
505 Oberlin Road
Suite 230
Raleigh, NC 27605
919-743-0204
800-442-2762
FAX: 919-743-0208
e-mail: dcoffey@autismsociety-nc.org
www.autismsociety-nc.org

Darla Coffey, Bookstore Manager
Jill Keel, Executive Director
Booklet addressing the description and implementation of visually aided communication. *$4.00*

8711 Getting Started with Facilitated Communication
Syracuse University, Institute on Communication
805 S Krouse
Syracuse, NY 13244
315-443-4485

Raymond Colton, Manager
Describes in detail how to help individuals with autism and/or severe communication difficulties to get started with facilitated communication.

Video

8712 Guide to Developing Language Competence in Handicapped Preschool Children
Charles C Thomas
2600 S 1st Street
Springfield, IL 62704
217-789-8980
800-258-8980
FAX: 217-789-9130
e-mail: books@ccthomas.com
www.ccthomas.com

Ennio Cipani
Michael Thomas, President
Job placement programs, remunerative work services and work adjustment training programs handicaps: teachers, administrators and parents. *$54.95*

268 pages Cloth 1991
ISBN 0-398057-48-6

8713 Hearing, Speech & Deafness Center (HSDC)
1625 19th Avenue
Seattle, WA 98122
206-323-5770
FAX: 206-328-6871
e-mail: hsdc@hsdc.org
www.hsdc.org

Susie Burdick, Development/Marketing Director
David Stoner, Editor
Mission is to enrich the lives of all adults and children who experience hearing loss, speech and language impairments, or who are deaf, by providing professional services and technology, and by promoting community awareness and accessibility. A not-for-profit United Way Agency.

16 pages Yearly 1937

8714 Hearing, Speech and Deafness Center (HSDC)
Hearing, Speech & Deafness Center (HSDC)
1625 19th Avenue
Seattle, WA 98122
206-323-5770
FAX: 206-328-6871
e-mail: hsdc@hsdc.org
www.hsdc.org

Susie Burdick, Executive Director
Our mission is to enrich lives of all adults and children who experience hearing loss, speech and language impairments or who are deaf, by providing professional services and by promoting community awareness and accessibility.

8715 **If Your Child Stutters: A Guide for Parents**
Stuttering Foundation of America
PO Box 11749
Suite 603
Memphis, TN 38111
901-452-7343
800-992-9392
FAX: 901-452-3931
e-mail: info@stutteringhelp.org
www.stutterhelp.org

Jane Fraser, President
A guide that enables parents to provide appropriate help to children who stutter. *$1.00*

8716 **Is the Child Really Stuttering? Questions & Answers About Disfluency**
Speech Bin
1965 25th Avenue
Vero Beach, FL 32960
772-770-0007
800-477-3324
FAX: 772-770-0006
www.speechbin.com
In a question and answer format concisely shows differences between normal developmental and abnorlam disfluency and motivates adult listeners to deal with problems speech behaviors in a positive way. Set of ten brochures. *$9.95*

8717 **Journal of Speech, Language and Hearing Re search**
American Speech-Language-Hearing Association
10801 Rockville Pike
Rockville, MD 20852
301-897-5700
800-638-8255
FAX: 301-897-7348
e-mail: irc@asha.org
www.asha.org

John E Berntah;, President
Arlene Pietranton, Executive Director
Joanne Jessen, Publications Director
Pertains broadly to studies of the processess and disorders of hearing, language, and speech diagnosis and treatment of such disorders.

8718 **Kitten Who Couldn't Purr**
William Morrow & Company
1350 Avenue of the Americas
New York, NY 10019
212-261-6500
FAX: 212-261-6925
Jonathan the kitten doesn't know how to purr to say thank you, so he sets off to find someone to teach him. *$12.95*
32 pages

8719 **Language Disabilities in Children and Adolescents**
McGraw-Hill School Publishing
220 East Danieldale Road
Desoto, TX 75115
972-224-1111
800-442-9685
FAX: 972-228-1982
www.mhschool.com

Joseph Gavigan, President
A comprehensive review of research in language disabilities.

8720 **Language and the Developing Child**
International Dyslexia Association
382 S Chester Street
Baltimore, MD 21231
800-ABC-D123
FAX: 410-296-0232
www.interdys.org
This collection of papers introduces a new generation of teachers, clinicians and parents to the work of one of the key figures in the search for the causes and treatment of dyslexia. *$15.00*

8721 **Language-Related Learning Disabilities: Their Nature and Treatment**
Brookes Publishing
PO Box 10624
Baltimore, MD 21285
410-337-9580
800-638-3775
FAX: 410-337-8539
e-mail: custserv@brookespublishing.com
www.brookespublishing.com

Paul Brooks, Owner
$47.00
464 pages Paperback
ISBN 1-55766-53-0

8722 **Late Talker: What to Do If Your Child Isn' t Talking Yet**
St Martin's Griffin

This handbook offers advice on ways to identify the warning signs of a speech disorder, information on how to get the right kind of evaluations and therapy, ways to obtain appropriate services through the school system and health insurance, at-home activities that parents can do with their child to stimulate speech, benefits of nutritional supplementation, and advice from experienced parents who've been there on what to expect and what you can do to be your child's best advocate. *$13.95*
256 pages Paperback 2004
ISBN 0-312309-24-4

8723 **Lollipop Lunch**
Speech Bin
1965 25th Avenue
Vero Beach, FL 32960
772-770-0007
800-477-3324
FAX: 772-770-0006
www.speechbin.com
Cleverly illustrated stories and activities for phonological and language development. *$19.95*
128 pages
ISBN 0-93785 -54-8

8724 **Motor Speech Disorders**
WB Saunders Company
1810 Creekside Lane
Darien, IL 60561
630-910-0749
FAX: 630-910-5789
www.wbsaunders.com
Professional text on rehabilitation techniques for motor speech disorders. *$74.00*
304 pages
ISBN 0-72162 -78-8

8725 **Motor Speech Disorders: Advances in Assessment and Treatment**
Brookes Publishing
PO Box 10624
Baltimore, MD 21285
410-337-9580
800-638-3775
FAX: 410-337-8539
e-mail: custserv@brookespublishing.com
www.brookespublishing.com

Paul Brooks, Owner
$38.00
288 pages Paperback
ISBN 1-55766 -37-5

8726 **Neuromotor Speech Disorders: Nature, Assessment, and Management**
Brookes Publishing
PO Box 10624
Baltimore, MD 21285
410-337-9580
800-638-3775
FAX: 410-337-8539
e-mail: custserv@brookespublishing.com
www.brookespublishing.com

Paul Brooks, Owner
Topics included in this book are: motor-speech imaging, anatomical structure and function in dysarthria, physiological and acoustic analyses of dysarthria intelligibility, dysphonia, and linguistic considerations in apraxia of speech. *$44.95*
320 pages Hardcover 1998
ISBN 1-55766 -26-2

8727 **Nonverbal Learning Disabilities at Home: A Parent's Guide**
Taylor & Francis Group

Explores the variety of daily life problems children with NLD may face, and provides practical strategies for parents to help them cope and grow, from preschool age through their challenging adolescent years. *$21.95*

267 pages Paperback 2001

ISBN 1-853029-40-8

8728 Perspectives: Whole Language Folio

Gallaudet University Bookstore
800 Florida Avenue NE
Washington, DC 20002
202-651-5000
800-451-1073
FAX: 202-651-5489

Erving Jordan, President

The 19 articles in this collection offer practical help to teachers seeking to emphasize whole language strategies in their classroom. *$9.95*

64 pages

8729 Promoting Communication in Infants and Young Children: 500 Ways to Succeed

Speech Bin
1965 25th Avenue
Vero Beach, FL 32960
772-770-0007
800-477-3324
FAX: 772-770-0006
www.speechbin.com

This practical reference for parents, caregivers and professional service providers how to promote communication development in infants and young children. Gives down-to-earth information and activities to help your youngest children succeed. It provides step-by-step suggestions for stimulationg children's speech and language skills. Paperback. *$14.95*

8730 Reading, Writing and Speech Problems in Children

International Dyslexia Association
382 S Chester Street
Baltimore, MD 21231
800-ABC-D123
FAX: 410-296-0232
www.interdys.org

A tribute to the man who more than any other aroused the attention of the scientific community and who provided the sound educational principles on which much teaching of dyslexics today is based. *$27.00*

ISBN 0-89079 -79-1

8731 Self-Therapy for the Stutterer

Stuttering Foundation of America
PO Box 11749
Memphis, TN 38111
901-452-7343
800-992-9392
FAX: 901-452-3931
e-mail: stutter@vantek.net
www.stutterhelp.org

Jane Fraser, President

A guide to help adults who stutter overcome the problem on their own. *$3.00*

191 pages Paperback

ISBN 0-933388-32-2

8732 Sound Connections for the Adolescent

Speech Bin
1965 25th Avenue
Vero Beach, FL 32960
772-770-0007
800-477-3324
FAX: 772-770-0006
www.speechbin.com

A resource to help older elementary and secondary students understand their sound systems an how it functions. It targets skills critical for academic achievement: phonological awareness, phonemic relationships, phonemic processing, listening and memory and teaches linguistic rules they need to succeed. *$19.95*

Paperback

8733 Stuttering

Federal Government
31 Center Drive Msc2320
Bethesda, MD 20892
800-241-1044
FAX: 301-402-0018
e-mail: nidcdinfo@nidcd.nih.gov
www.nidcd.nih.gov

Marin P Allen PhD, Chief OHCPL

Describes how speech is produced, treatments for stuttering and research supported by the federal government.

8734 Stuttering & Your Child: A Videotape for Parents

Stuttering Foundation of America
PO Box 11749
Memphis, TN 38111
901-452-7343
800-992-9392
FAX: 901-452-3931
e-mail: stutter@vantek.net
www.stutterhelp.org

Anne Edwards, Coordinator
Jane Fraser, President

Provides parents withup-to-date information on what stuttering is; what is thought to cause and worsen childhood stuttering; what parents can do to help their child. *$10.00*

8735 Talkable Tales

Speech Bin
1965 25th Avenue
Vero Beach, FL 32960
772-770-0007
800-477-3324
FAX: 772-770-0006
www.speechbin.com

Jan J Binney, Senior Editor

Read-a-rebus stories and pictures targeting most consonant phonemes for K-5 children. *$25.95*

128 pages

ISBN 0-93783 -44-0

8736 Traumatic Brain Injury: Mechanisms of Damage, Assessment & Intervention

Pro-Ed Publications
8700 Shoal Creek Boulevard
Austin, TX 78757
512-451-3246
800-897-3202
FAX: 800-397-7633
e-mail: feedback@proedinc.com
www.proedinc.com

Donald Hammill, Owner
Courtney King, Marketing Coordinator

Traumatic Brain Injury ranks as one of the most prevalent disorders with estimates ranging in hundreds of thousands of new cases each year. This book focuses on the mechanisms of acquired brain injury and the methods of assessment, along with treatment and outcome variables. *$41.00*

458 pages Hardcover

8737 Trouble with Explosives

Bradbury Press
135 S Mount Zion Road
Lebanon, IN 46052
800-257-5755
FAX: 800-882-8583

Polly moved regularly with her family, changing schools almost every year. This was especially difficult as she couldn't pronounce her explosive name, Polly Banks, without stuttering.

117 pages Hardcover

ISBN 0-87888 -94-1

8738 Understanding & Controlling Stuttering: A Comprehensive New Approach Based on the Valsa Hypo

National Stuttering Association

Demonstrates how physical and psychological factors may interact to stimulate and perpetuate stuttering through a Valsalva-Stuttering cycle. *$25.00*

176 pages 2000
ISBN 7-929773-01-3

8739 Vocal Rehabilitation: A Practice Book for Voice Improvement

Pro-Ed
8700 Shoal Creek Boulevard
Austin, TX 78757
512-451-3246
800-897-3202
FAX: 512-451-8542
e-mail: info@proedinc.com
www.proedinc.com

Donald Hammill, Owner

A complete program that clinicians can use to help clients eliminate vocal misuses or abuse and gain a healthy, proficient voice.

8740 What is Vocal Hoarseness?

Speech Bin
1965 25th Avenue
Vero Beach, FL 32960
772-770-0007
800-477-3324
FAX: 772-770-0006
www.speechbin.com

Brochures to teach parents, teachers and individuals with voice disorders about chronic hoarseness and what to do about it. Set of ten copies. *$16.95*

24 pages Package of 10
ISBN 0-93785 -55-6

Associations

8741 **ACB Government Employees**
American Council Of The Blind
1155 15th Street NW
Suite 1004
Washington, DC 20005
202-467-5081
800-424-8666
FAX: 202-467-5085
e-mail: tpacheco@acb.org
www.acb.org

Terry Pacheko, Membership Services Coordinator
Melanie Brunson, Executive Director
Members are present, former and retired employees of federal, state and local government agencies. Concerns of the organization include recruitment, placement and advancement of blind and visually impaired employees.

8742 **ACB Radio Amateurs**
American Council of the Blind
4911 Old Canton Road 239
Jackson, MS 39211
601-432-6293
800-424-8666
FAX: 601-982-6746
e-mail: 5xu@concentric.net
www.acb.org

Mike Duke, President
ACBRA is an organization of blind and sighted licensed radio amateurs who work together to make the hobby more accessible to people who are blind

8743 **ACB Social Service Providers**
American Council Of The Blind
1155 15th Street NW
Suite 1004
Washington, DC 20005
202-467-5081
800-424-8666
FAX: 202-467-5085
e-mail: info@acb.org
www.acb.org

Melanie Brunson, Executive Director
Blind and visually impaired social workers, social service professionals, students pursuing careers in social work and other interested persons are members of this organization. ACBSSP works to promote full participation by visually impaired social services professionals in the field of social welfare.

8744 **Achromatopsia Network**
PO Box 214
Berkeley, CA 94701
510-540-4700
FAX: 510-540-4767
e-mail: oscar@sinewave.com
www.achromat.org

Frances Futterman, President
The Achromatopsia Network is a nonprofit organization for individuals concerned with acrhomatopsia. It is committed to sharing information about achromatopsia and providing resources to meet the special needs of those affected by this eye condition; helping individuals and families concerned with achromatopsia to connect with one another; and promoting awareness and educating with a special emphasis on accomplishing this goal among those who provides services to the visually impaired.

8745 **American Academy of Ophthalmology**
PO Box 7424
San Francisco, CA 94120
415-561-8500
FAX: 415-561-8533
e-mail: aaoe@aao.org
www.aao.org

C.P. Wilkinson MD, President
H. Dunbar Hoskins Jr. MD, Trustee-At-Large
Keith D. Carter MD, Trustee-At-Large
Founded in 1896, but was incorporated as an independent organization in 1979 when the AAOO was divided into separate academies. The American Academy of Ophthalmology is the largest national membership association of Eye MDs. Eye MDs are ophthalmologists, medical doctors who provide comprehensive eye care, including medical, surgical and optical care. More than 90 percent of practicing US Eye MDs are Acadmey members, and the Academy has more than 7,000 international members.
1979

8746 **American Action Fund for Blind Children and Adults**
1800 Johnson Street
Suite 100
Baltimore, MD 21230
410-659-9315
FAX: 410-685-5653
e-mail: actionfund@nfb.org
www.actionfund.org

Jean Dyon Norris, Director
Marc Mauer, President
A service agency which specializes in providing to blind people help which is not readily available to them from government programs or other existing service systems. The services are planned especially to meet the needs of blind children, the elderly blind, and the deaf-blind.
1919

8747 **American Council of Blind Lions**
PO Box 2312
Fort Collins, CO 80522
970-484-2598
FAX: 970-484-2565
e-mail: info@acb.org
www.acb.org/acbl/

Alan Beatty, Contact
A wonderful combination of Lionism and visual impairment nurtures the American Council of Blind Lions. ACBL's mission is awareness and highlights the great activities of the Knights of the Blind. The goals are to assist all clubs in their understanding of issues surrounding blind and visually impaired individuals.
1971

8748 **American Council of the Blind**
1155 15th Street NW
Suite 1004
Washington, DC 20005
202-467-5081
800-424-8666
FAX: 202-467-5085
e-mail: info@acb.org
www.acb.org

Melanie Brunson, Executive Director
A national membership organization whose members are visually impaired and fully sighted individuals who are concerned about the dignity and well-being of blind people throughout America. Formed in 1961, the Council has become the largest organization of blind people in the US with over 70 state affiliates and special interest chapters.
1961

8749 **American Foundation for the Blind**
11 Penn Plaza
Suite 300
New York, NY 10001
212-502-7600
800-232-5463
FAX: 212-502-7777
e-mail: afbinfo@afb.net
www.afb.org

Carl R Augusto, President/CEO
The organizaton to which Helen Keller devoted her life, is a national nonprofit organization whose mission is to ensure that the ten million Americans who are blind or visually impaired enjoy the same rights and opportunities as other citizens.
1921

8750 **American Optometric Association**
243 N Lindbergh Boulevard
St Louis, MS 63141
314-991-4100
800-365-2219
FAX: 314-991-4101
e-mail: MDJones@aoa.org
www.aoanet.org

C. Thomas Crooks, III, O.D., President
Peter H. Kehoe, O.D., F.A.A.O, Vice President
Randolph E. Brooks, O.D., F.A.A.O, Secretary/Treasurer
the AOA is the acknowledged leader and recognised authority for the eye and vision care in the world. The objectives of the AOA are centered on improving the quality and availiability of eye and vision care. The AOA fulfills its missions in accordance with health care and public policy related to eye care will uniformly recognise optometrists as primary health care providers and ensure the public has acess to the full scope of optometric care.
1998

8751 American Printing House for the Blind
PO Box 6085
Louisville, KY 40206
502-895-2405
800-223-1839
FAX: 502-899-2274
e-mail: info@aph.org
www.aph.org

Tuck Tinsley, President
Bob Brasher, VP Advisory Services/Research
The world's largest nonprofit organization creating educational, workplace and independent living products and services for people who are visually impaired. Also promotes independence of the blind and visually impaired persons by providing specialized materials, products, and services needed for educationand life.
1958

8752 Associated Blind
315 5th Avenue
Suite 807
New York, NY 10016
212-683-4950
FAX: 212-683-4975
e-mail: memberservices@esightcareers.net
www.tabinc.org

Herbert R Brinberg, Chairman
Michelle Scott, Secretary
Theodore S Francavilla, Treasurer
Privately funded, non-profit agency, that was founded by a group of blind individuals as an organization promoting autonomy and self-determination. The mission is to assist individuals who are blind, visualy impaired or who have physical disabilities to become self-reliant and achieve financial independence through mainstream employment.
1938

8753 Associated Services for the Blind
919 Walnut Street
Philadelphia, PA 19107
215-627-0600
FAX: 215-922-0692
e-mail: asbinfo@asb.org
www.asb.org

Patricia C Johnson, CEO
Dolores Ferrara-Godzieba, Director
ASB, a non-private, non-profit organization, promotes self esteem, independence, and self-determination in people who are blind or visually impaired. ASB accomplishes this by providing support through education, training and resources, as well as through community action and public education, serving as a voice and advocate for the rights of all people who are blind or visually impaired.
1983

8754 Association for Education & Rehabilitation of the Blind & Visually Impaired
1703 N Beauregard Street
Suite 440
Alexandria, VA 22311
703-671-4500
877-492-2708
FAX: 703-671-6391
e-mail: aer@aerbvi.org
www.aerbvi.org

Sandra Ruconich, President
Jim Gandorf, Executive Director
Angela Booker, Associate For Exec. Support
The only international organization dedicated to rendering all possible support and assistance to the professionals who work in all phases of education and rehabilitation of blind and visually impaired children and adults. Our membership is comprised of more than 4,400 professionals who provide services to people with visual impairments.
1984

8755 Association for Macular Diseases
210 E 64th Street
8th Floor
New York, NY 10021
212-605-3777
800-622-8524
FAX: 212-605-3795
e-mail: foundation@retinal-research.org
www.macula.org

Lawrence A. Yannuzzi, President
Yale L. Fisher M.D., Vice President
Nina Y. Freund M.D. M.P.H, Secretary/Treasurer
The Macula Foundation, Inc., a not-for-profit organization was established in 1978 to support basic and clinical research in vitreous retinal and macular diseases, a major cause of blindness of all age groups. Since it was formed, the Foundation has distributed grants and awards of approximately 15 million dollars earmarked for important clinical and scientific research and related teaching programs. Numerous research projects have been successful as a result of the Foundation.
1978

8756 Blind Childrens Center
4120 Marathon Street
Los Angeles, CA 90029
323-664-2153
800-222-3566
FAX: 323-665-3828
e-mail: info@blindchildrenscenter.org
www.blindchildrenscenter.org

Midge Horton, Executive Director
A family centered agency which serves children with visual impairments from birth to school-age. The center-based and home-based programs and services help the children aquire skills and build their independence. The center utilizes its expertise and experience to serve families and professionals worldwide through support services, education, and research.
1938

8757 Blind Information Technology Specialists
American Council of the Blind
1155 15th Street NW
Suite 1004
Washington, DC 20005
202-467-5081
800-424-8666
202-467-5085
e-mail: earlene@earlenehughes.com
www.acb.org/bits

Earlene Hughes, President
John Farina, Vice President
Michael Malver, Secretary
Formerly the Visually Impaired Data Processors, BITS is a non profit organization which fosters the career development of blind computer professionals, promotes the use of computer technology by blind persons to improve the wualtiy of their personal and professional lives, and advocare for improved information access for all visually impaired people.

8758 Blinded Veterans Association
477 H Street NW
Washington, DC 20001
202-371-8880
800-669-7079
FAX: 202-371-8258
e-mail: bva@bva.org
www.bva.org

Larry Belote, National President
Dr. Sidney Ordway, National Secretary
Robert L. Campbell, Director District 2
To promote the welfare of blinded veterans so that, notwithstanding their disabilities, they may take their rightful place in the community and work with their fellow citizens toward the creation of a peaceful world. To preserve and strengthen a spirit of fellowship among blinded veterans so that they may give mutual aid and assistance to one another. To maintain and extend the institution of American freedom and encourage loyalty to the constitution and laws of the US and states which they live

1945

8759 Books for Blind and Physically Handicapped Individuals

Library of Congress
1291 Taylor Street NW
Washington, DC 20011
202-707-5100
888-657-7323
FAX: 202-707-0712
TTY: 202-707-0744
e-mail: nls@loc.gov
www.loc.gov/nls

Frank Kurt Cylke, Director
Marvine Wanamaker, Assistant Director
Administers a national library service that provides braille and recorded books and magazines on free loan to anyone who cannot read standard print because of visual of physical disabilities who are eligible residents of the Unites States of America citizens living abroad.
1931

8760 Braille Institute of America

741 N Vermont Avenue
Los Angeles, CA 90029
323-663-1111
800-272-4553
FAX: 323-663-0867
e-mail: la@brailleinstitute.org
www.brailleinstitute.org

James H. Jackson, Chairman, Board Of Directors
Leslie E Stocker, President
Provides an environment of hope and encouragement for people who are blind and visually impaired through integrated educational, social and recreational programs and services. Provides assistance at 5 regional centers in Southern California and through 200 community outreach programs. In 2005-06, the Institute provided these services to more than 55,000 people. The Institute is operated and funded almost entirely through private individual and foundation sources.
1929

8761 California State Library Braille and Talki ng Book Library

PO Box 942837
Sacramento, CA 94237
916-634-0640
800-952-5666
FAX: 916-654-1119
e-mail: btbl@library.ca.gov
www.library.ca.gov/html/pubser05.cfm

John Torkelson, Acting Head
Aimee Sgourakis, Senior Librarian
Mary Jane Kayes, Librarian
The State Library stands as one of California's great public research institutions with a five-fold mission:serving the needs of elected officials and state agency employees;preserving the state's cultural heritage by collecting historic materials on California and the West;assisting public libraries through financial aid and consulting services;offering special services to disadvantaged and handicapped clients;ensuring that the general public has convenient and consistent access to resources.
1950

8762 Canine Helpers for the Handicapped

5699 Ridge Road
Lockport, NY 14094
716-433-4035
FAX: 716-439-0822
e-mail: chhdogs@aol.com
www.caninehelpers.netfirms.com

Beverly Underwood, Executive Director
Colleen Underwood, Contact
Designed to unite deserving people with highly trained, disability specific dogs. The ultimate goal of this non-profit organization is to achieve a high degree of independence for the clients who have various physical and emotional challenges. Whether the need be for hearing, service, mobility (multi-service), seizure alert or therapy dogs, we are equipped to match a person with the right dog and train both to become an efficient team.
1983

8763 Caption Center

125 Western Avenue
Boston, MA 02134
617-300-3600
FAX: 617-300-1020
TTY:617-300-3600
e-mail: access@wgbh.org
www.icdri.org/dhhi/ccowgbh

Michael Burks, Chairman
Wen Lu, Secretary And Treasurer
Cynthia Waddell JD, President
Has been pioneering and delivering accessible media to disabled adults, students and their families, teachers and friends for over 30 years. Each year, the Center captions more than 10,000 hours worth of broadcast and cable programs, feature films, large-format and IMAX films, home videos, music videos, DVDs, teleconferences and CD-Roms.

8764 Chicago Lighthouse for People who are Blind and Visually Impaired

1850 W Roosevelt Road
Chicago, IL 60608
312-666-1331
FAX: 312-243-8539
TTY:312-666-8874
e-mail: support@chicagolighthouse.org
www.thechicagolighthouse.org

James Kesteloot, President
Mary Zabelski, Director Of Educational Sevices
A non profit agency committed to providing the highest quality educational, clinical, vocational, and rehabilitation services for children, youth and adults who are blind or visually impaired, including deaf blind and multi disabled. Also respects personal dignity and partners with individuals to enhance independent living and self sufficiency. This agency is a leader, innovator and advocate for people who are blind or visually impaired, enhancing the quality of life for all individuals.
1906

8765 Clovernook Center for the Blind and Visually Impaired

7000 Hamilton Avenue
Cincinnati, OH 45231
513-522-3860
888-234-7156
FAX: 513-728-3946
TTY:513-522-3860
e-mail: contact@clovernook.org
www.clovernook.org

Carol Friedman, LSW, Intake Specialist

8766 Clovernook Printing House, The Clovernook Center for the Blind and Visually Impaired

7000 Hamilton Avenue
Cincinnati, OH 45231
513-522-3860
FAX: 513-728-3950
e-mail: cvb@clovernook.org
www.clovernook.org

Charlotte Begley, Manager Clovernook Print House
Clovernook also offers Braille Transcription Services including: Literary Books, Literary Magazines, Religious Materials, Instructional Manuals, ADA Conformance Materials, Literary Textbook Materials, Menus, Braille Alphabet Cards, and Forms.
$145.00
591 pages
ISBN 1-930956-48-7

8767 College of Optometrists in Vision Development

215 W Garfield Road
Suite 210
Aurora, OH 44202
330-995-0718
888-268-3770
FAX: 330-995-0719
e-mail: info@covd.org
www.covd.org

Pamela R Happ, Executive Director
The College of Optometrists in Vision Development (COVD) is an international membership association of eye care professionals including optometrists, optometry students, and vision therapists. Members of COVD provide developmental vision care, vision therapy and vision rehabilitation services for children and adults.

8768 College of Syntonic Optometry
322 N Aurora Street
Ithaca, NY 14850
607-277-4749
FAX: 607-277-5216
www.syntonicphototherapy.com

Larry Wallace, President
Cathy Stern, Vice President
John Pulaski, Treasurer
An active and growing post-graduate educational organization. Established in 1933 its members include optometrists and other health professionals and supporters from around the world. Those who achieve a clinical level of experience and mastery are awarded the status of Fellow. Today, scientific as well as clinical verification of light's impact on health and healing and a growing public demand for functional and rehabilitative vision therapy continue to vitalise the college and its mission.

8769 Columbia Lighthouse for the Blind
1120 20th Street NW
Suite 750 S
Washington, DC 20036
202-454-6400
877-324-5252
FAX: 202-454-6401
e-mail: info@clb.org
www.clb.org

Dale Otto, CEO
Kim Zimmer, COO
Peter Mayo, President
Offer programs that enable individuals who are blind or visually impaired to obtain and maintain independence at home, school, work and in the community. The programs and services include asistive technology training, career services, rehabilitation services, comprehensive low vision care and a wide range of children's programs.
2000

8770 Council of Families with Visual Impairments
American Council of the Blind
6686 NE Capricorn Lane
Bremerton, WA 98311
202-467-5081
800-424-8666
FAX: 202-467-5085
e-mail: cindybur@comcast.net
www.acb.org

Cindy Van Winkle, President
Dennis Colley, First Vice President
Glenn McCully, Second Vice President
A network of parents with blind or visually impaired children that offers support and outreach, shares experiences in parent/child relationships, exchanges educational, cultural and medical information about child development and more.

8771 Deaf-Blind Division of the National Federation of the Blind
National Federation of the Blind
1800 Johnson Street
Baltimore, MD 21230
410-659-9314
FAX: 410-685-5653
e-mail: nfb@nfb.org
www.nfb.org

Marc Maurer, President
The nation's largest and most influential membership organization of blind persons, with a two-fold purpose: to help blind persons achieve self-confidence and self respect and to act as a vehicle for collective self-expression by the blind. The NFB improves blind people's lives through advocacy, education, research, technology, and programs encouraging independence and self-confidence. It is the leading force in the blindness field today and is the voice of the nations blind.
1940

8772 Eye Bank Association of America
1015 18th Street NW
Suite 1010
Washington, DC 20036
202-775-4999
FAX: 202-429-6036
e-mail: info@restoresight.org
www.restoresight.org

Patricia Acken-Oneil Esq., President/CEO
Joseph Kelly, Vice President
Amanda Nerone, Regulatory Officer
Established in 1961 by the American Academy of Ophthalmology's Committee on Eye Banks, the EBAA is a not-for-profit organization of eye banks dedicated to the restoration of sight through the promotion and advancement of eye banking. The EBAA has lead the transplantation field with the establishment of medical standards for the procurement and distribution of corneal tissue, accreditation of eye banks, and comprehensive education programs for doctors, technicians, and administrators.
1961

8773 Fidelco Guide Dog Foundation
103 Old Iron Ore Road
Bloomfield, CT 06002
860-243-5200
FAX: 860-243-7215
e-mail: apply@fidelco.org
www.fidelco.org

Roberta C Kaman, Chairman
Eliot D. Russman, Vice Chairman
Michael W. Hveem Esq., Secretary
More than just New England's only guide dog school, it is a family, a group of people tied together by their mission to help bring increased freedom and independence to men and women who are visually impaired. Also breeds, trains, and places the highest quality German Shepards with men and women across the Northeast.
1961

8774 Fight for Sight
381 Park Avenue S
Suite 809
New York, NY 10016
212-679-6060
FAX: 212-679-4466
e-mail: info@fightforsight.com
www.fightforsight.com

Kenneth R Barasch, President
Marlene Schiff, Vice President
Douglas Schwartz, Treasurer
The mission is to support vision research, to find causes and cures for blindness, and to help save the sight of children through support of pediatric eye centers.
1946

8775 Guide Dog Users
14311 Astrodome Drive
Silver Spring, MD 20906
301-598-5771
888-858-2481
FAX: 301-871-7591
e-mail: info@gdui.org
www.gdui.org

Sheila Styron, President
DeAnna Noriega, First Vice President
Kevin Chinn, Second Vice President
Guide Dog Users Inc, (GDUI) an affiliate of the American Council of the Blind, is the largest guide dog consumer driven group in the world. Since 1972, members can excercise the privilege of shaping the initiatives and issues that most profoundly affect guide dog handlers. GDUI has 19 affiliate organizations throughout the US where members can personally interact and work together on local as well as global issues.
1972

8776 Guide Dogs for the Blind
PO Box 151200
San Rafael, CA 94915
415-499-4000
800-295-4050
FAX: 415-499-4035
e-mail: information@guidedogs.com
www.guidedogs.com

Robert Phillips, CEO/President
Ralph Cechettini, Board Chair
Edward Schaefer, First Vice Chair
A nonprofit, charitable organization with a mission to provide Guide Dogs and training in their use to visually impaired people throughout the United States and Canada.

1942

8777 Guiding Eyes for the Blind

611 Granite Springs Road
Yorktown Heights, NY 10598
914-245-4024
800-942-0149
FAX: 914-245-1609
e-mail: info@guidingeyes.org
www.guidingeyes.org

William Badger, President/CEO
Carolyn Kihm, Director of Human Resources
Bev Klayman, Manager of Admissions Services

An internationally recognized guide dog school that is dedicated to enriching the lives of blind and visually impaired men and women by providing them with the freedom to travel safely, thereby assuring greater independence, dignity and new horizons of opportunity

1954

8778 Guiding Eyes for the Blind: Breeding and Placement Center

Guiding Eyes for the Blind
361 Route 164
Patterson, NY 12563
845-878-3330
FAX: 845-878-3749
e-mail: jrussenberger@guidingeyes.org
www.guidingeyes.org

Jane Russenberger, Executive Director
Janine Haughney, Director
Lee Nordin, Program Director

Provides the means for blind and visually impaired individuals to achieve mobility, independence and companionship through the use of our professionally bred and trained guide dogs. Each month Guiding Eyes graduates approximately 12 guide dog/student teams from all over the US, Canada, and internationally. The guide dogs, 26 day residential training program, special needs program and lifetime follow-up services are offered at no cost to the students. Also provides at home training at no cost.

1954

8779 Horizons for the Blind

2 N Williams Street
Crystal Lake, IL 60014
815-444-8800
FAX: 815-444-8830
e-mail: mail@horizons-blind.org
www.horizons-blind.org

Camille Cafarelli, Executive Director

A not for profit organization whose mission is to improve the quality of life for individuals who are blind and visually impaired, many who are senior citizens, by increasing accessibility to culture, education, recreation, employment and consumer information. Horizons enhances self-sufficiencey directly by providing braille, large print, and audio cassetts instruction in crafts, gardening, food preparation, and the operation of household appliances.

1977

8780 Independent Visually Impaired Enterprisers

American Council Of The Blind
1155 15th Street NW
Suite 1004
Washington, DC 20005
202-467-5081
800-424-8666
FAX: 202-467-5085
e-mail: info@acb.org
www.acb.org

Mary Susan Orester, President
James Radcliff, VP
Terry Pacheco, Membership Services Coordinator

Strives to broaden vocational opportunities in business for the visually impaired. Works to improve rehabilitation facilities for all types of business enterprises and publicizes the capabilities of blind and visually impaired business persons.

8781 Information Access Project: National Federation of the Blind

1800 Johnson Street
Baltimore, MD 21230
410-659-9314
FAX: 410-685-5653
e-mail: nfb@nfb.org
www.nfb.org

Marc Maurer, President
Joyce Scanlan, Program Director
John G. Pare' Jr., Director Of Public Relations

The nation's largest and most influential membership organization of blind persons. The purpose of the federation is to help blind persons achieve self confidence and self respect and to act as a vehicle for collective self expression by the blind. Members of the NFB strive to educate the public that the blind are normal individuals who can compete on terms of equality.

1940

8782 Institute for Families of Blind Children

4650 Sunset Boulevard
Mail Stop 111
Los Angeles, CA 90027
323-669-4649
FAX: 323-665-7869
e-mail: info@instituteforfamilies.org
www.instituteforfamilies.org

Nancy Mansfield, Executive Director

A non profit organization and all services are provided at no cost to families and professionals. Offers counseling and support to families facing the devastating diagnosis of visual impairment in their child and is there for every family member of the family during the many difficult days, weeks, and months of treatment.

1987

8783 International Association of Audio Information Services (IAAIS)

1102 W International Airport Road
Anchorage, AK 99518
412-434-6023
800-280-5325
e-mail: aiblink@ak.net
www.iaais.org

Heather Lusignan, President
Lori Kesigner, Administrative Assistant
Kim Walsh, First Vice President

A volunteer driven membership organization of services that turn text into speech for people who cannot see, hold or comprehend the printed word and who may be unable to access information due to a disability or health condition. IAAIS shall encourage and support the establishment and maintenance of audio information services that provide access to printed information for individuals who cannot read conventional print because of blindess or any other visual, physical or learning disability.

1977

8784 Jewish Braille Institute International

110 E 30th Street
New York, NY 10016
212-889-2525
800-433-1531
FAX: 212-689-3692
e-mail: admin@jbilibrary.org
www.jbilibrary.org

Ellen Isler, President
Israel Taub, Vice President/CFO
Judy E. Tenny, Chairman Of The Board

The JBI Library provides the visually impaired, blind, physically handicapped and reading disabled of all backgrounds and ages with books, magazines and cultural programs in Audio (in 7 languages) in Large Print and Braille. Its unique programs enrich the lives of 35,000 individuals in the United States, Israel and around the world. The JBI Library is an affiliated library of the Library of Congress and all of its services and materials are free of charge to those that are eligible.

1931

8785 Lighthouse International

Lighthouse International
111 E 59th Street
New York, NY 10022
212-821-9200
800-829-0500
FAX: 212-821-9707
e-mail: info@lighthouse.org
www.lighthouse.org

Roger O. Goldman, Chairman
Tara A. Cortes, RN, PhD, President/CEO
Eric S. Lamm, Vice Chair

Founded in 1905, lighthouse international is a leading non-profit organization that helps people of all ages overcome the challenges of vision loss. Through services, education, research and advocacy, the Lighthouse enables people with low vision and blindness to enjoy safe, independent and productive lives.

8786 Lions Clubs International
300 W 22nd Street
Oak Brook, IL 60523
630-571-5466
FAX: 630-571-8890
e-mail: it@lionsclubs.org
www.lionsclubs.org

Clement Kusiak, International President
Gary Lapentina, Chief Executive Officer
Lions are known for their service to persons who are blind and visually impaired. The Lions ambitious Sight First Program has restored sight through cataract surgeries, prevented serious vision loss and improved eye care services for hundreds of millions of adults and children. To continue and expand this effort, Lions have launced Campaign Sight First with a goal of raising at least $150 million dollars.
1917

8787 National Alliance of Blind Students NABS Liaison
American Council of the Blind
62 Marshall Road
Ridgefield, CT 06877
800-424-8666
e-mail: info@acb.org
www.blindstudents.org

Jennifer Barrow, President
A student affiliate of the American Council of the Blind which is a national organization of blind and visually impaired high school and college students who believe that every blind and visually impaired student has the right to an equal and accessible education. Also encourages blind and visually impaired students to challenge their limits and reach their potential.
1974

8788 National Association for Parents of Children with Visual Impairments (NAPVI)
PO Box 317
Watertown, MA 02471
617-972-7441
800-562-6265
FAX: 617-972-7444
e-mail: napvi@perkins.org
www.spedex.com/napvi

Mary Zabelski, President
Julie Urban, Vice President
D. Allison Rickerl, Secretary
A non profit organization of, by and for parents committed to providing support to the parents of children who have visual impairments . Also a national organization that enables parents to find information and resources for their children who are blind or visually impaired including those with additional disabilities. NAPVI also provides leadership, support, and training to assist parents in helping children reach their potential.

8789 National Association for Visually Handicapped
22 W 21st Street
Floor 6
New York, NY 10010
212-889-3141
FAX: 212-727-2931
e-mail: staff@navh.org
www.navh.org

Lorianie Marchi, CEO
The only nonprofit health organization in the world solely dedicated to providing assistance to the partially sighted whose mission is to help the hard of seeing worldwide cope with the psychological effects of visual impairment and to provide low vision services, visual aids and training to anyone in need of these services.

8790 National Association of Blind Educators
National Federation Of The Blind
1800 Johnson Street
Baltimore, MD 21230
410-659-9314
FAX: 410-685-5653
e-mail: nfb@nfb.org
www.nfb.org

Marc Maurer, President
Fredric Schroeder, First Vice President
Peggy Elliott, Second Vice President
Membership organization of blind teachers, professors and instructors in all levels of education. Provides support and information regarding professional responsibilities, classroom techniques, national testing methods and career obstacles. Publishes The Blind Educator, national magazine specifically for blind educators.

8791 National Association of Blind Lawyers
National Federation Of The Blind
1800 Johnson Street
Baltimore, MD 21230
410-659-9314
FAX: 410-685-5653
e-mail: nfb@nfb.org
www.nfb.org

Marc Mauer, President
Fredric Schroeder, First Vice President
Peggy Elliott, Second Vice President
Membership organization of blind attorneys, law students, judges and others in the law field. Provides support and information regarding employment, techniques used by the blind, advocacy, laws affecting the blind, current information about the American Bar Association and other issues for blind lawyers.

8792 National Association of Blind Secretaries and Transcribers
National Federation Of The Blind
1800 Johnson Street
Baltimore, MD 21230
410-659-9314
FAX: 410-685-5653
e-mail: nfb@nfb.org
www.nfb.org

Marc Maurer, President
Fredric Schroeder, First Vice President
Peggy Elliott, Second Vice President
Membership organization of blind secretaries and transcribers at all levels, including medical and paralegal transcription, office workers, customer-service personnel and many other similar fields. Addresses issues such as technology, accomodation, career planning and job training.

8793 National Association of Blind Students
National Federation of the Blind
1800 Johnson Street
Baltimore, MD 21230
410-659-9314
FAX: 410-685-5653
e-mail: sassywolf@ev1.net
www.nfbstudents.org

Marc Maurer, President
Joyce Scanlan, Program Director
The mission of the National Federation of the Blind is to achieve weidespread emotional acceptance and intellectual understanding that the real problem of blindness is not the loss of eyesight but the misconceptions and lack of information which exist. We do this by bringing blind people together to share success, to support each other in times of failure and to create imaginative solutions
1967

8794 National Association of Blind Teachers
American Council Of The Blind
1155 15th Street NW
Suite 1004
Washington, DC 20005
202-467-5081
800-424-8666
FAX: 202-467-5085
e-mail: info@acb.org
www.acb.org

Melanie Brunson, Executive Director
Works to advance the teaching profession for blind and visually impaired people, protects the interest of teachers, presents discussions and solutions for special problems encountered by blind teachers and publishes a directory of blind teachers in the US.

Monthly 1999

8795 **National Association of Guide Dog Users**
National Federation of the Blind
55 Delaware Avenue
Somerset, MA 02726 508-673-0218
e-mail: nfbmass@earthlink.net
www.nfb-nagdu.org

Priscilla Ferris, President
Marion Gwizdala, VP
Melissa Riccobono, Secretary
Provides information and support for guide dog users and works to secure high standards in guide dog training. Addresses issues of discrimination of guide dog users and offers public education about guide dog use.

8796 **National Association to Promote the Use of Braille**
National Federation of the Blind
5530 Corbin Avenue
Suite 330
Tarzana, CA 91356 818-342-6524
877-558-6524
FAX: 818-344-7930
e-mail: nfbcal@sbcglobal.net
www.nfbcal.org

Nadine Jacobson, President
Robert S. Jaquiss, First Vice President
Linda Mentink, Second Vice President
Dedicated to securing improved Braille instruction, increasing the number of braille materials available to the blind and providing information of braille in securing independence, education and employment for the blind.

8797 **National Braille Association**
3 Townline Circle
Rochester, NY 14623 585-427-8260
FAX: 585-427-0263
e-mail: nbaoffice@nationalbraille.org
www.nationalbraille.org

Diane Spence, President
Mary Ann Damm, Vice President
Jan Carrol, Secretary
Providing continuing education to those who prepare braille, and provides braille materials to persons who are visually impaired. Maintains collection of Braille textbooks, music, technical tables, and general interest items. Catalogs of the Braille collection in print or Braille are available on request.

8798 **National Braille Press**
88 Saint Stephen Street
Boston, MA 02115 617-266-6160
888-965-8965
888-965-8965
FAX: 617-437-0456
e-mail: orders@nbp.org
www.nbp.org

Paul V McLaughlin, Chairman
William Kilimanjaro, President
Richard H Willis, Treasurer
The guiding purposes of National Braille Press are to promote the literacy of blind children through braille, and to provide access to information that empowers blind people to actively engage in work, family, and commuity affairs.
1927

8799 **National Camp for Blind Children**
Christian Record Services
1300 King Street E
Po Box 31119
Oshawa Ontario, Canada, L1H 905-436-6938
FAX: 905-436-7102
e-mail: ppage@christianrecordservices.ca
www.crsblindservices.ca

Daniel Jackson, Chairman
Pat Page, Director
To enrich lives of those who are blind, visually impaired or physically challenged regardless of race, creed, economic status or gender. Also encourages each camper to achieve greater self-esteem and self confidence while seeking to excel in the use of his/her physical , mental, and spiritual capacities. Provides fee Christian publications and programs for people with visual impairments.

8800 **National Center for Vision and Child Development**
Lighthouse International
111 E 59th Street
New York, NY 10022 212-821-9200
800-829-0500
FAX: 212-821-9707
e-mail: info@lighthouse.org
www.lighthouse.org

Tara A Cortes PhD, RN, President/CEO
Roger O. Goldman, Chariman
Eric S. Lamm, Vice Chair
The worldwide leader in helping people of all ages who are blind or partially sighted overcome the challenges of vision loss.

8801 **National Diabetes Action Network for the Blind**
National Federation of the Blind
811 Cherry Street
Suite 309
Columbia, MO 65201 573-875-8911
FAX: 573-875-6184
e-mail: loiscares898@yahoo.com
www.nfb.org/nfb/diabetics.asp

Lois Williams, President
Leading support and information organization of persons losing vision due to diabetes. Provides personal contact and resource information with other blind diabetics about non-visual techniques of independently managing diabetes, monitoring glucose levels, measuring insulin and other matters concerning diabetes. Publishes Voice of the Diabetic, the leading publication about diabetes and blindness.

8802 **National Federation of the Blind**
1800 Johnson Street
Baltimore, MD 21230 410-659-9314
FAX: 410-685-5653
e-mail: nfb@nfb.org
www.nfb.org

Marc Maurer, President
Joyce Scanlan, Training Program Director
The largest membership organization of blind people in the nation, with chapters in every state and approximately 50,000 individual members. It seeks to integrate the blind into society on the basis of equality with the sighted so that the blind are seen as normal, participating citizens. Has 700 local chapters.
1940

8803 **National Federation of the Blind: Merchants Division**
National Federation of the Blind
1800 Johnson Street
Baltimore, MD 21230 410-659-9314
FAX: 410-685-5653
e-mail: nfb@nfb.org
www.nfb.org

Marc Maurer, President
Fred Schroeder, First Vice President
Peggy Elliott, Second Vice President
Membership organization of blind persons employed in either self-employment work or the Randolph-Sheppard vending program. Provides information regarding rehabilitation, social security, tax and other issues which directly affect blind merchants. Serves as advocacy and support group.

8804 **National Federation of the Blind: Blind Industrial Workers Division**
National Federation of the Blind
1800 Johnson Street
Baltimore, MD 21230 410-659-9314
FAX: 410-685-5653
e-mail: nfb@nfb.org
www.nfb.org

Marc Maurer, President
Fredric Schroeder, First Vice President
Peggy Elliott, Second Vice President
Membership organization of blind persons employed in industrial and manufacturing work or in government job programs for the blind. Dedicated to protecting the rights of blind workers in salary, job stability, advancement, and labor issues.

8805 National Federation of the Blind: Computer Science Division
National Federation of the Blind
1800 Johnson Street
Baltimore, MD 21230
410-659-9314
FAX: 410-685-5653
e-mail: nfb@nfb.org
www.nfb.org

Marc Maurer, President
Fredric Schroeder, First Vice President
Peggy Elliott, Second Vice President
National organization of blind persons knowledgeable in the computer science and technology fields. Works to develop new technologies, to secure access to current technology and to develop new ways of using current or new technologies by the blind.

8806 National Federation of the Blind: Human Services Division
1026 E 36th Street
Baltimore, MD 21218
410-235-3073
FAX: 410-235-3075
e-mail: humanser@nfbnet.org
www.nfb.org/nfbdvlst.htm

Melissa Riccobono, President
Membership organization of blind persons working in counseling, personnel, psychology, social work, psychiatry, rehabilitation, and other social science and human resource fields. Dedicated to improving employment opportunities and advancement for blind persons and provides resources regarding blindness-related techniques and methods used in these fields.

8807 National Federation of the Blind: Masonic Square Club
3110 Wisteria Avenue
Baltimore, MD 21214
410-598-0155
FAX: 410-598-2734
www.nfb.org

Fred Flowers, President
Blind individuals committed to sharing of Masonic experiences, goals and history.

8808 National Federation of the Blind: Public Employees Division
1800 Johnson Street
Baltimore, MD 21230
410-659-9314
FAX: 410-685-5653
e-mail: nfb@nfb.org
www.nfb.org

Marc Mauer, President
Fredric Schroeder, First Vice President
Peggy Elliott, Second Vice President
Organization of blind persons holding local, state or federal jobs. Focuses on issues such as changes in governmental hiring and retention practices, new job skills needed for the future, government employment downsizing, new electronic means of finding public sector jobs, self-advocacy and career planning strategies.

8809 National Federation of the Blind: Science and Engineering Division
National Federation of the Blind
1800 Johnson Street
Baltimore, MD 21230
410-659-9314
FAX: 410-685-5653
e-mail: nfb@nfb.org
www.nfb.org

Marc Maurer, President
Fredric Schroeder, First Vice President
Peggy Elliott, Second Vice President
Blind persons with expertise and experience in fields such as genetics, telecommunications, biology, chemistry, physics and nuclear physics or mechanical, electronic and chemical engineering. This is a strong support group to encourage blind persons in pursuit of these careers, many of which have been considered not possible for the blind in the past.

8810 National Federation of the Blind: Writers Division
National Federation of the Blind
1800 Johnson Street
Baltimore, MD 21230
410-659-9314
FAX: 410-685-5653
e-mail: nfb@nfb.org
www.nfb.org

Marc Maurer, President
Fredric Schroeder, First Vice President
Peggy Elliott, Second Vice President
Blind writers in all styles, including poetry, short story, fiction, non-fiction, magazine writing and theatrical work offer encouragement and support to blind writers and authors. Issues cover various aspects of this business, including selling your work, publishing, technology, motivation and discovering writing and publishing resources.

8811 National Industries for the Blind
1310 Braddock Place
Alexandria, VA 22314
703-310-0500
FAX: 703-998-8268
e-mail: info@nib.org
www.nib.org

John C. Peoples, Chairman
Dr. James A Kutsch Jr., Vice Chairman
William B. Johnson CPA, Treasurer
A nonprofit organization that represents over 100 associated industries serving people who are blind in thirty-six states. These agencies serve people who are blind or visually impaired and help them to reach their full potential. Services include job and family counseling, job skills training, instruction in Braille and other communication skills, children's programs and more.

8812 National Library Services for the Blind & Physically Handicapped
Library of Congress
1291 Taylor Street NW
Washington, DC 20011
202-707-5100
888-657-7323
FAX: 202-707-0712
TTY: 202-707-0744
e-mail: nls@loc.gov
www.loc.gov.nls

Frank Kurt Cylke, Director
Robert Fistick, Special Assistant
Michael Martys, Automation Officer
NLS is responsible for the selection, copyright clearance, and procurement of reading materials for blind and physically handicapped individuals. Distribution of the materials and relevant bibliographic information either directly or through cooperating state and local network libraries. Design, development, and procurement of sound reproduction equipment and its distribution either directly or through cooperating agencies.

8813 National Organization of Parents of Blind Children
National Federation of the Blind
1800 Johnson Street
Baltimore, MD 21230
410-659-9314
FAX: 410-685-5653
e-mail: nfb@nfb.org
www.nfb.org/nopbc.htm

Marc Maurer, President
Support information and advocacy organization of parents of blind or visually impaired children. Addresses issues ranging from help to parents of a newborn blind infant, mobility and braille instruction, education, social and community participation, development of self confidence and other vital factors involved in growth of a blind child.

8814 New Eyes for the Needy
PO Box 332
Short Hills, NJ 07078
973-376-4903
FAX: 973-376-3807

Clelia Biamonti, President
Jason Bernstein, Vice President
Katherine Coombs, Secretary

Non profit organization founded to improve the vision of the less fortunate throughout the world by providing assistance for the purchase of new eyeglasses in the United States and recycling used eyeglasses for distribution overseas. New Eyes is strengthned by our partnerships with thousands of social service agencies, optical dispensers, and vision missions.
1932

8815 Prevent Blindness America
211 W Wacker Drive
Suite 1700
Chicago, IL 60606
312-363-6001
800-331-2020
FAX: 847-843-8458
e-mail: info@preventblindness.org
www.preventblindness.org

John D. O'Neill Jr. Esq., Chair
James E. Anderson, Partner
Joanne Angle, Executive Director
The nation's leading volunteer eye health and safety organization dedicated to fighting blindness and saving sight. Also touches the lives of millions of people each year through public and professional education, advocacy, certified vision screening training, community and patient service programs and research.
1908

8816 Recording for the Blind & Dyslexic
20 Roszel Road
Princeton, NJ 08540
609-452-0606
866-732-3585
FAX: 609-750-1838
e-mail: custserv@rfbd.org
www.rfbd.org

Stephanie Campbell, Executive Director
John Kelly, Chief Executive Officer
Provides recorded and computerized textbooks, library services and other educational resources to people who cannot effectively read standard print because of visual impairment, dyslexia or other physical disability.

8817 Seeing Eye
PO Box 375
Morristown, NJ 07963
973-539-4425
FAX: 973-539-0922
e-mail: info@seeingeye.org
www.seeingeye.org

Kenneth Rosenthal, President
An organization that concentrates on its mission to enhance the independence, dignity, and self confidence of blind people through the use of seeing eye dogs. The Seeing Eye will be an organization that concentrates on its mission to enhance the independence, dignity, and self confidence of blind people through the use of Seeing Eye dogs, and on improving its ability to fulfill this mission. We will maintain and nuture the spirit of our founders and adhere to the highest standards of respect
1929

8818 Services for the Visually Impaired
8720 Georgia Avenue
Suite 210
Silver Spring, MD 20910
301-589-0894
FAX: 301-589-7281
e-mail: info@servicesvi.org
www.servicesvi.org

Ann Cook, Executive Director
Joel R Kahn, Business Manager
Gail Snider, Volunteer Coordinator
Provides skills and resources to DC area residents who are blind or experiencing vision loss, and are also committed to helping people regain their indepence and maintaining it.
1973

8819 Special Technologies Alternative Resources
210 McMorran Boulevard
Port Huron, MI 48060
810-982-3600
800-272-8570
FAX: 810-987-7327
TTY: 810-455-0200
e-mail: star@sccl.lib.mi.us
www.sccl.lib.mi.us/star.html

Stan Arnett Ii, Assistant Library Director
Mary Koch, Manager
Addresses the needs of a very unique diverse group of people by offering a full range of library services for people who cannot read standard print. Provides reading material in specialized formats that permit individuals with disabilities to have access to the written word, delivering to customer's mailboxes free of charge. Talking Book Machines, recorded books and magazines, descriptive videos, large print editions and braille books and magazines.

8820 Taping for the Blind
3935 Essex Lane
Houston, TX 77027
713-622-2767
FAX: 713-622-2772
e-mail: taping@hal-pc.org
www.tapingfortheblind.org

Randy De La Garza, President
Cynthia Franzetti, Executive Director
Jerry Hanlon, Vice President-Planning & Tech.
An independent non profit educational organization funded by corporations, listeners and individuals, with a mission to turn sight into sound, enriching the lives of individuals with visual, physical and learning disabilities. Founded in 1967 to read materials not availiable through other sources onto standard audio cassettes in our custom recording division. In 1978, Houston Taping fFor The Blind signed on the air. Reading several dozen popular magazines and best selling books on the air.
1967

8821 United States Association of Blind Athletes
33 N Institute Street
Colorado Springs, CO 80903
719-630-0422
FAX: 719-630-0616
e-mail: mlucas@usaba.org
www.usaba.org

Mark Lucas, Executive Director
Ryan Ortiz, Development Director
The mission is to increase the number and quality of grassroots through competitive, world class athletic opportunities for Americans who are blind or visually impaired. Also value the life enhancing aspects of sports and the opportunity to demonstrate the abilities of people who are blind and visually impaired.
1976

8822 Vermont Association for the Blind and Visually Impaired
37 Elmwood Avenue
Burlington, VT 05401
802-863-1358
800-639-5861
FAX: 802-863-1481
e-mail: general@vabvi.org
www.vabvi.org

Steven Pouliot, Executive Director
Carol Eaton, Adult Services Supervisor
Stephanie Bissonette, Teacher Visually Impaired
Founded from assistance with the Helen Keller and the American Foundation for the Blind with the mission to enable Vermonters with vision problems, whether blindness or impairment, to achieve and maintain independence. Also promotes self advocacy, independence, and coping skills through our education programsand adult services.
1926

8823 Vision World Wide
5707 Brockton Drive
Suite 302
Indianapolis, IN 46220
317-254-1332
800-431-1739
FAX: 317-251-6588
e-mail: info@visionww.org
www.visionww.org

William Corbin, Chairman
Patricia L Price, Founder/President
A non profit organization dedicated to improving the lives of the vision impaired through direct interaction and indirectly through the caregiving community. Also serve both the totally blind and those with various degrees and forms of vision loss.

1995

8824 **Visions/Services for the Blind & Visually Impaired**
500 Greenwich Street
Third Floor
New York, NY 10013
212-625-1616
888-245-8333
FAX: 212-219-4078
e-mail: info@visionsvcb.org
www.visionsvcb.org

Nancy Jones, President
Nancy D Miller, Ceo/Executive Director
Non profit rehabilitation and social service organization whose purpose is to develop and implement programs to assist blind and visually impaired people of all ages to lead independent and active lives in their homes and communities; and to educate the public to understand the capabilities and needs of people who are blind or visually impaired so that they might be integrated into all aspects of community life.

8825 **Visually Impaired Veterans of America**
American Council of the Blind
1075 N Rancho Avenue
Colton, CA 92324
909-825-3067
FAX: 909-213-8570
e-mail: bj2kiowa@worldnet.att.net
www.acb.org

John Fleming, President
Maintain, promote and foster the well bring and rehabilitation of all visually Impaired Veterans of the Armed Forces of the United States of America who are eligible to receive from the Veterans Administration; develops and encourages the practice of high standards of personal professional conduct among Visually Impaired Veterans; maintain, promote, and foster public confidence and awareness In Visually Impaired Veterans.

8826 **Washington Ear**
35 University Boulevard E
Silver Spring, MD 20901
301-681-6636
FAX: 301-681-5227
e-mail: information@washear.org
www.washear.org

Brother Hilary Mettes, Chairman
Margaret Pfanstiehl, President
George Long, Vice President
A non profit organization providing reading and information services for blind, visually impaired and physically disabled people who cannot effectively read print, see plays, watch television programs and films, or view museum exhibits. Ear free services strive to substitute hearing for seeing, improving the lives of people with limited or no vision by enabling them to be well-informed, fully productive members of their families, their communities and the working world.
1974

Camps

8827 **Camp Barakel**
PO Box 159
Fairview, MI 48621
989-848-2279
FAX: 989-848-2280
e-mail: info@campbarakel.org
www.campbarakel.org

Lee Brown, Program Director
Five-day Christian camp experience in mid-August for campers ages 13-55 who are physically disabled, visually impaired, upper trainable mentally impaired or educable mentally impaired, bus transportation provided from locations in Lansing, Flint and Bay City, Michigan.

8828 **Camp Challenge**
8914 US Highway 50 East
Bedford, IN 47421
812-834-5159
e-mail: campc@hpcisp.com
www.campc.org

Ralph Price, Director
Lyn Price, Assistant Director
Mike Corrence, Camp Director
One and two-week sessions for campers with developmental and or physical disabilities, hearing impairment and the blind/visually impaired. Ages 6-99 and families.

8829 **Camp Lawroweld**
Northern New England Conference
228 West Side Road
Weld, ME 04285
207-585-2984
FAX: 207-585-2895
www.lawroweld.org

Joseph Stagg Lawrence, Founder
Clarence Well, Founder
Harry Sabnani, Executive Director
Camp is located in Weld, Maine. Week sessions July for campers who are blind or visually impaired, all ages. Other camps coed, ages 9-16 and families, single adults, June - September.

8830 **Camp Lou Henry Hoover**
Girl Scouts of Washington Rock Council
201 Grove Street East
Westfield, NJ 07090
908-232-3236
FAX: 908-232-4508
e-mail: dhooker@gswrc.com.
www.camphoover.org

Deb Hooker, Camp Director
Coleen Hay, Camp Registrar
John Shabatura, Camp Ranger
Camp is located in Middleville, New Jersey. Sessions for girls who are blind/visually impaired, ages 7-18.

8831 **Camp Merrick**
PO Box 56
3650 Rick Hamilton Place
Nanjemoy, MD 20662
301-870-5858
FAX: 301-246-9108
e-mail: administrator@lionscampmerrick.org
www.lionscampmerrick.org

Robert Rainey, Administrator
Programs offered April-January for children who are blind/visually impaired, hearing impaired or diabetic. Coed, ages 6-15.

8832 **Christian Record Services/National Camps for Blind Children**
4444 South 52nd Street
Lincoln, NE 68516
402-488-0981
FAX: 402-488-7582
e-mail: info@christianrecord.org
www.christianrecord.org

Lawrence Pitcher, President
Ronald Welch, District Director
Dorothy Marston, District Director
Provides free Christian publications and programs, as well as new opportunities for people with visual impairments. Free services include subscription magazines available in braille, large print and audio cassette, full-vision books combining braille and print, lending library, gift bibles and study guides in braille, large print and audio cassette, national camps for blind children and scholarship assistance for blind young people trying to obtain a college education.

8833 **Columbia Lighthouse for the Blind Summer Camp**
Columbia Lighthouse for the Blind
1120 20th Street NW
Suite 750 South
Washington, DC 20036
202-454-6400
877-324-5252
FAX: 202-454-6401
e-mail: info@clb.org
www.clb.org

Peter Mayo, President
Antoine Johnson, Camp Programs Director
Michelle Tatro, Public Relations/Media

Helps enable the blind or visually impaired to obtain and maintain independence at home, school, work and in the community. Programs and services include early intervention services, training and consultation in assistive technology, career placement services, comprehensive low vision care and a wide range of rehabilitation services. Highly acclaimed summer camp, picnics and holiday activities encourage blind and visualy impaired children to make new friends and experience the joys of childhood.

8834 Directory of Camps for Blind and Visually Impaired Children & Adults

American Foundation for the Blind/AFB Press
PO Box 1020
Sewickley, PA 15143
412-741-1142
800-232-3044
FAX: 412-741-0609
e-mail: afborders@abdintl.com
www.afb.org

A guide to 200 sleepaway camps and day camps in the United States. Descriptions cover types of campers, age ranges, special activities offered, length of seasons and contact names. *$15.95*

34 pages Papberack
ISBN 0-891281-59-2

8835 Easter Seals Oklahoma

Easter Seals America
701 Northeast 13th Street
Oklahoma City, OK 73104
405-239-2525
FAX: 405-239-2278
e-mail: esok1@coxinet.net
www.eastersealsoklahoma.org

Patricia Filer, Executive Director

Providing services such as adult day services, child development center, OTIPT, speech therapy, reading/tutoring, vision and hearing screening.

8836 Enchanted Hills Camp for the Blind

Lighthouse for the Blind
214 Van Ness Avenue
San Francisco, CA 94102
415-431-1481
FAX: 415-863-7568
TTY:415-431-4572
e-mail: executive@lighthouse-sf.org
www.lighthouse-sf.org

Anita S Aaron, Executive Director
Anthony Fletcher, Director Community Services
Julie McCarthy, Facilities Manager

Camp is located in Napa, California. Half-week, one and two-week sessions for blind, deaf/blind children and adults, ages 5 and up. This program offers a basic camping experience. Activities include music, art, dance, hiking and riding. Camperships are available to California residents.

8837 Highbrook Lodge

Cleveland Sight Center
1909 East 101st Street
PO Box 1988
Cleveland, OH 44106
216-791-8118
FAX: 216-791-1101
www.clevelandsightcenter.org/camp

Michael Grady, President/Executive Director
James Sacher, Chair
Andrew Sikorovsky, Treasurer

Camp is located in Chardon, Ohio. Summer sessions for blind and disabled children, adults and families. There are seven sessions held annually during June, July and August with an entire range of outdoor camp activities. Camp activities focus on learning through play. Weekly rate: $100-$260 per week.

8838 Indian Creek Camp

Kentucky Tennessee Conference
PO Box 1088
Goodlettsville, TN 37070
615-859-1391
FAX: 615-859-2120
e-mail: info@indiancreekcamp.com
www.indiancreekcamp.com

Jerry Mahn, Director
Aaron Raines, Assistant Director
Richard Hallock, President

Camp is located in Liberty, Tennessee. Summer sessions for children and adults who are blind/visually impaired. Coed, ages 7-17, families and seniors.

8839 Kamp A-Komp-Plish

9035 Ironsides Road
Nanjemoy, MD 20622
301-870-3226
301-934-3590
FAX: 301-870-2620
e-mail: kampakomplish@melwood.org
www.kamakomplish.org/

Heidi Aldous, Camp Director
Doria Fleisher, Equestrian Manager
Earl Copus, Owner

Camp is located in Nanjemoy, Maryland. Half-week, one-week and two-week sessions for blind/visually impaired children and those with developmental disabilities and mobility limitation. Coed, ages 8-16.

8840 Kamp Kaleo

46872 Willow Springs Road
Burwell, NE 68823
308-346-5083
e-mail: kamp@micrord.com
www.kampkaleo.com/html/kampkaleo.html

Judie L Luther, Program Manager
Roddy Dunkerson, Religious Leader

Camp is located in Burwell, Nebraska. Summer sessions for campers who are blind/visually impaired or have developmental disabilities. Coed, ages 9-18 and families, seniors, single adults.

8841 Texas Lions Camp

PO Box 290247
Kerrville, TX 78029
830-896-8500
FAX: 830-896-3666
e-mail: tlc@ktc.com
www.lionscamp.com

Stephen S Mabry, Executive Director

The primary purpose of the League shall be to provide, without charge, a camp for physically disabled, hearing/vision impaired and diabetic children from the State of Texas, regardless of race, religion, or national origin. Our goal is to create an atmosphere wherein campers will learn the can do philosophy and be allowed to achieve maximum personal growth and self-esteem. The camp welcomes boys and girls ages 7-16.

8842 University of Iowa: Wendell Johnson Speech and Hearing Clinic

250 Hawkins Drive
Iowa City, IA 52242
319-335-1845
FAX: 319-335-8851
e-mail: wendy-fick@uiowa.edu
www.shc.uiowa.edu

Linda Louko, Clinic Director
Marlea O'Brien, Child Language Research Center
Dorothy Albright, Department Administration

The clinic offers assessment and remediation for communication disorders in adults and children. The clinic also offers a Intensive Summer Residential Clinic for school age children needing intervention services because of speech, language, hearing and/or reading problems.

8843 VISIONS Vacation Camp for the Blind

VISIONS/Services for the Blind & Visually Impaired
500 Greenwich Street
3rd Floor
New York, NY 10013
212-625-1616
FAX: 212-219-4078
e-mail: nnowak@visionsvcb.org
www.visionsvcb.org/camp.asp

Nancy T Jones, President
David Koch, Vice President
Burton M Strauss Jr, Treasurer

Is a non profit agency that promotes the independence of people of all ages who are blind or visually imparied.

8844 **Winnekeag**
34 Sawyer Street
PO Box 1169
South Lancaster, MA 01561
978-365-4551
FAX: 978-365-3838
e-mail: sneconference@sneconline.org
www.sneconline.org

Frank Tochterman, President/Religious Leader
Camp is located in Ashburnham, Massachusetts. Camping sessions for blind/visually impaired children. Coed, ages 8-16.

8845 **YMCA Camp Chingachgook on Lake George**
Capital District YMCA
1872 Pilot Knob Road
Kattskill Bay, NY 12844
518-656-9462
FAX: 518-656-9362
e-mail: chingachgook@cdymca.org
http://www.capitaldistrictymca.com/

George Painter, Executive Director
David Brown, President/CEO
Regina M Lagatta, VP Operations
Sailing programs for people with disabilities. Sessions for campers who are blind/visually impaired. Coed, ages 7-16, families, seniors and single adults.

Print & Non-Print Resources

8846 **AFB Directory of Services for Blind and Visually Impaired Persons in the US and Canada**
American Foundation for the Blind/AFB Press
PO Box 1020
Sewickley, PA 15143
412-741-1142
800-232-3044
FAX: 412-741-0609
e-mail: afborders@abdintl.com
www.afb.org

Stephanie Biagioli, Marketing Coordinator
Comprehensive CD-ROM and print resource containing more that 2,500 local, state, regional, and national services throughout the US and Canada for persons who are blind or visually impaired. *$74.95*
624 pages Hardcover/CDROM
ISBN 0-89128-00-5

8847 **AFB News**
American Foundation for the Blind/AFB Press
11 Penn Plaza
Suite 300
New York, NY 10001
212-502-7600
800-232-3044
FAX: 212-502-7777
e-mail: afborders@abdintl.com
www.afb.org

Carl Augusto, President
National newsletter for general readership about blindness and visual impairments featuring people, programs, services and activities.
12 pages Quarterly

8848 **About Children's Eyes**
National Association for Visually Handicapped
22 W 21st Street
Floor 6
New York, NY 10010
212-889-3141
FAX: 212-727-2931
e-mail: staff@navh.org
www.navh.org

Lorianie Marchi, Chief Executive Officer
How to identify the child with a visual problem.

8849 **About Children's Vision: A Guide for Parents**
National Association for Visually Handicapped
22 W 21st Street
Floor 6
New York, NY 10010
212-889-3141
FAX: 212-727-2931
e-mail: staff@navh.org
www.navh.org

Lorianie Marchi, Chief Executive Officer
Offers a better understanding of the normal and possible abnormal development of a child's eyesight. *$.50*

8850 **Access to Art: A Museum Directory for Blind and Visually Impaired People**
American Foundation for the Blind/AFB Press
PO Box 1020
Sewickley, PA 15143
412-741-1142
800-232-3044
FAX: 412-741-0609
e-mail: afborders@abdintl.com
www.afb.org
Details the access facilities of over 300 museums, galleries and exhibits in the United States. Also included are organizations offering art-related resources such as, art classes, competitions and traveling exhibits. *$19.95*
144 pages Large Print
ISBN 0-891281-56-8

8851 **African Americans in the Profession of Blindness Services**
Mississippi State University
PO Box 6189
Mississippi State, MS 39762
662-325-2001
800-675-7782
FAX: 662-325-8989
www.blind.msstate.edu

Kelly Schaefer, Dissemination Specialist
Elton Moore, Executive Director
This study investigated the level of participation by African Americans in vocational rehab. (VR) services to persons who are visually impaired. Using surveys and interviews with all state VR directors, national census data and national RSA data, it was found nationally that African Americans are substantially under-represented in the service provider ranks, yet over-represented as clients. *$20.00*
61 pages Paperback

8852 **Age-Related Macular Degeneration**
National Association for Visually Handicapped
22 W 21st Street
Floor 6
New York, NY 10010
212-889-3141
888-205-5951
FAX: 212-727-2931
e-mail: nauh@nauh.org
www.navh.org

Dr Lorraine H Marchi, Founder/CEO
Cesar Gomez, Executive Director
A large booklet offering information and up-to-date research on Macular Degeneration. Also available in Russian. Revised in 2007. *$4.00*

8853 **Aging and Vision: Declarations of Independence**
American Foundation for the Blind/AFB Press
PO Box 1020
Sewickley, PA 15143
412-741-1142
800-232-3044
FAX: 412-741-0609
e-mail: afborders@abdintl.com
www.afb.org
A very personal look at five older people who have successfully coped with visual impairmant and continue to lead active, satisfying lives. Their stories are not only inspirational, but also provide practical, down-to-earth suggestions for adapting to vision loss later in life. 18 minute video tape. Also available in PAL, $52.95, 0-89128-276-9. *$42.95*

VHS
ISBN 0-891282-20-3

8854 American Anals of the Deaf Reference
800 Florida Avenue NE
Washington, DC 20002
202-651-5488
FAX: 202-651-5489
e-mail: gupress@gallaudet.edu
http://gupress.gallaudet.edu

Donald F. Moores, Editor
The controlled scope of GUPress operations allows the continuance of a highly focused commitment to individual titles that has contributed significantly to its 20 years of leadership in publishing on Deaf issues. Gallaudet University Press brings unmatched experience and knowledge to the marketplace for books on and for the Deaf community, its advocates, and scholars invested in the study of deaf society.

8855 American Printing House for the Blind
PO Box 6085
Louisville, KY 40206
502-895-2405
800-223-1839
FAX: 502-899-2274
e-mail: info@aph.org
www.aph.org

Fred Gissoni, Customer Support
Tuck Tinsley, President
Devoted solely to producing products for people who are visually impaired. We manufacture books and magazines in braille, large type and recorded form from over 200 vendors across the U.S. We also make a wide range of educational and daily living aids, such as braille paper and styluses, talking book equipment, and synthetic speech computer products. APH also offers LOUIS, an electronic database that lists accessible books in all formats.

8856 Americans with Disabilities Act Guide for Places of Lodging: Serving Guests Who Are Blind
US Department of Justice
950 Pennsylvania Avenue NW Drs
- Nyav
Washington, DC 20530
202-586-5000
800-574-0301
FAX: 202-307-1197
www.ada.gov

Joanne Graham, Manager
A 12-page publication explaining what hotels, motels, and other places of transient lodging can do to accommodate guests who are blind or have low vision.

8857 Annual Report/Newsletter
National Accreditation Council for Agencies/Blind
15 E 40th Street
Room 1004
New York, NY 10016
212-683-5068
FAX: 212-683-4475

Ruth Westman, Executive Director
Provides standards and a program of accreditation for schools and organizations which serve children and adults who are blind or vision impaired.

8858 Art and Science of Teaching Orientation and Mobility to Persons with Visual Impairments
American Foundation for the Blind/AFB Press
PO Box 1020
Sewickley, PA 15143
412-741-1142
800-232-3044
FAX: 412-741-0609
e-mail: afborders@abdintl.com
www.afb.org
Comprehensive decription of the techniques of teaching orientation and mobility, presented along with considerations and strategies for sensitive and effective teaching. Hardcover. Paperback also available. *$48.00*

200 pages
ISBN 0-891282-45-9

8859 Association for Macular Diseases Newsletter
210 E 64th Street
8th Floor
New York, NY 10021
212-605-3719
FAX: 212-605-3795
e-mail: association@retinal-research.org
www.macula.org

Nikolai Stevenson, President
Walter Ross, Editor-in-Chief
Joan Daly, Treasurer
Not-for-profit organization promotes education and research in this scarcely explored field. Acts as a nationwide support group for individuals and their families endeavoring to adjust to the restrictions and changes brought about by macular disease. Offers hotline, educational materials, quarterly newsletter, support groups, referrals and seminars for persons and families affected by macular disease.
1978

8860 Awareness
NAPVI
PO Box 317
Watertown, MA 02471
617-972-7441
800-562-6265
FAX: 617-972-7444
e-mail: napvi@perkins.org
www.napvi.org

Susan LaVenture, Executive Director
Newsletter offering regional news, sports and activities, conferences, camps, legislative updates, book reviews, audio reviews, professional question and answer column and more for the visually impaired and their families.
Quarterly

8861 Awareness Training
Landmark Media
3450 Slade Run Drive
Falls Church, VA 22042
703-241-2030
800-342-4336
FAX: 703-536-9540
e-mail: landmarkmed@aol.com
www.landmarkmedia.com

Michael Hartogs, President
Covers disabilities of various types — vision, hearing, speech disorders, loss of limbs, loss of mobility, or mental/emotional limitations and how to integrate such individuals into various business and educational settings. It is a 4-part series designed to identify and enable others to interact effectively with those suffering such disabilities. *$495.00*
Set of 4

8862 Babycare Assistive Technology
Through the Looking Glass
2198 6th Street
Suite 100
Berkeley, CA 94710
510-848-1112
800-644-2666
FAX: 510-848-4445
e-mail: TLG@lookingglass.org
www.lookingglass.org

C Tuleja
A DeMoss
Megan Kirshbaum, Executive Director
Available in braille, large print or cassette. *$2.00*
8 pages

8863 Babycare Assistive Technology for Parents with Physical Disabilties
Through the Looking Glass
2198 6th Street
Suite 100
Berkeley, CA 94710
510-848-1112
800-644-2666
FAX: 510-848-4445
e-mail: TLG@lookingglass.org
www.lookingglass.org

Megan Kirshbaum, Executive Director

Relational, systems and Cultural perspectives. Available in braille, large print or cassette. *$2.00*
7 pages

8864 Basic Course in American Sign Language
TJ Publishers
2544 Tarpley Road
Suite 108
Carrollton, TX 75006
972-416-0800
800-999-1168
FAX: 301-585-5930
TTY: 301-585-4440
e-mail: TJPubinc@aol.com

Angela K Thames, President
Jerald A Murphy, VP
Accompanying videotapes and textbooks include voice translations. Hearing students can analyze sound for initial instruction, or opt to turn off the sound to sharpen visual acuity. Package includes the Basic Course in American Sign Language text, Student Study Guide, the original four 1-hour videotapes plus the ABCASI Vocabulary videotape. *$139.95*
280 pages Video

8865 Behavioral Vision Approaches for Persons with Physical Disabilities
Optometric Extension Program Foundation
2912 Daimler Street
Santa Ana, CA 92705
949-250-0846

A discussion of the behavioral vision/neuro-motor approach to providing directions for prescriptive and therapeutic services for the visually handicapped child or adult. *$49.50*
197 pages

8866 Belonging
Dial Books
375 Hudson Street
New York, NY 10014
212-366-2000
FAX: 212-414-3394
Meg attended special schools for the blind until she was ready for high school. She decided that she wanted to go to a regular high school. She and her mother practiced her walks to school and studied the layout of the building prior to school starting, but Meg was unprepared for the trip when there were 1,500 students. She adjusted quickly to the crowds and the pace of the new school.
200 pages Hardcover
ISBN 0-80370 -30-1

8867 Berthold Lowenfeld on Blindness and Blind People
American Foundation for the Blind/AFB Press
PO Box 1020
Sewickley, PA 15143
412-741-1142
800-232-3044
FAX: 412-741-0609
e-mail: afborders@abdintl.com
www.afb.org
These writings of the pioneering educator, author and advocate range over a forty-year period include various ground-breaking papers for the blind educator, a rememberance of Helen Keller and other essays on education, sociology and history. *$21.95*
254 pages Paperback
ISBN 0-891281-01-0

8868 Blind Educator
National Federation of the Blind
1800 Johnson Street
Baltimore, MD 21230
410-659-9314
FAX: 410-685-5653
e-mail: nfb@iamdigex.net
www.nfb.org

Marc Maurer, President
Magazine specifically for blind educators.

8869 Blind and Vision-Impaired Individuals
Mainstream
3 Bethesda Metro Center
Suite 830
Bethesda, MD 20814
301-961-9299
800-247-1380
FAX: 301-654-6714
e-mail: info@mainstreaminc.org

Charles Moster
Mainstreaming blind individuals into the workplace. *$ 2.50*
12 pages

8870 Blindness and Early Childhood Development Second Edition
American Foundation for the Blind/AFB Press
PO Box 1020
Sewickley, PA 15143
412-741-1142
800-232-3044
FAX: 412-741-0609
e-mail: afborders@abdintl.com
www.afb.org
A review of current knowledge on motor and locomotor development, perceptual development, language and cognitive processes, and social, emotional and personality development. Paperback. *$34.95*
384 pages
ISBN 0-891281-23-1

8871 Blindness, A Family Matter
American Foundation for the Blind/AFB Press
PO Box 1020
Sewickley, PA 15143
412-741-1142
800-232-3044
FAX: 412-741-0609
e-mail: afborders@abdintl.com
www.afb.org
A frank exploration of the effects of an individual's visual impairment on other members of the family and how those family members can play a positive role in the rehabilitation process. Features interviews with three families whose 'success stories' provide advice and encouragement, as well as interviews with newly blinded adults currently involved in a rehabilitation program. 23 minute video tape. Also available in PAL, $49.95, 0-89128-271-8. *$43.95*
VHS 1986
ISBN 0-891282-22-X

8872 Blindness: What it is, What it Does and How to Live with it
American Foundation for the Blind/AFB Press
PO Box 1020
Sewickley, PA 15143
412-741-1142
800-232-3044
FAX: 412-741-0609
e-mail: afborders@abdintl.com
www.afb.org
A classic work on how blindness affects self-perception and social interaction and what can be done to restore basic skills, mobility, daily living and an appreciation of life's pleasures. *$15.95*

396 pages Paperback
ISBN 0-891282-05-

8873 Books are Fun for Everyone
National Library Service for the Blind
1291 Taylor Street NW
Washington, DC 20542
202-707-5100
FAX: 202-707-0712
e-mail: nls@loc.gov
www.loc.gov/nls

Frank Cylke, Executive Director

8874 Braille Book Bank, Music Catalog
National Braille Association
3 Townline Circle
Rochester, NY 14623
585-427-8260

e-mail: nbaoffice@compuserve.com
www.nationalbraille.org

Angela Coffaro, Executive Director
Offers hundreds of musical titles in print form, braille and on cassette.

62 pages

8875 **Braille Book Review**
National Library Service for the Blind
1291 Taylor Street NW
Washington, DC 20542
202-707-5100
FAX: 202-707-0712
TTY:202-707-0744
e-mail: nls@loc.gov
www.loc.gov/nls

Robert Fistick, Head Publications/Media Section
Frank Cylke, Executive Director
New braille books and product news.
30 pages BiMonthly

8876 **Braille Documents**
Metrolina Association for the Blind
704 Louise Avenue
Charlotte, NC 28204
704-372-3870
800-926-5460
FAX: 704-372-3872

Robert Scheffel, Manager
This production shop creates Braille and large-print documents.

8877 **Braille Forum**
American Council of the Blind
1155 15th Street NW
Suite 1004
Washington, DC 20005
202-467-5081
800-424-8666
FAX: 202-467-5085
e-mail: slovering@acb.org
www.acb.org

Penny Reeder, Editor
Melanie Brunson, Executive Director
Offered in print, braille, cassette, IBM computer disk and e-mail. $25 per format per year for companies and non-US residents.
48 pages Magazine

8878 **Braille Monitor**
National Federation of the Blind
1800 Johnson Street
Baltimore, MD 21230
410-659-9314
FAX: 410-685-5653
e-mail: nfb@iamdigex.net
www.nfb.org

Marc Maurer, President
Leading publication in the blindness field, with a circulation of 30,000, this publication addresses issues of concern to the blind and the philosophy and activities of the National Federation of the Blind.
Monthly

8879 **Braille: An Extraordinary Volunteer Opportunity**
National Library Service for the Blind
1291 Taylor Street NW
Washington, DC 20542
202-707-5100
FAX: 202-707-0712
e-mail: nls@loc.gov
www.loc.gov/nls

Frank Cylke, Executive Director

8880 **Building Blocks: Foundations for Learning for Young Blind and Visually Impaired Children**
American Foundation for the Blind/AFB Press
PO Box 1020
Sewickley, PA 15143
412-741-1142
800-232-3044
FAX: 412-741-0609
e-mail: afborders@abdintl.com
www.afb.org

Presents the essential components of a successful early intervnetion program, including collaboration with family members, positive relationships between parents and professionals, public education, and attention to important programming components such as space exploration, braille readiness, orientation and mobility, play, cooking and music. Includes interviews with parents. Available in English or Spanish. 10 minute video tape. Also available in PAL, $33.95, 0-89128-268-8. *$26.95*
VHS
ISBN 0-891282-14-9

8881 **Bulletin**
National Association for Visually Handicapped
22 W 21st Street
New York, NY 10010
212-889-3141
FAX: 212-727-2931
e-mail: staff@navh.org
www.navh.org

Lorianie Marchi, Chief Executive Officer
Annual report offering information on Association activities and events, conferences, vision aids and resources for the visually impaired.

8882 **Burns Braille Transcription Dictionary**
American Foundation for the Blind/AFB Press
PO Box 1020
Sewickley, PA 15143
412-741-1142
800-232-3044
FAX: 412-741-0609
e-mail: afborders@abdintl.com
www.afb.org
A handy, portable guide that is a quick reference for anyone who needs to check print-to-braille and braille-to-print meanings and symbols. Paperback. *$19.95*
96 pages
ISBN 0-891292-32-7

8883 **Can't Your Child See? A Guide for Parents of Visually Impaired Children**
Pro-Ed Publications
8700 Shoal Creek Boulevard
Austin, TX 78757
512-451-3246
800-897-3202
FAX: 512-451-8542
e-mail: info@proedinc.com
www.proedinc.com

Donald Hammill, Owner
This second edition offers parents optimistic, practical guidelines for helping visually impaired children reach their full potential. *$26.00*
279 pages Paperback

8884 **Career Perspectives: Interviews with Blind and Visually Impaired Professionals**
American Foundation for the Blind/AFB Press
PO Box 1020
Sewickley, PA 15143
412-741-1142
800-232-3044
FAX: 412-741-0609
e-mail: afborders@abdintl.com
www.afb.org
Profiles of 20 successful archivers who describe in their own words what it takes to pursue and attain professional success in a sighted world. Available in large print, cassette and braille. *$16.95*
96 pages Large Print
ISBN 0-891281-70-3

8885 **Careers in Blindness Rehabilitation Services**
Mississippi State University
PO Box 6189
Mississippi State, MS 39762
662-325-2001
800-675-7782
FAX: 662-325-8989
www.blind.msstate.edu

Kelly Schaefer, Dissemination Specialist
Elton Moore, Executive Director
In a follow-up study in a series examining the substantial under-representation of African Americans as professionals in blindness services, researchers questioned college students about their knowledge, opinions and interests in blindness services. *$15.00*

54 pages Paperback

8886 Cataracts
National Association for Visually Handicapped
22 W 21st Street
Floor 6
New York, NY 10010
212-889-3141
FAX: 212-727-2931
e-mail: staff@navh.org
www.navh.org

Lorianie Marchi, Chief Executive Officer
A booklet offering information about Cataracts, diagnosis and treatment of this common condition. *$2.50*

8887 Characteristics, Services, & Outcomes of Rehab. Consumers who are Blind/Visually Impaired
Mississippi State University
PO Box 6189
Mississippi State, MS 39762
662-325-2001
800-675-7782
FAX: 662-325-8989
www.blind.msstate.edu

Brenda Cavenaugh, Principal Investigatorst
Steven J Pierce, Graduate Research Assistant
Kelly Schaefer, Dissemination Specialist
Issues regarding the efficacy of separate state agencies providing specialized vocational rehabilitation (VR) services to consumers who are blind have generated spirited discussions within the rehabilitation community throughout the history of the state-federal program. In this monograph, RRTC researches report results of their investigation of services provided to blind consumers in separate and general (combined) rehabilitation agencies. *$20.00*
45 pages Paperback

8888 Childhood Glaucoma: A Reference Guide for Families
NAPVI
PO Box 317
Watertown, MA 02471
617-972-7441
800-562-6265
FAX: 617-972-7444
e-mail: napvi@perkins.org
www.napvi.org

8889 Children with Visual Impairments Woodbine House
American Foundation for the Blind/AFB Press
11 Penn Plaza
Suite 300
New York, NY 10001
212-502-7600
800-232-3044
FAX: 301-897-5838
e-mail: afborder@abdintl.com
www.afb.org

Carl Augusto, President
Written by parents and professional, this book presents a comprehensive overview of the issues that are crucial to the healthy development of children with mild to severe visual impaiments. It also offers insight from parents about coping with the emotional aspects of raising a child with special needs. *$16.95*
416 pages
ISBN 0-933149-36-0

8890 Choice Magazine Listening
85 Channel Drive
Port Washington, NY 11050
516-883-8280
888-724-6423
888-724-6423
FAX: 516-944-6849
e-mail: choicemag@aol.com
www.choicemagazinelistening.org

Lois Miller, Office Manager
A free audio anthology is available bi-monthly to visually impaired/physically disabled or dislexic persons nationwide. Playable on the special free 4-track cassette playback equipment which is provided by the Library of Congress through the National Library Service. Each issue features eight hours of unabridged magazine articles, short stories, poetry and media selections from over 100 sources. College level and older. Bimonthly distribution.
Bi-Monthly

8891 Classification of Impaired Vision
National Association for Visually Handicapped
22 W 21st Street
Floor 6
New York, NY 10010
212-889-3141
FAX: 212-727-2931
e-mail: staff@navh.org
www.navh.org

Lorianie Marchi, Chief Executive Officer
Describes various degrees of impaired vision.

8892 Communication Skills for Visually Impaired Learners
Charles C Thomas
2600 S 1st Street
Springfield, IL 62704
217-789-8980
800-258-8980
FAX: 217-789-9130
e-mail: books@ccthomas.com
www.ccthomas.com

Michael Thomas, President
This book has been designed to provide a foundation for a better understanding of teaching reading, writing, and listening skills to students with visual impairments from preschool age through adult levels. The plan of the book incorporates the latest research findings with the practical experiences learned in the classroom. *$49.95*
322 pages Paperback 1997
ISBN 0-39806 -93-0

8893 Comprehensive Examination of Barriers to Employment Among Persons who are Blind or Impaired
Mississippi State University
PO Box 6189
Mississippi State, MS 39762
662-325-2001
800-675-7782
FAX: 662-325-8989
www.blind.msstate.edu

J Elton Moore, Author/Executive Director
Kelly Shaefer, Dissemination Specialist
A multi-phase research project designed to: identify barriers to employment; identify and develop innovative successful strategies to overcome these barriers; develop methods for others to utilize these strategies; disseminate this information to rehabilitation providers; replicate the use of selected strategies in other settings. *$20.00*
90 pages Paperback

8894 Concept Development for Visually Handicapped Children: A Resource Guide
American Foundation for the Blind/AFB Press
PO Box 1020
Sewickley, PA 15143
412-741-1142
800-232-3044
FAX: 412-741-0609
e-mail: afborders@abdintl.com
www.afb.org
A program for integrating such concepts as body imagery, gross motor movement, posture and tactile discrimination into the curriculum from kindergarten on. Paperback. *$16.95*
80 pages
ISBN 0-891280-18-9

8895 Contrasting Characteristics of Blind and Visually Impaired Clients
Mississippi State University
PO Box 6189
Mississippi State, MS 39762
662-325-2001
800-675-7782
FAX: 662-325-8989
www.blind.msstate.edu

Kelly Schaefer, Publications Manager
Elton Moore, Executive Director
This report examines cases in the National Blindness and Low Vision Employment Database to identify and profile environmental and personal characteristics of clients who are blind or visually impaired and who were achieving successful and unsuccessful retention of competitive jobs. A total of 787 cases were analyzed. *$15.00*

44 pages Paperback

8896 DVH Quarterly
University of Arkansas at Little Rock
2801 S University Avenue
Little Rock, AR 72204 501-569-3000

Bob Brasher, Editor
Mary Boaz, Manager
Offers information on upcoming events, conferences and workshops on and for visual disabilities. Book reviews, information on the newest resources and technology, educational programs, want ads and more.
Quarterly

8897 Dancing Cheek to Cheek
Blind Children's Center
4120 Marathon Street
Los Angeles, CA 90029 323-664-2153
800-222-3567
FAX: 323-665-3828
e-mail: info@blindchildrenscenter.org
www.blindchildrenscenter.org

Midge Horton, Executive Director
Beginning social, play and language interactions. *$ 10.00*
23 pages

8898 Data on Blindness and Visual Impairment in the US: A Resource Manual
American Foundation for the Blind/AFB Press
PO Box 1020
Sewickley, PA 15143 412-741-1142
800-232-3044
FAX: 412-741-0609
e-mail: afborders@abdintl.com
www.afb.org
Provides facts and figures for long-range planning, preparing grant proposals and legislative services. Paperback. *$47.00*
412 pages
ISBN 0-891281-52-5

8899 Deaf-Blind Perspective
Teaching Research
345 Monmouth Avenue
Monmouth, OR 97361 503-838-8391
800-438-9376
FAX: 503-838-8150
e-mail: dblink@tr.wou.edu
www.tr.wou.edu/dblink

John Reiman PhD, Director
Meredith Brodsky, Executive Director

8900 Descriptive Video Service
WGBH Educational Foundation
125 Western Avenue
Boston, MA 02134 617-300-2000
800-333-1203
FAX: 617-300-1011
e-mail: ncam@wgbh.org
www.wgbh.org

Sharon King, Outreach Director
Mary Ann Pack, Assistant Director
Henry Becton, Chief Executive Officer
A national service that makes PBS television programs, Hollywood movies on video and other visual media accessible to people who are blind or visually impaired. DVS provides narrated descriptions of the key visual elements without interfering with the audio or dialogue of a program or movie. The narration describes visual elements such as actions, settings, body language and graphics.

8901 Development of Social Skills by Blind and Visually Impaired Students
American Foundation for the Blind/AFB Press
PO Box 1020
Sewickley, PA 15143 412-741-1142
800-232-3044
FAX: 412-741-0609
e-mail: afborders@abdintl.com
www.afb.org
Offers an examination of the social interactions of blind and visually impaired children in mainstreamed settings and the community that highlights the need to teach social interaction skills to children and provide them with support. Paperback. *$39.95*
232 pages
ISBN 0-891282-17-3

8902 Diabetic Retinopathy
National Association for Visually Handicapped
22 W 21st Street
Floor 6
New York, NY 10010 212-889-3141
FAX: 212-727-2931
e-mail: staff@navh.org
www.navh.org

Lorianie Marchi, Chief Executive Officer
A booklet offering information about Diabetic Retinopathy.

8903 Dialogue Magazine
Blindskills
PO Box 5181
Salem, OR 97304 503-581-4224
800-860-4224
FAX: 503-581-0178
e-mail: info@blindskills.com
www.blindskills.com

Carol M McCarl, Executive Director
Karen Lynn Thomas, Editor
Publishes quarterly magazine in braille, large-type, cassette, e-mail and disk of news items, technology and articles of special interest to visually impaired youth and adults. $40.00 for not blind/legally blind. *$28.00*
Quarterly

8904 Dimensions: Visually Impaired Persons with Multiple Disabilities
American Foundation for the Blind/AFB Press
PO Box 1020
Sewickley, PA 15143 412-741-1142
800-232-3044
FAX: 412-741-0609
e-mail: afborders@abdintl.com
www.afb.org

Stephanie Biagioli, Marketing Coordinator
Twenty-one articles from the Journal of Visual Impairment and Blindness, present a wide range of approaches for working with persons with multiple disabilities. *$24.95*
116 pages Paperback
ISBN 0-89128 -63-0

8905 Diversity and Visual Impairment: The Influ ence of Race, Gender, Religion and Ethnicity
American Foundation for the Blind
11 Penn Plaza
Suite 300
New York, NY 10001 212-502-7600
800-232-5463
FAX: 212-502-7777
e-mail: afbinfo@afb.net
www.afb.org/store

Carl R Augusto, President/CEO
Cultural, social, ethnic, gender, and religious issues can influence the way an individual perceives and copes with a visual impairment. *$45.95*
480 pages 2001
ISBN 0-891283-83-8

8906 Do You Remember the Color Blue: And Other Questions Kids Ask About Blindness
Viking Books

The author answers thirteen thought-provoking questions that children have asked her over the years about being blind.

78 pages 2000
ISBN 0-670880-43-4

8907 **Dog Sponsorship Program**
Guide Dog Foundation for the Blind
371 E Jericho Tpke
Smithtown, NY 11787
631-265-2121
800-548-4337
FAX: 516-361-5192

Wells Jones, Executive Director
Offers information to an individual or an organization that wishes to sponsor a guide dog.

8908 **Don't Lose Sight of Cataracts**
National Eye Institute
Building 31
Bethesda, MD 20892
301-496-0417
800-869-2020
FAX: 301-402-1065
e-mail: 2020@nei.nih.gov
www.nei.nih.gov

8909 **Don't Lose Sight of Glaucoma**
National Eye Institute
Building 31
Bethesda, MD 20892
301-496-0417
800-869-2020
FAX: 301-402-1065
e-mail: 2020@nei.nih.gov
www.nei.nih.gov

8910 **Early Focus: Working with Young Blind and Visually Impaired Children**
American Foundation for the Blind/AFB Press
PO Box 1020
Sewickley, PA 15143
412-741-1142
800-232-3044
FAX: 412-741-0609
e-mail: afborders@abdintl.com
www.afb.org
Describes early intervention techniques used with blind and visually impaired children and stresses the benefits of family involvement and transdisciplinary teamwork. Paperback. *$32.95*
176 pages
ISBN 0-891282-15-7

8911 **Encyclopedia of Blindness and Vision Impairment Second Edition**
Facts on File
132 W 31st Street
Floor 17
New York, NY 10001
212-967-8800
800-322-8755
FAX: 212-967-9196
e-mail: jcchambers@factsonfile.com
www.factsonfile.com

James Chamber, Editor-in-Chief Arts/Humanities
Mark Donnell, President
Designed to provide both laymen and professionals with concise, practical information on the second most common disability in the U.S. *$65.00*
340 pages Hardbound
ISBN 6-810021-53-8

8912 **Equals in Partnership: Basic Rights for Families of Children with Blindness**
NAPVI
PO Box 317
Watertown, MA 02471
617-972-7441
800-562-6265
FAX: 617-972-7444
e-mail: napvi@perkins.org
www.napvi.org

8913 **Eye Research News Briefs**
Research to Prevent Blindness
645 Madison Avenue
Floor 21
New York, NY 10022
212-752-4333
800-621-0026
FAX: 212-688-6231
e-mail: info@rpbusa.org
www.rpbusa.org

James V Romano PhD, COO/Manager
Thomas Furlong, Director Public Information
Yearly publication from Research to Prevent Blindness. Free.
4 pages Yearly

8914 **Eye and Your Vision**
National Association for Visually Handicapped
22 W 21st Street
Floor 6
New York, NY 10010
212-889-3141
FAX: 212-727-2931
e-mail: staff@navh.org
www.navh.org

Lorianie Marchi, Chief Executive Officer
A large booklet offering information, with illustrations, on the eye. Includes information on protection of eyesight, how the eye works and vision disorders. Available in Russian and Spanish also. *$ 2.75*

8915 **Eye-Q Test**
National Association for Visually Handicapped
22 W 21st Street
Floor 6
New York, NY 10010
212-889-3141
FAX: 212-727-2931
e-mail: staff@navh.org
www.navh.org

Lorianie Marchi, Chief Executive Officer
Five questions and answers to assist in knowing more about vision. Also available in Spanish and Russian.

8916 **Facts: Books for Blind and Physically Handicapped Individuals**
National Library Service for the Blind
1291 Taylor Street NW
Washington, DC 20542
202-707-5100
e-mail: nls@loc.gov
www.loc.gov/nls

Frank Cylke, Executive Director
Annual

8917 **Family Context and Disability Culture Reframing: Through the Looking Glass**
Through the Looking Glass
2198 6th Street
Suite 100
Berkeley, CA 94710
510-848-1112
800-644-2666
FAX: 510-848-4445
e-mail: TLG@lookingglass.org
www.lookingglass.org

Mega Kirshbaum, Executive Director
Available in braille, large print or cassette. *$2.00*
5 pages

8918 **Family Guide to Vision Care**
American Optometric Association
243 N Lindbergh Boulevard
Saint Louis, MO 63141
314-991-4100
FAX: 314-991-4101
www.aoanet.org

Michael Jones, Executive Director
Offers information on the early developmental years of your vision, finding a family optometrist and how to take care of your eyesight through the learning years, the working years and the mature years.

8919 Family Guide: Growth & Development of the Partially Seeing Child
National Association for Visually Handicapped
22 W 21st Street
Floor 6
New York, NY 10010
212-889-3141
FAX: 212-727-2931
e-mail: staff@navh.org
www.navh.org

Lorianie Marchi, Chief Executive Officer
Offers information for parents and guidelines in raising a partially seeing child. *$.60*

8920 Fathers: A Common Ground
Blind Children's Center
4120 Marathon Street
Los Angeles, CA 90029
323-664-2153
800-222-3567
FAX: 323-665-3828
e-mail: info@blindchildrenscenter.org
www.blindchildrenscenter.org

Midge Horton, Executive Director
Exploring the concerns and roles of fathers of children with visual impairments. *$10.00*
50 pages

8921 Fighting Blindness News
RP Foundation Fighting Blindness
1401 W Mt Royal Avenue
4th Floor
Baltimore, MD 21217
410-225-9400
800-683-5555
FAX: 410-225-3936
TTY: 410-225-9409

Greg Vaughan, Manager
Offers information on medical updates, donor programs, assistive devices, resources and clinical trial information for persons with visual impariments, blindness and retinal degenerative diseases.
2x Year

8922 First Steps
Blind Children's Center
4120 Marathon Street
Los Angeles, CA 90029
323-664-2153
800-222-3567
FAX: 323-665-3828
e-mail: info@blindchildrenscenter.org
www.blindchildrenscenter.org

Midge Horton, Executive Director
A handbook for teaching young children who are visually impaired. Designed to assist students, professionals and parents working with children who are visually impaired. Visit our website for many publications addressing training very young children who are blind or visually impaired. *$35.00*
203 pages

8923 Focus
Visually Impaired Center
1422 W Court Street
Flint, MI 48503
313-235-2544

Laurie MacArthur, Executive Director
Newsletter offering information for the visually impaired person in the forms of legislative and law updates, ADA information, support groups, hotlines, and articles on the newest technology in the field.
Quarterly

8924 Foundations of Orientation and Mobility
American Foundation for the Blind/AFB Press
PO Box 1020
Sewickley, PA 15143
412-741-1142
800-232-3044
FAX: 412-741-0609
e-mail: afborders@abdintl.com
www.afb.org

This text has been updated and revised and includes current research from a variety of disciplines, an international perspective, and expanded contents on low vision, aging, multiple disabilities, accessibility, program design and adaptive technology from more that 30 eminent subject experts. *$68.95*
775 pages
ISBN 0-891289-46-1

8925 Foundations of Rehabilitation Counseling with Persons Who Are Blind
American Foundation for the Blind/AFB Press
PO Box 1020
Sewickley, PA 15143
412-741-1142
800-232-3044
FAX: 412-741-0609
e-mail: afborders@abdintl.com
www.afb.org

Rehabilitation professionals have long recognized that the needs of people who are blind or visually impaired are unique and requie a special knowledge and expertise to provide and corrdinate rehabilitation services. *$59.95*
477 pages
ISBN 0-891289-45-3

8926 Free Information/Membership Kit
National Association for Visually Handicapped
22 W 21st Street
New York, NY 10010
212-889-3141
FAX: 212-727-2931
e-mail: staff@navh.org
www.navh.org

Eva M Cohen, CEO Assistant
Lorianie H Marchi, Founder/CEO
A free packet describing brochures, pamphlets, and flyers available addressing the needs of the partially seeing, their families, friends and professionals who serve them: large print, visual aids, self-help, referrals. Includes information regarding vision dysfunction and coping with vision loss.
Quarterly

8927 Future Reflections
Natl. Organization for Parents of Blind Children
1800 Johnson Street
Baltimore, MD 21230
410-659-9314
FAX: 410-685-5653
e-mail: nfb@iamdigex.net

Marc Maurer, President
National magazine written specifically for parents and educators of blind children. Each issue addresses various topics important to blind children, their families and to school personnel.
Quarterly

8928 General Facts and Figures on Blindness
National Society to Prevent Blindness
500 E Remington Road
Schaumburg, IL 60173
800-331-2020

8929 Get a Wiggle On
American Alliance for Health, Phys. Ed. & Dance
1900 Association Drive
Reston, VA 20191
703-476-3400
FAX: 703-476-9527
e-mail: aaalf@aahperd.org

Michael Davis, Manager
Gives teachers and parents practical suggestions for helping blind and visually impaired infants grow and learn like other children. *$5.00*
80 pages
ISBN 0-88314 -77-2

8930 Gift of Sight
RP Foundation Fighting Blindness
1401 W Mt Royal Avenue
Baltimore, MD 21217
410-225-9409
800-683-5555
FAX: 410-225-3936
A pamphlet offering information on the Retina Donor Program, which studies diseased, human retinal tissue in their search for a cure of retinal degenerative diseases.

8931 Glaucoma
Glaucoma Research Foundation
251 Post Street
Suite 600
San Francisco, CA 94108
415-986-3162
800-826-6693
FAX: 415-986-3763
e-mail: info@glaucoma.org
www.glaucoma.org

Yuko Madono, Outreach/Public Relations
Tom Brunner, Chief Executive Officer
Offers information on what glaucoma is, the causes, treatments, types of glaucoma, eye exams and prevention.

8932 Glaucoma: The Sneak Thief of Sight
National Association for Visually Handicapped
22 W 21st Street
Floor 6
New York, NY 10010
212-889-3141
FAX: 212-727-2931
e-mail: staff@navh.org
www.navh.org

Lorianie Marchi, Chief Executive Officer
A pamphlet describing the disease, treatment and medications. Also available in Russian and Spanish. Revised in 1999. *$3.50*

8933 Gleams Newsletter
Glaucoma Research Foundation
251 Post Street
Suite 600
San Francisco, CA 94108
415-986-3162
800-826-6693
FAX: 415-986-3763
e-mail: info@glaucoma.org
www.glaucoma.org

Yuko Madono, Outreach/Public Relations
Tom Brunner, Chief Executive Officer
Offers updated medical & research information on glaucoma. Included are glaucoma treatmant and coping tips, legsilative information, professional articles and book reviews.
6 pages Quarterly 1982

8934 Good Employee Is Capable, Conscientious, Productive
American Foundation for the Blind/AFB Press
PO Box 1020
Sewickley, PA 15143
412-741-1142
800-232-3044
FAX: 412-741-0609
e-mail: afborders@abdintl.com
www.afb.org
Answers employers' questions about the blind and visually handicapped and provides assurance to employees with visual impairments can get to work, perform their jobs safely and require little in the way of special training.

ISBN 0-891289-19-4

8935 Guide Dog Foundation Flyer
Guide Dog Foundation for the Blind
371 E Jericho Tpke
Smithtown, NY 11787
631-265-2121
800-548-4337
FAX: 516-361-5192

Wells Jones, Executive Director
Offers information on the programs and services provided by the Foundation.

8936 Guidelines and Games for Teaching Efficient Braille Reading
American Foundation for the Blind/AFB Press
PO Box 1020
Sewickley, PA 15143
412-741-1142
800-232-3044
FAX: 412-741-0609
e-mail: afborders@abdintl.com
www.afb.org
Based on research in the areas of rapid reading and precision teaching, these guidelines represent a unique adaptation of a general reading program to the needs of braille readers. Paperback. *$ 24.95*
116 pages
ISBN 0-891281-05-3

8937 Guidelines for Comprehensive Low Vision Care
National Association for Visually Handicapped
22 W 21st Street
Floor 6
New York, NY 10010
212-889-3141
FAX: 212-727-2931
e-mail: staff@navh.org
www.navh.org

Lorianie Marchi, Chief Executive Officer
A description of the proper method to conduct a low vision evaluation. *$.50*

8938 Guideway
Guide Dog Foundation for the Blind
371 E Jericho Tpke
Smithtown, NY 11787
631-265-2121
800-548-4337
FAX: 516-361-5192

Wells Jones, Executive Director
Offers updates and information on the foundation's activities and guide dog programs. In print form but is also available on cassette.
Monthly

8939 Guild Audio Library
JGB Audio Library for the Blind
15 W 65th Street
New York, NY 10023
212-769-6331
800-284-4422
FAX: 212-769-6266
e-mail: info@JGB.org
www.JGB.org

Peter Williamson, Executive Director
Ken Satnley, Manager

8940 Guild Briefs
Catholic Guild for The Blind
180 N Michigan Avenue
Suite 1700
Chicago, IL 60601
312-243-8569
FAX: 312-236-8128
e-mail: guild@guildfortheblind.org
www.guildfortheblind.org

David Tabak, Executive Director
12 pages monthlyally

8941 Handbook for Itinerant and Resource Teachers of Blind Students
National Federation of the Blind
1800 Johnson Street
Baltimore, MD 21230
410-659-9314

e-mail: nfb@iamdigex.net

Marc Maurer, President
The Handbook provides help to teachers, school administrators or other school personnel that have experience with blind or visually impaired students. The Handbook devotes 45 pages to Braille and how to teach Braille for parents and teachers. There are other chapters offering information on the law, physical education, fitting in socially, testing and evaluation, home economics, daily living skills and more. *$23.00*
533 pages Softcover
ISBN 0-962412-20-1

8942 Handbook of Information for Members of the Achromatopsia Network
PO Box 214
Berkeley, CA 94701
510-540-4700
FAX: 510-540-4767
e-mail: futterman@achromat.org
www.achromat.org

8943 Health Care Professionals Who Are Blind or Visually Impaired
American Foundation for the Blind
11 Penn Plaza
Suite 300
New York, NY 10001
212-502-7600
800-232-5463
FAX: 212-502-7777
e-mail: afbinfo@afb.net
www.afb.org/store

Carl R Augusto, President/CEO
This resource is essential reading for older students and young adults who are blind or visually impaired, their families, and the professionals who work with them. *$21.95*
160 pages 2001
ISBN 0-891283-88-9

8944 Hearsay
Int'l Association of Audio Information Services
1102 W International Airport Road
Anchorage, AK 99518
412-434-6023
800-280-5325
e-mail: aiblink@ak.net
www.iaais.org
Newsletter for persons interested in radio reading services. *$7.00*
Quarterly

8945 Heart to Heart
Blind Children's Center
4120 Marathon Street
Los Angeles, CA 90029
323-664-2153
800-222-3567
FAX: 323-665-3828
e-mail: info@blindchildrenscenter.org
www.blindchildrenscenter.org

Midge Horton, Executive Director
Parents of children who are blind and partially sighted talk about their feelings. *$10.00*
12 pages

8946 Heartbreak of Being A Little Bit Blind
National Association for Visually Handicapped
22 W 21st Street
Floor 6
New York, NY 10010
212-889-3141
FAX: 212-727-2931
e-mail: staff@navh.org
www.navh.org

Lorianie Marchi, Chief Executive Officer
Summary of what it means to have impaired vision; includes illustrations.

8947 Helen Keller National Center Newsletter
111 Middle Neck Road
Sands Point, NY 11050
516-944-8900
800-225-0411
FAX: 516-944-7302
e-mail: hkncdir@aol.com
www.helenkeller.org/national

Joseph McNulty, Executive Director
The center provides evaluation and training in vocational skills, adaptive technology and computer skills, orientation and mobility, independent living, communication, speech-language skills, creative arts, fitness and leisure activities.

8948 Helping the Visually Impaired Child with Developmental Problems
Teachers College Press
Columbia University
New York, NY 10027
212-678-3929
800-575-6566
FAX: 212-678-4149

Mary Lynch, Manager
This book aims to explore the human consequences of severe visual problems combined with other handicaps. The application of child development research to educational interventions, the need for educational and rehabilitative services that serve the human and the special needs of children and their families and the promise of technology in helping to expand communicative possibilities are also discussed. *$18.95*
216 pages Paperback
ISBN 0-807729-02-7

8949 History and Use of Braille
American Council of the Blind
1155 15th Street NW
Suite 1004
Washington, DC 20005
202-467-5081
800-424-8666
FAX: 202-467-5085
e-mail: info@acb.org
www.acb.org

Melanie Brunson, Executive Director

8950 How Does a Blind Person Get Around?
American Foundation for the Blind/AFB Press
PO Box 1020
Sewickley, PA 15143
412-741-1142
800-232-3044
FAX: 412-741-0609
e-mail: afborders@abdintl.com
www.afb.org
Offers information on daily living as a blind person.

8951 How to Thrive, Not Just Survive
American Foundation for the Blind/AFB Press
PO Box 1020
Sewickley, PA 15143
412-741-1142
800-232-3044
FAX: 412-741-0609
e-mail: afborders@abdintl.com
www.afb.org

Stephanie Biagioli, Marketing Coordinator
Practical, hands-on guide for parents, teachers, and everyone involved in helping children develop the skills necessary for socialization, orientations and mobility, and leisure and recreational activities. Some of the subjects covered are eating, dressing, personal hygiene, self-esteem and etiquette. *$24.95*
104 pages Paperback
ISBN 0-89128 -48-7

8952 Hub
SPOKES Unlimited
415 Main Street
Klamath Falls, OR 97601
541-883-7547
FAX: 541-885-2469
e-mail: spokes@internetcds.com

Wendy Howard, Program Coordinator
Celeste Wolf, Clerical Support Specialist II
Newsletter on rehabilitation, peer counseling, blindness, visual impairments, information and referral.

8953 If Blindness Comes
National Federation of the Blind
1800 Johnson Street
Baltimore, MD 21230
410-659-9314
FAX: 410-685-5653
e-mail: nfb@iamdigex.net
www.nfb.org

Marc Maurer, President
An introduction to issues relating to vision loss and provides a positive, supportive philosophy about blindness. It is a general information book which includes answers to many common questions about blindness, information about services and programs for the blind and resource listings. Contact the Materials Center.

8954 **If Blindness Strikes Don't Strike Out**
Charles C Thomas
2600 S 1st Street
Springfield, IL 62704
217-789-8980
800-258-8980
FAX: 217-789-9130
e-mail: books@ccthomas.com
www.ccthomas.com

Michael Thomas, President
This book is a storehouse of information on daily life for the visually impaired and those around them. From opticons and laser canes to housekeeping to travel, the author describes how to successfully cope with the problems posed by visual impairment and blindness. Also available in cloth. *$36.95*
316 pages Paperback
ISBN 0-398064-34-2

8955 **Imagining the Possibilities: Creative Approaches to Orientation and Mobility Instruction**
American Foundation for the Blind
11 Penn Plaza
Suite 300
New York, NY 10001
212-502-7600
800-232-5463
FAX: 212-502-7777
e-mail: afbinfo@afb.net
www.afb.org/store

Carl R Augusto, President/CEO
Innovative and varied approaches to O&M techniques and teaching and dynamic suggestions on how to analyze learning styles are just some of the important topics included. *$49.95*
378 pages 2001
ISBN 0-891283-82-X

8956 **In the Mind of the Beholder.... a Video About Newly Blind Adults**
Aquarius Health Care Videos
PO Box 1159
Sherborn, MA 01770
508-650-6905
FAX: 508-650-4216
e-mail: aqvideos@tiac.net
Newly blind adults making the transition to using their non-visual senses. In a society in which most people are terrified of losing their vision- and yet know virtually nothing about vision loss- the blind are wrongly viewed as mysterious, pitiful or courageous. Produced by Karen Brown Davison, this film puts a human face and voice to blindness. By sharing the experience of losing their eyesight and relearning skills they once took for granted, the people in this film: nonvisual clues. *$195.00*

8957 **InTouch Networks: National Radio Reading Service**
JGB Audio Library for the Blind
15 W 65th Street
New York, NY 10023
212-769-6331
800-284-4422
FAX: 212-769-6266
e-mail: info@JGB.org
www.JGB.org

Peter Williamson, Director
Ken Stanley, Manager

8958 **Increasing Literacy Levels: Final Report**
Mississippi State University
PO Box 6189
Mississippi State, MS 39762
662-325-2001
800-675-7782
FAX: 662-325-8989
www.blind.msstate.edu

Kelly Schaefer, Dissemination Specialist
Elton Moore, Executive Director
This study is composed of three research projects to identify and analyze the appropriate use of and instruction in Braille, optical devices and other technologies as they relate to literacy and employment of individuals who are blind or visually impaired. *$20.00*
148 pages Paperback

8959 **Information Access Project**
National Federation of the Blind
1800 Johnson Street
Baltimore, MD 21230
410-659-9314
FAX: 410-685-5653
e-mail: nfb@iamdigex.net
www.nfb.org

Marc Maurer, President
Assists entities covered by the ADA in finding methods for converting visually displayed information, such as flyers, brochures and pamphlets, to formats accessible to individuals who are visually impaired.

8960 **Information on Glaucoma**
Glaucoma Research Foundation
251 Post Street
Suite 600
San Francisco, CA 94108
415-986-3162
800-826-6693
FAX: 415-986-3763
e-mail: info@glaucoma.org
www.glaucoma.org

Yuko Madono, Outreach/Public Releations
Tom Brunner, Chief Executive Officer

8961 **Inside the Beltway**
DC Regl Lib for the Blind & Physically Handicapped
901 G Street NW
Room 215
Washington, DC 20001
202-727-2142
FAX: 202-727-1129
TTY:202-727-2145
e-mail: lbphb_2000@yahoo.com
www.dclibrary.org

Grace J Lyons, Librarian
Phillip Long-Cross, Manager
Regional library/RPH is network library in the Library of Congress, National Library Services for the Blind and Physically Handicapped.
8 pages Quarterly

8962 **Insight**
United States Association of Blind Athletes
33 N Institute Street
Colorado Springs, CO 80903
719-630-0422
FAX: 719-630-0616
e-mail: media@usaba.org
www.usaba.org

Mark Lucas, Executive Director
Covers news, announcements and activities of the association.
20 pages Quarterly

8963 **Intervention Practices in the Retention of Competitive Employment**
Mississippi State University
PO Box 6189
Mississippi State, MS 39762
662-325-2001
800-675-7782
FAX: 662-325-8989
www.blind.msstate.edu

Kelly Schaefer, Dissemination Specialist
Elton Moore, Executive Director
This study investigated the methods by which an individual can retain competitive employment after the onset of a significant vision loss. Interviews were conducted with 89 rehabilitation counselors across the US Strategies that contribute to successful job retention were identified as well as best rehabilitation practices in job retention. *$15.00*
60 pages Paperback

8964 **JBI Voice**
Jewish Braille Institute of America
110 E 30th Street
New York, NY 10016
212-889-2525
800-433-1531
FAX: 212-689-3692
e-mail: admin@jbilibrary.org
www.jbilibrary.org

Ellen Isler MD, President
Israel A Taub, Associate Director
Monthly recorded magazine emphasizing Jewish current events and culture.
1931

8965 **Jewish Braille Review**
Jewish Braille Institute of America
110 E 30th Street
New York, NY 10016
212-889-2525
800-433-1531
FAX: 212-689-3692
e-mail: admin@jbilibrary.org
www.jbilibrary.org

Ellen Isler MD, President
Israel A Taub, Associate Director
The JBI seeks the integration of Jews who are blind, visually impaired and reading disabled into the Jewish community and society in general. More than 20,000 men, women and children in 50 countries receive a broad variety of JBI services.
1931

8966 **Jewish Heritage for the Blind**
1655 E 24th Street
Brooklyn, NY 11229
718-338-8200

Offers large print traditional prayer books for the High Holy days, festivals, fast days and daily rituals for those finding it difficult or impossible to read small print.

8967 **Journal of Visual Impairment and Blindness**
Sheridan Press, c/o FB
PO Box 465
Hanover, PA 17331
717-632-3535
800-352-2210
FAX: 717-633-8929
e-mail: pubsvc@tsp.sheridan.com
www.sheridanreprints.com

Sharon Shively, Managing Editor
Jane Erin, Editor-in-Chief
Joan Weisman, President
Published in braille, regular print and on ASC II disk and cassette, this journal contains a wide variety of subjects including rehabilitation, psychology, education, legislation, medicine, technology, employment, sensory aids and childhood development as they relate to visual impairments. $130 annual individual subscription, $180 annual institutional subscription.
64 pages Monthly
ISSN 0145-48 x

8968 **Juggler**
Beacon Press
25 Beacon Street
Boston, MA 02108
617-742-2110
FAX: 617-743-3097

Helen Atwan, Executive Director
Andre was the young son of a wealthy, early Quebec fur trader. Because he was almost totally blind, he was overly protected by his family, and his movement outside his home was very limited.
Film

8969 **Kernal Book Series**
National Federation of the Blind
1800 Johnson Street
Baltimore, MD 21230
410-659-9314
FAX: 410-685-5653
e-mail: nfb@iamdigex.net
www.nfb.org

Marc Maurer, President
A series of books written by the blind themselves. Each book is a collection of articles and stories about the real life experiences of blind persons. These books help educate the blind and the sighted alike about a positive philosophy regarding blindness. Contact the materials center.
$5 - $10 each

8970 **Know Your Eye**
American Council of the Blind
1155 15th Street NW
Suite 1004
Washington, DC 20005
202-467-5081
800-424-8666
FAX: 202-467-5085
e-mail: info@acb.org
www.acb.org

Melanie Brunson, Executive Director

8971 **Large Print Loan Library**
National Association for Visually Handicapped
22 W 21st Street
New York, NY 10010
212-889-3141
FAX: 212-727-2931
e-mail: staff@navh.org
www.navh.org

Lorianie Marchi, Chief Executive Officer
A huge large print catalog of all the publications, fiction and non-fiction, cassette tapes, books-on-tape and videos available for the visually impaired from the loan library of the National Association for the Visually Handicapped.
100 pages

8972 **Large Print Loan Library Catalog**
National Association for Visually Handicapped
22 W 21st Street
Floor 6
New York, NY 10010
212-889-3141
FAX: 212-727-2931
e-mail: staff@navh.org
www.navh.org

Lorianie Marchi, Chief Executive Officer
Listing of over 7,000 commercially published and NAVH large print books available through NAVH on a loan basis. Includes a limited selection of titles available for purchase. *$5.00*

8973 **Large Print Recipies for a Healthy Life**
123601 Wilshire
Los Angeles, CA 90025
310-826-8280
800-481-EYES
FAX: 310-458-8179

Judith Caditz, PhD, author
Dave Grill
$21.95
283 pages
ISBN 0-962236-82-9

8974 **Learning to Play**
Blind Children's Center
4120 Marathon Street
Los Angeles, CA 90029
323-664-2153
800-222-3567
FAX: 323-665-3828
e-mail: info@blindchildrenscenter.org
www.blindchildrenscenter.org

Midge Horton, Executive Director
Presenting play activities to the pre-school child who is visually impaired. *$10.00*
12 pages

8975 **Let's Eat**
Blind Children's Center
4120 Marathon Street
Los Angeles, CA 90029
323-664-2153
800-222-3567
FAX: 323-665-3828
e-mail: info@blindchildrenscenter.org
www.blindchildrenscenter.org

Midge Horton, Executive Director
Feeding a child with visual impairment. *$10.00*

28 pages

8976 **Let's Eat Video**
Blind Children's Center
4120 Marathon Street
Los Angeles, CA 90029
323-664-2153
800-222-3567
FAX: 323-665-3828
e-mail: info@blindchildrenscenter.org
www.blindchildrenscenter.org

Midge Horton, Executive Director
$35.00

8977 **Library Resources for the Blind and Physically Handicapped**
National Library Service for the Blind
1291 Taylor Street NW
Washington, DC 20542
202-707-5100
FAX: 202-707-0712
TTY:202-707-0744
e-mail: nls@loc.gov
www.loc.gov/nls

Frank Cylke, Executive Director
NLS administers a national library service that provides braille and recorded books and magazines on free loan to anyone who cannot read standard print because of visual or physical disabilities and who are eligible residents of the United States or American citizens living abroad. The directory describes the cooperating libaries. Online at www.loc.gov/reference/directories.html.
83 pages

8978 **Library Services for the Blind**
South Carolina State University
300 College Street NE
Orangeburg, SC 29117
803-536-7000
FAX: 803-536-8902
e-mail: bagingu@scsu.edu
library.scsu.edu

Mary L Small Dean, Library/Information Services
Andrew Hugine, President
News and information on developments in library services for readers who are blind and physically disabled.

8979 **Library Users of America Newsletter**
American Council of the Blind
1155 15th Street NW
Suite 1004
Washington, DC 20005
202-467-5081
800-424-8666
FAX: 202-467-5085
e-mail: info@acb.org
www.acb.org

Sharon Strzalkowski, President
Melanie Brunson, Executive Director
Published twice yearly, the newsletter contains much information about library services of particular interest to blind and visually impaired patrons, and is available in the following formats: Braille, audiocassette, large print and e-mail.

8980 **Lifestyles of Employed Legally Blind People**
Mississippi State University
PO Box 6189
Mississippi State, MS 39762
662-325-2001
800-675-7782
FAX: 662-325-8989
www.blind.msstate.edu

Lynn W McBroom PhD, Senior Research Scientist
Elton Moore, Executive Director
Results from a telephone survey show that visually impaired respondents are involved in a wide variety of activities with little restrictions on their range of activities. Sighted respondents tended to spend more time in child care, obtaining goods and services, attending to self-care activities and engaging in social activities, while visually impaired respondents spent more time in education and passive activities. This report is a study of expenditures and time use. *$ 10.00*

193 pages Paperback

8981 **Light the Way**
Blind Children's Center
4120 Marathon Street
Los Angeles, CA 90029
323-664-2153
800-222-3567
FAX: 323-665-3828
e-mail: info@blindchildrenscenter.org
www.blindchildrenscenter.org

Midge Horton, Executive Director
Newsletter of the Blind Childrens Center, a family-centered agency which serves children with visual impairments from birth to school-age. The center-based and home-based services help the children to acquire skills and build their independence. The center utilizes its expertise and experience to serve families and professionals worldwide through support services, education and research.

8982 **Lion**
Lion's Clubs International
300 W 22nd Street
Oak Brook, IL 60570
630-571-5466

Gary Lapetina, Chief Executive Officer
Publication for the blind.

8983 **Living with Achromatopsia**
PO Box 214
Berkeley, CA 94701
510-540-4700
FAX: 510-540-4767
e-mail: futterman@achromat.org
www.achromat.org

8984 **Long Cane News**
American Foundation for the Blind/AFB Press
PO Box 1020
Sewickley, PA 15143
412-741-1142
800-232-3044
FAX: 412-741-0609
e-mail: afborders@abdintl.com
www.afb.org

Liz Greco
SemiAnnual

8985 **Look Out for Annie**
Lighthouse International
111 E 59th Street
New York, NY 10022
212-821-9200
800-829-0500
FAX: 212-821-9706
e-mail: info@lighthouse.org

Joanna Mellor, VP Information Services
Tara Cortes, President
Depicts an older woman coping with her vision loss. It focuses on the emotional issues surrounding vision loss and conveys the idea that both the person with the vision disorder and their family and friends will need to make adjustments. *$25.00*
Video

8986 **Low Vision Questions and Answers: Definitions, Devices, Services**
American Foundation for the Blind/AFB Press
PO Box 1020
Sewickley, PA 15143
412-741-1142
800-232-3044
FAX: 412-741-0609
e-mail: afborders@abdintl.com
www.afb.org
What does low vision mean? What do low vision services cost? What diseases cause low vision? Answers to these and other questions are presented in a comprehensive format with accompanying photographs. $50.00/pack of 25.

21 pages
ISBN 0-891281-96-7

8987 Low Vision: Reflections of the Past, Issues for the Future
American Foundation for the Blind/AFB Press
PO Box 1020
Sewickley, PA 15143
412-741-1142
800-232-3044
FAX: 412-741-0609
e-mail: afborders@abdintl.com
www.afb.org

Background papers and a strategies section are used to identify the shifting needs of visually impaired persons and the resources that may be needed to address them. Paperback. *$29.95*

ISBN 0-891282-18-1

8988 Mainstreaming and the American Dream
American Foundation for the Blind/AFB Press
PO Box 1020
Sewickley, PA 15143
412-741-1142
800-232-3044
FAX: 412-741-0609
e-mail: afborders@abdintl.com
www.afb.org

Based on in-depth interviews with parents and professionals, this research monograph presents information on the needs and aspirations of parents of blind and visually impaired children. Paperback. *$34.95*
256 pages
ISBN 0-891281-91-6

8989 Mainstreaming the Visually Impaired Child
NAPVI
PO Box 317
Watertown, MA 02471
617-972-7441
800-562-6265
FAX: 617-972-7444
e-mail: napvi@perkins.org
www.napvi.org

A unique, informative guide for teachers and educational professionals that work with the visually impaired. *$10.00*
121 pages Paper

8990 Making Life More Livable
American Foundation for the Blind
11 Penn Plaza
Suite 300
New York, NY 10001
212-502-7600
800-232-5463
FAX: 212-502-7774
e-mail: afborder@abdintl.com
www.afb.org

Carl Augusto, President
Shows how simple adaptations in the home and environment can make a big difference in the lives of blind and visually impaired older persons. The suggestions offered are numerous and specific, ranging from how to mark food cans for greater visibility to how to get out of the shower safley. Large print. *$24.95*
128 pages 2001
ISBN 0-891283-87-0

8991 Meeting the Needs of People with Vision Loss: Multidisciplinary Perspective
Resources for Rehabilitation
33 Bedford Street
Suite 19a
Lexington, MA 02420
781-890-6371
FAX: 781-867-7517

Susan Greenblatt
Written by rehabilitation professionals, physicians, and a sociologist, this book discusses how to provide appropriate information and how to serve special populations. Chapters on the role of the family, diabetes and vision loss, special needs of children and adolescents, adults with hearing and vision loss. *$29.95*

ISBN 0-92971 -07-0

8992 Model Program Operation Manual: Business Enterprise Program Supervisors
Mississippi State University
PO Box 6189
Mississippi State, MS 39762
662-325-2001
800-675-7782
FAX: 662-325-8989
www.blind.msstate.edu

Kelly Schaefer, Publications Manager
Elton Moore, Executive Director
This monograph serves as a Model Program Operation Manual for Business Enterprise Program Supervisors who administer Randolph-Sheppard vending facilities under the Randolph-Sheppard Act. A wide variety of topics are covered including the role of the State Committee of Blind Venders, the role and responsibilities of the Vending Facility Operator, model qualification, for potential Facility Managers, guidelines for location of vending facilities and policies for closing vending facilities. *$20.00*
199 pages Paperback

8993 More Alike Than Different: Blind and Visually Impaired Children
American Foundation for the Blind/AFB Press
PO Box 1020
Sewickley, PA 15143
412-741-1142
800-232-3044
FAX: 412-741-0609
e-mail: afborders@abdintl.com
www.afb.org

Offers photographs of blind and visually impaired children around the world learning to read and write, travel independently and performing basic living skills. Covers the most recent technological advances and demonstrates the universality of educational needs and goals. Paperback. $100.00/pack of 25.

ISBN 0-891281-69-0

8994 Mothers with Visual Impairments who are Raising Young Children
Through the Looking Glass
2198 6th Street
Suite 100
Berkeley, CA 94710
510-848-1112
800-644-2666
FAX: 510-848-4445
e-mail: TLG@lookingglass.org
www.lookingglass.org

C Conley-Jung
R Olkin
Megan Kirshbaum, Executive Director
Available in braille, large print or cassette. *$2.00*
16 pages

8995 Move With Me
Blind Children's Center
4120 Marathon Street
Los Angeles, CA 90029
323-664-2153
800-222-3567
FAX: 323-665-3828
e-mail: info@blindchildrenscenter.org
www.blindchildrenscenter.org

Midge Horton, Executive Director
A parent's guide to movement development for babies who are visually impaired. *$10.00*
12 pages

8996 Musical Mainstream
National Library Service for the Blind
1291 Taylor Street NW
Washington, DC 20542
202-707-5100
FAX: 202-707-0712
e-mail: nls@loc.gov
www.loc.gov/nls

Frank Cylke, Executive Director
Articles selected from print music magazines.

Quarterly

8997 **Myotherapy**
Ballantine Books
1540 Broadway
New York, NY 10036 212-751-2600
FAX: 212-572-4949

Myotherapy explained as a technique.
1985

8998 **NBA Bulletin**
National Braille Association
3 Townline Circle
Rochester, NY 14623 585-427-8260
FAX: 585-427-0263
e-mail: nbaoffice@compuserve.com
www.nationalbraille.org

Joanna E Venneri, Editor
Angela Coffaro, Executive Director
Quarterly publication from the National Braille Association. *$50.00*
28-32 pages Quarterly

8999 **NLS News**
National Library Service for the Blind
1291 Taylor Street NW
Washington, DC 20542 202-707-5100
FAX: 202-707-0712
e-mail: nls@loc.gov
www.loc.gov/nls

Frank Cylke, Executive Director
Newsletter on current program developments.
Quarterly

9000 **NLS Update**
National Library Service for the Blind
1291 Taylor Street NW
Washington, DC 20542 202-707-5100
FAX: 202-707-0712
e-mail: nls@loc.gov
www.loc.gov/nls

Frank Cylke, Executive Director
Newsletter on the service's volunteer activities.
Quarterly

9001 **Newsline for the Blind**
National Federation of the Blind
1800 Johnson Street
Baltimore, MD 21230 410-659-9314
FAX: 410-685-5653
e-mail: nfb@iamdigex.net
www.nfb.org

Peggy Chong, Contact
Marc Maurer, President
Nation's only digital talking newspaper service for the blind. Allows the blind to read the full text of leading national and local newspapers by using a touch-tone telephone. Service is free of charge and available 24 hours a day, 7 days per week.

9002 **Not Without Sight**
American Foundation for the Blind/AFB Press
PO Box 1020
Sewickley, PA 15143 412-741-1142
800-232-3044
FAX: 412-741-0609
e-mail: afborders@abdintl.com
www.afb.org

This video describes the major types of visual impairment and their causes and effects on vision, while camera simulations approximate what people with each impairment actually see. Also demonstrates how people with low vision make the best use of the vision they have. 20 minute video tape. Also available in PAL, $52.95, 0-89128-272-6. *$42.95*
VHS 1975
ISBN 0-891282-27-0

9003 **One Two Three Sign with Me**
TJ Publishers
2544 Tarpley Road
Suite 108
Carrollton, TX 75006 972-416-0800
800-999-1168
FAX: 301-585-5930
e-mail: TJPubinc@aol.com

Angela K Thames, President
Jerald A Murphy, VP
Charming full color illustrations include basic shapes and counting. *$3.95*
24 pages Softcover

9004 **Opportunity**
National Industries for the Blind
1310 Braddock Place
Alexandria, VA 22314 703-998-0770
FAX: 703-998-8268
www.nib.org

George J Mertz, President/CEO
Offers information and articles on the newest technology, equipment, services and programs for blind and visually impaired persons.
Quarterly

9005 **Orientation and Mobility Primer for Families and Young Children**
American Foundation for the Blind/AFB Press
PO Box 1020
Sewickley, PA 15143 412-741-1142
800-232-3044
FAX: 412-741-0609
e-mail: afborders@abdintl.com
www.afb.org

Practical information for helping a child learn about his or her environment right from the start. Covers sensory training, concept development and orientation skills. Paperback. *$14.95*
48 pages
ISBN 0-891281-57-6

9006 **Out of Left Field**
American Foundation for the Blind/AFB Press
PO Box 1020
Sewickley, PA 15143 412-741-1142
800-232-3044
FAX: 412-741-0609
e-mail: afborders@abdintl.com
www.afb.org

Illustrates how youngsters who are blind or visually impaired integrated with their sighted peers in a variety of recreational and athletic activities. 17 minute video tape. Also available in PAL, $33.95, 0-89128-270-X. *$26.95*
VHS 1975
ISBN 0-891282-28-9

9007 **Out of the Corner of My Eye**
American Foundation for the Blind/AFB Press
PO Box 1020
Sewickley, PA 15143 412-741-1142
800-232-3044
FAX: 412-741-0609
e-mail: afborders@abdintl.com
www.afb.org

A personal account of students' vision loss and subsequent adjustment that is full of practical advice and cheerful encouragement, told by an 87 year old retired college teacher who has maintained her independence and zest for life. *$14.95*

ISBN 0-891281-93-2

9008 **Out of the Corner of My Eye: Living with Vision Loss in Later Life**
American Foundation for the Blind/AFB Press
PO Box 1020
Sewickley, PA 15143 412-741-1142
800-232-3044
FAX: 412-741-0609
e-mail: afborders@abdintl.com
www.afb.org

Stephanie Biagioli, Marketing Coordinator
A personal account of students' vision loss and subsequent adjustment that is full of practical advice and cheerful encouragement, told by an 87 year old retired college teacher who has maintained her independence and zest for life. Available in paperback or on audio cassette. *$23.95*
120 pages
ISBN 0-891281-82-1

9009 PB News
Prevent Blindness America
500 E Remington Road
Schaumburg, IL 60173
847-843-2020
800-331-2020
FAX: 847-843-8458
e-mail: info@preventblindness.org
www.preventblindness.org

Ken West, Director Marketing Comm.
$10.00
Quarterly

9010 PBA News
Prevent Blindness America
500 E Remington Road
Schaumburg, IL 60173
847-843-8458
800-331-2020
FAX: 847-843-2020
e-mail: info@preventblindness.org
www.preventblindness.org

Betsy van Die, Media Relations Director
Hugh R Parry, President/CEO
Daniel D Garrett, Senior VP
Publication offered three times yearly.
3 times yearly

9011 Parenting Preschoolers: Suggestions for Raising Young Blind Children
American Foundation for the Blind/AFB Press
PO Box 1020
Sewickley, PA 15143
412-741-1142
800-232-3044
FAX: 412-741-0609
e-mail: afborders@abdintl.com
www.afb.org
Provides practical answers to questions most frequently asked by parents and gives advice on what to expect, how to adapt to a child's situation and what to look for in early education programs. $50.00/pack of 25.
28 pages
ISBN 0-891289-98-4

9012 Patient's Guide to Visual Aids and Illumination
National Association for Visually Handicapped
22 W 21st Street
New York, NY 10010
212-889-3141
FAX: 212-727-2931
e-mail: staff@navh.org
www.navh.org

Lorianie Marchi, Chief Executive Officer
A reference booklet offering information on aids for the visually impaired.

9013 Pediatric Visual Diagnosis Fact Sheets
Blind Children's Center
4120 Marathon Street
Los Angeles, CA 90029
323-664-2153
800-222-3567
FAX: 323-665-3828
e-mail: info@blindchildrenscenter.org
www.blindchildrenscenter.org

Midge Horton, Executive Director
Fact sheets addressing commonly encountered eye conditions, diagnostic tests and materials. *$10.00*
10 pages

9014 Perkins Activity and Resource Guide: A Handbook for Teachers
Perkins School for the Blind
175 N Beacon Street
Watertown, MA 02472
617-924-3434
FAX: 781-926-2027
www.perkins.org

Steven Rothstein, President
This is a comprehensive, two volume guide with over 1,000 pages of activities, resources and instructional strategies for teachers and parents of students with visual and multiple disabilities. *$65.00*

9015 Personal Reader Update
Personal Reader Department
9 Centennial Drive
Peabody, MA 01960
978-977-2000
800-343-0311
FAX: 978-977-2409
Offers information on new services, assistive devices and technology for the blind.

9016 Picture is Worth a Thousand Words for Blind and Visually Impaired Persons Too!
American Foundation for the Blind/AFB Press
PO Box 1020
Sewickley, PA 15143
412-741-1142
800-232-3044
FAX: 412-741-0609
e-mail: afborders@abdintl.com
www.afb.org
Audiodescription - the art of describing in words for visually impaired viewers the visual aspects seen in television, film, etc. - is highlighted in this book for the blind and visually impaired person. *$7.95*
32 pages Large Print
ISBN 0-891282-12-2

9017 Popular Activities and Games for Blind, Visually Impaired & Disabled People
American Foundation for the Blind/AFB Press
PO Box 1020
Sewickley, PA 15143
412-741-1142
800-232-3044
FAX: 412-741-0609
e-mail: afborders@abdintl.com
www.afb.org
A manual of easy-to-follow instructions for more than 50 games and activities for blind and visually impaired persons of all ages, their families, recreation leaders and health care professionals. Large print. *$19.95*
64 pages
ISBN 0-959974-78-4

9018 Preschool Learning Activities for the Visually Impaired Child
NAPVI
PO Box 317
Watertown, MA 02471
617-972-7441
800-562-6265
FAX: 617-972-7444
e-mail: napvi@perkins.org
www.napvi.org
This guide for parents offers games and activities to keep visually impaired children active during the preschool years. *$8.00*
91 pages Paperback

9019 Providing Services for People with Vision Loss: Multidisciplinary Perspective
Resources for Rehabilitation
33 Bedford Street
Suite 19a
Lexington, MA 02420
781-862-6455
FAX: 781-861-7517
www.nfr.org
A collection of articles by ophthalmologists and rehabilitation professionals, including chapters on operating a low vision service, starting self-help programs, mental health services, aids and techniques that help people with vision loss. *$19.95*

136 pages
ISBN 0-929718-02-0

9020 Psychoeducational Assessment of Visually Impaired and Blind Students
Pro-Ed
8700 Shoal Creek Boulevard
Austin, TX 78757
512-451-3246
800-897-3202
FAX: 512-451-8542
e-mail: info@proedinc.com
www.proedinc.com

Donald Hammill, Owner
Professional reference book that addresses the problems specific to assessment of visually impaired and blind children. Of particular value to the practitioner are the extensive reviews of available tests, including ways to adapt those not designed for use with the visually handicapped. *$29.00*
140 pages Paperback
ISBN 0-890791-08-2

9021 Quarterly Update
National Association for Visually Handicapped
22 W 21st Street
Floor 6
New York, NY 10010
212-889-3141
FAX: 212-727-2931
e-mail: staff@navh.org
www.navh.org

Lorianie Marchi
Quarterly newsletter offering information on new products for the visually impaired, advances in medical treatments, new books available in the NAVH large print loan library and any new/updated booklets. Free. *$2.25*

9022 RP Messenger
Texas Association of Retinitis Pigmentosa
PO Box 8388
Corpus Christi, TX 78468
361-852-8515
FAX: 361-852-8515
e-mail: phstiefel@grande.com.nist
A bi-annual newsletter offering information on Retinitis Pigmentosa. *$15.00*
BiAnnual

9023 Raised Dot Computing Newsletter
Raised Dot Computing
408 S Baldwin Street
Madison, WI 53703
608-257-9595

e-mail: info@rdcbraille.com
Discusses braille computer techniques and devices for blind persons. *$7.00*

9024 Reaching, Crawling, Walking....Let's Get Moving
Blind Children's Center
4120 Marathon Street
Los Angeles, CA 90029
323-664-2153
800-222-3567
FAX: 323-665-3828
e-mail: info@blindchildrenscenter.org
www.blindchildrenscenter.org

Midge Horton, Executive Director
Orientation and mobility for preschool children who are visually imapired. *$10.00*
24 pages

9025 Reading Is for Everyone
National Library Service for the Blind
1291 Taylor Street NW
Washington, DC 20542
202-707-5100
FAX: 202-707-0712
e-mail: nls@loc.gov
www.loc.gov/nls

Frank Cylke, Executive Director

9026 Reading with Low Vision
National Library Service for the Blind
1291 Taylor Street NW
Washington, DC 20542
202-707-5100
FAX: 202-707-0712
e-mail: nls@loc.gov
www.loc.gov/nls

Frank Cylke, Executive Director

9027 Recording for the Blind News
Recording for the Blind
20 Roszel Road
Princeton, NJ 08540
609-452-0606
800-221-4792
FAX: 609-987-8116

John Kelly, Chief Executive Officer
A nonprofit organization that provides recorded books free of charge to blind and print-handicapped individuals.
3x Year

9028 Reference and Information Services From NLS
National Library Service for the Blind
1291 Taylor Street NW
Washington, DC 20542
202-707-5100
FAX: 202-707-0712
TTY:202-707-0744
e-mail: nls@loc.gov
www.loc.gov/nls

Frank Cylke, Executive Director

9029 Referring Blind and Low Vision Patients for Rehabilitation Services
American Foundation for the Blind/AFB Press
PO Box 1020
Sewickley, PA 15143
412-741-1142
800-232-3044
FAX: 412-741-0609
e-mail: afborders@abdintl.com
www.afb.org
Clear information on such basic topics as the objectives of low vision services, what's covered in the examinations, what rehabilitation services do and how to locate these services. Available in purchase of bulk quantity only.

ISBN 0-891289-13-5

9030 Resource List for Persons with Low Vision
American Council of the Blind
1155 15th Street NW
Suite 1004
Washington, DC 20005
202-467-5081
800-424-8666
FAX: 202-467-5085
e-mail: info@acb.org
www.acb.org

Melanie Brunson, Executive Director

9031 Resources for Family Centered Intervention for Infants, Toddlers, and Preschoolers
Hope
1856 N 1200 E
Logan, UT 84341
435-245-2888
FAX: 435-245-2888
e-mail: hope@hopepubl.com
www.hopepubl.com

Susan Watkins, Owner
Describes children with vision impairment in terms of characteristics, needs, and parent concerns. *$98.00*
Two volumes

9032 Rose-Colored Glasses
Human Sciences Press
233 Spring Street
New York, NY 10013
212-229-2859
800-221-9369
FAX: 212-463-0742

After a vacation, Deborah was excited about going back to school. Renewing old friendships, she met a classmate who seemed stuck up. Deborah learned that Melanie was in a recent accident resulting in impaired vision. She did not wish to wear her glasses, which were rose-colored and very funny looking. With Deborah's help, Miss Davis, the teacher showed a blurry film and then had Melanie speak about her impaired vision. When Melanie began to participate in the class they accepted her. *$16.95*

30 pages Hardcover
ISBN 0-87705 -08-8

9033 SCENE
Braille Institute
527 N Dale Avenue
Anaheim, CA 92801
714-821-5000
800-272-4553
FAX: 714-527-7621
www.brailleinstitute.org

Sheila Daily, Executive Director
Offers information on the organization, question and answer column, articles on the newest technology and more for visually impaired persons.

9034 Say it with Sign Videotape
Harris Communications
15155 Technology Drive
Eden Prairie, MN 55344
952-906-1180
800-825-6758
FAX: 952-906-1099
e-mail: mail@harriscomm.com
www.harriscomm.com

Bill Williams, National Sales Manager
Robert Harris, Owner
Contains both the serious and fun side of signing and provides the basic signs that might be needed in an emergency situation. *$39.95*
Video

9035 See A Bone
Facts on File
132 W 31st Street
Floor 17
New York, NY 10001
212-967-8800
800-322-8755
FAX: 212-967-9196
e-mail: jchambers@factsonfile.com
www.factsonfile.com

Mark Donnell, President
$65.00
352 pages
ISBN 0-816042-80-2

9036 See What I Feel
Britannica Film Company
345 4th Street
San Francisco, CA 94107
415-777-9876

A blind child tells her friends about her trip to the zoo. Each experience was explained as a blind child would experience it. A teacher's guide comes with this video.
Film

9037 See What I'm Saying
Fanlight Productions
4196 Washington Street
Suite 2
Boston, MA 02131
617-469-4999
800-937-4113
FAX: 617-469-3379
e-mail: fanlight@fanlight.com
www.fanlight.com

Karen McMillen, Marketing Director
Ben Achtenberg, Owner
This program illustrates how the acquisition of communication skill, particularly sign language, enhances a child's self esteem and family and peer relationship. The documentary follows Patricia, who is deaf and from a Spanish-speaking family, through her first year at the Kendall Demonstration Elementary School of Gallaudet University. *$195.00*

9038 See for Yourself
Lighthouse International
111 E 59th Street
New York, NY 10022
212-821-9200
800-829-0500
FAX: 212-821-9706
e-mail: info@lighthouse.org

Joanna Mellor, VP Information Services
Tara Cortes, President
This video features older adults with impaired vision who have been helped by vision rehabilitation. *$50.00*

9039 Seeing Eye Guide
Seeing Eye
PO Box 375
Morristown, NJ 07963
973-539-4425
FAX: 973-539-0922
e-mail: info@seeingeye.org
www.seeingeye.org

Kenneth Rosenthal, President
A quarterly publication from Seeing Eye.
Quarterly

9040 Seeing-Children Living with Blindness
Gareth Stevens
1555 N Rivercenter Drive
Milwaukee, WI 53212
414-332-3520
800-341-3569
FAX: 414-225-0377

Bob Famighetti, Publisher
Go with Thomas to a special school for children who can't see, where you will meet Andrew, Kate, Jordan, Katherine, Peter and Kent. Read what they told Thomas about being blind, about daily life, their feelings, the funny things, and the sad. *$10.95*

ISBN 1-555329-15-2

9041 Selecting a Program
Blind Children's Center
4120 Marathon Street
Los Angeles, CA 90029
323-664-2153
800-222-3567
FAX: 323-665-3828
e-mail: info@blindchildrenscenter.org
www.blindchildrenscenter.org

Midge Horton, Executive Director
A guide for parents of infants and preschoolers with visual impairments. *$10.00*
28 pages

9042 Shape Up 'n Sign
Gallaudet University Bookstore
11030 S Langley Avenue
Chicago, IL 60628
202-651-5488
800-621-2736
FAX: 202-651-5489
An aerobic exercise tape introducing the basic sign language for deaf and hearing children ages six to ten. *$22.95*
30 Minutes

9043 Shared Visions
Vista Center for the Blind & Visually Impaired
413 Laurel Street
Santa Cruz, CA 95060
831-458-9766
800-705-2970
FAX: 831-426-6233
www.vistacenter.org

Pam Brandin, Executive Director
Alice McGrath, CR Coordinator
A quarterly publication for Blind and Visually Impaired individuals from Vista Center for the Blind and Visually Impaired.

9044 Sharing Solutions: A Newsletter for Support Groups
Lighthouse International
111 E 59th Street
New York, NY 10022
212-821-9200
800-829-0500
FAX: 212-821-9706
e-mail: info@lighthouse.org
www.lighthouse.org

Joanna Mellor, VP Information Services
Tara Cortes, President
A newsletter for members and leaders of support groups for older adults with impaired vision. The letter provides a forum for support groups members to network and share information, printed in a very large type format.

9045 Show Me How: A Manual for Parents of Preschool Blind Children
American Foundation for the Blind/AFB Press
PO Box 1020
Sewickley, PA 15143 412-741-1142
800-232-3044
FAX: 412-741-0609
e-mail: afborders@abdintl.com
www.afb.org

A practical guide for parents, teachers and others who help preschool children attain age-related goals. Covers issues on playing precautions, appropriate toys and facilitating relationships with playmates. Paperback. *$12.95*
56 pages
ISBN 0-891281-13-4

9046 Sight by Touch
Landmark Media
3450 Slade Run Drive
Falls Church, VA 22042 703-241-2030
800-342-4336
FAX: 703-536-9540

Michael Hartogs, President
This video features the life and importance of Louis Braille. Vision-impaired performers and teachers demonstrate how Braille has benefitted their lives, and how improvements are constantly being made. *$195.00*
Video

9047 Sightings Newsletter
Schepens Eye Research Institute
20 Staniford Street
Boston, MA 02114 617-912-0100
FAX: 617-912-0110
e-mail: geninfo@@vision.eri.harvard.edu
www.eri.harvard.edu/default/htm

Michael Gilmore, President
Prominent center for research on eye, vision, and blinding diseases; dedicated to research that improves the understanding, management, and prevention of eye diseases and visual deficiencies; fosters collaboration among its faculty members; trains young scientists and clinicians from around the world; promotes communication with scientists in allied fields; leader in the worldwide dispersion of basic scientific knowledge of vision.

9048 Sign of the Times
Fanlight Productions
4196 Washington Street
Suite 2
Boston, MA 02131 617-469-4999
800-937-4113
FAX: 617-469-3379
e-mail: fanlight@fanlight.com
www.fanlight.com

Karen McMillen, Marketing Director
Ben Achtenberg, Owner
Profiles a public school in the heart of Los Angeles - an American microcosm where over 300 languages are spoken, and where cultures and races collide. Fairfax High, publicized as the site of gang activity and murder, has long been a focus for bad press. But something very right is going on in this school. A Sign of the Times offers a positive example of how the American dream and American education are still alive *$ 154.00*

9049 Smith Kettlewell Rehabilitation Engineering Research Center
Smith-Kettlewell Eye Research Institute
2318 Fillmore Street
San Francisco, CA 94115 415-345-2000
FAX: 415-345-8455
e-mail: rerc@ski.org
www.ski.org

Ruth S Poole, COO
Henry Metz, President
Reports on technology and devices for persons with visual impairments.

9050 Social Maturity Scale for Blind Preschool Children: A Guide to Its Use
American Foundation for the Blind/AFB Press
PO Box 1020
Sewickley, PA 15143 412-741-1142
800-232-3044
FAX: 412-741-0609
e-mail: afborders@abdintl.com
www.afb.org

An adaptation of the Vineland Social Maturity Scale for use with children from infancy to 6 years of age. *$9.95*
57 pages Paperback
ISBN 0-891280-59-6

9051 Specifications for Selecting a Vocabulary and Teaching Method/Braille Readers
American Foundation for the Blind/AFB Press
PO Box 1020
Sewickley, PA 15143 412-741-1142
800-232-3044
FAX: 412-741-0609
e-mail: afborders@abdintl.com
www.afb.org

Specifications for a reading series developing braille developed at the American Printing House For The Blind. Paperback. *$ 12.95*
84 pages
ISBN 0-891280-69-3

9052 Standing On My Own Two Feet
Blind Children's Center
4120 Marathon Street
Los Angeles, CA 90029 323-664-2153
800-222-3567
FAX: 323-665-3828
e-mail: info@blindchildrenscenter.org
www.blindchildrenscenter.org

Midge Horton, Executive Director
A guide to constructing mobility devices for children who are visually impaired. *$10.00*
38 pages

9053 Starting Points
Blind Children's Center
4120 Marathon Street
Los Angeles, CA 90029 323-664-2153
800-222-3567
FAX: 323-665-3828
e-mail: info@blindchildrenscenter.org
www.blindchildrenscenter.org

Midge Horton, Executive Director
Basic information for the clasroom teacher of 3 to 8 year olds whose multiple disabilities include visual impairment. *$35.00*
157 pages

9054 Step-By-Step Guide to Personal Management for Blind Persons
American Foundation for the Blind/AFB Press
PO Box 1020
Sewickley, PA 15143 412-741-1142
800-232-3044
FAX: 412-741-0609
e-mail: afborders@abdintl.com
www.afb.org

A manual of techniques in the areas of hygiene, grooming, clothing, shopping and child care. *$19.95*
136 pages Spiralbound
ISBN 0-891280-61-8

9055 Student Advocate
National Alliance of Blind Students
1010 Vermont Avenue NW
Suite 1100
Washington, DC 20005 202-783-2077
800-424-8666

Alan Kraut, Executive Director

A communication forum covering issues of concern to postsecondary students who are blind.

9056 Student Teaching Guide for Blind and Visually Impaired College Students
American Foundation for the Blind/AFB Press
PO Box 1020
Sewickley, PA 15143
412-741-1142
800-232-3044
FAX: 412-741-0609
e-mail: afborders@abdintl.com
www.afb.org

A comprehensive resource designed to enable the student to enter the classroom of a university or college with confidence. Large print. *$14.95*
52 pages
ISBN 0-891281-42-8

9057 Survey of Direct Labor Workers Who Are Blind & Employed by NIB
Mississippi State University
PO Box 6189
Mississippi State, MS 39762
662-325-2001
800-675-7782
FAX: 662-325-8989
www.blind.msstate.edu

Kelly Schaefer, Publications Manager
Elton Moore, Executive Director
This report is a follow-up to surveys by National Industries for the Blind in 1983 and 1987 and summarizes the results of a national survey of approximately 500 legally blind direct labor workers. *$10.00*
101 pages Paperback

9058 TBC Focus
400 S State Street
5
Chicago, IL 60605
312-747-4001
800-757-4654
e-mail: mgrady@ch.publib.org

Mamie Grady, Librarian
Published quarterly by the Chicago Public Library Talking Book Center. Free of charge.
4 pages Quarterly

9059 Talk to Me
Blind Children's Center
4120 Marathon Street
Los Angeles, CA 90029
323-664-2153
800-222-3567
FAX: 323-665-3828
e-mail: info@blindchildrenscenter.org
www.blindchildrenscenter.org

Midge Horton, Executive Director
A language guide for parents of children who are visually impaired. *$10.00*
11 pages

9060 Talk to Me II
Blind Children's Center
4120 Marathon Street
Los Angeles, CA 90029
323-664-2153
800-222-3567
FAX: 323-665-3828
e-mail: info@blindchildrenscenter.org
www.blindchildrenscenter.org

Midge Horton, Executive Director
$10.00
15 pages

9061 Talking Book Topics
National Library Services for the Blind
1291 Taylor Street NW
Washington, DC 20542
202-707-5100
FAX: 202-707-0712
e-mail: nls@loc.gov
www.loc.gov/nls

Frank Cylke, Executive Director
Offers hundreds of listings of books, fiction and nonfiction, for adults and children on cassette. Also offers listings on foreign language books on cassette, talking magazines and reviews.
BiMonthly

9062 Teaching Orientation and Mobility in the Schools: An Instructor's Companion
American Foundation for the Blind
11 Penn Plaza
Suite 300
New York, NY 10001
212-502-7600
800-232-5463
FAX: 212-502-7777
e-mail: afbinfo@afb.net
www.afb.org/store

Carl R Augusto, President/CEO
This book, with its useful forms, checklists, and tips, will help O&M instructors and teachers of visually impaired students master the arts of planning schedules, organizing equipment and work routines, working with school personnel and educational team members, and effectively providing instruction to children with diverse needs. *$ 39.95*
176 pages 2002
ISBN 0-891283-91-1

9063 Teaching Visually Impaired Children
Charles C Thomas
2600 S 1st Street
Springfield, IL 62704
217-789-8980
800-258-8980
FAX: 217-789-9130
e-mail: books@ccthomas.com
www.ccthomas.com

Michael Thomas, President
A comprehensive resource for the classroom teacher who is working with a visually impaired child for the first time, as well as a systematic overview of education for the specialist in visual disabilities. It approaches instructional challenges with clear explanations and practical suggestions, and it addresses common concerns of teachers in a reassuring and positive manner. Also available in cloth. *$35.95*
274 pages Paperback
ISBN 0-398065-96-9

9064 Textbook Catalog
National Braille Association
3 Townline Circle
Rochester, NY 14623
585-427-8260
e-mail: nbaoffice@compuserve.com
www.nationalbraille.org

Angela Coffaro, Executive Director
Lists hundreds of scholarly, college and professional textbooks offered in large print, braille or on cassette for visually impaired readers.
80 pages

9065 Three Rivers News
Carnegie Library of Pitts. Library for the Blind
4724 Baum Boulevard
Pittsburgh, PA 15213
412-687-2440
800-242-0586
FAX: 412-687-2442
e-mail: clbph@clpgh.org
www.clpgh.org/clp/LBPH

Sue Murdock, Director
Kathleen Kappel, Editor
Loans recorded books/magazines and playback equipment, large print books and described videos to western PA residents unable to use standard printed materials due to a visual, physical, or physically-based reading disability.
12 pages Quarterly

9066 To Love this Life: Quotations by Helen Keller
American Foundation for the Blind/AFB Press
11 Penn Plaza
Suite 300
New York, NY 10001
212-502-7600
800-232-5463
FAX: 212-502-7774
e-mail: aforder@abdintl.com
www.afb.org

Carl Augusto, President
Inspirational work that offers the penetrating observations of Helen Keller, the beloved deaf-blind champion of the rights of people with disabilities. Also available on cassette at $21.95 (ISBN# 0-89128-348-X) *$21.95*
144 pages Hardcover 2000
ISBN 0-891283-47-1

9067 Touch the Baby: Blind & Visually Impaired Children As Patients
American Foundation for the Blind/AFB Press
PO Box 1020
Sewickley, PA 15143
412-741-1142
800-232-3044
FAX: 412-741-0609
e-mail: afborders@abdintl.com
www.afb.org
A how-to manual for health care professionals working in hospitals, clinics and doctors' offices. Teaches the special communication and touch-related techniques needed to prevent blind and visually impaired patients from withdrawing from the healthcare workers and the outside world. $25.00/pack of 25.
13 pages
ISBN 0-891281-97-5

9068 Transition Activity Calendar for Students with Visual Impairments
Mississippi State University
PO Box 6189
Mississippi State, MS 39762
662-325-2001
800-675-7782
FAX: 662-325-8989
www.blind.msstate.edu

Kelly Schaefer, Dissemination Specialist
Elton Moore, Executive Director
The Transition Activity Calendar guides the student with a visual disability through the maze of college preparation. Beginning in junior high school, clearly written steps are listed for each grade level. Students planning to enter college after high school graduation can check-off their accomplishments each step of the way. The calendar helps students focus on their goals while providing reminders of tasks yet to be completed. It can be used in a self-directed manner or in a group format. *$4.25*
16 pages Paperback

9069 Transition to College for Students with Visual Impairments: Report
Mississippi State University
PO Box 6189
Mississippi State, MS 39762
662-325-2001
800-675-7782
FAX: 662-325-8989
www.blind.msstate.edu

Lynn McBroom PhD, Senior Research Scientist
Elton Moore, Executive Director
A report offering results from telephone interviews of college students with visual impairments and mail surveys of college officials which examines the transition experience of successful college students. General domains in the study include demographics, educational history, computers, specialized and adaptive equipment, resources, college preparation, problems adjusting to college and O&M skills. A literature review covers preparing for college, task timelines,and classroom, labs and tests. *$20.00*
151 pages Paperback

9070 Unseen Minority: A Social History of Blindness in the United States
American Foundation for the Blind/AFB Press
PO Box 1020
Sewickley, PA 15143
412-741-1142
800-232-3044
FAX: 412-741-0609
e-mail: afborders@abdintl.com
www.afb.org
A lively narrative, with anecdotes, that recounts how the blind overcame discrimination to gain full participation in the social, educational, economic and legislative spheres. Hardcover. *$40.00*
573 pages
ISBN 0-679505-39-3

9071 Upstate Update
New York State Talking Book & Braille Library
Empire State Plaza Cec
Albany, NY 12230
518-474-5935
FAX: 518-486-1957
TTY:518-474-7121
e-mail: tbbl@mail.nysed.gov
www.nysl.nysed.gov/tbbl

Jane Somers, Regional Librarian/Manager
Peter Douglas, Editor
Books on audio cassette, cassette players, braille books, summer reading programs, braille writer, magnifiers, closed-circuit T.V., large-print photocopier, cassette books and magazines, children's books on cassette, reference materials on blindness and other handicaps.
4 pages Quarterly

9072 Vision Enhancement
UN Printing
5707 Brockton Drive
Apt 302
Indianapolis, IN 46220
317-254-1332
800-431-1739
FAX: 317-251-6588
e-mail: info@visionww.org
www.visionww.org

Patricia L Price, President/Managing Editor
Designed to encourage and support individuals with vision loss, family members, and caregivers. *$25.00*
72-78 pages Quarterly

9073 Visual Aids and Informational Material
National Association for Visually Handicapped
22 W 21st Street
Floor 6
New York, NY 10010
212-889-3141
FAX: 212-727-2931
e-mail: staff@navh.org
www.navh.org

Lorianie Marchi, Chief Executive Officer
A complete listing of the visual aids NAVH carries such as magnifiers, talking clocks, large print playing cards, etc. *$2.50*
65 pages

9074 Visual Handicaps and Learning
Pro-Ed Publications
8700 Shoal Creek Boulevard
Austin, TX 78757
512-451-3246
800-897-3202
FAX: 512-451-8542
e-mail: info@proedinc.com
www.proedinc.com

Donald Hammill, Owner
The major focus of this new, third edition is to present a new way of thinking about individuals with visual impairment so that they are viewed as participating members of a seeing world despite their reduced visual functioning. *$28.00*
213 pages

9075 Visual Impairment: An Overview
American Foundation for the Blind/AFB Press
PO Box 1020
Sewickley, PA 15143
412-741-1142
800-232-3044
FAX: 412-741-0609
e-mail: afborders@abdintl.com
www.afb.org
An overall look at the most common forms of vision loss and their impact on the individual. Includes drawings as well as photographs that stimulate how people with vision loss see. Paperback. *$19.95*

56 pages
ISBN 0-891281-74-6

9076 Visually Handicapped Child in Your Class
Brookes Publishing
PO Box 10624
Baltimore, MD 21285
410-337-9580
800-638-3775
FAX: 410-337-8539
www.pbrookes.com

Paul Brooks, Owner
This book considers the theory and issues relating to the movement to integrate visually handicapped children into ordinary schools and offers practical suggestions to teachers to help such children participate fully in school life. *$21.50*
192 pages Paper
ISBN 0-304314-00-5

9077 Visually Structured Tasks
Autism Society of North Carolina Bookstore
505 Oberlin Road
Suite 230
Raleigh, NC 27605
919-743-0204
800-442-2762
FAX: 919-743-0208
e-mail: dcoffey@autismsociety-nc.org
www.autismsociety-nc.org

Darla Coffey, Bookstore Manager
Jill Keel, Executive Director
Independent activites for students with autism and other visual learners. *$24.95*

9078 Viva Vital News
5016 Silk Oak Drive
Sarasota, FL 34232

Membership service organization offering information for veterans and is an affiliate of the American Council of the Blind.

9079 Voice of Vision
GW Micro
725 Airport North Office Park
Fort Wayne, IN 46825
260-489-3671
FAX: 260-489-2608
e-mail: sales@gwmicro.com
www.gwmicro.com

Dan Weirich, Owner
Offers product reviews, product announcements, tips for making systems or applications more accessible, or explanations of concepts of interest to any computer user or would-be computer user. This association newsletter is available in braille, in large print, on audio cassette and on 3.5 or 5.25 IBM format diskette.
Quarterly

9080 Walking Alone and Marching Together
National Federation of the Blind
1800 Johnson Street
Baltimore, MD 21230
410-659-9314
FAX: 410-685-5653
e-mail: nfb@iamdigex.net
www.nfb.org

Marc Maurer, President
The history of the organized blind movement, this book spans more than 50 years of civil rights, social issues, attitudes and experiences of the blind. Published in 1990, it has been read by thousands of blind and sighted persons and is used in colleges, libraries and programs across the country as an important tool in understanding blindness and it's impact on both personal lives and the society at large. Braille $130, 2 track or 4 track cassette $40, Print $33.00. Contact Materials Center.

9081 We Can Do it Together!
American Foundation for the Blind/AFB Press
PO Box 1020
Sewickley, PA 15143
412-741-1142
800-232-3044
FAX: 412-741-0609
e-mail: afborders@abdintl.com
www.afb.org

This video illustrates a transdisciplinary team orientation and mobility program for students with severe visual and multiple impairments, covering both adapted communication systems used to teach mobility skills and basic indoor mobility in the school. For mobility instructors, administrators, teachers of the visually and severely handicapped, occupational, physical and speech therapists and parents. Discussion guide included. 10 minute video tape. Also available in PAL, $33.95, 0-89128-267-X. *$26.95*
VHS
ISBN 0-891282-13-0

9082 What Do You Do When You See a Blind Person - and What Don't You Do?
American Foundation for the Blind/AFB Press
PO Box 1020
Sewickley, PA 15143
412-741-1142
800-232-3044
FAX: 412-741-0609
e-mail: afborders@abdintl.com
www.afb.org
Examples of real-life situations that teach sighted persons how to interact effectively with blind persons. Topics covered include how to help someone across the street, how not to distract a guide dog and how to take leave of a blind person.
8 pages
ISBN 0-891281-95-9

9083 What Museum Guides Need to Know: Access for the Blind and Visually Impaired
American Foundation for the Blind/AFB Press
PO Box 1020
Sewickley, PA 15143
412-741-1142
800-232-3044
FAX: 412-741-0609
e-mail: afborders@abdintl.com
www.afb.org
Explains how blind and visually impaired museum-goers experience art and offers pointers on greeting people, asking if help is needed and teaching about a specific work of art. Contains information on access laws, resources, training guides and guidelines for preparing large print, cassette and braille materials. *$14.95*
64 pages Paperback
ISBN 0-891281-58-4

9084 Work Sight
Lighthouse International
111 E 59th Street
New York, NY 10022
212-821-9200
800-829-0500
FAX: 212-821-9706
e-mail: info@lighthouse.org

Joanna Mellor, VP Information Services
Tara Cortes, President
Intended for employers and employees who have concerns about vision loss and job performance. *$25.00*

9085 World Through Their Eyes
Lighthouse International
111 E 59th Street
New York, NY 10022
212-821-9200
800-829-0500
FAX: 212-821-9706
e-mail: info@lighthouse.org

Joanna Mellor, VP Information Services
Tara Cortes, President
Intended to help nursing home staff understand how residents with impaired vision perceive the world. Concrete suggestions help staff provide better care to visually impaired residents. *$25.00*

9086 You Seem Like a Regular Kid to Me
American Foundation for the Blind/AFB Press
PO Box 1020
Sewickley, PA 15143
412-741-1142
800-232-3044
FAX: 412-741-0609
e-mail: afborders@abdintl.com
www.afb.org
An interview with Jane, a blind child, tells other children what it's like to be blind. Jane explains how she gets around, takes care of herself, does her school work, spends her leisure time and even pays for things when she can't see money.

16 pages
ISBN 0-891289-21-6

Provides blind and vision impaired gold tournaments to members.

Sports

9087 **American Blind Bowling Association**
1735 Blaire Road SW
Roanoke, VA 24015 540-982-3838
http://www.ncpad.org/

Gary Robb, Executive Director
Promotes blind bowling throughout the US and Canada by sanctioning blind bowling leagues and conducting a National Tournament. Current membership exceeds 2,000 people in the United States and Canada.

9088 **Basketball: Beeping Foam**
Maxi Aids
42 Executive Boulevard
Farmingdale, NY 11735 631-752-0521
800-522-6294
FAX: 631-752-0689
TTY: 516-752-0738
e-mail: sales@maxiaids.com
www.maxiaids.com
This sound making basketball enables the visually impaired to play basketball or other games. *$29.95*

9089 **Blind Outdoor Leisure Development**
PO Box M
Aspen, CO 81612 970-923-0578
FAX: 970-923-7338
e-mail: possibilities@challengeaspen.com
www.challengeaspen.com

Houston Cowan, Executive Director
Outdoor recreation for the blind. Winter program of skiing with guides plus numerous summer programs for the visually impaired.

9090 **Challenge Golf**
Motivation Media
1245 Milwaukee Avenue
Glenview, IL 60025 847-827-9057
FAX: 847-297-6829

Dorothy Bauer, Coordinator
A plain-language video, Challenge Golf is packed with information for beginners or veterans. Peter Longo covers 5 handicaps (one-arm, one-leg, in a seated position, blind, and arthritis) clearly and concisely, on how to play golf with a physical disability. In color, complete with special effects, graphs and real handicapped golfers at play. *$38.95*
Home Edition

9091 **US Association of Blind Athletes**
33 N Institute Street
Colorado Springs, CO 80903 719-630-0422
FAX: 719-630-0616
e-mail: media@usaba.org
www.usaba.org

Mark Lucas, Executive Director
Nicole Jomantas, Communications Director
Susan Weeks, Development Director
Provides athletic opportunities and training in competitive sports for visually impaired and blind individuals throughout the US Competitions indlcude local, regional and national events, internation events, and the Winter and Summer Paralympic Games.

9092 **United States Blind Golf Association**
3094 Shamrock Street N
Tallahassee, FL 32309 615-885-2593

e-mail: roger.matas@internationalblindgolf.org
www.blindgolf.com

Phil Blackwell, President
Bruce Hooper, VP

Support Groups

9093 **Braille Institute Orange County Center**
527 N Dale Avenue
Anaheim, CA 92801 714-821-5000
800-272-4553
FAX: 714-527-7621
e-mail: oc@brailleinstitute.org
www.brailleinstitute.org

Sheila F. Daily, Regional Director
Gene Mathiowetz, Assistant Regional Director
Offers services, publications, information and programs free of charge to blind and visually impaired persons of all ages.

9094 **Consumer and Patient Information Hotline**
Prevent Blindness America
211 W Wacker Drive
Chicago, IL 60606 312-363-6001
800-331-2020
FAX: 847-843-2020
e-mail: info@preventblindness.org
www.preventblindness.org

Hugh Perry, Chief Executive Officer
Daniel Garrett, Senior VP
A toll-free line offering free information on a broad range of vision, eye health and safety topics including sports eye safety, diabetic retinopathy, glaucoma, cataracts, children's eye disorders and more.

9095 **Department of Ophthalmology Information Line**
Eye & Ear Infirmary
1855 W Taylor Street
Chicago, IL 60612 773-487-2862

Offers eye clinic and physician referrals to persons suffering from vision disorders as well as offers emergency information.

9096 **Lighthouse International Information and Resource Service**
111 E 59th Street
New York, NY 10022 212-821-9200
800-829-0500
FAX: 212-821-9705
e-mail: info@lighthouse.org
www.lighthouse.org

Tara A Cortes, President/CEO
Provides information about eye diseases, low vision, age-related vision loss, adaptive technology, optical devices, large print and braille publishers, helps people find low vision services, vision rehabilitation services, and support groups across the U.S.; offers large selection of consumer products.

9097 **National Association for Parents of Children with Visual Impairments (NAPVI)**
PO Box 317
Watertown, MA 02471 617-972-7441
800-562-6265
FAX: 617-972-7444
e-mail: napvi@perkins.org
www.napvi.org

Susan LaVenture, Executive Director
Mary Zabelski, President
Lars Anderson, VP
In 1979, a group of parents responding to their own needs founded NAPVI, the National Association for Parents of the Visually Impaired, Inc. Never before was there a self-help organization specific to the needs of families of children with visual impairments. Since that time, NAPVI has grown and helped families across the US and in other countries.

9098 Recorded Periodicals
Associated Services for the Blind
919 Walnut Street
Philadelphia, PA 19107
215-627-0600
FAX: 215-922-0692
www.ast.org

John Corrigan, Manager
Patricia Johnson, Chief Executive Officer
A subscription service of Associated Services for the Blind, these periodicals provide 21 magazines through this subscription service. A magazine list can be sent, in both large print and on audio cassette. *$18.00*

9099 VUE: Vision Use in Employment
Carroll Center for the Blind
770 Centre Street
Newton, MA 02458
617-969-6200
800-852-3131
FAX: 617-969-6204
www.carroll.org

Rachel Rosenbaum, President
Robert Mcgilliuray, Low Vision Administration
Provides engineering solutions plus training to help people keep jobs despite their vision loss.

9100 Washington Connection
American Council of the Blind
1155 15th Street NW
Suite 1004
Washington, DC 20005
202-467-5081
800-424-8666
FAX: 202-467-5085
www.acb.org

Day Al-Mohamed, Governmental Affairs Director
Melanie Brunson, Executive Director
Coverage of issues affecting blind people via legislative information, participates in law-making, legislative training seminars and networking of support resources across the US.

A

A-Solution, 524
A4 Tech (USA) Corporation, 1292
AACD Legal Series, 4280
AACRAO, 1847
AAN's Toll-Free Hotline, 8634
AAPD News, 4760
AARP, 1857
AARP Fulfillment, 4690, 4867, 4904, 4995, 7626, 7628, 7650, 7661
ABA Commission on Mental & Physical Disability Law, 4290, 4298, 4316, 4337
ABC Sign with Me, 7757
ABC Union, ACE, ANLV, Vegas Western Cab, 5352
ABC of Asthma, Allergies & Lupus, 8302
ABC's of Latex Allergy, 8303
ABCD Newsletter Volume Reprints, 4667
ABDA/ABMPP Workshop: The Art of Courtroom Testifying, 4281
ABLE Center for Independent Living, 4159
ABLE Program MCC-Longview, 2250
ABLEDATA, 1233
AC-ACLD/An Association for Children and Adults with Learning Disabilities, 5984
ACB Government Employees, 8741
ACB Radio Amateurs, 8742
ACB Social Service Providers, 8743
ACES/ACCESS Inclusion Program, 6533
ACPOC News, 8304
ACS Federal Healthcare, 722
ACT Assessment Test Preparation Reference Manual, 5827
ADA Business Brief: Restriping Parking Lots, 5105
ADA Business Brief: Service Animals, 5106
ADA Camp for Kids, 8180
ADA Guide for Small Businesses, 4761
ADA Guide for Small Towns, 4762
ADA Hotel Built-In Alerting System, 168
ADA Information Services, 4763
ADA Mandate for Social Change, 4282
ADA Pipeline, 4764
ADA Questions and Answers, 4739, 4765
ADA Tax Incentive Packet for Business, 4766
ADA Technical Assistance Program, 3099
ADA Teen Camp at Covenant Point, 8181
ADA Triangle D Camp, 8182
ADA and City Governments: Common Problems, 4767
ADA-TA: A Technical Assistance Update from the Department of Justice, 4768
ADD Challenge: A Practical Guide for Teachers, 1912
ADD Videos, 7364
ADD, Stepping Out of the Dark, 7364
ADD/ADHD Behavior-Change Resource Kit, 7365
ADD/ADHD Checklist, 7366
ADD: Helping Your Child, 7367
ADEC Resources for Independence, 5804
ADHD, 7368
ADHD Book of Lists: A Practical Guide for Helping Children and Teens with ADDs, 7369
ADHD Report, 7370
ADHD in Adults, 7371
ADHD in Schools: Assessment and Intervention Strategies, 7372
ADHD in the Classroom: Strategies for Teachers, 1913
ADHD in the Schools: Assessment and Intervention Strategies, 1914
ADHD with Comorbid Disorders: Clinical Assessment and Management, 7373
ADHD: Handbook for Diagnosis & Treatment, 7374
ADHD: What Can We Do?, 7375
ADHD: What Do We Know?, 7376
AEPS Child Progress Record: For Children Ages Three to Six, 1592
AEPS Child Progress Report: For Children Ages Birth to Three, 2191
AEPS Curriculum for Birth to Three Years, 1915
AEPS Curriculum for Three to Six Years, 1593
AEPS Data Recording Forms: For Children Ages Birth to Three, 2192
AEPS Data Recording Forms: For Children Ages Three to Six, 1594
AEPS Family Interest Survey, 1595
AEPS Family Report: For Children Ages Birth to Three, 4769
AEPS Family Report: For Children Ages Three to Six, 4972
AEPS Measurement for Birth to Three Years, 2193
AEPS Measurement for Three to Six Years, 2194
AFB Directory of Services for Blind and Visually Impaired Persons in the US and Canada, 8846
AFB News, 8847
AFB Press, 1766
AGS, 1617, 1640, 1672, 1691, 1709, 2213, 2214, 2215, 2217, 2221, 2223, 2224, 2225, 2239, 6195
AH! Asthma Camp, 8183
AHEAD, 1867, 4937
AHEAD Association, 723
AI Squared, 1316
AID Bulletin, 8305
AIDS 2nd Edition, 8306
AIDS Alert, 8307
AIDS Disease State Management Resource, 8308
AIDS Funding, 2917
AIDS Legal Council of Chicago, 4252
AIDS Project Los Angeles, 8314
AIDS Treatment Data Network, 1904
AIDS and Other Manifestations of HIV Infec tion, 8309
AIDS in the Twenty-First Century: Disease and Globalization, 8310
AIDS, What Does it Mean to You?, 8311
AIDS: The HIV Myth, 8312
AIDS: The Official Journal of the Internat ional AIDS Society, 8313
AIDSLAW of Louisiana, 4253
AIM Independent Living Center: Corning, 4028
AIM Independent Living Center: Elmira, 4029
AIMS Multimedia, 1336
AIR: Assessment of Interpersonal Relations, 2195
AJ Pappanikou Center, 1899, 1900
AJAO Newsletter, 7988
ALST: Adolescent Language Screening Test, 2196
AM Publishing, 8407
AMC Cancer Research Center, 4398
AMI, 292
ANCOR Wage and Hour Handbook, 4740
APLA Update, 8314
APSE Conference: Revitalizing Supported Employment, Climbing to the Future, 1527
APT Technology, 493
A AR P Fulfillment, 1583, 4323
ARC, 7291
ARC Fresno-Kelso Activity Center, 6381
ARC Gateway, 3082
ARC Of Cape Cod, 3884
The ARC Of San Diego-ARROW Center, 6507
The ARC Of San Diego-East County Training Center, 6508
The ARC Of San Diego-Rex Industries, 6509
ARC Of San-Diego-South Bay, 6382
ARC Of Southeast Los Angeles-Southeast Industries, 6383
ARC of Allen County, 5805
ARC of Gloucester County, 5909
ARC of Hunterdon County, 5910
ARC of Mercer County, 5911
ARC of Monmouth, 5912
ARC of Somerset County, 987
ARC's Government Report, 4770
ARC-Adult Vocational Program, 5648
ARC: VC Community Connections West, 6384
ARC: VC Ventura, 6385
ARCA - Dakota County Technical College, 4771
ARCA Newsletter, 4771
ARISE: Center for Independent Living: Oswe go, 4031
ARISE: Center for Independent Living: Syracuse, 4030
ARJO Inc., 121, 404
ARRISE, 7292
ASCCA, 8184
ASHA Leader, 7758, 8691
ASSETS School, 5769
ASSIST! to Independence, 3566
ASSISTECH, 153, 164, 165, 214
AT for Infants and Toddlers with Disabilities, 4668
AT for Parents with Disabilities, 4973
AT&T Foundation, 2646
ATLA, 3002
ATTAIN, 1234, 6142
ATV Solutions, 572, 578, 582
AU Kamp for Kids, 961
AUCD, 759
AVKO Dyslexia Research Foundation, 1721, 1634
AVKO Educational Research Foundation, 1689, 2178
Abacus, 1293
Abbot and Dorothy H Stevens Foundation, 2553
Abell-Hangar Foundation, 2831
Abilitations, 1695
Abilities Center of New Jersey, 5913
Abilities Unlimited, 961
Abilities in Motion, 4117
Abilities of Florida: An Affiliate of Service Source, 5736
Abilities of Northwest New Jersey, 5914
Abilities!, 724
Ability, 5091
Ability 1st, 3687
Ability Center, 50, 4022

Ability Center of Defiance, 4091
Ability Center of Greater Toledo, 1294, 4092
Ability First, 5649, 907
Ability First L.L. Frank Work Center, 6386
Ability Magazine, 4741
Ability Research, 1161
Ability Resources, 4102
Ability Works Incorporated, 5887
Abingdon Press, 5049
Able Trust, 2425
The Able Trust, 5759
Able to Laugh, 4772
AbleNet, 178, 205, 210, 289, 319, 340, 359, 362, 491, 492, 497, 513, 518, 1168, 1183, 1184, 1199, 1203, 1205, 1215, 1330, 1608, 1609, 1626, 1951, 5266, 5287
Abledata, 5187
Ablenet, 213
Ablewear Aids for Daily Living, 5188
Ablex Publishing Corporation, 2172
About Asthma, 8315
About Attention Disorder, 7377
About Children's Eyes, 8848
About Children's Vision: A Guide for Parents, 8849
Absorbent Dressing Powder, 293
Abstracts in Social Gerontology: Current Literature on Aging, 7603
Academic Press, 8309
Academic Press, Journals Division, 1872
Academic Software, 1163, 1164, 1197, 1217, 1383, 1396, 1416
Academy Eye Associates, 6911
Academy for Educational Development, 5189
Academy for Guided Imagery, 2251
Academy of Dentistry for Persons with Disabilities, 8124, 8583
Academy of Dispensing Audiologists, 7672
Academy of Rehabilitative Audiology, 7673, 7854
Acc-u-trol, 51
Accent Books & Products, 1577, 1587, 4683, 4745, 4864, 4866, 4868, 4899, 4915, 4936, 4951, 5006, 5125, 5299, 7556, 8053, 8069, 8106, 8357, 8455, 8554
Accent on Living Magazine, 4773
Accentcare, 6387
Access Alaska: ADA Partners Project, 3554
Access Alaska: Fairbanks, 3555
Access Alaska: Mat-Su, 3556
Access America, 5306
Access Center for Independent Living, 4093
Access Center of San Diego, 3582
Access Control Systems: NHX Nurse Call System, 169
Access Currents, 1573
Access Design Services: CILs as Experts, 4774
Access Equals Opportunity, 1574
Access For Disabled Americans, 5292
Access House, 1575
Access II Independent Living Center, 3967
Access II Independent Living Centers, 7632
Access Independence, 4199
Access Info, 4775
Access Living of Metropolitan Chicago, 3755
Access Mobility Systems, 92
Access Store Products for Barrier Free Environments, 425
Access Store.Com, 425
Access Systems International, 1220
Access To Independence Of Imperial Valley, 3583
Access To Independence Of North County, 3584
Access To Recreation, 406, 623, 660
Access Travel: Airports, 5294
Access Unlimited, 5190, 7943
Access Utah Network, 3478
Access Yosemite National Park, 5307
Access for 911 and Telephone Emergency Services, 4776
Access for All, 1576
Access for All: Integrating Deaf, Hard of Hearing and Hearing Preschoolers, 7759
Access to Art: A Museum Directory for Blind and Visually Impaired People, 8850
Access to Health Care: Number 1&2, 1916
Access to Health Care: Number 3&4, 1917
Access to Independence, 4775
Access to Independence of Cortland County, 4032
Access to Math, 1337
Access to Recreation, 426, 209
Access to Sailing, 8074
Access with Ease, 338, 588
Access-USA, 521
Accessibility Lift, 370
Accessible Home of Your Own, 1577
Accessible Journeys, 5328, 5329
Accessible Space, 3941
Accessible Stadiums, 5107
Accessnorth CIL of Northeastern MN: Aitkin, 3942
Accessnorth CIL of Northeastern MN: Duluth, 3943
Accesstotheplanet, 5329
Achieva, 1023
Achievement Centers For Children, 8203
Achievement Products, 427
Achieving Diversity and Independence, 4777
Achilles Track Club, 8075
Achromatopsia Network, 8744
Acid Maltase Deficiency Association (AMDA), 8125
Acorn Alcinda Foundation, 2774
Acrontech International, 1455
Acrylic Leg Warmers, 1077
Acting Blind, 5139
Action Products, 249
Action Toward Independence: Middletown, 4033
Action Toward Independence: Monticello, 4034
Active Re-Entry, 4183
Active Re-Entry: Vernal, 4184
Activities for Developing Pre-Skill Concepts In Children with Autism, 1799
Activities in Action, 7604
Activities with Developmentally Disabled Elderly and Older Adults, 7605
Activity-Based Approach to Early Intervention, 2nd Edition, 1918
Activity-Based Intervention: 2nd Edition, 4778
Acupressure Institute, 725
Ad Lib Drop-In Center: Consumer Management, Ownership and Empowerment, 4779
Ada S McKinley Vocational Services, 5780
Adaptable Housing: A Technical Manual for Implementing Adaptable Dwelling, 1578
Adapted Aquatics: Swimming for Persons with Physical or Mental Impairments, 8076
Adapted Physical Activity Programs, 1841, 4974
Adapted Physical Education and Sport, 8077
Adapted Physical Education for Students with Autism, 1919
Adaptek Systems, 170
Adapting Early Childhood Curricula for Children with Special Needs, 1920
Adapting Instruction for the Mainstream: A Sequential Approach to Teaching, 1921
Adaptivation, 1162
Adaptive Baby Care Equipment Video and Book, 5140
Adaptive Clothing: Adults, 428, 1092
Adaptive Design Shop, 122
Adaptive Device Locator System, 1163
Adaptive Education Strategies Building on Diversity, 1922
Adaptive Environments Center, 1565, 1580
Adaptive Environments Center Home Assessment Form, 1579
Adaptive Mainstreaming: A Primer for Teachers and Principals, 3rd Edition, 2197
Adaptive Sports Center, 8078, 8316
Adaptive Technology Catalog, 429
Adaptive Tracks, 8316
Addictive & Mental Disorders Division, 3256
Addie McBryde Rehabilitation Center for the Blind, 6851
Addison Point Specialized Services, 5852
Addison-Wesley Publishing Company, 4813, 7996, 7997, 8004, 8013, 8016
Address Book, 587
Adelante Development Center, 5943
Adjustable Bath Seat, 123
Adjustable Bed, 154
Adjustable Chair, 225
Adjustable Clear Acrylic Tray, 226
Adjustable Incline Board, 371
Adjustable Raised Toilet Seat & Guard, 124
Adjustable Rigid Chair, 227
Adjustable Tee Stool, 228
Adjustable Wedge, 250
Adjustment Training Center, 4142
Adlib Inc., 3885
Administration Building D HS S Campus, 3065
Administration for Children & Families, 1747
Administration on Children, Youth and Families, 2967
Administration on Developmental Disabilities, 2968
Administration on the Aging, 2969
Adobe News, 4780
Adolescents with Down Syndrome: Toward a More Fulfilling Life, 7378
Adolph Coors Foundation, 2381
Adrian's Closet, 1093
Adult ADD: The Complete Handbook: Everyt hing You Need to Know About How to Cope with ADD, 7379
Adult Absorbent Briefs, 1147
Adult Acorn Polartec Socks, 1078
Adult Acorn Slippers, 1079
Adult Bible Lessons for the Deaf, 7760
Adult Day Training, 3688
Adult Lap Shoulder Bodysuit, 1148
Adult Leukemia: A Comprehensive Guide for Patients and Families, 8317
Adult Life Skills, 2256
Adult Long Jumpsuit with Feet, 430, 1094
Adult Pull-On Feeding Bib, 1129
Adult Short Jumpsuit, 431, 1095
Adult Sleeveless Bodysuit, 1149
Adult Snap Front Sleeper, 1120

Adult Swim Diaper, 1150
Adult Tee Shoulder Bodysuit, 1151
Adult Waterproof Overpant, 1152
Adult Wet Wrap Swim Vest, 1153
Advance for Providers of Post-Acute Care, 1842
Advanced Breast Cancer: A Guide to Living with Metastic Disease, 8318
Advanced Diagnosis and Treatment for Neck and Back Pain, 8319
Advanced Language Tool Kit, 1596
Advanced Sign Language Vocabulary: A Resource Text for Educators, 1923, 7761
Advanced Technology Corporation, 559
Advances in Cardiac and Pulmonary Rehabilitation, 1924
Advantage Wheelchair & Walker Bags, 643
Adventure Day Camp, 8185
Adventure Learning Center at Eagle Village, 7310
Adventure Program, 901
Adventures in Fast Forward: Life, Love, a nd Work for the ADD Adult, 8320
Adventures in Musicland, 1359
Advocacy, 4254, 3472
Advocacy Center, 726
Advocacy Center for Persons with Disabilities, 727, 3083
Advocacy Services of Alaska, 3011
Advocado Press, 4330, 4944, 5083
Advocate, 4781
Advocate Christ Hospital and Medical Center, 6643
Advocate Christ Medical Center & Advocate Hope Children's Hospital, 6644
Advocate Illinois Masonic Medical Center, 6645
Advocate for Developmentally Disabled, 3181
Advocates for Children of New York, 728
Aerospace America, 546
Aerospace Compadre, 546
Aetna Foundation, 2392
Affix & Root Cards, 1597
African Americans in the Profession of Blindness Services, 8851
After School and More, 4782
After the Tears, 5046
Agassiz Village, 8186
Age Appropriate Puzzles, 5265
Age-Related Macular Degeneration, 8852
Agency of Human Services, 1289
Agent Orange & Spina Bifida, 8321
Ages & Stages Questionnaires, 2198
Aging & Vision News, 7606
Aging Brain, 1925
Aging Eye and Low Vision, 7607
Aging News Alert, 7608
Aging Process: Therapeutic Implications, 7609
Aging Research & Training News, 7610
Aging and Developmental Disability: Current Research, Programming, and Practice, 7611
Aging and Disabilities, 3495
Aging and Family Therapy: Practitioner Perspectives on Golden Pond, 7612
Aging and Our Families, 7613
Aging and Rehabilitation II, 1926
Aging and Vision News, 7614
Aging and Vision: Declarations of Independence, 8853
Aging in America, 7559
Aging in Stride, 7615
Aging in the Designed Environment, 7616
Aging with a Disability, 7617
Agnes M Lindsay Trust, 2621
Ahmanson Foundation, 2314
Ahnafield Corporation, 51, 57, 60, 66, 67, 81, 84, 95, 96, 97, 103, 108, 116, 117, 118, 120
Ai Squared, 1360, 5191
Aids for Arthritis Inc., 8003
Aiphone Corporation, 169
Air Lift Oxygen Carriers, 617
Air Lift Unlimited, 617
Air Products Foundation, 2775
AirLift Toileting System, 229
Akron Community Foundation, 2737
Akron Resources, 171
Akron Rotary Camp, 1009
Alabama Association of Homes and Services for the Aging, 7560
Alabama Council For Developmental Disabilities, 2990
Alabama Department of Education, 1785
Alabama Department of Education: Division of Special Education Services, 1785
Alabama Department of Public Health, 2991
Alabama Department of Rehabilitation Services, 2992, 6329
Alabama Department of Senior Services, 2993
Alabama Disabilities Advocacy Program, 2994
Alabama Division of Rehabilitation and Crippled Children, 2995
Alabama Easter Seal Society, 8184
Alabama Goodwill Industries, 6330
Alabama Institute for Deaf and Blind Library and Resource Center, 4359
Alabama Power Foundation, 2301
Alabama Public Library Service, 4361
Alabama Radio Reading Service Network (ARRS), 4360
Alabama Regional Library for the Blind and Physically Handicapped, 4361
Alabama School for Deaf, 7751
Alabama State Department of Human Resources, 2996
Alabama VA Regional Office, 5373
Alabama Veterans Facility, 5374
Alamitos-Belmont Rehab Hospital, 7062
Alante, 547
Alaska Center for the Blind and Visually Impaired, 6352
Alaska Commission on Aging, 3003
Alaska Department of Education: Office of Special Education, 1787
Alaska Department of Handicapped Children, 3004
Alaska Department of Labor, 5634
Alaska Division of Mental Health and Developmental Disabilities, 3005
Alaska Division of Vocational Rehabilitation, 3006
Alaska SILC, 3557
Alaska State Commission for Human Rights, 5635
Alaska State Library Talking Book Center, 4368
Alaska Veterans Facility, 6353
Alavi Foundation of New York, 2647
Albany County Department for Aging, 3320
Albany Talking Book Center, 4433
Albany VA Medical Center: Samuel S Stratton, 5506
Albany Vet Center, 5507
Albert & Bessie Mae Kronkosky Charitable Foundation, 2832
Albert G and Olive H Schlink Foundation, 2738
Albert L and Elizabeth T Tucker Foundation, 2410
Aldercrest Health and Rehabilitation Center, 7246
Aldersgate Center, 986, 1042
Aleda E Lutz VA Medical Center, 5467
Alert, 1881
Alerter, 7989
Alex Stern Family Foundation, 2734
Alex: The Life of a Child, 8322
Alexander Graham Bell Association, 1605, 1613, 1614, 1633, 1736, 1945, 2047, 2100, 2143, 5153, 7792, 7793, 7814, 7864, 7865, 7876, 7916, 7917, 7928, 7929, 7930
Alexander Graham Bell Association for the Deaf and Hard of Hearing, 1528, 7674
Alexander and Margaret Stewart Trust, 2411
Alexandria Community Y Head Start, 6022
Alexandria Library Talking Book Service, 4632
Alexandria VA Medical Center, 5450
Alexian Brothers Medical Center, 6646
Alfred Bersted Foundation, 2468
Alfred I DuPont Hospital for Children, 6548
Alice Tweed Touhy Foundation, 2315
Alive at 25: How I'm Beating Cystic Fibro sis, 8323
All About Attention Deficit Disorders, Revised, 5141, 7380
All About You: Appropriate Special Interactions and Self-Esteem, 1361
All Garden State Physical Therapy, 6877
All Kinds of Minds, 1598
All Star Review, 1362
All of Us: Talking Together, Sex Education for People with Developmental Disabilities, 4975
All the Way Up There, 8324
All-Turn-It Spinner, 5266
Allen County Public Library, 4467
Allen P & Josephine B Green Foundation, 2601
Allergies Sourcebook, 2nd Edition, 8325
Allergy Control Products, 8378
Allergy and Asthma Network Mothers of Asth matics, 5037
Allergy and Asthma Network Mothers of Asthmatics, 8634
Allergy and Asthma Network/Mothers of Asthmatics, 8433
Alliance House, 6758
Alliance for Disabled in Action, 4011
Alliance for Disabled in Action New Jersey, 5915
Alliance for Parental Involvement in Education, 1722, 5022, 7470
Alliance for People with Disabilities: Sea ttle, 4221
Alliance for Technology Access, 729, 1247
Alliance of People with Disabilities: Redmond, 4222
Allied Enterprises of Tupelo, 5887
Allied Services John Heinz Institute of Rehabilitation Medicine, 6244
Allied Services Rehabilitation Hospital, 6245

Allyn & Bacon, 1339, 2045, 2052, 2056, 2061, 2062, 2063, 2068, 2081, 2112, 2139, 2142, 2147, 2161, 2170, 2174, 2202, 2249, 7837
Allyn & Bacon Longman College Faculty, 2168
Aloha Nursing and Rehab Center, 7102
Aloha Special Technology Access Center, 1235
Alpha Home Royal Maid Association for the Blind, 3958
Alpha One: Aroostook, 3868
Alpha One: Augusta, 3869
Alpha One: Bangar, 3870
Alpha One: Main Office, 3871
Alpha One: South Portland, 3868
Alphabetic Phonics Curriculum, 1927
Alpine Alternatives, 8196
Alpine North Nursing and Rehabilitation Center, 6853
Alpine Nursing and Rehabilitation Center of Hershey, 6968
Alpine Ridge and Brandywood, 6969
Alta Bates Medical Center, 4391
Altarfire Publishing, 8474
Alternating Hemiplegia of Childhood Foundation, 2316
Alternative Approach to Allergies, 8326
Alternative Educational Delivery Systems, 1928
Alternative Medicine and Multiple Sclerosis, 8327
Alternative Teaching Strategies, 1929
Alternative Work Concepts, 1723
Alternatives for Growth: New Jersey, 5916
Alternatives in Education for the Hearing Impaired (AEHI), 5192
Altimate Medical, 384
Altman Foundation, 2648
AlumiRamp, 372
Aluminum Adjustable Support Canes for the Blind, 598
Aluminum Crutches, 618
Aluminum Walking Canes, 619
Alvin C York VA Medical Center, 5564
Alzheimer's Association, 2469
Alzheimer's Disease Education and Referral Center (ADEAR), 7561
Alzheimer's Store, 644
Amarillo VA Healthcare System, 5569
Amarillo Vet Center, 5570
Amateur Athletic Foundation of Los Angeles, 2317
Ambrose Monell Foundation, 2649
Ambulatory Cosmetology Technicians, 143
Amer. Assn. of Spinal Cord Injury Psych./Soc. Wks., 8571
America Civil Liberites Union, 8570
America West Airlines, 5308
American Academy for Cerebral Palsy and Developmental Medicine Annual Conference, 1529
American Academy of Allergy, Asthma and Immunology, 8328
American Academy of Audiology, 5193
American Academy of Child and Adolescent Psychiatry, 8126
American Academy of Environmental Medicine, 730
American Academy of Ophthalmology, 8745
American Academy of Ophthalmology Annual Meeting, 1530
American Academy of Osteopathy, 8127
American Academy of Otolaryngology: Head and Neck Surgery, 8128
American Academy of Pediatrics, 731
American Academy of Pediatrics Guide to Yo ur Child's Alleriges And Asthma, 8329
American Academy of Physical Medicine and Rehabilitation, 8129
American Action Fund for Blind Children and Adults, 8746
American Advertising Dist of Northern Virginia, 1846
American Alliance for Health, Phys. Ed. & Dance, 7638, 8929
American Amputee Foundation, 7545
American Anals of the Deaf Reference, 8854
American Annals of the Deaf, 7762
American Art Therapy Association, 5064
American Art Therapy Association (AATA), 1
American Assn. of Children's Residential Centers, 1547
American Association for Counseling & Development, 1767, 1874
American Association of Children's Residential Centers, 732
American Association of Homes and Services for the Aging, 7562
American Association of Music Therapy, 2
American Association of Oriental Medicine, 733
American Association of People with Disabilities, 734, 5194, 4760
American Association of Spinal Cord Injury Nurses, 8330, 8330
American Association of Spinal Cord Injury Psychologists & Social Workers, 7944
American Association of the Deaf-Blind, 7274
American Association of the Deaf-Blind (AADB), 7289
American Association of the Deaf-Blind National Conference, 1531
American Association on Mental Retardation, 7381
American Association on Mental Retardation AAMR Annual Meeting, 1532
American Back Society, 7945, 8319
American Baptist Churches Rhode Island, 1043
American Bar Association, 4283, 4332, 4343
American Blind Bowling Association, 9087
American Board for Certification in Orthotics & Prosthetics, 7546
American Board of Chelation Therapy, 735
American Board of Disability Analysts, 1533, 1551, 1563, 4281, 5071
American Board of Professional Disability Consultants, 736
American Botanical Council, 737, 5195
American Camping Association, 738, 1022, 8264
The American Camping Association, 967
American Cancer Society, 908, 8191, 8202, 8212
American Cancer Society Maryland, 8244
American Chai Trust, 2650
American Chemical Society, 5101
American Chiropractic Association, 739
American Cleft Palate-Cranifacial Association, 8384
American College Testing Program, 2199, 2042, 2231, 5827
American College of Advancement in Medicine, 740
American College of Nurse Midwives, 741
American College of Rheumatology Research and Education Foundation, 5196
American Counceling Association, 2092
American Council Of The Blind, 8741, 8743, 8780, 8794
American Council On Education, 7700
American Council for Headache Education (ACHE), 1724
American Council of Blind Lions, 8747
American Council of the Blind, 8748, 18, 8742, 8757, 8770, 8787, 8825, 8877, 8949, 8970, 8979, 9030, 9100
American Council of the Blind Annual Convention, 1534
American Counseling Association, 742, 1537, 1767, 1850, 1862, 1883, 1884, 2001, 4280, 4311, 6314
American Counselling Association, 1725
American Dance Therapy Association (ADTA), 3
American Diabetes Association, 8187, 1055, 8180, 8181, 8182, 8188, 8189, 8190, 8201, 8210, 8217, 8227, 8242, 8269, 8280, 8627
The American Diabetes Association, 8200
American Diabetes Association Annual Conference, 1535
American Diabetes Association Summer Camp, 8188
American Diabetes Association: Camp Grenada, 8189
American Diabetes Summer Camp, 1055, 8190
American Discount Medical, 432
American Express Foundation, 2623
American Falls Office: Living Independently for Everyone (LIFE), 3739
American Forensic Association, 8692
American Forensic Association Journal, 8692
American Foundation Corporation, 2739
American Foundation for Urologic Disease, 8428
American Foundation for the Blind, 2651, 8749, 2187, 8905, 8943, 8955, 8990, 9062
American Foundation for the Blind / AFB Press, 1766
American Foundation for the Blind-Midwest, 2470
American Foundation for the Blind/ AF B Press, 1268
American Foundation for the Blind/AFB Press, 7284, 7285, 7658, 7670, 8834, 8846, 8847, 8850, 8853, 8858, 8867, 8870, 8871, 8872, 8880, 8882, 8884, 8889, 8894, 8898, 8901, 8904, 8910, 8924, 8925, 8934, 8936, 8950, 8951, 8984, 8986, 8988, 8993, 9002, 9005, 9006, 9007, 9008, 9011, 9016, 9017, 9029, 9045, 9050, 9051, 9054, 9056, 9066, 9067, 9070, , 9075, 9081, 9082, 9083, 9086
American Foundation for the Blind: Southwest, 2833
American Group Psychotherapy Association, 8130
American Health Assistance Foundation, 2537
American Health Care Association, 5080
American Health Consultants, 8307
American Hearing Impaired Hockey Association, 7939
American Hearing Research Foundation, 7875

American Heart Association, 7547, 7557, 7949
American Heart Association Guide to Stroke Treatment, Recovery & Prevention, 8331
American Herb Association Newsletter, 4783
American Herbalists Guild, 743
American Holistic Medical Association, 744
American Hotel and Lodging Foundation, 5309
American Institute for Foreign Study, 2265
American Journal of Art Therapy, 4
American Journal of Audiology, 7763
American Journal of Orthopsychiatry, 8332
American Journal of Physical Medicine, 5060
American Journal of Psychiatry, 5061
American Journal of Public Health, 5062
American Journal of Speech-Language Pathology, 8693
American Journal on Mental Retardation, 7381
American Juvenile Arthritis Organization, 5108, 7988, 8039, 8066
American Juvenile Arthritis Organization (AJAO), 7946
American Juvenile Athritis Organization (AJAO), 8041
American Liver Foundation, 5197
American Lung Association, 8199, 8315, 8340, 8342, 8343, 8344, 8372, 8396, 8421, 8426, 8454, 8501, 8528, 8550, 8567, 8590, 8601, 8623
American Lung Association of Maryland, 957
American Lung Association of Oregon, 8204
American Massage Therapy Association, 745
American Medical Association, 4883, 8337
American Medical Industries, 294
American Mobility: Personal Mobility Solutions, 5198
American Music Therapy Association (AMTA), 5
American National Bank and Trust Company, 2471
American Network of Community Options & Resource, 4889
American Network of Community Options & Resources, 4740, 4831
American Occupational Therapy Association, 746, 5098
American Occupational Therapy Association (AOTA), 4820
American Occupational Therapy Foundation, 2538
American Optometric Association, 8750, 8918
American Organization for Bodywork Therapies of Asia, 747
American Orthopsychiatric Association, 1877, 8332
American Orthotic & Prosthetic Association, 1895
American Paraplegia Society, 7947
American Physical Therapy Association, 1536
American Printing House for the Blind, 8751, 8855
American Psychiatric Association, 8131
American Psychiatric Publishing, 5061
American Psychological Association, 1849
American Public Health Association, 748, 5062
American Red Cross, 8076
American Red Cross in Washington DC, 3886
American Red Cross of Cape Cod and Islands, 3886
American Red Cross: National Headquarters, 749
American Rehabilitation, 5063
American Rehabilitation Counseling Association, 1537
American SIDS Institute, 8635
American School for the Deaf, 7738
American School Counselor Association, 1725
American Self-Help Clearinghouse, 750
American Sign Language (ASL): Quick Facts, 7764
American Sign Language Handshape Cards, 1599
American Sign Language Handshape Dictionary, 7765
American Sign Language Phrase Book, 7766
American Sign Language: A Look at Its Structure & Community, 7767
American Social Health Association, 8132, 8141
American Society for Deaf Children, 7675
American Society for the Alexander Techniq ue, 751
American Society of Bariatric Physicians, 752
American Society of Clinical Hypnosis, 753
American Society of Teachers of the Alexander Technique, 754
American Speech-Language and Hearing Association, 5199
American Speech-Language-Hearing Association, 1538, 7676, 8674, 1648, 7758, 7763, 7855, 8691, 8693, 8717
American Spinal Injury Association, 7948
American Spinal Injury Association Annual Scientific Meeting, 1539
American Stroke Association, 7547, 7949
American Thermoform Corporation, 1224
American Tinnitus Association, 7677, 7924
American Universities International Programs, 2266
American Wheelchair Bowling Association, 8079
American-Scandinavian Foundation, 2267
Americans with Disabilities, 4742
Americans with Disabilities Act Checklist for New Lodging Facilities, 4784
Americans with Disabilities Act Guide for Places of Lodging: Serving Guests Who Are Blind, 8856
Americans with Disabilities Act Informatio n, 2970
Americans with Disabilities Act Manual, 4283
Americans with Disabilities Act: ADA Home Page, 5200
Americans with Disabilities Act: Questions and Answers, 4743
Americans with Disabilities Act: Selected Resources for Deaf, 4284
Ameritech Corporation Contributions Program, 2472
Amerock Corporation, 2473
Amigo Mobility International, 548, 401, 548
Amity Lodge, 6970
Amphibious ATV Distributors, 549, 549
Amplified Handsets, 172
Amplified Phones, 173
Amplified Portable Phone, 174
Amtrak, 5310
Amyotrophic Lateral Sclerosis: A Guide for Patients and Families, 8333
Amytrophic Lateral Sclerosis Association, 7950
Anaheim Veterans Center, 6388
Analog Switch Pad, 1164
Anchorage Job Training Center, 5633
Anchorage Regional Office, 5378
Andalusia Health Services, 2302
Andrews McMeel Publishing, 8338
Angel Fluff Diaper Company, 1155
Angel River Health and Rehabilitation, 7119
Angel View Crippled Children's Foundation, 906
Anglo California Travel Service, 5330
Anheuser-Busch Inc., 2602
Anixter Center, 5781
Ankylosing Spondylitis, 8334
Ann Arbor Area Community Foundation, 2570
Ann Arbor Center for Independent Living, 3906, 5881
Anna's Silent World, 7768
Annals Publishing Company, 8335
Annals of Dyslexia, 7382
Annals of Otology, Rhinology and Laryncology, 8335
Annandale at Suwanee, 6621
Anne and Henry Zarrow Foundation, 2766
Annual Report Sarkeys Foundation, 4786
Annual Report/Newsletter, 8857
Annuziata Sanguinetti Foundation, 2318
Anschutz Family Foundation, 2382
Answering Your Questions About Spina Bifid a, 8336
Antecedent Control: Innovative Approaches to Behavioral Support, 1930
Anthony Brothers Manufacturing, 5267
Anthracite Region Center for Independent Living, 4118
Antioch College, 2268
Aphasia, 8694
Aphasia: What is It?, 8695
Appalachian Center for Independent Living, 4233
Appalachian Independence Center, 4200
Apple Computer, 2319
Appliance 411, 5201
Applied Kinesiology: Muscle Response in Diagnosis, Therapy and Preventive Medicine, 4787
Applied Rehabilitation Counseling, 1931
Approaching Equality, 4285
Apria Healthcare, 433, 6534
Aquarius Health Care Videos, 4691, 4696, 4698, 4710, 4846, 4897, 4975, 5021, 5035, 5142, 5165, 5166, 5169, 5170, 5176, 5178, 5179, 5183, 7391, 7392, 7418, 7427, 7439, 7528, 7535, 8020, 8072, 8073, 8109, 8956
Aquatic Access, 399
Arbors East Subacute and Rehabilitation Center, 7196
Arbors at Canton Subacute And Rehabilitation Center, 7197
Arbors at Columbus, 6224
Arbors at Dayton, 7198
Arbors at Marietta, 7199
Arbors at Milford, 7200
Arbors at New Castle, 7080
Arbors at Sylvania, 7201
Arbors at Toledo Subacute and Rehab Centre, 7202
Arc Connection Newsletter, 4788, 7383

Arc Detroit, 3907
Arc Light, 7384
Arc Massachusetts, 2554, 4781
Arc Minnesota, 4757
The Arc Of Alabama, 3548
The Arc Of Alabama Inc., 6349
The Arc Of Anchorage, 2305
The Arc Of Arizonia, 2308
The Arc Of Georgia, 2460
Arc Of Meriden-Wallingford, Inc., 6535
Arc Of San Diego, 7326
Arc Of United States, 2903
Arc Putnam County, 2820
Arc South County Chapter, 2803
Arc of Alabama, 2303
Arc of Alaska, 2305
Arc of Anderson County, 2821
Arc of Arizona, 7384
Arc of Arkansas, 2310
Arc of Bergen and Passaic Counties, 5917
Arc of California, 2320
Arc of Colorado, 2383
Arc of Connecticut, 2393
Arc of Dane County, 2902
Arc of Davidson County, 2822
Arc of Delaware, 2407, 3070
Arc of Dunn County, 2903
Arc of Eau Claire, 2904
Arc of Florida, 2426
The Arc of Gloucester, 989
Arc of Hamilton County, 2823
Arc of Hawaii, 2461
Arc of Illinois The Illinois Life Span Project, 2474
Arc of Indiana, 2515
Arc of Iowa, 2522
Arc of Kansas, 2529
Arc of Kentucky, 2531
Arc of Louisiana, 2533
Arc of Maryland, 2539
Arc of Michigan, 2571
Arc of Minnesota, 2590
The Arc of Minnesota, 2590
Arc of Mississippi, 2600
Arc of Nebraska, 2612
Arc of New Jersey, 2624
The Arc of New Jersey, 992
Arc of New Mexico, 2642
Arc of North Carolina, 2723
Arc of North Dakota, 2735
Arc of Northern Rhode Island, 2804
Arc of Ohio, 2740
Arc of Oregon, 2769
Arc of Outagamie County, 2905
Arc of Pennsylvania, 2776
Arc of Racine County, 2906
Arc of South Carolina, 2816
Arc of Tennessee, 2822, 4788, 7383
The Arc of Tennessee, 2830
The Arc of Texas, 2873
Arc of U S, 5805
Arc of United Inc., 2303
Arc of United States, 2776, 2816, 2873
Arc of Utah, 2876
Arc of Virginia, 2881
Arc of Washington County, 2824
Arc of Washington State, 2891
Arc of Williamson County, 2825
Arc of Wisconsin Disability Association, 2907
Arc of Wyoming, 2916
Arc of the District of Columbia, 2412, 4770
Arc of the Farmington Valley, 6536
Arc of the United States, 5202
Arc-Down Syndrome Society of Rhode Island, 2805
Arc/Muskegon, 3908
Arcadia Foundation, 2777
Arcadia University, 2272
Arch and Stella Rowan Foundation, 2834
Architectural Barriers Action League, 5295
Archives of Neurology, 8337
Arcola Bus Sales, 89, 91
Arcola Mobility, 52
Arctic Access, 3558
Arden Rehabilitation And Healthcare Center, 7030
Arden Rehabilitation and Healthcare Center, 7247
Ardence, 6214
Ardmore Developmental Center, 5860
Area Access, 373
Area Cooperative Educational Services (ACES), 5709
Arena Stage, 6, 7275, 7678
Arista Surgical Supply Company, 618
Arista Surgical Supply Company/AliMed, 123, 132, 150, 622, 632, 698
Arizona State Department of Health Services, 1909
Arizona Association of Homes and Housing for the Aging, 7563
Arizona Braille and Talking Book Library, 4369
Arizona Bridge to Independent Living, 3567, 4803
Arizona Bridge to Independent Living: Mesa, 3569
Arizona Bridge to Independent Living: Phoenix, 3568
Arizona Camp Sunrise, 8191
Arizona Center for Disability Law, 3022
Arizona Center for the Blind and Visually Impaired, 6354
Arizona Civil Rights Division, 5638
Arizona Community Foundation, 2307
Arizona Department of Children's Rehabilitative Services, 3013
Arizona Department of Economic Security, 3014
Arizona Department of Education, 1789
Arizona Department of Family Health Services, 3015
Arizona Department of Handicapped Children, 3016
Arizona Department of Health Services, 1906, 1908, 1910, 1911, 2025
Arizona Division of Aging and Adult Services, 3017
Arizona Industries for the Blind, 6355
Arizona Rehabilitation State Services for the Blind and Visually Impaired, 3018
Arizonia Autism Resources, 2308
Arjo Inc., 139, 144, 232, 233, 400, 403
Arkansas Assistive Technology Projects, 3025
Arkansas Department of Human Services, 5647
Arkansas Department of Special Education, 1788
Arkansas Division of Aging & Adult Services, 3026
Arkansas Division of Developmental Disabilities Services, 3027
Arkansas Division of Services for the Blind, 3028
Arkansas Employment Security Department, 5643
Arkansas Employment Service Agency and Job Training Program, 5643
Arkansas Independent Living Council, 3576
Arkansas Lighthouse for the Blind, 6374
Arkansas Regional Library for the Blind and Physically Handicapped, 4377
Arkansas Rehabilitation Research and Training Center for the Deaf and Hard of Hearing, 7679
Arkansas School for the Blind, 4378
Arkasas Rehab Services, 5645
Arkenstone: The Benetech Initiative, 1165
Arlington County Department of Libraries, 4633
Arlington County Library, 4633
Arms Wide Open, 3719
Armstrong Medical, 434
Army and Air Force Exchange Services, 2269
Arnold A Schwartz Foundation, 2625
Aromatherapy Book: Applications and Inhalations, 4789
Aromatherapy for Common Ailments, 4790
Around the Clock: Parenting the Delayed AD HD Child, 7385
Arrowhead West, 6739
Art Therapy, 5064
Art Therapy SourceBook, 7
Art and Disabilities, 8
Art and Healing: Using Expressive Art to Heal Your Body, Mind, and Soul, 9
Art and Science of Teaching Orientation and Mobility to Persons with Visual Impairments, 8858
Art for All the Children: Approaches to Art Therapy for Children with Disabilities, 10
Art-Centered Education and Therapy for Children with Disabilities, 1932
Arthritis 101: Questions You Have Answers You Need, 7990
Arthritis Accent, 7991
Arthritis Answers: Basic Information About Arthritis, 7992
Arthritis Bible, 7993
Arthritis Consulting Services, 7951
Arthritis Foundation, 7952, 4907, 4908, 7552, 7946, 7992, 7998, 8005, 8007, 8008, 8011, 8014, 8021, 8023, 8025, 8027, 8028, 8036, 8045, 8046, 8050, 8052, 8055, 8056, 8061, 8064, 8071, 8123, 8334, 8451, 8517, 8565, 8568
Arthritis Foundation - Michigan Chapter, 8051
Arthritis Foundation Distribution Center, 5173, 7990, 8065, 8385, 8429, 8549
Arthritis Foundation Information Hotline, 8122
Arthritis Foundation Southern N.E. Chapter, 7991
Arthritis Foundation of Illinois News, 7994
Arthritis Foundation: Greater Southwest Chapter, 7995
Arthritis Helpbook, 7996
Arthritis Helpbook: A Tested Self-Management Program for Coping, 7997
Arthritis Information: Children, 7998
Arthritis News, 7999
Arthritis Observer, 8000
Arthritis Relief at Your Fingertips, 8001
Arthritis Reporter, 8002
Arthritis Self Help Products, 8003

Arthritis Self-Help Book, 8004
Arthritis Today, 8005
Arthritis and Diet, 8006
Arthritis and Employment: You Can Get the Job You Want, 8007
Arthritis and Pregnancy, 8008
Arthritis in Children, 8009
Arthritis in Children and La Artritis Infantojuvenil, 5108
Arthritis in Children: Resources for Children, Parents and Teachers, 8010
Arthritis on the Job: You Can Work with It, 8011
Arthritis, Rheumatic Diseases and Related Disorders, 8012
Arthritis: A Comprehensive Guide, 8013
Arthritis: Do You Know?, 8014
Arthritis: Stop Suffering, Start Moving, 8015
Arthritis: Taking Care of Yourself Health Guide for Understanding Your Arthritis, 8016
Arthritis: What Exercises Work, 8017
Arthritis: Your Complete Exercise Guide, 8018
Arthur Ross Foundation, 2652
Artic Business Vision (for DOS) and Artic WinVision (for Windows 95), 1319
Artic Technologies, 1216, 1319
Artificial Language Laboratory, 4524, 8705
Artificial Larynx, 175
Artists Fellowship, 2653
As I Am, 4791
Ascension Health, 6193
Asheville VA Medical Center, 5522
Ashton Memorial Nursing Home and Chemical Dependency Center, 6639
Ask the Doctor: Asthma, 8338
Aspen Publishers, 4706, 7665, 7666, 8473
Asperger's Syndrome: A Guide for Parents a nd Professionals, 8339
Assemblies of God Center for the Blind, 4550
Assessing Students with Special Needs, 2200
Assessing the Handicaps/Needs of Children, 1933
Assessment & Management of Mainstreamed Hearing-Impaired Children, 1934
Assessment Log & Developmental Progress Charts for the CCPSN, 1935, 2201
Assessment and Remediation of Articulatory and Phonological Disorders, 1936
Assessment in Mental Handicap: A Guide to Assessment Practices & Tests, 1937
Assessment of Children and Youth, 1938
Assessment of Individuals with Severe Disabilities, 1939
Assessment of Learners with Special Needs, 2202
Assessment of the Feasibility of Contracting with a Nominee Agency, 4286
Assessment of the Technology Needs of Vending Facilitiy Managers In Tennessee, 1940
Assessment: The Special Educator's Role, 1941
Assist.com, 5203
Assistance at Self-Serve Gas Stations, 5109
Assistech, 536
Assistive Software Products, 1363
Assistive Technology, 176, 145
Assistive Technology Advocacy Center (ATAC), 4009
Assistive Technology Center at NCEP: Nevada Community Enrichment Program, 3276
Assistive Technology Disabilities, 5204
Assistive Technology Educational Network of Florida, 3084
Assistive Technology Journal, 435
Assistive Technology News, 4792
Assistive Technology Resource Centers of Hawaii, 3111
Assistive Technology Resource Centers of Hawaii (ATRC), 4449
Assistive Technology Sourcebook, 436
Assistive Technology Training and Information Center (ATTIC), 3791
Assistive Technology for Older Persons, 7618
Assistive Technology for School Age, 4669
Assistive Technology in the Schools: A Guide for Idaho Educators, 1600
Assoc. on Handicapped Student Service Program, 4805
Associated Blind, 8752
Associated Services For The Blind & Visually Impaired, 4609
Associated Services for the Blind, 8753, 9098
Association for Applied Psychophysiology and Biofeedback, 755
Association for Education & Rehabilitation of the Blind & Visually Impaired, 1540, 8754
Association for International Practical Training, 2270
Association for Macular Diseases, 8755
Association for Macular Diseases Newsletter, 8859
Association for Network Care, 7953
Association for Neurologically Impaired Brain Injured Children, 7954
Association for Persons in Supported Employment, 756, 1527
Association for Persons with Severe Handicaps (TASH), 757
Association for Retarded Citizens of Jefferson County (The Arc), 6331
Association for Retarded Citizens: Alameda County, 6389
Association for the Blind, 6989
Association for the Cure of Cancer of the Prostate, 5205
Association of Children's Prosthetic/Orthotic Clinics, 7955
Association of Educational Therapists, 758
Association of Late-Deafened Adults, 7680
Association of Ohio Philanthropic Homes and Housing for Aging, 7564
Association of University Centers on Disabilities, 759
Association on Handicapped Student Service Program, 1881
Association on Higher Education and Disability, 1726
Association on Higher Education and Disability (AHEAD), 760
Assumption Activity Center, 6759
Asthma & Allergy Education for Worksite Clinicians, 2252
Asthma & Allergy Essentials for Children's Care Provider, 2253
Asthma Action Cards: Child Care Asthma/Allergy Action Card, 1601
Asthma Action Cards: Student Asthma Action Card, 1602
Asthma Alert, 8340
Asthma Care Training for Kids (ACT), 2254
Asthma Challenge, 8341
Asthma Handbook, 8342
Asthma Handbook Slides, 8343
Asthma Lifelines, 8344
Asthma Management and Education, 1942
Asthma Resource Directory, 8345
Asthma Sourcebook, 8346
Asthma and Allergy Answers: A Patient Education Library, 8347
Asthma and Allergy Foundation of America, 5206, 1601, 1602, 1668, 1677, 1942, 2252, 2253, 2254, 8303, 8341, 8347, 8456, 8490, 8596, 8672
Asthma and Exercise, 8348
Asthma in the School: Improving Control with Peak Flow Monitoring, 8349
Asthma in the Workplace, 8350
Aston-Patterning, 1943
At Home Among Strangers, 7769
At Home with Stickybear, 1364
Athena Rehab of Clayton, 7096
Atheneum, 8059, 8597
Athens Talking Book Center-Athens-Clarke County Regional Library, 4434
Atherton Family Foundation, 2462
Atkinson Foundation, 2321
Atlanta Institute of Medicine and Rehabilitation, 6622
Atlanta Regional Office, 5421
Atlanta VA Medical Center, 5422
Atlantic Coast Rehabilitation & Healthcare Center, 7168
Atlantis Community, 3650
Attainment Company, 1365, 447
Attention, 7386
Attention Deficit Disorder, 7387
Attention Deficit Disorder Association, 8430
Attention Deficit Disorder and Learning Disabilities, 7388
Attention Deficit Disorder in Adults Workbook, 7389
Attention Deficit Disorder in Children and Adolescents, 1944
Attention Deficit Disorder: A Different Perception, 7390
Attention Deficit Disorder: Adults, 7391
Attention Deficit Disorder: Children, 7392
Attention Deficit Disorders Association, Southern Region: Annual Conference, 1541
Attention Deficit Disorders: Assessment & Teaching, 7393
Attention Deficit-Hyperactivity Disorder: Is it a Learning Disability?, 5110
Attention Getter, 1366
Attention Teens, 1367
Attention-Deficit Hyperactivity Disorder: Symptoms and Suggestons for Treatment, 7394
Attention-Deficit/Hyperactivity Disorder, What Every Parent Wants to Know, 7395
Attitudes Toward Persons with Disabilities, 4793
Attorney General's Office: Disability Rights Bureau & Health Care Bureau, 3131
Audapter Speech System, 1320
Audio Book Contractors, 599
Audiogram/Clinical Records Manager, 1236
Audiology Foundation of America, 5207
Auditech: Classroom Amplification System Focus CFM802, 1603

Auditech: DirectEar Transmitter and Headset, 316
Auditech: Personal FM Educational System, 1604
Auditech: Personal PA Value Pack System, 317
Auditech: Pocketalker Pro, 318
Auditory Processing Disorders in Children: What Does It Mean?, 7770
Auditory-Verbal International, 5208, 7771
Auditory-Verbal Therapy for Parents and Professionals, 1605
Augmentative Communication Systems (AAC), 1166
Augmentative and Alternative Communication International Society For (ISAAC), 8696
Augmenting Basic Communciation in Natural Contexts, 7396
Augusta Rehabilitation Center, 7140
Augusta Talking Book Center, 4435
Augusta VA Medical Center, 5423
Aural Habilitation, 1945
Auricle, 7771
Aurora of Central New York, 7290
Austin Resource Center for Independent Living, 4160
Austin Resource Center: Round Rock, 4161
Austin Resource Center: San Marcos, 4162
Authoritative Guide to Self- Help Resource in Mental Health, 4794
Autism, 5142, 7397
Autism Handbook: Understanding & Treating Autism & Prevention Development, 7398
Autism Research Institute, 7399, 7400
Autism Research Review International, 7400
Autism Services Center, 7293, 7543
Autism Society Of North Carolina Bookstore, 7401
Autism Society of America, 7542, 7448
Autism Society of North Carolina, 7401, 7322, 7518
Autism Society of North Carolina Bookstore, 1799, 2043, 5117, 7397, 7402, 7403, 7406, 7409, 7411, 7414, 7417, 7436, 7445, 7452, 7458, 7459, 7481, 7497, 7506, 7514, 7515, 7517, 7532, 7534, 8710, 9077
Autism Treatment Center of America, 7294
Autism Treatment Guide, 7402
Autism and Asperger Syndrome, 7403
Autism and Learning, 7404
Autism in Adolescents and Adults, 7405
Autism...Nature, Diagnosis and Treatment, 7406
Autism: A Strange, Silent World, 7407
Autism: A World Apart, 7408
Autism: Explaining the Enigma, 7409
Autism: From Tragedy to Triumph, 7410
Autism: Identification, Education and Treatment, 7411
Autism: The Facts, 7412
Autistic Adults at Bittersweet Farms, 7413
Automated Functions, 1328
Automatic Card Shuffler, 5268
Automatic Wheelchair Anti-Rollback Device, 644
Automobile Lifts for Scooters, Wheelchairs and Powerchairs, 53
Automobility Program, 2577
Avacado Press, 4749
Avery Publishing Group, 8401, 8471, 8687
Avis Rent-A-Car, 5353
Avoid Eye Strain, Feel it T-Shirt, 1130
Avoiding Unfortunate Situations, 7414
AwareNews, 4795
Awareness, 8860
Awareness Posters, 8351
Awareness Training, 8861
Away We Ride, 1368
Away We Ride IntelliKeys Overlay, 1167
Away with Arthritis, 8019
Ayer Company Publishers, 2109
Ayurvedic Institute, 2255
Azure Acres Recovery Center, 6390

B

B AR C, 5650
B&H Reviews, 4849
A BA Commission on Mental & Physical Disability La, 4317, 4334
A BA Commission on Mental and Physical Disability, 2085
BA and Elinor Steinhagen Benevolent Trust, 2835
BCR Foundation, 2427
BESTspeech, 177
BG Industries, 162
BI-County Services, 5806
BIGmack Communication Aid, 1168
BIPAP S/T Ventilatory Support System, 295
BIT Talking Scale Bathroom Scale, 125
BOSC, 4979
BOSC: Directory of Facilities for People with Learning Disabilities, 1752
BPPV, 7772
BVA Bulletin, 5111
Baby Book for the Developmentally Challenged Child, 4976
Baby Jogger Company, 247
Babycare Assistive Technology, 8862
Babycare Assistive Technology for Parents with Physical Disabilties, 8863
Babyface: A Story of Heart and Bones, 4977
Bach Flower Therapy: Theory and Practice, 4796
Back Bay Books, 8600
Back Machine, 251
Back in the Saddle, 6391
Back in the Saddle Hippotherapy Program, 6647
Back-Huggar Pillow, 252
BackSaver, 230
BackSaver Products Company, 230
Backgammon Set: Deluxe, 5269
Backyards and Butterflies, 4978
Bad Axe Center for Independent Living, 3909
Bagel Holder, 335
The Bahmann Foundation, 2761
Bailey, 437
Bailey Manufacturing, 437
Bailey Manufacturing Company, 225, 226, 228, 244, 250, 371, 423, 488, 489, 490, 498, 499, 502, 511, 661
Bailey's Book House, 1369
Bain, Inc. Center For Independent Living, 3720
Bainbridge Subregional Library for the Blind & Physically Handicapped, 4436
Baker & Taylor, International, 7451
Baker Commodities Corporate Giving Program, 2322
Bakersfield Association for Retarded Citizens, 5650
Bakersfield Regional Rehabilitation Hospital, 6063
Balance Centers of America, 5807
Ball Bearing Spinner, 54
Ball Brothers Foundation, 2516
Ball Memorial Hospital, 6713
Ballantine Books, 4918, 8062, 8997
Ballard Rehabilitation Hospital, 6392
Baltimore Community Foundation, 2540, 2542
Baltimore Regional Office, 5455
Baltimore VA Medical Center, 5456
Bancroft NeuroHealth, 6878
Bancroft Rehabilitation Living Centers, 6760
Bangor Public Library, 4495
Bangor Veteran Center: Veterans Outreach Center, 5853
Bank One Texas N A, 2854
Bank One, Trust Group, 2521
Bank of America, 2855, 2862
Bank of America Client Foundation, 2428
Bank of America Foundation, 2323
Bank of Boston Corporation Charitable Foundation, 2555
Bank of the West, 2376
Bankers Trust Company, 2404
Banner Good Samaritan Medical Center, 6356
Bantam Books, 4953, 7437
Baptist Health Rehabilitation Institute, 3029
Baptist Heath, 3029
Bar 717 Ranch/Camp Trinity, 8192
Barbara Arnold, 1122
Barbara Chambers Children's Center, 6558
Barbara Olson Center of Hope, 6648
Bariatric Wheelchairs Regency FL, 662
Barnes-Jewish Hospital Washington University Medical Center, 7160
Baroco Corporation, 6796
Baron de Hirschmeyer Foundation, 2429
Barrier Free Education, 1606
Barron Collier Jr Foundation, 2430
Barron's Educational Series, 4675, 7475, 7476, 7477, 8477
Barrow Neurological Institute Rehab Center, 6058
Bartholomew County Public Library, 4468
Bartolucci Center, The- ILC Enterprises, 6649
Baruch College, 1249
Basic Course in American Sign Language, 5143, 8864
Basic Course in American Sign Language Package, 7773
Basic Course in Manual Communication, 7774
Basic Facts on Study Abroad, 2271
Basic Math Competency Skill Building, 1338
Basic Math: Detecting Special Needs, 1339
Basic Rear Closure Sweat Top, 1131
Basic Vocabulary: ASL for Parents and Children, 7775
Basketball School, 8080
Basketball: Beeping Foam, 9088
Bastyr University Natural Health Clinic, 761
Bath Fixtures, 126
Bath Products, 127
Bath Shower & Commode Chair, 128
Bath Supports, 129
Bath VA Medical Center, 5508
Bath and Shower Bench 3301B, 130

BathEase, 131
Bathtub Safety Rail, 132
Baton Rouge Area Foundation, 2534
Battenberg & Associates, 1370
Battery Device Adapter, 319
Battery Operated Cushion, 645
Battle Creek VA Medical Center, 5468
Baxter Healthcare Corporation, 6650, 293, 305
Bay Area Coalition for Independent Living, 3910
Bay Pine-Virginia Beach, 7021
Bay Pines VA Medical Center, 5415
Bay View Nursing and Rehabilitation Center, 7063
Bayfront Medical Center, 6565
Bayfront Rehabilitation Center, 6565
Baylor College of Medicine, 4621, 4623
Baylor College of Medicine Birth Defects Center, 4620
Baylor College of Medicine: Cullen Eye Institute, 4621
Baylor Institute for Rehabilitation, 6998
Bayshore Medical Center: Rehab, 6276
Bayview Nursing and Rehabilitation, 6393
Be Quiet, Marina!, 7415
BeOK Key Lever, 482
Beach Center on Families and Disability, 762, 3158
Beacon Foundation for the Mentally Retarded, 6357
Beacon Press, 8968
Beacon Therapeutic Diagnostic and Treatment Center, 6651
Beam, 7280
Bear River Ranch, 976
Beaumont Senior Center: Community Access Center, 3585
Beaver College, 2272
Becket Chimney Corners YMCA Outdoor Center, 8193
Beckley VA Medical Center, 5591
Bed Rails, 296
The Bedford School, 7354
Beebe Center, 5209
Beech Brook, 1010
Beechwood Rehabilitation Services A Community Integrated Brain Injury Program, 6971
Before and After Zachariah, 5047
Beginning ASL Video Course, 5144
Beginning Reading and Sign Language, 7776
Beginning Reasoning and Reading, 1607
Behavior Analysis in Education: Focus on Measurably Superior Instruction, 1946
Behavior Modification, 1947
Behavior Skills: Learning How People Should Act, 1371
Behavior Therapy and Research Society, 8133
Behavioral Disorders, 1948
Behavioral Vision Approaches for Persons with Physical Disabilities, 8865
Behind Special Education, 1949
Being Close, 8352
Belden Center, 6394
Beliefs, Values, and Principles of Self Advocacy, 4797
Beliefs: Pathways to Health and Well Being, 4798
Bell Atlantic Foundation, 2654, 2882
Bellefaire Jewish Children's Bureau, 6924
Bellingham Care Center, 7031
Bellingham Health Care and Rehabilitation Services, 7248
Belonging, 8866
Beltone Electronics Corporation, 7778
Ben B Cheney Foundation, 2892
Ben B and Iris M Margolis Foundation, 2877
Ben's Story: A Deaf Child's Right to Sign, 7777
Bench Marks, 4799
Benchmark Measures, 2203
Bend Work Activity Center, 5979
Benefis Healthcare, 6864
Benjamin Benedict Green-Field Foundation, 2475
Bennington School Summer Program, 1053
Benwood Foundation, 2826
Bergen Brunswig Corporation Contributions Program, 2324
Bergeron Health Care, 4035
Bergner Communications, 5126
Berkeley Planning Associates, 5092
Berkeley Speech Technologies, 177
Berklee Press Publications, 40
Berkley Publishing Group, 5016
Berkshire Meadows, 6797
Bernard McDonough Foundation, 2901
Berrien Community Foundation, 2572
Berthold Lowenfeld on Blindness and Blind People, 8867
Best 25 Catalog Resources for Making Life Easier, 438
Best Buddies, 7295
Best Center for Independent Living, 3848
BetaBed Pressure Pad, 253
Beth Abraham Health Services, 7175
Beth Abraham of Family Health Services, 7186
Bethel Mennonite Camp, 948
Bethy and the Mouse: A Father Remembers His Children with Disabilities, 5048
Better Back, 231
Better Hearing Institute, 7681
Better Sleep, 281
Betty Bacharach Rehabilitation Hospital, 6207
Between Friends, 7778
Beverly Enterprises Network, 6375
Beyond Baby Talk: From Sounds to Sentence s, a Parent's Guide to Language Development, 8697
Beyond Sight, Inc., 600
Beyond the Barriers, 8020
Bibs, 1096
Big Bold Timer Low Vision, 336
Big Bounder Power Wheelchair, 663
Big Lakes Developmental Center, 6740
Big Lamp Switch, 483
Big Number Pocket Sized Calculator, 601
Big Print Address Book, 588
Big Red Switch, 178
Bill Dvorak, Kayak and Rafting Expeditions, 5331
Bill T Smith Jr, 2431
Biloxi/Gulfport VA Medical Center, 5478
BioMedical Life Systems, 301, 579
Biology Concepts Through Discovery, 7416
Biology of the Autistic Syndromes, 7417
Biomedical Concerns in Persons with Down's Syndrome, 1950
Birdie Thornton Center, 3548
Birmingham Alliance for Technology Access Center, 1237
Birmingham Independent Living Center, 3549, 1237
Birmingham VA Medical Center, 5375
Birth Defect News, 4670
Birth Defect Research for Children, 763, 4667, 4670, 5121
Bishopswood, 7732
Bittersweet Chances: A Personal Journey o f Living and Learning in the Face of Illness, 8353
Black Hawk Center for Independent Living, 3804
Black Hills Workshop, 4143
Black Hills Workshop & Training Center, 4143
Blackstone Valley Center, 4131
Blackstone Valley Chapter RI Arc, 2806
Blazie Engineering, 1221, 1223
Blazing Toward a Cure Annual Conference, 1542
Blind & Vision Rehabilitation Services Of Pittsburgh, 6972
Blind Babies Foundation, 2325, 6395
Blind Children's Center, 5120, 5123, 5128, 5130, 5131, 5132, 5133, 5134, 5161, 8897, 8920, 8922, 8945, 8974, 8975, 8976, 8981, 8995, 9013, 9024, 9041, 9052, 9053, 9059, 9060
Blind Children's Fund, 2573
Blind Childrens Center, 8756
Blind Childrens Center Annual Meeting, 1543
Blind Educator, 8868
Blind Industries and Services of Maryland, 6784
Blind Information Technology Specialists, 8757
Blind Outdoor Leisure Development, 9089
Blind Service Association, 6652
Blind and Vision-Impaired Individuals, 5112, 8869
Blinded Veterans Association, 8758, 5111
Blinded Veterans Association National Convention, 1544
Blindness, 5145
Blindness and Early Childhood Development Second Edition, 8870
Blindness, A Family Matter, 8871
Blindness: What it is, What it Does and How to Live with it, 8872
Blindskills, 8903
Blinker Buddy II Electronic Turn Signal, 55
Blocks in Motion, 1372
Blooming Where You're Planted, 8354
Blount Foundation, 2304
Blowitz-Ridgeway Foundation, 2476
Blue Chip II, 458
Blue Ridge Independent Living Center, 4202
Blue Ridge Independent Living Center - Troutville, 4201
Blue Ridge Independent Living Center: Christianburg, 4203
Blue Ridge Independent Living Center: Low Moor, 4204
Blue Water CIL: Lapeer, 3911
Blue Water CIL: Port Huron, 3912
Blueberry Hill Healthcare, 6798
Bluebook: Explanation of the Contents of the ADA, 4287
Bluegrass Technology Center, 1238
Board Games: Snakes and Ladders, 5270
Board Games: Solitaire, 5271
Bob & Kay Timberlake Foundation, 2724

Bobby Dodd Institute (BDI), 6623
Boca Raton Rehabilitation Center, 7081
Bodman Foundation, 2655
Body Reflexology: Healing at Your Fingertips, 4800
Body Silent: The Different World of the Disabled, 4801
Body Suits, 439, 1097
Body of Knowledge/Hellerwork, 4802
Bodyline Comfort Systems, 252
Boggy Creek Gang Camp, 8194
Boise Health And Rehabilitation Center, 7103
Boise Regional Office, 5428
Boise VA Medical Center, 5429
Bold Line Paper, 589
Bold Tracks: Skiing for the Disabled, 8081
Bolton Manor Nursing Home, 7148
Bone Up on Arthritis, 8021
Bonfils-Stanton Foundation, 2384
Bonnie Prudden Myotherapy, 764
Book of Name Signs, 7779
Book of Possibilities: Elementary Edition, 1608
Book of Possibilities: Secondary Edition, 1609
Bookholder: Roberts, 484
Books are Fun for Everyone, 8873
Books for Blind and Physically Handicapped Individuals, 8759
Books for the Blind of Arizona, 4370
Books on Special Children, 4979, 1752, 1764, 1933, 4737, 6220, 7388, 7485, 7537
Boone County Community Network, 2517
Bootheel Area Independent Living Services, 3968
Booties with Non-Skid Soles, 1080
Boston Center for Independent Living, 3887
Boston Foundation, 2556
Boston Globe Foundation, 2557
Boston University, 4511, 6803
Boston University Arthritis Center, 4511
Boston University Center for Human Genetics, 4512
Boston University Hospital Vision Rehabilitation Services, 6799
Boston University Robert Dawson Evans Memorial Dept. of Clinical Research, 4513
Boston VA Regional Office, 5461
Bothin Foundation, 2326
Botsford Center For Rehabilitation & Health Improvement-Redford, 6828
Boulder Community Hospital, 6098
Boulder Community Hospital Mapleton Center, 7072
Boulder Park Terrace, 7158
Boulder Public Library, 4399
Boulder Vet Center, 5400
Bounder Plus Power Wheelchair, 709
Bounder Power Wheelchair, 710
Bowel Cancer, 8355
Bowel Continence & Spina Bifida, 8356
Bowel Management: A Manual of Ideas and Techniques, 8357
Bowling: Ball Ramp, 8082
Box Top Opener, 337
Boxlight, 1314
Boxlight Corporation, 1314
The Boy Inside, 5180
Boy Scouts of America, 4712
Boys Town National Research Hospital, 7682
Brachial Plexus Palsy Foundation, 2778
Bradbury Press, 7420, 8409, 8737
Bradford Regional Medical Center, 6973
Bradford Woods/Camp Riley, 935
Braille Blazer, 1221
Braille Book Bank, Music Catalog, 8874
Braille Book Review, 8875
Braille Circulating Library for the Blind, 4634
Braille Compass, 602
Braille Documents, 5146, 8876
Braille Forum, 8877
Braille Institute, 9033
Braille Institute Library, 4382
Braille Institute Orange County Center, 9093
Braille Institute Santa Barbara Center, 4383
Braille Institute Sight Center, 4384
Braille Institute of America, 8760
Braille Keyboard Labels, 1222
Braille Monitor, 8878
Braille N' Speak, 1223
Braille Notebook, 590
Braille Plates for Elevator, 603
Braille Playing Cards: Plastic, 5272
Braille Touch-Time Watches, 604
Braille and Talking Book Library, Perkins School for the Blind, 4514
Braille and Talking Book Library: Californ ia State Library, 4385
Braille: An Extraordinary Volunteer Opportunity, 8879
Braille: Bingo Cards, Boards and Call Numbers, 5273
Braille: Desk Calendar, 591
Braille: Greeting Cards, 592
Braille: Rook Cards, 5274
Brailon Thermoform Duplicator, 1224
Brain Allergies: The Psychonutrient, 8358
Brain Injury Association of America, 765, 7296
Brain Injury Association of New York State, 766, 7297
Brain Injury Association of Texas, 767, 7298
Brain Injury Rehabilitation Center Dr. P. Phillips, 6566, 6566
Brandecker Rehabilitation Center, 6653
Branden Publishing Company, 7410
Brandt Industries, 485
Braun Corporation, 56, 133, 63, 133, 417, 584
Bravo! + Three-Wheel Scooter, 550
Brawner Building, 2411
Brazoria County Center For Independent Living, 4163
Breaking Barriers, 1951
Breaking Ground, 8359
Breaking New Ground News Note, 8360
Breaking New Ground Resource Center, 8636
Breaking the Speech Barrier: Language Develpment Through Augmented Means, 8698
Breakthroughs: How to Reach Students with Autism, 7418
Breast Cancer Sourcebook, 8361
Breathe Easy Young People's Guide to Asthma, 8362
Breathe Free, 8363
Breathing Disorders: Your Complete Exercise Guide, 8364
Breathing Lessons: The Life and Work of Mark O'Brien, 8022
Breckenridge Outdoor Education Center, 915
Breezy, 664
Bremer Tower, 2594
Bremerton Convalescent and Rehabilitation Center, 7249
Brentwood Rehabilitation and Nursing Cente r, 7141
Brentwood Subacute Healthcare Center, 6654
Brevard County Libraries, 4415
Brevard County Library System, 4429
Brevard County Talking Books Library, 4415
Brewer Rehab And Living Center, 6179
Brian's House, 4119
Briarcliff Nursing Home & Rehab Facility, 6332
Briarwood Day Camp, 1024
Bridge Newsletter, 4803
Bridge Pointe Services & Goodwill of Southern Indiana, Inc, 5808
Bridgepark Center for Rehabilitation and Nursing Services, 7203
Bridges Beyond Sound, 7780
Bridging the Gap: A National Directory of Services for Women & Girls with Disabilities, 4804
Briefs, 1154
Briggs Foundation, 2327
Brigham Manor Nursing and Rehabilitation Center, 7149
Brigham and Women s Hospital, 4516
Brigham and Women's Hospital: Asthma and Allergic Disease Research Center, 4515
Brigham and Women's Hospital: Robert B Brigham Multipurpose Arthritis Center, 4516
Bright Horizons Summer Camp, 8195
Brighten Place, 6246
Brike International, 529
Bringing Out the Best, 5065
Bristol County Chapter Arc, 2807
Britannica Film Company, 4718, 5154, 7861, 8035, 8324, 9036
A Britsh Broadcasting Corporation Documentary, 7467
Broadcast Services for the Blind, 4386
Broadman and Holman, 7911
Broadmead, 3874
Broadview Multi-Care Center, 7204
Bronchial Asthma: Principles of Diagnosis and Treatment, 8365
Bronx Continuing Treatment Day Program, 6892
Bronx Independent Living Services, 4036
Bronx VA Medical Center, 5509
Brooke Publishing, 2159
Brookes Publishing, 1592, 1593, 1594, 1595, 1673, 1705, 1915, 1918, 1930, 1935, 1955, 1956, 1959, 1963, 1966, 1972, 1974, 1988, 1989, 1991, 2005, 2006, 2007, 2024, 2032, 2037, 2051, 2053, 2071, 2078, 2091, 2132, 2148, 2152, 2165, 2186, 2191, 2192, 2193, 2194, 2198, 2201, 2205, 2210, 2212, 4684, 4701, 4703, 4723, 4728, , 4729, 4750, 4769, 4778, 4823, 4830, 4843, 4845, 4893, 4932, 4955, 4957, 4972, 4980, 4982, 4985, 4986, 4987, 5002, 5012, 5018, 5027, 5029, 5038, 5039, 5054, 5068, 5069, 5073, 5074, 5078, 5160, 5181, 5181, 7288
Brookes Publishing Company, 1768, 1922, 1939, 1971, 2008, 2040, 2108, 2189
Brookings Institution, 4288, 7622, 7671

Brookline Books, 1769, 8, 15, 1635, 1657, 1660, 1661, 1707, 1708, 1937, 1952, 1970, 1986, 1990, 1995, 2017, 2049, 2133, 2135, 2150, 2153, 2156, 2158, 2171, 2176, 4678, 4724, 4797, 4835, 4840, 4895, 4902, 4916, 4941, 4978, 4981, 4984, 4994, 5008, 5024, 5044, 5048, 6188, 7419, 7482, 7505, 7509, 7531, 8466, 8522,
Brookline Books Publications, 2004
Brookline Books/Lumen Editions, 8566
Brooklyn Bureau of Community Service, 6893
Brooklyn Campus of the VA NY Harbor Healthcare System, 5510
Brooklyn Center for Independence of the Disabled, 4037
Brooklyn Home for Aged Men, 2656
Brooks / Cole Publishing Company, 1982
Brooks Memorial Hospital Rehabilitation Center, 6567
Brooks Publishing Company, 1941, 1946
Brooks/Cole Publishing Company, 1770, 7393
Brothers, Sisters, and Special Needs, 4980
Brotman Medical Center, 6396
Brotman Medical Center: RehabCare Unit, 6064, 6396
Broward County Talking Book Library, 4416
Brown County Library, 4660
Brown Foundation, 2836
Brown University Long Term Care Advisor, 5066
Brown-Heatly Library, 4622
Brown-Karhan Health Care, 6999
Broyhill Family Foundation, 2725
Bruno Independent Living Aids, 374, 53, 374, 379, 386, 387, 402, 414, 415, 419, 552, 570
Bryn Mawr Rehabilitation Hospital, 6974
Buck & Buck, 1068, 1069, 1070, 1071, 1072, 1074, 1075, 1076, 1077, 1080, 1081, 1084, 1085, 1086, 1087, 1088, 1101, 1107, 1110, 1112, 1116, 1121, 1123, 1124, 1126, 1127, 1128, 1131, 1132, 1133, 1134, 1136, 1137, 1144, 1145, 1146, 1156, 1157, 1158
Buck and Buck Clothing, 1098
Budget Cotton/Poly Open Back Gown, 1068
Budget Flannel Open Back Gown, 1069
Buffalo Hearing and Speech Center, 6894
Buffalo Regional Office, 5511
Buffalo State (SUNY), 2273
Build Rehabilitation Industries, 6397
Builders of Skills, 6133
Building Blocks: Foundations for Learning for Young Blind and Visually Impaired Children, 8880
Building Bridges: Including People with Disabilities in International Programs, 2274
Building Communicative Competence with Indiv. Who Use Augmentative & Alternative Commun., 8699
Building Owners and Managers Association International, 1566
Building the Healing Partnership: Parents, Professionals and Children, 1952, 4981
Bull Publishing, 8487
Bulletin, 8881
Bulletin Newsletter, 7781
Bulletin of the Association on the Handicapped, 4805
Burbank Rehabilitation Center, 6800
Bureau of Education for Exceptional Children, 3085
Bureau of Elderly & Adult Services, 3294
Bureau of Employment Programs Division of Workers' Compensation, 3522
Bureau of Rehabilitations Services, 4404
Burger School for the Autistic, 4525
Burke Rehabilitation Hospital, 6215
Burlington Northern Foundation, 2837
Burlington Northern Santa Fe Foundation, 2477
Burnett Foundation, 2838
Burnish Me Bright, 8700
Burns Braille Transcription Dictionary, 8882
Burns-Dunphy Foundation, 2328
Burnt Gin Camp, 1044
Bursitis, Tendonitis and Other Soft Tissue Rheumatic Syndromes, 8023
Bus Girl: Selected Poems, 7419
Bus and Taxi Sign, 486
Bushrod H Campbell and Ada F Hall Charity Fund, 2558
Business Publishers, 2963, 4328, 4336, 7610
Business as Usual, 5147
But I'm Ready to Go, 7420
Butler Adult Training Center, 6333
Butler VA Medical Center, 5544
Butlers Wheelchair Lifts, 375
Button Aid, 282
Buy!, 1610
Buying Time: The Media Role in Health Care, 5148
Bye-Bye Decubiti (BBD), 254
Bye-Bye Decubiti Air Mattress Overlay, 155

C

C D Publications, 1998, 2920, 2928, 2966
C FK R Career Materials, 1953
C&C Software, 1344
C-4 Work Center, 5782
C-CAD Center of United Cerebral Palsy of Metropolitan Dallas, 6009
C2ILMAX, 1169
CA Health and Human Services Agency, Dept of Rehab, 3040
CACLD, 5163, 7377, 7465, 7492, 7499, 7529
CAPCO Capability Corporation, 1459
CAPH Independent Living Center, 3586
CAPP National Parent Resource Center Federation for Children with Special Needs, 768
CAREERS & the disABLED Magazine, 5067
CAREsource Program Development, 7615, 7652
CARF International, 1727
CARF Rehabilitation Accreditation Commission, 769, 1727
CASA Inc., 4023
CC-M Productions, 8024
CD Publications, 7608
CDR Reports, 4806
CEC Catalog, 1843
CEC Div for Childrens' Communication Development, 5075
CEC-Division for Early Childhood, 1728
CEH, 5354
CH Foundation, 2839
CHAMP Camp, 7733
CHID Combined Health Information Database, 1239
CHOICES Center for Independent Living, 4024
CIL Options-One Stop Career Center: Royal Palm Beach, 3689
CIL of Central Florida, 3690
CIL of Florida Keys, 3691
CIL of Florida Keys-Key West, 3692
CIL of Mid-Michigan, 3913
CIL of North Central Florida, 3693
CINTEX: Speak to Your Appliances, 1373
CITE: Lighthouse for Central Florida, 1240
CKLS Headquarters, 4479
CNS Camp New Connections, 7311
CPB/WGBH National Center for Access Media, 6801
CREVT: Comprehensive Receptive and Expressive Vocabulary Test, 2204
CSD Spectrum, 7782
CV Mosby Company, 1889
Cabell County Public Library/Talking Book Department/Subregional Library for the Blind, 4652
Cabinet for Health Services, 3169
Caddo-Bossier Association for Retarded Citizens, 6761
Cadinal Hill Medical Center, 6749
California Association of Homes and Services for the Aging, 7565
California Community Care News Community Residential Care Association of CA, 4722
California Community Foundation, 2329
California Department of Aging, 3034
California Department of Education, 1729, 4387
California Department of Education: Special Education Division, 1790
California Department of Fair Employment & Housing, 5651, 4304, 4305, 4308
California Department of Handicapped Children, 3035
California Department of Rehabilitation, 3036
California Elwyn, 6398
California Endowment, 2330
California Eye Institute, 6399
California Financial Power of Attorney, 4807, 7619
California Foundation For Independent Living Centers, 3587
California Foundation for Independent Living Centers, 3588
California Governor's Committee on Employment of People with Disabilities, 3037
California Protection & Advocacy: (PAI) A Nonprofit Organization, 3038
California School Of Professional Psychology, 7725
California School of Professional Psychology, 4394
California State Council on Developmental Disabilities, 3039
California State Independent Living Council (SILC), 3589
California State Library Braille and Talki ng Book Library, 8761
California State Oriental Medical Association (CSOMA), 770
Cambridge Career Products Catalog, 440
Cambridge Educational, 440, 1420, 1516
Cambridge University Press, 8519, 8559
Camden Healthcare and Rehabilitation Center, 7223

Camiccia-Arnautou Charitable Foundation, 2431
Camp Seale Harris Southeastern Diabetes Education Services, 902
Camp AIM Lloyd Institute, 1025
Camp ARC Spencer, 1026
Camp Aldersgate, 994
Camp Allen, 982
Camp Allyn, 1011
Camp Alpine, 8196
Camp Baker, 7312
Camp Barakel, 8827
Camp Betsey Cox, 7313
Camp Birchwood, 8197
Camp Bon Coeur, 8198
Camp Breathe Easy, 8199
Camp Buckskin, 7314
Camp CAMP, 1048
Camp Can Do, 1027
Camp Candlelight, 8637
Camp Capella, 7734
Camp Carefree, 8200
Camp Carolina Trails for Children, 8201
Camp Catch-a-Rainbow, 8202
Camp Challenge, 951, 8828
Camp Chatterbox, 8683
Camp Cheerful, 8203
Camp Christmas Seal, 8204
Camp Civitan, 903
Camp Classen YMCA, 8205
Camp Comeca, 7735
Camp Conrad Chinnock, 8206
Camp Courage, 972
Camp Courage North, 8207
Camp Courageous, 1012
Camp Courageous of Iowa, 942
Camp Crosley YMCA, 8208
Camp Cub Creek Science Camp, 976
Camp Dartmouth-Hitchcock, 983
Camp Del Corazon, 8209
Camp Dickenson, 1056
Camp Discovery, 1046, 8210
Camp Dunmore, 1028
Camp Easter Seal: East/West, 1057
Camp Easter Seals, 980
Camp Eden Wood, 8211
Camp El Camino Pines, 7736
Camp Emanuel, 7737
Camp Enchantment, 8212
Camp Erdman YMCA, 927
Camp Esperanza Arthritis Foundation, 7978
Camp Fatima, 8213
Camp Fire U SA, 1062
Camp Floyd Rogers, 8214
Camp Forrest, 906
Camp Foundation, 2883
Camp Friendship, 973
Camp Fun in the Sun, 8215
Camp Glengarra, 8216
Camp Glyndon, 8217
Camp Gravatt, 1045
Camp Greentop, 955
Camp Harkness, 8218
Camp Hertko Hollow, 8219
Camp Hickory Hill, 8220
Camp Ho Mita Koda, 8221
Camp Hodia, 8222
Camp Holiday Trails, 1058
Camp Honor, 8223
Camp Horizons, 7315
Camp Huntington, 7316
Camp Independence, 8224
Camp Isola Bella, 7738
Camp J CC, 2262
Camp JCC, 956
Camp Jened, 8225
Camp Jewell YMCA Outdoor Center, 8226
Camp John Marc, 1049
Camp John Warvel, 8227
Camp Joslin, 8228
Camp Jotoni, 987
Camp Joy, 7739, 8229
Camp Kaleidoscope, 7317
Camp Keystone, 1029
Camp Killoqua, 1062
Camp Kostopulos, 1052
Camp L-Kee-Ta, 8230
Camp Lakewood, 977
Camp Lawroweld, 8829
Camp Lee Mar, 1030
Camp Libbey, 8231
Camp Little Giant, 928
Camp Lou Henry Hoover, 8830
Camp MITIOG, 8232
Camp Magruder, 8233
Camp Mark Seven, 7740
Camp Merrick, 8831
Camp Merry Heart, 988
Camp Millhouse, 936
Camp Mokuleia, 8234
Camp Nejeda Foundation, 8281
Camp New Hope, 929, 974
Camp Nissokone, 7318
Camp Northwood, 7319
Camp Not-A-Wheeze American Lung Association, 8235
Camp Nuhop, 7320
Camp Oakhurst, 7979
Camp Okizu, 8236
Camp Paha, 916
Camp Paivika, 907
Camp Rainbow, 8237
Camp Ramah in New England (Summer), 962
Camp Ramah in New England (Winter), 963
Camp Ramapo, 7321
Camp Rap-A-Hope Medical Society and the Alliance to the Medical, 8238
Camp Reach for the Sky, 908
Camp Recovery Center, 6400
Camp Roger, 967
Camp Ronald McDonald at Eagle Lake, 909
Camp Ronald McDonald for Good Times, 8239
Camp Royall, 7322
Camp Ruggles, 7323
Camp Setebaid, 8240
Camp Shady Brook, 8241
Camp Sioux, 8242
Camp Sisol, 7324
Camp Sky Ranch, 1006
Camp Smile-A-Mile, 8243
Camp Stepping Stone, 1013
Camp Summit, 1050
Camp Sun'N Fun, 989
Camp Sunrise, 8244
Camp Superkids, 957
Camp Surefoot, 1031
Camp Sweeney, 8245
Camp Tall Turf, 8246
Camp Taloali, 7741
Camp Tanager, 943
Camp Tekoa UMC, 7742
Camp Thorpe, 1054
Camp Thunderbird, 924
Camp Twin Lakes, 926
Camp Vacamas, 8247
Camp Venture, 995
Camp Virginia Jaycee, 1059
Camp Virginia Jaycee Newsletter, 1882
Camp Waban, 953
Camp Waziyatah, 8248
Camp Wheezeaway American Lung Association of Alabama, 8249
Camp Whitman on Seneca Lake, 996
Camp Winnebago, 975
Camp World Light, 7325
Camp Wyoming, 944
Camp for All, 1051
Camp-A-Lot, 7326
Campaign Math, 1340
Campbell Soup Foundation, 2626
Camping Unlimited, 910
Camping Unlimited for Children, 910
Campobello Chemical Dependency Recovery Center, 6401
Camps for Children & Teens with Diabetes, 8250
Can America Afford to Grow Old?, 4288
Can't Your Child See? A Guide for Parents of Visually Impaired Children, 8883
Can-Do Products Catalog, 134
Canandiagua VA Medical Center, 5512
Cancer Biotherapy Research Group, 5210
Cancer Care, 2657
Cancer Clinical Trials: Experimental Treatments and How They Can Help You, 5028
Cancer Immunology Research Foundation, 5211
Cancer Immunotherapy and Gene Therapy Institute, 5212
Cancer Information Service, 8638
Cancer Research Fund of Damon Runyon: Walter Winchell Foundation, 5213
Cancer Sourcebook, 8366
Cancer Victors Journal, 8367
Candlelighters Childhood Cancer Foundation, 2541
Candler General Hospital: Rehabilitation Unit, 6126
Canine Companions for Independence, 771
Canine Helpers for the Handicapped, 772, 8762
Canonicus Camp, 1043
Cape Coral Hospital, 7082
Cape Organization for Rights of the Disabled (CORD), 3888
Capital Area Center for Independent Living, 3914
Capital District Center for Independence, 4038
Capital District YMCA, 8845
Capitol Publications, 2930, 2937
Caprice Care Center, 7205
Capron Rehabilitation Center, 6517
Capscrew, 338
Caption Center, 4517, 7683, 8763
Captioned Media Program, 7684
Captions for Deaf and Hard-of-Hearing View ers, 7783
Car Builder, 1374
Card Holder Deluxe, 5275
Cardinal Hill Rehabilitation Hospital, 6167, 6749
Cards: Musical, 5276
Cards: UNO, 5277
Care Center East Health & Specialty Care Center, 7211

Care Electronics, 487
Care Master Medical Services, 6631
Career Achievement Center, 6866
Career Assessment & Planning Services, 5737
Career Assessment Inventories Learning Disabled, 1953
Career Connection Transition Program, 5652
Career Connections, 6031
Career Development Program (CDP), 5653
Career Education for Handicapped Individuals, 4744
Career Opportunity Development of New Jersey, 5918
Career Perspectives: Interviews with Blind and Visually Impaired Professionals, 8884
Careers in Blindness Rehabilitation Services, 8885
Caremark Healthcare Services, 6655
Carendo, 232
Carey Services, 5809
Carilion Health System, 7027
Carilion Rehabilitation: New River Valley, 7022
Caring and Sharing Center for Independent Living, 3694
Caring and Sharing Center: Pasco County, 3695
Caring and Sharing: Gulf Port, 3696
Caring for Alzheimer's Patients, 7620
Caring for America's Heroes, 4808
Caring for Children with Cerebral Palsy: A Team Approach, 8368
Caring for Children with Chronic Illness, 1954, 4671
Caring for Persons with Developmental Disabilities, 4809
Caring for Those You Love: A Guide to Compassionate Care for the Aged, 7621
Caring for the Disabled Elderly, 7622
Carl T Hayden VA Medical Center, 5380
Carl Vinson VA Medical Center, 5424
Carnegie Library of Pitts. Library for the Blind, 9065
Carnegie Library of Pittsburgh Library for the Blind & Physically Handicapped, 4610
Caro Center for Independent Living, 3915
Carolina Computer Access Center, 1241
Carolina Curriculum for Infants and Toddlers with Special Needs, 1955, 5038
Carolina Curriculum for Preschoolers with Special Needs, 1956, 2205
Carolyn's Catalog, 1099
Carolyn's Low Vision Products, 441
Carondelet Brain Injury Programs and Services (Bridges Now), 6358
Carpal Tunnel Syndrome, 7552
Carrie Estelle Doheny Foundation, 2331
Carroll Center for the Blind, 6802, 9099
Carroll School Summer Programs, 7327
Carson City Center for Independent Living, 4002
Cary Library, 4496
Casa Colina Center for Rehabilitation, 6404
Casa Colina Centers for Rehabilitation, 6402
Casa Colina Padua Village, 6403
Casa Colina Residential Services: Rancho Pino Verde, 6404
Casa Colina Transitional Living Center, 6405
Casa Colina Transitional Living Center: Pomona, 6406
Casa Colinas Centers for Rehabilitation, 6065
Casa Del Rey, 3570
Case Management Society of America, 773
Case Management in the Vocational Rehabilitation of Disabled Persons, 5092
Case Manager Magazine, 1844
Case Western Reserve University, 4596
Case Western Reserve University Northeast Ohio Multipurpose Arthritis Center, 4597
Casey Eye Institute, 4606
Casowasco Camp, Conference and Retreat Center, 7328
Castle Point Campus of the VA Hudson Valley Healthcare System, 5513
Catalog for Teaching Life Skills to Persons with Development Disability, 1611
Catalyst, 1845
The Catalyst, 1845
Cataracts, 5113, 8886
Cathedral Center for Independent Living, 3697
Catholic Charities Services, 1014, 1016
Catholic Guild for The Blind, 8940
Catholic Medical Center, 6873
Catholic Southwest, 6590
Catholic Youth Organization, 7747, 8260
Catskill Center for Independence, 4039
Cave Spring Rehabilitation Center, 6624
Cecil R Bomhr Rehabilitation Center of Nacogdoches Memorial Hospital, 6277
Cedar Ridge Camp, 8251
Cedar Spring Health and Rehabilitation Cen ter, 7258
Cedars of Marin, 6407
Centegra Northern Illinois Medical Center, 6656
Centennial Medical Center Tri Star Health System, 7224
Center Academy, 7299
Center Academy at Pinellas Park, 7329
Center For Independent Living- Kauai, 3733
Center Serving Persons with Mental Retardation, 4164
Center for Accessible Housing, 4077
Center for Accessible Living, 3849
Center for Accessible Living: Murray, 3850
Center for Accessible Technology, 1242
Center for Applied Special Technology, 1243
Center for Assistive Technology, 7566
Center for Assistive Technology & Env Access, 1606
Center for Assistive Technology & Inclusive Education Studies, 1244
Center for Assistive Technology and Environmental Access, 774, 6625
Center for Best Practices in Early Childhood, 1375
Center for Community Access, 3916
Center for Community Alternatives, 3851
Center for Community Re-entry, 8648
Center for Comprehensive Services, 6657
Center for Developmental Disabilities, 2817
Center for Disabilities Studies, 3474
Center for Disabilities and Development, 3151
Center for Disability Resources, 775, 1829
Center for Disability Rights, 3668
Center for Disability and Elder Law, 4255
Center for Educational Advancement New Jersey, 5919
Center for Handicapped Affairs, 3917
Center for Health Research: Eastern Washin gton University, 4810
Center for Health and Fitness, 8083
Center for Independence, 3651
Center for Independence Of The Disabled- Daly City, 3590
Center for Independence of the Disabled, 3591
Center for Independence of the Disabled of New York, 4040
Center for Independent Living, 3592, 3652
Center for Independent Living Options, 3852
Center for Independent Living SC, 3669
Center for Independent Living Southwest Kansas, 3813
Center for Independent Living for SW Kansas, 3814
Center for Independent Living in Central Florida - Advocacy Living Skills Peer Support, 3698
Center for Independent Living of Broward, 3699
Center for Independent Living of Central Nebraska, 3995
Center for Independent Living of Florida Keys, 3700
Center for Independent Living of Mid-Michigan, 3918
Center for Independent Living of Middle Tennessee, 4153
Center for Independent Living of N Central Florida, 3701
Center for Independent Living of N Florida, 3702
Center for Independent Living of NE Minnesota, 3944
Center for Independent Living of NW Florida, 3703
Center for Independent Living of North Central Florida, 3704
Center for Independent Living of S Florida, 3705
Center for Independent Living of SW Florida, 3706
Center for Independent Living of Western Wisconsin, 4237
Center for Independent Living: Action Towards Independence, 4041
Center for Independent Living: Amsterdam, 4042
Center for Independent Living: Camden, 4010
Center for Independent Living: E Hawaii, 3734
Center for Independent Living: Edison, 4011
Center for Independent Living: Fargo, 4085
Center for Independent Living: Kentucky Department for the Blind, 3853
Center for Independent Living: Long Branch, 4012
Center for Independent Living: Oakland, 3593
Center for Independent Living: Rochester, 4043
Center for Independent Living: South Jersey, 4013
Center for Independent Living: Tri-County, 3594
Center for Independent Living:Fresno, 3595
Center for Independent Living; East Oakland, 3596
Center for Independent Living; Oakland, 3597
Center for Interdisciplinary Research on Immunologic Diseases, 4518
Center for Learning, 6134
Center for Libraries and Educational Improvement, 4811

Center for Living & Working: Fitchburg, 3889
Center for Living & Working: Milford, 3890
Center for Living & Working: Worcester, 3891
Center for Mind/Body Studies, 776
Center for Neuro Skills, 6408, 7000
Center for Neuro-Rehabilitation, 6785
Center for Pain Control and Rehabilitation, 6568
Center for People with Disabilities, 3653
Center for People with Disabilities (CPWD), 3654
Center for People with Disabilities: Pueblo, 3655
Center for Psychiatric Rehabilitation, 6803
Center for Public Representation, 3200, 4346, 7596, 7631, 7646, 7647, 7660
Center for Rehabilitation Technology, 525
Center for Rehabilitation at Rush Presbyterian: Johnston R Bowman Health Center, 6658
Center for Research on Women with Disabilities, 4623
Center for Spine, Sports & Occupational Rehabilitation, 6659
Center for Universal Design, 777
Center for Vision Rehabilitation, 6911
Center for the Disabled, 997
Center for the Improvement of Human Functioning, 4480
Center for the Partially Sighted, 6409
Center for the Visually Impaired, 6626
Center of Independent Living: Visalia, 3598
Center on Deafness, 3756
Center on Education and Training for Employment, 6231
Center on Employment, 7685
Center on Evaluation of Assistive Technology, 1245
Center on Human Policy, 8649
Center on Human Policy: School of Education, 4571
Center on the Social & Emotional Foundations for Early Learning, 5214
Centering Corporation, 4825, 4856, 4997, 5046, 5058
Centers for Disease Control Public Health Service, 4812
Centers for Disease Control and Prevention, 4443, 8656
Central Alabama Veterans Healthcare System, 5376
Central Arkansas Rehab Hospital, 6054
Central Coast Center for IL: San Benito, 3599
Central Coast Center for Independent Living, 3600
Central Coast Center: Independent Living - Santa Cruz Office, 3601
Central Coast Neurobehavioral Center OPTIONS, 6410
Central Coast for Independent Living, 3602
Central Coast for Independent Living: Watsonville, 3603
Central Connecticut Association For Retarted Citizens Inc. (CCARC), 5710
Central Iowa Center for Independent Living, 3805, 4832
Central Island Healthcare, 7176
Central Library Downtown, 4660
Central Louisiana State Hospital Medical and Professional Library, 4491
Central Michigan University Summer Clinics, 7743
Central Missouri Diabetic Childrens Camp, 8220
Central Office D NA People Civil Services, 4257
Central Oregon Resources for Independent Living, 4107
Central Rappahannock Regional Library, 4635
Central Utah Independent Living Center, 4185
Centre City Tower, 2795
Century 50/60XR Sit, 233
Century College, 4543
Cerebral Palsy Association of Middlesex County, 5920
Cerebral Palsy Associations of New York State Annual Conference, 8134
Cerebral Palsy Center Summer Program, 990
Cerebral Palsy of Colorado, 6518
Cerebral Palsy of New Jersey, 990
Cerebral Palsy: A Complete Guide for Care giving, 8369
Cerebral Palsy: North County Center, 6411
Ceres Press, 1590
Cervical Support Pillow, 156
Chadder, 7421
The Chaddick Institute for Metropolitan Developmen, 2490
Chalet Village Health and Rehabilitation C enter, 7120
Challenge, 8370
Challenge Aspen, 917
Challenge Golf, 8084, 9090
Challenge Publications Limited, 8105
Challenge of Educating Together Deaf and Hearing Youth: Making Manistreaming Work, 1957
Challenged Scientists: Disabilities and the Triumph of Excellence, 1958
Chamois Shower Robe, 1121
Champ Camp American Lung Association of Alaska, 8252
Champion 1000, 665
Champion 2000, 666
Champion 3000, 667
Champlin Foundations, 2808
Change, 778
Change Your Brain, Change Your Life: The Breakthrough Program for Conquering Depression, 7422
Changing the Rules, 7784
Chapel Haven, 3670
Chapel Hill Rehabilitation and Healthcare Center, 7189
Characteristics, Services, & Outcomes of Rehab. Consumers who are Blind/Visually Impaired, 8887
Charles C Thomas, 24, 1932, 1944, 1957, 1978, 2009, 2011, 2014, 2018, 2019, 2039, 2041, 2064, 2076, 2079, 2124, 2140, 2163, 2190, 2240, 4693, 4998, 5013, 5085, 5288, 6141, 7800, 7805, 7926, 8712, 8892, 9063
Charles C Thomas Publications, 2169
Charles C Thomas Publisher, 1771, 1919, 1923
Charles Delmar Foundation, 2413
Charles G Thomas, Publisher, LTD., 6140
Charles W Skoien Jr, 4722
Charlotte Vet Center, 5523
Charlotte White Center, 6779
Chase Bank of Texas, 2835
Chatlos Foundation, 2432
Cheaha Mental Health, 6334
Checker Set: Deluxe, 5278
Cheever Publishing, 4773
Chelsea Community Hospital Rehabilitation Unit, 6829
Chelsea: The Story of a Signal Dog, 7785
Cheney's Liberty II, 376
Cherry Hills Health Care Center, 6519
Chesapeake Region Accessible Boating, 8085
Cheshire Occupational and Career Center, 5711
Chesity, 8371
Chess Set: Deluxe, 5279
Chestnut Hill Rehabilitation Hospital, 6247
Chevy Chase Nursing and Rehabilitation Cen ter, 7108
Chevy Lowered Floor, 57
Cheyenne VA Medical Center, 5601
Cheyenne Village, 5694
Chi Medical Library, 4526
Chicago Community Trust and Affiliates, 2478
Chicago Lawyers' Committee for Civil Rights Under Law, 4256
Chicago Lighthouse for People who are Blind and Visually Impaired, 8764
Chicago Public Library Talking Book Center, 4453
Child Care and the ADA: A Handbook for Inclusive Programs, 1959
Child Convertible Balance Beam Set, 488
Child Find/Early Childhood Disabilities Unit Montgomery County Public Schools, 6786
Child Neurology Service, 8135
Child Variable Balance Beam, 489
Child Who Never Grew Up, 7423
Child With Special Needs: Encouraging Inte llectual and Emotional Growth, 4813
Child and Adolescent Therapy: Cognitive-Be havioral Procedures, Second Edition, 7424
Child and Parent Resource Institute, 779
Child with Disabling Illness, 1960
Child's Mobility Crawler, 490
Childcare and the ADA, 4289
Childhood Asthma: A Matter of Control, 8372
Childhood Behavior Disorders: Applied Research & Educational Practice, 1961
Childhood Cancer Survivors: A Practical Guide to Your Future, 8373
Childhood Cancer: A Parent's Guide to Solid Tumor Cancers, 8374
Childhood Disablity and Family Systems, 1962
Childhood Glaucoma: A Reference Guide for Families, 8888
Childhood Leukemia: A Guide for Families, Friends & Caregivers, 8375
Childhood Speech, Language & Listening Pro blems, 8701
Children & Adults with ADHD, 7386
Children & Adults with Attention Deficit Disorder, 7421
Children With Cerebral Palsy: A Manual for Therapists, Parents and Community Workers, 8376
Children With Cerebral Palsy: A Parents' G uide, 8377
Children and Adolescents with Emotional and Behavioral Disorders, 1545

Children and Youth Assisted by Medical Technology in Educational Settings, 2nd Edition, 1963
Children of Aging Parents, 7567
Children of a Lesser God, 7786
Children s Hospital Boston, 3202
Children s Medical Program, 3248
Children with Acquired Brain Injury: Education and Supporting Families, 5029
Children with Asthma: A Manual for Parents, 8378
Children with Autism, 5030
Children with Cerebral Palsy, 8379
Children with Disabilities, 4982
Children with Facial Difference: A Parent' s Guide, 8380
Children with Mental Retardation, 7425
Children with Special Health Care Needs, 3528
Children with Spina Bifida: A Parents Guide, 8381
Children with Tourette Syndrome, 8382
Children with Visual Impairments Woodbine House, 8889
Children's Aid Society Summer Camps, 1005
Children's Alliance, 780
Children's Center for Neurodevelopmental Studies, 4371
Children's Fresh Air Society Fund, 2542
Children's Healthcare of Atlanta at Egleston, 6127
Children's Home and Aid Society of Illinois, 6660
Children's Hopes & Dreams Wish Foundation, 4682
Children's Hopes & Dreams Wish Fulfillment Foundation, 2627
Children's Hospital Central California Reh abilitation Center, 6412
Children's Hospital Los Angeles Rehabilitation Program, 6413
Children's Hospital Rehabilitation Center, 6096
Children's Medical Services, 3030
Children's National Medical Center, 781
Children's Needs Psychological Perspective, 1964
Children's Press, 4833
Children's Rehabilitation Service, 6335
Children's Specialized Hospital, 6208
Children's Specialized Hospital Medical Library - Parent Resource Center, 4564
Children's Therapy Center, 6414
Childrens Beach House, 7744, 8684
Childrens Hospital, 8680
Childrens Hospital Medical Center, 4518
Childs Spelling System: The Rules, 1612
Chiles Foundation, 2770
Chillicothe VA Medical Center, 5530
Chilton-Shelby Mental Health Center/ The Mitchell Center, 6336
Chinese Herbal Medicine, 4814
Choice Magazine Listening, 8890
Choice Switch Latch and Timer, 491
Choices for Work Program, 5738
Choices in Deafness, 7787
Choices, Choices 5.0, 1469
Choices: A Guide to Sex Counseling for the Physically Disabled Adult, 1965
Choose the Right Long Term Care: Home Care Assisted Living and Nursing Homes, 7623
Choosing Options and Accommodations for Children, 1966
Choosing Outcomes and Accommodations for Children (COACH), 5039
Choosing a Wheelchair: A Guide for Optimal Independence, 668
Christ Hospital Rehabilitation Unit, 6925
Christian Approach to Overcoming Disabilit y: A Doctor's Story, 4815
A Christian Approach to Overcoming Disability: A Doctor's Story, 4666
Christian Camps and Inner City Youth, 8246
Christian Education for the Blind, 4624
Christian Hospital Northeast, 6854
Christian Record Services, 8799
Christian Record Services/National Camps for Blind Children, 8832
Christmas Stories, 7788
Christopher & Dana Reeve Foundation Resource Center, 4565
Christopher & Dana Reeve Paralysis Resource Center, 7975
Christopher Reeve Paralysis Foundation, 7956, 4967, 7555, 8057
Chronic Fatigue Syndrome: Your Natural Gu ide To Healing with Diet, Herbs and Other Methods, 8383
Chronically Disabled Elderly in Society, 7624
Chronicle Guide to Grants, 2918, 2918
Chronimed Publishing, 8413
Church of the Nazarene, 4551
Cincinnati Children's Hospital Medical Center, 4598
Cincinnati VA Medical Center, 5531
Cincinnati Veterans Centers, 5532
Circletime Tales Deluxe, 1470
Circline Illuminated Magnifer, 605
City of Lakewood, 916
City of Lebanon New Hampshire, 7317
Civil Law Handbook on Psychiatric and Psyc hological Evidence and Testimony, 4290
Civil Rights Division/ Disability Rights Section, 2986
Civitan Acres, 1060
Civitan Foundation, 903
Clara Barton Diabetes Camp, 8253
Clara Barton For Girls With Diabetes, 8253
Clara Burke Nursing Home, 6975
Clare Branch, 6830
Claremont, 3643
Clarence & Grace Chamberlin Foundation, 2574
Clarence TC Ching Foundation, 2463
Clark Foundation, 2658
Clark House Nursing Center At Foxhill Village, 6804
Clark Memorial Hospital: RehabCare Unit, 6143
Clark-Winchcole Foundation, 2543
Clarke Health Care Products, 128
Clarkston Spec Healthcare Center, 6831
Classic, 58
Classification of Impaired Vision, 8891
Classique, 377
Classroom GOAL: Guide for Optimizing Auditory Learning Skills, 1613
Classroom Notetaker: How to Organize a Program Serving Students with Hearing Impairments, 1614
Classroom Success for the LD and ADHD Child, 1967
Claude Washington Benedum Foundation, 2779
Clausen House, 6415
Clay Center Adult Training Center, 5837
Clay Tree Society, 782
Clayton County Developmental Disabilities Board, 978
Clearbrook, 5783
Clearinghouse for Specialized Media and Technology, 1729, 4387
Clearinghouse on Disability Information: Office of Special Education & Rehab, 8639
Clearview-Brain Injury Center, 7259
Cleft Palate-Craniofacial Journal, 8384
Clement J Zablocki VA Medical Center, 5597
Cleo Of New York, 8082
Clerc: The Story of His Early Years, 7789
Cleveland Catholic Charities, 1015
Cleveland Clinic, 7206
Cleveland FES Center, 4599
Cleveland Foundation, 2741
Cleveland Public Library, 4600
Cleveland Regional Office, 5533
Cleveland Sight Center, 6926, 8837
Cleveland Society for the Blind, 6926
Client Assistance Program (CAP), 3132
Client Assistance Program: Alabama, 2997
Client Assistance Program: Alaska, 3007
Client Assistance Program: California, 3040
Clinch Independent Living Services, 4205
Clinical Applications of Music Therapy in Developmental Disability, Pediatrics and Neurology, 11
Clinical Care in Rheumatic Disease, 8385
Clinical Connection, 1846
Clinical Management of Childhood Stuttering, 2nd Edition, 1968
Clinician's Practical Guide to Attention-Deficit/Hyperactivity Disorder, 5068
Clinton County Rehabilitation Center d/b/a CCRC Community Link, 6661
Clip Board Notebook, 593
Clipper Ship Foundation, 2559
Clock, 1376
Clockworks, 5149
Clorox Company Foundation East Bay Community Foundation, 2332
Close Encounters of the Disabling Kind, 4816
Close-Up 6.5, 1170
Closer Look: The English Program at the Model Secondary School for the Deaf, 7790
Closing the Gap, 4817
Closing the Gap's Annual Conference, 1546
Cloth Diapers, 1155
Clothing Identification Kit, 283
Clothing Solutions, 1100
Clove Lakes Health Care and Rehabilitation Center, 7177
Clover Patch Camp, 997
Clovernook Center for the Blind and Visually Impaired, 8765
Clovernook Printing House, The Clovernook Center for the Blind and Visually Impaired, 8766
Club Foot & Other Foot Deformities Fact Sheet, 8386
Co:Writer, 1377
Coalition For Independence, 3815
Coalition For Independent Living Options Inc., 3707
Coalition for Independence, 4732
Coalition for Independence: Missouri Branch Office, 3969

Coalition for Independent Living Option, 3708
Coalition for Independent Living Options-One Stop Career Center, 3709
Coalition for the Education of Disabled Children, 4848
Coalition of Responsible Disabled, 4223
Coast to Coast Home Medical, 297
Coastal Disability Access, 4137
Coatesville VA Medical Center, 5545
Cobb Hospital and Medical Center: Rehab Ca re Center, 6128
Cochlear Implant Club International, 7686
Cochlear Implants, 7791
Cochlear Implants and Children, 7792
Cochlear Implants for Kids, 7793
Cockrell Foundation, 2840
Coeta and Donald Barker Foundation, 2333
Coffee County Training Center, 5605
Coffee in the Cereal: The First Year with Multiple Sclerosis, 8387
Cognition, Education and Deafness, 7794
Cognitive Approaches to Learning Disabilities, 1969
Cognitive Strategy Instruction That Really Improves Children's Academic Skills, 1970
Cogrehab, 7426
Coleman Tri- County Services, 3757
Collaborating for Comprehensive Services for Young Children and Families, 1971
Collaborative Teams for Students with Severe Disabilities, 1972
College Board, 1749
College Internship Program at the Berkshire Center, 6805
College Student's Guide to Merit and Other No-Need Funding, 2919
College and Career Programs for the Deaf, 7795
College and University, 1847
College of Maharishi Vedic Medicine Health Center, 783
College of Optometrists in Vision Development, 8767
College of Syntonic Optometry, 8768
Colleton Regional Hospital: RehabCare Unit, 6262
Colmery-O'Neil VA Medical Center, 5443
Colon & Rectal Cancer: A Comprehensive Guide for Patients & Families, 8388
Colon Health: Key to a Vibrant Life, 8389
Colonial Life and Accident Insurance Company Contributions Program, 2818
Colonial Manor Medical And Rehabilitation Center, 7051
Colonial Manor Medical and Rehabilitation Center, 7260
Colorado Association of Homes and Services for the Aging (CAHSA), 7568
Colorado Civil Rights Divsion, 5695
Colorado Department of Aging & Adult Servi ces, 3049
Colorado Department of Education, 1791
Colorado Department of Education: Special Education Service Unit, 1791
Colorado Developmental Disabilities Council, 3050
Colorado Division of Mental Health, 3051
Colorado Employment Service, 5696
Colorado Health Care Program for Children with Special Needs, 3052
Colorado Library for the Blind and Physically Handicapped, 4400
Colorado Lions Camp, 918
Colorado Springs Independence Center, 3656
Colorado Talking Book Library, 4400
Colorado/Wyoming VA Medical Center, 5401
Colton Redlands-Yucaipa Regional Occupational Programs, 5654
Columbia Disability Action Center, 4138
Columbia Foundation, 2544
Columbia Gas of Pennsylvania Corporate Giv ing, 2780
Columbia Gorge Center, 4108
Columbia Lighthouse for the Blind, 8769, 8833
Columbia Lighthouse for the Blind Summer Camp, 8833
Columbia Medical Center: Peninsula, 6578
Columbia Medical Manufacturing, 129
Columbia Regional Hospital: RehabCare Unit, 6196
Columbia Regional Office, 5558
Columbus Foundation and Affiliated Organizations, 2742
Columbus Health and Rehabilitation Center, 7121
Columbus McKinnon Corporation, 378
Columbus Rehabilitation And Subacute Institute, 7207
Columbus Speech and Hearing Center, 6927
Columbus Subregional Library For The Blind And Physically Handicapped, 4437
Comanche Pants, 1140
Combination File/Reference Carousel, 525
Come Back Jack: The Revealing Story of a Child Diagnosed with Autism, 7427
Come Sign with Us, 7796
Command Corporation, 1326
A Commitment to Inclusion: Outreach to Unserved/Underserved Populations, 4721
Committee for Purchase from People Who Are Blind or Severely Disabled, 2971
Commode, 135
Common ADA Errors and Omissions in New Construction and Alterations, 4291
Common ADA Problems at Newly Constructed Lodging Facilities, 5114
Commonly Asked Questions About Child Care Centers and the Americans with Disabilities Act, 4292
Commonly Asked Questions About Service Animals in Places of Business, 5115
Commonly Asked Questions About Title III of the ADA, 4293
Commonly Asked Questions About the ADA and Law Enforcement, 4294
Commonwealth Fund, 2659
Communi Care Health Services, 6928
CommuniCare of Clifton Nursing and Rehabilitation Center, 6928
Communicating with Deaf People: An Introduction, 7797
Communicating with Parents of Exceptional Children, 1973
Communicating with People Who Have Trouble Hearing & Seeing: A Primer, 7281
Communication & Language Acquisition: Discoveries from Atypical Development, 1974
Communication Aids for Children and Adults, 442
Communication Center/Minnesota State Services for the Blind, 4544
Communication Coloring Book, 8702
Communication Development and Disorders in African American Children, 8703
Communication Development in Children with Down Syndrome, 7428, 8704
Communication Disorders in Aging, 7625
Communication Options for Children Who are Deaf or Hard-of-Hearing, 7798
Communication Outlook, 8705
Communication Service for the Deaf (CSD), 7687, 7782
Communication Service for the Deaf: Rapid City, 4145
Communication Service for the Deaf: Yankton, 4144
Communication Skills for Visually Impaired Learners, 8892
Communication Skills for Working with Elders, 1975
Communication Unbound, 1976
Communication in Autism, 7429
Communique, 7799
Communities Actively Living Independent and Free, 3604
Communities Foundation of Texas, 2841
Community Access Center, 3605
Community Access Center: Indio Branch, 3606
Community Access Center: Perris, 3607
Community Alternatives, 4044
Community Connections of Southwest Michiga n, 3919
Community Enterprises, 784, 5712
Community Exploration, 1471
Community Foundation for Greater Atlanta, 2448
Community Foundation for Greater Buffalo, 2660
Community Foundation of Boone County, 2517
Community Foundation of Champaign County, 2479
Community Foundation of Greater Chattanooga, 2827
Community Foundation of Herkimer &, 2661
Community Foundation of Monroe County, 2575
Community Foundation of New Jersey, 2628
Community Foundation of Richmond & Central Virginia, 2884
Community Foundation of Santa Clara County, 2334
Community Foundation of Shreveport-Bossier, 2535
Community Foundation of Southeastern Connecticut, 2394
Community Foundation of Western Massachusetts, 2560
Community Foundation of the Capitol Region, 2662
Community Foundation of the Metropolitan Tarrant County, 2842
Community Gatepath, 6416
Community Health Funding Report, 2920
Community Health Network, 6714
Community Hospital Back and Conditioning Clinic, 6520
Community Hospital and Rehabilitation Center of Los Gatos-Saratoga, 6417
Community Hospital of Los Gatos Rehabilitation Services, 6066

Community Opportunities of East Ascension, 5847
Community Outpatient Rehabilitation Center, 5655
Community Outreach Program for the Deaf, 3571
Community Recreation and People with Disabilities: Strategies for Inclusion, 4723
Community Rehabilitation Services, 3608
Community Residential Alternative, 3757
Community Resources for Independence, 3609, 4120
Community Resources for Independence: Mendocino/Lake Branch, 3610
Community Resources for Independence: Napa Office, 3611
Community Resources for Independent Living, 3613
Community Resources for Independent Living Hayward, 3612
Community Service Center for the Deaf and Hard of Hearing, 4224
Community Service for the Blind, 1615
Community Services Building, 5628
Community Services for the Blind and Partially Sighted, 1615, 4225
Community Signs, 1616
Community Skills: Learning to Function in Your Neighborhood, 1378
Community Supports for People with Disabilities (CSP), 1810
Community Systems Inc., 6549
Commuter & Kid's Commuter, 700
Companion Activities, 1379
Compass Learning, 1358, 1376, 1412, 1434, 1445, 1446, 1447, 1452, 1471, 1478, 1505, 1506, 1507
Compass Learning Incorporated, 1525
Compassionate Friends, 8640
Complete Directory for Pediatric Disorders, 1753
Complete Directory for People with Chronic Illness, 1754
Complete Guide To Mercury Toxicity from De ntal Fillings, 8390
Complete Handbook of Children's Reading Disorders: You Can Prevent or Correct LDs, 1977
Complete IEP Guide: How to Advocate for Yo ur Special Ed Child, 4672, 5040
Complete Kid's Allergy and Asthma Guide: T he Parent's Handbook for Children of All Ages, 8391
Complete Learning Disabilities Directory, 1755
Complete Mental Health Directory, 1756
Complying with the Americans with Disabilities Act, 4295
Comprecare Foundation, 2385
Comprehensive Assessment in Special Education, 1978
Comprehensive Assessment of Spoken Language (CASL), 1617
Comprehensive Directory of Programs and Services, 4818
The Comprehensive Directory: Programs and Services And Special Needs In The Metro NY Area., 4709
Comprehensive Examination of Barriers to Employment Among Persons who are Blind or Impaired, 8893
Comprehensive Guide to ADD in Adults: Research, Diagnosis & Treatment, 7430
Comprehensive Pain Management Associates, 6906
Comprehensive Reference Manual for Signers and Interpreters, 7800
Comprehensive Rehabilitation Center at Lee Memorial Hospital, 6569
Comprehensive Rehabilitation Center of Naples Community Hospital, 6570
Comprehensive Signed English Dictionary, 7801
Compuserve: Handicapped Users' Database, 1246
Computer & Web Resources for People With Disabilities, 1247
Computer Access Center, 1248
Computer Access/Computer Learning, 1979
Computer Center for Visually Impaired People: Division of Continuing Studies, 1249
Computer Paper for Brailling, 1225
Computer and Web Resources for People with Disabilities, 1250
Computer-Enabling Drafting for People with Physical Disabilities, 1251
Computerized Speech Lab, 1321
Computers to Help People, 1252
Comsearch: Broad Topics, 2663
Concentration Cockpit: Explaining Attention Deficits, 7431
Concentration Video, 7432
Concept Development for Visually Handicapped Children: A Resource Guide, 8894
Concepts on the Move Advanced Overlay CD, 1171
Concepts on the Move Advanced Preacademics, 1380
Concepts on the Move Basic Overlay CD, 1172
Concerned Care Recreation Day Camp, 978
Conditional Love: Parents' Attitudes Toward Handicapped Children, 4983
Conditioning with Physical Disabilities, 8086
Conference Department, 1553
Conference of Educational Administrators Serving the Deaf, 7688
Conference of United Methodists, 8233, 8288
Confronting the Challenges of Spina Bifida, 8392
Conklin Center for the Blind, 6571
Connect, 7802, 8706
Connect Information Service, 5116
Connect Newsletter, 7803
Connecticut Association of Not-for-Profit Providers for the Aging, 7569
Connecticut Board of Education and Service for the Blind, 3057
Connecticut Braille Association, 4402
Connecticut Commission on Aging, 3058
Connecticut Department of Children and Youth Services, 3059
Connecticut Department of Education, 1792
Connecticut Department of Education: Bureau of Special Education, 1792
Connecticut Developmental Disabilities Council, 3060
Connecticut Governor's Committee on Employment of Disabled Persons, 5713
Connecticut Mutual Life Foundation, 2395
Connecticut Office of Protection and Advocacy for Persons with Disabilities, 3061
Connecticut State Board of Education and Services for the Blind, 1793
Connecticut State Government, 4403
Connecticut State Library, 4403
Connecticut Subacute Corporation, 6537
Connecticut Tech Act Project: Connecticut Department of Social Services, 4404
Connections Newsletter, 8393
Connections for Independent Living, 3657
Connelly Foundation, 2781
Conover Company, 1510, 1512
Conquering the Darkness: One Story of Reco vering from a Brain Injury, 8394
Conrad N Hilton Foundation, 2616
Constellations, 4819
Constructive Workshops, 5714
Consultants for Communication Technology, 1327, 1331
Consulting Psychologists Press, 1980
Consumer Buyer's Guide for Independent Living, 4820
Consumer Care Products, 260, 631, 637
Consumer Information Center, 5294, 7925
Consumer and Patient Information Hotline, 9094
Consumer's Guide to Home Adaptation, 1580
Contact Technologies, 50, 98
Contemporary Art Therapy with Adolescents, 12
Contemporary Issues in Behavioral Health Care, 1547
Continucare, A Service of the Rehab Institute of Chicago, 6662
Continuing Care, 1848
Contra Costa ARC, 6418
Contrasting Characteristics of Blind and Visually Impaired Clients, 8895
Control Your Child's Asthma, 8395
Controlling Asthma, 8396
Convaid, 669, 701
Convaid Products, 245, 551
Conversational Sign Language II, 7804
Conversations, 1472
Convert-Able Table, 234
Convert-O-Bike, 5267
Cooking Class: Learning About Food Preparation, 1381
Cool Handle, 339
Cooper Foundation, 2613
Coordinacion De Servicios Centrado En La Familia, 4984
Coping When a Parent Has Multiple Sclerosis, 8397
Coping and Caring: Living with Alzheimer's Disease, 7626
Coping and Prevailing with Multipe Scleros is and Other Life Struggles, 8398
Coping for Kids Who Stutter, 8707
Coping with ADD/ADHD, 7433
Coping with Asthma, 8399
Coping with Being Physically Challenged, 4673
Coping with Cerebral Palsy, 8400
Coping with Mild Traumatic Brain Surgery, 8401
Coping with Special Needs Classmates, 8402
Coping with a Physically Challenged Brother or Sister, 8403
Coping with the Multi-Handicapped Hearing Impaired: A Practical Approach, 7805
Coping+Plus: Dimensions of Disability, 4821
Cora Hoffman Center Day Program, 6895
Corcoran Physical Therapy, 6647

Cordless Big Red Switch, 492
Cordless Receiver, 340
Cordova Rehabilitation and Nursing Center, 7225
Core-Reading and Vocabulary Development, 1473
Corflex, 265
Cornelia de Lange Syndrome Foundation, 2396
Cornell Communications, 179
Cornerstone Services, 5784
Cornerstone Services Inc., 8641
Cornucopia, 5969
Cornucopia Software, 1509
Corona Regional Medical Center-Rehabiltation Center, 6419
Corporate Foundation Files, 2921
Corporate Foundation Profiles, 2922
Corporate Office, 5326, 6223
Costanoan, 911
Cottage Health System, 6442
Cotton Full-Back Vest, 1132
Cotton Stockings, 1101
Cotton/Poly Nancy Frocks, 1070
Council For Exceptional Children, 891
Council News, 4822
Council On International Educational Exchange, 5305
Council for Disability Rights, 4296, 4806
Council for Exceptional Children, 1730, 4636, 790, 1638, 1684, 1728, 1743, 1772, 1843, 1853, 1880, 1948, 2218, 4699
Council for Exceptional Children Annual Convention and Expo, 1548
Council for Extended Care, 7357
Council for Extended Care of Mentally Retarded Citizens, 7330
Council of American Instructors of the Deaf, 7689
Council of B BB s Foundation, 1574
Council of Families with Visual Impairments, 8770
Counseling Parents of Children with Chronic Illness or Disability, 5069
Counseling People with Diabetes, 8404
Counseling Persons with Communication Disorders and Their Families, 1981
Counseling Psychologist, 1849
Counseling Today, 1883
Counseling and Values, 1850
Counseling for Heart Disease, 8405
Counseling in Terminal Care & Bereavement, 4823
Counselor Education and Supervision, 1884
Count Us In, 7434
Counterpoint, 1885
Country Gardens Skilled Nursing and Rehabilitation Center, 7150
Country Manor Rehabilitation and Nursing C enter, 7151
County College of Morris, 1251
County of Santa Clara, 6085
Courage Center, 3945
Courage Center Headquarters, 972
Court-Related Needs of the Elderly and Persons with Disabilities, 4297
Covenant Health, 6272
Covenant Health Systems Owens White Outpatient Rehab Center, 6278
Covenant Healthcare Rehabilitation Program, 6189
Cowan Slavin Foundation, 2576
Cowles Charitable Trust, 2629
Cowley County Developmental Services, 3816
Craig Hospital, 6097
Crane Plumbing/Fiat Products, 126
Cranston Arc, 2809
Creating Positive Classroom Environments: Strategies for Behavior Management, 1982
Creating Wholeness: Self-Healing Workbook Using Dynamic Relaxation, Images and Thoughts, 4824
Creative Arts Resources Catalog, 13
Creative Arts Therapy Catalogs, 1618
Creative Care Package Catalog, 4825
Creative Designs, 1122
Creative Work Systems, 5854
Crescent Porter Hale Foundation, 2335
Crestfield Camp, 8254
Crestwood Communication Aids, 442
Crestwood Nursing & Rehabilitation Center, 7169
Crime and Justice, 2923
Criminal Law Handbook on Psychiatric & Psychological Evidence & Testimony, 4298
Cristo Rey Handicappers Program, 3920
Critical Air Medicine, 6420
Critical Voices on Special Education, 1983
Crockett Resource Center for Independent Living, 4165
Cross Roads Outdoor Ministries, 991
Crossing the River: Creating a Conceptual Revolution in Community & Disability, 4724
Crosslands Rehabilitation and Healthcare Center, 7237
Crossroads Industrial Services, 6715
Crossroads of Western Iowa, 6722
Crotched Mountain Adult Brain Injury Center, 6869
Crotched Mountain Foundation, 6869
Crown Point Community Foundation, 2518
Crown Publishing Group, 8406
Cruiser Bus Buggy 4MB, 551
Crutcher's Serenity House, 6421
Crutches, 620
Cub, SuperCub and Special Edition Scooters, 552
Cullen Foundation, 2843
Cultural Diversity, Families and the Special Education System, 1984
Culture, 4878
Culture and the Restructuring of Community Mental Health, 7435
Cunard Line, 5332
Curb-Sider Super XL, 379
Curing MS: How Science is Solving the Mys teries of Multiple Sclerosis, 8406
Curriculum Associates, 1462
Curriculum Decision Making for Students with Severe Handicaps, 1985
Cursive Writing Skills, 1619
Curtis & Doris K Hankamer Foundation, 2844
Curtis Instruments, 654
Custom, 670
Custom Durable, 671
Custom Earmolds, 320
Custom Lift Residential Elevators, 380
Cypress Pointe Rehabilitation and Healthca re Center, 7190
Cystic Fibrosis Foundation, 2545
Cystic Fibrosis in the 20th Century: Peop le, Events, and Progress, 8407
Cystic Fibrosis: Medical Care, 5070
Cystic Fibrosis: A Guide for Patient and F amily, 8408

D

D AR S, 3465
D C General Hospital, 3073
D C Office of Human Rights, 5731
D Sipp, 7741
DA Schulman, 645
DARCI, 1519
DAV Department of Alaska, 5379
DAV National Service Headquarters, 5364
DAYS: Depression and Anxiety in Youth Scale, 2206
DB-Link, 785
DC Public Library, Services to the Deaf, 7860
DC Regl Lib for the Blind & Physically Handicapped, 8961
DD Center/St Lukes: Roosevelt Hospital Center, 4045
DDDS/Georgetown Center, 6550
DE French Foundation, 2664
DEAF, 3892
DEP, Disabled Employment Program, 5093
DEUCE Environmental Control Unit, 493
DIRLINE, 1253
DMC Health Care Center-Novi, 6832
DNA People's Legal Services, 4257
DOCS: Developmental Observation Checklist System, 2207
DPS with BCP, 1456
DRAIL (Disability Resource Agency for Independent Living), 3614
DREAMMS for Kids, 4572, 1384, 1851
DRS Connection, 4826
DRTAC: Southeast ADA Center, 4764
DSHS/Aging & Adult Disability Services Administration, 3510
DSI, 136
DVH Quarterly, 8896
DW Auto & Home Mobility, 59
Dade Community Foundation, 2433
Dade County Talking Book Library, 4417
Daimler Chrysler, 2577
Dakota Center for Independent Living: Bism arck, 4087
Dakota Center for Independent Living: Dickinson, 4086
Dallas Academy, 7331
Dallas Foundation, 2845
Dallas Services for Visually Impaired Children, 7001
Damaco, 711
Damaco D90, 711
Daman Villa, 6976
Damar Homes Incorporated, 3792
The Dana Foundation The Dana Alliance For Brain Initiatives, 2717
Dancing Cheek to Cheek, 8897
Dancing from the Inside Out, 14
Daniel Freeman Rehabilitation Centers, 6422
Daniels And Fisher Tower, 2384
Danmar Products, 443
Danville Centre for Health and Rehabilitat ion, 7133
Darci Too, 1173
Dare Care Charity, 1882
Darrow Foundation, 2336

Dartmouth-Hitchcock Medical Center Pediatrics, 983
Data on Blindness and Visual Impairment in the US: A Resource Manual, 8898
Datahr Rehabilitation Institute, 6538
Daughters of Miriam Center/The Gallen Institute, 6879
David D & Nona S Payne Foundation, 2846
David Fulton Publishers, 7404
David J Green Foundation, 2665
David and Lucile Packard Foundation, 2337
Davidson College, 2275
Davidson College, Office of Study Abroad, 2275
Davis Center, 180
Davis Center for Hearing, Speech and Learning: Hearing Therapy, 7690, 8675
Davis Center for Rehabilitation Baptist Hospital of Miami, 6572
Davis Memorial Goodwill Industries, 5728
Dawn Enterprises, 3740
Dawnsign Press, 7921
Day at Play: A IKanDu Little Book, 1474
Dayle McIntosh Center: Laguna Niguel, 3615
Dayspring Associates, 444
Daytime Development Center, 2208
Dayton VA Medical Center, 5534
Dazor Manufacturing Corporation, 494, 605, 614
Deaf Action Center of GNO, 6762
Deaf Catholic, 7806
Deaf Children Signers, 5150
Deaf Culture Series, 5151
Deaf Empowerment: Emergence, Struggle and Rhetoric, 7807
Deaf Heritage: A Narrative History, 7808
Deaf History Unveiled: Interpretations from the New Scholarship, 7809
Deaf Like Me, 7810
Deaf Mosaic Series, 5152
Deaf Parents and Their Hearing Children, 7811
Deaf REACH, 7691
Deaf in America: Voices from a Culture, 7812
Deaf or Hard of Hearing Services New York State Education Department, 7745
The Deaf-Blind American, 7289
Deaf-Blind Division of the National Federation of the Blind, 8771
Deaf-Blind Perspective, 7282, 8899
Deafness Research Foundation, 7692
Deafness and Communicative Disorders Branch of Rehab Services Administration Office, 7693, 8676
Dean A McGee Eye Institute, 6956
Deciphering the System: A Guide for Families of Young Disabled Children, 1986
Deenie, 8409
Defining Rehabilitation Agency Types, 1987
Delano Regional Medical Center, 6423
Delaware Assistive Technology Initiative Center for Applied Science and Engineering, 3063, 4408
Delaware Association for the Blind, 6551
Delaware Client Assistance Program, 3064
Delaware Department of Health and Social Services, 3065
Delaware Department of Labor, 5725
Delaware Department of Public Instructing, 3066
Delaware Developmental Disability Council, 3067
Delaware Division for the Visually Impaired, 3068
Delaware Division of Vocational Rehabilitation- Department of Labor, 5724
Delaware Fair Employment Practice Agency, 5725
Delaware Industries for the Blind, 3069
Delaware Job Training Program Liaison, 5726
Delaware Library for the Blind and Physically Handicapped, 4409
Delaware Protection & Advocacy for Persons with Disabilities, 3070
Delaware VA Regional Office, 5408
Delaware Veterans Center, 6552
Delaware Workers Compensation Board, 3071
Delicate Threads, 4674
Dell Rapids Sportsmens Club, 5333
Delmar Learning, 8491
Delta Center, 6663
Delta Center for Independent Living, 3970
Delta Resource Center for Independent Living, 3577
Delta Society, 8659
Deluxe Bath Bench with Adjustable Legs, 137
Deluxe Convertible Exercise Staircase, 381
Deluxe Corporation, 2591
Deluxe Corporation Foundation, 2591
Deluxe Long Ring Low Vision Timer, 341
Deluxe Nova Wheeled Walker & Avant Wheeled Walker, 621
Deluxe Roller Knife, 342
Deluxe Signature Guide, 594
Deluxe Sock and Stocking Aid, 284
Deluxe Standard Wood Cane, 622
Demand Response Transportation Through a Rural ILC, 4827
Demos Medical Publishing, 4879, 7554, 8327, 8333, 8437, 8476, 8500, 8502, 8507, 8509, 8511, 8514, 8603
Demystifying Job Development: Field-Based Approaches to Job Development for the Disabled, 5094
Den-Mar Rehabilitation and Nursing Center, 7142
Dental Amalgam Syndrome (DAMS) Newsletter, 4388
Denver CIL, 3658
Denver Foundation, 2386
Denver VA Medical Center, 5402
Department Human Services, 3304
Department Of Health and Human Services, 3028
Department Of Human Services, 5876
Department Of Ophthalmalogy, 4430
Department Of Workforce Development, 5869
Department of Heath Education, 3328
Department of Aging and Independent Living, 4195
Department of Blind Rehabilitation, 3208
Department of Education, 1794, 1817, 3275, 3288, 4546, 5908, 6156
Department of Employment Security, 5787
Department of Health, 3115, 5093
Department of Health & Rehabilitative Services, 3086
Department of Health and Human Services, 3273, 3293, 5957
Department of Housing & Urban Development (HUD), 4875
Department of Human Rights, 3150
Department of Human Services, 3026, 3758, 3762, 5931, 6003
Department of Industrial Relations, 5608
Department of Justice ADA Mediation Program, 4299
Department of Labor, 3383, 3501, 5898, 5932
Department of Labor + Workforce Developments, 3012
Department of Labor and Employment, 5696
Department of Labor and Industrial Realtions, 3255
Department of Medicine and Surgery Veterans Administration, 5365
Department of Mental Health, 3251
Department of Mental Health, Retardation and Hospitals of Rhode Island, 3411
Department of Ophthalmology Information Line, 9095
Department of Ophthalmology and Visual Science, 4454
Department of Pennsylvania, 3402
Department of Physical Medicine & Rehabilitation at Sinai Hospital, 786
Department of Physical Medicine and Rehabilitation, 6870, 6564
Department of Public Health Human Services, 1814
Department of Public Instruction: Exceptional Children & Special Programs Division, 1794
Department of Services for the Blind, 6032
Department of Services for the Blind National Business & Disability Council, 6032
Department of Social & Health Services, 6033
Department of Social & Health Services National Business & Disability Council, 6033
Department of Social Services, 3182, 5723
Department of Social and Health, 6036
Department of Social and Health Services, 3515
Department of Veteran s Affairs, 5392
Department of Veterans Affairs, 5570
Department of Veterans Affairs Medical Center, 6347
Department of Veterans Affairs Regional Office - Vocational Rehab Division, 5366
Department of Veterans Affairs Vet Center #418, 6716
Department of Veterans Affairs of Washington DC, 6379
Department of Veterans Benefits, 5367
Des Moines Division-VA Central Iowa Health Care System, 6723
Des Moines VA Medical Center, 5438
Des Moines VA Regional Office, 5439
Des Moines YMCA Camp, 8255
Descriptive Video Service, 8900
Desert Haven Enterprises, 5656
Desert Life Rehabilitation & Care Center, 6359, 7056
Desert Regional Medical Center, 6424
Design for Acessibility, 1581
Designing and Using Assistive Technology: The Human Perspective, 1988
Designs for Comfort, 1106
Detecting Your Hidden Allergies, 8410

Determined to Win The Inspirational Story of Paradymic Athlete Jean Driscoll, 8411
Determined to Win: Children Living with Allergies and Asthma, 8412
Detroit Center for Independent Living, 3921
Deutsch Foundation, 2338
Developing Cross-Cultural Competence:Guide to Working with Young Children & Their Families, 1989
Developing Individualized Family Support Plans: A Training Manual, 1990
Developing Organized Coalitions and Strategic Plans, 4828
Developing Personal Safety Skills in Children with Disabilities, 4985
Developing Staff Competencies for Supporting People with Disabilities, 1991
Developing a Functional and Longitudinal Plan, 5117
Development of Language, 1992
Development of Social Skills by Blind and Visually Impaired Students, 8901
Developmental Disabilities Council, 1254
Developmental Disabilities Planning Council, 6144
Developmental Disabilities in Infancy and Childhood, 4986
Developmental Disabilities of Learning, 1993
Developmental Disabilities: A Handbook for Interdisciplinary Practice, 1995
Developmental Disabilities: A Handbook for Occupational Therapists, 1994
Developmental Disability Council: Arizona, 3019
Developmental Disability Council: Arkansas, 3031
Developmental Disability Services Section, 3352
Developmental Services Center, 2209
Developmental Services of Northwest Kansas, 6741
Developmental Training Services, 5697
Developmental Variation and Learning Disorders, 1996
Devereux, 6977
Devereux Center in New Jersey, 6880
Devereux Foundation, 6969, 6970, 6976
Devereux Foundation Health Services Center, 6978
Devereux Georgia Treatment Network, 6627
Devereux Santa Barbara, 6425
Devereux Texas Treatment Network Adult Community, 7002
Devereux's Kanner Center, 6979
Diabetes 101, 8413
Diabetes Action Network of the NFB, 8621
Diabetes Association Of Greater Cleveland, 8221
Diabetes Network of East Hawaii, 3112
Diabetes Self-Management, 8414
Diabetes Society of Santa Clara Valley, 8250
Diabetes: Caring for Your Emotions as Well as Your Health, 1757
Diabetic Cruise Desk, 5334
Diabetic Retinopathy, 8902
Diabetic Youth Foundation, 8256
Diabetic Youth Services, 8206
Diagnosis and Treatment of Autism, 7436
Diagnostic Report Writer, 1457
Dial Books, 8866
Dial-a-Hearing Screening Test, 7941
Dial: Disabled Information Awareness & Liv ing, 4014
Dialog Corporation, 1263
Dialogue Magazine, 8903
Dialysis at Sea Cruises, 5335
Dice: Jumbo Size, 5280
Dictionary of Congenital Malformations & Disorders, 4829
Dictionary of Developmental Disabilities Terminology, 4830, 4987
Dictionary of Special Education and Rehabilitation, 1758
Didlake, 6023
Diestco Manufacturing Company, 657
Diet and Arthritis, 8025
Different Heart, 8415
Difficult Child, 7437
Digest of Neurology and Psychiatry, 1997
Digi-Flex, 495
Digital Hearing Aids, 321
Digital Voice for Talking Database, 1322
Dilemma, 1382
Dimensions of State Mental Health Policy, 4300
Dimensions: Visually Impaired Persons with Multiple Disabilities, 8904
Dino-Games, 1383
Diocese of Maine Episcopal, 7732
Direct Center for Independence, 3572
Directions, 8416
Directions Unlimited Acccessible Tours, 5336
Directions: Technology in Special Education, 1384, 1851
Directory for Exceptional Children, 1759
Directory of Accessible Building Products, 1582
Directory of Accessible Van Rentals, 5296
Directory of Camps for Blind and Visually Impaired Children & Adults, 8834
Directory of Financial Aids for Women, 2924
Directory of Japanese Giving, 2925
Directory of Members, 4831
Directory of New and Emerging Foundations, 2926
Directory of Self-Help/Mutual Aid Support Groups for Older People, 7627
Directory of Travel Agencies for the Disabled, 5297
Directory of Venture Capital Firms, 2927
DisABILITY LINK NW, 3721
DisAbility Connections, 3922
DisAbility Resource Center: Knoxville, 4154
DisAbility Resource Connection: Everett, 4226
DisAbility Resources of Southwest Washington, 4731
Disabilities Network of Eastern Connecticut, 3671
Disabilities Sourcebook, 445
Disability Action Center NW, 3741
Disability Action Center for Georgia, 3722
Disability Action Center, NW, 3742
Disability Action Center-N.W., 3743
Disability Advocates of Kent County, 3923
Disability Analysis Handbook, 5071
Disability Analyst, 1533
Disability Awareness Guide, 4832
Disability Awareness Network, 4078
Disability Bookshop, 5296
Disability Bookshop Catalog, 446
Disability Center for Independent Living, 3659
Disability Coalition of Northern Kentucky, 3854
Disability Community Small Business Development Center, 787
Disability Compliance Bulletin, 4301
Disability Compliance for Higher Education, 1886
Disability Connection, 3924
Disability Connections, 3723
Disability Culture Perspective on Early Intervention, 7438
Disability Determination Section, 3523
Disability Determination Service: Birmingham, 2998
Disability Determination Services, 3000
Disability Funding News, 1998, 2928
Disability Information and Resources, 5215
Disability Law Center, 3488
Disability Law Center of Alaska, 3010
Disability Law Project, 3489
Disability Law in the United States, 4302
Disability Mall, 5216
Disability Net, 5217
Disability Network, 8642
Disability Network, Oakland/Macomb, 3925
Disability Policy Consortium, 3450
Disability Resource Agency for Independent Living: Modesto, 3616
Disability Resource Association, 3971
Disability Resource Center, 3710, 4206
Disability Resource Center of Fairfield County: Stratford Office, 3672
Disability Resource Center of SW Michigan, 3926
Disability Resources, 1887
Disability Resources Monthly, 1887
Disability Rights & Resources, 4079
Disability Rights Activist, 5218
Disability Rights Center, 3684
Disability Rights Center of Kansas, 3164
Disability Rights Education and Defense Fund, 4258, 4287, 4303, 5168
Disability Rights Movement, 4833
Disability Rights Now, 4303
Disability Rights Wisconsin: Milwaukee Office, 3532
Disability Services Division Of Montana Department Of Public Health, 6865
Disability Solutions for Independent Livin g, 3711
Disability Under the Fair Employment & Housing Act: What You Should Know About the Law, 4304
Disability and Communication Access Board, 3113
Disability and Health, National Center for Birth Defects and Developmental Disabilities, 8643
Disability and Rehabilitation, 1999
Disability and Social Performance: Using Drama to Achieve Successful Acts, 15
Disability and Sport, 8087
DisabilityResources.org, 5219
Disabled & Alone/Life Services for the Handicapped, 4892
Disabled Advocates Working for Northwest (DAWN), 4015
Disabled American Veterans, 5368
Disabled American Veterans, National Service & Legislative Headquarters, 5411
Disabled American Veterans: Ocean County, 5500
Disabled Children's Relief Fund, 788
Disabled Citizens Alliance for Independence, 3972

Disabled God: Toward a Liberatory Theology of Disability, 5049
Disabled People's International Fifth World Assembly as Reported by Two US Participants, 4834
Disabled Resource Services, 3660, 4826
Disabled Resources Center, 3617
Disabled Sports USA, 8088
Disabled Sports USA, Far West, 8089
Disabled Watersports Program Mission Bay Aquatic Center, 8090
Disabled We Stand, 4835
Disabled and Alone, 4996
Disabled and Alone/Life Services for the Handicapped, 789
Disabled, the Media, and the Information Age, 4836
Disablement in the Community, 4725
Disbled Resource Services, 3661
Discover Technology, 5220
Discovery Education, 1336
Discovery Newsletter, 4837
Discrimination is Against the Law, 4305
Discriptive Language Arts Development, 1458
Disorders of Motor Speech: Assessment, Treatment, and Clinical Characterization, 8708
District of Columbia Center for Independent Living, 3685
District of Columbia Department of Employment Services, 5729
District of Columbia Department of Handicapped Children, 3073
District of Columbia Dept. of Employment Services: Office of Workforce Development, 5730
District of Columbia Fair Employment Practice Agencies, 5731
District of Columbia General Hospital Physical Medicine & Rehab Services, 6559
District of Columbia Office on Aging, 3074
District of Columbia Public Library, 4411
District of Columbia Public Library: Services to the Deaf Community, 4411
District of Columbia Public Schools: Special Education Division, 1795
District of Columbia Regional Library for the Blind and Physically Handicapped, 4412
Diversified Opportunities, 6912
Diversity and Visual Impairment: The Influ ence of Race, Gender, Religion and Ethnicity, 8905
Divided Legacy: A History of the Schism in Medical Thought, The Bacteriological Era, 2000
Division 3 of Oakton College, 21
Division for Physical and Health Disabilities, 8136
Division for the Blind and Visually Impaired, 5859
Division of Birth Defects and Developmental Disabilities, 3100
Division of Blind Services, 6573
Division of Developmental Disabilities, 3299
Division of Disability Aging & Rehab Services, 1234
Division of Employment & Rehabilitation Services, 5641
Division of Employment & Training, 5955, 5726
Division of Graham-Field, 450
Division of Labor, 3056
Division of Mental Health and Substance Abuse, 3362
Division of Physical Medicine and Rehabilitation, 6426
Division of Rehabilitation, 6548
Division of Rehabilitation Service, 2999
Division of Rehabilitation Services, 3724, 3758, 3102, 6795
Division of Rehabilitation Services (DI RS), 5865
Division of Rehabilitation Services: Staff Library, 4653
Division of Rehabilitation-Education Services, University of Illinois, 6664
Division of Rehabilitative Services, 6006
Division of Special Education, 3451
Division of Vocational Rehabilitation Department of Social and Health Services, 7032
Division of Vocational Rehabilitation of Wyoming, 6042
Division of Workers Compensation, 3087
Dixie EMS, 409
Do You Hear That?, 5153
Do You Remember the Color Blue: And Other Questions Kids Ask About Blindness, 8906
Do-Able Renewable Home, 1583
Do-It-Leisure: Work Training Center, 5657
Doctor Yvonne Jones and Associates, 1731
Doctors Hospital, 6929
Dodd Hall at the Ohio State University Hospitals, 6930
Dodge Lowered Floor, 60
Dog Sponsorship Program, 8907
Dogs for the Deaf, 7694
Doing Things Together, 5154
Dolfinger-McMahon Foundation, 2782
Dollar Savings & Trust Company, 2765
Domestic Mistreatment of the Elderly: Towards Prevention, 7628
Don Johnston, 526, 1620, 1337, 1372, 1377, 1470, 1474, 1481, 1484, 1492, 1493, 1526
Don't Call Me Special: A First Look at Dis ability, 4675
Don't Feel Sorry for Paul, 7553, 8026
Don't Lose Sight of Cataracts, 8908
Don't Lose Sight of Glaucoma, 8909
Donaldsville Association for Retarded Citizens, 6763
Doorbell Signalers, 322
Dorma Architectural Hardware, 496
Double Gong Indoor/Outdoor Ringer, 323
Dougherty County Public Library, 4433
Dover Rehabilitation and Living Center, 7166
Down Syndrome, 7439
Downtown Neighborhood Learning Center, 5637
Doylestown Hospital Rehabilitation Center, 6248
Dr. Jack Widrich Foundation, 2434
Dr. Karen H Chao Developmental Optometry Karen H. Chao. O.D., 6427
Dr. Scholl Foundation, 2480
Dr. William O Benenson Rehabilitation Pavilion, 7178
Dream Catchers, 5155
Dreamer, 1295
Dresher Hill Health and Rehabilitation Cen ter, 7213
Dressing Stick, 285
Dressing Tips and Clothing Resources for Making Life Easier, 447
Drew Karol Industries, 298
Drive Master Company, 61, 65, 78, 88, 112, 114
Driven to Distraction, 7440
DuPage Center for Independent Living, 3759
Dual Brake Control, 62
Dual Brush with Suction Base, 343
Dual Relationships in Counseling, 2001
Dual Security Bed Rail, 157
Dual Switch Latch and Timer, 497
Dual-Mode Charger, 646
Duane Morrs Llt, 2800
Duchenne Muscular Dystrophy, 8417
Duchossois Foundation The Chamberlain Group Inc., 2481
Duke Endowment, 2726
Duke Medical Center, 4593
Duke University Medical Center, 6222
Duluth Public Library, 4545
Duracell & Rayovac Hearing Aid Batteries, 324
Duraline Medical Products, 299
Durham VA Medical Center, 5524
Duro-Med Industries, 300
Dusters, 1071
Dutch Neck T-Shirt, 1133
Duxbury Braille Translator, 1226
Duxbury Systems, 1226
Duxbury Systems Incorporated, 1231
Dwight D Eisenhower VA Medical Center, 5444
Dying and Disabled Children: Dealing with Loss and Grief, 5050
Dyna Vox Systems, 1323
DynaVox Devices & Software, 1323
Dynamic Dimensions, 5698
Dynamic Learning Center, 7300
Dynamic Living, 5221
Dynamic Systems, 255, 280
Dyslexia Training Program, 1621
Dyslexia over the Lifespan, 7441

E

E VA S, 1333
EASE, 7813
ECHO Housing: Recommended Construction and Installation Standards, 1584
EDI Camp, 8257
EIS Foundation, 2435
EL Darden Rehabilitation Center, 6337
EL Wiegand Foundation, 2617
ENDependence Center of Northern Virginia, 4207
ENVISION, 6742
EP Resource Guide, 4838
ERIC Clearinghouse on Disabilities and Special Education, 790
ESCIL Update Newsletter, 4839
ESI Master Resource Guide, 1385
ESS Work Center, 5658
EZ Access Roll-Up Ramp for Scooters, Wheel chairs, 382
EZ Dot, 1459
EZ Keys, 1386
EZ Keys for Windows, 1460
EZ Touch Panel, 1174

EZ-International, 550, 554, 558, 575, 585, 586
Eagle Hill School: Summer Program, 7332
Eagle Lake Children's Charities, 909
Eagle Pond Rehabilitation And Living Center, 6806
Eagle Sportschairs, 719
Ear Foundation, 7695
Early Childhood Intervention Clearinghouse, 1852
Early Childhood Reporter, 1888
Early Childhood Services, 6428
Early Communication Skills For Children with Down Syndrome, 2002
Early Focus: Working with Young Blind and Visually Impaired Children, 8910
Early Games for Young Children, 1387
Early Intervention, 1852
Early Intervention Program, 6669
Early Intervention, Implementing Child & Family Services for At-Risk Infants, 2003
Early Music Skills, 1388
Early Story of Alzheimer's Disease, 7629
Earning a Living, 4745
Earthware Computer Services, 1451
East Bay Community Foundation, 2339
East Bridge Building, 2595
East Brunswick Adult and Community Education Program, 2256
East Jefferson General Hospital Rehab Center, 6764
East King County Office, 4222
East Los Angeles Doctors Hospital, 6429
East Orange Campus of the VA New Jersey Healthcare System, 5501
East Penn Manufacturing Company, 720, 720
Easter Seal Camp Hemlocks, 923
Easter Seal Camp KYSOC, 949
Easter Seal Camp Wawbeek, 1065
Easter Seal Camp: New Hampshire, 984
Easter Seal Crossroads Rehabilitation Center, 937
Easter Seal Hackensack, 5921
Easter Seal Independent Living Center, 3676
Easter Seal Society of Dade County, 6574
Easter Seal Society of Mahoning, 6931
Easter Seal Society of New Jersey Highlands Workshop, 5922
Easter Seal Society of Washington, 7980
Easter Seal Work Center, 5644
Easter Seal of Greater Dallas, TX, 3452
Easter Seal of Ocean County, 5923
Easter Seal: Opportunity Center, 5606
Easter Seals, 6665, 8644, 930, 931, 4872, 4906, 4925, 5118, 5136, 5922, 8049
Easter Seals ARC of Northeast Indiana, 938
Easter Seals America, 7333, 7746, 8685, 8835
Easter Seals Arizona, 904
Easter Seals Broward County, 6575
Easter Seals Camp, 1047
Easter Seals Camp Fairlee Manor, 958
Easter Seals Camp Harmon, 912
Easter Seals Camp Stand by Me, 7980
Easter Seals Camp Sunnyside, 945
Easter Seals Central Alabama, 6338
Easter Seals Central California, 912
Easter Seals Colorado, 921
Easter Seals Colorado Rocky Mountain Villa, 919
Easter Seals DE/ MD Eastern Shore, 958
Easter Seals Delaware & Maryland's Eastern Shore, 6553
Easter Seals Disability Svcs: Bay Area, 6430
Easter Seals DuPage Dold Center for Children, 6666
Easter Seals East Georgia, 6628
Easter Seals Gilchrist-Marchman Rehab Center, 6667
Easter Seals Greater NW Texas, 3453
Easter Seals Iowa, 6724, 945
Easter Seals Jayne Shover Center, 6668
Easter Seals Massachusetts-Agassiz Village, 964
Easter Seals NH Camp Sno-Mo, 985
Easter Seals NH Camping Programs, 985
Easter Seals National, 6577, 6640, 6724
Easter Seals Nebraska, 980, 4876
Easter Seals New Jersey, 5924, 988
Easter Seals New York, 2666
Easter Seals Oklahoma, 7333, 7746, 8685, 8835
Easter Seals Oregon Camping Program, 1019
Easter Seals Project ACTION, 5311
Easter Seals Southeastern PA, 1027, 1028, 1031
Easter Seals Southwest Flordia, 6576
Easter Seals Superior California, 6431
Easter Seals Virginia, 1057
Easter Seals Wayne/Union Counties, 6145
Easter Seals West Alabama, 6339
Easter Seals Wisconsin, 1065
Easter Seals in Chicago, 6665
Easter Seals of Alabama, 5607
Easter Seals of Bartholomew County, 930
Easter Seals of Wayne & Union Counties, 939
Easter Seals-Goodwill Northern Rocky Mountains, 6640
Easter Seals: Achievement Center, 5607
Easter Seals: Arkansas, 6376
Easter Seals: UCP Timber Pointe Outdor Center, 931
Easter Seals: Volusia and Flagler Counties , FL, 6577
Eastern Blind Rehabilitation Center, 6539
Eastern Colorado Services for the Disabled, 3053
Eastern Idaho Regional Medical Center, 7104
Eastern Nebraska 4-H Camps and Centers, 981
Eastern Oregon Center for Independent Living, 4109
Eastern Paralyzed Veterans Association, 4573
Eastern Shore Center for Independent Living, 3875, 4839
Eastern Washington University, 4289
Eastside Rehabilitation and Living Center, 7143
Eastview Medical and Rehabilitation Center, 7261
Easy Access Housing, 5118
Easy Access to National Parks: The Sierra Club Guide for the Disabled, 5312
Easy Dressing Fashions: JC Penney, 1102
Easy Pivot Transfer Machine, 383
Easy Ply, 301
Easy Pour Locking Lid Pot, 344
Easy Stand, 384
Easy Things to Make Things Simple: Do It Yourself Modifications for Disabled Persons, 4840
EasyStand 6000 Glider, 623
Eating Disorders Sourcebook, 8418
Eating Out: Your Guide to More Enjoyable Dining, 8419
Eating Skills: Learning Basic Table Manners, 1389
Echo Grove Camp, 968
Echoing Hills, 8258
Ecology of Troubled Children, 2004
Econo-Float Water Flotation Cushion, 256
Econo-Float Water Flotation Mattress, 257
Economical Liberty, 385
Economics, Industry and Disability, 5095
Eden Acres Administrative Services, 5925
Edge, 672
Edge Effect: Achieve Total Health and Longevity with the Balanced Brain Advantage, 4841
Edgemoor Day Program, 6554
Edison Sheltered Workshop, 5926
Edith Nourse Rogers Memorial Veterans Hospital, 5462
Edmark Corporation, 1369
Edmonds Rehabilitation & Healthcare Centerer, 7250
Educating Children with Disabilities: A Transdisciplinary Approach, 3rd Edition, 2005
Educating Children with Multiple Disabilities: A Transdisciplinary Approach, 2006
Educating Inattentive Children, 7442
Educating Students Who Have Visual Impairments with Other Disabilities, 2007
Educating all Students in the Mainstream, 2008
Education and Auditory Research Foundation, 2828
Education of the Handicapped: Laws, Legislative Histories and Administrative Documents, 4306
Educational Accessibility Services, 791
Educational Activities, 1473
Educational Activities Software, 1338, 1346, 1382, 1398, 1458, 1472, 1476, 1488, 1494, 1514, 7416
Educational Audiology for the Limited Hearing Infant and Preschooler, 3rd Edition, 2009
Educational Care, 2010
Educational Equity Concepts, 1636, 2050, 4804
Educational Intervention for the Student with Multiple Disabilities, 2011
Educational Issues Among Children with Spina Bifida, 8420
Educational Media Corporation, 7456
Educational Prescriptions, 2012
Educational Productions, 44, 4704, 4714, 5138
Educational Referral Service, 1731
Educational Services for the Visually Impaired, 4379
Educational Software Institute, 1385
Educational Tutorial Consortium, 1710
Educators Publishing Service, 1596, 1597, 1598, 1607, 1612, 1619, 1621, 1623, 1624, 1629, 1630, 1631, 1639, 1641, 1642, 1643, 1644, 1646, 1647, 1650, 1652, 1653, 1654, 1655, 1659, 1671, 1674, 1678, 1679, 1680, 1681, 1683, 1686, 1688, 1692, 1693, 1694, 1697, 1698, 1699, 1700, 1701, 1702, 1703, 1712, 1713, 1714, 1715, 1716, 1719, , 1720, 1927, 1996, 2010, 2012, 2044, 2111, 2113, 2203, 2226, 2227, 2228, 2229, 2230, 2235, 7047, 7431, 7441
Educators Resource Directory, 1760
Edward Hines Jr Hospital, 5430

Edward John Noble Foundation, 2667
Edwin Mellen Press, 2035, 5009
Edyth Bush Charitable Foundation, 2436
Effective Instruction for Special Education, 2nd Edition, 2013
Effective Teaching Methods for Autistic Children, 2014
Effectively Educating Handicapped Students, 2015
Effectiveness of Cochlear Implants and Tactile Aids for Deaf Children, 7814
Efficacy of Asthma Education, Selected Abstracts, 8421
Eggleston Services, 1060
Ehrman Medical Library, 4574
Eight CAP, Inc. Head Start, 6833
El Paso Lighthouse for the Blind, 7003
El Paso Natural Gas Foundation, 2847
El Paso VA Healthcare Center, 5571
El Pomar Foundation, 2387
El Valle Community Parent Resource Center, 3454
El Valor Corporation, 6669
Elastic Shoelaces, 286
Elder Abuse, 7630
Elder Care, 7631
ElderLawAnswers.com, 4307, 5222
Elderly Guide to Budget Travel/Europe, 5298
Eleanora CU Alms Trust, 2743
Electra-Ride Elite, 386
Electra-Ride III, 387
Electric Can Opener & Knife Sharpener, 345
Electric Leg Bag Emptier and Tub Slide Shower Chair, 138
Electric Mobility Corporation, 553, 568, 569
Electronic Courseware Systems, 1390, 1359, 1388, 1402, 1404, 1435
Electronic House, 1585
Electronic House: Enhanced Lifestyles with Electronics, 1585
Electronic Speech Assistance Devices, 1324
Electronic Stethoscopes, 302
Elgin Rehabilitation Center, 6670
Eli Lilly & Co Corporate Contributions Pro, 2519
Elkhart Public Library for the Blind and Physiclly Handicapp, 4469
Elling Camps, 7334
Elmhurst Hospital Center, 6896
Elsevier Health, 1844
Elwyn Delaware, 4410, 6555
Embracing the Monster: Overcoming the Cha llenges of Hidden Disabilities, 7443
Emerging Leaders, 5156
Emmett Rehabilitation and Healthcare, 7105
Emory Autism Resource Center, 4438
Emory University, 4438
Emory University Laboratory for Ophthalmic Research, 4439
Emotional Problems of Childhood and Adolescence, 2016
Emotorsports, 530
Employment Development Department, 5659, 5665
Employment Discrimination Based on Disability, 4308
Employment Resources Program, 1255
Employment Service Division: Alabama, 5608
Employment Service: Alaska, 5634
Employment Service: California, 5659
Employment Standards Administration Department of Labor, 4309
Employment and Training Division, Region B, 5763
Employment for Individuals with Asperger S yndrome or Non-Verbal Learning Disability, 8709
Employment in the Mainstream, 4746
Empress Travel, 5336
EnTech: Enabling Technologies of Kentuckiana, 4488
Enabling & Empowering Families: Principles & Guidelines for Practice, 2017
Enabling Devices, 5281
Enabling News, 7632
Enabling Romance: A Guide to Love, Sex & Relationships for the Disabled, 4676
Enabling Technologies Company, 1227
Enchanted Hills Camp for the Blind, 8836
Encounters with Autistic States, 7444
Encyclopedia of AIDS: Social, Political, C ultural, and Scientific Record of the HIV Epidemic, 8422
Encyclopedia of Basic Employment and Daily Living Skills, 4747
Encyclopedia of Blindness and Vision Impairment Second Edition, 8911
Encyclopedia of Deafness and Hearing Disorders, 7815
Encyclopedia of Disability, 4842
Encyclopedia of Genetic Disorders & Birth Defects, 4988
Enforcing the ADA: A Status Report from th e Department of Justice, 4310
Englishton Park Academic Remediation, 7335
Englishton Park Presbyterian, 7335
Enhancer Cushion, 258
Enhancing Children's Communication: Research & Foundations, 1761
Enhancing Childrens Communication Research & Found, 1761
Enhancing Communication in Individuals with Autism Through Pictures/Words, 7445, 8710
Enhancing Self-Concepts and Achievement of Mildly Handicapped Students, 2018
Enrichments Catalog, 448
Entervan, 63
Environmental Dental Association, 792, 8390
Environmental Health Center: Dallas, 8137
Environmental Traveling Companions, 5337
Epilepsy Council of Greater Cincinnati, 3370
Epilepsy Foundation, 7548, 7957, 8138, 4506, 8425
Epilepsy Foundation for the National Capitol Area, 8645
Epilepsy Foundation of Greater North Texas, 2848
Epilepsy Foundation of Long Island, 2668
Epilepsy Foundation of Southeast Texas, 2849
Epilepsy Foundation: Central and South Texas, 2850
Epilepsy Society of New York, 2669
Epilepsy, 199 Answers: A Doctor Responds t o His Patients' Questions, 8423
Epilepsy: Patient and Family Guide, 8424
EpilepsyUSA, 8425
Episcopal Charities, 2670
Episcopal Church Of Hawaii, 8234
Episcopal Conference of the Deaf, 7696
Eplilepsy Foundation North and Central Alabama, 8637
Equal Access Center for Independence, 4208
Equal Employment Advisory Council, 4259
Equal Opportunity Employment Commission, 2972
Equal Opportunity Publications, 5067
Equal Treatment for People With Mental Ret ardation: Having and Raising Children, 7446
Equalizer 1000 Series, 647
Equalizer 5000 Home Gym, 648
Equals in Partnership: Basic Rights for Families of Children with Blindness, 8912
Equip for Equality, 3133
Equipment Shop, 449
Eric Clearinghouse on Disabilities and Gifted Education, 1772
Erie VA Medical Center, 5546
Erlanger Medical Center Baronness Campus, 7226
Ernest Health, 6299
Esalen Institute, 793
Escort II XL, 64
Esther A & Joseph Klingenstein Fund, 2671
Esu Memorial Union, 4481
Etac USA: F3 Wheelchair, 673
Ethical Conflicts in Management of Home Care, 5072
Ethical and Legal Issues in School Counseling, 4311
Eugene J Towbin Healthcare Center, 5383
Eugene and Agnes E Meyer Foundation, 2414
Eva L And Joseph M Bruening Foundation, 2744
Evac + Chair Corporation, 235
Evac + Chair Emergency Wheelchair, 235
Evacu-Trac, 674
Evaluation and Educational Programming of Deaf-Blind/Severly Multihandicapped Students, 2019
Evaluation and Treatment of the Psychogeriatric Patient, 2020
Evans Newton, 1750
Evansville Association for the Blind, 5810
Evelyn and Walter Hans Jr, 2340
Evenston Community Foundation, 2482
Everest & Jennings, 450, 676
Evergreen Healthcare, 7046
Evergreen Woods Health and Rehabilitation Center, 7083
Evert Conner Rights & Resources CIL, 3806
EveryBody's Different: Understanding and Changing Our Reactions to Disabilities, 4843
Everybody Counts Center for Independent Living, 3793
Everybody's Guide to Homeopathic Medicines, 4844
Everyday Social Interaction: A Program for People with Disabilities, 4845
Evio Plastics, 346
Exceed: A Division of Valley Resource Cent er, 6432
Exceptional Children, 1853
Exceptional Children in Focus, 2021
Exceptional Children: An Introductory Survey of Special Education, 1762
Exceptional Education, 1664, 1665, 1666, 1667, 2115
Exceptional Lives: Special Education in T oday's Schools, 4th Edition, 2022
Exceptional Parent Library, 4329, 4685, 4686, 4692, 4838, 4871, 4976, 5014, 5017, 5019, 5057, 5059, 5174, 7423, 7434, 7496, 8113, 8382

Exceptional Parent Magazine, 4989
Exceptional Student in the Regular Classroom, 5041
Exceptional Teaching Inc., 1622
Exercise Activities for the Elderly, 7633
Exercise and Your Arthritis, 8027
Exercise and the Older Adult, 7634
Exeter Hospital, 6870
Expanded Keyboard Emulator, 1175
Expendicare, 7211
Explode the Code Books 1-8, 1623
Explore Your Options, 7635
Explorer+ 4-Wheel Scooter, 554
Exploring Autism: A Look at the Genetics of Autism, 5223
Exploring the Bible: Bible Studies for the DEAF, 7816
Express Medical Supply, 451
Expressive and Receptive Fingerspelling, 7817
Exquisite Egronomic Protective Wear, 1103
Extendicare Health Services, Inc., 6324
Extensions for Independence, 527
Extra Loud Alarm with Lighter Plug, 606
Eye & Ear Infirmary, 9095
Eye Bank Association of America, 8772
Eye Bank Association of America Annual Meeting, 1549
Eye Foundation of Kansas City, 6863
Eye Institute of New Jersey, 4566
Eye Institute of the Medical College of Wisconsin and Froedtert Clinic, 4661
Eye Medical Center, 6433
Eye Medical Center of Fresno, 6433
Eye Relief Word Processing Software, 1520
Eye Research News Briefs, 8913
Eye and Your Vision, 8914
Eye-Centered: A Study of Spirituality of Deaf People, 7818
Eye-Q Test, 8915
Eyegaze Computer System, 1176

F

F Mason Perkins Trust, 2630
FA Davis Company, 8424
FAVRAH Senior Adult Enrichment Program, 6540
FCYD Camp, 8259
FDR Series of Low Vision Reading Aids, 1315
FM Kirby Foundation, 2631
FOR Community Services, 6807
FORE! Future Opportunity for Recreation and Employment for the Handicapped, 8091
FPL Group Foundation, 2437
FREED, 3618
FREED Center for Independent Living, 3619
FSSI, 2211
Face First, 5157
Face of Inclusion, 4990
Facilitating Self-Care Practices in the Elderly, 2023
Fact Sheet: Attention Deficit-Hyperactivit y Disorder, 7447
Fact Sheet: Autism Spectrum Disorders, 7448
Facts About Asthma, 8426
Facts on File, 4988, 8911, 9035
Facts: Books for Blind and Physically Handicapped Individuals, 5119, 8916
Facts: Music for Blind and Physically Handicapped Individuals, 16
Fair Employment Practice Agency, 5635
Fair Employment Practice Agency: Arizona, 5638
Fair Housing Design Guide for Accessibility, 1586
Fair Housing and Equal Employment, 5764
Fairacres Manor, 7073
Fairbanks Memorial Hospital/Denali Center, 7055
Fairfax County Public Library, 4642
Fairfield Center for Disabilities and Cerebral Palsy, 4094
Fairlawn Rehabilitation Hospital, 6808
Fairway Golf Cars, 528
Fairway Spirit Adaptive Golf Car: Model 4852, 528
Fairy Tales & Christmas Stories, 7819
Faith Mission Home, 7023
Fall Down, Laughing: How Squiggy Caught M ultiple Sclerosis and Didn't Tell Nobody, 8427
Fall Fun, 1391
Fall Fun IntelliKeys Overlay, 1177
Falling in Old Age, 7636
Families Magazine, 4991
Families in Recovery, 5073
Families of Spinal Muscular Atrophy, 8139
Families of Spinal Muscular Dystrophy, 8416
Families, Illness & Disability, 4992
Family Caregiver Alliance, 2380
Family Challenges: Parenting with a Disability, 4846
Family Context and Disability Culture Reframing: Through the Looking Glass, 8917
Family Counseling Center, 6671
Family Guide to Vision Care, 8918
Family Guide: Growth & Development of the Partially Seeing Child, 8919
Family Heritage Medical and Rehabilitation Center, 7262
Family Intervention Guide To Mental Illness, 7637
Family Interventions Throughout Disability, 4993
Family Matters, 6672
Family Resource Associates, 4016, 4677, 4702
Family Resource Center on Disabilities, 794
Family Resource Library/Center for Persons with Disabilities, 4629
Family Service Society, 6765
Family Support Project for the Developmentally Disabled, 8646
Family Therapy for ADHD: Treating Children , Adolescents and Adults, 7449
Family Urology, 8428
Family Voices, 795
Family-Centered Early Intervention with Infants and Toddlers, 2024
Family-Centered Service Coordination: A Manual for Parents, 4994
Family-Guided Activity-Based Intervention for Toddlers & Infants, 5074
Fanlight Productions, 14, 4717, 4719, 4772, 4791, 4927, 4969, 5020, 5139, 5147, 5148, 5157, 5162, 5164, 5167, 5171, 5172, 5175, 5180, 5185, 5186, 7408, 7530, 7852, 7942, 7986, 8022, 8040, 8415, 8462, 8475, 8587, 8612, 9037, 9048
Fannie E Rippel Foundation, 2632
Fantastic Series, 7820
Fargo VA Medical Center, 5528
Farmington Health Care Center, 6190
Farmington Valley ARC, 7450
Farnum Rehabilitation Center, 6871
Fashion Collection, 1109
Fashion Ease, 1104
Father Drumgoole Connelly Summer Camp, 7747, 8260
Fathers: A Common Ground, 8920
Favarh/Farmington Valley ARC, 796
Fay J Lindner Foundation, 2672
Faye McBeath Foundation, 2908
Fayetteville VA Medical Center, 5384, 5525
Feather River Industries, 5660
Featherlite, 555
Featherspring, 649
Featherweight Reachers, 287
Fedcap News, 4312
Fedcap Rehabilitation Services, 797, 4312
Federal Aviation Administration, 2975
Federal Benefits for Veterans and Dependents, 5369
Federal Communications Commission, 2973
Federal Consumer Information Center, 4742, 4743
Federal Funding to Fight AIDS, 2929
Federal Government, 3191, 7429, 7526, 7764, 7770, 7783, 7791, 7798, 7836, 8619, 8694, 8733
Federal Grants & Contracts Weekly, 2930
Federal Heights Rehabilitation and Nursing Center, 7238
Federal Laws of the Mentally Handicapped: Laws, Legislative Histories and Admin. Documents, 4313
Federal Resource Center for Special Education, 5224
Federal Student Aid Information Center, 2415
Federation Employment And Guidance Service (F-E-G-S), 6897
Federation For Children With Special Needs, 876
Federation for Children with Special Needs, 798, 5001, 5135
Federation of Families for Children's Mental Health, 799
Feeding Children with Special Needs, 2025
Feingold Association of the US, 800, 7503
Feldenkrais Guild of North America (FGNA), 801
Ferderal Government, 7918
Fibromyalgia Interval Training, 8429
Fidelco Guide Dog Foundation, 2397, 8773
Field Foundation of Illinois, 2483
Fifth Third Bank, 2743
Fight for Sight, 8774
Fighting Blindness News, 8921
Fighting for Darla: Challenges for Family Care & Professional Responsibility, 7451
Filmakers Library, 5158, 7407
Films & Videos on Aging and Sensory Change, 5159
Final Report: Adapting Through the Looking Glass, 5031
Final Report: Challenges and Strategies of Disabled Parents: Findings from a Survey, 5032
Financial Aid for Asian Americans, 2931
Financial Aid for Hispanic Americans, 2932
Financial Aid for Native Americans, 2933
Financial Aid for Research and Creative Ac tivities Abroad, 2934

Financial Aid for Study and Training Abroad, 2341
Financial Aid for Veterans, Military Personnel and their Dependents, 2935
Financial Aid for the Disabled and their Families, 2936
Finger Lakes Developmental Disabilities Service Office, 4575
Finger Lakes Independence Center, 4046
FingerFoniks, 1178
Fingerspelling: Expressive and Receptive Fluency, 7821
Fireman's Fund Foundation, 2342
Firemans Fund Insurance Companies, 2342
First Course in Phonic Reading, 1624
First Hill Care Center, 7033
First Manhattan Company, 2693
First National Bank of Chicago, 2499
First Occupational Center of New Jersey, 5927
First Security Bank of Utah, 2877
First State Senior Center, 6556
First Step Independent Living, 3620
First Steps, 8922
First Union Foundation, 2727
Fit for Work at Exeter Hospital, 5904
Fit to Work, 5661
Fitness Programming for Physical Disabilities, 8092
Five Green & Speckled Frogs, 1392
Five Green & Speckled Frogs IntelliKeys Overlay, 1179
Five Star Industries, 6673
FlagHouse Rehab Resources, 452
FlagHouse Special Populations, 453
Flagstaff City-Coconino County Public Library, 4372
Flannel Gowns, 1072
Flannel Pajamas, 1123
Flashing Lamp Telephone Ring Alerter, 181
Fleece Bed Jacket, 1088
Fleece Cape/Poncho, 1073
Fleece Robe, 1124
Flex-Air Pressure Relief System, 259
FlexShield Keyboard Protectors, 1296
Flinchbaugh Company, 375
Flint Michigan YMCA, 971
Flint Osteopathic Hospital: RehabCare Unit, 6191
Float Dress, 1074
Florence C and Harry L English Memorial Fund, 2449
Florence V Burden Foundation, 2673
Florida Adult Services, 3088
Florida Baptist Convention, 7325
Florida CORF, 6578
Florida Commission on Human Relations, 5740
Florida Community College at Jacksonville/ Services for Students with Disabilities, 6579
Florida Department of Education: Bureau of Exceptional Education And Student Services, 1797
Florida Department of Handicapped Children, 3089
Florida Department of Mental Health and Rehabilitative Services, 3090
Florida Developmental Disabilities Council, 3091
Florida Diabetes Camp, 8261
Florida Division of Blind Services, 4418
Florida Division of Vocational Rehabilitation, 3092, 5739
Florida Fair Employment Practice Agency, 5740
Florida Fund For Special Children, 924
Florida Hospital Rehabilitation Center, 6103
Florida Institute Of Rehabilitation Education (FIRE), 6580
Florida Institute for Neurologic Rehabilitation, Inc, 6581
Florida Instructional Materials Center for the Visually Handicapped, 4419
Florida Lions Camp, 925
Florida Rock Industries Foundation, 2438
Florida School for the Deaf and Blind, 7279
Florida Sheriffs Caruth Camp, 7336
Florida Sheriffs Youth Ranches, 7336
Florida's Protection and Advocacy Programs for Persons with Disabilities, 3093
Floyd Healthcare Resources, 6130
Floyd Rogers Foundation, 8214
Flushing Hospital, 6898
Flushing Manor Nursing and Rehab, 7179
Flute Song Magic, 7822
Flying Wheels Travel, 5338
Foam Decubitus Bed Pads, 158
Focal Group Psychotherapy, 2026
Focus, 8028, 8923
Focus Alternative Learning Center, 802, 7301
Focus Newsletter, 8430
Focus on Autism and Other Developmental Disabilities, 1854
Focus on Exceptional Children, 1855
Fold-Down 3-in-1 Commode, 303
Folding Chair with a Rigid Feel, 675
Folding Shower Chair By INVOCARE, 236
Folic Acid Counseling Pocket Card, 8431
Fontana Rehabilitation Workshop, 6434
Food Markers/Rubberbands, 347
Food!, 1625
Foot Inversion Tread, 498
Foot Placement Ladder, 499
Foot Snugglers, 1081
Foot Steering, 65
Foot Steering System, 66
Foothill Nursing and Rehab Center, 7064
Foothill Vocational Opportunities, 6435
For Hearing People Only, 7823
For Siblings Only, 4677
Force A Miracle, 4847
Ford Foundation, 2674
Ford Lowered Floor, 67
Forde's Functional Fashions, 1105
Formed Families: Adoption of Children with Handicaps, 4314
Formula Series Active Mobility Wheelchairs, 676
Forsyth Medical Center, 6913
Fort Howard VA Medical Center, 5457
Fort Lauderdale Vet Center, 6582
Fortis Foundation, 2675
Fortress, 652, 670, 672, 677, 684, 700, 703, 704, 705, 707, 714
Forum, 4848
Fosters Botanical and Herb Reviews, 4849
Fotheringhay Farms, 5715
Foundation & Corporate Grants Alert, 2937
Foundation 1000, 2938
Foundation Center, 2676, 2663, 2677, 2917, 2921, 2922, 2923, 2926, 2938, 2939, 2940, 2941, 2949, 2950, 2951, 2952, 2953, 2954, 2955, 2956, 2957, 2958, 2959, 2960, 2961, 2962, 2964, 4850
The Foundation Center, 2944
Foundation Center Library Services, 2677
Foundation Center's User-Friendly Guide, 2939
Foundation Directory, 2940
Foundation Fighting Blindness, 2546, 5225
Foundation Fundamentals for Nonprofit Organizations, 4850
Foundation Grants to Individuals, 2941
Foundation Industries, 6766
Foundation Managment Services, 2744
Foundation for Advancement in Cancer Therapy, 2678
Foundation for Children and Youth, 8259
Foundation for Seacoast Health, 2622
Foundation for the Advancement of Innovative Medicine, 2679
Foundation for the Carolinas, 2728
Foundations of Orientation and Mobility, 8924
Foundations of Rehabilitation Counseling with Persons Who Are Blind, 8925
Fountain Hills Lioness Braille Service, 4373
Four Oaks Center, 6932
Four Rivers Resource Services, 3794, 5811
Four-H Camp Howe, 965
Four-Ingredient Cookbook, 4851
Fourth and Long, 8029
Fowler Center, 969
Fox River Valley Center for Independent Living, 3760
Fox Subacute Center, 6980
Fraction Factory, 1341
Fragile Success: Nine Autistic Children, Childhood to Adulthood, 7452
Fragile X Family, 8432
Frames of Reference for the Assessment of Learning Disabilities, 2210
Francis Beidler Charitable Trust, 2484
Franciscan Rehabilitation Center, 6225
Frank & Mollie S VanDervoort Memorial Foun dation, 2578
Frank Mobility Systems, 650
Frank R and Elizabeth Simoni Foundation, 2561
Frank Stanley Beveridge Foundation, 2439
Franklin County Work Activity Center, 5828
Franklin Court Assisted Living, 4132
Franklin Skilled Nursing and Rehabilitation Center, 7152
Fraser, 4088
Frasier Rehabilitation Center Division of Clark Memorial Hospital, 6717
Frazier Rehab Institute, 6750
Fred & Lillian Deeks Memorial Foundation, 2745
Fred Finch Youth Center, 6436
Fred Gellert Foundation, 2343
Fred J Brunner Foundation, 2485
Free Appropriate Public Education, 4315
Free Hand: Enfranchising the Education of Deaf Children, 2027
Free Information/Membership Kit, 8926
Free Library of Philadelphia: Library for the Blind and Physically Handicapped, 4611
Free and User Supported Software for the IBM PC: A Resource Guide, 1393
Free to Breathe, 8433
Freedom Bath, 139
Freedom Center, 3876
Freedom Center for Independent Living, 3677
Freedom Resource Center for Independent Living: Fargo, 4089

Freedom Resource Center for Independent Living: Fergus Falls, 3946
Freedom Rider, 454, 454
Freedom Ryder Handcycles, 529
Freedom Scientific, 5226, 1482
Freedom Scientific Blind/ Low Vision Group, 1228
Freedom Three Wheel Walker, 624
Freedom Valley Disability Center, 4121
Freedom Wheelchair Lifts, 388
Freedom Wheels, 389
Freedom from Arthritis Through Nutrition & Help for Allergies, 8030
Freedom of Movement: IL History and Philosophy, 8031
Freedom to Create, 17
Freestone Rehabilitation Center, 6360
Freestyle II, 677
Fremont Area Foundation, 2579
Frequently Asked Questions About Multiple Chemical Sensitivity, 4852
Fresno City College, 5662
Fresno City College: Disabled Students Programs and Services, 5662
Fresno County Free Library Blind and Handicapped Services, 4389
Friday Afternoon, 1475
Friendly Ice Cream Corp Contributions Prog ram, 2562
Friends Academy Summer Camps, 8262
Friends of Disabled Adults and Children, 7958
Friends of Libraries for Deaf Action, 4508
Friends-In-Art, 18
Friendship Press, 4716
Friendship Ventures, 973, 8211
Frohock-Stewart, 124, 142, 146, 248
From Gesture to Language in Hearing and Deaf Children, 7824
From Mime to Sign Package, 7825
From Where I Sit: Making My Way wih Cereb ral Palsy, 8434
From the State Capitals: Public Health, 2942
Frost Foundation, 2643
Fulton County Rehab Center, 5785
Fun for Everyone, 1626
Functional Assessment Inventory Manual, 2028
Functional Electrical Stimulation for Ambulation by Paraplegics, 8032
Functional Fitness Assessment for Adults, 7638
Functional Forms, 260
Functional Literacy System, 1510
Functional Resources, 1256
Functional Restoration of Adults and Child ren with Upper Extremity Amputation, 7554
Functional Skills Screening Inventory, 1256
Fund for New Jersey, 2633
Fundamentals of Autism, 1627
Funnel, 348
Future Choices Independent Living Center, 3795
Future Horizons, 26
Future Reflections, 8927

G

G W Micro, 1335
GA and SK Etiquette, 7826
GA-SK, 7827
GAR Foundation, 2746
GE Foundation, 2398
GEICO Philanthropic Foundation Geico Corp., 2416
GM Mobility Program, 5313
GN Wilcox Trust, 2464
GO-MO Articulation Cards- Second Edition, 1628
A GS, 1718
GT Wheelchair Cushion, 261
GW Micro, 1180, 9079
Gabbi Talk Phone, 182
Gadabout Wheelchairs, 678, 678
Gainesville Division, North Florida/South Georgia Veterans Healthcare System, 5416
Gaining Access to IL, 3761
Gales Creek Camp Foundation, 1020
Gales Creek Diabetes Camp, 1020
Gallaudet Survival Guide to Signing, 7828
Gallaudet University, 843, 7697, 7717
Gallaudet University Alumni Association, 7697
Gallaudet University Bookstore, 2067, 2080, 2177, 4284, 5051, 7759, 7774, 7779, 7785, 7786, 7788, 7790, 7795, 7797, 7808, 7815, 7817, 7821, 7826, 7832, 7833, 7841, 7843, 7846, 7849, 7850, 7851, 7857, 7867, 7868, 7870, 7885, 7888, 7895, 7896, 7897, 7898, 7905, 7907, 7910, 7913, 7922, 7935, 8728, 9042
Gallaudet University Press, 1773, 5227, 2075, 2138, 4326, 7625, 7765, 7769, 7789, 7794, 7796, 7801, 7804, 7807, 7809, 7810, 7824, 7828, 7829, 7831, 7847, 7848, 7859, 7862, 7866, 7873, 7877, 7886, 7887, 7899, 7900, 7903, 7908, 7909, 7912, 7931, 7938
Gallaudet University Press Journal: Sign Language Studies, 7829
Gallaudet University-Denison House, 1773
Gallery Bookshop, 1977, 1993, 2060, 2083, 2090
Gallo Foundation, 2344
Gannett Foundation, 2885
Garaventa Canada, 674
Gareth Stevens, 4697, 8412, 8436, 8532, 9040
Garfield Medical Center, 6067
Garten Services, 6961
Gates Family Foundation, 2388
Gateway Arts Program, Crafts Store & Gallery, 5870
Gateway Center of Monterey County, 6437
Gateway Community Industries Inc.,, 6899
Gateway Industries: Castroville, 6438
Gateway Services/JCARC, 5812
Gaylord Hospital, 6541
Gaymar Industries, 262, 262, 681
Gazette International Networking Institute, 4945, 8469, 8552
Gebbie Foundation, 2680
Geer Adult Training Center, 6340
Gem Wheelchair & Scooter Service: Mobility & Homecare, 679
Gendron, 680, 662
General Electric Company, 2398
General Electric Foundation, 2399
General Facts and Figures on Blindness, 8928
General Mills Foundation, 2592
General Motors Mobility Program for Persons with Disabilities, 5313
Genesee Region Independent Living Center, 4047
Genesis Health System, 6725
Genesis Healthcare System, 6933
Genesis One Technologies, 1304
Genesis Regional Rehabilitation Center, 6725
Genetic Disorders Sourcebook, 4853
Genetic Nutritioneering, 4854
Genetics and Spina Bifida, 8435
Genova Diagnostics, 4591
Geo-Matt for High Risk Patients, 263
George A Martin Center, 6934
George Gund Foundation, 2747
George Hegyi Industrial Training Center, 5716
George J DePontis, 5091
George M Eisenberg Foundation for Charities, 2486
George Washington University Health Resource Center, 803
George Washington University Medical Center, 6560, 6560
George Wasserman Family Foundation, 2547
George Zoltan Lefton Company, 2487
George Zoltan Lefton Family Foundation, 2487
Georgetown University, 839
Georgetown University Center for Child and Human Development, 4413
Georgetown University, School of Medicine, 5110
Georgia Advocacy Office, 3101
Georgia Association of Homes and Services for the Aging, 7570
Georgia Client Assistance Program, 3102
Georgia Commission on Equal Opportunity, 5764
Georgia Department of Aging, 3103
Georgia Department of Handicapped Children, 3104
Georgia Department of Labor, 3724, 6624
Georgia Division of Mental Health, Developmental Disabilities & Addictive Diseases, 3105
Georgia Industries for the Blind, 6629
Georgia Library for the Blind and Physically Handicapped, 4440
Georgia Power, 2450
Georgia Public Library, 4440
Georgia State Board of Workers' Compensation, 3106
Georgia's SILC, 3725
Georgiana Institute, 7698
Geronimo, 712
Get Ready/Get Set/Go for the Code, 1629
Get a Wiggle On, 8929
Getting Better, 7830
Getting Our Heads Together, 7453
Getting Ready for the Outside World (G.R.O.W.), 1786
Getting Started with Facilitated Communication, 7454, 8711
Getting Together: A Head Start/School District Collaboration, 7455
Getting a Grip on ADD: A Kid's Guide to Understanding & Coping with ADD, 7456
Getting in Touch, 7283
Getting the Most Out of Consultation Services, 4726
Giant Food Foundation, 2417
Gift of Sight, 8930
Gil and Dody Weaver Foundation, 2851
Gillingham Manaual, 1630
Gilroy Workshop, 6439
Girl Scouts - Foothills Council, 8216

Girl Scouts of Delaware-Raritan, 7982
Girl Scouts of Shining Trail, 8230
Girl Scouts of Washington Rock Council, 8830
Glacier View Ranch, 920
Gladys Brooks Foundation, 2681
Glaser Foundation, 2893
Glaucoma, 8931
Glaucoma Laser Trial, 4527
Glaucoma Research Foundation, 2345, 4390, 5228, 8931, 8933, 8960
Glaucoma: The Sneak Thief of Sight, 8932
Gleams Newsletter, 8933
Glendale Adventist Medical Center, 6440
Glendale Memorial Hospital and Health Center, 6441
Glendale Memorial Hospital and Health Center Rehabilitation Unit, 6441
Glengariff Health Care Center, 7180
Glenkirk, 5786
Glens Falls Independent Living Center, 4048
Glenview Terrace Nursing Center, 7109
Glickenhaus Foundation, 2682
Global Assistive Devices, 166
Global Health Solutions, 8034, 8302
Global Perspectives on Disability: A Curriculum, 2029
Glossary of Terminology for Vocational Assessment/Evaluation/Work, 2030
GoalView: Special Education and RTI Studen t Management Information System., 1394
Goals and Objectives, 1461
Goals and Objectives IEP Program, 1462
Going Places, Children Living with Cerebral Palsy, 8436
Going to School with Facilitated Communication, 4855
Gold Violin, 635
Golden Eagle Passport, 5339
Golden Technologies, 237, 154, 547, 571, 574
Goldilocks and the Three Bears in Signed English, 7831
Goldman, Sachs & Company, 2488
Goleta Valley Cottage Hospital, 6442
Golf Xpress, 530
Gonzales Warm Springs Rehabilitation Hospital, 6279
Good Employee Is Capable, Conscientious, Productive, 8934
Good Grips Cutlery, 349
Good Samaritan Health System, 6981
Good Samaritan Health Systems, 8662
Good Samaritan Healthcare Physical Medicine and Rehabilitation, 6316
Good Samaritan Hospital, 6316, 6982
Good Samaritan Hospital-Health System Center, 6982
Good Shepherd Rehabilitation, 7214
Goodwill Easter Seals of the Gulf Coast, 6341
Goodwill Industries International, 804
Goodwill Industries of Central Indiana, 5813
Goodwill Industries of New Mexico, 5944
Goodwill Industries of North Georgia, 5763
Goodwill Industries of RI, 5992
Goodwill Industries of Southern New Jersey, 5928
Goodwill Industries- Suncoast, 3688, 5747, 5748, 5749, 5750, 5753, 5758
Goodwill Industries- Suncoast Incorporated, 5737
Goodwill Industries-Suncoast, 5738
Goodwill Industries-Suncoast Adult Day Training, 5741
Goodwill Industries-Suncoast Inc. Adult Day Training, 5742, 5743
Goodwill Industries-Suncoast Non-Residenti al Supports And Services Program, 5744
Goodwill Industries-Suncoast Supported Living, 5745
Goodwill Industries-Suncoast,Adult Day Training, 5746
Goodwill International, 5808
Goodwill Temporary Services, 5747
Govennor's Council on Developmental Disabilities, 4799
Govenors Coucil on Development Disabilities, 3107
Goverment of Rhode Isalnd, 3411
Government, 4409
Government Council on Developmental Disabilities, 4905
Government Information Services, 2929, 2943, 2945
Government Printing Office, 5369
Governor's Committee on Employment and Rehabilitation of People with Disabilities: Alaska, 3008
Governor's Committee on Employment of Persons with Disabilities, 2999
Governor's Council on Developmental Disabilities, 3020, 3107
Governor's Council on Disabilities and Special Education, 3009
Governor's Developmental Disability Council, 3147
Governor's Office oe Executive Policy & Programs, 3426
Gow School Summer Programs, 7337
Gpk, 241, 510
Grab Bars and Tub Rails, 304
Graduate Technological Education and the Human Experience of Disability, 2031
Grady Memorial Hospital, 6935
Graham Street Community Resources, 4139
Graham-Field, 658
Graham-Field Health Products, 240, 267, 405, 689
Grand Island VA Medical System, 5489
Grand Junction VA Medical Center, 5403
Grand Rapids Foundation, 2580
Grand Traverse Area Community Living Management Corporation, 3927
Grand Traverse Area Library for the Blind and Physically Handicapped, 4528
Grandmar, 639
Granger Foundation, 2581
Granite State Independent Living Foundation, 4008
Granny Good's Signs of Christmas, 7832
Graphic Controls Corporate Giving Program, 2683
Grassroots Consortium, 3455
Gray Street Workcenter, 5699
Grayson Foundation, 2451
Great Barrington Rehabilitation and Nursing Center, 7153
Great Big Safety Tub Mat, 140
Great Lakes Center for Independent Living, 3928
Great Lakes Regional Rehabilitation Center, 6226
Great Lakes/Macomb Rehabilitation Group, 3929
Great Oaks Joint Vocational School, 5970
Greater Baltimore Medical Center, 6787, 7147
Greater Cincinnati Foundation, 2748
Greater Detroit Agency for the Blind and Visually Impaired, 6834
Greater Enfield Association of Retarded Citizens, 5717
Greater Kansas City Community Foundation and Affiliated Trusts, 2603
Greater New Orleans Foundation, 4253
Greater Richmond ARC, 7312
Greater St. Louis Community Foundation, 2604
Greater Tacoma Community Foundation, 2894
Greater Wenatchee Community Foundation, 2895
Greater Worcester Community Foundation, 2563
Greeley Center for Independence, 3662
Green Bay Foundation, 2488
Green County Independent Living Resource Center, 4103
Green Door, 5732
Greenery Extended Care Center: Baltimore, 6788
Greenery Extended Care Center: Worcester, 6809
Greenery Rehabilitation & Skilled Nursing Center, 6810
Greenroots Consortium, 3455
Greenville Disability Action Center, 4140
Greenwood Publishing Group, 1774, 1958, 2036, 2048, 2073, 4295, 4300, 4320, 4321, 4333, 4341, 4680, 4821, 4836, 4858, 4877, 4949, 4964, 4983, 5005, 5010, 7435, 7624, 7640, 7649
Gresham Driving Aids, 68, 71, 72, 74, 82, 85, 87, 94, 100, 104, 105, 106, 107, 113
Grey House Publishing, 1775, 2927, 8114
Grief: What it is and What You Can Do, 4856
Griffin Area Resource Center Griffin Community Workshop Division, 5765
Groden Center, 5993
Grossberg Company, 2547
Grossmont Hospital Rehabilition Center, 6068
Grover Hermann Foundation, 2489
Growing Together Diabetes Camp, 8263
Growing Together: Information for Parents of Deaf Children, 7833
Growing Up with Epilepsy: A Pratical Guide for Parents, 8437
Guardianship Services Associates, 4260
Guest House of Slidell Sub-Acute and Rehab Center, 7138
Guide Dog Foundation Flyer, 8935
Guide Dog Foundation for the Blind, 2684, 8907, 8935, 8938
Guide Dog Users, 8775
Guide Dogs for the Blind, 8776
Guide Service of Washington, 5340
A Guide for People with Disabilities Seeking Employment, 4738, 5104
A Guide for the Wheelchair Traveler, 5292
Guide to ACA Accredited Camps, 8264
Guide to Developing Language Competence in Handicapped Preschool Children, 8712
A Guide to Disability Rights Law, 4756
Guide to Federal Funding for Child Care and Early Childhood Development, 2943

Guide to Federal Funding for Hospitals and Health Centers, 2944
Guide to Federal Funding for Volunteer Programs & Community Service, 2945
Guide to Hydrocephalus, 8438
Guide to Living With HIV Infection: Develo ped at the Johns Hoplins AIDS Clinic, 8439
Guide to Successful Employment for Individuals with Autism, 7457
Guide to Teaching Phonics, 1631
Guide to Wheelchair Sports and Recreation, 8093
Guide to the Selection of Musical Instruments, 19
A Guidebook on Consumer-Controlled Housing for Minnesotans with Disabilities, 4757
Guided Tour for Persons 17 & Over with Developmental and Physical Challenges, 5341
Guidelines and Games for Teaching Efficient Braille Reading, 8936
Guidelines for Comprehensive Low Vision Care, 8937
Guidelines for Helping Deaf-Blind Persons, 7834
Guidelines for Spina Bifida & Health Care Services Throughout Life, 8440
Guidelines on Disability, 4857
Guideway, 8938
Guiding Eyes for the Blind, 8777, 8778
Guiding Eyes for the Blind: Breeding and Placement Center, 8778
Guild Audio Library, 8939
Guild Briefs, 8940
Guild for the Blind, 4455
Guilford Press, 4794, 7370, 7371, 7372, 7373, 7375, 7376, 7385, 7424, 7449, 7520, 8483, 8488
Guilford Publication, 1913
Gulf Coast Independent Living Center, 3959

H

H AR C Mercantile, 1200
H UD U SE R, 1578
H&R Block Foundation, 2605
H.E.L.P. Knife, 350
HAC Hearing Aid Centers of America: HARC Mercantile, 455
The HANDYBAR, 110
HARC Mercantile, 55, 168, 172, 173, 174, 175, 188, 193, 194, 195, 196, 199, 201, 204, 207, 208, 211, 212, 215, 216, 217, 221, 223, 302, 310, 322, 323, 326, 327, 328, 329, 514, 515, 523, 606
HASL Independent Abilities Center, 4110
HCR Health Care Services, 6227
HCR Manor Care Foundation, 2749
HEAR Center, 7699
HELP, 1395
HIV Drug Book Revised, 8441
HIV Infection and Developmental Disabilities, 2032
HSC Pediatric Center, The, 6561
HSI Austin Center For Development, 6674
Hacienda La Puente Unified School District, 6443
Hacienda Rehabilitation and Care Center, 7057
Hackett Hill Nursing Center and Integrated Care, 6872
Haldimand-Norfolk Resource Education and C ounseling, 805
Halifax Hospital Medical Center Eye Clinic Professional Center, 6583
Hall County Library: East Hall Branch and Special Needs Library, 4441
Hall-Perrine Foundation, 2523
Halsted Terrace Nursing Center, 7110
Hamilton Adult Center, 6936
Hamilton Rehabilitation and Healthcare Cen ter, 7075
Hampton Public Library, 4637
Hampton Subregional Library for the Blind, 4637
Hampton VA Medical Center, 5582
Hand Brake Control Only, 69
Hand Control Systems, 70
Hand Dimmer Switch, 71
Hand Dimmer Switch with Horn Button, 72
Hand Gas & Brake Control, 73
Hand Operated Parking Brake, 74
Hand Parking Brake, 75
Handbook About Care in the Home, 4995
Handbook for Implementing Workshops for Siblings of Special Children, 2033
Handbook for Itinerant and Resource Teachers of Blind Students, 8941
Handbook for Speech Therapy, 2034
Handbook for the Special Education Administrator, 2035
Handbook of Adaptive Switches and Augmentative Communication Devices, 1396
Handbook of Assistive Devices for the Handicapped Elderly, 7639
Handbook of Autism and Pervasive Developmental Disorders, 7458
Handbook of Career Planning for Special Needs Students, 4748
Handbook of Career Planning for Students with Special Needs, 6010
Handbook of Chronic Fatigue Syndrome, 8442
Handbook of Developmental Education, 2036
Handbook of Epilepsy, 8443
Handbook of Information for Members of the Achromatopsia Network, 8942
Handbook of Services for the Handicapped, 4858
Handbook on Diability Discrimination Law, 4316
Handbook on Ethnicity, Aging and Mental Health, 7640
Handbook on Mental Disability Law, 4317
Handbook on Supported Education for People with Mental Illness, 2037
Handi Camp, 1032
Handi Home Lift, 390
Handi Prolift, 391
Handi Vangelism Ministries International, 1032
Handi-Kids, 966
Handi-Lift, 376, 377, 385, 390, 391, 398
Handi-Ramp, 392, 392
Handi-Works Productions, 6767
HandiWARE, 1397
Handicapped Driving Aids, 76
Handicapped Driving Aids of Michigan, 76
Handicapped Scuba Association, 8094
Handicapped Scuba Association International, 8094
Handicapped Student Program Postsecondary Education Association, 1550
Handicaps, 109
Hands-Free Controller, 5282
Handtalk Zoo, 7835
Handy-Helper Cutting Board, 351
Hang Gliding and Paragliding Mag, 8095
Happiness Bag, 940
Happiness Day at Parmadale, 1014
Happiness Day at St. Augustine Academy, 1015
Happiness Day at the Center for Pastoral Leadership, 1016
Happiness is Camping, 8265
Harborview Medical Center, 7034
Harborview Medical Center, Low Vision Aid Clinic, 7034
Hard Manufacturing Company, 159
Harden Foundation, 2346
Harlem Independent Living Center, 4049
Harmony Nursing and Rehabilitation Center, 7111
Harper Collins Publishers/ Basic Books, 1757
Harper Collins Publishers/Basic Books, 4862, 7667
Harper Perennial, 8326
HarperCollins, 7539, 8489
Harriet & Robert Heilbrunn Guild School, 2257
Harriet McDaniel Marshall Trust in Memory of Sanders McDaniel, 2452
Harrington House Nursing And Rehabilitation Center, 6811
Harris Communications, 325, 456, 203, 325, 456, 1649, 1690, 5143, 5144, 5150, 5151, 5152, 7776, 7819, 7820, 7823, 7858, 7880, 7884, 7904, 7920, 9034
Harris Methodist Fort Worth Hospital Mabee Rehabilitation Center, 6280
Harris Methodist Fort Worth/Mabee Rehabilitation Center, 7004
Harris and Eliza Kempner Fund, 2852
Harrison Center for the Arts, 6163
Harrison Health and Rehabilitation Centre, 7122
Harry C Moores Foundation, 2750
Harry C Trexler Trust, 2783
Harry F and Elaine Chaddick Foundation, 2490
Harry S Truman Memorial Veterans' Hospital, 5480
Harry and Grace Steele Foundation, 2347
Harry and Jeanette Weinberg Foundation, 2548
Hartford Foundation for Public Giving, 2400
Hartford Holiday Travel, 5334
Hartford Insurance Group, 2401
Hartford Regional Office, 5404
Hartford Vet Center, 5405
Harvard University Howe Laboratory of Ophthalmology, 4519
Harvard University Press, 7446
Harvey Randall Wickes Foundation, 2582
Hausmann Industries, 5929
Havirmill Foundation, 2583
Hawaii Assistive Technology Training and, 3114
Hawaii Center for Independent Living-Maui, 3735
Hawaii Centers for Independent Living, 3736
Hawaii Community Foundation, 2465

Hawaii Department for Children With Special Needs, 3115
Hawaii Department of Education, 1798
Hawaii Department of Education: Special Needs, 1798
Hawaii Department of Health, Adult Mental Health Division, 3116
Hawaii Department of Human Serv, 3117
Hawaii Department of Human Services, 3117
Hawaii Disability Compensation Division Department Labor and Industrial Relations, 3118
Hawaii Disability Rights Center, 3119
Hawaii Executive Office on Aging, 3120
Hawaii Fair Employment Practice Agency, 5770
Hawaii State Council on Developmental Disabilities, 3121
Hawaii State Library for the Blind and Physically Handicapped, 4450
Hawaii Veterans Centers, 5425
Hawaii Vocational Rehabilitation Division, 5771
Hawk Communication Device, 1325
Haworth Press, 1861, 1866, 1896, 1924, 1962, 1994, 2020, 2023, 2031, 2093, 2094, 2099, 2125, 2128, 4314, 4666, 4736, 4758, 4815, 4886, 4952, 5050, 5053, 5087, 5090, 6217, 7413, 7604, 7605, 7611, 7612, 7639, 7641, 7648, 7657, 7664, 7668, 7669, 8513, 8592
Haym Salomon Home for The Aged, 7181
Head Injury Hotline, 8647
Head Injury Rehabilitation: Children, 2038
Head Injury Treatment Program at Dover, 6203
Head Injury: The Facts: A Guide for Fami lies and Care-Givers, 8444
Headache Newsletter, 8445
Headlight Dimmer Switch, 77
Headliner, 1106
Headlines Support Group, 8648
Headmaster Plus, 183
Healing Arts Press, 7993, 8464, 8494, 8508
Healing Dressing for Pressure Sores, 305
Healing HIV: How To Rebuild Your Immune Sy stem, 8446
Healing Herbs, 4859
Health Action, 806
Health Alliance, 6235
Health Care Communications, 8626
Health Care Corporation of America, 6601
Health Care Financing Administration, 2974
Health Care Management in Physical Therapy, 2039
Health Care Professionals Who Are Blind or Visually Impaired, 8943
Health Care Quality Improvement Act of 1986, 4318
Health Care Solutions, 6249
Health Care for Students with Disabilities, 2040
Health Care of the Aged, 7641
Health Education AIDS Liason (HEAL), 8140
Health Promotion and Disease Prevention, 7642
Health Resource Center, 7700
Health Resource Center for Women with Disabilities, 807
Health Resources & Services Administration : State Bureau of Health, 3191
Health South Cane Creek Rehabilitation Center, 6266
Health South Corporation, 6166, 6266, 6444
Health South Corporation in Burmingham Alabama, 6588
Health South Corporation of Alabama, 6108
Health South of Nittany Valley, 6251
Health and Rehabilitation Products, 457
Health and Wellfare, 3126
HealthCare Solutions, 458
HealthQuest Subacute and Rehabilitation Programs, 6584
HealthSouth Rehabilitation Hospital, 6209
HealthSouth Central Georgia Rehabilitation Hospital, 6129
HealthSouth Chattanooga Rehabilitation Hospital, 6267
HealthSouth Emeral Coast Sports & Rehabilitation Center, 6585
HealthSouth Harmarville Rehabilitation Hospital, 6250
HealthSouth Hospital, 6059
HealthSouth Hospital Of Houston, 7005
HealthSouth Mountain View Regional Rehab Hospital, 6322
HealthSouth Nittany Valley Rehabilitation Hospital, 6251
HealthSouth Northern Kentucky Rehabilitation Hospital, 6751
HealthSouth Plano Rehabilitation Hospital, 6281
HealthSouth Regional Rehab Center/Florida, 6104
HealthSouth Rehab Center: Oklahoma, 6237
HealthSouth Rehab Hospital Of Arlington, 6282
HealthSouth Rehab Hospital Of Austin, 6283
HealthSouth Rehab Hospital Of Erie, 6252
HealthSouth Rehab Hospital Of Utah, 6305
HealthSouth Rehab Hospital: Largo, 6105
HealthSouth Rehab Hospital: South Carolina, 6263
HealthSouth Rehabilitation Center of Humble Texas, 6284
HealthSouth Rehabilitation Center: New Mexico, 6213
HealthSouth Rehabilitation Cntr/Tennessee, 6268
HealthSouth Rehabilitation Hospital, 6055, 6285
HealthSouth Rehabilitation Hospital Of Baton Rouge, 6768
HealthSouth Rehabilitation Hospital Of Fort Smith, 6377
HealthSouth Rehabilitation Hospital Of Miami, 6587
HealthSouth Rehabilitation Hospital Of Western Massachusetts, 6812
HealthSouth Rehabilitation Hospital of Altoona, 6253
HealthSouth Rehabilitation Hospital of Beaumont, 6286
HealthSouth Rehabilitation Hospital of North Alabama, 6046
HealthSouth Rehabilitation Hospital of Sarasota, 6588
HealthSouth Rehabilitation Hospital of Tallahassee, 6586
HealthSouth Rehabilitation Institute Of San Antonio, 6287
HealthSouth Rehabilitation of Louisville, 6168
HealthSouth Sea Pines Rehabilitation Hospital, 6589
HealthSouth Specialty Hospital Of North Louisiana, 6171
HealthSouth Sports Medicine & Rehabilitation Center, 6106
HealthSouth Sports Medicine Center, 6060
HealthSouth Sports Medicine and Rehabilitation Center, 6107
HealthSouth Treasure Coast Rehabilitation Hospital, 6108
HealthSouth Tri-State Rehabilitation Hospital, 6718
HealthSouth Tustin Rehabilitation Hospital, 6444
HealthSouth Valley Of The Sun Rehabilitation Hospital, 6361
HealthSouth Western Hills Regional Rehab Hospital, 6323
Healthcare Guidelines for Spina Bifida and Healthcare Services Throughout Life, 8447
Healthcare and Rehabilitation Center of Sanford, 7084
Healthfirst Press, 8446
Healthline, 1889
Healthsouth Corporation, 6586
Healthsouth Rehab Institute of Tucson, 6061
Healthsouth Rehabilitation Hospital of Greater Pittsburgh, 6254
Healthsouth Rehabilitation Hospital of Mechanicsburg, 6255
Healthsouth Rehabilitation Hospital of York, 6256
Healthsouth Rehabilitation at Sumner, 6269
Healthwin Specialized Care, 6719
Healthy Breathing, 8448
Hear Now, 7701
Hear You Are, 459
Hear to Listen & Learn: A Language Approach for Children with Ear Infections, 5160
Hearing Aid Batteries, 326
Hearing Aid Battery Testers, 327
Hearing Aid Dehumidifier, 328
Hearing Aids, 7836
Hearing Center, 455
Hearing Education and Awareness for Rockers, 7702
Hearing Impaired Employee, 7837
Hearing Loss Association Of America, 4752, 7838
Hearing Loss: The Journal of Self Help for Hard of Hearing People, 7838
Hearing, Speech & Deafness Center (HDSC), 477
Hearing, Speech & Deafness Center (HSDC), 7839, 8713, 7802, 7803, 7840, 8706, 8714
Hearing, Speech and Deafness Center (HSDC), 7840, 8714
Hearing-Impaired Children and Youth with Developmental Disabilities, 7841
Hearsay, 8944
The Heart Camp, 8198
Heart Disease in Persons with Down Syndrome, 8449
Heart of the Mind, 8450
Heart to Heart, 5120, 5161, 8945
Heartbreak of Being A Little Bit Blind, 8946
Hearth Day Treatment and Vocational Services, 5971
Heartland Opportunity Center, 5663
Heartspring, 6743

Heather Hill, 6228
Heather Hill Rehabilitation Hospital, 6228
Heavy Duty Sock Tuckers, 288
Heightened Independence and Progress: Hack ensack, 4017
Heightened Independence and Progress: Jers ey City, 4018
Heights Hospital Rehab Unit, 7006
Heldref Publications, 1865
Helen Bader Foundation, 2909
Helen Brach Foundation, 2491
Helen K and Arthur E Johnson Foundation, 2389
Helen Keller International, 4576
Helen Keller National Center, 5137, 7834, 7936
Helen Keller National Center Newsletter, 8947
Helen Keller National Center for Deaf-Blin d Youths and Adults (HKNC), 4577, 4860
Helen Steiner Rice Foundation, 2751
Helen and Teacher: The Story of Helen & Anne Sullivan Macy, 7284
Helm Distributing, 647, 648
Help Newsletter, 1890
Help Yourself Cookbook, 8451
Helping Children Understand Disabilities, 4678
Helping Hands, 1033, 5162
Helping Learning Disabled Gifted Children Learn Through Compensatory Play, 2041
Helping Others Breathe Easier, 8452
Helping People with Autism Manage Their Behavior, 7459
Helping Students Grow, 2042
Helping Your Child with Attention-Deficit Hyperactivity Disorder, 7460
Helping Your Hyperactive: Attention Deficit Child, 7461
Helping the Family Understand, 7842
Helping the Visually Impaired Child with Developmental Problems, 8948
Hemisphere Publishing Corporation, 1869
Hemophilia Association, 8223
Henkind Eye Institute Division of Montefiore Hospital, 6900
Henry & Tommy Lehmann Charitable Foundation, 2853
Henry Ford Health System, 6847
Henry Holt and Company, 8348
Henry J Kaiser Family Foundation, 2348
Henry Kaufmann Campgrounds Staten Island, 998
Henry L Hillman Foundation, 2784
Henry Nias Foundation, 2402
Henry W Bull Foundation, 2349
Henry and Lucy Moses Fund, 2685
Herb Research Foundation, 5229
Herbert W Hoover Foundation, 2752
Heritage Health and Rehabilitation Center, 7251
Herman Goldman Foundation, 2686
Herpes Resource Center, 8141
Herrick Health Sciences Library, 4391
Hesta Stuart Christian Charitable Trust, 2854
Hi-Desert Medical Center, 6445
HiRider, 681
Hidden Child: The Linwood Method for Reaching the Autistic Child, 7462
Hig's Manufacturing, 460
High Adventure Hang Gliding, 8096
High Profile Single Compartment Cushion, 264
High School Senior's Guide to Merit and Ot her No-Need Funding, 2946
High School Students Guide to Study, Travel, and Adventure Abroad, 2276
High Tech Center, 1257
High-Low Chair, 238
Highbrook Lodge, 8837
Higher Education Consortium for Urban Affairs (HECUA), 2277
Highland Pines Rehabilitation Center, 7085
Highland Unlimited Business Enterprises of CRI, 5972
Highlighter and Note Tape, 595
Hilcrest Medical Center: Kaiser Rehab Cent er, 6238
Hill School of Fort Worth, 7338
Hillcrest Baptist Medical Center, 7007
Hillcrest Baptist Medical Center: Rehab Care Unit, 6288
Hillcrest Foundation, 2855
Hillhaven Rehabilitation, 6630
Hillsborough County Talking Book Library Tampa-Hillsborough County Public Library, 4420
Hilo Vet Center, 5425
Hinsdale Hospital, 8664
Hip Function & Ambulation, 8453
His & Hers, 1125
History and Use of Braille, 8949
Hitchcock Rehabilitation Center, 6990
Hoblitzelle Foundation, 2856
Hockanum Greenhouse, 6542
Hockanum Industry, 6542
Hole in the Wall Gang Camp, 8266
Holiday Inn Boxborough Woods, 6813
Hollister Workshop, 5664
Hollywood Speaks, 7843
Holsten Conference Camping, 1056
Holy Cross Comprehensive Rehabilitation Center, 6069
Holy Cross Hospital, 6590
Holzer Clinic, 6937
Holzer Clinic Sycamore, 6938
Holzer Medical Center, 6938
Home Control of Allergies and Asthma, 8454
Home and Community Care for Chronically Ill Children, 4727
Home is in the Heart: Accommodating People with Disabilities in the Homestay Experience, 4861
Home of the Guiding Hands, 6446
HomeCare Magazine, 1856
Homecare Products EZ-Access Portable Ramps, 393
Homelink, 6726
Homemade Battery-Powered Toys, 1632
Homeopathic Educational Services, 808
Homer G Barr Trust, 2524
The Homestead Group Administrative Offices, 2804
Homestead Healthcare and Rehabilitation Ce nter, 7162
Homewaiter, 394
Honolulu VBA Regional Office, 5426
Hooleon Corp, 1187
Hooleon Corporation, 1229, 1222, 1232, 1296
Hope, 9031
Hope Center, 5700
Hope Community Resources, 3559
Hope Haven, 3807
Hope Network, 6835
Hope Network Rehabilitation Services, 6835
Hope Rehabilitation Services, 5664
Horace A Kimball and S Ella Kimball Foundation, 2810
Horace W Goldsmith Foundation, 2687
Horcher Lifting Systems, 395
Horizon Publishers, 7621
Horizon Rehabilitation Center, 6221
Horizons for the Blind, 4456, 8779
Horizontal Steering, 78
Horn Control Switch, 79
Hospice Alternative, 4862
Hospital Audiences, 1576
Hospital Environmental Control System, 500
Hospital For Special Care (HSC), 7076
Hospital of the Good Samaritan Acute Rehabilitation Unit, 6447
Hospitality Nursing Rehabilitation Center, 7263
Hospitalized Veterans Writing Project, 5370
Hostelling North America Hostelling International: American Youth Hostels, 5342
Houghton Mifflin, 8569
House Ear Institute, 7703
Housing Unlimited, 3877
Housing and Transportation of the Handicapped, 4319
Housing, Support, and Community, 4728
Houston Center for Independent Living, 4166
Houston Endowment, 2857
Houston Public Library: Access Center, 4625
Houston Regional Office, 5572
Houston VA Medical Center, 5573
Houston-Love Memorial Library, 4362
How Come You Walk Funny?, 8033
How Difficult Can This Be ? (Fat City), 5163
How Does a Blind Person Get Around?, 8950
How To Reach and Teach Children and Teens with Dyslexia, 7463
How We Play, 5164
How You Gonna Get to Heaven if You Can't Talk with Jesus?, 7844
How the Student with Hearing Loss Can Succeed in College, Second Edition, 1633
How to Conduct an Assessment, 2211
How to Deal with Back Pain and Rheumatoid Joint Pain, 8034
How to File a Title III Complaint, 4863
How to Find More About Your Child's Birth Defect or Disability, 5121
How to Live Longer with a Disability, 4864
How to Live with a Spinal Cord Injury, 8455
How to Outsmart Your Allergies, 8456
How to Own and Operate an Attention Deficit Disorder, 7464
How to Pay for Your Degree in Business & Related Fields, 2947
How to Pay for Your Degree in Education & Related Fields, 2948
How to Read for Everyday Living, 1476
How to Teach Autistic & Severely Handicapped Children, 2043
How to Teach Spelling/How to Spell, 2044
How to Thrive, Not Just Survive, 8951
How to Write for Everyday Living, 1398
Howard Heinz Endowment, 2785
Howard School, 2258
Howard University Child Development Center, 6562
Hoxie Harrison Smith Foundation, 2786
Hsbc Building, 2706
Hub, 8952
Hudson County CIL, 4018
Hug Just Isn't Enough, 5051

Hugh J Andersen Foundation, 2593
Hughen Center, 7981
Human Ecology Action League (HEAL), 809
Human Exceptionality: Society, School, and Family, 2045
Human Kinetics, 1841, 4974, 8077, 8086, 8087, 8092, 8098, 8112, 8115, 8364
Human Kinetics Press, 8018
Human Policy Press, 8649
Human Resource Management and the Americans with Disabilities Act, 4320
Human Rights Commission, 6008
Human Sciences Press, 2105, 4754, 5084, 7501, 7613, 7630, 7863, 9032
Human Services Building, 3237
Human Ware, 1317
HumanWare, 206
Humana Hospital: Morristown RehabCare, 6992
Humana Press, 8365
Hunter Holmes McGuire VA Medical Center, 5583
Hunter House, 8504
Hunter House Publishers, 1250, 8486
Huntington Health and Rehabilitation Cente r, 7227
Huntington Regional Office, 5592
Huntington VA Medical Center, 5593
Huntleigh Healthcare, 461, 253
Huntsville Subregional Library for the Blind & Physically Handicapped, 4363
Hutchinson Community Foundation, 2530
Hy-Tek Manufacturing Company, 1322
Hyams Foundation, 2564
Hyde Park-Woodlawn, 6675
Hydrocephalus: A Guide for Patients, Families & Friends, 8457
Hygienics Direct Company, 1159
Hyperactive Child, Adolescent, and Adult: ADD Through the Lifespan, 7465
Hyperactivity, Attention Deficits, and School Failure: Better Ways, 7466
Hyperion, 7493
Hypokalemic Periodic Paralysis Resource Page, 5230

I

I Can Do It, 8035
I ET Resources, 1365
I Have a Sister, My Sister is Deaf, 7845
I Heard That!, 2046
I Heard That!2, 2047
I Just Found Out I Have HIV... Now What?, 8458
I KNOW American History, 1399
I KNOW American History Overlay CD, 1400
A I Squared, 1318
I Want My Little Boy Back, 7467
I Wonder Who Else Can Help, 1857
I'm Not Disabled, 4865
IAL News, 8459
IBM Corporation, 2453
IBM National Support Center, 5766
IDEAMATICS, 184
IHS of Greater Pittsburgh, 6983
IKRON Institute for Rehabilitative and Psychological Services, 6939
IL Center: Cape Organization for Rights of the Disabled, 810
IL Resource Center: Ventura, 3621
IN Speechl Language-Hearing Association, 6146
IN-SIGHT Independent Living, 4133
IN-SOURCE, 6147
INVACARE IVC Tracer EX2 Wheelchair, 682
IPACHI, 3075
IRET Corporate Services Division, 5953
ISC, 4914
ISC: National Organization of People with Physical Disabilities, 8097
ITDG Publishing, 8376
Iberville Association for Retarded Citizens, 6769
Icon Health, 8529, 8530, 8531
Idaho Assistive Technology Project, 1258, 4451, 1600, 4668, 4669, 4973, 7618
Idaho Commission for the Blind & Visually Impaired, 5779
Idaho Commission for the Blind and Visually Impaired, 3744
Idaho Commission on Aging, 3125
Idaho Council on Developmental Disabilities, 3126, 4966
Idaho Department of Employment, 5775
Idaho Department of Handicapped Children, 3127
Idaho Disability Determinations Service, 3128
Idaho Elks Rehabilitation Hospital, 6641
Idaho Employment Service and Job Training Program Liaison, 5775
Idaho Fair Employment Practice Agency, 5776
Idaho Falls Office: Living Independently for Everyone (LIFE), 3745
Idaho Governor's Committee on Employment of People with Disabilities, 5777
Idaho Human Rights Commission, 5776
Idaho Industrial Commission, 3129
Idaho Mental Health Center, 3130
Idaho State Library: Talking Book Library, 4452
Idaho Vocational Rehabilitation Agency, 5778
Ideal-Phone, 184
Ideas for Easy Travel, 5299
Ideas for Kids on the Go, 4866
Ideas for Making Your Home Accessible, 1587
If Blindness Comes, 8953
If Blindness Strikes Don't Strike Out, 8954
If I Only Knew What to Say or Do, 4867
If Your Child Has Diabetes: An Answer Book for Parents, 8460
If Your Child Stutters: A Guide for Parents, 8715
If it Weren't for the Honor: I'd Rather Have Walked, 4868
If it is to Be, it is Up to Me, 1634
Illinois Assistive Technology Project, 3134
Illinois Center for Autism, 6676
Illinois Council on Developmental Disability, 3135
Illinois Department of Mental Health and Developmental Disabilities, 3136
Illinois Department of Rehab Services, 3762
Illinois Department of Rehabilitation, 3137
Illinois Department on Aging, 3138
Illinois Early Childhood Intervention Clearinghouse, 4457
Illinois Employment Service, 5787
Illinois Network of Centers for Independent Living, 3789
Illinois Regional Library for the Blind and Physically Handicapped, 4458
Illinois State Board of Education, 3132
Illinois State Board of Education: Department of Special Education, 1800
Illinois Valley Center for Independent Living, 3763
Illinois and Iowa Center for Independent Living, 3764
Image Systems, 1169
Imagery Procedures for People with Special Needs, 4869
Imagery in Healing Shamanism and Modern Medicine, 4870
Images of the Disabled, Disabling Images, 2048
Imagine!, 7468, 7468
Imagine: Innovative Resources for Cognitive & Physical Challenges, 5701
Imagining the Possibilities: Creative Approaches to Orientation and Mobility Instruction, 8955
Immune Deficiency Foundation, 8461
Immune Deficiency Foundation Newsletter, 8461
Imp Tricycle, 702
Impact Center for Independent Living, 3765
Impact: Ocala Vocational Services, 5748
Imperial, 7112
Implementing Cognitive Strategy Instruction Across the School, 1635
Implementing Family-Centered Services in Early Intervention, 2049
In Control, 8036
In Cube Pro Voice Command, 1326
In Search of Wings: A Journey Back from T raumatic Brain Injury, 7469
In Their Own Way, 7470
In This Sign, 7846
In Time and with Love: Caring for the Special Needs Infant and Toddler, 5052
In Touch Systems, 1305, 1306
In the Ear Hearing Aid Battery Extractor, 329
In the Middle, 8462
In the Mind of the Beholder.... a Video About Newly Blind Adults, 8956
In-Definite Arts Society, 20
In-Home Medical Care, 6631
In-Sight, 6987
InFocus, 1316
InTouch Networks: National Radio Reading Service, 8957
Inclinator Company of America, 370, 394, 396, 410, 413
Inclinette, 396
Include Us, 4871
Including All of Us: An Early Childhood Curriculum About Disability, 2050
Including Students with Severe and Multiple Disabilites in Typical Classrooms, 2051
Including Students with Special Needs: A Practical Guide for Classroom Teachers, 2052
Inclusive & Heterogeneous Schooling: Assessment, Curriculum, and Instruction, 2053, 2212
Inclusive Child Care for Infants and Toddlers: Meeting Individual and Special Needs, 4729
Inclusive Games, 8098

Inclusive Play People, 1636
Increasing Behaviors of Persons with Severe Retardation and Autism, 7471
Increasing Capabilities Access, 3025
Increasing Capabilities Access Network, 1259
Increasing Literacy Levels: Final Report, 8958
Increasing and Decreasing Behaviors of Persons with Severe Retardation and Autism, 1763
Independence, 3817, 4872
Independence First, 3818
Independence & Transition to Community Living: The Role of Independent Living Centers, 4730
Independence Associates, 3893
Independence CIL, 4933
Independence Empowerment Center, 4209
Independence First, 4238
Independence First: West Bend, 4239
Independence Northwest Center for Independent Living, 3673
Independence Now: Riverdale, 3878
Independence Now: Silver Spring, 3879
Independence Place, 3855
Independence Resource Center, 4210
Independence Unlimited, 3674
Independence Without Sight and Sound: Suggestions for Practitioners, 7285
Independent Connection, 3819
Independent Connection: Beloit, 3820
Independent Life Center, 3663
Independent Life Styles, 4167
Independent Living, 3678
Independent Living Aids, 134, 147, 181, 539, 540, 543, 544, 596, 597, 601, 604, 610, 615, 616
Independent Living Approach to Disability Policy Studies, 2054
Independent Living Center, 3558
Independent Living Center Network: Department of the Visually Handicapped, 4211
Independent Living Center Of Southern California, 3622
Independent Living Center of Alabaster, 3550
Independent Living Center of Eastern Indiana (ILCEIN), 3796
Independent Living Center of Jasper, 3551
Independent Living Center of Kern County, 3623
Independent Living Center of Lancaster, 3624
Independent Living Center of Mobile, 3552
Independent Living Center of Northeast Kan sas, 3821
Independent Living Center of SW Washington, 4227
Independent Living Center of Southeast Missouri, 3973
Independent Living Center of Starvos: Spri ngfield, 3895
Independent Living Center of Stavros: Gree nfield, 3896
Independent Living Center of the North Shore and Cape Ann, 3894
Independent Living Center of the Southeast, 3897
Independent Living Center: Massachusetts, 3898
Independent Living Center: Multi-Cultural Center of Boston, 3899
Independent Living Center: San Gabriel Valley, 3625
Independent Living Centers and Managed Care: Results of an ILRU Study on Involvement, 4873
Independent Living Challenges the Blues, 4874
Independent Living Matters, 4731
Independent Living Office, 4875, 3853
Independent Living Research Utilization, 4882
Independent Living Research Utilization I LR U, 4726
Independent Living Research Utilization ILRU, 4276, 4721, 4730, 4734, 4774, 4777, 4779, 4827, 4828, 4834, 4852, 4873, 4874, 4896, 4926, 4928, 4929, 4931, 4962, 4971, 5004, 5127, 7513, 7891, 8031
Independent Living Research Utilization Project, 4168
Independent Living Resource Center, 3822
Independent Living Resource Center, Inc., 3626, 3627
Independent Living Resource Center: San Francisco, 3628
Independent Living Resource Center: Santa Maria Office, 3629
Independent Living Resource of Contra Coast, 3630
Independent Living Resource of Fairfield, 3631
Independent Living Resource: Antioch, 3632
Independent Living Resource: Concord, 3633
Independent Living Resources, 4111
Independent Living Resources (ILR), 3634
Independent Living Service Northern California: Redding Office, 3635
Independent Living Services of Northern California, 3636
Independent Living: Iowa Everett Conner Center, 3808
Independent Mobility Systems, 101
Independent Newsletter, 4876
Independent Resource Georgetown, 3679
Independent Resources, 3680
Independent Resources: Dover, 3681
Independent Resources: Wilmington, 3682
Independent Visually Impaired Enterprisers, 8780
Indian Acres Camp for Boys, 7339
Indian Creek Camp, 8838
Indian Creek Health and Rehabilitation Center, 7123
Indian Creek Nursing Center, 6744
Indian Rivers, 6342
Indian Trails Camp, 970
Indiana Association of Homes for the Aging, 7571
Indiana Client Assistance Program, 3142
Indiana Congress of Parent and Teachers, 6148
Indiana Department of Education, 1801
Indiana Department of Education: Special Education Division, 1801
Indiana Developmental Disability Council, 3143
Indiana Employment Services and Job Training Program Liaison, 5814
Indiana Fair Employment Practice Agency, 5815
Indiana Institute on Disability and Community, 4470
Indiana Parent Information Association, 6149
Indiana Protection & Advocacy Services, 3144
Indiana Resource Center for Autism, 4470
Indiana Resource Center for Families with Special, 6147
Indiana State Commission for the Handicapped, 3145
Indiana University, 935
Indiana University: Multipurpose Arthritis Center, 4471
Indianapolis Regional Office, 5434
Indianapolis Resource Center For Independent Living, 3797
Individuals with Arthritis, 5122, 8037
Individuals with Cerebral Palsy, 8463
Industrial Accident Board de dept, 3071
Industrial Support Systems, 6434
Industries, 6848
Industries for the Blind of New York State, 6901
Industries of the Blind, 6914
Inflatable Back Pillow, 265
Infogrip: AdjustaCart, 531
Infogrip: BAT Personal Keyboard, 532
Infogrip: ErgoPOD Model 500, 1181
Infogrip: King Keyboard, 1297
Infogrip: Large Print Keyboard, 1298
Infogrip: Large Print/Braille Keyboard Labels, 1230
Infogrip: OnScreen, 1299
Informa Healthcare, 4829
Information & Referral Center, 2055
Information & Referral Services, 1342
Information + Referral Services, 1342
Information Access Project, 8959
Information Access Project: National Federation of the Blind, 8781
Information Service, 8678
Information Services for People with Developmental Disabilities, 4877
Information from HEATH Resource Center, 1776
Information on Glaucoma, 8960
Information, Protection & Advocacy for Persons with Disabilities, 3075
Information, Protection and Advocacy Center for Handicapped Individuals, 3076
Informed Touch, 8464
Informer, 8465
Infusion Therapies, 6109
Ingham Regional Medical Center, 4526
Injured Mind, Shattered Dreams: Brian's Survival from a Severe Head Injury, 8466
Inland North West Health Services, 8215
Inland Northwest Community Foundation, 2896
Innabah, 1034
Inner Traditions, 4787, 4796
Innerlip Plates, 352
Innovation Management Group, 5231, 1363
Innovative Industries, 5829
Innovative Practices for Teaching Sign Language Interpreters, 7847
Innovative Products, 683
Innovative Programs: An Example of How CILs Can Put Their Work in Context, 4878
Innoventions, 608
Inova Fairfax Hospital For Children, 8135
Inova Mount Vernon Hospital Rehabilitation Program, 6312
Inova Rehabilitation Center, 6312
Inpatient Pain Rehabilitation Program, 6902
Inside MS, 8467

Inside The Halo and Beyond: The Anatomy o f a Recovery, 8038
Inside the Beltway, 8961
Insight, 8962
Inspiration Ministries, 4240
Institute For Rehabilitation & Research, 4168
Institute for Basic Research in Developmental Disabilities, 4578
Institute for Driver Rehabilitation, 80
Institute for Families of Blind Children, 8782
Institute for Human Development, 3250, 6362
Institute for Rehabilitation & Research, 6289, 7008
Institute for Rehabilitation Research, 7749, 8686
Institute for Scientific Research, 811
Institute for Therapy Throughout the Arts, 21
Institute for Visual Sciences, 4579
Institute of Disability of the University of NH, 1819
Institute of Living: Hartford Hospital, 1997
Institute of Physical Medicine and Rehabilitation, 6135
Institute of Transpersonal Psychology, 812
Institute on Disability/UCED, 1732
Institution on Disability, 6051
Instruction of Persons with Severe Handicaps, 1637
Instructional Methods for Students, 2056
Instrumental Music for Dyslexics: A Teach ing Handbook, 22
Insurance Solutions: Plan Well, Live Better, 4879
Int'l Association of Audio Information Services, 8944
Integrated Health Services at Waterford Commons, 6940
Integrated Health Services of Amarillo, 7009
Integrated Health Services of Durham, 6222
Integrated Health Services of Michigan at Clarkston, 6192
Integrated Health Services of New Jersey at Somerset Valley, 6881
Integrated Health Services of Seattle, 7035
Integrated Health Services of St. Louis at Gravois, 6855
Integrating Transition Planning Into the IEP Process, 1638
Intelli Tools, 1182, 1186, 1300, 1301, 1309, 1401, 1521, 1524
IntelliKeys, 185, 1300
IntelliKeys IIe, 1182
IntelliKeys USB, 1301
IntelliPics Studio 3, 1401
IntelliTalk, 1521
IntelliTools, 185
Intensive Early Intervention and Beyond School-Based Inclusion Program, 4880
Interactions: Collaboration Skills for School Professionals, 2057
Interdisciplinary Clinical Assessment of Young Children with Developmental Disabilities, 8468
An Interdisciplinary Journal for the Socia l Study of Health, Illness and Medicine, 4785
Intermediate Conversational Sign Language, 7848
Internal I/O Port Adapter, 1183
International Academy of Biological Dentistry and Medicine, 8142
International Academy of Oral Medicine and Toxicology, 8143
International Association for Cancer Victors, 8367
International Association for Cancer Victors: Northern California Chapter, 8144
International Association of Audio Information Services (IAAIS), 8783
International Association of Laryngectomees, 8459
International Association of Machinists, 813
International Association of Parents and Professionals for Safe Alternatives in Childbirth, 1733
International Association of Professional Natural Hygientists, 8145
International Association of Yoga Therapists, 814
International Bio-Oxidative Medicine Foundation (IBOM), 2767
International Braille and Technology Center for the Blind, 8650
International Catholic Deaf Association, 7704, 7806
International Center for the Disabled, 1260
International Childbirth Education Association, 1734
International Chiropractors Association, 815
International Christian Youth Exchange, 2278
International Clinic of Biological Regeneration, 816
International College of Applied Kinesiology, 817
International Directory of Libraries for the Disabled, 4881
International Directory of Periodicals Related to Deafness, 7849
International Dyslexia Association, 1735, 3192, 3230, 3318, 3390, 7382, 7504, 8720, 8730
International Dyslexia Association of DC, 3077
International Dyslexia Association of NY: Buffalo Branch, 3321
International Dyslexia Association of New England, 3201
International Dyslexia Association: Arizona Branch, 3021
International Dyslexia Association: Austin Branch, 3456
International Dyslexia Association: Central California Branch, 3041
International Dyslexia Association: Central Ohio Branch, 3371
International Dyslexia Association: Florida Branch, 3094
International Dyslexia Association: Georgia Branch, 3108
International Dyslexia Association: Hawaii Branch, 3122
International Dyslexia Association: Illinois Branch, 3139
International Dyslexia Association: Indiana Branch, 3146
International Dyslexia Association: Iowa Branch, 3148
International Dyslexia Association: Kansas/West Missouri Branch, 3159
International Dyslexia Association: Maryland Branch, 3192
International Dyslexia Association: Minnesota Branch, 3230
International Dyslexia Association: Mississippi Branch, 3242
International Dyslexia Association: Nebraska Branch, 3266
International Dyslexia Association: New Jersey Branch, 3300
International Dyslexia Association: North Carolina Branch, 3353
International Dyslexia Association: Oregon Branch, 3390
International Dyslexia Association: Pennsylvania Branch, 3399
International Dyslexia Association: Rocky Mountain Branch, 3054
International Dyslexia Association: Tennessee Branch, 3440
International Dyslexia Association: Virginia Branch, 3502
International Dyslexia Association: Washington State Branch, 3511
International Dyslexia Association: Wisconsin Branch, 3533
International Education, 2271
International Encyclopedia of Foundations, 2949
International Handbook on Mental Health Policy, 4321
International Health Guide for Senior Citizen Travelers, 7643
International Hearing Dog, 7705, 7883
International Hearing Society, 7706
International Journal of Arts Medicine, 2058
International Lutheran Deaf Association, 7707
International Medical and Dental Hypnotherapy Association, 8146
International Organization for the Education of the Hearing Impaired, 1736
International Ozone Association, 8147
International Paper Company Foundation, 2688
International Partnership for Service-Learning and Leadership, 2279
International Rehabilitation Review, 1858
International Rett Syndrome Association, 8148
International Rolf Institute, 1891
International Telephone Directory, 7850
International University Partnerships, 2280
International Ventilator Users Network, 8469
International Women's Health Coalition, 818
Interpretation: A Sociolinguistic Model, 7851
Interpretations, 7852
Interpreting Disability: A Qualitative Reader, 2059
Interpreting: An Introduction, Revised Edition, 7853
Interstitial Cystitis Association, 5232
Intervention Practices in the Retention of Competitive Employment, 8963
Intervention Research in Learning Disabilities, 2060
Intervention in School and Clinic, 1859
Interwood Publications, 4335
Introduction to Learning Disabilities, 2nd Edition, 2061
Introduction to Mental Retardation, 2062
Introduction to Special Education: Teaching in an Age of Challenge, 4th Edition, 2063
Introduction to Spina Bifida, 8470
Introduction to the Nature and Needs of Students with Mild Disabilities, 2064
Introduction to the Profession of Counseling, 2065
Invacare Corporation, 306, 408, 556, 693

Invacare Fulfillment Center, 556
Invacare Top End, 721
Invisible Children, 4679
Iowa Association of Homes and Services for the Aging, 7572
Iowa Central Industries, 6727
Iowa Child Health Specialty Clinics, 3149
Iowa City VA Medical Center, 5440
Iowa Civil Rights Commission, 5830
Iowa Commission of Persons with Disabilities, 3150
Iowa Compass, 3151
Iowa Department for the Blind, 3152
Iowa Department for the Blind Library, 4476
Iowa Department of Economic Development, 5832
Iowa Department of Elder Affairs, 3153
Iowa Department of Human Services, 3154
Iowa Department of Public Instruction: Bureau of Special Education, 1802
Iowa Employment Service, 5831
Iowa Job Training Program Liaison, 5832
Iowa Protection & Advocacy for the Disabled, 3155
Iowa Registry for Congenital and Inherited Disorders, 4477
Iowa United Methodist Conference Center, 947
Iowa Valley Community College, 5833
Iowa Vocational Rehabilitation Services, 5834
Iredell Vocational Workshop, 5956
Iris Network for the Blind, 6780
Iron Horse Productions, 699
Iron Mountain VA Medical Center, 5469
Irvine Health Foundation, 2350
Irving Place Rehabilitation and Nursing Ce nter, 7139
Is the Child Really Stuttering? Questions & Answers About Disfluency, 8716
Isanogel Center, 941
Issues and Research in Special Education, 2066
Issues in Independent Living, 4882
Issues in Law and Medicine, 4322
It isn't Fair!: Siblings of Children with Disabilities, 4680
It's All in Your Head, 8471
It's Just Attention Disorder, 7472

J

J CC Of Baltimore, 960
J E Stewart Teaching Tools, 1670
J&T Corp, 8398
JADARA, 7856
JAMA: The Journal of the American Medical Association, 4883
JARC, 3930
JB Lippincott, 4689, 7553, 7768, 8026, 8306, 8588
JBI Voice, 8964
JCIL Advocate Times, 4884
JCYS Camp Red Leaf, 932
JE Stewart Teaching Tools, 1461, 1610, 1616, 1625, 1669, 1676, 1717
JFK Center for the Performing Arts, 48
JFK Johnson Rehab Institute, 6210
JGB Audio Library, 1737
JGB Audio Library for the Blind, 1748, 2257, 8939, 8957
JGB Cassette Library International, 4580
JIST Publishing, 6150
JOBS Administration Job Opportunities & Basic Skills, 5639
JOBS VI and SAGE, 5950
JRA and Me, 8039
Jack Eckerd Corporation Foundation, 2440
Jackets, 1089
Jackson Center for Independent Living, 3931, 4155, 4884
Jackson Cervipillo, 160
Jackson Foundation, 2771
Jackson Independent Living Center, 3960
Jackson Regional Office, 5479
Jackson Square Nursing and Rehabilitation Center, 7113
Jacksonville Area CIL: Havana, 3766
Jacksonville Area Center for Independent Living, 3767
Jacksonville Public Library, 4426
Jacob and Charlotte Lehrman Foundation, 2418
James A Haley VA Medical Center, 5417
James Branch Cabell Library, 4638
James E Van Zandt VA Medical Center, 5547
James H And Cecile C Quillen Rehabilitation Hospital, 6270
James Lawrence Kernan Hospital, 6789
James R Thorpe Foundation, 2594
James S McDonnell Foundation, 2606
Jane Coffin Childs Memorial Fund, 2403
Jane Coffin Childs Memorial Fund for Medical Research, 2403
Jane Phillips Medical Center, 6239, 6957, 6239
Janus of Santa Cruz, 6448
Japanese Corporate Connection: A Guide for Fundraisers, 2950
Jason & Nordic Publishers, 4885
Jason Aronson, 7444, 7510
Jawonio Vocational Center, 3322, 3322
Jay and Rose Phillips Family Foundation, 2595
Jedra Charitable Foundation, 2689
Jefferson Industries, 256, 257, 279
Jefferson Lee Ford III Memorial Foundation, 2441
Jelly Bean Switch, 1184
Jennifer Roberts Building, 3636
Jeremy P Tarcher, 4844, 8427, 8579
Jerry L Pettis Memorial VA Medical Center, 5387
Jersey Cape Diagnostic Training & Opportunity Center, 5930
Jessica Kingsley Publishers, 29, 30, 43
Jessie Ball duPont Fund, 2442
Jet 3 Ultra Power Wheelchair, 713
Jewish Braille Institute International, 8784
Jewish Braille Institute of America, 8964, 8965
Jewish Braille Review, 8965
Jewish Community Center of Greater Rochester/JCC, 7324
Jewish Community Center of Greater Washington JCC, 956
Jewish Council for Youth Services, 932
Jewish Guild for the Blind, 1737
Jewish Healthcare Foundation of Pittsburgh, 2787
Jewish Heritage for the Blind, 8966
Jewish Hospital of St. Louis: Department of Rehabilitation, 6197
Jewish Vocational Service of Jewish Family and Children's Services, 5882
Jewish Vocational Services, 5788
Jim Thorpe Rehabilitation Center at Southwest Medical Center, 6240
JoDavies Workshop, 5789
Job Accommodation Network, 819, 1738
Job Hunting Tips for the So-Called Handicapped, 6070
Job Opportunities for the Blind, 5861
Job Placement Digest, 6313
Job Search Handbook for People with Disabi lities, 6150
Job Service North Dakota, 5966
Job Training Program Liaison: California, 5665
Job Works NISH Food Service, 5749
Job Works NISH Postal Service, 5750
Jobri, 266
Jobs Information Business Service, 4741
Joe and Emily Lowe Foundation, 2443
John C Lincoln Hospital North Mountain, 6363
John D Dingell VA Medical Center, 5470
John D and Catherine T MacArthur Foundation, 2492
John E & Nellie J Bastien Memorial Foundation, 2444
John Edward Fowler Memorial Foundation, 2419
John F Blair Publishing, 1967
John G & Marie S Kennedy Memorial Foundati on, 2858
John H Dekker & Sons, 8350
John H Wellons Foundation, 2729
John H and Ethel G Nobel Charitable Trust, 2404
John H and Wilhelmina D Harland Charitable Foundation, 2454
John Hopkins University Pres, 8575
John J Pershing VA Medical Center, 5481
John L McClellan Memorial Hospital, 5385
John Muir Medical Center Rehabilitation Services, Therapy Center, 6449
John O Pastore Center, 3416
John P Murphy Foundation, 2753
John Randolph Foundation, 2886
John S Dunn Research Foundation, 2859
John Tracy Clinic, 7708
John W Anderson Foundation, 2520
Johns Hopkins Press Health Book, 8439
Johns Hopkins University Dana Center for Preventive Ophthalmology, 4502
Johns Hopkins University Press, 5086, 7490, 8043, 8301, 8369, 8516
Johns Hopkins University: Asthma and Allergy Center, 4503
Johnson Books: A Cordillera Press Guide, 8081
Johnson Controls Foundation, 2910
Johnson County Developmental Supports, 6745
Johnston County Industries, 6915
Joint Conference with ABMPP Annual Conference, 1551
Jonathan M Wainwright Memorial VA Medical Center, 5587
Joni and Friends, 820
Jordan's Motility Solutions: Adapt-Able Utensils, 353
Joseph Alexander Foundation, 2690
Joseph Drown Foundation, 2351
Joseph P Kennedy Jr Foundation, 2420

Joseph Willard Health Center, 2208
Joslin Diabetes Center, 8472, 8478
Joslin Guide to Diabetes, 8472
Jossey-Bass, 7365, 7366, 7369, 7463
Journal, 7854
Journal Of Spinal Cord Medicine, 7947
Journal for Vocational Special Needs Education, 1860
Journal of Applied School Psychology, 1861
Journal of Children's Communication Development, 5075
Journal of Cognitive Rehabilitation, 7473
Journal of Counseling & Development, 1862
Journal of Emotional and Behavioral Disorders, 1863
Journal of Employment Counseling, 6314
Journal of Head Trauma Rehabilitation, 8473
Journal of Learning Disabilities, 1864
Journal of Motor Behavior, 1865
Journal of Musculoskeletal Pain, 1866
Journal of Postsecondary Education & Disability, 1867
Journal of Prosthetics and Orthotics, 1868
Journal of Reading, Writing and Learning Disabled International, 1869
Journal of Religion, Disability & Health, 5053
Journal of School Health Association, 1870
Journal of Social Work in Disabilty & Rehabilitation, 4886
Journal of Special Education, 1871
Journal of Speech, Language and Hearing Re search, 7855, 8717
Journal of Visual Impairment and Blindness, 8967
Journal of Vocational Behavior, 1872
Journal of the American Deafness and Rehabilitation Association, 7856
Journal of the Association for Persons with Severe Handicaps, 4887
Journey, 7286
Journey to Well: Learning to Live After S pinal Cord Injury, 8474
Jouse, 1302
Joy of Signing, 7857
Joy of Signing Puzzle Book, 7858
Joy: A Shabazz Center for Independent Living, 4080
Joystick Driving Control, 81
Judevine Center for Autism, 4552
Judge David L Bazelon Center for Mental Health Law, 4261
Juggler, 8968
Juliet L Hillman Simonds Foundation, 2788
Julius and Betty Levinson Center, 6677
Jumpin' Johnny Get Back to Work, A Child's Guide to ADHD/Hyperactivity, 7474
Jumpsuits, 1141
Junction Center for Independent Living, 4212, 4213
Junior Blind of America, 2352
Junior National Association of the Deaf, 7709
Junior Wheelchair Sports Camp, 913
Jupiter Medical Center-Pavilion, 7086
Just Like Everyone Else, 4888
Just One Break (JOBS), 5951
Juvenile Diabetes Foundation International, 821

K

K-BIT: Kaufman Brief Intelligence Test, 2213
K-FAST: Kaufman Functional Academic Skills Test, 2214
K-SEALS: Kaufman Survey of Early Academic and Language Skills, 2215
KG Saur/Division of RR Bowker, 4881
KIDS (Keyboard Introductory Development Series), 1402
KLST-2: Kindergarten Language Screening Test Edition, 2nd Edition, 2216
Kachina Point Health Care & Rehabilitation Center, 7058
Kailua Kona Center for Independent Living: West Hawaii, 3737
Kalamazoo Center for Independent Living, 3932
Kaleidoscope Network, 8651
Kaleidoscope: Exploring the Experience of Disability Through Literature & the Fine Arts, 23
Kamp A-Komp-Plish, 8839
Kamp Kaleo, 8840
Kamp Kiwanis, 999
Kanawha County Public Library, 4654
Kansas Advocacy and Protective Services, 3160
Kansas Association of Homes for the Aging, 7573
Kansas City VA Medical Center, 5482
Kansas Client Assistance Program, 3161
Kansas Commission on Disability Concerns, 3162
Kansas Department on Aging, 3163, 7635
Kansas Developmental Disability Council, 3164
Kansas Fair Employment Practice Agency, 5838
Kansas Jaycees Cerebral Palsy Ranch, 8267
Kansas Rehabilitation Hospital, 6165
Kansas Services for the Blind & Visually Impaired, 3823
Kansas State Board of Education, 1803
Kansas State Board of Education: Special Education Outcomes Team, 1803
Kansas State Library, 4481
Kansas VA Regional Office, 5445
Kansas Vocational Rehabilitation Agency, 5839
Kate B Reynolds Charitable Trust, 2730
The Kate B Reynolds Charitable Trust, 2730
Kathleen Price and Joseph M Bryan Family Foundation, 2731
Katie's Farm, 1403
Kauai Center for Independent Living, 3738
Kaufman Test of Educational Achievement (K-TEA), 2217
Kay Elemetrics Corporation, 1321, 1463
Kayelemetrics Corporation, 1468
Keats Publishing, 4919, 8358
Keep the Promise: Managed Care and People with Disabilities, 4889
Keeping Ahead in School, 1639
Keeping Our Families Together, 4890
Keeping the Balance, 8475
Kelley Diversified, 5767
Kelly Services Foundation, 2584
Ken McRight Supplies, 155, 254
Ken-Crest Services, 1035
Kenai Peninsula IL Center, 3560
Kenai Peninsula IL Center: Seward, 3561
Kendall Demonstration Elementary School Curriculum Guides, 2067
Kendall/Hunt Publishing Company, 7634
Keni Peninsula-Central Peninsula, 3562
Kennebunk Nursing & Rehabilitation Center, 7144
Kennedy Center, 5718
Kennedy Job Training Center, 5790
Kennedy Park Medical Rehabilitation Center, 7264
Kenneth & Evelyn Lipper Foundation, 2691
Kenneth T and Eileen L Norris Foundation, 2353
Kenny Foundation, 5314
Kensington Publishing, 5026
Kent A Hall, 2525
Kent County Arc, 2811
Kent District Library for the Blind and Physically Handicapped, 4529
Kent Walderep National Paralysis Foundation, 8029
Kent Waldrep National Paralysis Foundation, 2860
Kentfield Rehabilitation Hospital & Outpatient Center, 6071
Kentucky Assistive Technology Service Network, 1261
Kentucky Association of Not-for-Profit Homes and Services for the Aging, 7574
Kentucky Chapter of the Arthritis Foundation, 8067
Kentucky Committee on Employment of People with Disabilities, 5840
Kentucky Council on Developmental Disability, 3165
Kentucky Department for Employment Service and Job Training Program Liaison, 5841
Kentucky Department for Mental Health and Mental Retardation Services, 3166
Kentucky Department for Mental Health:, 3167
Kentucky Department for the Blind, 3168, 5842
Kentucky Department of Education: Division of Exceptional Children's Services, 1804
Kentucky Easter Sales Society, 949
Kentucky Office For The Blind, 5843
Kentucky Office of Aging Services, 3169
Kentucky Protection & Advocacy Division, 3170
Kentucky Talking Book Library, 4489
Kentucky Tennessee Conference, 8838
Kentucky Vocational Rehabilitation Agency, 5844
Kernal Book Series, 8969
Kessler Institute for Rehabilitation, 7959, 8393
Kessler Institute for Rehabilitation, Welkind Facility, 6211
Ketch Industries, 6746
Ketogenic Diet: A Treatment for Epilepsy, 8476
Key Changes: A Portrait of Lisa Thorson, 8040
Key Holders, Ignition & Door Keys, 82
Key Tronic KB 5153 Touch Pad Keyboard, 1303
KeyMath Teach and Practice, 1640
KeyTronic, 1303
KeyWiz, 1185
Keyboard Tutor, Music Software, 1404

Keyboarding by Ability, 1405
Keyboarding for the Physically Handicapped, 1406
Keyboarding with One Hand, 1407
Keyguards for IntelliKeys, 1186
Keys to Independence, 4732
Keys to Parenting a Child with Attention Deficit Disorder, 7475
Keys to Parenting a Child with Cerebral Palsy, 8477
Keys to Parenting a Child with Downs Syndrome, 7476
Keys to Parenting the Child with Autism, 7477
Keywi, 1327
Kid Kare News, 4681
Kid's Custom, 703
Kid's Edge, 704
Kid's Liberty, 705
Kid-Friendly Chairs, 706
Kid-Friendly Parenting with Deaf and Hard of Hearing Children: A Treasury of Fun Activities, 7859
Kids Get Arthiritis Too!, 8041
Kids on the Block Arthritis Programs, 8123
Kidz Korner, 4682
Kim Marshall Series in English, 1641
Kim Marshall Series in Math, 1642
Kim Marshall Series in Reading, 1643
Kim Marshall Series in Vocabulary, 1644
Kindered Health Care, 7220
Kindred, 6519, 7060, 7265
Kindred Health Care, 7041, 7063, 7124, 7231, 7251, 7273
Kindred Health Care Center, 7061
Kindred Health Care Publications, 7239
Kindred Healthcare, 6804, 7056, 7105, 7212, 7219, 7241, 7250, 7264, 7272
Kindred Heights Nursing & Rehabilitation Center, 7219
Kindred Hospital-La Mirada, 6450
King's Daughter's Medical Center's Rehab Unit/Work Hardening Program, 6752
King's Rehabilitation Center, 5666
King's Rule, 1343
King's View Work Experience Center-Atwater, 6451
Kings Harbor Multicare Center, 7182
Kingstar International America, 251
Kiplinger Foundation, 2421
Kitsap Community Resources, 4228
Kitten Who Couldn't Purr, 8718
Kitzmiller-Bales Trust, 2390
Kiwanis Camp Wyman, 8268
Kiwanis Club of Montavilla, 1021
Kleinert's, 462
Kluge Children's Rehabilitation Center, 6315
Knee Socks, 1107
Kneelkar, 83
Knit Pants, 1142
Knock Light, 501
Know Your Diabetes, Know Yourself, 8478
Know Your Eye, 8970
Knowing Your Rights, 4323
Knox County Council for Developmental Disabilities, 5791
Knoxville VA Medical Center, 5441
Ko-Man-She, 8269
Koicheff Health Care Center, 6903
Kokomo Rehabilitation Hospital, 6151
Kolburne School, 6814
Konocti Industries: People Services, 5667
Koret Foundation, 2354
Kostopulos Dream Foundation, 1052
Kreider Services, 5792
Kresge Foundation, 2585
Krieger Publishing Company, 1965, 2154, 8032
Kroepke Kontrols, 54, 62, 69, 73, 75, 77, 79, 86
Kuhn Employment Oppurtunities, 6543
Kuschall North America, 227
Kuschall of America, 665, 666, 667, 675
Kuzell Institute for Arthritis and Infectious Diseases, 4392
Kweebec, 8270

L

LA Lions Camp for Disabled/Diabetic Youth, 952
LA Lions LPDCI Camp Pelican, 8271
LA Lions League Crippled Child, 952
LC Technologies, 1176
LCAR, 5816
LD Child and the ADHD Child: Ways Parents & Professionals Can Help, 7478
LDOnLine, 5233
LDS Hospital Rehabilitation Center, 6306
LIFE Center for Independent Living, 3768
LIFE of Central Mississippi, 3961
LIFE of South Mississippi, 3962
LIFE/ Run Centers for Independent Living, 4169
LIFE: Fort Hall, 3746
LINC-Monroe Randolph Center, 3769
LINK: Colby, 3824
LINK: Hays, 3825
LJ Skaggs and Mary C Skaggs Foundation, 2355
LK Whittier Foundation, 2356
LPB Communications, 186
LPDOS Deluxe, 1408
LRP Publications, 1886, 1888, 1902, 4301, 4327, 6122
LS&S, 463, 473
LSDC News, 7860
La Frontera Center, 6364
La Leche League International, 5056
La-Z-Boy, 397
La84 Foundation, 2317
LaBac Systems, 718
LaFayette-Walker Public Library, 4444
LaPalma Intercommunity Hospital, 6452
LaRabida Children's Hospital and Research Center, 6136
LaSalle Chicago Community Trust, 2493
Lab School of Washington, 7340
Labeling the Mentally Retarded, 7479
Laboure College Library, 4520
Ladacain Network, 6882
Ladybug Corner Chair, 239
Lafayette Nursing and Rehabilitation Center, 7097
Laffey-McHugh Foundation, 2408
Lake Charles Memorial Hospital, 6173
Lake County Center for Independent Living, 3770
Lake County Health Department, 6678
Lake County Public Library Talking Books Service, 4472
Lake Erie College, 2281
Lake Michigan Academy, 2259
Lake Ridge Campus, 8185
LakeMed Nursing and Rehabilitation Center, 7208
Lakeland Center, 6836
Lakemary Center, 6747
Lakeshore Center for Independent Living, 3933
Lakeshore Foundation, 8099, 901
Lakeshore Learning Materials, 1645
Lakeshore Rehabilitation Facility, 5609
Lakeshore Rehabilitation Hospital, 6047
Lakeside Milam Recovery Centers (LMRC), 7036
Lakeview NeuroRehabilitation Center, 6204
Lakeview Rehabilitation Hospital, 6169
Lakeview Subacute Care Center, 7170
Lakewood Health Care Center, 7037
Lambs Farm, 5793
Lambton County Developmental Services, 822
Lamplighter's Work Center, 5877
Lanakila Rehabilitation Center, 5772
Land of Lincoln Goodwill Industries, 5794
Landmark Media, 4865, 4960, 5145, 7286, 8861, 9046
Lane Community College, 2282
Language Arts: Detecting Special Needs, 2068
Language Disabilities in Children and Adolescents, 8719
Language Learning Practices with Deaf Children, 2069
Language Parts Catalog, 1646
Language Tool Kit, 1647
Language and Communication Disorders in Children, 2070
Language and the Developing Child, 8720
Language, Learning & Living, 187
Language, Speech and Hearing Services in School, 1648
Language-Related Learning Disabilities: Their Nature and Treatment, 8721
Lanting Foundation, 2586
Laptalker, 1328
Laradon Hall Society for Exceptional Children and Adults, 6521
Large Button Speaker Phone, 188
Large Print DOS, 1409
Large Print Keyboard Labels, 1187
Large Print Loan Library, 8971
Large Print Loan Library Catalog, 8972
Large Print Recipies for a Healthy Life, 8973
Large Print Telephone Dial, 189
Large Print Touch-Telephone Overlays, 190
Large Type, 1522
Las Animas County Rehabilitation Center, 5702
Las Vegas Healthcare And Rehabilitation Center, 6867
Las Vegas Healthcare and Rehabilitation Ce nter, 7165
Las Vegas Veterans Center, 5493
Las Vegas-Clark County Library District, 4561
Latchloc Automatic Wheelchair Tiedown, 84
Late Talker: What to Do If Your Child Isn' t Talking Yet, 8722
Latex Allergy in Spina Bifida Patients, 8479
Laugh with Accent, #3, 4683
Laureate Learning Systems, 1410
Laurel Designs, 643, 1073, 1082, 1090, 1108, 1138, 4851, 8047
Laurel Designs Catalog, 1108

Laurel Grove Hospital: Rehab Care Unit, 6072
Laurel Hill Center Independent Living Program, 4112
Law Center Newsletter, 4324
Lawrence Productions, 1403
Lazy Days RV Center, 102
Lead Poisoning in Childhood, 8480
League Serving People With Disabilities, 955
League for the Blind and Disabled, 3798
League for the Hard of Hearing, 7710
League of Human Dignity, 3809
League of Human Dignity: Lincoln, 3996
League of Human Dignity: Norfolk, 3997
League of Human Dignity: Omaha, 3998
Leaning Tower Y MC A, 8100
Leaning Tower YMCA: Conquerors Gym and Swim Program, 8100
Learn About the ADA in Your Local Library, 4891
Learning About Numbers, 1344
Learning Activity Packets, 1511
Learning American Sign Language, 1649
Learning Among Children with Spina Bifida, 8481
Learning Company, 1411, 1345, 1490
Learning Corporation of America, 4679, 5149
Learning Disabilities Association of America, 7368, 7447, 7460, 7464, 7466, 7484
Learning Disabilities Association of Arkansas, 1890
Learning Disabilities Consultants, 1892
Learning Disabilities Consultants Newsletter, 1892
Learning Disabilities, Literacy, and Adult Education, 2071
Learning Disabilities: Concepts and Characteristics, 2072
Learning Disability: Social Class and the Cons of Inequality In American Education, 2073
Learning English: Primary, 1477
Learning English: Rhyme Time, 1478
Learning Independence Through Computers, 1262
Learning Services Corporation, 6223
Learning Services of Northern California, 6453
Learning Services: Bear Creek, 6522
Learning Services: Carolina, 6916
Learning Services: Harris House Program, 6632
Learning Services: Morgan Hill, 6454
Learning Services: Shenandoah, 6024
Learning Services: Supported Living Programs, 6455
Learning Tools International, 1394
Learning a Living: A Guide to Planning Yo ur Career and Finding a Job for People with ADD, 7480
Learning and Individual Differences, 2074
Learning disAbilities Resources, 7432
Learning to Listen, 1650
Learning to Play, 5123, 8974
Learning to See: American Sign Language as a Second Language, 2075
Learning to Sign in My Neighborhood, 1651
Learning to Use Cursive Handwriting, 1652
Learning to Use Manuscript Handwriting, 1653
Lebanon VA Medical Center, 5548
Lectra-Lift, 397
Ledgewood Rehabilitation and Skilled Nursing Center, 7154
Lee County Library System: Talking Books Library, 4421
Lee Memorial Hospital, 6591
Left Foot Accelerator, 85
Left Foot Gas Pedal, 86
Left Hand Shift Lever, 87
Leg Elevation Board, 502
Legacy Emanuel Rehabilitation Center, 6962
Legal Action Center, 4262
Legal Center, 4263, 4325
Legal Center for People with Disabilities & Older People, 3055
Legal Center for the Elderly and Disabled, 4264
Legal Right: The Guide for Deaf and Hard of Hearing People, 4326
Legal Rights of Persons with Disabilities: An Analysis of Federal Law, 4327
Legal-Ethical Considerations, Restrictions and Obligations for Clinicians, 2076
Legislative Handbook for Parents, 4265
Legislative Network for Nurses, 4328
Legler Benbough Foundation, 2357
Lehigh Valley Center for Independent Living, 4122, 4894
Leisure Lift, 557, 557
Leisure-Lift, 562
Leo P La Chance Center for Rehabilitation and Nursing, 7155
Leo Yassenoff JCC Day Camps, 1017
Leon S Peters Rehabilitation Center, 6456
Les Turne Amyotrophic Laterial Sclerosis Foundation, 2494
Leslie G Ehmann Trust, 2772
Lester Electrical, 646
Lester H Higgins Adult Center, 6941
Let Community Employment be the Goal for Individuals with Autism, 7481
Let's Count Braille and Tactile Numbers Po ster, 5283
Let's Eat, 8975
Let's Eat Video, 8976
Let's Read: A Linguistic Reading Program, 1654
Let's Talk About Having Asthma, 8482
Let's be Friends, 7861
Letter Writing Guide, 596
Lettering Guide Value Pack, 597
Lettie Pate Whitehead Foundation, 2455
Leukemia & Lymphoma Society, 8149
Leukemia Society of America, 8150
Levenger, 609
Leveron, 503
Levi Strauss Foundation, 2358
Levindale Hebrew Geriatric Center, 6790
Lewiston Public Library, 4497
Lewiston Rehabilitation and Care Center, 7106
Lexia I, II and III Reading Series, 1479
Lexia Learning Systems, 1479, 1487
Lexington Center for Health and Rehabilita tion, 7134
Lexington School for the Deaf/Center for the Deaf, 7724
Lexington School for the Deaf: Center for the Deaf, 7711
Lexington VA Medical Center, 5447
Liaison Computer Work Station, 1304
Liberator, 191
Liberty, 684
Liberty LT, 398
Liberty Lightweight Aluminum Stroll Walker, 625
Liberty Resources, 4123
Library Commission for the Blind, 4478
Library Cooperative/ Library for the blind, 4535
Library Manager's Guide to Hiring and Serving Disabled Persons, 2077
Library Resources for the Blind and Physically Handicapped, 8977
Library Services for the Blind, 8978
Library Users of America Newsletter, 8979
Library for the Blind & Physically Handicapped, 4615
Library for the Blind and Physically Handicapped, 4405
Library for the Blind and Physically Handicapped SW Region of Arkansas, 4380
Library of Congress, 8759, 8812
Library of Michigan Service for the Blind, 4530
Life Adventure Camp, 950
Life Adventure Camp of the Bluegrass, 950
Life After Trauma: A Workbook for Healing, 8483
Life Beyond the Classroom: Transition Str ategies for Young People with Disabilities, 5096
Life Beyond the Classroom: Transition Strategies for Young People, 4684
Life Center for Independent Living, 3771
Life Centered Career Education: A Contemporary Based Approach, 4th Edition, 2218
Life Development Institute, 7302
Life Line, 8484
Life Planning Workbook, 4685
Life Planning for Adults with Developmental Disabilities, 7644
Life Science Associates, 7426
Life Sciences Press, 8581
Life Service Network of Illinois: Springfi eld, 7575
Life Services Network of Illinois, 7576
Life Skills Foundation, 3974
Life Skills Laundry Division, 6728
Life Skills for Vocational Success, 6048
Life Way Christian Resources Southern Baptist Conv, 2185
Life and Independence for Today, 4124
Life of North Mississippi: Greenville, 3963
Life of North Mississippi: Tupelo, 3964
Life of South Mississippi: Biloxi, 3965
Life on Wheels: For the Active Wheelchair User, 8042
Life-Span Approach to Nursing Care for Individuals with Developmental Disabilities, 2078
LifeLines, 4892, 4996
LifeQuest: Interdisciplinary Rehabilitation, 4249
LifeSkills Industries, 6753
LifeSpan, 6917
LifeWay Christian Resources Southern Baptist Conv., 2141, 5055, 7760
Lifecourse Rehabilitation Services, 6890
Lifelong Leisure Skills and Lifestyles for Persons with Developmental Disabilities, 4893
Lifestand, 650, 695
Lifestyles of Employed Legally Blind People, 8980

Lifeway Church Resources, 7816
Lifeworks Employment Services, 6815
Lifts for Swimming Pools and Spas, 399
Light the Way, 8981
Lighthouse Central Florida (Formerly C.I.T.E), 5751
Lighthouse Central Florida Inc., 3712
Lighthouse International, 8785, 464, 5159, 7606, 7607, 7627, 8785, 8800, 8985, 9038, 9044, 9084, 9085
Lighthouse International Information and Resource Service, 9096
Lighthouse Low Vision Products, 464
Lighthouse for the Blind, 8836
Lighthouse for the Blind in New Orleans, 6770
Lighthouse for the Blind of Palm Beach, 6592
Lighthouse for the Visually Impaired and Blind, 6593
Lighthouse of Houston, 7010
Lightweight Breezy, 685
Lilac Blind Foundation, 4229
Lincoln County Health System, 6994
Lincoln Regional Office, 5490
Lincoln VA Medical Center, 5491
Lincoln YMCA, 8297
Lindustries, 503
Linguistics of ASL: An Introduction, 7862
LinkPower 50, 1188
Linking Employment Ability Potential: Independent Living Center, 4095
Lion, 8982
Lion's Blind Center of Diablo Valley, 6457
Lion's Blind Center of Oakland, 6458
Lion's Clubs International, 8982
Lions Camp Merrick, 7748
Lions Camp Tatiyee, 905
Lions Club Industries for the Blind, 6918
Lions Clubs International, 2283, 8786
Lions Den Outdoor Learning Center, 7341
Lions Services Inc., 6919
Lions World Services for the Blind, 6378
Lions of Multiple District 35, 925
Lipomas & Lipomyelomeningocele, 8485
Lippincott Williams And Wilkins, 2098
Lippincott Williams & Wilkins, 8313, 8408
Lippincott, Williams & Wilkins, 1960, 2084, 2086, 2087, 2118, 5060, 5070, 7609, 7629, 7642, 7656, 7659, 8443, 8510
Lisa and Her Soundless World, 7863
Lisle, 2284
Listen to Me, 7864
Listening and Talking, 7865
Literacy & Your Deaf Child: What Every Pa rent Should Know, 7866
Literacy Program, 1655
Literature Based Reading, 1656
Literature Journal, 7867
Little Children, Big Needs, 4686
Little City Foundation, 2495
Little Friends, 6679
Little People of America, 8151
Little Red Hen, 1412
Little Rock Vet Center #0713, 6379
Live Independently Networking Center, 4081
Live Independently Networking Center: Hickory, 4082
Live Oaks Career Development Campus, 6942
Livin', 4894
Living Beyond Multiple Sclerosis: A Woman 's Guide, 8486
Living Independence Network Corporation, 3747
Living Independence Network Corporation: Canyon County Satelite, 3748
Living Independence for Everyone (LIFE), 3726
Living Independent for Everyone (LIFE): Pocatello Office, 3749
Living Independently Now Center (LINC), 3772
Living Independently Now Center Inc., Twin Falls, 3750
Living Independently Now Center, Inc., 3751
Living Independently for Everyone (LIFE): Blackfoot Office, 3752
Living Independently for Everyone (LIFE): Pocate, 3752
Living Independently for Everyone: Burley, 3753
Living Independently for Today and Tomorrow, 3989
Living Independently for Today and Tomorrow: Glendrive, 3988
Living Skills Center for the Visually Impaired, 6459
Living Waters, 1036
Living Well With HIV and AIDS, 8487
Living Well with Asthma, 8488
Living Well with Chronic Fatigue Syndrome and Fibromyalgia, 8489
Living an Idea: Empowerment and the Evolution of an Alternative School, 1657
Living in a State of Stuck, 4895
Living in the Community, 4896
Living with Achromatopsia, 8983
Living with Asthma and Allergies Brochure Series, 8490
Living with Brain Injury: A Guide for Fam ilies, 8491
Living with Rheumatoid Arthritis, 8043
Living with Spina Bifida: A Guide for Fam ilies and Professionals, 8492
Livingston Center for Independent Living, 3934
Lloyd Hearing Aid Corporation, 320, 321, 324, 333
LoSeCa Foundation, 823
Lodi Memorial Hospital, 6073
Lodi Memorial Hospital West, 6073
Lok-Tie Shoe Laces, 1082
Lola Wright Foundation, 2861
Lollipop Lunch, 8723
Loma Linda University Orthopedic and Rehabilitation Institute, 6460
Long Beach Department of Health and Human Services, 3042
Long Beach Memorial Medical Center Memorial Rehabilitation Hospital, 6074, 7065
Long Beach VA Medical Center, 5388
Long Cane News, 8984
Long Handled Bath Sponges, 141
Long Island Alzheimer's Foundation, 2692
Long Island Center for Independent Living, 4050
Long Island Talking Book Library System, 4588
Long Oven Mitts, 354
Longman Education/Addison Wesley, 1938, 2057
Longman Group, 2149
Longman Publishing Group, 2015, 2121, 2197, 2200, 5103, 7890
Longreach Reacher, 504
Longstreet Press, 8323
Longwood Foundation, 2409
Look Out for Annie, 8985
Look Who's Laughing, 4897
Look, Now Hear This: Combined Auditory Training and Speech-Reading Instruction, 2079
Looking Good: Learning to Improve Your Appearance, 1413
Loop Scissors, 505
Loop the Loop, 8044
Los Angeles County Department of Health Services, 3043
Los Angeles Regional Office, 5389
Loss for Words, 7868
Lost Tree Village Charitable Foundation, 2445
Lotus Press, 8363
Loud, Proud and Passionate, 4898
Loudoun County Local Government, 1061
Loudoun County Special Recreation Programs, 1061
Louis A Johnson VA Medical Center, 5594
Louis R Lurie Foundation, 2359, 2359
Louis Stokes VA Medical Center, 5535
Louis and Anne Abrons Foundation, 2693
Louis de la Parte Florida Mental Health Institute Research Library, 4422
Louisiana Assistive Technology Access Network, 3173
Louisiana Association of Homes and Service for the Aging, 7577
Louisiana Center for Dyslexia and Related Learning Disorders, 3174
Louisiana Center for the Blind, 6771
Louisiana Client Assistance Program, 3175
Louisiana Department of Aging, 3176
Louisiana Department of Education, 1805
Louisiana Department of Education: Office of Special Education Services, 1805
Louisiana Developmental Disability Council, 3177
Louisiana Division of Mental Health, 3178
Louisiana Employment Service and Job Training Program Liaison, 5848
Louisiana Learning Resources System, 3179
Louisiana Protection & Advocacy for Persons with Developmental Disabilities, 3180
Louisiana State Library, 4492
Louisiana State University Eye Center, 6772
Louisiana State University Genetics Section of Pediatrics, 4493
Louisiana Vocational Rehabilitation Agency, 5849
Louisville Free Public Library, 4490
Louisville VA Medical Center, 5448
Louisville VA Regional Office, 5449
Lourdes Regional Rehabilitation Center, 6883
Lousiana State University, 6772
Love Publishing Company, 1758, 1855, 1949, 1973, 2164, 2173, 4315, 7523
Love: Where to Find It, How to Keep It, 4899
Loving & Letting Go, 4997
Loving Justice, 4329
Low Effort and No Effort Steering, 88
Low Tech Assistive Devices: A Handbook for the School Setting, 1658
Low Vision Clinic/UAB School of Optometry, 6343
Low Vision Questions and Answers: Definitions, Devices, Services, 8986

Low Vision Services of Kentucky, 6754
Low Vision Telephones, 607
Low Vision: Reflections of the Past, Issues for the Future, 8987
Lowe's Syndrome Association Conference, 1552
Lucy Lee Hospital, 6858
Luke B Hancock Foundation, 2360
Lumex Cushions and Mattresses, 267
Lumex Recliner, 240
Luminaud, 465, 457, 1324
Lung Cancer: Making Sense of Diagnosis, Treatment, & Option, 8493
Lung Line Information Service, 8652
Lupus: Alternative Therapies That Work, 8494
Lutheran Charities Foundation of St. Louis, 2607
Lutheran Library for the Blind, 4553
Lutheran Retreats, 7736
Lutherans Outdoors South Dakota, 8279
Lutherdale Bible Camp, 1066
Lyme Disease Foundation, 5234
Lynchburg Area Center for Independent Living, 4214
Lynde and Harry Bradley Foundation, 2911
Lyons Campus of the VA New Jersey Healthcare System, 5502

M

M ER S Goodwill, 6856
M Evans and Company, 5003
M&M Health Care Apparel Company, 1109
MA Report, 1893
MAClown Vocational Rehabilitation Workshop, 5752
MADAMIST 50/50 PSI Air Compressor, 307
MAGIC Foundation for Children's Growth, 2496, 8495
MAGIC Touch, 8495
MAP Training Center, 6680
MARC Enterprises, 6344
MCC Supportive Care Services, 824
MDA Newsmagazine, 1873
MEDLINE, 1263
MIW, 6729
MMB Music, 13, 19, 32, 46, 1618, 1704, 2058
MN Governor's Council on Development Disabilities, 4924
MOMS Catalog, 466
MOOSE: A Very Special Person, 4900
MSFOCUS Magazine, 8496
MTA Readers, 1659
MVP+ 3-Wheel Scooter, 558
MacDonald Training Center, 6594
MacMillan Publishing Company, 7835, 8616
Macomb Library for the Blind and Physically Handicapped, 4531
Macon Library for the Blind and Physically Handicapped, 4442
Macon Resources, 6681
Mad Hatters: Theatre That Makes a World of Difference, 2260
Mada Medical Products, 130, 296, 303, 304, 307, 311, 315, 620, 624, 625, 628, 629, 630, 633, 638, 688, 696
Madden Open Hearts Camp, 8272
Madison County Hospital, 7131
Madison County Rehab Services, 7131
Madison Healthcare and Rehabilitation Center, 7228
Madonna Rehabilitation Hospital, 6201, 7163
Magee Rehabilitation Hospital, 6257
Magic Wand Keyboard, 1305
Magination Press, 8362
Magnetic Card Reader, 355
Magni-Cam & Primer, 608
Magnifier Bookweight, 609
Maharishi Ayur-Veda Medical Center, 825
Maine Assistive Technology Projects, 3184
Maine Bureau of Elder and Adult Services, 3185
Maine CITE, 1264
Maine Department Of Labor, 5855
Maine Department of Health and Human Services, 3186
Maine Developmental Disability Council, 3187
Maine Division for the Blind and Visually Impaired, 3188
Maine Governor's Committee on Employment of the Disabled, 5856
Maine Human Rights Commission, 5857, 5857
Maine State, 4498
Maine State Library, 4498
Maine VA Regional Office, 5453
Maine Workers' Compensation Board, 3189
Mainland Center Hospital RehabCare Unit, 7011
Mainstream, 826, 3578, 5862, 2088, 4746, 4816, 5097, 5112, 5122, 5867, 6049, 6182, 7488, 8037, 8054, 8463, 8869
Mainstream Magazine, 4901
Mainstream Online Magazine of the Able-Disabled, 5235
Mainstreaming Deaf and Hard of Hearing Students: Questions and Answers, 2080
Mainstreaming Exceptional Students: A Guide for Classroom Teachers, 4th Edition, 2081
Mainstreaming and the American Dream, 8988
Mainstreaming the Visually Impaired Child, 8989
Mainstreaming: A Practical Approach for Teachers, 2082
Majors Medical Equipment, 686
Make-a-Friend, 1037
Makemie Woods Camp, 8273
Makemie Woods Camp/Conference Retreat, 8274
Making Changes: Family Voices on Living Disabilities, 4902
Making Choices for Independent Living, 3880
Making Informed Medical Decisions: Where to Look and How to Use What You Find, 4903
Making Life More Livable, 8990
Making News, 4749
Making News: How to Get News Coverage of Disability Rights Issues, 4330
Making School Inclusion Work: A Guide to Everyday Practice, 1660
Making Self-Employment Work for People wit h Disabilities, 4750
Making Wise Decisions for Long-Term Care, 4904
Making a Difference, 4905
Making a Difference: A Wise Approach, 4906
Making the Workplace Accessible: Guidelines, Costs and Resources, 4751
Making the Writing Process Work, 7482
Making the Writing Process Work: Strategies for Composition and Self-Regulation, 1661
Man's Low-Vision Quartz Watches, 610
Management of Autistic Behavior, 7483, 8497
Management of Children and Adolescents with AD-HD, 7484
Management of Genetic Syndromes, 8498
Managing Aging and Human Services Agencies, 7645
Managing Attention Disorders in Children: A Guide for Practitioners, 7485
Managing Diagnostic Tool of Visual Perception, 2083
Managing Post-Polio Syndrome, 8499
Managing Your Activities, 4907
Managing Your Fatigue, 8045
Managing Your Health Care, 4908
Managing Your Pain, 8046
Managing Your Symptoms, 7869
Managing the Symptoms of Multiple Sclerosis, 8500
Manatee Springs Care & Rehabilitation Center, 6110
Manchester Regional Office, 5497
Manchester VA Medical Center, 5498
Mandy, 4687
Manhattan Public Library, 4482
Manisses Communications Group, 5066
Manor Care Health Services- Citrus Heights, 6461
Manor Care Health Services- Palm Desert, 6462
Manor Care Health Services-Fountain Valley, 6463
Manor Care Health Services-Hemet, 6464
Manor Care Health Services-Sunnyvale, 6465
Manor Care Health Services-Tacoma, 7038
Manor Care Health Services-Walnut Creek, 6466
Manor Care Nursing and Rehab Center: Tucson, 6365
Manor Care Nursing and Rehabilitation Center: Boulder, 6523
Manor Care Nursing: Denver, 6524
Manor Care Ohio, 6523
ManorCare Health Services-Arlington, 7024
ManorCare Health Services-Lynnwood, 7039
ManorCare Health Services-Spokane, 7040
Manual Alphabet Poster, 1662
Manual of Sequential Art Activities for Classified Children and Adolescents, 24
Many Faces of Asthma, 8501
Many Faces of Dyslexia, 1663
Maplebrook School, 7342
Mapleton Center, 6098
March of Dimes, 5124, 8386, 8535
March of Dimes Birth Defects Foundation, 827
Marcia & Otto Koehler Foundation, 2862
Marfan Syndrome Fact Sheet, 5124
Margaret L Wendt Foundation, 2694
Margaret T Morris Foundation, 2309
Marianjoy Rehabilitation Hospital and Clinics, 6137
Marin Center for Independent Living, 3637
Marin Community Foundation, 2361
Mariner Health Care: Connecticut, 6101
Mariner Health of Nashville, 7229

Marion VA Medical Center, 5431
Marist Brothers Mid-Hudson Valley Camp, 8275
Mark B Wallner Foundation, 2618
Mark Elmore Associates Architects, 1567
Mark Seven Deaf Foundation, 7740
Marketing Your Abilities: A Guide for the Disabled Job-Seeker, 6049
Marquis George MacDonald Foundation, 2695
Marriage & Disability, 5125
Marriner S Eccles Foundation, 2878
Marshall & Ilsley Trust Company, 2915
Marshall & Ilsley Trust of Florida, 2447
Marshall University College Of Educational & Human, 4657
Martin Luther Home Of Colorado, 3664
Martin Luther Home Society Inc., 4558
Martin Luther Homes of Beatrice, 3999
Martin Luther Homes of Delaware, 3683
Martin Luther Homes of Indiana, 3799
Martin Luther Homes of Iowa, 3810
Martin Luther Homes of Nebraska, 4000
Martin Luther Homes of Texas, 4170
Martin Luther Homes: Colorado Springs, 6525
Martin Technology, 636
Martinez Center for Rehab & Extended Care, 5390
Martinsburg VA Medical Center, 5595
Marvelwood School, 7343
Marvelwood Summer, 7343
Mary A Crocker Trust, 2362
Mary Bryant Home for the Blind, 6682
Mary Free Bed Rehabilitation Hospital, 6837
Mary Lanning Memorial Hospital, 7164
Mary Reynolds Babcock Foundation, 2732
Mary's Call, 2608
Maryland Client Assistance Program Division of Rehabilitation Services, 3193
Maryland Department of Aging, 3194
Maryland Department of Disabilities, 1265
Maryland Department of Handicapped Children, 3195
Maryland Developmental Disabilities Council, 3196
Maryland Division of Mental Health, 3197
Maryland Employment Services and Job Training Program Liaison, 5863
Maryland Fair Employment Practice Agency, 5864
Maryland National Capital Park and Planning Commission, 959
Maryland State Department of Education, 5865, 4504
Maryland State Department of Education: Division of Special Education, 1807
Maryland State Library for the Blind and Physically Handicapped, 4504
Maryland Technology Assistance Program, 1265
Maryland Veterans Centers, 5458
The Mask of Benevolence: Disabling the De af Community, 7921
Mask of Benevolence: Disabling the Deaf Community, 7870
MasoniCare Corporation, 7077
Masonic Healthcare Center, 7077
Massachusetts Aging Services Association, 7578
Massachusetts Assistive Technology Partnership, 3202
Massachusetts Client Assistance Program, 3203
Massachusetts Commission for the Blind, 3900
Massachusetts Department of Education, 1806
Massachusetts Department of Education: Program Quality Assurance, 1806
Massachusetts Department of Mental Health, 3204
Massachusetts Developmental Disabilities Council, 3205
Massachusetts Eye & Ear Infirmary, 4519
Massachusetts Eye and Ear Infirmary & Vision Rehabilitation Center, 6816
Massachusetts Fair Employment Practice Agency, 5871
Massachusetts Governor's Commission on Employment of Disabled Persons, 5872
Massachusetts Office on Disability, 3203
Massachusetts Rehabilitation Commission, 4521
Massena Center for Independent Living, 4051
Mastering the Medicare Maze, 7646
Mat Factory, 651
Match-Sort-Assemble Job Cards, 1664
Match-Sort-Assemble Pictures, 1665
Match-Sort-Assemble SCHEMATICS, 1666
Match-Sort-Assemble TOOLS, 1667
Math Rabbit, 1345
Math for Everyday Living, 1346
Math for Successful Living, 1347
Matheny School and Hospital, 7960
Maumee Valley GSC, 8231
Maxi Aids, 467, 110, 135, 137, 140, 149, 151, 157, 189, 190, 236, 282, 285, 291, 313, 314, 335, 336, 339, 341, 344, 345, 347, 350, 351, 355, 356, 363, 382, 483, 486, 535, 537, 538, 541, 542, 545, 565, 590, 591, 594, 598, 602, 603, 611, 612, 613, 619, 626, 641, , 682, 713, 1225, 5268, 5269, 5270, 5271, 5272, 5273, 5274, 5275, 5277, 5278, 5279, 5283, 5290, 5291, 9088
Maxi Marks, 533
Maxi Superior Cane, 626
Maxi-Aids Braille Timer, 356
Maynord's Chemical Dependency Recovery Centers, 6467
Maynord's Ranch for Men, 6468
Mayo Clinic Scottsdale, 7059
Mayor of the West Side, 4688
Mc Farland & Company, 2077
Mc Graw- Hill, School Publishing, 2157
McAlester Regional Health Center RehabCare Unit, 6958
McCune Charitable Foundation, 2644
McDonald's Corporation Contributions Program, 2497
McFarland & Company, 1393
McGraw-Hill Company, 1777, 7, 2107, 4854, 8611
McGraw-Hill School Publishing, 1637, 1762, 1765, 1920, 1921, 1936, 2016, 2021, 2065, 2072, 2082, 2106, 2144, 2146, 2166, 8719
McGraw-Hill School Publishn, 2070
McGraw-Hill, School Publishing, 1706, 1992, 4744, 5041, 7486, 7487
McInerny Foundation Bank Of Hawaii,Corporate Trustee, 2466
McKey Mouse, 1306
Mclean Hospital, 7311
Me, Too, 4689
Meadowbrook Manor, 6469
Meadowood Springs Speech and Hearing Camp, 7749, 8686
Meadows Foundation, 2863
Meadowvale Health and Rehabilitation Cente r, 7124
Meadowview Manor, 6470
Measure of Cognitive-Linguistic Abilities (MCLA), 2219
Measurement and Evaluation in Counseling and Development, 1874
Mecalift Sling Lifter, 400
Med Camps Coordinator, 994
Med Covers, 659
Med-Camps of Louisiana, 8276
Med-Sell, 5236
MedDev Corporation, 308
MedEscort International, 5315
Medem Network Societies American Academy of Opthamology, 5237
Medford Rehabilitation and Healthcare Cent er, 7212
Medi-Grip, 309
Medic Alert Foundation, International, 8653
Medicaid Information, 8654
Medical Aspects of Disability: A Handbook For The Rehabilitation Professional, 4909
Medical Herbalism, 5126
Medical Rehabilitation, 2084
Medical Research Institute Of San Francisco, 4392
Medical University of South Carolina Arthritis Clinical/Research Center, 4616
Medicare Information, 8655
Medicare Maximization, 7647
Medicare and Medicaid Patient and Program Protection Act of 1987, 4331
Medicenter of Tampa, 6595
Medina Foundation, 2897
Mediplex Rehab: Camden, 6212
Mediplex Rehab: Denver, 6099
Mediplex Rehabilitation Hospital, 6184
Mediplex of Colorado, 6526
Mednet, 83
Medpro, 268, 269, 276, 277
Medpro Static Air Chair Cushion, 268
Medpro Static Air Mattress Overlay, 269
Meeting Life's Challenges, 438, 8354
Meeting the Challenge of Progressive Multiple Sclerosis, 8502
Meeting the Needs of Employees with Disabilities, 4910
Meeting the Needs of People with Vision Loss: Multidisciplinary Perspective, 8991
Meeting-in-a-Box, 1668
Mega Wolf Communication Device, 1329
Melwood Access Adventures, 5316
Memorial Hospital of Gardenia, 6471
Memorial Regional Rehabilitation Center, 6152, 6720
Memory Castle, 1480
Memphis Center for Independent Living, 4156
Memphis VA Medical Center, 5565
Men's/Women's Low Vision Watches & Clocks, 611
Meniere's Disease, 8503
Menopause without Medicine, 8504
Mental & Physical Disability Law Digest, 2085
Mental & Physical Disability Law Reporter, 4332
Mental Disabilities and the Americans with Disabilities Act, 4333, 4334

Mental Health Association in Pennysylvania, 3400
The Mental Health Center: Riverside Courtyard, 6876
Mental Health Commission, 4297
Mental Health Concepts and Techniques for the Occupational Therapy Assistant, 2086
Mental Health Law News, 4335
Mental Health Law Reporter, 4336
Mental Health Unit, 6699
Mental Health and Mental Illness, 2087
Mental Retardation, 7486
Mental Retardation: A Life-Cycle Approach, 7487
Mental and Physical Disability Law Reporter, 4337
Mentally Disabled and the Law, 4338
Mentally Ill Individuals, 2088
Mentally Impaired Elderly: Strategies and Interventions to Maintain Function, 7648
Mentally Retarded Individuals, 5097, 7488
Mentor Network, 6657
The Mentor Network, 6991
Merck Company Foundation, 2634
Mercy Dubuque Physical Rehabilitation Unit, 6730
Mercy Hospital, 6472
Mercy Medical Center Mt. Shasta, 7066
Mercy Medical Center-Pain Services, 6731
Mercy Medical Group, 6472
Mercy Memorial Health Center-Rehab Center, 6241
Mercy Subacute Care, 7132
Meridan Medical Center For Subacute Care, 6791
Meridian Valley Clinical Laboratory, 4649
Merion Publications, 1842
Merrill Lynch & Company Foundation, 2635
Merwick Rehabilitation and Sub-Acute Care, 7171
MessageMate, 1189
Metametrix Clinical Laboratory, 828
Metamorphous Press, 4798
Methodist Hospital Rehabilitation Institute, 6153
Metro Health: St. Luke's Medical Center Pain Management Program, 6943
MetroHealth Medical Center, 6944
MetroWest Center for Independent Living, 3901
Metrolina Association for the Blind, 5146, 8876
Metropolitan Center for Independent Living, 3947
Metropolitan Employment & Rehabilitation Service, 6856
Metropolitan Washington Ear, 192
Metzger-Price Fund, 2696
The Meyer Foundation, 2414
Miami Childrens Hospital, 8292
Miami Dade Public Library System, 4417
Miami Heart Institute Adams Building, 6596
Miami Lighthouse for the Blind, 6597
Miami VA Medical Center, 5418
Miami-Dade County Disability Services and Independent Living (DSAIL), 3713
Michael Reese Health Trust, 2498
Michigan Association for Deaf Hard Of Hearing, 7799
Michigan Association for Deaf and Hard of Hearing, 3209, 7712
Michigan Association for Deaf, and Hard of Hearing, 3210
Michigan Association of Homes and Serivces for the Aging, 7579
Michigan Career And Technical Institute, 6838
Michigan Client Assistance Program, 3211
Michigan Coalition for Staff Development and School Improvement, 3212
Michigan Commission for the Blind, 3213, 3215
Michigan Commission for the Blind - Gaylord, 3214
Michigan Commission for the Blind Training Center, 3216, 6839
Michigan Commission for the Blind: Detroit, 3936
Michigan Commission for the Blind: Escanaba, 3217
Michigan Commission for the Blind: Flint, 3218
Michigan Commission for the Blind: Grand Rapids, 3219
Michigan Commission for the Blind: Independent Living Rehabilitation Program, 3935
Michigan Council of the Blind and Visually Impaired (MCBVI), 3220
Michigan Department of Civil Rights, 5879
Michigan Department of Community Health, 3221
Michigan Department of Education, 1808
Michigan Department of Education: Special Education Services, 1808
Michigan Department of Handicapped Children, 3222
Michigan Department of Labor and Economic Growth, 3215
Michigan Developmental Disability Council, 3223
Michigan Employment Service, 5878
Michigan Fair Employment Practice Agency, 5879
Michigan Office of Services to the Aging, 3224
Michigan Protection & Advocacy Service, 3225
Michigan Psychological Association, 1739
Michigan Rehabilitation Services, 3226
Michigan Rehabilitation Services: Dept of Labor And Economic Development, 5880
Michigan Resources, 5817
Michigan State University, 4524
Michigan VA Regional Office, 5471
Michigan's Assistive Technology Resource, 4532
Micro Audiometrics Corporation, 330
Microcomputer Evaluation of Careers & Academics (MECA), 1512
Microsoft Accessibility Technology for Everyone, 5238
Microsystems Software, 1397
Mid-America Rehabilitation Hospital HealthSouth, 6166
Mid-Atlantic LifeSpan, 7580
Mid-Illinois Talking Book Center, 4459
Mid-Iowa Health Foundation, 2526
Mid-Michigan Industries, 6840
Mid-Ohio Board for an Independent Living Environment (MOBILE), 4096
Mid-state Independent Living Consultants, 4241
Mid-state Independent Living Consultants: Stevens Point, 4242
Middlebury College Press, 8547
Middleton Village Nursing & Rehabilitation, 7265
Middletown Regional Hospital: Inpatient Rehabilitation Unit, 6945
Mideastern Michigan Library Co-op, 4533
Midland Center for Independent Living, 3937
Midland Empire Resources For Independent Living (MERIL), 3975
Midland Memorial Hospital & Medical Center, 6290
Midland Treatment Furniture, 2089
Midtown Sweep: Grassroots Advocacy at its Best, 5127
Milbank Foundation For Rehabilitation, 2697
Miles Away and Still Caring: A Guide for Long Distance Caregivers, 4690
Milldale Camp, 960
Milton Schamach Foundation, 2636
Milwaukee Foundation, 2912
Mind Matters, 8589
Mind-Body Clinic, 829
Mind/Body Health Services, 830
Mindplay, 1340, 1489
Mini Teleloop, 193
Mini-Bus and Mini-Vans, 89
Mini-Max Cushion, 270
Mini-Rider, 90
Minneapolis Foundation, 2596
Minneapolis VA Medical Center, 5474
Minneapolis YMCA Camping Services, 8296
Minnesota Assistive Technology Project, 3231
Minnesota Association of Centers for Independent Living, 3948
Minnesota Board on Aging, 3232
Minnesota Children with Special Needs, Minnesota Department of Health, 3233
Minnesota Department of Labor & Industry Workers Compensation Division, 3234
Minnesota Disability Law Center, 3235, 3238
Minnesota Employment Practice Agency, 5883
Minnesota Governor's Council on Developmental Disabilities GCDD, 3236
Minnesota Health and Housing Alliance, 7581
Minnesota Library for the Blind and Physically Handicapped, 4546
Minnesota Mental Health Division, 3237
Minnesota Protection & Advocacy for Persons with Disabilities, 3238
Minnesota Rehabilitation Services, 5884
Minnesota STAR Program, 1266, 4819
Minnesota State Council on Disability (MSCOD), 3239
Minnesota State Services for the Blind, 3240
Minority Outreach Project, 4052
A Miracle to Believe In, 5045, 7363
Miracle-Ear Children's Foundation, 2549
Mirror Go Lightly, 289
Mirrored Lives: Aging Children and Elderly Parents, 7649
Mississippi Assistive Technology Division, 3243
Mississippi Association of Homes and Services for the Aging, 7582
Mississippi Bureau of Mental Retardation, 3244
Mississippi Client Assistance Program, 3245
Mississippi Department Of Human Services, 3247
Mississippi Department of Education, 1813

Mississippi Department of Education: Office of Special Services, 1813
Mississippi Department of Mental Health, 3246
Mississippi Department of Rehabilitation Services, 5888, 3245
Mississippi Division of Aging and Adult Services, 3247
Mississippi Employment Secutity Commission, 5889
Mississippi Library Commission, 4548
Mississippi Library Commission\Talking Book and Braille Services, 4549
Mississippi Methodist Rehabilitation Center, 6852
Mississippi Project START, 1267
Mississippi Society for Disabilities, 831
Mississippi State Department of Health, 3248
Mississippi State Independent Living Center, 3966
Mississippi State University, 1940, 1987, 2055, 4286, 5890, 8851, 8885, 8887, 8893, 8895, 8958, 8963, 8980, 8992, 9057, 9068, 9069
Mississippi: Workers Compensation Commission, 3249
Missouri Association of Homes for the Aging, 7583
Missouri Department of Elementary and Secondary Ed, 1812, 1812
Missouri Division of Mental Retardation & Developmental Disabilities, 3251
Missouri Easter Seal Society: Southeast Region, 6857
Missouri Fair Employment Practice Agency, 5891, 5891
Missouri Governor's Council on Disability, 5892
Missouri Job Training Program Liaison, 5893
Missouri Protection & Advocacy Services, 3252
Missouri Rehabilitation Services for the Blind, 3253
Missouri Vocational Rehabilitation Agency, 5894
Mobile Care, 5355
Mobile Infirmary Medical Center: Rotary Rehabilitation Division, 6050
Mobility, 229
Mobility International U SA, 2029, 5293
Mobility International USA, 7961, 2274, 2298, 2299, 4759, 4861, 4898, 5156, 7987
Mobility Training for People with Disabilities, 4998
Mobility Vehicle Stairlifts and Ramps, 91
Model E-90W Hearing Aid, 331
Model F-188T Hearing Aid, 332
Model Program Operation Manual: Business Enterprise Program Supervisors, 8992
Modular QuadDesk, 241
Modular Wall Grab Bars, 142
Moen Foundation, 2499
Moisture Seekers, 8505
Molded Sock and Stocking Aid, 290
MonTECH, 3257, 4556
Monarch Mark 1-A, 92
Monkeys Jumping on the Bed, 1414
Monkeys Jumping on the Bed IntelliKeys Overlay, 1190
Monmouth Vans, Access and Mobility, 93
MonoMouse Electronic Magnifiers, 612
Monroe Center for Independent Living, 3938
Montana Advocacy Program, 3258
Montana Blind & Low Vision Services, 3259
Montana Council on Developmental Disabilit ies, 3260
Montana Department of Aging, 3261
Montana Department of Handicapped Children, 3262
Montana Fair Employment Practice Agency, 5896
Montana Governor's Committee on Employment of Disabled People, 5897
Montana Independent Living Project, 3990
Montana Protection & Advocacy for Persons with Disabilities, 3263
Montana State Fund, 3264
Montana State Library-Talking Book Library, 4557
Montana VA Regional Office, 5485
Montezuma Day Treatment, 5610
Montgomery County Arc, 2829
Montgomery County Department of Public Libraries/Special Needs Library, 4505
Montgomery Field, 6420
Montgomery Independent Living Center, 3553
Moody Foundation, 2864
Moonrise: One Family, Genetic Identity, a nd Muscular Dystrophy, 8506
More Alike Than Different: Blind and Visually Impaired Children, 8993
More Food!, 1669
More Than Just a Job, 6051
More Work!, 1670
Morgan Stanley Foundation, 2698
Morongo Basin Work Activity Center, 5668
Morris and Gwendolyn Cafritz Foundation, 2422
Morse Code Equalizer, 1191
Morse Code WSKE, 1415
Mosaic, 3799
Mosaic-Pontiac, 3773
Moss Rehabilitation Hospital, 6258, 5302
MossRehab ResourceNet, 5239
Mother Father Deaf: Living between Sound and Silence, 7871
Mother Lode Independent Living Center, 3638
Mother Lode Rehabilitation Enterprises, 5669
Mother to Be, 4999
Mothers with Visual Impairments who are Raising Young Children, 8994
Motion Design, 685
Motivation Media, 8084, 9090
Motivational Services, 3872
Motor Speech Disorders, 8724
Motor Speech Disorders: Advances in Assessment and Treatment, 8725
Motorized Stander, 559
Mount Carmel Health & Rehabilitation Center, 7266
Mount Carmel Medical and Rehabilitation Center, 7267
Mount Shepherd Retreat Center, 1007
Mount Sinai Medical Center, 2699
Mount Sinai Medical Center Rehabilitation Unit, 6598
Mountain Home VA Medical Center, 5566
Mountain State Center for Independent Living, 4234, 4235
Mountain Towers Healthcare & Rehabilitation Center, 7271
Mountain Valley Care and Rehabilitation Ce nter, 7107
Mountaineer Spina Bifida Camp, 8277
Mouthsticks, 1192
Move With Me, 5128, 8995
Moxie, 560
Mozart Effect: Tapping the Power of Music to Heal the Body, Strengthen the Mind, 25
Mt Hood Kiwanis Camp, 1021
Mt Sinai Medical Center, 4424
Mt. Carmel Guild, 6884
Mt. Sinai, 7118
Mt. Washington Pediatric Hospital, 6181
Muhlenberg County Opportunity Center, 6755
Mulholland Positioning Systems, 242
Multi Resource Centers, 5885
Multi-Marketing & Manufacturers, 366
Multi-Scan Single Switch Activity Center, 1416
MultiGrowth Resources, 7521
Multidisciplinary Assessment of Children With Learning Disabilities and Mental Retardation, 2090
Multiple Choices Center for Independent Living, 3727
Multiple Phone/Device Switch, 194
Multiple Sclerosis, 8507
Multiple Sclerosis Center of Oregon, 8152
Multiple Sclerosis Foundation, 8153, 8496
Multiple Sclerosis National Research Institute, 5240
Multiple Sclerosis Q&A: Reassuring Answer s to Frequently Asked Questions, 8687
Multiple Sclerosis and Having A Baby, 8508
Multiple Sclerosis: The Guide to Treatmen t and Management, 8509
Multiple Sclerosis: A Guide for Patients and Their Families, 8510
Multiple Sclerosis: A Guide for the Newly Diagnosed, 8511
Multisensory Teaching Approach, 1671
Multisensory Teaching of Basic Language Skills: Theory and Practice, 2091
Muncie Family YMCA, 8208
Muncie Health Care and Rehabilitation, 7125
Muppet Learning Keys, 1417
Muscular Dystrophies, 8512
Muscular Dystrophy Association, 832, 1873, 8287
Muscular Dystrophy Association (MDA), 8197
Muscular Dystrophy Association Free Camp, 8278
Muscular Dystrophy and Other Neuromuscular Diseases, 8513
Muscular Dystrophy in Children: A Guide fo r Families, 8514
Muscular Dystrophy: The Facts, 8515
Mushroom Inserts, 333
Music Therapy, 26
Music Therapy and Leisure for Persons with Disabilities, 27
Music Therapy for the Developmentally Disabled, 28
Music Therapy in Dementia Care, 29
Music Therapy, Sensory Integration and the Autistic Child, 30
Music and Dyslexia: Opening New Doors, 31
Music for the Hearing Impaired, 32
Music: Physician for Times to Come, 33
Musical Mainstream, 8996
Muskegon County Library for the Blind, 4534

Muskogee VA Medical Center, 5536
Muu Muu, 1075
My Body is Not Who I Am, 4691
My Buddy, 4692
My Country, 5165
My First Book of Sign, 7872
My House Is Killing Me! The Home Guide for Families With Allergies and Asthma, 8516
My Own Pain, 1418
My Signing Book of Numbers, 7873
Mycoclonus Research Foundation, 4567
Myositis, 8517
Myositis Association, 8154
Myotherapy, 8997
Myths and Facts, 4339

N

N AH B Research Center, 1582
NAD Broadcaster, 4340
NADS News, 7489
NAMI Indiana, 6154
NAMI Texas, 3457
NAPVI, 4265, 8860, 8888, 8912, 8989, 9018
NBA Bulletin, 8998
NC State University, 777
NCD Bulletin, 4911
NCDE Survival Strategies for Oversease Living for People with Disabilities, 4912
NCI Affiliates, 5670
NCOD, 7818
NEXUS Wheelchair Cushioning System, 271
NHIF Newsletter, 5076
NHeLP, 4266
NIH Osteoporosis and Related Bone Diseases National Resource Center, 7962
NISH, 6025
NLP Comprehensive, 7303
NLS News, 8999
NLS Update, 9000
NMDVR/NMTAP, 3315
NOD E-Newsletter, 4913
NOLO, 4342, 4807, 7619, 7623, 7663
NORESCO Workshop, 5703
NYALD News, 1894
NYS Commission on Quality of Care & Advocacy for Persons with Disabilities, 3323
NYS Independent Living Council, Inc., 4053
NYSARC, 3324
Nabisco Foundation, 2637
Nancy's Special Workout for the Physically Challenged, 8047
NanoPac, 1373
Nansemond Pointe Rehabilitation and Health care Center, 7242
Nantahala Outdoor Center, 5317
Napa County Mental Health Department, 6473
Napa Valley PSI Inc., 5671
Napa Valley Support Systems, 6474
Narcolepsy, 8518
Nasheville Regional Office, 5567
Nashville Rehabilitation Hospital, 6271
Nashville VA Medical Center, 5568
Nasometer, 1463
Nassau County Office for the Physically Challenged, 4054
Nassau Library System, 4581
Nat l Council for Community Behavioral Healthcare, 1876, 4344
Nat'l Council for Community Behavioral Healthcare, 2136, 7653
Nathaniel and Elizabeth P Stevens Foundation, 2565
National 4-H Council, 2285
National AIDS Fund, 8155
National AIDS Hotline, 8656
National Accreditation Council for Agencies/Blind, 8857
National Allergy and Asthma Network, 1893, 8345, 8349, 8452, 8544, 8614, 8622
National Alliance for the Mentally Ill, 7440
National Alliance for the Mentally Ill of NY State, 3325
National Alliance of Blind Students, 9055
National Alliance of Blind Students NABS Liaison, 8787
National Alliance of the Disabled (NAOTD), 5241
National Alliance on Mental Illness (NAMI), 7304
National Amputation Foundation, 7549
National Arts and Disability Center (NADC), 34
National Assoc. of State Directors of DD Services, 4935
National Association for Continence, 8156, 8562
National Association for Down Syndrome, 7305
National Association for Drama Therapy, 35
National Association for Holistic Aromatherapy, 833
National Association for Home Care, 8657
National Association for Parents of Children with Visual Impairments (NAPVI), 8788, 9097
National Association for Visually Handicapped, 5242, 8789, 7281, 8848, 8849, 8852, 8881, 8886, 8891, 8902, 8914, 8915, 8919, 8926, 8932, 8937, 8946, 8971, 8972, 9012, 9021, 9073
National Association of Blind Educators, 8790
National Association of Blind Lawyers, 8791
National Association of Blind Musicians, 37
National Association of Blind Secretaries and Transcribers, 8792
National Association of Blind Students, 8793
National Association of Blind Teachers, 8794
National Association of Colleges and Employers, 1740
National Association of Developmental Disabilities Councils, 834
National Association of Guide Dog Users, 8795
National Association of Private Special Education Centers, 1741
National Association of Protection and Advocacy Systems, 835
National Association of School Psychologists, 1778, 1928, 1964, 2074, 2232
National Association of State Directors of Developmental Disabilities Services (NASDDDS), 836
National Association of State Directors of Special, 1885
National Association of the Deaf, 7713, 4340, 7684, 7756
National Association of the Physically Handicapped, 837
National Association to Advance Fat Acceptance, 8157
National Association to Promote the Use of Braille, 8796
National Ataxia Foundation, 8158
National Autism Hotline, 7543
National Black Deaf Advocates, 7714
National Brachial Plexus/Erb's Palsy Association, 8159
National Braille Association, 4582, 8797, 4582, 8874, 8998, 9064
National Braille Press, 8798
National Brain Tumor Foundation, 5243
National Business & Disability Council, 838, 5244
National Call Center, 1535
National Camp for Blind Children, 8799
National Cancer Institute, 8638
National Captioning Institute, 7715
National Car Rental System, 5356
National Catholic Office of the Deaf, 7716, 7927
National Center for Accessible Media, 8677
National Center for Education in Maternal and Child Health, 839
National Center for Homeopathy, 1742
National Center for Learning Disabilities, 1875
National Center for State Courts, 4267
National Center for Vision and Aging, 7614
National Center for Vision and Child Development, 8800
National Center for Youth Law, 4268
National Center on Birth Defects and Developmental Disabilities, 4443
National Cerebral Palsy of American, 3477
National Clearinghouse for Professions in Special Education, 1743
National Clearinghouse of Rehabilitation Materials, 7511
National Clearinghouse of Rehabilitation Training Materials, 5077
National Clearinghouse on Disability and Exchange, 4912
National Clearinghouse on Family Support and Children's Mental Health, 1796
National Clearinghouse on Postsecondary Education, 1776
National Coalition of Federal Aviation Employees with Disabilities, 2975
National College of Naturopathic Medicine, 840, 882
National Conference on Building Codes and Standards, 1568
National Council of Architectural Registration Boards (NCARB), 1569
National Council on Disability, 841, 2976, 4351, 4911
National Council on Independent Living, 842, 3686, 4230
National Council on Multifamily Housing Industry, 1586
National Council on Rehabilitation Education, 1744
National Council on the Aging, 7603, 7655
National Council on the Aging Conference, 1553
National Cued Speech Association, 8678
National Data Book of Foundations, 2951
National Deaf Bowling Association, 7874
National Deaf Education Network and Clearinghouse, 843, 7717

National Diabetes Action Network for the Blind, 8801
National Diabetes Information Clearinghouse, 8160
National Digestive Diseases Information Clearinghouse, 8161
National Directory of Corporate Giving, 2952
National Disability Sports Alliance, 8101
National Dissemination Center for Children and Youth with Disabilities (NICHCY), 844
National Division of the Blind and Visually Impaired, 2977
National Down Syndrome Congress, 7306
National Down Syndrome Society, 7307
National Early Childhood Technical Assistance Center, 845
National Easter Seal Society, 846
National Easter Seals, 939
National Easter Seals Chicago, 6931
National Education Association of the United States, 1745
National Endowment for the Arts Office, 1581
National Endowment for the Arts: Office for AccessAbility, 36
National Epilepsy Library (NEL), 4506
National Eye Institute, 5113, 8908, 8909
National Eye Research Foundation (NERF), 2500, 4460
National Family Association for Deaf-Blind, 7276, 7287
National Federation Of The Blind, 8790, 8791, 8792
National Federation of the Blind, 2550, 8802, 847, 848, 849, 851, 852, 5861, 8650, 8771, 8793, 8795, 8796, 8801, 8803, 8804, 8805, 8809, 8810, 8813, 8868, 8878, 8941, 8953, 8959, 8969, 9001, 9080
National Federation of the Blind: Blind Industrial Workers Division, 848, 8804
National Federation of the Blind: Computer Science Division, 849, 8805
National Federation of the Blind: Human Services Division, 8806
National Federation of the Blind: Masonic Square Club, 8807
National Federation of the Blind: Merchants Division, 847, 8803
National Federation of the Blind: Music Division, 37
National Federation of the Blind: Public Employees Division, 850, 8808
National Federation of the Blind: Science and Engineering Division, 851, 8809
National Federation of the Blind: Writers Division, 852, 8810
National Foundation for Facial Reconstruction, 2700
National Foundation of Wheelchair Tennis, 2363
National Fragile X Foundation, 8162
National Fraternal Society of the Deaf, 7718
National Guide to Funding Religion, 2953
National Guide to Funding for Children, Youth & Families, 2954
National Guide to Funding for Elementary & Secondary Education, 2955
National Guide to Funding for Libraries and Information Services, 2956
National Guide to Funding for Women and Girls, 2957
National Guide to Funding in Aging, 2958
National Guide to Funding in Arts and Culture, 2959
National Guide to Funding in Health, 2960
National Guide to Funding in Higher Education, 2961
National Guild of Hypnotists, 853
National Head Injury Foundation, 5076
National Headache Foundation, 2501
National Health Information Center, 7544
National Health Law Program, 4266
National Hemophilia Foundation, 2701, 8163
National Hookup, 4914
National Hydrocephalus Foundation, 8484
National Industries for the Blind, 8811, 9004
National Information Center for Children, 854
National Information Center for Children and Youth with Disabilities (NICHCY), 7277
National Information Clearinghouse on Children who are Deaf-Blind, 7278
National Institue Health, 4510
National Institute of Art and Disabilities, 17
National Institute of Arthritis, 8006, 8009, 8010, 8012, 8058, 8060
National Institute of Arthritis and Musculoskeletal and Skin Diseases, 7963
National Institute of Child Health and Human Development, 8658
National Institute of Health, 1239
National Institute of Neurological Disorders and Stroke, 7964
National Institute on Deafness and Other Communication Disorders (NIDCD), 7719
National Institute on Disability and Rehabilitation Research, 855, 4414
National Institutes of Health: National Eye Institute, 2978
National Jewish Center for Immunology, 8352, 8448, 8523, 8613, 8629, 8652
National Jewish Medical & Research Center, 4401
National Kidney and Urologic Diseases Information Clearinghouse, 8164
National Legal Center for the Medically Dependent, 4269, 4322
National Lekotek Center, 4461, 5284
National Library Office, 4601
National Library Service for the Blind, 16, 5119, 8873, 8875, 8879, 8916, 8977, 8996, 8999, 9000, 9025, 9026, 9028
National Library Service in Washington, 4602
National Library Services for the Blind, 9061
National Library Services for the Blind & Physically Handicapped, 8812
National Library of Medicine, 1253
National Managed Health Care Congress, 1554
National Maternal and Child Health Bureau, 856
National Mental Health Association, 857, 8165
National Mobility Equipment Dealers Association, 7965
National Multiple Sclerosis Society, 7966, 5733, 8467
National Neurofibromatosis Foundation The Childrens Tumor Foundation, 2702
National Offices, 771
National Organization of Parents of Blind Children, 8813
National Organization of the Senior Blind, 7584
National Organization on Disability, 858, 5245, 4733, 4913
National Parkinson Foundation, 7967, 1542, 1564, 8545
National Rehabilitation Association (NRA), 859, 5079, 6313
National Rehabilitation Center, 5246
National Rehabilitation Hospital, 6102, 1245
National Rehabilitation Information Center, 4507
National Rehabilitation Information Center (NARIC), 860, 7720
National Respite Locator Service, 861
National Right to Work Legal Defense and Education Foundation, 4270
National Service Dog Center, 8659
National Skeet Shooting Association, 8102
National Society for Experiential Education, 1746
National Society to Prevent Blindness, 8928
National Spinal Cord Injury Association, 8572, 8586
National Sports Center for the Disabled, 8103, 8631
National Stroke Association, 7550
National Stuttering Association, 8738
National Survey Of Americans With Disabilities, 4733
National Technical Institute For The Deaf (NTID), 7685
National Technical Institute for the Deaf, 7721
National Technology Database, 1268
National Theatre Workshop of the Handicapped (NTWH), 38
National Theatre of the Deaf, 39, 7722
National Vaccine Information Center, 862
National Voluntary Organizations for Independent Living for the Aging, 7585
National Wheelchair Poolplayers Association, 8104
National Women's Health Information Center, 5247
National Women's Health Network, 863
National-Louis University, 6134
Nationwide Foundation, 2754
Native American Advocacy Program for Perso ns with Disabilities, 4146
Native American Protection and Advocacy, 864
Natl. Clearinghouse for Alcohol & Drug Information, 2188
Natl. Organization for Parents of Blind Children, 8927
Natural Access, 687
Navarro Hospital, 6291
Navarro Regional Hospital: RehabCare Unit, 6291
Nazarene Publishing House, 4551
NeSoDak Bible Camp/Klein Ranch, 8279
Neal Freeling, 3220
Nebraska Advocacy Services, 3267
Nebraska Assistive Technology Partnership Nebraska Department of Education, 4559
Nebraska Association of Homes for the Aging, 7586
Nebraska Client Assistance Program, 3268
Nebraska Commission for the Blind & Visually Impaired, 3269
Nebraska Department of Education: Special Populations Office, 1817

Nebraska Department of Health & Human Services of Medically Handicapped Children's Prgm, 3270
Nebraska Department of Health and Human Services, Division of Aging Services, 3271
Nebraska Department of Mental Health, 3272
Nebraska Employment Services, 5898
Nebraska Fair Employment Practice Agency, 5899
Nebraska Library Commission: Talking Book and Braille Service, 4560
Nebraska Planning Council on Developmental Disabilities, 3273
Nebraska Vocational Rehabilitation Agency, 5900
Nebraska Workers' Compensation Court, 3274
NeckEase, 161
Needlepoint Daypoint, 8280
Negotiating the Disability Maze, 4693
Negotiating the Special Education Maze: A Guide for Parents and Teachers, 4694, 5033, 5042
Neisloss Family Foundation, 2703
Nejeda, 8281
Nek-Lo, Nek-Lo Hot and Cold Pillow-Perfect, Body Buddy, Hugg-L-O Pillow, 272
Nell J Redfield Foundation, 2619
Nelson Publications, 7541
NeuroControl Corporation, 5248
Neurobiology of Autism, 7490
Neuromotor Speech Disorders: Nature, Assessment, and Management, 8726
Neuropsychiatric Pain Rehabilitation Clinic, 6599
Neuropsychiatry of Epilepsy, 8519
Neuroscience Publishers, 7473
Nevada Assistive Technology Project, 3277
Nevada Bureau of Services to the Blind and Visually Impaired, 3278
Nevada Department of Education: Special Eduction Branch, 1822
Nevada Developmental Disability Council, 3279
Nevada Disability Advocacy and Law Center -Sparks/Reno Office, 3280
Nevada Division for Aging: Carson City, 3281
Nevada Division for Aging: Las Vegas, 3282
Nevada Division of Mental Health and Devel opmental Services, 3283
Nevada Fair Employment Practice Agency, 5901
Nevada Governor's Committee on Employment of Persons with Disabilities, 5902
Nevada State Library and Archives, 4562
Nevalyn F Nevil, Marna L Beatty & David Moxley, 4954
New Beginnings: The Blind Children's Center, 4393
New Courier Travel, 5343
New Directions Travel, 5344
New Directions for People with Disabilities, 2286
New England Center for Children, 6817
New England Regional Genetics Group, 4499
New England Rehabilitation Hospital of Portland, 6180
New England Rehabilitation Hospital: Massachusetts, 6185
New Eyes for the Needy, 8814
New Focus, 5835
New Hampshire Assistive Technology Partnership Project, 3288
New Hampshire Client Assistance Program, 3289
New Hampshire Commission for Human Rights, 3290
New Hampshire Department of Education, 1818
New Hampshire Department of Education: Bureau for Special Education Services, 1818
New Hampshire Department of Mental Health, 3291
New Hampshire Developmental Disabilities Council, 3292
New Hampshire Division of Developmental Services, 3293
New Hampshire Division of Elderly and Adult Services, 3294
New Hampshire Employment Security, 5905
New Hampshire Fair Employment Practice Agency, 5906
New Hampshire Governor's Commission on Disability, 3295
New Hampshire Job Training Program Liaison, 5907
New Hampshire Protection & Advocacy for Persons with Disabilities, 3296
New Hampshire Rehabilitation and Sports Medicine, 6873
New Hampshire State Library: Talking Book Services, 4563
New Hampshire Technology Partnership Project: Institute on Disability, 1819
New Hampshire Veterans Centers, 5499
New Hampshire Workers Compensation Board, 3287
New Harbinger Publications, 2026, 7637, 7644
New Hope Services, 5818
New Horizons Independent Living Center, 4695
New Horizons Rehabilitation, 5819
New Horizons Village, 3675
New Horizons in Sexuality, 4915
New Horizons: Alexandria, 3858
New Horizons: Monroe, 3859
New Horizons: Prescott Valley, 3573
New Horizons: Shreveport, 3860
New Jersey Association of Nonprofit Homes for the Aging, 7587
New Jersey Camp Jaycee, 992
New Jersey Center for Outreach and Services for the Autism Community (COSAC), 4568
New Jersey Commission for the Blind and Visually Impaired, 3301, 5931
New Jersey Council on Developmental Disabilities, 4930
New Jersey Department of Aging, 3302
New Jersey Department of Education, 1820
New Jersey Department of Education: Office of Special Education Program, 1820
New Jersey Department of Health and Senior Service, 3303
New Jersey Department of Health/Special Child Health Services, 3303
New Jersey Department of Labor & Workforce Development, 1269
New Jersey Developmental Disabilities Council, 4991
New Jersey Division of Mental Health Services, 3304
New Jersey Employment Service and Job Training Program Services, 5932
New Jersey Governor's Liaison to the Office of Disability Employment Policy, 3305
New Jersey Library for the Blind and Handicapped, 4569
New Jersey Medical School, 4566
New Jersey Protection & Advocacy for Persons with Disabilities, 3306
New Jersey Protection and Advocacy, 4009
New Jersey YMHA/YWHA Camps Milford, 7344
New Language of Toys: Teaching Communicati on Skills to Children with Special Needs, 5000, 5285
New Medico Community Re-Entry Service, 6841
New Medico Rehabilitation and Skilled Nursing Center at Lewis Bay, 6818
New Medico, Highwatch Rehabilitation Center, 6874
New Mexico Aging and Long-Term Services Department, 3309
New Mexico Client Assistance Program, 3310
New Mexico Commission for the Blind, 3311
New Mexico Department of Health: Children's Medical Services, 3312
New Mexico Employment Services and Job Training Liaison, 5945
New Mexico Governor's Committee on Concerns of the Handicapped, 3313
New Mexico Protection & Advocacy for Persons with Disabilities, 3314
New Mexico State Department Of Education, 4025
New Mexico State Department of Education, 1821, 1270
New Mexico State Library for the Blind and Physically Handicapped, 4570
New Mexico Technology Assistance Program, 1270, 3315, 4025
New Mexico VA Healthcare System, 5504
New Mexico Veterans Centers, 5505
New Mexico Workers Compensation Administration, 3316
New Mobility, 8048
New Music Therapist's Handbook, 40
New Orleans Resources for Independent Living, 3861
New Orleans Speech and Hearing Center, 6773
New Orleans VA Medical Center, 5451
New Quad Grip, 94
New State Office of Mental Health Agency, 3326
New Ventures, 5768
New Vision Enterprises, 6756
New Vision Store, 468, 5280
New Vistas, 4026
New Voices: Self Advocacy By People with Disabilities, 4916
New World Library, 8598
New York Association for the Learning Disabled, 1894
New York Association of Homes and Services for the Aging, 7588
New York Chapter of the Arthritis Foundation, 8002
New York City Campus of the VA NY Harbor Healthcare System, 5514
New York Client Assistance Program, 3327
New York Community Trust, 2704

New York Department of Handicapped Children, 3328
New York District Kiwanis, 999
New York Families for Autistic Children, 7491
New York Foundation, 2705
New York Public Library, 4583
New York Public Library: Andrew Heiskell Library for the Blind and Physically Handicapped, 4583
New York Regional Office, 5515
New York Service for the Handicapped, 7979
New York State Commisionon Qualityof Careand Advoc, 3334
New York State Commission for the Blind, 3329
New York State Commission on Quality of Care, 3330
New York State Congress of Parents and Teachers, 3331
New York State Department of Health, 1002, 1003
New York State Department of Labor, 5952
New York State Education Department, 1823, 1001, 3348
New York State Foundations, 2962
New York State Office of Advocates for Persons with Disabilities, 3332
New York State Office of Mental Health, 3333
New York State TRAID Project, 3334
New York State Talking Book & Braille Library, 4584, 9071
New York Therapeutic Riding Center, 865
New York University Medical Center, 4574
New York-Presbyterian Hospital, 6904
Newark Healthcare Center, 6946
Newark Regional Office, 5503
Newburgh Center for Independent Living, 4055
Newmarket Press, 5052
Newport County Arc, 2812
Newport County Chapter of Retarded Citizens, 5994
Newport Hospital, 6988
Newport News Public Library System, 4639
News from Advocates for Deaf-Blind, 7287
NewsLine, 5001
Newsletter of American Hearing Research Foundation, 7875
Newsletter of PA's AT Lending Library, 5129
Newsline for the Blind, 9001
Nexus Health Systems, 6303
Niagara Frontier Center for Independent Living, 4056
Nick Joins In, 8520
Nightshirts, 1126
Nine Lives Press, 516
Ninety-Second Street Y Camps Nesher Program, 1000
Nintendo, 5282
Nishna Productions-Shenandoah Work Center, 6732
No Barriers, 5166
No Boundaries, 555, 560
No Longer Disabled: The Federal Courts, 4341
No Longer Immune: A Counselor's Guide to AIDS, 2092
No More Allergies, 8521
No More Job Interviews!: Self-Employment Strategies for People with Disabilities, 6216
No Time for Jello: One Family's Experience, 8522
No-Run Nylon Stockings, 1110
NoBody's Perfect....Educating Children about Disabilities, 4696
Noble Centers, 5820
Nobody is Burning Wheelchairs, 8049
Nobody's Perfect: Living and Growing with Children Who Have Special Needs, 5054
Nocturnal Asthma, 8523
Nolo's Guide to Social Security Disability, 4342
Non-Hodgkin's Lymphomas: Making Sense of Diagnosis, Treatment & Options, 8524
Non-Traditional Casting Project, 41
Nonverbal Learning Disabilities at Home: A Parent's Guide, 8727
Norcliffe Foundation, 2898
Nordson Corporate Giving Program, 2755
Norfolk Foundation, 2887
Norman Marcus Pain Institute, 6905
North America Riding for the Handicapped Associati, 866, 8116
North Atlantic Books, 2000, 4789
North Auburn Rehabilitation And Health Center, 7252
North Broward Medical Center, 7087, 6600
North Broward Rehab Unit, 6600
North Carolina Accessibility Code, 1588
North Carolina Assistive Technology Project, 3355
North Carolina Association of Nonprofits for the Aging, 7589
North Carolina Children & Youth Branch, 3356
North Carolina Client Assistance Program, 3357
North Carolina Department of Insurance, 1588
North Carolina Department of Public Instruction: Exceptional Children Division, 1815
North Carolina Developmental Disabilities, 3358
North Carolina Division of Aging, 3359
North Carolina Division of Services for the Blind, 5957
North Carolina Industrial Commission, 3360
North Carolina Library for the Blind and Physically Handicapped, 4592
North Carolina Publc of Health, 3356
North Carolina State University, 4077
North Carolina Workers Compensation Board, 3354
North Central Alabama Mental Retardation Authority, 6345
North Central Florida Citrus County, 3714
North Central Independent Living Services, 3991
North Chicago VA Medical Center, 5432
North Coast Rehabilitation Center, 6075
North Country Center for Independent Livin g, 4057
North Country Independent Living, 4243
North Country Independent Living: Ashland, 4244
North Dakota Client Assistance Program, 3364
North Dakota Community Foundation, 2736
North Dakota Department of Aging, 3365
North Dakota Department of Education: Special Education, 1816
North Dakota Department of Human Services, 3366
North Dakota Department of Labor, Equal Employment Opportunity Division, 5965
North Dakota Employment Service and Job Training Program Liaison, 5966
North Dakota Governor's Committee on Employment of Disabled Persons, 5967
North Dakota State Library Talking Book Services, 4595, 4837
North Dakota VA Regional Office, 5529
North Dakota Vocational Rehabilitation Agency, 5968
North Dakota Workers Compensation Board, 3363
North District Independent Living Program, 3728
North Georgia Talking Book Center, 4444
North Hastings Community Integration Assoc iation, 867
North Hills Hospital, 7235
North Little Rock Regional Office, 5386
North Ridge Medical and Rehabilitation Cen ter, 7268
North Star Community Services, 4917
North Texas Rehabilitation Center, 7012
North Valley Rehabilitation Hospital, 6076
North Valley Services, 6475
Northampton VA Medical Center, 5463
Northeast Independent Living Program, 3902
Northeast Independent Living Services, 3976
Northeast Occupational Exchange, 5858
Northeast Rehabilitation Clinic, 7167
Northeast Rehabilitation Hospital, 6205
Northeastern Pennsylvania Center for Independent Living, 4125
Northern Arizona University, 6362
Northern Arizona VA Health Center, 5381
Northern Cartographic, 5306
Northern Illinois Center for Adaptive Technology, 1271
Northern Illinois Special Recreation Association (NISRA), 6683
Northern Nevada Center for Independent Living, 4822
Northern Nevada Center for Independent Living: Fallon, 4003
Northern Nevada Center for Independent Living: Reno, 4004
Northern New England Association of Homes and Services for the Aging, 7590
Northern New England Conference, 8829
Northern New Hampshire Mental Health and Developmental Services, 6875
Northern New York Community Foundation, 2706
Northern Regional Center for Independent Living: Lowville, 4058
Northern Regional Center for Independent Living: Watertown, 4059
Northern Utah Center for Independent Living, 4186
Northern Virginia Resource Center for Deaf and Hard of Hearing Persons, 4640
Northern West Virginia Center for Independent Living, 4236
Northland Library Cooperative, 4535
Northport VA Medical Center, 5516
Northridge Hospital Medical Center, 6077, 7067

Northridge Hospital Medical Center Rehabiltation Medicine, 6476
Northridge Hospital Medical Center: Center for Rehabilitation Medicine, 6477
Northside Mental Health Center, 1575
Northstar Community Services, 6733
Northview Developmental Services, 6748
Northwest Alabama Easter Seals Children's Clinic Rehabilitation Center, 6346
Northwest Arkansas Rehabilitation Hospital, 6056
Northwest Continuum Care Center, 7041
Northwest Hospital Center for Medical Rehabilitation, 6317
Northwest Kansas Library System Talking Books, 4483
Northwest Kiwanis Camp, 8282
Northwest Limousine Service, 5357
Northwest Medical Center, 6601
Northwest Ozarks Regional Library for the Blind and Handicapped, 4381
Northwestern Mutual Life Foundation, 2913
Northwestern University Multipurpose Arthritis & Musculoskeletal Center, 4462
Northwoods Lodge, 7253
Northwoods of Cortland, 7183
Norton- Lambert Corporation, 1170
Norwalk Hospital Section Of Physical Medicine And Rehabilitation, 6544
Norwalk Press, 8389
Norway Rehabilitation and Living Center, 7145
Norwegian Cruise Line, 5345
Nosey Cup, 357
Not Deaf Enough: Raising a Child Who is Hard of Hearing, 7876
Not Without Sight, 9002
Nothing is Impossible: Reflections on a N ew Life, 4918
Nova Care, 6366
Novartis Pharmaceuticals Division, 7500
Now Where Did I Put My Keys?, 7650
Nurse Healers: Professional Associates International, 868
Nursery Rhymes from Mother Goose, 7877
Nutritional Desk Reference, 4919
Nutritional Influences on Illness:, 4920
Nylon Snip Slip, 1156
Nylon Stretch Bra, 1157

O

O&P Almanac, 1895
O'Reilly, 8524
OASYS, 1513
OCCK, 1272
OMRON Foundation Omron Electronics Llc, 2502
ONLINE, 2220
OPTIONS, 3949
OPTIONS for Independence, 4186
OPTIONS for Independence: Brigham Satellit e, 4187
OR/ID Conference of United Methodist Church, 8286
OT Practice, 5098
OWLS: Oral and Written Language Scales LC/OE & WE, 2221
Oak Forest Hospital of Cook County, 6684
Oak Hill Nursing and Rehabilitation Center, 7220
Oak Leyden Developmental, 7292
Oak Spring Program, 7982
Oakcrest Care Center, 6963
Oakhill-Senior Program, 6964
Oakland County Library for the Visually & Physically Impaired, 4536
Oakland School & Camp, 7345
Oakland VA Regional Office, 5391
Oakland Work Activity Area, 5672
Oaks at Avon Nursing and Rehabilitation Ce nter, 7088
Oakwood Rehabilitation and Nursing Center, 7156
Oberkotter Foundation, 2789
Obesity, 8525
Obesity Sourcebook, 8526
Occulta, 8527
Occupational Asthma: Lung Hazards on the Job, 8528
Occupational Center of Hudson County, 5933
Occupational Center of Union County, 5934
Occupational Outlook Quarterly, 6318
Occupational Therapy Across Cultural Boundaries, 2093
Occupational Therapy Approaches to Traumatic Brain Injury, 2094
Occupational Therapy Strategies and Adaptations for Independent Daily Living, 6217
Occupational Therapy in Health Care, 1896
Occupational Training Center of Burlington County, 5935
Occuptational Training Center of Camden County, New Jersey, 5936
Ocean State Center for Independent Living, 4134
Oconee Regional Library, 4445
Office Of Grants Managment, 2492
Office Of Library & Information Services for the Blind and Physically Handicapped, 4614
Office for Students with Disabilities, University of Texas at Arlington, 4171
Office of Disability and Employment Policy, 1738
Office of Elderly Affairs, 3176
Office of Juvenile Justice and Delinquency Prevention, 5249
Office of Mental Health, 3326
Office of Policy, 2979
Office of Rehabilitation Services, 4135, 5995
Office of Special Education Programs: Department of Education, 2980
Office of State Coordinator of Vocational Education for Students with Disability, 5821
Office of Vocational Rehabilitation, 5985
Office of Vocational Rehabilitation Servic es (OVRS), 3391
Office of the Commissioner, 1269
Office of the Governor, 3430
Official Patient's Sourcebook on Cystic Fi brosis, 8529
Official Patient's Sourcebook on Muscular Dystrophy, 8530
Official Patient's Sourcebook on Post-Poli o Syndrome: A Revised and Updated Directory, 8531
Ohio Bureau for Children with Medical Hand icaps, 3372
Ohio Bureau of Worker's Compensation, 3373
Ohio Civil Rights Commission, 5973
Ohio Client Assistance Program, 3374
Ohio Coalition for the Education of Children with Disabilities, 1897
Ohio Commission On Minority Health, 5974
Ohio County Public Library Services for the Blind and Physically Handicapped, 4655
Ohio Department of Aging, 3375
Ohio Department of Education, 1824
Ohio Department of Education: Division of Special Education, 1824
Ohio Department of Health, 3372
Ohio Department of Mental Health, 3376
Ohio Developmental Disability Council, 3377
Ohio Governor's Council on People with Disabilities, 3378
Ohio Legal Rights Service, 3379
Ohio Regional Library for the Blind and Physically Handicapped, 4601
Ohio Rehabilitation Services Commission, 3380
Ohio Statewide Independent Living Council, 4097
Ohio and W Virginia Y MC A, 8295
Okada Specialty Guide Dogs, 8166
Okizu Foundation, 8236
Oklahoma Association of Homes and Services for the Aging, 7591
Oklahoma City VA Medical Center, 5537, 4808
Oklahoma Client Assistance Program, 3384
Oklahoma Department of Children with Disabilities, 3385
Oklahoma Department of Human Services Aging Services Division, 3386
Oklahoma Department of Mental Health & Substance Abuse Services, 3387
Oklahoma Department of Rehabilitation Services, 3388
Oklahoma Department of Rehabilitation Services (DRS), 5976
Oklahoma Employment Services and Job Training Program Liaison, 5977
Oklahoma Governor's Committee on Employment of People with Disabilities, 5978
Oklahoma League for the Blind, 6959
Oklahoma Library for the Blind & Physically Handicapped, 4603
Oklahoma Medical Research Foundation, 4604
Oklahoma State Department of Education, 1825
Oklahoma Veterans Centers Vet Center, 5538
Oklahoma Workers Compensation Board, 3383
Oklahomans for Independent Living, 4104
Old Adobe Developmental Services, 6478, 6485
Old Adobe Developmental Services-Rohnert Park Services (Behavioral), 6479
Old MacDonald's Farm Deluxe, 1419
Old MacDonald's Farm IntelliKeys Overlay, 1193
Older Adults with Developmental Disabilities: Optimizing Choice and Change, 7651
Omnicare Foundation, 2532
Omnigraphics, 445, 4853, 8325, 8346, 8361, 8366, 8418, 8526, 8537
On My Own, 3977
On Our Own Terms: Children Living with Physical Disabilities, 4697
On The Spectrum, 5167

On Your Behalf, 7652
On a Green Bus: A UKanDu Little Book, 1481
On the Edge of Deaf Culture: An Annotated Bibliography of Hearing Children/Deaf Parents, 7878
On the Level, 7879
On the Road to Autonomy: Promoting Self-Competence in Children & Youth with Disabilities, 5002
Once Upon a Time...Children's Classics Retold in American Sign Language, 7880
One Day at a Time: Children Living with Leukemia, 8532
One Thousand FS, 652, 714
One Two Three Sign with Me, 9003
One for All Lift All, 401
One-Step Communicator, 1330
One-Stop Service, 5753
Open Back Nightshirts, 1127
Open Back T-Shirts, 1134
Open Book, 1482
Open Road, 42, 5318
Open for Business, 5168
Open to the Public, 5169
Opening the Courthouse Door: An ADA Access Guide for State Courts, 4343
Operation Help: A Mental Health Advocate Guide to Medicaid, 7653
Operation Help: A Mental Health Advocate's Guide to Medicaid, 4344
Operation Job Match, 5733
Ophthalmic Research Laboratory Eye Institute/First Hill Campus, 4650
Oppenstein Brothers Foundation, 2609
Opportunities for Access: A Center for Independent Living, 3774
Opportunities for Independent Living, 4147
Opportunities for the Handicapped, 5673
Opportunity, 9004
Opportunity Center, 5727
Opportunity East Rehabilitation Services for the Blind, 6993
Opportunity Plus of NC, 869
Optelec U S, 1315, 1408, 1409
Optimum Resource, 1348, 1353, 1354, 1355, 1356, 1357, 1364, 1374, 1429, 1430, 1431, 1432, 1433, 1486, 1491, 1495, 1496, 1497, 1498, 1499, 1500, 1501, 1502, 1503, 1504, 1508, 1515
Optimum Resource Educational Software, 1348
Optimum Resource Software, 1483
Option Indigo Press, 4705, 5045, 7363
Options, 5099, 8533
Options Center For Independent Living: Bourbonnais, 3775
Options Center for Independent Living: Watseka, 3776
Options Interstate Resource Center for Independent Living, 3950
Options for Independence: Auburn, 4060
Options for Independence: Seneca Falls, 4061
Options for Independent Living: Fond du Lac, 4245
Options of Linn County, 6734
Options: Revolutionary Ideas in the War on Cancer, 8534
Optometric Extension Program Foundation, 2364, 8865
Oral/Facial Clefts Fact Sheet, 8535
Orange County ARC, 5674
Orange County Library System: Audio-Visual Department, 4423
Orchard Village, 5795
Ordean Foundation, 2597
Oregon Advocacy Center, 3392
Oregon Association of Homes for the Aging, 7592
Oregon Bureau of Labor & Industry, 5980
Oregon Clarion, 4921
Oregon Client Assistance Program, 3393
Oregon Commission for the Blind, 3394, 4113
Oregon Department of Education:, 1826
Oregon Department of Education: Office of Special Education, 1826
Oregon Department of Mental Health, 3395
Oregon Developmental Disability Council, 4921
Oregon Fair Employment Practice Agency, 5980
Oregon Health & Sciences University, 8152
Oregon Health Sciences University, 5539
Oregon Health Sciences University, Elks' Children's Eye Clinic, 4606
Oregon Nursing And Rehabilitation Center, 7209
Oregon Talking Book & Braille Services, 4607
Oregon Technology Access for Life, 3396
Organ Transplants: Making the Most of Your Gift of Life, 4922
Orientation and Mobility Primer for Families and Young Children, 9005
Oris B Hastings Charitable Foundation, 2503
Orthopedic Products Corporation, 231
Orthotics and Prosthetics Almanac, 8536
Orthotics and Prosthetics National Office, 8536
Oryx Press, 1779, 1656
Osage City Resource Center for Independent Living, 3826
Osborn Medical Corporation, 312
Oshkosh Medical and Rehabilitation Center, 7269
Ostberg Foundation, 2638
Osteoarthritis, 8050
Osteogenesis Imperfecta Foundation, 5250
Osteoporosis Sourcebook, 8537
Osterguard Enterprises c/o Jim's Shop, 655
Otitos Media in Young Children: Medical, Developmental, & Educational Considerations, 7881
Otto Bremer Foundation, 2598
Our Lady of Lourdes Medical Center, 6883
Our Lady of Lourdes Rehabilitation Center, 6172
Our Own Road, 5170
Our Way, 3579
Our World, 1875
Out and About: A UKanDu Little Book, 1484
Out of Darkness, 7492
Out of Left Field, 9006
Out of the Corner of My Eye, 9007
Out of the Corner of My Eye: Living with Vision Loss in Later Life, 9008
Out of the Fog: Treatment Options and Cop ing Strategies for ADD, 7493
Out-N-About American Walker, 627
Out-Of-Sync Child: Recognizing and Coping With Sensory Integration Dysfunction, 7494
Out-Sider III, 402
Outdoor Independence, 561
Outside in School, 7346
Outsider: The Life and Art of Judith Scott, 5171
Outsiders in a Hearing World, 7882
Oval Window Audio, 334
Over the Rainbow Disabled Travel Services & Wheelers Accessible Van Rentals, 5358
Overcoming Dyslexia, 7495
Overcoming Dyslexia in Children, Adolescents and Adults, 2095
Overcoming Mobility Barriers International, 1570
Overcoming Rheumatoid Arthritis, 8051
Overeaters Anonymous World Service Office, 8167
Overlook Lodge, 7735
Owl Publishing, 8395
Oxford Journals, 5081
Oxford Textbook of Geriatric Medicine, 2096
Oxford University Press, 2096, 2134, 2145, 4725, 4727, 4950, 7398, 7412, 8355, 8417, 8444, 8512, 8515, 8574, 8607
Ozark Independent Living, 3978

P

P A Department of Labor and Industry, 5986
P CI Education Publishing, 1389
P CI Educational Publishing, 1361, 1611
P ES CO International, 5950
PAC Unit, 95
PACE Center for Independent Living, 3777
PACE II, 8052
PACER Center (Parent Advocacy Coalition for Educational Rights), 870
PAL News, 4345
PALAESTRA: Forum of Sport/PE/Recreation for Those with Disabilities, 8105
PALS Support Groups, 8660
PARI Independent Living Center, 4136
PAT-3: Photo Articulation Test, 2222
PB News, 9009
PBA News, 9010
PCI, 5286
PDF News, 8538
PDF Newsletter, 8539
PDP Products, 8540
PEAK Parent Center, 871, 1780, 4923
PECO Energy Company Contributions Program, 2790
PEERS Program, 6078
PIRS Hotsheet, 6079
PKU for Children: Learning to Measure, 2097
PNC Bank Foundation, 2791
POZ Magazine, 8541
A PP A, 1589
PRIDE Industries, 5675, 6480
PRO-ED, 6053
PSP Advocate, 8542
PSS CogRehab Software, 1464
PVA Sports and Recreation Program, 5412
PWI Forum, 5885
PWI Profile, 5866
PXE International, 8661
Pac-All Carriers, 653
Pac-All Wheelchair Carrier, 653
Pace Saver Plus II, 562
Pacific Century Trust, 2464

Pacific Hospital Of Long Beach-Neuro Care Unit, 6481
Pacific Institute of Aromatherapy, 872
Pacific Islands Health Care System, 5427
Pacific Specialty & Rehabilitation Center r, 7254
Pacific Spine and Pain Center, 6965
Pacing Yourself, 8053
Paducah Centre For Health and Rehabilitati on, 7135
Pain Alleviation Center, 6906
Pain Centers: A Revolution in Health Care, 2098
Pain Control & Rehabilitation Institute of Georgia, 6633
Pain Erasure, 5003
Pain Institute of Tampa, 6602
Pain Treatment Center, Baptist Hospital of Miami, 6603
Palestine Resource Center for Independent Living, 4172
Palgrav Macmillan, 8310
Palm Beach County Library, 4428
Palm Beach Habilitation Center, 5754
Palmer & Dodge, 2558
Palmer Independence, 563
Palmer Industries, 561, 563, 564
Palmer Twosome, 564
Panhandle Action Center for Independent Living Skills, 4173
Panhandle Independent Living Services, 4001
Pantheon Books, 8700
Panties, 1158
Pants & Slacks, 1143
Paradigm Design Group, 1571
Paradise Vally Hospital-South Bay Rehabilitation Center, 6482
Paragon House, 8394
Parallels in Time, 4924
Paralysis Society of America, 5319
Paralyzed Veterans Of America, 5319
Paralyzed Veterans of America, 7968, 1571, 5300, 5412, 8093
Paraplegics and Quadriplegics, 8054
Paraquad, 3979
Parent Assistance Network, 8662
Parent Centers and Independent Living Centers: Collectively We're Stronger, 5004
Parent Connection, 3458
Parent Magic, 5141, 7380
Parent Professional Advocacy League, 873, 4345, 8660
Parent Survival Manual, 7496
Parent Teacher Packet, 5043, 8543
Parent as Parnters in Education of Alabama, 8663
Parent to Parent, 874
Parent to Parent of New York State, 3335
Parent's Guide to Allergies and Asthma, 8544
Parent's Guide to Autism, 7497
Parent's Guide to Down Syndrome: Toward a Brighter Future, 7498
Parent-Child Interaction and Developmental Disabilities, 5005
Parental Concerns in College Student Mental Health, 2099
Parenting, 5006
Parenting Attention Deficit Disordered Teens, 7499
Parenting Preschoolers: Suggestions for Raising Young Blind Children, 9011
Parenting with a Disability, 5007
Parents And Friends, Inc, 5676
Parents Helping Parents (PHP), 875
Parents Helping Parents: A Directory of Support Groups for ADD, 7500
Parents Supporting Parents Network, 3459
Parents and Friends, 6483
Parents and Teachers, 2100
Parents for Residential Reform, 876
Parents, Let's Unite for Kids, 1273
Paring Boards, 358
Park DuValle Community Health Center, 6757
Park Health And Rehabilitation Center, 7159
Park Manor Convalescent Center, 7042
Parker Bath, 403
Parker Foundation, 2365
Parker Publishing Company, 4800
Parker-Hannifin Foundation, 2756
Parkinson's Disease Foundation, 2504, 2707, 8538, 8539
Parkinsons Report, 8545
Parkview Acres Care and Rehabilitation Cen ter, 7161
Parkview Regional Rehabilitation Center, 6155
Parma Community General Hospital Acute Rehabilitation Center, 6229, 6947
Parrot Easy Language Simple Anaylsis, 1465
Parrot Software, 1457, 1465, 1485
Part B News, 7654
Part Two: A Preview of Independence and Transition to Community Living, 4734
Part of the Team, 4925
Partial Seizure Disorders: Help for Patients and Families, 8546
Partnering with Public Health: Funding & Advocacy Opportunities for CILs and SILCs, 4926
Partners Resource Network, 3460
Partners in Everyday Communicative Exchanges, 5078
Pasadena Foundation, 2366
Passion for Justice, 4927
Pathfinder, 1274
Pathfinder Parent Training and Information Center, 1274
Pathfinder Publishing, 8387
Pathfinder Village, 6907
Pathfinders for Independent Living, 3856
Pathways Brain Injury Program, 7136
Pathways for the Future, 4083
Pathways to Better Living, 8055
Pathways to Independence, 5937
Patient Lifting & Injury Prevention, 404
Patient Transport Chair, 688
Patient and Family Education, 2101
Patient's Guide to Visual Aids and Illumination, 9012
Patient-Centered Guides, 668, 4903, 4922, 5028, 5034, 5036, 8042, 8373, 8374, 8375, 8388, 8457, 8493, 8546, 8609
Patients-Centered Guides, 8317, 8318
Patricia Neal Rehab Center : Ft. Sanders R egional Medical Center, 6272
Patrick Rehab Wellness Center, 6994
Patrick and Anna M Cudahy Fund, 2914
Patriot Extra Wide Folding Walkers, 628
Patriot Folding Walker Series, 629
Patriot Reciprocal Folding Walkers, 630
Patterson-Barclay Memorial Foundation, 2456
Paul H Brookes Publishing Company, 1950, 2102, 4282, 5095, 5096, 5100, 5102, 6183, 7443
Paul and Annetta Himmelfarb Foundation, 2423
Paws for Silence, 7883
Peabody Articulation Decks, 1672
Peabody Early Experiences Kit (PEEK), 2223
Peabody Individual Achievement Test-Revised Normative Update (PIAT-R-NU), 2224
Peabody Language Development Kits (PLDK), 2225
Pearle Vision Foundation, 2865
Pearlman Biomedical Research Institute, 4424
Pearson, 2248
Pearson Education, 2022
Pearson Performance Solutions, 469
Pearson Reid London House, 470
Pedal Ease, 96
Pedal-in-Place Exerciser, 506
Pediatric Center at Plymouth Meeting Integrated Health Services, 6984
Pediatric Early Elementary (PEEX II) Examination, 2226
Pediatric Exam of Educational-PEERAMID Readiness at Middle Childhood, 2227
Pediatric Examination of Educational Readiness, 2228
Pediatric Extended Examination at-PEET Three, 2229
Pediatric Rehabilitation Department, JFK Medical Center, 6885
Pediatric Rheumatology Clinic, 4593
Pediatric Seating System, 273
Pediatric Visual Diagnosis Fact Sheets, 9013
Peer Counseling: Roles, Functions, Boundaries, 4928
Peer Mentor Volunteers: Empowering People for Change, 4929
Pegasus LITE, 1523
Peidmont Independent Living Center, 4215
Pencil/Pen Weighted Holders, 534
Penguin Books, 8422
Peninsula Center for Independent Living, 4216
Penitent, With Poses: An HIV+ Mother Refle cts, 8547
Penn State Milton S. Hershey Medical Center College Of Medicine, 6985
Penn West Conference Ucc, 1036
Pennstate, 6968
Pennsylvania Association of Nonprofit Homes for the Aging, 7593
Pennsylvania Bureau of Blindness, 3402
Pennsylvania Client Assistance Program, 3403
Pennsylvania College of Optometry Eye Institute, 4612
Pennsylvania Council on Independent Living, 4118
Pennsylvania Department of Aging, 3404
Pennsylvania Department of Children with Disabilities, 3405
Pennsylvania Department of Education: Bureau of Special Education, 1827
Pennsylvania Developmental Disabilities Council, 3406
Pennsylvania Employment Services and Job Training, 5986
Pennsylvania Governor's Committee on Employment of Disabled Persons, 5987
Pennsylvania Human Relations Commission Agency, 5988

Pennsylvania Pain Rehabilitation Center, 6986
Pennsylvania Protection & Advocacy for Persons with Disabilities, 3407
Pennsylvania Veterans Centers, 5549
Pennsylvania Workers Compensation Board, 3401
Pennsylvania's Initiative on Assistive Technology, 1275, 4126
Penrose Hospital/ St. Francis Healthcare System, 6517
People Against Cancer, 8168, 8548, 8533, 8534
People First International, 877
People First of Canada, 878
People Services, 6484
People and Families, 4930
People and Places, 5346
People to People International, 2287
People with Disabilities & Abuse: Implications for Center for Independent Living, 4931
People with Disabilities Who Challenge the System, 4932
People with Hearing Loss and the Workplace Guide for Employers/ADA Compliances, 4752
People's Voice, 4933
People-to-People Committee for the Handicapped, 879
People-to-People Committee on Disability, 880
People-to-People International: Committee for the Handicapped, 881
Peoria Area Blind People's Center, 6685
Peoria Area Community Foundation, 2505
Peoria Association for Retarded Citizens, 6686
Perennial Currents, 25
Perfect Solutions, 1194
Perigee Books, 7494
Perigee Visual Dictionary of Signing, 7884
Perkins Activity and Resource Guide: A Handbook for Teachers, 9014
Perkins Brailler, 535
Perkins School for the Blind, 9014
Perkins-Ponder Foundation, 2457
Permaflex Home Care Mattress, 162
Permobil, 715, 716
Permobil Max 90, 715
Permobil Super 90, 716
Perry Health Facility, 6111
Perry Point VA Medical Center, 5459
Perry Rehabilitation Center, 6367
Perry River Home Care, 3951
Perseus Publishing, 4715
Person to Person: Guide for Professionals Working with the Disabled, 2nd Edition, 2102
Personal Data Systems, 1320
Personal FM Systems, 195
Personal Guide to Living Well with Fibromyalgia, 8549
Personal Infrared Listening System, 196
Personal Perspectives on Personal Assistance Services, 4934
Personal Reader Department, 1291, 9015
Personal Reader Update, 9015
Personality and Emotional Disturbance, 2103
Perspective on Aging, 7655
Perspective: Parent-Child Folio, 7885
Perspectives, 4935
Perspectives on Prevention and Treatment of Cancer in the Elderly, 7656
Perspectives on a Parent Movement, 5008
Perspectives: Whole Language Folio, 8728
Pervasive Developmental Disorders; Finding a Diagnosis and Getting Help, 5034
Petaluma Recycling Center, 6485
Peter A Towne Physical Therapy Center, 6948
Peterson's Guide to Colleges with Programs for Learning Disabled Students, 2104
Pettigrew Rehabilitation and Healthcare Center, 7191
Phantom Compact Size Scooter, 565
Phantom Lake YMCA Camp, 8283
PharmaThera, 6995
Pharmacologic Therapy of Pediatric Asthma, 8550
Phelps School Summer School, 7347
Phenomenology of Depressive Illness, 2105
Philadelphia Foundation, 2792
Philadelphia Regional Office and Insurance Center, 5550
Philadelphia VA Medical Center, 5551
Phillip Roy, 1195
Philomatheon Society of the Blind, 6949
Phoenix Childrens Hospital (PCH), 8237
Phoenix Dance, 5172
Phoenix Veterans Center, 6368
Phone Manager, 1331
Phone of Our Own: The Deaf Insurrection Against Ma Bell, 7886
Phone-TTY, 197
PhoneMax Amplified Telephone, 536
Phonemic Awareness in Young Children: A Classroom Curriculum, 1673
Phonics for Thought, 1674
Phonological Awareness Training for Reading, 1675
Physical & Occupational Therapy in Geriatrics...Current Trends in Geriatrics Rehab, 7657
Physical Disabilities and Health Impairments: An Introduction, 2106
Physical Education and Sports for Exceptional Students, 2107
Physical Management of Multiple Handicaps: A Professional's Guide, 2108
Physically Handicapped in Society, 2109
Physically Impaired Association of Michigan, 4532
Pickens County Arc, 2819
Picture is Worth a Thousand Words for Blind and Visually Impaired Persons Too!, 9016
Piece of Cake Math, 1349
Pied Piper: Musical Activities to Develop Basic Skills, 43
Piedmont Living Center, 4215
Pilgrim Pines Camp, 914
Pillow Talk, 167
Pilot Books, 5298, 7643
Pilot Industries: Ellenville, 6908
Pine Castle, 6604
Pine Meadows Healthcare and Rehabilitation Center, 7230
Pine Tree Camp, 954
Pine Tree Society, 954
Pinecrest Rehabilitation Hospital and Outpatient Centers, 6112
Pinellas Talking Book Library for the Blind and Physically Handicapped, 4425
Pines Residential Treatment Center, 7025
Pioneer Center of McHenry County, 6687
Pioneer Vocational/Industrial Services, 5845
Pittsburgh Foundation, 2793
Pittsburgh Presbytery, 8254
Pittsburgh Regional Office, 5552
A Place for Me, 5138
Place of Their Own: Creating the Deaf Community in America, 7887
Place to Live, 4936
Placer Independent Resource Services, 3639, 6079
Places for People, 3980
Plan Ahead: Do What You Can, 8551
Planning Reasonable Accommodations: A Cost Effective Guide in a Legal Framework, 4271
Plastic Card Holder, 507
Platte River Industries, 6527
Play!, 1676
Please Don't Say Hello, 7501
Please Understand Me: Software Program and Books, 1420
Plenum Publishing Corporation, 4824, 7405, 7620
Plum Enterprises, 509, 1103
Plume, 8419
Pocatello Regional Medical Center, 6132
Pocket, 8441
Pocket Guide to the ADA: Accessibility Gu idelines for Buildings and Facilities, 4272
Pocket Otoscope, 310
Polaris Industries, 566
Polaris Trail Blazer, 566
Polio Connection of America, 8499
Polio Health International, 7969
Polio Network News, 8552
Polio Society, 7970
Polk Brothers Foundation, 2506
Polk County Association for Handicapped Citizens, 6605
Polyester Nancy Frocks, 1076
Polymyalgia Rheumatica and Giant Cell Arthritis, 8553
Pomerado Rehabilitation Outpatient Service, 6486
Pomona Valley Workshop, 5677
Pompano Rehabilitation and Nursing Center, 7089
Pond, 1421
Pool Exercise Program, 5173
Poplar Bluff RehabCare Program, 6858
Popular Activities and Games for Blind, Visually Impaired & Disabled People, 9017
Port City Enterprises, 6774
Port Jefferson Health Care Facility, 7184
PortaPower Plus, 1307
Portable Hand Controls, 97
Portable Large Print Computer, 1317
Portable Shampoo Bowl, 143
Portable Vehicle Controls, 98
Porter Sargent Publishers, 1759
Porterville Sheltered Workshop, 5678
Portland Naturopathic Clinic: NCNM National Health Centers Eastside Clinic, 882
Portland Public Library, 4500
Portland Regional Office, 5540
Portland VA Medical Center, 5541
Portneuf Medical Center Rehabilitation, 6642
Post Polio, 8554
Post-Polio Health, 8555
Post-Polio Health International, 7971, 8555, 8620

Post-Polio Support Group, 8664
Post-Polio Syndrome Information Book, 8556
Post-Polio Syndrome: A Guide for Polio Su rvivors and Their Families, 8557
Postgraduate Center for Mental Health, 4585
Posture-Glide Lounger, 689
Potomac Technology, 471
Potty Learning for Children who Experience Delay, 5174
Power Breathing Program, 1677
Power Door, 508
Power Seat Base (6-Way), 99
Power for Off-Pavement, 717
Power of Attorney for Health Care, 4346
PowerLink 2 Control Unit, 359
A Practical Guide to Art Therapy Groups, 4758
Practicing Rehabilitation with Geriatric Clients, 2110
Prader-Willi Alliance of New York, 8169
Prader-Willi Alliance of New York Annual Conference, 1555
Prader-Willi Alliance of New York Monthly Newsletter, 8558
Prader-Willi Syndrome Association USA, 8170
Prader-Willi Syndrome: Development and Ma nifestations, 8559
Pragmatic Approach, 2111
Prairie Cruiser, 690
Prairie Freedom Center for Independent Living, 4149, 4150
Prairie Freedom Center for Independent Living of Yankton, 4148
Prairie IL Resource Center, 3827
Prairie Independent Living Resource Center, 3828
Pre-Reading Screening Procedures, 2230
PreReading Strategies, 7888
Prelude, 144
Prentke Romich Company, 198, 183, 187, 191, 219, 220, 224, 500, 1302, 1453
Prentke Romich Company Product Catalog, 472
Preparation and Employment of Students, 5100
Preparing for ACT Assessment, 2231
Presby, 7217
Presbytery of Eastern Virginia, 8273, 8274
Preschool Learning Activities for the Visually Impaired Child, 9018
Preschoolers with Special Needs: Children At-Risk, Children with Disabilities, 2nd Edition, 2112
Prescott Public Library, 4374
Prescriptions for Independence, 7658
President's Committee for People with Intellectual Disabilities, 1747
President's Committee on Employment of Employment of the Disabled, 5796
President's Committee on People with Disabilities: Arkansas, 3032
President's Committee on People with Intellecutual Disabilities, 2981
Prevent Blindness America, 8815, 9009, 9010, 9094
Prevent Blindness Connecticut, 4406
Prevent Child Abuse of Metropolitan Washington, 8665
Preventable Brain Damage, 7502
Preventing Academic Failure, 2113
Preventing School Dropouts, 2114
Preventing Secondary Conditions Associated with Spina Bifida or Cerebral Palsy, 8560
Prevocational Assessment, 2115
Pride Industries: Grass Valley, 6487
Prima Publishing, 7379, 7461, 8383, 8697
Primacy Healthcare and Rehabilitation Cent er, 7231
Primary Children's Medical Center, 6307
Primary Phonics, 1678
Prime Engineering, 243, 243
Primer on the Rheumatic Diseases, 8056
Primrose Supported Employment Programs, 5755
Principal Financial Group Foundation, 2527
Print, Play & Learn #1 Old Mac's Farm, 1422
Print, Play & Learn #7: Sampler, 1423
Printed Rear Closure Sweat Top, 1135
Pro- Ed Publications, 2123, 2207, 2242, 2247, 6010
Pro- Max/ Division Of Bow- Flex Of America, 421
Pro-Ed, 1781, 1864, 1871, 2119, 2216, 7387, 8497, 8739, 9020
Pro-Ed Publication, 1903
Pro-Ed Publications, 28, 1628, 1675, 1854, 1859, 1863, 1879, 1934, 1961, 1968, 1969, 1981, 2003, 2013, 2069, 2095, 2114, 2117, 2120, 2155, 2160, 2167, 2180, 2181, 2183, 2195, 2196, 2204, 2206, 2222, 2234, 2243, 2244, 2245, 2246, 4748, 7483, 7527, 7889, 8400, 8736, 8883, 9074
Proceedings, 4937
Products for People with Disabilities, 473
Professional Books/Future Health, 8410
Professional Development Programs, 1811
Professional Fit Clothing, 1111
Professional Report, 5079
Profex Medical Products, 158
Programmed Phonics Books 1-2 & Cassettes, 1679
Programming Concepts, 1371, 1378, 1381, 1413, 1454, 1518
Programs for Aphasia and Cognitive Disorders, 1485
Programs for Children 3 to 5 with Disabili lities, 1001
Programs for Children Birth to 2 with Disa abilities, 1002
Programs for Children with Disabilities: Ages 3 through 5, 6156
Programs for Children with Special Health Care Needs, 1003, 6157
Programs for Infants and Toddlers with Disabilities: Ages Birth through 2, 6158
Progress Center South, 3778
Progress Center for Independent Living, 3779
Progress Valley: Phoenix, 6369
Progress Without Punishment: Approaches for Learners with Behavior Problems, 2116
Progress in Research, 7555, 8057
Progressive Center for Independent Living, 4019
Progressive Independence, 4105
Progressive Options, 4114
Project AID Resource Center, 8305
Project Freedom, 4020
Project Independence Supported Employment, 5679
Project LINK, 5867
Project LINK Guidebook, 6182
Projects W Industry Goodwill Industries of America, 5866
Promoting Communication in Infants and Young Children: 500 Ways to Succeed, 8729
Promoting Postsecondary Education for Students with Learning Disabilities, 2117
Prone Support Walker, 631
Prosthetics and Orthotics Center in Blue Island, 6688
ProtectaCap, ProtectaCap+PLUS, ProtectaChin Guard and ProtectaHip, 509
Protecting Against Latex Allergy, 8561
Protection & Advocacy Project, 3367
Protection & Advocacy System: Alaska, 3010
Protection & Advocacy for People with Disabilities, 3423
Protection & Advocacy for Persons with Developmental Disabilities: Alaska, 3011
Protection & Advocacy for Persons with with Disabilities: Arizona, 3022
Protection & Advocacy of Individual Rights, 3181
Protection and Advocacy (PA I), 3038
Protection and Advocacy Agency of Indiana, 6159
Protection and Advocacy Agency of NY, 3336
Protection and Advocacy System, 3544
Protestant Guild Learning Center, 6819
Providence Health System, 6080
Providence Holy Cross Medical Center, 6080
Providence Hospital Work, 6950
Providence Medical Center, 6319
Providence Regional Office, 5556
Providence Rehabilitation Services, 6320, 6320
Providence Speech and Hearing Center, 8679
Providence VA Medical Center, 5557
Provider Magazine, 5080
Providing Services for People with Vision Loss: Multidisciplinary Perspective, 9019
Prudential Financial, 2639
Prudential Foundation, 2639
Psoriatic Arthritis, 8058
Psy-Ed Corp, 4989
Psychiatric Institute of Washington, 6563
Psychiatric Mental Health Nursing, 2118
Psychiatric Services, 8131
Psychiatric Staffing Crisis in Community Mental Health, 1876
Psycho-Educational Assessment of Preschool Children, 2232
Psychoeducational Assessment of Hearing-Impaired Students, 7889
Psychoeducational Assessment of Visually Impaired and Blind Students, 2119, 9020
Psychological & Educational Publications, 2034, 2236, 2238
Psychological & Social Impact of Disabilit y, 4938
Psychological Software Services, 1464
Psychology and Health, 4939
Psychology of Deafness, 7890
Psychology of Disability, 4940
Public Health Reports, 5081
Public Health/State Capitols, 5082
Public Interest Law Center of Philadelphia, 3408, 4324
Public Law 101-336, 4273
Public Library Of Anniston-Calhoun County, 4364
Public Technology, 5359
Public Welfare Foundation, 2424
PublishAmerica, 8353

Publishers Group West, 8630
Publix Super Market Corporation Office, 2446
Publix Super Markets Charities, 2446
Pueblo Diversified Industries, 6528
Pueblo Goodwill Industries, 3665
Puget Sound Healthcare Center, 7255
Punctuation Rules, 1486
Purdue University, 8360, 8636
Pure Facts, 7503
Push to Talk Amplified Handset, 199
Push-Button Quad Cane, 632
Pushin' Forward, 5175
Putnam County Comprehensive Services, 5822
Putnam Publishing Group, 8460
Puzzle Games: Cooking, Eating, Community and Grooming, 5286
Puzzle Power: Sampler, 1424
Puzzle Power: Zoo & School Days, 1425
Puzzle Tanks, 1350

Q

Quad Canes, 633
Quad City Deaf & Hard of Hearing Youth Group: Tomorrow's Leaders for our Community, 7891
Quad Commander, 510
Quad Grip with Pin, 100
Quadtro Cushion, 274
Quaezar, 5719
Quality Care Newsletter, 8562
Quality Health Care Foundation of Wyoming, 7594
Quality of Life for Persons with Disabilities, 4941
Quan Yin Healing Arts Center, 883
Quantum Books, 4968
Quantum Technology, 5251
Quarterly Update, 9021
Queen Anne Health Care, 7043, 7043
Queen of Angels/Hollywood Presbyterian Medical Center, 6081
Queen of the Valley Hospital, 6082
Queens Independent Living Center, 4062
Quest, 6606
Quest Books, 33
Quest Camp, 7348
Questar Corporation Contributions Program, 2879
Questions and Answers: The ADA and Hiring Police Officers, 4274
Questions and Answers: The ADA and Persons with HIV/AIDS, 8563
Queue, 1341
Queue Inc., 1349
Queue Incorporated, 1387
Quick Reading Test, Phonics Based Reading, Reading SOS (Strategies for Older Students), 1487
Quick Talk, 1488
Quickie 2, 567
Quilted Waterproof Bib, 1112
Quincy Rehabilitation Institute of Holy Cross Hospital, 7018

R

RA Bloch Cancer Foundation, 2610
RA Rapaport Publishing, 8414
RAIL, 3981
RAMP Regional Access and Mobility Project, 3780
RB King Counseling Center, 6689
RC Baker Foundation, 2367
A RC Community Support Systems, 6672
A RC of Beaver county, 1026
RCI, 5946
RD Equipment, 138, 152
REACH Rehabilitation Program: Leader Nursing and Rehabilitation Center, 6886
REACH Rehabilitation and Catastrophic Long-Term Care, 6887
REACH of Dallas Resource Center on Independent Living, 4174
REACH of Dallas Resource on Independent Living, 4942
REACH of Denton Resource Center on Independent Living, 4175
REACH/Resource Center on Independent Living, 4176, 4275
REACHing Out Newsletter, 4942
REHAB Products and Services, 6690
RESNA Annual Conference, 1556
RET Project: (Rehabilitation Engineering Technology San Francisco State University, 8666
RI Services for the Blind and Visually Impaired, 5996
RIC Northshore, 6691
RIC Prosthetics and Orthotics Center, 6692
RIC Windermere House, 6693
RIC and Swedish Covenant Hospital Rehabilitation Services, 6694
RISE, 6735
RISE-Resource: Information, Support and Empowerment, 4177
ROHO, 270, 271, 273, 274
ROHO Group, 258, 264
ROW Adventures, 5347
RP Foundation Fighting Blindness, 8921, 8930
RP Messenger, 9022
RSA Union Building, 2990
RTC Connection, 4943
RULES: Revised, 2233
Race the Clock, 1489
Ragged Edge Magazine, 5083
Ragged Edge: The Disability Experience, 4944
Ragtime Industries, 6736
Rain Poncho, 1090
Rainier Vista Care Center, 7044
Raised Dot Computing, 1231, 9023
Raised Dot Computing Newsletter, 9023
Raised Line Drawing Kit, 537
Raising Kids with Special Needs, 5035
Rajesh, 8059
Raleigh Rehabilitation and Healthcare Cent er, 7192
Ralph H Johnson VA Medical Center, 5559
Ralph M Parsons Foundation, 2368
Ramah in the Poconos, 7750
Ramplette Telescoping Ramp, 405
Rampvan, 101
Rancho Adult Day Care Center, 6488
Rancho Los Amigos Medical Center, 6488
Rancho Los Amigos National Rehabilitation Center, 6083
Rand-Scot, 634, 383
Random House, 8331
Ranger All Seasons Corporation, 573, 576
Ransom Fidelity Company Foundation, 2587
Rascal 3-Wheeler, 568
Rascal ConvertAble, 569
Rasmuson Foundation, 2306
Rasmussen's Syndrome and Hemispherectomy Support Network Newsletter, 8171, 8564
Rational Effectiveness Training Systems, 5953
Raven Rock Lutheran Camp, 7349
Ray Graham Association for People with Disabilities, 6695
Raynaud's Phenomenon, 8565
Raytheon Company Contributions Program, 2566
Reach Rehabilitation Program: Americana Healthcare, 6696
Reaching the Autistic Child: A Parent Trai ning Program, 8566
Reaching, Crawling, Walking....Let's Get Moving, 5130, 9024
Reader Rabbit, 1490
Reader's Digest Foundation, 2708
Readers Digest Association, 2708
Reading Comprehension Series, 1491
Reading Is for Everyone, 9025
Reading Rehabilitation Hospital, 4613
Reading and Deafness, 2120
Reading for Content, 1680
Reading from Scratch, 1681
Reading in the Workplace, 1514
Reading with Low Vision, 9026
Reading, Writing and Speech Problems in Children, 7504, 8730
Readings on Research in Stuttering, 2121
Readings: A Journal of Reviews and Commentary in Mental Health, 1877
Readjusment Counciling Service Western Mountain Re, 5488
Real People Press, 8450
Reality of Dyslexia, 7505
Rear Closure Shirts, 1136
Rear Closure T-Shirt, 1137
Reasoning and Reading Levels I and II, 1682
Rebound Head Injury Recovery Services of the Carolinas, 6264
Rebound: Northeast Methodist Hospital, 6292
Rebsamen Rehabilitation Center, 6057
Receptive-Expressive Emergent-REEL-2 Language Test, 2nd Edition, 2234
Recipe for Reading, 1683
Reclining Power Wheelchairs, 718
Recognizing Children with Special Needs, 4698
Record Book for Individuals with Autism, 7506
Recorded Periodicals, 9098
Recording for the Blind, 9027
Recording for the Blind & Dyslexic, 8816
Recording for the Blind News, 9027
Recreation & Sports, 8106
Recreation Activities for the Elderly, 2122
Recreation Unlimited, 1018
Recreation Vehicles, 102
Red Notebook, 4508
Red Rock Center for Independence, 4188
Red Rock Center for Independence: Fillmore, 4189

Redman Apache, 691
Redman Crow Line, 692
Redman Powerchair, 246, 691, 692, 712, 717
Reduced Effort Steering, 103
Reference Manual for Communicative Sciences and Disorders, 2123
Reference Service Press, 2341, 2919, 2924, 2931, 2932, 2933, 2934, 2935, 2936, 2946, 2947, 2948
Reference and Information Services From NLS, 9028
Referring Blind and Low Vision Patients for Rehabilitation Services, 9029
Reflections on Growing Up Disabled, 4699
Regal Scooters, 570
Regent, 571
Regenta Park, 6584
Regional ADA Technical Assistance Center, 3307
Regional ADA Technical Assitance Agency, 6138
Regional Access and Mobilization Project (RAMP), 3781
Regional Access and Mobilization Project: DeKalb, 3782
Regional Assessment and Training Center, 5704
Regional Center for Rehabilitation, 6489
Regional Early Childhood Director Center, 3337
Regional Library, 4418
Regional Rehabilitation Center Pitt County Memorial Hospital, 6920
Regis College, 7360
Registry of Interpreters for the Deaf, 7723, 7892
Regular Kid, 8567
Rehab Care, 6775, 6957
Rehab Home Care, 6921
Rehab Institute at Florence Nightingale He alth Center, 7185
Rehab Pro, 1878
Rehab and Educational Aids for Living, 234, 238, 239
RehabCare, 6776
Rehabiliation Engineering Center for Personal Licensed Transportation, 5360
Rehabilitation & Healthcare Center Of Birmingham, 7054
Rehabilitation Achievement Center, 6697
Rehabilitation Associates, 6545
Rehabilitation Center Baptist Hospital, 6273
Rehabilitation Center at McFarland Hospital, 6274
Rehabilitation Center at Thibodeaux Regional, 6775
Rehabilitation Center for Children and Adults, 6607
Rehabilitation Center of Lake Charles Memorial Hospital, 6173
Rehabilitation Center of Palm Beach, 7090
Rehabilitation Counseling and Services: Profession and Process, 2124
Rehabilitation Engineering & Assistive Technology Society of North America (RESNA), 1276
Rehabilitation Engineering Research Center on Hearing Enhancement and Assistive Devices, 7724
Rehabilitation Engineering and Assistive Technology Society of North America (RESNA), 474
Rehabilitation Enterprises of North Easter n Wyoming: Newcastle, 4250
Rehabilitation Enterprises of Washington, 7045
Rehabilitation Gazette, 4945
Rehabilitation Hospital of Colorado Springs, 6100
Rehabilitation Hospital of Indiana, 7126
Rehabilitation Hospital of the Pacific, 6638
Rehabilitation Institute of Chicago, 807, 4735, 6691, 8083
Rehabilitation Institute of Chicago Learning Resource Center, 8107
Rehabilitation Institute of Chicago's Virginia Wadsworth Sports Program, 8632
Rehabilitation Institute of Chicago: Alexian Brothers Medical Center, 6698
Rehabilitation Institute of Ohio at Miami Valley Hospital, 6230
Rehabilitation Institute of Santa Barbara, 6490
Rehabilitation Institute of Sarasota, 6113
Rehabilitation Institute of Southern California, 6491
Rehabilitation International, 884, 1557, 1858
Rehabilitation Interventions for the Institutionalized Elderly, 2125
Rehabilitation Nursing for the Neurological Patient, 2126
Rehabilitation Opportunities, 6792
Rehabilitation Research & Training Center for Persons Who Are Hard of Hearing or Deafened, 7725
Rehabilitation Research Library, 4586
Rehabilitation Research and Development Center, 5392
Rehabilitation Resource Manual: VISION, 2127
Rehabilitation Resource University, 2030
Rehabilitation Service of North Central Ohio, 4098
Rehabilitation Services, 885, 6933
Rehabilitation Services Administration, 5734, 6370, 5063
Rehabilitation Services Administration of the District of Columbia, 886
Rehabilitation Specialists, 6888
Rehabilitation Technology, 2128
Rehabilitation Technology Association Conference, 1558
Rehabilitation and Healthcare Center of Almanace, 7193
Rehabilitation and Healthcare Center of Mo nroe, 7194
Rehabilitation and Healthcare Center of Ta mpa, 7091
Rehabilitation and Research Center Virginia Commonwealth University, 7243
Rehabilitation in the Aging, 7659
Rehabilitative Services Administration, 2982
Reinberger Foundation, 2757
Reiter's Syndrome, 8568
Reizen Braille Labeler, 538
Relationship Development Intervention with Young Children, 7507
Relax-A-Flex, 259, 261
Relaxation Techniques for People with Special Needs, 4946
Relaxation: A Comprehensive Manual for Adults and Children with Special Needs, 4947
Reliance House, 6546
Religious Signing: A Comprehensive Guide for All Faiths, 7893
Remedial and Special Education, 1879
Removing the Barriers: Accessibility Guidelines and Specifications, 1589
Renaissance Center, 6608
Renaissance Clubhouse, 3903
Renaissance at 87th Street, 7114
Renaissance at Hillside, 7115
Renaissance at Midway, 7116
Renaissance at South Shore, 7117
Reno Regional Office, 5494
Report Writing in Assessment and Evaluation, 2129
Report on Disability Programs, 2963
Research & Training Center on Mental Health for Hard of Hearing Persons, 4394
Research Press, 1782, 1763, 1912, 2137, 4809, 4869, 4880, 4946, 4947, 4959, 5065, 7283, 7471
Research and Training Center, 4943
Research for Rett Foundation, 4365
Research to Prevent Blindness, 2709, 8913
Research!America, 5252
Resource Center for Accessible Living, 4063
Resource Center for Independent Living, 1277
Resource Center for Independent Living of Osage, 3832
Resource Center for Independent Living: Bu rlington, 3830
Resource Center for Independent Living: El Dorado, 3831
Resource Center for Independent Living: Emporia, 3829
Resource Center for Independent Living: Fo rt Scott, 3832
Resource Center for Independent Living: Minot, 4090
Resource Center for Independent Living: Ot tawa, 3833
Resource Center for the Handicapped, 4231
Resource List for Persons with Low Vision, 9030
Resourceful Woman, 4735
Resources for Children with Special Needs, 4709, 4711, 4782, 4818, 7512
Resources for Family Centered Intervention for Infants, Toddlers, and Preschoolers, 9031
Resources for Independence, 3881
Resources for Independent Living, 3640, 3882, 4217
Resources for Independent Living: Baton Ro ge, 3862
Resources for Independent Living: Baton Rouge, 3861
Resources for Independent Living: Metairie, 3863
Resources for People with Disabilities and Chronic Conditions, 4948
Resources for Rehabilitation, 2130, 2127, 4910, 4948, 8991, 9019
Resources in Special Education, 1901
Resourcing: Handbook for Special Education Resource Teachers, 1684
Respiratory Health Association, 5320
Respironics, 295
Restructuring High Schools for All Students: Taking Inclusion to the Next Level, 2131
Restructuring for Caring and Effective Education: Administrative Guide, 2132
Resurrection Children's Center, 7026

Retaining At-Risk Students: The Role of Career and Vocational Education, 6231
Retarded Isn't Stupid, Mom!, 7508
Rethinking Attention Deficit Disorder, 7509
Retirement Research Foundation, 2507
Rewarding Speech, 1685
Rheumatoid Arthritis, 8060
Rhode Island Arc, 2813
Rhode Island Association of Facilities for the Aging, 7595
Rhode Island Department Health, 3412
Rhode Island Department of Education: Office of Special Needs, 1828
Rhode Island Department of Elderly Affairs, 3413
Rhode Island Department of Mental Health, 3414
Rhode Island Developmental Disabilities Council, 3415
Rhode Island Disability Law Center, 3418
Rhode Island Foundation, 2814
Rhode Island Governor's Commission on Disabilities, 3416
Rhode Island Parent Information Network, 3417
Rhode Island Protection & Advocacy for Persons with Disabilities, 3418
Rhode Island Services for the Blind and Visually Impaired, 3419
Rhodes Hearing, 331, 332
Rich Foundation, 2458
Richard L Roudebush VA Medical Center, 5435
Richard W Higgins Charitable Foundation M And I Marshall And Ilsley Bank, 2447
Richmond Research Training Center, 6026
Rickshaw Exerciser, 406
Ricon, 58, 90, 99
Ricon Corporation, 407
Riddle of Autism: A Psychological Analysis, 7510
Ride the Red Cycle, 8569
Rifin Family/Daughters of Israel, 1748
Right Hand Turn Signal Switch Lever, 104
Right Turn, 1351
Right at Home, 5176
Rights of People Who Are HIV Positive, 8570
Rigid Aluminum Cane with Golf Grip, 613
Riley Child Development Center, 6160
Rimland Services for Autistic Citizens, 7350
Ring-a-Lite, 200
Rinz-L-O Pillow Company, 272
Rio Vista Rehabilitation Hospital, 6293
Ripley Healthcare and Rehabilitation Cente r, 7232
Rita J and Stanley H Kaplan Foundation, 2710
River Odysseys West: ROW, 5348
River View School, 1786
The River: A Journey to the Source of HIV and AIDS, 8600
Riverdeep Incorporated, 1449
Riverside Community Hospital, 7068
Riverside Lutheran Bible Camp, 946
Riverside Medical Center, 6699
Road Ahead: Transition to Adult Life for Persons with Disabilities, 4753
Roadster 20, 572
Roanoke City Public Library System, 4641
Roanoke Memorial Hospital, 7027
Roanoke Regional Office, 5584
Robert Campeau Family Foundation, 2758
Robert Ellis Simon Foundation, 2369
Robert J Dole VA Medical Center, 5446
Robert Rose, 8391
Robert Scheuer, 2405
Robert Sterling Clark Foundation, 2711
Robert Wood Johnson Foundation, 2640
Robert Young Mental Health Center Division of Trinity Regional Haelth System, 6700
Robey W Estes Family Foundation, 2888
Robey W Estes Jr, 2888
RoboMath, 1352
Rochester Area Foundation, 2599
Rochester Institute Of Technology, 4589
Rochester Rotary Club, 1004
Rochester Rotary Sunshine Camp, 1004
Rocker Balance Square, 511
Rockland Independent Living Center, 4064
Rockwell Foundation, 2866
Rocky Mountain Chapter of the Arthritis Foundation, 8000
Rocky Mountain Conference of the, 920
Rocky Mountain Resource & Training Institute, 6052
Rocky Mountain Village, 921
Rodale Press, 4859
Rodeo, 1426
Rodeo IntelliKeys Overlay, 1196
Roger Randall Center, 6781
Role Portrayal and Stereotyping on Television, 4949
Rolf Institute, 887
Roll Chair, 244
Rollin M Gerstacker Foundation, 2588
Rolling Along with Goldilocks and the Thre e Bears, 4700
Rolling Hills Country Day Camp, 7351
Rolling Start, 3641
Rolling Start: Victorville, 3642
Rolls 2000 Series, 693
Rome Subregional Library for the Blind and Physically Handicapped, 4446
Ronald McDonald House, 888
Ronald McDonald House of California, 8239
Room Valet Visual-Tactile Alerting System, 201
Rosalind Russell Medical Research Center for Arthritis, 4395
Rose-Colored Glasses, 9032
Roseburg VA Medical Center, 5542
Rosen Publishing Group, 4673, 7433, 8397, 8399, 8402, 8403
Rosen Publishing Group's PowerKids Press, 8482
Rosewood Center, 6793
Rosomoff Comprehensive Pain Center, The, 6609
Rotary International, 2288
Rotary Youth Exchange, 2288
Route 52 Salisbury Turnpike, 7321
Rowan Community, 7074
Rowan County Vocational Workshop, 5958
Roy and Christine Sturgis Charitable Trust, 2311
Ruben Center for Independent Living, 3800
Rubicon Programs, 6492
Rule-ette, 1686
Rural Center for Independent Living, 4005
Rush Copley Medical Center-Rehab Neuro Physical Unit, 6139
Rush Hayward Masonic Fund, 2508
Rusk Institute of Rehabilitation Medicine, 6218
Rutherford Vocational Workshop, 5959
Rutland Mental Health Services, 7020
Rutledge Hill Press, 8322
Ryland Group Corporate Giving Program, 2551

S

S W Georgia Regional Library, 4436
SACC Assistive Technoloy Center, 1278
SAILS, 4178
SAMHSA News, 1898
SAYdee Posters, 1687
SB Waterman & E Blade Charitable Foundation, 2915
SC Department of Health and Environmental Control, 1044
SC Independent Living Council, 4141
SCARC, Inc Evaluation, Training + Emplomen t Center, 5756
SCCIL at Titusville, 3715
SCENE, 9033
SCI Psychosocial Process, 8571
SCI/LIFE, 8572
SCI: Six County, 6951
SE Alaska ILC: Ketchikan, 3563
SE Alaska Independent Living Center (SAIL), 3564
SE Alaska Independent Living: Sitka, 3565
SEE Center for the Advancement of Deaf Children, 7726
SHALOM Denver, 6529
SILC Department of Vocational Rehabilitation, 3857
SILC, Indiana Council on Independent Living (ICOIL), 3801
SILO: Cental Islip, 4065
SILO: Hauppauge, 4066
SL Stuart and Associates, 6034
SLIDER Bathing System, 145
SMILES, 3952
SOAR Summer Adventures, 7352
SPIN Early Childhood Care & Education Cntr, 6530
SPINabilities: A Young Person's Guide to Spina Bifida, 8573
SPOKES Unlimited, 4115, 8952
SS-Access Single Switch Interface for PC's with MS-DOS, 1197
SSD (Services for Students with Disabilities), 1749
STAR, 3231
Sacramento Center & Regional Offices, 6431
Sacramento Medical Center, 5393
Sacramento Vocational Services, 5680
Sacremento State, 1257
Safari Scooter, 573
Safari Tilt, 245
Safe and Dry-Feel and Sure-Toddler Dry, 1159
Sagamore Publishing, 27
Sage Publications, 1947, 4785, 4842
Sailing Fascination, 8108
Saint Clares Hospital, 750
Saint Joseph Regional Medical Center- South Bend, 6721
Saint Jude Medical Center, 7069
Salem VA Medical Center, 5585
The Salvation Army, 968
Sammons Preston Enrichments Catalog, 475

Sammons Preston Rolyan, 360, 337, 342, 343, 354, 367, 368, 381, 448, 475, 482, 621, 642, 1192, 2089
Sampson-Katz Center, 6701
Samuel S Johnson Foundation, 2773
Samuel W Bell Home for Sightless, 4099
San Antonio Area Foundation, 2867
San Antonio Warm Springs Rehabilitation Hospital, 6294
San Bernardino Valley Lighthouse for the Blind, 6493
San Diego Area Chapter of the Arthritis Foundation, 7989
San Diego VA Regional Office, 5394
San Francisco Foundation, 2370
San Francisco Public Library for the Blind and Print Handicapped, 4396
San Francisco VA Medical Center, 5395
San Francisco Vocational Services, 5681
San Joaquin General Hospital, 6426
San Joaquin Valley Rehabilitation Hospital, 6084
San Jose State University Library, 4397
San Juan Center for Independence, 4027
San Luis Medical and Rehabilitation Center, 7270
Sandhills Academy, 2261
Sandra Beasley Independent Living Center, 4106
Sanilac County Community Mental Health, 6842
Santa Barbara Bank & Trust, 2349
Santa Barbara Foundation, 2371, 4780
Santa Barbara Parks and Recreation Department, 913, 1559
Santa Barbara Wheelchair Sports Conference, 1559
Santa Clara Valley Blind Center, Inc., 6494
Santa Clara Valley Medical Center, 6085
Santa Fe Community Foundation, 2645
Santa Fe Mountain Center, 993
Sarasota Memorial Hospital/Comprehensive Rehabilitation Unit, 6610
Sarkeys Foundation, 2768
Savannah Association for the Blind, 6634
Savannah Rehabilitation and Nursing Center, 7098
Say What, 291
Say it with Sign Videotape, 9034
Scandinavian Seminar, 2289
Scanmaster, 1310
Scanning WSKE, 1311
Schaefer Enterprises, 6531
Schepens Eye Research Institute, 4522, 9047
Scheuer Associates Foundation, 2405
Schnurmacher Center for Rehabilitation and Nursing, 7186
Scholastic, 8434
School Based Assessment of Attention Deficit Disorders, 7511
School Of Medicine, Rheumatology Division, 4471
School of Piano Technology for the Blind, 6035
Schools And Services For Children With Autism Spectrum Disorders., 3338
Schools for Children with Autism Spectrum Disorders, 7512
Schroth School & Technical Education Center, 6882
Schwab Rehabilitation Hospital, 7118
Scientific Health Solutions, 8172
Scoffolding Student Learning, 2133
Scoota Bug, 574
Scooter & Wheelchair Battery Fuel Gauges and Motor Speed Controllers, 654
Scott Sign Systems, 512
Scottish Rite Center for Childhood Language Disorders, 8680
Screening in Chronic Disease, 4950, 8574
Scribner, 7540
Scripps Memorial Hospital Encinitas, 6086
Scripps Memorial Hospital at La Jolla, 6087
Scripps Memorial Hospital: Pain Center, 6495
Sea Pines Rehabilitation Hospital, 6114, 6589
Seacrest Village Nursing Center, 7172
Seagull Industries for the Disabled, 5757
Sears-Roebuck Foundation, 2509
Seat-A-Robics, 5177
Seattle Medical and Rehabilitation Center, 7046
Seattle Regional Office, 5588
Sebasticook Farms-Great Bay Foundation, 6782
Second Course in Phonic Reading, 1688
Second Time Around, 5836
Secret Agent Walking Stick, 635
Secretary State Office, 4555
Sedgwick County Workshop, 5705
Sedgwick Press/Grey House Publishing, 1753, 1754, 1755, 1756, 1760
See A Bone, 9035
See What I Feel, 9036
See What I'm Saying, 9037
See for Yourself, 9038
Seeing Eye, 8817, 9039
Seeing Eye Guide, 9039
Seeing Voices: A Journey into the World of the Deaf, 7894
Seeing-Children Living with Blindness, 9040
Seizures and Epilepsy in Childhood: A Guid e, 8575
Selecting a Program, 5131, 9041
Selective Nontreatment of Handicapped, 2134
Self Help for Hard of Hearing People, 7727
Self Reliance, 3716
Self-Therapy for the Stutterer, 8731
Sellersburg Health and Rehabilitation Cent re, 7127
Senior Citizens and the Law, 7596, 7660
Senior Health Care Management, 7089
Senior Program for Teens and Young Adults with Special Needs, 2262
Sense-Sations, 125, 182, 283, 288, 348, 519, 587, 589, 592, 593, 1130, 1139, 5276
Sequanota, 8688
Sequential Spelling I-VII, 1689
Serape, 1138
Series Adapter, 513
Sertoma Centre, 5797
Service Center for Independent Living: Covina Office, 3643
Service Club for the Blind, 6859
Service Coordination for Early Intervention: Parents and Friends, 2135
ServiceSource, 6027
Services Maximizing Independent Living and Empowerment (SMILE), 3574
Services for Independent Living, 3982, 4100, 4795
Services for Students with Disabilities, 1809
Services for the Blind, 4544
Services for the Blind and Visually Impaired, 3420
Services for the Seriously Mentally Ill: A Survey of Mental Health Centers, 2136
Services for the Visually Impaired, 8818
Serving Adults with Cognitive Disabilities, 7513
Setebaid Services, 8240
Seven Fifty-Five FS, 707
Sex Education: Issues for the Person with Autism, 7514
Sexual Adjustment, 4951
Sexuality After Spinal Cord Injury: Answers to Your Questions, 8576
Sexuality and Disabilities: A Guide for Human Service Practitioners, 4952
Sexuality and Disability, 5084
Sexuality and the Developmentally Handicapped, 5009
Sexuality and the Person with Spina Bifida, 8577
Shady Oaks Camp, 8284
Shalom House, Inc, 3873
Shambhala Publications, 4814, 4870
Shands Rehab Hospital, 7092
Shannon Medical Center: RehabCare Unit, 6295
Shape Up 'n Sign, 9042
Share, 8232
Shared Visions, 9043
Sharing Solutions: A Newsletter for Support Groups, 9044
Sharp Calculator with Illuminated Numbers, 539
Sharp Coronado Hospital, 6496
Shasta County Opportunity Center, 5682
Shattered Dreams-Lonely Choices: Birth Parents of Babies with Disabilities, 5010
Shaughnessy-Kaplan Rehabilitation Hospital, 6820
Shawmut Bank, 2406
Shelby County Community Services, 6702
Shelby Pines Rehabilitation and Healthcare Center, 7233
Shell Oil Company Foundation, 2868
Sheltered Occupational Center of Virginia, 6028
Shenandoah Valley Workforce Investment Board, 4218
Shenango Valley Foundation, 2794
Shepherd Center for Treatment of Spinal Injuries, 6635
Sheridan Press, c/o FB, 8967
Sheridan VA Medical Center, 5602
Sherman Lake YMCA Outdoor Center, 7353, 8285
Shilo Inns & Resorts, 5321
Shiloh Senior Citizens Center, 7597
Shining Bright: Head Start Inclusion, 4701
Shirley Spero, 2567
Shoebox Tasks: Work Activities, 7515
Shop Talk, 2137
Shop Til You Drop, 1427
Shore Community Services, 5798
Shore Training Center, 5798
Shore Village Rehabilitation & Nursing Center, 7146
Show Me How: A Manual for Parents of Preschool Blind Children, 9045
Shreveport VA Medical Center, 5452
Shriners Burn Institute: Cincinnati Unit, 6232
Shriners Burn Institute: Galveston Unit, 6296
Shriners Burns Hospital: Boston, 6186

Shriners Hospital Springfield Unit Springfield Unit for Crippled Children, 6187
Shriners Hospital for Children-Shreveport, 6174
Shriners Hospital for Children: Honolulu, 6131
Shriners Hospitals, 6321
Shriners Hospitals For Children-Northern California, 6497
Shriners Hospitals for Children, 6498
Shriners Hospitals for Children Cincinnati, 6232
Shriners Hospitals for Children St. Louis, 6860
Shriners Hospitals for Children, Erie, 6260
Shriners Hospitals for Children, Greenville, 6265
Shriners Hospitals for Children, Houston, 6297
Shriners Hospitals for Children, Lexington, 6170
Shriners Hospitals for Children, Philadelphia, 6259
Shriners Hospitals for Children: Intermountain, 6308
Shriners Hospitals for Children: Portland, 6243
Shriners Hospitals for Children: Spokane, 6321
Shriners Hospitals for Children: Tampa, 6115
Shriners Hospitals for Children: Twin Cities, 6849
Shriners Hospitals, Philadelphia Unit, for Crippled Children, 6261
Shrinners Hospital sfor Children, 6265
Shrinners Hospitals for Children, 6259
Sibling Forum, 4702
Sibling Information Network Newsletter, 1899
Siboney Learning Group, 1347
Sibpage, 1900
Sibshops: Workshops for Siblings of Children with Special Needs, 4703
Sickened: The Memoir of a Muchausen by Pro xy Childhood, 4953
Sickle Cell Disease Association of Illinois, 8195
Side Velcro Slacks, 1144
Side-Zip Sweat Pants, 1145
Sidney Stern Memorial Trust, 2372
Sierra 3000/4000, 575
Sierra Club Books, 5312
Sierra Health Foundation, 2373
Sierra Pain Institute, 6868
Sight by Touch, 9046
Sightings Newsletter, 9047
Sign Language Coloring Books, 7895
Sign Language Feelings, 7896
Sign Language Interpreters and Interpreting, 7897
Sign of the Times, 9048
Sign with Me Books, 7898
Signaling Wake-Up Devices, 514
Signature and Address Self-Inking Stamps, 540
Signed English Schoolbook, 2138
Signed English Starter, 7899
Signing Family: What Every Parent Should Know About Sign Communication, 7900
Signing Naturally Curriculum, 1690
Signing for Reading Success, 7901
Signing: How to Speak with Your Hands, 7902
Signs Across America, 7903
Signs Everywhere, 7904
Signs for Computing Terminology, 7905
Signs for Me: Basic Sign Vocabulary for Children, Parents & Teachers, 7906
Signs for Sexuality: A Resource Manual, 7907
Signs of the Times, 7908
Silent Call Communications, 202
Silent Garden: Raising Your Deaf Child, 7909
Silicon Valley Community Foundation, 2374
Silicon Valley Independent Living Center, 3645
Silicon Valley Independent Living Center: Gilroy Office, 3644
Silicone Padding, 275
Silvercrest Center for Nursing & Rehabilitation, 6219
Simon & Schuster, 4790
Simon Foundation, 8465
Simon Foundation for Continence, 8578
Simon Sounds it Out, 1492
Simon Spells, 1493
Simonton Cancer Center, 8173
Simplicity, 1198
Simultaneous Communication, ASL, and Other Communication Modes, 7910
Sinai Hospital of Detroit: Dept. of Opthalmology, 4527
Since Owen, A Parent-to-Parent Guide for Care of the Disabled Child, 5011
Sing Praise Hymnal, 7911
Singeria/Metropolitan Parent Center, 3339
Single Switch Latch and Timer, 5287
Single-Handed: A Book for Persons with the Use of Only One Hand, 7556
Sinus Survival, 8579
Sioux Falls VA Medical Center, 5561
Siouxland Community Foundation, 2528
Siragusa Foundation, 2510
Siskin Hospital For Physical Rehabilitation, 6996
Siskin Hospital for Physical Rehabilitation, 7234
Sisler McFawn Foundation, 2759
Sister Cities International, 2290
Sister Kenny Institute, 6194
Sjogren's Syndrome Foundation, 2552, 8505
Skadden Fellowship Foundation, 2712
SkiSoft Publishing Corporation, 1520
Skills Inc., 5799
Skills Unlimited, 6909
Skin and Dental Dysfunction Foundation, 5253
Skokie Accessible Library Services, 4463
Skokie Public Library, 4463
Sky Ranch Lutheran Camp, 922
Skyway, 694
Skyway Machine, 694
Sleep Better! A Guide to Improving Sleep for Children with Special Needs, 5012
SleepSafe Beds, 163
Sleeping Beauty, 7912
Sleeping Beauty Videotape, 7913
Slicing Aid, 361
Slim Armstrong Mounting System, 1199
Slim Line Brake Only, 105
Slim Line Control, 106
Slim Line Control: Brake and Throttle, 107
Slingerland Institute for Literacy, 7047
Slingerland Screening Tests, 2235
Slosburg Family Charitable Trust, 2614
Slosson Educational Publications, 1627, 2151, 7394
Slow Motion/Sea Legs, 8109
Small Appliance Receiver, 362
Small Business Development Center, 5881
Small Differences, 5178
Small Wonder, 1691
Smart + Strong, 8541
Smart Kitchen/How to Design a Comfortable, Safe & Friendly Workplace, 1590
Smart Leg, 408
Smart Modem, 1200
Smith Kettlewell Rehabilitation Engineering Research Center, 9049
Smith-Kettlewell Eye Research Institute, 9049
Smoke Detector with Strobe, 515
Smooth Mover, 409
Snug Seat, 127, 361
So Many of My Friends Have Moved Away or Died, 7661
Social Development and the Person with Spi na Bifida, 8580
Social Learning Center, 6783
Social Maturity Scale for Blind Preschool Children: A Guide to Its Use, 9050
Social Perceptions of People with Disabilities in History, 5085
Social Security, 3045, 3096, 3097, 3123, 3171, 3172, 3421, 3441, 3479, 3512, 3524, 3541
Social Security Administration, 2983, 3095, 3227, 3308, 2979, 3098, 3156
Social Security Admission, 3023
Social Security Bulletin, 7662
Social Security Library, 4509
Social Security Online, 5254
Social Security, Medicare, and Pensions, 7663
Social Security: Albany Disability Determination, 3340
Social Security: Arkansas Disability Determination Services, 3033
Social Security: Atlanta Disability Determination, 3109
Social Security: Austin Disability Determination, 3461
Social Security: Baltimore Disability Determination, 3198
Social Security: Baton Rouge Disability Determination, 3182
Social Security: Bismarck Disability Determination, 3368
Social Security: Boston Disability Determination, 3206
Social Security: California Disability Determination Services, 3044
Social Security: Carson City Disability Determination, 3284
Social Security: Charleston Disability Determination, 3524
Social Security: Cheyenne Disability Determination, 3541
Social Security: Columbus Disability Determination, 3381
Social Security: Concord Disability Determination, 3297
Social Security: Decatur Disability Determination, 3110

Social Security: Des Moines Disability Determination, 3156
Social Security: Frankfort Disability Determination, 3171
Social Security: Fresno Disability Determination Services, 3045
Social Security: Harrisburg Disability Determination, 3409
Social Security: Hartford Area Office, 3062
Social Security: Helena Disability Determination, 3265
Social Security: Honolulu Disability Determination, 3123
Social Security: Jefferson City Disability Determination, 3254
Social Security: Lincoln Disability Determination, 3275
Social Security: Louisville Disability Determination, 3172
Social Security: Madison Disability Determination, 3534
Social Security: Maine Disability Determination, 3190
Social Security: Miami Disability Determination, 3096
Social Security: Mobile Disability Determination Services, 3000
Social Security: Nashville Disability Determination, 3441
Social Security: Oakland Disability Determination Services, 3046
Social Security: Olympia Disability Determination, 3512
Social Security: Orlando Disability Determination, 3097
Social Security: Phoenix Disability Determination Services, 3023
Social Security: Providence Disability Determination, 3421
Social Security: Raleigh Disability Determination, 3361
Social Security: Sacramento Disability Determination Services, 3047
Social Security: Salem Disability Determination, 3397
Social Security: Salt Lake City Disability Determination, 3479
Social Security: San Diego Disability Determination Services, 3048
Social Security: Santa Fe Disability Determination, 3317
Social Security: Springfield Disability Determination, 3140
Social Security: St. Paul Disability Determination, 3241
Social Security: Tampa Disability Determination, 3098
Social Security: Tucson Disability Determination Services, 3024
Social Security: Vermont Disability Determination Services, 3490
Social Security: West Columbia Disability Determination, 3424
Social Security: Wilmington Disability Determination, 3072
Social Skills on the Job, 6195
Social Studies: Detecting and Correcting Special Needs, 2139
Social Vocational Services, 5683
Social and Emotional Development of Exceptional Students: Handicapped, 2140
Socialization Games for Persons with Disabilities, 4954, 5288
Society State of Alabama, 8238
Society for Equal Access: Independent Living Center, 4101
Society for Progressive Supranuclear Palsy, 8542
Society for Progressive Supranuclear Palsy (SPSP), 7972
Society for Rehabilitation, 6952
Society for the Blind, 6499
Society's Assets: Elkhorn, 4246
Society's Assets: Kenosha, 4247
Society's Assets: Racine, 4248
Soft Touch, 1167, 1171, 1172, 1177, 1179, 1190, 1193, 1196, 1201, 1202, 1204, 1206, 1208, 1209, 1210, 1211, 1212, 1213, 1366, 1367, 1368, 1379, 1380, 1391, 1392, 1399, 1400, 1414, 1418, 1419, 1423, 1425, 1426, 1427, 1428, 1436, 1437, 1438, 1439, 1440, 1441, 1442, 1443, 1444, 1448, 1450
Soft Touch Incorporated, 1207, 1422
Soft-Touch Convertible Flotation Mattress, 276
Soft-Touch Gel Flotation Cushion, 277
SoftTouch Favorites IntelliKeys Overlay, 1201
Solo Scooter, 576
SoloRider Industries, 577
Solutions at Santa Barbara: Transitional Living Center, 6500
Solving Language Difficulties: Remedial Routines, 1692
Solving the Puzzle of Chronic Fatigue, 8581
Someday's Child, 4704
Somerset Training and Employment Program, 5938
Something Magical, 44
Something's Wrong with My Child, 5013
Sometimes I Get All Scribbly, 5014
Sometimes You Just Want to Feel Like a Human Being, 4955
Son-Rise Program, 6821, 8667
Son-Rise: The Miracle Continues, 5015, 7516, 8582
Songs I Sing at Preschool, 1428
Songs I Sing at Preschool IntelliKeys Over lay, 1202
Sonic Alert, 203
Sonic Alert Bed Shaker, 164
Sonora Area Foundation, 2375
Sonoran Rehabilitation and Care Center, 7060
Soon Will Come the Light, 7517
Sophie Russell Testamentary Trust Bank Of Hawaii, 2467
Souderton Special Needs Day Camp, 1038
Sound & Fury, 5179
Sound Connections for the Adolescent, 8732
Sound Induction Receiver, 204
Sound Sentences, 1494
Sound Workbook, 1693
Sound, Listening, and Learning Center, 7728
Sound-Off 1-5, 1694
Source Book Profiles, 2964
Source of Help and Hope Newsletter, 8061
Sources for Community IL Services, 3580
South Arlington Medical Center: Rehab Care Unit, 6298
South Bay Vocational Center, 5684
South Carolina Assistive Technology Program (SCATP), 1829
South Carolina Assistive Technology Project, 3425, 4792
South Carolina Association of Nonprofit Homes for the Aging, 7598
South Carolina Client Assistance Program, 3426
South Carolina Commission for the Blind, 3427
South Carolina Department of Children with Disabilities, 3428
South Carolina Department of Education: Office of Exceptional Children, 1830
South Carolina Department of Mental Health and Mental Retardation, 3429
South Carolina Developmental Disabilities Council, 3430
South Carolina Employment Security Commission South Carolina Center, 5997
South Carolina Governor's Committee on Employment of the Handicapped, 5998
South Carolina Services Information System, 3431
South Carolina State Library, 4617
South Carolina State University, 8978
South Carolina Vocational Rehabilitation Department, 5999
South Central Iowa Center for Independent Living, 3811
South Central Kansas Library System, 4484
South Central Pennsylvania Center for Inde pendence Living, 4127
South Central Technical College (SCTC), 1810
South Central Wyoming Healthcare and Rehabilitation, 7272
South Coast Medical Center, 6088, 7070
South Dakota Advocacy Services, 3433
South Dakota Assistive Technology Project, 4151
South Dakota Department of Aging, 3434
South Dakota Department of Children's Special Health Services, 3435
South Dakota Department of Education & Cultural Affairs: Office of Special Education, 1831
South Dakota Department of Human Services Division of Mental Health, 3436
South Dakota Department of Human Services: Computer Technology Services, 1279
South Dakota Developmental Disability Council, 3437
South Dakota Division of Rehabilitation, 3438
South Dakota Governor's Advisory Committee on Employment of the Disabled, 6002
South Dakota State Department of Health, 3435
South Dakota State Library, 4618
South Dakota State Vocational Rehabilitati on, 6003
South Dakota VA Regional Office, 5562
South Dakota Veterans Centers, 5563
South Dakota Workforce Investment Act Training Programs, 6004
South Dakota of Human Services, 3436
South Georgia Regional Library-Valdosta Talking Book Center, 4447
South Louisiana Rehabilitation Hospital, 6175
South Miami Hospital, 6116
South Shore Healthcare, 7187
South Texas Charitable Foundation, 2869
South Texas Lighthouse for the Blind, 7013
South Texas Rehabilitation Hospital, 6299
South Texas Veterans Healthcare System, 5574

Southeast Center for Independent Living, 3904
Southeast Disability & Business Technical Assist., 3099
Southeast Kansas Independent Living, 3835
Southeast Kansas Independent Living: Colum bus, 3837
Southeast Kansas Independent Living: Pittsburg, 3836
Southeast Kansas Independent Living: Yates Center, 3834
Southeast Kansas: Chanute, 3838
Southeast Kansas: Fredonia, 3839
Southeast Ohio Sight Center, 6953
Southeastern Blind Rehabilitation Center, 6347
Southeastern Michigan Commission for the Blind, 3939
Southeastern Minnesota Center for Independent Living: Rochester, 3953, 3954
Southeastern Missouri Alliance for Independence (SEMO Alliance), 3983
Southeastern Paralyzed Veterans Of America (PVA), 3729
Southern Adirondack Independent Living, 4067
Southern Arizona VA Healthcare System, 5382
Southern California Chapter, 7978
Southern California Golf Association, 8091
Southern California Rehabilitation Services, 3646
Southern Illinois Talking Book Center, 4464
Southern Illinois University, 928
Southern Illinois University at Carbondale, 2291
Southern Indiana Center for Independent Living, 3802
Southern Indiana Resource Solutions, 5823
Southern Maryland Center for LIFE, 3883
Southern Minnesota Independent Living Enterprises and Services, 3955
Southern Nevada Center for Independent Living: Las Vegas, 4007
Southern Nevada Center for Independent Living: North Las Vegas, 4006
Southern New England Rehab Center, 7221
Southern Tier Independence Center, 4068
Southern Worcester County Rehabilitation Inc., 6822
Southside Virginia Training Center, 7028
Southwest Branch of the International Dyslexia Association, 3318
Southwest Center for Independence, 3666
Southwest Center for Independence: Cortez, 3667
Southwest Center for Independent Living (SWCIL), 3984
Southwest Communication Resource, 6891
Southwest District Independent Living Program, 3730
Southwest Louisiana Independence Center: L ake Charles, 3864
Southwest Louisians Independence Center: Lafayette, 3865
Southwest Medical Center, 6240
Southwestern Center for Independent Living, 3956
Southwestern Diabetic Fund, 8245
Southwestern Idaho Housing Authority, 3754
Southwestern Independent Living Center, 4069
Soyland Access To Independent Living, 3783
Soyland Access to IL, 3784
Soyland Access to Independent Living (SAIL), 3785
Soyland Access to Independent Living: Charleston, 3786
Spa Area Independent Living Services, 3581
Space Coast CIL News, 4956
Space Coast Center for Independent Living, 3717, 4956
Spalding Rehab Hospital West Unit, 6532
Spalding Rehabilitation Hospital at Memorial Hospital of Laramie, 6328
Span-America Medical Systems, 263
Spatial Orientation and Sequencing Development Remedial Activities, 2236
Spatial Tilt Custom Chair, 246
Spaulding University, 4488
SpeakEasy Communication Aid, 205
Speakwriter 2000, 206
Special Assistance Services (SAS), 5322
Special Camps for Special Kids, 1049
Special Care in Dentistry, 8583
Special Children, 8668
Special Children/Special Solutions, 4705
Special Clothes, 428, 430, 431, 439, 1078, 1079, 1089, 1091, 1092, 1094, 1095, 1096, 1097, 1113, 1114, 1117, 1120, 1129, 1141, 1142, 1143, 1147, 1148, 1149, 1150, 1151, 1152, 1153, 1154
Special Clothes Adult Catalogue, 1113
Special Clothes for Special Children, 1114, 5255
Special Edge, 1901
Special Education Action Commette, 8669
Special Education And Rehab Services, 7693, 8676
Special Education Report, 1902, 4706
Special Education Teacher Packet, 5055
Special Education Today, 2141
Special Education and Vocational Rehabilitation Agency: New York, 5954
Special Education for Today, 2142
Special Format Books for Children and Youth Ages 3-19, 4707
Special Format Books for Children and Youth: Ages 3-19.Serving New York City/Long Island, 4708
Special Kids Need Special Parents: A Resou rce for Parents of Children With Special Needs, 5016
Special Kind of Parenting, 5056
Special Needs 5, 247
Special Needs Center/Phoenix Public Library, 4375
Special Needs Project, 1783, 436, 1632, 1929, 1979, 2033, 2104, 4990, 5011, 5047, 5307, 6070, 7617
Special Needs Systems, 5766
Special Olympics, 8110
Special Olympics International, 8111
Special Parent, Special Child, 5017
Special Populations Division, 959
Special Services Division: Indiana State Library, 4473
Special Services/Talking Books, 4642
Special Siblings: Growing Up With Someone with A Disability, 4957
Special Technologies Alternative Resources, 8819
Special Tree Rehabilitation System, 6843
Special U, 4547
Specialty Care Shoppe, 1115
Specialty Hospital, 6130, 7099
Specifications for Selecting a Vocabulary and Teaching Method/Braille Readers, 9051
SpectraLift, 410
Spectrum, 7518
Spectrum Aquatics, 411
Spectrum Products, 412
Spectrum Products Catalog, 412
Speech Bin, 1695, 2237, 1685, 1687, 2219, 2233, 5289, 7524, 7934, 8695, 8702, 8707, 8716, 8723, 8729, 8732, 8735, 8740
Speech Discrimination Unit, 207
Speech and the Hearing-Impaired Child, 2143
Speech-Language Delights, 1696
Speech-Language Pathology and Audiology: An Introduction, 2144
Speechmaker-Personal Speech Amplifier, 208
Spell of Words, 1697
Spellbinding 2, 1698
Spellbound, 1699
Spelling Dictionary, 1700
Spelling Rules, 1495
Spelling Test Generator, 1496
Spelling Workbooks Emphasizing Rules and Generalization for Corrective Drill, 1701
Spenco Medical Group, 278, 275
Spero Charitable Foundation, 2567
Spina Bifida, 8584
Spina Bifida Association of America, 8174, 4271, 4672, 4676, 4694, 4700, 4713, 4751, 4970, 4977, 5000, 5033, 5040, 5042, 5043, 5285, 7533, 8321, 8336, 8351, 8356, 8370, 8371, 8381, 8392, 8411, 8420, 8431, 8435, 8438, 8440, 8453, 8470, 8479, 8481, 8485, 8520, 8525, 8527, 8543, 8551, 8560, 8561, 8573, 8577, 8580, 8584, 8591, 8593, 8595, , 8599, 8610, 8618, 8628
Spina Bifida Program of DC Children's Hospital, 6564
Spinabilities: A Young Person's Guide to Spina Bifida, 8585
Spinal Cord Dysfunction, 2145
Spinal Cord Injury Life, 8586
Spinal Cord Injury Series, 8587
Spinal Cord Society (SCS), 7973
Spinal Network: The Total Wheelchair Reso urce Book, 516
Spine, 8588
Spirit of Lo: An Ordinary Family's Extraor dinary Journey, 8589
Spokane VA Medical Center, 5589
Sport Science Review: Adapted Physical Activity, 8112
Sportaid, 476
Sports & Recreation for the Disabled, 8113
Sports Market Place Directory, 8114
Sports and Exercise for Children with Chronic Health Conditions, 8115
Sports n' Spokes Magazine, 5300
Sportster 10, 578
Spring Dell Center, 7914
Springer Publishing Company, 1926, 1975, 2101, 2110, 2122, 2126, 2175, 2182, 4671, 4793, 4909, 4938, 4939, 4940, 4993, 5072, 7502, 7633, 7636, 7645
Springer Publishing Compn, 1931
Springfield Center for Independent Living, 3787
Square D Foundation, 2511
Squirrel Hollow Summer Camp, 7354
St Elizabeth Hospital Physical Rehabilitation Unit In-Patient/CARFT Certified, 6703
St Frances Cabrini Hospital, 6176

St Lukes Roosevelt, 4045
St Martin's Griffin, 8722
St Vincent Children s Specialty Hospital, 7733
St. Anne's Nursing Center, 6117
St. Anthony Hospital, 6242
St. Anthony Hospital: Rehabilitation Unit, 6242
St. Anthony Memorial Hospital: Rehab Unit, 6161
St. Anthony's Hospital, 6118, 7093
St. Anthony's Rehabilitation Hospital, 6119
St. Camillus Health and Rehabilitation Cen ter, 7188
St. Catherine's Hospital, 6325
St. Catherine's Rehabilitation Hospital and Villa Maria Nursing Center, 6120
St. Clair County Library Special Technologies Alternative Resources (S.T.A.R.), 4537
St. Cloud VA Medical Center, 5475
St. David s Medical Center, 6300
St. David's Rehabilitation Center, 6300
St. Frances Cabrini Hospital: Rehab Unit, 6176
St. Francis Health Care Centre, 6233
St. Francis Rehabilitation Hospital, 6954
St. George Care and Rehabilitation Center, 7239
St. George's Society of New York, 2713
St. James Association for Retarded Citizens, 5850
St. John Hospital: North Shore, 6193
St. John Valley Associates, 7308
St. John of God Community Services Vocational Rehabilitation, 5939
St. John's Nursing Center, 6121
St. John's Pleasant Valley Hospital Neuro Care Unit, 6501
St. John's Regional Medica Center-Industrial Therapy Center, 6502
St. Joseph Health System, 6089
St. Joseph Hospital, 6326
St. Joseph Hospital Rehabilitation, 6206
St. Joseph Hospital Rehabilitation Center, 4474
St. Joseph Hospital and Medical Center, 6062
St. Joseph Rehabilitation Center, 6089
St. Joseph Rehabilitation Hospital and Outpatient Center, 6214
St. Jude Brain Injury Network, 6090
St. Jude Hospital, 6090
St. Jude Medical Center, 6091
St. Lawrence Rehabilitation Center, 7173
St. Louis Regional Office, 5483
St. Louis Society for the Blind and Visually Impaired, 6861
St. Louis VA Medical Center, 5484
St. Mark's Hospital, 7240
St. Martin's Press, 8017, 8312, 8506
St. Mary Medical Center, 6092
St. Mary's Medical Center: RehabCare Center, 6275
St. Mary's Regional Rehabilitation Center, 6198
St. Mary's RehabCare Center, 6997
St. Patrick Hospital: Rehab Unit, 6177
St. Patrick RehabCare Unit, 6776
St. Paul Abilities Network, 889
St. Paul Regional Office, 5476
St. Petersburg Regional Office, 5419
St. Rita's Medical Center Rehabilitation Services, 6234
St. Vincent Hospital and Health Center, 6200
Stae Agency, 3509
StairClimber, 636
StairLIFT SC & SL, 413
Stairway Elevators, 414
Stamford Hospital, 7078
Stand-Up Wheelchairs, 695
Standard 3-in-1 Commode, 311
Standard Search: Oral Health Care for People with Developmental Disabilities, 5256
Standard Touch Turner Sip & Puff Switch, 209
Standard Wheelchair, 696
Standards for the Diagnosis and Care of Patients with Asthma, 8590
Standing Aid Frame with Rear Entry, 637
Standing On My Own Two Feet, 5132, 9052
Stanley W Metcalf Foundation, 2714
Star Bright Books, 7415
Star Center, 1280
Stark Community Foundation, 2760
Start with the Arts, 45
Starting Over, 1702
Starting Points, 9053
Starting and Sustaining Genetic Support Gr oups, 5086
State Agency for the Blind and Visually Impaired, 3341
State Department of Wyoming, 3545
State Division of Vocational Rehabilitation, 6162
State Education Agency Rural Representative, 3342
State Library of Louisiana: Services for the Blind and Physically Handicapped, 4494
State Library of Ohio: Talking Book Program, 4602
State Mental Health Representative for Children and Youth, 3343
State Mental Retardation Program, 3344
State Office Building, 3194
State Office of Wisconsin, 3536
State Planning Council on Developmental Disabilities, 3124
State University of New York, 2292
State University of New York Health Sciences Center, 4587
State University of New York Press, 1983
State of Arizona, 1789
State of Connecticut Agency, 1793
State of Illinois Center, 3135
State of Maine, 3185
State of Massachusetts, 5869
State of Michigan, 2571
State of Michigan/Bureau of Workers' Disability Compensation, 3228
State of Nebraska, 3274
State of Nevada, 5903
State of Nevada Client Assistance Program, 3285
State of Oregon Office of Vocational Rehabilitation Service, 5981
State of Vermont Department of Aging and Disabilities, 6018
State of Washington, 3521
State of West Virginia, 3522
Staten Island Center for Independent Living, 4070
Statesman Health and Rehabilitation Center, 7215
Statewide Information at Texas School for the Deaf, 3462
Staunton Farm Foundation, 2795
Staunton Public Library Talking Book Center, 4643
Stay Tuned, 7942
Steady Write, 541
Steel Food Guard, 363
Steelcase Foundation, 2589
Steele, 517
SteeleVest, 517
Steering Backup System, 108
Stella B Gross Charitable Trust, 2376
Step on It! Computer Control Pedals, 1308
Step-By-Step Guide to Personal Management for Blind Persons, 9054
Step-by-Step Communicator, 210
Stepping Stones, 1064
Stepping Stones Center, 1011, 1013
Steps to Independence: Teaching Everyday S kills to Children with Special Needs, 8591
Sterling Press, 4841
Sterling Ranch, 3575
Sterling Ranch: Residence for Special Women, 3575
Sterling-Turner Foundation, 2870
Stevens Publishing Corporation, 1848
Stewardship Foundation, 2899
Stewart Huston Charitable Trust, 2796
Stewart Rehabilitation Center: McKay Dee Hospital, 6309
Stick Canes, 638
Stickybear Math, 1353
Stickybear Numbers, 1354
Stickybear Parts of Speech, 1497
Stickybear Reading, 1498
Stickybear Reading Comprehension, 1499
Stickybear Spellgrabber, 1500
Stickybear Spelling, 1501
Stickybear Spelling Rules, 1502
Stickybear Town Builder, 1429
Stickybear Typing, 1430, 1515
Stickybear Word Problems, 1355
Stickybear's Early Learning Activities, 1431
Stickybear's Kindergarden Activities, 1432
Stickybear's Math Splash, 1356
Stickybear's Math Town, 1357
Stickybear's Reading Fun Park, 1503
Stickybear's Reading Room, 1504
Stickybear's Science Fair: Light, 1433
Still Me, 8062
The Stocker Foundation, 2762
Stone Mountain School, 1008
Stone-Hayes Center for Independent Living, 3788
Stonewall Community Foundation, 2715
Stop-Leak Gel Flotation Mattress, 279
Store @ HDSC Product Catalog, 477
Storybook Maker Deluxe, 1434
Stout Vocational Rehab Institute, 2028, 2129, 2184, 6327
Straight and Custom Curved Stairlifts, 415
Strategies for Teaching Learners with Special Needs, 2146
Strategies for Teaching Students with Learning and Behavior Problems, 2147
Strategies for Working with Families of Young Children with Disabilities, 5018
Streator Unlimited, 6704
Strength for the Journey, 8286
Strengthening the Roles of Independent Living Centers Through Implementing Legal Services, 4276
Stretch-View Wide-View Rectangular Illuminated Magnifier, 614

Stricken: Voices from the Hidden Epidemic of Chronic Fatigue Syndrome, 8592
Strider, 312
Strides Magazine, 8116
String Switch, 1203
Strive Physical Therapy Centers, 6611
Strobe Light Signalers, 211
Stroke Connection, 7557
Structure of Words, 1703
Student Advocate, 9055
Student Guide, 2965
Student Independent Living Experience Massachusetts Hospital School, 3905
Student Teaching Guide for Blind and Visually Impaired College Students, 9056
Students with Acquired Brain Injury: The School's Response, 2148
Students with Disabilities Office, 1281
Students with Mild Disabilities in the Secondary School, 2149
Studio 49 Catalog, 1704
Study Power: Study Skills to Improve Your Learning and Your Grades: A Workbook, 5044
Stuttering, 8733
Stuttering & Your Child: A Videotape for Parents, 8734
Stuttering Foundation of America, 8681, 8715, 8731, 8734
Stuttering Severity Instrument for Children and Adults, 2238
Sub-Acute Saratoga Hospital, 6503
SubAcute Care: American SubAcute Care Association Annual Convention/Expo, 1560
Substance Abuse Funding News, 2966
Substance Abuse and Physical Disability, 5087
Successful Job Accommodation Strategies, 6122
Successful Job Search Strategies for the D sabled: Understanding the ADA, 7519
Successful Models of Community Long Term Care Services for the Elderly, 7664
Suffolk Cooperative Library System: Long Island Talking Book Library, 4588
Suffolk Independent Living Organization (SILO), 4071
Summer Camp for Children with Muscular Dystrophy, 8287
Summer Day Camp, 7355
Summer Enrichment Camp, 7751
Summer Wheelchair Sports Camp, 7983
Summeries of Legal Precedents and Law Review Articles concern Parents with Disabilities, 4277
Summit Camp, 7356
Summit Independent Living Center: Hamilton, 3993
Summit Independent Living Center: Kalipsell, 3992
Summit Independent Living Center: Missoula, 3994
Summit Ridge Center, 6889
Summit Ridge Center Genesis Eldercare, 7174
Sun Trust Bank Atlanta, 2449, 2452, 2459
Sun-Mate Seat Cushions, 280
SunTrust Bank, Atlanta Foundation, 2459
Sunbridge Care and Rehabilitation, 6612
Suncoast Center for Independent Living, 3718
Sundial Special Vacations, 5349, 5349
Sunnyhill Adventure Center, 7357
Sunnyside Nursing Center, 6093
Sunrise Medical/Quickie Designs, 567, 664
Sunset View Castle Nursing Homes Castle Nursing Homes, 7210
Sunshine Services, 6737
Super Challenger, 1435
Super Stretch Socks, 1116
Superarm Lift, 109
Superintendent of Documents, 5303
Superintendent of Public Instruction: Special Education Section, 1838
Superior Alliance for Independent Living (SAIL), 3940
Superkids, 8063, 8063
Support Group for Brachial Plexus Injury, 8175
Support Plus, 1160
Support Works, 8670
Supported Employment Program, 5758
Supported Employment for Disabled People, 4754
Supporting Young Adults Who are Deaf-Blind in Their Communities, 7288
Supporting and Strengthening Families, 2150
Surdna Foundation, 2716
SureHands Lift & Care Systems, 416
Suregrip Bathtub Rail, 146
Surf Chair, 697
Survey of Direct Labor Workers Who Are Blind & Employed by NIB, 9057
Survival Strategies for Going Abroad, A Guide for People with Disabilites, 5301
Suttle Lake United Methodist Camp, 8288
Swalm Foundation, 2871
Swimwear, 1117
Swindells Charitable Foundation Trust, 2406
Swing-A-Way, 417
Switch Basics, 1436
Switch Basics IntelliKeys Overlay, 1204
Sycamore Rehabilitation Services, 5824
Symbi-Key Computer Switch Interface, 1205
Symptomatic Chiari Malformation, 8593
Synapse Adaptive, 429
Synergos Neurological Center: Hayward, 6504
Synergos Neurological Center: Mission Hills, 6505
Syracuse Community-Referenced Curriculum Guide for Students with Disabilties, 1705
Syracuse University, 4571
Syracuse University, Institute on Communication, 7454, 8711
Syracuse University, School of Education, 4855
Syracuse VA Medical Center, 5517
System 2000/Versa, 1312
Systems 2000, 579
Systems Unlimited/LIFE Skills, 5184

T

T AF KI D, 5518
T HI Brentwood, 6654
T J Publishers, 1651, 4285, 7773
T J Publishers, Distributor, 1599
T Shirt is Done in Braille: Read Gently, 1139
TAC Industries, 6955
TASH Connections, 4278
TASK Team of Advocates for Special Kids, 1282
TBC Focus, 9058
TCRC Sight Center, 6705
TDI National Directory & Resource Guide: Blue Book, 7915
TEACCH, 7309
TEAM Vocational Program, 5720
TERI, 4958
TERRA-JET USA, 580
TESTS, 2151
TETRA Corporation, 5640
TJ Publishers, 1662, 2027, 7757, 7766, 7767, 7775, 7777, 7784, 7812, 7822, 7825, 7844, 7845, 7853, 7872, 7893, 7894, 7902, 7906, 7937, 8864, 9003
The TJX Companies, 2568
The TJX Foundation, 2568
TLC: Treatment and Learning Centers, 6794
TLL Temple Foundation, 2872
TMX Tricycle, 708
TOVA, 1466
TRIAID, 581, 583, 702, 708
TRU-Mold Shoes, 1083
TS Micro Tech, 1295
TSA CT Kid's Summer Event, 8289
TSA Newsletter, 8594
TTAP Outreach: Technology Team Assessment Process, 1467
TTY's: Telephone Device for the Deaf, 212
TV & VCR Remote, 518
Tacoma Area Coalition of Individuals with Disabilities, 4232
Taconic Resources for Independence, 4072
Tactile Thermostat, 519
Tahoe Adaptive Ski School, 8089
Take a Chance, 5289
Taking Charge, 8595
Taking Charge of ADHD Complete Authoritative Guide for Parents, 7520
Taking Part: Introducing Social Skills to Young Children, 2239
Talisman Summer Camp, 7358
Talk to Me, 5133, 9059
Talk to Me II, 5134, 9060
Talk with Me, 7916
TalkTrac Wearable Communicator, 213
Talkable Tales, 8735
Talking Bathroom Scale, 147
Talking Book & Braille Services Oregon State Library, 4608
Talking Book Center Brunswick-Glynn County Regional Library, 4448
Talking Book Department, Parkersburg and Wood County Public Library, 4656
Talking Book Library at Worcester Public Library, 4523
Talking Book Library-Jacksonville Public Libraries, 4426
Talking Book Program, 4626
Talking Book Program/Texas State Library, 4626
Talking Book Service: Mantatee County Central Library, 4427
Talking Book Topics, 9061
Talking Book and Braille Service, 4560
Talking Books Library for the Blind and Physically Handicapped, 4428
Talking Books Plus, 4615
Talking Books Service Evansville Vanderburgh County Public Library, 4475
Talking Books/Homebound Services, 4429
Talking Bookz/ Sckls, 4484

Talking Calculators, 214
Talking Clinical Thermometer, 313
Talking Clocks, 215
Talking Desktop Calculators, 542
Talking Electronic Organizers, 543
Talking Screen, 1332
Talking Thermometers, 314
Talking Watches, 216
Tampa Bay Academy, 6613
Tampa General Rehabilitation Center, 6123, 6614
Tampa Lighthouse for the Blind, 6615
Taping for the Blind, 8820
Target Teach, 1750
Tarjan Center at UCLA, 34
Taylor & Francis, 11, 12, 1999, 2038, 2103, 7430, 7919, 7923, 8320, 8709
Taylor & Francis Group, 1925, 7507, 8339, 8727
Taylor Publishing Company, 7389
Tazewell County Resource Center, 6706
Teach Me Phonemics Blends Overlay CD, 1206
Teach Me Phonemics Medial Overlay CD, 1207
Teach Me Phonemics Overlay Series Bundle, 1208
Teach Me Phonemics Series Bundle, 1437
Teach Me Phonemics Super Bundle, 1438
Teach Me Phonemics: Blends, 1439
Teach Me Phonemics: Final, 1440
Teach Me Phonemics: Initial, 1441
Teach Me Phonemics: Medial, 1442
Teach Me to Talk, 1443
Teach Me to Talk Overlay CD, 1209
Teach Me to Talk: USB-Overlay CD, 1210
Teach and Reach Students with Attention Deficit Disorders, 7521
Teacher Preparation and Special Education, 890
A Teacher's Guide to HCU, 1906
Teacher's Guide to Including Students with Disabilities in Regular Physical Education, 2152
A Teacher's Guide to Isovaleric Acidemia, 1907
A Teacher's Guide to MSUD, 1908
A Teacher's Guide to Methylmalonic Acidemia, 1909
A Teacher's Guide to PKU, 1910
A Teacher's Guide to Propionic Acidemia, 1911
Teachers Institute for Special Education, 1407
Teachers College Press, 1976, 1984, 1985, 2059, 2066, 2116, 2179, 8948
Teachers Institute for Special Education, 1405, 1406
Teachers Working Together, 2153
Teaching Adults with Learning Disabilities, 2154
Teaching Basic Guitar Skills to Special Learners, 46
Teaching Chemistry to Students with Disabilities, 5101
Teaching Children with Autism: Strategies for Initiating Positive Interactions, 7522
Teaching Disturbed and Disturbing Students: An Integrative Approach, 2155
Teaching Dressing Skills: Buttons, Bows and More, 7558
Teaching Every Child Every Day: Integrated Learning in Diverse Classrooms, 2156
Teaching Exceptional Children, 1880
Teaching Individuals with Physical and Multiple Disabilities, 1706
Teaching Infants and Preschoolers with Handicaps, 2157
Teaching Language-Disabled Children: A Communication/Games Intervention, 2158
Teaching Learners with Mild Disabilities: Integrating Research and Practice, 2159
Teaching Mathematics to Students with Learning Disabilities, 2160
Teaching Mildly and Moderately Handicapped Students, 2161
Teaching Orientation and Mobility in the Schools: An Instructor's Companion, 9062
Teaching People with Developmental Disabilities, 4959
Teaching Reading to Children with Down Syndrome: A Guide for Parents and Teachers, 2162
Teaching Reading to Disabled and Handicapped Learners, 2163
Teaching Reading to Handicapped Children, 2164
Teaching Research, 785, 7278, 7282, 8899
Teaching Self-Determination to Students with Disabilities, 2165
Teaching Social Skills to Hearing-Impaired Students, 7917
Teaching Social Skills to Youngsters with Disabilities, 5135
Teaching Special Students in Mainstream, 1764
Teaching Students Ways to Remember, 1707
Teaching Students with Learning Problems, 2166
Teaching Students with Learning and Behavior Problems, 2167
Teaching Students with Mild and Moderate Learning Problems, 2168
Teaching Students with Moderate/Severe Disabilities, Including Autism, 2169
Teaching Students with Special Needs in Inclusive Settings, 2170
Teaching Test-Taking Skills: Helping Students Show What They Know, 1708
Teaching Visually Impaired Children, 9063
Teaching Young Children to Read, 2171
Teaching and Mainstreaming Autistic Children, 7523
Teaching the Bilingual Special Education Student, 2172
Teaching the Learning Disabled Adolescent, 2173
Teaching the Mentally Retarded Student: Curriculum, Methods, and Strategies, 2174
TeamRehab Report, 5088
Tech Connection, 1283
Tech-Able, 1284
Technical Aids & Assistance for the Disabled Center, 1285
Techniques for Aphasia Rehab: (TARGET) Generating Effective Treatment, 7524
Technology Access Center of Tucson, 1286
Technology Assistance for Special Consumers, 1287, 4366
Technology and Handicapped People, 2175
Technology and Media Division, 891
Technology for the Disabled, 4960
Teen Tunes Plus, 1444
Teen Tunes Plus IntelliKeys Overlay, 1211
Teenagers with ADD, 7525
Teens Talk to Teens about Asthma, 8596
Teichert Foundation, 2377
Telecaption Adapter, 217
Telecommunication Relay Services, 7918
Telecommunications for the Deaf, 7827, 7915
Telecommunications for the Deaf (TDI), 7729, 7813
Teleflex Foundation, 2797
Telephone Communication and Hearing Impaired, 7919
Television Remote Controls with Large Numbers, 544
Telling Stories, 7920
Tellus Business Services, 200
Tempered Wind, 8597
Temple Community Hospital, 6506
Temple University, 1275, 4126
Temple University Institute on Disabilities, 5129
Temple University Medical School, 8133
Ten Things I Learned from Bill Porter, 8598
Tenco Industries, 6738
Tenet South Florida, 6112
Tennessee Assistive Technology Projects, 3442
Tennessee Association of Homes for the Aging, 7599
Tennessee Client Assistance Program, 3443
Tennessee Commission on Aging and Disability, 3444
Tennessee Council on Developmental Disabilities, 3445, 8359
Tennessee Department Human Services, 6006
Tennessee Department of Children with Disabilities, 3446
Tennessee Department of Education, 1832
Tennessee Department of Labor: Job Training Program Liaison, 6007
Tennessee Department of Mental Health and Developmental Disabilities, 3447
Tennessee Division of Rehabilitation, 3448
Tennessee Fair Employment Practice Agency, 6008
Tennessee Jaycee Fund, 1046
Tennessee Library for the Blind and Physically Handicapped, 4619
Tennessee Protection and Advocacy, 3443
Tennessee Technology Access Program (TTAP), 4157
Tennessee Valley Rehabilitation, 6348
Tennis in a Wheelchair, 8117
Teratogen and Birth Defects Information Project, 8671
Terra-Jet: Utility Vehicle, 580
Terrier Tricycle, 581
Terry-Wash Mitt: Medium Size, 148
Terrycloth Robes, 1128
Terrycloth Slippers, 1084
Test Accommodations for Students with Disabilities, 2240
Test Critiques: Volumes I-X, 2241
Test of Early Reading Ability Deaf or Hard of Hearing, 2242
Test of Language Development: Primary, 2243
Test of Mathematical Abilities, 2nd Editio n, 2244
Test of Nonverbal Intelligence, 3rd Editio n, 2245
Test of Phonological Awareness, 2246
Test of Written Spelling, 3rd Edition, 2247
Tethering Cord, 8599
Texas Advocates Supporting Kids with Disabilities, 3463

Texas Association of Homes and Services for the Aging, 7600
Texas Association of Retinitis Pigmentosa, 9022
Texas Commission for the Blind, 3464
Texas Commission for the Deaf and Hard of Hearing, 3465
Texas Council for Developmental Disabilities, 3466
Texas Department of Human Services, 3467
Texas Department of Mental Health & Mental Retardation, 3468
Texas Department on Aging, 3469
Texas Education Agency, 1833
Texas Education Agency: Special Education Unit, 1834
Texas Employment Services and Job Training Program Liaison, 6011
Texas Federation of Families for Children's Mental Health, 3470
Texas Governor's Committee on People with Disabilities, 3471
Texas Lions Camp, 7752, 8290, 8841
Texas NeuroRehab Center, 6301
Texas Protection & Advocacy Services for Disabled Persons, 3472
Texas Rehabilitation Commission Independent Living Services, 4179
Texas Respite Resource Network, 3473
Texas School of the Deaf, 1835
Texas Specialty Hospital at Dallas, 6302, 7014
Texas Speech-Language-Hearing Association, 8682
Texas Technology Access Project, 3474
Texas UAP for Developmental Disabilities, 3475
Texas Workers Compensation Commission, 3476
Texas Workforce Commission, 6011
Textbook Catalog, 9064
Textbooks and the Student Who Can't Read Them: A Guide for Teaching Content, 2176
That All May Worship, 5057
That's My Child, 5019
Theatre Without Limits, 47
Theoretical Issues in Sign Language Research, 7922
Therapeutic Interventions in Alzheimer's, 7665
Therapeutic Nursery Program, 2209
Therapro, 141, 148, 284, 286, 287, 290, 309, 349, 352, 357, 358, 364, 365, 369, 484, 495, 504, 505, 507, 520, 534, 595, 7558
Therapro Inc., 1658
Therapy Putty, 520
There are Solutions for the Student with Asthma, 8601
There are Tyrannosaurs Trying on Pants in My Bedroom, 1445
There's a Hearing Impaired Child in My Class, 2177
They Don't Come with Manuals, 5020
They Grow in Silence, 7923
They're Just Kids, 5021
Thibodaux Hospital: Regional Rehabilitatio n Center, 6178
Thick-n-Easy, 364
Thinking About Tomorrow: A Career Guide for Teens with Arthritis, 8064
Thinking Big, 8602
Third Line Press, 4920
Thoele Manufacturing, 506
Thomasville Rehabilitation Center, 5611
Thoms Rehabilitation Hospital, 6922, 6922, 7453
Three Billy Goats Gruff, 1446
Three Hundred Tips for Making Life with Multiple Sclerosis Easier, 8603
Three Little Pigs, 1447
Three R's for Special Education: Rights, Resources, Results, 5181
Three Rivers Center for Independent Living, 3812, 4128
Three Rivers Health Care, 6199
Three Rivers IL Center, 3840
Three Rivers Independent Living Center: Centralia, 3841
Three Rivers Independent Resource Center, 3842
Three Rivers News, 9065
Three Rivers Press, 9, 7422
Thresholds AMISS, 5800
Thresholds Bridge Deaf North, 6707
Thresholds Psychiatric Rehabilitation Centers, 892, 6707
Thresholds South Suburbs, 6708
Through the Looking Glass, 3647, 4277, 4890, 4992, 4999, 5007, 5025, 5031, 5032, 5089, 5140, 5182, 7438, 7811, 7871, 7878, 8862, 8863, 8917, 8994
Thumb Industries, 6844
Thumbs Up Cup, 365
Thyssen Krupp Access, 418
Tic Tac Toe, 5290
Tidewater Center for Technology Access Special Education Annex, 1288
Tilt-N-Table, 655
Tim's Trim, 111
Timber Ridge Ranch NeuroRestorative Services, 6380
Timberland Opportunities Association, 7048
Timbertop Nature Adventure Camp, 7359
Times Mirror Foundation, 2378
Timex Easy Reader, 615
Tinnitus Today, 7924
Tirr System, 6289
Tisch Foundation, 2719
Title II & III Regulation Amendment Regarding Detectable Warnings, 4347
Title II Complaint Form, 4348
Title II Highlights, 4349
Title III Technical Assistance Manual and Supplement, 4350
To Live with Grace and Dignity, 4961
To Love this Life: Quotations by Helen Keller, 9066
To Teach a Dyslexic, 2178
To a Different Drumbeat, 5022
Togus VA Medical Center, 5454
Tohatchi Area of Opportunity & Services, 5947
Toilet Guard Rail, 149
Toledo Community Foundation, 2763
Toll-Free Information Line, 8672
Tom Snyder Productions, 1362, 1469
Tomah VA Medical Center, 5598
Tomorrow's Promise: Language Arts, 1505
Tomorrow's Promise: Mathematics, 1358
Tomorrow's Promise: Reading, 1506
Tomorrow's Promise: Spelling, 1507
Tools for Students, 4710
Tools for Transition, 1709
Topeka & Shawnee County Public Library Talking Book Service, 4485
Topeka Independent Living Resource Center, 3843
Topics in Early Childhood Special Education, 1903
Topics in Geriatric Rehabilitation, 7666
Torah Alliance of Families of Kids with Disabilities, 5518
Torso Support, 639
Total Living Center, 4021
Touch Turner Company, 218
Touch Turner-Page Turning Devices, 218
Touch of Nature Environmental Center, 933
Touch the Baby: Blind & Visually Impaired Children As Patients, 9067
Touch/Ability Connects People with Disabilities & Alternative Health Care Pract., 4962
TouchCorders, 1448
TouchCorders Holder, 1212
TouchWindow Touch Screen, 1449
Touchdown Keytop/Keyfront Kits, 1232
Touchstone Neurorecovery Center, 6303
Tourette Syndrome Association, 8176, 8594
Tourette Syndrome Association Annual Medical Letter, 8604
Tourette Syndrome Association Children's Newsletter, 8605
Tourette Syndrome Association Conference, 1561
Tourette Syndrome Association Newsletter, 8606
Tourette Syndrome Association of Connecticut (TSA), 8289
Tourette Syndrome Camp Organization, 934
Tourette Syndrome: The Facts, 8607
Tourette's Syndrome - Tics, Obsessions, Co mpulsions: Developmental Psychopathology, 8608
Tourette's Syndrome: Finding Answers and Getting Help, 8609
Touro Rehabilitation Center, 6777
Toward Effective Public School Program for Deaf Students, 2179
Toward Independence, 4351
Tower Program at Regis College, 7360
Toyei Industries, 6371
Trabant North Knox, 2521
Trace Research and Development Center, 4662
Trager International, 893
Training Module: Adaptive Baby Care Equipment, 5182
Training Resource Network, 4753, 5094, 6216
Training, Resource & Assistive-Technology, 6778
Trans Health Incorporated, 6221
Transcription Services, 521
Transfer Bench, 315
Transfer Bench with Back, 248
Transfer Tub Bench, 150
Transition Activity Calendar for Students with Visual Impairments, 9068
Transition Matters: from School to Independence: A Guide and Directory of Services, 4711
Transition from School to Work, 5102
Transition from School to Work for Persons with Disabilities, 5103
Transition in Adolescence, 8610
Transition to College for Students with Visual Impairments: Report, 9069
Transitional Hospitals Corporation, 6636

Transitional Learning Center at Galveston, 7015
Transitioning Exceptional Children and Youth Into the Community, 4736
Transitions to Adult Life, 4737
Transportation Equipment for People with Disabilities, 112
Transylvania Vocational Services, 5960
Traumatic Brain Injury: Cognitive & Communication Disorders, 7526
Traumatic Brain Injury: Mechanisms of Damage, Assessment & Intervention, 7527, 8736
Travel Information Service/Moss Rehab Hospital, 5302
Travelers Aid Society, 5323
Treating Cerebral Palsy for Clinicians by Clinicians, 2180
Treating Disordered Speech Motor Control, 2181
Treating Epilepsy Naturally: A Guide to A lternative and Adjunct Therapies, 8611
Treating Families of Brain Injury Survivors, 2182
Treatment Review, 1904
Treatment and Learning Centers (TLC), 5868
Tree of Life Publications, 8030
Treemont Nursing And Rehabilitation Center, 7016
Trekker 40, 582
Tri-County Center for Independent Living, 3985
Tri-County Independent Living Center, 3648, 4190, 5685
Tri-County Patriots for Independent Living, 4129
Tri-Grip Bathtub Rail, 151
Tri-Lo's, 583
Tri-Post Steering Wheel Spinner, 113
Tri-State Resource and Advocacy Corporation, 4158
Tri-Wheelers, 584
Triangle Community Foundation, 2733
Triangle Y Ranch YMCA, 7361
Trimedia Publications, 1856
Trinity Health Foundation, 6700
Trisha's of Acton, 1118
Triumph 3000/4000, 585
Triumph Scooter, 586
Trouble with Explosives, 8737
Truman Neurological Center, 6862
Trumbull Park, 6709
Trunks, 1146
Tub Slide Shower Chair, 152
Tucson Association for the Blind and Visually Imparied, 6372
Tufts-New England Medical Center, 6823
Tulare County Training Center Able Industries, 5686
Tulsa City- County Library System, 4605
Tulsa City-County Library System: Outreach Services, 4605
Tunnell Center for Rehab, 6510
Tuomey Healthcare System, 7222
Turnabout Game, 5291
Turning Automotive Seating (TAS), 419
Turnkey Computer Systems for the Visually, Physically, and Hearing Impaired, 1333
Turtle Teasers, 1450
Turtle Teasers IntelliKeys Overlay, 1213
Tuscaloosa Subregional Library for the Blind & Physically Handicapped, 4367
Tuscaloosa VA Medical Center, 5377
Tustin Rehabilitation Hospital, 6094
Twin Lakes Camp, 7984, 8291
Twin Peaks Press, 5297
Twin-Rest Seat Cushion & Glamour Pillow, 281
Twitch and Shout, 8612
Two Hundred Fifty Tips for Making Life with Arthritis Easier, 8065

U

U CL A Medical Center, 6095
U S Department of Education/ NI DR R, 6142
U S Department of Education, 2415, 2985, 4414, 8639
U S Department of Health, 7544
U S Department of Health and Human Services, 1898, 2967, 2968, 2969, 2981, 3072
U S Department of Justice, 4347, 4348, 4349, 4350
U S Department of the Interior, National Park Serv, 5339
U S Hang Gliding Association, 8095
U S Social Security Administration, 4509
U-Control II, 1214
UCLA Medical Center: Department of Anesthesiology, Acute Pain Services, 6095
UCP National, 1751
UN Printing, 9072
UNUM Charitable Foundation Maine Association Of Non Profits, 2536
UPMC Braddock, 7216
UPMC McKeesport, 7217
UPMC Passavant, 7218
US Association of Blind Athletes, 9091
US Department Veterans Affairs Beckley Vet Center, 5596
US Department of Education, 2965
US Department of Education: Office of Civil Rights, 2984, 2985
US Department of Health and Human Services, 4812
US Department of Health and Human Services Office for Civil Rights, 4352
US Department of Housing & Urban Development, 4857
US Department of Justice, 2986, 2970, 4273, 4274, 4291, 4292, 4293, 4294, 4299, 4310, 4339, 4738, 4739, 4756, 4761, 4762, 4763, 4765, 4766, 4767, 4768, 4776, 4784, 4863, 4891, 5104, 5105, 5106, 5107, 5109, 5114, 8563, 8856
US Department of Labor, 4353, 3078
US Department of Labor Office of Federal Contract Compliance Programs, 4354
US Department of Labor/Bureau of Labor Stats, 6318
US Department of Labor: Office of Federal Contract Programs, 2987
US Department of Transportation, 2988, 5359
US Department of Veterans Affairs National Headquarters, 5371
US Government TTY Directory, 7925
US Hang Gliding Association Jayne Defanfils, 8118
US Healthworks, 5989
US Office of Personnel Management, 2989
US Paralympics, 8633
US Role in International Disability Activities: A History, 4963
US Servas, 5324
US Social Security Administration, 7662
US Veteran's Affairs, 5372
USA Deaf Sports Federation, 7940
USX Foundation, 2798
Ukiah Valley Association for Habilitation, 6511
Ultra-Lite XL Hand Control, 114
Ultratec, 478
Umpqua Valley Disabilities Network, 4116
Un-Skru, 366
Uncommon Fathers, 5023
Undercounter Lid Opener, 367
Understanding, 5136
Understanding & Controlling Stuttering: A Comprehensive New Approach Based on the Valsa Hypo, 8738
Understanding ADHD, 7528
Understanding Asthma, 8613
Understanding Asthma: The Blueprint for Breathing, 8614
Understanding Attention Deficit Disorder, 7529
Understanding Autism, 7530
Understanding Cub Scouts with Disabilities, 4712
Understanding Cystic Fibrosis, 8615
Understanding Deafness Socially, 7926
Understanding Down Syndrome: An Introduction for Parents, 7531
Understanding Juvenile Rheumatoid Arthritis, 8066
Understanding Multiple Sclerosis, 8616
Understanding and Accommodating Physical Disabilities: Desk Reference, 4964
Understanding and Coping with Achromatopsia, 8617
Understanding and Teaching Emotionally Disturbed Children & Adolescents, 2183
Understanding the Nature of Autism, 7532
Underwood-Miller, 7390, 7538
Uni-Turner, 368
Unicorn Keyboards, 1309
Union Pacific Foundation, 2615
Unisex Low Vision Watch, 616
United Cerebral Palsy, 4358
United Cerebral Palsy Association, 8177, 3064, 4356
United Cerebral Palsy Association Development Conference, 1562
United Cerebral Palsy Association New York, 8225
United Cerebral Palsy Association of New York State, 8178
United Cerebral Palsy Associations of New Jersey, 5940, 3307
United Cerebral Palsy Research and Educational Foundation, 1751
United Cerebral Palsy of Maine, 7734
United Cerebral Palsy of Texas, 3477
United Cerebral Palsy of Western New York, 6910
United Church Of Christ, 914
United Communications Group, 7654
United Disability Services, 23
United Foundation for Disabled Archers, 8119
United Spinal Association, 1591
United States Access Board, 1572, 1573
United States Association of Blind Athletes, 8821, 8962

United States Blind Golf Association, 9092
United States Department of the Interior National Park Service, 5303
United States Tennis Association, 8117
United We Stand of New York, 3345
Unity, 219
Univ. of DE/Alfred I duPont Hospital for Children, 3063
Univ. of Delaware/duPont Hospital for Children, 4408
Universal Attention Disorders, 1466
Universal Hand Cuff, 369
Universal Institute: Rehab & Fitness Center, 8179
Universal Pediatric Services, 894
Universal Switch Mounting System, 1215
University Afiliated Program/Rose F Kennedy Center, 3346
University Healthcare-Rehabilitation Center, 6310
University Legal Services AT Program, 4355
University Medical Center, 6202, 6274
University Of Arkansas, 7679
University Of Cincinnati Uap, 4598
University Of Virginia School Of Engineering, 5360
University Press of Mississippi, 8615
University at Buffalo, 7566
University of Alabama, 2994
University of Arkansas at Little Rock, 8896
University of California Press, 7479
University of Cincinnati Hospital, 6235
University of Colorado Health Sciences Center, 6096
University of Idaho, 4451
University of Illinois Medical Center, 6710
University of Illinois at Chicago, 4465
University of Illinois at Chicago: Lions of Illinois Eye Research Institute, 4465
University of Illinois/Division of Rehab Education, 7983
University of Iowa, 4477
University of Iowa: Wendell Johnson Speech and Hearing Clinic, 7362, 7753, 8689, 8842
University of Kansas, 762, 3158
University of Maine at Augusta, 1264, 3184
University of Miami, 6124
University of Miami: Bascom Palmer Eye Institute, 4430
University of Miami: Jackson Memorial Rehabilitation Center, 6124
University of Miami: Mailman Center for Child Development, 4431
University of Michigan, 1809, 4538
University of Michigan: Orthopaedic Research Laboratories, 4538
University of Minnesota, 4547
University of Minnesota at Crookston, 2293
University of Missouri, 4554
University of Missouri-Kansas City, 3250
University of Missouri: Columbia Arthritis Center, 4554
University of Montana, 4556
University of Nebraska, 981
University of New Hampshire, 1732
University of New Hampshire: Inst on Disability, 5155
University of North Carolina at Chapel Hill, 7309, 8492
University of North Carolina at Chapel Hill: Neuroscience Research Building, 4594
University of Oregon, 2294
University of Oregon International Service, 2295
University of Pennsylvania, 2280
University of Rochester Medical Center, 3347
University of South Carolina, 775, 2817
University of South Dakota, 8671
University of South Florida, 4422
University of Texas, 3475
University of Texas Southwestern Medical Center/Allergy & Immunology, 4627
University of Texas at Austin, 1281
University of Texas at Austin Library, 4628
University of Virginia, 6315
University of Virginia Health System General Clinical Research Group, 4644
University of Virginia, Rehab Engineering Centers, 656
University of Washington PKU Clinic, 2097
University of Wisconsin, 1860
University of Wisconsin-Madison, 4662
Unlocking Potenial: College and Other Choi ces for People with LD and AD/HD, 7533
Unloving Care, 7667
Unseen Minority: A Social History of Blindness in the United States, 9070
Until Tomorrow: A Family Lives with Autism, 7534
Unyeway, 5687
Up and Running, 1524
Upledger Institute, 895
Upper Peninsula Library for the Blind, 4539
Upper Pinellas Association for Retarded Citizens, 6616
Upper Valley Medical/Rehab Services, 6236
Uppertone, 522
Upstate Update, 9071
Upward Bound Camp: Evans Creek, 1022
Urologic Care of the Child with Spina Bifida, 8618
Usher Syndrome, 8619
Using the Dictionary of Occupational Titles in Career Decision Making, 2184
Utah Assistive Technology Program (UTAP) Utah State University, 4191
Utah Assistive Technology Projects, 3480
Utah Client Assistance Program, 3481
Utah Department of Aging, 3482
Utah Department of Human Services, 3483, 3484
Utah Department of Human Services: Division of Services for People with Disabilities, 3483
Utah Department of Mental Health, 3484
Utah Division of Services for the Disabled, 3485
Utah Division of Veterans Affairs, 5578, 5578
Utah Employment Services, 6013
Utah Governor's Committee on Employment of the Handicapped, 6014
Utah Governor's Council for People with Disabilities, 3486
Utah Independent Living Center, 4192
Utah Independent Living Center: Minersville, 4193
Utah Independent Living Center: Tooele, 4194
Utah Labor Commission, 3487
Utah Protection & Advocacy Services for Persons with Disabilities, 3488
Utah State Library Division: Program for the Blind and Disabled, 4630
Utah State Office of Education, 1836
Utah State Office of Education: At-Risk and Special Education Service Unit, 1836
Utah State Office of Rehabilitation, 6016
Utah State University, 3480
Utah Veterans Centers, 6015
Utah Vocational Rehabilitation Agency, 6016

V

V A Department Veterans Affairs, 5523
V A Montana Healthcare System, 5486
V Foundation for Cancer Research, 5257
V Hunter Trust, 2391
V OR T Corporation, 1395, 1456
V XI Corporation Incorporated, 1334
V-Bar Enterprises, 5688
VA Ann Arbor Healthcare System, 5472
VA Boston Healthcare System: Brockton Division, 5464
VA Boston Healthcare System: Jamaica Plain Campus, 5465
VA Boston Healthcare System: West Roxbury Division, 5466
VA Central California Health Care Syste, 5396
VA Central Iowa Health Care System, 5442
VA Connecticut Healthcare System: Newington Division, 5406
VA Connecticut Healthcare System: West Haven, 5407
VA Greater Los Angeles Healthcare System, 5397
VA Hudson Valley Health Care System, 5519
VA Illiana Health Care System, 5433
VA Maryland Health Care System, 5460
VA Medical Center, Washington DC, 5413
VA Montana Healthcare System, 5487
VA Nebraska-Western Iowa Health Care System, 5492
VA North Indiana Health Care System: Fort Wayne Campus, 5436
VA North Texas Health Veterans Affairs Car e System: Dallas VA Medical Center, 5575
VA Northern California Healthcare System, 5398
VA Northern Indiana Health Care System: Marion Campus, 5437
VA Pittsburgh Healthcare System, Highland Drive Division, 5554
VA Pittsburgh Healthcare System, University Drive Division, 5553
VA Puget Sound Health Care System, 5590
VA Salt Lake City Healthcare System, 5579
VA San Diego Healthcare System, 5399
VA Sierra Nevada Healthcare System, 5495
VA Southern Nevada Healthcare System, 5496
VA Western NY Healthcare System, Batavia, 5520
VA Western NY Healthcare System, Buffalo, 5521
VACC Camp, 8292
VAK Tasks Workbook: Visual, Auditory and Kinesthetic, 1710
VBS Special Education Teaching Guide, 2185
VCT/A Job Retention Skill Training Program, 5645
VESID, 3348
VIP Newsletter, 1905
VISION, 1216

VISIONS Vacation Camp for the Blind, 8843
VISIONS/Services for the Blind & Visually Impaired, 8843
VOLAR Center for Independent Living, 4180
VSA Arts, 48
VSA Arts of Indiana, 6163
VSA Arts of Maine, 47
VSA Arts of New York City, 3349
VUE: Vision Use in Employment, 9099
Vacamas Program for Youth, 8247
Val J Halomandaris, 8657
Vale-Asche Foundation, 2874
Valley Associates for Independent Living (VAIL), 4218
Valley Associates for Independent Living: Lexington, 4219
Valley Association for Independent Living (VAIL), 4181
Valley Association for Independent Living: Harlingen, 4182
Valley Center for the Blind, 6512
Valley Forge Specialized Educational Services, 2263
Valley Garden Health Care and Rehabilitati on Center, 7071
Valley Health Care and Rehabilitation Cent er, 7061
Valley Industries, 5706
Valley Light Industries, 5689
Valley Memorial Health Center, 5721
Valley Regional Medical Center, 7236
Valley Regional Medical Center: RehabCare Unit, 6304
Valley View Regional Hospital-RehabCare Unit, 6960
Valpar International, 1517
ValueOptions, 5258
Van Ameringen Foundation, 2720
Van G Miller & Associates, 6726
VanMatre Rehabilitation Center, 6711
Vancouver Health & Rhabilitation Center, 7256
Vancouver Health and Rehabilitation Center, 7049
Vanderbilt Rehabilitation Center, 6988
Vangater, Vangater II, Mini-Vangater, 420
Vanguard School, 2263
Vantage, 220
Vantage Mini-Vans, 115, 115
Vantage Press, 8019
Variety Club Camp, 1039
Vaughn-Blumberg Services, 6350
Vector Mobility, 706
Velcro Booties, 1085
Velcro Sneaker, 1086
Ventilator-Assisted Living, 8620
Ventura Enterprises, 640
Ventures Travel, 5350
Vermont Achievement Center, 6311
Vermont Assistive Technology Project: Department of Aging & Disabilities, 1289, 4195
Vermont Assistive Technology Projects, 3491
Vermont Association for the Blind and Visually Impaired, 8822
Vermont Back Research Center, 7974
Vermont Center for Independent Living, 4197
Vermont Center for Independent Living: Bennington, 4198
Vermont Center for Independent Living: Brattleboro, 4196
Vermont Client Assistance Program, 3492
Vermont College of Norwich University, 4
Vermont Community Foundation, 2880
Vermont Department Of Health, 3496
Vermont Department of Aging, 3493
Vermont Department of Developmental and, 3494
Vermont Department of Disabilities, Aging and Independent Living, 3495
Vermont Department of Health: Children with Special Health Needs, 3496
Vermont Department of Libraries/Special Services Unit, 4631
Vermont Developmental Disabilities Council, 3497
Vermont Division for the Blind and Visually Impaired, 3498
Vermont Division of Disability & Aging Services, 3499
Vermont Employment Services and Job Training, 6019
Vermont Governor's Committee on Employment of People with Disabilities, 6020
Vermont Interdependent Services Team Approach (VISTA), 2186
Vermont Protection and Advocacy, 3500
Vermont VA Regional Office Center, 5580
Vermont Veterans Centers, 5581
Versatrainer, 421
Vertek, 1513
Vertical Home Lift Sales, 422
Vestibular Board, 423
Vestibular Disorder Association, 7772
Vestibular Disorders Association, 4965, 7730, 4965, 7730, 7830, 7842, 7869, 7879, 7933, 8503
Vet Center, 5477, 5488
Vet Center Readjustment Counseling Service, 5473
Vet Health Administration U S Department of VA, 5526
Veterans Benefits Administration, 5511
Veterans Benefits Administration U S Deparment of, 5552
Veterans Benefits Administration U S Department V, 5580
Veterans Benefits Administration U S Department of, 5404, 5434, 5588
Veterans Benefits Administration U S Dept. of V A, 5391, 5401, 5408
Veterans Benefits Administration U S Deptartment o, 5494
Veterans Benefits Administration, U S Dept. of V A, 5373, 5378, 5386, 5389, 5394, 5419, 5421, 5426, 5428, 5439, 5445, 5449, 5453, 5455, 5461, 5471, 5476, 5479, 5483, 5490, 5497, 5503, 5515, 5527, 5529, 5533, 5536, 5540, 5550, 5556, 5558, 5567, 5572, 5576, 5584, 5592, 5600, 5604
Veterans Health Administration U S Department of V, 5393, 5431, 5534, 5560, 5597
Veterans Health Administration U S Department. of, 5406
Veterans Health Administration U S Dept. of V A, 5375
Veterans Health Administration U S Deptartment of, 5397, 5462, 5508
Veterans Health Administration, U S Department of, 5519, 5549
Veterans Health Administration, U S Dept. of V A, 5377, 5380, 5382, 5383, 5387, 5388, 5390, 5396, 5398, 5399, 5402, 5403, 5407, 5414, 5415, 5416, 5417, 5418, 5420, 5422, 5423, 5424, 5429, 5430, 5432, 5433, 5435, 5436, 5437, 5438, 5440, 5443, 5444, 5446, 5447, 5448, 5450, 5451, 5452, 5454, 5456, 5457, 5459, 5463, 5464, 5465, 5466, 5467, 5468, 5469, , 5470, 5472, 5474, 5475, 5478, 5480, 5481, 5482, 5484, 5487, 5489, 5491, 5492, 5495, 5496, 5498, 5502, 5506, 5509, 5510, 5512, 5513, 5514, 5516, 5517, 5520, 5521, 5522, 5524, 5525, 5528, 5530, 5531, 5531, 5535
Veterans Health Administration, US Dept. of VA, 5376, 5381, 5384, 5385, 5395, 5409, 5427, 5501, 5504, 5566, 5568
Via Rehabilitation Services, 911
Vibes Bed Shaker, 165
Vibra Health Care, 6099
Vibration Watch/Countdown Timer, 166
Vibrotactile Personal Alerting System, 221
Vicki La Rue, 1051
Victims of Dementia: Services, Support and Care, 7668
Victor E Speas Foundation, 2611
Victoria Foundation, 2641
Video Guide to Disability Awareness, 5183
Video Intensive Parenting, 5184
Views from Our Shoes, 4713
Viewstar, 222, 222
Viking Books, 8906
Villa Esperanza Services, 6513
Village Square Nursing Center, 6514
Villard Books, 8329
Villiard Books, 8521
Vinfen Corporation, 6824
Vinland Center Lake Independence, 3957
Vinsen Corporation, 5870
Vintage, 7495
Virginia Autism Resource Center, 4645
Virginia Beach Foundation, 2889
Virginia Beach Public Library Special Services Library, 4646
Virginia Chapter of the Arthtitis Foundation, 4647
Virginia Commonwealth University, 4638
Virginia Commonwealth University, Medical College, 1545
Virginia Department Of Education, 1837
Virginia Department for the Blind and Vision Impaired, 3503
Virginia Department of Education: Division of Pre & Early Adolescent Education, 1837
Virginia Department of Mental Health, 3504
Virginia Department of Veterans Services, 5586
Virginia Developmental Disability Council, 3505
Virginia Office Protection and Advocacy for People with Disabilities, 3506
Virginia Office for Protection & Advocacy, 3507
Virginia Office for Protection and Advocacy, 3508
Virginia State Library for the Visually and Physically Handicapped, 4648
Virginia's Developmental Disabilities Plan ning Council, 3509
Visalia Workshop, 5690
Visi-Pitch III, 1468
Vision, 7927
Vision Enhancement, 9072

Vision Foundation, 2569
Vision Loss Resources, 6850
Vision Northwest, 6966
Vision Rehabilitation Service, 6823
Vision World Wide, 8823
Vision and Aging: Issues in Social Work Practice, 7669
Visions & Values, 4966
Visions/Services for the Blind & Visually Impaired, 4073, 8824
Visiting Nurse Association of America, 8673
Visiting Nurse Association of North Shore, 6825
Vista Center for the Blind & Visually Impaired, 6515, 9043
Vista Wheelchair, 698
Visual Aids and Informational Material, 9073
Visual Alerting Guest Room Kit, 523
Visual Handicaps and Learning, 9074
Visual Impairment: An Overview, 9075
Visual Independence Program, 6863
Visually Handicapped Child in Your Class, 9076
Visually Impaired Center, 6845, 8923
Visually Impaired Persons of Southwest Florida, 6617
Visually Impaired Seniors as Senior Companions: A Reference Guide, 7670
Visually Impaired Veterans of America, 8825
Visually Structured Tasks, 9077
Vital Signs: Crip Culture Talks Back, 5185
Viva Vital News, 9078
Vocabulary Development, 1508
Vocal Rehabilitation: A Practice Book for Voice Improvement, 8739
Vocational Counseling for Special Populations, 6140
Vocational Evaluation and Traumatic Brain Injury: A Procedural Manual, 6327
Vocational Interest Profile Report, 1516
Vocational Rehabilitation Agency, 5873, 5948
Vocational Rehabilitation Service Opelika, 5612
Vocational Rehabilitation Service: Dothan, 5614
Vocational Rehabilitation Service: Gadsden, 5615
Vocational Rehabilitation Service: Homewoo d, 5616
Vocational Rehabilitation Service: Huntsvi lle, 5617
Vocational Rehabilitation Service: Jackson, 5618
Vocational Rehabilitation Service: Jasper, 5619
Vocational Rehabilitation Service: Mobile, 5620
Vocational Rehabilitation Service: Muscle Shoals, 5621
Vocational Rehabilitation Service: Scottsboro, 5613
Vocational Rehabilitation Service: Selma, 5622
Vocational Rehabilitation Service: Tallade ga, 5623
Vocational Rehabilitation Service: Troy, 5624
Vocational Rehabilitation Service: Tuscalo osa, 5625
Vocational Rehabilitation Services: Andalu sa, 5626
Vocational Rehabilitation Services: Annist on, 5627
Vocational Rehabilitation and Employment, 6220
Vocational Rehabilitation and Supported Employment, 6183
Vocational Rehabilitation, Division of Department of Workforce Services, 6043
Vocational Training and Employment of the Autistic Adolescent, 6141
Vocational and Rehabilitation Agency, 5636, 5707, 5722, 5773, 5779, 5801, 5825, 5859, 5886, 5903, 5908, 5941, 5949, 5961, 5975, 5982, 5990, 6021, 6029, 6001, 6012
Vocational and Rehabilitation Agency Department of Education, 5760
Vocational and Rehabilitation Agency Division of Services for the Blind, 5646
Vocational and Rehabilitation Agency Massachusetts Commission for the Blind, 5874
Vocational and Rehabilitation Agency Rehabilitation Services Administrations, 5641
Vocational and Rehabilitation Agency for Persons Who Are Visually Impaired, 5647
Vocational and Rehabilitation Agency: Commision for the Blind, 5983
Vocational and Rehabilitation Agency: Commission for the Blind, 6001
Vocational and Rehabilitation Agency: Department for the Blind/Visually Impaired, 6030
Vocational and Rehabilitation Agency: Department of Human Services, 5962, 5991, 5996
Vocational and Rehabilitation Agency: Divi sion of Services to the Blind/Visually Impaired, 6005
Vocational and Rehabilitation Agency: Division of Vocational Rehabilitation, 5761, 6017, 6036
Vocational and Rehabilitation Agency: State Department of Social Services, 5723
Vocational and Rehabilitation Agency: State Rehabilitation Commission, 6012
Vocational and Rehabilitation Agency: Vocational Rehabilitation Department, 6000
Vocational and Rehabilitation Service Columbiana, 5628
Vocational and Rehabilitation Service: Decatur, 5629
Vocational and Rehabilitation Services: Montgomery, 5630
Vocational and Rehabilitation: Division of Wisconsin, 6040
Vocational-Educational Services for Individuals, 7745
Voice Amplified Handsets, 223
Voice Choice, 116
Voice Scan, 117
Voice of Vision, 9079
Voice of the Diabetic, 8621
Voice-It, 1334
Voices for Independence, 4130
Voices of Vision Talking Book Center at DuPage Library System, 4466
Volasuca Volunteers of America, 1063
Volcanoes, 1451
Volta Review, 7928
Volta Voices, 7929
Volunteer Transcribing Services, 1711
Volunteer Voice, 8067
Volunteers of America, 1063
Volunteers of America Supported Living Program, 3866

W

W Alton Jones Foundation, 2890
W GB H Educational Foundation, 6801
W Troy Cole Independent Living Specialist, 3867
WA & NEWS, 8068
WA Department of Services for the Blind, 3513
WAVE Work, Achievement, Value, & Education, 5735
WB Saunders Company, 8724
WCI/Weitbrecht Communications, 479
WCIB Heavy-Duty Folding Cane, 641
WG Hefner VA Medical Center, 5526
WGBH Educational Foundation, 8900
WINGS for Learning, 1343, 1350, 1351, 1417, 1421, 1480
WM Keck Foundation, 2379
WORK, 4755
WP and HB White Foundation, 2512
WRAD, 7731
WW Norton & Company, 4801, 8038
WW Smith Charitable Trust, 2799
WX: Work Capacities, 5895
WY Department of Health: Mental Health and Substance Abuse Service Division, 3542
Wabash Independent Living Center & Learning Center (WILL), 3803
Wabash/Employability Center, 5826
Waco Regional Office, 5576
Wage and Hour Division of the Employment Standards Administration, 3078
Wagon Road Camp, 1005
Wahiawa Family, 5774
Wakeman/ Walworth, 2942
Wakeman/Walworth, 5082
Walden Rehabilitation and Nursing Center, 7157
Walgreens Home Medical Center, 480
Walker Leg Support, 642
Walker Publishing Company, 8015, 8311
WalkerTalker, 224
Walking Alone and Marching Together, 9080
Walking Tomorrow, 4967, 7975
Wallace Memorial Library, 4589
Walton Option for Independent Living, 3731
Walton Options For Independent Living (Warrington), 3732
Walton Rehabilitation Health System, 6637, 7100
Walton Way Medical, 481
War Memorial Hospital, 7257
Wardrobe Wagon: The Special Needs Clothing Store, 5259
Warner Books, 7367, 8001, 8624
Warner Robins Rehabilitation and Nursing C enter, 7101
Warp Drive, 118
Warren Achievement Center, 6712
Warren Grant Magnuson Clinical Center, 4510
Warren Memorial Hospital, 7244
Wasatch Valley Rehabilitation, 7241
Wasatch Vision Clinic, 7019
Washable Shoes, 1087

Washington Association of Housing and Services for the Aging, 7601
Washington Client Assistance Program, 3514
Washington Connection, 9100
Washington County Disability, Aging and Veteran Services, 3398
Washington County Vocational Workshop, 5802
Washington DC VA Medical Center, 5414
Washington Department of Mental Health, 3515
Washington Developmental Disability, 3516
Washington Ear, 8826
Washington Governor's Committee on Disability Issues & Employment, 3517
Washington Hearing and Speech Society, 3079
Washington Memorial Library, 4442
Washington Office of Superintendent of Public Instruction, 3518
Washington Protection & Advocacy System, 3519
Washington Square Health Foundation, 2513
Washington State Developmental Disabilities Council, 3520
Washington Talking Book and Braille Library, 4651
Washington Technology Access Center, 1290
Washington Watch, 4356
Washtenaw County Library for the Blind & Physically Handicapped, 4540
Waterfront Books, 8625
Waterfront Books Publishing Company, 1784
Waterproof Sheet-Topper Mattress and Chair Pad, 167
Waterville Public Library, 4501
Waupaca Elevator Company, 380
Waushers Industries, 7052
Wayne County Regional Educational Service Agency, 1325, 1329
Wayne County Regional Library for the Blind, 4541
Wayne State University, 791
Wayne State University: CS Mott Center for Human Genetics and Development, 4542
We Are PHAMALY, 49
We CAN Hear and Speak, 7930
We Can Do it Together!, 9081
We Can Speak for Ourselves: Self Advocacy by Mentally Handicapped People, 5024
We Magazine, 5260
We Media, 5261
We're Not Stupid, 7535
WebABLE, 5262
Webster Enterprises of Jackson County, 5963
Week the World Heard Gallaudet, 7931
Weiner's Herbal, 4968
Welcome Homes Retirement Community for the Visually Impaired, 6846
Weldon Center for Rehabilitation, 6826
Well Mind Association of Greater Washington, 3080
Wellsouth Health Systems, 7135
Wes Test Engineering Corporation, 1519
WesTest Engineering Corporation, 1173
Wesley Woods, 1040
Wesley Woods Camp & Retired Center, 947
West Central Alabama Easter Seals Rehabilitation Center, 6351
West Central Illinois Center for Independent Living, 3789
West Central Independent Living Solutions, 3986
West Essex Rehab Center, 5942
West Florida Hospital: The Rehabilitation Institute, 6618
West Florida Regional Library, 4432
West Gables Health Care Center, 6619
West Michigan Learning Disabilities Foundation, 2259
West Palm Beach VA Medical Center, 5420
West Suburban Hospital Medical Center, 6662
West Texas Lighthouse for the Blind, 7017
West Texas VA Healthcare System, 5577
West Virginia Advocates, 3525, 3526
West Virginia Autism Training Center, 4657
West Virginia Client Assistance Program, 3526
West Virginia Department of Aging, 3527
West Virginia Department of Children with Disabilities, 3528
West Virginia Department of Education: Office of Special Education, 1839
West Virginia Department of Health, 3529, 3535
West Virginia Developmental Disabilities Council, 3530
West Virginia Division of Rehabilitation Services, 3531, 6037
West Virginia Employment Services and Job Training Programs Liaison, 6038
West Virginia Hospital Association, 896
West Virginia Library Commission, 4658
West Virginia Rehabilitation Center, 7050
West Virginia Research and Training Center, 2220
West Virginia School for the Blind Library, 4659
West Virginia Vocational Rehabilitation, 6039
Westbank Sheltered Workshop, 5851
Westchester County Independent Living Center, 4074
Westchester Disabled on the Move, 4075
Westchester Institute for Human Development, 3350
Westerly Chariho Arc, 2815
Western Alliance Center for Independent Living, 4084
Western Michigan University, 3208
Western NC Conference/United Methodist Church, 7742
Western New York Foundation, 2721
Western Psychological Services, 7374, 7442, 7472, 7536
Western Regional Vocational Rehabilitation Facility Clifford File, Jr., 5964
Western Resources for dis-ABLED Independence, 4152
Western Washington University, 2296
Westin Hotels and Resorts, 5325
Westpark Rehabilitation Center, 7128
Westside Center for Independent Living, 3649
Westside Opportunity Workshop, 5691
Westside Parents Work Activity Center, 5803
Westview Nursing and Rehabilitation Center, 7129
Weyerhaeuser Company Foundation, 2900
Wgbh Educational Foundation, 8677
What About Me?, 4714
What About Me? Growing Up with a Developme ntally Disabled Sibling, 4715
What Can Baby Hear?: Auditory Tests and In terventions for Infants with Multiple Disabilities, 7932
What Do You Do When You See a Blind Person - and What Don't You Do?, 9082
What Everyone Needs to Know About Asthma, 8622
What It's Like to be Me, 4716
What Museum Guides Need to Know: Access for the Blind and Visually Impaired, 9083
What Psychotherapists Should Know about Disabilty, 5089
What School Personnel Should Know About Asthma, 8623
What Was That!, 1452
What You Need To Know, 7933
What Your Doctor May Not Tell You About Ch ildren's Allergies and Asthma, 8624
What is Auditory Processing?, 7934
What is Vocal Hoarseness?, 8740
What's a Virus, Anyway? The Kid's Book About AIDS, 8625
Wheat Ridge Ministries, 2514
Wheel Life News, 656
Wheelchair Access, 7976, 8068
Wheelchair Accessories, 657
Wheelchair Activity/Computer Table, 545
Wheelchair Aide, 658
Wheelchair Back Pack and Tote Bag, 659
Wheelchair Batteries, 8069
Wheelchair Carrier, 424
Wheelchair Getaways, 5351
Wheelchair Getaways Wheelchair/Scooter Accessible Van Rentals, 5361
Wheelchair Motorcycle Association, 8120
Wheelchair Ponchos, 1091
Wheelchair Roller, 660
Wheelchair Sports, USA, 8121
Wheelchair Work Table, 661
A Wheelchair for Petronilia, 7986
Wheelchair with Shock Absorbers, 699
WheelchairNet, 5263
Wheelchairs of Kansas, 690
Wheelers, 5362
Wheelers Accessible Van Rentals, 119, 5326, 5363, 5304
Wheelies Manufacturing, 1140
Wheelin Around, 5304
Wheelin' Around, 8070
When Billy Broke His Head...and Other Tales of Wonder, 4717
When I Grow Up, 4718
When Parents Can't Fix It, 4719
When You Have a Visually Impaired Student in Your Classroom: A Guide for Teachers, 2187
When Your Student Has Arthritis: A Guide for Teachers, 8071
When the Brain Goes Wrong, 4969
When the Mind Hears, 7935
When the Road Turns: Inspirational Storie s About People with MS, 8626
Where to Stay USA, 5305
White Cane and Wheels, 5186
White City VA Domiciliary, 5543
Whittier High School District, 5652
Whittier Trust Company Foundations Office, 2356
Whole Person, 3987
Whole Person: Nortonville, 3844
Whole Person: Olathe, 3845
Whole Person: Prairie Village, 3846

Whole Person: Tonganoxie, 3847
Whoops, 1509
Whurr Publishers, 22, 31
Why Mine?, 5058
Why My Child, 4720
Why Won't My Child Pay Attention?, 7536
Wichita Public Library, 4486, 4487
Wichita Public Library/Talking Book Service, 4487
Wilderness Inquiry, 5327
Wiley Publishing, 4272, 7519, 8442, 8608, 8701
Wiley-Liss, 8498
Wilkes-Barre VA Medical Center, 5555
Will Grundy Center for Independent Living, 3790
Will of Stewart Huston, 2796
Willam G Gilmore Foundation, 2380
Willamette Valley Rehabilitation Center, 6967
William B Dietrich Foundation, 2800
William H Honor Rehabilitation Center Henry Ford Wyanclotte Hospital, 6847
William Hein & Company, 4302, 4306, 4313, 4318, 4319, 4331, 4338
William J and Dorothy K O'Neill Foundation, 2764
William Jennings Bryan Dorn VA Medical Center, 5560
William Morrow & Company, 4687, 8044, 8602, 8718
William N and Pennington Foundation, 2620
The William Randolph Hearst Foundations, 2718
William S Hein & Company, 4357
William S Middleton Memorial VA Hospital Center, 5599
William Stamps Farish Fund, 2875
William T Grant Foundation, 2722
William Talbott Hillman Foundation, 2801
William V and Catherine A McKinney Charitable Foundation, 2802
Willough at Naples, 6620
Wilmer Ophthalmology Institute, 4502
Wilmington VA Medical, 5409
Wilmington Vet Center, 5410
WinSCAN: The Single Switch Interface for PC's with Windows, 1217
Winchester Centre For Health & Rehabilitation, 7137
Winchester Rehabilitation Center, 7245
Wind River Healthcare and Rehabilitation Center, 7273
Window-Ease, 524
Window-Eyes, 1335
Windsor Estates Health and Rehab Center, 7130
Windsor Rehabilitation and Healthcare Cent er, 7079
Wings Press, 7469
Winifred Law Opportunity Center, 4279
Winkler Court, 7094
Winnekeag, 8844
Winston-Salem Industries for the Blind, 6923
Winston-Salem Regional Office, 5527
Winston-Salem Rehabilitation and Healthcar e Center, 7195
Winter Conference, 1563
Winter Park Memorial Hospital, 6125, 7095
Winthrop Rockefeller Foundation, 2312
Winways, 6516
Wiregrass Rehabilitation Center, 5631
Wisconsin Association of Homes & Services for the Aging, 7602
Wisconsin Badger Camp, 1067
Wisconsin Bureau of Aging, 3536
Wisconsin Chapter of the Arthritis Foundation, 7999
Wisconsin Coalition for Advocacy: Madison Office, 3537
Wisconsin Council on Developmental Disabilities (WCDD), 3538
Wisconsin Governor's Committee for People with Disabilities, 3539
Wisconsin Lions Camp, 8293
Wisconsin Lions Foundation, 8293
Wisconsin Regional Library for the Blind & Physically Handicapped, 4663
Wisconsin VA Regional Office, 5600
Wisconsin Vocational Rehabilitation Agency, 6041
Wise Enterprises, 156, 160, 161
Wishing Wells Clothing Collection, 1119
Wishing Wells Collection, 1125
Wiswall Center for Independent Living, 4076
With Standing Ovation, 8072
Without Pity, 8073
Without Reason: A Family Copes with Autism, 7537
Without Sight and Sound, 5137, 7936
Wivik 3, 1453
Wolfner Library for the Blind, 4555
A Woman's Guide To Living With HIV Infecti on, 8301
Women to Women, 897
Women with Attention Deficit Disorder: Em bracing Disorganization at Home and Work, 7538
Women with Physical Disabilities: Achievin g & Maintaining Health & Well-Being, 4970
Women with Visible & Invisible Disabilitie es: Multiple Intersections, Issues, Therapies, 5090
Wonderland Camp Foundation, 979
Woodbine House, 2002, 2162, 4674, 5023, 5030, 7425, 7462, 7480, 7525, 7787, 8377, 8379, 8380, 8585
Woodcock Reading Mastery Tests, 2248
Woodlands, 1041
Woodrow Wilson Rehabilitation Center, 7029
Woodrow Wilson Rehabilitation Center Training Program, 4220
Woodside Day Program, 6557
Woodstock Health and Rehabilitation Center, 7053
Word Attack Manual, 1712
Word Demons, 1713
Word Elements: How They Work Together, 1714
Word Mastery, 1715
Word from Washington, 4358
Wordly Wise A,B,C, 1716
Words Plus, 1175, 1218
Words+, 1185, 1188, 1189, 1191, 1198, 1214, 1219, 1307, 1311, 1312, 1332, 1386, 1415, 1460, 1523
Words+ Equalizer, 1218
Words+ IST (Infrared, Sound, Touch), 1219
Words- Plus, 1178
Work Enhancement Center of Western Kentucky, 5846
Work Exploration Center, 5762
Work Inc., 5875
Work Sight, 9084
Work Training Center for the Handicapped, 5692
Work Training Programs, 5693
Work and Disability: Issues and Strategie s in Career Development and Job Placement, 6053
Work in the Context of Disability Culture, 4971
Work!, 1717
Work, Health and Income Among the Elderly, 7671
Work-Related Vocational Assessment Systems, 1517
Workers Compensation, 3012
Workers Compensation Agency, 3229
Workers Compensation Board Alabama, 3001
Workers Compensation Board Colorado, 3056
Workers Compensation Board Illinois, 3141
Workers Compensation Board Iowa, 3157
Workers Compensation Board Louisiana, 3183
Workers Compensation Board Maryland, 3199
Workers Compensation Board Massachusetts, 3207
Workers Compensation Board Missouri, 3255
Workers Compensation Board Nevada, 3286
Workers Compensation Board New Hampshire, 3298
Workers Compensation Board New Mexico, 3319
Workers Compensation Board New York, 3351
Workers Compensation Board North Dakota, 3369
Workers Compensation Board Ohio, 3382
Workers Compensation Board Oklahoma, 3389
Workers Compensation Board Pennsylvania, 3410
Workers Compensation Board Rhode Island, 3422
Workers Compensation Board Tennessee, 3449
Workers Compensation Board Vermont, 3501
Workers Compensation Board Washington, 3521
Workers Compensation Board Wisconsin, 3540
Workers Compensation Board Wyoming, 3543
Workers Compensation Board: District of Columbia, 3081
Workers Compensation Board: South Carolina, 3432
Workers Compensation Board: South Dakota, 3439
Workforce and Technology Center, 6795
Working Bibliography on Behavioral and Emotional Disorders, 2188
Working Together & Taking Part, 1718
Working Together with Children and Families: Case Studies, 2189
Working Together: Workplace Culture, Employment and Disabilities, 6188
Working with Visually Impaired Young Students: A Curriculum Guide, 2190
Workplace Skills: Learning How to Function on the Job, 1518
Workshops, 6048
Workshops Inc., 5632

Worksight, 5890
World Association of Persons with Disabilities, 5264
A World Awaits You, 4759, 5293, 7987
World Chiropractic Alliance, 7551, 7977
World Experience, 2297
World Institute on Disability, 898, 1916, 1917, 2054, 4888, 4934, 4961, 4963
World Research Foundation, 4376
World Through Their Eyes, 9085
World Without AIDS: The Controvertial Holistic Health, 7539
World of Options, 2298
World of Options: A Guide to International Educational Exchange, 2299
World's Best Books from the Diabetes Experts: Publications Catalog, 8627
Worldwide Disability Solutions Group, 2319
Worldwide Mobility Products, 64
Worst Loss: How Families Heal from the Death of a Child, 5059
Worthmore Academy, 2264
Wright-Way, 70
Write This Way, 1525
Write: OutLoud, 1526
Writer's Showcase Press, 4847
Writing Skills 1 and 2, 1719
Writing Skills for the Adolescent, 1720
Wyman Center, 8257, 8268
Wyoming Client Assistance Program, 3544
Wyoming Department of Aging, 3545
Wyoming Department of Education, 1840, 4664
Wyoming Department of Employment Unemployment Insurance, 6044
Wyoming Department of Workforce Services, 6042
Wyoming Developmental Disability Council, 3546
Wyoming Governor's Committee on Employment of the Handicapped, 6045
Wyoming Institute for Disabilities (WIND), 899
Wyoming Protection & Advocacy for Persons with Disabilities, 3547
Wyoming Services for Independent Living, 4251
Wyoming Services for the Visually Impaired, 4664
Wyoming Veterans Centers, 5603
Wyoming's New Options in Technology (WYNOT) - University of Wyoming, 4665
Wyoming/Colorado VA Regional Office, 5604

X

XL Steering, 120
Xavier Society for the Blind, 4590
Xerox Imaging Systems/Adaptive Products Department, 1291

Y

Y MC A of Greater Seattle, 8298
Y MC A of Tri- County mtero mil, 7361
Y WC A of Greater Portland, 7755
YAI: National Institute for People with Disabilities, 900
YMCA Camp Chingachgook on Lake George, 8845
YMCA Camp Copneconic, 971
YMCA Camp Duncan, 934
YMCA Camp Fitch, 7754, 7985, 8294, 8690
YMCA Camp Glacier Hollow, 7359
YMCA Camp H R Erdman, 927
YMCA Camp Horseshoe, 8295
YMCA Camp Ihduhapi, 8296
YMCA Camp Kitaki, 8297
YMCA Camp Orkila, 8298
YMCA Camp Weona, 8299
YMCA Camp of Maine, 8183
YMCA Camping Services, 7318
YMCA Of Greater Des Moines, 8255
YMCA Outdoor Center Campbell Gard, 8300
YMCA of Greater Buffalo, 8299
YMCA of Greater Hartford, 8226
YMCA of Greater Oklahoma City, 8205
YMCA of the Ozarks, 977
YMCA of the Pikes Peak Region (PPYMCA), 8241
YWCA Camp Westwind, 7755
Yale New Haven Health System-Bridgeport Hospital, 6547
Yale University Press, 8557
Yale University: Vision Research Center, 4407
Yavapai Regional Medical Center-West, 5642
Yorba Linda Placentia Farm YMCA, 7355
You And Your Deaf Child, 7937
You May Be Able to Adopt, 5025
You Mean I'm Not Lazy, Stupid or Crazy?!: A Self-Help Book for Adults with ADD, 7540
You Seem Like a Regular Kid to Me, 9086
You Tell Me: Learning Basic Information, 1454
You Will Dream New Dreams, 5026
You and Your ADD Child, 7541
You and Your Deaf Child: A Self-Help Guide for Parents of Deaf and Hard of Hearing Children, 7938
Young Children with Special Needs, 1765
Young Children with Special Needs: A Developmentally Appropriate Approach, 2249
Young Onset Parkinson Conference, 1564
Young Person's Guide to Spina Bifida, 8628
Youngstown Foundation, 2765
Youngstown YMCA, 7754, 7985, 8294, 8690
Younker Rehabilitation Center of Iowa Methodist Medical Center, 6164
Your Child Has a Disability: A Complete So urcebook of Daily and Medical Care, 5027
Your Child and Asthma, 8629
Your Child in the Hospital: A Practical Guide for Parents, 5036
Your Cleft-Affected Child, 8630
Youth Leadership Camp, 7756
Youth for Understanding International Exchange, 2300
Youville Hospital & Rehab Center, 6827
Yuma Center for the Visually Impaired, 6373
Yuma County Workshop, 5708

Z

ZoomText, 1318
Zygo Industries, 1313

Alabama

Adventure Program, 901
Alabama Institute for Deaf and Blind Library and Resource Center, 4359
Alabama Power Foundation, 2301
Alabama Radio Reading Service Network (ARRS), 4360
Alabama Regional Library for the Blind and Physically Handicapped, 4361
Alabama VA Regional Office, 5373
Alabama Veterans Facility, 5374
Andalusia Health Services, 2302
Arc of Alabama, 2303
Birdie Thornton Center, 3548
Birmingham Independent Living Center, 3549
Birmingham VA Medical Center, 5375
Blount Foundation, 2304
Camp Seale Harris Southeastern Diabetes Education Services, 902
Central Alabama Veterans Healthcare System, 5376
Coffee County Training Center, 5605
Easter Seal: Opportunity Center, 5606
Easter Seals: Achievement Center, 5607
Employment Service Division: Alabama, 5608
Houston-Love Memorial Library, 4362
Huntsville Subregional Library for the Blind & Physically Handicapped, 4363
Independent Living Center of Alabaster, 3550
Independent Living Center of Jasper, 3551
Independent Living Center of Mobile, 3552
Lakeshore Rehabilitation Facility, 5609
Montezuma Day Treatment, 5610
Montgomery Independent Living Center, 3553
Public Library Of Anniston-Calhoun County, 4364
Research for Rett Foundation, 4365
Technology Assistance for Special Consumers, 4366
Thomasville Rehabilitation Center, 5611
Tuscaloosa Subregional Library for the Blind & Physically Handicapped, 4367
Tuscaloosa VA Medical Center, 5377
Vocational Rehabilitation Service Opelika, 5612
Vocational Rehabilitation Service: Dothan, 5614
Vocational Rehabilitation Service: Gadsden, 5615
Vocational Rehabilitation Service: Homewoo d, 5616
Vocational Rehabilitation Service: Huntsvi lle, 5617
Vocational Rehabilitation Service: Jackson, 5618
Vocational Rehabilitation Service: Jasper, 5619
Vocational Rehabilitation Service: Mobile, 5620
Vocational Rehabilitation Service: Muscle Shoals, 5621
Vocational Rehabilitation Service: Scottsboro, 5613
Vocational Rehabilitation Service: Selma, 5622
Vocational Rehabilitation Service: Tallade ga, 5623
Vocational Rehabilitation Service: Troy, 5624
Vocational Rehabilitation Service: Tuscalo osa, 5625
Vocational Rehabilitation Services: Andalu sa, 5626
Vocational Rehabilitation Services: Annist on, 5627
Vocational and Rehabilitation Service Columbiana, 5628
Vocational and Rehabilitation Service: Decatur, 5629
Vocational and Rehabilitation Services: Montgomery, 5630
Wiregrass Rehabilitation Center, 5631
Workshops Inc., 5632

Alaska

Access Alaska: ADA Partners Project, 3554
Access Alaska: Fairbanks, 3555
Access Alaska: Mat-Su, 3556
Alaska SILC, 3557
Alaska State Library Talking Book Center, 4368
Anchorage Job Training Center, 5633
Anchorage Regional Office, 5378
Arc of Alaska, 2305
Arctic Access, 3558
DAV Department of Alaska, 5379
Employment Service: Alaska, 5634
Fair Employment Practice Agency, 5635
Hope Community Resources, 3559
Kenai Peninsula IL Center, 3560
Kenai Peninsula IL Center: Seward, 3561
Keni Peninsula-Central Peninsula, 3562
Rasmuson Foundation, 2306
SE Alaska ILC: Ketchikan, 3563
SE Alaska Independent Living Center (SAIL), 3564
SE Alaska Independent Living: Sitka, 3565

Arizona

ASSIST! to Independence, 3566
Arizona Braille and Talking Book Library, 4369
Arizona Bridge to Independent Living, 3567
Arizona Bridge to Independent Living: Mesa, 3569
Arizona Bridge to Independent Living: Phoenix, 3568
Arizona Community Foundation, 2307
Arizonia Autism Resources, 2308
Bonnie Prudden Myotherapy, 764
Books for the Blind of Arizona, 4370
CARF Rehabilitation Accreditation Commission, 769
Camp Civitan, 903
Carl T Hayden VA Medical Center, 5380
Casa Del Rey, 3570
Children's Center for Neurodevelopmental Studies, 4371
Community Outreach Program for the Deaf, 3571
Direct Center for Independence, 3572
Downtown Neighborhood Learning Center, 5637
Easter Seals Arizona, 904
Fair Employment Practice Agency: Arizona, 5638
Flagstaff City-Coconino County Public Library, 4372
Fountain Hills Lioness Braille Service, 4373
International Association of Yoga Therapists, 814
JOBS Administration Job Opportunities & Basic Skills, 5639
Lions Camp Tatiyee, 905
Margaret T Morris Foundation, 2309
Muscular Dystrophy Association, 832
Native American Protection and Advocacy, 864
New Horizons: Prescott Valley, 3573
Northern Arizona VA Health Center, 5381
Prescott Public Library, 4374
Services Maximizing Independent Living and Empowerment (SMILE), 3574
Southern Arizona VA Healthcare System, 5382
Special Needs Center/Phoenix Public Library, 4375
Sterling Ranch: Residence for Special Women, 3575
TETRA Corporation, 5640
Vocational and Rehabilitation Agency Rehabilitation Services Administrations, 5641
Wheelers, 5362
Wheelers Accessible Van Rentals, 5363
World Research Foundation, 4376
Yavapai Regional Medical Center-West, 5642

Arkansas

Arc of Arkansas, 2310
Arkansas Employment Service Agency and Job Training Program, 5643
Arkansas Independent Living Council, 3576
Arkansas Regional Library for the Blind and Physically Handicapped, 4377
Arkansas School for the Blind, 4378
Case Management Society of America, 773
Delta Resource Center for Independent Living, 3577
Easter Seal Work Center, 5644
Educational Services for the Visually Impaired, 4379
Eugene J Towbin Healthcare Center, 5383
John L McClellan Memorial Hospital, 5385
North Little Rock Regional Office, 5386
Northwest Ozarks Regional Library for the Blind and Handicapped, 4381
Our Way, 3579
Roy and Christine Sturgis Charitable Trust, 2311
Sources for Community IL Services, 3580
Spa Area Independent Living Services, 3581
VCT/A Job Retention Skill Training Program, 5645
Vocational and Rehabilitation Agency Division of Services for the Blind, 5646
Vocational and Rehabilitation Agency for Persons Who Are Visually Impaired, 5647
Winthrop Rockefeller Foundation, 2312

California

ARC-Adult Vocational Program, 5648

Ability First, 5649
Access Center of San Diego, 3582
Access To Independence Of Imperial Valley, 3583
Access To Independence Of North County, 3584
Acupressure Institute, 725
Ahmanson Foundation, 2314
Alice Tweed Touhy Foundation, 2315
Alliance for Technology Access, 729
Alternating Hemiplegia of Childhood Foundation, 2316
Amateur Athletic Foundation of Los Angeles, 2317
American Academy of Ophthalmology Annual Meeting, 1530
American Association of Oriental Medicine, 733
American College of Advancement in Medicine, 740
Anglo California Travel Service, 5330
Annuziata Sanguinetti Foundation, 2318
Apple Computer, 2319
Arc of California, 2320
Association of Educational Therapists, 758
Atkinson Foundation, 2321
Baker Commodities Corporate Giving Program, 2322
Bakersfield Association for Retarded Citizens, 5650
Bank of America Foundation, 2323
Beaumont Senior Center: Community Access Center, 3585
Bergen Brunswig Corporation Contributions Program, 2324
Blind Babies Foundation, 2325
Blind Childrens Center Annual Meeting, 1543
Bothin Foundation, 2326
Braille Institute Library, 4382
Braille Institute Santa Barbara Center, 4383
Braille Institute Sight Center, 4384
Braille and Talking Book Library: California State Library, 4385
Briggs Foundation, 2327
Broadcast Services for the Blind, 4386
Burns-Dunphy Foundation, 2328
CAPH Independent Living Center, 3586
California Community Foundation, 2329
California Department of Fair Employment & Housing, 5651
California Endowment, 2330
California Foundation For Independent Living Centers, 3587
California Foundation for Independent Living Centers, 3588
California State Independent Living Council (SILC), 3589
California State Oriental Medical Association (CSOMA), 770
Camp Forrest, 906
Camp Paivika, 907
Camp Reach for the Sky, 908
Camp Ronald McDonald at Eagle Lake, 909
Camping Unlimited, 910
Canine Companions for Independence, 771
Career Connection Transition Program, 5652
Career Development Program (CDP), 5653
Carrie Estelle Doheny Foundation, 2331
Center for Independence Of The Disabled-Daly City, 3590
Center for Independence of the Disabled, 3591
Center for Independent Living: Oakland, 3593
Center for Independent Living: Tri-County, 3594
Center for Independent Living:Fresno, 3595
Center for Independent Living; East Oakland, 3596
Center for Independent Living; Oakland, 3597
Center of Independent Living: Visalia, 3598
Central Coast Center for IL: San Benito, 3599
Central Coast Center for Independent Living, 3600
Central Coast Center: Independent Living - Santa Cruz Office, 3601
Central Coast for Independent Living, 3602
Central Coast for Independent Living: Watsonville, 3603
Clearinghouse for Specialized Media and Technology, 4387
Clorox Company Foundation East Bay Community Foundation, 2332
Coeta and Donald Barker Foundation, 2333
College Student's Guide to Merit and Other No-Need Funding, 2919
Colton Redlands-Yucaipa Regional Occupational Programs, 5654
Communities Actively Living Independent and Free, 3604
Community Access Center, 3605
Community Access Center: Indio Branch, 3606
Community Access Center: Perris, 3607
Community Foundation of Santa Clara County, 2334
Community Outpatient Rehabilitation Center, 5655
Community Rehabilitation Services, 3608
Community Resources for Independence: Mendocino/Lake Branch, 3610
Community Resources for Independence: Napa Office, 3611
Community Resources for Independent Living, 3613
Community Resources for Independent Living Hayward, 3612
Costanoan, 911
Crescent Porter Hale Foundation, 2335
DRAIL (Disability Resource Agency for Independent Living), 3614
Darrow Foundation, 2336
David and Lucile Packard Foundation, 2337
Dayle McIntosh Center: Laguna Niguel, 3615
Desert Haven Enterprises, 5656
Deutsch Foundation, 2338
Directory of Financial Aids for Women, 2924
Disability Resource Agency for Independent Living: Modesto, 3616
Disabled Resources Center, 3617
Do-It-Leisure: Work Training Center, 5657
ESS Work Center, 5658
East Bay Community Foundation, 2339
Easter Seals Camp Harmon, 912
Employment Service: California, 5659
Environmental Dental Association, 792
Environmental Traveling Companions, 5337
Esalen Institute, 793
Evelyn and Walter Hans Jr, 2340
FREED, 3618
FREED Center for Independent Living, 3619
Feather River Industries, 5660
Financial Aid for Asian Americans, 2931
Financial Aid for Hispanic Americans, 2932
Financial Aid for Native Americans, 2933
Financial Aid for Research and Creative Activities Abroad, 2934
Financial Aid for Study and Training Abroad, 2341
Financial Aid for Veterans, Military Personnel and their Dependents, 2935
Financial Aid for the Disabled and their Families, 2936
Fireman's Fund Foundation, 2342
First Step Independent Living, 3620
Fit to Work, 5661
Fred Gellert Foundation, 2343
Fresno City College: Disabled Students Programs and Services, 5662
Fresno County Free Library Blind and Handicapped Services, 4389
Gallo Foundation, 2344
Glaucoma Research Foundation, 2345, 4390
Harden Foundation, 2346
Harry and Grace Steele Foundation, 2347
Health Action, 806
Heartland Opportunity Center, 5663
Henry J Kaiser Family Foundation, 2348
Henry W Bull Foundation, 2349
Herrick Health Sciences Library, 4391
High School Senior's Guide to Merit and Other No-Need Funding, 2946
Hollister Workshop, 5664
Homeopathic Educational Services, 808
How to Pay for Your Degree in Business & Related Fields, 2947
How to Pay for Your Degree in Education & Related Fields, 2948
IL Resource Center: Ventura, 3621
Independent Living Center Of Southern California, 3622
Independent Living Center of Kern County, 3623
Independent Living Center of Lancaster, 3624
Independent Living Center: San Gabriel Valley, 3625
Independent Living Resource Center, Inc., 3626, 3627
Independent Living Resource Center: San Francisco, 3628
Independent Living Resource Center: Santa Maria Office, 3629
Independent Living Resource of Contra Coast, 3630
Independent Living Resource of Fairfield, 3631
Independent Living Resource: Antioch, 3632
Independent Living Resource: Concord, 3633
Independent Living Resources (ILR), 3634
Independent Living Service Northern California: Redding Office, 3635
Independent Living Services of Northern California, 3636
Institute of Transpersonal Psychology, 812
Irvine Health Foundation, 2350
Jerry L Pettis Memorial VA Medical Center, 5387
Job Training Program Liaison: California, 5665
Joni and Friends, 820
Joseph Drown Foundation, 2351
Junior Blind of America, 2352
Junior Wheelchair Sports Camp, 913
Kenneth T and Eileen L Norris Foundation, 2353
King's Rehabilitation Center, 5666
Konocti Industries: People Services, 5667

Koret Foundation, 2354
Kuzell Institute for Arthritis and Infectious Diseases, 4392
LJ Skaggs and Mary C Skaggs Foundation, 2355
LK Whittier Foundation, 2356
Legler Benbough Foundation, 2357
Levi Strauss Foundation, 2358
Long Beach VA Medical Center, 5388
Los Angeles Regional Office, 5389
Louis R Lurie Foundation, 2359
Luke B Hancock Foundation, 2360
Marin Center for Independent Living, 3637
Marin Community Foundation, 2361
Mark B Wallner Foundation, 2618
Martinez Center for Rehab & Extended Care, 5390
Mary A Crocker Trust, 2362
Morongo Basin Work Activity Center, 5668
Mother Lode Independent Living Center, 3638
Mother Lode Rehabilitation Enterprises, 5669
NCI Affiliates, 5670
Napa Valley PSI Inc., 5671
National Foundation of Wheelchair Tennis, 2363
New Beginnings: The Blind Children's Center, 4393
New Directions Travel, 5344
New Directions for People with Disabilities, 2286
Oakland VA Regional Office, 5391
Oakland Work Activity Area, 5672
Opportunities for the Handicapped, 5673
Optometric Extension Program Foundation, 2364
Orange County ARC, 5674
PRIDE Industries, 5675
Pacific Institute of Aromatherapy, 872
Parents And Friends, Inc, 5676
Parents Helping Parents (PHP), 875
Parker Foundation, 2365
Pasadena Foundation, 2366
Pilgrim Pines Camp, 914
Placer Independent Resource Services, 3639
Pomona Valley Workshop, 5677
Porterville Sheltered Workshop, 5678
Project Independence Supported Employment, 5679
Quan Yin Healing Arts Center, 883
RC Baker Foundation, 2367
Ralph M Parsons Foundation, 2368
Rehabilitation Research and Development Center, 5392
Research & Training Center on Mental Health for Hard of Hearing Persons, 4394
Robert Ellis Simon Foundation, 2369
Rolling Start, 3641
Rolling Start: Victorville, 3642
Rosalind Russell Medical Research Center for Arthritis, 4395
Sacramento Medical Center, 5393
Sacramento Vocational Services, 5680
San Diego VA Regional Office, 5394
San Francisco Foundation, 2370
San Francisco Public Library for the Blind and Print Handicapped, 4396
San Francisco VA Medical Center, 5395
San Francisco Vocational Services, 5681
San Jose State University Library, 4397
Santa Barbara Foundation, 2371
Santa Barbara Wheelchair Sports Conference, 1559
Service Center for Independent Living: Covina Office, 3643
Shasta County Opportunity Center, 5682
Sidney Stern Memorial Trust, 2372
Sierra Health Foundation, 2373
Silicon Valley Community Foundation, 2374
Silicon Valley Independent Living Center, 3645
Silicon Valley Independent Living Center: Gilroy Office, 3644
Social Vocational Services, 5683
Sonora Area Foundation, 2375
South Bay Vocational Center, 5684
Southern California Rehabilitation Services, 3646
Stella B Gross Charitable Trust, 2376
Teichert Foundation, 2377
Through the Looking Glass, 3647
Times Mirror Foundation, 2378
Tri-County Independent Living Center, 3648, 4190, 5685, 5685
Tulare County Training Center Able Industries, 5686
Unyeway, 5687
V-Bar Enterprises, 5688
VA Central California Health Care Syste, 5396
VA Greater Los Angeles Healthcare System, 5397
VA Northern California Healthcare System, 5398
VA San Diego Healthcare System, 5399
Valley Light Industries, 5689
Visalia Workshop, 5690
WM Keck Foundation, 2379
Westside Center for Independent Living, 3649
Westside Opportunity Workshop, 5691
Willam G Gilmore Foundation, 2380
Work Training Center for the Handicapped, 5692
Work Training Programs, 5693
World Experience, 2297
World Institute on Disability, 898

Canada

Child and Parent Resource Institute, 779
Clay Tree Society, 782
Haldimand-Norfolk Resource Education and C ounseling, 805
Lambton County Developmental Services, 822
LoSeCa Foundation, 823
MCC Supportive Care Services, 824
North Hastings Community Integration Assoc iation, 867
People First of Canada, 878
St. Paul Abilities Network, 889

Colorado

AMC Cancer Research Center, 4398
Adolph Coors Foundation, 2381
American Society of Bariatric Physicians, 752
American Universities International Programs, 2266
Anschutz Family Foundation, 2382
Arc of Colorado, 2383
Association for Applied Psychophysiology and Biofeedback, 755
Atlantis Community, 3650
Bill Dvorak, Kayak and Rafting Expeditions, 5331
Bonfils-Stanton Foundation, 2384
Boulder Public Library, 4399
Boulder Vet Center, 5400
Breckenridge Outdoor Education Center, 915
Camp Paha, 916
Center for Independence, 3651
Center for Independent Living, 3592, 3652
Center for People with Disabilities, 3653
Center for People with Disabilities (CPWD), 3654
Center for People with Disabilities: Pueblo, 3655
Challenge Aspen, 917
Cheyenne Village, 5694
Colorado Civil Rights Divsion, 5695
Colorado Employment Service, 5696
Colorado Library for the Blind and Physically Handicapped, 4400
Colorado Lions Camp, 918
Colorado Springs Independence Center, 3656
Colorado/Wyoming VA Medical Center, 5401
Comprecare Foundation, 2385
Connections for Independent Living, 3657
Denver CIL, 3658
Denver Foundation, 2386
Denver VA Medical Center, 5402
Developmental Training Services, 5697
Disability Center for Independent Living, 3659
Disabled Resource Services, 3660
Disbled Resource Services, 3661
Dynamic Dimensions, 5698
Easter Seals Colorado Rocky Mountain Villa, 919
El Pomar Foundation, 2387
Gates Family Foundation, 2388
Glacier View Ranch, 920
Grand Junction VA Medical Center, 5403
Gray Street Workcenter, 5699
Greeley Center for Independence, 3662
Helen K and Arthur E Johnson Foundation, 2389
Hope Center, 5700
Imagine: Innovative Resources for Cognitive & Physical Challenges, 5701
Independent Life Center, 3663
Kitzmiller-Bales Trust, 2390
Las Animas County Rehabilitation Center, 5702
Martin Luther Home Of Colorado, 3664
Mind/Body Health Services, 830
NORESCO Workshop, 5703
National Jewish Medical & Research Center, 4401
North America Riding for the Handicapped Association, 866
PEAK Parent Center, 871
Pueblo Goodwill Industries, 3665
Regional Assessment and Training Center, 5704
Rocky Mountain Village, 921
Rolf Institute, 887
Sedgwick County Workshop, 5705
Sky Ranch Lutheran Camp, 922
Southwest Center for Independence, 3666

Southwest Center for Independence: Cortez, 3667
V Hunter Trust, 2391
Valley Industries, 5706
Wyoming/Colorado VA Regional Office, 5604
Yuma County Workshop, 5708

Connecticut

Aetna Foundation, 2392
American Herbalists Guild, 743
American Institute for Foreign Study, 2265
Arc of Connecticut, 2393
Area Cooperative Educational Services (ACES), 5709
Center for Disability Rights, 3668
Center for Independent Living SC, 3669
Central Connecticut Association For Retarted Citizens Inc. (CCARC), 5710
Chapel Haven, 3670
Cheshire Occupational and Career Center, 5711
Community Enterprises, 784, 5712
Community Foundation of Southeastern Connecticut, 2394
Connecticut Braille Association, 4402
Connecticut Governor's Committee on Employment of Disabled Persons, 5713
Connecticut Mutual Life Foundation, 2395
Connecticut State Library, 4403
Connecticut Tech Act Project: Connecticut Department of Social Services, 4404
Constructive Workshops, 5714
Cornelia de Lange Syndrome Foundation, 2396
Disabilities Network of Eastern Connecticut, 3671
Disability Resource Center of Fairfield County: Stratford Office, 3672
Easter Seal Camp Hemlocks, 923
Favarh/Farmington Valley ARC, 796
Fidelco Guide Dog Foundation, 2397
Focus Alternative Learning Center, 802
Fotheringhay Farms, 5715
GE Foundation, 2398
General Electric Foundation, 2399
George Hegyi Industrial Training Center, 5716
Greater Enfield Association of Retarded Citizens, 5717
Hartford Foundation for Public Giving, 2400
Hartford Insurance Group, 2401
Hartford Regional Office, 5404
Hartford Vet Center, 5405
Henry Nias Foundation, 2402
Independence Northwest Center for Independent Living, 3673
Independence Unlimited, 3674
Jane Coffin Childs Memorial Fund for Medical Research, 2403
John H and Ethel G Nobel Charitable Trust, 2404
Kennedy Center, 5718
Library for the Blind and Physically Handicapped, 4380, 4405
New Horizons Village, 3675
Prevent Blindness Connecticut, 4406
Quaezar, 5719
Scheuer Associates Foundation, 2405
Swindells Charitable Foundation Trust, 2406
TEAM Vocational Program, 5720
VA Connecticut Healthcare System: Newington Division, 5406
VA Connecticut Healthcare System: West Haven, 5407
Valley Memorial Health Center, 5721
Vocational and Rehabilitation Agency: State Department of Social Services, 5723
Yale University: Vision Research Center, 4407

Delaware

Arc of Delaware, 2407
Delaware Assistive Technology Initiative Center for Applied Science and Engineering, 4408
Delaware Division of Vocational Rehabilitation- Department of Labor, 5724
Delaware Fair Employment Practice Agency, 5725
Delaware Job Training Program Liaison, 5726
Delaware Library for the Blind and Physically Handicapped, 4409
Delaware VA Regional Office, 5408
Easter Seal Independent Living Center, 3676
Elwyn Delaware, 4410
Freedom Center for Independent Living, 3677
Independent Living, 3678
Independent Resource Georgetown, 3679
Independent Resources, 3680
Independent Resources: Dover, 3681
Independent Resources: Wilmington, 3682
Laffey-McHugh Foundation, 2408
Longwood Foundation, 2409
Martin Luther Homes of Delaware, 3683
Opportunity Center, 5727
Wilmington VA Medical, 5409
Wilmington Vet Center, 5410

District of Columbia

Albert L and Elizabeth T Tucker Foundation, 2410
Alexander Graham Bell Association for the Deaf and Hard of Hearing Annual Conference, 1528
Alexander and Margaret Stewart Trust, 2411
American Association of People with Disabilities, 734
American Association on Mental Retardation AAMR Annual Meeting, 1532
American Council of the Blind Annual Convention, 1534
American Public Health Association, 748
American Red Cross: National Headquarters, 749
Arc of the District of Columbia, 2412
Association for Persons with Severe Handicaps (TASH), 757
Blinded Veterans Association National Convention, 1544
Center for Mind/Body Studies, 776
Change, 778
Charles Delmar Foundation, 2413
Children's National Medical Center, 781
Chronicle Guide to Grants, 2918
DAV National Service Headquarters, 5364
Davis Memorial Goodwill Industries, 5728
Department of Medicine and Surgery Veterans Administration, 5365
Department of Veterans Benefits, 5367
Disability Rights Center, 3684
Disabled American Veterans, National Service & Legislative Headquarters, 5411
District of Columbia Center for Independent Living, 3685
District of Columbia Department of Employment Services, 5729
District of Columbia Dept. of Employment Services: Office of Workforce Development, 5730
District of Columbia Fair Employment Practice Agencies, 5731
District of Columbia Public Library: Services to the Deaf Community, 4411
District of Columbia Regional Library for the Blind and Physically Handicapped, 4412
Eugene and Agnes E Meyer Foundation, 2414
Eye Bank Association of America Annual Meeting, 1549
Federal Benefits for Veterans and Dependents, 5369
Federal Grants & Contracts Weekly, 2930
Federal Student Aid Information Center, 2415
Foundation & Corporate Grants Alert, 2937
George Washington University Health Resource Center, 803
Georgetown University Center for Child and Human Development, 4413
Giant Food Foundation, 2417
Golden Eagle Passport, 5339
Green Door, 5732
Guide Service of Washington, 5340
Jacob and Charlotte Lehrman Foundation, 2418
John Edward Fowler Memorial Foundation, 2419
Joseph P Kennedy Jr Foundation, 2420
Kiplinger Foundation, 2421
Morris and Gwendolyn Cafritz Foundation, 2422
National Association of Protection and Advocacy Systems, 835
National Center for Education in Maternal and Child Health, 839
National Council on Disability, 841
National Council on the Aging Conference, 1553
National Deaf Education Network and Clearinghouse, 843
National Dissemination Center for Children and Youth with Disabilities (NICHCY), 844
National Information Center for Children, 854
National Institute on Disability and Rehabilitation Research, 855, 4414
National Organization on Disability, 858
National Women's Health Network, 863
Operation Job Match, 5733
PVA Sports and Recreation Program, 5412
Paul and Annetta Himmelfarb Foundation, 2423
Public Technology, 5359
Public Welfare Foundation, 2424
Rehabilitation Services Administration, 5734
Rehabilitation Services Administration of the District of Columbia, 886
Sister Cities International, 2290

Student Guide, 2965
SubAcute Care: American SubAcute Care Association Annual Convention/Expo, 1560
Teacher Preparation and Special Education, 890
US Department of Veterans Affairs National Headquarters, 5371
US Veteran's Affairs, 5372
United Cerebral Palsy Association Development Conference, 1562
VA Medical Center, Washington DC, 5413
WAVE Work, Achievement, Value, & Education, 5735
Washington DC VA Medical Center, 5414

Florida

Abilities of Florida: An Affiliate of Service Source, 5736
Ability 1st, 3687
Able Trust, 2425
Adult Day Training, 3688
Advocacy Center for Persons with Disabilities, 727
Arc of Florida, 2426
BCR Foundation, 2427
Bank of America Client Foundation, 2428
Baron de Hirschmeyer Foundation, 2429
Barron Collier Jr Foundation, 2430
Bay Pines VA Medical Center, 5415
Birth Defect Research for Children, 763
Blazing Toward a Cure Annual Conference, 1542
Brevard County Talking Books Library, 4415
Broward County Talking Book Library, 4416
CEH, 5354
CIL Options-One Stop Career Center: Royal Palm Beach, 3689
CIL of Central Florida, 3690
CIL of Florida Keys, 3691
CIL of Florida Keys-Key West, 3692
CIL of North Central Florida, 3693
Camiccia-Arnautou Charitable Foundation, 2431
Camp Thunderbird, 924
Career Assessment & Planning Services, 5737
Caring and Sharing Center for Independent Living, 3694
Caring and Sharing Center: Pasco County, 3695
Caring and Sharing: Gulf Port, 3696
Cathedral Center for Independent Living, 3697
Center for Independent Living in Central Florida - Advocacy Living Skills Peer Support, 3698
Center for Independent Living of Broward, 3699
Center for Independent Living of Florida Keys, 3700
Center for Independent Living of N Central Florida, 3701
Center for Independent Living of N Florida, 3702
Center for Independent Living of NW Florida, 3703
Center for Independent Living of North Central Florida, 3704
Center for Independent Living of S Florida, 3705
Center for Independent Living of SW Florida, 3706
Chatlos Foundation, 2432
Choices for Work Program, 5738
Coalition For Independent Living Options Inc., 3707
Coalition for Independent Living Option, 3708
Coalition for Independent Living Options-One Stop Career Center, 3709
Cunard Line, 5332
Dade Community Foundation, 2433
Dade County Talking Book Library, 4417
Dialysis at Sea Cruises, 5335
Disability Solutions for Independent Livin g, 3711
Dr. Jack Widrich Foundation, 2434
EIS Foundation, 2435
Edyth Bush Charitable Foundation, 2436
FPL Group Foundation, 2437
Florida Division of Blind Services, 4418
Florida Division of Vocational Rehabilitation, 5739
Florida Fair Employment Practice Agency, 5740
Florida Instructional Materials Center for the Visually Handicapped, 4419
Florida Lions Camp, 925
Florida Rock Industries Foundation, 2438
Frank Stanley Beveridge Foundation, 2439
Gainesville Division, North Florida/South Georgia Veterans Healthcare System, 5416
Goodwill Industries-Suncoast Adult Day Training, 5741
Goodwill Industries-Suncoast Inc. Adult Day Training, 5742, 5743
Goodwill Industries-Suncoast Non-Residenti al Supports And Services Program, 5744
Goodwill Industries-Suncoast Supported Living, 5745
Goodwill Industries-Suncoast,Adult Day Training, 5746
Goodwill Temporary Services, 5747
Hillsborough County Talking Book Library Tampa-Hillsborough County Public Library, 4420
Impact: Ocala Vocational Services, 5748
Jack Eckerd Corporation Foundation, 2440
James A Haley VA Medical Center, 5417
Jefferson Lee Ford III Memorial Foundation, 2441
Jessie Ball duPont Fund, 2442
Job Works NISH Food Service, 5749
Job Works NISH Postal Service, 5750
Joe and Emily Lowe Foundation, 2443
John E & Nellie J Bastien Memorial Foundation, 2444
Lee County Library System: Talking Books Library, 4421
Lighthouse Central Florida (Formerly C.I.T.E), 5751
Lighthouse Central Florida Inc., 3712
Lost Tree Village Charitable Foundation, 2445
Louis de la Parte Florida Mental Health Institute Research Library, 4422
MAClown Vocational Rehabilitation Workshop, 5752
Miami VA Medical Center, 5418
Miami-Dade County Disability Services and Independent Living (DSAIL), 3713
National Car Rental System, 5356
North Central Florida Citrus County, 3714
Norwegian Cruise Line, 5345
One-Stop Service, 5753
Orange County Library System: Audio-Visual Department, 4423
Palm Beach Habilitation Center, 5754
Pearlman Biomedical Research Institute, 4424
Pinellas Talking Book Library for the Blind and Physically Handicapped, 4425
Primrose Supported Employment Programs, 5755
Publix Super Markets Charities, 2446
Richard W Higgins Charitable Foundation M And I Marshall And Ilsley Bank, 2447
SCARC, Inc Evaluation, Training + Emplomen t Center, 5756
SCCIL at Titusville, 3715
Seagull Industries for the Disabled, 5757
Self Reliance, 3716
Space Coast Center for Independent Living, 3717
St. Petersburg Regional Office, 5419
Suncoast Center for Independent Living, 3718
Supported Employment Program, 5758
Talking Book Library-Jacksonville Public Libraries, 4426
Talking Book Service: Mantatee County Central Library, 4427
Talking Books Library for the Blind and Physically Handicapped, 4428
Talking Books/Homebound Services, 4429
The Able Trust, 5759
University of Miami: Bascom Palmer Eye Institute, 4430
University of Miami: Mailman Center for Child Development, 4431
Upledger Institute, 895
Vocational and Rehabilitation Agency Department of Education, 5760
West Florida Regional Library, 4432
West Palm Beach VA Medical Center, 5420
Work Exploration Center, 5762
Young Onset Parkinson Conference, 1564

Georgia

Albany Talking Book Center, 4433
American Spinal Injury Association Annual Scientific Meeting, 1539
Arms Wide Open, 3719
Athens Talking Book Center-Athens-Clarke County Regional Library, 4434
Atlanta Regional Office, 5421
Atlanta VA Medical Center, 5422
Augusta Talking Book Center, 4435
Augusta VA Medical Center, 5423
Bain, Inc. Center For Independent Living, 3720
Bainbridge Subregional Library for the Blind & Physically Handicapped, 4436
Camp Twin Lakes, 926
Carl Vinson VA Medical Center, 5424
Center for Assistive Technology and Environmental Access, 774
Columbus Subregional Library For The Blind And Physically Handicapped, 4437
Community Foundation for Greater Atlanta, 2448

DisABILITY LINK NW, 3721
Disability Action Center for Georgia, 3722
Disability Connections, 3723
Emory Autism Resource Center, 4438
Emory University Laboratory for Ophthalmic Research, 4439
Employment and Training Division, Region B, 5763
Fair Housing and Equal Employment, 5764
Florence C and Harry L English Memorial Fund, 2449
Georgia Library for the Blind and Physically Handicapped, 4440
Georgia Power, 2450
Georgia's SILC, 3725
Grayson Foundation, 2451
Griffin Area Resource Center Griffin Community Workshop Division, 5765
Hall County Library: East Hall Branch and Special Needs Library, 4441
Harriet McDaniel Marshall Trust in Memory of Sanders McDaniel, 2452
Human Ecology Action League (HEAL), 809
IBM Corporation, 2453
IBM National Support Center, 5766
John H and Wilhelmina D Harland Charitable Foundation, 2454
Kelley Diversified, 5767
Lettie Pate Whitehead Foundation, 2455
Living Independence for Everyone (LIFE), 3726
Macon Library for the Blind and Physically Handicapped, 4442
Metametrix Clinical Laboratory, 828
Multiple Choices Center for Independent Living, 3727
National Center on Birth Defects and Developmental Disabilities, 4443
New Ventures, 5768
North District Independent Living Program, 3728
North Georgia Talking Book Center, 4444
Oconee Regional Library, 4445
Parent to Parent, 874
Patterson-Barclay Memorial Foundation, 2456
Perkins-Ponder Foundation, 2457
Rich Foundation, 2458
Rome Subregional Library for the Blind and Physically Handicapped, 4446
South Georgia Regional Library-Valdosta Talking Book Center, 4447
Southeastern Paralyzed Veterans Of America (PVA), 3729
Southwest District Independent Living Program, 3730
SunTrust Bank, Atlanta Foundation, 2459
Talking Book Center Brunswick-Glynn County Regional Library, 4448
The Arc Of Georgia, 2460
Walton Option for Independent Living, 3731
Walton Options For Independent Living (Warrington), 3732

Hawaii

ASSETS School, 5769
Arc of Hawaii, 2461
Assistive Technology Resource Centers of Hawaii (ATRC), 4449
Atherton Family Foundation, 2462
Camp Erdman YMCA, 927
Center For Independent Living- Kauai, 3733
Center for Independent Living: E Hawaii, 3734
Clarence TC Ching Foundation, 2463
GN Wilcox Trust, 2464
Hawaii Center for Independent Living-Maui, 3735
Hawaii Centers for Independent Living, 3736
Hawaii Community Foundation, 2465
Hawaii Fair Employment Practice Agency, 5770
Hawaii State Library for the Blind and Physically Handicapped, 4450
Hawaii Veterans Centers, 5425
Hawaii Vocational Rehabilitation Division, 5771
Honolulu VBA Regional Office, 5426
Kailua Kona Center for Independent Living: West Hawaii, 3737
Kauai Center for Independent Living, 3738
Lanakila Rehabilitation Center, 5772
McInerny Foundation Bank Of Hawaii,Corporate Trustee, 2466
Over the Rainbow Disabled Travel Services & Wheelers Accessible Van Rentals, 5358
Pacific Islands Health Care System, 5427
Sophie Russell Testamentary Trust Bank Of Hawaii, 2467
Wahiawa Family, 5774

Idaho

American Falls Office: Living Independently for Everyone (LIFE), 3739
Boise Regional Office, 5428
Boise VA Medical Center, 5429
Dawn Enterprises, 3740
Disability Action Center NW, 3741
Disability Action Center, NW, 3742
Disability Action Center-N.W., 3743
Idaho Assistive Technology Project, 4451
Idaho Commission for the Blind and Visually Impaired, 3744
Idaho Employment Service and Job Training Program Liaison, 5775
Idaho Fair Employment Practice Agency, 5776
Idaho Falls Office: Living Independently for Everyone (LIFE), 3745
Idaho Governor's Committee on Employment of People with Disabilities, 5777
Idaho State Library: Talking Book Library, 4452
Idaho Vocational Rehabilitation Agency, 5778
LIFE: Fort Hall, 3746
Living Independence Network Corporation, 3747
Living Independence Network Corporation: Canyon County Satelite, 3748
Living Independent for Everyone (LIFE): Pocatello Office, 3749
Living Independently Now Center Inc., Twin Falls, 3750
Living Independently Now Center, Inc., 3751
Living Independently for Everyone (LIFE): Blackfoot Office, 3752
Living Independently for Everyone: Burley, 3753
ROW Adventures, 5347
River Odysseys West: ROW, 5348
Southwestern Idaho Housing Authority, 3754

Illinois

Access Living of Metropolitan Chicago, 3755
Ada S McKinley Vocational Services, 5780
Alfred Bersted Foundation, 2468
Alzheimer's Association, 2469
American Academy of Pediatrics, 731
American Board of Chelation Therapy, 735
American Massage Therapy Association, 745
American National Bank and Trust Company, 2471
American Society of Clinical Hypnosis, 753
Ameritech Corporation Contributions Program, 2472
Amerock Corporation, 2473
Anixter Center, 5781
Arc of Illinois The Illinois Life Span Project, 2474
Benjamin Benedict Green-Field Foundation, 2475
Blowitz-Ridgeway Foundation, 2476
Burlington Northern Santa Fe Foundation, 2477
C-4 Work Center, 5782
Camp Little Giant, 928
Center on Deafness, 3756
Chicago Community Trust and Affiliates, 2478
Chicago Public Library Talking Book Center, 4453
Clearbrook, 5783
Community Foundation of Champaign County, 2479
Community Residential Alternative, 3757
Cornerstone Services, 5784
Department of Ophthalmology and Visual Science, 4454
Division of Rehabilitation Services, 3724, 3758
Dr. Scholl Foundation, 2480
DuPage Center for Independent Living, 3759
Duchossois Foundation The Chamberlain Group Inc., 2481
Easter Seals of Bartholomew County, 930
Easter Seals: UCP Timber Pointe Outdor Center, 931
Edward Hines Jr Hospital, 5430
Evenston Community Foundation, 2482
Family Resource Center on Disabilities, 794
Field Foundation of Illinois, 2483
Fox River Valley Center for Independent Living, 3760
Francis Beidler Charitable Trust, 2484
Fred J Brunner Foundation, 2485
Fulton County Rehab Center, 5785
Gaining Access to IL, 3761
George M Eisenberg Foundation for Charities, 2486
George Zoltan Lefton Family Foundation, 2487
Glenkirk, 5786
Green Bay Foundation, 2488
Grover Hermann Foundation, 2489
Guild for the Blind, 4455
Harry F and Elaine Chaddick Foundation, 2490

Health Resource Center for Women with Disabilities, 807
Helen Brach Foundation, 2491
Horizons for the Blind, 4456
Illinois Department of Rehab Services, 3762
Illinois Early Childhood Intervention Clearinghouse, 4457
Illinois Employment Service, 5787
Illinois Regional Library for the Blind and Physically Handicapped, 4458
Illinois Valley Center for Independent Living, 3763
Illinois and Iowa Center for Independent Living, 3764
Impact Center for Independent Living, 3765
Jacksonville Area CIL: Havana, 3766
Jacksonville Area Center for Independent Living, 3767
Jewish Council for Youth Services, 932
Jewish Vocational Services, 5788
JoDavies Workshop, 5789
John D and Catherine T MacArthur Foundation, 2492
Kennedy Job Training Center, 5790
Knox County Council for Developmental Disabilities, 5791
Kreider Services, 5792
LIFE Center for Independent Living, 3768
LINC-Monroe Randolph Center, 3769
LaSalle Chicago Community Trust, 2493
Lake County Center for Independent Living, 3770
Lambs Farm, 5793
Land of Lincoln Goodwill Industries, 5794
Les Turne Amyotrophic Laterial Sclerosis Foundation, 2494
Life Center for Independent Living, 3771
Lions Clubs International, 2283
Little City Foundation, 2495
Living Independently Now Center (LINC), 3772
MAGIC Foundation for Children's Growth, 2496
Marion VA Medical Center, 5431
McDonald's Corporation Contributions Program, 2497
Michael Reese Health Trust, 2498
Mid-Illinois Talking Book Center, 4459
Moen Foundation, 2499
Mosaic-Pontiac, 3773
National Easter Seal Society, 846
National Eye Research Foundation (NERF), 2500, 4460
National Headache Foundation, 2501
National Lekotek Center, 4461
New Courier Travel, 5343
North Chicago VA Medical Center, 5432
Northwest Limousine Service, 5357
Northwestern University Multipurpose Arthritis & Musculoskeletal Center, 4462
OMRON Foundation Omron Electronics Llc, 2502
Opportunities for Access: A Center for Independent Living, 3774
Options Center For Independent Living: Bourbonnais, 3775
Options Center for Independent Living: Watseka, 3776
Orchard Village, 5795
Oris B Hastings Charitable Foundation, 2503
PACE Center for Independent Living, 3777
Peoria Area Community Foundation, 2505
Polk Brothers Foundation, 2506
President's Committee on Employment of Employment of the Disabled, 5796
Progress Center South, 3778
Progress Center for Independent Living, 3779
RAMP Regional Access and Mobility Project, 3780
Regional Access and Mobilization Project (RAMP), 3781
Regional Access and Mobilization Project: DeKalb, 3782
Retirement Research Foundation, 2507
Rotary Youth Exchange, 2288
Rush Hayward Masonic Fund, 2508
Sears-Roebuck Foundation, 2509
Sertoma Centre, 5797
Shore Training Center, 5798
Siragusa Foundation, 2510
Skills Inc., 5799
Skokie Accessible Library Services, 4463
Southern Illinois Talking Book Center, 4464
Southern Illinois University at Carbondale, 2291
Soyland Access To Independent Living, 3783
Soyland Access to IL, 3784
Soyland Access to Independent Living (SAIL), 3785
Soyland Access to Independent Living: Charleston, 3786
Springfield Center for Independent Living, 3787
Square D Foundation, 2511
Stone-Hayes Center for Independent Living, 3788
Thresholds AMISS, 5800
Thresholds Psychiatric Rehabilitation Centers, 892
Touch of Nature Environmental Center, 933
University of Illinois at Chicago: Lions of Illinois Eye Research Institute, 4465
VA Illiana Health Care System, 5433
Voices of Vision Talking Book Center at DuPage Library System, 4466
WP and HB White Foundation, 2512
Washington County Vocational Workshop, 5802
Washington Square Health Foundation, 2513
West Central Illinois Center for Independent Living, 3789
Westside Parents Work Activity Center, 5803
Wheat Ridge Ministries, 2514
Will Grundy Center for Independent Living, 3790
YMCA Camp Duncan, 934

Indiana

ADEC Resources for Independence, 5804
ARC of Allen County, 5805
Allen County Public Library, 4467
American Camping Association, 738
Arc of Indiana, 2515
Assistive Technology Training and Information Center (ATTIC), 3791
BI-County Services, 5806
Balance Centers of America, 5807
Ball Brothers Foundation, 2516
Bartholomew County Public Library, 4468
Bradford Woods/Camp Riley, 935
Bridge Pointe Services & Goodwill of Southern Indiana, Inc, 5808
Camp Millhouse, 936
Carey Services, 5809
Community Foundation of Boone County, 2517
Crown Point Community Foundation, 2518
Damar Homes Incorporated, 3792
Easter Seal Crossroads Rehabilitation Cent er, 937
Easter Seals ARC of Northeast Indiana, 938
Easter Seals of Wayne & Union Counties, 939
Eli Lilly & Co Corporate Contributions Pro, 2519
Elkhart Public Library for the Blind and Physiclly Handicapp, 4469
Evansville Association for the Blind, 5810
Everybody Counts Center for Independent Living, 3793
Four Rivers Resource Services, 3794, 5811
Future Choices Independent Living Center, 3795
Gateway Services/JCARC, 5812
Goodwill Industries of Central Indiana, 5813
Happiness Bag, 940
Independent Living Center of Eastern Indiana (ILCEIN), 3796
Indiana Employment Services and Job Training Program Liaison, 5814
Indiana Fair Employment Practice Agency, 5815
Indiana Resource Center for Autism, 4470
Indiana University: Multipurpose Arthritis Center, 4471
Indianapolis Regional Office, 5434
Indianapolis Resource Center For Independent Living, 3797
Isanogel Center, 941
John W Anderson Foundation, 2520
LCAR, 5816
Lake County Public Library Talking Books Service, 4472
League for the Blind and Disabled, 3798
Martin Luther Homes of Indiana, 3799
Michigan Resources, 5817
New Hope Services, 5818
New Horizons Rehabilitation, 5819
Noble Centers, 5820
Office of State Coordinator of Vocational Education for Students with Disability, 5821
Putnam County Comprehensive Services, 5822
Richard L Roudebush VA Medical Center, 5435
Ruben Center for Independent Living, 3800
SILC, Indiana Council on Independent Living (ICOIL), 3801
Southern Indiana Center for Independent Living, 3802
Southern Indiana Resource Solutions, 5823
Special Services Division: Indiana State Library, 4473
St. Joseph Hospital Rehabilitation Center, 4474
Sycamore Rehabilitation Services, 5824
Talking Books Service Evansville Vanderburgh County Public Library, 4475
Trabant North Knox, 2521
VA North Indiana Health Care System: Fort Wayne Campus, 5436
VA Northern Indiana Health Care System: Marion Campus, 5437
Wabash Independent Living Center & Learning Center (WILL), 3803

Wabash/Employability Center, 5826

Iowa

ACT Assessment Test Preparation Reference Manual, 5827
Arc of Iowa, 2522
Black Hawk Center for Independent Living, 3804
Camp Courageous of Iowa, 942
Camp Tanager, 943
Camp Wyoming, 944
Central Iowa Center for Independent Living, 3805
College of Maharishi Vedic Medicine Health Center, 783
Des Moines VA Medical Center, 5438
Des Moines VA Regional Office, 5439
Easter Seals Camp Sunnyside, 945
Evert Conner Rights & Resources CIL, 3806
Franklin County Work Activity Center, 5828
Hall-Perrine Foundation, 2523
Homer G Barr Trust, 2524
Hope Haven, 3807
Independent Living: Iowa Everett Conner Center, 3808
Innovative Industries, 5829
Iowa City VA Medical Center, 5440
Iowa Civil Rights Commission, 5830
Iowa Department for the Blind Library, 4476
Iowa Employment Service, 5831
Iowa Job Training Program Liaison, 5832
Iowa Registry for Congenital and Inherited Disorders, 4477
Iowa Valley Community College, 5833
Iowa Vocational Rehabilitation Services, 5834
Kent A Hall, 2525
Knoxville VA Medical Center, 5441
League of Human Dignity, 3809
Library Commission for the Blind, 4478
Maharishi Ayur-Veda Medical Center, 825
Martin Luther Homes of Iowa, 3810
Mid-Iowa Health Foundation, 2526
New Focus, 5835
Principal Financial Group Foundation, 2527
Riverside Lutheran Bible Camp, 946
Second Time Around, 5836
Siouxland Community Foundation, 2528
South Central Iowa Center for Independent Living, 3811
Universal Pediatric Services, 894
VA Central Iowa Health Care System, 5442
Wesley Woods Camp & Retired Center, 947

Kansas

American Academy of Environmental Medicine, 730
Arc of Kansas, 2529
Beach Center on Families and Disability, 762
CKLS Headquarters, 4479
Center for Independent Living Southwest Kansas, 3813
Center for Independent Living for SW Kansas, 3814
Center for the Improvement of Human Functioning, 4480
Clay Center Adult Training Center, 5837
Coalition For Independence, 3815
Colmery-O'Neil VA Medical Center, 5443
Cowley County Developmental Services, 3816
Dwight D Eisenhower VA Medical Center, 5444
Hospitalized Veterans Writing Project, 5370
Hutchinson Community Foundation, 2530
Independence, 3817
Independence First, 3818
Independent Connection, 3819
Independent Connection: Beloit, 3820
Independent Living Center of Northeast Kan sas, 3821
Independent Living Resource Center, 3822
International College of Applied Kinesiology, 817
Kansas Fair Employment Practice Agency, 5838
Kansas Services for the Blind & Visually Impaired, 3823
Kansas State Library, 4481
Kansas VA Regional Office, 5445
Kansas Vocational Rehabilitation Agency, 5839
LINK: Colby, 3824
LINK: Hays, 3825
Manhattan Public Library, 4482
Northwest Kansas Library System Talking Books, 4483
Osage City Resource Center for Independent Living, 3826
Prairie IL Resource Center, 3827
Prairie Independent Living Resource Center, 3828
Resource Center for Independent Living: Bu rlington, 3830
Resource Center for Independent Living: El Dorado, 3831
Resource Center for Independent Living: Emporia, 3829
Resource Center for Independent Living: Fo rt Scott, 3832
Resource Center for Independent Living: Ot tawa, 3833
Robert J Dole VA Medical Center, 5446
South Central Kansas Library System, 4484
Southeast Kansas Independent Living, 3835
Southeast Kansas Independent Living: Colum bus, 3837
Southeast Kansas Independent Living: Pittsburg, 3836
Southeast Kansas Independent Living: Yates Center, 3834
Southeast Kansas: Chanute, 3838
Southeast Kansas: Fredonia, 3839
Three Rivers IL Center, 3840
Three Rivers Independent Living Center: Centralia, 3841
Three Rivers Independent Resource Center, 3842
Topeka & Shawnee County Public Library Talking Book Service, 4485
Topeka Independent Living Resource Center, 3843
Whole Person: Nortonville, 3844
Whole Person: Prairie Village, 3846
Whole Person: Tonganoxie, 3847
Wichita Public Library, 4486
Wichita Public Library/Talking Book Service, 4487

Kentucky

Arc of Kentucky, 2531
Best Center for Independent Living, 3848
Bethel Mennonite Camp, 948
Center for Accessible Living, 3849
Center for Accessible Living: Murray, 3850
Center for Independent Living Options, 3852
Center for Independent Living: Kentucky Department for the Blind, 3853
Children's Alliance, 780
Disability Coalition of Northern Kentucky, 3854
Easter Seal Camp KYSOC, 949
EnTech: Enabling Technologies of Kentuckiana, 4488
Independence Place, 3855
Kentucky Committee on Employment of People with Disabilities, 5840
Kentucky Department for Employment Service and Job Training Program Liaison, 5841
Kentucky Department for the Blind, 5842
Kentucky Office For The Blind, 5843
Kentucky Talking Book Library, 4489
Kentucky Vocational Rehabilitation Agency, 5844
Lexington VA Medical Center, 5447
Life Adventure Camp, 950
Louisville Free Public Library, 4490
Louisville VA Medical Center, 5448
Louisville VA Regional Office, 5449
Omnicare Foundation, 2532
Pathfinders for Independent Living, 3856
Pioneer Vocational/Industrial Services, 5845
SILC Department of Vocational Rehabilitation, 3857
Wheelchair Getaways, 5351
Wheelchair Getaways Wheelchair/Scooter Accessible Van Rentals, 5361
Work Enhancement Center of Western Kentucky, 5846

Louisiana

Alexandria VA Medical Center, 5450
Arc of Louisiana, 2533
Baton Rouge Area Foundation, 2534
Camp Challenge, 951
Central Louisiana State Hospital Medical and Professional Library, 4491
Community Foundation of Shreveport-Bossier, 2535
Community Opportunities of East Ascension, 5847
LA Lions Camp for Disabled/Diabetic Youth, 952
Louisiana Employment Service and Job Training Program Liaison, 5848
Louisiana State Library, 4492
Louisiana State University Genetics Section of Pediatrics, 4493
Louisiana Vocational Rehabilitation Agency, 5849
New Horizons: Alexandria, 3858
New Horizons: Monroe, 3859
New Horizons: Shreveport, 3860
New Orleans VA Medical Center, 5451
Resources for Independent Living: Baton Ro ge, 3862

Resources for Independent Living: Baton Rouge, 3861
Resources for Independent Living: Metairie, 3863
Shreveport VA Medical Center, 5452
Southwest Louisiana Independence Center: L ake Charles, 3864
Southwest Louisians Independence Center: Lafayette, 3865
St. James Association for Retarded Citizens, 5850
State Library of Louisiana: Services for the Blind and Physically Handicapped, 4494
Volunteers of America Supported Living Program, 3866
W Troy Cole Independent Living Specialist, 3867
Westbank Sheltered Workshop, 5851

Maine

Addison Point Specialized Services, 5852
Alpha One: Aroostook, 3868
Alpha One: Augusta, 3869
Alpha One: Bangar, 3870
Alpha One: Main Office, 3871
Bangor Public Library, 4495
Bangor Veteran Center: Veterans Outreach Center, 5853
Camp Waban, 953
Cary Library, 4496
Creative Work Systems, 5854
High School Students Guide to Study, Travel, and Adventure Abroad, 2276
Lewiston Public Library, 4497
Maine Department Of Labor, 5855
Maine Governor's Committee on Employment of the Disabled, 5856
Maine Human Rights Commission, 5857
Maine State Library, 4498
Maine VA Regional Office, 5453
Motivational Services, 3872
Northeast Occupational Exchange, 5858
Pine Tree Camp, 954
Portland Public Library, 4500
Shalom House, Inc, 3873
Togus VA Medical Center, 5454
UNUM Charitable Foundation Maine Association Of Non Profits, 2536
Waterville Public Library, 4501
Women to Women, 897

Maryland

American Association of the Deaf-Blind National Conference, 1531
American College of Nurse Midwives, 741
American Health Assistance Foundation, 2537
American Occupational Therapy Association, 746
American Occupational Therapy Foundation, 2538
American Speech-Language-Hearing Association, 1538
Arc of Maryland, 2539
Ardmore Developmental Center, 5860
Association for International Practical Training, 2270
Association of University Centers on Disabilities, 759
Baltimore Community Foundation, 2540
Baltimore Regional Office, 5455
Baltimore VA Medical Center, 5456
Broadmead, 3874
Camp Greentop, 955
Camp JCC, 956
Camp Superkids, 957
Candlelighters Childhood Cancer Foundation, 2541
Children's Fresh Air Society Fund, 2542
Clark-Winchcole Foundation, 2543
Columbia Foundation, 2544
Community Health Funding Report, 2920
Cystic Fibrosis Foundation, 2545
Department of Physical Medicine & Rehabilitation at Sinai Hospital, 786
Disability Funding News, 2928
Easter Seals Camp Fairlee Manor, 958
Eastern Shore Center for Independent Living, 3875
Federation of Families for Children's Mental Health, 799
Fort Howard VA Medical Center, 5457
Foundation Fighting Blindness, 2546
Freedom Center, 3876
GEICO Philanthropic Foundation Geico Corp., 2416
George Wasserman Family Foundation, 2547
Goodwill Industries International, 804
Harry and Jeanette Weinberg Foundation, 2548
Hostelling North America Hostelling International: American Youth Hostels, 5342
Housing Unlimited, 3877
Independence Now: Riverdale, 3878
Independence Now: Silver Spring, 3879
International Association of Machinists, 813
Job Opportunities for the Blind, 5861
Johns Hopkins University Dana Center for Preventive Ophthalmology, 4502
Johns Hopkins University: Asthma and Allergy Center, 4503
Mainstream, 826, 3578, 5862, 5862
Making Choices for Independent Living, 3880
Maryland Employment Services and Job Training Program Liaison, 5863
Maryland Fair Employment Practice Agency, 5864
Maryland National Capital Park and Planning Commission, 959
Maryland State Department of Education, 5865
Maryland State Library for the Blind and Physically Handicapped, 4504
Maryland Veterans Centers, 5458
Milldale Camp, 960
Mobile Care, 5355
Montgomery County Department of Public Libraries/Special Needs Library, 4505
National 4-H Council, 2285
National Epilepsy Library (NEL), 4506
National Federation of the Blind, 2550
National Federation of the Blind: Blind Industrial Workers Division, 848
National Federation of the Blind: Computer Science Division, 849
National Federation of the Blind: Merchants Division, 847
National Federation of the Blind: Public Employees Division, 850
National Federation of the Blind: Science and Engineering Division, 851
National Federation of the Blind: Writers Division, 852
National Rehabilitation Information Center, 4507
National Rehabilitation Information Center (NARIC), 860
PWI Profile, 5866
People-to-People Committee for the Handicapped, 879
Perry Point VA Medical Center, 5459
Project LINK, 5867
Red Notebook, 4508
Report on Disability Programs, 2963
Resources for Independence, 3881
Ryland Group Corporate Giving Program, 2551
Sjogren's Syndrome Foundation, 2552
Social Security Library, 4509
Southern Maryland Center for LIFE, 3883
Substance Abuse Funding News, 2966
Treatment and Learning Centers (TLC), 5868
VA Maryland Health Care System, 5460
Warren Grant Magnuson Clinical Center, 4510
Youth for Understanding International Exchange, 2300

Massachusetts

ARC Of Cape Cod, 3884
AU Kamp for Kids, 961
Abbot and Dorothy H Stevens Foundation, 2553
Adlib Inc., 3885
American Red Cross of Cape Cod and Islands, 3886
American Society for the Alexander Techniq ue, 751
American Society of Teachers of the Alexander Technique, 754
Arc Massachusetts, 2554
Bank of Boston Corporation Charitable Foundation, 2555
Boston Center for Independent Living, 3887
Boston Foundation, 2556
Boston Globe Foundation, 2557
Boston University Arthritis Center, 4511
Boston University Center for Human Genetics, 4512
Boston University Robert Dawson Evans Memorial Dept. of Clinical Research, 4513
Boston VA Regional Office, 5461
Braille and Talking Book Library, Perkins School for the Blind, 4514
Brigham and Women's Hospital: Asthma and Allergic Disease Research Center, 4515
Brigham and Women's Hospital: Robert B Brigham Multipurpose Arthritis Center, 4516
Bushrod H Campbell and Ada F Hall Charity Fund, 2558
CAPP National Parent Resource Center Federation for Children with Special Needs, 768
Camp Ramah in New England (Summer), 962

Camp Ramah in New England (Winter), 963
Cape Organization for Rights of the Disabled (CORD), 3888
Caption Center, 4517
Center for Interdisciplinary Research on Immunologic Diseases, 4518
Center for Living & Working: Fitchburg, 3889
Center for Living & Working: Milford, 3890
Center for Living & Working: Worcester, 3891
Clipper Ship Foundation, 2559
Community Foundation of Western Massachusetts, 2560
DEAF, 3892
Department Of Workforce Development, 5869
Easter Seals Massachusetts-Agassiz Village, 964
Edith Nourse Rogers Memorial Veterans Hospital, 5462
Federation for Children with Special Needs, 798
Four-H Camp Howe, 965
Frank R and Elizabeth Simoni Foundation, 2561
Friendly Ice Cream Corp Contributions Prog ram, 2562
Gateway Arts Program, Crafts Store & Gallery, 5870
Greater Worcester Community Foundation, 2563
Handi-Kids, 966
Harvard University Howe Laboratory of Ophthalmology, 4519
Hyams Foundation, 2564
IL Center: Cape Organization for Rights of the Disabled, 810
Independence Associates, 3893
Independent Living Center of Starvos: Spri ngfield, 3895
Independent Living Center of Stavros: Gree nfield, 3896
Independent Living Center of the North Shore and Cape Ann, 3894
Independent Living Center of the Southeast, 3897
Independent Living Center: Massachusetts, 3898
Independent Living Center: Multi-Culural Center of Boston, 3899
Laboure College Library, 4520
Massachusetts Commission for the Blind, 3900
Massachusetts Fair Employment Practice Agency, 5871
Massachusetts Governor's Commission on Employment of Disabled Persons, 5872
Massachusetts Rehabilitation Commission, 4521
MetroWest Center for Independent Living, 3901
Mind-Body Clinic, 829
Nathaniel and Elizabeth P Stevens Foundation, 2565
National Managed Health Care Congress, 1554
New England Regional Genetics Group, 4499
Northampton VA Medical Center, 5463
Northeast Independent Living Program, 3902
Parent Professional Advocacy League, 873
Parents for Residential Reform, 876
Raytheon Company Contributions Program, 2566
Renaissance Clubhouse, 3903
Scandinavian Seminar, 2289
Schepens Eye Research Institute, 4522
Southeast Center for Independent Living, 3904
Spero Charitable Foundation, 2567
Student Independent Living Experience Massachusetts Hospital School, 3905
Talking Book Library at Worcester Public Library, 4523
The TJX Foundation, 2568
VA Boston Healthcare System: Brockton Division, 5464
VA Boston Healthcare System: Jamaica Plain Campus, 5465
VA Boston Healthcare System: West Roxbury Division, 5466
Vocational and Rehabilitation Agency Massachusetts Commission for the Blind, 5874
Work Inc., 5875

Michigan

Aleda E Lutz VA Medical Center, 5467
Ann Arbor Area Community Foundation, 2570
Ann Arbor Center for Independent Living, 3906
Arc Detroit, 3907
Arc of Michigan, 2571
Arc/Muskegon, 3908
Artificial Language Laboratory, 4524
Bad Axe Center for Independent Living, 3909
Battle Creek VA Medical Center, 5468
Bay Area Coalition for Independent Living, 3910
Berrien Community Foundation, 2572
Blind Children's Fund, 2573
Blue Water CIL: Lapeer, 3911
Blue Water CIL: Port Huron, 3912
Burger School for the Autistic, 4525
CIL of Mid-Michigan, 3913
Camp Roger, 967
Capital Area Center for Independent Living, 3914
Caro Center for Independent Living, 3915
Center for Community Access, 3916
Center for Handicapped Affairs, 3917
Center for Independent Living of Mid-Michigan, 3918
Chi Medical Library, 4526
Clarence & Grace Chamberlin Foundation, 2574
Community Connections of Southwest Michiga n, 3919
Community Foundation of Monroe County, 2575
Cowan Slavin Foundation, 2576
Cristo Rey Handicappers Program, 3920
Daimler Chrysler, 2577
Department Of Human Services, 5876
Detroit Center for Independent Living, 3921
DisAbility Connections, 3922
Disability Advocates of Kent County, 3923
Disability Community Small Business Development Center, 787
Disability Connection, 3924
Disability Network, Oakland/Macomb, 3925
Disability Resource Center of SW Michigan, 3926
Echo Grove Camp, 968
Educational Accessibility Services, 791
Fowler Center, 969
Frank & Mollie S VanDervoort Memorial Foun dation, 2578
Fremont Area Foundation, 2579
Glaucoma Laser Trial, 4527
Grand Rapids Foundation, 2580
Grand Traverse Area Community Living Management Corporation, 3927
Grand Traverse Area Library for the Blind and Physically Handicapped, 4528
Granger Foundation, 2581
Great Lakes Center for Independent Living, 3928
Great Lakes/Macomb Rehabilitation Group, 3929
Harvey Randall Wickes Foundation, 2582
Havirmill Foundation, 2583
Indian Trails Camp, 970
Iron Mountain VA Medical Center, 5469
JARC, 3930
John D Dingell VA Medical Center, 5470
Kalamazoo Center for Independent Living, 3932
Kelly Services Foundation, 2584
Kent District Library for the Blind and Physically Handicapped, 4529
Kresge Foundation, 2585
Lakeshore Center for Independent Living, 3933
Lamplighter's Work Center, 5877
Lanting Foundation, 2586
Library of Michigan Service for the Blind, 4530
Livingston Center for Independent Living, 3934
Macomb Library for the Blind and Physically Handicapped, 4531
Michigan Commission for the Blind: Detroit, 3936
Michigan Commission for the Blind: Independent Living Rehabilitation Program, 3935
Michigan Employment Service, 5878
Michigan Fair Employment Practice Agency, 5879
Michigan Rehabilitation Services: Dept of Labor And Economic Development, 5880
Michigan VA Regional Office, 5471
Michigan's Assistive Technology Resource, 4532
Mideastern Michigan Library Co-op, 4533
Midland Center for Independent Living, 3937
Monroe Center for Independent Living, 3938
Muskegon County Library for the Blind, 4534
Northland Library Cooperative, 4535
Oakland County Library for the Visually & Physically Impaired, 4536
Ransom Fidelity Company Foundation, 2587
Rehabilitation Services, 885
Rollin M Gerstacker Foundation, 2588
Small Business Development Center, 5881
Southeastern Michigan Commission for the Blind, 3939
St. Clair County Library Special Technologies Alternative Resources (S.T.A.R.), 4537
Steelcase Foundation, 2589

Superior Alliance for Independent Living (SAIL), 3940
University of Michigan: Orthopaedic Research Laboratories, 4538
Upper Peninsula Library for the Blind, 4539
VA Ann Arbor Healthcare System, 5472
Vet Center Readjustment Counseling Service, 5473
Washtenaw County Library for the Blind & Physically Handicapped, 4540
Wayne County Regional Library for the Blind, 4541
Wayne State University: CS Mott Center for Human Genetics and Development, 4542
YMCA Camp Copneconic, 971

Minnesota

Accessible Space, 3941
Accessnorth CIL of Northeastern MN: Aitkin, 3942
Accessnorth CIL of Northeastern MN: Duluth, 3943
Arc of Minnesota, 2590
Camp Courage, 972
Camp Friendship, 973
Camp New Hope, 929, 974
Camp Winnebago, 975
Center for Independent Living of NE Minnesota, 3944
Century College, 4543
Closing the Gap's Annual Conference, 1546
Communication Center/Minnesota State Services for the Blind, 4544
Courage Center, 3945
Deluxe Corporation Foundation, 2591
Duluth Public Library, 4545
Flying Wheels Travel, 5338
General Mills Foundation, 2592
Higher Education Consortium for Urban Affairs (HECUA), 2277
Hugh J Andersen Foundation, 2593
James R Thorpe Foundation, 2594
Jay and Rose Phillips Family Foundation, 2595
Jewish Vocational Service of Jewish Family and Children's Services, 5882
Metropolitan Center for Independent Living, 3947
Minneapolis Foundation, 2596
Minneapolis VA Medical Center, 5474
Minnesota Association of Centers for Independent Living, 3948
Minnesota Employment Practice Agency, 5883
Minnesota Library for the Blind and Physically Handicapped, 4546
Minnesota Rehabilitation Services, 5884
Miracle-Ear Children's Foundation, 2549
OPTIONS, 3949
Options Interstate Resource Center for Independent Living, 3950
Ordean Foundation, 2597
Otto Bremer Foundation, 2598
PACER Center (Parent Advocacy Coalition for Educational Rights), 870
PWI Forum, 5885
Perry River Home Care, 3951
Rochester Area Foundation, 2599
SMILES, 3952
Southeastern Minnesota Center for Independent Living: Rochester, 3953, 3954
Southern Minnesota Independent Living Enterprises and Services, 3955
Southwestern Center for Independent Living, 3956
Special U, 4547
St. Cloud VA Medical Center, 5475
St. Paul Regional Office, 5476
University of Minnesota at Crookston, 2293
Ventures Travel, 5350
Vinland Center Lake Independence, 3957

Mississippi

Allied Enterprises of Tupelo, 5887
Alpha Home Royal Maid Association for the Blind, 3958
Arc of Mississippi, 2600
Biloxi/Gulfport VA Medical Center, 5478
Gulf Coast Independent Living Center, 3959
Jackson Independent Living Center, 3960
Jackson Regional Office, 5479
LIFE of Central Mississippi, 3961
LIFE of South Mississippi, 3962
Life of North Mississippi: Greenville, 3963
Life of North Mississippi: Tupelo, 3964
Life of South Mississippi: Biloxi, 3965
Mississippi Department of Rehabilitation Services, 5888
Mississippi Employment Secutity Commission, 5889
Mississippi Library Commission, 4548
Mississippi Library Commission\Talking Book and Braille Services, 4549
Mississippi Society for Disabilities, 831
Mississippi State Independent Living Center, 3966
Worksight, 5890

Missouri

Access II Independent Living Center, 3967
Allen P & Josephine B Green Foundation, 2601
Anheuser-Busch Inc., 2602
Assemblies of God Center for the Blind, 4550
Bootheel Area Independent Living Services, 3968
Camp Cub Creek Science Camp, 976
Camp Lakewood, 977
Church of the Nazarene, 4551
Coalition for Independence: Missouri Branch Office, 3969
Concerned Care Recreation Day Camp, 978
Delta Center for Independent Living, 3970
Disability Resource Association, 3971
Disabled Citizens Alliance for Independence, 3972
Greater Kansas City Community Foundation and Affiliated Trusts, 2603
Greater St. Louis Community Foundation, 2604
H&R Block Foundation, 2605
Harry S Truman Memorial Veterans' Hospital, 5480
Independent Living Center of Southeast Missouri, 3973
International Clinic of Biological Regeneration, 816
James S McDonnell Foundation, 2606
John J Pershing VA Medical Center, 5481
Judevine Center for Autism, 4552
Kansas City VA Medical Center, 5482
Life Skills Foundation, 3974
Lutheran Charities Foundation of St. Louis, 2607
Lutheran Library for the Blind, 4553
Mary's Call, 2608
Midland Empire Resources For Independent Living (MERIL), 3975
Missouri Fair Employment Practice Agency, 5891
Missouri Governor's Council on Disability, 5892
Missouri Job Training Program Liaison, 5893
Missouri Vocational Rehabilitation Agency, 5894
Northeast Independent Living Services, 3976
On My Own, 3977
Oppenstein Brothers Foundation, 2609
Ozark Independent Living, 3978
Paraquad, 3979
People to People International, 2287
People-to-People Committee on Disability, 880
People-to-People International: Committee for the Handicapped, 881
Places for People, 3980
RA Bloch Cancer Foundation, 2610
RAIL, 3981
Southeastern Missouri Alliance for Independence (SEMO Alliance), 3983
Southwest Center for Independent Living (SWCIL), 3984
St. Louis Regional Office, 5483
St. Louis VA Medical Center, 5484
Tri-County Center for Independent Living, 3985
University of Missouri: Columbia Arthritis Center, 4554
Victor E Speas Foundation, 2611
WX: Work Capacities, 5895
West Central Independent Living Solutions, 3986
Whole Person, 3987
Whole Person: Olathe, 3845
Wolfner Library for the Blind, 4555
Wonderland Camp Foundation, 979

Montana

Living Independently for Today and Tomorrow, 3989
Living Independently for Today and Tomorrow: Glendrive, 3988
MonTECH, 4556
Montana Fair Employment Practice Agency, 5896
Montana Governor's Committee on Employment of Disabled People, 5897
Montana Independent Living Project, 3990
Montana State Library-Talking Book Library, 4557
Montana VA Regional Office, 5485
North Central Independent Living Services, 3991
Summit Independent Living Center: Hamilton, 3993

Summit Independent Living Center: Kalipsell, 3992
Summit Independent Living Center: Missoula, 3994
V A Montana Healthcare System, 5486
VA Montana Healthcare System, 5487
Vet Center, 5477, 5488

Nebraska

Arc of Nebraska, 2612
Camp Easter Seals, 980
Center for Independent Living of Central Nebraska, 3995
Cooper Foundation, 2613
Eastern Nebraska 4-H Camps and Centers, 981
Grand Island VA Medical System, 5489
League of Human Dignity: Lincoln, 3996
League of Human Dignity: Norfolk, 3997
League of Human Dignity: Omaha, 3998
Lincoln Regional Office, 5490
Lincoln VA Medical Center, 5491
Martin Luther Home Society Inc., 4558
Martin Luther Homes of Beatrice, 3999
Martin Luther Homes of Nebraska, 4000
Nebraska Assistive Technology Partnership Nebraska Department of Education, 4559
Nebraska Employment Services, 5898
Nebraska Fair Employment Practice Agency, 5899
Nebraska Library Commission: Talking Book and Braille Service, 4560
Nebraska Vocational Rehabilitation Agency, 5900
Panhandle Independent Living Services, 4001
Slosburg Family Charitable Trust, 2614
Union Pacific Foundation, 2615
VA Nebraska-Western Iowa Health Care System, 5492

Nevada

ABC Union, ACE, ANLV, Vegas Western Cab, 5352
Carson City Center for Independent Living, 4002
Conrad N Hilton Foundation, 2616
EL Wiegand Foundation, 2617
Las Vegas Veterans Center, 5493
Las Vegas-Clark County Library District, 4561
Nell J Redfield Foundation, 2619
Nevada Fair Employment Practice Agency, 5901
Nevada Governor's Committee on Employment of Persons with Disabilities, 5902
Nevada State Library and Archives, 4562
Northern Nevada Center for Independent Living: Reno, 4003, 4004
Reno Regional Office, 5494
Rural Center for Independent Living, 4005
Southern Nevada Center for Independent Living: Las Vegas, 4006, 4007
VA Sierra Nevada Healthcare System, 5495
VA Southern Nevada Healthcare System, 5496
William N and Pennington Foundation, 2620

New Hampshire

Agnes M Lindsay Trust, 2621
Camp Allen, 982
Camp Dartmouth-Hitchcock, 983
Easter Seal Camp: New Hampshire, 984
Easter Seals NH Camp Sno-Mo, 985
Fit for Work at Exeter Hospital, 5904
Foundation for Seacoast Health, 2622
Granite State Independent Living Foundation, 4008
Manchester Regional Office, 5497
Manchester VA Medical Center, 5498
National Guild of Hypnotists, 853
New Hampshire Employment Security, 5905
New Hampshire Fair Employment Practice Agency, 5906
New Hampshire Job Training Program Liaison, 5907
New Hampshire State Library: Talking Book Services, 4563
New Hampshire Veterans Centers, 5499

New Jersey

ARC of Gloucester County, 5909
ARC of Hunterdon County, 5910
ARC of Mercer County, 5911
ARC of Monmouth, 5912
Abilities Center of New Jersey, 5913
Abilities of Northwest New Jersey, 5914
Alliance for Disabled in Action New Jersey, 5915
Alternatives for Growth: New Jersey, 5916
American Organization for Bodywork Therapies of Asia, 747
American Self-Help Clearinghouse, 750
Arc of Bergen and Passaic Counties, 5917
Arc of New Jersey, 2624
Arnold A Schwartz Foundation, 2625
Assistive Technology Advocacy Center (ATAC), 4009
Avis Rent-A-Car, 5353
Camp Jotoni, 987
Camp Merry Heart, 988
Camp Sun'N Fun, 989
Campbell Soup Foundation, 2626
Career Opportunity Development of New Jersey, 5918
Center for Educational Advancement New Jersey, 5919
Center for Independent Living: Camden, 4010
Center for Independent Living: Edison, 4011
Center for Independent Living: Long Branch, 4012
Center for Independent Living: South Jersey, 4013
Cerebral Palsy Association of Middlesex County, 5920
Cerebral Palsy Center Summer Program, 990
Children's Hopes & Dreams Wish Fulfillment Foundation, 2627
Children's Specialized Hospital Medical Library - Parent Resource Center, 4564
Christopher & Dana Reeve Foundation Resource Center, 4565
Community Foundation of New Jersey, 2628
Cowles Charitable Trust, 2629
Cross Roads Outdoor Ministries, 991
Dial: Disabled Information Awareness & Living, 4014
Disabled Advocates Working for Northwest (DAWN), 4015
Disabled American Veterans: Ocean County, 5500
East Orange Campus of the VA New Jersey Healthcare System, 5501
Easter Seal Hackensack, 5921
Easter Seal Society of New Jersey Highlands Workshop, 5922
Easter Seal of Ocean County, 5923
Easter Seals New Jersey, 5924
Eden Acres Administrative Services, 5925
Edison Sheltered Workshop, 5926
Eye Institute of New Jersey, 4566
F Mason Perkins Trust, 2630
FM Kirby Foundation, 2631
Family Resource Associates, 4016
Fannie E Rippel Foundation, 2632
First Occupational Center of New Jersey, 5927
Fund for New Jersey, 2633
Goodwill Industries of Southern New Jersey, 5928
Hausmann Industries, 5929
Heightened Independence and Progress: Hack ensack, 4017
Heightened Independence and Progress: Jers ey City, 4018
Jersey Cape Diagnostic Training & Opportunity Center, 5930
Lyons Campus of the VA New Jersey Healthcare System, 5502
Merck Company Foundation, 2634
Milton Schamach Foundation, 2636
Mycoclonus Research Foundation, 4567
Nabisco Foundation, 2637
New Jersey Camp Jaycee, 992
New Jersey Center for Outreach and Services for the Autism Community (COSAC), 4568
New Jersey Commission for the Blind and Visually Impaired, 5931
New Jersey Employment Service and Job Training Program Services, 5932
New Jersey Library for the Blind and Handicapped, 4569
Newark Regional Office, 5503
Occupational Center of Hudson County, 5933
Occupational Center of Union County, 5934
Occupational Training Center of Burlington County, 5935
Occuptational Training Center of Camden County, New Jersey, 5936
Ostberg Foundation, 2638
Pathways to Independence, 5937
Progressive Center for Independent Living, 4019
Project Freedom, 4020
Prudential Foundation, 2639
Robert Wood Johnson Foundation, 2640
Somerset Training and Employment Program, 5938
St. John of God Community Services Vocational Rehabilitation, 5939
Total Living Center, 4021
United Cerebral Palsy Associations of New Jersey, 5940
Victoria Foundation, 2641
West Essex Rehab Center, 5942

New Mexico

Ability Center, 4022
Adelante Development Center, 5943
Arc of New Mexico, 2642
CASA Inc., 4023
CHOICES Center for Independent Living, 4024
Dental Amalgam Syndrome (DAMS) Newsletter, 4388
Family Voices, 795
Frost Foundation, 2643
Goodwill Industries of New Mexico, 5944
McCune Charitable Foundation, 2644
New Mexico Employment Services and Job Training Liaison, 5945
New Mexico State Library for the Blind and Physically Handicapped, 4570
New Mexico Technology Assistance Program, 4025
New Mexico VA Healthcare System, 5504
New Mexico Veterans Centers, 5505
New Vistas, 4026
RCI, 5946
San Juan Center for Independence, 4027
Santa Fe Community Foundation, 2645
Santa Fe Mountain Center, 993
Tohatchi Area of Opportunity & Services, 5947
Vocational Rehabilitation Agency, 5873, 5948

New York

AIDS Funding, 2917
AIM Independent Living Center: Corning, 4028
AIM Independent Living Center: Elmira, 4029
ARISE: Center for Independent Living: Oswe go, 4031
ARISE: Center for Independent Living: Syracuse, 4030
AT&T Foundation, 2646
Abilities!, 724
Access to Independence of Cortland County, 4032
Action Toward Independence: Middletown, 4033
Action Toward Independence: Monticello, 4034
Advocacy Center, 726
Advocates for Children of New York, 728
Alavi Foundation of New York, 2647
Albany VA Medical Center: Samuel S Stratton, 5506
Albany Vet Center, 5507
Altman Foundation, 2648
Ambrose Monell Foundation, 2649
American Chai Trust, 2650
American Express Foundation, 2623
American Foundation for the Blind, 2651
American Foundation for the Blind-Midwest, 2470
American-Scandinavian Foundation, 2267
Arthur Ross Foundation, 2652
Artists Fellowship, 2653
Basic Facts on Study Abroad, 2271
Bath VA Medical Center, 5508
Bergeron Health Care, 4035
Bodman Foundation, 2655
Brain Injury Association of New York State, 766
Bronx Independent Living Services, 4036
Bronx VA Medical Center, 5509
Brooklyn Campus of the VA NY Harbor Healthcare System, 5510
Brooklyn Center for Independence of the Disabled, 4037
Brooklyn Home for Aged Men, 2656
Buffalo Regional Office, 5511
Buffalo State (SUNY), 2273
Camp Aldersgate, 994
Camp Venture, 995
Camp Whitman on Seneca Lake, 996
Canandiagua VA Medical Center, 5512
Cancer Care, 2657
Canine Helpers for the Handicapped, 772
Capital District Center for Independence, 4038
Castle Point Campus of the VA Hudson Valley Healthcare System, 5513
Catskill Center for Independence, 4039
Center for Community Alternatives, 3851
Center for Independence of the Disabled of New York, 4040
Center for Independent Living: Action Towards Independence, 4041
Center for Independent Living: Amsterdam, 4042
Center for Independent Living: Rochester, 4043
Center on Human Policy: School of Education, 4571
Clark Foundation, 2658
Clover Patch Camp, 997
Commonwealth Fund, 2659
Community Alternatives, 4044
Community Foundation for Greater Buffalo, 2660
Community Foundation of Herkimer &, 2661
Community Foundation of the Capitol Region, 2662
Comsearch: Broad Topics, 2663
Corporate Foundation Files, 2921
Corporate Foundation Profiles, 2922
Crime and Justice, 2923
DD Center/St Lukes: Roosevelt Hospital Center, 4045
DE French Foundation, 2664
DREAMMS for Kids, 4572
David J Green Foundation, 2665
Diabetic Cruise Desk, 5334
Directions Unlimited Acccessible Tours, 5336
Directory of Japanese Giving, 2925
Directory of New and Emerging Foundations, 2926
Directory of Venture Capital Firms, 2927
Disabled Children's Relief Fund, 788
Disabled and Alone/Life Services for the Handicapped, 789
Easter Seals New York, 2666
Eastern Paralyzed Veterans Association, 4573
Edward John Noble Foundation, 2667
Ehrman Medical Library, 4574
Epilepsy Foundation of Long Island, 2668
Epilepsy Society of New York, 2669
Episcopal Charities, 2670
Esther A & Joseph Klingenstein Fund, 2671
Fay J Lindner Foundation, 2672
Fedcap Rehabilitation Services, 797
Feingold Association of the US, 800
Finger Lakes Developmental Disabilities Service Office, 4575
Finger Lakes Independence Center, 4046
Florence V Burden Foundation, 2673
Ford Foundation, 2674
Fortis Foundation, 2675
Foundation 1000, 2938
Foundation Center, 2676
Foundation Center Library Services, 2677
Foundation Center's User-Friendly Guide, 2939
Foundation Directory, 2940
Foundation Grants to Individuals, 2941
Foundation for Advancement in Cancer Therapy, 2678
Foundation for the Advancement of Innovative Medicine, 2679
Gebbie Foundation, 2680
Genesee Region Independent Living Center, 4047
Gladys Brooks Foundation, 2681
Glens Falls Independent Living Center, 4048
Glickenhaus Foundation, 2682
Graphic Controls Corporate Giving Program, 2683
Guide Dog Foundation for the Blind, 2684
Guide to Federal Funding for Hospitals and Health Centers, 2944
Harlem Independent Living Center, 4049
Helen Keller International, 4576
Helen Keller National Center for Deaf-Blin d Youths and Adults (HKNC), 4577
Henry Kaufmann Campgrounds Staten Island, 998
Henry and Lucy Moses Fund, 2685
Herman Goldman Foundation, 2686
Horace W Goldsmith Foundation, 2687
Institute for Basic Research in Developmental Disabilities, 4578
Institute for Visual Sciences, 4579
International Christian Youth Exchange, 2278
International Encyclopedia of Foundations, 2949
International Paper Company Foundation, 2688
International Partnership for Service-Learning and Leadership, 2279
International Women's Health Coalition, 818
JGB Cassette Library International, 4580
JOBS VI and SAGE, 5950
Japanese Corporate Connection: A Guide for Fundraisers, 2950
Jedra Charitable Foundation, 2689
Joseph Alexander Foundation, 2690
Just One Break (JOBS), 5951
Juvenile Diabetes Foundation International, 821
Kamp Kiwanis, 999
Kenneth & Evelyn Lipper Foundation, 2691
Long Island Alzheimer's Foundation, 2692
Long Island Center for Independent Living, 4050
Louis and Anne Abrons Foundation, 2693
March of Dimes Birth Defects Foundation, 827
Margaret L Wendt Foundation, 2694
Marquis George MacDonald Foundation, 2695
Massena Center for Independent Living, 4051
Merrill Lynch & Company Foundation, 2635
Metzger-Price Fund, 2696
Milbank Foundation For Rehabilitation, 2697
Minority Outreach Project, 4052

Morgan Stanley Foundation, 2698
Mount Sinai Medical Center, 2699
NYS Independent Living Council, Inc., 4053
Nassau County Office for the Physically Challenged, 4054
Nassau Library System, 4581
National Braille Association, 4582
National Business & Disability Council, 838
National Data Book of Foundations, 2951
National Directory of Corporate Giving, 2952
National Foundation for Facial Reconstruction, 2700
National Guide to Funding Religion, 2953
National Guide to Funding for Children, Youth & Families, 2954
National Guide to Funding for Elementary & Secondary Education, 2955
National Guide to Funding for Libraries and Information Services, 2956
National Guide to Funding for Women and Girls, 2957
National Guide to Funding in Aging, 2958
National Guide to Funding in Arts and Culture, 2959
National Guide to Funding in Health, 2960
National Guide to Funding in Higher Education, 2961
National Hemophilia Foundation, 2701
National Neurofibromatosis Foundation The Childrens Tumor Foundation, 2702
Neisloss Family Foundation, 2703
New York City Campus of the VA NY Harbor Healthcare System, 5514
New York Community Trust, 2704
New York Foundation, 2705
New York Public Library: Andrew Heiskell Library for the Blind and Physically Handicapped, 4583
New York Regional Office, 5515
New York State Department of Labor, 5952
New York State Foundations, 2962
New York State Talking Book & Braille Library, 4584
New York Therapeutic Riding Center, 865
Newburgh Center for Independent Living, 4055
Niagara Frontier Center for Independent Living, 4056
Ninety-Second Street Y Camps Nesher Program, 1000
North Country Center for Independent Livin g, 4057
Northern New York Community Foundation, 2706
Northern Regional Center for Independent Living: Watertown, 4058, 4059
Northport VA Medical Center, 5516
Nurse Healers: Professional Associates International, 868
Options for Independence: Auburn, 4060
Options for Independence: Seneca Falls, 4061
Parkinson's Disease Foundation, 2504, 2707
People and Places, 5346
Postgraduate Center for Mental Health, 4585
Prader-Willi Alliance of New York Annual Conference, 1555
Programs for Children 3 to 5 with Disabili lities, 1001
Programs for Children Birth to 2 with Disa abilities, 1002
Programs for Children with Special Health Care Needs, 1003
Queens Independent Living Center, 4062
Rational Effectiveness Training Systems, 5953
Reader's Digest Foundation, 2708
Rehabilitation International, 884, 1557
Rehabilitation Research Library, 4586
Research to Prevent Blindness, 2709
Resource Center for Accessible Living, 4063
Rita J and Stanley H Kaplan Foundation, 2710
Robert Sterling Clark Foundation, 2711
Rochester Rotary Sunshine Camp, 1004
Rockland Independent Living Center, 4064
SILO: Cental Islip, 4065
SILO: Hauppauge, 4066
Skadden Fellowship Foundation, 2712
Source Book Profiles, 2964
Southern Adirondack Independent Living, 4067
Southern Tier Independence Center, 4068
Southwestern Independent Living Center, 4069
Special Education and Vocational Rehabilitation Agency: New York, 5954
St. George's Society of New York, 2713
Stanley W Metcalf Foundation, 2714
State University of New York, 2292
State University of New York Health Sciences Center, 4587
Staten Island Center for Independent Living, 4070
Stonewall Community Foundation, 2715
Suffolk Cooperative Library System: Long Island Talking Book Library, 4588
Suffolk Independent Living Organization (SILO), 4071
Surdna Foundation, 2716
Syracuse VA Medical Center, 5517
Taconic Resources for Independence, 4072
The Dana Foundation The Dana Alliance For Brain Initiatives, 2717
The William Randolph Hearst Foundations, 2718
Tisch Foundation, 2719
Torah Alliance of Families of Kids with Disabilities, 5518
Tourette Syndrome Association Conference, 1561
VA Hudson Valley Health Care System, 5519
VA Western NY Healthcare System, Batavia, 5520
VA Western NY Healthcare System, Buffalo, 5521
Van Ameringen Foundation, 2720
Visions/Services for the Blind & Visually Impaired, 4073
Wagon Road Camp, 1005
Wallace Memorial Library, 4589
Westchester County Independent Living Center, 4074
Westchester Disabled on the Move, 4075
Western New York Foundation, 2721
William T Grant Foundation, 2722
Wiswall Center for Independent Living, 4076
Xavier Society for the Blind, 4590
YAI: National Institute for People with Disabilities, 900

North Carolina

AHEAD Association, 723
Arc of North Carolina, 2723
Asheville VA Medical Center, 5522
Association on Higher Education and Disability (AHEAD), 760
Bob & Kay Timberlake Foundation, 2724
Broyhill Family Foundation, 2725
Camp Sky Ranch, 1006
Center for Accessible Housing, 4077
Center for Universal Design, 777
Charlotte Vet Center, 5523
Davidson College, Office of Study Abroad, 2275
Disability Awareness Network, 4078
Disability Rights & Resources, 4079
Division of Employment & Training, 5955
Duke Endowment, 2726
Durham VA Medical Center, 5524
Fayetteville VA Medical Center, 5384, 5525
First Union Foundation, 2727
Foundation for the Carolinas, 2728
Genova Diagnostics, 4591
Handicapped Student Program Postsecondary Education Association, 1550
Iredell Vocational Workshop, 5956
John H Wellons Foundation, 2729
Joy: A Shabazz Center for Independent Living, 4080
Kate B Reynolds Charitable Trust, 2730
Kathleen Price and Joseph M Bryan Family Foundation, 2731
Live Independently Networking Center, 4081
Live Independently Networking Center: Hickory, 4082
Mary Reynolds Babcock Foundation, 2732
Mount Shepherd Retreat Center, 1007
National Early Childhood Technical Assistance Center, 845
National Respite Locator Service, 861
North Carolina Division of Services for the Blind, 5957
North Carolina Library for the Blind and Physically Handicapped, 4592
Opportunity Plus of NC, 869
Pathways for the Future, 4083
Pediatric Rheumatology Clinic, 4593
Rowan County Vocational Workshop, 5958
Rutherford Vocational Workshop, 5959
Stone Mountain School, 1008
Transylvania Vocational Services, 5960
Triangle Community Foundation, 2733
University of North Carolina at Chapel Hill: Neuroscience Research Building, 4594
WG Hefner VA Medical Center, 5526
Webster Enterprises of Jackson County, 5963
Western Alliance Center for Independent Living, 4084
Western Regional Vocational Rehabilitation Facility Clifford File, Jr., 5964
Winston-Salem Regional Office, 5527

North Dakota

Alex Stern Family Foundation, 2734
Arc of North Dakota, 2735
Center for Independent Living: Fargo, 4085
Dakota Center for Independent Living: Bism arck, 4087
Dakota Center for Independent Living: Dickinson, 4086
Fargo VA Medical Center, 5528
Fraser, 4088

Freedom Resource Center for Independent Living: Fargo, 3946, 4089
North Dakota Community Foundation, 2736
North Dakota Department of Labor, Equal Employment Opportunity Division, 5965
North Dakota Employment Service and Job Training Program Liaison, 5966
North Dakota Governor's Committee on Employment of Disabled Persons, 5967
North Dakota State Library Talking Book Services, 4595
North Dakota VA Regional Office, 5529
North Dakota Vocational Rehabilitation Agency, 5968
Resource Center for Independent Living: Minot, 4090

Ohio

Ability Center of Defiance, 4091
Ability Center of Greater Toledo, 4092
Access Center for Independent Living, 4093
Akron Community Foundation, 2737
Akron Rotary Camp, 1009
Albert G and Olive H Schlink Foundation, 2738
American Foundation Corporation, 2739
Antioch College, 2268
Arc of Ohio, 2740
Beech Brook, 1010
Camp Allyn, 1011
Camp Courageous, 1012
Camp Stepping Stone, 1013
Case Western Reserve University, 4596
Case Western Reserve University Northeast Ohio Multipurpose Arthritis Center, 4597
Chillicothe VA Medical Center, 5530
Cincinnati Children's Hospital Medical Center, 4598
Cincinnati VA Medical Center, 5531
Cincinnati Veterans Centers, 5532
Cleveland FES Center, 4599
Cleveland Foundation, 2741
Cleveland Public Library, 4600
Cleveland Regional Office, 5533
Columbus Foundation and Affiliated Organizations, 2742
Cornucopia, 5969
Dayton VA Medical Center, 5534
Disabled American Veterans, 5368
Eleanora CU Alms Trust, 2743
Eva L And Joseph M Bruening Foundation, 2744
Fairfield Center for Disabilities and Cerebral Palsy, 4094
Fred & Lillian Deeks Memorial Foundation, 2745
GAR Foundation, 2746
George Gund Foundation, 2747
Great Oaks Joint Vocational School, 5970
Greater Cincinnati Foundation, 2748
HCR Manor Care Foundation, 2749
Happiness Day at Parmadale, 1014
Happiness Day at St. Augustine Academy, 1015
Happiness Day at the Center for Pastoral Leadership, 1016
Harry C Moores Foundation, 2750
Hearth Day Treatment and Vocational Services, 5971
Helen Steiner Rice Foundation, 2751
Herbert W Hoover Foundation, 2752
Highland Unlimited Business Enterprises of CRI, 5972
John P Murphy Foundation, 2753
Lake Erie College, 2281
Leo Yassenoff JCC Day Camps, 1017
Linking Employment Ability Potential: Independent Living Center, 4095
Louis Stokes VA Medical Center, 5535
Mid-Ohio Board for an Independent Living Environment (MOBILE), 4096
National Association of the Physically Handicapped, 837
Nationwide Foundation, 2754
Nordson Corporate Giving Program, 2755
Ohio Civil Rights Commission, 5973
Ohio Commission On Minority Health, 5974
Ohio Regional Library for the Blind and Physically Handicapped, 4601
Ohio Statewide Independent Living Council, 4097
Parker-Hannifin Foundation, 2756
Recreation Unlimited, 1018
Rehabilitation Service of North Central Ohio, 4098
Reinberger Foundation, 2757
Robert Campeau Family Foundation, 2758
Samuel W Bell Home for Sightless, 4099
Services for Independent Living, 3982, 4100
Sisler McFawn Foundation, 2759
Society for Equal Access: Independent Living Center, 4101
Stark Community Foundation, 2760
State Library of Ohio: Talking Book Program, 4602
The Bahmann Foundation, 2761
The Stocker Foundation, 2762
Toledo Community Foundation, 2763
Trager International, 893
William J and Dorothy K O'Neill Foundation, 2764
Youngstown Foundation, 2765

Oklahoma

Ability Resources, 4102
Anne and Henry Zarrow Foundation, 2766
Green County Independent Living Resource Center, 4103
International Bio-Oxidative Medicine Foundation (IBOM), 2767
Muskogee VA Medical Center, 5536
Oklahoma City VA Medical Center, 5537
Oklahoma Department of Rehabilitation Services (DRS), 5976
Oklahoma Employment Services and Job Training Program Liaison, 5977
Oklahoma Governor's Committee on Employment of People with Disabilities, 5978
Oklahoma Library for the Blind & Physically Handicapped, 4603
Oklahoma Medical Research Foundation, 4604
Oklahoma Veterans Centers Vet Center, 5538
Oklahomans for Independent Living, 4104
Progressive Independence, 4105
Sandra Beasley Independent Living Center, 4106
Sarkeys Foundation, 2768
Tulsa City-County Library System: Outreach Services, 4605

Oregon

Arc of Oregon, 2769
Bend Work Activity Center, 5979
Building Bridges: Including People with Disabilities in International Programs, 2274
Central Oregon Resources for Independent Living, 4107
Chiles Foundation, 2770
Columbia Gorge Center, 4108
DB-Link, 785
Easter Seals Oregon Camping Program, 1019
Eastern Oregon Center for Independent Living, 4109
Feldenkrais Guild of North America (FGNA), 801
Gales Creek Diabetes Camp, 1020
HASL Independent Abilities Center, 4110
Independent Living Resources, 4111
Jackson Foundation, 2771
Lane Community College, 2282
Laurel Hill Center Independent Living Program, 4112
Leslie G Ehmann Trust, 2772
Mt Hood Kiwanis Camp, 1021
National College of Naturopathic Medicine, 840
Oregon Commission for the Blind, 4113
Oregon Fair Employment Practice Agency, 5980
Oregon Health Sciences University, 5539
Oregon Health Sciences University, Elks' Children's Eye Clinic, 4606
Oregon Talking Book & Braille Services, 4607
People First International, 877
Portland Naturopathic Clinic: NCNM National Health Centers Eastside Clinic, 882
Portland Regional Office, 5540
Portland VA Medical Center, 5541
Progressive Options, 4114
Roseburg VA Medical Center, 5542
SPOKES Unlimited, 4115
Samuel S Johnson Foundation, 2773
State of Oregon Office of Vocational Rehabilitation Service, 5981
Sundial Special Vacations, 5349
Talking Book & Braille Services Oregon State Library, 4608
Umpqua Valley Disabilities Network, 4116
University of Oregon, 2294
University of Oregon International Service, 2295
Upward Bound Camp: Evans Creek, 1022
Vocational and Rehabilitation Agency: Commision for the Blind, 5983
White City VA Domiciliary, 5543
World of Options, 2298
World of Options: A Guide to International Educational Exchange, 2299

Pennsylvania

AC-ACLD/An Association for Children and Adults with Learning Disabilities, 5984
Abilities in Motion, 4117
Accessible Journeys, 5328
Accesstotheplanet, 5329
Achieva, 1023
Acorn Alcinda Foundation, 2774
Air Products Foundation, 2775
Anthracite Region Center for Independent Living, 4118
Arc of Pennsylvania, 2776
Arcadia Foundation, 2777
Associated Services For The Blind & Visually Impaired, 4609
Beaver College, 2272
Brachial Plexus Palsy Foundation, 2778
Brian's House, 4119
Briarwood Day Camp, 1024
Butler VA Medical Center, 5544
Camp AIM Lloyd Institute, 1025
Camp ARC Spencer, 1026
Camp Can Do, 1027
Camp Dunmore, 1028
Camp Keystone, 1029
Camp Lee Mar, 1030
Camp Surefoot, 1031
Carnegie Library of Pittsburgh Library for the Blind & Physically Handicapped, 4610
Claude Washington Benedum Foundation, 2779
Coatesville VA Medical Center, 5545
Columbia Gas of Pennsylvania Corporate Giv ing, 2780
Community Resources for Independence, 3609, 4120
Connelly Foundation, 2781
Dolfinger-McMahon Foundation, 2782
Erie VA Medical Center, 5546
Free Library of Philadelphia: Library for the Blind and Physically Handicapped, 4611
Freedom Valley Disability Center, 4121
Guided Tour for Persons 17 & Over with Developmental and Physical Challenges, 5341
Handi Camp, 1032
Harry C Trexler Trust, 2783
Helping Hands, 1033
Henry L Hillman Foundation, 2784
Howard Heinz Endowment, 2785
Hoxie Harrison Smith Foundation, 2786
Innabah, 1034
International University Partnerships, 2280
James E Van Zandt VA Medical Center, 5547
Jewish Healthcare Foundation of Pittsburgh, 2787
Juliet L Hillman Simonds Foundation, 2788
Ken-Crest Services, 1035
Lebanon VA Medical Center, 5548
Lehigh Valley Center for Independent Living, 4122
Liberty Resources, 4123
Life and Independence for Today, 4124
Living Waters, 1036
Make-a-Friend, 1037
Northeastern Pennsylvania Center for Independent Living, 4125
Oberkotter Foundation, 2789
Office of Vocational Rehabilitation, 5985
PECO Energy Company Contributions Program, 2790
PNC Bank Foundation, 2791
Pennsylvania College of Optometry Eye Institute, 4612
Pennsylvania Employment Services and Job Training, 5986
Pennsylvania Governor's Committee on Employment of Disabled Persons, 5987
Pennsylvania Human Relations Commission Agency, 5988
Pennsylvania Veterans Centers, 5549
Pennsylvania's Initiative on Assistive Technology, 4126
Philadelphia Foundation, 2792
Philadelphia Regional Office and Insurance Center, 5550
Philadelphia VA Medical Center, 5551
Pittsburgh Foundation, 2793
Pittsburgh Regional Office, 5552
Reading Rehabilitation Hospital, 4613
Shenango Valley Foundation, 2794
Souderton Special Needs Day Camp, 1038
South Central Pennsylvania Center for Inde pendence Living, 4127
Staunton Farm Foundation, 2795
Stewart Huston Charitable Trust, 2796
Teleflex Foundation, 2797
Three Rivers Center for Independent Living, 3812, 4128
Tri-County Patriots for Independent Living, 4129
US Healthworks, 5989
USX Foundation, 2798
VA Pittsburgh Healthcare System, Highland Drive Division, 5554
VA Pittsburgh Healthcare System, University Drive Division, 5553
Variety Club Camp, 1039
Voices for Independence, 4130
WW Smith Charitable Trust, 2799
Wesley Woods, 1040
Wilkes-Barre VA Medical Center, 5555
William B Dietrich Foundation, 2800
William Talbott Hillman Foundation, 2801
William V and Catherine A McKinney Charitable Foundation, 2802
Woodlands, 1041

Rhode Island

Aldersgate Center, 986, 1042
Arc South County Chapter, 2803
Arc of Northern Rhode Island, 2804
Arc-Down Syndrome Society of Rhode Island, 2805
Blackstone Valley Center, 4131
Blackstone Valley Chapter RI Arc, 2806
Bristol County Chapter Arc, 2807
Canonicus Camp, 1043
Champlin Foundations, 2808
Cranston Arc, 2809
Department of Veterans Affairs Regional Office - Vocational Rehab Division, 5366
Franklin Court Assisted Living, 4132
Goodwill Industries of RI, 5992
Groden Center, 5993
Horace A Kimball and S Ella Kimball Foundation, 2810
IN-SIGHT Independent Living, 4133
Kent County Arc, 2811
Newport County Arc, 2812
Newport County Chapter of Retarded Citizens, 5994
Ocean State Center for Independent Living, 4134
Office Of Library & Information Services for the Blind and Physically Handicapped, 4614
Office of Rehabilitation Services, 4135, 5995
PARI Independent Living Center, 4136
Providence Regional Office, 5556
Providence VA Medical Center, 5557
Rhode Island Arc, 2813
Rhode Island Foundation, 2814
Talking Books Plus, 4615
Westerly Chariho Arc, 2815

South Carolina

Arc of South Carolina, 2816
Burnt Gin Camp, 1044
Camp Gravatt, 1045
Center for Developmental Disabilities, 2817
Center for Disability Resources, 775
Coastal Disability Access, 4137
Colonial Life and Accident Insurance Company Contributions Program, 2818
Columbia Disability Action Center, 4138
Columbia Regional Office, 5558
Graham Street Community Resources, 4139
Greenville Disability Action Center, 4140
Medical University of South Carolina Arthritis Clinical/Research Center, 4616
Pickens County Arc, 2819
Ralph H Johnson VA Medical Center, 5559
SC Independent Living Council, 4141
South Carolina Employment Security Commission South Carolina Center, 5997
South Carolina Governor's Committee on Employment of the Handicapped, 5998
South Carolina State Library, 4617
South Carolina Vocational Rehabilitation Department, 5999
Vocational and Rehabilitation Agency: Commission for the Blind, 6001
Vocational and Rehabilitation Agency: Vocational Rehabilitation Department, 6000
William Jennings Bryan Dorn VA Medical Center, 5560

South Dakota

Adjustment Training Center, 4142
Black Hills Workshop & Training Center, 4143
Communication Service for the Deaf: Rapid City, 4145
Communication Service for the Deaf: Yankton, 4144
Dell Rapids Sportsmens Club, 5333
Native American Advocacy Program for Perso ns with Disabilities, 4146
Opportunities for Independent Living, 4147
Prairie Freedom Center for Independent Living, 4148, 4149, 4150, 4150
Sioux Falls VA Medical Center, 5561
South Dakota Assistive Technology Project, 4151

South Dakota Governor's Advisory Committee on Employment of the Disabled, 6002
South Dakota State Library, 4618
South Dakota State Vocational Rehabilitati on, 6003
South Dakota VA Regional Office, 5562
South Dakota Veterans Centers, 5563
South Dakota Workforce Investment Act Training Programs, 6004
Vocational and Rehabilitation Agency: Divi sion of Services to the Blind/Visually Impaired, 6005
Western Resources for dis-ABLED Independence, 4152

Tennessee

Alvin C York VA Medical Center, 5564
American Board of Disability Analysts, 1533
Arc Putnam County, 2820
Arc of Anderson County, 2821
Arc of Davidson County, 2822
Arc of Hamilton County, 2823
Arc of Washington County, 2824
Arc of Williamson County, 2825
Benwood Foundation, 2826
Camp Discovery, 1046
Center for Independent Living of Middle Tennessee, 4153
Community Foundation of Greater Chattanooga, 2827
DisAbility Resource Center: Knoxville, 4154
Division of Rehabilitative Services, 6006
Easter Seals Camp, 1047
Education and Auditory Research Foundation, 2828
Jackson Center for Independent Living, 3931, 4155
Joint Conference with ABMPP Annual Conference, 1551
Memphis Center for Independent Living, 4156
Memphis VA Medical Center, 5565
Montgomery County Arc, 2829
Mountain Home VA Medical Center, 5566
Nasheville Regional Office, 5567
Nashville VA Medical Center, 5568
Tennessee Department of Labor: Job Training Program Liaison, 6007
Tennessee Fair Employment Practice Agency, 6008
Tennessee Library for the Blind and Physically Handicapped, 4619
Tennessee Technology Access Program (TTAP), 4157
The Arc of Tennessee, 2830
Tri-State Resource and Advocacy Corporation, 4158
Vision Foundation, 2569
Winter Conference, 1563

Texas

ABLE Center for Independent Living, 4159
Abell-Hangar Foundation, 2831
Albert & Bessie Mae Kronkosky Charitable Foundation, 2832
Amarillo VA Healthcare System, 5569
Amarillo Vet Center, 5570
American Botanical Council, 737
American Foundation for the Blind: Southwest, 2833
Arch and Stella Rowan Foundation, 2834
Army and Air Force Exchange Services, 2269
Attention Deficit Disorders Association, Southern Region: Annual Conference, 1541
Austin Resource Center for Independent Living, 4160
Austin Resource Center: Round Rock, 4161
Austin Resource Center: San Marcos, 4162
BA and Elinor Steinhagen Benevolent Trust, 2835
Baylor College of Medicine Birth Defects Center, 4620
Baylor College of Medicine: Cullen Eye Institute, 4621
Brain Injury Association of Texas, 767
Brazoria County Center For Independent Living, 4163
Brown Foundation, 2836
Brown-Heatly Library, 4622
Burlington Northern Foundation, 2837
Burnett Foundation, 2838
C-CAD Center of United Cerebral Palsy of Metropolitan Dallas, 6009
CH Foundation, 2839
Camp CAMP, 1048
Camp John Marc, 1049
Camp Summit, 1050
Camp for All, 1051
Center Serving Persons with Mental Retardation, 4164
Center for Research on Women with Disabilities, 4623
Christian Education for the Blind, 4624
Cockrell Foundation, 2840
Communities Foundation of Texas, 2841
Community Foundation of the Metropolitan Tarrant County, 2842
Crockett Resource Center for Independent Living, 4165
Cullen Foundation, 2843
Curtis & Doris K Hankamer Foundation, 2844
Dallas Foundation, 2845
David D & Nona S Payne Foundation, 2846
El Paso Natural Gas Foundation, 2847
El Paso VA Healthcare Center, 5571
Epilepsy Foundation of Greater North Texas, 2848
Epilepsy Foundation of Southeast Texas, 2849
Epilepsy Foundation: Central and South Texas, 2850
Gil and Dody Weaver Foundation, 2851
Handbook of Career Planning for Students with Special Needs, 6010
Harris and Eliza Kempner Fund, 2852
Henry & Tommy Lehmann Charitable Foundation, 2853
Hesta Stuart Christian Charitable Trust, 2854
Hillcrest Foundation, 2855
Hoblitzelle Foundation, 2856
Houston Center for Independent Living, 4166
Houston Endowment, 2857
Houston Public Library: Access Center, 4625
Houston Regional Office, 5572
Houston VA Medical Center, 5573
Independent Life Styles, 4167
Independent Living Research Utilization Project, 4168
John G & Marie S Kennedy Memorial Foundati on, 2858
John S Dunn Research Foundation, 2859
Kent Waldrep National Paralysis Foundation, 2860
LIFE/ Run Centers for Independent Living, 4169
Lisle, 2284
Lola Wright Foundation, 2861
Lowe's Syndrome Association Conference, 1552
Marcia & Otto Koehler Foundation, 2862
Martin Luther Homes of Texas, 4170
Meadows Foundation, 2863
Moody Foundation, 2864
Office for Students with Disabilities, University of Texas at Arlington, 4171
Palestine Resource Center for Independent Living, 4172
Panhandle Action Center for Independent Living Skills, 4173
Pearle Vision Foundation, 2865
REACH of Dallas Resource Center on Independent Living, 4174
REACH of Denton Resource Center on Independent Living, 4175
REACH/Resource Center on Independent Living, 4176
RISE-Resource: Information, Support and Empowerment, 4177
Rockwell Foundation, 2866
SAILS, 4178
San Antonio Area Foundation, 2867
Shell Oil Company Foundation, 2868
South Texas Charitable Foundation, 2869
South Texas Veterans Healthcare System, 5574
Sterling-Turner Foundation, 2870
Swalm Foundation, 2871
TLL Temple Foundation, 2872
Talking Book Program/Texas State Library, 4626
Texas Employment Services and Job Training Program Liaison, 6011
Texas Rehabilitation Commission Independent Living Services, 4179
The Arc of Texas, 2873
University of Texas Southwestern Medical Center/Allergy & Immunology, 4627
University of Texas at Austin Library, 4628
VA North Texas Health Veterans Affairs Car e System: Dallas VA Medical Center, 5575
VOLAR Center for Independent Living, 4180
Vale-Asche Foundation, 2874
Valley Association for Independent Living (VAIL), 4181
Valley Association for Independent Living: Harlingen, 4182
Vocational and Rehabilitation Agency: State Rehabilitation Commission, 6012
Waco Regional Office, 5576
West Texas VA Healthcare System, 5577
William Stamps Farish Fund, 2875

Utah

Active Re-Entry, 4183
Active Re-Entry: Vernal, 4184
Arc of Utah, 2876

Ben B and Iris M Margolis Foundation, 2877
Camp Kostopulos, 1052
Central Utah Independent Living Center, 4185
Family Resource Library/Center for Persons with Disabilities, 4629
Marriner S Eccles Foundation, 2878
OPTIONS for Independence, 4186
OPTIONS for Independence: Brigham Satellit e, 4187
Questar Corporation Contributions Program, 2879
Red Rock Center for Independence, 4188
Red Rock Center for Independence: Fillmore, 4189
Utah Assistive Technology Program (UTAP) Utah State University, 4191
Utah Division of Veterans Affairs, 5578
Utah Employment Services, 6013
Utah Governor's Committee on Employment of the Handicapped, 6014
Utah Independent Living Center, 4192
Utah Independent Living Center: Minersville, 4193
Utah Independent Living Center: Tooele, 4194
Utah State Library Division: Program for the Blind and Disabled, 4630
Utah Veterans Centers, 6015
Utah Vocational Rehabilitation Agency, 6016
VA Salt Lake City Healthcare System, 5579

Vermont

Bennington School Summer Program, 1053
Camp Thorpe, 1054
State of Vermont Department of Aging and Disabilities, 6018
Vermont Assistive Technology Project: Department of Aging & Disabilities, 4195
Vermont Center for Independent Living, 4197
Vermont Center for Independent Living: Bennington, 4198
Vermont Center for Independent Living: Brattleboro, 4196
Vermont Community Foundation, 2880
Vermont Department of Libraries/Special Services Unit, 4631
Vermont Employment Services and Job Training, 6019
Vermont Governor's Committee on Employment of People with Disabilities, 6020
Vermont VA Regional Office Center, 5580
Vermont Veterans Centers, 5581

Virginia

ACS Federal Healthcare, 722
APSE Conference: Revitalizing Supported Employment, Climbing to the Future, 1527
Access Independence, 4199
Alexandria Community Y Head Start, 6022
Alexandria Library Talking Book Service, 4632
American Board of Professional Disability Consultants, 736
American Chiropractic Association, 739
American Counseling Association, 742
American Diabetes Association Annual Conference, 1535
American Diabetes Summer Camp, 1055
American Physical Therapy Association, 1536
American Rehabilitation Counseling Association, 1537
Appalachian Independence Center, 4200
Arc of Virginia, 2881
Arlington County Department of Libraries, 4633
Association for Education & Rehabilitation of the Blind & Visually Impaired Intl Conference, 1540
Association for Persons in Supported Employment, 756
Bell Atlantic Foundation, 2654, 2882
Blue Ridge Independent Living Center, 4202
Blue Ridge Independent Living Center - Troutville, 4201
Blue Ridge Independent Living Center: Christianburg, 4203
Blue Ridge Independent Living Center: Low Moor, 4204
Braille Circulating Library for the Blind, 4634
Brain Injury Association of America, 765
Camp Dickenson, 1056
Camp Easter Seal: East/West, 1057
Camp Foundation, 2883
Camp Holiday Trails, 1058
Camp Virginia Jaycee, 1059
Central Rappahannock Regional Library, 4635
Children and Adolescents with Emotional and Behavioral Disorders, 1545
Civitan Acres, 1060
Clinch Independent Living Services, 4205
Community Foundation of Richmond & Central Virginia, 2884
Council for Exceptional Children, 4636
Council for Exceptional Children Annual Convention and Expo, 1548
Didlake, 6023
Disability Resource Center, 3710, 4206
ENDependence Center of Northern Virginia, 4207
ERIC Clearinghouse on Disabilities and Special Education, 790
Equal Access Center for Independence, 4208
Federal Funding to Fight AIDS, 2929
From the State Capitals: Public Health, 2942
Gannett Foundation, 2885
Guide to Federal Funding for Child Care and Early Childhood Development, 2943
Guide to Federal Funding for Volunteer Programs & Community Service, 2945
Hampton Subregional Library for the Blind, 4637
Hampton VA Medical Center, 5582
Hunter Holmes McGuire VA Medical Center, 5583
Independence Empowerment Center, 4209
Independence Resource Center, 4210
Independent Living Center Network: Department of the Visually Handicapped, 4211
International Chiropractors Association, 815
James Branch Cabell Library, 4638
John Randolph Foundation, 2886
Junction Center for Independent Living, 4212, 4213
Learning Services: Shenandoah, 6024
Loudoun County Special Recreation Programs, 1061
Lynchburg Area Center for Independent Living, 4214
NISH, 6025
National Association of Developmental Disabilities Councils, 834
National Association of State Directors of Developmental Disabilities Services (NASDDDS), 836
National Council on Independent Living, 842, 3686, 4230, 4230
National Maternal and Child Health Bureau, 856
National Mental Health Association, 857
National Rehabilitation Association (NRA), 859
National Vaccine Information Center, 862
Newport News Public Library System, 4639
Norfolk Foundation, 2887
Northern Virginia Resource Center for Deaf and Hard of Hearing Persons, 4640
Peidmont Independent Living Center, 4215
Peninsula Center for Independent Living, 4216
RESNA Annual Conference, 1556
Rehabiliation Engineering Center for Personal Licensed Transportation, 5360
Resources for Independent Living, 3640, 3882, 4217, 4217
Richmond Research Training Center, 6026
Roanoke City Public Library System, 4641
Roanoke Regional Office, 5584
Robey W Estes Family Foundation, 2888
Salem VA Medical Center, 5585
ServiceSource, 6027
Sheltered Occupational Center of Virginia, 6028
Special Services/Talking Books, 4642
Staunton Public Library Talking Book Center, 4643
Technology and Media Division, 891
University of Virginia Health System General Clinical Research Group, 4644
Valley Associates for Independent Living (VAIL), 4218
Valley Associates for Independent Living: Lexington, 4219
Virginia Autism Resource Center, 4645
Virginia Beach Foundation, 2889
Virginia Beach Public Library Special Services Library, 4646
Virginia Chapter of the Arthtitis Foundation, 4647
Virginia Department of Veterans Services, 5586
Virginia State Library for the Visually and Physically Handicapped, 4648
Vocational and Rehabilitation Agency, 5636, 5707, 5722, 5722, 5773, 5779, 5801, 5825, 5859, 5886, 5903, 5908, 5941, 5949, 5961, 5975, 5982
Vocational and Rehabilitation Agency: Department for the Blind/Visually Impaired, 5962, 5991, 5996, 5996, 6030
W Alton Jones Foundation, 2890
Woodrow Wilson Rehabilitation Center Training Program, 4220

Washington

Alliance for People with Disabilities: Sea ttle, 4221
Alliance of People with Disabilities: Redmond, 4222
American Holistic Medical Association, 744
Arc of Washington State, 2891
Bastyr University Natural Health Clinic, 761
Ben B Cheney Foundation, 2892
Camp Killoqua, 1062
Career Connections, 6031
Coalition of Responsible Disabled, 4223
Community Service Center for the Deaf and Hard of Hearing, 4224
Community Services for the Blind and Partially Sighted, 4225
Department of Services for the Blind National Business & Disability Council, 6032
Department of Social & Health Services National Business & Disability Council, 6033
DisAbility Resource Connection: Everett, 4226
Glaser Foundation, 2893
Greater Tacoma Community Foundation, 2894
Greater Wenatchee Community Foundation, 2895
Independent Living Center of SW Washington, 4227
Inland Northwest Community Foundation, 2896
Jonathan M Wainwright Memorial VA Medical Center, 5587
Kitsap Community Resources, 4228
Lilac Blind Foundation, 4229
Medina Foundation, 2897
Meridian Valley Clinical Laboratory, 4649
National Association for Holistic Aromatherapy, 833
Norcliffe Foundation, 2898
Ophthalmic Research Laboratory Eye Institute/First Hill Campus, 4650
Resource Center for the Handicapped, 4231
SL Stuart and Associates, 6034
School of Piano Technology for the Blind, 6035
Seattle Regional Office, 5588
Spokane VA Medical Center, 5589
Stewardship Foundation, 2899
Tacoma Area Coalition of Individuals with Disabilities, 4232
VA Puget Sound Health Care System, 5590
Vocational and Rehabilitation Agency: Division of Vocational Rehabilitation, 5761, 6017, 6036, 6036
Volasuca Volunteers of America, 1063
Washington Talking Book and Braille Library, 4651
Western Washington University, 2296
Weyerhaeuser Company Foundation, 2900

West Virginia

Appalachian Center for Independent Living, 4233
Beckley VA Medical Center, 5591
Bernard McDonough Foundation, 2901
Cabell County Public Library/Talking Book Department/Subregional Library for the Blind, 4652
Division of Rehabilitation Services: Staff Library, 4653
Huntington Regional Office, 5592
Huntington VA Medical Center, 5593
Institute for Scientific Research, 811
Job Accommodation Network, 819
Kanawha County Public Library, 4654
Louis A Johnson VA Medical Center, 5594
Martinsburg VA Medical Center, 5595
Mountain State Center for Independent Living, 4234, 4235
Northern West Virginia Center for Independent Living, 4236
Ohio County Public Library Services for the Blind and Physically Handicapped, 4655
Rehabilitation Technology Association Conference, 1558
Ronald McDonald House, 888
Stepping Stones, 1064
Talking Book Department, Parkersburg and Wood County Public Library, 4656
US Department Veterans Affairs Beckley Vet Center, 5596
West Virginia Autism Training Center, 4657
West Virginia Division of Rehabilitation Services, 6037
West Virginia Employment Services and Job Training Programs Liaison, 6038
West Virginia Hospital Association, 896
West Virginia Library Commission, 4658
West Virginia School for the Blind Library, 4659
West Virginia Vocational Rehabilitation, 6039

Wisconsin

American Academy for Cerebral Palsy and Developmental Medicine Annual Conference, 1529
American Association of Children's Residential Centers, 732
Arc of Dane County, 2902
Arc of Dunn County, 2903
Arc of Eau Claire, 2904
Arc of Outagamie County, 2905
Arc of Racine County, 2906
Arc of Wisconsin Disability Association, 2907
Brown County Library, 4660
Center for Independent Living of Western Wisconsin, 4237
Clement J Zablocki VA Medical Center, 5597
Contemporary Issues in Behavioral Health Care, 1547
Easter Seal Camp Wawbeek, 1065
Eye Institute of the Medical College of Wisconsin and Froedtert Clinic, 4661
Faye McBeath Foundation, 2908
Helen Bader Foundation, 2909
Independence First, 4238
Independence First: West Bend, 4239
Inspiration Ministries, 4240
Johnson Controls Foundation, 2910
Lutherdale Bible Camp, 1066
Lynde and Harry Bradley Foundation, 2911
Mid-state Independent Living Consultants, 4241
Mid-state Independent Living Consultants: Stevens Point, 4242
Milwaukee Foundation, 2912
North Country Independent Living, 4243
North Country Independent Living: Ashland, 4244
Northwestern Mutual Life Foundation, 2913
Options for Independent Living: Fond du Lac, 4245
Patrick and Anna M Cudahy Fund, 2914
SB Waterman & E Blade Charitable Foundation, 2915
Society's Assets: Elkhorn, 4246
Society's Assets: Kenosha, 4247
Society's Assets: Racine, 4248
Tomah VA Medical Center, 5598
Trace Research and Development Center, 4662
Vocational and Rehabilitation: Division of Wisconsin, 6040
William S Middleton Memorial VA Hospital Center, 5599
Wisconsin Badger Camp, 1067
Wisconsin Regional Library for the Blind & Physically Handicapped, 4663
Wisconsin VA Regional Office, 5600
Wisconsin Vocational Rehabilitation Agency, 6041

Wyoming

Arc of Wyoming, 2916
Cheyenne VA Medical Center, 5601
Division of Vocational Rehabilitation of Wyoming, 6042
LifeQuest: Interdisciplinary Rehabilitation, 4249
Rehabilitation Enterprises of North Easter n Wyoming: Newcastle, 4250
Sheridan VA Medical Center, 5602
Vocational Rehabilitation, Division of Department of Workforce Services, 6043
Wyoming Department of Employment Unemployment Insurance, 6044
Wyoming Governor's Committee on Employment of the Handicapped, 6045
Wyoming Institute for Disabilities (WIND), 899
Wyoming Services for Independent Living, 4251
Wyoming Services for the Visually Impaired, 4664
Wyoming Veterans Centers, 5603
Wyoming's New Options in Technology (WYNOT) - University of Wyoming, 4665

AIDS

AID Bulletin, 8305
AIDS 2nd Edition, 8306
AIDS Alert, 8307
AIDS Disease State Management Resource, 8308
AIDS Funding, 2917
AIDS Legal Council of Chicago, 4252
AIDS and Other Manifestations of HIV Infec tion, 8309
AIDS in the Twenty-First Century: Disease and Globalization, 8310
AIDS, What Does it Mean to You?, 8311
AIDS: The HIV Myth, 8312
AIDS: The Official Journal of the Internat ional AIDS Society, 8313
AIDSLAW of Louisiana, 4253
APLA Update, 8314
Beliefs: Pathways to Health and Well Being, 4798
Cancer Immunology Research Foundation, 5211
Children with Disabilities, 4982
Encyclopedia of AIDS: Social, Political, C ultural, and Scientific Record of the HIV Epidemic, 8422
Federal Funding to Fight AIDS, 2929
Guide to Living With HIV Infection: Develo ped at the Johns Hoplins AIDS Clinic, 8439
HIV Drug Book Revised, 8441
HIV Infection and Developmental Disabilities, 2032
Healing HIV: How To Rebuild Your Immune Sy stem, 8446
Health Education AIDS Liason (HEAL), 8140
I Just Found Out I Have HIV... Now What?, 8458
Legislative Network for Nurses, 4328
Levi Strauss Foundation, 2358
Living Well With HIV and AIDS, 8487
Living Well with Chronic Fatigue Syndrome and Fibromyalgia, 8489
Michigan Association for Deaf, and Hard of Hearing, 3210
Moonrise: One Family, Genetic Identity, a nd Muscular Dystrophy, 8506
National AIDS Fund, 8155
National AIDS Hotline, 8656
No Longer Immune: A Counselor's Guide to AIDS, 2092
POZ Magazine, 8541
Penitent, With Poses: An HIV+ Mother Refle cts, 8547
Public Health/State Capitols, 5082
Questions and Answers: The ADA and Persons with HIV/AIDS, 8563
Rights of People Who Are HIV Positive, 8570
The River: A Journey to the Source of HIV and AIDS, 8600
Sight by Touch, 9046
Strength for the Journey, 8286
What's a Virus, Anyway? The Kid's Book About AIDS, 8625
World Without AIDS: The Controvertial Holistic Health, 7539

Accupressure

Acupressure Institute, 725

Aging

Abstracts in Social Gerontology: Current Literature on Aging, 7603
Activities in Action, 7604
Activities with Developmentally Disabled Elderly and Older Adults, 7605
Administration on the Aging, 2969
Adventures in Fast Forward: Life, Love, a nd Work for the ADD Adult, 8320
Aging & Vision News, 7606
Aging Brain, 1925
Aging Eye and Low Vision, 7607
Aging News Alert, 7608
Aging Process: Therapeutic Implications, 7609
Aging Research & Training News, 7610
Aging and Developmental Disability: Current Research, Programming, and Practice, 7611
Aging and Family Therapy: Practitioner Perspectives on Golden Pond, 7612
Aging and Our Families, 7613
Aging and Vision News, 7614
Aging and Vision: Declarations of Independence, 8853
Aging in America, 7559
Aging in Stride, 7615
Aging in the Designed Environment, 7616
Aging with a Disability, 7617
Alabama Association of Homes and Services for the Aging, 7560
Alabama Department of Senior Services, 2993
Alabama VA Regional Office, 5373
Alaska Commission on Aging, 3003
Albany County Department for Aging, 3320
Albany VA Medical Center: Samuel S Stratton, 5506
Aleda E Lutz VA Medical Center, 5467
Alexandria VA Medical Center, 5450
Alive at 25: How I'm Beating Cystic Fibro sis, 8323
Alternative Medicine and Multiple Sclerosis, 8327
Alvin C York VA Medical Center, 5564
Alzheimer's Association, 2469
Alzheimer's Disease Education and Referral Center (ADEAR), 7561
Amarillo VA Healthcare System, 5569
American Association of Homes and Services for the Aging, 7562
Amyotrophic Lateral Sclerosis: A Guide for Patients and Families, 8333
Anchorage Regional Office, 5378
Arizona Association of Homes and Housing for the Aging, 7563
Arizona Division of Aging and Adult Services, 3017
Arkansas Division of Aging & Adult Services, 3026
Asheville VA Medical Center, 5522
Assistive Technology for Older Persons, 7618
Association for International Practical Training, 2270
Association of Ohio Philanthropic Homes and Housing for Aging, 7564
Atlanta Regional Office, 5421
Atlanta VA Medical Center, 5422
Augusta VA Medical Center, 5423
Baltimore Regional Office, 5455
Baltimore VA Medical Center, 5456
Bath VA Medical Center, 5508
Battle Creek VA Medical Center, 5468
Bay Pines VA Medical Center, 5415
Beckley VA Medical Center, 5591
BetaBed Pressure Pad, 253
Biloxi/Gulfport VA Medical Center, 5478
Birmingham VA Medical Center, 5375
Blindness, A Family Matter, 8871
Boise Regional Office, 5428
Boise VA Medical Center, 5429
Boston VA Regional Office, 5461
Bronx VA Medical Center, 5509
Brooklyn Campus of the VA NY Harbor Healthcare System, 5510
Brooklyn Home for Aged Men, 2656
Buffalo Regional Office, 5511
Building Blocks: Foundations for Learning for Young Blind and Visually Impaired Children, 8880
Butler VA Medical Center, 5544
California Association of Homes and Services for the Aging, 7565
California Department of Aging, 3034
California Financial Power of Attorney, 7619
Can America Afford to Grow Old?, 4288
Canandiagua VA Medical Center, 5512
Caring for Alzheimer's Patients, 7620
Caring for Those You Love: A Guide to Compassionate Care for the Aged, 7621
Caring for the Disabled Elderly, 7622
Carl T Hayden VA Medical Center, 5380
Carl Vinson VA Medical Center, 5424
Castle Point Campus of the VA Hudson Valley Healthcare System, 5513
Center for Disability and Elder Law, 4255
Central Alabama Veterans Healthcare System, 5376
Cheyenne VA Medical Center, 5601
Children of Aging Parents, 7567
Chillicothe VA Medical Center, 5530
Choose the Right Long Term Care: Home Care Assisted Living and Nursing Homes, 7623
Chronically Disabled Elderly in Society, 7624
Cincinnati VA Medical Center, 5531
Clement J Zablocki VA Medical Center, 5597
Cleveland Regional Office, 5533
Coatesville VA Medical Center, 5545
Colmery-O'Neil VA Medical Center, 5443
Colorado Association of Homes and Services for the Aging (CAHSA), 7568
Colorado Department of Aging & Adult Servi ces, 3049
Colorado/Wyoming VA Medical Center, 5401
Columbia Regional Office, 5558
Communication Disorders in Aging, 7625
Communication Skills for Working with Elders, 1975
Connecticut Association of Not-for-Profit Providers for the Aging, 7569
Connecticut Commission on Aging, 3058
Coping and Caring: Living with Alzheimer's Disease, 7626
Court-Related Needs of the Elderly and Persons with Disabilities, 4297
DSHS/Aging & Adult Disability Services Administration, 3510
Dayton VA Medical Center, 5534

Delaware VA Regional Office, 5408
Denver VA Medical Center, 5402
Des Moines VA Medical Center, 5438
Des Moines VA Regional Office, 5439
Directory of Self-Help/Mutual Aid Support Groups for Older People, 7627
District of Columbia Office on Aging, 3074
Domestic Mistreatment of the Elderly: Towards Prevention, 7628
Duchenne Muscular Dystrophy, 8417
Durham VA Medical Center, 5524
Dwight D Eisenhower VA Medical Center, 5444
Early Story of Alzheimer's Disease, 7629
East Orange Campus of the VA New Jersey Healthcare System, 5501
Edith Nourse Rogers Memorial Veterans Hospital, 5462
Edward Hines Jr Hospital, 5430
El Paso VA Healthcare Center, 5571
Elder Abuse, 7630
Elder Care, 7631
ElderLawAnswers.com, 4307
Employment for Individuals with Asperger S yndrome or Non-Verbal Learning Disability, 8709
Enabling News, 7632
Erie VA Medical Center, 5546
Eugene J Towbin Healthcare Center, 5383
Exercise Activities for the Elderly, 7633
Exercise and the Older Adult, 7634
Explore Your Options, 7635
Facilitating Self-Care Practices in the Elderly, 2023
Falling in Old Age, 7636
Family Intervention Guide To Mental Illness, 7637
Fargo VA Medical Center, 5528
Fayetteville VA Medical Center, 5384, 5525
Films & Videos on Aging and Sensory Change, 5159
Florida Adult Services, 3088
Fort Howard VA Medical Center, 5457
Functional Fitness Assessment for Adults, 7638
Gainesville Division, North Florida/South Georgia Veterans Healthcare System, 5416
Georgia Association of Homes and Services for the Aging, 7570
Georgia Department of Aging, 3103
Get Ready/Get Set/Go for the Code, 1629
Golf Xpress, 530
Grand Island VA Medical System, 5489
Grand Junction VA Medical Center, 5403
Hampton VA Medical Center, 5582
Handbook of Assistive Devices for the Handicapped Elderly, 7639
Handbook on Ethnicity, Aging and Mental Health, 7640
Harry S Truman Memorial Veterans' Hospital, 5480
Hartford Regional Office, 5404
Hawaii Executive Office on Aging, 3120
Head Injury: The Facts: A Guide for Fami lies and Care-Givers, 8444
Health Care of the Aged, 7641
Health Promotion and Disease Prevention, 7642
Highlighter and Note Tape, 595
Honolulu VBA Regional Office, 5426
Houston Regional Office, 5572
Houston VA Medical Center, 5573
Hunter Holmes McGuire VA Medical Center, 5583
Huntington Regional Office, 5592
Huntington VA Medical Center, 5593
Idaho Commission on Aging, 3125
Illinois Department on Aging, 3138
Increasing and Decreasing Behaviors of Persons with Severe Retardation and Autism, 1763
Independent Living Matters, 4731
Independent Living Office, 4875
Indiana Association of Homes for the Aging, 7571
Indianapolis Regional Office, 5434
Insurance Solutions: Plan Well, Live Better, 4879
International Health Guide for Senior Citizen Travelers, 7643
Interstitial Cystitis Association, 5232
Iowa Association of Homes and Services for the Aging, 7572
Iowa City VA Medical Center, 5440
Iowa Department of Elder Affairs, 3153
Iron Mountain VA Medical Center, 5469
Jackson Regional Office, 5479
James A Haley VA Medical Center, 5417
James E Van Zandt VA Medical Center, 5547
Jerry L Pettis Memorial VA Medical Center, 5387
John D Dingell VA Medical Center, 5470
John J Pershing VA Medical Center, 5481
John L McClellan Memorial Hospital, 5385
Jonathan M Wainwright Memorial VA Medical Center, 5587
Kansas Association of Homes for the Aging, 7573
Kansas City VA Medical Center, 5482
Kansas Department on Aging, 3163
Kansas VA Regional Office, 5445
Kentucky Association of Not-for-Profit Homes and Services for the Aging, 7574
Kentucky Office of Aging Services, 3169
Knoxville VA Medical Center, 5441
Lebanon VA Medical Center, 5548
Legal Center, 4263, 4325
Legal Center for the Elderly and Disabled, 4264
Lexington VA Medical Center, 5447
Life Planning for Adults with Developmental Disabilities, 7644
Life Service Network of Illinois: Springfi eld, 7575
Life Services Network of Illinois, 7576
Lighthouse International, 8785
Lincoln Regional Office, 5490
Lincoln VA Medical Center, 5491
Long Beach VA Medical Center, 5388
Los Angeles Regional Office, 5389
Louis A Johnson VA Medical Center, 5594
Louis Stokes VA Medical Center, 5535
Louisiana Association of Homes and Service for the Aging, 7577
Louisiana Department of Aging, 3176
Louisville VA Medical Center, 5448
Louisville VA Regional Office, 5449
Lyons Campus of the VA New Jersey Healthcare System, 5502
Maine VA Regional Office, 5453
Making Wise Decisions for Long-Term Care, 4904
Managing Aging and Human Services Agencies, 7645
Managing the Symptoms of Multiple Sclerosis, 8500
Manchester Regional Office, 5497
Manchester VA Medical Center, 5498
Marion VA Medical Center, 5431
Martinez Center for Rehab & Extended Care, 5390
Martinsburg VA Medical Center, 5595
Maryland Department of Aging, 3194
Massachusetts Aging Services Association, 7578
Mastering the Medicare Maze, 7646
MedEscort International, 5315
Medicare Information, 8655
Medicare Maximization, 7647
Meeting the Challenge of Progressive Multiple Sclerosis, 8502
Memphis VA Medical Center, 5565
Mentally Impaired Elderly: Strategies and Interventions to Maintain Function, 7648
Miami VA Medical Center, 5418
Michigan Association of Homes and Serivces for the Aging, 7579
Michigan Office of Services to the Aging, 3224
Michigan Psychological Association, 1739
Michigan VA Regional Office, 5471
Mid-Atlantic LifeSpan, 7580
Miles Away and Still Caring: A Guide for Long Distance Caregivers, 4690
Minneapolis VA Medical Center, 5474
Minnesota Board on Aging, 3232
Minnesota Health and Housing Alliance, 7581
Mirrored Lives: Aging Children and Elderly Parents, 7649
Mississippi Association of Homes and Services for the Aging, 7582
Mississippi Division of Aging and Adult Services, 3247
Missouri Association of Homes for the Aging, 7583
Montana Department of Aging, 3261
Mountain Home VA Medical Center, 5566
Multiple Sclerosis: The Guide to Treatmen t and Management, 8509
Muscular Dystrophies, 8512
Muscular Dystrophy in Children: A Guide fo r Families, 8514
Muscular Dystrophy: The Facts, 8515
Muskogee VA Medical Center, 5536
Nasheville Regional Office, 5567
Nashville VA Medical Center, 5568
National Council on the Aging Conference, 1553
National Guide to Funding in Aging, 2958
National Organization of the Senior Blind, 7584
National Voluntary Organizations for Independent Living for the Aging, 7585
Nebraska Association of Homes for the Aging, 7586
Nebraska Department of Health and Human Services, Division of Aging Services, 3271
Nevada Division for Aging: Carson City, 3281
Nevada Division for Aging: Las Vegas, 3282

New Hampshire Division of Elderly and Adult Services, 3294
New Jersey Association of Nonprofit Homes for the Aging, 7587
New Jersey Department of Aging, 3302
New Mexico Aging and Long-Term Services Department, 3309
New Mexico VA Healthcare System, 5504
New Orleans VA Medical Center, 5451
New York Association of Homes and Services for the Aging, 7588
New York City Campus of the VA NY Harbor Healthcare System, 5514
New York Regional Office, 5515
Newark Regional Office, 5503
North Carolina Association of Nonprofits for the Aging, 7589
North Carolina Division of Aging, 3359
North Chicago VA Medical Center, 5432
North Dakota Department of Aging, 3365
North Dakota VA Regional Office, 5529
North Little Rock Regional Office, 5386
Northampton VA Medical Center, 5463
Northern Arizona VA Health Center, 5381
Northern New England Association of Homes and Services for the Aging, 7590
Northport VA Medical Center, 5516
Not Without Sight, 9002
Now Where Did I Put My Keys?, 7650
Oakland VA Regional Office, 5391
Ohio Department of Aging, 3375
Oklahoma Association of Homes and Services for the Aging, 7591
Oklahoma City VA Medical Center, 5537
Oklahoma Department of Human Services Aging Services Division, 3386
Older Adults with Developmental Disabilities: Optimizing Choice and Change, 7651
On Your Behalf, 7652
Operation Help: A Mental Health Advocate Guide to Medicaid, 7653
Oregon Association of Homes for the Aging, 7592
Oxford Textbook of Geriatric Medicine, 2096
PSP Advocate, 8542
Pacific Islands Health Care System, 5427
Part B News, 7654
Passion for Justice, 4927
Pennsylvania Association of Nonprofit Homes for the Aging, 7593
Pennsylvania Department of Aging, 3404
Perry Point VA Medical Center, 5459
Perspective on Aging, 7655
Perspectives on Prevention and Treatment of Cancer in the Elderly, 7656
Philadelphia Regional Office and Insurance Center, 5550
Philadelphia VA Medical Center, 5551
Physical & Occupational Therapy in Geriatrics...Current Trends in Geriatrics Rehab, 7657
Pittsburgh Regional Office, 5552
Portland Regional Office, 5540
Portland VA Medical Center, 5541
Practicing Rehabilitation with Geriatric Clients, 2110
Prescriptions for Independence, 7658
Providence Regional Office, 5556
Providence VA Medical Center, 5557
Quality Health Care Foundation of Wyoming, 7594
Ralph H Johnson VA Medical Center, 5559
Recreation Activities for the Elderly, 2122
Rehabilitation Interventions for the Institutionalized Elderly, 2125
Rehabilitation Research and Development Center, 5392
Rehabilitation in the Aging, 7659
Reno Regional Office, 5494
Retirement Research Foundation, 2507
Rhode Island Association of Facilities for the Aging, 7595
Rhode Island Department of Elderly Affairs, 3413
Richard L Roudebush VA Medical Center, 5435
Roanoke Regional Office, 5584
Robert J Dole VA Medical Center, 5446
Role Portrayal and Stereotyping on Television, 4949
Roseburg VA Medical Center, 5542
Sacramento Medical Center, 5393
Salem VA Medical Center, 5585
San Diego VA Regional Office, 5394
San Francisco VA Medical Center, 5395
Seattle Regional Office, 5588
Senior Citizens and the Law, 7596, 7660
Sheridan VA Medical Center, 5602
Shiloh Senior Citizens Center, 7597
Shreveport VA Medical Center, 5452
Sioux Falls VA Medical Center, 5561
Sister Cities International, 2290
So Many of My Friends Have Moved Away or Died, 7661
Social Security Bulletin, 7662
Social Security, Medicare, and Pensions, 7663
South Carolina Association of Nonprofit Homes for the Aging, 7598
South Carolina Services Information System, 3431
South Dakota Department of Aging, 3434
South Dakota VA Regional Office, 5562
South Texas Veterans Healthcare System, 5574
Southern Arizona VA Healthcare System, 5382
Spokane VA Medical Center, 5589
St. Cloud VA Medical Center, 5475
St. Louis Regional Office, 5483
St. Louis VA Medical Center, 5484
St. Paul Regional Office, 5476
St. Petersburg Regional Office, 5419
State of Vermont Department of Aging and Disabilities, 6018
Strategies for Teaching Students with Learning and Behavior Problems, 2147
Successful Models of Community Long Term Care Services for the Elderly, 7664
Syracuse VA Medical Center, 5517
Teaching Special Students in Mainstream, 1764
Tennessee Association of Homes for the Aging, 7599
Tennessee Commission on Aging and Disability, 3444
Texas Association of Homes and Services for the Aging, 7600
Texas Department on Aging, 3469
Therapeutic Interventions in Alzheimer's, 7665
Three Hundred Tips for Making Life with Multiple Sclerosis Easier, 8603
Togus VA Medical Center, 5454
Tomah VA Medical Center, 5598
Topics in Geriatric Rehabilitation, 7666
Tourette Syndrome: The Facts, 8607
Tuscaloosa VA Medical Center, 5377
US Department of Veterans Affairs National Headquarters, 5371
US Servas, 5324
Unloving Care, 7667
Utah Department of Aging, 3482
Utah Division of Veterans Affairs, 5578
V A Montana Healthcare System, 5486
VA Ann Arbor Healthcare System, 5472
VA Boston Healthcare System: Brockton Division, 5464
VA Boston Healthcare System: Jamaica Plain Campus, 5465
VA Boston Healthcare System: West Roxbury Division, 5466
VA Central California Health Care Syste, 5396
VA Connecticut Healthcare System: Newington Division, 5406
VA Connecticut Healthcare System: West Haven, 5407
VA Greater Los Angeles Healthcare System, 5397
VA Illiana Health Care System, 5433
VA Montana Healthcare System, 5487
VA Nebraska-Western Iowa Health Care System, 5492
VA North Indiana Health Care System: Fort Wayne Campus, 5436
VA Northern California Healthcare System, 5398
VA Northern Indiana Health Care System: Marion Campus, 5437
VA Pittsburgh Healthcare System, Highland Drive Division, 5554
VA Pittsburgh Healthcare System, University Drive Division, 5553
VA Puget Sound Health Care System, 5590
VA Salt Lake City Healthcare System, 5579
VA San Diego Healthcare System, 5399
VA Sierra Nevada Healthcare System, 5495
VA Southern Nevada Healthcare System, 5496
VA Western NY Healthcare System, Batavia, 5520
VA Western NY Healthcare System, Buffalo, 5521
Vermont Department of Disabilities, Aging and Independent Living, 3495
Vermont VA Regional Office Center, 5580
Vision and Aging: Issues in Social Work Practice, 7669
Visiting Nurse Association of America, 8673
Visually Impaired Seniors as Senior Companions: A Reference Guide, 7670
WG Hefner VA Medical Center, 5526
Waco Regional Office, 5576
Washington Association of Housing and Services for the Aging, 7601
Washington County Disability, Aging and Veteran Services, 3398
Washington DC VA Medical Center, 5414
We Can Do it Together!, 9081

West Palm Beach VA Medical Center, 5420
West Texas VA Healthcare System, 5577
West Virginia Department of Aging, 3527
West Virginia Hospital Association, 896
White City VA Domiciliary, 5543
Wilkes-Barre VA Medical Center, 5555
William Jennings Bryan Dorn VA Medical Center, 5560
William S Middleton Memorial VA Hospital Center, 5599
Wilmington VA Medical, 5409
Winston-Salem Regional Office, 5527
Wisconsin Association of Homes & Services for the Aging, 7602
Wisconsin Bureau of Aging, 3536
Wisconsin VA Regional Office, 5600
Work Exploration Center, 5762
Work, Health and Income Among the Elderly, 7671
Wyoming Department of Aging, 3545
Wyoming/Colorado VA Regional Office, 5604

Alternative Therapies

Academy for Guided Imagery, 2251
American Academy of Osteopathy, 8127
American Association of Oriental Medicine, 733
American Board of Chelation Therapy, 735
American College of Advancement in Medicine, 740
American College of Nurse Midwives, 741
American Council for Headache Education (ACHE), 1724
American Herb Association Newsletter, 4783
American Holistic Medical Association, 744
American Social Health Association, 8132
American Society for the Alexander Techniq ue, 751
American Society of Clinical Hypnosis, 753
American Society of Teachers of the Alexander Technique, 754
Aromatherapy Book: Applications and Inhalations, 4789
Aromatherapy for Common Ailments, 4790
Association for Applied Psychophysiology and Biofeedback, 755
Association on Higher Education and Disability, 1726
Ayurvedic Institute, 2255
Bach Flower Therapy: Theory and Practice, 4796
Bastyr University Natural Health Clinic, 761
Beliefs, Values, and Principles of Self Advocacy, 4797
Brain Allergies: The Psychonutrient, 8358
California State Oriental Medical Association (CSOMA), 770
Center for Mind/Body Studies, 776
Chinese Herbal Medicine, 4814
Chronic Fatigue Syndrome: Your Natural Gu ide To Healing with Diet, Herbs and Other Methods, 8383
College of Maharishi Vedic Medicine Health Center, 783
Colon Health: Key to a Vibrant Life, 8389
Coping with Mild Traumatic Brain Surgery, 8401
Creating Wholeness: Self-Healing Workbook Using Dynamic Relaxation, Images and Thoughts, 4824
Curing MS: How Science is Solving the Mys teries of Multiple Sclerosis, 8406
Designing and Using Assistive Technology: The Human Perspective, 1988
Detecting Your Hidden Allergies, 8410
Divided Legacy: A History of the Schism in Medical Thought, The Bacteriological Era, 2000
Edge Effect: Achieve Total Health and Long evity with the Balanced Brain Advantage, 4841
Environmental Health Center: Dallas, 8137
Esalen Institute, 793
Everybody's Guide to Homeopathic Medicines, 4844
Fall Down, Laughing: How Squiggy Caught M ultiple Sclerosis and Didn't Tell Nobody, 8427
Feldenkrais Guild of North America (FGNA), 801
Fosters Botanical and Herb Reviews, 4849
Foundation for the Advancement of Innovative Medicine, 2679
Handbook of Chronic Fatigue Syndrome, 8442
Headache Newsletter, 8445
Healing Herbs, 4859
Health Action, 806
Heart of the Mind, 8450
Herb Research Foundation, 5229
Homeopathic Educational Services, 808
Human Ecology Action League (HEAL), 809
Imagery in Healing Shamanism and Modern Medicine, 4870
Informed Touch, 8464
Institute of Transpersonal Psychology, 812
International Association of Parents and Professionals for Safe Alternatives in Childbirth, 1733
International Association of Professional Natural Hygientists, 8145
International Association of Yoga Therapists, 814
International Bio-Oxidative Medicine Foundation (IBOM), 2767
International Childbirth Education Association, 1734
International Clinic of Biological Regeneration, 816
International College of Applied Kinesiology, 817
International Ozone Association, 8147
It's All in Your Head, 8471
Living Beyond Multiple Sclerosis: A Woman 's Guide, 8486
Living an Idea: Empowerment and the Evolution of an Alternative School, 1657
Long Beach Department of Health and Human Services, 3042
Los Angeles County Department of Health Services, 3043
Lupus: Alternative Therapies That Work, 8494
Maharishi Ayur-Veda Medical Center, 825
Medical Herbalism, 5126
Menopause without Medicine, 8504
Mind-Body Clinic, 829
Mind/Body Health Services, 830
Myotherapy, 8997
National Association for Holistic Aromatherapy, 833
National Association to Advance Fat Acceptance, 8157
National Center for Homeopathy, 1742
National College of Naturopathic Medicine, 840
National Guild of Hypnotists, 853
National Headache Foundation, 2501
National Vaccine Information Center, 862
Nothing is Impossible: Reflections on a N ew Life, 4918
Nurse Healers: Professional Associates International, 868
Nutritional Desk Reference, 4919
Nutritional Influences on Illness:, 4920
Optometric Extension Program Foundation, 2364
PACER Center (Parent Advocacy Coalition for Educational Rights), 870
Pacific Institute of Aromatherapy, 872
Pain Erasure, 5003
Pocket Guide to the ADA: Accessibility Gu idelines for Buildings and Facilities, 4272
Portland Naturopathic Clinic: NCNM National Health Centers Eastside Clinic, 882
Quan Yin Healing Arts Center, 883
Rolf Institute, 887
Scientific Health Solutions, 8172
Small Wonder, 1691
Solving the Puzzle of Chronic Fatigue, 8581
Tourette's Syndrome - Tics, Obsessions, Co mpulsions: Developmental Psychopathology, 8608
Trager International, 893
Upledger Institute, 895
Weiner's Herbal, 4968

Amputation

American Amputee Foundation, 7545
Breaking New Ground Resource Center, 8636
Functional Restoration of Adults and Child ren with Upper Extremity Amputation, 7554
National Amputation Foundation, 7549
Rajesh, 8059
Single-Handed: A Book for Persons with the Use of Only One Hand, 7556
With Standing Ovation, 8072

Amythrophic Lateral Sclerosis

Amytrophic Lateral Sclerosis Association, 7950
Les Turne Amyotrophic Laterial Sclerosis Foundation, 2494

Art & Music Therapies

Academy of Dentistry for Persons with Disabilities, 8124
American Art Therapy Association (AATA), 1
American Association of Music Therapy, 2
Art Therapy SourceBook, 7

Art and Disabilities, 8
Art and Healing: Using Expressive Art to Heal Your Body, Mind, and Soul, 9
Art for All the Children: Approaches to Art Therapy for Children with Disabilities, 10
Art-Centered Education and Therapy for Children with Disabilities, 1932
Clinical Applications of Music Therapy in Developmental Disability, Pediatrics and Neurology, 11
Contemporary Art Therapy with Adolescents, 12
Creative Arts Resources Catalog, 13
Creative Arts Therapy Catalogs, 1618
Dancing from the Inside Out, 14
Facts: Music for Blind and Physically Handicapped Individuals, 16
Freedom to Create, 17
Friends-In-Art, 18
Guide to the Selection of Musical Instruments, 19
In-Definite Arts Society, 20
Institute for Therapy Throughout the Arts, 21
Instrumental Music for Dyslexics: A Teach ing Handbook, 22
International Journal of Arts Medicine, 2058
Kaleidoscope: Exploring the Experience of Disability Through Literature & the Fine Arts, 23
Mad Hatters: Theatre That Makes a World of Difference, 2260
Manual of Sequential Art Activities for Classified Children and Adolescents, 24
Mozart Effect: Tapping the Power of Music to Heal the Body, Strengthen the Mind, 25
Music Therapy, 26
Music Therapy and Leisure for Persons with Disabilities, 27
Music Therapy for the Developmentally Disabled, 28
Music Therapy in Dementia Care, 29
Music Therapy, Sensory Integration and the Autistic Child, 30
Music and Dyslexia: Opening New Doors, 31
Music for the Hearing Impaired, 32
Music: Physician for Times to Come, 33
National Arts and Disability Center (NADC), 34
National Endowment for the Arts: Office for AccessAbility, 36
National Federation of the Blind: Music Division, 37
New Music Therapist's Handbook, 40
Open Road, 42, 5318
Pied Piper: Musical Activities to Develop Basic Skills, 43
Special Care in Dentistry, 8583
Start with the Arts, 45
Teaching Basic Guitar Skills to Special Learners, 46
VSA Arts, 48
We Are PHAMALY, 49

Arthritis

AJAO Newsletter, 7988
Alerter, 7989
American College of Rheumatology Research and Education Foundation, 5196
American Juvenile Arthritis Organization (AJAO), 7946
Ankylosing Spondylitis, 8334
Arthritis 101: Questions You Have Answers You Need, 7990
Arthritis Accent, 7991
Arthritis Answers: Basic Information About Arthritis, 7992
Arthritis Bible, 7993
Arthritis Consulting Services, 7951
Arthritis Foundation, 7952
Arthritis Foundation Information Hotline, 8122
Arthritis Foundation of Illinois News, 7994
Arthritis Foundation: Greater Southwest Chapter, 7995
Arthritis Helpbook, 7996
Arthritis Helpbook: A Tested Self-Management Program for Coping, 7997
Arthritis Information: Children, 7998
Arthritis News, 7999
Arthritis Observer, 8000
Arthritis Relief at Your Fingertips, 8001
Arthritis Reporter, 8002
Arthritis Self Help Products, 8003
Arthritis Self-Help Book, 8004
Arthritis Today, 8005
Arthritis and Diet, 8006
Arthritis and Employment: You Can Get the Job You Want, 8007
Arthritis and Pregnancy, 8008
Arthritis in Children, 8009
Arthritis in Children and La Artritis Infantojuvenil, 5108
Arthritis in Children: Resources for Children, Parents and Teachers, 8010
Arthritis on the Job: You Can Work with It, 8011
Arthritis, Rheumatic Diseases and Related Disorders, 8012
Arthritis: A Comprehensive Guide, 8013
Arthritis: Do You Know?, 8014
Arthritis: Stop Suffering, Start Moving, 8015
Arthritis: Taking Care of Yourself Health Guide for Understanding Your Arthritis, 8016
Arthritis: What Exercises Work, 8017
Arthritis: Your Complete Exercise Guide, 8018
Away with Arthritis, 8019
Big Lamp Switch, 483
Body Reflexology: Healing at Your Fingertips, 4800
Bone Up on Arthritis, 8021
Bursitis, Tendonitis and Other Soft Tissue Rheumatic Syndromes, 8023
Camp Esperanza Arthritis Foundation, 7978
Card Holder Deluxe, 5275
Challenge Golf, 8084, 9090
Checker Set: Deluxe, 5278
Child With Special Needs: Encouraging Inte llectual and Emotional Growth, 4813
Clinical Care in Rheumatic Disease, 8385
Diet and Arthritis, 8025
Exercise and Your Arthritis, 8027
Freedom from Arthritis Through Nutrition & Help for Allergies, 8030
Help Yourself Cookbook, 8451
How to Deal with Back Pain and Rheumatoid Joint Pain, 8034
In Control, 8036
Individuals with Arthritis, 5122, 8037
JRA and Me, 8039
Kids on the Block Arthritis Programs, 8123
Living with Rheumatoid Arthritis, 8043
Managing Your Activities, 4907
Managing Your Fatigue, 8045
Managing Your Health Care, 4908
Managing Your Pain, 8046
Myositis, 8517
National Institute of Arthritis and Musculoskeletal and Skin Diseases, 7963
Osteoarthritis, 8050
Overcoming Rheumatoid Arthritis, 8051
PACE II, 8052
Pathways to Better Living, 8055
Polymyalgia Rheumatica and Giant Cell Arthritis, 8553
Primer on the Rheumatic Diseases, 8056
Psoriatic Arthritis, 8058
Raynaud's Phenomenon, 8565
Reiter's Syndrome, 8568
Rheumatoid Arthritis, 8060
Source of Help and Hope Newsletter, 8061
Thinking About Tomorrow: A Career Guide for Teens with Arthritis, 8064
Thumbs Up Cup, 365
Two Hundred Fifty Tips for Making Life with Arthritis Easier, 8065
Understanding Juvenile Rheumatoid Arthritis, 8066
When Your Student Has Arthritis: A Guide for Teachers, 8071

Asthma

AAN's Toll-Free Hotline, 8634
ABC of Asthma, Allergies & Lupus, 8302
ABC's of Latex Allergy, 8303
AH! Asthma Camp, 8183
About Asthma, 8315
Allergy and Asthma Network Mothers of Asth matics, 5037
American Academy of Allergy, Asthma and Immunology, 8328
American Academy of Pediatrics Guide to Yo ur Child's Alleriges And Asthma, 8329
Ask the Doctor: Asthma, 8338
Asthma & Allergy Education for Worksite Clinicians, 2252
Asthma & Allergy Essentials for Children's Care Provider, 2253
Asthma Action Cards: Child Care Asthma/Allergy Action Card, 1601
Asthma Action Cards: Student Asthma Action Card, 1602
Asthma Alert, 8340
Asthma Care Training for Kids (ACT), 2254
Asthma Challenge, 8341
Asthma Handbook, 8342
Asthma Handbook Slides, 8343
Asthma Lifelines, 8344
Asthma Management and Education, 1942
Asthma Resource Directory, 8345
Asthma Sourcebook, 8346

Asthma and Allergy Answers: A Patient Education Library, 8347
Asthma and Allergy Foundation of America, 5206
Asthma and Exercise, 8348
Asthma in the School: Improving Control with Peak Flow Monitoring, 8349
Asthma in the Workplace, 8350
Breathe Easy Young People's Guide to Asthma, 8362
Bronchial Asthma: Principles of Diagnosis and Treatment, 8365
Camp Not-A-Wheeze American Lung Association, 8235
Camp Vacamas, 8247
Camp Wheezeaway American Lung Association of Alabama, 8249
Childhood Asthma: A Matter of Control, 8372
Children with Asthma: A Manual for Parents, 8378
Complete Kid's Allergy and Asthma Guide: T he Parent's Handbook for Children of All Ages, 8391
Control Your Child's Asthma, 8395
Controlling Asthma, 8396
Coping with Asthma, 8399
Determined to Win: Children Living with Allergies and Asthma, 8412
Efficacy of Asthma Education, Selected Abstracts, 8421
Facts About Asthma, 8426
Free to Breathe, 8433
Helping Others Breathe Easier, 8452
Home Control of Allergies and Asthma, 8454
How to Outsmart Your Allergies, 8456
Let's Talk About Having Asthma, 8482
Living Well with Asthma, 8488
Living with Asthma and Allergies Brochure Series, 8490
MA Report, 1893
Many Faces of Asthma, 8501
Meeting-in-a-Box, 1668
My House Is Killing Me! The Home Guide for Families With Allergies and Asthma, 8516
Nocturnal Asthma, 8523
Parent's Guide to Allergies and Asthma, 8544
Pharmacologic Therapy of Pediatric Asthma, 8550
Power Breathing Program, 1677
Regular Kid, 8567
Standards for the Diagnosis and Care of Patients with Asthma, 8590
Teens Talk to Teens about Asthma, 8596
There are Solutions for the Student with Asthma, 8601
Toll-Free Information Line, 8672
Understanding Asthma, 8613
Understanding Asthma: The Blueprint for Breathing, 8614
What Everyone Needs to Know About Asthma, 8622
What School Personnel Should Know About Asthma, 8623
What Your Doctor May Not Tell You About Ch ildren's Allergies and Asthma, 8624
Your Child and Asthma, 8629

Attention Deficit Disorder

ADD Challenge: A Practical Guide for Teachers, 1912
ADD, Stepping Out of the Dark, 7364
ADD: Helping Your Child, 7367
ADHD Report, 7370
ADHD in Adults, 7371
ADHD in the Classroom: Strategies for Teachers, 1913
ADHD with Comorbid Disorders: Clinical Assessment and Management, 7373
ADHD: Handbook for Diagnosis & Treatment, 7374
ADHD: What Do We Know?, 7376
ALST: Adolescent Language Screening Test, 2196
ASHA Leader, 7758, 8691
About Attention Disorder, 7377
Adapted Physical Education for Students with Autism, 1919
Adventure Learning Center at Eagle Village, 7310
All About Attention Deficit Disorders, Revised, 5141, 7380
Around the Clock: Parenting the Delayed AD HD Child, 7385
Attention, 7386
Attention Deficit Disorder, 7387
Attention Deficit Disorder in Adults Workbook, 7389
Attention Deficit Disorder in Children and Adolescents, 1944
Attention Deficit Disorder: A Different Perception, 7390
Attention Deficit Disorder: Adults, 7391
Attention Deficit Disorder: Children, 7392
Attention Deficit Disorders Association, Southern Region: Annual Conference, 1541
Attention Deficit Disorders: Assessment & Teaching, 7393
Attention-Deficit Hyperactivity Disorder: Symptoms and Suggestons for Treatment, 7394
Attention-Deficit/Hyperactivity Disorder, What Every Parent Wants to Know, 7395
Braille Book Bank, Music Catalog, 8874
Burnish Me Bright, 8700
Camp Betsey Cox, 7313
Camp Buckskin, 7314
Camp Kaleidoscope, 7317
Camp Northwood, 7319
Camp Ruggles, 7323
Camp World Light, 7325
Casowasco Camp, Conference and Retreat Center, 7328
Chadder, 7421
Clinical Connection, 1846
Clinical Management of Childhood Stuttering, 2nd Edition, 1968
Clinician's Practical Guide to Attention-Deficit/Hyperactivity Disorder, 5068
Cogrehab, 7426
Communication & Language Acquisition: Discoveries from Atypical Development, 1974
Community Signs, 1616
Comprehensive Assessment of Spoken Language (CASL), 1617
Comprehensive Guide to ADD in Adults: Research, Diagnosis & Treatment, 7430
Concentration Cockpit: Explaining Attention Deficits, 7431
Coping for Kids Who Stutter, 8707
Coping with ADD/ADHD, 7433
Counseling Persons with Communication Disorders and Their Families, 1981
Development of Language, 1992
Disorders of Motor Speech: Assessment, Treatment, and Clinical Characterization, 8708
Driven to Distraction, 7440
Educating Inattentive Children, 7442
Englishton Park Academic Remediation, 7335
Fact Sheet: Attention Deficit-Hyperactivit y Disorder, 7447
Family Therapy for ADHD: Treating Children , Adolescents and Adults, 7449
Florida Sheriffs Caruth Camp, 7336
Focus Newsletter, 8430
GO-MO Articulation Cards- Second Edition, 1628
Getting a Grip on ADD: A Kid's Guide to Understanding & Coping with ADD, 7456
Gillingham Manaual, 1630
Handbook for Speech Therapy, 2034
Helping Your Hyperactive: Attention Deficit Child, 7461
How to Own and Operate an Attention Deficit Disorder, 7464
Hyperactive Child, Adolescent, and Adult: ADD Through the Lifespan, 7465
Hyperactivity, Attention Deficits, and School Failure: Better Ways, 7466
If Your Child Stutters: A Guide for Parents, 8715
Indian Acres Camp for Boys, 7339
Is the Child Really Stuttering? Questions & Answers About Disfluency, 8716
It's Just Attention Disorder, 7472
Jumpin' Johnny Get Back to Work, A Child's Guide to ADHD/Hyperactivity, 7474
K-SEALS: Kaufman Survey of Early Academic and Language Skills, 2215
KLST-2: Kindergarten Language Screening Test Edition, 2nd Edition, 2216
Lollipop Lunch, 8723
Loudoun County Special Recreation Programs, 1061
Management of Children and Adolescents with AD-HD, 7484
Managing Attention Disorders in Children: A Guide for Practitioners, 7485
Maplebrook School, 7342
Model Program Operation Manual: Business Enterprise Program Supervisors, 8992
New Jersey YMHA/YWHA Camps Milford, 7344
Out of the Corner of My Eye, 9007
Outside in School, 7346
Parenting Attention Deficit Disordered Teens, 7499
Parenting Preschoolers: Suggestions for Raising Young Blind Children, 9011
Parents Helping Parents: A Directory of Support Groups for ADD, 7500
Readings on Research in Stuttering, 2121

Reference Manual for Communicative Sciences and Disorders, 2123
Rethinking Attention Deficit Disorder, 7509
Rolling Hills Country Day Camp, 7351
Rose-Colored Glasses, 9032
School Based Assessment of Attention Deficit Disorders, 7511
Seeing-Children Living with Blindness, 9040
Sharing Solutions: A Newsletter for Support Groups, 9044
Slingerland Screening Tests, 2235
Solving Language Difficulties: Remedial Routines, 1692
Speech Bin, 1695, 2237
Speech-Language Pathology and Audiology: An Introduction, 2144
Stuttering, 8733
Stuttering & Your Child: A Videotape for Parents, 8734
Stuttering Foundation of America, 8681
Stuttering Severity Instrument for Children and Adults, 2238
Summit Camp, 7356
Survey of Direct Labor Workers Who Are Blind & Employed by NIB, 9057
Taking Charge of ADHD Complete Authoritative Guide for Parents, 7520
Teach and Reach Students with Attention Deficit Disorders, 7521
Teenagers with ADD, 7525
Triangle Y Ranch YMCA, 7361
Trouble with Explosives, 8737
Understanding ADHD, 7528
Understanding Attention Deficit Disorder, 7529
Why Won't My Child Pay Attention?, 7536
Women with Attention Deficit Disorder: Embracing Disorganization at Home and Work, 7538
You Seem Like a Regular Kid to Me, 9086
You and Your ADD Child, 7541

Autism

ARRISE, 7292
Activities for Developing Pre-Skill Concepts In Children with Autism, 1799
Autism, 5142, 7397
Autism Handbook: Understanding & Treating Autism & Prevention Development, 7398
Autism Research Institute, 7399
Autism Research Review International, 7400
Autism Services Center, 7293
Autism Society of America, 7542
Autism Society of North Carolina, 7401
Autism Treatment Center of America, 7294
Autism Treatment Guide, 7402
Autism and Asperger Syndrome, 7403
Autism and Learning, 7404
Autism in Adolescents and Adults, 7405
Autism...Nature, Diagnosis and Treatment, 7406
Autism: A Strange, Silent World, 7407
Autism: A World Apart, 7408
Autism: Explaining the Enigma, 7409
Autism: From Tragedy to Triumph, 7410
Autism: Identification, Education and Treatment, 7411
Autism: The Facts, 7412
Autistic Adults at Bittersweet Farms, 7413
Avoiding Unfortunate Situations, 7414
Biology of the Autistic Syndromes, 7417
Breakthroughs: How to Reach Students with Autism, 7418
CNS Camp New Connections, 7311
Camp Baker, 7312
Camp Horizons, 7315
Camp Royall, 7322
Camp Sisol, 7324
Camp-A-Lot, 7326
Children with Autism, 5030
Come Back Jack: The Revealing Story of a Child Diagnosed with Autism, 7427
Communication Unbound, 1976
Communication in Autism, 7429
Developing a Functional and Longitudinal Plan, 5117
Diagnosis and Treatment of Autism, 7436
Effective Teaching Methods for Autistic Children, 2014
Encounters with Autistic States, 7444
Enhancing Communication in Individuals with Autism Through Pictures/Words, 7445, 8710
Exploring Autism: A Look at the Genetics of Autism, 5223
Fact Sheet: Autism Spectrum Disorders, 7448
Fighting for Darla: Challenges for Family Care & Professional Responsibility, 7451
Filmakers Library, 5158
Focus on Autism and Other Developmental Disabilities, 1854
Fragile Success: Nine Autistic Children, Childhood to Adulthood, 7452
Fundamentals of Autism, 1627
Gateway Arts Program, Crafts Store & Gallery, 5870
Getting Started with Facilitated Communication, 7454, 8711
Going to School with Facilitated Communication, 4855
Guide to Successful Employment for Individuals with Autism, 7457
Handbook of Autism and Pervasive Developmental Disorders, 7458
Helping People with Autism Manage Their Behavior, 7459
Hidden Child: The Linwood Method for Reaching the Autistic Child, 7462
How to Teach Autistic & Severely Handicapped Children, 2043
Increasing Behaviors of Persons with Severe Retardation and Autism, 7471
Intensive Early Intervention and Beyond School-Based Inclusion Program, 4880
Keys to Parenting the Child with Autism, 7477
Let Community Employment be the Goal for Individuals with Autism, 7481
Living with Spina Bifida: A Guide for Families and Professionals, 8492
Management of Autistic Behavior, 7483, 8497
Mount Sinai Medical Center, 2699
National Autism Hotline, 7543
Neurobiology of Autism, 7490
New Jersey Camp Jaycee, 992
New York Families for Autistic Children, 7491
Ninety-Second Street Y Camps Nesher Program, 1000
Parent Survival Manual, 7496
Parent's Guide to Autism, 7497
Pervasive Developmental Disorders; Finding a Diagnosis and Getting Help, 5034
Please Don't Say Hello, 7501
Reaching the Autistic Child: A Parent Training Program, 8566
Record Book for Individuals with Autism, 7506
Riddle of Autism: A Psychological Analysis, 7510
Rimland Services for Autistic Citizens, 7350
Schools for Children with Autism Spectrum Disorders, 7512
Sex Education: Issues for the Person with Autism, 7514
Shoebox Tasks: Work Activities, 7515
Son-Rise Program, 8667
Son-Rise: The Miracle Continues, 7516, 8582
Soon Will Come the Light, 7517
Spectrum, 7518
Sunnyhill Adventure Center, 7357
TEACCH, 7309
Teaching Children with Autism: Strategies for Initiating Positive Interactions, 7522
Teaching and Mainstreaming Autistic Children, 7523
Transition Matters: from School to Independence: A Guide and Directory of Services, 4711
Treating Disordered Speech Motor Control, 2181
Uncommon Fathers, 5023
Understanding Autism, 7530
Understanding the Nature of Autism, 7532
Until Tomorrow: A Family Lives with Autism, 7534
Vanguard School, 2263
Visually Structured Tasks, 9077
Without Reason: A Family Copes with Autism, 7537
YMCA Outdoor Center Campbell Gard, 8300

Behavioral Disorders

Alternative Teaching Strategies, 1929
American Academy of Child and Adolescent Psychiatry, 8126
Behavior Analysis in Education: Focus on Measurably Superior Instruction, 1946
Behavior Modification, 1947
Behavior Therapy and Research Society, 8133
Behavioral Disorders, 1948
Childhood Behavior Disorders: Applied Research & Educational Practice, 1961
Children and Adolescents with Emotional and Behavioral Disorders, 1545
Contemporary Issues in Behavioral Health Care, 1547
Creating Positive Classroom Environments: Strategies for Behavior Management, 1982

Journal of Emotional and Behavioral Disorders, 1863
Journal of Motor Behavior, 1865
Journal of Vocational Behavior, 1872
Life Adventure Camp, 950
Progress Without Punishment: Approaches for Learners with Behavior Problems, 2116
Teaching Students with Learning and Behavior Problems, 2167
Touch of Nature Environmental Center, 933
ValueOptions, 5258
Working Bibliography on Behavioral and Emotional Disorders, 2188

Birth Defects

ABCD Newsletter Volume Reprints, 4667
Birth Defect News, 4670
Birth Defect Research for Children, 763
Camp Bon Coeur, 8198
Camp Del Corazon, 8209
Club Foot & Other Foot Deformities Fact Sheet, 8386
Cornelia de Lange Syndrome Foundation, 2396
Counseling for Heart Disease, 8405
Dictionary of Congenital Malformations & Disorders, 4829
Different Heart, 8415
Division of Birth Defects and Developmental Disabilities, 3100
Don't Feel Sorry for Paul, 7553, 8026
How to Find More About Your Child's Birth Defect or Disability, 5121
Madden Open Hearts Camp, 8272
Management of Genetic Syndromes, 8498
March of Dimes Birth Defects Foundation, 827
Marfan Syndrome Fact Sheet, 5124
National Fragile X Foundation, 8162
Oral/Facial Clefts Fact Sheet, 8535
Teratogen and Birth Defects Information Project, 8671
Why My Child, 4720

Blind/Deaf

American Association of the Deaf-Blind, 7274
American Association of the Deaf-Blind National Conference, 1531
Beam, 7280
Communicating with People Who Have Trouble Hearing & Seeing: A Primer, 7281
Florida School for the Deaf and Blind, 7279
National Family Association for Deaf-Blind, 7276
National Information Center for Children and Youth with Disabilities (NICHCY), 7277
National Information Clearinghouse on Children who are Deaf-Blind, 7278

Brain Injuries

Before and After Zachariah, 5047
Brain Injury Association of America, 765, 7296
Brain Injury Association of New York State, 766, 7297
Brain Injury Association of Texas, 767, 7298
Headlines Support Group, 8648
Living with Brain Injury: A Guide for Fam ilies, 8491
Measure of Cognitive-Linguistic Abilities (MCLA), 2219
NHIF Newsletter, 5076
Rasmussen's Syndrome and Hemispherectomy Support Network Newsletter, 8171, 8564
Ride the Red Cycle, 8569
Students with Acquired Brain Injury: The School's Response, 2148
Traumatic Brain Injury: Mechanisms of Damage, Assessment & Intervention, 7527, 8736
When Billy Broke His Head...and Other Tales of Wonder, 4717

Cancer

Adult Leukemia: A Comprehensive Guide for Patients and Families, 8317
Advanced Breast Cancer: A Guide to Living with Metastic Disease, 8318
Alexander and Margaret Stewart Trust, 2411
Arizona Camp Sunrise, 8191
Association for the Cure of Cancer of the Prostate, 5205
Bowel Cancer, 8355
Breast Cancer Sourcebook, 8361
Camp Catch-a-Rainbow, 8202
Camp Enchantment, 8212
Camp Jewell YMCA Outdoor Center, 8226
Camp Magruder, 8233
Camp Mokuleia, 8234
Camp Okizu, 8236
Camp Rainbow, 8237
Camp Rap-A-Hope Medical Society and the Alliance to the Medical, 8238
Camp Reach for the Sky, 908
Camp Ronald McDonald for Good Times, 8239
Camp Smile-A-Mile, 8243
Camp Sunrise, 8244
Cancer Biotherapy Research Group, 5210
Cancer Care, 2657
Cancer Clinical Trials: Experimental Treatments and How They Can Help You, 5028
Cancer Immunotherapy and Gene Therapy Institute, 5212
Cancer Information Service, 8638
Cancer Research Fund of Damon Runyon: Walter Winchell Foundation, 5213
Cancer Sourcebook, 8366
Cancer Victors Journal, 8367
Candlelighters Childhood Cancer Foundation, 2541
Childhood Cancer Survivors: A Practical Guide to Your Future, 8373
Childhood Cancer: A Parent's Guide to Solid Tumor Cancers, 8374
Colon & Rectal Cancer: A Comprehensive Guide for Patients & Families, 8388
Conquering the Darkness: One Story of Reco vering from a Brain Injury, 8394
Foundation for Advancement in Cancer Therapy, 2678
Happiness is Camping, 8265
Hole in the Wall Gang Camp, 8266
International Association for Cancer Victors: Northern California Chapter, 8144
Jane Coffin Childs Memorial Fund for Medical Research, 2403
Leukemia & Lymphoma Society, 8149
Leukemia Society of America, 8150
Non-Hodgkin's Lymphomas: Making Sense of Diagnosis, Treatment & Options, 8524
One Day at a Time: Children Living with Leukemia, 8532
Options, 8533
Options: Revolutionary Ideas in the War on Cancer, 8534
People Against Cancer, 8168, 8548
Psychology and Health, 4939
RA Bloch Cancer Foundation, 2610
Simonton Cancer Center, 8173
V Foundation for Cancer Research, 5257
YMCA Camp Horseshoe, 8295

Cerebral Palsy

All the Way Up There, 8324
American Academy for Cerebral Palsy and Developmental Medicine Annual Conference, 1529
Caring for Children with Cerebral Palsy: A Team Approach, 8368
Cerebral Palsy Associations of New York State Annual Conference, 8134
Cerebral Palsy Center Summer Program, 990
Cerebral Palsy: A Complete Guide for Care giving, 8369
Children With Cerebral Palsy: A Manual for Therapists, Parents and Community Workers, 8376
Children With Cerebral Palsy: A Parents' G uide, 8377
Children with Cerebral Palsy, 8379
Coping with Cerebral Palsy, 8400
Echoing Hills, 8258
From Where I Sit: Making My Way wih Cereb ral Palsy, 8434
Individuals with Cerebral Palsy, 8463
Kansas Jaycees Cerebral Palsy Ranch, 8267
Keys to Parenting a Child with Cerebral Palsy, 8477
Matheny School and Hospital, 7960
No Time for Jello: One Family's Experience, 8522
Preventing Secondary Conditions Associated with Spina Bifida or Cerebral Palsy, 8560
Ten Things I Learned from Bill Porter, 8598
Treating Cerebral Palsy for Clinicians by Clinicians, 2180
United Cerebral Palsy Association, 8177
United Cerebral Palsy Association Development Conference, 1562
United Cerebral Palsy Association of New York State, 8178
United Cerebral Palsy Research and Educational Foundation, 1751

Chiropractics

American Chiropractic Association, 739
International Chiropractors Association, 815

Chronic Disabilities

Access to Health Care: Number 1&2, 1916
Access to Health Care: Number 3&4, 1917
Brothers, Sisters, and Special Needs, 4980
Burnt Gin Camp, 1044
Camp Holiday Trails, 1058
Caring for Children with Chronic Illness, 1954, 4671
Counseling Parents of Children with Chronic Illness or Disability, 5069
Developing Cross-Cultural Competence:Guide to Working with Young Children & Their Families, 1989
Family Interventions Throughout Disability, 4993
Home and Community Care for Chronically Ill Children, 4727
National Hemophilia Foundation, 2701, 8163
Screening in Chronic Disease, 4950, 8574
Usher Syndrome, 8619
Woodlands, 1041

Cleft Palate

Children with Facial Difference: A Parent' s Guide, 8380
Cleft Palate-Craniofacial Journal, 8384
Your Cleft-Affected Child, 8630

Cognitive Disorders

ADD/ADHD Behavior-Change Resource Kit, 7365
ADD/ADHD Checklist, 7366
ADHD, 7368
ADHD Book of Lists: A Practical Guide for Helping Children and Teens with ADDs, 7369
ADHD in Schools: Assessment and Intervention Strategies, 7372
ADHD: What Can We Do?, 7375
Adult ADD: The Complete Handbook: Everyt hing You Need to Know About How to Cope with ADD, 7379
Annals of Dyslexia, 7382
Arc Connection Newsletter, 4788, 7383
Arc Light, 7384
Attention Deficit Disorder and Learning Disabilities, 7388
Augmenting Basic Communciation in Natural Contexts, 7396
Be Quiet, Marina!, 7415
Best Buddies, 7295
Biology Concepts Through Discovery, 7416
But I'm Ready to Go, 7420
Camp Easter Seal: East/West, 1057
Camp Nissokone, 7318
Camp Nuhop, 7320
Camp Ramapo, 7321
Center Academy, 7299
Center Academy at Pinellas Park, 7329
Change Your Brain, Change Your Life: The Breakthrough Program for Conquering Depression, 7422
Child and Adolescent Therapy: Cognitive-Be havioral Procedures, Second Edition, 7424
Concentration Video, 7432
Count Us In, 7434
Dallas Academy, 7331
Difficult Child, 7437
Disability Culture Perspective on Early Intervention, 7438
Dynamic Learning Center, 7300
Elling Camps, 7334
Embracing the Monster: Overcoming the Cha llenges of Hidden Disabilities, 7443
Equal Treatment for People With Mental Ret ardation: Having and Raising Children, 7446
Evaluation and Treatment of the Psychogeriatric Patient, 2020
Focus Alternative Learning Center, 7301
Getting Our Heads Together, 7453
Getting Together: A Head Start/School District Collaboration, 7455
Gow School Summer Programs, 7337
Helping Your Child with Attention-Deficit Hyperactivity Disorder, 7460
Hill School of Fort Worth, 7338
How To Reach and Teach Children and Teens with Dyslexia, 7463
I Want My Little Boy Back, 7467
Imagine!, 7468
In Search of Wings: A Journey Back from T raumatic Brain Injury, 7469
In Their Own Way, 7470
Journal of Cognitive Rehabilitation, 7473
Keys to Parenting a Child with Attention Deficit Disorder, 7475
LD Child and the ADHD Child: Ways Parents & Professionals Can Help, 7478
Lab School of Washington, 7340
Life Development Institute, 7302
Making the Writing Process Work, 7482
Marvelwood Summer, 7343
A Miracle to Believe In, 7363
NLP Comprehensive, 7303
Oakland School & Camp, 7345
Out of Darkness, 7492
Out of the Fog: Treatment Options and Cop ing Strategies for ADD, 7493
Out-Of-Sync Child: Recognizing and Coping With Sensory Integration Dysfunction, 7494
Overcoming Dyslexia, 7495
Phelps School Summer School, 7347
Preventable Brain Damage, 7502
Pure Facts, 7503
Quest Camp, 7348
Relationship Development Intervention with Young Children, 7507
SOAR Summer Adventures, 7352
Serving Adults with Cognitive Disabilities, 7513
Squirrel Hollow Summer Camp, 7354
Successful Job Search Strategies for the D sabled: Understanding the ADA, 7519
Summer Day Camp, 7355
Talisman Summer Camp, 7358
Techniques for Aphasia Rehab: (TARGET) Generating Effective Treatment, 7524
Timbertop Nature Adventure Camp, 7359
Tower Program at Regis College, 7360
Traumatic Brain Injury: Cognitive & Communication Disorders, 7526
You Mean I'm Not Lazy, Stupid or Crazy?!: A Self-Help Book for Adults with ADD, 7540

Cystic Fibrosis

Alex: The Life of a Child, 8322
Bittersweet Chances: A Personal Journey o f Living and Learning in the Face of Illness, 8353
Cystic Fibrosis Foundation, 2545
Cystic Fibrosis in the 20th Century: Peop le, Events, and Progress, 8407
Cystic Fibrosis: A Guide for Patient and F amily, 8408
Official Patient's Sourcebook on Cystic Fi brosis, 8529
Spirit of Lo: An Ordinary Family's Extraor dinary Journey, 8589
Understanding Cystic Fibrosis, 8615
YMCA Camp Kitaki, 8297

Dementia

Victims of Dementia: Services, Support and Care, 7668

Dental Issues

Complete Guide To Mercury Toxicity from De ntal Fillings, 8390
Environmental Dental Association, 792
International Academy of Biological Dentistry and Medicine, 8142
International Academy of Oral Medicine and Toxicology, 8143
International Medical and Dental Hypnotherapy Association, 8146
Standard Search: Oral Health Care for People with Developmental Disabilities, 5256

Depression

Coping with Being Physically Challenged, 4673
DAYS: Depression and Anxiety in Youth Scale, 2206
Focal Group Psychotherapy, 2026
Phenomenology of Depressive Illness, 2105

Developmental Disabilities

Administration on Developmental Disabilities, 2968
American Association on Mental Retardation AAMR Annual Meeting, 1532
As I Am, 4791
Association of University Centers on Disabilities, 759
Baby Book for the Developmentally Challenged Child, 4976
Breaking Ground, 8359
Camp ARC Spencer, 1026
Camp Cheerful, 8203
Camp Courageous, 1012
Camp Cub Creek Science Camp, 976
Camp Dickenson, 1056
Camp Fatima, 8213
Camp Killoqua, 1062
Camp Lee Mar, 1030
Camp New Hope, 974

Camp Sun'N Fun, 989
Camp Thunderbird, 924
Camp Whitman on Seneca Lake, 996
Camp Winnebago, 975
Caring for Persons with Developmental Disabilities, 4809
Catalog for Teaching Life Skills to Persons with Development Disability, 1611
Center for Developmental Disabilities, 2817
Center for Disability Resources, 775
Cheyenne Village, 5694
Civitan Acres, 1060
Clay Tree Society, 782
Communication Development and Disorders in African American Children, 8703
Community Opportunities of East Ascension, 5847
Concerned Care Recreation Day Camp, 978
Cross Roads Outdoor Ministries, 991
DOCS: Developmental Observation Checklist System, 2207
Developmental Disabilities in Infancy and Childhood, 4986
Developmental Disabilities: A Handbook for Interdisciplinary Practice, 1995
Developmental Services Center, 2209
Dictionary of Developmental Disabilities Terminology, 4830, 4987
Directory for Exceptional Children, 1759
East Brunswick Adult and Community Education Program, 2256
Enhancing Children's Communication: Research & Foundations, 1761
Family Support Project for the Developmentally Disabled, 8646
Family-Centered Service Coordination: A Manual for Parents, 4994
Fragile X Family, 8432
Glenkirk, 5786
Handbook of Developmental Education, 2036
Happiness Day at Parmadale, 1014
Happiness Day at the Center for Pastoral Leadership, 1016
Helping Hands, 1033
Information Services for People with Developmental Disabilities, 4877
Innabah, 1034
Jewish Council for Youth Services, 932
Ken-Crest Services, 1035
Knox County Council for Developmental Disabilities, 5791
Lambs Farm, 5793
Lambton County Developmental Services, 822
Language, Learning & Living, 187
Lead Poisoning in Childhood, 8480
Life Beyond the Classroom: Transition Str ategies for Young People with Disabilities, 5096
Life-Span Approach to Nursing Care for Individuals with Developmental Disabilities, 2078
Lifelong Leisure Skills and Lifestyles for Persons with Developmental Disabilities, 4893
Living Waters, 1036
LoSeCa Foundation, 823
Lutherdale Bible Camp, 1066
MAGIC Foundation for Children's Growth, 2496
MAGIC Touch, 8495
Measurement and Evaluation in Counseling and Development, 1874
Mount Shepherd Retreat Center, 1007
National Association of Developmental Disabilities Councils, 834
National Association of State Directors of Developmental Disabilities Services (NASDDDS), 836
Parallels in Time, 4924
People First International, 877
Pilgrim Pines Camp, 914
Professional Fit Clothing, 1111
Relaxation Techniques for People with Special Needs, 4946
Richmond Research Training Center, 6026
Sexuality and the Developmentally Handicapped, 5009
Sibpage, 1900
Spring Dell Center, 7914
TERI, 4958
Teaching People with Developmental Disabilities, 4959
Wesley Woods Camp & Retired Center, 947
Young Children with Special Needs: A Developmentally Appropriate Approach, 2249

Diabetes

ADA Camp for Kids, 8180
ADA Teen Camp at Covenant Point, 8181
ADA Triangle D Camp, 8182
American Diabetes Association, 8187
American Diabetes Association Annual Conference, 1535
American Diabetes Association Summer Camp, 8188
American Diabetes Association: Camp Grenada, 8189
American Diabetes Summer Camp, 1055, 8190
Bar 717 Ranch/Camp Trinity, 8192
Camp Carefree, 8200
Camp Carolina Trails for Children, 8201
Camp Classen YMCA, 8205
Camp Conrad Chinnock, 8206
Camp Discovery, 1046, 8210
Camp Floyd Rogers, 8214
Camp Fun in the Sun, 8215
Camp Glyndon, 8217
Camp Hertko Hollow, 8219
Camp Hickory Hill, 8220
Camp Ho Mita Koda, 8221
Camp Hodia, 8222
Camp John Warvel, 8227
Camp Joslin, 8228
Camp Setebaid, 8240
Camp Sioux, 8242
Camp Sweeney, 8245
Camp Waziyatah, 8248
Camps for Children & Teens with Diabetes, 8250
Cedar Ridge Camp, 8251
Clara Barton Diabetes Camp, 8253
Counseling People with Diabetes, 8404
Crestfield Camp, 8254
Des Moines YMCA Camp, 8255
Diabetes 101, 8413
Diabetes Network of East Hawaii, 3112
Diabetes Self-Management, 8414
Diabetes: Caring for Your Emotions as Well as Your Health, 1757
Diabetic Cruise Desk, 5334
Diabetic Youth Foundation, 8256
EDI Camp, 8257
Eating Out: Your Guide to More Enjoyable Dining, 8419
FCYD Camp, 8259
Florida Diabetes Camp, 8261
Friends Academy Summer Camps, 8262
Gales Creek Diabetes Camp, 1020
Growing Together Diabetes Camp, 8263
If Your Child Has Diabetes: An Answer Book for Parents, 8460
Joslin Guide to Diabetes, 8472
Juvenile Diabetes Foundation International, 821
Kiwanis Camp Wyman, 8268
Know Your Diabetes, Know Yourself, 8478
Ko-Man-She, 8269
Kweebec, 8270
Makemie Woods Camp, 8273
Makemie Woods Camp/Conference Retreat, 8274
Meeting the Needs of People with Vision Loss: Multidisciplinary Perspective, 8991
National Diabetes Action Network for the Blind, 8801
National Diabetes Information Clearinghouse, 8160
National Digestive Diseases Information Clearinghouse, 8161
NeSoDak Bible Camp/Klein Ranch, 8279
Needlepoint Daypoint, 8280
Nejeda, 8281
No More Allergies, 8521
Voice of the Diabetic, 8621
Wisconsin Lions Camp, 8293
World's Best Books from the Diabetes Experts: Publications Catalog, 8627
YMCA Camp Copneconic, 971
YMCA Camp Fitch, 7754, 7985, 8294, 8690
YMCA Camp Orkila, 8298

Diet & Nutrition

Feingold Association of the US, 800
Metametrix Clinical Laboratory, 828

Down Syndrome

Adolescents with Down Syndrome: Toward a More Fulfilling Life, 7378
Arc-Down Syndrome Society of Rhode Island, 2805
Biomedical Concerns in Persons with Down's Syndrome, 1950
Bus Girl: Selected Poems, 7419
Clockworks, 5149
Communication Development in Children with Down Syndrome, 7428, 8704
Down Syndrome, 7439
Early Communication Skills For Children wi th Down Syndrome, 2002
Keys to Parenting a Child with Downs Syndrome, 7476
Learning a Living: A Guide to Planning Yo ur Career and Finding a Job for People with ADD, 7480
NADS News, 7489

National Association for Down Syndrome, 7305
National Down Syndrome Congress, 7306
National Down Syndrome Society, 7307
Parent's Guide to Down Syndrome: Toward a Brighter Future, 7498
Spinabilities: A Young Person's Guide to Spina Bifida, 8585
Teaching Reading to Children with Down Syndrome: A Guide for Parents and Teachers, 2162
Understanding Down Syndrome: An Introduction for Parents, 7531

Dyslexia

ASSETS School, 5769
Dyslexia Training Program, 1621
Dyslexia over the Lifespan, 7441
International Dyslexia Association, 1735
International Dyslexia Association of DC, 3077
International Dyslexia Association of NY: Buffalo Branch, 3321
International Dyslexia Association of New England, 3201
International Dyslexia Association: Arizona Branch, 3021
International Dyslexia Association: Austin Branch, 3456
International Dyslexia Association: Central California Branch, 3041
International Dyslexia Association: Central Ohio Branch, 3371
International Dyslexia Association: Florida Branch, 3094
International Dyslexia Association: Georgia Branch, 3108
International Dyslexia Association: Hawaii Branch, 3122
International Dyslexia Association: Illinois Branch, 3139
International Dyslexia Association: Indiana Branch, 3146
International Dyslexia Association: Iowa Branch, 3148
International Dyslexia Association: Kansas/West Missouri Branch, 3159
International Dyslexia Association: Maryland Branch, 3192
International Dyslexia Association: Minnesota Branch, 3230
International Dyslexia Association: Mississippi Branch, 3242
International Dyslexia Association: Nebraska Branch, 3266
International Dyslexia Association: New Jersey Branch, 3300
International Dyslexia Association: North Carolina Branch, 3353
International Dyslexia Association: Oregon Branch, 3390
International Dyslexia Association: Pennsylvania Branch, 3399
International Dyslexia Association: Rocky Mountain Branch, 3054
International Dyslexia Association: Tennessee Branch, 3440
International Dyslexia Association: Virginia Branch, 3502
International Dyslexia Association: Washington State Branch, 3511
International Dyslexia Association: Wisconsin Branch, 3533
Language and the Developing Child, 8720
Louisiana Center for Dyslexia and Related Learning Disorders, 3174
Many Faces of Dyslexia, 1663
Overcoming Dyslexia in Children, Adolescents and Adults, 2095
Pre-Reading Screening Procedures, 2230
Reading, Writing and Speech Problems in Children, 7504, 8730
Reality of Dyslexia, 7505
Recording for the Blind & Dyslexic, 8816
Sandhills Academy, 2261
Southwest Branch of the International Dyslexia Association, 3318
TESTS, 2151
To Teach a Dyslexic, 2178
We're Not Stupid, 7535

Education & Counseling

ACS Federal Healthcare, 722
Acid Maltase Deficiency Association (AMDA), 8125
Adventure Program, 901
Advocacy Center, 726
Advocates for Children of New York, 728
American Counseling Association, 742
American Occupational Therapy Association, 746
American Red Cross: National Headquarters, 749
American Self-Help Clearinghouse, 750
Association for Persons in Supported Employment, 756
Association on Higher Education and Disability (AHEAD), 760
Breckenridge Outdoor Education Center, 915
CAPP National Parent Resource Center Federation for Children with Special Needs, 768
CARF Rehabilitation Accreditation Commission, 769
Camp Chatterbox, 8683
Camp Dartmouth-Hitchcock, 983
Camp Easter Seals, 980
Camp Independence, 8224
Camp Lakewood, 977
Camp Thorpe, 1054
Camp Waban, 953
Case Management Society of America, 773
Center for Assistive Technology and Environmental Access, 774
Challenge Aspen, 917
Colorado Lions Camp, 918
Community Enterprises, 784
Easter Seal Camp: New Hampshire, 984
Easter Seal Crossroads Rehabilitation Cent er, 937
Easter Seals, 8644
Easter Seals ARC of Northeast Indiana, 938
Easter Seals Massachusetts-Agassiz Village, 964
Easter Seals of Bartholomew County, 930
Educational Accessibility Services, 791
Favarh/Farmington Valley ARC, 796
George Washington University Health Resource Center, 803
Handi Camp, 1032
IL Center: Cape Organization for Rights of the Disabled, 810
Institute for Scientific Research, 811
Mainstream, 826
Med-Camps of Louisiana, 8276
National Council on Disability, 841
National Easter Seal Society, 846
National Kidney and Urologic Diseases Information Clearinghouse, 8164
National Organization on Disability, 858
National Rehabilitation Association (NRA), 859
National Respite Locator Service, 861
Native American Protection and Advocacy, 864
People-to-People Committee for the Handicapped, 879
People-to-People International: Committee for the Handicapped, 881
Pine Tree Camp, 954
Professional Development Programs, 1811
Teacher Preparation and Special Education, 890
Technology and Media Division, 891

Emergency Alert

Cornell Communications, 179
Sidney Stern Memorial Trust, 2372
Step-by-Step Communicator, 210
TalkTrac Wearable Communicator, 213

Environmental Disorders

Allergies Sourcebook, 2nd Edition, 8325
Alternative Approach to Allergies, 8326
Protecting Against Latex Allergy, 8561

Epilepsy

Acting Blind, 5139
The Boy Inside, 5180
Camp Candlelight, 8637
Easter Seals Camp Harmon, 912
Epilepsy Council of Greater Cincinnati, 3370
Epilepsy Foundation, 7548, 7957, 8138
Epilepsy Foundation for the National Capitol Area, 8645
Epilepsy Foundation of Greater North Texas, 2848
Epilepsy Foundation of Long Island, 2668
Epilepsy Foundation of Southeast Texas, 2849
Epilepsy Foundation: Central and South Texas, 2850
Epilepsy Society of New York, 2669
Epilepsy, 199 Answers: A Doctor Responds t o His Patients' Questions, 8423
Epilepsy: Patient and Family Guide, 8424
EpilepsyUSA, 8425
Father Drumgoole Connelly Summer Camp, 7747, 8260
Growing Up with Epilepsy: A Pratical Guide for Parents, 8437
Ketogenic Diet: A Treatment for Epilepsy, 8476
Narcolepsy, 8518
Neuropsychiatry of Epilepsy, 8519
On The Spectrum, 5167
Outsider: The Life and Art of Judith Scott, 5171

Phantom Lake YMCA Camp, 8283
Phoenix Dance, 5172
Pushin' Forward, 5175
Seizures and Epilepsy in Childhood: A Guid e, 8575
Twin Lakes Camp, 7984, 8291
Vibration Watch/Countdown Timer, 166
When the Brain Goes Wrong, 4969
White Cane and Wheels, 5186
YMCA Camp Weona, 8299

Head & Neck Injuries

Annals of Otology, Rhinology and Laryncology, 8335
Cervical Support Pillow, 156
Guide to Hydrocephalus, 8438
Head Injury Hotline, 8647
Head Injury Rehabilitation: Children, 2038
Health and Rehabilitation Products, 457
IAL News, 8459
Injured Mind, Shattered Dreams: Brian's Survival from a Severe Head Injury, 8466
Jackson Cervipillo, 160
Journal of Head Trauma Rehabilitation, 8473
Life Line, 8484
NeckEase, 161

Hearing Impairments

ABC Sign with Me, 7757
ADA Hotel Built-In Alerting System, 168
ASSISTECH, 153
Academy of Dispensing Audiologists, 7672
Academy of Rehabilitative Audiology, 7673
Access for All: Integrating Deaf, Hard of Hearing and Hearing Preschoolers, 7759
Addison Point Specialized Services, 5852
Adult Bible Lessons for the Deaf, 7760
Advanced Sign Language Vocabulary: A Resource Text for Educators, 1923, 7761
Akron Resources, 171
Alexander Graham Bell Association for the Deaf and Hard of Hearing, 1528, 7674
Alternatives in Education for the Hearing Impaired (AEHI), 5192
American Academy of Audiology, 5193
American Academy of Environmental Medicine, 730
American Action Fund for Blind Children and Adults, 8746
American Annals of the Deaf, 7762
American Hearing Impaired Hockey Association, 7939
American Journal of Audiology, 7763
American Sign Language (ASL): Quick Facts, 7764
American Sign Language Handshape Cards, 1599
American Sign Language Handshape Dictionary, 7765
American Sign Language Phrase Book, 7766
American Sign Language: A Look at Its Structure & Community, 7767
American Society for Deaf Children, 7675
American Speech-Language and Hearing Association, 5199
Americans with Disabilities Act: Selected Resources for Deaf, 4284
Amplified Handsets, 172
Amplified Phones, 173
Amplified Portable Phone, 174
Anna's Silent World, 7768
Approaching Equality, 4285
Arena Stage, 6, 7275, 7678
Arkansas Rehabilitation Research and Training Center for the Deaf and Hard of Hearing, 7679
Assessment & Management of Mainstreamed Hearing-Impaired Children, 1934
Association of Late-Deafened Adults, 7680
At Home Among Strangers, 7769
Audiology Foundation of America, 5207
Auditech: Personal FM Educational System, 1604
Auditech: Personal PA Value Pack System, 317
Auditory-Verbal Therapy for Parents and Professionals, 1605
Aural Habilitation, 1945
Auricle, 7771
Aurora of Central New York, 7290
BPPV, 7772
Basic Course in American Sign Language, 5143, 8864
Basic Course in American Sign Language Package, 7773
Basic Course in Manual Communication, 7774
Basic Vocabulary: ASL for Parents and Children, 7775
Bath and Shower Bench 3301B, 130
Battery Device Adapter, 319
Bed Rails, 296
Beebe Center, 5209
Beginning ASL Video Course, 5144
Beginning Reading and Sign Language, 7776
Belonging, 8866
Ben's Story: A Deaf Child's Right to Sign, 7777
Better Hearing Institute, 7681
Between Friends, 7778
Bishopswood, 7732
Book of Name Signs, 7779
Boys Town National Research Hospital, 7682
Bridges Beyond Sound, 7780
Bulletin Newsletter, 7781
CHAMP Camp, 7733
CSD Spectrum, 7782
Camp Capella, 7734
Camp Comeca, 7735
Camp Courage, 972
Camp El Camino Pines, 7736
Camp Emanuel, 7737
Camp Isola Bella, 7738
Camp Mark Seven, 7740
Camp Taloali, 7741
Camp Tekoa UMC, 7742
Captioned Media Program, 7684
Captions for Deaf and Hard-of-Hearing View ers, 7783
Center on Employment, 7685
Challenge of Educating Together Deaf and Hearing Youth: Making Manistreaming Work, 1957
Changing the Rules, 7784
Chelsea: The Story of a Signal Dog, 7785
Children of a Lesser God, 7786
Choices in Deafness, 7787
Christmas Stories, 7788
Clark-Winchcole Foundation, 2543
Classroom GOAL: Guide for Optimizing Auditory Learning Skills, 1613
Classroom Notetaker: How to Organize a Program Serving Students with Hearing Impairments, 1614
Clerc: The Story of His Early Years, 7789
Closer Look: The English Program at the Model Secondary School for the Deaf, 7790
Cochlear Implant Club International, 7686
Cochlear Implants, 7791
Cochlear Implants and Children, 7792
Cochlear Implants for Kids, 7793
Cognition, Education and Deafness, 7794
College and Career Programs for the Deaf, 7795
Come Sign with Us, 7796
Communicating with Deaf People: An Introduction, 7797
Communication Options for Children Who are Deaf or Hard-of-Hearing, 7798
Communication Service for the Deaf (CSD), 7687
Communique, 7799
Comprehensive Reference Manual for Signers and Interpreters, 7800
Comprehensive Signed English Dictionary, 7801
Conference of Educational Administrators Serving the Deaf, 7688
Connect, 7802, 8706
Connect Newsletter, 7803
Conversational Sign Language II, 7804
Coping with the Multi-Handicapped Hearing Impaired: A Practical Approach, 7805
Council of American Instructors of the Deaf, 7689
Crutches, 620
Custom Earmolds, 320
DB-Link, 785
Davis Center, 180
Deaf Catholic, 7806
Deaf Children Signers, 5150
Deaf Culture Series, 5151
Deaf Empowerment: Emergence, Struggle and Rhetoric, 7807
Deaf Heritage: A Narrative History, 7808
Deaf History Unveiled: Interpretations from the New Scholarship, 7809
Deaf Like Me, 7810
Deaf Mosaic Series, 5152
Deaf Parents and Their Hearing Children, 7811
Deaf REACH, 7691
Deaf in America: Voices from a Culture, 7812
Deaf or Hard of Hearing Services New York State Education Department, 7745
Deaf-Blind Division of the National Federation of the Blind, 8771
Deaf-Blind Perspective, 7282, 8899
Deafness Research Foundation, 7692
Deafness and Communicative Disorders Branch of Rehab Services Administration Office, 7693, 8676
Dial-a-Hearing Screening Test, 7941
Digital Hearing Aids, 321
Do You Hear That?, 5153

Dogs for the Deaf, 7694
Doorbell Signalers, 322
Double Gong Indoor/Outdoor Ringer, 323
Duracell & Rayovac Hearing Aid Batteries, 324
EASE, 7813
Ear Foundation, 7695
Education and Auditory Research Foundation, 2828
Education of the Handicapped: Laws, Legislative Histories and Administrative Documents, 4306
Effectively Educating Handicapped Students, 2015
Effectiveness of Cochlear Implants and Tactile Aids for Deaf Children, 7814
Enchanted Hills Camp for the Blind, 8836
Encyclopedia of Deafness and Hearing Disorders, 7815
Episcopal Conference of the Deaf, 7696
Evaluation and Educational Programming of Deaf-Blind/Severly Multihandicapped Students, 2019
Exploring the Bible: Bible Studies for the DEAF, 7816
Expressive and Receptive Fingerspelling, 7817
Eye-Centered: A Study of Spirituality of Deaf People, 7818
Fairy Tales & Christmas Stories, 7819
Fantastic Series, 7820
Final Report: Adapting Through the Looking Glass, 5031
Fingerspelling: Expressive and Receptive Fluency, 7821
Flashing Lamp Telephone Ring Alerter, 181
Flute Song Magic, 7822
Fold-Down 3-in-1 Commode, 303
For Hearing People Only, 7823
Foundation Fighting Blindness, 2546, 5225
Free Hand: Enfranchising the Education of Deaf Children, 2027
Freedom Three Wheel Walker, 624
From Gesture to Language in Hearing and Deaf Children, 7824
From Mime to Sign Package, 7825
GA and SK Etiquette, 7826
GA-SK, 7827
Gallaudet Survival Guide to Signing, 7828
Gallaudet University Alumni Association, 7697
Gallaudet University Press, 1773, 5227
Gallaudet University Press Journal: Sign Language Studies, 7829
General Motors Mobility Program for Persons with Disabilities, 5313
Georgiana Institute, 7698
Getting Better, 7830
Getting in Touch, 7283
Going Places, Children Living with Cerebral Palsy, 8436
Goldilocks and the Three Bears in Signed English, 7831
Grab Bars and Tub Rails, 304
Granny Good's Signs of Christmas, 7832
Growing Together: Information for Parents of Deaf Children, 7833
Guidelines for Helping Deaf-Blind Persons, 7834
HAC Hearing Aid Centers of America: HARC Mercantile, 455
HEAR Center, 7699
Handtalk Zoo, 7835
Harris Communications, 325, 456
Hartford Foundation for Public Giving, 2400
Healing Dressing for Pressure Sores, 305
Health Resource Center, 7700
Hear Now, 7701
Hear You Are, 459
Hear to Listen & Learn: A Language Approach for Children with Ear Infections, 5160
Hearing Aid Batteries, 326
Hearing Aid Battery Testers, 327
Hearing Aid Dehumidifier, 328
Hearing Aids, 7836
Hearing Education and Awareness for Rockers, 7702
Hearing Impaired Employee, 7837
Hearing Loss: The Journal of Self Help for Hard of Hearing People, 7838
Hearing, Speech & Deafness Center (HSDC), 7839, 8713
Hearing, Speech and Deafness Center (HSDC), 7840, 8714
Hearing-Impaired Children and Youth with Developmental Disabilities, 7841
Helen Keller National Center Newsletter, 8947
Helping the Family Understand, 7842
Hollywood Speaks, 7843
House Ear Institute, 7703
How You Gonna Get to Heaven if You Can't Talk with Jesus?, 7844
How the Student with Hearing Loss Can Succeed in College, Second Edition, 1633
How to Thrive, Not Just Survive, 8951
Human Policy Press, 8649
I Have a Sister, My Sister is Deaf, 7845
I Heard That!, 2046
I Heard That!2, 2047
In This Sign, 7846
In the Ear Hearing Aid Battery Extractor, 329
Independence Without Sight and Sound: Suggestions for Practitioners, 7285
Innovative Practices for Teaching Sign Language Interpreters, 7847
Intermediate Conversational Sign Language, 7848
International Catholic Deaf Association, 7704
International Directory of Periodicals Related to Deafness, 7849
International Hearing Dog, 7705
International Hearing Society, 7706
International Lutheran Deaf Association, 7707
International Organization for the Education of the Hearing Impaired, 1736
International Telephone Directory, 7850
Interpretation: A Sociolinguistic Model, 7851
Interpretations, 7852
Interpreting: An Introduction, Revised Edition, 7853
Invisible Children, 4679
Jason & Nordic Publishers, 4885
John Tracy Clinic, 7708
Journal, 7854
Journal of the American Deafness and Rehabilitation Association, 7856
Journey, 7286
Joy of Signing, 7857
Joy of Signing Puzzle Book, 7858
Junior National Association of the Deaf, 7709
Kid-Friendly Parenting with Deaf and Hard of Hearing Children: A Treasury of Fun Activities, 7859
Knock Light, 501
LPB Communications, 186
LSDC News, 7860
Language Learning Practices with Deaf Children, 2069
League for the Hard of Hearing, 7710
Learning American Sign Language, 1649
Learning to See: American Sign Language as a Second Language, 2075
Learning to Sign in My Neighborhood, 1651
Legal Right: The Guide for Deaf and Hard of Hearing People, 4326
Let's be Friends, 7861
Lexington School for the Deaf: Center for the Deaf, 7711
Liberty Lightweight Aluminum Stroll Walker, 625
Linguistics of ASL: An Introduction, 7862
Lions Camp Merrick, 7748
Lisa and Her Soundless World, 7863
Listen to Me, 7864
Listening and Talking, 7865
Literacy & Your Deaf Child: What Every Pa rent Should Know, 7866
Literature Journal, 7867
Look, Now Hear This: Combined Auditory Training and Speech-Reading Instruction, 2079
Loss for Words, 7868
MADAMIST 50/50 PSI Air Compressor, 307
Mainstreaming Deaf and Hard of Hearing Students: Questions and Answers, 2080
Managing Your Symptoms, 7869
Mandy, 4687
Marist Brothers Mid-Hudson Valley Camp, 8275
The Mask of Benevolence: Disabling the De af Community, 7921
Mask of Benevolence: Disabling the Deaf Community, 7870
Meniere's Disease, 8503
Michigan Association for Deaf and Hard of Hearing, 3209, 7712
Michigan Commission for the Blind, 3213, 3215
Michigan Commission for the Blind - Gaylord, 3214
Michigan Commission for the Blind Training Center, 3216
Michigan Commission for the Blind: Escanaba, 3217
Michigan Commission for the Blind: Flint, 3218
Michigan Commission for the Blind: Grand Rapids, 3219
Micro Audiometrics Corporation, 330
Mini Teleloop, 193
Miracle-Ear Children's Foundation, 2549
Model E-90W Hearing Aid, 331
Model F-188T Hearing Aid, 332
Mother Father Deaf: Living between Sound and Silence, 7871
Mushroom Inserts, 333
My First Book of Sign, 7872

My Signing Book of Numbers, 7873
NAD Broadcaster, 4340
National Association of Blind Educators, 8790
National Association of Blind Lawyers, 8791
National Association of Blind Secretaries and Transcribers, 8792
National Association of the Deaf, 7713
National Black Deaf Advocates, 7714
National Captioning Institute, 7715
National Catholic Office of the Deaf, 7716
National Center for Accessible Media, 8677
National Deaf Bowling Association, 7874
National Deaf Education Network and Clearinghouse, 843, 7717
National Division of the Blind and Visually Impaired, 2977
National Federation of the Blind: Merchants Division, 847, 8803
National Federation of the Blind: Science and Engineering Division, 851, 8809
National Federation of the Blind: Writers Division, 852, 8810
National Fraternal Society of the Deaf, 7718
National Institute on Deafness and Other Communication Disorders (NIDCD), 7719
National Rehabilitation Information Center (NARIC), 860, 7720
National Technical Institute for the Deaf, 7721
National Theatre of the Deaf, 39, 7722
News from Advocates for Deaf-Blind, 7287
Newsletter of American Hearing Research Foundation, 7875
Not Deaf Enough: Raising a Child Who is Hard of Hearing, 7876
Nursery Rhymes from Mother Goose, 7877
Okada Specialty Guide Dogs, 8166
On the Edge of Deaf Culture: An Annotated Bibliography of Hearing Children/Deaf Parents, 7878
On the Level, 7879
Once Upon a Time...Children's Classics Retold in American Sign Language, 7880
One Two Three Sign with Me, 9003
Otitos Media in Young Children: Medical, Developmental, & Educational Considerations, 7881
Outsiders in a Hearing World, 7882
Oval Window Audio, 334
Parents and Teachers, 2100
Patient Transport Chair, 688
Patriot Extra Wide Folding Walkers, 628
Patriot Folding Walker Series, 629
Patriot Reciprocal Folding Walkers, 630
Paws for Silence, 7883
People with Disabilities Who Challenge the System, 4932
People with Hearing Loss and the Workplace Guide for Employers/ADA Compliances, 4752
Perigee Visual Dictionary of Signing, 7884
Personal FM Systems, 195
Personal Infrared Listening System, 196
Perspective: Parent-Child Folio, 7885
Phone of Our Own: The Deaf Insurrection Against Ma Bell, 7886
Phone-TTY, 197
PhoneMax Amplified Telephone, 536
Place of Their Own: Creating the Deaf Community in America, 7887
Pocket Otoscope, 310
Potomac Technology, 471
PreReading Strategies, 7888
Products for People with Disabilities, 473
Psychoeducational Assessment of Hearing-Impaired Students, 7889
Psychology of Deafness, 7890
Push to Talk Amplified Handset, 199
Quad Canes, 633
Quad City Deaf & Hard of Hearing Youth Group: Tomorrow's Leaders for our Community, 7891
Ramah in the Poconos, 7750
Reading and Deafness, 2120
Registry of Interpreters for the Deaf, 7723, 7892
Rehabilitation Engineering Research Center on Hearing Enhancement and Assistive Devices, 7724
Rehabilitation Research & Training Center for Persons Who Are Hard of Hearing or Deafened, 7725
Religious Signing: A Comprehensive Guide for All Faiths, 7893
Ring-a-Lite, 200
SEE Center for the Advancement of Deaf Children, 7726
Say it with Sign Videotape, 9034
See What I'm Saying, 9037
Seeing Voices: A Journey into the World of the Deaf, 7894
Self Help for Hard of Hearing People, 7727
Shape Up 'n Sign, 9042
Show Me How: A Manual for Parents of Preschool Blind Children, 9045
Sign Language Coloring Books, 7895
Sign Language Feelings, 7896
Sign Language Interpreters and Interpreting, 7897
Sign of the Times, 9048
Sign with Me Books, 7898
Signaling Wake-Up Devices, 514
Signed English Schoolbook, 2138
Signed English Starter, 7899
Signing Family: What Every Parent Should Know About Sign Communication, 7900
Signing Naturally Curriculum, 1690
Signing for Reading Success, 7901
Signing: How to Speak with Your Hands, 7902
Signs Across America, 7903
Signs Everywhere, 7904
Signs for Computing Terminology, 7905
Signs for Me: Basic Sign Vocabulary for Children, Parents & Teachers, 7906
Signs for Sexuality: A Resource Manual, 7907
Signs of the Times, 7908
Silent Call Communications, 202
Silent Garden: Raising Your Deaf Child, 7909
Simultaneous Communication, ASL, and Other Communication Modes, 7910
Sing Praise Hymnal, 7911
Sleeping Beauty, 7912
Sleeping Beauty Videotape, 7913
Smoke Detector with Strobe, 515
Sonic Alert, 203
Sonic Alert Bed Shaker, 164
Sound & Fury, 5179
Sound Induction Receiver, 204
Sound, Listening, and Learning Center, 7728
Speech and the Hearing-Impaired Child, 2143
Standard 3-in-1 Commode, 311
Standard Wheelchair, 696
Stay Tuned, 7942
Stick Canes, 638
Strobe Light Signalers, 211
Summer Enrichment Camp, 7751
Supporting Young Adults Who are Deaf-Blind in Their Communities, 7288
TDI National Directory & Resource Guide: Blue Book, 7915
TTY's: Telephone Device for the Deaf, 212
Talk with Me, 7916
Talking Thermometers, 314
Teaching Social Skills to Hearing-Impaired Students, 7917
Telecaption Adapter, 217
Telecommunication Relay Services, 7918
Telecommunications for the Deaf (TDI), 7729
Telephone Communication and Hearing Impaired, 7919
Telling Stories, 7920
Test of Early Reading Ability Deaf or Hard of Hearing, 2242
Texas School of the Deaf, 1835
Theoretical Issues in Sign Language Research, 7922
There's a Hearing Impaired Child in My Class, 2177
They Grow in Silence, 7923
To Love this Life: Quotations by Helen Keller, 9066
Toward Effective Public School Program for Deaf Students, 2179
Transcription Services, 521
Transfer Bench, 315
US Government TTY Directory, 7925
USA Deaf Sports Federation, 7940
Ultratec, 478
Understanding Deafness Socially, 7926
Vestibular Disorders Association, 7730
Vibes Bed Shaker, 165
Vibrotactile Personal Alerting System, 221
Vision, 7927
Visual Alerting Guest Room Kit, 523
Volta Review, 7928
Volta Voices, 7929
WCI/Weitbrecht Communications, 479
WRAD, 7731
We CAN Hear and Speak, 7930
Week the World Heard Gallaudet, 7931
What You Need To Know, 7933
What is Auditory Processing?, 7934
When the Mind Hears, 7935
Without Sight and Sound, 5137, 7936
YWCA Camp Westwind, 7755
You And Your Deaf Child, 7937
You and Your Deaf Child: A Self-Help Guide for Parents of Deaf and Hard of Hearing Children, 7938
Youth Leadership Camp, 7756

Hemophilia

Bright Horizons Summer Camp, 8195
Camp Honor, 8223

Herbal Medicine

American Botanical Council, 737
American Herbalists Guild, 743

Human Interaction Disabilities

Asperger's Syndrome: A Guide for Parents a nd Professionals, 8339
Carroll School Summer Programs, 7327
Eagle Hill School: Summer Program, 7332
Taking Part: Introducing Social Skills to Young Children, 2239

Immune Deficiencies

Camp Shady Brook, 8241
Immune Deficiency Foundation Newsletter, 8461
Legal Action Center, 4262
Suttle Lake United Methodist Camp, 8288

Incontinence

Adaptive Clothing: Adults, 428, 1092
Adult Absorbent Briefs, 1147
Care Electronics, 487
Duraline Medical Products, 299
Fashion Ease, 1104
Informer, 8465
Kleinert's, 462
MOMS Catalog, 466
National Association for Continence, 8156
Quality Care Newsletter, 8562
Safe and Dry-Feel and Sure-Toddler Dry, 1159
Simon Foundation for Continence, 8578
Specialty Care Shoppe, 1115
Waterproof Sheet-Topper Mattress and Chair Pad, 167

Language Disorders

American Forensic Association Journal, 8692
American Speech-Language-Hearing Association, 1538, 7676, 8674
Auditory Processing Disorders in Children: What Does It Mean?, 7770
Beyond Baby Talk: From Sounds to Sentence s, a Parent's Guide to Language Development, 8697
Building Communicative Competence with Indiv. Who Use Augmentative & Alternative Commun., 8699
Guide to Developing Language Competence in Handicapped Preschool Children, 8712
Language Arts: Detecting Special Needs, 2068
Language Disabilities in Children and Adolescents, 8719
Language and Communication Disorders in Children, 2070
OWLS: Oral and Written Language Scales LC/OE & WE, 2221
PAT-3: Photo Articulation Test, 2222
Peabody Early Experiences Kit (PEEK), 2223
Peabody Language Development Kits (PLDK), 2225
Perspectives: Whole Language Folio, 8728
RULES: Revised, 2233
Receptive-Expressive Emergent-REEL-2 Language Test, 2nd Edition, 2234
Test of Language Development: Primary, 2243
Test of Phonological Awareness, 2246
Woodcock Reading Mastery Tests, 2248

Learning Disabilities

AC-ACLD/An Association for Children and Adults with Learning Disabilities, 5984
ADHD in the Schools: Assessment and Intervention Strategies, 1914
AEPS Child Progress Record: For Children Ages Three to Six, 1592
AEPS Child Progress Report: For Children Ages Birth to Three, 2191
AEPS Curriculum for Birth to Three Years, 1915
AEPS Curriculum for Three to Six Years, 1593
AEPS Data Recording Forms: For Children Ages Birth to Three, 2192
AEPS Data Recording Forms: For Children Ages Three to Six, 1594
AEPS Family Interest Survey, 1595
AEPS Family Report: For Children Ages Birth to Three, 4769
AEPS Measurement for Birth to Three Years, 2193
AEPS Measurement for Three to Six Years, 2194
AHEAD Association, 723
AIR: Assessment of Interpersonal Relations, 2195
AVKO Dyslexia Research Foundation, 1721
Activity-Based Approach to Early Intervention, 2nd Edition, 1918
Adaptive Education Strategies Building on Diversity, 1922
Adaptive Mainstreaming: A Primer for Teachers and Principals, 3rd Edition, 2197
Advanced Language Tool Kit, 1596
Affix & Root Cards, 1597
Ages & Stages Questionnaires, 2198
All Kinds of Minds, 1598
Alphabetic Phonics Curriculum, 1927
Alternative Educational Delivery Systems, 1928
American College Testing Program, 2199
American School Counselor Association, 1725
Arkansas Department of Special Education, 1788
Assessing Students with Special Needs, 2200
Assessment Log & Developmental Progress Charts for the CCPSN, 1935, 2201
Assessment of Learners with Special Needs, 2202
Assessment: The Special Educator's Role, 1941
Assistive Technology, 176
Attention Deficit-Hyperactivity Disorder: Is it a Learning Disability?, 5110
BOSC: Directory of Facilities for People with Learning Disabilities, 1752
Beginning Reasoning and Reading, 1607
Behind Special Education, 1949
Benchmark Measures, 2203
Book of Possibilities: Elementary Edition, 1608
Book of Possibilities: Secondary Edition, 1609
Books on Special Children, 4979
Buy!, 1610
CEC Catalog, 1843
CREVT: Comprehensive Receptive and Expressive Vocabulary Test, 2204
Carolina Curriculum for Infants and Toddlers with Special Needs, 2nd Edition, 1955
Carolina Curriculum for Preschoolers with Special Needs, 1956
Catalyst, 1845
Childs Spelling System: The Rules, 1612
Christian Approach to Overcoming Disabilit y: A Doctor's Story, 4815
A Christian Approach to Overcoming Disability: A Doctor's Story, 4666
Clovernook Printing House, The Clovernook Center for the Blind and Visually Impaired, 8766
Cognitive Approaches to Learning Disabilities, 1969
Colorado Department of Education: Special Education Service Unit, 1791
A Commitment to Inclusion: Outreach to Unserved/Underserved Populations, 4721
Communicating with Parents of Exceptional Children, 1973
Communication Coloring Book, 8702
Complete Directory for Pediatric Disorders, 1753
Complete Directory for People with Chronic Illness, 1754
Complete Handbook of Children's Reading Disorders: You Can Prevent or Correct LDs, 1977
Complete Learning Disabilities Directory, 1755
Comprehensive Assessment in Special Education, 1978
Computer Access/Computer Learning, 1979
Coping with Special Needs Classmates, 8402
Council for Exceptional Children, 1730
Critical Voices on Special Education, 1983
Daytime Development Center, 2208
Department of Public Health Human Services, 1814
Developmental Disabilities of Learning, 1993
Developmental Variation and Learning Disorders, 1996
Early Childhood Reporter, 1888
Early Intervention, 1852
Educating all Students in the Mainstream, 2008
Educational Care, 2010
Educational Prescriptions, 2012
Educational Referral Service, 1731
Educators Resource Directory, 1760
Effective Instruction for Special Education, 2nd Edition, 2013
Exceptional Children: An Introductory Survey of Special Education, 1762
Explode the Code Books 1-8, 1623
Feeding Children with Special Needs, 2025
First Course in Phonic Reading, 1624

Florida Department of Education: Bureau of Exceptional Education And Student Services, 1797
Focus on Exceptional Children, 1855
Food!, 1625
Frames of Reference for the Assessment of Learning Disabilities, 2210
Global Perspectives on Disability: A Curriculum, 2029
Graduate Technological Education and the Human Experience of Disability, 2031
Guide to Teaching Phonics, 1631
Handbook for Implementing Workshops for Siblings of Special Children, 2033
Handbook for the Special Education Administrator, 2035
Hawaii Department of Education: Special Needs, 1798
Help Newsletter, 1890
Helping Learning Disabled Gifted Children Learn Through Compensatory Play, 2041
Helping Students Grow, 2042
How to Teach Spelling/How to Spell, 2044
Howard School, 2258
Human Exceptionality: Society, School, and Family, 2045
If it is to Be, it is Up to Me, 1634
Illinois State Board of Education: Department of Special Education, 1800
Implementing Cognitive Strategy Instruction Across the School, 1635
Including Students with Special Needs: A Practical Guide for Classroom Teachers, 2052
Indiana Department of Education: Special Education Division, 1801
Instructional Methods for Students, 2056
Intervention Research in Learning Disabilities, 2060
Intervention in School and Clinic, 1859
Introduction to Learning Disabilities, 2nd Edition, 2061
Introduction to Special Education: Teaching in an Age of Challenge, 4th Edition, 2063
Issues and Research in Special Education, 2066
Journal of Applied School Psychology, 1861
Journal of Children's Communication Development, 5075
Journal of Learning Disabilities, 1864
Journal of Postsecondary Education & Disability, 1867
Journal of Reading, Writing and Learning Disabled International, 1869
Journal of Social Work in Disabilty & Rehabilitation, 4886
Journal of Special Education, 1871
K-BIT: Kaufman Brief Intelligence Test, 2213
K-FAST: Kaufman Functional Academic Skills Test, 2214
Kansas State Board of Education: Special Education Outcomes Team, 1803
Kaufman Test of Educational Achievement (K-TEA), 2217
Keeping Ahead in School, 1639
Kendall Demonstration Elementary School Curriculum Guides, 2067
Kentucky Department of Education: Division of Exceptional Children's Services, 1804
KeyMath Teach and Practice, 1640
Kim Marshall Series in English, 1641
Kim Marshall Series in Math, 1642
Kim Marshall Series in Reading, 1643
Kim Marshall Series in Vocabulary, 1644
LDOnLine, 5233
Lakeshore Learning Materials, 1645
Language-Related Learning Disabilities: Their Nature and Treatment, 8721
Learning Disabilities Consultants Newsletter, 1892
Learning Disabilities, Literacy, and Adult Education, 2071
Learning Disabilities: Concepts and Characteristics, 2072
Learning Disability: Social Class and the Cons of Inequality In American Education, 2073
Learning and Individual Differences, 2074
Learning to Listen, 1650
Learning to Use Cursive Handwriting, 1652
Learning to Use Manuscript Handwriting, 1653
Leo Yassenoff JCC Day Camps, 1017
Let's Read: A Linguistic Reading Program, 1654
Life Beyond the Classroom: Transition Strategies for Young People, 4684
Life Centered Career Education: A Contemporary Based Approach, 4th Edition, 2218
Literacy Program, 1655
Literature Based Reading, 1656
MTA Readers, 1659
Mainstreaming Exceptional Students: A Guide for Classroom Teachers, 4th Edition, 2081
Making School Inclusion Work: A Guide to Everyday Practice, 1660
Making Self-Employment Work for People wit h Disabilities, 4750
Making the Writing Process Work: Strategie s for Composition and Self-Regulation, 1661
Managing Diagnostic Tool of Visual Perception, 2083
Manual Alphabet Poster, 1662
Maryland State Department of Education: Division of Special Education, 1807
Match-Sort-Assemble Job Cards, 1664
Match-Sort-Assemble TOOLS, 1667
McGraw-Hill Company, 1777
Michigan Department of Education: Special Education Services, 1808
Mississippi Department of Education: Office of Special Services, 1813
Missouri Department of Elementary and Secondary Education: Special Education Programs, 1812
More Food!, 1669
More Work!, 1670
Multisensory Teaching Approach, 1671
Multisensory Teaching of Basic Language Skills: Theory and Practice, 2091
National Clearinghouse for Professions in Special Education, 1743
National Clearinghouse on Family Support and Children's Mental Health, 1796
National Education Association of the United States, 1745
Nebraska Department of Education: Special Populations Office, 1817
New Hampshire Department of Education: Bureau for Special Education Services, 1818
New Mexico State Department of Education, 1821
New York State Education Department, 1823
North Dakota Department of Education: Special Education, 1816
Ohio Department of Education: Division of Special Education, 1824
Oklahoma State Department of Education, 1825
Oregon Department of Education: Office of Special Education, 1826
Our World, 1875
Peabody Articulation Decks, 1672
Peabody Individual Achievement Test-Revised Normative Update (PIAT-R-NU), 2224
Pennsylvania Department of Education: Bureau of Special Education, 1827
Phonemic Awareness in Young Children: A Classroom Curriculum, 1673
Phonics for Thought, 1674
Phonological Awareness Training for Reading, 1675
Play!, 1676
A Practical Guide to Art Therapy Groups, 4758
Pragmatic Approach, 2111
Preschoolers with Special Needs: Children At-Risk, Children with Disabilities, 2nd Edition, 2112
Preventing School Dropouts, 2114
Prevocational Assessment, 2115
Primary Phonics, 1678
Pro-Ed, 1781
Programmed Phonics Books 1-2 & Cassettes, 1679
Promoting Postsecondary Education for Students with Learning Disabilities, 2117
Reading for Content, 1680
Reading from Scratch, 1681
Reasoning and Reading Levels I and II, 1682
Recipe for Reading, 1683
Remedial and Special Education, 1879
Resourcing: Handbook for Special Education Resource Teachers, 1684
Rewarding Speech, 1685
Rhode Island Department of Education: Office of Special Needs, 1828
Rule-ette, 1686
SAYdee Posters, 1687
Second Course in Phonic Reading, 1688
Sequential Spelling I-VII, 1689
Shop Talk, 2137
Social Studies: Detecting and Correcting Special Needs, 2139
Sound Workbook, 1693
Sound-Off 1-5, 1694
South Carolina Department of Education: Office of Exceptional Children, 1830
Spatial Orientation and Sequencing Development Remedial Activities, 2236
Special Education Report, 1902
Special Education Today, 2141

Special Education for Today, 2142
Special Siblings: Growing Up With Someone with A Disability, 4957
Spell of Words, 1697
Spellbinding 2, 1698
Spellbound, 1699
Spelling Dictionary, 1700
Spelling Workbooks Emphasizing Rules and Generalization for Corrective Drill, 1701
Starting Over, 1702
Strategies for Teaching Learners with Special Needs, 2146
Stricken: Voices from the Hidden Epidemic of Chronic Fatigue Syndrome, 8592
Structure of Words, 1703
Students with Mild Disabilities in the Secondary School, 2149
Studio 49 Catalog, 1704
Syracuse Community-Referenced Curriculum Guide for Students with Disabilties, 1705
Teaching Adults with Learning Disabilities, 2154
Teaching Chemistry to Students with Disabilities, 5101
Teaching Every Child Every Day: Integrated Learning in Diverse Classrooms, 2156
Teaching Exceptional Children, 1880
Teaching Infants and Preschoolers with Handicaps, 2157
Teaching Learners with Mild Disabilities: Integrating Research and Practice, 2159
Teaching Mathematics to Students with Learning Disabilities, 2160
Teaching Mildly and Moderately Handicapped Students, 2161
Teaching Reading to Handicapped Children, 2164
Teaching Students Ways to Remember, 1707
Teaching Students with Mild and Moderate Learning Problems, 2168
Teaching Students with Special Needs in Inclusive Settings, 2170
Teaching Test-Taking Skills: Helping Students Show What They Know, 1708
Teaching Young Children to Read, 2171
Teaching the Bilingual Special Education Student, 2172
Tennessee Department of Education, 1832
Test Accommodations for Students with Disabilities, 2240
Test Critiques: Volumes I-X, 2241
Test of Mathematical Abilities, 2nd Editio n, 2244
Test of Nonverbal Intelligence, 3rd Editio n, 2245
Test of Written Spelling, 3rd Edition, 2247
Texas Education Agency, 1833
Textbooks and the Student Who Can't Read Them: A Guide for Teaching Content, 2176
Tools for Transition, 1709
Topics in Early Childhood Special Education, 1903
Treatment and Learning Centers (TLC), 5868
Unlocking Potenial: College and Other Choi ces for People with LD and AD/HD, 7533
Utah State Office of Education: At-Risk and Special Education Service Unit, 1836
VAK Tasks Workbook: Visual, Auditory and Kinesthetic, 1710
Virginia Department of Education: Division of Pre & Early Adolescent Education, 1837
West Virginia Department of Education: Office of Special Education, 1839
Word Attack Manual, 1712
Word Demons, 1713
Word Elements: How They Work Together, 1714
Word Mastery, 1715
Wordly Wise A,B,C, 1716
Work!, 1717
Working Together & Taking Part, 1718
Worthmore Academy, 2264
Writing Skills 1 and 2, 1719
Writing Skills for the Adolescent, 1720
Wyoming Department of Education, 1840
Young Children with Special Needs, 1765

Lowe's Syndrome

Lowe's Syndrome Association Conference, 1552

Lung Disorders

Adventure Day Camp, 8185
Aldersgate Center, 986, 1042
BIPAP S/T Ventilatory Support System, 295
Becket Chimney Corners YMCA Outdoor Center, 8193
Being Close, 8352
Breathe Free, 8363
Camp Breathe Easy, 8199
Camp Christmas Seal, 8204
Camp Crosley YMCA, 8208
Camp Glengarra, 8216
Camp L-Kee-Ta, 8230
Camp Libbey, 8231
Camp Tall Turf, 8246
Canonicus Camp, 1043
Coast to Coast Home Medical, 297
Glacier View Ranch, 920
Healthy Breathing, 8448
Heart Disease in Persons with Down Syndrome, 8449
Keeping the Balance, 8475
LA Lions LPDCI Camp Pelican, 8271
Lung Cancer: Making Sense of Diagnosis, Treatment, & Option, 8493
Lung Line Information Service, 8652
Occupational Asthma: Lung Hazards on the Job, 8528
Respiratory Health Association, 5320
YMCA Camp Ihduhapi, 8296

Massage Therapy

American Massage Therapy Association, 745
American Organization for Bodywork Therapies of Asia, 747
Bonnie Prudden Myotherapy, 764

Mental Disabilities

Addictive & Mental Disorders Division, 3256
Aging and Rehabilitation II, 1926
Agnes M Lindsay Trust, 2621
Ahmanson Foundation, 2314
Alaska Division of Mental Health and Developmental Disabilities, 3005
American Group Psychotherapy Association, 8130
American Journal of Art Therapy, 4
American Music Therapy Association (AMTA), 5
American Psychiatric Association, 8131
Authoritative Guide to Self- Help Resource in Mental Health, 4794
Beech Brook, 1010
Bennington School Summer Program, 1053
Children's Needs Psychological Perspective, 1964
Colorado Division of Mental Health, 3051
Community Foundation of Santa Clara County, 2334
Complete Mental Health Directory, 1756
Consulting Psychologists Press, 1980
Cornerstone Services, 5784
Cornerstone Services Inc., 8641
Counseling Psychologist, 1849
Criminal Law Handbook on Psychiatric & Psychological Evidence & Testimony, 4298
Culture and the Restructuring of Community Mental Health, 7435
Department of Mental Health, Retardation and Hospitals of Rhode Island, 3411
Developmental Disability Services Section, 3352
Dimensions of State Mental Health Policy, 4300
Division of Mental Health and Substance Abuse, 3362
Eating Disorders Sourcebook, 8418
Ecology of Troubled Children, 2004
Emotional Problems of Childhood and Adolescence, 2016
Eugene and Agnes E Meyer Foundation, 2414
Florida Department of Mental Health and Rehabilitative Services, 3090
Georgia Division of Mental Health, Developmental Disabilities & Addictive Diseases, 3105
Giant Food Foundation, 2417
Green Door, 5732
Handbook on Mental Disability Law, 4317
Handbook on Supported Education for People with Mental Illness, 2037
Hawaii Department of Health, Adult Mental Health Division, 3116
Idaho Mental Health Center, 3130
Illinois Department of Mental Health and Developmental Disabilities, 3136
International Handbook on Mental Health Policy, 4321
Journal of Counseling & Development, 1862
Judge David L Bazelon Center for Mental Health Law, 4261
Kentucky Department for Mental Health and Mental Retardation Services, 3166

Law Center Newsletter, 4324
Louisiana Division of Mental Health, 3178
Louisiana Employment Service and Job Training Program Liaison, 5848
Maine Department of Health and Human Services, 3186
Maryland Division of Mental Health, 3197
Massachusetts Department of Mental Health, 3204
Mental & Physical Disability Law Digest, 2085
Mental Disabilities and the Americans with Disabilities Act, 4333, 4334
Mental Health Association in Pennsylvania, 3400
Mental Health Concepts and Techniques for the Occupational Therapy Assistant, 2086
Mental Health Law News, 4335
Mental Health Law Reporter, 4336
Mental Health and Mental Illness, 2087
Mentally Disabled and the Law, 4338
Mentally Ill Individuals, 2088
Michigan Department of Community Health, 3221
Minnesota Mental Health Division, 3237
NAMI Texas, 3457
National Alliance on Mental Illness (NAMI), 7304
National Association of School Psychologists, 1778
National Mental Health Association, 857, 8165
Nebraska Department of Mental Health, 3272
Nevada Division of Mental Health and Devel opmental Services, 3283
New Hampshire Department of Mental Health, 3291
New Jersey Division of Mental Health Services, 3304
New State Office of Mental Health Agency, 3326
New York State Office of Mental Health, 3333
Occupational Center of Union County, 5934
Office of Rehabilitation Services, 5995
Ohio Department of Mental Health, 3376
Oklahoma Department of Mental Health & Substance Abuse Services, 3387
Operation Help: A Mental Health Advocate's Guide to Medicaid, 4344
Oregon Department of Mental Health, 3395
Overeaters Anonymous World Service Office, 8167
Parent Professional Advocacy League, 873
Parental Concerns in College Student Mental Health, 2099
Personality and Emotional Disturbance, 2103
Providing Services for People with Vision Loss: Multidisciplinary Perspective, 9019
Psychiatric Mental Health Nursing, 2118
Psychiatric Staffing Crisis in Community Mental Health, 1876
Psycho-Educational Assessment of Preschool Children, 2232
Readings: A Journal of Reviews and Commentary in Mental Health, 1877
Rhode Island Department of Mental Health, 3414
SAMHSA News, 1898
Services for the Seriously Mentally Ill: A Survey of Mental Health Centers, 2136
Social and Emotional Development of Exceptional Students: Handicapped, 2140
South Carolina Department of Mental Health and Mental Retardation, 3429
South Dakota Department of Human Services Division of Mental Health, 3436
State Mental Health Representative for Children and Youth, 3343
Stone Mountain School, 1008
Supported Employment for Disabled People, 4754
Teaching Disturbed and Disturbing Students: An Integrative Approach, 2155
Tennessee Department of Mental Health and Developmental Disabilities, 3447
Texas Department of Mental Health & Mental Retardation, 3468
Texas Federation of Families for Children's Mental Health, 3470
Thresholds AMISS, 5800
Thresholds Psychiatric Rehabilitation Centers, 892
Treating Families of Brain Injury Survivors, 2182
Understanding and Teaching Emotionally Disturbed Children & Adolescents, 2183
Utah Department of Mental Health, 3484
VA Maryland Health Care System, 5460
Virginia Department of Mental Health, 3504
Vocational and Rehabilitation Agency: Department of Human Services, 5996
WY Department of Health: Mental Health and Substance Abuse Service Division, 3542
Washington Department of Mental Health, 3515
We Can Speak for Ourselves: Self Advocacy by Mentally Handicapped People, 5024
Well Mind Association of Greater Washington, 3080
Wesley Woods, 1040

Mental Retardation

ANCOR Wage and Hour Handbook, 4740
ARC, 7291
ARC Gateway, 3082
ARC's Government Report, 4770
American Journal on Mental Retardation, 7381
Arc Massachusetts, 2554
Arc Putnam County, 2820
Arc South County Chapter, 2803
Arc of Alabama, 2303
Arc of Alaska, 2305
Arc of Anderson County, 2821
Arc of Arkansas, 2310
Arc of Bergen and Passaic Counties, 5917
Arc of California, 2320
Arc of Colorado, 2383
Arc of Connecticut, 2393
Arc of Dane County, 2902
Arc of Davidson County, 2822
Arc of Delaware, 2407
Arc of Dunn County, 2903
Arc of Eau Claire, 2904
Arc of Florida, 2426
Arc of Hamilton County, 2823
Arc of Hawaii, 2461
Arc of Illinois The Illinois Life Span Project, 2474
Arc of Indiana, 2515
Arc of Iowa, 2522
Arc of Kansas, 2529
Arc of Kentucky, 2531
Arc of Louisiana, 2533
Arc of Maryland, 2539
Arc of Michigan, 2571
Arc of Minnesota, 2590
Arc of Mississippi, 2600
Arc of Nebraska, 2612
Arc of New Jersey, 2624
Arc of New Mexico, 2642
Arc of North Carolina, 2723
Arc of North Dakota, 2735
Arc of Northern Rhode Island, 2804
Arc of Ohio, 2740
Arc of Oregon, 2769
Arc of Outagamie County, 2905
Arc of Pennsylvania, 2776
Arc of Racine County, 2906
Arc of South Carolina, 2816
The Arc of Tennessee, 2830
The Arc of Texas, 2873
Arc of Utah, 2876
Arc of Virginia, 2881
Arc of Washington County, 2824
Arc of Washington State, 2891
Arc of Williamson County, 2825
Arc of Wisconsin Disability Association, 2907
Arc of Wyoming, 2916
Arc of the District of Columbia, 2412
Arc of the United States, 5202
Ardmore Developmental Center, 5860
Arizonia Autism Resources, 2308
Assessing the Handicaps/Needs of Children, 1933
Assessment in Mental Handicap: A Guide to Assessment Practices & Tests, 1937
Blackstone Valley Chapter RI Arc, 2806
Breaking the Speech Barrier: Language Develpment Through Augmented Means, 8698
Bristol County Chapter Arc, 2807
Camp Huntington, 7316
Camp Joy, 7739, 8229
Camp Virginia Jaycee, 1059
Camp Virginia Jaycee Newsletter, 1882
Child Who Never Grew Up, 7423
Children with Mental Retardation, 7425
Connecticut Office of Protection and Advocacy for Persons with Disabilities, 3061
Cornucopia, 5969
Council for Extended Care of Mentally Retarded Citizens, 7330
Cranston Arc, 2809
Developmental Disabilities: A Handbook for Occupational Therapists, 1994
Directory of Members, 4831
Farmington Valley ARC, 7450
Federal Laws of the Mentally Handicapped: Laws, Legislative Histories and Admin. Documents, 4313
Happiness Day at St. Augustine Academy, 1015
Introduction to Mental Retardation, 2062

Introduction to the Nature and Needs of Students with Mild Disabilities, 2064
Joseph P Kennedy Jr Foundation, 2420
Keep the Promise: Managed Care and People with Disabilities, 4889
Kennedy Center, 5718
Kent County Arc, 2811
Labeling the Mentally Retarded, 7479
Lions Den Outdoor Learning Center, 7341
Little City Foundation, 2495
Match-Sort-Assemble Pictures, 1665
Match-Sort-Assemble SCHEMATICS, 1666
Me, Too, 4689
Mental Retardation, 7486
Mental Retardation: A Life-Cycle Approach, 7487
Mentally Retarded Individuals, 7488
Mississippi Bureau of Mental Retardation, 3244
Mississippi Department of Mental Health, 3246
Missouri Division of Mental Retardation & Developmental Disabilities, 3251
Montezuma Day Treatment, 5610
Montgomery County Arc, 2829
Multidisciplinary Assessment of Children With Learning Disabilities and Mental Retardation, 2090
Newport County Arc, 2812
Orange County ARC, 5674
Orchard Village, 5795
Pickens County Arc, 2819
President's Committee for People with Intellectual Disabilities, 1747
President's Committee on People with Intellecutual Disabilities, 2981
Quaezar, 5719
Raven Rock Lutheran Camp, 7349
Retarded Isn't Stupid, Mom!, 7508
Rhode Island Arc, 2813
Sometimes You Just Want to Feel Like a Human Being, 4955
Special Education Teacher Packet, 5055
St. John Valley Associates, 7308
State Mental Retardation Program, 3344
TASH Connections, 4278
Teaching the Mentally Retarded Student: Curriculum, Methods, and Strategies, 2174
VBS Special Education Teaching Guide, 2185
Ventures Travel, 5350
Westerly Chariho Arc, 2815

Multiple Disabilities

AU Kamp for Kids, 961
Akron Rotary Camp, 1009
Alternative Work Concepts, 1723
American Association of People with Disabilities, 734
Bethel Mennonite Camp, 948
Bradford Woods/Camp Riley, 935
Briarwood Day Camp, 1024
Bringing Out the Best, 5065
Camp AIM Lloyd Institute, 1025
Camp Aldersgate, 994
Camp Allen, 982
Camp Allyn, 1011
Camp Alpine, 8196
Camp CAMP, 1048
Camp Can Do, 1027
Camp Civitan, 903
Camp Courageous of Iowa, 942
Camp Dunmore, 1028
Camp Eden Wood, 8211
Camp Forrest, 906
Camp Friendship, 973
Camp Greentop, 955
Camp JCC, 956
Camp John Marc, 1049
Camp Keystone, 1029
Camp Kostopulos, 1052
Camp Little Giant, 928
Camp Merry Heart, 988
Camp Millhouse, 936
Camp Paha, 916
Camp Paivika, 907
Camp Roger, 967
Camp Ronald McDonald at Eagle Lake, 909
Camp Sky Ranch, 1006
Camp Stepping Stone, 1013
Camp Summit, 1050
Camp Surefoot, 1031
Camp Tanager, 943
Camp Twin Lakes, 926
Camp Venture, 995
Camp Wyoming, 944
Camp for All, 1051
Camping Unlimited, 910
Children with Acquired Brain Injury: Education and Supporting Families, 5029
Clover Patch Camp, 997
Clovernook Center for the Blind and Visually Impaired, 8765
Costanoan, 911
Cultural Diversity, Families and the Special Education System, 1984
Disability and Health, National Center for Birth Defects and Developmental Disabilities, 8643
Division for Physical and Health Disabilities, 8136
Easter Seal Camp Hemlocks, 923
Easter Seal Camp Wawbeek, 1065
Easter Seals Camp, 1047
Easter Seals Camp Fairlee Manor, 958
Easter Seals Camp Sunnyside, 945
Easter Seals Colorado Rocky Mountain Villa, 919
Easter Seals Oklahoma, 7333, 7746, 8685, 8835
Easter Seals Oregon Camping Program, 1019
Easter Seals of Wayne & Union Counties, 939
Easter Seals: UCP Timber Pointe Outdor Center, 931
Educating Children with Multiple Disabilities: A Transdisciplinary Approach, 2006
Educating Students Who Have Visual Impairments with Other Disabilities, 2007
Florida Lions Camp, 925
Foundations of Orientation and Mobility, 8924
Four-H Camp Howe, 965
Handi-Kids, 966
Henry Kaufmann Campgrounds Staten Island, 998
Including All of Us: An Early Childhood Curriculum About Disability, 2050
Interdisciplinary Clinical Assessment of Young Children with Developmental Disabilities, 8468
Journal for Vocational Special Needs Education, 1860
Kamp Kiwanis, 999
Lions Camp Tatiyee, 905
Make-a-Friend, 1037
Maryland National Capital Park and Planning Commission, 959
Milldale Camp, 960
Mt Hood Kiwanis Camp, 1021
National Association for Parents of Children with Visual Impairments (NAPVI), 8788, 9097
Northwest Kiwanis Camp, 8282
PDP Products, 8540
Perkins Activity and Resource Guide: A Handbook for Teachers, 9014
Physical Management of Multiple Handicaps: A Professional's Guide, 2108
Programs for Children 3 to 5 with Disabili lities, 1001
Recreation Unlimited, 1018
Rochester Rotary Sunshine Camp, 1004
Senior Program for Teens and Young Adults with Special Needs, 2262
Shady Oaks Camp, 8284
Starting Points, 9053
Stepping Stones, 1064
Teaching Students with Moderate/Severe Disabilities, Including Autism, 2169
Texas Speech-Language-Hearing Association, 8682
Upward Bound Camp: Evans Creek, 1022
Variety Club Camp, 1039
Volasuca Volunteers of America, 1063
Wagon Road Camp, 1005
What Can Baby Hear?: Auditory Tests and In terventions for Infants with Multiple Disabilities, 7932

Multiple Sclerosis

Blooming Where You're Planted, 8354
Coffee in the Cereal: The First Year with Multiple Sclerosis, 8387
Coping When a Parent Has Multiple Sclerosis, 8397
Coping and Prevailing with Multipe Scleros is and Other Life Struggles, 8398
Dressing Tips and Clothing Resources for Making Life Easier, 447
Inside MS, 8467
MSFOCUS Magazine, 8496
Multiple Sclerosis, 8507
Multiple Sclerosis Center of Oregon, 8152
Multiple Sclerosis Foundation, 8153
Multiple Sclerosis National Research Institute, 5240
Multiple Sclerosis Q&A: Reassuring Answer s to Frequently Asked Questions, 8687
Multiple Sclerosis and Having A Baby, 8508
Multiple Sclerosis: A Guide for Patients and Their Families, 8510
Multiple Sclerosis: A Guide for the Newly Diagnosed, 8511
National Multiple Sclerosis Society, 7966
Understanding Multiple Sclerosis, 8616
When the Road Turns: Inspirational Storie s About People with MS, 8626

Muscular Dystrophy

Camp Birchwood, 8197
MDA Newsmagazine, 1873
Muscular Dystrophy Association, 832
Muscular Dystrophy Association Free Camp, 8278
Muscular Dystrophy and Other Neuromuscular Diseases, 8513
Official Patient's Sourcebook on Muscular Dystrophy, 8530
Summer Camp for Children with Muscular Dystrophy, 8287

Neurological Impairments

Archives of Neurology, 8337
Association for Neurologically Impaired Brain Injured Children, 7954
Child Neurology Service, 8135
Digest of Neurology and Psychiatry, 1997
National Institute of Neurological Disorders and Stroke, 7964

Obesity

American Society of Bariatric Physicians, 752
Obesity Sourcebook, 8526

Orthopedical Disabilities

American Board for Certification in Orthotics & Prosthetics, 7546
American Journal of Orthopsychiatry, 8332
Doing Things Together, 5154
Orthotics and Prosthetics Almanac, 8536
Osteoporosis Sourcebook, 8537

Pain Management

AMI, 292
Acrylic Leg Warmers, 1077
Fibromyalgia Interval Training, 8429
Foot Snugglers, 1081
Personal Guide to Living Well with Fibromyalgia, 8549
TRU-Mold Shoes, 1083

Parkinson Disease

Allen P & Josephine B Green Foundation, 2601
Blazing Toward a Cure Annual Conference, 1542
National Parkinson Foundation, 7967
PDF News, 8538
PDF Newsletter, 8539
Parkinson's Disease Foundation, 2504, 2707
Parkinsons Report, 8545
Young Onset Parkinson Conference, 1564

Pediatric Issues

American Academy of Pediatrics, 731
American Association of Children's Residential Centers, 732
American SIDS Institute, 8635
Assessment of Children and Youth, 1938
Child and Parent Resource Institute, 779
Child with Disabling Illness, 1960
Childcare and the ADA, 4289
Children's Alliance, 780
Children's National Medical Center, 781
Choosing Options and Accommodations for Children, 1966
Commonly Asked Questions About Child Care Centers and the Americans with Disabilities Act, 4292
Cystic Fibrosis: Medical Care, 5070
Disabilities Sourcebook, 445
Disabled Children's Relief Fund, 788
Family Voices, 795
Federation for Children with Special Needs, 798
Federation of Families for Children's Mental Health, 799
Formed Families: Adoption of Children with Handicaps, 4314
Handbook of Epilepsy, 8443
Inclusive Child Care for Infants and Toddlers: Meeting Individual and Special Needs, 4729
It isn't Fair!: Siblings of Children with Disabilities, 4680
National Center for Education in Maternal and Child Health, 839
National Center for Youth Law, 4268
National Dissemination Center for Children and Youth with Disabilities (NICHCY), 844
National Early Childhood Technical Assistance Center, 845
National Information Center for Children, 854
National Maternal and Child Health Bureau, 856
Parent to Parent, 874
Parents Helping Parents (PHP), 875
Parents for Residential Reform, 876
Pediatric Early Elementary (PEEX II) Examination, 2226
Pediatric Exam of Educational-PEERAMID Readiness at Middle Childhood, 2227
Pediatric Examination of Educational Readiness, 2228
Pediatric Extended Examination at-PEET Three, 2229
Programs for Children Birth to 2 with Disa abilities, 1002
Ronald McDonald House, 888
Transitioning Exceptional Children and Youth Into the Community, 4736
Universal Pediatric Services, 894

Phenylketonuria

PKU for Children: Learning to Measure, 2097
A Teacher's Guide to PKU, 1910

Physical Disabilities

ABC Union, ACE, ANLV, Vegas Western Cab, 5352
ACPOC News, 8304
ARJO Inc., 121
Abilities!, 724
Ability Center, 50
Abledata, 5187
Ablewear Aids for Daily Living, 5188
Access America, 5306
Access Design Services: CILs as Experts, 4774
Access Info, 4775
Access Store Products for Barrier Free Environments, 425
Access Travel: Airports, 5294
Access Unlimited, 5190, 7943
Access Yosemite National Park, 5307
Access to Sailing, 8074
Accessibility Lift, 370
Accessible Journeys, 5328
Achievement Products, 427
Achieving Diversity and Independence, 4777
Achilles Track Club, 8075
Action Products, 249
Ad Lib Drop-In Center: Consumer Management, Ownership and Empowerment, 4779
Adapted Aquatics: Swimming for Persons with Physical or Mental Impairments, 8076
Adapted Physical Activity Programs, 1841
Adapted Physical Education and Sport, 8077
Adaptive Design Shop, 122
Adaptive Sports Center, 8078
Adaptive Tracks, 8316
Address Book, 587
Adjustable Bath Seat, 123
Adjustable Bed, 154
Adjustable Chair, 225
Adjustable Clear Acrylic Tray, 226
Adjustable Incline Board, 371
Adjustable Raised Toilet Seat & Guard, 124
Adjustable Rigid Chair, 227
Adjustable Tee Stool, 228
Advanced Diagnosis and Treatment for Neck and Back Pain, 8319
Advantage Wheelchair & Walker Bags, 643
Advocacy Center for Persons with Disabilities, 727
Aerospace Compadre, 546
Air Lift Oxygen Carriers, 617
Alante, 547
Albany Vet Center, 5507
Alert, 1881
All of Us: Talking Together, Sex Education for People with Developmental Disabilities, 4975
Alliance for Technology Access, 729
AlumiRamp, 372
Aluminum Crutches, 618
Aluminum Walking Canes, 619
America West Airlines, 5308
American Academy of Otolaryngology: Head and Neck Surgery, 8128
American Academy of Physical Medicine and Rehabilitation, 8129
American Back Society, 7945
American Board of Professional Disability Consultants, 736
American Camping Association, 738
American Discount Medical, 432
American Hotel and Lodging Foundation, 5309
American Mobility: Personal Mobility Solutions, 5198
American Physical Therapy Association, 1536

American Wheelchair Bowling Association, 8079
Americans with Disabilities, 4742
Americans with Disabilities Act: Questions and Answers, 4743
Amigo Mobility International, 548
Amtrak, 5310
Anglo California Travel Service, 5330
Appliance 411, 5201
Applied Kinesiology: Muscle Response in Diagnosis, Therapy and Preventive Medicine, 4787
Apria Healthcare, 433
Architectural Barriers Action League, 5295
Arcola Mobility, 52
Area Access, 373
Armstrong Medical, 434
Assist.com, 5203
Assistive Technology Disabilities, 5204
Assistive Technology Sourcebook, 436
Association of Children's Prosthetic/Orthotic Clinics, 7955
Automobile Lifts for Scooters, Wheelchairs and Powerchairs, 53
Avis Rent-A-Car, 5353
BIT Talking Scale Bathroom Scale, 125
Back Machine, 251
Back-Huggar Pillow, 252
BackSaver, 230
Backyards and Butterflies, 4978
Bagel Holder, 335
Bailey, 437
Ball Bearing Spinner, 54
Bariatric Wheelchairs Regency FL, 662
Basketball School, 8080
Bath Products, 127
Bath Shower & Commode Chair, 128
Bath Supports, 129
BathEase, 131
Bathtub Safety Rail, 132
Battery Operated Cushion, 645
BeOK Key Lever, 482
Behavioral Vision Approaches for Persons with Physical Disabilities, 8865
Best 25 Catalog Resources for Making Life Easier, 438
Better Back, 231
Beyond the Barriers, 8020
Big Bounder Power Wheelchair, 663
Big Red Switch, 178
Blinker Buddy II Electronic Turn Signal, 55
Bold Tracks: Skiing for the Disabled, 8081
Bookholder: Roberts, 484
Boulder Vet Center, 5400
Bounder Plus Power Wheelchair, 709
Bounder Power Wheelchair, 710
Bowel Management: A Manual of Ideas and Techniques, 8357
Bowling: Ball Ramp, 8082
Box Top Opener, 337
Braun Corporation, 56, 133
Bravo! + Three-Wheel Scooter, 550
Breaking New Ground News Note, 8360
Breezy, 664
Bruno Independent Living Aids, 374
Bus and Taxi Sign, 486
Butlers Wheelchair Lifts, 375
Button Aid, 282
Bye-Bye Decubiti (BBD), 254
Bye-Bye Decubiti Air Mattress Overlay, 155
CC-M Productions, 8024
CEH, 5354
Camp Jotoni, 987
Camp Ramah in New England (Summer), 962
Camp Ramah in New England (Winter), 963
Canine Companions for Independence, 771
Capscrew, 338
Carendo, 232
Carpal Tunnel Syndrome, 7552
Center for Assistive Technology, 7566
Center for Health and Fitness, 8083
Center for Libraries and Educational Improvement, 4811
Center for Universal Design, 777
Century 50/60XR Sit, 233
Champion 1000, 665
Champion 2000, 666
Champion 3000, 667
Charlotte Vet Center, 5523
Cheney's Liberty II, 376
Chesapeake Region Accessible Boating, 8085
Chevy Lowered Floor, 57
Child Convertible Balance Beam Set, 488
Child Variable Balance Beam, 489
Child's Mobility Crawler, 490
Childhood Leukemia: A Guide for Families, Friends & Caregivers, 8375
Choice Switch Latch and Timer, 491
Choosing a Wheelchair: A Guide for Optimal Independence, 668
Classic, 58
Classique, 377
Clearinghouse on Disability Information: Office of Special Education & Rehab, 8639
Clip Board Notebook, 593
Clothing Identification Kit, 283
Clothing Solutions, 1100
Columbus McKinnon Corporation, 378
Combination File/Reference Carousel, 525
Commode, 135
Communication Aids for Children and Adults, 442
Commuter & Kid's Commuter, 700
Conditioning with Physical Disabilities, 8086
Consumer Buyer's Guide for Independent Living, 4820
Convaid, 669, 701
Convert-Able Table, 234
Cool Handle, 339
Coping with a Physically Challenged Brother or Sister, 8403
Cordless Big Red Switch, 492
Cordless Receiver, 340
Crescent Porter Hale Foundation, 2335
Cruiser Bus Buggy 4MB, 551
Cub, SuperCub and Special Edition Scooters, 552
Cunard Line, 5332
Cursive Writing Skills, 1619
Custom, 670
Custom Durable, 671
Custom Lift Residential Elevators, 380
DSI, 136
DW Auto & Home Mobility, 59
Damaco D90, 711
Danmar Products, 443
Dayspring Associates, 444
Deenie, 8409
Deluxe Bath Bench with Adjustable Legs, 137
Deluxe Convertible Exercise Staircase, 381
Deluxe Nova Wheeled Walker & Avant Wheeled Walker, 621
Deluxe Roller Knife, 342
Deluxe Signature Guide, 594
Deluxe Sock and Stocking Aid, 284
Deluxe Standard Wood Cane, 622
Demand Response Transportation Through a Rural ILC, 4827
Developing Organized Coalitions and Strategic Plans, 4828
Dialysis at Sea Cruises, 5335
Digi-Flex, 495
Directions Unlimited Acccessible Tours, 5336
Directory of Accessible Van Rentals, 5296
Directory of Travel Agencies for the Disabled, 5297
Disability Bookshop Catalog, 446
Disability Community Small Business Development Center, 787
Disability Mall, 5216
Disability and Sport, 8087
DisabilityResources.org, 5219
Disabled Sports USA, 8088
Disabled Sports USA, Far West, 8089
Disabled Watersports Program Mission Bay Aquatic Center, 8090
Discover Technology, 5220
Dodge Lowered Floor, 60
Dorma Architectural Hardware, 496
Dressing Stick, 285
Drew Karol Industries, 298
Drive Master Company, 61
Dual Brake Control, 62
Dual Brush with Suction Base, 343
Dual Security Bed Rail, 157
Dual Switch Latch and Timer, 497
Dual-Mode Charger, 646
Duro-Med Industries, 300
Dynamic Living, 5221
Dynamic Systems, 255
ERIC Clearinghouse on Disabilities and Special Education, 790
EZ Access Roll-Up Ramp for Scooters, Wheel chairs, 382
Eagle Sportschairs, 719
East Penn Manufacturing Company, 720
Easter Seals Camp Stand by Me, 7980
Easter Seals Project ACTION, 5311
Easy Access Housing, 5118
Easy Access to National Parks: The Sierra Club Guide for the Disabled, 5312
Easy Pour Locking Lid Pot, 344
Easy Stand, 384
Easy Things to Make Things Simple: Do It Yourself Modifications for Disabled Persons, 4840
Econo-Float Water Flotation Cushion, 256
Econo-Float Water Flotation Mattress, 257
Economical Liberty, 385
Edge, 672
Elastic Shoelaces, 286
Elderly Guide to Budget Travel/Europe, 5298
Electric Can Opener & Knife Sharpener, 345
Electric Leg Bag Emptier and Tub Slide Shower Chair, 138
Electric Mobility Corporation, 553
Enhancer Cushion, 258

Enrichments Catalog, 448
Environmental Traveling Companions, 5337
Equalizer 1000 Series, 647
Equipment Shop, 449
Escort II XL, 64
Etac USA: F3 Wheelchair, 673
Evacu-Trac, 674
Everest & Jennings, 450
Evio Plastics, 346
Explorer+ 4-Wheel Scooter, 554
Express Medical Supply, 451
Extensions for Independence, 527
FORE! Future Opportunity for Recreation and Employment for the Handicapped, 8091
Fairway Spirit Adaptive Golf Car: Model 4852, 528
Family Resource Center on Disabilities, 794
Family Urology, 8428
Featherspring, 649
Featherweight Reachers, 287
Fedcap Rehabilitation Services, 797
Fitness Programming for Physical Disabilities, 8092
FlagHouse Special Populations, 453
Flex-Air Pressure Relief System, 259
Florence C and Harry L English Memorial Fund, 2449
Flying Wheels Travel, 5338
Foam Decubitus Bed Pads, 158
Folding Chair with a Rigid Feel, 675
Folding Shower Chair By INVOCARE, 236
Foot Inversion Tread, 498
Foot Steering, 65
Foot Steering System, 66
Ford Lowered Floor, 67
Formula Series Active Mobility Wheelchairs, 676
Four-Ingredient Cookbook, 4851
Freedom Bath, 139
Freedom Ryder Handcycles, 529
Freedom Wheels, 389
Freedom of Movement: IL History and Philosophy, 8031
Freestyle II, 677
Frequently Asked Questions About Multiple Chemical Sensitivity, 4852
Friends of Disabled Adults and Children, 7958
Functional Forms, 260
Funnel, 348
GT Wheelchair Cushion, 261
Gabbi Talk Phone, 182
Gadabout Wheelchairs, 678
Gaymar Industries, 262
Gem Wheelchair & Scooter Service: Mobility & Homecare, 679
Gendron, 680
Genetic Nutritioneering, 4854
Geo-Matt for High Risk Patients, 263
Geronimo, 712
Getting the Most Out of Consultation Services, 4726
Golden Technologies, 237
Good Grips Cutlery, 349
Great Big Safety Tub Mat, 140
Gresham Driving Aids, 68
Guide Service of Washington, 5340
A Guide for the Wheelchair Traveler, 5292
Guide to ACA Accredited Camps, 8264
Guide to Wheelchair Sports and Recreation, 8093
Guided Tour for Persons 17 & Over with Developmental and Physical Challenges, 5341
Guidelines on Disability, 4857
H.E.L.P. Knife, 350
The HANDYBAR, 110
Hand Brake Control Only, 69
Hand Dimmer Switch, 71
Hand Dimmer Switch with Horn Button, 72
Hand Gas & Brake Control, 73
Hand Operated Parking Brake, 74
Hand Parking Brake, 75
Handi Home Lift, 390
Handi Prolift, 391
Handi-Ramp, 392
Handicapped Driving Aids, 76
Handicapped Scuba Association International, 8094
Handy-Helper Cutting Board, 351
Hang Gliding and Paragliding Mag, 8095
Hard Manufacturing Company, 159
Hartford Vet Center, 5405
Headmaster Plus, 183
Health Care Management in Physical Therapy, 2039
HealthCare Solutions, 458
Heavy Duty Sock Tuckers, 288
Helping Children Understand Disabilities, 4678
HiRider, 681
Hig's Manufacturing, 460
High Adventure Hang Gliding, 8096
High Profile Single Compartment Cushion, 264
High-Low Chair, 238
Hip Function & Ambulation, 8453
Home is in the Heart: Accommodating People with Disabilities in the Homestay Experience, 4861
Homecare Products EZ-Access Portable Ramps, 393
Homemade Battery-Powered Toys, 1632
Homewaiter, 394
Horcher Lifting Systems, 395
Horizontal Steering, 78
Horn Control Switch, 79
Hospital Environmental Control System, 500
Hostelling North America Hostelling International: American Youth Hostels, 5342
How Come You Walk Funny?, 8033
How We Play, 5164
Hughen Center, 7981
Huntleigh Healthcare, 461
Hydrocephalus: A Guide for Patients, Families & Friends, 8457
I Can Do It, 8035
INVACARE IVC Tracer EX2 Wheelchair, 682
ISC: National Organization of People with Physical Disabilities, 8097
Ideal-Phone, 184
Ideas for Kids on the Go, 4866
Imp Tricycle, 702
Inclinette, 396
Inclusive Games, 8098
Independence & Transition to Community Living: The Role of Independent Living Centers, 4730
Independent Living Centers and Managed Care: Results of an ILRU Study on Involvement, 4873
Independent Living Challenges the Blues, 4874
Indian Trails Camp, 970
Inflatable Back Pillow, 265
Innerlip Plates, 352
Innovative Products, 683
Innovative Programs: An Example of How CILs Can Put Their Work in Context, 4878
Inside The Halo and Beyond: The Anatomy o f a Recovery, 8038
Institute for Driver Rehabilitation, 80
International Association of Machinists, 813
Invacare Corporation, 306
Invacare Fulfillment Center, 556
Invacare Top End, 721
Isanogel Center, 941
Issues in Independent Living, 4882
Jet 3 Ultra Power Wheelchair, 713
Job Accommodation Network, 819
Jobri, 266
Jordan's Motility Solutions: Adapt-Able Utensils, 353
Journal of Musculoskeletal Pain, 1866
Journal of Prosthetics and Orthotics, 1868
Joystick Driving Control, 81
Just Like Everyone Else, 4888
Kenny Foundation, 5314
Key Changes: A Portrait of Lisa Thorson, 8040
Key Holders, Ignition & Door Keys, 82
Kid's Custom, 703
Kid's Edge, 704
Kid's Liberty, 705
Kid-Friendly Chairs, 706
Kids Get Arthiritis Too!, 8041
Kneelkar, 83
Koret Foundation, 2354
Ladybug Corner Chair, 239
Lakeshore Foundation, 8099
Land of Lincoln Goodwill Industries, 5794
Large Button Speaker Phone, 188
Large Print Touch-Telephone Overlays, 190
Latchloc Automatic Wheelchair Tiedown, 84
Leaning Tower YMCA: Conquerors Gym and Swim Program, 8100
Lectra-Lift, 397
Left Foot Accelerator, 85
Left Hand Shift Lever, 87
Leg Elevation Board, 502
Leisure Lift, 557
Letter Writing Guide, 596
Lettering Guide Value Pack, 597
Leveron, 503
Liberty, 684
Liberty LT, 398
Life on Wheels: For the Active Wheelchair User, 8042
Lifestand, 650
Lifts for Swimming Pools and Spas, 399
Lightweight Breezy, 685
Little People of America, 8151
Living in the Community, 4896
Long Handled Bath Sponges, 141
Long Oven Mitts, 354
Longreach Reacher, 504
Loop Scissors, 505

Loop the Loop, 8044
Low Effort and No Effort Steering, 88
Low Tech Assistive Devices: A Handbook for the School Setting, 1658
Lumex Cushions and Mattresses, 267
Lumex Recliner, 240
MVP+ 3-Wheel Scooter, 558
Majors Medical Equipment, 686
Making Informed Medical Decisions: Where to Look and How to Use What You Find, 4903
Marriage & Disability, 5125
Maryland State Department of Education, 5865
Mat Factory, 651
Maxi Superior Cane, 626
Med-Sell, 5236
MedDev Corporation, 308
Medi-Grip, 309
Medicaid Information, 8654
Medpro Static Air Chair Cushion, 268
Medpro Static Air Mattress Overlay, 269
Meeting the Needs of Employees with Disabilities, 4910
Mental and Physical Disability Law Reporter, 4337
Midland Treatment Furniture, 2089
Midtown Sweep: Grassroots Advocacy at its Best, 5127
Mini-Max Cushion, 270
Mini-Rider, 90
Mirror Go Lightly, 289
Mobile Care, 5355
Mobility International USA, 7961
Mobility Training for People with Disabilities, 4998
Modular QuadDesk, 241
Modular Wall Grab Bars, 142
Molded Sock and Stocking Aid, 290
Monarch Mark 1-A, 92
Monmouth Vans, Access and Mobility, 93
MonoMouse Electronic Magnifiers, 612
Mulholland Positioning Systems, 242
NEXUS Wheelchair Cushioning System, 271
NIH Osteoporosis and Related Bone Diseases National Resource Center, 7962
Nancy's Special Workout for the Physically Challenged, 8047
Nantahala Outdoor Center, 5317
National Association of the Physically Handicapped, 837
National Car Rental System, 5356
National Disability Sports Alliance, 8101
National Hookup, 4914
National Library Services for the Blind & Physically Handicapped, 8812
National Mobility Equipment Dealers Association, 7965
National Skeet Shooting Association, 8102
National Sports Center for the Disabled, 8103, 8631
National Wheelchair Poolplayers Association, 8104
Natural Access, 687
Nek-Lo, Nek-Lo Hot and Cold Pillow-Perfect, Body Buddy, Hugg-L-O Pillow, 272
New Courier Travel, 5343
New Directions Travel, 5344
New Hampshire Veterans Centers, 5499
New Mobility, 8048
Nick Joins In, 8520
No Barriers, 5166
Nobody is Burning Wheelchairs, 8049
Northwest Limousine Service, 5357
Norwegian Cruise Line, 5345
Nosey Cup, 357
O&P Almanac, 1895
Oak Spring Program, 7982
One Thousand FS, 652, 714
One for All Lift All, 401
Open for Business, 5168
Open to the Public, 5169
Operation Job Match, 5733
Opportunity Plus of NC, 869
Organ Transplants: Making the Most of Your Gift of Life, 4922
Out-N-About American Walker, 627
Outdoor Independence, 561
PAC Unit, 95
PALAESTRA: Forum of Sport/PE/Recreation for Those with Disabilities, 8105
Pac-All Wheelchair Carrier, 653
Pace Saver Plus II, 562
Pacing Yourself, 8053
Pain Centers: A Revolution in Health Care, 2098
Palmer Independence, 563
Palmer Twosome, 564
Paraplegics and Quadriplegics, 8054
Parent Centers and Independent Living Centers: Collectively We're Stronger, 5004
Paring Boards, 358
Parker Bath, 403
Part Two: A Preview of Independence and Transition to Community Living, 4734
Partial Seizure Disorders: Help for Patients and Families, 8546
Partnering with Public Health: Funding & Advocacy Opportunities for CILs and SILCs, 4926
Patient Lifting & Injury Prevention, 404
Pedal Ease, 96
Pediatric Seating System, 273
Peer Counseling: Roles, Functions, Boundaries, 4928
Peer Mentor Volunteers: Empowering People for Change, 4929
Pencil/Pen Weighted Holders, 534
People and Places, 5346
People with Disabilities & Abuse: Implications for Center for Independent Living, 4931
People-to-People Committee on Disability, 880
Permaflex Home Care Mattress, 162
Permobil Max 90, 715
Permobil Super 90, 716
Personal Perspectives on Personal Assistance Services, 4934
Phantom Compact Size Scooter, 565
Physical Disabilities and Health Impairments: An Introduction, 2106
Physical Education and Sports for Exceptional Students, 2107
Physically Handicapped in Society, 2109
Plastic Card Holder, 507
Polaris Trail Blazer, 566
Polio Health International, 7969
Portable Hand Controls, 97
Portable Shampoo Bowl, 143
Portable Vehicle Controls, 98
Posture-Glide Lounger, 689
Power Door, 508
Power Seat Base (6-Way), 99
Power for Off-Pavement, 717
PowerLink 2 Control Unit, 359
Prairie Cruiser, 690
Prelude, 144
Prime Engineering, 243
Prone Support Walker, 631
ProtectaCap, ProtectaCap+PLUS, ProtectaChin Guard and ProtectaHip, 509
Protection & Advocacy for People with Disabilities, 3423
Push-Button Quad Cane, 632
Quad Commander, 510
Quadtro Cushion, 274
Quickie 2, 567
ROW Adventures, 5347
Raised Line Drawing Kit, 537
Ramplette Telescoping Ramp, 405
Rampvan, 101
Rascal 3-Wheeler, 568
Rascal ConvertAble, 569
Reclining Power Wheelchairs, 718
Recreation & Sports, 8106
Recreation Vehicles, 102
Redman Apache, 691
Redman Crow Line, 692
Reduced Effort Steering, 103
Regal Scooters, 570
Regent, 571
Rehabiliation Engineering Center for Personal Licensed Transportation, 5360
Rehabilitation Engineering and Assistive Technology Society of North America (RESNA), 474
Rehabilitation Gazette, 4945
Rehabilitation Institute of Chicago Learning Resource Center, 8107
Rehabilitation Institute of Chicago's Virginia Wadsworth Sports Program, 8632
Rehabilitation Services, 885
Ricon Corporation, 407
Right Hand Turn Signal Switch Lever, 104
Rocker Balance Square, 511
Roll Chair, 244
Rolls 2000 Series, 693
Room Valet Visual-Tactile Alerting System, 201
Safari Scooter, 573
Safari Tilt, 245
Sailing Fascination, 8108
Sammons Preston Enrichments Catalog, 475
Sammons Preston Rolyan, 360
Santa Barbara Wheelchair Sports Conference, 1559
Scoota Bug, 574
Scooter & Wheelchair Battery Fuel Gauges and Motor Speed Controllers, 654
Scott Sign Systems, 512
Seven Fifty-Five FS, 707
Sexual Adjustment, 4951
Sexuality and Disabilities: A Guide for Human Service Practitioners, 4952
Shilo Inns & Resorts, 5321
Sierra 3000/4000, 575
Signature and Address Self-Inking Stamps, 540
Silicone Padding, 275
Skyway, 694

Slicing Aid, 361
Slim Line Brake Only, 105
Slim Line Control, 106
Slim Line Control: Brake and Throttle, 107
Slow Motion/Sea Legs, 8109
Small Appliance Receiver, 362
Smart Leg, 408
Smooth Mover, 409
Society for Progressive Supranuclear Palsy (SPSP), 7972
Soft-Touch Convertible Flotation Mattress, 276
Soft-Touch Gel Flotation Cushion, 277
Solo Scooter, 576
SoloRider Industries, 577
Spatial Tilt Custom Chair, 246
Speakwriter 2000, 206
Special Assistance Services (SAS), 5322
Special Children, 8668
Special Clothes for Special Children, 5255
Special Needs 5, 247
Special Olympics, 8110
Special Olympics International, 8111
SpectraLift, 410
Spenco Medical Group, 278
Sport Science Review: Adapted Physical Activity, 8112
Sportaid, 476
Sports & Recreation for the Disabled, 8113
Sports Market Place Directory, 8114
Sports and Exercise for Children with Chronic Health Conditions, 8115
StairClimber, 636
StairLIFT SC & SL, 413
Stairway Elevators, 414
Standard Touch Turner Sip & Puff Switch, 209
Standing Aid Frame with Rear Entry, 637
Steady Write, 541
Steel Food Guard, 363
Steering Backup System, 108
Still Me, 8062
Stop-Leak Gel Flotation Mattress, 279
Straight and Custom Curved Stairlifts, 415
Strengthening the Roles of Independent Living Centers Through Implementing Legal Services, 4276
Strides Magazine, 8116
Substance Abuse and Physical Disability, 5087
Summer Wheelchair Sports Camp, 7983
Superarm Lift, 109
Superkids, 8063
SureHands Lift & Care Systems, 416
Suregrip Bathtub Rail, 146
Surf Chair, 697
Swing-A-Way, 417
Systems 2000, 579
TMX Tricycle, 708
TV & VCR Remote, 518
Talking Bathroom Scale, 147
Teaching Dressing Skills: Buttons, Bows and More, 7558
Teaching Individuals with Physical and Multiple Disabilities, 1706
Technology and Handicapped People, 2175
Television Remote Controls with Large Numbers, 544
Tempered Wind, 8597
Terra-Jet: Utility Vehicle, 580
Terrier Tricycle, 581
Terry-Wash Mitt: Medium Size, 148
Texas Governor's Committee on People with Disabilities, 3471
Therapy Putty, 520
They Don't Come with Manuals, 5020
Thick-n-Easy, 364
Thinking Big, 8602
Three Rivers News, 9065
Thyssen Krupp Access, 418
Tilt-N-Table, 655
Tim's Trim, 111
Toilet Guard Rail, 149
Torso Support, 639
Touch Turner-Page Turning Devices, 218
Touch/Ability Connects People with Disabilities & Alternative Health Care Pract., 4962
Tourette's Syndrome: Finding Answers and Getting Help, 8609
Transfer Bench with Back, 248
Transfer Tub Bench, 150
Transportation Equipment for People with Disabilities, 112
Travel Information Service/Moss Rehab Hospital, 5302
Travelers Aid Society, 5323
Treating Epilepsy Naturally: A Guide to A lternative and Adjunct Therapies, 8611
Tri-Grip Bathtub Rail, 151
Tri-Lo's, 583
Tri-Post Steering Wheel Spinner, 113
Tri-Wheelers, 584
Triumph 3000/4000, 585
Triumph Scooter, 586
Twin-Rest Seat Cushion & Glamour Pillow, 281
US Department Veterans Affairs Beckley Vet Center, 5596
US Hang Gliding Association Jayne Defanfils, 8118
US Paralympics, 8633
Ultra-Lite XL Hand Control, 114
Un-Skru, 366
Undercounter Lid Opener, 367
Understanding and Accommodating Physical Disabilities: Desk Reference, 4964
Uni-Turner, 368
United Foundation for Disabled Archers, 8119
Universal Hand Cuff, 369
Uppertone, 522
Utah Veterans Centers, 6015
Vangater, Vangater II, Mini-Vangater, 420
Vantage Mini-Vans, 115
Ventura Enterprises, 640
Vermont Back Research Center, 7974
Vertical Home Lift Sales, 422
Vestibular Board, 423
Vista Wheelchair, 698
Voice Choice, 116
Voice Scan, 117
Volunteer Voice, 8067
WA & NEWS, 8068
WA Department of Services for the Blind, 3513
WCIB Heavy-Duty Folding Cane, 641
Walgreens Home Medical Center, 480
Walker Leg Support, 642
Walking Tomorrow, 4967, 7975
Wardrobe Wagon: The Special Needs Clothing Store, 5259
Warp Drive, 118
Westin Hotels and Resorts, 5325
Westside Parents Work Activity Center, 5803
Wheel Life News, 656
Wheelchair Access, 7976
Wheelchair Accessories, 657
Wheelchair Activity/Computer Table, 545
Wheelchair Aide, 658
Wheelchair Back Pack and Tote Bag, 659
Wheelchair Batteries, 8069
Wheelchair Carrier, 424
Wheelchair Getaways, 5351
Wheelchair Getaways Wheelchair/Scooter Accessible Van Rentals, 5361
Wheelchair Motorcycle Association, 8120
Wheelchair Sports, USA, 8121
Wheelchair Work Table, 661
A Wheelchair for Petronilia, 7986
Wheelchair with Shock Absorbers, 699
WheelchairNet, 5263
Wheelers, 5362
Wheelers Accessible Van Rentals, 5326, 5363
Wheelin' Around, 8070
Where to Stay USA, 5305
Wilderness Inquiry, 5327
Window-Ease, 524
Wonderland Camp Foundation, 979
Work in the Context of Disability Culture, 4971
Workshops Inc., 5632
A World Awaits You, 4759, 7987
World Chiropractic Alliance, 7551, 7977
World of Options, 2298
World of Options: A Guide to International Educational Exchange, 2299
XL Steering, 120
Your Child in the Hospital: A Practical Guide for Parents, 5036

Polio

Breathing Lessons: The Life and Work of Mark O'Brien, 8022
Managing Post-Polio Syndrome, 8499
Official Patient's Sourcebook on Post-Poli o Syndrome: A Revised and Updated Directory, 8531
Polio Network News, 8552
Polio Society, 7970
Post Polio, 8554
Post-Polio Health, 8555
Post-Polio Health International, 7971
Post-Polio Support Group, 8664
Post-Polio Syndrome Information Book, 8556
Post-Polio Syndrome: A Guide for Polio Su rvivors and Their Families, 8557
Ventilator-Assisted Living, 8620
Without Pity, 8073

Prader-Willi Syndrome

Prader-Willi Alliance of New York, 8169
Prader-Willi Alliance of New York Annual Conference, 1555
Prader-Willi Alliance of New York Monthly Newsletter, 8558
Prader-Willi Syndrome Association USA, 8170
Prader-Willi Syndrome: Development and Ma nifestations, 8559

Rare Disabilities

Alternating Hemiplegia of Childhood Foundation, 2316
Brachial Plexus Palsy Foundation, 2778
International Rett Syndrome Association, 8148
National Ataxia Foundation, 8158
National Brachial Plexus/Erb's Palsy Association, 8159
National Neurofibromatosis Foundation The Childrens Tumor Foundation, 2702
Support Group for Brachial Plexus Injury, 8175
A Teacher's Guide to HCU, 1906
A Teacher's Guide to Isovaleric Acidemia, 1907
A Teacher's Guide to Methylmalonic Acidemia, 1909
A Teacher's Guide to Propionic Acidemia, 1911

Respiratory Disorders

Advances in Cardiac and Pulmonary Rehabilitation, 1924
Breathing Disorders: Your Complete Exercise Guide, 8364
Champ Camp American Lung Association of Alaska, 8252
International Ventilator Users Network, 8469
Sinus Survival, 8579
VACC Camp, 8292

Riding Programs

North America Riding for the Handicapped Association, 866

Severe Disabilites

Assessment of Individuals with Severe Disabilities, 1939
Association for Persons with Severe Handicaps (TASH), 757
Camp Jened, 8225
Collaborative Teams for Students with Severe Disabilities, 1972
Curriculum Decision Making for Students with Severe Handicaps, 1985
Including Students with Severe and Multiple Disabilites in Typical Classrooms, 2051
Instruction of Persons with Severe Handicaps, 1637
Journal of the Association for Persons with Severe Handicaps, 4887
Life After Trauma: A Workbook for Healing, 8483
Partners in Everyday Communicative Exchanges, 5078
Preparation and Employment of Students, 5100
Transitions to Adult Life, 4737
Vocational and Rehabilitation Agency, 5722, 5779, 5825, 5908, 5961, 6029

Sexual Abuse & Related Conditions

Herpes Resource Center, 8141
Prevent Child Abuse of Metropolitan Washington, 8665
Shining Bright: Head Start Inclusion, 4701
Wilmington Vet Center, 5410

Sjogren's Syndrome

Moisture Seekers, 8505
Sjogren's Syndrome Foundation, 2552

Speech Disorders

Adaptive Technology Catalog, 429
American Journal of Speech-Language Pathology, 8693
Annuziata Sanguinetti Foundation, 2318
Aphasia, 8694
Artificial Larynx, 175
Assessment and Remediation of Articulatory and Phonological Disorders, 1936
Augmentative and Alternative Communication International Society For (ISAAC), 8696
Awareness Training, 8861
Central Michigan University Summer Clinics, 7743
Childhood Speech, Language & Listening Pro blems, 8701
Childrens Beach House, 7744, 8684
Communication Outlook, 8705
Davis Center for Hearing, Speech and Learning: Hearing Therapy, 7690, 8675
Journal of Speech, Language and Hearing Re search, 7855, 8717
Kitten Who Couldn't Purr, 8718
Language Parts Catalog, 1646
Language Tool Kit, 1647
Language, Speech and Hearing Services in School, 1648
Late Talker: What to Do If Your Child Isn' t Talking Yet, 8722
Liberator, 191
Luminaud, 465
Meadowood Springs Speech and Hearing Camp, 7749, 8686
Mississippi Society for Disabilities, 831
Motor Speech Disorders, 8724
Motor Speech Disorders: Advances in Assessment and Treatment, 8725
National Cued Speech Association, 8678
Neuromotor Speech Disorders: Nature, Assessment, and Management, 8726
Nonverbal Learning Disabilities at Home: A Parent's Guide, 8727
Prentke Romich Company Product Catalog, 472
Promoting Communication in Infants and Young Children: 500 Ways to Succeed, 8729
Providence Speech and Hearing Center, 8679
Scottish Rite Center for Childhood Language Disorders, 8680
Sequanota, 8688
Sound Connections for the Adolescent, 8732
SpeakEasy Communication Aid, 205
Speech Discrimination Unit, 207
Speechmaker-Personal Speech Amplifier, 208
Take a Chance, 5289
Talkable Tales, 8735
Talking Desktop Calculators, 542
Understanding & Controlling Stuttering: A Comprehensive New Approach Based on the Valsa Hypo, 8738
Unity, 219
University of Iowa: Wendell Johnson Speech and Hearing Clinic, 7362, 7753, 8689, 8842
Vantage, 220
Vocal Rehabilitation: A Practice Book for Voice Improvement, 8739
Voice Amplified Handsets, 223
WalkerTalker, 224
What is Vocal Hoarseness?, 8740

Spina Bifida

ASCCA, 8184
Agassiz Village, 8186
Agent Orange & Spina Bifida, 8321
Answering Your Questions About Spina Bifid a, 8336
Awareness Posters, 8351
Babyface: A Story of Heart and Bones, 4977
Boggy Creek Gang Camp, 8194
Bowel Continence & Spina Bifida, 8356
Camp Harkness, 8218
Camp MITIOG, 8232
Camp Oakhurst, 7979
Challenge, 8370
Chesity, 8371
Children with Spina Bifida: A Parents Guide, 8381
Confronting the Challenges of Spina Bifida, 8392
Determined to Win The Inspirational Story of Paradymic Athlete Jean Driscoll, 8411
Educational Issues Among Children with Spi na Bifida, 8420
Genetics and Spina Bifida, 8435
Guidelines for Spina Bifida & Health Care Services Throughout Life, 8440
Healthcare Guidelines for Spina Bifida and Healthcare Services Throughout Life, 8447
In the Middle, 8462
Introduction to Spina Bifida, 8470
Latex Allergy in Spina Bifida Patients, 8479
Learning Among Children with Spina Bifida, 8481
Lipomas & Lipomyelomeningocele, 8485
Mountaineer Spina Bifida Camp, 8277
Obesity, 8525
Occulta, 8527
On Our Own Terms: Children Living with Physical Disabilities, 4697
Parent Teacher Packet, 5043, 8543
Plan Ahead: Do What You Can, 8551
SPINabilities: A Young Person's Guide to Spina Bifida, 8573
Sexuality and the Person with Spina Bifida, 8577
Sherman Lake YMCA Outdoor Center, 7353, 8285
Social Development and the Person with Spi na Bifida, 8580
Spina Bifida, 8584
Spina Bifida Association of America, 8174
Steps to Independence: Teaching Everyday S kills to Children with Special Needs, 8591

Symptomatic Chiari Malformation, 8593
Taking Charge, 8595
Transition in Adolescence, 8610
Urologic Care of the Child with Spina Bifida, 8618
Young Person's Guide to Spina Bifida, 8628

Spinal Cord Injuries

American Association of Spinal Cord Injury Nurses, 8330
American Association of Spinal Cord Injury Psychologists & Social Workers, 7944
American Paraplegia Society, 7947
American Spinal Injury Association, 7948
American Spinal Injury Association Annual Scientific Meeting, 1539
Association for Network Care, 7953
Baptist Health Rehabilitation Institute, 3029
Christopher Reeve Paralysis Foundation, 7956
Connections Newsletter, 8393
Directions, 8416
Families of Spinal Muscular Atrophy, 8139
Functional Electrical Stimulation for Ambulation by Paraplegics, 8032
How to Live with a Spinal Cord Injury, 8455
Journey to Well: Learning to Live After S pinal Cord Injury, 8474
NeuroControl Corporation, 5248
Paralysis Society of America, 5319
Paralyzed Veterans of America, 7968
Progress in Research, 7555, 8057
Resources for People with Disabilities and Chronic Conditions, 4948
SCI Psychosocial Process, 8571
SCI/LIFE, 8572
Sexuality After Spinal Cord Injury: Answers to Your Questions, 8576
Spinal Cord Dysfunction, 2145
Spinal Cord Injury Life, 8586
Spinal Cord Injury Series, 8587
Spinal Cord Society (SCS), 7973
Spine, 8588
Sports n' Spokes Magazine, 5300
Tethering Cord, 8599
VA North Texas Health Veterans Affairs Car e System: Dallas VA Medical Center, 5575

Stroke

American Heart Association Guide to Stroke Treatment, Recovery & Prevention, 8331
American Stroke Association, 7547, 7949
Aphasia: What is It?, 8695
Fourth and Long, 8029
Kent Waldrep National Paralysis Foundation, 2860
Kessler Institute for Rehabilitation, 7959
National Stroke Association, 7550
Pedal-in-Place Exerciser, 506
Stroke Connection, 7557
Tennis in a Wheelchair, 8117
Universal Institute: Rehab & Fitness Center, 8179

Theater & Dance Therapies

American Dance Therapy Association (ADTA), 3
Disability and Social Performance: Using Drama to Achieve Successful Acts, 15
National Association for Drama Therapy, 35
National Theatre Workshop of the Handicapped (NTWH), 38
Non-Traditional Casting Project, 41
Something Magical, 44
Theatre Without Limits, 47

Tinnitus

American Tinnitus Association, 7677
Tinnitus Today, 7924

Tourette Syndrome

Children with Tourette Syndrome, 8382
TSA CT Kid's Summer Event, 8289
TSA Newsletter, 8594
Tourette Syndrome Association, 8176
Tourette Syndrome Association Annual Medical Letter, 8604
Tourette Syndrome Association Children's Newsletter, 8605
Tourette Syndrome Association Conference, 1561
Tourette Syndrome Association Newsletter, 8606
Twitch and Shout, 8612
YMCA Camp Duncan, 934

Visual Impairments

ACB Government Employees, 8741
ACB Radio Amateurs, 8742
ACB Social Service Providers, 8743
AFB Directory of Services for Blind and Visually Impaired Persons in the US and Canada, 8846
AFB News, 8847
AFB Press, 1766
About Children's Eyes, 8848
About Children's Vision: A Guide for Parents, 8849
Access to Art: A Museum Directory for Blind and Visually Impaired People, 8850
Achromatopsia Network, 8744
Adaptek Systems, 170
African Americans in the Profession of Blindness Services, 8851
Age-Related Macular Degeneration, 8852
Ai Squared, 5191
Aluminum Adjustable Support Canes for the Blind, 598
American Academy of Ophthalmology, 8745
American Academy of Ophthalmology Annual Meeting, 1530
American Anals of the Deaf Reference, 8854
American Blind Bowling Association, 9087
American Council of Blind Lions, 8747
American Council of the Blind, 8748
American Council of the Blind Annual Convention, 1534
American Foundation for the Blind, 2651, 8749
American Foundation for the Blind-Midwest, 2470
American Foundation for the Blind: Southwest, 2833
American Optometric Association, 8750
American Printing House for the Blind, 8751, 8855
Americans with Disabilities Act Guide for Places of Lodging: Serving Guests Who Are Blind, 8856
Amerock Corporation, 2473
Annual Report/Newsletter, 8857
Arizona Rehabilitation State Services for the Blind and Visually Impaired, 3018
Art and Science of Teaching Orientation and Mobility to Persons with Visual Impairments, 8858
Associated Blind, 8752
Associated Services for the Blind, 8753
Association for Education & Rehabilitation of the Blind & Visually Impaired, 1540, 8754
Association for Macular Diseases, 8755
Association for Macular Diseases Newsletter, 8859
Avoid Eye Strain, Feel it T-Shirt, 1130
Awareness, 8860
BESTspeech, 177
BVA Bulletin, 5111
Babycare Assistive Technology, 8862
Babycare Assistive Technology for Parents with Physical Disabilties, 8863
Backgammon Set: Deluxe, 5269
Basketball: Beeping Foam, 9088
Berthold Lowenfeld on Blindness and Blind People, 8867
Beyond Sight, Inc., 600
Big Bold Timer Low Vision, 336
Big Number Pocket Sized Calculator, 601
Big Print Address Book, 588
Bill Dvorak, Kayak and Rafting Expeditions, 5331
Blind Babies Foundation, 2325
Blind Children's Fund, 2573
Blind Childrens Center, 8756
Blind Childrens Center Annual Meeting, 1543
Blind Educator, 8868
Blind Information Technology Specialists, 8757
Blind Outdoor Leisure Development, 9089
Blind and Vision-Impaired Individuals, 5112, 8869
Blinded Veterans Association, 8758
Blinded Veterans Association National Convention, 1544
Blindness, 5145
Blindness and Early Childhood Development Second Edition, 8870
Blindness: What it is, What it Does and How to Live with it, 8872
Board Games: Solitaire, 5271
Bold Line Paper, 589
Books are Fun for Everyone, 8873
Books for Blind and Physically Handicapped Individuals, 8759
Braille Book Review, 8875
Braille Compass, 602
Braille Documents, 5146, 8876
Braille Forum, 8877
Braille Institute Orange County Center, 9093
Braille Institute of America, 8760

Braille Monitor, 8878
Braille Notebook, 590
Braille Plates for Elevator, 603
Braille Playing Cards: Plastic, 5272
Braille Touch-Time Watches, 604
Braille: An Extraordinary Volunteer Opportunity, 8879
Braille: Bingo Cards, Boards and Call Numbers, 5273
Braille: Desk Calendar, 591
Braille: Greeting Cards, 592
Braille: Rook Cards, 5274
Bulletin, 8881
Bureau of Education for Exceptional Children, 3085
Burns Braille Transcription Dictionary, 8882
Burns-Dunphy Foundation, 2328
California Department of Education: Special Education Division, 1790
California State Library Braille and Talki ng Book Library, 8761
Camp Barakel, 8827
Camp Challenge, 951, 8828
Camp Courage North, 8207
Camp Lawroweld, 8829
Camp Lou Henry Hoover, 8830
Camp Merrick, 8831
Can't Your Child See? A Guide for Parents of Visually Impaired Children, 8883
Canine Helpers for the Handicapped, 772, 8762
Caption Center, 7683, 8763
Cards: Musical, 5276
Cards: UNO, 5277
Career Perspectives: Interviews with Blind and Visually Impaired Professionals, 8884
Careers in Blindness Rehabilitation Services, 8885
Carolyn's Catalog, 1099
Carolyn's Low Vision Products, 441
Cataracts, 5113, 8886
Characteristics, Services, & Outcomes of Rehab. Consumers who are Blind/Visually Impaired, 8887
Chicago Lighthouse for People who are Blind and Visually Impaired, 8764
Childhood Glaucoma: A Reference Guide for Families, 8888
Children with Visual Impairments Woodbine House, 8889
Choice Magazine Listening, 8890
Christian Record Services/National Camps for Blind Children, 8832
Circline Illuminated Magnifer, 605
Classification of Impaired Vision, 8891
College of Optometrists in Vision Development, 8767
College of Syntonic Optometry, 8768
Columbia Lighthouse for the Blind, 8769
Columbia Lighthouse for the Blind Summer Camp, 8833
Committee for Purchase from People Who Are Blind or Severely Disabled, 2971
Communication Skills for Visually Impaired Learners, 8892
Community Services for the Blind and Partially Sighted Store: Sight Connection, 1615
Comprehensive Examination of Barriers to Employment Among Persons who are Blind or Impaired, 8893
Concept Development for Visually Handicapped Children: A Resource Guide, 8894
Connecticut Board of Education and Service for the Blind, 3057
Consumer and Patient Information Hotline, 9094
Contrasting Characteristics of Blind and Visually Impaired Clients, 8895
Council of Families with Visual Impairments, 8770
DVH Quarterly, 8896
Dancing Cheek to Cheek, 8897
Darrow Foundation, 2336
Data on Blindness and Visual Impairment in the US: A Resource Manual, 8898
Dazor Manufacturing Corporation, 494
Defining Rehabilitation Agency Types, 1987
Delaware Division for the Visually Impaired, 3068
Delaware Industries for the Blind, 3069
Deluxe Long Ring Low Vision Timer, 341
Department Of Human Services, 5876
Department of Medicine and Surgery Veterans Administration, 5365
Department of Ophthalmology Information Line, 9095
Descriptive Video Service, 8900
Deutsch Foundation, 2338
Development of Social Skills by Blind and Visually Impaired Students, 8901
Diabetic Retinopathy, 8902
Dialogue Magazine, 8903
Dice: Jumbo Size, 5280
Dimensions: Visually Impaired Persons with Multiple Disabilities, 8904
Directory of Camps for Blind and Visually Impaired Children & Adults, 8834
Diversity and Visual Impairment: The Influ ence of Race, Gender, Religion and Ethnicity, 8905
Division of Vocational Rehabilitation of Wyoming, 6042
Do You Remember the Color Blue: And Other Questions Kids Ask About Blindness, 8906
Dog Sponsorship Program, 8907
Don't Lose Sight of Cataracts, 8908
Don't Lose Sight of Glaucoma, 8909
Early Focus: Working with Young Blind and Visually Impaired Children, 8910
Encyclopedia of Blindness and Vision Impairment Second Edition, 8911
Equals in Partnership: Basic Rights for Families of Children with Blindness, 8912
Exceptional Teaching Inc., 1622
Extra Loud Alarm with Lighter Plug, 606
Eye Bank Association of America, 8772
Eye Bank Association of America Annual Meeting, 1549
Eye Research News Briefs, 8913
Eye and Your Vision, 8914
Eye-Q Test, 8915
Facts: Books for Blind and Physically Handicapped Individuals, 5119, 8916
Family Context and Disability Culture Reframing: Through the Looking Glass, 8917
Family Guide to Vision Care, 8918
Family Guide: Growth & Development of the Partially Seeing Child, 8919
Fathers: A Common Ground, 8920
Fidelco Guide Dog Foundation, 2397, 8773
Fight for Sight, 8774
Fighting Blindness News, 8921
First Occupational Center of New Jersey, 5927
First Steps, 8922
Focus, 8028, 8923
Food Markers/Rubberbands, 347
Foundations of Rehabilitation Counseling with Persons Who Are Blind, 8925
Free Information/Membership Kit, 8926
Freedom Scientific, 5226
Future Reflections, 8927
General Facts and Figures on Blindness, 8928
Get a Wiggle On, 8929
Gift of Sight, 8930
Glaucoma, 8931
Glaucoma Research Foundation, 2345, 5228
Glaucoma: The Sneak Thief of Sight, 8932
Gleams Newsletter, 8933
Good Employee Is Capable, Conscientious, Productive, 8934
Guide Dog Foundation Flyer, 8935
Guide Dog Foundation for the Blind, 2684
Guide Dog Users, 8775
Guide Dogs for the Blind, 8776
Guidelines and Games for Teaching Efficient Braille Reading, 8936
Guidelines for Comprehensive Low Vision Care, 8937
Guideway, 8938
Guiding Eyes for the Blind, 8777
Guiding Eyes for the Blind: Breeding and Placement Center, 8778
Guild Audio Library, 8939
Guild Briefs, 8940
Handbook for Itinerant and Resource Teachers of Blind Students, 8941
Handbook of Information for Members of the Achromatopsia Network, 8942
Hawaii Department of Human Services, 3117
Health Care Professionals Who Are Blind or Visually Impaired, 8943
Hearsay, 8944
Heart to Heart, 5120, 5161, 8945
Heartbreak of Being A Little Bit Blind, 8946
Helen and Teacher: The Story of Helen & Anne Sullivan Macy, 7284
Helping the Visually Impaired Child with Developmental Problems, 8948
Henry W Bull Foundation, 2349
Highbrook Lodge, 8837
History and Use of Braille, 8949
Horizons for the Blind, 8779
Hospitalized Veterans Writing Project, 5370
How Does a Blind Person Get Around?, 8950
Hub, 8952
If Blindness Comes, 8953
If Blindness Strikes Don't Strike Out, 8954
Imagining the Possibilities: Creative Approaches to Orientation and Mobility Instruction, 8955

In the Mind of the Beholder.... a Video About Newly Blind Adults, 8956
InTouch Networks: National Radio Reading Service, 8957
Increasing Literacy Levels: Final Report, 8958
Independent Visually Impaired Enterprisers, 8780
Indian Creek Camp, 8838
Information & Referral Center, 2055
Information Access Project, 8959
Information Access Project: National Federation of the Blind, 8781
Information on Glaucoma, 8960
Inside the Beltway, 8961
Insight, 8962
Institute for Families of Blind Children, 8782
International Association of Audio Information Services (IAAIS), 8783
International Braille and Technology Center for the Blind, 8650
International Directory of Libraries for the Disabled, 4881
Intervention Practices in the Retention of Competitive Employment, 8963
Iowa Department for the Blind, 3152
JBI Voice, 8964
Jewish Braille Institute International, 8784
Jewish Braille Review, 8965
Jewish Guild for the Blind, 1737
Jewish Heritage for the Blind, 8966
Job Opportunities for the Blind, 5861
Journal of Visual Impairment and Blindness, 8967
Juggler, 8968
Junior Blind of America, 2352
Kaleidoscope Network, 8651
Kamp A-Komp-Plish, 8839
Kamp Kaleo, 8840
Kenneth T and Eileen L Norris Foundation, 2353
Kentucky Office For The Blind, 5843
Kernal Book Series, 8969
Know Your Eye, 8970
LS&S, 463
Large Print Loan Library, 8971
Large Print Loan Library Catalog, 8972
Large Print Recipies for a Healthy Life, 8973
Learning to Play, 5123, 8974
Let's Eat, 8975
Let's Eat Video, 8976
Library Resources for the Blind and Physically Handicapped, 8977
Library Services for the Blind, 8978
Library Users of America Newsletter, 8979
Lifestyles of Employed Legally Blind People, 8980
Light the Way, 8981
Lighthouse Central Florida (Formerly C.I.T.E), 5751
Lighthouse International Information and Resource Service, 9096
Lighthouse Low Vision Products, 464
Lion, 8982
Lions Clubs International, 2283, 8786
Living with Achromatopsia, 8983
Long Cane News, 8984
Look Out for Annie, 8985
Low Vision Questions and Answers: Definitions, Devices, Services, 8986
Low Vision Telephones, 607
Low Vision: Reflections of the Past, Issues for the Future, 8987
Magnetic Card Reader, 355
Magni-Cam & Primer, 608
Maine Division for the Blind and Visually Impaired, 3188
Mainstreaming and the American Dream, 8988
Mainstreaming the Visually Impaired Child, 8989
Making Life More Livable, 8990
Man's Low-Vision Quartz Watches, 610
Maxi Aids, 467
Maxi Marks, 533
Maxi-Aids Braille Timer, 356
Medem Network Societies American Academy of Opthamology, 5237
Medic Alert Foundation, International, 8653
Men's/Women's Low Vision Watches & Clocks, 611
Metropolitan Washington Ear, 192
Michigan Council of the Blind and Visually Impaired (MCBVI), 3220
Minnesota State Services for the Blind, 3240
Missouri Rehabilitation Services for the Blind, 3253
More Alike Than Different: Blind and Visually Impaired Children, 8993
Mothers with Visual Impairments who are Raising Young Children, 8994
Move With Me, 5128, 8995
Musical Mainstream, 8996
NBA Bulletin, 8998
NISH, 6025
NLS News, 8999
NLS Update, 9000
National Alliance of Blind Students NABS Liaison, 8787
National Association for Visually Handicapped, 5242, 8789
National Association of Blind Students, 8793
National Association of Blind Teachers, 8794
National Association of Guide Dog Users, 8795
National Association to Promote the Use of Braille, 8796
National Braille Association, 8797
National Braille Press, 8798
National Camp for Blind Children, 8799
National Center for Vision and Child Development, 8800
National Eye Research Foundation (NERF), 2500
National Federation of the Blind, 2550, 8802
National Federation of the Blind: Blind Industrial Workers Division, 848, 8804
National Federation of the Blind: Computer Science Division, 849, 8805
National Federation of the Blind: Human Services Division, 8806
National Federation of the Blind: Masonic Square Club, 8807
National Federation of the Blind: Public Employees Division, 850, 8808
National Industries for the Blind, 8811
National Organization of Parents of Blind Children, 8813
National Service Dog Center, 8659
Nebraska Commission for the Blind & Visually Impaired, 3269
Nevada Bureau of Services to the Blind and Visually Impaired, 3278
New Eyes for the Needy, 8814
New Jersey Commission for the Blind and Visually Impaired, 3301, 5931
New Mexico Commission for the Blind, 3311
New Vision Store, 468
New York State Commission for the Blind, 3329
Newsline for the Blind, 9001
North Carolina Division of Services for the Blind, 5957
North Dakota Vocational Rehabilitation Agency, 5968
Oklahoma Department of Rehabilitation Services, 3388
Opportunity, 9004
Oregon Commission for the Blind, 3394
Oregon Health Sciences University, 5539
Orientation and Mobility Primer for Families and Young Children, 9005
Out of Left Field, 9006
Out of the Corner of My Eye: Living with Vision Loss in Later Life, 9008
PB News, 9009
PBA News, 9010
PXE International, 8661
Patient's Guide to Visual Aids and Illumination, 9012
Pearle Vision Foundation, 2865
Pediatric Visual Diagnosis Fact Sheets, 9013
Pennsylvania Bureau of Blindness, 3402
Perkins Brailler, 535
Personal Reader Update, 9015
Picture is Worth a Thousand Words for Blind and Visually Impaired Persons Too!, 9016
Popular Activities and Games for Blind, Visually Impaired & Disabled People, 9017
Preschool Learning Activities for the Visually Impaired Child, 9018
Prevent Blindness America, 8815
Psychoeducational Assessment of Visually Impaired and Blind Students, 2119, 9020
Quantum Technology, 5251
Quarterly Update, 9021
RP Messenger, 9022
Raised Dot Computing Newsletter, 9023
Reaching, Crawling, Walking....Let's Get Moving, 9024
Reading Is for Everyone, 9025
Reading with Low Vision, 9026
Recorded Periodicals, 9098
Recording for the Blind News, 9027
Reference and Information Services From NLS, 9028
Referring Blind and Low Vision Patients for Rehabilitation Services, 9029
Rehabilitation Resource Manual: VISION, 2127
Reizen Braille Labeler, 538
Research to Prevent Blindness, 2709
Resource List for Persons with Low Vision, 9030
Resources for Family Centered Intervention for Infants, Toddlers, and Preschoolers, 9031

Rhode Island Services for the Blind and Visually Impaired, 3419
Rigid Aluminum Cane with Golf Grip, 613
Robert Ellis Simon Foundation, 2369
Roy and Christine Sturgis Charitable Trust, 2311
SCENE, 9033
Say What, 291
School of Piano Technology for the Blind, 6035
See A Bone, 9035
See What I Feel, 9036
See for Yourself, 9038
Seeing Eye, 8817
Seeing Eye Guide, 9039
Selecting a Program, 5131, 9041
Self-Therapy for the Stutterer, 8731
Services for the Blind and Visually Impaired, 3420
Services for the Visually Impaired, 8818
Shared Visions, 9043
Sharp Calculator with Illuminated Numbers, 539
Sightings Newsletter, 9047
Smith Kettlewell Rehabilitation Engineering Research Center, 9049
Social Maturity Scale for Blind Preschool Children: A Guide to Its Use, 9050
South Carolina Commission for the Blind, 3427
Special Technologies Alternative Resources, 8819
Specifications for Selecting a Vocabulary and Teaching Method/Braille Readers, 9051
Standing On My Own Two Feet, 5132, 9052
Step-By-Step Guide to Personal Management for Blind Persons, 9054
Stretch-View Wide-View Rectangular Illuminated Magnifier, 614
Student Advocate, 9055
Student Teaching Guide for Blind and Visually Impaired College Students, 9056
T Shirt is Done in Braille: Read Gently, 1139
TBC Focus, 9058
Tactile Thermostat, 519
Talk to Me, 5133, 9059
Talk to Me II, 5134, 9060
Talking Book Topics, 9061
Talking Calculators, 214
Talking Clinical Thermometer, 313
Talking Clocks, 215
Talking Watches, 216
Taping for the Blind, 8820
Teaching Orientation and Mobility in the Schools: An Instructor's Companion, 9062
Teaching Visually Impaired Children, 9063
Texas Commission for the Blind, 3464
Texas Lions Camp, 7752, 8290, 8841
Textbook Catalog, 9064
Tic Tac Toe, 5290
Timex Easy Reader, 615
Touch the Baby: Blind & Visually Impaired Children As Patients, 9067
Transition Activity Calendar for Students with Visual Impairments, 9068
Transition to College for Students with Visual Impairments: Report, 9069
Turnabout Game, 5291
US Association of Blind Athletes, 9091
Understanding and Coping with Achromatopsia, 8617
Unisex Low Vision Watch, 616
United States Association of Blind Athletes, 8821
United States Blind Golf Association, 9092
Unseen Minority: A Social History of Blindness in the United States, 9070
Upstate Update, 9071
Utah Division of Services for the Disabled, 3485
VIP Newsletter, 1905
VISIONS Vacation Camp for the Blind, 8843
VUE: Vision Use in Employment, 9099
Vermont Association for the Blind and Visually Impaired, 8822
Vermont Division for the Blind and Visually Impaired, 3498
Viewstar, 222
Virginia Department for the Blind and Vision Impaired, 3503
Vision Enhancement, 9072
Vision Foundation, 2569
Vision World Wide, 8823
Visions/Services for the Blind & Visually Impaired, 8824
Visual Aids and Informational Material, 9073
Visual Handicaps and Learning, 9074
Visual Impairment: An Overview, 9075
Visually Handicapped Child in Your Class, 9076
Visually Impaired Veterans of America, 8825
Viva Vital News, 9078
Vocational and Rehabilitation Agency Massachusetts Commission for the Blind, 5874
Vocational and Rehabilitation Agency: State Rehabilitation Commission, 6012
Vocational and Rehabilitation: Division of Wisconsin, 6040
Voice of Vision, 9079
Volunteer Transcribing Services, 1711
WP and HB White Foundation, 2512
Walking Alone and Marching Together, 9080
Washington Connection, 9100
Washington Ear, 8826
West Virginia Vocational Rehabilitation, 6039
What Do You Do When You See a Blind Person - and What Don't You Do?, 9082
What Museum Guides Need to Know: Access for the Blind and Visually Impaired, 9083
When You Have a Visually Impaired Student in Your Classroom: A Guide for Teachers, 2187
Winnekeag, 8844
Work Sight, 9084
Working with Visually Impaired Young Students: A Curriculum Guide, 2190
World Through Their Eyes, 9085
YMCA Camp Chingachgook on Lake George, 8845

Women

Health Resource Center for Women with Disabilities, 807
International Women's Health Coalition, 818
National Women's Health Network, 863
A Woman's Guide To Living With HIV Infecti on, 8301
Women to Women, 897

Grey House Publishing
Education Directories

The Complete Learning Disabilities Directory, 2007

The Complete Learning Disabilities Directory is the most comprehensive database of Programs, Services, Curriculum Materials, Professional Meetings & Resources, Camps, Newsletters and Support Groups for teachers, students and families concerned with learning disabilities. This information-packed directory includes information about Associations & Organizations, Schools, Colleges & Testing Materials, Government Agencies, Legal Resources and much more. For quick, easy access to information, this directory contains four indexes: Entry Name Index, Subject Index and Geographic Index. With every passing year, the field of learning disabilities attracts more attention and the network of caring, committed and knowledgeable professionals grows every day. This directory is an invaluable research tool for these parents, students and professionals.

"Due to its wealth and depth of coverage, parents, teachers and others... should find this an invaluable resource." -Booklist

900 pages; Softcover ISBN 1-59237-122-1, $145.00 ◆ Online Database $195.00 ◆ Online Database & Directory Combo $280.00

Educators Resource Directory, 2007/08

Educators Resource Directory is a comprehensive resource that provides the educational professional with thousands of resources and statistical data for professional development. This directory saves hours of research time by providing immediate access to Associations & Organizations, Conferences & Trade Shows, Educational Research Centers, Employment Opportunities & Teaching Abroad, School Library Services, Scholarships, Financial Resources, Professional Consultants, Computer Software & Testing Resources and much more. Plus, this comprehensive directory also includes a section on Statistics and Rankings with over 100 tables, including statistics on Average Teacher Salaries, SAT/ACT scores, Revenues & Expenditures and more. These important statistics will allow the user to see how their school rates among others, make relocation decisions and so much more. For quick access to information, this directory contains four indexes: Entry & Publisher Index, Geographic Index, a Subject & Grade Index and Web Sites Index. *Educators Resource Directory* will be a well-used addition to the reference collection of any school district, education department or public library.

"Recommended for all collections that serve elementary and secondary school professionals." –Choice

1,000 pages; Softcover ISBN 1-59237-179-5, $145.00 ◆ Online Database $195.00 ◆ Online Database & Directory Combo $280.00

Grey House Publishing
General Reference Titles

The Value of a Dollar 1600-1859, The Colonial Era to The Civil War

Following the format of the widely acclaimed, T*he Value of a Dollar, 1860-2004, The Value of a Dollar 1600-1859, The Colonial Era to The Civil War* records the actual prices of thousands of items that consumers purchased from the Colonial Era to the Civil War. Our editorial department had been flooded with requests from users of our Value of a Dollar for the same type of information, just from an earlier time period. This new volume is just the answer – with pricing data from 1600 to 1859. Arranged into five-year chapters, each 5-year chapter includes a Historical Snapshot, Consumer Expenditures, Investments, Selected Income, Income/Standard Jobs, Food Basket, Standard Prices and Miscellany. There is also a section on Trends. This informative section charts the change in price over time and provides added detail on the reasons prices changed within the time period, including industry developments, changes in consumer attitudes and important historical facts. This fascinating survey will serve a wide range of research needs and will be useful in all high school, public and academic library reference collections.

600 pages; Hardcover ISBN 1-59237-094-2, $135.00

The Value of a Dollar 1860-2004, Third Edition

A guide to practical economy, *The Value of a Dollar* records the actual prices of thousands of items that consumers purchased from the Civil War to the present, along with facts about investment options and income opportunities. This brand new Third Edition boasts a brand new addition to each five-year chapter, a section on Trends. This informative section charts the change in price over time and provides added detail on the reasons prices changed within the time period, including industry developments, changes in consumer attitudes and important historical facts. Plus, a brand new chapter for 2000-2004 has been added. Each 5-year chapter includes a Historical Snapshot, Consumer Expenditures, Investments, Selected Income, Income/Standard Jobs, Food Basket, Standard Prices and Miscellany. This interesting and useful publication will be widely used in any reference collection.

"Recommended for high school, college and public libraries." –ARBA

600 pages; Hardcover ISBN 1-59237-074-8, $135.00

To preview any of our Directories Risk-Free for 30 days, call (800) 562-2139 or fax to (518) 789-0556

Working Americans 1880-1999
Volume I: The Working Class, Volume II: The Middle Class, Volume III: The Upper Class

Each of the volumes in the *Working Americans 1880-1999* series focuses on a particular class of Americans, The Working Class, The Middle Class and The Upper Class over the last 120 years. Chapters in each volume focus on one decade and profile three to five families. Family Profiles include real data on Income & Job Descriptions, Selected Prices of the Times, Annual Income, Annual Budgets, Family Finances, Life at Work, Life at Home, Life in the Community, Working Conditions, Cost of Living, Amusements and much more. Each chapter also contains an Economic Profile with Average Wages of other Professions, a selection of Typical Pricing, Key Events & Inventions, News Profiles, Articles from Local Media and Illustrations. The *Working Americans* series captures the lifestyles of each of the classes from the last twelve decades, covers a vast array of occupations and ethnic backgrounds and travels the entire nation. These interesting and useful compilations of portraits of the American Working, Middle and Upper Classes during the last 120 years will be an important addition to any high school, public or academic library reference collection.

"These interesting, unique compilations of economic and social facts, figures and graphs will support multiple research needs. They will engage and enlighten patrons in high school, public and academic library collections." –Booklist

Volume I: The Working Class ◆ 558 pages; Hardcover ISBN 1-891482-81-5, $145.00 ◆ Volume II: The Middle Class ◆ 591 pages; Hardcover ISBN 1-891482-72-6; $145.00 ◆ Volume III: The Upper Class ◆ 567 pages; Hardcover ISBN 1-930956-38-X, $145.00

Working Americans 1880-1999 Volume IV: Their Children

This Fourth Volume in the highly successful *Working Americans 1880-1999* series focuses on American children, decade by decade from 1880 to 1999. This interesting and useful volume introduces the reader to three children in each decade, one from each of the Working, Middle and Upper classes. Like the first three volumes in the series, the individual profiles are created from interviews, diaries, statistical studies, biographies and news reports. Profiles cover a broad range of ethnic backgrounds, geographic area and lifestyles – everything from an orphan in Memphis in 1882, following the Yellow Fever epidemic of 1878 to an eleven-year-old nephew of a beer baron and owner of the New York Yankees in New York City in 1921. Chapters also contain important supplementary materials including News Features as well as information on everything from Schools to Parks, Infectious Diseases to Childhood Fears along with Entertainment, Family Life and much more to provide an informative overview of the lifestyles of children from each decade. This interesting account of what life was like for Children in the Working, Middle and Upper Classes will be a welcome addition to the reference collection of any high school, public or academic library.

600 pages; Hardcover ISBN 1-930956-35-5, $145.00

Working Americans 1880-2003 Volume V: Americans At War

Working Americans 1880-2003 Volume V: Americans At War is divided into 11 chapters, each covering a decade from 1880-2003 and examines the lives of Americans during the time of war, including declared conflicts, one-time military actions, protests, and preparations for war. Each decade includes several personal profiles, whether on the battlefield or on the homefront, that tell the stories of civilians, soldiers, and officers during the decade. The profiles examine: Life at Home; Life at Work; and Life in the Community. Each decade also includes an Economic Profile with statistical comparisons, a Historical Snapshot, News Profiles, local News Articles, and Illustrations that provide a solid historical background to the decade being examined. Profiles range widely not only geographically, but also emotionally, from that of a girl whose leg was torn off in a blast during WWI, to the boredom of being stationed in the Dakotas as the Indian Wars were drawing to a close. As in previous volumes of the *Working Americans* series, information is presented in narrative form, but hard facts and real-life situations back up each story. The basis of the profiles come from diaries, private print books, personal interviews, family histories, estate documents and magazine articles. For easy reference, *Working Americans 1880-2003 Volume V: Americans At War* includes an in-depth Subject Index. The *Working Americans* series has become an important reference for public libraries, academic libraries and high school libraries. This fifth volume will be a welcome addition to all of these types of reference collections.

600 pages; Hardcover ISBN 1-59237-024-1; $145.00
Five Volume Set (Volumes I-V), Hardcover ISBN 1-59237-034-9, $675.00

Working Americans 1880-2005 Volume VI: Women at Work

Unlike any other volume in the *Working Americans* series, this Sixth Volume, is the first to focus on a particular gender of Americans. *Volume VI: Women at Work*, traces what life was like for working women from the 1860's to the present time. Beginning with the life of a maid in 1890 and a store clerk in 1900 and ending with the life and times of the modern working women, this text captures the struggle, strengths and changing perception of the American woman at work. Each chapter focuses on one decade and profiles three to five women with real data on Income & Job Descriptions, Selected Prices of the Times, Annual Income, Annual Budgets, Family Finances, Life at Work, Life at Home, Life in the Community, Working Conditions, Cost of Living, Amusements and much more. For even broader access to the events, economics and attitude towards women throughout the past 130 years, each chapter is supplemented with News Profiles, Articles from Local Media, Illustrations, Economic Profiles, Typical Pricing, Key Events, Inventions and more. This important volume illustrates what life was like for working women over time and allows the reader to develop an understanding of the changing role of women at work. These interesting and useful compilations of portraits of women at work will be an important addition to any high school, public or academic library reference collection.

600 pages; Hardcover ISBN 1-59237-063-2; $145.00

Working Americans 1880-2005 Volume VII: Social Movements

The newest addition to the widely-successful *Working Americans* series, *Volume VII: Social Movements* explores how Americans sought and fought for change from the 1880s to the present time. Following the format of previous volumes in the Working Americans series, the text examines the lives of 34 individuals who have worked — often behind the scenes — to bring about change. Issues include topics as diverse as the Anti-smoking movement of 1901 to efforts by Native Americans to reassert their long lost rights. Along the way, the book will profile individuals brave enough to demand suffrage for Kansas women in 1912 or demand an end to lynching during a March on Washington in 1923. Each profile is enriched with real data on Income & Job Descriptions, Selected Prices of the Times, Annual Incomes & Budgets, Life at Work, Life at Home, Life in the Community, along with News Features, Key Events, and Illustrations. The depth of information contained in each profile allow the user to explore the private, financial and public lives of these subjects, deepening our understanding of how calls for change took place in our society. A must-purchase for the reference collections of high school libraries, public libraries and academic libraries.

600 pages; Hardcover ISBN 1-59237-101-9; $145.00
Seven Volume Set (Volumes I-VII), Hardcover ISBN 1-59237-133-7, $945.00

The Encyclopedia of Warrior Peoples & Fighting Groups

Many military groups throughout the world have excelled in their craft either by fortuitous circumstances, outstanding leadership, or intense training. This new second edition of The Encyclopedia of Warrior Peoples and Fighting Groups explores the origins and leadership of these outstanding combat forces, chronicles their conquests and accomplishments, examines the circumstances surrounding their decline or disbanding, and assesses their influence on the groups and methods of warfare that followed. This edition has been completely updated with information through 2005 and contains over 20 new entries. Readers will encounter ferocious tribes, charismatic leaders, and daring militias, from ancient times to the present, including Amazons, Buffalo Soldiers, Green Berets, Iron Brigade, Kamikazes, Peoples of the Sea, Polish Winged Hussars, Sacred Band of Thebes, Teutonic Knights, and Texas Rangers. With over 100 alphabetical entries, numerous cross-references and illustrations, a comprehensive bibliography, and index, the Encyclopedia of Warrior Peoples and Fighting Groups is a valuable resource for readers seeking insight into the bold history of distinguished fighting forces.

"This work is especially useful for high school students, undergraduates, and general readers with an interest in military history." –Library Journal

Pub. Date: May 2006; Hardcover ISBN 1-59237-116-7; $135.00

The Encyclopedia of Invasions & Conquests, From the Ancient Times to the Present

Throughout history, invasions and conquests have played a remarkable role in shaping our world and defining our boundaries, both physically and culturally. This second edition of the popular Encyclopedia of Invasions & Conquests, a comprehensive guide to over 150 invasions, conquests, battles and occupations from ancient times to the present, takes readers on a journey that includes the Roman conquest of Britain, the Portuguese colonization of Brazil, and the Iraqi invasion of Kuwait, to name a few. New articles will explore the late 20th and 21st centuries, with a specific focus on recent conflicts in Afghanistan, Kuwait, Iraq, Yugoslavia, Grenada and Chechnya. Categories of entries include countries, invasions and conquests, and individuals. In addition to covering the military aspects of invasions and conquests, entries cover some of the political, economic, and cultural aspects, for example, the effects of a conquest on the invade country's political and monetary system and in its language and religion. The entries on leaders – among them Sargon, Alexander the Great, William the Conqueror, and Adolf Hitler – deal with the people who sought to gain control, expand power, or exert religious or political influence over others through military means. Revised and updated for this second edition, entries are arranged alphabetically within historical periods. Each chapter provides a map to help readers locate key areas and geographical features, and bibliographical references appear at the end of each entry. Other useful features include cross-references, a cumulative bibliography and a comprehensive subject index. This authoritative, well-organized, lucidly written volume will prove invaluable for a variety of readers, including high school students, military historians, members of the armed forces, history buffs and hobbyists.

"Engaging writing, sensible organization, nice illustrations, interesting and obscure facts, and useful maps make this book a pleasure to read." –ARBA

Pub. Date: March 2006; Hardcover ISBN 1-59237-114-0; $135.00

Encyclopedia of Prisoners of War & Internment

This authoritative second edition provides a valuable overview of the history of prisoners of war and interned civilians, from earliest times to the present. Written by an international team of experts in the field of POW studies, this fascinating and thought-provoking volume includes entries on a wide range of subjects including the Crusades, Plains Indian Warfare, concentration camps, the two world wars, and famous POWs throughout history, as well as atrocities, escapes, and much more. Written in a clear and easily understandable style, this informative reference details over 350 entries, 30% larger than the first edition, that survey the history of prisoners of war and interned civilians from the earliest times to the present, with emphasis on the 19th and 20th centuries. Medical conditions, international law, exchanges of prisoners, organizations working on behalf of POWs, and trials associated with the treatment of captives are just some of the themes explored. Entries range from the Ardeatine Caves Massacre to Kurt Vonnegut. Entries are arranged alphabetically, plus illustrations and maps are provided for easy reference. The text also includes an introduction, bibliography, appendix of selected documents, and end-of-entry reading suggestions. This one-of-a-kind reference will be a helpful addition to the reference collections of all public libraries, high schools, and university libraries and will prove invaluable to historians and military enthusiasts.

"Thorough and detailed yet accessible to the lay reader. Of special interest to subject specialists and historians; recommended for public and academic libraries." - Library Journal

Pub. Date: March 2006; Hardcover ISBN 1-59237-120-5; $135.00

The Religious Right, A Reference Handbook

Timely and unbiased, this third edition updates and expands its examination of the religious right and its influence on our government, citizens, society, and politics. From the fight to outlaw the teaching of Darwin's theory of evolution to the struggle to outlaw abortion, the religious right is continually exerting an influence on public policy. This text explores the influence of religion on legislation and society, while examining the alignment of the religious right with the political right. A historical survey of the movement highlights the shift to "hands-on" approach to politics and the struggle to present a unified front. The coverage offers a critical historical survey of the religious right movement, focusing on its increased involvement in the political arena, attempts to forge coalitions, and notable successes and failures. The text offers complete coverage of biographies of the men and women who have advanced the cause and an up to date chronology illuminate the movement's goals, including their accomplishments and failures. This edition offers an extensive update to all sections along with several brand new entries. Two new sections complement this third edition, a chapter on legal issues and court decisions and a chapter on demographic statistics and electoral patterns. To aid in further research, The Religious Right, offers an entire section of annotated listings of print and non-print resources, as well as of organizations affiliated with the religious right, and those opposing it. Comprehensive in its scope, this work offers easy-to-read, pertinent information for those seeking to understand the religious right and its evolving role in American society. A must for libraries of all sizes, university religion departments, activists, high schools and for those interested in the evolving role of the religious right.

" Recommended for all public and academic libraries." - Library Journal

Pub. Date: November 2006; Hardcover ISBN 1-59237-113-2; $135.00

From Suffrage to the Senate, America's Political Women

From Suffrage to the Senate is a comprehensive and valuable compendium of biographies of leading women in U.S. politics, past and present, and an examination of the wide range of women's movements. Up to date through 2006, this dynamically illustrated reference work explores American women's path to political power and social equality from the struggle for the right to vote and the abolition of slavery to the first African American woman in the U.S. Senate and beyond. This new edition includes over 150 new entries and a brand new section on trends and demographics of women in politics. The in-depth coverage also traces the political heritage of the abolition, labor, suffrage, temperance, and reproductive rights movements. The alphabetically arranged entries include biographies of every woman from across the political spectrum who has served in the U.S. House and Senate, along with women in the Judiciary and the U.S. Cabinet and, new to this edition, biographies of activists and political consultants. Bibliographical references follow each entry. For easy reference, a handy chronology is provided detailing 150 years of women's history. This up-to-date reference will be a must-purchase for women's studies departments, high schools and public libraries and will be a handy resource for those researching the key players in women's politics, past and present.

"An engaging tool that would be useful in high school, public, and academic libraries looking for an overview of the political history of women in the US." –Booklist

Pub. Date: October 2006; Two Volume Set; Hardcover ISBN 1-59237-117-5; $195.00

An African Biographical Dictionary

This landmark second edition is the only biographical dictionary to bring together, in one volume, cultural, social and political leaders – both historical and contemporary – of the sub-Saharan region. Over 800 biographical sketches of prominent Africans, as well as foreigners who have affected the continent's history, are featured, 150 more than the previous edition. The wide spectrum of leaders includes religious figures, writers, politicians, scientists, entertainers, sports personalities and more. Access to these fascinating individuals is provided in a user-friendly format. The biographies are arranged alphabetically, cross-referenced and indexed. Entries include the country or countries in which the person was significant and the commonly accepted dates of birth and death. Each biographical sketch is chronologically written; entries for cultural personalities add an evaluation of their work. This information is followed by a selection of references often found in university and public libraries, including autobiographies and principal biographical works. Appendixes list each individual by country and by field of accomplishment – rulers, musicians, explorers, missionaries, businessmen, physicists – nearly thirty categories in all. Another convenient appendix lists heads of state since independence by country. Up-to-date and representative of African societies as a whole, An African Biographical Dictionary provides a wealth of vital information for students of African culture and is an indispensable reference guide for anyone interested in African affairs.

"An unquestionable convenience to have these concise, informative biographies gathered into one source, indexed, and analyzed by appendixes listing entrants by nation and occupational field." –Wilson Library Bulletin

Pub. Date: July 2006; Hardcover ISBN 1-59237-112-4; $125.00

American Environmental Leaders, From Colonial Times to the Present

A comprehensive and diverse award winning collection of biographies of the most important figures in American environmentalism. Few subjects arouse the passions the way the environment does. How will we feed an ever-increasing population and how can that food be made safe for consumption? Who decides how land is developed? How can environmental policies be made fair for everyone, including multiethnic groups, women, children, and the poor? American Environmental Leaders presents more than 350 biographies of men and women who have devoted their lives to studying, debating, and organizing these and other controversial issues over the last 200 years. In addition to the scientists who have analyzed how human actions affect nature, we are introduced to poets, landscape architects, presidents, painters, activists, even sanitation engineers, and others who have forever altered how we think about the environment. The easy to use A–Z format provides instant access to these fascinating individuals, and frequent cross references indicate others with whom individuals worked (and sometimes clashed). End of entry references provide users with a starting point for further research.

"Highly recommended for high school, academic, and public libraries needing environmental biographical information." –Library Journal/Starred Review

Two Volume Set; Hardcover ISBN 1-57607-385-8 $175.00

World Cultural Leaders of the Twentieth Century

An expansive two volume set that covers 450 worldwide cultural icons, World Cultural Leaders of the Twentieth Century includes each person's works, achievements, and professional careers in a thorough essay. Who was the originator of the term "documentary"? Which poet married the daughter of the famed novelist Thomas Mann in order to help her escape Nazi Germany? Which British writer served as an agent in Russia against the Bolsheviks before the 1917 revolution? These and many more questions are answered in this illuminating text. A handy two volume set that makes it easy to look up 450 worldwide cultural icons: novelists, poets, playwrights, painters, sculptors, architects, dancers, choreographers, actors, directors, filmmakers, singers, composers, and musicians. World Cultural Leaders of the Twentieth Century provides entries (many of them illustrated) covering the person's works, achievements, and professional career in a thorough essay and offers interesting facts and statistics. Entries are fully cross-referenced so that readers can learn how various individuals influenced others. A thorough general index completes the coverage.

"Fills a need for handy, concise information on a wide array of international cultural figures."-ARBA

Two Volume Set; Hardcover ISBN 1-57607-038-7 $175.00

To preview any of our Directories Risk-Free for 30 days, call (800) 562-2139 or fax to (518) 789-0556

Grey House Publishing
Business Directories

The Directory of Business Information Resources, 2007

With 100% verification, over 1,000 new listings and more than 12,000 updates, this 2007 edition of *The Directory of Business Information Resources* is the most up-to-date source for contacts in over 98 business areas – from advertising and agriculture to utilities and wholesalers. This carefully researched volume details: the Associations representing each industry; the Newsletters that keep members current; the Magazines and Journals - with their "Special Issues" - that are important to the trade, the Conventions that are "must attends," Databases, Directories and Industry Web Sites that provide access to must-have marketing resources. Includes contact names, phone & fax numbers, web sites and e-mail addresses. This one-volume resource is a gold mine of information and would be a welcome addition to any reference collection.

"This is a most useful and easy-to-use addition to any researcher's library." –The Information Professionals Institute

2,500 pages; Softcover ISBN 1-59237-146-9, $195.00 ▯ Online Database $495.00

Nations of the World, 2007/08 A Political, Economic and Business Handbook

This completely revised edition covers all the nations of the world in an easy-to-use, single volume. Each nation is profiled in a single chapter that includes Key Facts, Political & Economic Issues, a Country Profile and Business Information. In this fast-changing world, it is extremely important to make sure that the most up-to-date information is included in your reference collection. This edition is just the answer. Each of the 200+ country chapters have been carefully reviewed by a political expert to make sure that the text reflects the most current information on Politics, Travel Advisories, Economics and more. You'll find such vital information as a Country Map, Population Characteristics, Inflation, Agricultural Production, Foreign Debt, Political History, Foreign Policy, Regional Insecurity, Economics, Trade & Tourism, Historical Profile, Political Systems, Ethnicity, Languages, Media, Climate, Hotels, Chambers of Commerce, Banking, Travel Information and more. Five Regional Chapters follow the main text and include a Regional Map, an Introductory Article, Key Indicators and Currencies for the Region. As an added bonus, an all-inclusive CD-ROM is available as a companion to the printed text. Noted for its sophisticated, up-to-date and reliable compilation of political, economic and business information, this brand new edition will be an important acquisition to any public, academic or special library reference collection.

"A useful addition to both general reference collections and business collections." –RUSQ

1,700 pages; Print Version Only Softcover ISBN 1-59237-177-9, $155.00

The Directory of Venture Capital & Private Equity Firms, 2007

This edition has been extensively updated and broadly expanded to offer direct access to over 2,800 Domestic and International Venture Capital Firms, including address, phone & fax numbers, e-mail addresses and web sites for both primary and branch locations. Entries include details on the firm's Mission Statement, Industry Group Preferences, Geographic Preferences, Average and Minimum Investments and Investment Criteria. You'll also find details that are available nowhere else, including the Firm's Portfolio Companies and extensive information on each of the firm's Managing Partners, such as Education, Professional Background and Directorships held, along with the Partner's E-mail Address. *The Directory of Venture Capital & Private Equity Firms* offers five important indexes: Geographic Index, Executive Name Index, Portfolio Company Index, Industry Preference Index and College & University Index. With its comprehensive coverage and detailed, extensive information on each company, *The Directory of Venture Capital & Private Equity Firms* is an important addition to any finance collection.

"The sheer number of listings, the descriptive information provided and the outstanding indexing make this directory a better value than its principal competitor, Pratt's Guide to Venture Capital Sources. Recommended for business collections in large public, academic and business libraries." –Choice

1,300 pages; Softcover ISBN 1-59237-176-0, $565.00/$450.00 Library ▯ Online Database (includes a free copy of the directory) $889.00

To preview any of our Directories Risk-Free for 30 days, call (800) 562-2139 or fax to (518) 789-0556

The Directory of Mail Order Catalogs, 2007

Published since 1981, the *Directory of Mail Order Catalogs* is the premier source of information on the mail order catalog industry. It is the source that business professionals and librarians have come to rely on for the thousands of catalog companies in the US. New for 2007, The Directory of Mail Order Catalogs has been combined with its companion volume, *The Directory of Business to Business Catalogs*, to offer all 13,000 catalog companies in one easy-to-use volume. Section I: Consumer Catalogs, covers over 9,000 consumer catalog companies in 44 different product chapters from Animals to Toys & Games. Section II: Business to Business Catalogs, details 5,000 business catalogs, everything from computers to laboratory supplies, building construction and much more. Listings contain detailed contact information including mailing address, phone & fax numbers, web sites, e-mail addresses and key contacts along with important business details such as product descriptions, employee size, years in business, sales volume, catalog size, number of catalogs mailed and more. Three indexes are included for easy access to information: Catalog & Company Name Index, Geographic Index and Product Index. *The Directory of Mail Order Catalogs*, now with its expanded business to business catalogs, is the largest and most comprehensive resource covering this billion-dollar industry. It is the standard in its field. This important resource is a useful tool for entrepreneurs searching for catalogs to pick up their product, vendors looking to expand their customer base in the catalog industry, market researchers, small businesses investigating new supply vendors, along with the library patron who is exploring the available catalogs in their areas of interest.

"This is a godsend for those looking for information." –Reference Book Review

1,700 pages; Softcover ISBN 1-59237-156-6 $350.00/$250.00 Library □ Online Database (includes a free copy of the directory) $495.00

Sports Market Place Directory, 2007

For over 20 years, this comprehensive, up-to-date directory has offered direct access to the Who, What, When & Where of the Sports Industry. With over 20,000 updates and enhancements, the *Sports Market Place Directory* is the most detailed, comprehensive and current sports business reference source available. In 1,800 information-packed pages, *Sports Market Place Directory* profiles contact information and key executives for: Single Sport Organizations, Professional Leagues, Multi-Sport Organizations, Disabled Sports, High School & Youth Sports, Military Sports, Olympic Organizations, Media, Sponsors, Sponsorship & Marketing Event Agencies, Event & Meeting Calendars, Professional Services, College Sports, Manufacturers & Retailers, Facilities and much more. *The Sports Market Place Directory* provides organization's contact information with detailed descriptions including: Key Contacts, physical, mailing, email and web addresses plus phone and fax numbers. Plus, nine important indexes make sure that you can find the information you're looking for quickly and easily: Entry Index, Single Sport Index, Media Index, Sponsor Index, Agency Index, Manufacturers Index, Brand Name Index, Facilities Index and Executive/Geographic Index. For over twenty years, *The Sports Market Place Directory* has assisted thousands of individuals in their pursuit of a career in the sports industry. Why not use "THE SOURCE" that top recruiters, headhunters and career placement centers use to find information on or about sports organizations and key hiring contacts.

1,800 pages; Softcover ISBN 1-59237-189-2, $225.00 □ Online Database $479.00

Food and Beverage Market Place, 2007

Food and Beverage Market Place is bigger and better than ever with thousands of new companies, thousands of updates to existing companies and two revised and enhanced product category indexes. This comprehensive directory profiles over 18,000 Food & Beverage Manufacturers, 12,000 Equipment & Supply Companies, 2,200 Transportation & Warehouse Companies, 2,000 Brokers & Wholesalers, 8,000 Importers & Exporters, 900 Industry Resources and hundreds of Mail Order Catalogs. Listings include detailed Contact Information, Sales Volumes, Key Contacts, Brand & Product Information, Packaging Details and much more. *Thomas Food and Beverage Market Place* is available as a three-volume printed set, a subscription-based Online Database via the Internet, on CD-ROM, as well as mailing lists and a licensable database.

"An essential purchase for those in the food industry but will also be useful in public libraries where needed. Much of the information will be difficult and time consuming to locate without this handy three-volume ready-reference source." –ARBA

8,500 pages, 3 Volume Set; Softcover ISBN 1-59237-152-3, $595.00 □ Online Database $795.00 □ Online Database & 3 Volume Set Combo, $995.00

To preview any of our Directories Risk-Free for 30 days, call (800) 562-2139 or fax to (518) 789-0556

The Grey House Homeland Security Directory, 2007

This updated edition features the latest contact information for government and private organizations involved with Homeland Security along with the latest product information and provides detailed profiles of nearly 1,000 Federal & State Organizations & Agencies and over 3,000 Officials and Key Executives involved with Homeland Security. These listings are incredibly detailed and include Mailing Address, Phone & Fax Numbers, Email Addresses & Web Sites, a complete Description of the Agency and a complete list of the Officials and Key Executives associated with the Agency. Next, *The Grey House Homeland Security Directory* provides the go-to source for Homeland Security Products & Services. This section features over 2,000 Companies that provide Consulting, Products or Services. With this Buyer's Guide at their fingertips, users can locate suppliers of everything from Training Materials to Access Controls, from Perimeter Security to BioTerrorism Countermeasures and everything in between – complete with contact information and product descriptions. A handy Product Locator Index is provided to quickly and easily locate suppliers of a particular product. Lastly, an Information Resources Section provides immediate access to contact information for hundreds of Associations, Newsletters, Magazines, Trade Shows, Databases and Directories that focus on Homeland Security. This comprehensive, information-packed resource will be a welcome tool for any company or agency that is in need of Homeland Security information and will be a necessary acquisition for the reference collection of all public libraries and large school districts.

"Compiles this information in one place and is discerning in content. A useful purchase for public and academic libraries." –Booklist

800 pages; Softcover ISBN 1-59237-151-5, $195.00 ▯ Online Database (includes a free copy of the directory) $385.00

The Grey House Transportation Security Directory & Handbook

This brand new title is the only reference of its kind that brings together current data on Transportation Security. With information on everything from Regulatory Authorities to Security Equipment, this top-flight database brings together the relevant information necessary for creating and maintaining a security plan for a wide range of transportation facilities. With this current, comprehensive directory at the ready you'll have immediate access to: Regulatory Authorities & Legislation; Information Resources; Sample Security Plans & Checklists; Contact Data for Major Airports, Seaports, Railroads, Trucking Companies and Oil Pipelines; Security Service Providers; Recommended Equipment & Product Information and more. Using the *Grey House Transportation Security Directory & Handbook*, managers will be able to quickly and easily assess their current security plans; develop contacts to create and maintain new security procedures; and source the products and services necessary to adequately maintain a secure environment. This valuable resource is a must for all Security Managers at Airports, Seaports, Railroads, Trucking Companies and Oil Pipelines.

800 pages; Softcover ISBN 1-59237-075-6, $195

The Grey House Safety & Security Directory, 2007

The Grey House Safety & Security Directory is the most comprehensive reference tool and buyer's guide for the safety and security industry. Arranged by safety topic, each chapter begins with OSHA regulations for the topic, followed by Training Articles written by top professionals in the field and Self-Inspection Checklists. Next, each topic contains Buyer's Guide sections that feature related products and services. Topics include Administration, Insurance, Loss Control & Consulting, Protective Equipment & Apparel, Noise & Vibration, Facilities Monitoring & Maintenance, Employee Health Maintenance & Ergonomics, Retail Food Services, Machine Guards, Process Guidelines & Tool Handling, Ordinary Materials Handling, Hazardous Materials Handling, Workplace Preparation & Maintenance, Electrical Lighting & Safety, Fire & Rescue and Security. The Buyer's Guide sections are carefully indexed within each topic area to ensure that you can find the supplies needed to meet OSHA's regulations. Six important indexes make finding information and product manufacturers quick and easy: Geographical Index of Manufacturers and Distributors, Company Profile Index, Brand Name Index, Product Index, Index of Web Sites and Index of Advertisers. This comprehensive, up-to-date reference will provide every tool necessary to make sure a business is in compliance with OSHA regulations and locate the products and services needed to meet those regulations.

"Presents industrial safety information for engineers, plant managers, risk managers, and construction site supervisors…" –Choice

1,500 pages, 2 Volume Set; Softcover ISBN 1-59237-160-4, $225.00

The Grey House Biometric Information Directory

The Biometric Information Directory is the only comprehensive source for current biometric industry information. This 2006 edition is the first published by Grey House. With 100% updated information, this latest edition offers a complete, current look, in both print and online form, of biometric companies and products – one of the fastest growing industries in today's economy. Detailed profiles of manufacturers of the latest biometric technology, including Finger, Voice, Face, Hand, Signature, Iris, Vein and Palm Identification systems. Data on the companies include key executives, company size and a detailed, indexed description of their product line. Plus, the Directory also includes valuable business resources, and current editorial make this edition the easiest way for the business community and consumers alike to access the largest, most current compilation of biometric industry information available on the market today. The new edition boasts increased numbers of companies, contact names and company data, with over 700 manufacturers and service providers. Information in the directory includes: Editorial on Advancements in Biometrics; Profiles of 700+ companies listed with contact information; Organizations, Trade & Educational Associations, Publications, Conferences, Trade Shows and Expositions Worldwide; Web Site Index; Biometric & Vendors Services Index by Types of Biometrics; and a Glossary of Biometric Terms. This resource will be an important source for anyone who is considering the use of a biometric product, investing in the development of biometric technology, support existing marketing and sales efforts and will be an important acquisition for the business reference collection for large public and business libraries.

800 pages; Softcover ISBN 1-59237-121-3, $225

The Rauch Guide to the US Adhesives & Sealants, Cosmetics & Toiletries, Ink, Paint, Plastics, Pulp & Paper and Rubber Industries

The Rauch Guides are known worldwide for their comprehensive marketing information. Acquired by Grey House Publishing in 2005, new updated and revised editions will be published throughout 2005 and 2006. Each Guide provides market facts and figures in a highly organized format, ideal for today's busy personnel, serving as ready-references for top executives as well as the industry newcomer. *The Rauch Guides* save time and money by organizing widely scattered information and providing estimates for important business decisions, some of which are available nowhere else. Each Guide is organized into several information-packed chapters. After a brief introduction, the ECONOMICS section provides data on industry shipments; long-term growth and forecasts; prices; company performance; employment, expenditures, and productivity; transportation and geographical patterns; packaging; foreign trade; and government regulations. Next, TECHNOLOGY & RAW MATERIALS provide market, technical, and raw material information for chemicals, equipment and related materials, including market size and leading suppliers, prices, end uses, and trends. PRODUCTS & MARKETS provide information for each major industry product, including market size and historical trends, leading suppliers, five-year forecasts, industry structure, and major end uses. For easy access, each *Guide* contains a chapter on INDUSTRY ACTIVITIES, ORGANIZATIONS & SOURCES OF INFORMATION with detailed information on meetings, exhibits, and trade shows, sources of statistical information, trade associations, technical and professional societies, and trade and technical periodicals. Next, the COMPANY DIRECTORY profiles major industry companies, both public and private. Generally several hundred companies are analyzed. Information includes complete contact information, web address, estimated total and domestic sales, product description, and recent mergers and acquisitions. Each Guide also contains several APPENDICES that provide a cross-reference of suppliers, subsidiaries and divisions. The Rauch Guides will prove to be an invaluable source of market information, company data, trends and forecasts that anyone in these fast-paced industries.

The Rauch Guide to the U.S. Paint Industry Softcover ISBN 1-59237-127-2 $595 ♦ The Rauch Guide to the U.S. Plastics Industry Softcover ISBN 1-59237-128-0 $595 ♦ The Rauch Guide to the U.S. Adhesives and Sealants Industry Softcover ISBN 1-59237-129-9 $595 ♦ The Rauch Guide to the U.S. Ink Industry Softcover ISBN 1-59237-126-4 $595 ♦ The Rauch Guide to the U.S. Rubber Industry Softcover ISBN 1-59237-130-2 $595 ♦ The Rauch Guide to the U.S. Pulp and Paper Industry Softcover ISBN 1-59237-131-0 $595 ♦ The Rauch Guide to the U.S. Cosmetic and Toiletries Industry Softcover ISBN 1-59237-132-9 $895

The Grey House Performing Arts Directory, 2007

The Grey House Performing Arts Directory is the most comprehensive resource covering the Performing Arts. This important directory provides current information on over 8,500 Dance Companies, Instrumental Music Programs, Opera Companies, Choral Groups, Theater Companies, Performing Arts Series and Performing Arts Facilities. Plus, this edition now contains a brand new section on Artist Management Groups. In addition to mailing address, phone & fax numbers, e-mail addresses and web sites, dozens of other fields of available information include mission statement, key contacts, facilities, seating capacity, season, attendance and more. This directory also provides an important Information Resources section that covers hundreds of Performing Arts Associations, Magazines, Newsletters, Trade Shows, Directories, Databases and Industry Web Sites. Five indexes provide immediate access to this wealth of information: Entry Name, Executive Name, Performance Facilities, Geographic and Information Resources. *The Grey House Performing Arts Directory* pulls together thousands of Performing Arts Organizations, Facilities and Information Resources into an easy-to-use source – this kind of comprehensiveness and extensive detail is not available in any resource on the market place today.

"Immensely useful and user-friendly ... recommended for public, academic and certain special library reference collections." –Booklist

1,500 pages; Softcover ISBN 1-59237-138-8, $185.00 ♦ Online Database $335.00

To preview any of our Directories Risk-Free for 30 days, call (800) 562-2139 or fax to (518) 789-0556

New York State Directory, 2007/08

The New York State Directory, published annually since 1983, is a comprehensive and easy-to-use guide to accessing public officials and private sector organizations and individuals who influence public policy in the state of New York. *The New York State Directory* includes important information on all New York state legislators and congressional representatives, including biographies and key committee assignments. It also includes staff rosters for all branches of New York state government and for federal agencies and departments that impact the state policy process. Following the state government section are 25 chapters covering policy areas from agriculture through veterans' affairs. Each chapter identifies the state, local and federal agencies and officials that formulate or implement policy. In addition, each chapter contains a roster of private sector experts and advocates who influence the policy process. The directory also offers appendices that include statewide party officials; chambers of commerce; lobbying organizations; public and private universities and colleges; television, radio and print media; and local government agencies and officials.

New York State Directory - 800 pages; Softcover ISBN 1-59237-190-6; $145.00
New York State Directory with Profiles of New York – 2 volumes; 1,600 pages; Softcover ISBN 1-59237-191-4; $225

Profiles of New York ♦ Profiles of Florida ♦ Profiles of Texas ♦ Profiles of Illinois ♦ Profiles of Michigan ♦ Profiles of Ohio ♦ Profiles of New Jersey ♦ Profiles of Massachusetts ♦ Profiles of Pennsylvania ♦ Profiles of Wisconsin ♦ Profiles of Connecticut ♦ Profiles of Indiana ♦ Profiles of North Carolina ♦ Profiles of Virginia ♦ Profiles of California

Packed with over 50 pieces of data that make up a complete, user-friendly profile of each state, these directories go even further by then pulling selected data and providing it in ranking list form for even easier comparisons between the 100 largest towns and cities! The careful layout gives the user an easy-to-read snapshot of every single place and county in the state, from the biggest metropolis to the smallest unincorporated hamlet. The richness of each place or county profile is astounding in its depth, from history to weather, all packed in an easy-to-navigate, compact format. No need for piles of multiple sources with this volume on your desk. Here is a look at just a few of the data sets you'll find in each profile: History, Geography, Climate, Population, Vital Statistics, Economy, Income, Taxes, Education, Housing, Health & Environment, Public Safety, Newspapers, Transportation, Presidential Election Results, Information Contacts and Chambers of Commerce. As an added bonus, there is a section on Selected Statistics, where data from the 100 largest towns and cities is arranged into easy-to-use charts. Each of 22 different data points has its own two-page spread with the cities listed in alpha order so researchers can easily compare and rank cities. A remarkable compilation that offers overviews and insights into each corner of the state, *Profiles of New York*, *Profiles of Florida* and *Profiles of Texas* go beyond Census statistics, beyond metro area coverage, beyond the 100 best places to live. Drawn from official census information, other government statistics and original research, you will have at your fingertips data that's available nowhere else in one single source. Data will be published on additional states in 2006 and 2007.

Each Profiles of… title ranges from 400-800 pages, priced at $149.00 each

Research Services Directory: Commercial & Corporate Research Centers

This Ninth Edition provides access to well over 8,000 independent Commercial Research Firms, Corporate Research Centers and Laboratories offering contract services for hands-on, basic or applied research. *Research Services Directory* covers the thousands of types of research companies, including Biotechnology & Pharmaceutical Developers, Consumer Product Research, Defense Contractors, Electronics & Software Engineers, Think Tanks, Forensic Investigators, Independent Commercial Laboratories, Information Brokers, Market & Survey Research Companies, Medical Diagnostic Facilities, Product Research & Development Firms and more. Each entry provides the company's name, mailing address, phone & fax numbers, key contacts, web site, e-mail address, as well as a company description and research and technical fields served. Four indexes provide immediate access to this wealth of information: Research Firms Index, Geographic Index, Personnel Name Index and Subject Index.

"An important source for organizations in need of information about laboratories, individuals and other facilities." –ARBA

1,400 pages; Softcover ISBN 1-59237-003-9, $395.00 ♦ Online Database (includes a free copy of the directory) $850.00

International Business and Trade Directories

Completely updated, the Third Edition of *International Business and Trade Directories* now contains more than 10,000 entries, over 2,000 more than the last edition, making this directory the most comprehensive resource of the worlds business and trade directories. Entries include content descriptions, price, publisher's name and address, web site and e-mail addresses, phone and fax numbers and editorial staff. Organized by industry group, and then by region, this resource puts over 10,000 industry-specific business and trade directories at the reader's fingertips. Three indexes are included for quick access to information: Geographic Index, Publisher Index and Title Index. Public, college and corporate libraries, as well as individuals and corporations seeking critical market information will want to add this directory to their marketing collection.

"Reasonably priced for a work of this type, this directory should appeal to larger academic, public and corporate libraries with an international focus." –Library Journal

1,800 pages; Softcover ISBN 1-930956-63-0, $225.00 ♦ Online Database (includes a free copy of the directory) $450.00

To preview any of our Directories Risk-Free for 30 days, call (800) 562-2139 or fax to (518) 789-0556

Directory of Libraries in Canada, 2007/08

The Directory of Libraries in Canada brings together almost 7,000 listings including libraries and their branches, information resource centers, archives and library associations and learning centers. The directory offers complete and comprehensive information on Canadian libraries, resource centers, business information centers, professional associations, regional library systems, archives, library schools and library technical programs. The Directory of Libraries in Canada includes important features of each library and service, including library information; personnel details, including contact names and e-mail addresses; collection information; services available to users; acquisitions budgets; and computers and automated systems. Useful information on each library's electronic access is also included, such as Internet browser, connectivity and public Internet/CD-ROM/subscription database access. The directory also provides powerful indexes for subject, location, personal name and Web site/e-mail to assist researchers with locating the crucial information they need. The Directory of Libraries in Canada is a vital reference tool for publishers, advocacy groups, students, research institutions, computer hardware suppliers, and other diverse groups that provide products and services to this unique market.

850 pages; Hardcover ISBN 978-1-59237-222-5; $315.00

Canadian Environmental Directory, 2007/08

The Canadian Environmental Directory is Canada's most complete and only national listing of environmental associations and organizations, government regulators and purchasing groups, product and service companies, special libraries, and more! The extensive Products and Services section provides detailed listings enabling users to identify the company name, address, phone, fax, e-mail, Web address, firm type, contact names (and titles), product and service information, affiliations, trade information, branch and affiliate data. The Government section gives you all the contact information you need at every government level – federal, provincial and municipal. We also include descriptions of current environmental initiatives, programs and agreements, names of environment-related acts administered by each ministry or department PLUS information and tips on who to contact and how to sell to governments in Canada. The Associations section provides complete contact information and a brief description of activities. Included are Canadian environmental organizations and international groups including industry, commercial and professional associations, registered charities, special interest and common interest organizations. All the Information you need about the Canadian environmental industry: directory of products and services, special libraries and resource, conferences, seminars and tradeshows, chronology of environmental events, law firms and major Canadian companies, The Canadian Environmental Directory is ideal for business, government, engineers and anyone conducting research on the environment.

Hardcover ISBN 978-1-59237-218-8; 900 pages; $315.00

The Asian Databook: Statistics for all US Counties & Cities with Over 10,000 Population

This is the first-ever resource that compiles statistics and rankings on the US Asian population. *The Asian Databook* presents over 20 statistical data points for each city and county, arranged alphabetically by state, then alphabetically by place name. Data reported for each place includes Population, Languages Spoken at Home, Foreign-Born, Educational Attainment, Income Figures, Poverty Status, Homeownership, Home Values & Rent, and more. Next, in the Rankings Section, the top 75 places are listed for each data element. These easy-to-access ranking tables allow the user to quickly determine trends and population characteristics. This kind of comparative data can not be found elsewhere, in print or on the web, in a format that's as easy-to-use or more concise. A useful resource for those searching for demographics data, career search and relocation information and also for market research. With data ranging from Ancestry to Education, *The Asian Databook* presents a useful compilation of information that will be a much-needed resource in the reference collection of any public or academic library along with the marketing collection of any company whose primary focus in on the Asian population.

1,000 pages; Softcover ISBN 1-59237-044-6 $150.00

The Hispanic Databook: Statistics for all US Counties & Cities with Over 10,000 Population

Previously published by Toucan Valley Publications, this second edition has been completely updated with figures from the latest census and has been broadly expanded to include dozens of new data elements and a brand new Rankings section. The Hispanic population in the United States has increased over 42% in the last 10 years and accounts for 12.5% of the total US population. For ease-of-use, *The Hispanic Databook* presents over 20 statistical data points for each city and county, arranged alphabetically by state, then alphabetically by place name. Data reported for each place includes Population, Languages Spoken at Home, Foreign-Born, Educational Attainment, Income Figures, Poverty Status, Homeownership, Home Values & Rent, and more. Next, in the Rankings Section, the top 75 places are listed for each data element. These easy-to-access ranking tables allow the user to quickly determine trends and population characteristics. This kind of comparative data can not be found elsewhere, in print or on the web, in a format that's as easy-to-use or more concise. A useful resource for those searching for demographics data, career search and relocation information and also for market research. With data ranging from Ancestry to Education, *The Hispanic Databook* presents a useful compilation of information that will be a much-needed resource in the reference collection of any public or academic library along with the marketing collection of any company whose primary focus in on the Hispanic population.

"This accurate, clearly presented volume of selected Hispanic demographics is recommended for large public libraries and research collections."-Library Journal

1,000 pages; Softcover ISBN 1-59237-008-X, $150.00

Ancestry in America: A Comparative Guide to Over 200 Ethnic Backgrounds

This brand new reference work pulls together thousands of comparative statistics on the Ethnic Backgrounds of all populated places in the United States with populations over 10,000. Never before has this kind of information been reported in a single volume. Section One, Statistics by Place, is made up of a list of over 200 ancestry and race categories arranged alphabetically by each of the 5,000 different places with populations over 10,000. The population number of the ancestry group in that city or town is provided along with the percent that group represents of the total population. This informative city-by-city section allows the user to quickly and easily explore the ethnic makeup of all major population bases in the United States. Section Two, Comparative Rankings, contains three tables for each ethnicity and race. In the first table, the top 150 populated places are ranked by population number for that particular ancestry group, regardless of population. In the second table, the top 150 populated places are ranked by the percent of the total population for that ancestry group. In the third table, those top 150 populated places with 10,000 population are ranked by population number for each ancestry group. These easy-to-navigate tables allow users to see ancestry population patterns and make city-by-city comparisons as well. Plus, as an added bonus with the purchase of *Ancestry in America*, a free companion CD-ROM is available that lists statistics and rankings for all of the 35,000 populated places in the United States. This brand new, information-packed resource will serve a wide-range or research requests for demographics, population characteristics, relocation information and much more. *Ancestry in America: A Comparative Guide to Over 200 Ethnic Backgrounds* will be an important acquisition to all reference collections.

"This compilation will serve a wide range of research requests for population characteristics ... it offers much more detail than other sources." –Booklist

1,500 pages; Softcover ISBN 1-59237-029-2, $225.00

The American Tally: Statistics & Comparative Rankings for U.S. Cities with Populations over 10,000

This important statistical handbook compiles, all in one place, comparative statistics on all U.S. cities and towns with a 10,000+ population. *The American Tally* provides statistical details on over 4,000 cities and towns and profiles how they compare with one another in Population Characteristics, Education, Language & Immigration, Income & Employment and Housing. Each section begins with an alphabetical listing of cities by state, allowing for quick access to both the statistics and relative rankings of any city. Next, the highest and lowest cities are listed in each statistic. These important, informative lists provide quick reference to which cities are at both extremes of the spectrum for each statistic. Unlike any other reference, *The American Tally* provides quick, easy access to comparative statistics – a must-have for any reference collection.

"A solid library reference." -Bookwatch

500 pages; Softcover ISBN 1-930956-29-0, $125.00

The Environmental Resource Handbook, 2007/08

The Environmental Resource Handbook is the most up-to-date and comprehensive source for Environmental Resources and Statistics. Section I: Resources provides detailed contact information for thousands of information sources, including Associations & Organizations, Awards & Honors, Conferences, Foundations & Grants, Environmental Health, Government Agencies, National Parks & Wildlife Refuges, Publications, Research Centers, Educational Programs, Green Product Catalogs, Consultants and much more. Section II: Statistics, provides statistics and rankings on hundreds of important topics, including Children's Environmental Index, Municipal Finances, Toxic Chemicals, Recycling, Climate, Air & Water Quality and more. This kind of up-to-date environmental data, all in one place, is not available anywhere else on the market place today. This vast compilation of resources and statistics is a must-have for all public and academic libraries as well as any organization with a primary focus on the environment.

"...the intrinsic value of the information make it worth consideration by libraries with environmental collections and environmentally concerned users." –Booklist

1,000 pages; Softcover ISBN 1-59237-195-7, $155.00 ▯ Online Database $300.00

Weather America, A Thirty-Year Summary of Statistical Weather Data and Rankings

This valuable resource provides extensive climatological data for over 4,000 National and Cooperative Weather Stations throughout the United States. *Weather America* begins with a new Major Storms section that details major storm events of the nation and a National Rankings section that details rankings for several data elements, such as Maximum Temperature and Precipitation. The main body of *Weather America* is organized into 50 state sections. Each section provides a Data Table on each Weather Station, organized alphabetically, that provides statistics on Maximum and Minimum Temperatures, Precipitation, Snowfall, Extreme Temperatures, Foggy Days, Humidity and more. State sections contain two brand new features in this edition – a City Index and a narrative Description of the climatic conditions of the state. Each section also includes a revised Map of the State that includes not only weather stations, but cities and towns.

"Best Reference Book of the Year." –Library Journal

2,013 pages; Softcover ISBN 1-891482-29-7, $175.00

Crime in America's Top-Rated Cities

This volume includes over 20 years of crime statistics in all major crime categories: violent crimes, property crimes and total crime. *Crime in America's Top-Rated Cities* is conveniently arranged by city and covers 76 top-rated cities. *Crime in America's Top-Rated Cities* offers details that compare the number of crimes and crime rates for the city, suburbs and metro area along with national crime trends for violent, property and total crimes. Also, this handbook contains important information and statistics on Anti-Crime Programs, Crime Risk, Hate Crimes, Illegal Drugs, Law Enforcement, Correctional Facilities, Death Penalty Laws and much more. A much-needed resource for people who are relocating, business professionals, general researchers, the press, law enforcement officials and students of criminal justice.

"Data is easy to access and will save hours of searching." –Global Enforcement Review

832 pages; Softcover ISBN 1-891482-84-X, $155.00

Sedgwick Press
Health Directories

The Complete Directory for People with Disabilities, 2007

A wealth of information, now in one comprehensive sourcebook. Completely updated, this edition contains more information than ever before, including thousands of new entries and enhancements to existing entries and thousands of additional web sites and e-mail addresses. This up-to-date directory is the most comprehensive resource available for people with disabilities, detailing Independent Living Centers, Rehabilitation Facilities, State & Federal Agencies, Associations, Support Groups, Periodicals & Books, Assistive Devices, Employment & Education Programs, Camps and Travel Groups. Each year, more libraries, schools, colleges, hospitals, rehabilitation centers and individuals add *The Complete Directory for People with Disabilities* to their collections, making sure that this information is readily available to the families, individuals and professionals who can benefit most from the amazing wealth of resources cataloged here.

"No other reference tool exists to meet the special needs of the disabled in one convenient resource for information." –Library Journal

1,200 pages; Softcover ISBN 1-59237-147-7, $165.00 ▯ Online Database $215.00 ▯ Online Database & Directory Combo $300.00

The Complete Directory for People with Chronic Illness, 2007/08

Thousands of hours of research have gone into this completely updated 2005/06 edition – several new chapters have been added along with thousands of new entries and enhancements to existing entries. Plus, each chronic illness chapter has been reviewed by an medical expert in the field. This widely-hailed directory is structured around the 90 most prevalent chronic illnesses – from Asthma to Cancer to Wilson's Disease – and provides a comprehensive overview of the support services and information resources available for people diagnosed with a chronic illness. Each chronic illness has its own chapter and contains a brief description in layman's language, followed by important resources for National & Local Organizations, State Agencies, Newsletters, Books & Periodicals, Libraries & Research Centers, Support Groups & Hotlines, Web Sites and much more. This directory is an important resource for health care professionals, the collections of hospital and health care libraries, as well as an invaluable tool for people with a chronic illness and their support network.

"A must purchase for all hospital and health care libraries and is strongly recommended for all public library reference departments." –ARBA

1,200 pages; Softcover ISBN 1-59237-183-3, $165.00 ▯ Online Database $215.00 ▯ Online Database & Directory Combo $300.00

The Complete Mental Health Directory, 2006/07

This is the most comprehensive resource covering the field of behavioral health, with critical information for both the layman and the mental health professional. For the layman, this directory offers understandable descriptions of 25 Mental Health Disorders as well as detailed information on Associations, Media, Support Groups and Mental Health Facilities. For the professional, *The Complete Mental Health Directory* offers critical and comprehensive information on Managed Care Organizations, Information Systems, Government Agencies and Provider Organizations. This comprehensive volume of needed information will be widely used in any reference collection.

"... the strength of this directory is that it consolidates widely dispersed information into a single volume." –Booklist

800 pages; Softcover ISBN 1-59237-124-8, $165.00 ▯ Online Database $215.00 ▯ Online & Directory Combo $300.00

To preview any of our Directories Risk-Free for 30 days, call (800) 562-2139 or fax to (518) 789-0556

Older Americans Information Directory, 2006/07

Completely updated for 2006/07, this sixth edition has been completely revised and now contains 1,000 new listings, over 8,000 updates to existing listings and over 3,000 brand new e-mail addresses and web sites. You'll find important resources for Older Americans including National, Regional, State & Local Organizations, Government Agencies, Research Centers, Libraries & Information Centers, Legal Resources, Discount Travel Information, Continuing Education Programs, Disability Aids & Assistive Devices, Health, Print Media and Electronic Media. Three indexes: Entry Index, Subject Index and Geographic Index make it easy to find just the right source of information. This comprehensive guide to resources for Older Americans will be a welcome addition to any reference collection.

"Highly recommended for academic, public, health science and consumer libraries…" –Choice

1,200 pages; Softcover ISBN 1-59237-136-1, $165.00 ◆ Online Database $215.00 ◆ Online Database & Directory Combo $300.00

The Complete Directory for Pediatric Disorders, 2007

This important directory provides parents and caregivers with information about Pediatric Conditions, Disorders, Diseases and Disabilities, including Blood Disorders, Bone & Spinal Disorders, Brain Defects & Abnormalities, Chromosomal Disorders, Congenital Heart Defects, Movement Disorders, Neuromuscular Disorders and Pediatric Tumors & Cancers. This carefully written directory offers: understandable Descriptions of 15 major bodily systems; Descriptions of more than 200 Disorders and a Resources Section, detailing National Agencies & Associations, State Associations, Online Services, Libraries & Resource Centers, Research Centers, Support Groups & Hotlines, Camps, Books and Periodicals. This resource will provide immediate access to information crucial to families and caregivers when coping with children's illnesses.

"Recommended for public and consumer health libraries." –Library Journal

1,200 pages; Softcover ISBN 1-59237-150-7 $165.00 ◆ Online Database $215.00 ◆ Online Database & Directory Combo $300.00

The Directory of Drug & Alcohol Residential Rehabilitation Facilities

This brand new directory is the first-ever resource to bring together, all in one place, data on the thousands of drug and alcohol residential rehabilitation facilities in the United States. *The Directory of Drug & Alcohol Residential Rehabilitation Facilities* covers over 1,000 facilities, with detailed contact information for each one, including mailing address, phone and fax numbers, email addresses and web sites, mission statement, type of treatment programs, cost, average length of stay, numbers of residents and counselors, accreditation, insurance plans accepted, type of environment, religious affiliation, education components and much more. It also contains a helpful chapter on General Resources that provides contact information for Associations, Print & Electronic Media, Support Groups and Conferences. Multiple indexes allow the user to pinpoint the facilities that meet very specific criteria. This time-saving tool is what so many counselors, parents and medical professionals have been asking for. *The Directory of Drug & Alcohol Residential Rehabilitation Facilities* will be a helpful tool in locating the right source for treatment for a wide range of individuals. This comprehensive directory will be an important acquisition for all reference collections: public and academic libraries, case managers, social workers, state agencies and many more.

"This is an excellent, much needed directory that fills an important gap…" –Booklist

300 pages; Softcover ISBN 1-59237-031-4, $135.00

Sedgwick Press
Hospital & Health Plan Directories

The Comparative Guide to American Hospitals, 2007

This is the first ever resource to compare all of the nation's hospitals by 17 measures of quality in the treatment of heart attack, heart failure and pneumonia. This data is based on the Hospital Compare study, produced by Medicare, and is available in print and in a unique and user-friendly format from Grey House Publishing, along with extra contact information from Grey House's *Directory of Hospital Personnel. The Comparative Guide to American Hospitals* provides a snapshot profile of each of the nations 6,000 hospitals. These informative profiles illustrate how the hospital rates in 17 important areas: Heart Attack Care (% who receive Aspirin at Arrival, Aspirin at Discharge, ACE Inhibitor for LVSD, Beta Blocker at Arrival, Beta Blocker at Discharge, Thrombolytic Agent Received, PTCA Received and Adult Smoking Cessation Advice); Heart Failure (% who receive LVF Assessment, ACE Inhibitor for LVSD, Discharge Instructions, Adult Smoking Cessation Advice); and Pneumonia (% who receive Initial Antibiotic Timing, Pneumococcal Vaccination, Oxygenation Assessment, Blood Culture Performed and Adult Smoking Cessation Advice). Each profile includes the raw percentage for that hospital, the state average, the US average and data on the top hospital. For easy access to contact information, each profile includes the hospitals address, phone and fax numbers, email and web addresses, type and accreditation along with 5 top key administrations. These profiles will allow the user to quickly identify the quality of the hospital and have the necessary information at their fingertips to make contact with that hospital. Most importantly, *The Comparative Guide to American Hospitals* provides an easy-to-use Ranking Table for each of the data elements to allow the user to quickly locate the hospitals with the best level of service. This brand new title will be a must for the reference collection at all public, medical and academic libraries.

2,500 pages; Softcover ISBN 1-59237-182-5; $225.00

The Directory of Hospital Personnel, 2007

The Directory of Hospital Personnel is the best resource you can have at your fingertips when researching or marketing a product or service to the hospital market. A "Who's Who" of the hospital universe, this directory puts you in touch with over 150,000 key decision-makers. With 100% verification of data you can rest assured that you will reach the right person with just one call. Every hospital in the U.S. is profiled, listed alphabetically by city within state. Plus, three easy-to-use, cross-referenced indexes put the facts at your fingertips faster and more easily than any other directory: Hospital Name Index, Bed Size Index and Personnel Index. *The Directory of Hospital Personnel* is the only complete source for key hospital decision-makers by name. Whether you want to define or restructure sales territories… locate hospitals with the purchasing power to accept your proposals… keep track of important contacts or colleagues… or find information on which insurance plans are accepted, *The Directory of Hospital Personnel* gives you the information you need – easily, efficiently, effectively and accurately.

"Recommended for college, university and medical libraries." -ARBA

2,500 pages; Softcover ISBN 1-59237-178-7 $325.00 ◆ Online Database $545.00 ◆ Online Database & Directory Combo, $650.00

The Directory of Health Care Group Purchasing Organizations, 2006

This comprehensive directory provides the important data you need to get in touch with over 800 Group Purchasing Organizations. By providing in-depth information on this growing market and its members, *The Directory of Health Care Group Purchasing Organizations* fills a major need for the most accurate and comprehensive information on over 800 GPOs – Mailing Address, Phone & Fax Numbers, E-mail Addresses, Key Contacts, Purchasing Agents, Group Descriptions, Membership Categorization, Standard Vendor Proposal Requirements, Membership Fees & Terms, Expanded Services, Total Member Beds & Outpatient Visits represented and more. Five Indexes provide a number of ways to locate the right GPO: Alphabetical Index, Expanded Services Index, Organization Type Index, Geographic Index and Member Institution Index. With its comprehensive and detailed information on each purchasing organization, *The Directory of Health Care Group Purchasing Organizations* is the go-to source for anyone looking to target this market.

"The information is clearly arranged and easy to access…recommended for those needing this very specialized information." –ARBA

1,000 pages; Softcover ISBN 1-59237-0091-8, $325.00 ◆ Online Database, $650.00 ◆ Online Database & Directory Combo, $750.00

To preview any of our Directories Risk-Free for 30 days, call (800) 562-2139 or fax to (518) 789-0556

The HMO/PPO Directory, 2007

The HMO/PPO Directory is a comprehensive source that provides detailed information about Health Maintenance Organizations and Preferred Provider Organizations nationwide. This comprehensive directory details more information about more managed health care organizations than ever before. Over 1,100 HMOs, PPOs, Medicare Advantage Plans and affiliated companies are listed, arranged alphabetically by state. Detailed listings include Key Contact Information, Prescription Drug Benefits, Enrollment, Geographical Areas served, Affiliated Physicians & Hospitals, Federal Qualifications, Status, Year Founded, Managed Care Partners, Employer References, Fees & Payment Information and more. Plus, five years of historical information is included related to Revenues, Net Income, Medical Loss Ratios, Membership Enrollment and Number of Patient Complaints. Five easy-to-use, cross-referenced indexes will put this vast array of information at your fingertips immediately: HMO Index, PPO Index, Other Providers Index, Personnel Index and Enrollment Index. *The HMO/PPO Directory* provides the most comprehensive data on the most companies available on the market place today.

"Helpful to individuals requesting certain HMO/PPO issues such as co-payment costs, subscription costs and patient complaints. Individuals concerned (or those with questions) about their insurance may find this text to be of use to them." -ARBA

600 pages; Softcover ISBN 1-59237-158-2, $325.00 ▯ Online Database, $495.00 ▯ Online Database & Directory Combo, $600.00

Medical Device Register, 2007

The only one-stop resource of every medical supplier licensed to sell products in the US. This award-winning directory offers immediate access to over 13,000 companies - and more than 65,000 products – in two information-packed volumes. This comprehensive resource saves hours of time and trouble when searching for medical equipment and supplies and the manufacturers who provide them. Volume I: The Product Directory, provides essential information for purchasing or specifying medical supplies for every medical device, supply, and diagnostic available in the US. Listings provide FDA codes & Federal Procurement Eligibility, Contact information for every manufacturer of the product along with Prices and Product Specifications. Volume 2 - Supplier Profiles, offers the most complete and important data about Suppliers, Manufacturers and Distributors. Company Profiles detail the number of employees, ownership, method of distribution, sales volume, net income, key executives detailed contact information medical products the company supplies, plus the medical specialties they cover. Four indexes provide immediate access to this wealth of information: Keyword Index, Trade Name Index, Supplier Geographical Index and OEM (Original Equipment Manufacturer) Index. Medical Device Register, 2007 is the only one-stop source for locating suppliers and products; looking for new manufacturers or hard-to-find medical devices; comparing products and companies; know who's selling what and who to buy from cost effectively. This directory has become the standard in its field and will be a welcome addition to the reference collection of any medical library, large public library, university library along with the collections that serve the medical community.

"A wealth of information on medical devices, medical device companies… and key personnel in the industry is provide in this comprehensive reference work... A valuable reference work, one of the best hardcopy compilations available." -Doody Publishing

3,000 pages Two Volumes; Hardcover ISBN 1-59237-181-7; $325.00

The Directory of Independent Ambulatory Care Centers

This first edition of *The Directory of Independent Ambulatory Care Centers* provides access to detailed information that, before now, could only be found scattered in hundreds of different sources. This comprehensive and up-to-date directory pulls together a vast array of contact information for over 7,200 Ambulatory Surgery Centers, Ambulatory General and Urgent Care Clinics, and Diagnostic Imaging Centers that are not affiliated with a hospital or major medical center. Detailed listings include Mailing Address, Phone & Fax Numbers, E-mail and Web Site addresses, Contact Name and Phone Numbers of the Medical Director and other Key Executives and Purchasing Agents, Specialties & Services Offered, Year Founded, Numbers of Employees and Surgeons, Number of Operating Rooms, Number of Cases seen per year, Overnight Options, Contracted Services and much more. Listings are arranged by State, by Center Category and then alphabetically by Organization Name. Two indexes provide quick and easy access to this wealth of information: Entry Name Index and Specialty/Service Index. *The Directory of Independent Ambulatory Care Centers* is a must-have resource for anyone marketing a product or service to this important industry and will be an invaluable tool for those searching for a local care center that will meet their specific needs.

"Among the numerous hospital directories, no other provides information on independent ambulatory centers. A handy, well-organized resource that would be useful in medical center libraries and public libraries." –Choice

986 pages; Softcover ISBN 1-930956-90-8, $185.00 ▯ Online Database, $365.00 ▯ Online Database & Directory Combo, $450.00